The commentary text in this Handbook is written to assist users in understanding and applying *Code* provisions. The commentary explains the reasoning behind *Code* requirements and provides numerous examples, table, photographs, and illustrations. The commentary text is shaded green to distinguish it from the text of the *Code*. Please note that the commentary is not part of the *Code* and therefore is not enforceable.



upper floor or more than 50 percent of the egress capacity of any upper floor. Exit stair C discharges into an area on the discharge level that is sprinklered and separated from the remainder of the floor and the basement, which are not sprinklered. The hourly fire resistance rating of the floor slab and the separating fire barrier are the same as required for the enclosure of exit stair C [e.g., a 2-hour rating if the stair is new and serves four or more stories in accordance with 7.1.3.2.1(2)]. Exit stair D discharges into a wired-glass foyer in the nonsprinklered portion of the floor in accordance with 7.7.2.5.

**7.7.3 Arrangement and Marking of Exit Discharge.**

**7.7.3.1** Where more than one exit discharge is required, exit discharges shall be arranged to meet the remoteness criteria of 7.5.1.3.

**7.7.3.2** The exit discharge shall be arranged and marked to

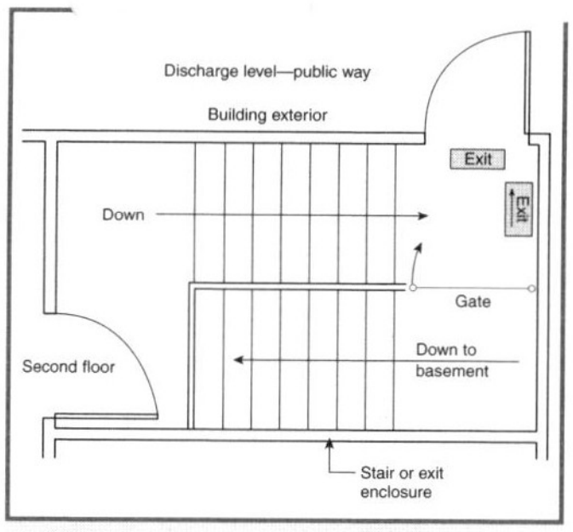


*Exhibit 7.103 Interruption of exit stair at LED.*

Calculations interspersed within the commentary show how *Code* requirements are applied.



the first floor use door assemblies directly to the outside (not shown) for egress. The means of egress system is designed for half of the occupant load of floors 2 through 14 to use the stair at the left of the exhibit, and for the other half to use the stair at the right of the exhibit. The sum of the 150 persons from each of floors 2 through 14 is considered the total cumulative occupant load assigned to each of the two stairs for purposes of applying 7.2.2.2.1.2(B). The total cumulative occupant load assigned to each of the two stairs is calculated as follows:

$$\frac{13 \text{ floors} \times 150 \text{ persons}}{\text{per floor per stair}} = 1950 \text{ persons per stair}$$

Thus, the 2000-person threshold of Table 7.2.2.2.1.2(B) is not reached. No part of either stair is required to be increased to a minimum width of 56 in. (1420 mm). The stairs must be at least 44 in. (1120 mm)

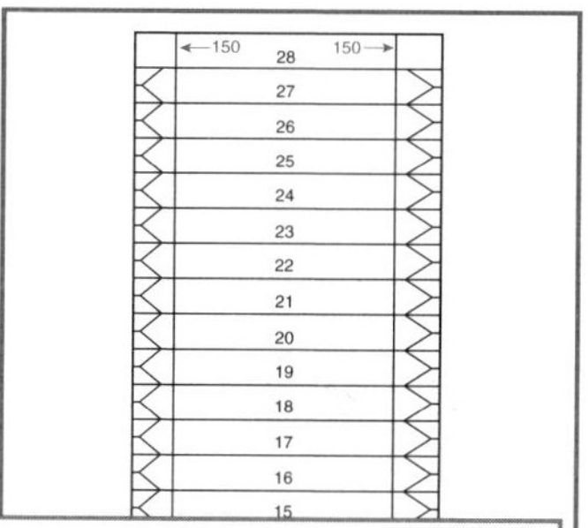




(2) The force that, when applied to the operating device in the direction of egress, is required to operate the door leaf is not more than 15 lbf (67 N).
(3) The force required to operate the door leaf in the direction of travel is not more than 30 lbf (133 N) to set the leaf in motion and is not more than 15 lbf (67 N) to close the leaf or open it to the minimum required width.
(4) The door leaf is operable using a force of not more than 50 lbf (222 N) when a force of 250 lbf (1100 N) is applied perpendicularly to the leaf adjacent to the operating device, unless the door opening is an existing horizontal-sliding exit access door assembly serving an area with an occupant load of fewer than 50.
(5) The door assembly complies with the fire protection rating, if required, and, where rated, is self-closing or automatic-closing by means of smoke detection in accordance with 7.2.1.8 and is installed in accordance with NFPA 80, *Standard for Fire Doors and Other Opening Protectives*.

The special type of horizontal-sliding door assembly addressed by 7.2.1.14 is different from a traditional horizontal-sliding door assembly. When force is applied in the direction of egress travel to the door actuator, the door leaf must slide to the side to allow passage. This concept is illustrated in Exhibit 7.24.

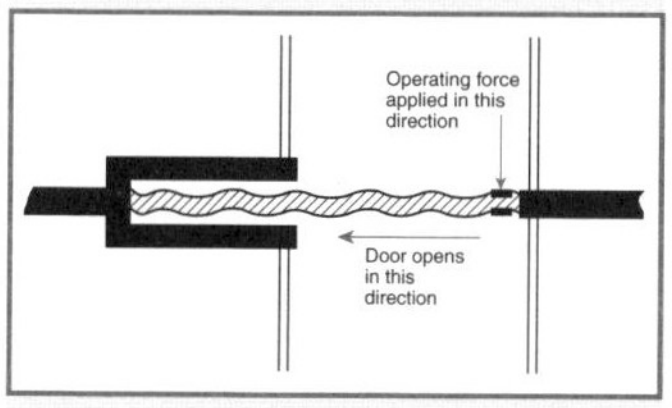


*Exhibit 7.24 Horizontal-sliding door assembly operation.*

Although the provisions of 7.2.1.14 do not require specific occupancy chapter permission for use of horizontal-sliding door assemblies, some occupancy chapters impose additional restrictions. For example, 28.2.2.2.4 prohibits the installation of these door assemblies across a corridor in a new hotel or dormitory.

The requirements for the installation of horizontal-sliding door assemblies address the following:

1. Simple method of operation from either side without special knowledge or effort
2. Force necessary to operate the door assembly
3. Fire protection rating applicable to door assembly location and purpose
4. Automatic-closing means by smoke detection or means for self-closing

The force requirements of 7.2.1.14(3) and (4) help to ensure that the door assembly can be operated if the usual method of operation required by 7.2.1.14(2) fails.

It is important that sliding door assemblies, other than those addressed by 7.2.1.4.1(4)(c), be evaluated for compliance with all the requirements of 7.2.1.14. Traditional sliding door assemblies do not comply with these requirements; an example of a type of door assembly that does comply is shown in Exhibit 7.25.

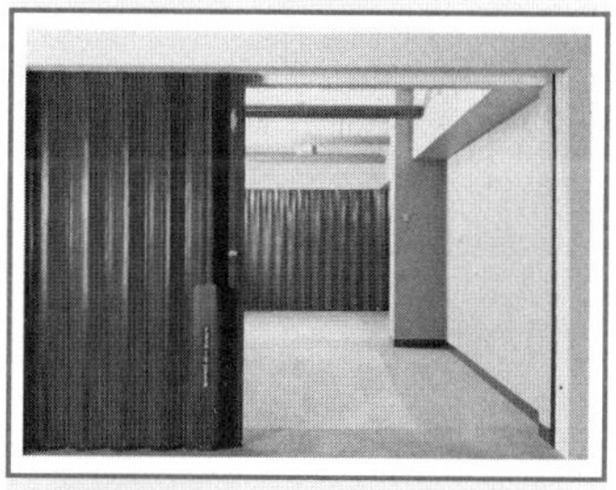

*Exhibit 7.25 Horizontal-sliding door assembly addressed by 7.2.1.14. (Photo courtesy of Won-Door Corp.)*

**7.2.1.15 Inspection of Door Openings.**

**7.2.1.15.1** Where required by Chapters 11 through 43, door assemblies for which the door leaf is required to swing in the direction of egress travel shall be inspected and tested not less than annually in accordance with 7.2.1.15.2 through 7.2.1.15.8.

The provisions of 7.2.1.15 are new to the 2009 edition of the *Code* and address the inspection and testing of door openings. The criteria for the inspection and testing of door openings apply only where specifically required by another portion of the *Code*, typically an occupancy chapter.



Commentary exhibits, including both drawings and photographs, provide detailed views of *Code* concepts. These exhibits are enclosed in green boxes and numbered sequentially throughout each chapter. Green shading over the caption also makes these exhibits easily discernible.

# Contents

# Preface

For more than 80 years, the National Fire Protection Association has been the developer and publisher of the *Life Safety Code*®. Formerly known as the *Building Exits Code,* the *Code* is prepared by the NFPA Committees on Safety to Life — 14 of the more than 200 technical committees operating within the framework of NFPA's consensus standards-development system. The members of the Committees on Safety to Life bring to the committee deliberations their knowledge and competence in the design and construction of buildings and structures, in the manufacture and testing of building components and accessories, and in the enforcement of regulations pertaining to life safety from fire and other related hazards encountered in buildings and structures. The committee members also participate in the development of *NFPA 5000*®, *Building Construction and Safety Code*®, which is processed in the same revision cycle as NFPA *101*®. There are many similarities between the two codes, especially within the occupancy chapters.

The *Life Safety Code* is a unique document; its contents address specific requirements that have a direct influence on safety to life in both new construction *and* existing buildings — not new construction alone. Moreover, although the *Code*'s paramount concern is life safety and not protection of property per se, there are also — by observance of the *Code*'s requirements — ancillary benefits to mission continuity and property protection.

The impact that application of the *Code* can have on saving lives is difficult to measure; however, it is reasonable to assume that its influence is extremely significant. For example, of the many fatal public building fires investigated by NFPA, invariably one or more of the building features contributing to loss of life from fire were in violation of the requirements of the *Code.*

NFPA recognizes that a code suitable for enforcement must, by the nature of its purpose, be concise and without explanatory text. In addition, a code cannot be written to cover every situation that will be encountered; thus, it must be applied with judgment and used with good sense and with an awareness of the rationale for the requirements to be enforced. A little help and counsel along the way can make the job a lot easier; hence, NFPA has also developed this *Life Safety Code Handbook.*

This handbook gives users of the *Life Safety Code* background information on the reasons for certain *Code* provisions. It also provides some suggestions, through its text and illustrations, on how some *Code* requirements can be implemented effectively. This kind of information is intended to provide users of the *Code* with a better understanding of, and appreciation for, the requirements contained in the *Code.* The net result should be buildings and structures that are increasingly more fire safe. The reader is cautioned, however, to look upon the commentary that appears in the handbook as the views of the editors and — where commentary reads relatively the same as in earlier editions — the contributors to earlier editions of the handbook. The commentary does not necessarily reflect the official position of NFPA.

Where a pair of occupancy chapters addresses a given occupancy (for example, Chapter 12 for new assembly occupancies and Chapter 13 for existing assembly occupancies), the *Code* text for both chapters is presented in side-by-side columns to permit easy comparison. Further, the accompanying commentary points out differences between the provisions applicable to new construction and to existing buildings.

Annex B, Elevators for Occupant-Controlled Evacuation Prior to Phase I Emergency Recall Operations, and Annex C, Supplemental Evacuation Equipment, are new to the 2009 edition of the *Code.* The *Code* text and accompanying commentary are new to this handbook. David de Vries of Firetech Engineering Inc. drafted the commentary, and tracked down the associated photographs, for Annex C.

For this edition of the handbook, Gregory Harrington revised the commentary for Chapters 8 through 11, 24, 26, 28 through 33, 36 through 40, and 42; Ron Coté revised the commentary for Chapters 1 through 7, 12 through 23, and 43, wrote the commentary for Annex B, and finalized the commentary for Annex C.

Ron Coté, P.E.
Principal Life Safety Engineer
NFPA

Gregory E. Harrington, P.E.
Principal Fire Protection Engineer
NFPA

# About the Editors

Ron Coté, P.E., is the principal life safety engineer in the Building Fire Protection and Life Safety group at NFPA. He joined the NFPA staff in 1981 and serves as staff liaison and secretary to several Safety to Life and Building Code technical committees. Prior to his employment with NFPA, Ron worked for seven years as a fire protection engineer for Factory Mutual Research Corporation. Ron is a registered Professional Engineer in the discipline of Fire Protection in the Commonwealth of Massachusetts.

Gregory E. Harrington, P.E., is a principal fire protection engineer in the NFPA Building Fire Protection and Life Safety group and serves as staff liaison and secretary to several Safety to Life and Building Code technical committees. Following the publication of the 2009 edition of NFPA 1, *Fire Code*, he assumed staff responsibility for that project as well. Prior to joining NFPA in 1996, Greg spent three years as a fire protection engineer with the San Antonio, Texas, Fire Department and also worked as a consulting engineer with Schirmer Engineering Corporation. He holds the degree of Master of Science in Fire Protection Engineering from Worcester Polytechnic Institute and is a registered Professional Engineer in the discipline of Fire Protection in the State of Connecticut.

**PART ONE**

# *Life Safety Code*® and Commentary

Part One of this handbook includes the complete text of the 2009 *Life Safety Code*®, which is made up of mandatory chapters (Chapters 1 through 43) and nonmandatory annex material. The 14 committees on safety to life prepared the mandatory provisions found in Chapters 1 through 43 within the framework of NFPA's consensus standards–development system. Because these provisions are designed to be suitable for adoption into law, or for reference by other codes and standards, the text is concise, without extended explanation.

The committees on safety to life also developed the material found in Annex A, Annex B, and Annex C of the *Code*. The material in Annex A is designed to assist users in interpreting the mandatory *Code* provisions. It is not considered to be part of the requirements of the *Code*; it is advisory or informational. An asterisk (*) following a *Code* paragraph number indicates that nonmandatory material pertaining to that paragraph appears in Annex A. For readers' convenience, in this handbook, Annex A material has been interspersed to appear immediately following its base paragraph in the body of the mandatory *Code* text. The material in Annex B and Annex C is written in mandatory language, but applies only where specifically adopted.

The handbook editors — Ron Coté, P.E., and Gregory Harrington, P.E. — prepared the explanatory commentary that accompanies the *Code,* Annex B, and Annex C. The commentary follows the *Code* text it discusses and is easily identified by green shading. Designed to help users understand and apply *Code* provisions, the commentary gives detailed explanations of the reasoning behind *Code* requirements, examples of calculations, applications of requirements, and tables of useful information. More than 400 drawings and photographs show practical applications of specific *Code* provisions. Used together with the *Code*, the commentary provides a rich resource for assessing the level of life safety from fires in buildings.

# CHAPTER 1

# Administration

NFPA *101*®, *Life Safety Code*®, is an occupancy-based document that is written and formatted so the user may go directly to the applicable occupancy chapter (i.e., Chapters 12 through 42), provided that the user is familiar enough with the occupancy classification criteria of Section 6.1 to classify the occupancy correctly. The applicable occupancy chapter provides a complete road map to direct the user to all needed portions of the core chapters, which develop the basic life safety concepts and offer a host of protection tools, systems, and features. The core chapters are positioned at the front of the *Code* in Chapters 1 through 11 and in Chapter 43 on building rehabilitation. A student of the *Code* might read and study the *Code* in chapter order, but the average user will typically consult an occupancy chapter first and then reference only those portions of the core chapters that apply to the project at hand as directed by the occupancy chapter.

The basic philosophy and core requirements of the *Code* are presented in Chapters 1 through 11 and Chapter 43. The scope, purpose, and application of the *Code* are positioned in Chapter 1 to allow the building blocks or fundamentals of the *Code* to be described, understood, and correctly applied.

Although any part of this handbook might be relevant and directly applicable to a specific type of structure or occupancy, the user is encouraged to develop a sound understanding of the rudimentary concepts of occupant life safety. Such understanding includes recognizing where the *Code* applies and the extent to which the designer, authority having jurisdiction, or both, should apply the *Code* requirements for new versus existing buildings. See, for example, 1.3.1 and its associated annex material.

The long-standing recognition of "equivalency" (see Section 1.4) is also an important concept, not only in NFPA *101* but also in the NFPA codes and standards used in combination with NFPA *101*. The equivalency concept allows for innovative approaches to life safety and fire safety. Although the *Code* is a comprehensive document, it is conceivable that a situation that the *Code* does not contemplate might arise. Equivalency considerations allow for such a situation to be evaluated and for a mutually agreeable solution to be developed that would provide the same or better level of life safety than that which would result from strict compliance with the prescriptive requirements.

## 1.1* Scope

### 1.1.1 Title.

NFPA *101*, *Life Safety Code*, shall be known as the *Life Safety Code*®, is cited as such, and shall be referred to herein as "this *Code*" or "the *Code*."

The title of the *Code* was changed from *Building Exits Code* to *Code for Safety to Life from Fire in Buildings and Structures* in 1966. The change in title expanded the scope of the *Code* from a specification-based code for stairs, doors, and fire escapes to a performance- and specification-based code that addresses the myriad factors that affect life safety in the event of fire.

From 1966 through 2002, the *Code* was referred to by its shortened name, *Life Safety Code*®. In 2003, the *Code* was officially renamed *Life Safety Code*.

The change in title reflects the *Code*'s ever-changing content. In some cases, the *Code* addresses non-fire, day-to-day, building occupant use issues. For example, in 12.2.5.4.3 and 13.2.5.4.3, which apply to assembly occupancies, access and egress routes are required to be maintained so that crowd management, security, and emergency medical personnel are able to reach any individual at any time without undue hindrance.

**A.1.1** The following is a suggested procedure for determining the *Code* requirements for a building or structure:

(1) Determine the occupancy classification by referring to the occupancy definitions in Chapter 6 and the occupancy Chapters 12 through 42. *(See 6.1.14 for buildings with more than one use.)*
(2) Determine if the building or structure is new or existing. *(See the definitions in Chapter 3.)*
(3) Determine the occupant load. *(See 7.3.1.)*
(4) Determine the hazard of contents. *(See Section 6.2.)*
(5) Refer to the applicable occupancy chapter of the *Code*, Chapters 12 through 42. *[See Chapters 1 through 4 and Chapters 6 through 11, as needed, for general information (such as definitions) or as directed by the occupancy chapter.]*
(6) Determine the occupancy subclassification or special use condition, if any, by referring to Chapters 16 and 17, day-care occupancies; Chapters 18 and 19, health care occupancies; Chapters 22 and 23, detention and correctional occupancies; Chapters 28 and 29, hotels and dormitories; Chapters 32 and 33, residential board and care occupancies; Chapters 36 and 37, mercantile occupancies; and Chapter 40, industrial occupancies, which contain subclassifications or special use definitions.
(7) Proceed through the applicable occupancy chapter to verify compliance with each referenced section, subsection, paragraph, subparagraph, and referenced codes, standards, and other documents.
(8) Where two or more requirements apply, refer to the occupancy chapter, which generally takes precedence over the base Chapters 1 through 4 and Chapters 6 through 11.
(9) Where two or more occupancy chapters apply, such as in a mixed occupancy *(see 6.1.14)*, apply the most restrictive requirements.

The steps outlined in A.1.1 were developed to help the user determine which *Code* requirements might apply to a given building if the more prevalent, prescriptive, specification-based life safety systems option is used. If the performance-based option is used, see 4.4.3.

Because specific occupancy requirements are detailed in separate chapters, the *Code* user should first identify the proper occupancy classification for a building. Guidance on classifying occupancy is presented in Section 6.1. The *Code* user will then be able to determine the appropriate chapter(s) for that occupancy.

***Example 1: Determining Code Requirements***

A jewelry retail sales operation (i.e., a jewelry store) occupying all of the twelfth floor of a multitenant building uses 5000 ft$^2$ (465 m$^2$), or 95 percent, of the floor area for sales purposes. Using the occupancy classification criteria and definitions found in Section 6.1, the jewelry store should be classified as a mercantile occupancy (see 6.1.10.1). In determining that the floor is a mercantile occupancy, the *Code* user narrows the range of choice of applicable occupancy chapters from Chapters 12 through 42 to the two that specifically address mercantile occupancies — Chapters 36 and 37.

Using the definition of *existing building* found in 3.3.32.5, the user can determine whether the building is subject to the requirements for new construction or for existing buildings. If the jewelry store used in this example was occupied subsequent to the adoption of the *Code* currently being enforced, the user determines that the life safety features required are those that apply to new construction. Thus, the user could narrow the applicable occupancy requirements to those for new mercantile occupancies as detailed in Chapter 36.

The *Code* user next identifies the subclassification of the mercantile occupancy (see 36.1.4.2) as Class A, Class B, or Class C on the basis of the 5000 ft$^2$ (465 m$^2$) floor area used for sales purposes. Because the jewelry store occupies more than 3000 ft$^2$ (280 m$^2$), but less than 30,000 ft$^2$ (2800 m$^2$), it is classified as a Class B mercantile occupancy. The user then locates the requirements of Chapter 36 that specifically apply to Class B mercantile occupancies and those requirements that apply across all subclassifications of mercantile occupancies. The user notes that Chapter 36 does not repeat the requirements found in Chapters 1 through 4 and Chapters 6 through 10, because the *Code* mandatorily references the use of those chapters. Because the jewelry store is located in the high-rise portion of the building, 36.4.2 requires compliance with a portion of the high-rise building requirements of Chapter 11 — specifically, the automatic sprinkler system provisions of 11.8.3.1.

In this example, the *Code* user recognizes that the requirements of Chapters 1 through 4, Chapters 6 through 10, a portion of Chapter 11, and Chapter 36 apply and are required to be met. This selection process is outlined in Exhibit 1.1.

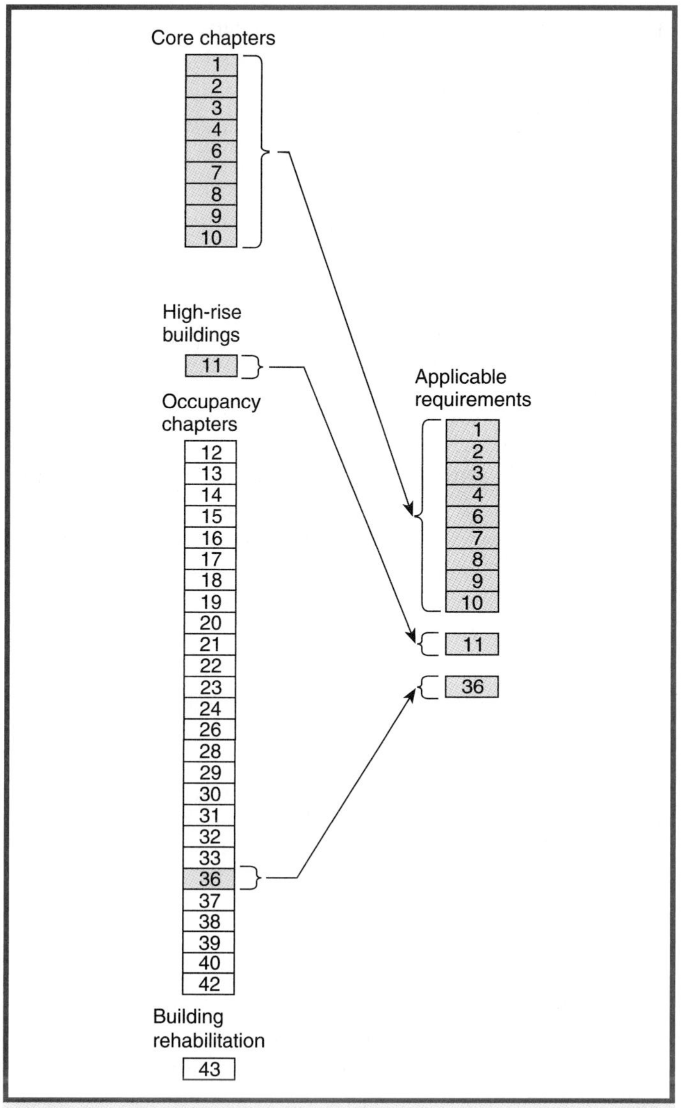


***Exhibit 1.1*** *Selecting specification-based Code requirements that apply to a given occupancy; in this case, a new mercantile occupancy on the twelfth floor of a multitenant building.*

***Example 2: Determining Code Requirements***

Consider a two-story mall building where two tenant spaces formerly occupied by a shoe store and a children's clothing store [each with 5000 $ft^2$ (465 $m^2$) of floor area for sales purposes] are to be gutted, combined in area, and outfitted for a new tenant that will sell sporting goods. The new tenant will occupy 10,000 $ft^2$ (929 $m^2$) of floor area for sales purposes. The *Code* user first identifies that the rehabilitation work will require compliance with the provisions of Chapter 43, Building Rehabilitation, and that such work falls into the rehabilitation category of Change of Use (see 43.2.2.1.5 and 43.7.1). The rehabilitation work also falls into the rehabilitation category of Modification, as explained further in this example. The user also notes that the occupancy involved is mercantile.

Next, the *Code* user consults the mercantile occupancy subclassification criteria of 36.1.4.2 or 37.1.4.2. The previous tenants each were Class B mercantile occupancies. The new tenant that will occupy the combined spaces of the previous tenants will be a Class B mercantile occupancy. The modification does not involve a change in mercantile subclassification, so the provisions of 36.1.1.4 and 37.1.1.4 do not mandate compliance with the requirements for new construction.

Chapter 43 is consulted to learn whether Chapter 36 for new mercantile occupancies or Chapter 37 for existing mercantile occupancies is to be used. Per 43.7.1, the change of use must be further classified as repair, renovation, modification, or reconstruction work. The reconfiguration of the space leads to classifying the work as a modification (see 43.2.2.1.3). Per 43.1.2.1(1), for a modification, the requirements of the applicable existing occupancy chapter must be met. Thus, the provisions of Chapter 37 for existing mercantile occupancies are required as the base requirements for starting the rehabilitation of the tenant space.

Per 43.5.1.3, newly constructed elements, components, and systems must comply with the requirements of other sections of the *Code* applicable to new construction. So, portions of Chapter 36 for new mercantile occupancies also will apply.

As explained in Example 1, the requirements of Chapters 1 through 4 and Chapters 6 through 10 must be met.

In Example 2, the *Code* user recognizes that the requirements of Chapters 1 through 4, Chapters 6 through 10, some portions of Chapter 36, Chapter 37, and some portions of Chapter 43 apply and are required to be met. This selection process is outlined in Exhibit 1.2.

## 1.1.2 Danger to Life from Fire.

The *Code* addresses those construction, protection, and occupancy features necessary to minimize danger to life from the effects of fire, including smoke, heat, and toxic gases created during a fire.

Subsection 1.1.2 does not list panic as a danger arising from the effects of a fire that needs to be addressed specifically via *Code* requirements. Panic is not a

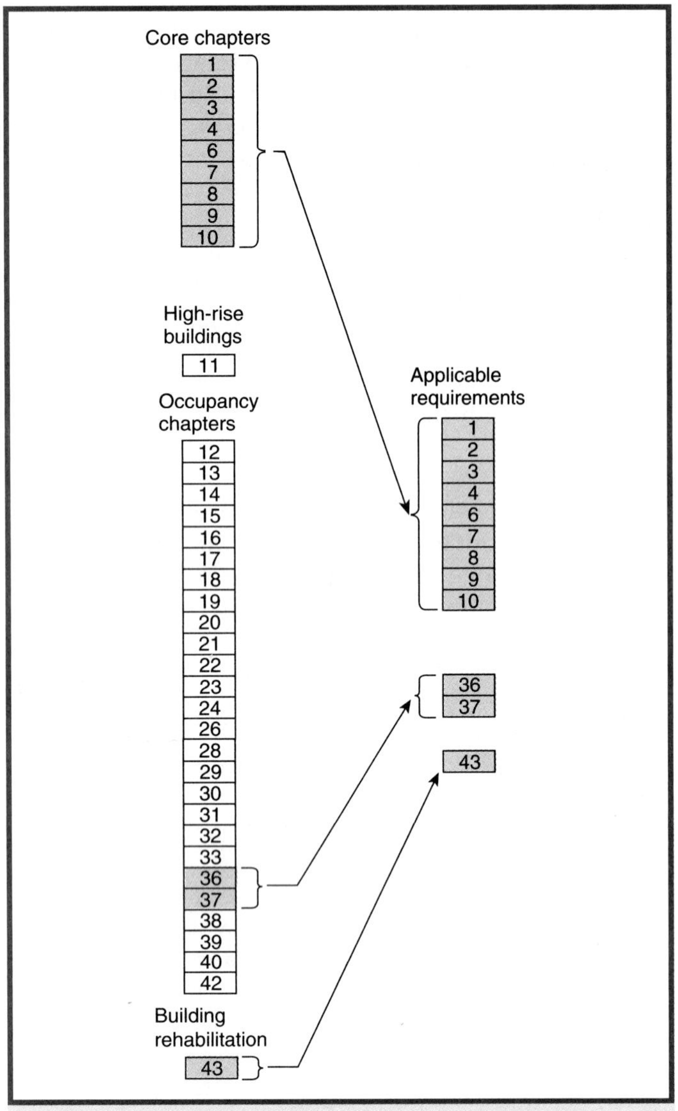


***Exhibit 1.2*** *Selecting specification-based Code requirements that apply to a given occupancy; in this case, a new mercantile tenant fit-out in a mall building space formerly occupied by two mercantile tenants.*

typical reaction of occupants in a burning building that at least comes close to being *Code* compliant. Studies of building fires indicate that occupants typically exhibit altruistic behavior toward others. Human response to a threatening situation might follow one of a variety of behaviors. Individuals might choose to investigate, sound an alarm, assist with rescue, seek help, or flee. Such actions constitute normal behavior, even when taken collectively. Most people avoid direct contact with a fire while undertaking another action.

In February of 2003, a fire at The Station nightclub in West Warwick, Rhode Island, claimed 100 patrons' lives. The fire began when pyrotechnics ignited the exposed, acoustical foamed plastic panels that lined the walls and ceiling of a platform serving as a stage for the musical group performing to a capacity crowd. Patrons died as the fire spread faster than they could egress the building. More than 30 bodies were found blocking the main entrance/exit. Some reviewers of the disaster might judge the patrons as having panicked, while others might say the patrons behaved rationally in trying to move toward the exits but were hindered when their actions created a crowd crush. Patron behavior was not the problem. The problem stemmed from the facility being far from *Code* compliant. The pyrotechnic devices (gerbs) used were designed for a venue with a much higher ceiling. The exposed foamed plastic panels lining the walls and ceiling of the performers' platform were a prohibited material and noted as a distinct hazard by existing *Code* requirements applicable to interior wall and ceiling finish.

Crowd behavior in large assembly occupancy venues is difficult to predict and manage. The life safety evaluation required of large assembly occupancies by the provisions of Chapters 12 and 13 deals not only with fire but also with storm, collapse, crowd behavior, and other related factors, a list of which is provided in A.12.4.1.3 and A.13.4.1.3.

### 1.1.3 Egress Facilities.

The *Code* establishes minimum criteria for the design of egress facilities so as to allow prompt escape of occupants from buildings or, where desirable, into safe areas within buildings.

Relocating building occupants to safe areas within a building might include moving them to one of the following locations:

1. Into an area of refuge
2. Through doors in a horizontal exit into another fire compartment
3. Through doors in a smoke barrier into another smoke compartment

In some cases, an egress system that relies on total evacuation to the exterior is not practical. For example, in a health care occupancy, building evacuation might expose patients to conditions more dangerous than those encountered in relocating the patients from a fire compartment to a safe smoke compartment on the same floor. For most occupancies, the *Code* provisions permit the designer to choose whether the egress system relies on full evacuation. For occupancies such as health care, a protect-in-place strategy is used that requires the subdivision of floors into two or more smoke compartments, regardless of the presence of fire exit stairs.

For high-rise buildings, egress systems have traditionally been implemented so as to rely on partial building evacuation/relocation. Occupants on the fire floor and the floors immediately above and below the fire floor are asked to relocate to floors a few levels below the fire floor. This procedure is intended to preclude having to direct all building occupants to evacuate immediately to ground level until the fire conditions dictate such action. Following the September 11, 2001, collapse of the World Trade Center towers in New York City, occupants of high-rise buildings have reported a reluctance to stay behind at the first hint of a fire or similar problem. Building managers and code consultants need to re-evaluate high-rise building emergency plans that rely on partial evacuation or relocation. See A.4.8.2.1(3) for detailed guidance on occupant evacuation strategies.

### 1.1.4 Other Fire-Related Considerations.

The *Code* addresses other considerations that are essential to life safety in recognition of the fact that life safety is more than a matter of egress. The *Code* also addresses protective features and systems, building services, operating features, maintenance activities, and other provisions in recognition of the fact that achieving an acceptable degree of life safety depends on additional safeguards to provide adequate egress time or protection for people exposed to fire.

### 1.1.5* Considerations Not Related to Fire.

The *Code* also addresses other considerations that, while important in fire conditions, provide an ongoing benefit in other conditions of use, including non-fire emergencies.

**A.1.1.5** Life safety in buildings includes more than safety from fire. Although fire safety has been the long-standing focus of NFPA *101*, its widely known title, *Life Safety Code*, and its technical requirements respond to a wider range of concerns, including, for example, crowd safety.

Numerous elements affect the overall level of life safety. The *Code* addresses many of these factors, including combustibility of interior finishes and the evacuation preparedness of occupants. However, other areas are not addressed, such as the influence of public education on fire safety. See 1.1.6 and related commentary for more information on factors not covered by the *Code*.

### 1.1.6 Areas Not Addressed.

The *Code* does not address the following:

(1)* General fire prevention or building construction features that are normally a function of fire prevention codes and building codes

**A.1.1.6(1)** This *Code* is intended to be adopted and used as part of a comprehensive program of building regulations that include building, mechanical, plumbing, electrical, fuel gas, fire prevention, and land use regulations.

(2) Prevention of injury incurred by an individual due to that individual's failure to use reasonable care
(3) Preservation of property from loss by fire

The *Code* is not intended to be either a building code or a fire prevention code. However, in the interest of public safety, the *Code* does contain provisions typically associated with a building code or fire prevention code. For example, although construction requirements are typically considered the domain of a building code, Chapters 18 and 19 provide minimum, fire-rated construction requirements for buildings housing health care occupancies. The construction requirements are provided to ensure the structural integrity of the building for the period of time required for staff to evacuate those occupants incapable of self-preservation.

Similarly, the provisions of Chapters 12 and 13 — for assembly occupancies — require fire-rated building construction, depending on the number of occupants and the levels of the building occupied as assembly occupancies. The requirement recognizes the lengthy time periods necessary to evacuate large numbers of persons, especially from floors above the level of exit discharge. Thus, fire-rated building construction is intended to ensure the structural integrity of the building for the period of time required for occupants to evacuate.

Although preventative measures are typically associated with a fire prevention code, the operating features sections located at the end of most of the occupancy chapters contain requirements that do the following:

1. Limit the flammability of contents introduced into certain occupancies
2. Require the training of facility employees in emergency duties

3. Require occupants to practice emergency egress and relocation

These operational requirements, when combined with egress and other specific occupancy chapter requirements, provide an appropriate life safety package.

The *Code* intentionally excludes traditional building code topics such as wind loads, seismic considerations, and exterior exposure protection.

Although the *Code* requirements were developed to provide life safety from fire, adherence to its requirements might assist in property conservation and prevention of personal injuries. For example, the automatic sprinkler systems required for life safety purposes provide substantial property protection benefits as well.

## 1.2* Purpose

The purpose of this *Code* is to provide minimum requirements, with due regard to function, for the design, operation, and maintenance of buildings and structures for safety to life from fire. Its provisions will also aid life safety in similar emergencies.

This *Code* specifies the minimum requirements that collectively help to ensure safety to occupants from fires and similar emergencies to the degree specified by the objectives stated in Section 4.2. However, it is not the *Code*'s intent to prevent the user from exceeding the specified minimum requirements. See also 4.6.9.

**A.1.2** The *Code* endeavors to avoid requirements that might involve unreasonable hardships or unnecessary inconvenience or interference with the normal use and occupancy of a building but provides for fire safety consistent with the public interest.

Protection of occupants is achieved by the combination of prevention, protection, egress, and other features, with due regard to the capabilities and reliability of the features involved. The level of life safety from fire is defined through requirements directed at the following:

(1) Prevention of ignition
(2) Detection of fire
(3) Control of fire development
(4) Confinement of the effects of fire
(5) Extinguishment of fire
(6) Provision of refuge or evacuation facilities, or both
(7) Staff reaction
(8) Provision of fire safety information to occupants

Buildings are normally designed to accommodate a specific functional need. The *Code* considers the normal occupancy of a building and attempts not to interfere with its regular use or to set requirements that cause unreasonable hardship or unnecessary inconvenience to its normal functioning. For example, although self-closing devices on doors help to ensure continuous fire and smoke compartmentation, the health care occupancy provisions of this *Code* do not require self-closing devices on patient room doors because of the day-to-day functional need for staff to monitor conditions, which necessitates that doors remain open. The health care occupancy chapters achieve the intended minimum level of life safety, without unduly interfering with normal operation of the facility, by combining other features and protection schemes. For example, 18.7.2 and 19.7.2, which apply to new and existing health care occupancies, respectively, require that staff establish procedures to be followed in case of fire, including closing doors to isolate the fire area and confine the effects of the fire.

In addressing life safety from fire and similar emergencies, the *Code* focuses on the movement of people in an emergency. However, many of the building features that assist with the safe movement of people in an emergency also provide increased safety during normal building use. For example, new stairs are not permitted to have a riser height that exceeds 7 in. (180 mm) or to provide a tread depth less than 11 in. (280 mm) to reduce the potential to trip under emergency egress use. This safe stair geometry also reduces the potential of tripping whenever the stair is used.

The occupancy chapters make varying use of any or all of the protection features in A.1.2(1) through (8). A business occupancy located in a single-story building uses fewer of the protection features to accomplish the intended minimum level of life safety than does a health care occupancy. A health care occupancy accomplishes its minimum level of life safety by extensively applying the features of A.1.2(1) through (7) using a defend-in-place strategy. This strategy recognizes that some occupants of a health care occupancy are both incapable of self-preservation and difficult to move, particularly to other floors or to the exterior of the building. The provision of A.1.2(8) for providing safety information to occupants is not an important requirement for a health care occupancy, because it is expected that staff will direct any needed relocation or evacuation so as to relieve the patients from having to know how to relocate or evacuate by themselves.

## 1.3 Application

### 1.3.1* New and Existing Buildings and Structures.

The *Code* shall apply to both new construction and existing buildings and existing structures.

**A.1.3.1** Various chapters contain specific provisions for existing buildings and structures that might differ from those for new construction.

In order to provide a minimum level of life safety to all occupancies in all structures, the *Code* applies to both new construction and existing buildings. Provisions exist throughout the *Code* that apply specifically to existing buildings. Such provisions should be thought of as applying to existing conditions. Also, the *Code* contains requirements for new construction that have been modified to apply to existing buildings. The modifications were made to limit the resulting disruption and financial impact on existing buildings while providing the intended minimum level of life safety. The requirements applicable to new construction are often more stringent than those for existing buildings, because providing appropriate life safety requirements is considered less disruptive and more cost-effective during construction. If no modification for existing buildings appears within a *Code* requirement, the same provision applies for new construction and existing buildings.

See also 4.6.5, 4.6.6, and 4.6.10 and the definitions of *existing* and *existing building* in 3.3.73 and 3.3.32.5, respectively.

### 1.3.2 Vehicles and Vessels.

The *Code* shall apply to vehicles, vessels, or other similar conveyances, as specified in Section 11.6, in which case such vehicles and vessels shall be treated as buildings.

## 1.4* Equivalency

Nothing in this *Code* is intended to prevent the use of systems, methods, or devices of equivalent or superior quality, strength, fire resistance, effectiveness, durability, and safety over those prescribed by this *Code*.

**A.1.4** Before a particular mathematical fire model or evaluation system is used, its purpose and limitations need to be known. The technical documentation should clearly identify any assumptions included in the evaluation. Also, it is the intent of the Committee on Safety to Life to recognize that future editions of this *Code* are a further refinement of this edition and earlier editions. The changes in future editions will reflect the continuing input of the fire protection/life safety community in its attempt to meet the purpose stated in this *Code*.

Section 1.4, Equivalency, presents a powerful design alternative that permits individual and multiple specification-based requirements to be satisfied by components and systems that the authority having jurisdiction is convinced meet the goals, objectives, and intended level of life safety of the *Code*. Where all life safety systems, rather than individual and multiple specification-based systems, are engineered to meet the goals and objectives of the *Code*, true performance-based design is permitted in accordance with Chapter 5. In other words, equivalency deals with discrete, manageable pieces of the overall life safety system; performance-based design treats the system as a whole. See Section 4.4.

With each new edition, the *Code* continues its evolution from a specification-based code to a performance-oriented code. Section 4.4 permits a complete performance-based design approach in accordance with Chapter 5. However, the traditional, widely accepted, specification-based approach is maintained as an option. The vast majority of building projects will continue to use this traditional approach. The performance-based design approach is complex and expensive and, therefore, feasible for megasized developments.

Section 1.4 recognizes that, although the majority of the *Code* uses specification language as the basis for enforcement, it should not inhibit the use of alternate or equivalent systems or design approaches to comply with *Code*-specified performance criteria. It is stipulated, however, that equivalency must be demonstrated by appropriate technical documentation. The evaluation and approval of such systems and approaches is the responsibility of the authority having jurisdiction.

The *Code* contemplates the several forms of equivalency that follow.

1. *Code-specified alternative.* In some instances, the *Code* presents a written requirement and then provides an alternate method of obtaining the desired level of protection, usually via an exemption. For example, for new educational occupancies, 14.3.6 requires that interior corridors be constructed of 1-hour fire resistance-rated assemblies. However, 14.3.6(2) allows the 1-hour rating requirement to be reduced to that of a nonrated smoke partition if the building is protected throughout by an approved, supervised automatic sprinkler

system. Thus, the *Code* specifies that the combination of smoke partitions and sprinkler protection is the equivalent of 1-hour fire resistance–rated corridor walls for new educational occupancies.

**2.** *NFPA 101A equivalency methods.* NFPA 101A, *Guide on Alternative Approaches to Life Safety,*[1] provides a set of equivalency methods that can be used to assess equivalency for health care occupancies, detention and correctional occupancies, board and care occupancies, business occupancies, and educational occupancies. Each system awards high point values for providing a building with strong life safety and fire protection features and assesses low point values for unsafe conditions. Factors are weighted with respect to their impact on life safety principles. High point to low point values are assigned. The completed evaluations are presented to the authority having jurisdiction for review and approval.

In addition to the fire safety evaluation systems, NFPA 101A contains a procedure for determining the evacuation capability for residents of existing residential board and care occupancies. Use of this method is also subject to the review and approval of the authority having jurisdiction. The requirements of Chapter 33, applicable to existing residential board and care occupancies, vary depending on the evacuation capability of the residents and staff working together as a group.

**3.** *More recent edition of the Code.* As explained in A.1.4, future editions of the *Code* are considered refinements of earlier editions because they clarify intent with respect to the revised topics. Use of a newer edition in its entirety should be considered as equivalent to use of an earlier edition.

Caution must be exercised when applying the concept of equivalency. It is important to recognize that specific provisions are part of a carefully crafted set of requirements that result in a desired level of life safety. A revision to one portion of the *Code* might be a part of, or the result of, changes to other parts of the *Code*. Therefore, it would be inappropriate to refer only to a specific section of a more recent edition of the *Code* that reflects a less stringent requirement than previous editions without taking into account any associated provisions that may have become more stringent to compensate for that more relaxed provision.

It is not the intent of the *Code* to limit the user to the three specified methods of judging equivalency. It is the intent to allow emerging technology to be used to satisfy the prescribed performance requirements. Fire modeling (see 3.3.92) has developed to the stage that authorities having jurisdiction are routinely approving equivalency on the basis of such technology. Additionally, the results of fire tests and other documented forms of engineering analysis have prompted the approval of authorities having jurisdiction.

### 1.4.1 Technical Documentation.

Technical documentation shall be submitted to the authority having jurisdiction to demonstrate equivalency.

### 1.4.2 Approval.

The system, method, or device shall be approved for the intended purpose by the authority having jurisdiction.

### 1.4.3* Equivalent Compliance.

Alternative systems, methods, or devices approved as equivalent by the authority having jurisdiction shall be recognized as being in compliance with this *Code*.

**A.1.4.3** An equivalent method of protection provides an equal or greater level of safety. It is not a waiver or deletion of a *Code* requirement.

The prescriptive provisions of this *Code* provide specific requirements for broad classifications of buildings and structures. These requirements are stated in terms of fixed values, such as maximum travel distance, minimum fire resistance ratings, and minimum features of required systems, such as detection, alarm, suppression, and ventilation, and not in terms of overall building or system performance.

However, the equivalency clause in 1.4.3 permits the use of alternative systems, methods, or devices to meet the intent of the prescribed code provisions where approved as being equivalent. Equivalency provides an opportunity for a performance-based design approach. Through the rigor of a performance-based design, it can be demonstrated whether a building design is satisfactory and complies with the implicit or explicit intent of the applicable code requirement.

When employing the equivalency clause, it is important to clearly identify the prescriptive-based code provision being addressed (scope), to provide an interpretation of the intent of the provision (goals and objectives), to provide an alternative approach (proposed design), and to provide appropriate support for the suggested alternative (evaluation of proposed designs).

Performance resulting from proposed designs can be compared to the performance of the design features required by this *Code*. Using prescribed features as a baseline for comparison, it can then be demonstrated in the evaluation whether a proposed design offers the intended level of performance. A comparison of safety provided can be used as the basis for establishing equivalency.

Subsection 1.4.3 emphasizes that there is more than one way to achieve *Code* compliance. A building either follows the specification criteria, achieves equivalency, or meets the requirements that apply to a full performance-based design. Where the equivalency option is used and the authority having jurisdiction has judged the alternative approach to life safety as providing equivalency to the *Code* requirements, a building is considered to be *Code* compliant. Compliance through equivalency does not differ from compliance through strict adherence to the specification-based requirements; however, compliance through equivalency does differ from a waiver that permits continued use of a noncomplying building. The *Code* provisions do not recognize the concept of waivers, but instead require that a level of safety is provided that is equivalent to that required by the prescriptive-based provisions.

## 1.5 Units and Formulas

### 1.5.1 SI Units.

Metric units of measurement in this *Code* are in accordance with the modernized metric system known as the International System of Units (SI).

### 1.5.2 Primary Values.

The inch-pound value for a measurement, and the SI value given in parentheses, shall each be acceptable for use as primary units for satisfying the requirements of this *Code*.

In the *Code*, inch-pound values for measurements appear first, and metric (SI) values are given within parentheses, as permitted by the NFPA *Manual of Style for NFPA Technical Committee Documents.*[2] The 2003 edition of the *Code* experimented with presenting SI units first and following with inch-pound values within parentheses in an attempt to give the *Code* more international appeal. As a result, well-established criteria changed in format. For example, the requirement for new hospital and nursing home corridors to be a minimum of 8 ft (2440 mm) wide was changed to express that width as 2440 mm (96 in.). The average user could not readily identify with the large magnitude inch specifications, which required mentally converting 96 in. to 8 ft. The experiment with the change in units failed. The 2006 edition returned the formatting to that used in earlier editions of the *Code*.

As permitted by 1.5.2, the inch-pound value and the SI value are each acceptable for use as primary values for satisfying the requirements of this *Code*. The metric values are calculated by taking the inch-pound values, applying conversion factors, and rounding to a specified number of significant digits. Thus, the SI values might not represent the nominal dimensions to which products are manufactured for use in countries using SI units.

## 1.6 Enforcement

This *Code* shall be administered and enforced by the authority having jurisdiction designated by the governing authority.

NFPA publishes Chapters 1 through 43 of the *Code* using mandatory language suitable for adoption for regulatory purposes. Section 1.6 establishes the authority having jurisdiction (AHJ) (see definition in 3.2.2) as the entity responsible for administering and enforcing the *Code*. The role of the AHJ is further defined in 4.6.1.

### References Cited in Commentary

1. NFPA 101A, *Guide on Alternative Approaches to Life Safety*, 2007 edition, National Fire Protection Association, Quincy, MA. (Note: The 2007 edition of NFPA 101A is calibrated to measure equivalency against the requirements of the 2006 edition of the *Code*. The 2010 edition of NFPA 101A will measure equivalency against the requirements of the 2009 edition of the *Code*. NFPA 101A is published one year after its companion edition of the *Code*, since it is necessary to have the *Code* revisions finalized before calibrating the NFPA 101A fire safety evaluation systems.)
2. NFPA *Manual of Style for NFPA Technical Committee Documents*, National Fire Protection Association, Quincy, MA, 2004.

CHAPTER 2

# Referenced Publications

Chapter 2 lists mandatory referenced publications. By positioning the information immediately after Chapter 1, Administration, the *Code* user is presented with the complete list of publications needed for effective use of the *Code* before reading the "meat" of the requirements. The provisions of the publications that are mandated by the *Code* are also requirements in the same way, for example, that the provisions of Chapter 7, Means of Egress, are mandated. Regardless of whether a requirement actually resides within the *Code* or is mandatorily referenced and appears only in the referenced publication, the requirement must be met to achieve compliance with the *Code*. Annex D lists nonmandatory referenced publications.

The *Life Safety Code* achieves its intended level of occupant safety by mandating the installation of various building features and systems. Where specific equipment and systems are required, their proper installation and maintenance are important. Rather than develop its own installation criteria, the *Code* mandates the use of expert documents. The referenced document becomes a legally enforceable part of NFPA *101*.

The level of reference to a particular document varies. For example, although *NFPA 72®, National Fire Alarm Code®*,[1] permits numerous occupant notification measures, NFPA *101* might limit the options that can be used for an occupancy. Paragraphs 14.3.4.3.1.2 and 15.3.4.3.1.2 permit positive alarm sequence notification for new and existing educational occupancies; however, rather than specifying the role of positive alarm sequence, those paragraphs refer to 9.6.3.4. Paragraph 9.6.3.4 points the user to *NFPA 72* for the detailed criteria applicable to positive alarm sequence, provided that the occupancy chapter has given permission for its use.

Another occupant notification method, the presignal system, as described in *NFPA 72*, is addressed by the *Code*. Once again, though, an occupancy chapter must permit the presignal system as detailed in 9.6.3.3. A presignal system is not permitted for use in educational occupancies. Therefore, even though it is recognized in *NFPA 72*, this occupant notification method is not permitted for schools. Thus, not all of the options offered by a referenced document can be used. The user of the *Code* must be aware of the reference and of any limitations or caveats on use of the referenced documents.

NFPA *101*, like other NFPA codes and standards, can mandate the use of a referenced document only if that document is an ANSI-accredited, consensus-based code or standard, provided that such an ANSI-accredited document exists. NFPA policy does not permit mandating the use of a referenced document that has not been developed under consensus procedures, nor does it permit reference to those documents developed by committees whose membership is not balanced with respect to user interests. A code or standard written by a committee dominated by an interest group has too great a potential for bias.

The documents listed in Chapter 2 are mandatory only to the extent called for in the *Code*. For example, the inclusion of NFPA 13, *Standard for the Installation of Sprinkler Systems*,[2] does not mean that all buildings must be sprinklered. Rather, where the *Code* requires buildings, other than small residential occupancies, to be sprinklered, NFPA 13 is to be used for sprinkler installation. See 9.7.1.1(1) as an example of *Code* language that mandatorily references the use of other NFPA documents.

The *Code* recognizes that existing installations need not be continuously upgraded as new editions of the referenced standards are adopted. This is specified in 4.6.7.

## 2.1 General

The documents or portions thereof listed in this chapter are referenced within this code and shall be considered part of the requirements of this document.

## 2.2 NFPA Publications

National Fire Protection Association, 1 Batterymarch Park, Quincy, MA 02169-7471.

NFPA 1, *Fire Code,* 2009 edition.

NFPA 10, *Standard for Portable Fire Extinguishers,* 2007 edition.

NFPA 11, *Standard for Low-, Medium-, and High-Expansion Foam,* 2005 edition.

NFPA 12, *Standard on Carbon Dioxide Extinguishing Systems,* 2008 edition.

NFPA 12A, *Standard on Halon 1301 Fire Extinguishing Systems,* 2009 edition.

NFPA 13, *Standard for the Installation of Sprinkler Systems,* 2007 edition.

NFPA 13D, *Standard for the Installation of Sprinkler Systems in One- and Two-Family Dwellings and Manufactured Homes,* 2007 edition.

NFPA 13R, *Standard for the Installation of Sprinkler Systems in Residential Occupancies up to and Including Four Stories in Height,* 2007 edition.

NFPA 14, *Standard for the Installation of Standpipe and Hose Systems,* 2007 edition.

NFPA 15, *Standard for Water Spray Fixed Systems for Fire Protection,* 2007 edition.

NFPA 16, *Standard for the Installation of Foam-Water Sprinkler and Foam-Water Spray Systems,* 2007 edition.

NFPA 17, *Standard for Dry Chemical Extinguishing Systems,* 2009 edition.

NFPA 17A, *Standard for Wet Chemical Extinguishing Systems,* 2009 edition.

NFPA 25, *Standard for the Inspection, Testing, and Maintenance of Water-Based Fire Protection Systems,* 2008 edition.

NFPA 30, *Flammable and Combustible Liquids Code,* 2008 edition.

NFPA 30B, *Code for the Manufacture and Storage of Aerosol Products,* 2007 edition.

NFPA 31, *Standard for the Installation of Oil-Burning Equipment,* 2006 edition.

NFPA 40, *Standard for the Storage and Handling of Cellulose Nitrate Film,* 2007 edition.

NFPA 45, *Standard on Fire Protection for Laboratories Using Chemicals,* 2004 edition.

NFPA 54, *National Fuel Gas Code,* 2009 edition.

NFPA 58, *Liquefied Petroleum Gas Code,* 2008 edition.

*NFPA 70®, National Electrical Code®*, 2008 edition.

*NFPA 72®, National Fire Alarm Code®*, 2007 edition.

NFPA 80, *Standard for Fire Doors and Other Opening Protectives,* 2007 edition.

NFPA 82, *Standard on Incinerators and Waste and Linen Handling Systems and Equipment,* 2004 edition.

NFPA 88A, *Standard for Parking Structures,* 2007 edition.

NFPA 90A, *Standard for the Installation of Air-Conditioning and Ventilating Systems,* 2009 edition.

NFPA 90B, *Standard for the Installation of Warm Air Heating and Air-Conditioning Systems,* 2009 edition.

NFPA 91, *Standard for Exhaust Systems for Air Conveying of Vapors, Gases, Mists, and Noncombustible Particulate Solids,* 2004 edition.

NFPA 92A, *Standard for Smoke-Control Systems Utilizing Barriers and Pressure Differences,* 2009 edition.

NFPA 92B, *Standard for Smoke Management Systems in Malls, Atria, and Large Spaces,* 2009 edition.

NFPA 96, *Standard for Ventilation Control and Fire Protection of Commercial Cooking Operations,* 2008 edition.

NFPA 99, *Standard for Health Care Facilities,* 2005 edition.

NFPA 101A, *Guide on Alternative Approaches to Life Safety,* 2007 edition.

NFPA 105, *Standard for the Installation of Smoke Door Assemblies and Other Opening Protectives,* 2007 edition.

NFPA 110, *Standard for Emergency and Standby Power Systems,* 2005 edition.

NFPA 111, *Standard on Stored Electrical Energy Emergency and Standby Power Systems,* 2005 edition.

NFPA 160, *Standard for the Use of Flame Effects Before an Audience,* 2006 edition.

NFPA 170, *Standard for Fire Safety and Emergency Symbols,* 2006 edition.

NFPA 204, *Standard for Smoke and Heat Venting,* 2007 edition.

NFPA 211, *Standard for Chimneys, Fireplaces, Vents, and Solid Fuel–Burning Appliances,* 2006 edition.

NFPA 220, *Standard on Types of Building Construction,* 2009 edition.

NFPA 221, *Standard for High Challenge Fire Walls, Fire Walls, and Fire Barrier Walls,* 2009 edition.

NFPA 241, *Standard for Safeguarding Construction, Alteration, and Demolition Operations,* 2004 edition.

NFPA 251, *Standard Methods of Tests of Fire Resistance of Building Construction and Materials,* 2006 edition.

NFPA 252, *Standard Methods of Fire Tests of Door Assemblies,* 2008 edition.

NFPA 253, *Standard Method of Test for Critical Radi-*

*ant Flux of Floor Covering Systems Using a Radiant Heat Energy Source,* 2006 edition.

NFPA 255, *Standard Method of Test of Surface Burning Characteristics of Building Materials,* 2006 edition.

NFPA 256, *Standard Methods of Fire Tests of Roof Coverings,* 2003 edition.

NFPA 257, *Standard on Fire Test for Window and Glass Block Assemblies,* 2007 edition.

NFPA 259, *Standard Test Method for Potential Heat of Building Materials,* 2008 edition.

NFPA 260, *Standard Methods of Tests and Classification System for Cigarette Ignition Resistance of Components of Upholstered Furniture,* 2009 edition.

NFPA 261, *Standard Method of Test for Determining Resistance of Mock-Up Upholstered Furniture Material Assemblies to Ignition by Smoldering Cigarettes,* 2009 edition.

NFPA 265, *Standard Methods of Fire Tests for Evaluating Room Fire Growth Contribution of Textile Coverings on Full Height Panels and Walls,* 2007 edition.

NFPA 286, *Standard Methods of Fire Tests for Evaluating Contribution of Wall and Ceiling Interior Finish to Room Fire Growth,* 2006 edition.

NFPA 288, *Standard Methods of Fire Tests of Floor Fire Door Assemblies Installed Horizontally in Fire Resistance–Rated Floor Systems,* 2007 edition.

NFPA 415, *Standard on Airport Terminal Buildings, Fueling Ramp Drainage, and Loading Walkways,* 2008 edition.

NFPA 418, *Standard for Heliports,* 2006 edition.

NFPA 430, *Code for the Storage of Liquid and Solid Oxidizers,* 2004 edition.

NFPA 432, *Code for the Storage of Organic Peroxide Formulations,* 2002 edition.

NFPA 434, *Code for the Storage of Pesticides,* 2002 edition.

NFPA 701, *Standard Methods of Fire Tests for Flame Propagation of Textiles and Films,* 2004 edition.

NFPA 703, *Standard for Fire Retardant–Treated Wood and Fire-Retardant Coatings for Building Materials,* 2009 edition.

NFPA 750, *Standard on Water Mist Fire Protection Systems,* 2006 edition.

NFPA 914, *Code for Fire Protection of Historic Structures,* 2007 edition.

NFPA 1124, *Code for the Manufacture, Transportation, Storage, and Retail Sales of Fireworks and Pyrotechnic Articles,* 2006 edition.

NFPA 1126, *Standard for the Use of Pyrotechnics Before a Proximate Audience,* 2006 edition.

NFPA 1971, *Standard on Protective Ensembles for Structural Fire Fighting and Proximity Fire Fighting,* 2007 edition.

NFPA 2001, *Standard on Clean Agent Fire Extinguishing Systems,* 2008 edition.

It is NFPA policy that the edition of the NFPA publications referenced be the most current at the time the *Code* is issued. The life safety technical committees do not have to act to update the edition of referenced NFPA publications. The updating occurs editorially.

The publications by organizations other than NFPA, listed in Section 2.3, carry an edition date adopted by the life safety technical committees via the normal revision process involving proposals and comments and public review via the Report on Proposals (ROP) and Report on Comments (ROC). This means the technical committees must take deliberate action to adopt a specific edition of the publications by organizations other than NFPA. This is done to assure that the provisions of those documents, mandated for use with the *Code,* are appropriate.

## 2.3 Other Publications

### 2.3.1 ACI Publications.

American Concrete Institute, P.O. Box 9094, Farmington Hills, MI 48333. www.concrete.org

ACI 216.1/TMS 0216.1, *Standard Method for Determining Fire Resistance of Concrete and Masonry Construction Assemblies*, 1997.

### 2.3.2 ANSI Publications.

American National Standards Institute, Inc., 25 West 43rd Street, 4th floor, New York, NY 10036.

ANSI A14.3, *Safety Requirements for Fixed Ladders*, 1992.

ICC/ANSI A117.1, *American National Standard for Accessible and Usable Buildings and Facilities*, 2003.

BHMA/ANSI A156.19, *American National Standard for Power Assist and Low Energy Power Operated Doors*, 2002.

ANSI Z22-3.1, *National Fuel Gas Code*, 2006.

### 2.3.3 ASCE Publications.

American Society of Civil Engineers, 1801 Alexander Bell Drive, Reston, VA 20191-4400. www.asce.org

ASCE/SFPE 29, *Standard Calculation Methods for Structural Fire Protection*, 1999.

### 2.3.4 ASME Publications.

American Society of Mechanical Engineers, Three Park Avenue, New York, NY 10016-5990. www.asme.org

ASME A17.1/CSA B44, *Safety Code for Elevators and Escalators*, 2007.

ASME A17.3, *Safety Code for Existing Elevators and Escalators*, 2005.

### 2.3.5 ASSE Publications.

American Society of Safety Engineers, 1800 East Oakton Street, Des Plaines, IL 60018.

ANSI/ASSE A1264.1, *Safety Requirements for Workplace Floor and Wall Openings, Stairs and Railing Systems*, 2007.

### 2.3.6 ASTM Publications.

ASTM International, 100 Barr Harbor Drive, P.O. Box C700, West Conshohocken, PA 19428-2959. www.astm.org

ASTM D 1929, *Standard Test Method for Determining Ignition Temperatures of Plastic*, 2001.

ASTM D 2859, *Standard Test Method for Ignition Characteristics of Finished Textile Floor Covering Materials*, 2004.

ASTM D 2898, *Standard Test Methods for Accelerated Weathering of Fire-Retardant-Treated Wood for Fire Testing*, 1994 (1999).

ASTM E 84, *Standard Test Method for Surface Burning Characteristics of Building Materials*, 2004.

ASTM E 108, *Standard Test Methods for Fire Tests of Roof Coverings*, 2004.

ASTM E 119, *Standard Test Methods for Fire Tests of Building Construction and Materials*, 2007a.

ASTM E 136, *Standard Test Method for Behavior of Materials in a Vertical Tube Furnace at 750 Degrees C*, 2004.

ASTM E 648, *Standard Test Method for Critical Radiant Flux of Floor Covering Systems Using a Radiant Heat Energy Source,* 2006.

ASTM E 814, *Standard Test Method for Fire Tests of Through-Penetration Fire Stops*, 2002.

ASTM E 1352, *Standard Test Method for Cigarette Ignition Resistance of Mock-Up Upholstered Furniture Assemblies*, 2002.

ASTM E 1353, *Standard Test Methods for Cigarette Ignition Resistance of Components of Upholstered Furniture*, 2002.

ASTM E 1537, *Standard Test Method for Fire Testing of Upholstered Furniture*, 2002.

ASTM E 1590, *Standard Test Method for Fire Testing of Mattresses*, 2002.

ASTM E 1591, *Standard Guide for Obtaining Data for Deterministic Fire Models*, 2000.

ASTM E 1966, *Standard Test Method for Fire-Resistive Joint Systems*, 2001.

ASTM E 2010, *Standard Test Method for Positive Pressure Fire Tests of Window Assemblies*, 2001.

ASTM E 2073, *Standard Test Method for Photopic Luminance of Photoluminescent (Phosphorescent) Markings*, 2007.

ASTM E 2074, *Standard Test Method for Fire Tests of Door Assemblies, Including Positive Pressure Testing of Side-Hinged and Pivoted Swinging Door Assemblies*, 2000e1.

ASTM E 2307, *Standard Test Method for Determining Fire Resistance of Perimeter Fire Barrier Systems Using Intermediate-Scale, Multi-Story Test Apparatus*, 2004.

ASTM F 851, *Standard Test Method for Self-Rising Seat Mechanisms*, 2000.

ASTM F 1577, *Standard Test Methods for Detention Locks for Swinging Doors*, 2001.

ASTM G 155, *Standard Practice for Operating Xenon Arc Light Apparatus for Exposure of Non-Metallic Materials*, 2000ae1.

### 2.3.7 FMGR Publications.

FM Global Research, FM Global, 1301 Atwood Avenue, P.O. Box 7500, Johnston, RI 02919. www.fmglobal.com

FM 4880, *Approval Standard for Class I Insulated Wall or Wall and Roof/Ceiling Panels; Plastic Interior Finish Materials; Plastic Exterior Building Panels; Wall/Ceiling Coating Systems; Interior or Exterior Finish Systems*, 1994.

### 2.3.8 UL Publications.

Underwriters Laboratories Inc., 333 Pfingsten Road, Northbrook, IL 60062-2096. www.ul.com

ANSI/UL 9, *Standard for Fire Tests of Window Assemblies*, 2000, Revised 2005.

ANSI/UL 10B, *Standard for Fire Tests of Door Assemblies*, 1997, Revised 2001.

ANSI/UL 10C, *Standard for Positive Pressure Fire Tests of Door Assemblies*, 1998, Revised 2001.

ANSI/UL 263, *Standard for Fire Tests of Building Construction and Materials*, 2003.

UL 294, *Standard for Access Control System Units*, 2004.

ANSI/UL 555, *Standard for Fire Dampers*, 2006.

ANSI/UL 555S, *Standard for Smoke Dampers*, 2006.

ANSI/UL 723, *Standard for Test for Surface Burning Characteristics of Building Materials*, 2003, Revised 2005.

ANSI/UL 790, *Test Methods for Fire Tests of Roof Coverings*, 2004.

ANSI/UL 924, *Standard for Emergency Lighting and Power Equipment*, 2006.

ANSI/UL 1040, *Standard for Fire Test of Insulated Wall Construction*, 1996, Revised 2001.

ANSI/UL 1479, *Standard for Fire Tests of Through-Penetration Firestops*, 2003, Revised 2007.

ANSI/UL 1715, *Standard for Fire Test of Interior Finish Material*, 1997, Revised 2004.

ANSI/UL 1784, *Standard for Air Leakage Tests for Door Assemblies*, 2001, Revised 2004.

UL 1975, *Standard for Fire Tests for Foamed Plastics Used for Decorative Purposes*, 2006.

UL 1994, *Standard for Luminous Egress Path Marking Systems*, 2004, Revised 2005.

ANSI/UL 2079, *Standard for Tests for Fire Resistance of Building Joint Systems*, 2004, Revised 2006.

### 2.3.9 U.S. Government Publications.

U.S. Government Printing Office, Washington, DC 20402. www.access.gpo.gov

Title 16, Code of Federal Regulations, Part 1500 and Part 1507.

Title 16, Code of Federal Regulations, Part 1632, "Standard for the Flammability of Mattresses and Mattress Pads" (FF 4-72).

### 2.3.10 Other Publication.

*Webster's Third New International Dictionary of the English Language, Unabridged*, Merriam-Webster, Inc., Springfield, MA, 2002.

## 2.4 References for Extracts in Mandatory Sections

NFPA 1, *Fire Code,* 2009 edition.

*NFPA 72*®, *National Fire Alarm Code*®, 2007 edition.

NFPA 80, *Standard for Fire Doors and Other Opening Protectives,* 2007 edition.

NFPA 88A, *Standard for Parking Structures,* 2007 edition.

NFPA 252, *Standard Methods of Fire Tests of Door Assemblies,* 2008 edition.

NFPA 288, *Standard Methods of Fire Tests of Floor Fire Door Assemblies Installed Horizontally in Fire Resistance–Rated Floor Systems,* 2007 edition.

NFPA 301, *Code for Safety to Life from Fire on Merchant Vessels,* 2008 edition.

NFPA 415, *Standard on Airport Terminal Buildings, Fueling Ramp Drainage, and Loading Walkways,* 2008 edition.

NFPA 914, *Code for Fire Protection of Historic Structures,* 2007 edition.

NFPA 921, *Guide for Fire and Explosion Investigations,* 2008 edition.

*NFPA 5000*®, *Building Construction and Safety Code*®, 2009 edition.

ASCE 7, *Minimum Design Loads for Buildings and Other Structures*, 2002.

This chapter contains mandatory references to other documents. As noted in the commentary that follows the chapter title, the extent to which these documents are mandatory is specified within the *Code.*

The reasons for locating all mandatory references in a single chapter are, first, to simplify use of the *Code* and, second, to make it easier for adopting jurisdictions to update the references in only one location rather than throughout the *Code.* The editions of the referenced publications listed in Chapter 2 are legally referenced editions, unless the jurisdiction, when adopting the *Code,* has updated the list of codes and standards.

### References Cited in Commentary

1. *NFPA 72*®, *National Fire Alarm Code*®, 2007 edition, National Fire Protection Association, Quincy, MA.
2. NFPA 13, *Standard for the Installation of Sprinkler Systems*, 2007 edition, National Fire Protection Association, Quincy, MA.

CHAPTER 3

# Definitions

Anyone who has ever participated in a code-development process — whether it be NFPA's or that of another organization — knows of the many hours spent deliberating whether the language is clear and easily understood and whether it expresses the committee's intent. Establishing the requirements for a code is not an easy task. During committee meetings, the question is usually asked regarding whether everyone will understand the limits or application of a particular rule. Invariably, the same questions are asked about select words or terms.

When words or terms used in the *Code* fall outside of generally accepted meanings or dictionary definitions — or otherwise require a clarification — they are defined in Chapter 3. When a word is not defined, the *Code* intends for the user to employ the dictionary definition — in this case, *Webster's Third New International Dictionary of the English Language, Unabridged.*[1] See Section 3.1.

For example, the word *exit* has numerous meanings in the dictionary. Included is the definition "goes off the stage," used as a stage direction for a specified actor to leave the stage. Another definition includes the following three meanings:

1. "The act of going out or going away"
2. "Death"
3. "A passage" or "a way out"

To the layperson, "passage" or "a way out" is probably what is understood when hearing the term *exit* used or seeing an exit sign. The NFPA *101* definition, however, is somewhat more detailed and is used to fix the limits on what actually constitutes an exit. The NFPA *101* definition in 3.3.75 reads as follows:

> **Exit.** That portion of a means of egress that is separated from all other spaces of a building or structure by construction or equipment as required to provide a protected way of travel to the exit discharge.

This is but one of the more than 250 terms defined in Chapter 3 of the *Code*. The definitions of the occupancy classifications (e.g., assembly occupancy, mercantile occupancy, industrial occupancy) appear in Chapter 3 and are repeated in their entirety in Chapter 6 to assist the user of the *Code* in properly classifying an occupancy.

The final point about defined terms in NFPA documents is that the definitions should not contain any requirements. To the extent possible, defined terms merely provide the meaning of a term within the context of the *Code* requirements.

## 3.1 General

The definitions contained in this chapter shall apply to the terms used in this *Code*. Where terms are not included, common usage of the terms shall apply. The following terms, for the purposes of this *Code*, shall have the meanings given in this chapter, if not otherwise modified by another chapter. Words used in the present tense shall include the future; words used in the masculine gender shall include the feminine and neuter; the singular number shall include the plural, and the plural number shall include the singular. Where terms are not defined in this chapter or within another chapter, they shall be defined using their ordinarily accepted meanings within the context in which they are used. *Webster's Third New International Dictionary of the English Language, Unabridged*, shall be a source for ordinarily accepted meaning.

## 3.2 NFPA Official Definitions

**3.2.1* Approved.** Acceptable to the authority having jurisdiction.

**A.3.2.1 Approved.** The National Fire Protection Association does not approve, inspect, or certify any installations, procedures, equipment, or materials; nor does it approve or evaluate testing laboratories. In determining the acceptability of installations, procedures, equipment, or materials, the authority having jurisdiction may base acceptance on compliance with NFPA or other appropriate standards. In the absence of such standards, said authority may require evidence of proper installation, procedure, or use. The authority having jurisdiction may also refer to the listings or labeling practices of an organization that is concerned with product evaluations and is thus in a position to determine compliance with appropriate standards for the current production of listed items.

**3.2.2* Authority Having Jurisdiction (AHJ).** An organization, office, or individual responsible for enforcing the requirements of a code or standard, or for approving equipment, materials, an installation, or a procedure.

**A.3.2.2 Authority Having Jurisdiction (AHJ).** The phrase "authority having jurisdiction," or its acronym AHJ, is used in NFPA documents in a broad manner, since jurisdictions and approval agencies vary, as do their responsibilities. Where public safety is primary, the authority having jurisdiction may be a federal, state, local, or other regional department or individual such as a fire chief; fire marshal; chief of a fire prevention bureau, labor department, or health department; building official; electrical inspector; or others having statutory authority. For insurance purposes, an insurance inspection department, rating bureau, or other insurance company representative may be the authority having jurisdiction. In many circumstances, the property owner or his or her designated agent assumes the role of the authority having jurisdiction; at government installations, the commanding officer or departmental official may be the authority having jurisdiction.

**3.2.3* Code.** A standard that is an extensive compilation of provisions covering broad subject matter or that is suitable for adoption into law independently of other codes and standards.

**A.3.2.3 Code.** The decision to designate a standard as a "code" is based on such factors as the size and scope of the document, its intended use and form of adoption, and whether it contains substantial enforcement and administrative provisions.

**3.2.4 Labeled.** Equipment or materials to which has been attached a label, symbol, or other identifying mark of an organization that is acceptable to the authority having jurisdiction and concerned with product evaluation, that maintains periodic inspection of production of labeled equipment or materials, and by whose labeling the manufacturer indicates compliance with appropriate standards or performance in a specified manner.

**3.2.5* Listed.** Equipment, materials, or services included in a list published by an organization that is acceptable to the authority having jurisdiction and concerned with evaluation of products or services, that maintains periodic inspection of production of listed equipment or materials or periodic evaluation of services, and whose listing states that either the equipment, material, or service meets appropriate designated standards or has been tested and found suitable for a specified purpose.

**A.3.2.5 Listed.** The means for identifying listed equipment may vary for each organization concerned with product evaluation; some organizations do not recognize equipment as listed unless it is also labeled. The authority having jurisdiction should utilize the system employed by the listing organization to identify a listed product.

**3.2.6 Shall.** Indicates a mandatory requirement.

**3.2.7 Should.** Indicates a recommendation or that which is advised but not required.

## 3.3 General Definitions

**3.3.1 Accessible Area of Refuge.** See 3.3.20.1.

**3.3.2 Accessible Means of Egress.** See 3.3.161.1.

**3.3.3 Accessible Route.** A continuous unobstructed path that complies with this *Code* and ICC/ANSI A117.1, *American National Standard for Accessible and Usable Buildings and Facilities*.

**3.3.4* Actuating Member or Bar.** The activating mechanism of a panic hardware or fire exit hardware device located on the egress side of a door.

**A.3.3.4 Actuating Member or Bar.** The active surface of the actuating bar needs to be visually and physically distinct from the rest of the device. The actuating bar is also called a cross bar or push pad.

**3.3.5 Addition.** An increase in building area, aggregate floor area, building height, or number of stories of a structure.

**3.3.6 Air Traffic Control Tower.** See 3.3.262.1.

**3.3.7 Aircraft Loading Walkway.** An aboveground device through which passengers move between a point in an airport terminal building and an aircraft. Included in this category are walkways that are essentially fixed and permanently placed, or walkways that are essentially mobile in nature and that fold, telescope, or pivot from a fixed point at the airport terminal building. [**415,** 2008]

**3.3.8 Air-Inflated Structure.** See 3.3.254.1.

**3.3.9 Airport Terminal Building.** See 3.3.32.1.

**3.3.10 Air-Supported Structure.** See 3.3.254.2.

**3.3.11* Aisle Accessway.** The initial portion of an exit access that leads to an aisle.

**A.3.3.11 Aisle Accessway.** *Aisle accessway* is the term used for the previously unnamed means of egress component leading to an aisle or other means of egress. For example, circulation space between parallel rows of seats having a width of 12 in. to 24 in. (305 mm to 610 mm) and a length not exceeding 100 ft (30 m) is an aisle accessway. Some of the circulation space between tables or seats in restaurants might be considered aisle accessway.

Depending on the width of aisle accessway, which is influenced by its length and expected utilization, the movement of a person through the aisle accessway might require others to change their individual speed of movement, alter their postures, move their chairs out of the way, or proceed ahead of the person.

**3.3.12 Alarm.**

***3.3.12.1 Single Station Alarm.*** A detector comprising an assembly that incorporates a sensor, control components, and an alarm notification appliance in one unit operated from a power source either located in the unit or obtained at the point of installation. [*72,* 2007]

***3.3.12.2 Smoke Alarm.*** A single- or multiple-station alarm responsive to smoke. [*72,* 2007]

**3.3.13 Alternative Calculation Procedure.** A calculation procedure that differs from the procedure originally employed by the design team but that provides predictions for the same variables of interest.

**3.3.14 Ambulatory Health Care Occupancy.** See 3.3.178.1.

**3.3.15 Analysis.**

***3.3.15.1 Sensitivity Analysis.*** An analysis performed to determine the degree to which a predicted output will vary given a specified change in an input parameter, usually in relation to models.

***3.3.15.2 Uncertainty Analysis.*** An analysis performed to determine the degree to which a predicted value will vary.

**3.3.16 Anchor Building.** See 3.3.32.2.

**3.3.17 Apartment Building.** See 3.3.32.3.

**3.3.18 Approved Existing.** See 3.3.73.1.

**3.3.19 Area.**

***3.3.19.1 Detention and Correctional Residential Housing Area.*** Sleeping areas and any contiguous day room, group activity space, or other common space for customary access of residents.

***3.3.19.2 Floor Area.***

***3.3.19.2.1* Gross Floor Area.*** The floor area within the inside perimeter of the outside walls of the building under consideration with no deduction for hallways, stairs, closets, thickness of interior walls, columns, or other features.

***A.3.3.19.2.1 Gross Floor Area.*** Where the term *floor area* is used, it should be understood to be gross floor area, unless otherwise specified.

***3.3.19.2.2 Net Floor Area.*** The floor area within the inside perimeter of the outside walls, or the outside walls and fire walls of the building under consideration with deductions for hallways, stairs, closets, thickness of interior walls, columns, or other features.

***3.3.19.3 Gross Leasable Area.*** The total floor area designated for tenant occupancy and exclusive use. The area of tenant occupancy is measured from the centerlines of joint partitions to the outside of the tenant walls. All tenant areas, including areas used for storage, are part of the gross leasable area.

***3.3.19.4* Hazardous Area.*** An area of a structure or building that poses a degree of hazard greater than that normal to the general occupancy of the building or structure.

***A.3.3.19.4 Hazardous Area.*** Hazardous areas include areas for the storage or use of combustibles or flammables; toxic, noxious, or corrosive materials; or heat-producing appliances.

***3.3.19.5 Living Area.*** Any normally occupiable space in a residential occupancy, other than sleeping rooms or rooms that are intended for combination sleeping/living, bathrooms, toilet compartments, kitchens, closets, halls, storage or utility spaces, and similar areas.

***3.3.19.6 Occupiable Area.*** An area of a facility occupied by people on a regular basis.

***3.3.19.7 Rehabilitation Work Area.*** That portion of a building affected by any renovation, modification, or reconstruction work as initially intended by the owner, and indicated as such in the permit, but excluding other portions of the building where incidental work entailed by the intended work must be performed, and excluding portions of the building where work not initially intended by the owner is specifically required.

**3.3.20* Area of Refuge.** An area that is either (1) a story in a building where the building is protected throughout by an approved, supervised automatic sprinkler system and has not less than two accessible rooms or spaces separated from each other by smoke-resisting partitions; or (2) a space located in a path of travel leading to a public way that is protected from the effects of fire, either by means of separation from other spaces in the same building or by virtue of location, thereby permitting a delay in egress travel from any level.

**A.3.3.20 Area of Refuge.** An area of refuge has a temporary use during egress. It generally serves as a staging area that provides relative safety to its occupants while potential emergencies are assessed, decisions are made, and mitigating activities are begun. Taking refuge within such an area is, thus, a stage of the total egress process, a stage between egress from the immediately threatened area and egress to a public way.

An area of refuge might be another building connected by a bridge or balcony, a compartment of a subdivided story, an elevator lobby, or an enlarged story-level exit stair landing. An area of refuge is accessible by means of horizontal travel or, as a minimum, via an accessible route meeting the requirements of ICC/ANSI A117.1, *American National Standard for Accessible and Usable Buildings and Facilities*.

This *Code* recognizes any floor in a building protected throughout by an approved, supervised automatic sprinkler system as an area of refuge. This recognition acknowledges the ability of a properly designed and functioning automatic sprinkler system to control a fire at its point of origin and to limit the production of toxic products to a level that is not life threatening.

The requirement for separated rooms or spaces can be met on an otherwise undivided floor by enclosing the elevator lobby with ordinary glass or other simple enclosing partitions that are smoke resisting.

For some occupancies, one accessible room or space is permitted.

***3.3.20.1 Accessible Area of Refuge.*** An area of refuge that complies with the accessible route requirements of ICC/ANSI A117.1, *American National Standard for Accessible and Usable Buildings and Facilities.*

**3.3.21 Assembly.**

***3.3.21.1 Door Assembly.*** Any combination of a door, frame, hardware, and other accessories that is placed in an opening in a wall that is intended primarily for access or for human entrance or exit. [**252**, 2008]

The definition of the term *door assembly* is new to the 2009 edition of the *Code*. In prior editions, the term *door* appeared more than 225 times in Chapter 7. The term *door* did not, by itself, make clear whether the term related to the overall door assembly, the door leaf, or the door opening. During preparation of this edition, each occurrence of the term *door* in Chapter 7 was scrutinized, and revised as needed, to clarify its meaning. The work was done through the normal revision process involving the Report on Proposals and Report on Comments by volunteer committee members representing the Door and Hardware Institute and the Builders Hardware Manufacturers Association. It is a credit to the NFPA codes and standards process that volunteers will undertake such tasks with enthusiasm in the name of making the *Code* more usable. In many cases, the term *door* was changed to the term *door assembly*. The definition of *door assembly* in 3.3.21.1 was extracted from the expert NFPA document on the subject, NFPA 252, *Standard Methods of Fire Tests of Door Assemblies*.[2]

***3.3.21.1.1 Fire Door Assembly.*** Any combination of a fire door, a frame, hardware, and other accessories that together provide a specific degree of fire protection to the opening. [**80,** 2007]

***3.3.21.1.1.1 Floor Fire Door Assembly.*** A combination of a fire door, a frame, hardware, and other accessories installed in a horizontal plane, which together provide a specific degree of fire protection to a through-opening in a fire resistance–rated floor. [**288,** 2007]

***3.3.21.2 Fire Window Assembly.*** A window or glass block assembly having a fire protection rating. [**80,** 2007]

**3.3.22 Assembly Occupancy.** See 3.3.178.2.

**3.3.23 Atmosphere.**

***3.3.23.1 Common Atmosphere.*** The atmosphere that exists between rooms, spaces, or areas within a building that are not separated by an approved smoke barrier.

***3.3.23.2 Separate Atmosphere.*** The atmosphere that exists between rooms, spaces, or areas that are separated by an approved smoke barrier.

**3.3.24* Atrium.** A large-volume space created by a floor opening or series of floor openings connecting two or more stories that is covered at the top of the series of openings and is used for purposes other than an enclosed stairway; an elevator hoistway; an escalator opening; or as a utility shaft used for plumbing, electrical, air-conditioning, or communications facilities.

**A.3.3.24 Atrium.** As defined in NFPA 92B, *Standard for Smoke Management Systems in Malls, Atria, and Large Spaces*, a large-volume space is an uncompartmented space, generally two or more stories high, within which smoke from a fire either in the space or in a communicating space can move and accumulate without restriction. Atria and covered malls are examples of large-volume spaces.

**3.3.25*** **Attic.** The space located between the ceiling of a story and the roof directly above that habitable story.

**A.3.3.25 Attic.** The attic space might be used for storage. The concealed rafter space between the ceiling membrane and the roof sheathing that are attached to the rafters is not considered an attic.

**3.3.26 Automatic.** That which provides a function without the necessity of human intervention.

**3.3.27 Barrier.**

***3.3.27.1* Fire Barrier.*** A continuous membrane or a membrane with discontinuities created by protected openings with a specified fire protection rating, where such membrane is designed and constructed with a specified fire resistance rating to limit the spread of fire, that also restricts the movement of smoke.

***A.3.3.27.1 Fire Barrier.*** A fire barrier might be vertically or horizontally aligned, such as a wall or floor assembly.

***3.3.27.2* Smoke Barrier.*** A continuous membrane, or a membrane with discontinuities created by protected openings, where such membrane is designed and constructed to restrict the movement of smoke.

***A.3.3.27.2 Smoke Barrier.*** A smoke barrier might be vertically or horizontally aligned, such as a wall, floor, or ceiling assembly. A smoke barrier might or might not have a fire resistance rating. Application of smoke barrier criteria where required elsewhere in the *Code* should be in accordance with Section 8.3.

***3.3.27.3* Thermal Barrier.*** A material that limits the average temperature rise of an unexposed surface to not more than 250°F (139°C) for a specified fire exposure complying with the standard time-temperature curve of NFPA 251, *Standard Methods of Tests of Fire Resistance of Building Construction and Materials.*

***A.3.3.27.3 Thermal Barrier.*** Finish ratings, as published in the UL *Fire Resistance Directory,* are one way of determining thermal barrier.

**3.3.28 Basement.** Any story of a building wholly or partly below grade plane that is not considered the first story above grade plane. *(See also 3.3.115.1, First Story Above Grade Plane.)*

The definition of the term *basement* is new to the 2009 edition of the *Code*. The addition is part of a major revision of text throughout the *Code* related to terminology used to describe building height and number of stories relative to grade plane, finished ground level, and level of exit discharge. See 3.3.115, *Grade Plane;* 3.3.85, *Finished Ground Level;* and 3.3.77.1, *Level of Exit Discharge.*

**3.3.29*** **Birth Center.** A facility in which low-risk births are expected following normal, uncomplicated pregnancies, and in which professional midwifery care is provided to women during pregnancy, birth, and postpartum.

**A.3.3.29 Birth Center.** A birth center is a low-volume service for healthy, childbearing women, and their families, who are capable of ambulation in the event of fire or fire-threatening events. Birth center mothers and babies have minimal analgesia, receive no general or regional anesthesia, and are capable of ambulation, even in second-stage labor.

**3.3.30 Bleachers.** A grandstand in which the seats are not provided with backrests.

**3.3.31 Board and Care.** See 3.3.178.12, Residential Board and Care Occupancy.

**3.3.32*** **Building.** Any structure used or intended for supporting or sheltering any use or occupancy.

**A.3.3.32 Building.** The term *building* is to be understood as if followed by the words *or portions thereof. (See also Structure, A.3.3.254.)*

***3.3.32.1 Airport Terminal Building.*** A structure used primarily for air passenger enplaning or deplaning, including ticket sales, flight information, baggage handling, and other necessary functions in connection with air transport operations. This term includes any extensions and satellite buildings used for passenger handling or aircraft flight service functions. Aircraft loading walkways and "mobile lounges" are excluded. [**415,** 2008]

***3.3.32.2 Anchor Building.*** A building housing any occupancy having low or ordinary hazard contents and having direct access to a mall building, but having all required means of egress independent of the mall.

***3.3.32.3* Apartment Building.*** A building or portion thereof containing three or more dwelling units with independent cooking and bathroom facilities.

***A.3.3.32.3 Apartment Building.*** The *Code* specifies that, wherever there are three or more living units in a building, the building is considered an apartment building and is required to comply with either Chapter 30 or Chapter 31, as appropriate. Townhouse units are considered to be apartment buildings if there are three or more units in the building. The type of wall required between units in order to consider them to be separate buildings is normally established by the authority having jurisdiction.

If the units are separated by a wall of sufficient fire resistance and structural integrity to be considered as separate buildings, then the provisions of Chapter 24 apply to each townhouse. Condominium status is a form of ownership, not occupancy; for example, there are condominium warehouses, condominium apartments, and condominium offices.

***3.3.32.4 Bulk Merchandising Retail Building.*** A building in which the sales area includes the storage of combustible materials on pallets, in solid piles, or in racks in excess of 12 ft (3660 mm) in storage height.

***3.3.32.5* Existing Building.*** A building erected or officially authorized prior to the effective date of the adoption of this edition of the *Code* by the agency or jurisdiction.

***A.3.3.32.5 Existing Building.*** With respect to judging whether a building should be considered existing, the deciding factor is not when the building was designed or when construction started but, rather, the date plans were approved for construction by the appropriate authority having jurisdiction.

***3.3.32.6* Flexible Plan and Open Plan Educational or Day-Care Building.*** A building or portion of a building designed for multiple teaching stations.

***A.3.3.32.6 Flexible Plan and Open Plan Educational or Day-Care Building.*** Flexible plan buildings have movable corridor walls and movable partitions of full-height construction with doors leading from rooms to corridors. Open plan buildings have rooms and corridors delineated by tables, chairs, desks, bookcases, counters, low-height partitions, or similar furnishings. It is the intent that low-height partitions not exceed 60 in. (1525 mm).

***3.3.32.7* High-Rise Building.*** A building where the floor of an occupiable story is greater than 75 ft (23 m) above the lowest level of fire department vehicle access.

***A.3.3.32.7 High-Rise Building.*** It is the intent of this definition that, in determining the level from which the highest occupiable floor is to be measured, the enforcing agency should exercise reasonable judgment, including consideration of overall accessibility to the building by fire department personnel and vehicular equipment. Where a building is situated on a sloping terrain and there is building access on more than one level, the enforcing agency might select the level that provides the most logical and adequate fire department access.

***3.3.32.8* Historic Building.*** A building or facility deemed to have historical, architectural, or cultural significance by a local, regional, or national jurisdiction.

***A.3.3.32.8 Historic Building.*** Designation for a historic building might be in an official national, regional, or local historic register, listing, or inventory.

***3.3.32.9* Mall Building.*** A single building enclosing a number of tenants and occupancies wherein two or more tenants have a main entrance into one or more malls. For the purpose of this *Code*, anchor buildings shall not be considered as a part of the mall building.

***A.3.3.32.9 Mall Building.*** A mall building might enclose one or more uses, such as retail and wholesale stores, drinking and dining establishments, entertainment and amusement facilities, transportation facilities, offices, and other similar uses.

***3.3.32.10* Special Amusement Building.*** A building that is temporary, permanent, or mobile and contains a device or system that conveys passengers or provides a walkway along, around, or over a course in any direction as a form of amusement arranged so that the egress path is not readily apparent due to visual or audio distractions or an intentionally confounded egress path, or is not readily available due to the mode of conveyance through the building or structure.

***A.3.3.32.10 Special Amusement Building.*** Special amusement buildings include amusements such as a haunted house, a roller coaster–type ride within a building, a multilevel play structure within a building, a submarine ride, and similar amusements where the occupants are not in the open air.

**3.3.33 Bulk Merchandising Retail Building.** See 3.3.32.4.

**3.3.34 Business Occupancy.** See 3.3.178.3.

**3.3.35 Categories of Rehabilitation Work.** The nature and extent of rehabilitation work undertaken in an existing building.

**3.3.36* Cellular or Foamed Plastic.** A heterogeneous system comprised of not less than two phases, one of which is a continuous, polymeric, organic material, and the second of which is deliberately introduced for the purpose of distributing gas in voids throughout the material.

**A.3.3.36 Cellular or Foamed Plastic.** Cellular or foamed plastic might contain foamed and unfoamed polymeric or monomeric precursors (prepolymer, if used), plasticizers, fillers, extenders, catalysts, blowing agents, colorants, stabilizers, lubricants, surfactants, pigments, reaction control agents, processing aids, and flame retardants.

**3.3.37 Change of Occupancy Classification.** The change in the occupancy classification of a structure or portion of a structure.

**3.3.38 Change of Use.** A change in the purpose or level of activity within a structure that involves a change in application of the requirements of the *Code*.

**3.3.39 Combustible (Material).** See 3.3.160.1.

**3.3.40 Combustion.** A chemical process of oxidation that occurs at a rate fast enough to produce heat and usually light in the form of either a glow or a flame.

**3.3.41 Common Atmosphere.** See 3.3.23.1.

**3.3.42* Common Path of Travel.** The portion of exit access that must be traversed before two separate and distinct paths of travel to two exits are available.

**A.3.3.42 Common Path of Travel.** Common path of travel is measured in the same manner as travel distance but terminates at that point where two separate and distinct routes become available. Paths that merge are common paths of travel.

**3.3.43 Compartment.**

***3.3.43.1* Fire Compartment.*** A space within a building that is enclosed by fire barriers on all sides, including the top and bottom.

***A.3.3.43.1 Fire Compartment.*** Additional fire compartment information is contained in 8.2.2.

In the provisions for fire compartments utilizing the outside walls of a building, it is not intended that the outside wall be specifically fire resistance rated, unless required by other standards. Likewise, it is not intended that outside windows or doors be protected, unless specifically required for exposure protection by another section of this *Code* or by other standards.

***3.3.43.2* Smoke Compartment.*** A space within a building enclosed by smoke barriers on all sides, including the top and bottom.

***A.3.3.43.2 Smoke Compartment.*** Where smoke compartments using the outside walls or the roof of a building are provided, it is not intended that outside walls or roofs, or any openings therein, be capable of resisting the passage of smoke. Application of smoke compartment criteria where required elsewhere in the *Code* should be in accordance with Section 8.5.

**3.3.44* Consumer Fireworks, 1.4G.** *(Formerly known as Class C, Common Fireworks.)* Any small fireworks device designed primarily to produce visible effects by combustion that complies with the construction, chemical composition, and labeling regulations of the U.S. Consumer Product Safety Commission, as set forth in 16 CFR, Parts 1500 and 1507. Some small devices designed to produce audible effects are included, such as whistling devices, ground devices containing 0.8 gr (50 mg) or less of explosive composition (salute powder), and aerial devices containing 2 gr (130 mg) or less of explosive composition (salute powder) per explosive unit.

**A.3.3.44 Consumer Fireworks, 1.4G.** Consumer Fireworks, 1.4G contain limited quantities of pyrotechnic composition per unit and do not pose a mass explosion hazard where stored; therefore, they are not required to be stored in a magazine.

Consumer Fireworks, 1.4G are normally classed as Explosive, 1.4G and described as Fireworks UN0336 by the U.S. Department of Transportation (U.S. DOT). *(See Annex C of* NFPA 1124, *Code for the Manufacture, Transportation, Storage, and Retail Sales of Fireworks and Pyrotechnic Articles.)*

**3.3.45 Contents and Furnishings.** Any movable objects in a building for functional, operational, or decorative reasons, excluding parts of the building structure, building service equipment, and items meeting the definition of interior finish.

**3.3.46 Court.** An open, uncovered, unoccupied space, unobstructed to the sky, bounded on three or more sides by exterior building walls.

***3.3.46.1 Enclosed Court.*** A court bounded on all sides by the exterior walls of a building or by the exterior walls and lot lines on which walls are permitted.

***3.3.46.2 Food Court.*** A public seating area located in a mall that serves adjacent food preparation tenant spaces.

**3.3.47* Critical Radiant Flux.** The level of incident radiant heat energy on a floor-covering system at the most distant flameout point.

**A.3.3.47 Critical Radiant Flux.** Critical radiant flux is the property determined by the test procedure of NFPA 253, *Standard Method of Test for Critical Radiant Flux of Floor Covering Systems Using a Radiant Heat Energy Source*. The unit of measurement of critical radiant flux is watts per square centimeter ($W/cm^2$).

**3.3.48 Data Conversion.** The process of developing the input data set for the assessment method of choice.

**3.3.49 Day-Care Home.** See 3.3.131.1.

**3.3.50 Day-Care Occupancy.** See 3.3.178.4.

**3.3.51 Design Fire Scenario.** See 3.3.96.1.

**3.3.52 Design Specification.** See 3.3.244.1.

**3.3.53 Design Team.** A group of stakeholders including, but not limited to, representatives of the architect, client, and any pertinent engineers and other designers.

**3.3.54 Detention and Correctional Occupancy.** See 3.3.178.5.

**3.3.55 Detention and Correctional Residential Housing Area.** See 3.3.19.1.

**3.3.56 Device.**

***3.3.56.1 Multiple Station Alarm Device.*** Two or more single station alarm devices that can be interconnected so that actuation of one causes all integral or separate audible alarms to operate; or one single station alarm device having connections to other detectors or to a manual fire alarm box. [*72,* 2007]

***3.3.56.2* Stair Descent Device.*** A portable device, incorporating a means to control the rate of descent, used to transport a person with a severe mobility impairment downward on stairs during emergency egress.

***A.3.3.56.2 Stair Descent Device.*** A stair descent device typically requires the assistance of a trained operator.

**3.3.57 Door.**

***3.3.57.1 Elevator Lobby Door.*** A door between an elevator lobby and another building space other than the elevator shaft.

***3.3.57.2 Fire Door.*** The door component of a fire door assembly.

**3.3.58 Door Assembly.** See 3.3.21.1.

**3.3.59* Dormitory.** A building or a space in a building in which group sleeping accommodations are provided for more than 16 persons who are not members of the same family in one room, or a series of closely associated rooms, under joint occupancy and single management, with or without meals, but without individual cooking facilities.

**A.3.3.59 Dormitory.** Rooms within dormitories intended for the use of individuals for combined living and sleeping purposes are guest rooms or guest suites. Examples of dormitories are college dormitories, fraternity and sorority houses, and military barracks.

**3.3.60 Draft Stop.** A continuous membrane used to subdivide a concealed space to resist the passage of smoke and heat.

**3.3.61* Dwelling Unit.** One or more rooms arranged for complete, independent housekeeping purposes with space for eating, living, and sleeping; facilities for cooking; and provisions for sanitation.

**A.3.3.61 Dwelling Unit.** It is not the intent of the *Code* that the list of spaces in the definition of the term *dwelling unit* in 3.3.61 is to be all inclusive. It is the intent of the *Code* that the list of spaces is a minimal set of criteria that must be provided to be considered a dwelling unit and, therefore, the dwelling unit can contain other spaces that are typical to a single-family dwelling.

***3.3.61.1* One- and Two-Family Dwelling Unit.*** A building that contains not more than two dwelling units with independent cooking and bathroom facilities.

**Formal Interpretation**
**NFPA *101*®**
***Life Safety Code*®**
**2009 edition**

**Reference 3.3.61**

**F.I. No. 101-03-2**

*Background:* There are several locations in the *Code,* where a stair can be open or provided with a door to a dwelling unit but must be separated from all other portions of the building with no door therein. For example: 30.2.4.2(3) allows an apartment to have access to a single exit provided that the stair serves only that unit and is separated from all other portions of the building by a 1-hr fire barrier with no openings therein. The definition of "dwelling unit" in 3.3.61 states that a dwelling unit is "one or more rooms arranged for complete, independent housekeeping purposes with space for eating, living, and sleeping; facilities for cooking; and provisions for sanitation." There have been interpretations of this definition that if a space is not on the list, it is not part of the dwelling unit. In other words libraries, studies, sun rooms, private offices, and private garages would not be considered part of the dwelling unit and under paragraphs such as 30.2.4.2(3) would have to be separated from the stair and no door would be allowed in the separation. It is recognized that under the building code, there are other requirements to separate a garage from a dwelling unit but would permit doors in the separation.

*Question No 1:* Is it the intent of the *Code* that the list of spaces in the 3.3.61 definition of *Dwelling Unit* be an all inclusive list and that other spaces are not part of the dwelling unit?

*Answer:* No.

*Question No 2:* Is it the intent of the *Code* that the list of spaces in the 3.3.61 definition of *Dwelling Unit* is a minimal set of criteria that must be provided to be considered a dwelling unit and therefore the dwelling unit can contain other spaces that are typical to a single-family dwelling?

*Answer:* Yes.

*Issue Edition:* 2003
*Reference:* 3.3.50
*Issue Date:* August 18, 2004
*Effective Date:* September 7, 2004

*A.3.3.61.1 One- and Two-Family Dwelling Unit.* The application statement of 24.1.1.1 limits each dwelling unit to being "occupied by members of a single family with not more than three outsiders." The *Code* does not define the term *family*. The definition of family is subject to federal, state, and local regulations and might not be restricted to a person or a couple (two people) and their children. The following examples aid in differentiating between a single-family dwelling and a lodging or rooming house:

(1) An individual or a couple (two people) who rent a house from a landlord and then sublease space for up to three individuals should be considered a family renting to a maximum of three outsiders, and the house should be regulated as a single-family dwelling in accordance with Chapter 24.
(2) A house rented from a landlord by an individual or a couple (two people) in which space is subleased to 4 or more individuals, but not more than 16, should be considered and regulated as a lodging or rooming house in accordance with Chapter 26.
(3) A residential building that is occupied by 4 or more individuals, but not more than 16, each renting from a landlord, without separate cooking facilities, should be considered and regulated as a lodging or rooming house in accordance with Chapter 26.

*3.3.61.2 One-Family Dwelling Unit.* A building that consists solely of one dwelling unit with independent cooking and bathroom facilities.

*3.3.61.3 Two-Family Dwelling Unit.* A building that consists solely of two dwelling units with independent cooking and bathroom facilities.

**3.3.62 Educational Occupancy.** See 3.3.178.6.

**3.3.63* Electroluminescent.** Refers to a light-emitting capacitor in which alternating current excites phosphor atoms placed between electrically conductive surfaces and produces light.

**A.3.3.63 Electroluminescent.** This light source is typically contained inside the device.

**3.3.64 Elevator Evacuation System.** A system, including a vertical series of elevator lobbies and associated elevator lobby doors, an elevator shaft(s), and a machine room(s), that provides protection from fire effects for elevator passengers, people waiting to use elevators, and elevator equipment so that elevators can be used safely for egress.

**3.3.65 Elevator Lobby.** A landing from which occupants directly enter an elevator car(s) and into which occupants directly enter upon leaving an elevator car(s).

The definition of the term *elevator lobby* is new to the 2009 edition of the *Code*. The term was defined to help support the new criteria of 7.2.1.6.3 on elevator lobby exit access door locking.

**3.3.66 Elevator Lobby Door.** See 3.3.57.1.

**3.3.67 Enclosed Court.** See 3.3.46.1.

**3.3.68 Equipment or Fixture.** Any plumbing, heating, electrical, ventilating, air-conditioning, refrigerating, and fire protection equipment; and elevators, dumbwaiters, escalators, boilers, pressure vessels, or other mechanical facilities or installations related to building services.

**3.3.69 Equivalency.** An alternative means of providing an equal or greater degree of safety than that afforded by strict conformance to prescribed codes and standards.

**3.3.70* Evacuation Capability.** The ability of occupants, residents, and staff as a group either to evacuate a building or to relocate from the point of occupancy to a point of safety.

**A.3.3.70 Evacuation Capability.** The evacuation capability of the residents and staff is a function of both the ability of the residents to evacuate and the assistance provided by the staff. It is intended that the evacuation capability be determined by the procedure acceptable to the authority having jurisdiction. It is also intended that the timing of drills, the rating of residents, and similar actions related to determining the evacuation capability be performed by persons approved by or acceptable to the authority having jurisdiction. The evacuation capability can be determined by the use of the definitions in 3.3.70, the application of NFPA 101A, *Guide on Alternative Approaches to Life Safety*, Chapter 6, or a program of drills (timed).

Where drills are used in determining evacuation capability, it is suggested that the facility conduct and record fire drills six times per year on a bimonthly basis, with a minimum of two drills conducted during the night when residents are sleeping, and that the facility conduct the drills in consultation with the authority having jurisdiction. Records should indicate the time taken to reach a point of safety, date and time of day, location of simulated fire origin, escape paths used, and comments relating to residents who resisted or failed to participate in the drills.

Translation of drill times to evacuation capability is determined as follows:

(1) 3 minutes or less — prompt
(2) Over 3 minutes, but not in excess of 13 minutes — slow
(3) More than 13 minutes — impractical

Evacuation capability, in all cases, is based on the time of day or night when evacuation of the facility would be most difficult, such as when residents are sleeping or fewer staff are present.

Evacuation capability determination is considered slow if the following conditions are met:

(1) All residents are able to travel to centralized dining facilities without continuous staff assistance.
(2) There is continuous staffing whenever there are residents in the facility.

*3.3.70.1* ***Impractical Evacuation Capability.*** The inability of a group to reliably move to a point of safety in a timely manner.

*3.3.70.2* ***Prompt Evacuation Capability.*** The ability of a group to move reliably to a point of safety in a timely manner that is equivalent to the capacity of a household in the general population.

*3.3.70.3* ***Slow Evacuation Capability.*** The ability of a group to move reliably to a point of safety in a timely manner, but not as rapidly as members of a household in the general population.

**3.3.71 Exhibit.** A space or portable structure used for the display of products or services.

**3.3.72 Exhibitor.** An individual or entity engaged in the display of the products or services offered.

**3.3.73* Existing.** That which is already in existence on the date this edition of the *Code* goes into effect.

**A.3.3.73 Existing.** See *Existing Building*, A.3.3.32.5.

*3.3.73.1* ***Approved Existing.*** That which is already in existence on the date this edition of the *Code* goes into effect and is acceptable to the authority having jurisdiction.

**3.3.74 Existing Building.** See 3.3.32.5.

**3.3.75* Exit.** That portion of a means of egress that is separated from all other spaces of a building or structure by construction or equipment as required to provide a protected way of travel to the exit discharge.

**A.3.3.75 Exit.** Exits include exterior exit doors, exit passageways, horizontal exits, exit stairs, and exit ramps. In the case of a stairway, the exit includes the stair enclosure, the door to the stair enclosure, the stairs and landings inside the enclosure, the door from the stair enclosure to the outside or to the level of exit discharge, and any exit passageway and its associated doors, if such are provided, so as to discharge the stair directly to the outside. In the case of a door leading directly from the street floor to the street or open air, the exit comprises only the door.

Doors of small individual rooms, as in hotels, while constituting exit access from the room, are not referred to as exits, except where they lead directly to the outside of the building from the street floor.

*3.3.75.1** ***Horizontal Exit.*** A way of passage from one building to an area of refuge in another building on approximately the same level, or a way of passage through or around a fire barrier to an area of refuge on approximately the same level in the same building that affords safety from fire and smoke originating from the area of incidence and areas communicating therewith.

*A.3.3.75.1* ***Horizontal Exit.*** Horizontal exits should not be confused with egress through doors in smoke barriers. Doors in smoke barriers are designed only for temporary protection against smoke, whereas horizontal exits provide protection against serious fire for a relatively long period of time in addition to providing immediate protection from smoke. *(See 7.2.4.)*

**3.3.76 Exit Access.** That portion of a means of egress that leads to an exit.

**3.3.77 Exit Discharge.** That portion of a means of egress between the termination of an exit and a public way.

*3.3.77.1** ***Level of Exit Discharge.*** The story that is either (1) the lowest story from which not less than 50 percent of the required number of exits and not less than 50 percent of the required egress capacity from such a story discharge directly outside at the finished ground level; or (2) where no story meets the conditions of item (1), the story that is provided with one or more exits that discharge directly to the outside to the finished ground level via the smallest elevation change.

The definition of the term *level of exit discharge* was revised for the 2009 edition of the *Code*. The changes to the definition are part of a major revision of text throughout the *Code* related to terminology used to describe building height and number of stories relative to grade plane, finished ground level, and level of exit discharge. See 3.3.115, *Grade Plane*, and 3.3.85, *Finished Ground Level*. The term *level of exit discharge* is used in the commentary accompanying 4.6.3, which specifies how to determine stories in height.

The definition of *level of exit discharge* provides no allowance for having more than one level of exit discharge for a building. There is no primary or secondary level of exit discharge — only the level of exit discharge. The level designated as the level of exit discharge is used, for example, as the lowest floor for purposes of determining stories in height (see 4.6.3). Requirements related to minimum construction type are based on the number of stories in height used for a particular occupancy (see the __.1.6 subsection of most of the occupancy chapters — for example, 12.1.6 for new assembly occupancies). The examples that follow demonstrate the application of the definition of the term *level of exit discharge* to a variety of building exit discharge arrangements.

***Example 1***

Exhibit 3.1 depicts a four-story building. The finished ground level varies little in elevation from building side to building side. The first story is the lowest story from which not less than 50 percent of the required number of means of egress and not less than 50 percent of the required egress capacity from that story discharge directly outside at the finished ground level. As such, it is designated as the level of exit discharge (LED).

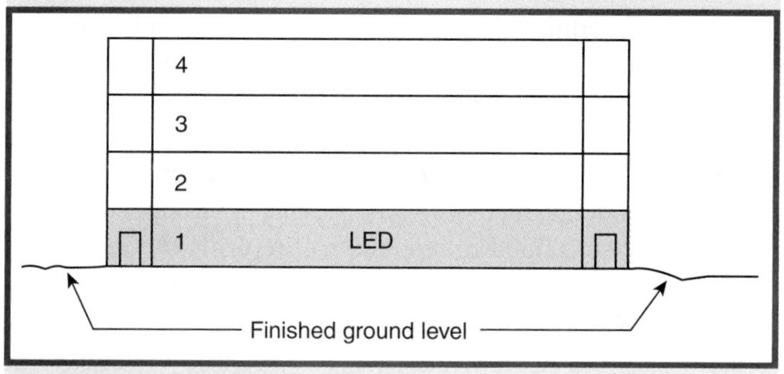


***Exhibit 3.1*** *Level of exit discharge at story with common finished ground level.*

***Example 2***

Exhibit 3.2 depicts a four-story building similar to that described in Example 1. The finished ground level varies in elevation from building side to building side. Both the first story and the second story are stories from which not less than 50 percent of the required number of means of egress and not less than 50 percent of the required egress capacity from that story discharge directly outside at the finished ground level. The definition of *level of exit discharge* causes the *Code* user to designate the lowest such story with the

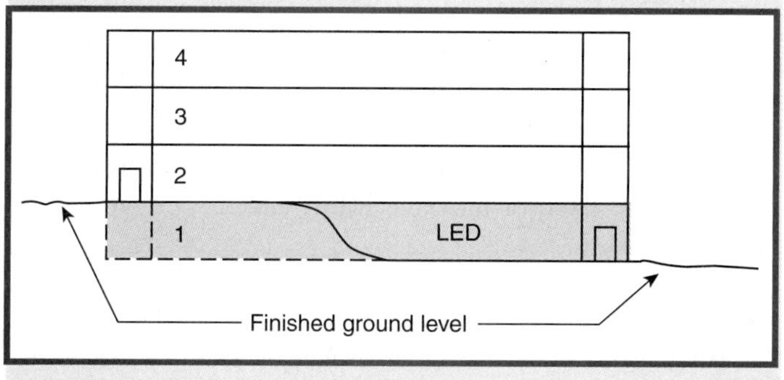


***Exhibit 3.2*** *Level of exit discharge at lowest story.*

resultant classification of the lowest story (designated in Exhibit 3.2 as story 1) as the level of exit discharge.

***Example 3***

Exhibit 3.3 depicts a four-story building where the finished ground level varies significantly in elevation such that three of the floors have exits that discharge to finished ground level. Based on occupant load, each floor requires three means of egress that are supplied by three equally sized exit stairs. Each of the three exit discharge floors has less than 50 percent of the required number of means of egress discharging from that floor, so that the specification of item (1) of the definition of *level of exit discharge* in 3.3.77.1 is not met. Per item (2) of 3.3.77.1, the level of exit discharge is that exit discharge story with the smallest elevation change needed to reach the finished ground level. The floors designated in Exhibit 3.3 as 1 and 3 require travel over stairs to reach the finished ground level. The floor designated as 2 discharges directly at finished ground level and is classified as the level of exit discharge.

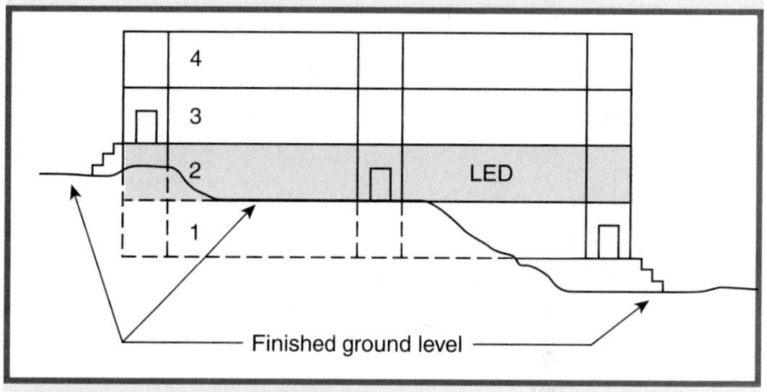


***Exhibit 3.3*** *Level of exit discharge at exit story with least elevation difference from finished ground level.*

***A.3.3.77.1 Level of Exit Discharge.*** Low occupancy, ancillary spaces with exit doors discharging directly to the outside, such as mechanical equipment rooms or storage areas, that are located on levels other than main occupiable floors should not be considered in the determination of level of exit discharge.

The text of A.3.3.77.1 advises that low occupancy spaces with exit doors discharging directly to the outside, such as mechanical equipment rooms that are located on levels other than main occupiable floors, should not be considered in the determination of level of exit discharge. Exhibit 3.4 depicts a building where the lowest floor (designated as −1) is occupied only for housing mechanical equipment and other building service equipment. It is the lowest story from which not less than 50 percent of the required number of means of egress and not less than 50 percent of the required egress capacity from that story discharge directly outside at the finished ground level and meets the definition of *level of exit discharge*. The annex text advises that the next to lowest floor (designated in Exhibit 3.4 as 1) should be considered the level of exit discharge. The annex text was written in recognition of the fact that a floor level with few occupants and an exit door installed more for accommodating equipment moves than egress should not penalize the building operators in the application of provisions that rely on determination of level of exit discharge, as might be done when considering the number of stories in height for purposes of applying minimum construction requirements.

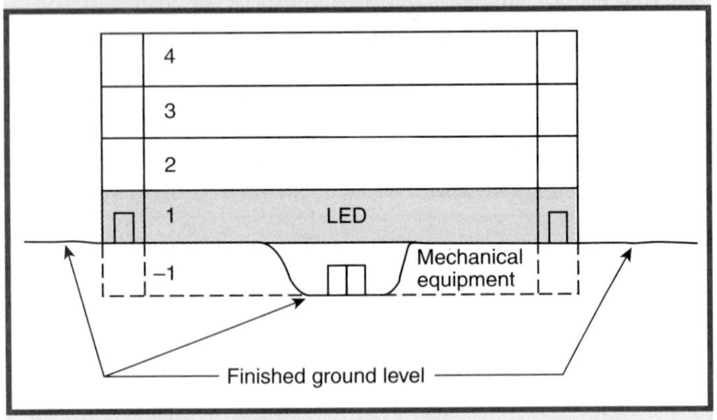


***Exhibit 3.4*** *Mechanical equipment floor disregarded in determination of level of exit discharge.*

**3.3.78 Exposition.** An event in which the display of products or services is organized to bring together the provider and user of the products or services.

**3.3.79 Exposition Facility.** See 3.3.82.1.

**3.3.80* Exposure Fire.** A fire that starts at a location that is remote from the area being protected and grows to expose that which is being protected.

**A.3.3.80 Exposure Fire.** An exposure fire usually refers to a fire that starts outside a building, such as a wildlands fire or vehicle fire, and that, consequently, exposes the building to a fire.

**3.3.81 Externally Illuminated.** See 3.3.135.1.

**3.3.82 Facility.**

***3.3.82.1 Exposition Facility.*** A convention center, hotel, or other building at which exposition events are held.

***3.3.82.2* Limited Care Facility.*** A building or portion of a building used on a 24-hour basis for the housing of four or more persons who are incapable of self-preservation because of age; physical limitations due to accident or illness; or limitations such as mental retardation/developmental disability, mental illness, or chemical dependency.

***A.3.3.82.2 Limited Care Facility.*** Limited care facilities and residential board and care occupancies both provide care to people with physical and mental limitations. However, the goals and programs of the two types of occupancies differ greatly. The requirements in this *Code* for limited care facilities are based on the assumption that these are medical facilities, that they provide medical care and treatment, and that the patients are not trained to respond to the fire alarm; that is, the patients do not participate in fire drills but, rather, await rescue. *(See Section 18.7.)*

The requirements for residential board and care occupancies are based on the assumption that the residents are provided with personal care and activities that foster continued independence, that the residents are encouraged and taught to overcome their limitations, and that most residents, including all residents in prompt and slow homes, are trained to respond to fire drills to the extent they are able. Residents are required to participate in fire drills. *(See Section 32.7.)*

**3.3.83 Festival Seating.** See 3.3.221.1.

**3.3.84 Finish.**

***3.3.84.1 Interior Ceiling Finish.*** The interior finish of ceilings.

***3.3.84.2* Interior Finish.*** The exposed surfaces of walls, ceilings, and floors within buildings.

***A.3.3.84.2 Interior Finish.*** Interior finish is not intended to apply to surfaces within spaces such as those that are concealed or inaccessible. Furnishings that, in some cases, might be secured in place for functional reasons should not be considered as interior finish.

***3.3.84.3* Interior Floor Finish.*** The interior finish of floors, ramps, stair treads and risers, and other walking surfaces.

***A.3.3.84.3 Interior Floor Finish.*** Interior floor finish includes coverings applied over a normal finished floor or stair treads and risers.

***3.3.84.4 Interior Wall Finish.*** The interior finish of columns, fixed or movable walls, and fixed or movable partitions.

**3.3.85 Finished Ground Level (Grade).** The level of the finished ground (earth or other surface on ground). *(See also 3.3.115, Grade Plane.)*

The definition of the term *finished ground level* is new to the 2009 edition of the *Code*. The addition is part of a major revision of text throughout the *Code* related to terminology used to describe building height and number of stories relative to grade plane, finished ground level, and level of exit discharge. See 3.3.115, *Grade Plane*. See the commentary associated with 3.3.77.1, *Level of Exit Discharge*, where the term *finished ground level* is used in determining the level of exit discharge for a variety of exit discharge arrangements.

**3.3.86 Fire Barrier.** See 3.3.27.1.

**3.3.87 Fire Barrier Wall.** See 3.3.268.1.

**3.3.88 Fire Compartment.** See 3.3.43.1.

**3.3.89 Fire Door.** See 3.3.57.2.

**3.3.90 Fire Door Assembly.** See 3.3.21.1.1.

**3.3.91 Fire Exit Hardware.** See 3.3.124.1.

**3.3.92* Fire Model.** A structured approach to predicting one or more effects of a fire.

**A.3.3.92 Fire Model.** Due to the complex nature of the principles involved, models are often packaged as computer software. Any relevant input data, assumptions, and limitations needed to properly implement the model will be attached to the fire models.

**3.3.93 Fire Protection Rating.** See 3.3.206.1.

**3.3.94 Fire Resistance Rating.** See 3.3.206.2.

**3.3.95 Fire Safety Functions.** Building and fire control functions that are intended to increase the level of life safety for occupants or to control the spread of the harmful effects of fire. [*72,* 2007]

**3.3.96* Fire Scenario.** A set of conditions that defines the development of fire, the spread of combustion products throughout a building or portion of a building, the reactions of people to fire, and the effects of combustion products.

**A.3.3.96 Fire Scenario.** A fire scenario defines the conditions under which a proposed design is expected to meet the fire safety goals. Factors typically include fuel characteristics, ignition sources, ventilation, building characteristics, and occupant locations and characteristics. The term *fire scenario* includes more than the characteristics of the fire itself but excludes design specifications and any characteristics that do not vary from one fire to another; the latter are called assumptions. The term *fire scenario* is used here to mean only those specifications required to calculate the fire's development and effects, but, in other contexts, the term might be used to mean both the initial specifications and the subsequent development and effects (i.e., a complete description of fire from conditions prior to ignition to conditions following extinguishment).

***3.3.96.1 Design Fire Scenario.*** A fire scenario selected for evaluation of a proposed design. [**914,** 2007]

**3.3.97 Fire Watch.** The assignment of a person or persons to an area for the express purpose of notifying the fire department, the building occupants, or both of an emergency; preventing a fire from occurring; extinguishing small fires; or protecting the public from fire or life safety dangers. [**1,** 2009]

**3.3.98 Fire Window Assembly.** See 3.3.21.2.

**3.3.99 Fire-Retardant-Treated Wood.** A wood product impregnated with chemical by a pressure process or other means during manufacture, which is tested in accordance with NFPA 255, has a listed flame spread of 25 or less, and shows no evidence of significant progressive combustion when the test is continued for an additional 20-minute period; nor does the flame front progress more than 10.5 ft (3.2 m) beyond the centerline of the burners at any time during the test.

**3.3.100 First Story Above Grade Plane.** See 3.3.115.1.

**3.3.101 Fixed Seating.** See 3.3.221.2.

**3.3.102* Flame Spread.** The propagation of flame over a surface.

**A.3.3.102 Flame Spread.** See Section 10.2.

**3.3.103 Flame Spread Index.** See 3.3.138.1.

**3.3.104 Flashover.** A transition phase in the development of a compartment fire in which surfaces exposed to thermal radiation reach ignition temperature more or less simultaneously and fire spreads rapidly throughout the space, resulting in full room involvement or total involvement of the compartment or enclosed space. [**921,** 2008]

**3.3.105 Flexible Plan and Open Plan Educational or Day-Care Building.** See 3.3.32.6.

**3.3.106 Floor Fire Door Assembly.** See 3.3.21.1.1.1.

**3.3.107 Flow Time.** A component of total evacuation time that is the time during which there is crowd flow past a point in the means of egress system.

**3.3.108 Fly Gallery.** A raised floor area above a stage from which the movement of scenery and operation of other stage effects are controlled.

**3.3.109 Folding and Telescopic Seating.** See 3.3.221.3.

**3.3.110 Food Court.** See 3.3.46.2.

**3.3.111 Fuel Load.** See 3.3.153.1.

**3.3.112 General Industrial Occupancy.** See 3.3.178.8.1.

**3.3.113 Goal.** A nonspecific overall outcome to be achieved that is measured on a qualitative basis.

**3.3.114 Grade.** See 3.3.85, Finished Ground Level (Grade).

**3.3.115 Grade Plane.** A reference plane representing the average of the finished ground level adjoining the building at all exterior walls. When the finished ground level slopes down from the exterior walls, the grade plane is established by the lowest points within the area between the building and the lot line or, when the lot line is more than 6 ft (1830 mm) from the building, between the building and a point 6 ft (1830 mm) from the building.

***3.3.115.1 First Story Above Grade Plane.*** Any story having its finished floor surface entirely above grade plane, except that a basement is to be considered as a first story above grade plane where the finished surface of the floor above the basement is (1) more than 6 ft (1830 mm) above grade plane or (2) more than 12 ft (3660 mm) above the finished ground level at any point.

The definition of the terms *grade plane* and *first story above grade plane* are new to the 2009 edition of the *Code*. The additions are part of a major revision of text throughout the *Code* related to terminology used to describe building height and number of stories relative to grade plane, finished ground level, and level of exit discharge. See 3.3.85, *Finished Ground Level*, and 3.3.77.1, *Level of Exit Discharge*.

Exhibit 3.5 demonstrates application of the definition of the term *grade plane*. The length and width of the building are each 200 ft (61 m). The finished ground level varies significantly in elevation from building side to building side. The average finished ground level elevation at each building side is as follows:

North side: +30 ft (+9.1 m)

East side: +26 ft (+7.9 m)

South side: +2 ft (0.6 m)

West side: +22 ft (+6.7 m)

The average of the finished ground level elevation around the four sides of the building is the average of the four sides' average finished ground level, as the length and width are equal. If two sides of the building were twice as long as the other two sides, the two longer sides would have twice the effect in calculating the grade plane as the two shorter sides. In the example where all four sides are the same length, the average of the finished ground level is calculated as [30 ft + 26 ft + 2 ft +22 ft]/4 = 20 ft ([9.1 m + 7.9 m + 0.6 m +6.7 m]/4 = 6.1 m). The grade plane is established as the elevation of 20 ft (6.1 m). The grade plane and the first story above grade plane (as defined in 3.3.115.1) are illustrated in Exhibit 3.6.

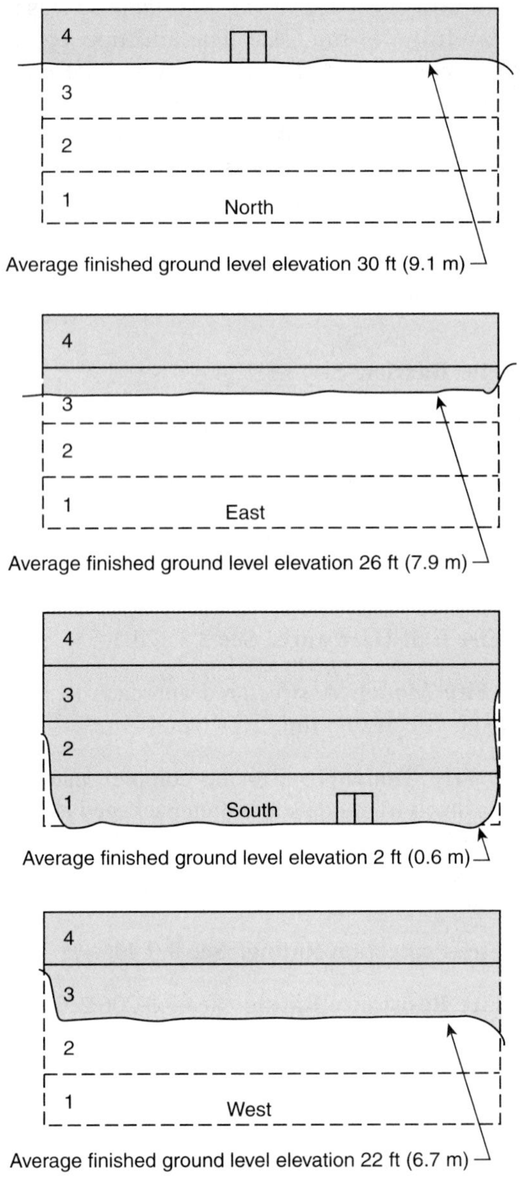


***Exhibit 3.5*** *Grade plane determined in relation to finished ground level.*

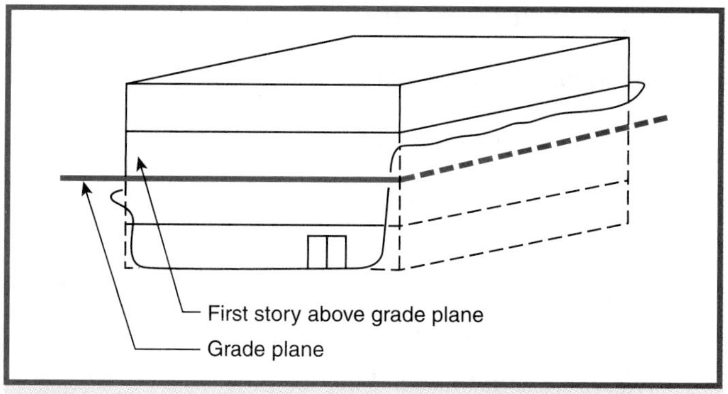


***Exhibit 3.6*** *Grade plane and first story above grade plane.*

**3.3.116* Grandstand.** A structure that provides tiered or stepped seating.

**A.3.3.116 Grandstand.** Where the term *grandstand* is preceded by an adjective denoting a material, it means a grandstand the essential members of which, exclusive of seating, are of the material designated.

**3.3.117 Gridiron.** The structural framing over a stage supporting equipment for hanging or flying scenery and other stage effects.

**3.3.118 Gross Floor Area.** See 3.3.19.2.1.

**3.3.119 Gross Leasable Area.** See 3.3.19.3.

**3.3.120 Guard.** A vertical protective barrier erected along exposed edges of stairways, balconies, and similar areas.

**3.3.121 Guest Room.** An accommodation combining living, sleeping, sanitary, and storage facilities within a compartment.

**3.3.122 Guest Suite.** See 3.3.255.1.

**3.3.123 Handrail.** A bar, pipe, or similar member designed to furnish persons with a handhold.

**3.3.124 Hardware.**

***3.3.124.1 Fire Exit Hardware.*** A door-latching assembly incorporating an actuating member or bar that releases the latch bolt upon the application of a force in the direction of egress travel and that additionally provides fire protection where used as part of a fire door assembly.

***3.3.124.2 Panic Hardware.*** A door-latching assembly incorporating an actuating member or bar that releases the latch bolt upon the application of a force in the direction of egress travel.

**3.3.125 Hazardous Area.** See 3.3.19.4.

**3.3.126 Health Care Occupancy.** See 3.3.178.7.

**3.3.127* Heat Release Rate (HRR).** The rate at which heat energy is generated by burning. [**921,** 2008]

**A.3.3.127 Heat Release Rate (HRR).** The heat release rate of a fuel is related to its chemistry, physical form, and availability of oxidant and is ordinarily expressed as British thermal units per second (Btu/s) or kilowatts (kW).

Chapters 40 and 42 include detailed provisions on high hazard industrial and storage occupancies.

**3.3.128 High Hazard Industrial Occupancy.** See 3.3.178.8.2.

**3.3.129 High-Rise Building.** See 3.3.32.7.

**3.3.130 Historic Building.** See 3.3.32.8.

**3.3.131 Home.**

***3.3.131.1* Day-Care Home.*** A building or portion of a building in which more than 3 but not more than 12 clients receive care, maintenance, and supervision, by other than their relative(s) or legal guardians(s), for less than 24 hours per day.

***A.3.3.131.1 Day-Care Home.*** A day-care home is generally located within a dwelling unit.

***3.3.131.2 Nursing Home.*** A building or portion of a building used on a 24-hour basis for the housing and nursing care of four or more persons who, because of mental or physical incapacity, might be unable to provide for their own needs and safety without the assistance of another person.

**3.3.132 Horizontal Exit.** See 3.3.75.1.

**3.3.133 Hospital.** A building or portion thereof used on a 24-hour basis for the medical, psychiatric, obstetrical, or surgical care of four or more inpatients.

**3.3.134* Hotel.** A building or groups of buildings under the same management in which there are sleeping accommodations for more than 16 persons and primarily used by transients for lodging with or without meals.

**A.3.3.134 Hotel.** So-called apartment hotels should be classified as hotels, because they are potentially subject to the same transient occupancy as hotels. Transients are those who occupy accommodations for less than 30 days.

**3.3.135 Illuminated.**

***3.3.135.1* Externally Illuminated.*** Refers to an illumination source that is contained outside of the device or sign legend area that is to be illuminated.

***A.3.3.135.1 Externally Illuminated.*** The light source is typically a dedicated incandescent or fluorescent source.

*3.3.135.2* **Internally Illuminated.*** Refers to an illumination source that is contained inside the device or legend that is illuminated.

*A.3.3.135.2 **Internally Illuminated.*** The light source is typically incandescent, fluorescent, electroluminescent, photoluminescent, light-emitting diodes, or self-luminous.

**3.3.136 Impractical Evacuation Capability.** See 3.3.70.1.

**3.3.137 Incapacitation.** A condition under which humans do not function adequately and become unable to escape untenable conditions.

**3.3.138 Index.**

*3.3.138.1 **Flame Spread Index.*** A comparative measure, expressed as a dimensionless number, derived from visual measurements of the spread of flame versus time for a material tested in accordance with ASTM E 84, *Standard Test Method for Surface Burning Characteristics of Building Materials*, or ANSI/UL 723, *Standard for Test for Surface Burning Characteristics of Burning Materials*.

*3.3.138.2 **Smoke Developed Index.*** A comparative measure, expressed as a dimensionless number, derived from measurements of smoke obscuration versus time for a material tested in accordance with ASTM E 84, *Standard Test Method for Surface Burning Characteristics of Building Materials*, or ANSI/UL 723, *Standard for Test for Surface Burning Characteristics of Burning Materials*.

**3.3.139 Industrial Occupancy.** See 3.3.178.8.

**3.3.140 Input Data Specification.** See 3.3.244.2.

**3.3.141 Interior Ceiling Finish.** See 3.3.84.1.

**3.3.142 Interior Finish.** See 3.3.84.2

**3.3.143 Interior Floor Finish.** See 3.3.84.3.

**3.3.144 Interior Wall Finish.** See 3.3.84.4.

**3.3.145 Internally Illuminated.** See 3.3.135.2.

**3.3.146 Legitimate Stage.** See 3.3.246.1.

**3.3.147 Level of Exit Discharge.** See 3.3.77.1.

**3.3.148 Life Safety Evaluation.** A written review dealing with the adequacy of life safety features relative to fire, storm, collapse, crowd behavior, and other related safety considerations.

**3.3.149 Limited Access Structure.** See 3.3.254.3.

**3.3.150 Limited Care Facility.** See 3.3.82.2.

**3.3.151 Limited-Combustible (Material).** See 3.3.160.2.

**3.3.152 Living Area.** See 3.3.19.5.

**3.3.153 Load.**

*3.3.153.1* **Fuel Load.*** The total quantity of combustible contents of a building, space, or fire area.

*A.3.3.153.1 **Fuel Load.*** Fuel load includes interior finish and trim.

*3.3.153.2 **Occupant Load.*** The total number of persons that might occupy a building or portion thereof at any one time.

**3.3.154 Load-Bearing Element.** Any column, girder, beam, joist, truss, rafter, wall, floor, or roof sheathing that supports any vertical load in addition to its own weight, or any lateral load.

**3.3.155 Lock-Up.** An incidental use area in other than a detention and correctional occupancy where occupants are restrained and such occupants are mostly incapable of self-preservation because of security measures not under the occupants' control.

The definition of the term *lockup* was revised for the 2009 edition of the *Code*. The words "an area" were changed to "an incidental use area" to prevent *Code* users from incorrectly using the term *lockup* for a building predominantly used for the detention of persons but for which the provisions of 22.4.5.1.1 or 23.4.5.1.1 would not impose a classification of detention and correctional occupancy because the number of detainees does not exceed 49. Where the predominant use of the building is the detention of persons, the occupancy should be classified as detention and correctional and subject to the full provisions of Chapter 22 or Chapter 23, not to the lockup provisions of 22.4.5 or 23.4.5. The lockup provisions of 22.4.5 and 23.4.5 are meant to be applied to detention areas where the predominant use is something other than detention — as might occur, for example, at immigration control at an international airport or the security office at a sports stadium or mercantile mall building.

**3.3.156 Lodging or Rooming House.** A building or portion thereof that does not qualify as a one- or two-family dwelling, that provides sleeping accommodations for a total of 16 or fewer people on a transient or permanent basis, without personal care services, with or without meals, but without separate cooking facilities for individual occupants.

**3.3.157 Major Tenant.** A tenant space, in a mall building, with one or more main entrances from the exterior that also serve as exits and are independent of the mall.

The definition of the term *major tenant* is new to the 2009 edition of the *Code*. The term was defined to help support the new criteria of 36.4.4.3.6 and 37.4.4.3.6, which permit each major tenant of a mercantile mall to provide a maximum of one-half of its means of egress independent of the mall, thus reducing the overall occupant load for which the mall's egress system must be sized.

**3.3.158 Mall.** A roofed or covered common pedestrian area within a mall building that serves as access for two or more tenants and does not exceed three levels that are open to each other.

**3.3.159 Mall Building.** See 3.3.32.9.

**3.3.160 Material.**

***3.3.160.1 Combustible (Material).*** A material that, in the form in which it is used and under the conditions anticipated, will ignite and burn; a material that does not meet the definition of noncombustible or limited-combustible.

***3.3.160.2* Limited-Combustible (Material).*** Refers to a building construction material not complying with the definition of noncombustible *(see 3.3.160.3)* that, in the form in which it is used, has a potential heat value not exceeding 3500 Btu/lb (8141 kJ/kg), where tested in accordance with NFPA 259, *Standard Test Method for Potential Heat of Building Materials*, and includes either of the following: (1) materials having a structural base of noncombustible material, with a surfacing not exceeding a thickness of $^1/_8$ in. (3.2 mm) that has a flame spread index not greater than 50; (2) materials, in the form and thickness used, having neither a flame spread index greater than 25 nor evidence of continued progressive combustion, and of such composition that surfaces that would be exposed by cutting through the material on any plane would have neither a flame spread index greater than 25 nor evidence of continued progressive combustion.

***A.3.3.160.2 Limited-Combustible (Material).*** Materials subject to increase in combustibility or flame spread index beyond the limits herein established through the effects of age, moisture, or other atmospheric condition are considered combustible. *(See* NFPA 259, *Standard Test Method for Potential Heat of Building Materials, and* NFPA 220, *Standard on Types of Building Construction.)*

***3.3.160.3 Noncombustible (Material).*** A material that, in the form in which it is used and under the conditions anticipated, will not ignite, burn, support combustion, or release flammable vapors, when subjected to fire or heat. Materials that are reported as passing ASTM E 136, *Standard Test Method for Behavior of Materials in a Vertical Tube Furnace at 750 Degrees C*, shall be considered noncombustible materials.

***3.3.160.4 Weathered-Membrane Material.*** Membrane material that has been subjected to a minimum of 3000 hours in a weatherometer in accordance with ASTM G 155, *Standard Practice for Operating Xenon Arc Light Apparatus for Exposure of Non-Metallic Materials*, or approved equivalent.

**3.3.161* Means of Egress.** A continuous and unobstructed way of travel from any point in a building or structure to a public way consisting of three separate and distinct parts: (1) the exit access, (2) the exit, and (3) the exit discharge.

**A.3.3.161 Means of Egress.** A means of egress comprises the vertical and horizontal travel and includes intervening room spaces, doorways, hallways, corridors, passageways, balconies, ramps, stairs, elevators, enclosures, lobbies, escalators, horizontal exits, courts, and yards.

***3.3.161.1 Accessible Means of Egress.*** A means of egress that provides an accessible route to an area of refuge, a horizontal exit, or a public way.

**3.3.162 Means of Escape.** A way out of a building or structure that does not conform to the strict definition of means of egress but does provide an alternate way out.

**3.3.163* Membrane.** A thin layer of construction material.

**A.3.3.163 Membrane.** For the purpose of fire protection features, a membrane can consist of materials such as gypsum board, plywood, glass, or fabric. For the purpose of membrane structures, a membrane consists of thin, flexible, water-impervious material capable of being supported by an air pressure of $1^1/_2$ in. (38 mm) water column.

**3.3.164 Membrane Structure.** See 3.3.254.4.

**3.3.165 Mercantile Occupancy.** See 3.3.178.9.

**3.3.166 Mezzanine.** An intermediate level between the floor and the ceiling of any room or space.

**3.3.167 Mixed Occupancy.** See 3.3.178.10.

**3.3.168* Modification.** The reconfiguration of any space; the addition or elimination of any door or window; the addition or elimination of load-bearing elements; the reconfiguration or extension of any system; or the installation of any additional equipment.

**A.3.3.168 Modification.** Modification does not include repair or replacement of interior finishes.

**3.3.169 Multilevel Play Structure.** See 3.3.254.5.

**3.3.170 Multiple Occupancy.** See 3.3.178.11.

**3.3.171 Multiple Station Alarm Device.** See 3.3.56.1.

**3.3.172 Multipurpose Assembly Occupancy.** See 3.3.178.2.1.

**3.3.173 Net Floor Area.** See 3.3.19.2.2.

**3.3.174 Noncombustible (Material).** See 3.3.160.3.

**3.3.175 Non-Sleeping Suite (Health Care Occupancies).** See 3.3.255.2.1.

**3.3.176 Nursing Home.** See 3.3.131.2.

**3.3.177* Objective.** A requirement that needs to be met to achieve a goal.

**A.3.3.177 Objective.** Objectives define a series of actions necessary to make the achievement of a goal more likely. Objectives are stated in more specific terms than goals and are measured on a more quantitative, rather than qualitative, basis.

**3.3.178 Occupancy.** The purpose for which a building or other structure, or part thereof, is used or intended to be used. [**ASCE/SEI 7:**1.2]

***3.3.178.1* Ambulatory Health Care Occupancy.*** An occupancy used to provide services or treatment simultaneously to four or more patients that provides, on an outpatient basis, one or more of the following: (1) treatment for patients that renders the patients incapable of taking action for self-preservation under emergency conditions without the assistance of others; (2) anesthesia that renders the patients incapable of taking action for self-preservation under emergency conditions without the assistance of others; (3) emergency or urgent care for patients who, due to the nature of their injury or illness, are incapable of taking action for self-preservation under emergency conditions without the assistance of others.

***A.3.3.178.1 Ambulatory Health Care Occupancy.*** It is not the intent that occupants be considered to be incapable of self-preservation just because they are in a wheelchair or use assistive walking devices, such as a cane, a walker, or crutches. Rather, it is the intent to address emergency care centers that receive patients who have been rendered incapable of self-preservation due to the emergency, such as being rendered unconscious as a result of an accident or being unable to move due to sudden illness.

***3.3.178.2* Assembly Occupancy.*** An occupancy (1) used for a gathering of 50 or more persons for deliberation, worship, entertainment, eating, drinking, amusement, awaiting transportation, or similar uses; or (2) used as a special amusement building, regardless of occupant load.

***A.3.3.178.2 Assembly Occupancy.*** Assembly occupancies might include the following:

(1) Armories
(2) Assembly halls
(3) Auditoriums
(4) Bowling lanes
(5) Club rooms
(6) College and university classrooms, 50 persons and over
(7) Conference rooms
(8) Courtrooms
(9) Dance halls
(10) Drinking establishments
(11) Exhibition halls
(12) Gymnasiums
(13) Libraries
(14) Mortuary chapels
(15) Motion picture theaters
(16) Museums
(17) Passenger stations and terminals of air, surface, underground, and marine public transportation facilities
(18) Places of religious worship
(19) Pool rooms
(20) Recreation piers
(21) Restaurants
(22) Skating rinks
(23) Special amusement buildings, regardless of occupant load
(24) Theaters

Assembly occupancies are characterized by the presence or potential presence of crowds with attendant panic hazard in case of fire or other emergency. They are generally open or occasionally open to the public, and the occupants, who are present voluntarily, are not ordinarily subject to discipline or control. Such buildings are ordinarily occupied by able-bodied persons and are not used for sleeping purposes. Special conference rooms, snack areas, and other areas incidental to, and under the control of, the management of other occupancies, such as offices, fall under the 50-person limitation.

Restaurants and drinking establishments with an occupant load of fewer than 50 persons should be classified as mercantile occupancies.

For special amusement buildings, see 12.4.7 and 13.4.7.

*3.3.178.2.1 Multipurpose Assembly Occupancy.* An assembly room designed to accommodate temporarily any of several possible assembly uses.

*3.3.178.3* Business Occupancy.* An occupancy used for the transaction of business other than mercantile.

*A.3.3.178.3 Business Occupancy.* Business occupancies include the following:

(1) Air traffic control towers (ATCTs)
(2) City halls
(3) College and university instructional buildings, classrooms under 50 persons, and instructional laboratories
(4) Courthouses
(5) Dentists' offices
(6) Doctors' offices
(7) General offices
(8) Outpatient clinics (ambulatory)
(9) Town halls

Doctors' and dentists' offices are included, unless of such character as to be classified as ambulatory health care occupancies. *(See 3.3.178.1.)*

Birth centers should be classified as business occupancies if they are occupied by fewer than four patients, not including infants, at any one time; do not provide sleeping facilities for four or more occupants; and do not provide treatment procedures that render four or more patients, not including infants, incapable of self-preservation at any one time. For birth centers occupied by patients not meeting these parameters, see Chapter 18 or Chapter 19, as appropriate.

Service facilities common to city office buildings, such as newsstands, lunch counters serving fewer than 50 persons, barber shops, and beauty parlors are included in the business occupancy group.

City halls, town halls, and courthouses are included in this occupancy group, insofar as their principal function is the transaction of public business and the keeping of books and records. Insofar as they are used for assembly purposes, they are classified as assembly occupancies.

*3.3.178.4* Day-Care Occupancy.* An occupancy in which four or more clients receive care, maintenance, and supervision, by other than their relatives or legal guardians, for less than 24 hours per day.

*A.3.3.178.4 Day-Care Occupancy.* Day-care occupancies include the following:

(1) Adult day-care occupancies, except where part of a health care occupancy
(2) Child day-care occupancies
(3) Day-care homes
(4) Kindergarten classes that are incidental to a child day-care occupancy
(5) Nursery schools

In areas where public schools offer only half-day kindergarten programs, many child day-care occupancies offer state-approved kindergarten classes for children who need full-day care. Because these classes are normally incidental to the day-care occupancy, the requirements of the day-care occupancy should be followed.

*3.3.178.5* Detention and Correctional Occupancy.* An occupancy used to house one or more persons under varied degrees of restraint or security where such occupants are mostly incapable of self-preservation because of security measures not under the occupants' control.

*A.3.3.178.5 Detention and Correctional Occupancy.* Detention and correctional occupancies include the following:

(1) Adult and juvenile substance abuse centers
(2) Adult and juvenile work camps
(3) Adult community residential centers
(4) Adult correctional institutions
(5) Adult local detention facilities
(6) Juvenile community residential centers
(7) Juvenile detention facilities
(8) Juvenile training schools

See A.22.1.1.1.4 and A.23.1.1.1.4.

*3.3.178.6* Educational Occupancy.* An occupancy used for educational purposes through the twelfth grade by six or more persons for 4 or more hours per day or more than 12 hours per week.

*A.3.3.178.6 Educational Occupancy.* Educational occupancies include the following:

(1) Academies
(2) Kindergartens
(3) Schools

An educational occupancy is distinguished from an assembly occupancy in that the same occupants are regularly present.

*3.3.178.7* Health Care Occupancy.* An occupancy used to provide medical or other treatment or care simultaneously to four or more patients on an inpatient basis, where such patients are mostly incapable of self-preservation due to age, physical or mental disability, or because of security measures not under the occupants' control.

*A.3.3.178.7 Health Care Occupancy.* Health care occupancies include the following:

(1) Hospitals
(2) Limited care facilities
(3) Nursing homes

Occupants of health care occupancies typically have physical or mental illness, disease, or infirmity. They also include infants, convalescents, or infirm aged persons.

***3.3.178.8* Industrial Occupancy.*** An occupancy in which products are manufactured or in which processing, assembling, mixing, packaging, finishing, decorating, or repair operations are conducted.

***A.3.3.178.8 Industrial Occupancy.*** Industrial occupancies include the following:

(1) Drycleaning plants
(2) Factories of all kinds
(3) Food processing plants
(4) Gas plants
(5) Hangars (for servicing/maintenance)
(6) Laundries
(7) Power plants
(8) Pumping stations
(9) Refineries
(10) Sawmills
(11) Telephone exchanges

In evaluating the appropriate classification of laboratories, the authority having jurisdiction should treat each case individually, based on the extent and nature of the associated hazards. Some laboratories are classified as occupancies other than industrial; for example, a physical therapy laboratory or a computer laboratory.

***3.3.178.8.1* General Industrial Occupancy.*** An industrial occupancy in which ordinary and low hazard industrial operations are conducted in buildings of conventional design suitable for various types of industrial processes.

***A.3.3.178.8.1 General Industrial Occupancy.*** General industrial occupancies include multistory buildings where floors are occupied by different tenants or buildings suitable for such occupancy and, therefore, are subject to possible use for types of industrial processes with a high density of employee population.

***3.3.178.8.2* High Hazard Industrial Occupancy.*** An industrial occupancy in which industrial operations that include high hazard materials, processes, or contents are conducted.

***A.3.3.178.8.2 High Hazard Industrial Occupancy.*** A high hazard industrial occupancy includes occupancies where gasoline and other flammable liquids are handled, used, or stored under such conditions that involve possible release of flammable vapors; where grain dust, wood flour or plastic dust, aluminum or magnesium dust, or other explosive dusts are produced; where hazardous chemicals or explosives are manufactured, stored, or handled; where materials are processed or handled under conditions that might produce flammable flyings; and where other situations of similar hazard exist. Chapters 40 and 42 include detailed provisions on high hazard industrial and storage occupancies.

***3.3.178.8.3 Special-Purpose Industrial Occupancy.*** An industrial occupancy in which ordinary and low hazard industrial operations are conducted in buildings designed for, and suitable only for, particular types of operations, characterized by a relatively low density of employee population, with much of the area occupied by machinery or equipment.

***3.3.178.9* Mercantile Occupancy.*** An occupancy used for the display and sale of merchandise.

***A.3.3.178.9 Mercantile Occupancy.*** Mercantile occupancies include the following:

(1) Auction rooms
(2) Department stores
(3) Drugstores
(4) Restaurants with fewer than 50 persons
(5) Shopping centers
(6) Supermarkets

Office, storage, and service facilities incidental to the sale of merchandise and located in the same building should be considered part of the mercantile occupancy classification.

***3.3.178.10 Mixed Occupancy.*** A multiple occupancy where the occupancies are intermingled.

***3.3.178.11 Multiple Occupancy.*** A building or structure in which two or more classes of occupancy exist.

***3.3.178.12* Residential Board and Care Occupancy.*** An occupancy used for lodging and boarding of four or more residents, not related by blood or marriage to the owners or operators, for the purpose of providing personal care services.

***A.3.3.178.12 Residential Board and Care Occupancy.*** The following are examples of facilities that are classified as residential board and care occupancies:

(1) Group housing arrangement for physically or mentally handicapped persons who normally attend school in the community, attend worship in the community, or otherwise use community facilities
(2) Group housing arrangement for physically or mentally handicapped persons who are undergoing training in preparation for independent living, for paid employment, or for other normal community activities
(3) Group housing arrangement for the elderly that provides personal care services but that does not provide nursing care
(4) Facilities for social rehabilitation, alcoholism, drug abuse, or mental health problems that contain a group housing arrangement and that provide personal care services but do not provide acute care

(5) Assisted living facilities
(6) Other group housing arrangements that provide personal care services but not nursing care

***3.3.178.13* Residential Occupancy.*** An occupancy that provides sleeping accommodations for purposes other than health care or detention and correctional.

***A.3.3.178.13 Residential Occupancy.*** Residential occupancies are treated as separate occupancies in this *Code* as follows:

(1) One- and two-family dwellings (Chapter 24)
(2) Lodging or rooming houses (Chapter 26)
(3) Hotels, motels, and dormitories (Chapters 28 and 29)
(4) Apartment buildings (Chapters 30 and 31)

***3.3.178.14 Separated Occupancy.*** A multiple occupancy where the occupancies are separated by fire resistance–rated assemblies.

***3.3.178.15* Storage Occupancy.*** An occupancy used primarily for the storage or sheltering of goods, merchandise, products, or vehicles.

***A.3.3.178.15 Storage Occupancy.*** Storage occupancies include the following:

(1) Barns
(2) Bulk oil storage
(3) Cold storage
(4) Freight terminals
(5) Grain elevators
(6) Hangars (for storage only)
(7) Parking structures
(8) Truck and marine terminals
(9) Warehouses

Storage occupancies are characterized by the presence of relatively small numbers of persons in proportion to the area.

**3.3.179 Occupant Characteristics.** The abilities or behaviors of people before and during a fire.

**3.3.180 Occupant Load.** See 3.3.153.2.

**3.3.181 Occupiable Area.** See 3.3.19.6.

**3.3.182 Occupiable Story.** See 3.3.251.1.

**3.3.183 One- and Two-Family Dwelling Unit.** See 3.3.61.1.

**3.3.184 One-Family Dwelling Unit.** See 3.3.61.2.

**3.3.185 Open Parking Structure.** See 3.3.254.6.

**3.3.186 Open Structure.** See 3.3.254.7.

**3.3.187 Open-Air Mercantile Operation.** An operation conducted outside of all structures, with the operations area devoid of all walls and roofs except for small, individual, weather canopies.

**3.3.188* Outside Stair.** A stair with not less than one side open to the outer air.

**A.3.3.188 Outside Stair.** See 7.2.2.6.

**3.3.189 Panic Hardware.** See 3.3.124.2.

**3.3.190* Performance Criteria.** Threshold values on measurement scales that are based on quantified performance objectives.

**A.3.3.190 Performance Criteria.** Performance criteria are stated in engineering terms. Engineering terms include temperatures, radiant heat flux, and levels of exposure to fire products. Performance criteria provide threshold values used to evaluate a proposed design.

**3.3.191 Permanent Structure.** See 3.3.254.8.

**3.3.192* Personal Care.** The care of residents who do not require chronic or convalescent medical or nursing care.

**A.3.3.192 Personal Care.** Personal care involves responsibility for the safety of the resident while inside the building. Personal care might include daily awareness by management of the resident's functioning and whereabouts, making and reminding a resident of appointments, the ability and readiness for intervention in the event of a resident experiencing a crisis, supervision in the areas of nutrition and medication, and actual provision of transient medical care.

**3.3.193* Photoluminescent.** Having the ability to store incident electromagnetic radiation typically from ambient light sources, and release it in the form of visible light. [**301,** 2008]

**A.3.3.193 Photoluminescent.** The released light is normally visible for a limited time if the ambient light sources are removed or partially obscured.

**3.3.194 Pinrail.** A rail on or above a stage through which belaying pins are inserted and to which lines are fastened.

**3.3.195* Platform.** The raised area within a building used for the presentation of music, plays, or other entertainment.

**A.3.3.195 Platform.** Platforms also include the head tables for special guests; the raised area for lecturers and speakers; boxing and wrestling rings; theater-in-the-round; and for similar purposes wherein there are no overhead drops, pieces of scenery, or stage effects other than lighting and a screening valance.

A platform is not intended to be prohibited from using a curtain as a valance to screen or hide the electric conduit, lighting track, or similar fixtures, nor is a platform prohibited from using curtains that are used to obscure the back wall of the stage; from using a curtain between the auditorium and the stage (grand or house curtain); from using a maximum of four leg drops; or from using a valance to screen light panels, plumbing, and similar equipment from view.

*3.3.195.1 Temporary Platform.* A platform erected within an area for not more than 30 days.

**3.3.196 Plenum.** A compartment or chamber to which one or more air ducts are connected and that forms part of the air-distribution system.

**3.3.197 Point of Safety.** A location that (a) is exterior to and away from a building; or (b) is within a building of any construction type protected throughout by an approved automatic sprinkler system and that is either (1) within an exit enclosure meeting the requirements of this *Code,* or (2) within another portion of the building that is separated by smoke barriers in accordance with Section 8.5 having a minimum $^1/_2$-hour fire resistance rating, and that portion of the building has access to a means of escape or exit that conforms to the requirements of this *Code* and does not necessitate return to the area of fire involvement; or (c) is within a building of Type I, Type II(222), Type II(111), Type III(211), Type IV, or Type V(111) construction *(see 8.2.1.2)* and is either (1) within an exit enclosure meeting the requirements of this *Code*, or (2) within another portion of the building that is separated by smoke barriers in accordance with Section 8.5 having a minimum $^1/_2$-hour fire resistance rating, and that portion of the building has access to a means of escape or exit that conforms to the requirements of this *Code* and does not necessitate return to the area of fire involvement.

**3.3.198 Previously Approved.** That which was acceptable to the authority having jurisdiction prior to the date this edition of the *Code* went into effect.

**3.3.199 Private Party Tent.** See 3.3.260.1.

**3.3.200 Professional Engineer.** A person registered or licensed to practice engineering in a jurisdiction, subject to all laws and limitations imposed by the jurisdiction.

**3.3.201 Prompt Evacuation Capability.** See 3.3.70.2.

**3.3.202* Proposed Design.** A design developed by a design team and submitted to the authority having jurisdiction for approval.

**A.3.3.202 Proposed Design.** The design team might develop a number of trial designs that will be evaluated to determine whether they meet the performance criteria. One of the trial designs will be selected from those that meet the performance criteria for submission to the authority having jurisdiction as the proposed design.

The proposed design is not necessarily limited to fire protection systems and building features. It also includes any component of the proposed design that is installed, established, or maintained for the purpose of life safety, without which the proposed design could fail to achieve specified performance criteria. Therefore, the proposed design often includes emergency procedures and organizational structures that are needed to meet the performance criteria specified for the proposed design.

**3.3.203 Proscenium Wall.** See 3.3.268.2.

**3.3.204 Public Way.** A street, alley, or other similar parcel of land essentially open to the outside air deeded, dedicated, or otherwise permanently appropriated to the public for public use and having a clear width and height of not less than 10 ft (3050 mm).

**3.3.205* Ramp.** A walking surface that has a slope steeper than 1 in 20.

**A.3.3.205 Ramp.** See 7.2.5.

**3.3.206 Rating.**

***3.3.206.1 Fire Protection Rating.*** The designation indicating the duration of the fire test exposure to which a fire door assembly or fire window assembly was exposed and for which it met all the acceptance criteria as determined in accordance with NFPA 252, *Standard Methods of Fire Tests of Door Assemblies*, or NFPA 257, *Standard on Fire Test for Window and Glass Block Assemblies*, respectively.

***3.3.206.2 Fire Resistance Rating.*** The time, in minutes or hours, that materials or assemblies have withstood a fire exposure as determined by the tests, or methods based on tests, prescribed by this *Code*.

**3.3.207* Reconstruction.** The reconfiguration of a space that affects an exit or a corridor shared by more than one occupant space; or the reconfiguration of a space such that the rehabilitation work area is not permitted to be occupied because existing means of egress and fire protection systems, or their equivalent, are not in place or continuously maintained.

**A.3.3.207 Reconstruction.** It is not the intent that a corridor, aisle, or circulation space within a suite be considered as a corridor that is shared by more than one occupant space. The suite should be considered as only one occupant space. The following situations should be considered to involve more than one occupant space:

(1) Work affecting a corridor that is common to multiple guest rooms on a floor of a hotel occupancy
(2) Work affecting a corridor that is common to multiple living units on a floor of an apartment building occupancy

(3) Work affecting a corridor that is common to multiple tenants on a floor of a business occupancy

**3.3.208 Registered Architect.** A person licensed to practice architecture in a jurisdiction, subject to all laws and limitations imposed by the jurisdiction.

**3.3.209 Registered Design Professional (RDP).** An individual who is registered or licensed to practice his/her respective design profession as defined by the statutory requirements of the professional registration laws of the state or jurisdiction in which the project is to be constructed.

**3.3.210 Regular Stage.** See 3.3.246.2.

**3.3.211 Rehabilitation Work Area.** See 3.3.19.7

**3.3.212 Renovation.** The replacement in kind or strengthening of load-bearing elements; or the refinishing, replacement, bracing, strengthening, or upgrading of existing materials, elements, equipment, or fixtures, without involving the reconfiguration of spaces.

**3.3.213 Repair.** The patching, restoration, or painting of materials, elements, equipment, or fixtures for the purpose of maintaining such materials, elements, equipment, or fixtures in good or sound condition.

**3.3.214 Residential Board and Care Occupancy.** See 3.3.178.12.

**3.3.215 Residential Board and Care Resident.** A person who receives personal care and resides in a residential board and care facility.

**3.3.216 Residential Occupancy.** See 3.3.178.13.

**3.3.217 Safe Location.** A location remote or separated from the effects of a fire so that such effects no longer pose a threat.

**3.3.218 Safety Factor.** A factor applied to a predicted value to ensure that a sufficient safety margin is maintained.

**3.3.219 Safety Margin.** The difference between a predicted value and the actual value where a fault condition is expected.

**3.3.220 Sally Port (Security Vestibule).** A compartment provided with two or more doors where the intended purpose is to prevent continuous and unobstructed passage by allowing the release of only one door at a time.

**3.3.221 Seating.**

***3.3.221.1* Festival Seating.*** A form of audience/spectator accommodation in which no seating, other than a floor or finished ground level, is provided for the audience/spectators gathered to observe a performance.

***A.3.3.221.1 Festival Seating.*** Festival seating describes situations in assembly occupancies where live entertainment events are held that are expected to result in overcrowding and high audience density that can compromise public safety. It is not the intent to apply the term *festival seating* to exhibitions; sports events; dances; conventions; and bona fide political, religious, and educational events. Assembly occupancies with 15 $ft^2$ (1.4 $m^2$) or more per person should not be considered festival seating.

***3.3.221.2 Fixed Seating.*** Seating that is secured to the building structure.

***3.3.221.3 Folding and Telescopic Seating.*** A structure that is used for tiered seating of persons and whose overall shape and size can be reduced, without being dismantled, for purposes of moving or storing.

***3.3.221.4 Smoke-Protected Assembly Seating.*** Seating served by means of egress that is not subject to smoke accumulation within or under the structure.

**3.3.222 Self-Closing.** Equipped with an approved device that ensures closing after opening.

**3.3.223* Self-Luminous.** Illuminated by a self-contained power source and operated independently of external power sources.

**A.3.3.223 Self-Luminous.** An example of a self-contained power source is tritium gas. Batteries do not qualify as a self-contained power source. The light source is typically contained inside the device.

**3.3.224* Self-Preservation (Day-Care Occupancy).** The ability of a client to evacuate a day-care occupancy without direct intervention by a staff member.

**A.3.3.224 Self-Preservation (Day-Care Occupancy).** Examples of clients who are incapable of self-preservation include infants, clients who are unable to use stairs because of confinement to a wheelchair or other physical disability, and clients who cannot follow directions or a group to the outside of a facility due to mental or behavioral disorders. It is the intent of this *Code* to classify children under the age of 24 months as incapable of self-preservation. Examples of direct intervention by staff members include carrying a client, pushing a client outside in a wheelchair, and guiding a client by direct hand-holding or continued bodily contact. If clients cannot exit the building by themselves with minimal intervention from staff members, such as verbal orders, classification as incapable of self-preservation should be considered.

**3.3.225 Sensitivity Analysis.** See 3.3.15.1.

**3.3.226 Separate Atmosphere.** See 3.3.23.2.

**3.3.227 Separated Occupancy.** See 3.3.178.14.

**3.3.228 Severe Mobility Impairment.** The ability to move to stairs but without the ability to use the stairs.

**3.3.229 Single Station Alarm.** See 3.3.12.1.

**3.3.230* Situation Awareness.** The perception of the elements in the environment within a volume of time and space, the comprehension of their meaning, and the projection of their status in the near future.

The definition of the term *situation awareness* is new to the 2009 edition of the *Code*. The term was defined to help support the new criteria of 4.5.5, which add situation awareness to the fundamental requirements of Section 4.5. See 4.5.5 and A.4.5.5 for examples of systems that are currently required by the *Code* and that help to provide situation awareness.

**A.3.3.230 Situation Awareness.** Situation awareness (also called situational awareness), described in a simpler fashion, is being aware of what is happening around you and understanding what that information means to you now and in the future. This definition, and the more formal definition, come from the extensive work of human factors (ergonomics) experts in situation awareness, most notably Mica R. Endsley (Endsley, Bolte and Jones, *Designing for Situation Awareness: An approach to user-centered design*, CRC Press, Taylor and Francis, Boca Raton, FL, 2003). Within the *Code*, and the standards it references, are long-standing requirements for systems and facilities that enhance situation awareness. Included are fire/smoke detection, alarm, and communication systems plus the system status panels in emergency command centers; supervisory systems for various especially critical components (e.g., certain valves) of fire protection systems; waterflow indicators; certain signs; and the availability of trained staff, notably in health care occupancies. Serious failures of situation awareness have been identified as central to unfortunate outcomes in various emergencies; for example, typical responses of people to developing fires also exhibit situation awareness problems as incorrect assumptions are made about the rapidity of fire growth or the effect of opening a door. Good situation awareness is critical to decision making, which, in turn, is critical to performance during an emergency.

**3.3.231 Sleeping Suite (Health Care Occupancies).** See 3.3.255.2.2.

**3.3.232 Slow Evacuation Capability.** See 3.3.70.3.

**3.3.233 Smoke Alarm.** See 3.3.12.2.

**3.3.234 Smoke Barrier.** See 3.3.27.2.

**3.3.235 Smoke Compartment.** See 3.3.43.2.

**3.3.236 Smoke Detector.** A device that detects visible or invisible particles of combustion. [*72,* 2007]

**3.3.237 Smoke Developed Index.** See 3.3.138.2.

**3.3.238* Smoke Partition.** A continuous membrane that is designed to form a barrier to limit the transfer of smoke.

**A.3.3.238 Smoke Partition.** A smoke partition is not required to have a fire resistance rating.

**3.3.239* Smokeproof Enclosure.** An enclosure designed to limit the movement of products of combustion produced by a fire.

**A.3.3.239 Smokeproof Enclosure.** For further guidance, see the following publications:

(1) ASHRAE *Handbook and Product Directory — Fundamentals*
(2) *Principles of Smoke Management*, by Klote and Milke
(3) NFPA 105, *Standard for the Installation of Smoke Door Assemblies and Other Opening Protectives*

**3.3.240 Smoke-Protected Assembly Seating.** See 3.3.221.4.

**3.3.241 Special Amusement Building.** See 3.3.32.10.

**3.3.242 Special Inspection.** Services provided by a qualified person, retained by the owner and approved by the authority having jurisdiction, who observes the installation and witnesses the pretesting and operation of the system or systems.

**3.3.243 Special-Purpose Industrial Occupancy.** See 3.3.178.8.3.

**3.3.244 Specification.**

***3.3.244.1* Design Specification.*** A building characteristic and other conditions that are under the control of the design team.

***A.3.3.244.1 Design Specification.*** Design specifications include both hardware and human factors, such as the conditions produced by maintenance and training. For purposes of performance-based design, the design specifications of interest are those that affect the ability of the building to meet the stated goals and objectives.

***3.3.244.2 Input Data Specification.*** Information required by the verification method.

**3.3.245 Staff (Residential Board and Care).** Persons who provide personal care services, supervision, or assistance.

**3.3.246 Stage.** A space within a building used for entertainment and utilizing drops or scenery or other stage effects.

*3.3.246.1 Legitimate Stage.* A stage with a height greater than 50 ft (15 m) measured from the lowest point on the stage floor to the highest point of the roof or floor deck above.

*3.3.246.2 Regular Stage.* A stage with a height of 50 ft (15 m) or less measured from the lowest point on the stage floor to the highest point of the roof or floor deck above.

**3.3.247 Stair Descent Device.** See 3.3.56.2.

**3.3.248 Stakeholder.** An individual, or representative of same, having an interest in the successful completion of a project.

**3.3.249 Storage Occupancy.** See 3.3.178.15.

**3.3.250* Stories in Height.** The story count starting with the level of exit discharge and ending with the highest occupiable story containing the occupancy considered.

**A.3.3.250 Stories in Height.** Stories below the level of exit discharge are not counted as stories for determining the stories in height of a building.

**3.3.251 Story.** The portion of a building located between the upper surface of a floor and the upper surface of the floor or roof next above.

*3.3.251.1* Occupiable Story.* A story occupied by people on a regular basis.

*A.3.3.251.1 Occupiable Story.* Stories used exclusively for mechanical equipment rooms, elevator penthouses, and similar spaces are not occupiable stories.

**3.3.252 Street.** A public thoroughfare that has been dedicated for vehicular use by the public and can be used for access by fire department vehicles.

**3.3.253* Street Floor.** A story or floor level accessible from the street or from outside the building at the finished ground level, with the floor level at the main entrance located not more than three risers above or below the finished ground level, and arranged and utilized to qualify as the main floor.

**A.3.3.253 Street Floor.** Where, due to differences in street levels, two or more stories are accessible from the street, each is a street floor. Where there is no floor level within the specified limits for a street floor above or below the finished ground level, the building has no street floor.

**3.3.254* Structure.** That which is built or constructed.

**A.3.3.254 Structure.** The term *structure* is to be understood as if followed by the words *or portion thereof. (See also Building, A.3.3.32.)*

*3.3.254.1 Air-Inflated Structure.* A structure whose shape is maintained by air pressure in cells or tubes forming all or part of the enclosure of the usable area and in which the occupants are not within the pressurized area used to support the structure.

*3.3.254.2* Air-Supported Structure.* A structure where shape is maintained by air pressure and in which occupants are within the elevated pressure area.

*A.3.3.254.2 Air-Supported Structure.* A cable-restrained air-supported structure is one in which the uplift is resisted by cables or webbing that is anchored by various methods to the membrane or that might be an integral part of the membrane. An air-supported structure is not a tensioned-membrane structure.

*3.3.254.3 Limited Access Structure.* A structure or portion of a structure lacking emergency openings.

*3.3.254.4 Membrane Structure.* A building or portion of a building incorporating an air-inflated, air-supported, tensioned-membrane structure; a membrane roof; or a membrane-covered rigid frame to protect habitable or usable space.

*3.3.254.5 Multilevel Play Structure.* A structure that consists of tubes, slides, crawling areas, and jumping areas that is located within a building and is used for climbing and entertainment, generally by children.

*3.3.254.6 Open Parking Structure.* A parking structure that, at each parking level, has wall openings open to the atmosphere, for an area of not less than 1.4 $ft^2$ for each linear foot (0.4 $m^2$ for each linear meter) of its exterior perimeter. Such openings are distributed over at least 40 percent of the building perimeter or uniformly over two opposing sides. Interior wall lines and column lines are at least 20 percent open, with openings distributed to provide ventilation.

*3.3.254.7* Open Structure.* A structure that supports equipment and operations not enclosed within building walls.

*A.3.3.254.7 Open Structure.* Open structures are often found in oil refining, chemical processing, or power plants. Roofs or canopies without enclosing walls are not considered an enclosure.

*3.3.254.8 Permanent Structure.* A building or structure that is intended to remain in place for a period of more than 180 days in any consecutive 12-month period.

*3.3.254.9 Temporary Structure.* A building or structure not meeting the definition of *permanent structure. (See also 3.3.254.8, Permanent Structure.)*

*3.3.254.10 Tensioned-Membrane Structure.* A membrane structure incorporating a membrane and a structural support system such as arches, columns and cables, or beams wherein the stresses developed in the tensioned membrane interact with those in the structural support so that the entire assembly acts together to resist the applied loads.

*3.3.254.11* Underground Structure.* A structure or portions of a structure in which the floor level is below the level of exit discharge.

*A.3.3.254.11 Underground Structure.* In determining openings in exterior walls, doors or access panels are permitted to be included. Windows are also permitted to be included, provided that they are openable or provide a breakable glazed area.

*3.3.254.12 Water-Surrounded Structure.* A structure fully surrounded by water.

**3.3.255 Suite.**

*3.3.255.1 Guest Suite.* An accommodation with two or more contiguous rooms comprising a compartment, with or without doors between such rooms, that provides living, sleeping, sanitary, and storage facilities.

*3.3.255.2 Suite (Health Care Occupancies).* A series of rooms or spaces or a subdivided room separated from the remainder of the building by walls and doors.

*3.3.255.2.1 Non-Sleeping Suite (Health Care Occupancies).* A suite without patient beds intended for overnight sleeping.

*3.3.255.2.2 Sleeping Suite (Health Care Occupancies).* A suite containing one or more patient beds intended for overnight sleeping.

**3.3.256 Technically Infeasible.** A change to a building that has little likelihood of being accomplished because the existing structural conditions require the removal or alteration of a load-bearing member that is an essential part of the structural frame, or because other existing physical or site constraints prohibit modification or addition of elements, spaces, or features that are in full and strict compliance with applicable requirements.

**3.3.257 Temporary Platform.** See 3.3.195.1.

**3.3.258 Temporary Structure.** See 3.3.254.9.

**3.3.259 Tensioned-Membrane Structure.** See 3.3.254.10.

**3.3.260* Tent.** A temporary structure, the covering of which is made of pliable material that achieves its support by mechanical means such as beams, columns, poles, or arches, or by rope or cables, or both.

**A.3.3.260 Tent.** A tent might also include a temporary tensioned-membrane structure.

*3.3.260.1 Private Party Tent.* A tent erected in the yard of a private residence for entertainment, recreation, dining, a reception, or similar function.

**3.3.261 Thermal Barrier.** See 3.3.27.3.

**3.3.262 Tower.** An enclosed independent structure or portion of a building with elevated levels for support of equipment or occupied for observation, control, operation, signaling, or similar limited use.

*3.3.262.1 Air Traffic Control Tower.* An enclosed structure or building at airports with elevated levels for support of equipment and occupied for observation, control, operation, and signaling of aircraft in flight and on the ground.

The definition of the term *air traffic control tower* is new to the 2009 edition of the *Code*. The term was defined to help support the new criteria of 11.3.4, which impose on air traffic control towers requirements that exceed those for other towers addressed by Section 11.3.

**3.3.263 Two-Family Dwelling Unit.** See 3.3.61.3.

**3.3.264 Uncertainty Analysis.** See 3.3.15.2.

**3.3.265 Underground Structure.** See 3.3.254.11.

**3.3.266 Verification Method.** A procedure or process used to demonstrate or confirm that the proposed design meets the specified criteria.

**3.3.267* Vertical Opening.** An opening through a floor or roof.

**A.3.3.267 Vertical Opening.** Vertical openings might include items such as stairways; hoistways for elevators, dumbwaiters, and inclined and vertical conveyors; shaftways used for light, ventilation, or building services; or expansion joints and seismic joints used to allow structural movements.

**3.3.268 Wall.**

*3.3.268.1 Fire Barrier Wall.* A wall, other than a fire wall, that has a fire resistance rating.

*3.3.268.2 Proscenium Wall.* The wall that separates the stage from the auditorium or house.

**3.3.269 Water-Surrounded Structure.** See 3.3.254.12.

**3.3.270 Weathered-Membrane Material.** See 3.3.160.4.

**3.3.271 Yard.** An open, unoccupied space other than a court, unobstructed from the finished ground level to the sky on the lot on which a building is situated.

## References Cited in Commentary

1. *Webster's Third New International Dictionary of the English Language, Unabridged,* Merriam-Webster, Inc., Springfield, MA, 2002.
2. NFPA 252, *Standard Methods of Fire Tests of Door Assemblies,* 2008 edition, National Fire Protection Association, Quincy, MA.

# CHAPTER 4

# General

Chapter 1 contains general administration provisions, including title, scope, purpose, application, equivalency, units and formulas, and enforcement. Chapter 4 contains all remaining general *Code* provisions.

Within Chapter 4, Sections 4.1, 4.2, and 4.3 address goals, objectives, and assumptions and apply to prescriptive-based and performance-based life safety designs.

Section 4.4 offers building designers and owners the prerogative of following the prescriptive requirements of the *Code* or developing an acceptable performance-based design in accordance with Chapter 5 and in careful consultation with the authority having jurisdiction (AHJ).

Section 4.5 includes fundamental requirements that present a qualitative summary of what the other specific requirements, in total, are supposed to achieve.

Section 4.6 presents the philosophy associated with enforcement of the *Code* — namely, who enforces it and when it applies to special conditions. Paragraph 4.6.10.2 mandates a warrant of fitness for buildings that have utilized the performance-based option. The warrant of fitness verifies for the AHJ that the terms and conditions that were part of the performance-based design have not been modified to the point that the building is unsafe.

Section 4.7 presents the operational details associated with emergency egress and relocation drills.

Section 4.8 rounds out the chapter by presenting emergency plan requirements.

## 4.1* Goals

**A.4.1** The goals in Section 4.1 reflect the scope of this *Code (see Section 1.1)*. Other fire safety goals that are outside the scope of this *Code* might also need to be considered, such as property protection and continuity of operations. Compliance with this *Code* can assist in meeting goals outside the scope of the *Code*.

The goals in Section 4.1 apply regardless of whether the prescriptive-based option of 4.4.1(1) and 4.4.2 or the performance-based option of 4.4.1(2) and 4.4.3 is used. For prescriptive-based life safety systems, compliance with the specifications of Chapter 4 and Chapters 6 through 43 provides a level of life safety that meets the goals of Section 4.1. For performance-based life safety systems, compliance with the goals needs to be demonstrated in the required documentation package, with consideration given not only to the goals but also to the objectives (see Section 4.2) and performance criteria (see Section 5.2) associated with specific design fire scenarios (see Section 5.5).

### 4.1.1* Fire.

A goal of this *Code* is to provide an environment for the occupants that is reasonably safe from fire by the following means:

(1)* Protection of occupants not intimate with the initial fire development

(2) Improvement of the survivability of occupants intimate with the initial fire development

**A.4.1.1(1)** The phrase "intimate with the initial fire development" refers to the person(s) at the ignition source or first materials burning, not to all persons within the same room or area.

The example that follows illustrates the level of safety intended by compliance with the requirement of 4.1.1(1) to protect occupants not intimate with initial fire development.

***Example: Protection of Occupants Not Intimate with Initial Fire Development***

Consider a two-person patient sleeping room in a hospital, such as the one shown in Exhibit 4.1. One patient, Patient 1, occupies a bed near the room door to the corridor. The other patient, Patient 2, occupies a bed near the outside wall with a window.

Assume that Patient 1 is smoking in bed, contrary to hospital policy, and ignites her sleeping gown and bedding. Patient 1 is considered to be intimate with initial fire development. Patient 2 is located approximately 48 in. (1220 mm) from Patient 1 and is not considered intimate with initial fire development. To meet the goal of 4.1.1, the prescriptive requirements applicable to hospitals via the health care occupancy provisions of Chapters 18 and 19 work together to save the life of Patient 2. Note that Patient 2's egress route involves passing the fire in Patient 1's bed. Therefore, the applicable *Code* requirements combine a host of building features, systems, and staff actions to save Patient 2. In doing so, the level of safety offered to Patient 2 has the effect required by 4.1.1(2) of improving the survivability of Patient 1, who is intimate with initial fire development. Compliance with 4.1.1(2) is more a consequence of having met 4.1.1(1) rather than a deliberate protection scheme.

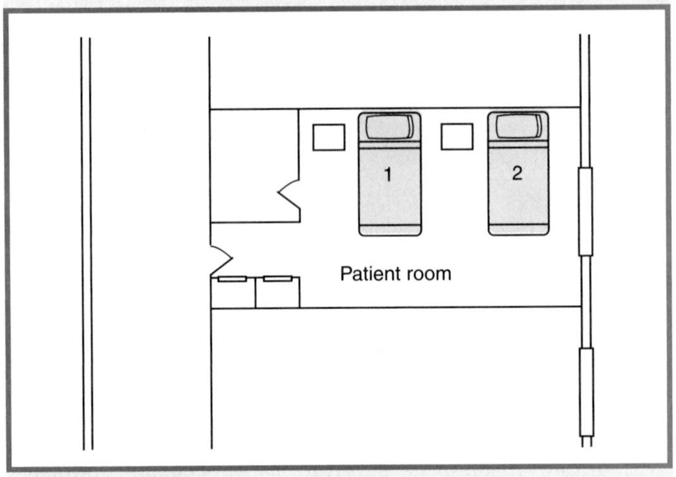


***Exhibit 4.1*** *Protection of occupant not intimate with initial fire development.*

**A.4.1.1** Reasonable safety risk is further defined by subsequent language in this *Code.*

### 4.1.2* Comparable Emergencies.

An additional goal is to provide life safety during emergencies that can be mitigated using methods comparable to those used in case of fire.

**A.4.1.2** Emergencies that are comparable to fires refers to incidents where the hazard involves thermal attributes similar to fires or airborne contaminants similar to smoke, such that features mandated by this *Code* can be expected to mitigate the hazard. Examples of such incidents might be explosions and hazardous material releases. The *Code* recognizes that features mandated by this *Code* might be less effective against such hazards than against fires.

The provision of 4.1.1 in the 2006 edition was titled Fire and Similar Emergency. In the 2009 edition, the provision was split into 4.1.1, Fire, and 4.1.2, Comparable Emergencies, as the term *similar emergencies* was not explained. The new 4.1.2 and A.4.1.2 clarify the subject; provide examples of comparable emergencies; and recognize that features required by the *Code* might not be as effective in mitigating such hazards, as the *Code*'s primary focus is protection against fire.

### 4.1.3* Crowd Movement.

An additional goal is to provide for reasonably safe emergency crowd movement and, where required, reasonably safe nonemergency crowd movement.

**A.4.1.3** An assembly occupancy is an example of an occupancy where the goal of providing for reasonably safe emergency and nonemergency crowd movement has applicability. A detention or correctional occupancy is an example of an occupancy where emergency and nonemergency crowd movement is better addressed by detention and correctional facilities specialists than by this *Code.*

An example of a requirement for nonemergency crowd movement appears in 12.2.5.4.3 and 13.2.5.4.3, which apply to assembly occupancies, where access and egress routes are required to be maintained so that crowd management, security, and emergency medical personnel are able to move to any individual at any time without undue hindrance. However, almost all other occupancy chapters remain silent on the subject of nonemergency crowd movement — some because the committee has made a conscious decision to omit such information, and others because the subject has not been discussed at technical committee meetings. For example, the detention and correctional occupancies chapters deliberately remain silent on the subject because professionals who are involved in the daily operation of such facilities are best qualified to address the movement of residents in occupancies where security concerns are paramount. It is important to note that, per the purpose statement in Section 1.2, the minimum requirements of this *Code* were developed with due regard for function. The *Code* endeavors to avoid requirements that might interfere with the normal use and occupancy of a building.

## 4.2 Objectives

As in the case of application of the goals of Section 4.1, the objectives of Section 4.2 apply regardless of whether the prescriptive-based option of 4.4.1(1) and 4.4.2 or the performance-based option of 4.4.1(2) and 4.4.3 is used. For prescriptive-based life safety systems, compliance with the specifications of Chapter 4 and Chapters 6 through 43 provides a level of life safety that meets the objectives of Section 4.2. For performance-based life safety systems, compliance with the objectives needs to be demonstrated in the required documentation, with consideration given not only to the objectives but also to the goals (see Section 4.1) and performance criteria (see Section 5.2) associated with specific design fire scenarios (see Section 5.5).

The objectives present requirements that must be satisfied to achieve the goals of Section 4.1. Objectives are stated in more specific terms than goals and tend to be more quantitative than qualitative. The goals of Section 4.1 are general enough to apply to numerous NFPA documents. The objectives of Section 4.2 are more specific to the *Life Safety Code* itself. Goals and objectives, taken together, form the initial targets at which a performance-based life safety system can take aim. The goals and objectives alone do not provide sufficient detail to develop and measure the performance of a design. Rather, the performance criteria and other elements of Chapter 5, Performance-Based Option, are needed to flesh out the subject in sufficient detail.

### 4.2.1 Occupant Protection.

A structure shall be designed, constructed, and maintained to protect occupants who are not intimate with the initial fire development for the time needed to evacuate, relocate, or defend in place.

### 4.2.2 Structural Integrity.

Structural integrity shall be maintained for the time needed to evacuate, relocate, or defend in place occupants who are not intimate with the initial fire development.

### 4.2.3 Systems Effectiveness.

Systems utilized to achieve the goals of Section 4.1 shall be effective in mitigating the hazard or condition for which they are being used, shall be reliable, shall be maintained to the level at which they were designed to operate, and shall remain operational.

## 4.3* Assumptions

**A.4.3** Additional assumptions that need to be identified for a performance-based design are addressed in Chapter 5.

### 4.3.1* General.

The protection methods of this *Code* are based on the hazards associated with fire and other events that have comparable impact on a building and its occupancy.

**A.4.3.1** Protection against certain terrorist acts will generally require protection methods beyond those required by this *Code*.

### 4.3.2 Single Fire Source.

The fire protection methods of this *Code* assume a single fire source.

The protection methods referenced in 4.3.1 are expressed in the requirements applicable to any given occupancy. The committees on safety to life have traditionally discussed proposed *Code* changes in the context of mitigating the hazards associated with fire. With the revision to Section 4.1 that splits out the goals associated with fire from those associated with comparable emergencies, the technical committees now evaluate changes based on protection from fire and comparable emergencies.

The text of A.4.3.1 advises that the *Code* does not prescribe protection methods against certain terrorist acts. Society's behavior might have changed following the September 11, 2001, collapse of the World Trade Center towers in New York City, as evidenced by the reluctance of occupants of high-rise buildings to stay behind at the first hint of fire or similar problem. Yet, society has not demanded, for example, that unlimited resources be expended to make a high-rise building immune to a direct strike by an airliner. It is not practical to protect against all terrorist acts.

For the user of the traditional, prescriptive, specification-based requirements, the single fire source assumption of 4.3.2 is a piece of explanatory material and not a requirement. The assumption explains that the *Code* authors developed the requirements with the challenge of a single fire source in mind. Thus, most occupancy chapters require a minimum of two means of egress; if the single fire blocks one, then the other should be available for egress. Had the *Code* been written to protect against fires that begin in two locations, then it probably would be common to find occupancy chapter requirements for a minimum of three means of egress, even for small buildings with small occupant loads. Historically, the *Code*'s approach to protecting against a single-source fire has proved to meet society's expectations.

## 4.4 Life Safety Compliance Options

### 4.4.1 Options.

Life safety meeting the goals and objectives of Sections 4.1 and 4.2 shall be provided in accordance with either of the following:

(1) Prescriptive-based provisions per 4.4.2
(2) Performance-based provisions per 4.4.3

*Code* editions prior to 2000 required compliance with the prescriptive, specification-based requirements and offered some additional design flexibility via the equivalency concept contained in Section 1.4. The newer editions offer the option of designing the life safety systems using an *in toto* performance-based approach. Both the prescriptive-based and performance-based options are tied to the goals and objectives of Sections 4.1 and 4.2, respectively.

The prescriptive-based and performance-based options are offered as equivalents, with neither option designated as the preferred method. Given that performance-based design is new to most *Code* users, and that it is complicated to use, most traditional buildings will probably continue to be designed and built to comply with the prescriptive requirements. The performance-based approach will be reserved for use on large, complicated structures where the additional costs associated with such a design can be offset by savings on prescriptive features that can be omitted from the design. The performance-based option also is to be used for innovative designs that are likely to be prohibited by the prescriptive requirements. For example, many years ago, before atria were specifically addressed in the *Code*, a designer proposing to build an atrium building would likely have been challenged by the authority having jurisdiction, who might view the atrium as a hole in the building's floors through which smoke and other products of combustion could be spread. In subsequent editions of the *Code*, the inclusion of provisions for atria showed that, with full building sprinkler and smoke control systems, the atrium could be turned into a fire and life safety asset — one that serves as a smoke dispersion and accumulation chamber early in the fire, so as to allow exit access through the atrium. The performance-based approach offers a host of new tools that are used to prove the efficacy of unique designs and unusual, functionally dictated space arrangements.

### 4.4.2 Prescriptive-Based Option.

**4.4.2.1** A prescriptive-based life safety design shall be in accordance with Chapters 1 through 4, Chapters 6 through 11, Chapter 43, and the applicable occupancy chapter, Chapters 12 through 42.

A prescriptive-based life safety design is the traditional norm. Each applicable requirement is met individually, and the resultant level of life safety is deemed to meet the goals and objectives of Sections 4.1 and 4.2, respectively. The requirements are chosen, depending on occupancy classification, from a wide host of possible *Code* chapters, namely, any and all chapters except Chapter 5, Performance-Based Option.

**4.4.2.2** Prescriptive-based designs meeting the requirements of Chapters 1 through 3, Sections 4.5 through 4.8, and Chapters 6 through 43 of this *Code* shall be deemed to satisfy the provisions of Sections 4.1 and 4.2.

**4.4.2.3** Where specific requirements contained in Chapters 11 through 43 differ from general requirements contained in Chapters 1 through 4, and Chapters 6 through 10, the requirements of Chapters 11 through 43 shall govern.

The *Life Safety Code* is formatted such that Chapters 1 through 4 and Chapters 6 through 10 contain administrative provisions and fundamental requirements establishing minimum acceptable criteria for all types of occupancies. Chapters 12 through 42 of the *Code* establish criteria for life safety based on the characteristic needs of specific occupancies. Chapter 11 further modifies those provisions if unusual situations exist or the building is windowless, underground, or high-rise. Chapter 43 on existing building rehabilitation was added to the *Code* in 2006 and serves the dual role of being a core chapter and a chapter that has requirements specific to certain occupancies. Where requirements differ between the general provisions of Chapters 1 through 4 and Chapters 6 through 10 and the more specific provisions of Chapters 11 through 43, the requirements contained in Chapters 11 through 43 take precedence.

To avoid conflicts, if an occupancy chapter exempts itself from a requirement of a core chapter, the core chapter will usually specify that the deviation from the requirement is permitted. For example, although 7.2.2.3.3.1 requires treads of stairs and landing surfaces to be solid, 7.2.2.3.3.4 permits noncombustible grated stair treads and landings in various specified occupancies, including industrial occupancies as provided in Chapter 40. Paragraph 40.2.2.3.1(1) confirms the exemption for noncombustible grated stair treads and landings in industrial occupancies.

### 4.4.3 Performance-Based Option.

A performance-based life safety design shall be in accordance with Chapters 1 through 5.

A performance-based life safety design is exempt from the myriad prescriptive, specification-based requirements of the *Code* but must meet the administrative and general requirements of Chapters 1 through 4. The design must adhere to the definitions of Chapter 3 so that the authority having jurisdiction that judges the performance of the design can communicate with the designer in terminology that is common to all *Code* users. More important, the performance-based design must meet the provisions contained in Chapter 5, Performance-Based Option. Chapter 5 contains a limited number of prescriptive provisions that have been retained from Chapter 7, Means of Egress, for applicability to the performance-based design. See Section 5.3.

## 4.5 Fundamental Requirements

Section 4.5 outlines the fundamental concepts that are addressed in detail by the requirements contained in the other chapters of the *Code*. The fundamental concepts briefly detailed in this section apply both to prescriptive-based and performance-based life safety designs. Achieving the life safety fundamentals that follow helps to ensure a reasonable level of life safety in building design and arrangement.

1. Provide for adequate safety without dependence on any single safeguard.
2. Provide an appropriate degree of life safety considering the size, shape, and nature of the occupancy.
3. Provide for backup or redundant egress arrangements.
4. Ensure that the egress paths are clear, unobstructed, and unlocked.
5. Ensure that the exits and egress routes are clearly marked to avoid confusion and provide the cues needed for their effective use.
6. Provide adequate lighting.
7. Ensure prompt occupant response by providing early warning of fire.
8. Ensure that required systems facilitate and enhance situation awareness.
9. Ensure the suitable enclosure of vertical openings.
10. Ensure compliance with applicable installation standards.
11. Maintain all required features in proper working order.

### 4.5.1 Multiple Safeguards.

The design of every building or structure intended for human occupancy shall be such that reliance for safety to life does not depend solely on any single safeguard. An additional safeguard(s) shall be provided for life safety in case any single safeguard is ineffective due to inappropriate human actions or system failure.

### 4.5.2 Appropriateness of Safeguards.

Every building or structure shall be provided with means of egress and other fire and life safety safeguards of the kinds, numbers, locations, and capacities appropriate to the individual building or structure, with due regard to the following:

(1) Character of the occupancy, including fire load
(2) Capabilities of the occupants
(3) Number of persons exposed
(4) Fire protection available
(5) Capabilities of response personnel
(6) Height and construction type of the building or structure
(7) Other factors necessary to provide occupants with a reasonable degree of safety

### 4.5.3 Means of Egress.

**4.5.3.1 Number of Means of Egress.** Two means of egress, as a minimum, shall be provided in every building or structure, section, and area where size, occupancy, and arrangement endanger occupants attempting to use a single means of egress that is blocked by fire or smoke. The two means of egress shall be arranged to minimize the possibility that both might be rendered impassable by the same emergency condition.

**4.5.3.2 Unobstructed Egress.** In every occupied building or structure, means of egress from all parts of the building shall be maintained free and unobstructed. Means of egress shall be accessible to the extent necessary to ensure reasonable safety for occupants having impaired mobility.

**4.5.3.3 Awareness of Egress System.** Every exit shall be clearly visible, or the route to reach every exit shall be conspicuously indicated. Each means of egress, in its entirety, shall be arranged or marked so that the way to a place of safety is indicated in a clear manner.

**4.5.3.4 Lighting.** Where artificial illumination is needed in a building or structure, egress facilities shall be included in the lighting design.

### 4.5.4* Occupant Notification.

In every building or structure of such size, arrangement, or occupancy that a fire itself might not provide adequate occupant warning, fire alarm systems shall be provided where necessary to warn occupants of the existence of fire.

**A.4.5.4** Fire alarms alert occupants to initiate emergency procedures, facilitate orderly conduct of fire drills, and initiate response by emergency services.

### 4.5.5* Situation Awareness.

Systems used to achieve the goals of Section 4.1 shall be effective in facilitating and enhancing situation awareness, as appropriate, by building management, other occupants and emergency responders of the functionality or state of critical building systems, the conditions that might warrant emergency response, and the appropriate nature and timing of such responses.

**A.4.5.5** Systems encompass facilities or equipment and people. Included are fire/smoke detection, alarm, and communication systems plus the system status panels in emergency command centers; supervisory systems for various especially critical components (e.g., certain valves) of fire protection systems; certain signs; and the availability of trained staff, notably in health care occupancies.

The provision of 4.5.5 applicable to situation awareness is new to the 2009 edition of the *Code*. It adds no new requirement but recognizes that many of the systems required by the *Code* enhance situation awareness. Examples of such systems are provided in A.4.5.5. The term *situation awareness* is defined in 3.3.230.

### 4.5.6 Vertical Openings.

Every vertical opening between the floors of a building shall be suitably enclosed or protected, as necessary, to afford reasonable safety to occupants while using the means of egress and to prevent the spread of fire, smoke, or fumes through vertical openings from floor to floor before occupants have entered exits.

### 4.5.7 System Design/Installation.

Any fire protection system, building service equipment, feature of protection, or safeguard provided to achieve the goals of this *Code* shall be designed, installed, and approved in accordance with applicable NFPA standards.

### 4.5.8 Maintenance.

Whenever or wherever any device, equipment, system, condition, arrangement, level of protection, or any other feature is required for compliance with the provisions of this *Code*, such device, equipment, system, condition, arrangement, level of protection, or other feature shall thereafter be maintained, unless the *Code* exempts such maintenance.

## 4.6 General Requirements

### 4.6.1 Authority Having Jurisdiction.

The authority having jurisdiction (AHJ) is the person or office enforcing the *Code*. In cases where the *Code* is legally enforced, the AHJ is usually a fire marshal or building official. The AHJ can also be a safety office, insurance engineering department, accreditation service, other agency, or specified personnel within those groups, especially where the *Code* is enforced at other than a governmental level.

The term *authority having jurisdiction* is used extensively across all NFPA codes and standards. As such, its definition (see 3.2.2) is an NFPA official definition that must be adopted without change for each code and standard. The NFPA official definitions appear in Section 3.2 and the *Code*-specific definitions in Section 3.3.

It is common for multiple authorities having jurisdiction to review the same project while enforcing this *Code*, other codes, or both. For example, under the *Code*, several agencies — such as state and local fire marshals; federal, state, and local health care licensing agencies; Joint Commission (formerly the Joint Commission on Accreditation of Healthcare Organizations, or JCAHO) accreditation personnel; insurance inspectors; and building inspectors — perform inspections in health care facilities.

**4.6.1.1** The authority having jurisdiction shall determine whether the provisions of this *Code* are met.

**4.6.1.2** Any requirements that are essential for the safety of building occupants and that are not specifically provided for by this *Code* shall be determined by the authority having jurisdiction.

The provisions of Section 4.6 give the authority having jurisdiction the final determination of whether adequate life safety is provided in a building. When the authority having jurisdiction determines that the *Code* has not specifically addressed a particular life safety situation, the authority can supplement the requirements in the *Code* to address the situation. The power to supplement requirements is an important responsibility, because the *Code* cannot anticipate every type of building and occupancy configuration.

**4.6.1.3** Where it is evident that a reasonable degree of safety is provided, any requirement shall be permitted to be modified if, in the judgment of the authority having jurisdiction, its application would be hazardous under normal occupancy conditions.

The provision of 4.6.1.3 gives the authority having jurisdiction latitude in permitting a requirement to be modified if the strict enforcement of the provision would otherwise create more of a hazard and, thus, less overall life safety than would be achieved by modification. For example, the *Code* requires an exit sign at an exit and, via the provisions of 7.10.1.2, requires that the sign be readily visible from any direction of exit access. If the exit door in question were installed in the plane of a corridor wall, the exit sign would need to be positioned perpendicular to the corridor wall. If there is limited headroom at the door, perhaps due to a ceiling projection such as a beam running across the corridor at that point, the exit sign might create the potential for occupants to bump their heads. This provision permits the authority having jurisdiction to allow the exit sign to be mounted flush against the corridor wall, based on judgment that a reasonable degree of safety is provided.

### 4.6.2 Previously Approved Features.

Where another provision of this *Code* exempts a previously approved feature from a requirement, the exemption shall be permitted, even where the following conditions exist:

(1) The area is being modernized, renovated, or otherwise altered.
(2) A change of occupancy has occurred, provided that the feature's continued use is approved by the authority having jurisdiction.

The term *previously approved* is defined in 3.3.198 as "that which was acceptable to the authority having jurisdiction prior to the date this edition of the *Code* went into effect." In a relatively few cases, the responsible technical committees have earmarked specific features that can be continued in use if such features were previously approved. For example, in 40.2.2.8, regarding existing, previously approved escalators in industrial occupancies, the message to the current AHJ is that if an AHJ of an earlier period judged the escalator as adequate for use within the means of egress, the escalator should continue to be approved for use. The AHJ that gave the original approval had detailed criteria in the *Code* at that time. The criteria no longer exist, because new escalators are not permitted to comprise any of the required means of egress. The current AHJ is expected to continue recognizing the earlier approval. However, if there is a change of occupancy, the previously approved feature must also receive the current approval of the AHJ, because the feature that had been acceptable in the original occupancy might not be acceptable for the new occupancy. See 4.6.2(2).

Contrast the preceding example with the treatment of existing stairs in 7.2.2.1.2(2) where approved, existing noncomplying stairs are recognized in lieu of stairs complying with the detailed criteria of 7.2.2. The term *approved existing*, which is different from the term *previously approved*, is defined in 3.3.73.1 as "that which is already in existence on the date this edition of the *Code* goes into effect and is acceptable to the authority having jurisdiction." In this case, it does not matter how an earlier AHJ ruled on the acceptability of the stair. The current AHJ must evaluate the noncomplying stair and determine whether it is acceptable for continued use.

### 4.6.3 Stories in Height.

Unless otherwise specified in another provision of this *Code*, the stories in height of a building for locating an occupancy shall be determined as follows:

(1) The stories in height shall be counted starting with the level of exit discharge and ending with the highest occupiable story containing the occupancy considered.
(2) Stories below the level of exit discharge shall not be counted as stories.
(3) Interstitial spaces used solely for building or process systems directly related to the level above or below shall not be considered a separate story.
(4) A mezzanine shall not be counted as a story for the purpose of determining the allowable stories in height.
(5) Where a maximum one-story abovegrade parking structure, enclosed, open, or a combination thereof, of Type I or Type II (222) construction or open Type IV

construction, with grade entrance, is provided under a building of occupancies other than assembly, health care, detention and correctional, and ambulatory health care occupancies, the number of stories shall be permitted to be measured from the floor above such a parking area.

The provisions of 4.6.3 are new to the 2009 edition of the *Code* and were developed to support consistent use of the term *stories in height* in other sections of the *Code*. Criteria typically presented in the __.1.6 subsection of an occupancy chapter, related to minimum construction requirements, use stories in height as thresholds for requiring specific building construction types. The examples that follow demonstrate application of the provisions of 4.6.3.

*Example 1*

Exhibit 4.2 depicts a six-story existing building. Floors 1 and 2 are occupied as an assembly occupancy. Floors 3 through 6 are occupied as a business occupancy. The first story, which is used as an assembly occupancy, is the level of exit discharge, as it is the lowest story from which not less than 50 percent of the required number of means of egress and not less than 50 percent of the required egress capacity from that story discharge directly outside at the finished ground level (see definition of *level of exit discharge* in 3.3.77.1). The provision of 4.6.3(1) directs that the stories in height are to be counted starting at the level of exit discharge and ending at the highest occupiable story containing the occupancy considered. The second story is the highest occupiable story containing the assembly occupancy. The sixth story is the highest occupiable story containing the business occupancy. This leads to classifying the building as being two stories in height for the assembly occupancy and six stories in height for the business occupancy.

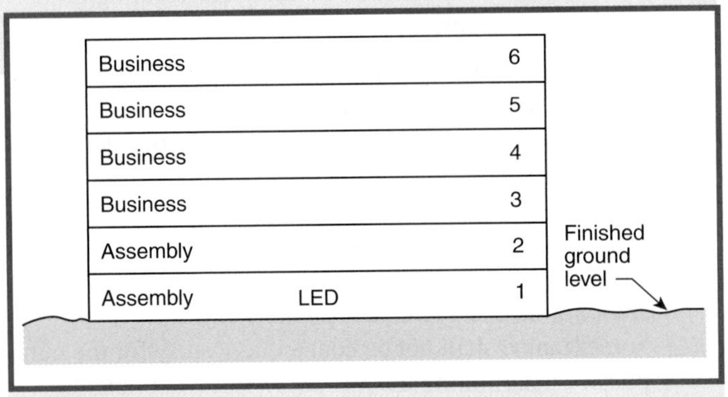


**Exhibit 4.2** *An assembly occupancy two stories in height and a business occupancy six stories in height.*

*Example 2*

Exhibit 4.3 depicts the building addressed in Example 1 but has two additional floor levels, both located below the level of exit discharge. The provision of 4.6.3(2) directs that stories below the level of exit discharge are not to be counted as stories for purposes of determining stories in height. This leads to classifying the building as being two stories in height for the assembly occupancy and six stories in height for the business occupancy, as was done in Example 1 where no basement levels were present.

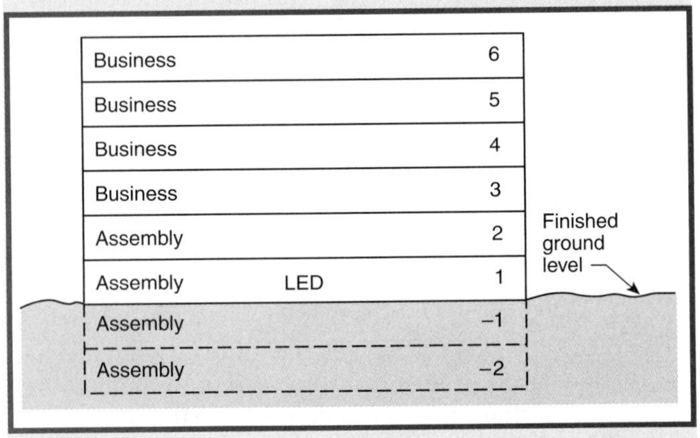


**Exhibit 4.3** *Another assembly occupancy two stories in height and a business occupancy six stories in height.*

*Example 3*

Exhibit 4.4 depicts a building similar to that addressed in Example 1, but the first story assembly occupancy has a higher ceiling height and a mezzanine along the exterior walls. The provision of 4.6.3(4) directs that a mezzanine is not to be counted as a story for purposes of determining stories in height. This leads to classifying the building as being one story in height for the as-

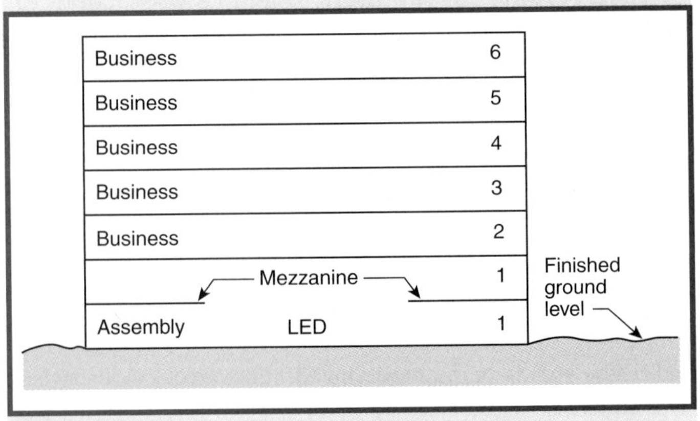


**Exhibit 4.4** *An assembly occupancy one story in height and a business occupancy six stories in height.*

sembly occupancy and six stories in height for the business occupancy.

*Example 4*

Exhibit 4.5 depicts a building similar to that addressed in Example 1, but the first two stories, which are used as an assembly occupancy, have an interstitial space above their ceilings used to house mechanical equipment serving those two floors. The provision of 4.6.3(3) directs that interstitial spaces used solely for building or process systems directly related to the level above or below are not to be counted as separate stories for purposes of determining stories in height. This leads to classifying the building as being two stories in height for the assembly occupancy and six stories in height for the business occupancy.

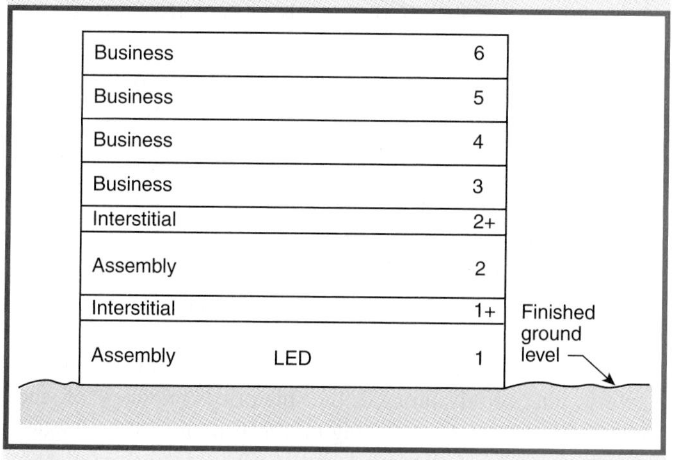


***Exhibit 4.5*** *An assembly occupancy two stories in height and a business occupancy six stories in height.*

*Example 5*

Exhibit 4.6 depicts a building similar to that addressed in Example 1, but the first story is used as a parking structure, as are the two levels below the level of exit discharge. The entire building is of Type II(222) construction (see Table A.8.2.1.2). The provision of 4.6.3(5) directs that where a maximum one-story abovegrade parking structure, whether enclosed, open, or a combination thereof, of Type I or Type II(222) construction or of open Type IV construction, with grade entrance, is provided under a building of occupancies other than assembly, health care, detention and correctional, or ambulatory health care, the number of stories used in determining stories in height is permitted to be measured from the floor above such parking area. The presence of the assembly occupancy precludes the level of exit discharge used as parking from being excluded from the count of stories in height for the assembly occupancy, but does not preclude such for the business occupancy. This leads to classifying the building as being two stories in height for the assembly occupancy and five stories in height for the business occupancy.

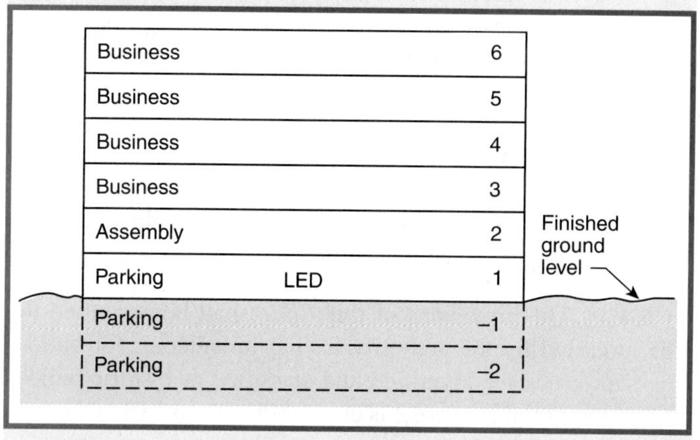


***Exhibit 4.6*** *An assembly occupancy two stories in height and a business occupancy five stories in height.*

*Example 6*

Exhibit 4.7 depicts a building similar to that addressed in Example 5, but the second story is used as a mercantile occupancy. The entire building is of Type II(222) construction (see Table A.8.2.1.2). The provision of 4.6.3(5) directs that where a maximum one-story abovegrade parking structure, whether enclosed, open, or a combination thereof, of Type I or Type II(222) construction or of open Type IV construction, with grade entrance, is provided under a building of occupancies other than assembly, health care, detention and correctional, or ambulatory health care, the number of stories used in determining stories in height

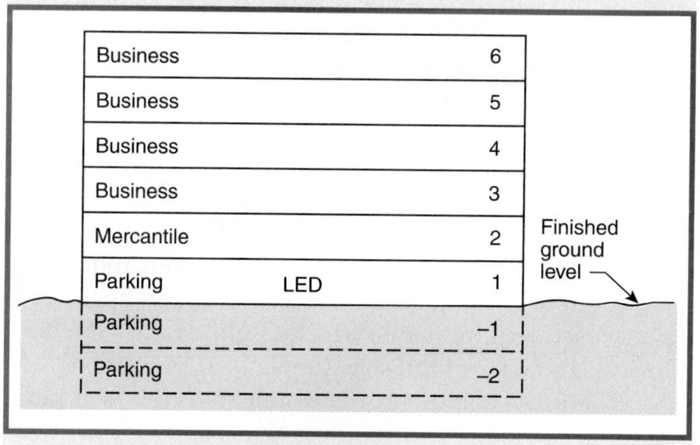


***Exhibit 4.7*** *A mercantile occupancy one story in height and a business occupancy five stories in height.*

is permitted to be measured from the floor above such parking area. Given that the occupancies involved (i.e., mercantile and business) are not assembly, health care, detention and correctional, or ambulatory health care, the floor used for parking at the level of exit discharge can be discounted in determining the stories in height. This leads to classifying the building as being one story in height for the mercantile occupancy and five stories in height for the business occupancy.

### 4.6.4 Historic Buildings.

**4.6.4.1** Rehabilitation projects in historic buildings shall comply with Chapter 43.

**4.6.4.2*** The provisions of this *Code* shall be permitted to be modified by the authority having jurisdiction for buildings or structures identified and classified as historic buildings or structures where it is evident that a reasonable degree of safety is provided.

**A.4.6.4.2** See A.4.6.5.

Rather than providing historic buildings with a blanket exemption from *Code* requirements, the provision of 4.6.4.2 reinforces the concept that existing buildings, as well as new construction, need to meet minimum life safety criteria. This provision permits the authority having jurisdiction to offer some leniency — as long as the AHJ judges that a reasonable degree of safety is provided, compliance with modified requirements is adequate.

Historic buildings might have numerous design defects, such as open stair shafts or highly combustible interior finishes. Rather than waiving requirements, the authority having jurisdiction might require that the facility attain a level of safety equivalent to, or nearly equivalent to, that mandated by the *Code*. For example, the AHJ might require the use of sprinkler systems, smoke detection systems, voice alarm systems for staged evacuation, smoke control systems, or other appropriate features to overcome the existing life safety defects. The use of such alternatives could raise the building's life safety to levels many times greater than those that previously existed without requiring the rebuilding of the structure to the *Code*'s specification-based requirements, which might destroy the historical character of the structure.

The provision of 4.6.4.2, which gives the AHJ permission to modify *Code* requirements, applies only to a historic building for which there is no ongoing rehabilitation. Where historic buildings are rehabilitated, the provisions of Chapter 43 must be met as required by 4.6.4.1. See Chapter 43, Building Rehabilitation, especially Section 43.10.

### 4.6.5* Modification of Requirements for Existing Buildings.

Where it is evident that a reasonable degree of safety is provided, the requirements for existing buildings shall be permitted to be modified if their application would be impractical in the judgment of the authority having jurisdiction.

**A.4.6.5** In existing buildings, it is not always practical to strictly apply the provisions of this *Code*. Physical limitations can cause the need for disproportionate effort or expense with little increase in life safety. In such cases, the authority having jurisdiction needs to be satisfied that reasonable life safety is ensured.

In existing buildings, it is intended that any condition that represents a serious threat to life be mitigated by the application of appropriate safeguards. It is not intended to require modifications for conditions that do not represent a significant threat to life, even though such conditions are not literally in compliance with the *Code*.

An example of what is intended by 4.6.5 would be a historic ornamental guardrail baluster with spacing that does not comply with the 4 in. (100 mm) requirement. Because reducing the spacing would have minimal impact on life safety but could damage the historic character of the guardrail, the existing spacing might be approved by the authority having jurisdiction.

The provisions of 4.6.5 give the authority having jurisdiction some leeway in applying the *Code* to existing buildings. The *Code* recognizes that there might be situations where applying the requirements to existing situations is not practical, so the provisions of 4.6.5 give the authority having jurisdiction the authority to modify those requirements. However, the *Code* reemphasizes that a reasonable degree of safety must be provided.

### 4.6.6 Time Allowed for Compliance.

A limited but reasonable time, commensurate with the magnitude of expenditure, disruption of services, and degree of hazard, shall be allowed for compliance with any part of this *Code* for existing buildings.

In some cases, appreciable costs — in terms of actual monetary expenditures and disruption of daily activities — might be involved in immediately bringing an existing building into *Code* compliance. Where this is true, it is appropriate for the operator or owner of the facility to formulate a schedule, approved by the authority having jurisdiction, that allows suitable periods of time for correcting various deficiencies. However, the degree of hazard is an important consideration in this instance; if the degree of hazard is serious enough, it might be necessary to close the building to occupancy while renovations are made to bring the building features associated with the serious hazard into compliance. Once the building is reoccupied, the AHJ might permit some reasonable, additional time for bringing the remaining deficient features into *Code* compliance with the requirements that apply specifically to existing buildings.

**4.6.7* Referenced Publications.**

Existing buildings or installations that do not comply with the provisions of the standards referenced in this document *(see Chapter 2)* shall be permitted to be continued in service, provided that the lack of conformity with these standards does not present a serious hazard to the occupants as determined by the authority having jurisdiction.

**A.4.6.7** The Committee on Safety to Life recognizes that it is sometimes impractical to continually upgrade existing buildings or installations to comply with all the requirements of the referenced publications included in Chapter 2.

The *Code* mandates that the fire and life safety systems used for compliance are to be installed in accordance with the requirements of approximately 70 NFPA codes and standards and more than 45 documents developed by other organizations. Mandatorily referenced documents are listed in Chapter 2, and specific editions are cited.

In recognition that it is impractical to expect systems to be continually upgraded to meet the newest edition of an installation standard, the *Code* allows the authority having jurisdiction to permit continued use of a system whose lack of compliance with the cited edition of a referenced standard does not present a serious hazard.

**4.6.8 Building Rehabilitation.**

Editions of the *Code* prior to 2006 required modernizations, renovations, additions, and changes of occupancy to comply with the requirements for new construction. Chapter 43, Building Rehabilitation, was added in 2006 and carried forward into this edition. It was written to encourage the adaptive reuse of existing structures. It relaxes the former requirement that rehabilitation projects must comply with the requirements for new construction. It imposes those requirements necessary to achieve the intended level of life safety in lieu of requiring strict compliance with the requirements applicable to new buildings.

The provisions of Chapter 43 are permitted to be used only if the existing building is brought into compliance with the occupancy chapter requirements applicable to the existing occupancy. See 43.1.2.1(1). For example, if an existing business occupancy is to undergo renovation, the provisions of Chapter 43 are permitted to be used only if the existing building is brought into compliance with the requirements of Chapter 39, Existing Business Occupancies. Thus, the existing business occupancy building undergoing the renovation is held, as a starting point, to the same requirements that apply to any other existing business occupancy building. Then, per 43.1.2.1(2), requirements related to the renovation work being undertaken are added.

Some of the occupancy chapters have requirements that supplement those of Chapter 43 and impose the requirements for new construction on existing buildings that are being rehabilitated, including those situations in which the use is changed so as to increase the occupant load. For example, mercantile occupancies are further subclassified as a Class A, Class B, or Class C mercantile occupancy, based on the floor area used for sales purposes. For the purposes of this example, consider that the rehabilitation project involves an addition to an existing mercantile occupancy. If consideration of the combined space created by the addition and the existing portion of the building results in a change of mercantile occupancy subclassification (e.g., a reclassification from Class C to Class B or from Class B to Class A), the existing portion of the building must also meet the requirements applicable to new construction. See 36.1.1.3.3 and 37.1.1.3.3.

For assembly occupancies, the same concept exists, but its application criteria are specified differently, given that assembly occupancies no longer use the subclassification scheme of editions earlier than 1997 (i.e., Class A, Class B, and Class C). The existing portion of the assembly occupancy building is required to meet the provisions that apply to new construction under either of the following conditions (see 13.1.1.6):

1. The occupant load of the combined space created by the addition and the existing assembly area

increases from less than 500 to more than 500, so as to require a third exit.

2. The occupant load of the combined space created by the addition and the existing assembly area increases from less than 1000 to more than 1000, so as to require a fourth exit.

Chapter 43 addresses change of use or change of occupancy as categories of rehabilitation subject to the requirements of the chapter. In addition, for mercantile occupancies, 36.1.1.4 and 37.1.1.4(2) mandate that a change from Class C to Class A or Class B, or from Class B to Class A, must meet the provisions applicable to new construction.

**4.6.8.1** Rehabilitation work on existing buildings shall be classified as one of the following work categories in accordance with 43.2.2.1:

(1) Repair
(2) Renovation
(3) Modification
(4) Reconstruction
(5) Change of use or occupancy classification
(6) Addition

**4.6.8.2** Rehabilitation work on existing buildings shall comply with Chapter 43.

**4.6.8.3** Except where another provision of this *Code* exempts a previously approved feature from a requirement, the resulting feature shall be not less than that required for existing buildings.

**4.6.8.4*** Existing life safety features that exceed the requirements for new buildings shall be permitted to be decreased to those required for new buildings.

**A.4.6.8.4** In some cases, the requirements for new construction are less restrictive, and it might be justifiable to permit an existing building to use the less restrictive requirements. However, extreme care needs to be exercised when granting such permission, because the less restrictive provision might be the result of a new requirement elsewhere in the *Code*. For example, in editions of the *Code* prior to 1991, corridors in new health care occupancies were required to have a 1-hour fire resistance rating. Since 1991, such corridors have been required only to resist the passage of smoke. However, this provision is based on the new requirement that all new health care facilities be protected throughout by automatic sprinklers. *(See A.4.6.8.5.)*

**4.6.8.5*** Existing life safety features that do not meet the requirements for new buildings, but that exceed the requirements for existing buildings, shall not be further diminished.

**A.4.6.8.5** An example of what is intended by 4.6.8.4 and 4.6.8.5 follows. In a hospital that has 6 ft (1830 mm) wide corridors, such corridors cannot be reduced in width, even though the provisions for existing hospitals do not require 6 ft (1830 mm) wide corridors. However, if a hospital has 10 ft (3050 mm) wide corridors, they are permitted to be reduced to 8 ft (2440 mm) in width, which is the requirement for new construction. If the hospital corridor is 36 in. (915 mm) wide, it would have to be increased to 48 in. (1220 mm), which is the requirement for existing hospitals.

The intent behind 4.6.8.4 and 4.6.8.5 is to prevent existing life safety features that exceed the requirement for existing buildings from being decreased to a level less than that required for new construction. For example, a new hospital is constructed with 8 ft (2440 mm) wide corridors for compliance with 18.2.3.4. In subsequent years the building becomes an existing hospital subject to the provisions of Chapter 19, Existing Health Care Occupancies. The minimum corridor width required by 19.2.3.4 for an existing hospital is 48 in. (1220 mm). The minimum 48 in. (1220 mm) criterion is meant to apply to existing situations, but is not intended to permit the existing 8 ft (2440 mm) corridor to be decreased in width. This example is addressed in additional detail in A.4.6.8.5.

For a similar concept related to the removal of existing life safety features, see 4.6.13.2.

### 4.6.9 Provisions in Excess of *Code* Requirements.

Nothing in this *Code* shall be construed to prohibit a better building construction type, an additional means of egress, or an otherwise safer condition than that specified by the minimum requirements of this *Code*.

Although the *Life Safety Code* is a minimum requirement code, it does not prohibit the use of a design that exceeds the provisions of the *Code*. Although, in practice, economic considerations usually discourage the use of a design that exceeds minimum requirements, there have been instances where money was saved or additional money was generated when *Code* provisions were exceeded. For example, a hotel was constructed with full automatic sprinkler protection, although such protection was not required by the *Code* in effect at the time. Sprinklering the building permitted a third stairway to be eliminated because of the increased travel distance permitted in a sprinklered building. The construction cost of the stair was saved, and additional revenue-producing guest rooms were built in the space that the stair otherwise would have occupied.

### 4.6.10 Conditions for Occupancy.

**4.6.10.1** No new construction or existing building shall be occupied in whole or in part in violation of the provisions of this *Code*, unless the following conditions exist:

(1) A plan of correction has been approved.
(2) The occupancy classification remains the same.
(3) No serious life safety hazard exists as judged by the authority having jurisdiction.

From an enforcement standpoint, 4.6.10.1 is probably one of the most important requirements in the *Code*, because it states that a building, whether new or existing, cannot be occupied if it is in violation of the provisions of the *Code*.

Because the *Code* applies retroactively, 4.6.10.1 prohibits the use of existing, nonconforming facilities. However, 4.6.10.1 does permit the building to continue to be used, provided that the occupancy classification remains the same and there is no serious life safety hazard, as judged by the authority having jurisdiction, that would constitute an imminent threat. Such permission does not exempt the building from compliance with the *Code*. A limited, but reasonable, time (see 4.6.6) for bringing the building into compliance with the *Code* to the extent deemed necessary by the AHJ under 4.6.5 must be established and fulfilled.

**4.6.10.2** Where compliance with this *Code* is effected by means of a performance-based design, the owner shall annually certify compliance with the conditions and limitations of the design by submitting a warrant of fitness acceptable to the authority having jurisdiction. The warrant of fitness shall attest that the building features, systems, and use have been inspected and confirmed to remain consistent with design specifications outlined in the documentation required by Section 5.8 and that such features, systems, and use continue to satisfy the goals and objectives specified in Sections 4.1 and 4.2. *(See Chapter 5.)*

Traditional, specification-based life safety systems rely on the combined effect of all required features, systems, and arrangements to provide the intended level of life safety. This overlap of protection schemes and the resulting redundancy in protection methods, which are mandated by the prescriptive requirements, have historically provided flexibility for a building to undergo changes in how its space is configured and used. For example, a business occupancy floor arranged to provide executives with private offices could be renovated by removing the office walls, installing modular furniture and cubicles, and creating an open-office floor plan for use by telemarketers. The occupancy would remain a business occupancy, and compliance with the provisions of Section 43.7 applicable to change of use would have a minor effect on upgrading the level of life safety that existed prior to the renovation.

However, had the original executive office floor been designed using the performance-based option, the removal of office walls would need to be analyzed with respect to its effect on the life safety systems. The performance-based design might have been based on a scenario in which a fire would not propagate beyond one of the private offices due to fire-rated compartmentation. Removing the office walls and creating an open floor plan would result in the loss of the performance-based design's compartmentation premise. Further analysis would be needed to determine whether the original life safety systems continued to meet the goals and objectives after the renovation.

Although the example cited in this commentary centers on a substantial renovation that involves removal of office walls, subtle changes that "creep" into a building over time might also adversely affect a life safety system designed using the performance-based option. For this reason, 4.6.10.2 requires annual certification via a warrant of fitness.

The provisions of 4.6.10.2 are located in Chapter 4 in the hope that the requirement will be noticed and enforced. If the requirement were to appear in Chapter 5, Performance-Based Option, it might go unnoticed after the performance-based design is completed and the certificate of occupancy issued.

### 4.6.11 Construction, Repair, and Improvement Operations.

**4.6.11.1*** Buildings, or portions of buildings, shall be permitted to be occupied during construction, repair, alterations, or additions only where required means of egress and required fire protection features are in place and continuously maintained for the portion occupied or where alternative life safety measures acceptable to the authority having jurisdiction are in place.

**A.4.6.11.1** Fatal fires have occurred when, for example, a required stair has been closed for repairs or removed for rebuilding, or when a required automatic sprinkler system has been shut off to change piping.

The provisions of 4.6.11.1 help to control a relatively common practice — the occupation of completed portions of a partially completed structure. The *Code* permits such occupation if certain conditions are met. For example, the *Code* requires that egress features for the portion occupied be complete and maintained to be usable. In many cases, the egress facilities, although completed, are not usable because they are blocked with stored building materials and equipment needed for the ongoing construction, or doors are locked to limit access to parts of the building still under construction. In such cases, occupancy is prohibited.

The *Code* also requires that fire protection features be in place and be continuously maintained. The incidence of fire is more frequent, and therefore more likely, during construction or rehabilitation. Extra caution and concern need to be exercised to ensure adequate egress capacity and arrangement during periods of construction in any occupied building.

Paragraph 4.6.11.1 recognizes that, in lieu of strict adherence to the egress and fire protection features, alternative life safety measures might make the building safe enough to be occupied. As usual, the authority having jurisdiction is charged with judging whether the alternative measures provide an acceptable remedy. Paragraph 4.6.11.1 is conceptually similar to 4.6.10.1.

**4.6.11.2*** In buildings under construction, adequate escape facilities shall be maintained at all times for the use of construction workers. Escape facilities shall consist of doors, walkways, stairs, ramps, fire escapes, ladders, or other approved means or devices arranged in accordance with the general principles of the *Code* insofar as they can reasonably be applied to buildings under construction.

**A.4.6.11.2** See also NFPA 241, *Standard for Safeguarding Construction, Alteration, and Demolition Operations.*

**4.6.11.3** Flammable or explosive substances or equipment for repairs or alterations shall be permitted in a building while the building is occupied if the condition of use and safeguards provided do not create any additional danger or impediment to egress beyond the normally permissible conditions in the building.

### 4.6.12 Change of Use or Occupancy Classification.

In any building or structure, whether or not a physical alteration is needed, a change from one use or occupancy classification to another shall comply with 4.6.8.

Change of use or change of occupancy classification is treated as a category of rehabilitation. Such changes are required by 4.6.8 to comply with the provisions of Chapter 43, Building Rehabilitation.

### 4.6.13 Maintenance, Inspection, and Testing.

**4.6.13.1** Whenever or wherever any device, equipment, system, condition, arrangement, level of protection, fire-resistive construction, or any other feature is required for compliance with the provisions of this *Code*, such device, equipment, system, condition, arrangement, level of protection, fire-resistive construction, or other feature shall thereafter be continuously maintained. Maintenance shall be provided in accordance with applicable NFPA requirements or requirements developed as part of a performance-based design, or as directed by the authority having jurisdiction.

Paragraph 4.6.13.1 emphasizes the importance of maintaining items required by the *Code*. It is useless to have an egress door that will not open, a self-closing device that does not close the door, or a sprinkler system with no water.

**4.6.13.2** No existing life safety feature shall be removed or reduced where such feature is a requirement for new construction.

Paragraph 4.6.13.2 is similar to 4.6.8.4 and 4.6.8.5 in that it is intended to prevent existing life safety features that exceed the requirement for existing buildings from being decreased to a level less than that required for new construction. For example, a new hospital is constructed with automatic sprinkler protection for compliance with 18.3.5.1. In subsequent years the building becomes an existing hospital subject to the provisions of Chapter 19. Based on minimum construction type and number of stories, many existing hospitals are exempted from sprinkler requirements. The sprinkler exemption is meant to apply to existing situations, but it is not intended to permit the existing sprinkler system to be removed.

**4.6.13.3*** Existing life safety features obvious to the public, if not required by the *Code*, shall be either maintained or removed.

**A.4.6.13.3** Examples of such features include automatic sprinklers, fire alarm systems, standpipes, and portable fire extinguishers. The presence of a life safety feature, such as sprinklers or fire alarm devices, creates a reasonable expectation by the public that these safety features are functional. When systems are inoperable or taken out of service but the devices remain, they present a false sense of safety. Also, before taking any life safety features out of service, extreme care needs to be exercised to ensure that the feature is not required, was not originally provided as an alternative or equivalent, or is no longer required due to other new requirements in the current *Code*. It is not intended that the entire system or protection feature be removed. Instead, components such as sprinklers, initiating devices, notification appliances, standpipe hose, and exit systems should be removed to reduce the likelihood of relying on inoperable systems or features.

The *Code* directs that nonrequired life safety features that are obvious to the public be either maintained or removed to prevent false expectations or a false sense of security by building occupants. For example, if the water supply to a nonrequired wet standpipe system were permanently shut off because the system piping leaked, but the hose and nozzle for occupant use were left attached to the standpipe, an occupant could be endangered while attempting to use the system. If the nonrequired standpipe system were turned off and abandoned, it would be necessary, as a minimum, to remove all hose and nozzles and to place prominent signage at each outlet station advising that the system is out of service. The standpipe system piping, however, would not have to be removed.

**4.6.13.4** Any device, equipment, system, condition, arrangement, level of protection, fire-resistive construction, or any other feature requiring periodic testing, inspection, or operation to ensure its maintenance shall be tested, inspected, or operated as specified elsewhere in this *Code* or as directed by the authority having jurisdiction.

**4.6.13.5** Maintenance, inspection, and testing shall be performed under the supervision of a responsible person who shall ensure that testing, inspection, and maintenance are made at specified intervals in accordance with applicable NFPA standards or as directed by the authority having jurisdiction.

Subsection 4.6.13 stresses that the application of maintenance, inspection, and testing requires a three-component approach. None of the three components — maintenance, inspection, or testing — applied alone, or applied in tandem with only one of the other two, will ensure that the life safety features and systems will continue to work as required.

## 4.7* Fire Drills

**A.4.7** The purpose of emergency egress and relocation drills is to educate the participants in the fire safety features of the building, the egress facilities available, and the procedures to be followed. Speed in emptying buildings or relocating occupants, while desirable, is not the only objective. Prior to an evaluation of the performance of an emergency egress and relocation drill, an opportunity for instruction and practice should be provided. This educational opportunity should be presented in a nonthreatening manner, with consideration given to the prior knowledge, age, and ability of audience.

The usefulness of an emergency egress and relocation drill, and the extent to which it can be performed, depends on the character of the occupancy.

In buildings where the occupant load is of a changing character, such as hotels or department stores, no regularly organized emergency egress and relocation drill is possible. In such cases, the emergency egress and relocation drills are to be limited to the regular employees, who can be thoroughly schooled in the proper procedure and can be trained to properly direct other occupants of the building in case of emergency evacuation or relocation. In occupancies such as hospitals, regular employees can be rehearsed in the proper procedure in case of fire; such training is always advisable in all occupancies, regardless of whether regular emergency egress and relocation drills can be held.

Subsections 4.7.1 through 4.7.6 and the associated material from Annex A serve as a primer on how to conduct an emergency egress and relocation drill. The ____.7 section, Operating Features, of some of the occupancy chapters provides emergency egress and relocation drill details that directly correlate a drill with the characteristics of the occupancy. An understanding of how the drill details have been matched to the needs of the occupants can be gained by comparing 14.7.2 (new educational occupancies emergency egress drills) with 18.7.1 (new health care occupancies evacuation and relocation plan and fire drills).

### 4.7.1 Where Required.

Emergency egress and relocation drills conforming to the provisions of this *Code* shall be conducted as specified by the provisions of Chapters 11 through 43, or by appropriate action of the authority having jurisdiction. Drills shall be designed in cooperation with the local authorities.

### 4.7.2* Drill Frequency.

Emergency egress and relocation drills, where required by Chapters 11 through 43 or the authority having jurisdiction, shall be held with sufficient frequency to familiarize occupants with the drill procedure and to establish conduct of the drill as a matter of routine. Drills shall include suitable procedures to ensure that all persons subject to the drill participate.

**A.4.7.2** If an emergency egress and relocation drill is considered merely as a routine exercise from which some persons are allowed to be excused, there is a grave danger that, in an actual emergency, the evacuation and relocation will not be successful. However, there might be circumstances under which all occupants do not participate in an emergency egress and relocation drill; for example, infirm or bedridden patients in a health care occupancy.

### 4.7.3 Orderly Evacuation.

When conducting drills, emphasis shall be placed on orderly evacuation rather than on speed.

### 4.7.4* Simulated Conditions.

Drills shall be held at expected and unexpected times and under varying conditions to simulate the unusual conditions that can occur in an actual emergency.

**A.4.7.4** Fire is always unexpected. If the drill is always held in the same way at the same time, it loses much of its value. When, for some reason during an actual fire, it is not possible to follow the usual routine of the emergency egress and relocation drill to which occupants have become accustomed, confusion and panic might ensue. Drills should be carefully planned to simulate actual fire conditions. Not only should drills be held at varying times, but different means of exit or relocation areas should be used, based on an assumption that fire or smoke might prevent the use of normal egress and relocation avenues.

### 4.7.5 Relocation Area.

Drill participants shall relocate to a predetermined location and remain at such location until a recall or dismissal signal is given.

**4.7.6*** A written record of each drill shall be completed by the person responsible for conducting the drill and maintained in an approved manner.

**A.4.7.6** The written record required by this paragraph should include such details as the date, time, participants, location, and results of that drill.

## 4.8 Emergency Plan

### 4.8.1 Where Required.

Emergency plans shall be provided as follows:

(1) Where required by the provisions of Chapters 11 through 42
(2) Where required by action of the authority having jurisdiction

The requirement for an emergency plan can take either of the following forms:

1. An occupancy chapter can require an emergency plan; for example, see 18.7.1.1 and 18.7.2.2, applicable to new health care occupancies.
2. The authority having jurisdiction can require such plans in accordance with 4.8.1(2).

### 4.8.2 Plan Requirements.

**4.8.2.1*** Emergency plans shall include the following:

(1) Procedures for reporting of emergencies
(2) Occupant and staff response to emergencies
(3)* Evacuation procedures appropriate to the building, its occupancy, and emergencies *(see Section 4.3)*
(4) Appropriateness of the use of elevators
(5) Design and conduct of fire drills
(6) Type and coverage of building fire protection systems
(7) Other items required by the authority having jurisdiction

**A.4.8.2.1(3)** It is assumed that a majority of buildings will use a total evacuation strategy during a fire. It should be noted that evacuation from a building could occur for reasons other than a fire, but such other reasons are not the primary focus of the *Code*. As used herein, total evacuation is defined as the process in which all, or substantially all, occupants leave a building or facility in either an unmanaged or managed sequence or order. An alternative to total evacuation, is partial evacuation, which can be defined as the process in which a select portion of a building or facility is cleared or emptied of its occupants while occupants in other portions mostly carry on normal activity. In either case, the evacuation process can be ordered or managed in accordance with an established priority in which some or all occupants of a building or facility clear their area and utilize means of egress routes. This is typically done so that the more-endangered occupants are removed before occupants in less-endangered areas. Alternative terms describing this sequencing or ordering of evacuation are *staged evacuation* and *phased evacuation*.

Table A.4.8.2.1(3) illustrates options for extent of management and extent of evacuation. Some of the options shown might not be appropriate. As noted in Table A.4.8.2.1(3), either total or partial evacuation can include staged (zoned) evacuation or phased evacuation, which is referred to as managed or controlled evacuation. It should also be noted that the evacuation process might not include relocation to the outside of the building but might instead include relocation to an area of refuge or might defend the occupants in place to minimize the need for evacuation.

The different methods of evacuation are also used in several contexts throughout the *Code*. Though most of the methods of evacuation are not specifically defined or do not have established criteria, various sections of the *Code* promulgate them as alternatives to total evacuation. The following sections discuss these alternatives in more detail:

(1) Section 4.7 — Provides requirements for fire and relocation drills
(2) 7.2.12 — Provides requirements for area of refuge
(3) 7.2.4 — Provides requirements for horizontal exits
(4) 9.6.3.6 — Provides the alarm signal requirements for different methods of evacuation
(5) 9.6.3.9 — Permits automatically transmitted or live voice evacuation or relocation instructions to occupants and requires them in accordance with *NFPA 72, National Fire Alarm Code*
(6) 14.3.4.2.3 (also Chapter 15) — Describes alternative protection systems in educational occupancies
(7) 18.1.1.2/18.1.1.3/Section 18.7 (also Chapter 19) — Provide methods of evacuation for health care occupancies
(8) Chapters 22 and 23 — Provide methods of evacuation for detention and correctional occupancies, including the five groups of resident user categories
(9) Chapters 32 and 33 — Provide method of evacuation for residential board and care occupancies
(10) 32.1.4/33.1.4 — For residential board and care occupancies, state that "no means of escape or means of egress shall be considered as complying with the minimum criteria for acceptance, unless emergency evacuation drills are regularly conducted"
(11) 40.2.5.1.2 — For industrial occupancies, states that "ancillary facilities in special-purpose industrial occupancies where delayed evacuation is anticipated shall have not less than a 2-hour fire resistance–rated separation from the predominant industrial occupancy and shall have one means of egress that is separated from the predominant industrial occupancy by 2-hour fire resistance–rated construction"

The method of evacuation should be accomplished in the context of the physical facilities, the type of activities undertaken, and the provisions for the capabilities of occupants (and staff, if available). Therefore, in addition to meeting the requirements of the *Code*, or when establishing an equivalency or a performance-based design, the following recommendations and general guidance information should be taken into account when designing, selecting, executing, and maintaining a method of evacuation:

(1) When choosing a method of evacuation, the available safe egress time (ASET) must always be greater than the required safe egress time (RSET).
(2) The occupants' characteristics will drive the method of evacuation. For example, occupants might be incapable of evacuating themselves because of age, physical or mental disabilities, physical restraint, or a combination thereof. However, some buildings might be staffed with people who could assist in evacuating. Therefore, the method of evacuation is dependent on the ability of occupants to move as a group, with or without assistance. For more information, see the definitions under the term *Evacuation Capability* in Chapter 3.
(3) An alternative method of evacuation might or might not have a faster evacuation time than a total evacuation.

***Table A.4.8.2.1(3) Occupant Evacuation Strategies***

| | Extent of Management | |
|---|---|---|
| **Extent of Evacuation** | **Managed Sequence** | **Unmanaged Sequence** |
| No evacuation | No movement — remain in place upon direction | No movement — remain in place per prior instruction |
| Partial evacuation | Managed or controlled partial evacuation<br>In-building relocation on same floor<br>In-building relocation to different floors<br>Occupants of some floors leave building | Unmanaged or uncontrolled partial evacuation |
| Total evacuation | Managed or controlled total evacuation | Unmanaged or uncontrolled total evacuation |

However, the priority of evacuation should be such that the occupants in the most danger are given a higher priority. This prioritization will ensure that occupants more intimate with the fire will have a faster evacuation time.

(4) Design, construction, and compartmentation are also variables in choosing a method of evacuation. The design, construction, and compartmentation should limit the development and spread of a fire and smoke and reduce the need for occupant evacuation. The fire should be limited to the room or compartment of fire origin. Therefore, the following factors need to be considered:
   (a) Overall fire resistance rating of the building
   (b) Fire-rated compartmentation provided with the building
   (c) Number and arrangement of the means of egress
(5) Fire safety systems should be installed that compliment the method of evacuation, and should include consideration of the following:
   (a) Detection of fire
   (b) Control of fire development
   (c) Confinement of the effects of fire
   (d) Extinguishment of fire
   (e) Provision of refuge or evacuation facilities, or both
(6) One of the most important fire safety systems is the fire alarm and communication system, particularly the notification system. The fire alarm system should be in accordance with *NFPA 72, National Fire Alarm Code*, and should take into account the following:
   (a) Initial notification of only the occupants in the affected zone(s) (e.g., zone of fire origin and adjacent zones)
   (b) Provisions to notify occupants in other unaffected zones to allow orderly evacuation of the entire building
   (c) Need for live voice communication
   (d) Reliability of the fire alarm and communication system
(7) The capabilities of the staff assisting in the evacuation process should be considered in determining the method of evacuation.
(8) The ability of the fire department to interact with the evacuation should be analyzed. It is important to determine if the fire department can assist in the evacuation or if fire department operations hinder the evacuation efforts.
(9) Evacuation scenarios for hazards that are normally outside of the scope of the *Code* should be considered to the extent practicable. (*See 4.3.1.*)
(10) Consideration should be given to the desire of the occupants to self-evacuate, especially if the nature of the building or the fire warrants evacuation in the minds of the occupants. Self-evacuation might also be initiated by communication between the occupants themselves through face-to-face contact, mobile phones, and so forth.
(11) An investigation period, a delay in the notification of occupants after the first activation of the fire alarm, could help to reduce the number of false alarms and unnecessary evacuations. However, a limit to such a delay should be established before a general alarm is sounded, such as positive alarm sequence as defined in *NFPA 72, National Fire Alarm Code*.
(12) Consideration should be given to the need for an evacuation that might be necessary for a scenario other than a fire (e.g., bomb threat, earthquake).
(13) Contingency plans should be established in the event the fire alarm and communication system fail, which might facilitate the need for total evacuation.
(14) The means of egress systems should be properly maintained to ensure the dependability of the method of evacuation.
(15) Fire prevention policies or procedures, or both, should be implemented that reduce the chance of a fire (e.g., limiting smoking or providing fire-safe trash cans).
(16) The method of evacuation should be properly documented, and written forms of communication should be provided to all of the occupants, which might include sign postings throughout the building. Consideration should be given to the development of documentation for an operation and maintenance manual or a fire emergency plan, or both.
(17) Emergency egress drills should be performed on a regular basis. For more information, see Section 4.7.
(18) The authority having jurisdiction should also be consulted when developing the method of evacuation.

Measures should be in place and be employed to sequence or control the order of a total evacuation, so that such evacuations proceed in a reasonably safe, efficient manner. Such measures include special attention to the evacuation capabilities and needs of occupants with disabilities, either permanent or temporary. For comprehensive guidance on facilitating life safety for such populations, go to www.nfpa.org. For specific guidance on stair descent devices, see A.7.2.12.2.3(2).

In larger buildings, especially high-rise buildings, it is recommended that all evacuations — whether partial or total — be managed to sequence or control the order in which certain occupants are evacuated from their origin areas and to make use of available means of egress. In high-rise buildings, the exit stairs, at any level, are designed to accommodate the egress flow of only a very small portion of the occupants — from only one or a few stories, and within a relatively short time period — on the order of a few minutes. In case of a fire, only the immediately affected floor(s) should be given priority use of the means of egress serving that floor(s). Other floors should then be given priority use of the means of egress, depending on the anticipated spread of the fire and its combustion products, and to clear certain floors to facilitate eventual fire service operations. Typically, this means that the one or two floors above and below a fire floor will have secondary priority immediately after the fire floor. Depending on where combustion products move, for example, upwards through a building with cool-weather stack effect, the next priority floors will be the uppermost occupied floors in the building.

Generally, in order to minimize evacuation time for most or all of a relatively tall building to be evacuated, occupants from upper floors should have priority use of exit stairs. For people descending many stories of stairs, this priority will maximize their opportunity to take rest stops without unduly extending their overall time to evacuate a building. Thus, the precedence behavior of evacuees should be that people already in an exit stair should normally not defer to people attempting to enter the exit stair from lower floors, except for those lower floors most directly impacted by a fire or other imminent danger. Notably, this is contrary to the often observed behavior of evacuees in high-rise building evacuations where lower floor precedence behavior occurs. (Similarly, in the most commonly observed behavior of people normally disembarking a passenger airliner, people within the aisle defer to people entering the aisle, so that the areas closest to the exit typically clear first.) Changing, and generally managing, the sequence or order within which egress occurs will require effectively informing building occupants and evaluating resulting performance in a program of education, training, and drills.

When designing the method of evacuation for a complex building, all forms of egress should be considered. For example, consideration could be given to an elevator evacuation system. An elevator evacuation system involves an elevator design that provides protection from fire effects so that elevators can be used safely for egress. See 7.2.13 and A.7.2.12.2.4 for more information.

For further guidance, see the following publications:

(1) *NFPA Fire Protection Handbook*, 19th edition, Section 2, Chapter 2, which provides good methodology for managing exposures and determining the method of evacuation
(2) *NFPA Fire Protection Handbook*, 19th edition, Section 13, which provides further commentary on methods of evacuation for different occupancies
(3) *SFPE Handbook of Fire Protection Engineering*, Section 3, Chapter 13, which provides an overview of some of the research on methods of evacuation

The text of A.4.8.2.1(3) is new to the 2009 edition of the *Code*. The text serves as a primer on the subject of evacuation strategies. A wide range of strategies is offered, running the gamut from total evacuation to partial evacuation to sheltering in place without evacuation. For any given building and its occupants, no one evacuation strategy fits all possible emergencies. An effective plan calls for more than one evacuation strategy and a way to communicate to occupants at the time of an emergency the strategy that is to be employed.

**A.4.8.2.1** Items to be considered in preparing an emergency plan should include the following:

(1) Purpose of plan
(2) Building description, including certificate of occupancy
(3) Appointment, organization, and contact details of designated building staff to carry out the emergency duties
(4) Identification of events (man-made and natural) considered life safety hazards impacting the building
(5) Responsibilities matrix (role-driven assignments)
(6) Policies and procedures for those left behind to operate critical equipment
(7) Specific procedures to be used for each type of emergency
(8) Requirements and responsibilities for assisting people with disabilities
(9) Procedures for accounting for employees
(10) Training of building staff, building emergency response teams, and other occupants in their responsibilities
(11) Documents, including diagrams, showing the type, location, and operation of the building emergency features, components, and systems
(12) Practices for controlling life safety hazards in the building
(13) Inspection and maintenance of building facilities that provide for the safety of occupants
(14) Conducting fire and evacuation drills
(15) Interface between key building management and emergency responders
(16) Names or job titles of persons who can be contacted for further information or explanation of duties
(17) Post-event (including drill) critique/evaluation, as addressed in 5.14 of NFPA 1600, *Standard on Disaster/Emergency Management and Business Continuity Programs*
(18) Means to update the plan, as necessary

The text of A.4.8.2.1 is new to the 2009 edition of the *Code*. A lesson learned from the September 11, 2001, terrorist attacks on the World Trade Center towers in New York City and the Pentagon building in Arlington, Virginia, is the importance of having a detailed emergency plan that is tailored to the building and its occupants. The 18 topics listed in A.4.8.2.1 as requiring attention in the development of an emergency plan broadly cover the needed facets of such a plan.

**4.8.2.2** Required emergency plans shall be submitted to the authority having jurisdiction for review.

**4.8.2.3** Emergency plans shall be reviewed and updated as required by the authority having jurisdiction.

No one generic emergency plan can adequately address the needs of all buildings. The AHJ has great latitude in establishing requirements that will result in the creation and upkeep of an emergency plan tailored to the needs of the facility.

CHAPTER 5

# Performance-Based Option

Chapter 5 provides a performance-based alternative to the prescriptive provisions. This performance-based option is a process that can be used to determine whether the building design satisfies the fire safety goals and objectives specified in the *Code*. This chapter is not intended to replace the prescriptive *Code;* however, it can be used instead of the prescriptive requirements. The performance-based option provides for design flexibility.

Examples of performance-based design include the development of fire safety designs for unique architectural problems not anticipated by the current *Code*. The performance-based option requires the designer and the authority having jurisdiction (AHJ) to agree on the interpretation of the *Code* in terms of goals, objectives, desired levels of safety, appropriate fire scenarios, assumptions, and safety factors. The performance-based option in this chapter addresses these issues explicitly while also presenting information regarding the selection of appropriate calculation methods and input values. Additionally, this chapter outlines a documentation procedure that improves the transmission of information from the designer to the AHJ, thereby aiding in the approval of safe, cost-effective designs.

Many of the concepts in this chapter have never been addressed in earlier codes or standards. For this reason, simple illustrative examples are provided to give the user a better idea of the concepts being discussed. The examples are generally based on specific building occupancies, but the concepts and ideas presented should be applicable across a range of occupancies.

## 5.1 General Requirements

### 5.1.1* Application.

The requirements of this chapter shall apply to life safety systems designed to the performance-based option permitted by 4.4.1 and 4.4.3.

**A.5.1.1** Chapter 5 provides requirements for the evaluation of a performance-based life safety design. The evaluation process is summarized in Figure A.5.1.1.

*Code Criteria.* On the left side of Figure A.5.1.1 is input from the *Code*. The life safety goals have been stated in Section 4.1. The objectives necessary to achieve these goals are stated in Section 4.2. Section 5.2 specifies the performance criteria that are to be used to determine whether the objectives have been met.

*Input.* At the top of Figure A.5.1.1 is the input necessary to evaluate a life safety design.

The design specifications are to include certain retained prescriptive requirements, as specified in Section 5.3. All assumptions about the life safety design and the response of the building and its occupants to a fire are to be clearly stated as indicated in Section 5.4. Scenarios are used to assess the adequacy of the design. Eight sets of initiating events are specified for which the ensuing outcomes are to be satisfactory.

*Performance Assessment.* Appropriate methods for assessing performance are to be used per Section 5.6. Safety factors are to be applied to account for uncertainties in the assessment, as stated in Section 5.7. If the resulting predicted outcome of the scenarios is bounded by the performance criteria, the objectives have been met, and the life safety design is considered to be in compliance with this

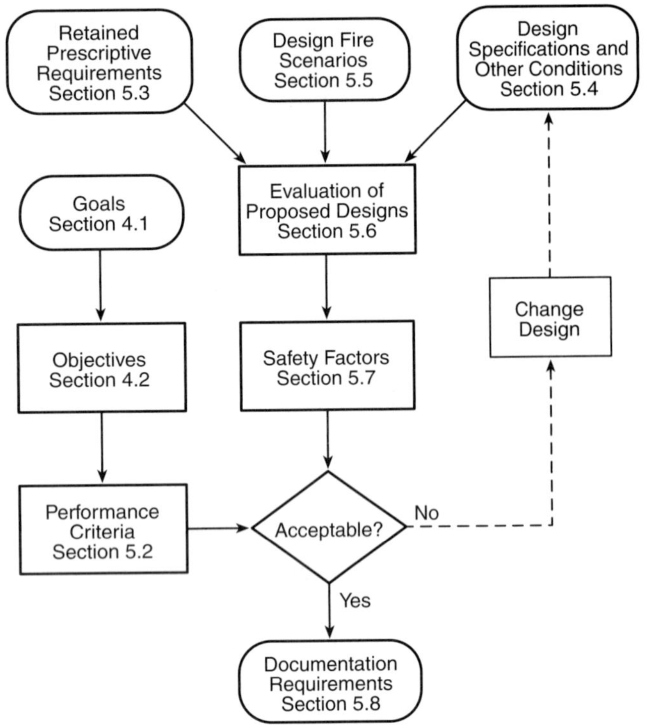


***Figure A.5.1.1*** *Performance-Based Life Safety Code Compliance Process.*

*Code*. Although not part of this *Code*, a design that fails to comply can be changed and reassessed, as indicated on the right side of Figure A.5.1.1.

*Documentation.* The approval and acceptance of a life safety design are dependent on the quality of the documentation of the process. Section 5.8 specifies a minimum set of documentation that is to accompany a submission.

The performance option of this *Code* establishes acceptable levels of risk to occupants of buildings and structures as addressed in Section 1.1. While the performance option of this *Code* does contain goals, objectives, and performance criteria necessary to provide an acceptable level of risk to occupants, it does not describe how to meet the goals, objectives, and performance criteria. Design and engineering are needed to develop solutions that meet the provisions of Chapter 5. The *SFPE Engineering Guide to Performance-Based Fire Protection Analysis and Design of Buildings* provides a framework for these assessments. Other useful references include the *Australian Fire Engineering Guidelines* and the *British Standard Firesafety Engineering in Buildings*.

Exhibit 5.1 provides a tool for guidance through a performance-based design. Exhibit 5.1 follows the same pattern as Figure A.5.1.1, with the *Code*-specified goals, objectives, and criteria on the left side of the chart, but it provides more detail on how the general and specific requirements included in this *Code* are used to formulate the various aspects of the design input. Several aspects of the design input are covered in various sections of this chapter, while others are developed or determined by the design team on the basis of the proposed building design. Once completed, the design input is then used with the chosen verification methods to obtain design output, to which a safety factor is applied. After applying the safety factor, the output can be compared to the fire safety criteria to determine whether the design passes or fails, after which the building design either is submitted for approval or is re-evaluated after modifications are made to satisfy the criteria.

### 5.1.2 Goals and Objectives.

The performance-based design shall meet the goals and objectives of this *Code* in accordance with Sections 4.1 and 4.2.

### 5.1.3 Qualifications.

The performance-based design shall be prepared by a registered design professional.

The qualifications needed by designers who develop performance-based designs are varied. Currently no certification or credential exists that formally identifies an individual as being capable of adequately developing performance-based designs. The best a code can do is to require performance-based designs to be prepared by a registered design professional. It is then left to the states and other governmental bodies to regulate the responsibilities of each registered design professional.

### 5.1.4* Independent Review.

The authority having jurisdiction shall be permitted to require an approved, independent third party to review the proposed design and provide an evaluation of the design to the authority having jurisdiction.

**A.5.1.4** A third-party reviewer is a person or group of persons chosen by the authority having jurisdiction to review proposed performance-based designs. The *SFPE Guidelines for Peer Review in the Fire Protection Design Process* provides a method for the initiation, scope, conduct, and report of a peer review of a fire protection engineering design.

The owner or developer may include a fee for third-party review in the budget for a performance-based

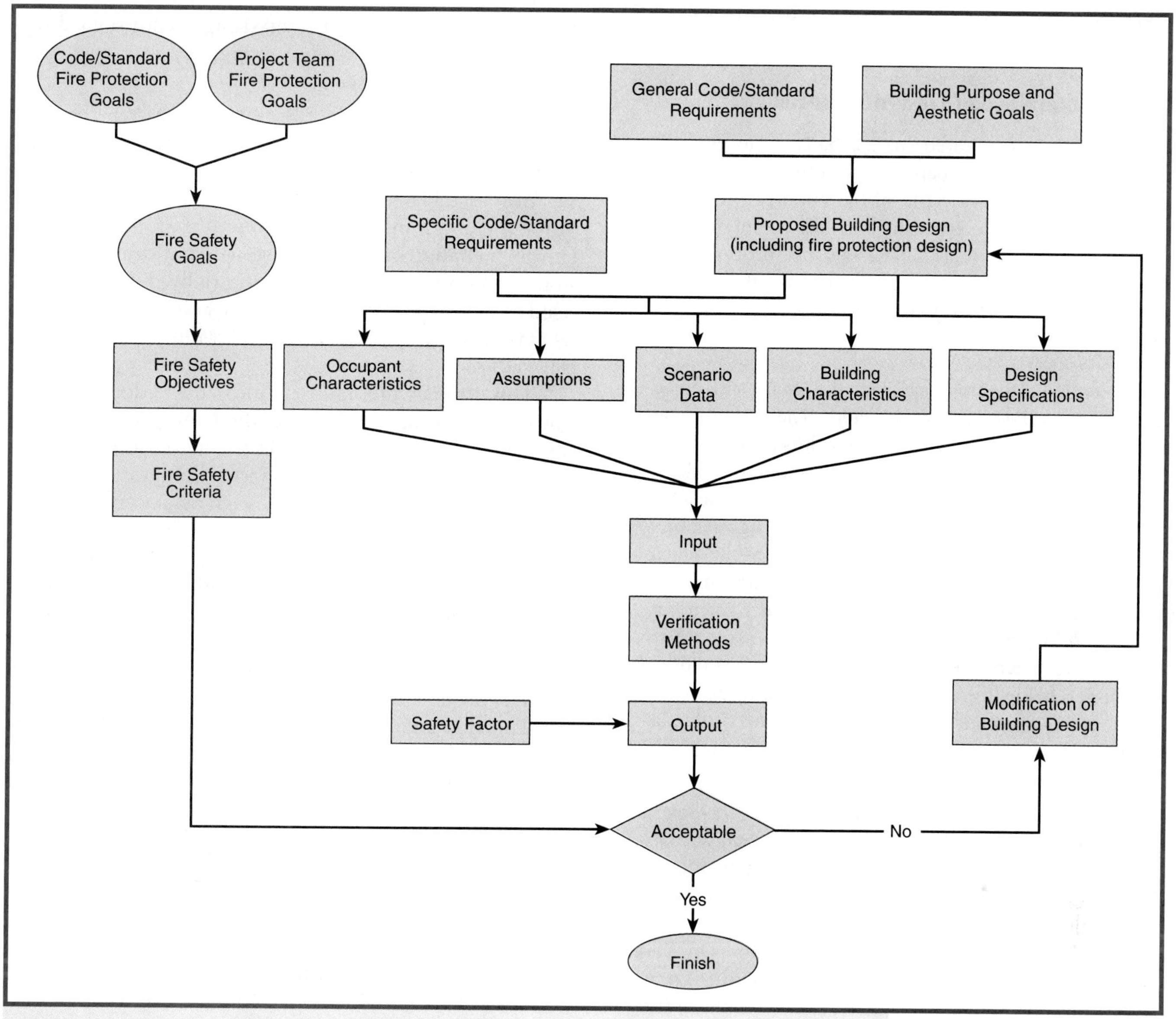


***Exhibit 5.1*** *Performance-based design process.*

project. This fee does not indicate that the third-party reviewer is responsible or beholden to the owner. The owner provides the funds for the authority having jurisdiction to hire a third-party reviewer, who then provides all findings to the AHJ.

### 5.1.5 Sources of Data.

Data sources shall be identified and documented for each input data requirement that must be met using a source other than a design fire scenario, an assumption, or a building design specification. The degree of conservatism reflected in such data shall be specified, and a justification for the source shall be provided.

### 5.1.6* Final Determination.

The authority having jurisdiction shall make the final determination as to whether the performance objectives have been met.

**A.5.1.6** For guidance on reviewing performance-based designs, see the *SFPE Enforcer's Guide to Performance-Based Design Review*. Additional guidance on reviewing designs in which fire risk assessment is used can be found in NFPA 551, *Guide for the Evaluation of Fire Risk Assessments*.

### 5.1.7* Maintenance of Design Features.

The design features required for the building to continue to meet the performance goals and objectives of this *Code* shall be maintained for the life of the building. Such performance goals and objectives shall include complying with all documented assumptions and design specifications. Any variations shall require the approval of the authority having jurisdiction prior to the actual change. *(See also 4.6.10.2.)*

**A.5.1.7** Continued compliance with the goals and objectives of the *Code* involves many factors. The building construction — including openings, interior finish, and fire- and smoke-resistive construction — and the building and fire protection systems need to retain at least the same level of performance as is provided for the original design parameters. The use and occupancy should not change to the degree that assumptions made about the occupant characteristics, combustibility of furnishings, and existence of trained personnel are no longer valid. In addition, actions provided by other personnel, such as emergency responders, should not be diminished below the documented assumed levels. Also, actions needed to maintain reliability of systems at the anticipated level need to meet the initial design criteria.

The long-term maintenance of a performance-based design is an issue that has been deemed noteworthy but for which a general solution has not been identified, due to the limited experience with performance-based designs to date. Long-term maintenance is essentially a management-of-change issue. On approval of the performance-based (building) design, it becomes a *de facto* building-specific code. As such, the provisions of the design must be maintained for the lifetime of the building. New Zealand has dealt with this issue by using independent qualified persons (IQPs) who annually certify whether a building remains compliant after a certificate of occupancy has been issued. See 4.6.10.2, which requires a yearly warrant of fitness for buildings for which performance-based design was utilized.

*Example: Maintenance of Design Features*

In 5.1.7, the *Code* requires that the design features of the building be maintained for the life of the building. The design features that might be modified include the following:

1. Occupancy and use of the structure
2. Design specifications
3. Assumptions made by the design team regarding the building conditions, emergency response personnel, or staff assistance
4. Characteristics of the building and occupants

The example that follows shows how great an impact a minor change can have on the design input of a performance-based design. The example does not involve a change in the occupancy of the building, but simply a change in building use. The building in question is an educational facility, originally designed and used as a high school but currently being modified for use as a kindergarten through grade 3 elementary school.

This type of change in building use does not require major modifications to the building structure; however, the shops and labs in the high school would have to be converted into spaces that normally are used in an elementary school, such as classrooms, offices, or storage space. Outside of these modified spaces, the design specifications remain the same. Additionally, many of the assumptions remain unchanged, such as the worst-case time for ignition, the ambient temperature, or the status of the ventilation system. However, changes are required in the characteristics used as design input.

The designer overseeing the change in building use needs to re-evaluate occupant characteristics, based on the fact that the building was designed with the typical occupant falling into the 14- to 18-year-old category. Now the typical occupant age will range from about 4 to 8 years old. This change may lead to differences in movement speed, reaction time, and type of reaction. Additionally, the designer might have to make modifications in the location and number of occupants considered in the evaluation, based on the new use. Additional changes would have to be made regarding the need for, and level of, staff assistance.

Modifications might also be required in building characteristics, such as the fuel load. The change in building use could lead to differences in the amount and type of fuel. More items geared toward young children might or might not mean additional faster-burning materials. The building might no longer contain shop or lab areas, which act as a fire hazard, but it might have additional storage space, which can add significantly to the fuel load. The designer should investigate the impact of the different fuel loads in the two building uses.

Based on the specific building, there may be additional factors that have to be modified in the design input before the building is re-evaluated. No matter how small the modification might be, the building stakeholders should ensure that the building performance remains at a level that meets the performance goals and objectives. This re-evaluation might simply entail verifying that the new value for part of the design input is still within the allowable range, or it might entail a complete re-evaluation of the structure. In either case, the authority having jurisdiction needs to be consulted before any changes are made.

### 5.1.8 Special Definitions.

A list of special terms used in this chapter follows:

(1) **Alternative Calculation Procedure.** See 3.3.13.
(2) **Data Conversion.** See 3.3.48.
(3) **Design Fire Scenario.** See 3.3.96.1.
(4) **Design Specification.** See 3.3.244.1.
(5) **Design Team.** See 3.3.53.
(6) **Exposure Fire.** See 3.3.80.
(7) **Fire Model.** See 3.3.92.
(8) **Fire Scenario.** See 3.3.96.
(9) **Fuel Load.** See 3.3.153.1.
(10) **Incapacitation.** See 3.3.137.
(11) **Input Data Specification.** See 3.3.244.2.
(12) **Occupant Characteristics.** See 3.3.179.
(13) **Performance Criteria.** See 3.3.190.
(14) **Proposed Design.** See 3.3.202.
(15) **Safe Location.** See 3.3.217.
(16) **Safety Factor.** See 3.3.218.
(17) **Safety Margin.** See 3.3.219.
(18) **Sensitivity Analysis.** See 3.3.15.1.
(19) **Stakeholder.** See 3.3.248.
(20) **Uncertainty Analysis.** See 3.3.15.2.
(21) **Verification Method.** See 3.3.266.

## 5.2 Performance Criteria

### 5.2.1 General.

A design shall meet the objectives specified in Section 4.2 if, for each design fire scenario, assumption, and design specification, the performance criterion in 5.2.2 is met.

### 5.2.2* Performance Criterion.

Any occupant who is not intimate with ignition shall not be exposed to instantaneous or cumulative untenable conditions.

**A.5.2.2** One of the methods that follow can be used to avoid exposing occupants to untenable conditions.

**Method 1.** The design team can set detailed performance criteria that ensure that occupants are not incapacitated by fire effects. The *SFPE Engineering Guide to Performance-Based Fire Protection Analysis and Design of Buildings* describes a process of establishing tenability limits.

The guide references D. A. Purser, "Toxicity Assessment of Combustion Products," Chapter 2/6, *SFPE Handbook of Fire Protection Engineering*, which describes a fractional effective dose (FED) calculation approach, which is also contained in NFPA 269, *Standard Test Method for Developing Toxic Potency Data for Use in Fire Hazard Modeling*. FED addresses the effects of carbon monoxide, hydrogen cyanide, carbon dioxide, hydrogen chloride, hydrogen bromide, and anoxia. It is possible to use the test data, combined with laboratory experience, to estimate the FED value that leads to the survival of virtually all people. This value is about 0.8.

There is a relationship between exposures leading to death and those leading to incapacitation. Kaplan [Kaplan and Hartzell, *Journal of Fire Sciences*, 2:286–305 (1984)] found that rodent susceptibility is similar to that of humans and that for the narcotic gases, CO and HCN, incapacitation is estimated to occur at one-third to one-half of the lethal exposure. A set of very large statistical studies on human lethality associated with carbon monoxide involving almost 5000 fatalities (Hirschler et al., "Carbon monoxide and human lethality: Fire and non-fire studies," Elsevier, 1993) showed that the vast majority of fire deaths are attributable to carbon monoxide poisoning, which results in lethality at levels as low as 25 percent carboxyhemoglobin (much lower than previously believed) without requiring the effect of additional toxicants. This work was also confirmed by Gann [Gann et al., *Fire and Materials,* 18:193 (1994)], who also found that carbon monoxide dominates the lethality of fire smoke, since most fire deaths occur remote from the fire room in fires that have proceeded past flashover. Thus, if an FED value of 0.8 were used for a nonlethal exposure, an FED of 0.3 would be reasonable for a nonincapacitating exposure.

If the authority having jurisdiction or the design professional is concerned with potential toxic fire effects, other than those addressed by the FED procedure as documented, the calculation procedure can be expanded by adding additional terms to the FED equation, with each term expressed as a ratio. The numerator of the ratio is the cumulative exposure to that fire effect, measured as an integral of the product of instantaneous exposure (concentration for toxic products) and time. The denominator of the ratio is the quantity of cumulative exposure for which FED equals the chosen threshold value (i.e., 0.8 or 0.3) based on that fire effect alone. A complete analysis of tenability requires consideration of tenability criteria for thermal effects (convected heat and radiated heat) and smoke obscuration, as well as those for smoke toxicity, and an example of the application of such criteria is shown in ASTM E 2280, *Standard Guide for Fire Hazard Assessment of the Effect of Upholstered Seating Furniture Within Patient Rooms of Health Care Facilities*.

For buildings where an unusually large fraction of the occupants are especially vulnerable, the calculation procedure for the smoke toxicity incapacitating criterion should be modified to use FED values lower than 0.8 or 0.3.

**Method 2.** For each design fire scenario and the design specifications, conditions, and assumptions, the design team can demonstrate that each room or area will be fully evacuated before the smoke and toxic gas layer in that room descends to a level lower than 6 ft (1830 mm) above the floor. The timing of such an evacuation means that no occupant is exposed to fire effects. Such an evacuation requires calculation of the locations, movement, and behavior of occupants, because fire effects and occupants are separated by moving the occupants. A level of 60 in. (1525 mm) is often used in calculations, but, at that level, a large fraction of the population would not be able to stand, walk, or run normally and still avoid inhalation of toxic gases. They would have to bend over or otherwise move their heads closer to the floor level.

**Method 3.** For each design fire scenario and the design specifications and assumptions, the design team can demonstrate that the smoke and toxic gas layer will not descend to a level lower than 6 ft (1830 mm) above the floor in any occupied room. The advantage of this procedure is that it conservatively ensures that no occupant is exposed to fire effects, regardless of where occupants are located or where they move. This eliminates the need for calculations regarding occupants, including those for their behavior, movement locations, pre-fire characteristics, and reactions to fire effects. This procedure is even more conservative and simpler than the procedure in Method 2, because it does not allow fire effects in occupied rooms to develop to a point where people could be affected at any time during the fire.

**Method 4.** For each design fire scenario and the design specifications and assumptions, the design team can demonstrate that no fire effects will reach any occupied room. The advantage of this procedure is that it eliminates the need for calculations regarding occupants, including those for their behavior, movement, locations, pre-fire characteristics, and reactions to fire effects. A further advantage is that it also eliminates the need for some of the modeling of fire effects, because it is not necessary to model the filling of rooms, only the spread of fire effects to those rooms. This procedure is even more conservative and simpler than the procedures in Methods 2 and 3, because it does not allow any fire effects in occupied rooms.

The methods described in A.5.2.2 provide an indication of the variety of ways of demonstrating that a proposed design meets the performance criteria and, therefore, the objectives. The methods also illustrate how different approaches can result in different margins of safety. Specifically, Methods 2, 3, and 4 are all similar in their approach — they deal with smoke filling a room. Method 2 concentrates on evacuating people before the smoke level reaches 6 ft (1830 mm) above the floor. This method presumes that the smoke will eventually reach a lower level and could, therefore, expose people crawling under the smoke layer. This method results in a relatively small margin of safety. Method 3 has a presumably more proactive design in that its intent is to prevent the smoke layer from descending any lower than 6 ft (1830 mm) above the floor. The intent of this method is to prevent exposure to occupants without their leaving the room, unless they are taller than 6 ft (1830 mm) and unwilling or unable to bend over. This method produces a greater margin of safety than that of Method 2. The margin of safety for Method 4 is the greatest — excluding the room of fire origin — because it requires the proposed design to prevent smoke from reaching any occupied room.

Three additional points are relevant to these methods. The first is that the final performance criteria might be the result of an agreement with the authority having jurisdiction, which might require or accept a threshold other than the 6 ft (1830 mm) threshold cited. In both Methods 2 and 3, a value of 7 ft (2135 mm), 6 ft 6 in. (1980 mm), or 5 ft (1525 mm) might be justified instead, based on the use of different fractions of the population requiring protection — given that some people are taller than 6 ft (1830 mm) — or the use of different safety margins based on the uncertainty calculation of the smoke layer height. The threshold for smoke layer height and other thresholds need to be a subject of discussion before beginning the performance-based design.

The second point is that Method 4 presumes that the room of fire origin is unoccupied. Depending on the facility and the scenario, this might not be a reasonable assumption. If it is not, the criteria for safety for the room of fire origin need to be set separately.

The final point, outlined in the discussion that follows, demonstrates the differences among Methods 2, 3, and 4 with respect to the level of analysis required, not with regard to their use as a specification for performing an analysis or determining whether the design meets the performance criterion for the method. Depending on the method selected for use in the evaluation, the designer needs to perform different types and levels of analysis. If it is decided to use Method 2, which states that the smoke and toxic gas will not descend to a level lower than 6 ft (1830 mm) before the area is fully evacuated, the designer needs to model both the fire and smoke spread in the building to determine the time each space becomes untenable. Additionally, the designer needs to model each occupant's egress from the building, determining the times at which each space is occupied or fully evacuated. The models and the levels of fire and smoke spread and occupant egress can then be compared to determine if the toxic gas level and smoke descend beyond the specified level before the area is fully evacuated. This analysis path requires detailed modeling of both the toxic gas spread and the evacuation of the occupants. Care must be taken to ensure that the modeling is completed conservatively and accurately, because Method 2 does not provide a large margin for error inherent in the design.

If Method 3, which states that the smoke and toxic gas layer will not descend below 6 ft (1830 mm) in any occupied room, is selected, the analysis becomes both less complicated and more conservative. After identifying each occupied space in the building, including spaces that will be occupied during occupant egress, the analysis will consist of a determination of when and whether the smoke and toxic gas layer will descend below the specified level in these areas. While the design still needs a detailed analysis of the fire and the spread of the products of combustion to determine the level of filling in each occupied area, such an analysis need not consider the building occupants or any actions they might take before or during the emergency.

If the stakeholders wish to design the building to satisfy Method 4, which states that no fire effects will reach any occupied area, the analysis becomes even less complicated and more conservative than that of Method 3. The designer should evaluate the building for each fire scenario to determine only if the smoke and toxic products of combustion will spread beyond the room of origin to occupied areas. This process often requires less complicated design tools and verification methods, because the rate and degree of smoke movement in the building is irrelevant as long as the designer can determine whether the smoke or toxic gas will travel into occupied areas.

## 5.3 Retained Prescriptive Requirements

### 5.3.1* Systems and Features.

All fire protection systems and features of the building shall comply with applicable NFPA standards for those systems and features.

**A.5.3.1** This requirement applies both to systems and features required by the *Code* that reference applicable standards and to any additional systems or features included in the design at the discretion of the design team. The referenced standards are hereby expected to state maintenance, testing, and other requirements needed to provide positive assurance of an acceptable level of reliability. The referenced standards themselves might be prescriptive- or performance-based.

### 5.3.2 Means of Egress.

The design shall comply with the following requirements in addition to the performance criteria of Section 5.2 and the methods of Sections 5.4 through 5.8:

(1) Changes in level in means of egress — 7.1.7
(2) Guards — 7.1.8
(3) Doors — 7.2.1
(4) Stairs — 7.2.2, excluding the provisions of 7.2.2.5.1, 7.2.2.5.2, 7.2.2.6.2, 7.2.2.6.3, and 7.2.2.6.4
(5) Ramps — 7.2.5, excluding the provisions of 7.2.5.3.1, 7.2.5.5, and 7.2.5.6.1
(6) Fire escape ladders — 7.2.9
(7) Alternating tread devices — 7.2.11
(8) Capacity of means of egress — Section 7.3, excluding the provisions of 7.3.3 and 7.3.4
(9) Impediments to egress — 7.5.2
(10) Illumination of means of egress — Section 7.8
(11) Emergency lighting — Section 7.9
(12) Marking of means of egress — Section 7.10

The prescriptive provisions listed in 5.3.2 for the means of egress do not readily lend themselves to performance-based calculation. However, these requirements cannot be excluded from the design. Therefore, these prescriptive provisions are retained for performance-based designs. For example, prescriptive exit sign requirements help to ensure the effectiveness of the means of egress; emergency lighting along the egress path provides prescriptive reliability for the illumination needed for effective exiting. A rationale for retaining these prescriptive requirements is that existing models of evacuation behavior are not sophisticated enough to quantify the effect of signs or lighting on the speed and effectiveness of exiting behavior.

### 5.3.3 Equivalency.

Equivalent designs for the features covered in the retained prescriptive requirements mandated by 5.3.2 shall be addressed in accordance with the equivalency provisions of Section 1.4.

## 5.4 Design Specifications and Other Conditions

### 5.4.1* Clear Statement.

Design specifications and other conditions used in the performance-based design shall be clearly stated and shown to be realistic and sustainable.

**A.5.4.1** The design specifications and other conditions form the input to evaluation of proposed designs *(see Section 5.6)*. Where a specification or condition is not known, a reasonable estimation is permitted. However, the design team must take steps to ensure that the estimation is valid during the life of the building. Any estimations need to be documented. *(See Section 5.8.)*

An example of an estimation could be a material property value needed as input by a computer fire model. Typically, computer fire models allow a single value to be input for material properties. However, if the material property varies with temperature, there is a question as to which single value adequately characterizes the material. The single value used to estimate the behavior of the material over the entire temperature range that might be experienced during the course of a fire needs to be conservatively selected and documented.

See A.5.6 for more information on computer fire models.

### 5.4.2 Assumptions and Design Specifications Data.

**5.4.2.1** Each assumption and design specification used in the design shall be accurately translated into input data specifications, as appropriate for the method or model.

The documentation of the performance-based analysis needs to clearly indicate the process for converting assumptions and design specifications into input data specifications. In some cases, the conversion process is straightforward. For example, room dimensions are explicitly stated in the design specification and can be used as input data without modification. However, if the designer assumes that a certain material will be the fuel consumed by the fire, then the process of converting that assumption into a heat release rate curve, a mass loss curve, toxic potency values, a flame spread rate, or other data for modeling needs to be described.

The source of much of the input data for the verification methods is the design specifications for the building. The design specifications are to include all the information from the building design that affects the ability of the building to meet the stated goals and objectives. In addition to the building plans and drawings, the design specification information is to be presented for use by the designer and the authority having jurisdiction. Both parties then review the information and implement it as input data specifications.

The simple example that follows illustrates the type of information that should be included with the design specifications.

***Example: Design Specifications***

This example is based on a hypothetical, four-story business occupancy building. The example building plan is shown in Exhibit 5.2, which is not drawn to scale. The fire protection and egress features for the building are not designed to meet the prescriptive *Code* requirements, with the exception of those items listed in 5.3.2. Additionally, the building has not been analyzed using the methods in Chapter 5. To conserve time and space, the systems, features, and construction details specified in this example are not explained in full detail, since this information is available from a variety of other sources. However, when completing an actual performance-based design, detailed information on each system and construction feature, such as an automatic sprinkler system or a fire barrier wall, needs to be compiled and presented for use by the designer and the authority having jurisdiction.

A description of the layout and dimensions of the building is to be developed. This description is to include a breakdown of each area to be considered in the performance-based design, as well as a description of the building as a whole.

*Building Specifications*

Building footprint — 100 ft × 250 ft (30 m × 76 m)

Building height — 50 ft (15 m)

Story height (top of floor slab to bottom of slab on next floor) — 12 ft (3660 mm)

Floor height (below false ceiling) — 10 ft (3050 mm)

Steel frame construction (interior columns) — W8 × 28 steel columns protected by two layers of gypsum wallboard — total 1 in. (25 mm) thick; include design and construction details for column protection

Poured-on-deck concrete slab — 6 in. (150 mm) thick, supported by prefabricated joists

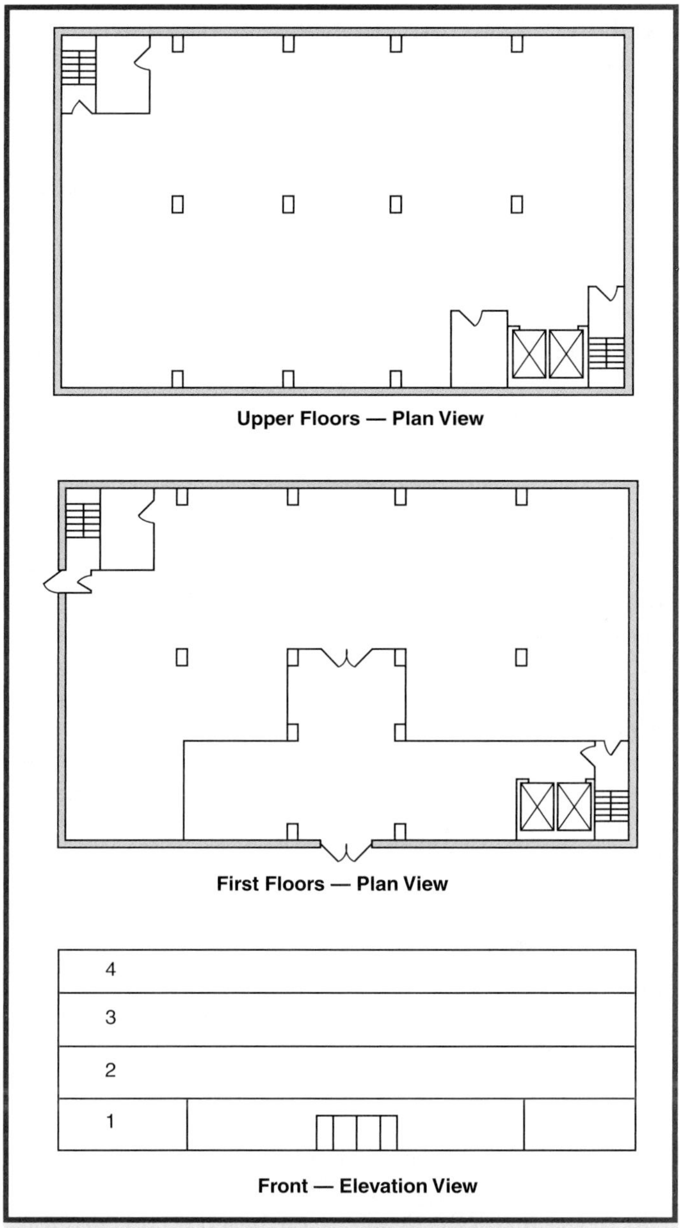


***Exhibit 5.2** Four-story business occupancy building.*

Interior finish material — gypsum wallboard

Ceiling construction — include design and fabrication details for ceiling construction and materials

Automatic sprinkler system — installed throughout per NFPA 13, *Standard for the Installation of Sprinkler Systems*[1]; include all specifications for sprinkler system normally included in a prescriptive system design [e.g., information relative to design density, response time index (RTI), spacing]

Alarm system — initiation by means of waterflow alarm incorporated into sprinkler system that operates when flow of water is equal to or greater than that from single sprinkler; waterflow alarm activates evacuation signal designed per *NFPA 72®, National Fire Alarm Code®*[2]; include all specification and design information for alarm system normally provided for a prescriptive design

HVAC system — designed and installed per NFPA 90A, *Standard for the Installation of Air-Conditioning and Ventilating Systems*,[3] and applicable regional plumbing and mechanical code

*Stairs*

Two exit stair enclosures located in opposite corners of building

Stair enclosures — 10 ft × 25 ft (3050 mm × 7620 mm)

Stair riser height — 6 in. (150 mm)

Stair tread depth — 12 in. (305 mm)

Stair clear width — 48 in. (1220 mm)

Stairs enclosed with 2-hour fire resistance–rated barrier walls (provide design and construction details)

$1\frac{1}{2}$-hour fire protection–rated, self-closing, 32 in. (810 mm) clear width doors

*Elevators*

Two 12 ft × 12 ft (3660 mm × 3660 mm) elevators separated from rest of building by 2-hour fire resistance–rated barrier walls (provide design and construction details)

Elevator installation per ASME A17.1/CSA B44, *Safety Code for Elevators and Escalators*[4]

*Storage Room — Located on Upper Floors Next to Elevator Lobby*

Dimensions — 20 ft × 25 ft (6100 mm × 7620 mm)

Nonbearing walls constructed of gypsum wallboard mounted on metal studs

32 in. (810 mm) clear width self-closing door

*Rest Room — Located Adjacent to Second Stair Enclosure*

Dimensions — 15 ft × 25 ft (4570 mm × 7620 mm)

Nonbearing walls constructed of gypsum wallboard mounted on metal studs

32 in. (810 mm) clear width self-closing door

*Entranceway (Ground Floor)*

Separated from remainder of first floor by 2-hour fire resistance–rated barrier walls (provide design and construction details)

Two main doors for entry into office space on ground floor — $1\frac{1}{2}$-hour fire protection-rated, self-closing, 40 in. (1015 mm) clear width

Two exterior exit doors off lobby — self-closing, 40 in. (1015 mm) clear width

Dimensions to be indicated on drawing

Emergency lighting and marking of means of egress — specify details and design per *Code*'s prescriptive requirements.

***Example: Assumptions***

In addition to compiling building specifications, a variety of assumptions needs to be made by the designer in developing a performance-based design. These assumptions are to remain constant and consistent throughout the analysis of the building. This example is included to provide information relating to the types of assumptions that might be made for a hypothetical 15-story hotel occupancy building. Similar to the design specifications example, this information is provided in a list format. Certain assumptions made by the design team can be included with different sections of the design input, such as assumptions regarding the location of the occupants, which would be included with the occupant characteristics. Additionally, any assumptions that do not remain constant across the various scenarios cannot be classified as assumptions — they instead become scenario-related data. The breakdown of information should be agreed on with the AHJ before a design is submitted.

**Status of Ventilation System.** Information relating to the ventilation system and its status at the time of ignition should be included among the assumptions. While the design and construction information pertaining to the ventilation system would be included in the design specifications, the assumptions relating to this system would relate purely to its status at the time of the fire — mainly whether it was on or off. Additionally, information relating to whether the ventilation system would remain on throughout the fire scenarios — or whether an automatic device would shut down the system — could be included in this data. This example assumes that the ventilation system is on and operating normally at the time of ignition.

**Ambient Temperature.** Ambient temperature is based on the anticipated condition of the building at the time of ignition. For most modern buildings, ambient temperature is dependent on the occupancy classification, since many buildings now incorporate heating/ventilation systems that maintain a constant temperature. For this example, the ambient temperature is 70°F (21°C).

**Ignition Time.** Assume worst-case time of day for the various fire scenarios. In the case of a hotel, the worst-case time is in the evening or very early morning hours, when the occupants are expected to be sleeping.

**Egress Paths.** Assumptions are to be made regarding the condition of the egress ways and whether they are clear of debris. These assumptions are generally dependent on the anticipated use of the building, as certain building types are more likely than others to have objects stored or placed in the egress paths. In this example, the assumption that each stairway is clear of clutter and debris is based on daily verification by a hotel employee. However, the lobby area — which might be used as a primary means of egress — is often cluttered with items such as luggage or chairs, and the designer needs to estimate a usable egress width.

**Mobility Impairment.** Assume one mobility-impaired occupant per floor of the structure. The mobility impairments affect the occupant characteristics of the building. The actual number of mobility-impaired individuals using the building might be based on one of the following:

1. Severity of the impairments
2. Local jurisdictional requirements
3. Selection by the design team, based on the location of the structure and the anticipated clientele
4. Number of rooms properly equipped to house mobility-impaired individuals

**Occupant Age Distribution.** Assumptions regarding the age distribution of occupants are to be made. Research has shown that groups of occupants separated by age have different movement speeds, and the design team needs to conservatively estimate the number of middle-aged adults, elderly, and children who will be located within the structure.

**System Performance.** Assume that all systems perform as designed, unless the scenario specifically mandates a system failure.

**Egress Path Selection.** Assume that all occupants will attempt to egress via the exit most familiar to them or that they will attempt to use the path followed when entering the building. Since most occupants will probably have used the elevator, assume occupants will use the first exit stair encountered in moving toward the elevators.

**Fire Fighter Staging.** Depending on the time that passes until fire fighter arrival, assume that the speed of occupant movement on stairs will be reduced by half for the stairs that the fire department uses as a staging area.

**5.4.2.2** Any assumption and design specifications that the design analyses do not explicitly address or incorporate and that are, therefore, omitted from input data specifications shall be identified, and a sensitivity analysis of the consequences of that omission shall be performed.

The term *design analyses*, as used in 5.4.2.2, means the baseline analyses of the proposed design. The design analyses are compiled into a report and submitted to the authority having jurisdiction for approval. Design specifications and assumptions would not be included in the baseline analyses if, for example, the designer originally considered incorporating an automatic suppression system into the building design or designing the building to rely on manual suppression if a fire occurs. In such a case, the designer would perform an analysis on each of those options and include in the proposed design the analysis that best satisfies the performance criteria at the lowest cost. The rejected option would be included as an appendix in the submittal to the AHJ. The appendix would indicate why the rejected option was not included in the analyses, as well as how the building performance would change if the rejected option were to be incorporated into the design.

**5.4.2.3** Any assumption and design specifications modified in the input data specifications, because of limitations in test methods or other data-generation procedures, shall be identified, and a sensitivity analysis of the consequences of the modification shall be performed.

For example, new and innovative designs for detection systems, suppression systems, or overall building layout and egress systems might be incorporated into a performance-based design. Unfortunately, while the design team may feel that these systems and modifications provide a marked improvement in the performance of the building, they might not be quantifiable in the models used to analyze the structure. If the design specifications and assumptions are such that they cannot be directly implemented into a model, the design team needs to provide justification for selection of input values to be used for the specifications and assumptions. This justification needs to include the following:

1. Detailed description of the new or modified system
2. Rationale behind the selection of the system for incorporation into the building design
3. Reason for not incorporating specifications and assumptions directly into the model input
4. Anticipated level of performance
5. Improvements expected from the system
6. Means of specifying input values in the input data specifications

Due to the level of uncertainty involved in this type of input data specification development, the design team needs to perform a sensitivity analysis on any of the input values formulated using this procedure. An example of a type of system whose design specification cannot be directly incorporated into the input data specifications is a new detection and alarm system that has not been fully tested in the arrangement and layout of the proposed building. If the design team can provide justification that the model cannot accurately predict the system's performance, then modifications should be made to the input data specification to account for the differences in the results of the analysis and the performance of the system.

### 5.4.3 Building Characteristics.

Characteristics of the building or its contents, equipment, or operations that are not inherent in the design specifications, but that affect occupant behavior or the rate of hazard development, shall be explicitly identified.

Building characteristics that are not classified as design specifications tend to be limited to particular spaces within the building, occupancy- or purpose-driven, or long-term or transitory adjustments by occupants to problems in the functionality of the basic design. The building characteristics depend largely on the materials used to decorate and furnish the building and on the anticipated layout of such materials. The identification of building characteristics needs to take into account the intended use of the building and potential aging effects on the materials used. The identification of building characteristics of concern requires considerable experience with the hazard-related consequences of both typical and problematic operations in occupancies of the type proposed.

Examples of building characteristics include the anticipated layout, fuel load, and burning characteristics of a work area composed of cubicles in a business occupancy. In addition to the flammability characteristics of the interior lining materials of a structure, an additional modification could be included with the building characteristics to account for the potential buildup of combustible dust or hydrocarbon residue on the material in an industrial complex. Buildings in which there is a high rate of occupant turnover and movement, such as educational facilities or dormitories, might include doors — and more importantly, fire doors — that are routinely blocked open, allowing the uninhibited passage of smoke and other fire products of combustion. Designers of a mercantile occupancy might deliberately or inadvertently create a maze-like effect, which not only affects evacuation times but might also lead to anxiety and confusion in the occupants during an emergency.

The description of the building characteristics is to include all of the information related to the building and its various contents and features that is not included with the design specifications. Various examples of building characteristics are provided in this commentary. However, the example that follows includes a more detailed description of the types of items that should be included with the building characteristics when developing a performance-based design. Additionally, this example presents differences in, and modifications that would be required for, the building characteristics if the intended use is changed from a business occupancy to a mercantile occupancy. The different occupancy types can lead to large differences in smoke production and spread throughout the structure, as well as differences in evacuation time. The designer needs to carefully select and document the characteristics of the specific building. The designer also needs to use conservative estimates of the various building characteristics, particularly if there is a possibility that the owner might change the building type or occupancy.

***Example: Building Characteristics***

The building in question is a three-story office building that is being converted into a three-level department store. The specifications that follow provide a description of the building characteristics that might be used in the original performance-based design for the business occupancy.

**Office Space.** The space is divided throughout by work cubicles. A baseline case office setup for cubicle arrangement is to be specified. Arrangements are to be analyzed using sensitivity analysis to determine the allowable level of variance in office setup.

**Fuel Load.** The fuel load is dependent on office setup. A fixed fuel load is to be used, as limited types of materials are available for consumption. The fuel load will consist of materials such as office furniture, computers, cubicle finishing materials, and paper. Tests that measure the burning rate of office cubicles and different office setups are to be consulted to determine the total combined fuel load. The flammability of each potential fuel item in the area of ignition is to be estimated. Other potential sources of fuel in a business occupancy include the interior finish materials and paper or office equipment in storage areas.

The flammability information for the fuel sources, such as the heat release rate, rate of flame spread, and mass loss rate, can be determined from several sources. The flammability data for the fuels in question might be available in typical fire protection texts, such as the NFPA *Fire Protection Handbook,*[5] the *SFPE Handbook of Fire Protection Engineering,*[6] and Drysdale's *An Introduction to Fire Dynamics.*[7] This information can also be estimated using the results from small-scale tests, such as those from a cone calorimeter or a LIFT (lateral ignition and flamespread test) apparatus. A more accurate determination of the flammability characteristics can be produced in large-scale testing of the fuels in question. This is not to suggest that the designer conduct large-scale testing of the anticipated fuel sources for each design; however, a review of large-scale tests completed on items similar to those in question at fire testing labs such as the National Institute of Standards and Technology (NIST) Building and Fire Research Laboratory might provide accurate estimates of the required material properties. NIST has compiled this research in reports such as "A Survey of Fuel Loads in Contemporary Office Buildings" by Caro and Milke.[8] These reports are available for downloading on NIST's web site or at its research library. The flammability of the specific items in question should be documented as accurately as possible.

**Egress Paths.** Despite the variability of the office setup, business occupancies typically will have clear, fixed paths of egress. The egress paths will generally consist of a perimeter loop around the office core, along with multiple aisleways leading from the interior offices to the perimeter loop. Based on the type of business occupying the structure, the designer should determine whether the egress paths are likely to remain clear of clutter and debris. This facet of the building characteristics could also be included with the design assumptions.

**Fire Doors.** The condition of the fire doors in the structure is to be specified with the building characteristics. Business occupancies generally keep fire doors in the structure closed due to the limited need to block the doors open, since, generally, occupant turnover is not large and movement of furniture is periodic.

The building characteristics described in this commentary are assumptions relating to the building's function. These business occupancy characteristics can be compared to those identified for the department store to determine which characteristics can be replaced with new values for the new occupancy. Generally, some differences exist; if the new characteristics vary significantly, the designer might have to reevaluate the performance of the structure completely.

The paragraphs that follow present the types of information that are to be included with the building characteristics for the renovated mercantile occupancy spaces.

**Mercantile Space.** As in the case of the business occupancy, a base case setup of the mercantile space is to be specified. However, a mercantile occupancy generally modifies the arrangement and setup of the building contents more frequently than a business occupancy does, based on the type of store involved. The design is to be sufficiently robust so that almost every typical arrangement of the mercantile occupancy is permitted, with the exception of extreme cases utilizing highly volatile or flammable substances.

**Fuel Load.** The fuel load for a mercantile occupancy is based primarily on the intended merchandise. The fuel load could consist of items ranging from electronics, plastics, and food products to wood materials, upholstered furniture, and seasonal decorations. The fuel load can vary greatly, depending on the type of store and even the time of year. The design is to be based on the worst-case fuel load that the designer believes might be contained in the building at any time.

**Egress Paths.** Many mercantile establishments either inadvertently or deliberately create maze-like paths that run through the store. While such paths might keep shoppers in the store for longer periods, causing them to view more of the merchandise, they will also cause longer evacuation times and can lead to anxiety during emergencies. Additionally, due to restocking operations and the moving of merchandise, the egress paths and aisleways in a mercantile occupancy might be partially or fully blocked.

**Fire Doors.** Mercantile occupancies are frequently moving items and storing contents and may have large occupant loads moving between different spaces. These practices might result in the fire doors within the structure being blocked open, potentially allowing smoke and other products of combustion to spread uninhibited throughout the structure. The evaluation should consider this issue, or the designer should take steps to ensure that the fire doors remain closed.

### 5.4.4* Operational Status and Effectiveness of Building Features and Systems.

The performance of fire protection systems, building features, and emergency procedures shall reflect the documented performance and reliability of the components of those systems or features, unless design specifications are incorporated to modify the expected performance.

**A.5.4.4** Systems addressed by this requirement include automatic fire suppression systems and fire alarm systems. Performance issues that need to be documented might include response time indexes, discharge densities, and distribution patterns. Calculations should not include an unlimited supply of extinguishing agent if only a limited supply will be provided in the actual structure or building.

Emergency procedures addressed by this requirement might be of two types. The design team could include documentation from buildings that are operationally very similar, along with documented operational performance measures tied to the recruitment and training of emergency team personnel. Where such data are unavailable, or where the proposed design differs significantly from other buildings, the design could be based on detailed analyses of the decisions and tasks that need to be performed by emergency personnel, using plausible conservative assumptions about the occupant characteristics and training of those personnel.

Subsection 5.4.4 and A.5.4.4 are meant to help ensure that the performance-based design analysis is realistic and reflects the anticipated operation of the systems, including people-oriented systems like emergency procedures. In other words, the analysis must consider that the systems installed in buildings are limited — they are not like Hollywood guns that never run out of bullets. Designers need to make sure that the analysis deals with the systems in a practical manner and is representative of how the systems will be installed in the building.

Subsection 5.4.4 addresses inherent performance limitations more than reliability concerns, which are separately addressed in 5.5.3.8, through mandatory analysis of scenarios with systems and features rendered unavailable. For example, there are different modes of fire detection (such as ionization smoke detectors, photoelectric smoke detectors, fixed-temperature heat detectors, and rate-of-rise heat detectors) that provide different speeds of response to different fire scenarios. Also, automatic fire sprinklers use varying design densities of different agents, resulting in different speeds and degrees of effectiveness, depending on the fire scenario. Fire doors are rated for different durations and are expected to withstand different levels of heat impact before failing. Additionally, fire barrier walls are expected to exhibit various performance levels, particularly if one wall extends from the floor to the roof while another extends to a level below the roof. Systems related to emergency procedures are not of the "one size fits all" character. Such emergency procedures must be tailored to the specific building and occupant population.

### 5.4.5 Occupant Characteristics.

**5.4.5.1* General.** The selection of occupant characteristics to be used in the design calculations shall be approved by the authority having jurisdiction and shall provide an accurate reflection of the expected population of building users. Occupant characteristics shall represent the normal occupant profile, unless design specifications are used to modify the expected occupant features. Occupant characteristics shall not vary across fire scenarios, except as authorized by the authority having jurisdiction.

**A.5.4.5.1** Examples of design features that might be incorporated to modify expected occupant characteristics include training, use of staff to assist with notification and movement, or type of notification appliance used.

**5.4.5.2* Response Characteristics.** The basic response characteristics of sensibility, reactivity, mobility, and susceptibility shall be evaluated. Such evaluation shall include the expected distribution of characteristics of a population appropriate to the use of the building. The source of data for these characteristics shall be documented.

**A.5.4.5.2** The four basic characteristics — sensibility, reactivity, mobility, and susceptibility — comprise a minimum, exhaustive set of mutually exclusive performance characteristics of people in buildings that can affect a fire safety system's ability to meet life safety objectives. The characteristics are briefly described as follows:

(1) Sensibility to physical cues, which is the ability to sense the sounding of an alarm and can also include discernment and discrimination of visual and olfactory cues in addition to auditory emanations from the fire itself
(2) Reactivity, which is the ability to interpret cues correctly and take appropriate action and can be a function of cognitive capacity, speed of instinctive reaction, or group dynamics; might need to consider reliability or likelihood of a wrong decision, as in situations where familiarity with the premises influences wayfinding
(3) Mobility (speed of movement), which is determined by individual capabilities, as well as crowding phenomena, such as arching at doorways
(4) Susceptibility to products of combustion, which includes metabolism, lung capacity, pulmonary disease, allergies, or other physical limitations that affect survivability in a fire environment

In application, as with the use of computer evacuation models, assumptions can address a larger number of factors that are components of the basic performance characteristics, including the following:

(1) Alertness — condition of being awake/asleep, can depend on time of day
(2) Responsiveness — ability to sense cues and react
(3) Commitment — degree to which occupant is committed to an activity underway before the alarm
(4) Focal point — point at which an occupant's attention is focused (e.g., to front of classroom, stage, or server in business environment)
(5) Physical and mental capabilities — influence on ability to sense, respond, and react to cues; might be related to age or disability
(6) Role — influence on whether occupant will lead or follow others
(7) Familiarity — influence of time spent in building or participation in emergency training
(8) Social affiliation — extent to which an occupant will act/react as an individual or as a member of a group
(9) Condition over the course of the fire — effects, both physiological and psychological, of the fire and its combustion products on each occupant

For a more detailed explanation of occupant characteristics, see the *SFPE Engineering Guide to Human Behavior in Fire*. Occupant characteristics that are discussed in the guide include the following:

(1) Population numbers and density
(2) Condition of being alone or with others
(3) Familiarity with the building
(4) Distribution and activities
(5) Alertness
(6) Physical and cognitive ability
(7) Social affiliation
(8) Role and responsibility
(9) Location
(10) Commitment
(11) Focal point
(12) Occupant condition
(13) Gender
(14) Culture
(15) Age

**5.4.5.3 Location.** It shall be assumed that, in every normally occupied room or area, at least one person shall be located at the most remote point from the exits.

All occupant locations at the beginning of the fire must be specified. This information is critical for egress analysis, since travel distances to the exits must be known. Depending on the scenarios of interest, conditions within selected egress paths must be analyzed. However, the conditions in the room of fire origin always need to be determined.

**5.4.5.4* Number of Occupants.** The design shall be based on the maximum number of people that every occupied room or area is expected to contain. Where the success or failure of the design is contingent on the number of occupants not exceeding a specified maximum, operational controls shall be used to ensure that the maximum number of occupants is not exceeded.

**A.5.4.5.4** The number of people expected to be contained in a room or area should be based on the occupant load factor specified in Table 7.3.1.2 or other approved sources.

An example of another approved source for occupant load factors is zoning regulations. Also, the authority having jurisdiction might specify a higher occupant load than that calculated using the occupant load factors of Table 7.3.1.2 to provide an additional safety margin.

The occupant characteristics specified for a performance-based design need to provide an accurate representation of the abilities and behaviors of the building occupants before and during a fire. This information is critical to a performance-based design if the design is to be based on and compared with Method 2 of A.5.2.2. The selection of Method 2 requires that each room or area be fully evacuated before the smoke layer in that room descends below 6 ft (1830 mm) above the floor. To show that each space is clear before the smoke layer reaches this level, the designer must document the spread of fire, its products of combustion, and the movement of people throughout the building during the emergency as accurately as possible using current verification methods. To model the evacuation of the building, characteristics of the occupants of that building must be formulated. The overall function of occupant characteristics is the estimation of the time required to evacuate the building. Therefore, the designer also needs to formulate response characteristics, which dictate how the occupants perceive the fire threat, the time required to respond to this threat, and the time to evacuate the building once the decision has been made to leave. Additionally, the designer needs to determine the number and location of people occupying the structure at the time of fire initiation. Staff assistance and emergency response, which also have an impact on evacuation time, are presented in separate examples in the commentary on this chapter.

***Example: Response Characteristics, Location, and Number of Occupants***

This example presents a sample of occupant characteristics that could be used as the basis for an egress analysis. It is critical that the designer account for premovement activities when completing an egress analysis, as occupants will often spend as much time, if not far more, deciding and preparing to leave than they actually do while moving through the building.[9] The list of occupant characteristics is based on a hypothetical, three-story apartment building as shown in Exhibit 5.3. This building has two enclosed exit stairs located in proximity to two of the opposite corners of the structure. The stair on the bottom right-hand side of Exhibit 5.3 is assumed to be the main, front stairway for the structure — the egress path most familiar to the majority of the people in the building. The building is laid out such that there are 16 one-bedroom apartments (2–5, 8–11, 13–16, and 18–21) and 6 three-bedroom apartments (1, 6, 7, 12, 17, and 22), as follows:

*16 Small Apartments (2–5, 8–11, 13–16, and 18–21)*

Single bedroom
Two people per apartment

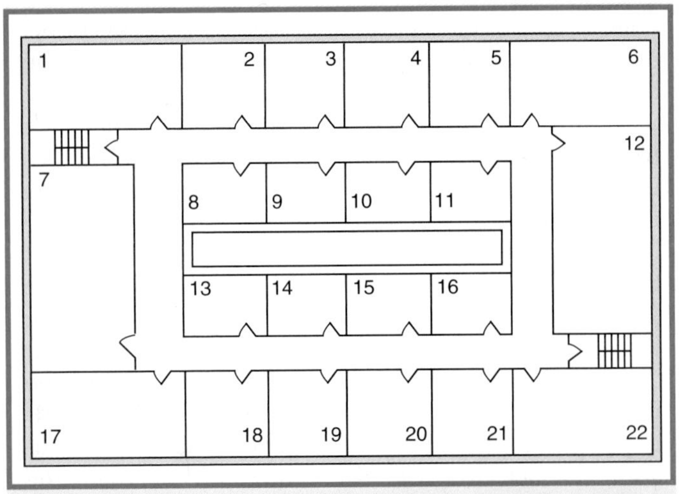


**Exhibit 5.3** *Three-story apartment building — typical floor plan.*

Two mobility-impaired people (walking disabled) per floor; base case locations, apartments 3 and 14 — subject to sensitivity analysis

*6 Large Apartments (1, 6, 7, 12, 17, and 22)*

Three bedrooms

Three apartments with two adults and two children; three apartments with two adults and three children; base case locations, five-person apartments 7, 12, and 17

Distribution of four- and five-person apartments subject to sensitivity analysis

**Notification Time.** Notification time is the time from ignition until the sounding of the alarm. Notification time depends on the fire scene and design specification of the detection and alarm system.

**Reaction Time.** Assume everyone in the building is sleeping at the time of alarm. This state of sensibility presents a delay in the reaction time of the occupants. Additionally, average reaction time is highly influenced by the performance of the detection and alarm system. Research has shown that the performance of an alarm system and the occupants' response to the sounding of the alarm have a dramatic effect on the average delay time.[10] The average reaction time of adult occupants is determined on the basis of the condition of occupants at the time of alarm (sleeping), the design features and audibility of the alarm system, and any local regulation relating to delay times to be used in egress analysis. This example assumes that children will not react and prepare to evacuate without prompting from adults; therefore, only an estimate for adults is to be provided. The predicted range of reaction time is to be provided.

**Pre-Evacuation Time.** An additional factor that needs to be considered when performing egress analyses is activities that occupants engage in before leaving the building. These activities range from gathering children or pets to getting dressed and packing up valuable belongings. The climate of the building location might factor into the delay time, as occupants are more reluctant to go outside in particularly cold weather, and — before they do — more time will be spent finding and donning jackets and other clothing. In the case of mobility-impaired individuals who require mobility aids, delay time will also include the time required to find, gather, and begin using these devices. An average time for pre-evacuation activities is to be specified for each of the apartment groups. For this example, the apartments housing two adults and no children have pre-evacuation times based on the time required to get dressed; gather items such as a jacket, keys, shoes, and a wallet; and then begin to egress the building. An additional amount of time should be added for those apartments housing mobility-impaired individuals. For those apartments housing children, an additional time factor should be added for the time required to get the children together, dressed, and ready to move out of the building. Information on reaction time and pre-evacuation activities is critical for the completion of an accurate egress analysis. This information can be found in the NFPA *Fire Protection Handbook,* the *SFPE Handbook of Fire Protection Engineering*, or tests, such as those cited in the Proulx and Fahy paper.[10]

In summary, the following pre-evacuation times are also to be included in the egress analysis:

1. Adult apartments pre-evacuation time — provide predicted range based on specific occupant characteristics and available literature and test data
2. Adult apartments for mobility-impaired individuals pre-evacuation time — provide predicted range
3. Apartments with children pre-evacuation time — provide predicted range

**Travel Time.** The final component of an egress analysis is the calculation of the time required for occupants to leave the structure once they begin to evacuate. This travel time is primarily based on the location of the occupants and the speed at which they can navigate through the building. Depending on the structure in question, the occupants' ability to move might be affected by crowding phenomena and unfamiliarity with the structure. Other factors that influence travel time are as follows:

1. Families remain in a group throughout evacuation and move at the speed of the slowest member.
2. Occupants have varied familiarity with the structure.
3. Occupants egress via the most familiar path, unless fire or products of combustion block that path; assume occupants from apartments 1, 2, 3, 7, 8, 9, and 17 attempt to use the stairway in the upper left-hand corner of Exhibit 5.3, while the rest of the occupants use the stairway in the bottom right-hand corner of the exhibit.

Occupant movement speeds are available from several sources, including the NFPA *Fire Protection Handbook*, the *SFPE Handbook of Fire Protection Engineering*, and Fruin's *Pedestrian Planning and* Design,[11] or from tests on different samples of the population.

Movement speeds for the following are to be included in the egress analysis:

1. Adults on floor — provide predicted range based on available literature and test data
2. Adults on stairs — provide predicted range
3. Families with children on floor — provide predicted range
4. Families with children on stairs — provide predicted range
5. Mobility-impaired adults on floor — provide predicted range
6. Mobility-impaired adults on stairs — provide predicted range

Egress time is calculated as follows:

$$\text{Egress time} = t_n + t_r + t_p + t_t$$

where:

$t_n$ = notification time
$t_r$ = reaction time
$t_p$ = pre-evacuation time
$t_t$ = travel time

**5.4.5.5* Staff Assistance.** The inclusion of trained employees as part of the fire safety system shall be identified and documented.

**A.5.4.5.5** For example, in hospitals, staff characteristics such as number, location, quality, and frequency of training should be considered.

Certain occupancies or building types might require that staff assistance be provided during the evacuation procedure in order for the occupants to evacuate the building safely. The assistance of trained staff in public places, such as department stores, shopping malls, theaters, arenas, or similar buildings, can help occupants unfamiliar with the building find emergency exits, accelerating their departure and reducing the overall evacuation time. However, it is important that staff members who are accounted for in a design be properly trained and drilled so that they are familiar with their role in the evacuation of the building.

Other examples of occupancies where staff assistance might be required are nursing homes, hospitals, and residential board and care facilities. In facilities housing the elderly or mentally or physically impaired individuals, occupants might be slow to react to warning or alarm systems and might be slow in moving as well. Depending on the severity of the impairment of the occupants, evacuation time might be extremely prolonged without the incorporation of staff assistance. Take, for example, a nursing home that houses nonambulatory occupants incapable of self-preservation. The range of impairments of the occupants might include the following:

1. Inability to hear an alarm
2. Inability to comprehend the significance of an alarm
3. Inability to walk unassisted
4. Inability to move at all without the use of a wheelchair

Due to the varied nature of the occupants in such a setting, the designer will most likely be unable to predict the types of impairments that the occupants of that building will have at any specific time.

***Example: Staff Assistance***

The hypothetical building for this example is a two-story nursing home with 6 occupant rooms, an entrance/waiting room, a desk/office area, and a cafeteria/lounge on the first floor; and 12 occupant rooms on the second floor. Exhibit 5.4 shows a plan view for each floor.

There are a total of 18 rooms, each housing 2 patients, for a total permanent occupancy of 36 patients. These people might suffer from a variety of impairments, which will greatly affect their ability to egress the building in a timely manner in the event of an emergency. This example assumes that any occupant confined to a wheelchair is housed on the ground floor. The occupant characteristics for this building are not discussed in detail for this example, as occupant characteristics and their impact were addressed in the commentary to A.5.4.5.4. However, this example briefly presents the impact of staff assistance on the various time components that can be used to determine the total egress time.

It is assumed that the occupants of the building are sleeping. Because there is a fairly high likelihood that some of the occupants of this building are hearing impaired or might be unable to comprehend and react to an alarm, the reaction time for this component of the population could be infinite. Additionally, elderly occupants might take more time getting dressed and preparing to leave, further lengthening the pre-evacuation time. There is a high likelihood that some of the occupants of this structure suffer from mobility or mental impairments, which would also affect their travel time. Some of the occupants might be unable to move without assistance, so their travel time will be infinite, while others might simply move at a very slow pace.

Staff assistance can be factored into a design to negate some of the effects of various impairments on egress time. The actual level of staff required in a structure of this type might be restricted by local jurisdictions and individual company specifications. For this example, it is assumed that the building is staffed full-time with three nurses, seven aides, and a desk clerk. Two of the nurses and four of the aides are located on the second floor. The designer should work with the building owner and stakeholders to develop a written facility fire safety plan that outlines each person's responsibility in the event of a fire. For this example, it is assumed that, upon alarm and confirmation of a fire, the desk clerk is to notify and interact with the fire department, while the nurses and aides help the occupants to evacuate the building.

The designer must make certain assumptions regarding the facility staff and the degree to which they will affect the occupant response characteristics and evacuation. There must be a basis for each assumption made by the designer regarding staff assistance, and each should be documented. Assumptions might include the following:

1. All patients are under 24-hour supervision and their location is always known.
2. Wheelchair-bound patients are located on the first floor only, and the occupants either are seated in, or located near, their wheelchairs.
3. The facility has an emergency evacuation plan that is practiced twice a year.
4. Each nurse and aide is assigned a patient or group of patients who they must ensure escapes safely from the building.
5. Upon hearing an alarm, the staff verifies that there is a fire, notifies each of the occupants, and proceeds to take the following actions:
   a. The staff closes the door to each room upon leaving to prevent smoke from entering that room.
   b. The staff begins helping those in need of assistance in moving through the building.

The effects of staff assistance on the time to evacuation can be stated with each component of the egress analysis time, based on the assumptions made. The first component of the egress time calculation is the time to notification. This component is generally based on the sounding of the alarm, but one of the assumptions for this example is that the staff verifies the existence of a fire before helping to notify the occupants. This action introduces a time delay in the notification time. The second and third components of the egress time calculation are the reaction and pre-evacuation times. As previously discussed, these times might be dramatically affected by hearing, mental, or physical impairments. When the staff is notifying the occupants of the fire, they need to ensure that each occupant capable of evacuating without assistance begins to react, or staff is to help them to begin evacuating the structure. This might include getting each occupant dressed and prepared to leave, as well as placing the occupants into wheelchairs, if necessary.

The delay estimate for staff assistance must include consideration of the fact that each member of the staff might be responsible for more than one person and that there might be delays associated with each person. For the example presented here, the average staff member is assigned three or four people, and an average delay developed depends on the anticipated

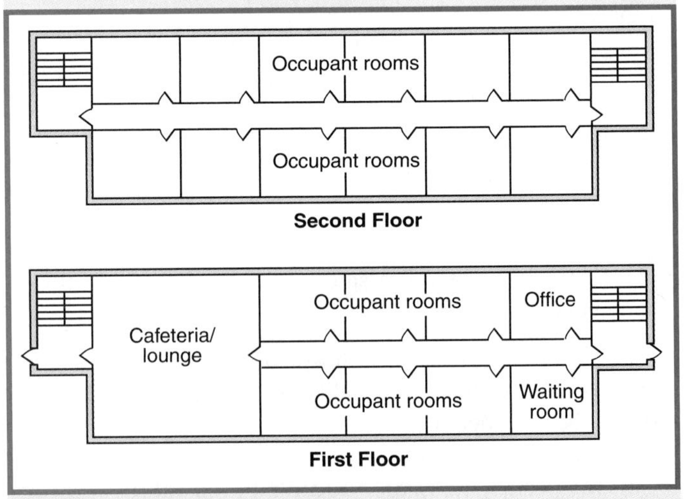


*Exhibit 5.4 Two-story nursing home.*

level of impairment associated with each person. These actions introduce further delays in the reaction and pre-evacuation activities.

Finally, the staff aids the occupants in moving through the building. This might include wheeling them out of the building, walking next to them throughout the egress process, or simply directing them out of the building. Initially, estimates are to be made for each of these delays, and these estimates are to be confirmed by the evacuation drills.

### 5.4.6 Emergency Response Personnel.

Design characteristics or other conditions related to the availability, speed of response, effectiveness, roles, and other characteristics of emergency response personnel shall be specified, estimated, or characterized sufficiently for evaluation of the design.

Depending on the design in question, it might be desirable to omit the operations of emergency response personnel. If this is the case, this assumption is to be documented as part of the final design.

Depending on the type of occupancy and the use of the building, the designer might wish to incorporate the actions of emergency personnel into the evaluation of the structure. The design team needs to make many assumptions regarding the time to arrival and overall capabilities of the response personnel, and these assumptions must be incorporated into the design documentation. The designer cannot simply assume that the fire department will arrive 30 seconds after the initial fire alarm and suppress the fire immediately upon arrival. The example that follows is provided to present the type of questions that should be addressed regarding emergency response personnel, as well as some of the assumptions that might be made.

#### *Example: Emergency Response Personnel*

The facility in this example is an industrial occupancy located on the outskirts of a suburban town. The facility manufactures plastic products and runs two shifts per day. There are two buildings on the campus. One building houses the administrative personnel and design team offices as well as a cafeteria and lounge; all of the manufacturing takes place in the other building. The processes used in manufacturing the product are hazardous and involve the use of toxic and flammable chemicals. The town has two full-time fire stations, both with the same resources. One is located 5 mi (8 km) from the facility; the other is 10 mi (16 km) from the facility.

When determining the assumptions that can be made about the emergency response personnel, it might be useful for the designer to develop a list of questions to ask the owner and authority having jurisdiction or fire department representative on the design team. The answers to such questions can help assess the level of dependence the design should have on the arrival of the fire department. The following are sample questions:

1. Is there a fire brigade on-site?
2. What is the brigade's level of training?
3. What is the estimated response time of the local fire department?
4. How many response personnel will respond with the first arriving company?
5. How many response personnel will respond with the second arriving company?
6. Is the local fire department familiar with, and trained to respond to, emergencies at the facility?
7. When an alarm is sounded, does the signal go straight to the local fire department or to a security station on-site?
8. Who will assess the situation before calling the local fire department?
9. What types of hazards exist on-site, and where are they located?
10. Do these hazards pose health threats to the surrounding community, to the employees, or to the fire fighters?
11. Does the local fire department have the equipment to respond to the types of fire incidents that could develop?
12. Does the municipality or the plant supply the equipment specified in item 11?
13. If supplied by the company, is the equipment stored on-site?
14. What type of access does the fire department have to the site?
15. How long will it take the fire fighters to set up for suppression efforts at a range of locations on the campus?

All assumptions regarding the fire department's response time need to be verified as feasible by the fire department. The overall intention of these questions regarding the fire department and its capabilities is to determine the time to arrival, the time to agent application, and the time to suppression, which can then be incorporated into the building evaluation. These various times should take into consideration not just the fire department but also the building, as the designer should be aware that certain building designs present more challenging situations than others.

When emergency response personnel are to be an important part of the fire safety design, the designer needs to try to make the building as friendly to the fire department as possible. To facilitate this process, the designer should consult with the fire department early in and throughout the process to ensure that the design is optimized for fire-fighting operations and that any assumptions made regarding the fire department are accurate.

### 5.4.7* Post-Construction Conditions.

Design characteristics or other conditions related to activities during the life of a building that affect the ability of the building to meet the stated goals and objectives shall be specified, estimated, or characterized sufficiently for evaluation of the design.

**A.5.4.7** Design proposals need to state explicitly any design specifications or estimations regarding building fire safety plans, inspection programs, or other ongoing programs whose performance is necessary for the building, when occupied and operational, to meet the stated goals and objectives. Programs of interest include any maintenance, training, labeling, or certification programs required to ensure operational status or reliability in building systems or features.

Subsection 5.4.7 relates to the management-of-change issues discussed in 5.1.7. One design characteristic that typically changes post-construction is the fuel load. The design basis fuel load must anticipate such changes, no matter what their size. Increased quantities of fuel load that involve materials that are easier to ignite and that involve higher and faster growing heat release rates, with higher smoke generation rates, could have a significant impact on the performance-based design. Neither the designer nor the authority having jurisdiction will want to reanalyze the design's acceptability fully whenever post-construction conditions change slightly. To avoid that need while maintaining safety, the designer must use assumptions that are more conservative than the conditions actually anticipate and also identify those conditions of greatest sensitivity that must be maintained or reanalyzed.

### 5.4.8 Off-Site Conditions.

Design characteristics or other conditions related to resources or conditions outside the property being designed that affect the ability of the building to meet the stated goals and objectives shall be specified, estimated, or characterized sufficiently for evaluation of the design.

Off-site conditions are considered to be outside the property line and out of the control of the owner/operator. One example of an off-site condition is the status of the public water main. If the fire protection design relies on a sprinkler system fed by the public water main, then the analysis should consider the possibility that the public water main won't deliver the required amount of water.

### 5.4.9* Consistency of Assumptions.

The design shall not include mutually inconsistent assumptions, specifications, or statements of conditions.

**A.5.4.9** The design elements required to be excluded by 5.4.9 include those regarding the interrelations between the performance of building elements and systems, occupant behavior, or emergency response actions that conflict with each other. For each fire scenario, care needs to be taken to ensure that conflicts in actions do not occur. Typical conflicts could include the following:

(1) Assuming a fire door will remain closed during the fire to contain smoke while this same door is used by occupants during egress from the area
(2) Assuming fire apparatus will arrive immediately from a distant location to provide water to fire department connections and similar situations

For example, an assumption that compartmentation blocking the passage of fire and smoke will be maintained at the door to a stairwell cannot be paired with an assumption that evacuation through that door will extend over many minutes.

### 5.4.10* Special Provisions.

Additional provisions that are not covered by the design specifications, conditions, estimations, and assumptions provided in Section 5.4, but that are required for the design to comply with the performance objectives, shall be documented.

**A.5.4.10** The provisions required by 5.4.10 to be documented include those that are in excess of basic requirements covered by referenced codes and standards, typical design requirements, and operating procedures. It includes provisions such as the following:

(1) More frequent periodic testing and maintenance to increase the reliability of fire protection systems
(2) Redundant systems to increase reliability
(3) On-site guard service to enhance detection of fires and aid in fire response procedures
(4) Staff training
(5) Availability and performance of emergency response personnel
(6) Other factors

## 5.5* Design Fire Scenarios

**A.5.5** Design fire scenarios define the challenge a building is expected to withstand. Design fire scenarios capture and limit value judgments on the type and severity of the fire challenge to which a proposed fire safety system needs to respond. The system includes any and all aspects of the proposed design that are intended to mitigate the effects of a fire, such as egress system, automatic detection and suppression, barriers, staff training, and placement of manual extinguishers.

Design fire scenarios come from two sources: those that are specified in 5.5.3.1 through 5.5.3.8, and those that are developed by the design team based on the unique characteristics of the building as required by 5.5.2. In most, if not all, cases, more than one design fire scenario will be developed to meet the requirements of 5.5.2.

Once the set of design fire scenarios is established, both those specified by 5.5.3.1 through 5.5.3.8 and those that are developed as required by 5.5.2, they need to be quantified into a format that can be used for the evaluation of proposed designs. The *SFPE Engineering Guide to Performance-Based Fire Protection Analysis and Design of Buildings* outlines a process and identifies tools and references that can be used at each step of this process.

### 5.5.1 Approval of Parameters.

The authority having jurisdiction shall approve the parameters involved in design fire scenarios. The proposed design shall be considered to meet the goals and objectives if it achieves the performance criteria for each required design fire scenario. *(See 5.5.3.)*

### 5.5.2* Evaluation.

Design fire scenarios shall be evaluated using a method acceptable to the authority having jurisdiction and appropriate for the conditions. Each design fire scenario shall be as challenging as any that could occur in the building, but shall be realistic, with respect to at least one of the following scenario specifications:

(1) Initial fire location
(2) Early rate of growth in fire severity
(3) Smoke generation

**A.5.5.2** The protection systems and features used to meet the challenge of the design fire scenario should be typical of, and consistent with, those used for other similar areas of the building. They should not be designed to be more effective in the building area addressed than in similar areas not included and that are, therefore, not explicitly evaluated.

Paragraph A.5.5 indicates that 5.5.2 will typically force one or more scenarios to be considered in addition to the eight specified in 5.5.3.1 through 5.5.3.8. The specified scenarios are to be considered for all performance-based designs, but they do not necessarily represent a comprehensive set of scenarios. There might be additional scenarios truly unique to the proposed facility that need to be analyzed. The intent of including nonspecific scenarios (as opposed to the specific scenarios of 5.5.3) is to capture those scenarios in which initial fire location, early rate of growth in fire severity, or smoke generation (see 5.5.2) poses a greater problem than those conditions captured by the scenarios in 5.5.3. However, there are also other conditions that may require development of scenarios — overcrowding of a specific space being just one example. The authority having jurisdiction might also specify additional scenarios to account for a historical, local fire that the AHJ is determined will not recur.

The discussion that follows suggests how suitable scenarios may be developed.

### Introduction

To provide a comprehensive design (i.e., to demonstrate how the fire safety system will respond to a variety of fires), more than one scenario should be considered. It is suggested that, at a minimum, the following three types of scenarios be considered:

1. High-frequency, low-consequence scenario (typical)
2. Low-frequency, high-consequence scenario (high-challenge)
3. Special problems scenario

The scenario in item 1 is used to demonstrate that the fire safety system can manage fires that start as relatively small fires but are frequent (e.g., a wastebasket fire). The scenario in item 2 should present a greater challenge to the fire safety system (e.g., fire in an egress path). The intent is to consider a larger fire, but not one that is so unrealistically large that it ensures the proposed design (or any other) will not perform adequately. The first two scenario types tacitly assume that the fire safety system will function as designed. However, the scenario in item 3 is included to account for those situations in which some aspect of the fire safety system might be compromised (e.g., improperly closed valve on a sprinkler system, detection/alarm system temporarily out of service, degradation of egress system after an earthquake or other natural disaster). The scenario in item 3 can also be used to consider the reliability of the fire safety system design.

Commentary Table 5.1 provides general scenarios — those that may be experienced by most, if not all, occupancies. Commentary Table 5.1 presents examples

**Commentary Table 5.1 General Scenarios**

| Fire Type | Scenario: Occupant in Room of Fire Origin but Not Intimate | Scenario: Room of Fire Origin Normally Unoccupied |
|---|---|---|
| Slow-developing fire | • Cigarette ignition of upholstered furniture<br>• Electrical ignition of small appliance or lighting, or overloaded outlet | • Overloaded or failed wiring igniting switch gear, electrical devices, or insulation, followed by ignition of wooden structural members |
| Moderate-developing fire | • Kitchen/cooking fire<br>• Trash can fire<br>• Open flame ignition of upholstered furniture | • Wildland or exposure fire (e.g., from a neighboring building or parked car)<br>• Lightning-induced ignition of building roof<br>• Laundry room fire |
| Fast-developing fire | • Flammable liquids | • Flammable liquid storage |
| Shielded from systems, or other problems present | • Fire with impaired "first line of defense"<br>• Shielded flaming fires; limited fuel and larger | • External trash collection or trash chute fire<br>• Flammable liquid storage<br>• Room of fire origin door open<br>• Fire in egress path |

of typical and high-challenge fires, based on slow-, moderate-, and fast-developing fires that expose people in the room of origin who are not intimate with ignition, and based on when the room of origin is unoccupied. The table also presents examples of special problem fires for these same individuals.

The left column of Commentary Table 5.1 indicates a general fire type, characterized by the rate at which a potential fire hazard might develop. Fire development is defined by a heat release rate curve (HRRC). An additional factor in defining the type of fire is the peak heat release rate, which must be severe enough to challenge the fire safety system but not so severe that no design can effectively reduce the hazards of the postulated fires. The peak heat release rate is a function of the amount of fuel of the first item ignited, if the fire doesn't spread beyond that first item, or the maximum amount of fuel within the room of origin (e.g., the room goes to flashover).

### Scenario Components

At a minimum, a fire scenario consists of the following:

1. Ignition factors (source, location, and material; other items ignited if applicable)
2. At least one heat release rate curve (HRRC)
3. Occupant locations (see 5.4.5.3)
4. Occupant characteristics (see 5.4.5.2)
5. Special factors (shielded, systems unreliable, open door)

**Ignition Factors.** Ignition factors include the source of ignition; the material that is first ignited and, if it is a solid, where it is ignited; and whether other items are also ignited. Ignition factors to consider when constructing a fire scenario are shown in Commentary Table 5.2.

**Ignition Source.** Ignition sources are of primary interest when considering the frequency of design fires. Possible sources of ignition include the following:

1. Smoking
2. Open flame
3. Electrical source
4. Incendiary
5. Hot surface
6. Spontaneous combustion
7. Radiant source

Various electrical ignition scenarios are possible, and historical data should be consulted to determine which is most appropriate for the occupancy being considered. In addition to smoking-related ignitions and open flames, another example of incendiary ignition would be a "runaway" industrial reaction. Hot surfaces are most often associated with either cooking (stoves, hot plates) or industrial processes (engines, furnaces). Spontaneous combustion is essentially an uncontrolled exothermic chemical reaction, due to either a buildup of flammable vapors (e.g., due to improper storage or decomposition) or accidental mixing of reactive chemicals (e.g., some cleaning fluids). A common radiant source is a portable heater.

*First Item Ignited.* The first item ignited is somewhat dependent on the ignition source. For example, an overheated electrical wire is most likely to ignite its own insulation; cooking fires usually ignite items close to the flames, not structural assemblies (e.g., wall or ceiling finish materials). The first item ignited is of interest for two reasons. First, it may pose either a thermal or a nonthermal hazard by itself (e.g., an occupied mattress or the toxic products resulting from its combustion). Second, the first item might ignite a second item that poses an additional or greater hazard. Examples of second items include merchandise, structural assemblies, and carpets capable of releasing toxic combustion products. There may be no need to consider the "second item ignited" column of Commentary Table 5.2 if the first item ignited presents enough of a hazard by itself. Certain types of upholstered furniture fall into this category because of the toxic combustion products they release and their relatively high heat release rate.

*Second Item Ignited.* Ignition of a second item is important in scenarios involving flashover or where structural stability is an issue. Ignition of a second item should be reflected in the heat release rate curve for the room of origin. Ignition of a second item can have the following two effects on the room heat release rate curve:

1. The peak heat release rate might be increased.
2. The growth phase of the fire might be accelerated.

The possibility of both phenomena occurring might apply to certain scenarios (e.g., if the second item involves flammable liquids or gases).

**Heat Release Rate Curves.** Heat release rate curves can be constructed by referring to the *SFPE Handbook of Fire Protection Engineering* and Drysdale's *An Introduction to Fire Dynamics.*

**Special Factors.** The following are several additional factors that might be critical to the development of scenarios.

*Ignition Location.* The location of the point of ignition can affect the eventual course and spread of a fire. In some cases, specifying a location also implies additional items in the scenario. For example, a kitchen fire could actually be a cooking fire that involves a burner igniting loose clothing or a grease fire igniting "ordinary" combustibles nearby.

*Fire Spread.* With regard to fire spread, the point of ignition is significant because it might, in part, determine the severity of the fire. An aspect of this issue is

***Commentary Table 5.2 Ignition Factors***

| Ignition Source | First Item Ignited | Second Item Ignited |
|---|---|---|
| Cigarette | Electrical equipment[1] | Structural assembly[2] |
| Electrical lighting | Wiring | Library book stack |
| Incendiary | Seating | Merchandise display |
| Spontaneous combustion | Sets and decorations | Carpets |
| Stove/hot plate | Exhibit displays | Curtains |
| Process-inherent[3] | Upholstered furniture | |
| | Electrical appliance | |
| | Trash | |
| | Ordinary combustibles[4] | |
| | Gas leaks | |
| | Flammable liquids | |
| | Mattress | |
| | Medical equipment | |

[1]Includes, but is not limited to, dust collectors, uninterruptible power supplies, generators, HVAC equipment, dryers, and freezers

[2]Consists of exterior/interior wall or ceiling finish, wall studs, ceiling joists, and insulation

[3]Applies primarily to industrial settings

[4]Includes mixtures of paper, common plastics, and other materials

the availability of oxygen. If the first item ignited is an upholstered chair, two different scenarios result, depending on whether the ignition location is on the outside (e.g., by a wastebasket fire) or on the inside (e.g., a cigarette between a seat cushion and the arm of the chair). In the former case, a flaming fire is likely to occur; in the latter, a smoldering fire with copious amounts of products of combustion results. Additionally, the point of origin might be conducive to localized flashover. Localized flashover has been observed in experiments involving bunk beds and desks with enclosed leg wells (modesty panels). These geometries tend to concentrate heat energy such that an intense fire is created in a relatively small area.

*Relative Location.* Relative location is somewhat related to the localized flashover. These fires are characterized by the ignition point being shielded from fire protection systems. The problem is that the initial fire development is not sensed by the fire detection system. This results in a larger fire at the time of detection and a commensurate decrease in the time to evacuate. A common scenario involving shielded fires is a fire in warehouse rack storage.

*Interference with Evacuation.* The loss or degradation of any one egress path (e.g., when a fire originates in some aspect of the egress system) can place a significant burden on the fire safety system of a facility. If more than two exits exist, the loss of one will have a lesser impact than if only one or two exits are initially available. If a fire originates in a location shared by more than one egress path (e.g., where two egress paths merge into a single corridor or a dead-end corridor), the impact is greater than if the fire originates in one of several parallel egress routes.

*Compartmentation Barriers.* This situation involves the fire breaching a barrier or originating in a concealed space or on an exterior surface. When the fire breaches a barrier, the potential for a severe fire increases. The problem with fire originating in a concealed space or on an exterior surface is similar to that addressed under the factor "relative location" (fire shielded from detection or suppression systems).

## General Design Scenarios

The general design scenarios shown in Commentary Table 5.3 are recommended as a starting point, since they encompass the issues addressed in earlier commentary. For those instances in which Commentary Table 5.3 does not apply, a process is provided for selecting components for site-specific scenarios that address the concepts of these general scenarios.

## Development of Scenarios

The guidelines that follow are for use in specifying fire scenarios.

## Typical Scenarios

Typical scenarios can be specified partly through routine statistical analysis of fire experience in similar buildings. An advantage of common or typical scenarios is that they provide a good prediction of the building's performance if fire occurs. Such scenarios also tend to fit easily within the scope of available fire models and calculation methods. This means the authority having jurisdiction can review the results for these scenarios to obtain a basic sense of the building's level of safety and the appropriateness of the calculations.

***Commentary Table 5.3 General Design Scenarios***

| Typical Scenario | High-Challenge Scenario | Special Problem Scenario |
|---|---|---|
| Fast growth in room contents | Flammable liquids in means of egress | Ordinary fire in typical unoccupied room with sprinklers or detectors out of commission |
| Ordinary fire in attic or "challenging" concealed space | Largest room fire, fastest growth consistent with use; worst occupant characteristics | |
| Ordinary fire in typical occupied room with people not intimate with ignition | Worst flame spread fire, if area critical to egress; or flammable room linings or decorations | |
| Slow-developing fire in typical occupied room with worst-case occupant characteristics | | |

## High-Challenge Scenarios

High-challenge scenarios are any scenarios that pose unusual fire challenges to the building design. High-challenge scenarios can be developed by refining common scenarios (e.g., changing the area of fire origin) to create a greater challenge. Also, high-challenge scenarios can be developed by reducing the challenge in scenarios previously identified as beyond the design expectations (i.e., too severe to use as the basis for evaluation).

The illustrative techniques that follow are to be used for developing high-challenge scenarios from typical scenarios.

**1.** *Change the area of fire origin.* Consider an area (e.g., a bedroom) where occupants are likely to be particularly vulnerable. Consider an area (e.g., a concealed space, an external surface) where fire can develop outside the effective range of key fire protection features (such as detectors or sprinklers). Consider an area (e.g., an egress corridor) that is critical to occupant movement to safety.

**2.** *Increase the initial size or speed of the development of the fire.* This might be done by adjusting the parameters in a fire growth model (e.g., increasing the alpha value in a *t*-squared modeled fire; creating a scenario that reflects a fast or ultrafast fire; increasing the peak heat release rate value for the fire) or by increasing the assumed room fuel load or decreasing the space between major combustible items.

**3.** *Assume common degradations in design assumptions.* For example, assume the doors are blocked open, allowing the passage of fire effects to secondary spaces; or assume an unlimited oxygen supply for fire growth that could result from open doors, broken windows, or other circumstances.

**4.** *Increase the toxicity or yields of products of combustion.*

Developing high-challenge scenarios from scenarios beyond design expectations involves less-challenging quantitative assumptions. For example, if the bomb used in the New York City World Trade Center incident of 1993 were to be deemed too severe for a high-rise office building, how small a bomb would constitute an appropriate high-challenge test? To pose another example, if the *Code* cannot ensure protection of occupants who are intimate with initial fire development, how close can occupants be without being considered intimate?

### 5.5.3* Required Design Fire Scenarios.

Design fire scenarios shall comply with the following:

(1) Scenarios selected as design fire scenarios shall include, but shall not be limited to, those specified in 5.5.3.1 through 5.5.3.8.
(2) Design fire scenarios demonstrated by the design team to the satisfaction of the authority having jurisdiction as inappropriate for the building use and conditions shall not be required to be evaluated fully.

**A.5.5.3** It is desirable to consider a wide variety of different fire scenarios to evaluate the complete life safety capabilities of the building or structure. Fire scenarios should not be limited to a single or a couple of worst-case fire scenarios.

The descriptive terms used to indicate the rate of fire growth for the scenarios are intended to be generic. Use of *t*-squared fires is not required for any scenario.

One or more of the required eight design fire scenarios specified in 5.5.3.1 through 5.5.3.8 might not apply. For instance, if the designer is analyzing a building that serves primarily as a warehouse but also has limited office space, and that building does not have any concealed wall or ceiling spaces, then Design Fire Scenario 4 (see 5.5.3.4) might not be applicable.

Another example of a situation in which one of the required scenarios might not apply to a particular design is a building isolated from any possible exposure to outside fire sources, which eliminates the need to evaluate the building using Design Fire Scenario 7 (see 5.5.3.7). The possible ignition or fuel sources for an exposure fire might include trees or vegetation, cars, delivery trucks, or dumpsters. If the designer can show the authority having jurisdiction that the building is designed such that there would be no vegetation around the perimeter; that no personnel or delivery vehicles could park next to, or even within, a certain distance of the building; and that no man-made flammable objects would be placed around the perimeter of the building, then this scenario might not be applicable.

Each of the theoretical examples would be very rare, and justifying the inappropriateness of any of the scenarios could be very difficult for the designer. The majority of buildings to which one or more of the required scenarios do not apply will generally be very specialized cases, such as an aircraft hangar with no concealed spaces or a research lab with no external fuel sources that could lead to an exposure fire. If the designer believes that one or more of the scenarios do not apply to the building in question, the designer should consult the authority having jurisdiction early in the evaluation process and provide written justification for why the scenarios do not apply.

**5.5.3.1* Design Fire Scenario 1.** Design Fire Scenario 1 shall be described as follows:

(1) It is an occupancy-specific fire representative of a typical fire for the occupancy.
(2) It explicitly accounts for the following:
   (a) Occupant activities
   (b) Number and location
   (c) Room size
   (d) Furnishings and contents
   (e) Fuel properties and ignition sources
   (f) Ventilation conditions
   (g) Identification of the first item ignited and its location

**A.5.5.3.1** An example of Design Fire Scenario 1 for a health care occupancy would involve a patient room with two occupied beds with a fire initially involving one bed and the room door open. This is a cursory example in that much of the explicitly required information indicated in 5.5.3.1 can be determined from the information provided in the example. Note that it is usually necessary to consider more than one scenario to capture the features and conditions typical of an occupancy.

The idea behind Design Fire Scenario 1 is to ensure that the types of fires most likely in a given occupancy type — that is, the statistically most significant scenarios — are considered in the design analysis. These scenarios have a great degree of variety, from the small fires experienced weekly at aluminum rolling mills to the kitchen fires in high-rise apartment buildings (i.e., residences).

**5.5.3.2* Design Fire Scenario 2.** Design Fire Scenario 2 shall be described as follows:

(1) It is an ultrafast-developing fire, in the primary means of egress, with interior doors open at the start of the fire.
(2) It addresses the concern regarding a reduction in the number of available means of egress.

**A.5.5.3.2** Design Fire Scenario 2 examples include a fire involving ignition of gasoline as an accelerant in a means of egress, clothing racks in corridors, renovation materials, or other fuel configurations that can cause an ultrafast fire. The means of egress chosen is the doorway with the largest egress capacity among doorways normally used in the ordinary operation of the building. The baseline occupant characteristics for the property are assumed. At ignition, doors are assumed to be open throughout the building.

Design Fire Scenario 2 is intended to provide information on the maximum potential spread of fire effects, mostly smoke and toxic products. It answers the question "What is the maximum extent of smoke that may be experienced if an egress path is blocked?"

**5.5.3.3* Design Fire Scenario 3.** Design Fire Scenario 3 shall be described as follows:

(1) It is a fire that starts in a normally unoccupied room, potentially endangering a large number of occupants in a large room or other area.
(2) It addresses the concern regarding a fire starting in a normally unoccupied room and migrating into the space that potentially holds the greatest number of occupants in the building.

**A.5.5.3.3** An example of Design Fire Scenario 3 is a fire in a storage room adjacent to the largest occupiable room in the building. The contents of the room of fire origin are specified to provide the largest fuel load and the most rapid growth in fire severity consistent with the normal use of the room. The adjacent occupiable room is assumed to be filled to capacity with occupants. Occupants are assumed to be somewhat impaired in whatever form is most consistent with the intended use of the building. At ignition, doors from both rooms are assumed to be open. Depending on the design, doorways connect the two rooms or they connect via a common hallway or corridor.

For purposes of this scenario, an occupiable room is a room that might contain people; that is, a location within a building where people are typically found.

**5.5.3.4* Design Fire Scenario 4.** Design Fire Scenario 4 shall be described as follows:

(1) It is a fire that originates in a concealed wall or ceiling space adjacent to a large occupied room.
(2) It addresses the concern regarding a fire originating in a concealed space that does not have either a detection system or a suppression system and then spreading into the room within the building that potentially holds the greatest number of occupants.

**A.5.5.3.4** An example of Design Fire Scenario 4 is a fire originating in a concealed wall or ceiling space adjacent to a large, occupied function room. Ignition involves concealed combustibles, including wire or cable insulation and thermal or acoustical insulation. The adjacent function room is assumed to be occupied to capacity. The baseline occupant characteristics for the property are assumed. At ignition, doors are assumed to be open throughout the building.

**5.5.3.5* Design Fire Scenario 5.** Design Fire Scenario 5 shall be described as follows:

(1) It is a slowly developing fire, shielded from fire protection systems, in close proximity to a high occupancy area.
(2) It addresses the concern regarding a relatively small ignition source causing a significant fire.

**A.5.5.3.5** An example of Design Fire Scenario 5 is a cigarette fire in a trash can. The trash can is close enough to room contents to ignite more substantial fuel sources but is not close enough to any occupant to create an intimate-with-ignition situation. If the intended use of the property involves the potential for some occupants to be incapable of movement at any time, the room of origin is chosen as the type of room likely to have such occupants, filled to capacity with occupants in that condition. If the intended use of the property does not involve the potential for some occupants to be incapable of movement, the room of origin is chosen to be an assembly or function area characteristic of the use of the property, and the trash can is placed so that it is shielded by furniture from suppression systems. At ignition, doors are assumed to be open throughout the building.

**5.5.3.6* Design Fire Scenario 6.** Design Fire Scenario 6 shall be described as follows:

(1) It is the most severe fire resulting from the largest possible fuel load characteristic of the normal operation of the building.
(2) It addresses the concern regarding a rapidly developing fire with occupants present.

**A.5.5.3.6** An example of Design Fire Scenario 6 is a fire originating in the largest fuel load of combustibles possible in normal operation in a function or assembly room, or in a process/manufacturing area, characteristic of the normal operation of the property. The configuration, type, and geometry of the combustibles are chosen so as to produce the most rapid and severe fire growth or smoke generation consistent with the normal operation of the property. The baseline occupant characteristics for the property are assumed. At ignition, doors are assumed to be closed throughout the building.

This scenario includes everything from a big couch fire in a small dwelling to a rack fire in combustible liquids stock in a big box retail store.

The Dupont Plaza Hotel fire of 1986 in San Juan, Puerto Rico,[12] is an example of Design Fire Scenario 6. The storage of chairs was part of the normal operating procedures of the hotel. The location and potential heat release of the chairs were evidently considered a small threat due to the lack of an ignition source. Unfortunately, a source was supplied, with tragic results.

**5.5.3.7* Design Fire Scenario 7.** Design Fire Scenario 7 shall be described as follows:

(1) It is an outside exposure fire.
(2) It addresses the concern regarding a fire starting at a location remote from the area of concern and either spreading into the area, blocking escape from the area, or developing untenable conditions within the area.

**A.5.5.3.7** An example of Design Fire Scenario 7 is an exposure fire. The initiating fire is the closest and most severe fire possible consistent with the placement and type of adjacent properties and the placement of plants and combustible adornments on the property. The baseline occupant characteristics for the property are assumed.

This category includes wildlands/urban interface fires and exterior wood shingle problems, where applicable.

**5.5.3.8* Design Fire Scenario 8.** Design Fire Scenario 8 shall be described as follows:

(1) It is a fire originating in ordinary combustibles in a room or area with each passive or active fire protection system independently rendered ineffective.
(2) It addresses concerns regarding the unreliability or unavailability of each fire protection system or fire protection feature, considered individually.
(3)* It is not required to be applied to fire protection systems for which both the level of reliability and the design performance in the absence of the system are acceptable to the authority having jurisdiction.

**A.5.5.3.8(3)** The exemption is applied to each active or passive fire protection system individually and requires two different types of information to be developed by analysis and approved by the authority having jurisdiction. System reliability is to be analyzed and accepted. Design performance in the absence of the system is also to be analyzed and accepted, but acceptable performance does not require fully meeting the stated goals and objectives. It might not be possible to meet fully the goals and objectives if a key system is unavailable, and yet no system is totally reliable. The authority having jurisdiction will determine which level of performance, possibly short of the stated goals and objectives, is acceptable, given the very low probability (i.e., the system's unreliability probability) that the system will not be available.

**A.5.5.3.8** Design Fire Scenario 8 addresses a set of conditions with a typical fire originating in the building with any one passive or active fire protection system or feature being ineffective. Examples include unprotected openings between floors or between fire walls or fire barrier walls, failure of rated fire doors to close automatically, shutoff of sprinkler system water supply, nonoperative fire alarm system, inoperable smoke management system, or automatic smoke dampers blocked open. This scenario should represent a reasonable challenge to the other building features provided by the design and presumed to be available.

The concept of a fire originating in ordinary combustibles is intentionally selected for this scenario. This fire, although presenting a realistic challenge to the building and the associated building systems, does not represent the worst-case scenario or the most challenging fire for the building. Examples include the following:

(1) Fire originating in ordinary combustibles in the corridor of a patient wing of a hospital under the following conditions:
 (a) Staff is assumed not to close any patient room doors upon detection of fire.
 (b) The baseline occupant characteristics for the property are assumed, and the patient rooms off the corridor are assumed to be filled to capacity.
 (c) At ignition, doors to patient rooms are not equipped with self-closing devices and are assumed to be open throughout the smoke compartment.

(2) Fire originating in ordinary combustibles in a large assembly room or area in the interior of the building under the following conditions:
 (a) The automatic suppression systems are assumed to be out of operation.
 (b) The baseline occupant characteristics for the property are assumed, and the room of origin is assumed to be filled to capacity.
 (c) At ignition, doors are assumed to be closed throughout the building.

(3) Fire originating in ordinary combustibles in an unoccupied small function room adjacent to a large assembly room or area in the interior of the building under the following conditions:
 (a) The automatic detection systems are assumed to be out of operation.
 (b) The baseline occupant characteristics for the property are assumed, the room of origin is assumed to be unoccupied, and the assembly room is assumed to be filled to capacity.
 (c) At ignition, doors are assumed to be closed throughout the building.

Design Fire Scenario 8 provides information to the authority having jurisdiction by answering a series of "What if . . . ?" questions. For example, what if the hotel sprinkler system is out of service when a fire occurs? What might be the extent of the fire and smoke and their subsequent effects on the egress system? Similar questions can be posed for other fire protection system components and subsystems.

### 5.5.4 Design Fire Scenarios Data.

**5.5.4.1** Each design fire scenario used in the performance-based design proposal shall be translated into input data specifications, as appropriate for the calculation method or model.

**5.5.4.2** Any design fire scenario specifications that the design analyses do not explicitly address or incorporate and that are, therefore, omitted from input data specifications shall be identified, and a sensitivity analysis of the consequences of that omission shall be performed.

Paragraph 5.5.4.2 is included to remind the designer that even if every design fire specification cannot be incorporated into a specific design tool or verification method, each must be addressed in the analysis in some manner. For example, an evacuation model that does not address crowding or queuing effects does not address the particular delay hazard initiated by Design Fire Scenario 2, which reduces the means of egress from the building. Additionally, many fire effects models do not address barrier breach, and, therefore, fail to incorporate the defining characteristics of Design Fire Scenario 4, a concealed space fire threatening an adjacent, occupied space.

Despite the fact that these models do not incorporate particular aspects of the design fire scenario specifications, those aspects must be addressed in the design, either through conservative assumptions supported by accepted technical resources or test data or by comparative techniques that will conservatively account for these effects. A sensitivity analysis should be performed on the omission of these aspects, as well as the techniques used to account for their omission.

**5.5.4.3** Any design fire scenario specifications modified in input data specifications, because of limitations in test methods or other data-generation procedures, shall be identified, and a sensitivity analysis of the consequences of the modification shall be performed.

Paragraph 5.5.4.3 essentially expresses the same concern as 5.5.4.2; however, the concern arises more from a limitation of available data than from a limitation of the model. Typically, both types of limitations will be present. When analyzing Design Fire Scenario 2, there may not be a model available that accounts for crowding or queuing, or there may be only a model that assumes uniform speeds and sizes of occupants due to lack of data on expected ranges of occupant characteristics. These effects will tend to produce results for an estimated speed of evacuation, in the absence of turbulence, that are unrealistically fast. Additionally, with regard to Design Fire Scenario 4, there may be no model to determine time to barrier breach and insufficient data on burn-through or failure behavior of the materials and assemblies proposed in the design.

## 5.6* Evaluation of Proposed Designs

**A.5.6** The *SFPE Engineering Guide to Performance-Based Fire Protection Analysis and Design of Buildings* outlines a process for evaluating whether trial designs meet the performance criteria during the design fire scenarios. Additional information on reviewing the evaluation of a performance-based design can be found in the *SFPE Enforcer's Guide to Performance-Based Design Review*.

The procedures described in Sections 5.2 and 5.4 identify required design fire scenarios among the design fire scenarios within which a proposed fire safety design is required to perform and the associated untenable conditions that are to be avoided in order to maintain life safety. Section 5.6 discusses methods that form the link from the scenarios and criteria to the goals and objectives.

Assessment methods are used to demonstrate that the proposed design will achieve the stated goals/objectives by providing information indicating that the performance criteria of Section 5.2 can be adequately met. Assessment methods are permitted to be either tests or modeling.

*Tests.* Test results can be directly used to assess a fire safety design when they accurately represent the scenarios developed by using Section 5.4 and provide output data matching the performance criteria in Section 5.2. Because the performance criteria for this *Code* are stated in terms of human exposure to lethal fire effects, no test will suffice. However, tests will be needed to produce data for use in models and other calculation methods.

*Standardized Tests.* Standardized tests are conducted on various systems and components to determine whether they meet some predetermined, typically prescriptive criteria. Results are given on a pass/fail basis — the test specimen either does or does not meet the pre-established criteria. The actual performance of the test specimen is not usually recorded.

*Scale.* Tests can be either small, intermediate, or full scale. Small-scale tests are used to test activation of detection and suppression devices and the flammability and toxicity of materials. Usually, the item to be tested is placed within the testing device or apparatus. Intermediate-scale tests can be used to determine the adequacy of system components — for example, doors and windows — as opposed to entire systems. The difference between small- and intermediate-scale tests is usually one of definition provided by those conducting the test. Full-scale tests are typically used to test building and structural components or entire systems. The difference between intermediate- and large-scale tests is also subject to the definition of those performing the test. Full-scale tests are intended to most closely depict performance of the test subject as installed in the field; that is, most closely represent real world performance.

Full-scale building evacuations can provide information on how the evacuation of a structure is likely to occur for an existing building with a given population without subjecting occupants to the real physical or psychological effects of a fire.

*Data Uses.* The data obtained from standardized tests have three uses for verification purposes. First, the test results can be used instead of a model. This use is typically the role of full-scale test results. Second, the test results can be used as a basis for validating the model. The model predictions match well with the test results. Therefore, the model can be used in situations similar to the test scenario. Third, the test results can be used as input to models. This is typically the use of small-scale tests, specifically flammability tests.

*Start-Up Test.* Start-up test results can be used to demonstrate that the fire safety system performs as designed. The system design might be based on modeling. If the start-up test indicates a deficiency, the system needs to be adjusted and retested until it can be demonstrated that the design can meet the performance criteria. Typically, start-up tests apply only to the installation to which they are designed.

*Experimental Data.* Experimental data from nonstandardized tests can be used when the specified scenario and the experimental setup are similar. Typically, experimental data are applicable to a greater variety of scenarios than are standardized test results.

*Human and Organizational Performance Tests.* Certain tests determine whether inputs used to determine human performance criteria remain valid during the occupancy of a building. Tests of human and organizational performance might include any of the following:

(1) Measuring evacuation times during fire drills
(2) Querying emergency response team members to determine whether they know required procedures
(3) Conducting field tests to ensure that emergency response team members can execute tasks within predetermined times and accuracy limits

Design proposals should include descriptions of any tests needed to determine whether stated goals, objectives, and performance criteria are being met.

*Modeling.* Models can be used to predict the performance criteria for a given scenario. Because of the limitations on using only tests for this purpose, models are expected to be used in most, if not all, performance-based design assessments.

The effect of fire and its toxic products on the occupants can be modeled, as can the movement and behavior of occupants during the fire. The term *evacuation model* will be used to describe models that predict the location and movements of occupants, and the term *tenability model* will be used to describe models that predict the effects on occupants of specified levels of exposure to fire effects.

*Types of Fire Models.* Fire models are used to predict fire-related performance criteria. Fire models can be either probabilistic or deterministic. Several types of deterministic models are available: computational fluid dynamics (CFD or field) models, zone models, purpose-built models, and hand calculations. Probabilistic fire models are also available but are less likely to be used for this purpose.

Probabilistic fire models use the probabilities as well as the severity of various events as the basis of evaluation. Some probabilistic models incorporate deterministic models, but are not required to do so. Probabilistic models attempt to predict the likelihood or probability that events or severity associated with an unwanted fire will occur, or they predict the "expected loss," which can be thought of as the probability-weighted average severity across all possible scenarios. Probabilistic models can be manifested as fault or event trees or other system models that use frequency or probability data as input. These models tend to be manifested as computer software, but are not required to do so. Furthermore, the discussion that follows under "Sources of Models" can also be applied to probabilistic models, although it concentrates on deterministic models.

CFD models can provide more accurate predictions than other deterministic models, because they divide a given space into many smaller volumes. However, since they are still models, they are not absolute in their depiction of reality. In addition, they are much more expensive to use, because they are computationally intensive. Because of their expense, complexity, and intensive computational needs, CFD models require much greater scrutiny than do zone models.

It is much easier to assess the sensitivity of different parameters with zone models, because they generally run much faster and the output is much easier to interpret. Prediction of fire growth and spread has a large number of variables associated with it.

Purpose-built models (also known as stand-alone models) are similar to zone models in their ease of use. However, purpose-built models do not provide a comprehensive model. Instead, they predict the value of one variable of interest. For example, such a model can predict the conditions of a ceiling jet at a specified location under a ceiling, but a zone model would "transport" those conditions throughout the enclosure.

Purpose-built models might or might not be manifested as computer software. Models that are not in the form of software are referred to as hand calculations. Purpose-built models are, therefore, simple enough that the data management capabilities of a computer are not necessary. Many of the calculations are found in the *SFPE Handbook of Fire Protection Engineering*.

*Types of Evacuation Models.* Four categories of evacuation models can be considered: single-parameter estimation methods, movement models, behavioral simulation models, and tenability models.

*Single-parameter estimation methods* are generally used for simple estimates of movement time. They are usually based on equations derived from observations of movement in nonemergency situations. They can be hand calculations or simple computer models. Examples include calculation methods for flow times based on widths of exit paths and travel times based on travel distances. Sources for these methods include the *SFPE Handbook of Fire Protection Engineering* and the NFPA *Fire Protection Handbook*.

*Movement models* generally handle large numbers of people in a network flow similar to water in pipes or ball bearings in chutes. They tend to optimize occupant behavior, resulting in predicted evacuation times that can be unrealistic and far from conservative. However, they can be useful in an overall assessment of a design, especially in early evaluation stages where an unacceptable result with this sort of model indicates that the design has failed to achieve the life safety objectives.

*Behavioral simulation models* take into consideration more of the variables related to occupant movement and behavior. Occupants are treated as individuals and can have unique characteristics assigned to them, allowing a more realistic simulation of the design under consideration. However, given the limited availability of data for the development of these models, for their verification by their authors, or for input when using them, their predictive reliability is questionable.

*Tenability Models.* In general, tenability models will be needed only to automate calculations for the time-of-exposure effect equations referenced in A.5.2.2.

*Other Models.* Models can be used to describe combustion (as noted, most fire models only characterize fire effects), automatic system performance, and other elements of the calculation. There are few models in common use for these purposes, so they are not further described here.

*Sources of Models.* A compendia of computer fire models are found in the *SFPE Computer Software Directory* and in Olenick, S. and Carpenter, D., "An Updated International Survey of Computer Models for Fire and Smoke," *Journal of Fire Protection Engineering*, 13, 2, 2003, pp. 87–110. Within these references are models that were developed by the Building Fire Research Laboratory of the National Institute of Standards and Technology, which can be downloaded from the Internet at http://www.bfrl.nist.gov/864/fmabs.html. Evacuation models are discussed in the *SFPE Handbook of Fire Protection Engineering* and the NFPA *Fire Protection Handbook.*

*Validation.* Models undergo limited validation. Most can be considered demonstrated only for the experimental results they were based on or the limited set of scenarios to which the model developers compared the model's output, or a combination of both.

The Society of Fire Protection Engineers has a task group that independently evaluates computer models. In January 1998, they finished their first evaluation and had chosen a second model for evaluation. Until more models can be independently evaluated, the model user has to rely on the available documentation and previous experience for guidance regarding the appropriate use of a given model.

The design professional should present the proposal, and the authority having jurisdiction, when deciding whether to approve a proposal, should consider the strength of the evidence presented for the validity, accuracy, relevance, and precision of the proposed methods. An element in establishing the strength of scientific evidence is the extent of external review and acceptance of the evidence by peers of the authors of that evidence.

Models have limitations. Most are not user friendly, and experienced users are able to construct more reasonable models and better interpret output than are novices. For these reasons, the third-party review and equivalency provisions of 5.1.4 and 5.3.3 are provided. The intent is not to discourage the use of models, only to indicate that they should be used with caution by those who are well versed in their nuances.

*Input Data.* The first step in using a model is to develop the input data. The heat release rate curve specified by the user is the driving force of a fire effects model. If this curve is incorrectly defined, the subsequent results are not usable. In addition to the smoldering and growth phases that will be specified as part of the scenario definition, two additional phases are needed to complete the input heat release rate curve — steady burning and burnout.

Steady burning is characterized by its duration, which is a function of the total amount of fuel available to be burned. In determining the duration of this phase, the designer needs to consider how much fuel has been assumed to be consumed in the smoldering and growth phases and how much is assumed to be consumed in the burnout phase that follows. Depending on the assumptions made regarding the amount of fuel consumed during burnout, the time at which this phase starts is likely to be easy to determine.

The preceding discussion assumes that the burning objects are solid (for example, tables and chairs). If liquid or gaseous fuels are involved, the shape of the curve will be different. For example, smoldering is not relevant for burning liquids or gases, and the growth period is very short, typically measured in seconds. Peak heat release rate can depend primarily on the rate of release, on the leak rate (gases and liquid sprays), or on the extent of spill (pooled liquids). The steady burning phase is once again dependent on the amount of fuel available to burn. Like the growth phase, the burnout phase is typically short (for example, closing a valve), although it is conceivable that longer times might be appropriate, depending on the extinguishment scenario.

Material properties are usually needed for all fuel items, both initial and secondary, and the enclosure surfaces of involved rooms or spaces.

For all fires of consequence, it is reasonable to assume that the fire receives adequate ventilation. If there is insufficient oxygen, the fire will not be sustained. An overabundance of oxygen is only a concern in special cases (for example, hermetically sealed spaces) when a fire might not occur due to dilution of the fuel (that is, a flammable mixture is not produced). Therefore, given that the scenarios of interest will occur in nonhermetically sealed enclosures, it is reasonable to assume that adequate ventilation is available and that, if a fire starts, it will continue to burn until it either runs out of fuel or is extinguished by other means. The only variable that might need to be assumed is the total vent width.

Maximum fire extent is affected by two geometric aspects: burning object proximity to walls and overall enclosure dimensions.

The room dimensions affect the time required for a room to flashover. For a given amount and type of fuel, under the same ventilation conditions, a small room will flashover before a large room. In a large room with a small amount of fuel, a fire will behave as if it is burning outside — that is, adequate oxygen for burning and no concentration of heat exist. If the fuel package is unchanged but the dimensions of the room are decreased, the room will begin to have an affect on the fire, assuming adequate ventilation. The presence of the relatively smaller enclosure results in the buildup of a hot layer of smoke and other products of combustion under the ceiling. This buildup, in turn, feeds more heat back to the seat of the fire, which results in an increase in the pyrolysis rate of the fuel and, thus, increases the amount of heat energy released by the fire. The room enclosure surfaces themselves also contribute to this radiation feedback effect.

Probabilistic data are expressed as either a frequency (units of inverse time) or a probability (unitless, but applicable to a stated period of time). An example of the former is the expected number of failures per year and the range of the latter is between zero and one, inclusive. Probabilities can be either objective or subjective. Subjective probabilities express a degree of belief that an event will occur. Objective probabilities are based on historical data and can be expressed as a reliability of an item, such as a component or a system.

### 5.6.1 General.

A proposed design's performance shall be assessed relative to each performance objective in Section 4.2 and each applicable scenario in 5.5.3, with the assessment conducted through the use of appropriate calculation methods. The authority having jurisdiction shall approve the choice of assessment methods.

The verification process starts with the submittal of a proposed design to the authority having jurisdiction. If the AHJ does not consider itself qualified to perform an adequate review of the performance-based design, the AHJ might specify a qualified third-party reviewer. The owner typically incurs the expense associated with the third-party review process.

The first step of the verification process is to identify the goals and the objectives relating to those goals. Attention must be paid to both those objectives that apply to the facility as a whole and those that apply only to limited aspects of the facility. The AHJ's purpose in this review is to determine whether the designer/owner's objectives are commensurate with the community's objectives. Next, the AHJ reviews the performance criteria that relate to each of the objectives for consistency and reasonableness. Do the objectives form a comprehensive package? Are they realistic? The next step involves the characteristics of that which is being protected — people, property, and so on. Once again, a comprehensive, cohesive set of assumptions is sought.

Essentially, the verification process ensures that the logic flow and justification for the choices made are sound; the links between the components are checked to ensure that the design process flows — objectives are to be met by demonstrating that criteria have been achieved through the judicious use of verification methods. Assumptions need to be reasonable, consistent, comprehensive, cohesive, and supported by adequate references.

Presumably, the designer's proposal ensures that all criteria are met for all scenarios. Ultimately, the AHJ is interested in determining whether the designer did a credible job so that the predicted results provide a sufficient margin of safety to allow the design to be approved. Because of the complexity involved in determining credibility, many discussions can be anticipated between the AHJ, the designer, and, if used, the third-party reviewer.

### 5.6.2 Use.

The design professional shall use the assessment methods to demonstrate that the proposed design will achieve the goals and objectives, as measured by the performance criteria in light of the safety margins and uncertainty analysis, for each scenario, given the assumptions.

The choice of which model to select depends on the objectives, the performance criteria to be predicted, and the scenarios to be considered. The model selected should use most, if not all, of the input data specifications and must produce design output that can be directly compared to the performance criteria selected as a baseline for the analysis. Two criteria are usually of greatest interest: the upper layer temperature and the height of the smoke layer interface. If the objective is to reduce property damage in a telephone vault, then a purpose-built model that predicts smoke filling is adequate. If the objective is the life safety of those not intimate with the fire — both within the room of origin and along adjacent egress paths — in a rectilinear room, then a zone model is adequate. If life safety is the objective and the fire occurs in a more geometrically challenging configuration (e.g., an amusement park fun house or enclosed amusement ride), then a field model is appropriate. If the effects on occupants are to be estimated, an evacuation or toxicity model needs to be used.

### 5.6.3 Input Data.

**5.6.3.1 Data.** Input data for computer fire models shall be obtained in accordance with ASTM E 1591, *Standard Guide for Obtaining Data for Deterministic Fire Models.* Data for use in analytical models that are not computer-based fire models shall be obtained using appropriate measurement, recording, and storage techniques to ensure the applicability of the data to the analytical method being used.

**5.6.3.2 Data Requirements.** A complete listing of input data requirements for all models, engineering methods, and other calculation or verification methods required or proposed as part of the performance-based design shall be provided.

Documentation of the assumptions made by the model user while developing the input data is critical. If the model user does not explicitly state the values used and the references from which they are taken, the credibility of the analysis is decreased.

**5.6.3.3* Uncertainty and Conservatism of Data.** Uncertainty in input data shall be analyzed and, as determined appropriate by the authority having jurisdiction, addressed through the use of conservative values.

**A.5.6.3.3** Procedures used to develop required input data need to preserve the intended conservatism of all scenarios and assumptions. Conservatism is only one means to address the uncertainty inherent in calculations and does not eliminate the need to consider safety factors, sensitivity analysis, and other methods of dealing with uncertainty. The *SFPE Engineering Guide to Performance-Based Fire Protection Analysis and Design of Buildings* outlines a process for identifying and treating uncertainty.

### 5.6.4* Output Data.

The assessment methods used shall accurately and appropriately produce the required output data from input data, based on the design specifications, assumptions, and scenarios.

**A.5.6.4** An assessment method translates input data, which might include test specifications, parameters, or variables for modeling, or other data, into output data, which are measured against the performance criteria. Computer fire models should be evaluated for their predictive capability in accordance with ASTM E 1355, *Standard Guide for Evaluating the Predictive Capability of Deterministic Fire Models*.

The design team selects verification methods that produce output data that can be directly compared to the performance criteria. Any additional output data needs to be included with the analysis results and submitted to the authority having jurisdiction for review.

### 5.6.5 Validity.

Evidence shall be provided to confirm that the assessment methods are valid and appropriate for the proposed building, use, and conditions.

If the chosen assessment method is a computer model, then the validity of the model, with regard to the scenario being modeled, might be in question. By choosing a particular model, the designer is tacitly assuming that the model is valid for the particular scenario. Two situations are possible: either the assumption is correct (and there's nothing to worry about) or the assumption is not correct. If the assumption is not correct, this does not immediately invalidate the entire analysis. Part of the argument for using a particular model is that it is the only tool available (i.e., choice is constrained by the available resources) that can be used. If a sensitivity analysis is also performed, this will go a long way in demonstrating that a range of conditions has been considered and the "real" answer has been adequately bounded by the results of the sensitivity analysis.

## 5.7* Safety Factors

Approved safety factors shall be included in the design methods and calculations to reflect uncertainty in the assumptions, data, and other factors associated with the performance-based design.

**A.5.7** The assessment of precision required in 5.8.2 will require a sensitivity and uncertainty analysis, which can be translated into safety factors.

*Sensitivity Analysis.* The first run a model user makes should be labeled as the base case, using the nominal values of the various input parameters. However, the model user should not rely on a single run as the basis for any performance-based fire safety system design. Ideally, each variable or parameter that the model user made to develop the nominal input data should have multiple runs associated with it, as should combinations of key variables and parameters. Thus, a sensitivity analysis should be conducted that provides the model user with data that indicate how the effects of a real fire might vary and how the response of the proposed fire safety design might also vary.

The interpretation of a model's predictions can be a difficult exercise if the model user does not have knowledge of fire dynamics or human behavior.

In addition to justification of the base case input data specification values, the design team should include an allowable range of values determined using a sensitivity analysis. The design team should investigate the effects of varying key components and variables independently and in combination and should document the effects of this variation.

*Reasonableness Check.* The model user should first try to determine whether the predictions actually make sense; that is, whether they do not upset intuition or preconceived expectations. Most likely, if the results do not pass this test, an input error has been committed.

Sometimes the predictions appear to be reasonable but are, in fact, incorrect. For example, a model can predict higher temperatures farther from the fire than closer to it. The values themselves might be reasonable; for example, they are not hotter than the fire, but they do not "flow" down the energy as expected.

A margin of safety can be developed using the results of the sensitivity analysis in conjunction with the performance criteria to provide the possible range of time during which a condition is estimated to occur.

Safety factors and margin of safety are two concepts used to quantify the amount of uncertainty in engineering analyses. Safety factors are used to provide a margin of safety and represent, or address, the gap in knowledge between the theoretically perfect model — reality — and the engineering models that can only partially represent reality.

Safety factors can be applied either to the predicted level of a physical condition or to the time at which the condition is predicted to occur. Thus, a physical or a temporal safety factor, or both, can be applied to any predicted condition. A predicted condition (that is, a parameter's value) and the time at which it occurs are best represented as distributions. Ideally, a computer fire model predicts the expected or nominal value of the distribution. Safety factors are intended to represent the spread of the distributions.

Given the uncertainty associated with data acquisition and reduction, and the limitations of computer modeling, any condition predicted by a computer model can be thought of as an expected or nominal value within a broader range. For example, an upper layer temperature of 1110°F (600°C) is predicted at a given time. If the modeled scenario is then tested (that is, full-scale experiment based on the computer model's input data), the actual temperature at that given time could be 1185°F or 1085°F (640°C or 585°C). Therefore, the temperature should be reported as 1110°F + 75°F/−25°F (600°C + 40°C/−15°C) or as a range of 1085°F to 1185°F (585°C to 640°C).

Ideally, predictions are reported as a nominal value, a percentage, or an absolute value. As an example, an upper layer temperature prediction could be reported as "1110°F (600°C), 55°F (30°C)" or "1110°F (600°C), 5 percent." In this case, the physical safety factor is 0.05 (i.e., the amount by which the nominal value should be degraded and enhanced). Given the state-of-the-art of computer fire modeling, this is a very low safety factor. Physical safety factors tend to be on the order of tens of percent. A safety factor of 50 percent is not unheard of.

Part of the problem in establishing safety factors is that it is difficult to state the percentage or range that is appropriate. These values can be obtained when the computer model predictions are compared to test data. However, using computer fire models in a design mode does not facilitate this comparison, due to the following:

(1) The room being analyzed has not been built yet.
(2) Test scenarios do not necessarily depict the intended design.

A sensitivity analysis should be performed, based on the assumptions that affect the condition of interest. A base case that uses all nominal values for input parameters should be developed. The input parameters should be varied over reasonable ranges, and the variation in predicted output should be noted. This output variation can then become the basis for physical safety factors.

The temporal safety factor addresses the issue of when a condition is predicted and is a function of the rate at which processes are expected to occur. If a condition is predicted to occur 2 minutes after the start of the fire, this prediction can be used as a nominal value. A process similar to that already described for physical safety factors can also be employed to develop temporal safety factors. In such a case, however, the rates (e.g., rates of heat release and toxic product generation) will be varied instead of absolute values (e.g., material properties).

The margin of safety can be thought of as a reflection of societal values and can be imposed by the authority having jurisdiction for that purpose. Because the time for which a condition is predicted will most likely be the focus of the authority having jurisdiction (e.g., the model predicts that occupants will have 5 minutes to safely evacuate), the margin of safety will be characterized by temporal aspects and tacitly applied to the physical margin of safety.

Escaping the harmful effects of fire (or mitigating them) is, effectively, a race against time. When assessing fire safety system designs based on computer model predictions, the choice of an acceptable time is important. When an authority having jurisdiction is faced with the predicted time of untenability, a decision needs to be made regarding whether sufficient time is available to ensure the safety of building occupants. The authority having jurisdiction is assessing the margin of safety. Is there sufficient time to get everyone out safely? If the authority having jurisdiction feels that the predicted egress time is too close to the time of untenability, the authority having jurisdiction can impose an additional period of time that the designer will have to incorporate into the system design. In other words, the authority having jurisdiction can impose a greater margin of safety than that originally proposed by the designer.

## 5.8 Documentation Requirements

### 5.8.1* General.

All aspects of the design, including those described in 5.8.2 through 5.8.14, shall be documented. The format and content of the documentation shall be acceptable to the authority having jurisdiction.

**A.5.8.1** The *SFPE Engineering Guide to Performance-Based Fire Protection Analysis and Design of Buildings* describes the documentation that should be provided for a performance-based design.

Proper documentation of a performance-based design is critical to design acceptance and construction. Proper documentation will also ensure that all parties involved understand the factors necessary for the implementation, maintenance, and continuity of the fire protection design. If attention to details is maintained in the documentation, there should be little dispute during approval, construction, start-up, and use.

Poor documentation could result in rejection of an otherwise good design, poor implementation of the design, inadequate system maintenance and reliability, and an incomplete record for future changes or for testing the design forensically.

### 5.8.2* Technical References and Resources.

The authority having jurisdiction shall be provided with sufficient documentation to support the validity, accuracy, relevance, and precision of the proposed methods. The engineering standards, calculation methods, and other forms of scientific information provided shall be appropriate for the particular application and methodologies used.

**A.5.8.2** The sources, methodologies, and data used in performance-based designs should be based on technical references that are widely accepted and used by the appropriate professions and professional groups. This acceptance is often based on documents that are developed, reviewed, and validated under one of the following processes:

(1) Standards developed under an open consensus process conducted by recognized professional societies, codes or standards organizations, or governmental bodies
(2) Technical references that are subject to a peer review process and published in widely recognized peer-reviewed journals, conference reports, or other publications
(3) Resource publications, such as the *SFPE Handbook of Fire Protection Engineering*, which are widely recognized technical sources of information

The following factors are helpful in determining the acceptability of the individual method or source:

(1) Extent of general acceptance in the relevant professional community, including peer-reviewed publication, widespread citation in the technical literature, and adoption by or within a consensus document
(2) Extent of documentation of the method, including the analytical method itself, assumptions, scope, limitations, data sources, and data reduction methods
(3) Extent of validation and analysis of uncertainties, including comparison of the overall method with experimental data to estimate error rates, as well as analysis of the uncertainties of input data, uncertainties and limitations in the analytical method, and uncertainties in the associated performance criteria
(4) Extent to which the method is based on sound scientific principles
(5) Extent to which the proposed application is within the stated scope and limitations of the supporting information, including the range of applicability for which there is documented validation, and considering factors such as spatial dimensions, occupant characteristics, and ambient conditions, which can limit valid applications

In many cases, a method will be built from, and will include, numerous component analyses. Such component analyses should be evaluated using the same acceptability factors that are applied to the overall method, as outlined in items (1) through (5).

A method to address a specific fire safety issue, within documented limitations or validation regimes, might not exist. In such a case, sources and calculation methods can be used outside of their limitations, provided that the design team recognizes the limitations and addresses the resulting implications.

The technical references and methodologies to be used in a performance-based design should be closely evaluated by the design team and the authority having jurisdiction, and possibly by a third-party reviewer. The strength of the technical justification should be judged using criteria in items (1) through (5). This justification can be strengthened by the presence of data obtained from fire testing.

### 5.8.3 Building Design Specifications.

All details of the proposed building design that affect the ability of the building to meet the stated goals and objectives shall be documented.

### 5.8.4 Performance Criteria.

Performance criteria, with sources, shall be documented.

### 5.8.5 Occupant Characteristics.

Assumptions about occupant characteristics shall be documented.

### 5.8.6 Design Fire Scenarios.

Descriptions of design fire scenarios shall be documented.

### 5.8.7 Input Data.

Input data to models and assessment methods, including sensitivity analyses, shall be documented.

### 5.8.8 Output Data.

Output data from models and assessment methods, including sensitivity analyses, shall be documented.

### 5.8.9 Safety Factors.

The safety factors utilized shall be documented.

### 5.8.10 Prescriptive Requirements.

Retained prescriptive requirements shall be documented.

### 5.8.11* Modeling Features.

**A.5.8.11** Documentation for modeling should conform to ASTM E 1472, *Standard Guide for Documenting Computer Software for Fire Models*, although most, if not all, models were originally developed before this standard was promulgated. Information regarding the use of the model DETACT-QS can be found in the *SFPE Engineering Guide–the Evaluation of the Computer Fire Model DETACT-QS*.

**5.8.11.1** Assumptions made by the model user, and descriptions of models and methods used, including known limitations, shall be documented.

**5.8.11.2** Documentation shall be provided to verify that the assessment methods have been used validly and appropriately to address the design specifications, assumptions, and scenarios.

### 5.8.12 Evidence of Modeler Capability.

The design team's relevant experience with the models, test methods, databases, and other assessment methods used in the performance-based design proposal shall be documented.

### 5.8.13 Performance Evaluation.

The performance evaluation summary shall be documented.

### 5.8.14 Use of Performance-Based Design Option.

Design proposals shall include documentation that provides anyone involved in the ownership or management of the building with notification of the following:

(1) Approval of the building as a performance-based design with certain specified design criteria and assumptions
(2) Need for required re-evaluation and reapproval in cases of remodeling, modification, renovation, change in use, or change in established assumptions

## References Cited in Commentary

1. NFPA 13, *Standard for the Installation of Sprinkler Systems*, 2007 edition, National Fire Protection Association, Quincy, MA.
2. *NFPA 72®, National Fire Alarm Code®*, 2007 edition, National Fire Protection Association, Quincy, MA.
3. NFPA 90A, *Standard for the Installation of Air-Conditioning and Ventilating Systems*, 2009 edition, National Fire Protection Association, Quincy, MA.
4. ASME A17.1/CSA B44, *Safety Code for Elevators and Escalators*, American Society of Mechanical Engineers, New York, NY, 2007.
5. Cote, A. E., ed., NFPA *Fire Protection Handbook*, 20th edition, National Fire Protection Association, Quincy, MA, 2008.
6. DiNenno, P. J., ed., *SFPE Handbook of Fire Protection Engineering*, 3rd edition, National Fire Protection Association, Quincy, MA, 2002.
7. Drysdale, D., *An Introduction to Fire Dynamics*, 2nd ed., John Wiley & Sons, Chichester, UK, 1999.
8. Caro, T. and Milke, J., NIST-GCR-96-697, "A Survey of Fuel Loads in Contemporary Office Buildings," Gaithersburg, MD: National Institute of Standards and Technology, September 1996.
9. Proulx, G., "Evacuation Time and Movement in Apartment Buildings," *Fire Safety Journal*, 24, No. 3 (1995), 229–246.
10. Proulx, G. and Fahy, R., "The Time Delay to Start Evacuation: Review of Five Case Studies," *Proceedings of the Fifth International Symposium on Fire Safety Science*, International Association for Fire Safety Science, 1997.
11. Fruin, J. J., *Pedestrian Planning and Design*, ed. George R. Strakosch, Metropolitan Association of Urban Designers and Environmental Planners, Inc., New York, 1987.
12. Klem, T., "Investigation Report on the Dupont Plaza Hotel Fire, San Juan, Puerto Rico, December 31, 1986," NFPA LS-11, 1987.

CHAPTER 6

# Classification of Occupancy and Hazard of Contents

Chapter 6 addresses the following considerations needed for accurately determining which *Code* provisions apply to a specific building:

1. Classification of occupancy
2. Choice of treating multiple occupancies as either mixed occupancies or separated occupancies
3. Categorization of the relative hazard presented by the contents or use of the building

Proper classification of the occupancy is crucial; since the *Code* is not a "one size fits all" document, the selection of the proper occupancy is of paramount importance to ensure that the correct chapters and sections of the *Code* are used. The occupancy classification scheme uses general descriptions of each occupancy (e.g., assembly, educational, day-care, or health care). The annex text that accompanies each of the occupancy classifications provides lists of the most common building uses for each classification.

Occupancy classification of a building often encompasses more than one category. It is common for multiple occupancy types to coexist within a single building. For example, a hotel often consists of a multiple occupancy that includes hotel, assembly, mercantile, and business occupancies. Paragraph 6.1.14.1.1 permits multiple occupancies to be treated as either mixed occupancies or separated occupancies. An office building with a newsstand and sundries shop located off the main lobby might be classified wholly as a business occupancy by considering the mercantile use as incidental to the predominant business use as permitted by 6.1.14.1.3(1), thus avoiding the provisions applicable to a multiple occupancy.

Hazard of contents, as addressed in Section 6.2, describes the relative hazard associated with the contents and operational aspects of the building. *Hazard of contents* is a relative term that is used to describe the potential threat to occupants from a fire that occurs in building contents in a given occupancy type.

## 6.1 Classification of Occupancy

Each of the occupancy groupings addressed by Chapter 6 was developed to reflect the design features, usage patterns, and unique life safety needs of occupants who are characteristic of a given occupancy. This approach was used to assess the degree to which the features contained in the core chapters need to be combined to achieve the minimum level of life safety necessary for an occupancy. It is extremely important that the correct occupancy classification be made, because the *Code* requirements differ for each type of occupancy. Improper classification might result in an inadequate level of life safety or overspending on nonrequired items. The occupancy groupings are as follows:

**1.** *Assembly.* Assembly occupancies generally contain large numbers of people who are unfamiliar with the space and are, therefore, subject to indecision regarding the best means of egress in an emergency.

**2.** *Educational.* Educational occupancies primarily include the large numbers of young people found in school buildings.

**3.** *Day-care.* Day-care occupancies contain both young and adult clients who are under the supervision of adults other than their relatives or legal guardians. In cases where day-care occupancies cater to preschool age children, the occupants might need to be carried out of the facility during evacuation.

**4.** *Health care.* Health care occupancies are characterized by occupants who are incapable of self-preservation and occupy the occupancy on an inpatient basis. For occupancies that provide health care services on an outpatient basis, see the description that follows on ambulatory health care occupancies. In a health care occupancy, the occupants may not be able to use exits, regardless of the number of exits provided. Occupants might be immobile, connected to monitoring equipment, debilitated, or recovering from surgery; or they might be disabled in some other way. The *Code,* in this instance, calls for a defend-in-place design strategy that uses horizontal movement and compartmentation. It recognizes that the occupants are to be provided enough protection to enable them to survive the fire by remaining in the structure, at least temporarily.

**5.** *Ambulatory health care.* Ambulatory health care occupancies are similar to health care occupancies in that the occupants are generally incapable of self-preservation, but, unlike health care occupancies, the patients receive medical care on an outpatient basis. In many cases, the treatment causes the patient to be incapable of self-preservation. In other cases, a procedure, such as administering general anesthesia that is needed in conjunction with a treatment, renders the patient incapable of self-preservation. In yet other cases, the patient arrives at the ambulatory health care facility incapable of self-preservation due to an injury or illness, as is common in an emergency or urgent care outpatient facility. The ambulatory health care occupancy operates on an outpatient basis, so no individual patient occupies the building for a period of 24 hours or more.

**6.** *Detention and correctional.* Detention and correctional occupancies, as in the case of health care occupancies, house occupants who are incapable of self-preservation. In a detention and correctional occupancy, however, the incapability for self-preservation is due to the security imposed on the occupants. Because doors are not unlocked to allow free egress to the public way, the defend-in-place design strategy is used.

**7.** *Residential.* Residential occupancies are characterized by occupants who are asleep for a portion of the time they occupy the building. The sleeping that takes place is for normal restorative rest, as opposed to the sleeping that takes place in a hospital or residential board and care facility where caretakers are present. Sleeping occupants might be unaware of an incipient fire and might be trapped before egress can occur, thus creating a need for early warning smoke alarms. This occupancy group is further divided into one- and two-family dwellings, lodging or rooming houses, hotels and dormitories, and apartment buildings. Each occupancy in the group has characteristic needs that differ from the others. For this reason, separate chapters of the *Code* address each of these subgroups.

**8.** *Residential board and care.* Residential board and care occupancies, as in the case of residential occupancies, provide sleeping accommodations. However, the residents also receive personal care services by caretakers who live with the residents. Personal care includes assistance with many of the activities of daily living, such as bathing and dressing. Personal care does not include medical care.

**9.** *Mercantile.* Mercantile occupancies, as in the case of assembly occupancies, are characterized by large numbers of people who gather in a space that is relatively unfamiliar to them. In addition, mercantile occupancies often contain sizable quantities of combustible contents and use circuitous egress paths that are deliberately arranged to force occupants to travel around displays of materials that are available for sale.

**10.** *Business.* Business occupancies generally have a lower occupant density than mercantile occupancies, and the occupants are usually more familiar with their surroundings. However, confusing and indirect egress paths are often developed due to office layouts and the arrangement of tenant spaces. The *Code* requirements for such occupancies address the needs of visitors unfamiliar with the building.

**11.** *Industrial.* Industrial occupancies expose occupants to a wide range of processes and materials of varying hazard. Special-purpose industrial occupancies, which are characterized by large installations of equipment that dominate the space, are addressed separately from general-purpose industrial facilities, which have higher densities of human occupancy.

**12.** *Storage.* Storage occupancies are characterized by relatively low human occupancy in comparison to building size and by varied hazards associated with the materials stored.

### 6.1.1 General.

**6.1.1.1 Occupancy Classification.** The occupancy of a building or structure, or portion of a building or structure, shall be classified in accordance with 6.1.2 through 6.1.13. Occupancy classification shall be subject to the ruling of the authority having jurisdiction where there is a question of proper classification in any individual case.

Because the appropriate occupancy classification is not always easily determined, the *Code* assigns the authority having jurisdiction the responsibility of determining whether the designer, owner's representative, or other applicable person has correctly classified the occupancy.

**6.1.1.2 Special Structures.** Occupancies in special structures shall conform to the requirements of the specific occupancy chapter, Chapters 12 through 43, except as modified by Chapter 11.

The provision of 6.1.1.2 clarifies that placing an occupancy in a special structure — such as a limited access, underground, water-surrounded, or high-rise building — does not create a unique occupancy. Rather, the occupancy is classified as one of those addressed by Chapters 12 through 42. Chapter 11 is then consulted to identify any permitted modifications that apply to the special structure.

### 6.1.2 Assembly.

For requirements, see Chapters 12 and 13.

**6.1.2.1* Definition — Assembly Occupancy.** An occupancy (1) used for a gathering of 50 or more persons for deliberation, worship, entertainment, eating, drinking, amusement, awaiting transportation, or similar uses; or (2) used as a special amusement building, regardless of occupant load.

**A.6.1.2.1 Assembly Occupancy.** Assembly occupancies might include the following:

(1) Armories
(2) Assembly halls
(3) Auditoriums
(4) Bowling lanes
(5) Club rooms
(6) College and university classrooms, 50 persons and over
(7) Conference rooms
(8) Courtrooms
(9) Dance halls
(10) Drinking establishments
(11) Exhibition halls
(12) Gymnasiums
(13) Libraries
(14) Mortuary chapels
(15) Motion picture theaters
(16) Museums
(17) Passenger stations and terminals of air, surface, underground, and marine public transportation facilities
(18) Places of religious worship
(19) Pool rooms
(20) Recreation piers
(21) Restaurants
(22) Skating rinks
(23) Special amusement buildings, regardless of occupant load
(24) Theaters

Assembly occupancies are characterized by the presence or potential presence of crowds with attendant panic hazard in case of fire or other emergency. They are generally or occasionally open to the public, and the occupants, who are present voluntarily, are not ordinarily subject to discipline or control. Such buildings are ordinarily not used for sleeping purposes. Special conference rooms, snack areas, and other areas incidental to, and under the control of, the management of other occupancies, such as offices, fall under the 50-person limitation.

Restaurants and drinking establishments with an occupant load of fewer than 50 persons should be classified as mercantile occupancies.

Occupancy of any room or space for assembly purposes by fewer than 50 persons in another occupancy, and incidental to such other occupancy, should be classified as part of the other occupancy and should be subject to the provisions applicable thereto.

For special amusement buildings, see 12.4.7 and 13.4.7.

**6.1.2.2 Other. (Reserved)**

The definition of *assembly occupancy* in 6.1.2.1(1) is an example of an occupancy classification definition that utilizes thresholds that must be met in order to fall into the occupancy classification described. In the case of assembly occupancies, the thresholds relate to number of occupants and use of the space. Both the occupant number and use thresholds must be met [except for special amusement buildings, as addressed in item (2) of 6.1.2.1, for which the number of occupants is not germane] in order to create an assembly occupancy. For example, the situation where 40 persons gather for entertainment fits one of the listed assembly use criteria but not the minimum 50-person criterion, so such assemblage of persons is not an assembly occupancy. Similarly, the situation where 60 persons occupy work cubicles in an office setting fits the minimum 50-person criterion but not any of the assembly use criteria, so such assemblage of persons is not an assembly occupancy.

Item (2) of 6.1.2.1 clarifies that a special amusement building is an assembly occupancy, even if the occupant load is fewer than 50 persons. If this were not the case, the house of horror amusement building at a carnival, for example, could be treated as a business occupancy, because it does not have the minimum

50-person occupant load typically associated with an assembly occupancy, and the necessary level of life safety might not be provided. As an assembly occupancy, a special amusement building is subject to the provisions of Chapter 12 or Chapter 13. Because such buildings purposely confound the egress path and further confuse the occupants with sound and lighting effects, they need to meet the special requirements of 12.4.7 or 13.4.7.

For other than special amusement buildings, the threshold at which an assembly use becomes an assembly occupancy is the 50-person occupant load.

There is no *Code*-sanctioned occupancy called a *small assembly occupancy*. An occupancy used for the purposes in item (1) of 6.1.2.1 either is or is not an assembly occupancy based on the 50-person criterion [except for special amusement buildings, as addressed in item (2) of 6.1.2.1]. As the fourth paragraph of A.6.1.2.1 advises, small assembly uses are considered part of the predominant occupancy [see 6.1.14.1.3(2)]. Except for special amusement buildings, as addressed in item (2) of 6.1.2.1, there are no assembly occupancies with occupant loads fewer than 50 persons.

### 6.1.3 Educational.

For requirements, see Chapters 14 and 15.

**6.1.3.1* Definition — Educational Occupancy.** An occupancy used for educational purposes through the twelfth grade by six or more persons for 4 or more hours per day or more than 12 hours per week.

**A.6.1.3.1 Educational Occupancy.** Educational occupancies include the following:

(1) Academies
(2) Kindergartens
(3) Schools

An educational occupancy is distinguished from an assembly occupancy in that the same occupants are regularly present.

**6.1.3.2 Other Occupancies.** Other occupancies associated with educational institutions shall be in accordance with the appropriate parts of this *Code*.

**6.1.3.3 Incidental Instruction.** In cases where instruction is incidental to some other occupancy, the section of this *Code* governing such other occupancy shall apply.

An elementary school classroom used for the requisite hours detailed in 6.1.3.1, with an occupant load of 50 or more, is classified as an educational occupancy, not an assembly occupancy. The assembly occupancy criteria of 6.1.2.1 involve not just the minimum 50-person criterion but also the use criterion of gathering for deliberation, worship, entertainment, eating, drinking, amusement, awaiting transportation, or similar use. See 14.2.5.4 and 15.2.5.4, which require a second exit access door from any educational occupancy room with an occupant load of more than 50 persons.

Educational occupancies are limited to facilities used for educational purposes through the twelfth grade. A college classroom does not meet this criterion and is classified as a business occupancy or, where the college classroom has an occupant load of 50 or more, as an assembly occupancy.

Incidental instruction, as addressed in 6.1.3.3, conducted in some other occupancy is permitted to be considered part of that other occupancy and is subject to the provisions applicable to such other occupancy. For example, a developer of learning software might have a test lab where students, under the direction of teaching specialists, test the effectiveness of such software. The laboratory experience does not substitute for the students' normal schooling. The instruction is incidental to the building functioning as a business occupancy. The occupancy is classified as a business occupancy and is subject to the provisions of Chapter 38 or Chapter 39.

### 6.1.4 Day Care.

For requirements, see Chapters 16 and 17.

**6.1.4.1* Definition — Day-Care Occupancy.** An occupancy in which four or more clients receive care, maintenance, and supervision, by other than their relatives or legal guardians, for less than 24 hours per day.

**A.6.1.4.1 Day-Care Occupancy.** Day-care occupancies include the following:

(1) Adult day-care occupancies, except where part of a health care occupancy
(2) Child day-care occupancies
(3) Day-care homes
(4) Kindergarten classes that are incidental to a child day-care occupancy
(5) Nursery schools

In areas where public schools offer only half-day kindergarten programs, many child day-care occupancies offer state-approved kindergarten classes for children who need full-day care. As these classes are normally incidental to the day-care occupancy, the requirements of the day-care occupancy should be followed.

**6.1.4.2 Other. (Reserved)**

Day-care occupancies have some similarities to educational occupancies. However, in lieu of educational activity with classroom occupants and teachers, there are activities with clients and staff, with staff serving as caretakers. The clients of a day-care occupancy might be adults. It has become fairly common for elderly adults to attend a day-care facility.

The provision of 6.1.14.1.3(2) permits a nonresidential use with an occupant load fewer than that established by Section 6.1 for the occupancy threshold to be considered part of the predominant occupancy where such nonresidential use is incidental to the predominant occupancy. Consider a day-care center for 10 clients where such center occupies less than 1000 $ft^2$ (93 $m^2$) in a 100,000 $ft^2$ (9300 $m^2$) office building. The day-care center is a nonresidential use. The occupancy threshold for day-care occupancy classification is four or more clients per 6.1.4.1. The day-care center occupies less than 1 percent of the building area, but it cannot be considered incidental to the business use. Per 6.1.4.1 and 6.1.14.1.3(2), it must be classified as a day-care occupancy. Thus, the building is classified as a multiple occupancy comprised of both a business occupancy and a day-care occupancy. The building must meet the provisions of 6.1.14, including protection as either separated occupancies or mixed occupancies. In other words, the provisions for day-care occupancies must be applied, even though the day-care center is small in comparison to the remainder of the building. Otherwise, the day-care clients would not be adequately protected.

### 6.1.5 Health Care.

For requirements, see Chapters 18 and 19.

**6.1.5.1* Definition — Health Care Occupancy.** An occupancy used to provide medical or other treatment or care simultaneously to four or more patients on an inpatient basis, where such patients are mostly incapable of self-preservation due to age, physical or mental disability, or because of security measures not under the occupants' control.

**A.6.1.5.1 Health Care Occupancy.** Health care occupancies include the following:

(1) Hospitals
(2) Limited care facilities
(3) Nursing homes

Occupants of health care occupancies typically have physical or mental illness, disease, or infirmity. They also include infants, convalescents, or infirm aged persons.

**6.1.5.2 Other. (Reserved)**

Chapters 18 and 19 address hospitals, nursing homes, and limited care facilities as health care occupancies. These subclassifications of health care occupancies are defined in 3.3.133, 3.3.131.2, and 3.3.82.2, respectively. The definitions specify that each type of facility accommodate four or more persons. Because 24.1.1.1 permits a living unit housing a family and up to three outsiders to be classified as a one-family dwelling, a home with three or fewer persons incapable of self-preservation does not constitute a health care occupancy.

The definition of *health care occupancy* in 6.1.5.1 was changed for the 2009 edition to clarify that it applies to patient care on an inpatient basis. In earlier editions, the *Code* user learned this clarification by inference after reading the definition of *ambulatory health care occupancy,* which clearly stipulates the outpatient criterion. See 18.1.1.1.3, 18.1.1.1.7, 19.1.1.1.3, and 19.1.1.1.7 for criteria related to providing sleeping accommodations for more than 24 hours (i.e., the inpatient criterion). Health care occupancies, if they are to be protected by the provisions of Chapter 18 or Chapter 19, must have at least four inpatients. A health care facility used only for outpatients is addressed by 6.1.6.1 as an ambulatory health care occupancy and is subject to the provisions of Chapter 20 or Chapter 21.

A definition of *birth center* appears in 3.3.29. Also, guidance for whether a birth center is to be classified as a business occupancy or as a health care occupancy is provided in the third paragraph of A.6.1.11.1.

### 6.1.6 Ambulatory Health Care.

For requirements, see Chapters 20 and 21.

**6.1.6.1* Definition — Ambulatory Health Care Occupancy.** An occupancy used to provide services or treatment simultaneously to four or more patients that provides, on an outpatient basis, one or more of the following:

(1) Treatment for patients that renders the patients incapable of taking action for self-preservation under emergency conditions without the assistance of others
(2) Anesthesia that renders the patients incapable of taking action for self-preservation under emergency conditions without the assistance of others
(3) Emergency or urgent care for patients who, due to the nature of their injury or illness, are incapable of taking action for self-preservation under emergency conditions without the assistance of others

**A.6.1.6.1 Ambulatory Health Care Occupancy.** It is not the intent that occupants be considered to be incapable of self-preservation just because they are in a wheelchair or use assistive walking devices, such as a cane, a walker, or crutches. Rather, it is the intent to address emergency care centers that receive patients who have been rendered incapable of self-preservation due to the emergency, such as being rendered unconscious as a result of an accident or being unable to move due to sudden illness.

**6.1.6.2 Other. (Reserved)**

Note that the definition of *ambulatory health care occupancy* in 6.1.6.1 stipulates an outpatient criterion, and that the definition of *health care occupancy* in 6.1.5.1 stipulates an inpatient criterion. A health care facility used only for outpatients is addressed by 6.1.6.1 as an ambulatory health care occupancy and is subject to the provisions of Chapter 20 or Chapter 21. Health care occupancies, if they are to be protected by the provisions of Chapter 18 or Chapter 19, must have at least four inpatients. See 18.1.1.1.3, 18.1.1.1.7, 19.1.1.1.3, and 19.1.1.1.7 for criteria related to providing sleeping accommodations for more than 24 hours (i.e., the inpatient criterion).

Chapters 20 and 21 address the outpatient form of a health care occupancy. The requirements draw heavily from those applicable to business occupancies but supplement them with special provisions that address the fact that some patients in such occupancies are incapable of self-preservation. As is the case with other health care occupancies, the facility must accommodate at least four persons. The provisions of 6.1.6.1 (1) through (3) further define the treatment, care, and initial condition of the patient that can render the patient incapable of self-preservation.

Dialysis treatment centers that accommodate four or more patients at one time generally fall under the classification of ambulatory health care occupancy based on 6.1.6.1(1). The blood-filtering treatment often wreaks havoc with the patients' blood pressure. Even if the patients are provided with instructions on how to clamp and cut their blood-filtering tubing, there is no assurance that they have the capability of immediately evacuating the facility without the assistance of others.

Day-surgery centers that accommodate four or more patients at one time generally fall under the classification of ambulatory health care occupancy based on 6.1.6.1(2). The anesthesia used prevents the patients from taking action for self-preservation under emergency conditions without the assistance of others.

Urgent-care centers that accommodate four or more patients at one time generally fall under the classification of ambulatory health care occupancy based on 6.1.6.1(3). The nature of the injury, illness, or condition present when the patients arrive for treatment prevents the patients from taking action for self-preservation under emergency conditions without the assistance of others.

The four-person criterion of 6.1.6.1 is meant to be applied independently on an area-by-area basis within a building. For example, it is common practice for individual health care practitioners to rent their own tenant space within a multitenant office building. Assume three dentists, each specializing in tooth extraction where the patients are under general anesthesia, have their own tenant spaces. Each of the three dentists does not have more than two patients under anesthesia or recovering from the effects of anesthesia at any time. Although, collectively, the three dentists might have six patients simultaneously rendered incapable of self-preservation due to anesthesia, the four-person criterion is not satisfied within any tenant space considered alone. Each dentist's office would be considered a business occupancy and not an ambulatory health care occupancy.

### 6.1.7 Detention and Correctional.

For requirements, see Chapters 22 and 23.

**6.1.7.1* Definition — Detention and Correctional Occupancy.** An occupancy used to house one or more persons under varied degrees of restraint or security where such occupants are mostly incapable of self-preservation because of security measures not under the occupants' control.

**A.6.1.7.1 Detention and Correctional Occupancy.** Detention and correctional occupancies include the following:

(1) Adult and juvenile substance abuse centers
(2) Adult and juvenile work camps
(3) Adult community residential centers
(4) Adult correctional institutions
(5) Adult local detention facilities
(6) Juvenile community residential centers
(7) Juvenile detention facilities
(8) Juvenile training schools

See A.22.1.1.1.4 and A.23.1.1.1.4.

**6.1.7.2* Nonresidential Uses.** Within detention and correctional facilities, uses other than residential housing shall be in accordance with the appropriate chapter of the *Code*. *(See 22.1.2.3 and 23.1.2.3.)*

**A.6.1.7.2** Chapters 22 and 23 address the residential housing areas of the detention and correctional occupancy as defined in 3.3.178.5. Examples of uses, other than residential housing, include gymnasiums or industries.

The definition of *detention and correctional occupancy* (see 6.1.7.1) was changed for the 2006 edition of the *Code* to apply at the threshold of one or more persons. Formerly, the threshold was four or more persons. This change was made for correlation with the provisions for lockups in other than detention and correctional occupancies, as addressed in 22.4.5 and 23.4.5, which were added to the *Code* in 2006. The provisions for lockups are needed for application even when only one person is detained, as the locked doors characteristic of such detention deny the occupant free egress as required by 7.2.1.5. A lockup in an occupancy other than detention and correctional that detains any individual for more than 24 hours is required to be classified as a detention and correctional occupancy (see 22.4.5.1.2 and 23.4.5.1.2) and is subject to the provisions of Chapter 22 or Chapter 23. Thus, the provisions of Chapters 22 and 23 needed to be made applicable to one or more residents.

Chapters 22 and 23 are intended to apply only to those areas of detention and correctional facilities used for occupant housing, such as sleeping and day activity areas. Other occupied spaces within the facility are to receive an occupancy classification representative of their use and are to be regulated by the applicable provisions of Chapters 12 through 21 and Chapters 24 through 42. For example, cafeterias are regulated using the assembly occupancy chapters, and metal shops follow the requirements of the industrial occupancy chapter. The authority having jurisdiction usually modifies the occupancy requirements of those chapters due to special security needs.

### 6.1.8 Residential.

For requirements, see Chapters 24 through 31.

**6.1.8.1 Definition — Residential Occupancy.** An occupancy that provides sleeping accommodations for purposes other than health care or detention and correctional.

**6.1.8.1.1* Definition — One- and Two-Family Dwelling Unit.** A building that contains not more than two dwelling units with independent cooking and bathroom facilities.

**A.6.1.8.1.1 One- and Two-Family Dwelling Unit.** The application statement of 24.1.1.1 limits each dwelling unit to being "occupied by members of a single family with not more than three outsiders." The *Code* does not define the term *family*. The definition of family is subject to federal, state, and local regulations and might not be restricted to a person or a couple (two people) and their children. The following examples aid in differentiating between a single-family dwelling and a lodging or rooming house:

(1) An individual or a couple (two people) who rent a house from a landlord and then sublease space for up to three individuals should be considered a family renting to a maximum of three outsiders, and the house should be regulated as a single-family dwelling in accordance with Chapter 24.
(2) A house rented from a landlord by an individual or a couple (two people) in which space is subleased to 4 or more individuals, but not more than 16, should be considered and regulated as a lodging or rooming house in accordance with Chapter 26.
(3) A residential building that is occupied by 4 or more individuals, but not more than 16, each renting from a landlord, without separate cooking facilities, should be considered and regulated as a lodging or rooming house in accordance with Chapter 26.

**6.1.8.1.2 Definition — Lodging or Rooming House.** A building or portion thereof that does not qualify as a one- or two-family dwelling, that provides sleeping accommodations for a total of 16 or fewer people on a transient or permanent basis, without personal care services, with or without meals, but without separate cooking facilities for individual occupants.

**6.1.8.1.3* Definition — Hotel.** A building or groups of buildings under the same management in which there are sleeping accommodations for more than 16 persons and primarily used by transients for lodging with or without meals.

**A.6.1.8.1.3 Hotel.** So-called apartment hotels should be classified as hotels, because they are potentially subject to the same transient occupancy as hotels. Transients are those who occupy accommodations for less than 30 days.

**6.1.8.1.4* Definition — Dormitory.** A building or a space in a building in which group sleeping accommodations are provided for more than 16 persons who are not members of the same family in one room, or a series of closely associated rooms, under joint occupancy and single management, with or without meals, but without individual cooking facilities.

**A.6.1.8.1.4 Dormitory.** Rooms within dormitories intended for the use of individuals for combined living and sleeping purposes are guest rooms or guest suites. Examples of dormitories include college dormitories, fraternity and sorority houses, and military barracks.

**6.1.8.1.5 Definition — Apartment Building.** A building or portion thereof containing three or more dwelling units with independent cooking and bathroom facilities.

**6.1.8.2 Other. (Reserved)**

Residential occupancies are characterized by occupants who are asleep for a portion of the time they occupy the building. The sleeping that takes place is for normal restorative rest, as opposed to the sleeping that takes place in a hospital or residential board and care facility where caretakers are present. Sleeping occupants might be unaware of an incipient fire and might be trapped before egress can occur. This occupancy group is further divided into one- and two-family dwellings, lodging or rooming houses, hotels and dormitories, and apartment buildings. Each occupancy in the group has characteristic needs that differ from the others. For this reason, separate chapters of the *Code* address each of these subgroups or subclassifications.

The residential occupancy subclassifications of one- and two-family dwellings, lodging or rooming houses, hotels, dormitories, and apartment buildings are defined in 6.1.8.1.1 through 6.1.8.1.5.

The definition of *apartment building* in 6.1.8.1.5 is copied from that in 3.3.32.3, which has advisory text in A.3.3.32.3. The text of A.3.3.32.3 clarifies that town house–type apartments — particularly those under condominium ownership — are to be classified as apartment buildings. It is often mistakenly believed that condominiums are a form of occupancy rather than a form of ownership.

Although people sleep in health care occupancies and detention and correctional occupancies, they occupy such facilities for other than normal residential purposes. Because the occupants of these facilities are incapable of self-preservation — in one case due to illness or infirmity and, in the other, as a result of security measures — the provisions that apply to normal residential occupancies might not provide the necessary level of life safety. The user is referred to Chapters 18 and 19 for health care occupancies and Chapters 22 and 23 for detention and correctional occupancies. See also 6.1.5 and 6.1.7.

### 6.1.9 Residential Board and Care.

For requirements, see Chapters 32 and 33.

**6.1.9.1* Definition — Residential Board and Care Occupancy.** An occupancy used for lodging and boarding of four or more residents, not related by blood or marriage to the owners or operators, for the purpose of providing personal care services.

**A.6.1.9.1 Residential Board and Care Occupancy.** The following are examples of facilities classified as residential board and care occupancies:

(1) Group housing arrangement for physically or mentally handicapped persons who normally attend school in the community, attend worship in the community, or otherwise use community facilities
(2) Group housing arrangement for physically or mentally handicapped persons who are undergoing training in preparation for independent living, for paid employment, or for other normal community activities
(3) Group housing arrangement for the elderly that provides personal care services but that does not provide nursing care
(4) Facilities for social rehabilitation, alcoholism, drug abuse, or mental health problems that contain a group housing arrangement and that provide personal care services but do not provide acute care
(5) Assisted living facilities
(6) Other group housing arrangements that provide personal care services but not nursing care

**6.1.9.2 Other. (Reserved)**

Residential board and care occupancies, as in the case of residential occupancies, provide sleeping accommodations. However, the residents also receive personal care services by caretakers who live with the residents. Personal care includes assistance with many of the activities of daily living, such as bathing and dressing. Personal care does not include medical care.

The provision of personal care services to residents of residential board and care facilities is an indicator that the residents might have special needs. The requirements of Chapters 32 and 33 credit the combined abilities of staff and residents to evacuate the building or relocate to a point of safety.

### 6.1.10 Mercantile.

For requirements, see Chapters 36 and 37.

**6.1.10.1* Definition — Mercantile Occupancy.** An occupancy used for the display and sale of merchandise.

**A.6.1.10.1 Mercantile Occupancy.** Mercantile occupancies include the following:

(1) Auction rooms
(2) Department stores
(3) Drugstores
(4) Restaurants with fewer than 50 persons
(5) Shopping centers
(6) Supermarkets

Office, storage, and service facilities incidental to the sale of merchandise and located in the same building should be considered part of the mercantile occupancy classification.

**6.1.10.2 Other. (Reserved)**

Mercantile occupancies, as in the case of assembly occupancies, are characterized by large numbers of people who gather in a space that is relatively unfamiliar to them. In addition, mercantile occupancies often contain sizable quantities of combustible contents and use circuitous egress paths that are deliberately arranged to force occupants to travel around displays of materials that are available for sale.

Mall buildings, while predominantly occupied by mercantile occupancies, typically have assembly occupancies within them (e.g., food courts or cinemas) making the mall building a multiple occupancy building. In 12.1.2.3 and 13.1.2.3, applicable to new and existing assembly occupancies, the provisions of Chapters 12 and 13 are made applicable to the assembly occupancy tenant space, but the specialized mall criteria of 36.4.4 and 37.4.4 from the mercantile occupancy chapters are made applicable to the space outside the assembly occupancy tenant space, as that space might be used for egress by the occupants of the assembly occupancy.

Bulk merchandising retail buildings, which characteristically consist of a warehouse-type building occupied for sales purposes, are a subclass of mercantile occupancy with a greater potential for hazards than more traditional mercantile operations. See also 36.4.5 and 37.4.5.

## 6.1.11 Business.

For requirements, see Chapters 38 and 39.

**6.1.11.1* Definition — Business Occupancy.** An occupancy used for the transaction of business other than mercantile.

**A.6.1.11.1 Business Occupancy.** Business occupancies include the following:

(1) Air traffic control towers (ATCTs)
(2) City halls
(3) College and university instructional buildings, classrooms under 50 persons, and instructional laboratories
(4) Courthouses
(5) Dentists' offices
(6) Doctors' offices
(7) General offices
(8) Outpatient clinics (ambulatory)
(9) Town halls

Doctors' and dentists' offices are included, unless of such character as to be classified as ambulatory health care occupancies. *(See 3.3.178.1.)*

Birth centers should be classified as business occupancies if they are occupied by fewer than four patients, not including infants, at any one time; do not provide sleeping facilities for four or more occupants; and do not provide treatment procedures that render four or more patients, not including infants, incapable of self-preservation at any one time. For birth centers occupied by patients not meeting these parameters, see Chapter 18 or Chapter 19, as appropriate.

Service facilities common to city office buildings, such as newsstands, lunch counters serving fewer than 50 persons, barber shops, and beauty parlors are included in the business occupancy group.

City halls, town halls, and courthouses are included in this occupancy group, insofar as their principal function is the transaction of public business and the keeping of books and records. Insofar as they are used for assembly purposes, they are classified as assembly occupancies.

**6.1.11.2 Other. (Reserved)**

Business occupancies generally have a lower occupant density than mercantile occupancies, and the occupants are usually more familiar with their surroundings. However, confusing and indirect egress paths are often developed due to office layouts and the arrangement of tenant spaces. The *Code* requirements for such occupancies address the needs of visitors unfamiliar with the building.

Depending on the characteristics of a laboratory, it may be classified as a business occupancy, industrial occupancy, or other occupancy.

Paragraph A.6.1.11.1 provides guidance in classifying a birth center as a business occupancy or a health care occupancy. The definition of *birth center* appears in 3.3.29. Also see A.3.3.29, Birth Center.

A medical office that provides treatment or performs procedures that render patients incapable of self-preservation might be classified as an ambulatory health care occupancy or as a business occupancy. Guidance on the subject appears in the commentary that follows 6.1.6.2.

## 6.1.12 Industrial.

For requirements, see Chapter 40.

**6.1.12.1* Definition — Industrial Occupancy.** An occupancy in which products are manufactured or in which processing, assembling, mixing, packaging, finishing, decorating, or repair operations are conducted.

**A.6.1.12.1 Industrial Occupancy.** Industrial occupancies include the following:

(1) Drycleaning plants
(2) Factories of all kinds
(3) Food processing plants
(4) Gas plants
(5) Hangars (for servicing/maintenance)
(6) Laundries
(7) Power plants
(8) Pumping stations
(9) Refineries
(10) Sawmills
(11) Telephone exchanges

In evaluating the appropriate classification of laboratories, the authority having jurisdiction should treat each case individually, based on the extent and nature of the associated hazards. Some laboratories are classified as occupancies other than industrial; for example, a physical therapy laboratory or a computer laboratory.

**6.1.12.2 Other. (Reserved)**

Industrial occupancies expose occupants to a wide range of processes and materials of varying hazard. Special-purpose industrial occupancies, which are characterized by large installations of equipment that dominate the space, are addressed separately from general-purpose industrial facilities, which have higher densities of human occupancy.

Industrial occupancy buildings, along with storage occupancy buildings, are more likely than any other occupancy to have contents with a wide range of hazards. Where industrial operations in a special-purpose industrial occupancy or general-purpose industrial occupancy include high hazard materials, processes, or contents (see 6.2.2.4), the occupancy is to be classified as a high hazard industrial occupancy, not as a special-purpose or general-purpose industrial occupancy

Depending on the characteristics of a laboratory, it may be classified as a business occupancy, industrial occupancy, or other occupancy.

### 6.1.13 Storage.

For requirements, see Chapter 42.

**6.1.13.1* Definition — Storage Occupancy.** An occupancy used primarily for the storage or sheltering of goods, merchandise, products, or vehicles.

**A.6.1.13.1 Storage Occupancy.** Storage occupancies include the following:

(1) Barns
(2) Bulk oil storage
(3) Cold storage
(4) Freight terminals
(5) Grain elevators
(6) Hangars (for storage only)
(7) Parking structures
(8) Truck and marine terminals
(9) Warehouses

Storage occupancies are characterized by the presence of relatively small numbers of persons in proportion to the area.

**6.1.13.2 Other. (Reserved)**

Storage occupancies are characterized by relatively low human occupancy in comparison to building size and by varied hazards associated with the materials stored.

Storage occupancy buildings, along with industrial occupancy buildings, are more likely than any other type of occupancy to have contents with a wide range of hazards.

Bulk merchandising retail buildings, which characteristically consist of a warehouse-type building occupied for sales purposes, are a subclass of mercantile occupancy rather than a storage occupancy. See 36.4.5 and 37.4.5.

In prior editions of the *Code*, the sheltering of animals was one of the examples of a storage occupancy included in the definition of *storage occupancy*. The phrase "sheltering of animals" was deleted, as not all facilities housing animals are storage occupancies. See NFPA 150, *Standard on Fire and Life Safety in Animal Housing Facilities.*[1]

### 6.1.14 Multiple Occupancies.

**6.1.14.1 General.**

**6.1.14.1.1** Multiple occupancies shall comply with the requirements of 6.1.14.1 and one of the following:

(1) Mixed occupancies — 6.1.14.3
(2) Separated occupancies — 6.1.14.4

Classifying a building simply as a multiple occupancy is an incomplete classification, as the options for occupancy classification are limited to assembly, educational, day-care, health care, ambulatory health care, residential (one- and two-family dwellings, lodging or rooming houses, hotels and dormitories, or apartment buildings), residential board and care, mercantile, business, industrial, and storage. Rather, a classification of multiple occupancy needs to include mention of the occupancy types involved. For example, a multiple occupancy building with spaces used for sales and spaces used for storage should be classified as a multiple occupancy that is part mercantile occupancy and part storage occupancy.

Once a building is classified as a multiple occupancy and the occupancy types present are identified, the provisions of 6.1.14.1.1 are applied. Paragraph 6.1.14.1.1 offers the option of protecting multiple occupancies via the mixed occupancy requirements of 6.1.14.3 or via the separated occupancy requirements of 6.1.14.4.

If the mixed occupancy option of 6.1.14.3 is chosen for the protection of the multiple occupancy, the *Code* provisions for all occupancy types present must be compared. For each subject area addressed, the more stringent requirement from the applicable occupancy chapters must be identified and followed. Consider, for example, a new multiple occupancy building that is part ordinary hazard mercantile occupancy and part ordinary hazard storage occupancy for which the mixed occupancy form of protection is to be provided. In comparing the requirements of Chapter 36 for new mercantile occupancies and Chapter 42 for ordinary hazard storage occupancies, it becomes evident that neither occupancy is consistently stricter than the other on all features and systems addressed by the occupancy chapter. For example, both occupancies are permitted to use access-controlled egress doors in accordance with 7.2.1.6.2, but mercantile occupancies are permitted to do so only if the entire building is protected throughout by either a fire detection system or a sprinkler system (see 36.2.2.2.6 and 42.2.2.2.3). Mercantile occupancies are permitted to use horizontal or vertical security grilles or doors in accordance with 7.2.1.4.1(3) (see 36.2.2.2.7), but no such permission is given for storage occupancies in 42.2.2.2. In each case, the more stringent provision must be followed in the multiple occupancy being protected as a mixed occupancy.

If the separated occupancy option of 6.1.14.4 is chosen for the protection of the multiple occupancy, the *Code* user must identify the appropriate cell or cells of Table 6.1.14.4.1(a) or Table 6.1.14.4.1(b) to determine the minimum hourly fire resistance rating needed between the occupancies.

**6.1.14.1.2** Where exit access from an occupancy traverses another occupancy, the multiple occupancy shall be treated as a mixed occupancy.

Paragraph 6.1.14.1.2 was new to the 2006 edition of the *Code* and is carried forward into the 2009 edition. It was added to clarify the original intent, which was not fully explained when the provisions for multiple occupancies were added to the 2003 edition. Users incorrectly believed they could satisfy the provisions for multiple occupancies protected as separated occupancies by complying with the following two-step approach:

1. Separate the multiple occupancies from each other by the fire resistance–rated construction required by Table 6.1.14.4.1(a) or Table 6.1.14.4.1(b).
2. Provide egress paths from one of the occupancies to involve travel through doors in the separating construction into the other occupancy (meaning that the two occupancies would share a common corridor). See Exhibit 6.1.

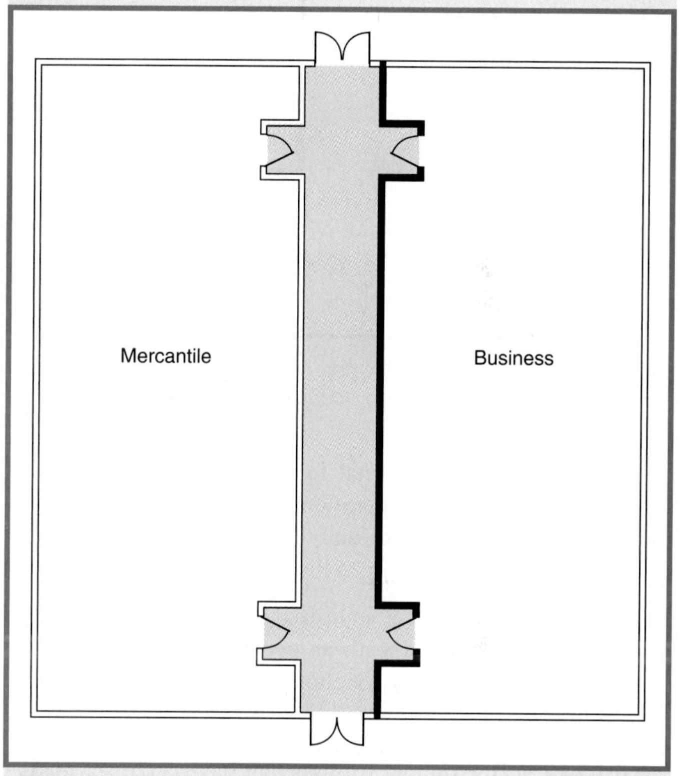


***Exhibit 6.1*** *Multiple occupancy building with shared egress corridor, which prohibits it from protection via the separated occupancy provisions.*

The shared corridor system does not permit the multiple occupancy to be protected as separated occupancies. Instead, the multiple occupancy must be protected as a mixed occupancy.

In Exhibit 6.2, the two required means of egress for the business occupancy are provided by two remotely located doors opening directly to the outside. The door openings to the corridor, located in the fire resistance–rated separation, are convenient extras not required by the *Code*. With this arrangement, the multiple occupancy is permitted to be protected as separated occupancies.

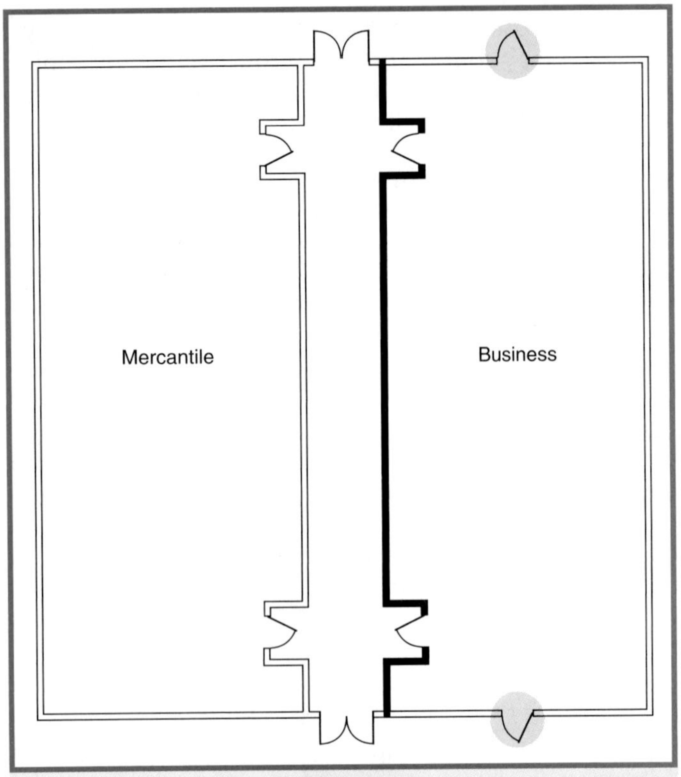


***Exhibit 6.2*** *Multiple occupancy building permitted to be protected via the separated occupancy provisions.*

**6.1.14.1.3*** Where incidental to another occupancy, areas used as follows shall be permitted to be considered part of the predominant occupancy and shall be subject to the provisions of the *Code* that apply to the predominant occupancy:

(1) Mercantile, business, industrial, or storage use
(2)* Nonresidential use with an occupant load fewer than that established by Section 6.1 for the occupancy threshold

**A.6.1.14.1.3(2)** Examples of uses that have occupant loads below the occupancy classification threshold levels include the following:

(1) Assembly use with fewer than 50 persons within a business occupancy
(2) Educational use with fewer than 6 persons within an apartment building.

Paragraph 6.1.14.1.3 clarifies that some, but not all, incidental uses can be considered part of the predominant occupancy. Incidental residential uses, regardless of the number of persons for whom sleeping accommodations are provided, are classified as residential occupancies and are subject to the appropriate residential occupancy chapter requirements. For example, if there are sleeping facilities for five fire fighters in a fire station, the *Code* does not permit the building to be classified simply as a storage occupancy where motor vehicles are sheltered. Rather, the proper classification is a multiple occupancy that is part storage occupancy and part residential occupancy (i.e., lodging/rooming house in this case). The requirements that apply to both occupancies need to be compared, with the more stringent provisions applied in accordance with 6.1.14.3, or the occupancies need to be separated from each other by fire resistance–rated construction in accordance with 6.1.14.4, in which case each occupancy is prohibited from sharing the other occupancy's means of egress per 6.1.14.1.2.

In addition, a day-care use with more than three clients is not exempted by either of the criteria of 6.1.14.1.3. For example, a small day-care center with 14 clients located in a high-rise office building is not part of the predominant business occupancy. The more stringent of the requirements that apply to day-care occupancies and business occupancies need to be implemented in accordance with 6.1.14.3, or the occupancies need to be separated from each other by fire resistance–rated construction in accordance with 6.1.14.4, in which case each occupancy is prohibited from sharing the other occupancy's means of egress per 6.1.14.1.2.

If the day-care use in the high-rise office building addressed in the preceding paragraph had only three clients, that number of clients would be less than the threshold number of four clients at which a day-care use becomes a day-care occupancy (see 6.1.4.1). The day-care use could, therefore, be classified as incidental to the business occupancy as permitted by 6.1.14.1.3(2).

**A.6.1.14.1.3** Examples of uses that might be incidental to another occupancy include the following:

(1) Newsstand (mercantile) in an office building
(2) Giftshop (mercantile) in a hotel
(3) Small storage area (storage) in any occupancy
(4) Minor office space (business) in any occupancy
(5) Maintenance area (industrial) in any occupancy

**6.1.14.2 Definitions.**

**6.1.14.2.1 Multiple Occupancy.** A building or structure in which two or more classes of occupancy exist.

**6.1.14.2.2 Mixed Occupancy.** A multiple occupancy where the occupancies are intermingled.

**6.1.14.2.3 Separated Occupancy.** A multiple occupancy where the occupancies are separated by fire resistance–rated assemblies.

**6.1.14.3 Mixed Occupancies.**

**6.1.14.3.1** Each portion of the building shall be classified as to its use in accordance with Section 6.1.

**6.1.14.3.2** The means of egress facilities, construction type, protection, and other safeguards in the building shall comply with the most restrictive fire and life safety requirements of the occupancies involved.

An example of a multiple occupancy building that is protected as a mixed occupancy is illustrated in Exhibit 6.3. Because the assembly occupancy (i.e., the auditorium) shares the internal corridor egress system with the educational occupancy classrooms and shops, separating the individual occupancies from each other so that they do not share any common exit access is impractical. Therefore, the provision of 6.1.14.1.2 requires that the multiple occupancy be protected as a mixed occupancy.

In the building depicted in Exhibit 6.3, assume that the office space (business occupancy) is considered incidental to the predominant occupancies of educational (i.e., the classrooms and shops) and assembly (i.e., the auditorium) as permitted by 6.1.14.1.3(1). Assuming also that the building is new, the occupancy requirements of Chapter 12 for new assembly occupancies are compared with those of Chapter 14 for new educational occupancies for each of the subjects addressed by the *Code*. In each comparison of requirements between the applicable occupancy chapters, the more stringent requirement is chosen as having applicability to the multiple occupancy.

For example, the 6 ft (1830 mm) minimum corridor width requirement of 14.2.3.2 for educational occupancies is stricter than the 44 in. (1120 mm) minimum requirement of 12.2.3.8 for assembly occupancies and, thus, applies throughout the floor. The panic hardware requirement of 12.2.2.2.3 for assembly occupancies is identical to that in 14.2.2.2.2 for educational occupancies; therefore, this common requirement applies to all doors provided with latches or locks throughout the multiple occupancy. With regard to travel distance, in assembly occupancies, travel distance to the nearest exit is limited by 12.2.6.2 to a maximum of 200 ft (61 m) in a nonsprinklered building or 250 ft (76 m) in a sprinklered building; educational occupancies are limited by 14.2.6.2 and 14.2.6.3 to a 150 ft (46 m) travel distance in a nonsprinklered building and 200 ft (61 m) in a sprinklered building. So, the stricter travel distance requirement from the educational occupancy chapter applies to the multiple occupancy.

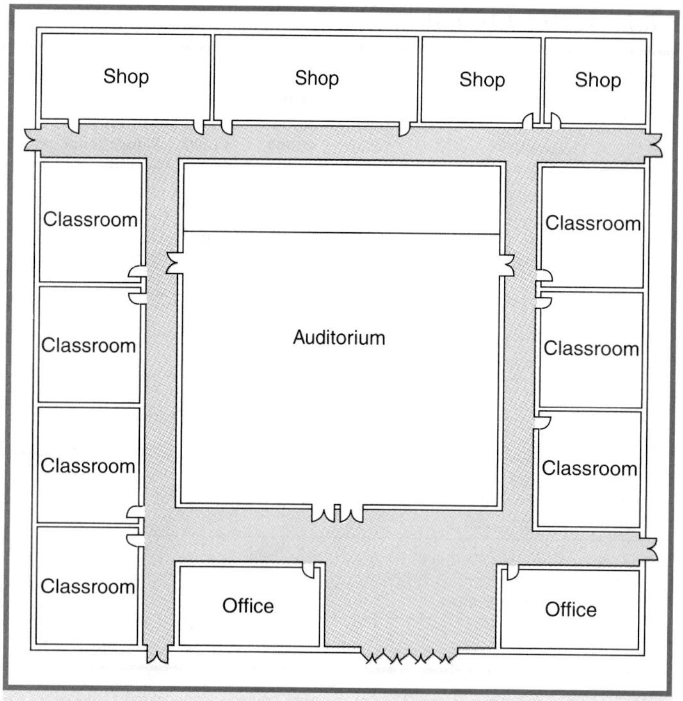


***Exhibit 6.3** Multiple occupancy building protected via the mixed occupancy provisions.*

**6.1.14.4 Separated Occupancies.**

**6.1.14.4.1** Where separated occupancies are provided, each part of the building comprising a distinct occupancy, as described in this chapter, shall be completely separated from other occupancies by fire-resistive assemblies, as specified in 6.1.14.4.2, 6.1.14.4.3, Table 6.1.14.4.1(a), and Table 6.1.14.4.1(b), unless separation is provided by approved existing separations.

**6.1.14.4.2** Occupancy separations shall be classified as 3-hour fire resistance–rated, 2-hour fire resistance–rated, or 1-hour fire resistance–rated and shall meet the requirements of Chapter 8.

**6.1.14.4.3** The minimum fire resistance rating specified in Table 6.1.14.4.1(a) and Table 6.1.14.4.1(b) shall be permitted to be reduced by 1 hour, but in no case shall it be reduced to less than 1 hour, where the building is protected throughout by an approved automatic sprinkler system in accordance with 9.7.1.1(1) and supervised in accordance with 9.7.2, unless prohibited by the double-dagger footnote entries in the tables.

**6.1.14.4.4** Occupancy separations shall be vertical, horizontal, or both or, when necessary, of such other form as required to provide complete separation between occupancy divisions in the building.

*Table 6.1.14.4.1(a) Required Separation of Occupancies (hours),[†] Part 1*

| Occupancy | Assembly ≤ 300 | Assembly >300 to ≤1000 | Assembly >1000 | Educational | Day-Care >12 Clients | Day-Care Homes | Health Care | Ambulatory Health Care | Detention & Correctional | One- & Two-Family Dwellings | Lodging or Rooming Houses | Hotels & Dormitories |
|---|---|---|---|---|---|---|---|---|---|---|---|---|
| Assembly ≤ 300 | — | 0 | 0 | 2 | 2 | 1 | 2[‡] | 2 | 2[‡] | 2 | 2 | 2 |
| Assembly >300 to ≤1000 | | — | 0 | 2 | 2 | 2 | 2[‡] | 2 | 2[‡] | 2 | 2 | 2 |
| Assembly >1000 | | | — | 2 | 2 | 2 | 2[‡] | 2 | 2[‡] | 2 | 2 | 2 |
| Educational | | | | — | 2 | 2 | 2[‡] | 2 | 2[‡] | 2 | 2 | 2 |
| Day-Care>12 Clients | | | | | — | 1 | 2[‡] | 2 | 2[‡] | 2 | 2 | 2 |
| Day-Care Homes | | | | | | — | 2[‡] | 2 | 2[‡] | 2 | 2 | 2 |
| Health Care | | | | | | | — | 2[‡] | 2[‡] | 2[‡] | 2[‡] | 2[‡] |
| Ambulatory Health Care | | | | | | | | — | 2[‡] | 2 | 2 | 2 |
| Detention & Correctional | | | | | | | | | — | 2[‡] | 2[‡] | 2[‡] |
| One- & Two-Family Dwellings | | | | | | | | | | — | 1 | 1 |
| Lodging or Rooming Houses | | | | | | | | | | | — | 1 |
| Hotels & Dormitories | | | | | | | | | | | | — |

[†]*Minimum Fire Resistance Rating.* The fire resistance rating is permitted to be reduced by 1 hour, but in no case to less than 1 hour, where the building is protected throughout by an approved automatic sprinkler system in accordance with 9.7.1.1(1) and supervised in accordance with 9.7.2.

[‡]The 1-hour reduction due to the presence of sprinklers in accordance with the single-dagger footnote is not permitted.

Note that 6.1.14.4.1 requires the fire-rated construction separating occupancies protected as separated occupancies to have the minimum fire resistance rating specified in Table 6.1.14.4.1(a) and Table 6.1.14.4.1(b), unless separation is provided by approved existing separations. The phrase "unless separation is provided by approved existing separations" does not mean that existing separations are exempt from the requirements of Table 6.1.14.4.1(a) and Table 6.1.14.4.1(b). An approved existing separation is a separation approved by the current authority having jurisdiction (AHJ) and is different from a previously approved separation. See 3.3.73.1 for the definition of *approved existing* and 3.3.198 for the definition of *previously approved.* If the current AHJ refuses to approve an existing separation, the provisions of Table 6.1.14.4.1(a) and Table 6.1.14.4.1(b) can be invoked, as applicable. For example, where an existing separation stops at the underside of a suspended ceiling, the AHJ can withhold approval of the existing separation and require compliance with Table 6.1.14.4.1(a) and Table 6.1.14.4.1(b). In another example, the existing separation in a sprinklered building is judged to have approximately 45 minutes of fire resistance rating, but Table 6.1.14.4.1(a) and Table 6.1.14.4.1(b) require a minimum 1-hour rating in such building. The AHJ judges the existing separation acceptable and approves it. The existing separation becomes an approved existing separation not subject to the requirements of Table 6.1.14.4.1(a) and Table 6.1.14.4.1(b).

Exhibit 6.4 illustrates a simple example of a multiple occupancy building where the individual occupancies can easily be protected as separated occupancies. Because each individual-use space is arranged to meet its egress requirements independently of its neighbors, meeting only the requirements that apply to the occupancy of that individual-use space is adequate to protect each space if the fire resistance–rated separations required by Table 6.1.14.4.1(a) or Table 6.1.14.4.1(b) are provided.

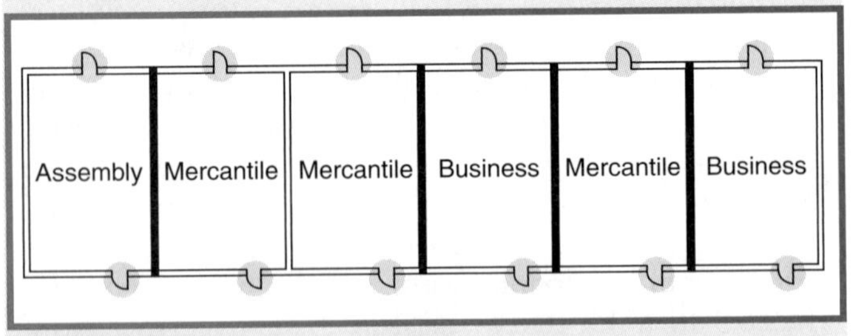


***Exhibit 6.4*** *Multiple occupancy building protected via the separated occupancy provisions.*

Table 6.1.14.4.1(b) includes a cell where mercantile occupancies (located under column 1) intersect with

*Table 6.1.14.4.1(b) Required Separation of Occupancies (hours)*†*, Part 2*

| Occupancy | Apartment Buildings | Board & Care, Small | Board & Care, Large | Mercantile | Mercantile, Mall | Mercantile, Bulk Retail | Business | Industrial, General Purpose | Industrial, Special-Purpose | Industrial, High Hazard | Storage, Low & Ordinary Hazard | Storage, High Hazard |
|---|---|---|---|---|---|---|---|---|---|---|---|---|
| Assembly ≤ 300 | 2 | 2 | 2 | 2 | 2 | 3 | 1 | 2 | 2 | 3 | 2 | 3 |
| Assembly >300 to ≤1000 | 2 | 2 | 2 | 2 | 2 | 3 | 2 | 2 | 2 | 3 | 2 | 3 |
| Assembly >1000 | 2 | 2 | 2 | 2 | 2 | 3 | 2 | 3 | 2 | 3 | 3 | 3 |
| Educational | 2 | 2 | 2 | 2 | 2 | 3 | 2 | 3 | 3 | 3 | 3 | 3 |
| Day-Care >12 Clients | 2 | 2 | 2 | 2 | 2 | 3 | 2 | 3 | 3 | 3 | 3 | 3 |
| Day-Care Homes | 2 | 2 | 2 | 2 | 2 | 3 | 2 | 3 | 3 | 3 | 2 | 3 |
| Health Care | 2‡ | 2‡ | 2‡ | 2‡ | 2‡ | 2‡ | 2‡ | 2‡ | 2‡ | 2‡ | 2‡ | 2‡ |
| Ambulatory Health Care | 2 | 2 | 2 | 2 | 2 | 2‡ | 1 | 2 | 2 | 2‡ | 2 | 2‡ |
| Detention & Correctional | 2‡ | 2‡ | 2‡ | 2‡ | 2‡ | 2‡ | 2‡ | 2‡ | 2‡ | NP | 2‡ | NP |
| One- & Two- Family Dwellings | 1 | 1 | 2 | 2 | 2 | 3 | 2 | 2 | 2 | 3 | 2 | 3 |
| Lodging or Rooming Houses | 1 | 2 | 2 | 2 | 2 | 3 | 2 | 2 | 2 | 3 | 2 | 3 |
| Hotels & Dormitories | 1 | 2 | 2 | 2 | 2 | 3 | 2 | 2 | 2 | 3 | 2 | 3 |
| Apartment Buildings | — | 2 | 2 | 2 | 2 | 3 | 2 | 2 | 2 | 3 | 2 | 3 |
| Board & Care, Small | | — | 1 | 2 | 2 | 3 | 2 | 3 | 3 | 3 | 3 | 3 |
| Board & Care, Large | | | — | 2 | 2 | 3 | 2 | 3 | 3 | 3 | 3 | 3 |
| Mercantile | | | | — | 0 | 3 | 2 | 2 | 2 | 3 | 2 | 3 |
| Mercantile, Mall | | | | | — | 3 | 2 | 3 | 3 | 3 | 2 | 3 |
| Mercantile, Bulk Retail | | | | | | — | 2 | 2 | 2 | 3 | 2 | 2 |
| Business | | | | | | | — | 2 | 2 | 2 | 2 | 2 |
| Industrial, General Purpose | | | | | | | | — | 1 | 1 | 1 | 1 |
| Industrial, Special-Purpose | | | | | | | | | — | 1 | 1 | 1 |
| Industrial, High Hazard | | | | | | | | | | — | 1 | 1 |
| Storage, Low & Ordinary Hazard | | | | | | | | | | | — | 1 |
| Storage, High Hazard | | | | | | | | | | | | — |

NP: Not permitted.

†*Minimum Fire Resistance Rating.* The fire resistance rating is permitted to be reduced by 1 hour, but in no case to less than 1 hour, where the building is protected throughout by an approved automatic sprinkler system in accordance with 9.7.1.1(1) and supervised in accordance with 9.7.2.

‡The 1-hour reduction due to the presence of sprinklers in accordance with the single-dagger footnote is not permitted.

business occupancies (located under column 8). To find the intersection of business occupancies with mercantile occupancies, the user would identify the cell where business occupancies (under column 1) intersect with mercantile occupancies (under column 5). This particular intersection is an empty cell in Table 6.1.14.4.1(b). An empty cell for table locations other than where an occupancy intersects with itself (e.g., where apartment buildings located under column 1 intersect with apartment buildings under column 2) does not mean that no separation is required. Rather, it means that the user needs to use column 1 to find the other occupancy first and then locate the remaining occupancy from one of the corresponding columns 2 through 13. For the case of a multiple occupancy that is part mercantile occupancy and part business occupancy, the order of using the table is to locate mercantile under column 1 and business under column 8.

In the case of the multiple occupancy that is part mercantile occupancy and part business occupancy, the corresponding cell specifies that a 2-hour fire resistance–rated separation is required to achieve protection of the multiple occupancy as separated occupancies if the building is not sprinklered. If the multiple occupancy building is sprinklered, the 2-hour fire resistance–rated separation is permitted to be reduced to 1 hour per the dagger symbol footnote to Table 6.1.14.4.1(b).

### Combining the Mixed Occupancy and Separated Occupancy Forms of Protection

It is not the intent of 6.1.14.1.1 or any other portion of 6.1.14 to prohibit a portion of a multiple occupancy building from being protected as a mixed occupancy and another portion of the same multiple occupancy building to be separated from the mixed occupancies by fire-rated barriers as required by Table 6.1.14.4.1(a) or Table 6.1.14.4.1(b) so as to be considered a separated occupancy.

In Exhibit 6.5, assume that the building is new; the building is protected throughout by an approved automatic sprinkler system in accordance with 9.7.1.1(1) and supervised in accordance with 9.7.2; and the office space (business occupancy) is considered incidental to the predominant occupancies of educational (i.e., the classrooms), assembly (i.e., the auditorium, which, in this case, has an occupant load exceeding 300), and day-care, as permitted by 6.1.14.1.3(1). The day-care occupancy space satisfies all required egress features via the two sets of doors that discharge directly outside; the doors from the day-care space to the corridor are convenience doors provided in excess of *Code* requirements. The day-care occupancy space is separated from the combined assembly occupancy and educational occupancy spaces by 1-hour fire resistance-rated construction in compliance with Table 6.1.14.4.1(a) so as to meet the separated occupancies form of protection. Table 6.1.14.4.1(a) was used to establish the minimum 1-hour fire-rated separation as follows:

1. In the first column, in the row for assembly >300 to ≤1000, the user moves across the table to the column for day-care >12 clients, noting the required fire rating of 2 hours.
2. In the first column, in the row for educational, the user moves across the table to the column for day-care >12 clients, noting the required fire rating of 2 hours.
3. In the title of Table 6.1.14.4.1(a), the user notes the dagger symbol and references the footnote. The building is protected throughout by an approved automatic sprinkler system in accordance with 9.7.1.1(1) and supervised in accordance with 9.7.2, so the required fire-rated separation values of 2 hours from the applicable table cells are reduced to 1 hour.

Returning to Exhibit 6.5, the assembly occupancy space, which is landlocked at the center of the building, shares its exit access with that of the educational occupancy spaces. The provision of 6.1.14.1.2 requires that the portion of the multiple occupancy building that houses the assembly occupancy and the educational occupancy be protected as a mixed occupancy. The occupancy requirements of Chapter 12 for new assembly occupancies are compared with those of Chapter 14 for new educational occupancies for each of the subjects addressed by the *Code*. In each comparison of requirements between the applicable occupancy chapters, the more stringent requirement is chosen as having applicability to the portion of the multiple occupancy building housing the assembly occupancy and educational occupancy spaces being protected as mixed occupancies.

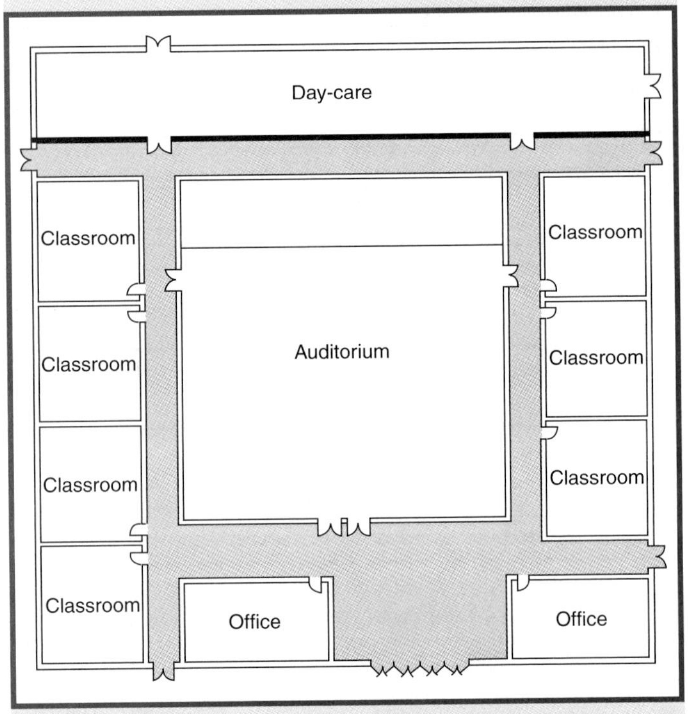


***Exhibit 6.5*** *Multiple occupancy building protected via combination of the mixed occupancy and separated occupancy provisions.*

## 6.2 Hazard of Contents

### 6.2.1 General.

**6.2.1.1** For the purpose of this *Code*, the hazard of contents shall be the relative danger of the start and spread of fire, the danger of smoke or gases generated, and the danger of explosion or other occurrence potentially endangering the lives and safety of the occupants of the building or structure.

The classification of hazard of contents is based on the potential threat to life presented by the contents. A fuel load that might be considered as *light hazard* contents in terms of its ease of extinguishment by a sprinkler system might, in fact, produce enough smoke and other products of combustion to threaten the lives of the occupants. In this case, the *Code* requires the material to be classified as *ordinary hazard* contents or as *high hazard* contents.

The *Code*'s method of classifying hazard of contents is based on life safety. For this reason, the *Code*'s provisions are not readily incorporated into the design criteria of other codes or standards where hazard classification is based on property preservation. Many light hazard materials, in terms of extinguishment characteristics, are required to be treated as ordinary hazard under the *Code*. For example, a business occupancy might be classified as light hazard contents by NFPA 13, *Standard for the Installation of Sprinkler Systems,*[2] for purposes of sprinkler system design but be considered ordinary hazard contents for purposes of applying *Life Safety Code* requirements.

The *Life Safety Code* classifies contents based on the threat of fire, explosions, and other similar events. It does not specifically consider the danger posed by toxic chemicals, etiologic contamination, or similar hazards.

**6.2.1.2** Hazard of contents shall be classified by the registered design professional (RDP) or owner and submitted to the authority having jurisdiction for review and approval on the basis of the character of the contents and the processes or operations conducted in the building or structure.

The provision of 6.2.1.2 places the task of tentatively determining the hazard of contents on the building owner or registered design professional (RDP). The authority having jurisdiction (AHJ) then receives the owner's or RDP's recommended classification, reviews it on the basis of the character of the contents and operations present, and either approves or disapproves such classification. In most cases, a tentative classification of ordinary hazard contents will receive the AHJ's approval. In cases where there is nothing combustible, a safe classification is that of light hazard contents, but the contents of few spaces are limited to such materials. Where rapid fire spread is expected or there is potential for explosion, the logical tentative classification for presentation to the AHJ is that of high hazard contents.

**6.2.1.3*** For the purpose of this *Code*, where different degrees of hazard of contents exist in different parts of a building or structure, the most hazardous shall govern the classification, unless hazardous areas are separated or protected as specified in Section 8.7 and the applicable sections of Chapters 11 through 43.

**A.6.2.1.3** Under the provision of 6.2.1.3, any violation of the requirements of Chapters 11 through 42 for separation or protection of hazardous operation or storage would inherently involve violation of the other sections of the *Code*, unless additional egress facilities appropriate to high hazard contents were provided.

The presence of a high hazard contents area on a floor does not have to result in classification of the entire floor as a high hazard contents area if separation or protection is provided in accordance with the requirements of Section 8.7. Once the potential hazard has been mitigated either by automatic sprinkler protection or via isolation from the remainder of the floor by fire resistance–rated construction, the remainder of the floor, if it has ordinary hazard contents, is permitted to be treated as an ordinary hazard contents area. For example, in an industrial occupancy where an area is used for the dispensing and transfer of flammable liquids from large containers to smaller containers, and such area is separated by fire resistance–rated construction in accordance with Section 8.7, the requirements for high hazard contents areas apply only within the high hazard contents area. The remainder of the floor is not penalized by the presence of the high hazard contents area, provided that the requisite separation is present. For details on the limitations imposed on areas having high hazard contents — such as maximum 75 ft (23 m) travel distance — see Section 7.11.

Paragraph 6.2.1.3 references the separation or protection provisions of Section 8.7, as do the requirements of the __.3.2 subsection of the occupancy chapters, related to protection from hazards, which leads the user to the mistaken belief that the terms *hazardous (contents) area* and *high hazard contents area* are synonymous. Building areas requiring protection by the __.3.2 subsection of an occupancy chapter are not necessarily high hazard areas. Often such areas are occupied by ordinary hazard materials in quantities exceeding those typically associated with the occupancy. For example, a storage room for office supplies in a business occupancy might be required to be protected as a hazardous area in accordance with Section 8.7. Yet, the materials stored are the same ordinary hazard materials dispensed throughout the office area. See the differentiation made between hazardous areas and high hazard contents areas in 38.3.2.1 and 38.3.2.2 or 39.3.2.1 and 39.3.2.2. Each occupancy chapter's __.3.2 subsection is concerned with relative hazards — typically the presence of combustible materials in quantities exceeding those typical of the occupancy.

## 6.2.2 Classification of Hazard of Contents.

**6.2.2.1* General.** The hazard of contents of any building or structure shall be classified as low, ordinary, or high in accordance with 6.2.2.2, 6.2.2.3, and 6.2.2.4.

**A.6.2.2.1** These classifications do not apply to the application of sprinkler protection classifications. *(See* NFPA 13, *Standard for the Installation of Sprinkler Systems.)*

**6.2.2.2* Low Hazard Contents.** Low hazard contents shall be classified as those of such low combustibility that no self-propagating fire therein can occur.

**A.6.2.2.2** Chapter 42 recognizes storage of noncombustible materials as low hazard. In other occupancies, it is assumed that, even where the actual contents hazard is normally low, there is sufficient likelihood that some combustible materials or hazardous operations will be introduced in connection with building repair or maintenance, or some psychological factor might create conditions conducive to panic, so that the egress facilities cannot safely be reduced below those specified for ordinary hazard contents.

Very few occupancies qualify as having low hazard contents. When pressed for an example of low hazard contents, the cautious offer "pig iron ingots stored underwater." A more realistic and useful example of low hazard contents might be metal parts stored in metal containers on metal — not wood — pallets supported by metal shelving. If the same metal parts stored in metal containers were placed on wood pallets, the pallets would be capable of sustaining a self-propagating fire, and the hazard of contents classification would be ordinary.

**6.2.2.3* Ordinary Hazard Contents.** Ordinary hazard contents shall be classified as those that are likely to burn with moderate rapidity or to give off a considerable volume of smoke.

**A.6.2.2.3** Ordinary hazard classification represents the conditions found in most buildings and is the basis for the general requirements of this *Code*.

The fear of poisonous fumes or explosions is necessarily a relative matter to be determined on a judgment basis. All smoke contains some toxic fire gases but, under conditions of ordinary hazard, there should be no unduly dangerous exposure during the period necessary to escape from the fire area, assuming there are proper exits.

**6.2.2.4* High Hazard Contents.** High hazard contents shall be classified as those that are likely to burn with extreme rapidity or from which explosions are likely. *(For means of egress requirements, see Section 7.11.)*

**A.6.2.2.4** High hazard contents include occupancies where flammable liquids are handled or used or are stored under conditions involving possible release of flammable vapors; where grain dust, wood flour or plastic dust, aluminum or magnesium dust, or other explosive dusts are produced; where hazardous chemicals or explosives are manufactured, stored, or handled; where materials are processed or handled under conditions producing flammable flyings; and other situations of similar hazard.

Chapters 40 and 42 include detailed provisions on high hazard contents.

Occupancies containing low hazard or high hazard contents are rare. In deciding which hazard classification applies, users need to ask the following questions:

1. Do the contents qualify for a low hazard classification?
2. Do the contents qualify for a high hazard classification?

If the answer to each of these questions is "no," then the hazard of contents classification is ordinary.

Once an ordinary hazard of contents classification is made, the application of *Code* requirements becomes simple, because the vast majority of the provisions are written to apply to ordinary hazard contents without mentioning ordinary hazard specifically. Generally, specialized requirements apply to high hazard contents, such as those specified in Section 7.11, and to the few exceptions for which application is limited to low hazard contents, such as the unlimited travel distance permitted in low hazard storage occupancies by Table 42.2.6.

### References Cited in Commentary

1. NFPA 150, *Standard on Fire and Life Safety in Animal Housing Facilities,* 2007 edition, National Fire Protection Association, Quincy, MA.
2. NFPA 13, *Standard for the Installation of Sprinkler Systems,* 2007 edition, National Fire Protection Association, Quincy, MA.

CHAPTER 7

# Means of Egress

The earliest editions of the *Life Safety Code* were titled the *Building Exits Code*. This title made it evident that one of the main themes addressed in the *Code* was that sufficient exits are needed to allow building occupants to leave a building safely during a fire or similar emergency.

The term *means of egress* is defined in 3.3.161 as "a continuous and unobstructed way of travel from any point in a building or structure to a public way consisting of three separate and distinct parts: (1) the exit access, (2) the exit, and (3) the exit discharge." The concept of the three-part means of egress was made part of the *Code* in 1956. Since that time, this concept has been well understood, and its philosophy has been implemented by code officials and building designers.

This chapter is segmented to describe the key elements that are typical of egress features.

Separation of the means of egress from other use areas is important to ensure a route of safe passage for the occupants. Subsection 7.1.3 establishes a set of basic principles concerning the separation and segregation of exits to achieve this objective.

Section 7.2 establishes criteria applicable to a variety of components that might constitute a part of the means of egress — from door assemblies and stairs (which are permitted by all occupancy chapters) to specialized components such as alternating tread devices (which are permitted by the occupancy chapters only within the constraints applied by this chapter, such as for the purposes of providing access to unoccupied roof spaces).

The method used to determine the number of occupants who can safely move through any of these individual components is addressed in Section 7.3, which deals with the capacity of the means of egress. Part of this approach also involves establishing how many people can reasonably be expected to occupy a given area; Section 7.3 also presents occupant load factors.

Sections 7.4 through 7.7 relate to the number, arrangement, measurement, and discharge of the means of egress. These four sections not only address the proper number of exits and exit access points, they also control the distance to the exits and the placement of the exits with respect to one another.

The illumination of the means of egress, emergency lighting, and the marking of the means of egress with appropriate signage are related topics. The portions of this chapter that address these subjects were written in recognition of the fact that simply having enough exits that are properly arranged does not guarantee that the exits are readily apparent in a variety of circumstances. Section 7.8 governs normal illumination for the means of egress, while emergency lighting provisions, which address the reillumination of means of egress routes upon loss of normal power, are covered in Section 7.9. Section 7.10 establishes the requirements for proper marking of the means of egress with various types of exit signs and directional exit signs.

Sections 7.11 and 7.12 provide general rules for egress arrangement for high hazard areas and for mechanical equipment rooms.

## 7.1 General

The purpose of Chapter 7 is to establish minimum requirements for the means of egress for application to all occupancy classifications. In agreement with the

1.3.1 application statement, Chapter 7 presents requirements that apply to both new construction and existing buildings. Where the requirements of this chapter are unsuitable for a specific occupancy or impose an unreasonable burden on an existing facility, exemptions are provided as part of the text.

Sometimes the exemptions take the form of a concise statement that refers the user to the specific occupancy chapter. Only by consulting the complete text in the specific occupancy chapter does the user learn the details of the exemption from the Chapter 7 requirements. For example, where 7.2.1.5.1 requires that egress door assemblies remain unlocked, 7.2.1.5.3 cues the user to the fact that, for health care occupancies and detention and correctional occupancies, locked door assemblies are permitted under certain conditions. Paragraph 7.2.1.5.3 uses the phrase "where otherwise provided in Chapters 18 through 23" to refer the user to chapters in which the details of the exemption's conditions can be found. For example, 18.2.2.2.5.1 permits locked door assemblies in health care occupancies where the clinical needs of the patients require specialized security measures for their safety or where patients pose a security threat, with the provision that staff must be able to readily unlock the door assemblies at all times in accordance with the criteria of 18.2.2.2.6.

In addition to specifying means of egress features that are required to be provided in all occupancies, Chapter 7 presents other features that, although not required, are permitted to be part of the means of egress if specified conditions are met. Recognizing that some provisions detailed in this chapter might not be suitable to a particular occupancy, the *Code* often introduces such features using the wording "where permitted in Chapters 11 through 43." For example, door assemblies in means of egress can be equipped with the access-controlled entrance and egress locking system addressed in 7.2.1.6.2 only where specifically permitted by an occupancy chapter. New business occupancies are permitted to use such a system via 38.2.2.2.6, which reads "access-controlled egress doors complying with 7.2.1.6.2 shall be permitted." If an occupancy chapter is silent on the use of access-controlled egress door assemblies, such door assemblies are prohibited within the required means of egress serving that type of occupancy.

Chapter 7 also presents features that are mandatory only when another part of the *Code* specifically requires the use of that component, system, or arrangement. Recognizing that some of the features detailed in this way in Chapter 7 might not be necessary for a particular occupancy, the *Code* often introduces such features using the wording "where required in Chapters 11 through 43." For example, Section 7.10 provides details for exit signs but does not require such signs. Section 7.10 is written to include all the criteria necessary for providing exit signs if another part of the *Code* — typically an occupancy chapter — requires exit signs in accordance with Section 7.10. New assembly occupancies require exit signs per 12.2.10.1, which reads "means of egress shall be provided with signs in accordance with Section 7.10."

Thus, some of the provisions of Chapter 7 are absolute requirements that apply to all occupancies, unless specific exemptions are presented; some provisions are permitted to be used only if another part of the *Code* — typically an occupancy chapter — specifically includes language permitting such use; and some provisions apply only where another part of the *Code* — typically an occupancy chapter — specifically includes language requiring the use of that feature.

### 7.1.1* Application.

Means of egress for both new and existing buildings shall comply with this chapter. *(See also 5.5.3.)*

Means of egress are to comply with the requirements of this chapter and those detailed in Chapter 11, Chapters 12 through 42 for the appropriate occupancy, and Chapter 43. To avoid creating conflicting requirements, the occupancy chapters, Chapters 12 through 42, are permitted to establish provisions or requirements less stringent than those in Chapter 7 only if correlating language is added to the Chapter 7 requirement to which the exemption applies. However, if a provision of Chapters 11 through 43 is written to be more stringent than Chapter 7, it only needs to include the stricter requirement. In accordance with 4.4.2.3, where the specific requirements of Chapters 11 through 43 differ from the general requirements contained in Chapters 1 through 4 and Chapters 6 through 10, the more specific requirements of Chapters 11 through 43 govern. See also the commentary following 4.4.2.3.

**A.7.1.1** An installation of supplemental evacuation equipment is not recognized as a means of egress. Consequently, such equipment does not satisfy any requirement for minimum number of, capacity of, travel distance to, or remoteness of, means of egress.

Annex C, Supplemental Evacuation Equipment, is new to the 2009 edition of the *Code*. It is not part of Chapter 7, Means of Egress, because supplemental evacuation equipment, including platform rescue systems and controlled descent devices, is not credited with meeting any of the requirements for means of egress. Supplemental evacuation equipment is provided voluntarily to supplement the egress systems. Annex C helps to ensure that such equipment does not provide a false sense of security or interfere with the use of the required egress systems. See the commentary associated with new Annex C.

### 7.1.2 Special Definitions.

The occupants of a building must be protected from obstacles to safe egress. To achieve this goal, the protection of each component in the egress system is to be considered. Clear and concise definitions of the terms in 7.1.2 appear in Chapter 3. These definitions help explain the special features of each component. The term *means of egress* has been used for many years, but it was not until the late 1950s that its definition was expanded to comprise three separate and distinct parts: (1) the exit access, (2) the exit, and (3) the exit discharge. Prior to that, the term *exit* was used more often than the term *means of egress*, a fact evidenced by the *Code*'s original title, the *Building Exits Code.*

A list of special terms used in this chapter follows:

(1) **Accessible Area of Refuge.** See 3.3.20.1.

For an area of refuge to be considered an accessible area of refuge, it must be capable of being reached by a person in a wheelchair without traveling over stairs or other obstacles. ICC/ANSI A117.1, *American National Standard for Accessible and Usable Buildings and Facilities,*[1] provides additional details on accessible routes. This edition of the *Life Safety Code* references the 2003 edition of ICC/ANSI A117.1, which was processed in an effort to achieve harmony with the *Americans with Disabilities Act Accessibility Guidelines for Buildings and Facilities* (ADAAG),[2] which has since been revised to become *ADA and ABA Accessibility Guidelines for Buildings and Facilities* (ADA-ABA-AG).[3]

(2) **Accessible Means of Egress.** See 3.3.161.1.

A means of egress is considered an accessible means of egress if it meets one of the following criteria:

1. A wheelchair-bound person is able to travel unassisted through the exit access, exit, and exit discharge to a public way (i.e., ramp-type travel and not stair-type travel if elevation differences are involved).
2. A wheelchair-bound person is able to travel unassisted through that portion of the exit access necessary to reach an area of refuge.

The area of refuge specified in item 2 serves as a temporary haven from the effects of the fire. A person with severe mobility impairment must have the ability to travel from the area of refuge to the public way, although such travel might depend on the assistance of others. If elevation differences are involved, a special, protected elevator might be used, or the person might be carried on an extra-wide stair. See also 7.5.4.

(3) **Area of Refuge.** See 3.3.20.

The definition of *area of refuge* in 3.3.20 establishes the provisions that would create an area of refuge. Item (1) in 3.3.20 recognizes the combination of a sprinklered building and any story providing access to two accessible rooms or spaces separated from each other by smoke-resisting partitions. Some occupancy chapters exempt their occupancy from the criterion for the two accessible rooms or spaces separated from each other by smoke-resisting partitions. Those occupancy chapters recognize each story of a sprinklered building as being an area of refuge under the premise that it might be frightening to be left behind on such a floor without the ability to move to another room, but it is not dangerous, because the sprinkler system is designed to control the fire. See, for example, 28.2.2.12.2, 30.2.2.12.2, 36.2.2.12.2, and 38.2.2.12.2 for hotels and dormitories, apartment buildings, mercantile occupancies, and business occupancies, respectively.

(4) **Common Path of Travel.** See 3.3.42.

Common path of travel involves providing only one egress path for the initial portion of the exit access. The occupant does not have a choice of independent directions to travel. Common path of travel is addressed in 7.5.4.1.4 and the __.2.5 subsection of the occupancy chapters. The occupancy chapter limitations on common path of travel are summarized in Table A.7.6.

(5) **Electroluminescent.** See 3.3.63.
(6) **Elevator Evacuation System.** See 3.3.64.
(7) **Elevator Lobby.** See 3.3.65.
(8) **Elevator Lobby Door.** See 3.3.57.1.

The terms *elevator evacuation system*, *elevator lobby*, and *elevator lobby door* are defined for purposes of applying

7.2.13. Although elevators are addressed in 7.2.13 as a component of a means of egress system, the restrictions imposed recognize the elevator only as a second means of egress from a tower with limited occupant load, without access by the general public, with sprinkler protection throughout the tower building, and with other detailed features. See also 11.3.2.2.2.

Annex B, Elevators for Occupant-Controlled Evacuation Prior to Phase I Emergency Recall Operations, is new to the 2009 edition of the *Code*. It is not part of Chapter 7, Means of Egress, because there is no assurance that the elevators will remain in service for the time needed to evacuate the building. Where elevators are used for occupant-controlled evacuation in accordance with the provisions of Annex B, the full complement of egress elements, routes, and systems must be provided as required by the provisions of Chapter 7 and the applicable occupancy chapter.

(9) **Exit.** See 3.3.75.

The term *exit* is defined by 3.3.75 as that portion of a means of egress that is separated from other building spaces by enclosing it within construction, the fire resistance of which is specified by 7.1.3.2, with limited openings through the enclosing construction and protection of such openings. The exit might include door assemblies, stairs, ramps, smokeproof enclosures, exit passageways, and outside balconies. In each case, the exit components are required to conform to the *Code* specifications for fire protection, dimensions, and arrangement. In its simplest form, an exit is a doorway or a door opening directly to the exterior at grade. Such doorway or door opening provides the requisite protected way of travel to the exit discharge without the need for fire-rated, separating construction. An exit other than a door opening directly to the outside must provide a protected path of travel.

In the case of a stairway, the exit includes the door assembly into the stairway enclosure, the stair enclosure, the stairs and landings inside the enclosure, and the door assembly from the enclosure to the exterior or interior exit discharge.

The entrance to an exit enclosure is part of the exit and usually consists of a fire protection–rated door assembly that provides a protected entrance into a protected area. A fire door assembly, however, does not always signal an entrance to an exit. A door assembly or fire door assembly between a hotel room and a corridor or a fire door assembly across a corridor or lobby is part of exit access and not part of an exit, unless the corridor or lobby and all other openings into the corridor or lobby are separated and protected as required for an exit in accordance with 7.1.3.2, as might be accomplished using an exit passageway (see 7.2.6). Such protection is seldom provided for corridors, because, although it might be technically and monetarily feasible at the time the exit passageway is constructed, it would be difficult to maintain over the life of the building, as penetrations for communications cabling and other rehabilitation projects dimish the protection features.

Various building features — where properly arranged and constructed — might constitute an exit. Examples include an exterior exit door assembly, an exit passageway, a horizontal exit, an exit stair, or an exit ramp.

Several types of exits that might occur are shown in Exhibit 7.1 as shaded areas. On the second floor, exits include the following:

1. Two exit stairs enclosed by fire resistance–rated barriers, including a fire protection–rated, self-closing door assembly
2. Horizontal exit consisting of a fire resistance–rated barrier, including a pair of fire protection-rated, self-closing cross-corridor door assemblies that completely divide the floor into two fire compartments

On the first floor, exits include the following:

1. Two door assemblies from the corridor directly to the outside at grade level
2. Horizontal exit that is a vertical extension of, and, therefore, similar to, the horizontal exit located immediately above on the second floor
3. Exit passageway that connects one of the second-floor exit stair enclosures directly with the outside and is separated from the remainder of the first floor by fire resistance–rated barriers, including fire protection–rated, self-closing door assemblies for other than the door assembly to the outside

Note that the spiral stair connecting the first- and second-floor rooms at the upper right corner of the second floor in Exhibit 7.1 is not an exit. The spiral stair does not provide the separated and protected travel path required of an exit by 7.1.3.2.1. The spiral stair shown might have been installed in accordance with 8.6.8.2, with permission of the applicable occupancy chapter [e.g., see 38.3.1.1(1) for new business occupancies]. The spiral stair is a convenience opening that is prohibited by 8.6.8.2(5) from serving as a required means of egress.

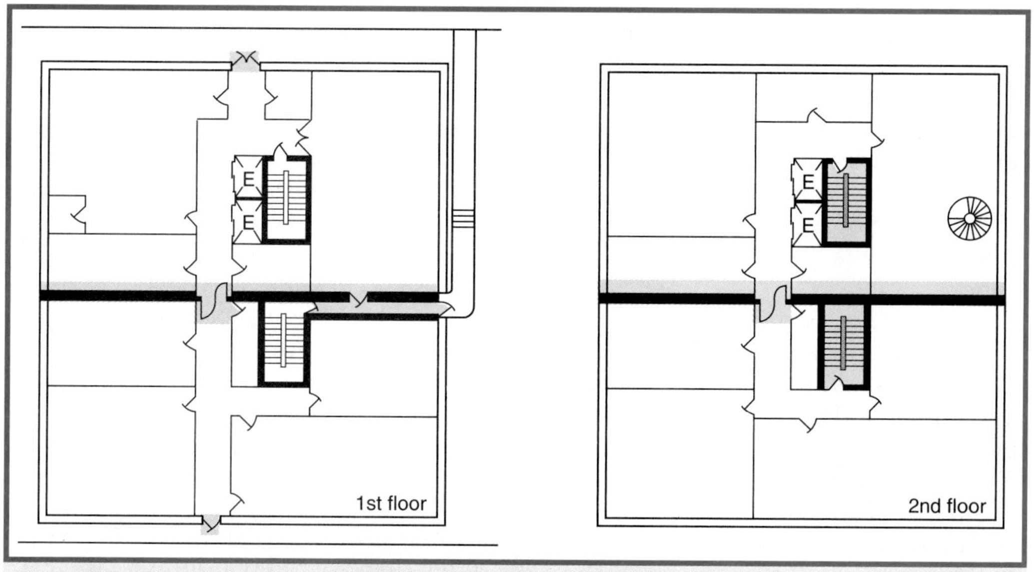


**Exhibit 7.1** *Various forms of exits.*

For detailed requirements for a horizontal exit, see 7.2.4. For detailed requirements for an exit passageway, see 7.2.6.

(10) **Exit Access.** See 3.3.76.

The exit access includes the rooms and building spaces people occupy and the door assemblies, aisles, corridors, unenclosed stairs, and unenclosed ramps that are traversed to reach an exit. Spaces constituting exit access are shown in Exhibit 7.2 as shaded areas. All spaces occupied and traversed in reaching an exit are considered the exit access portion of the means of egress. The shading shown in the exhibit indicates that exit access comprises more floor area than either of the other components of means of egress — the exit and exit discharge.

The small closet in the room at the upper left corner of the first floor in Exhibit 7.2 is judged to be not occupiable and, therefore, is not part of the exit access. Similarly, if an HVAC shaft were running up through the building, it too would be considered nonoccupiable and not part of the exit access.

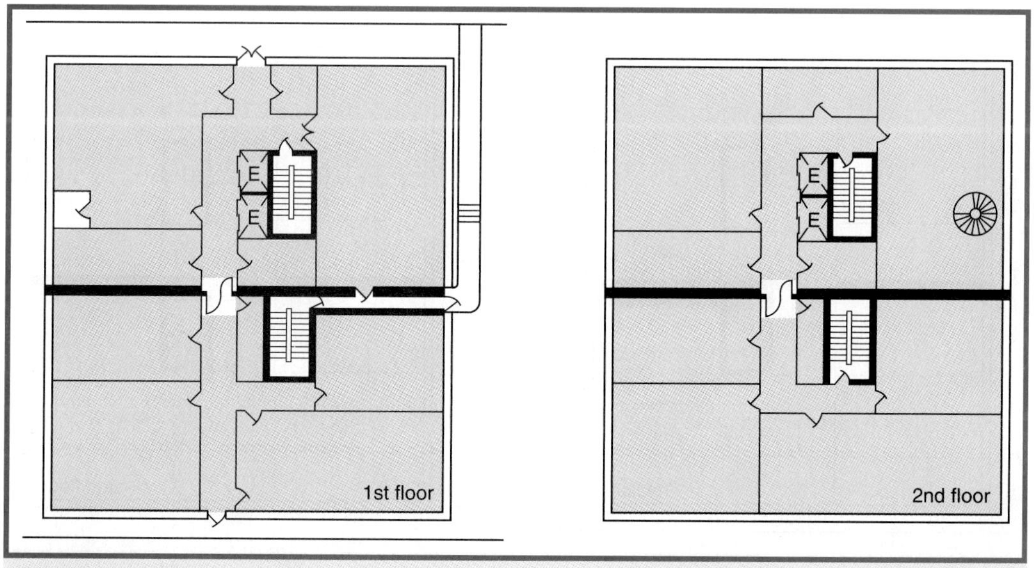


**Exhibit 7.2** *Spaces constituting exit access.*

Note that the two elevators are shaded so as to denote they are within the exit access. The elevators are not permitted to serve as components of the means of egress system. The building occupants must be provided with egress components and paths independent of the elevators. Yet, the travel across the elevator floor to the corridor is exit access for the building occupants who find themselves on the elevator at the time the fire emergency is called to their attention.

The spiral stair connecting the first- and second-floor rooms at the upper right corner of the second floor in Exhibit 7.2 is not an exit, as explained in the commentary associated with 7.1.2(9), as it does not provide the separated and protected travel path required of an exit by 7.1.3.2.1. The spiral stair shown might have been installed in accordance with 8.6.8.2, with permission of the applicable occupancy chapter [e.g., see 38.3.1.1(1) for new business occupancies]. The spiral stair is a convenience opening that is prohibited by 8.6.8.2(5) from serving as a required means of egress. Yet, travel on the spiral stair to reach an exit access path provided on the first floor or the second floor is exit access for the building occupants who find themselves on the spiral stair at the time the fire emergency is called to their attention.

(11) **Exit Discharge.** See 3.3.77.

Because some exits do not discharge directly into a public way, the exit discharge is defined as providing building occupants with a path of travel from the termination of an exit to a public way. This path of travel might be inside the building, as permitted by 7.7.2, or outside. Where an exit opens onto an alley, court, or yard, a safe path of travel is required to be provided to a public way or some equivalent safe area. This portion of the means of egress is the exit discharge. See also 7.7.1.

Forms of exit discharge are shown in Exhibit 7.3 as shaded areas. Because occupants leave the building at the first floor only, no exit discharge occurs on the second floor. The first-floor exit discharge includes the following:

1. Exterior space beginning at the exit door assemblies from the corridor and continuing to the public way (street)
2. Exterior walkway along the side of the building beginning at the door assembly from the exit passageway and continuing to the public way
3. Interior path of travel from the second-floor exit stair discharging through a portion of the first-floor corridor

A portion of the first floor through which an occupant of the second floor needs to travel is considered exit discharge, because the occupant reaches a required exit on the second floor (i.e., the enclosed exit stair) and then is forced to leave that protected area after traveling through the stair enclosure door opening on the first floor. However, an occupant of the first floor who travels across the same space, the space considered exit discharge for the person whose exit access

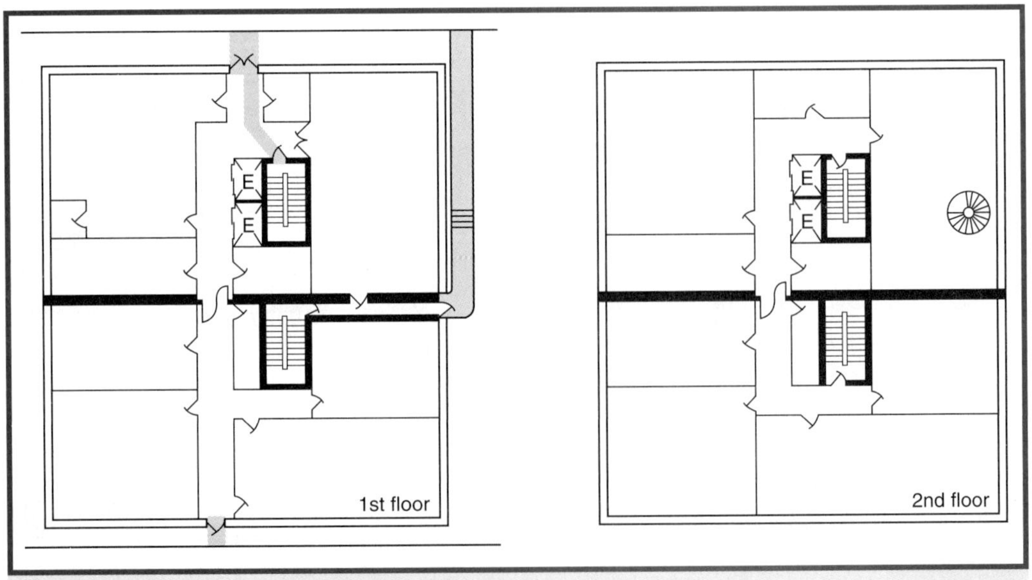


***Exhibit 7.3*** *Spaces constituting exit discharge.*

travel began on the second floor, is considered to be within exit access and still en route to finding an exit, which occurs upon reaching the door opening to the outside. See also 7.7.2.

(12) **Externally Illuminated.** See 3.3.135.1.
(13) **Horizontal Exit.** See 3.3.75.1.

A horizontal exit is a fire barrier with fire door assemblies that provides passage from one fire compartment of a building to another fire compartment in the same building or in an adjoining building on approximately the same level. Substantial fire separations are required, because the area to which egress is made serves as a temporary safe haven. The horizontal exit might be a combination of a 2-hour fire resistance–rated barrier separating a building into two areas with $1\frac{1}{2}$-hour fire protection–rated door assemblies that allow travel from one side of the barrier to the other; or the horizontal exit might be a bridge or balcony that allows travel to an adjoining building. An example of a horizontal exit is depicted in Exhibit 7.1 by the barrier running across the center of the building, which provides a continuous separation from outside wall to opposite outside wall.

Horizontal exits are particularly useful in health care occupancies and in detention and correctional occupancies where they are important components of an effective defend-in-place strategy. Horizontal exits make it possible to move nonambulatory patients horizontally to a temporary safe area rather than vertically down flights of stairs. They also provide added safety to residents of detention and correctional occupancies by allowing those residents to relocate within a building, rather than requiring that they rely on staff to unlock door assemblies to allow them to evacuate to the outside. For details on horizontal exits, see 7.2.4.

(14) **Internally Illuminated.** See 3.3.135.2.
(15) **Means of Egress.** See 3.3.161.

A means of egress, by definition, provides a path of egress travel to a public way. In effect, the *Code* emphasizes the need to move building occupants to a safe place. In means of egress arrangements on university campuses, military bases, resorts, and other large complexes, there are numerous areas a building occupant could reach before reaching a public way that afford the intended level of safety from a building fire. It is the *Code*'s intent that occupants have the ability to move to a safe place from which they can continue to move away from the burning building, as necessary. At that safe point, *Code* requirements cease to apply. This concept provides the basis for A.7.8.1.1, which is applicable to illumination of means of egress. This annex text states that the extent to which illumination needs to be provided outside the building — that is, within the exit discharge portion of the means of egress — should be to either a public way or a distance away from the building that is considered safe, whichever is closest to the building being evacuated.

From every location in a building, a means of egress or path of travel is required over which a person can move to gain access to the outside or to a place of safety. Any persons who gain entrance to a building usually have available to them that ingress route by which to egress. However, one important consideration makes egressing more than just reversing one's route of entry, especially if emergency conditions exist. This reverse route might consist of features that, although not obstacles upon entrance, prove to be such upon egress. For example, a door leaf hinged to swing in the direction of entry can become an obstacle when one attempts to leave the building in the opposite direction. The door leaf swings against the flow of traffic — a flow that, during emergency egress, is greatly increased, as compared with the leisurely flow of people entering a building. As another example, in assembly occupancies where turnstiles are used to meter ingress, reversing one's route often is not possible if additional openings independent of the turnstiles are not provided.

A basic principle of the *Code* requires that every component of a means of egress be operable by, and under the control of, the occupants attempting egress. Where the *Code* makes exemptions to this basic concept — for example, in health care occupancies where locked door assemblies are permitted if it is necessary for the clinical needs of the patients — it does so by substituting requirements adequate to achieve the same level of life safety as would be provided if the means of egress system were fully under the control of the building occupants. For example, in the case of health care occupancy door assemblies that are locked for the clinical needs of the patients, staff is required to carry the keys needed to unlock those door assemblies at all times.

(16) **Photoluminescent.** See 3.3.193.

Photoluminescent materials have been used effectively as internally illuminated exit and directional exit signs in accordance with 7.10.7 and as floor proximity egress path marking in accordance with 7.10.1.7.

The provisions of 7.2.2.5.5 on exit stair path markings are new to the 2009 edition of the *Code*. Photoluminescent or self-luminous materials will typically be used to satisfy the requirements for exit stair path markings. See 7.2.2.5.5.10.

(17) **Ramp.** See 3.3.205.

Requirements for ramps used in a means of egress are found in 7.2.5.

(18) **Self-Luminous.** See 3.3.223.

See the commentary on photoluminescent and self-luminous materials that follows 7.1.2(16).

(19) **Severe Mobility Impairment.** See 3.3.228.

See also 7.5.4.1, which requires new areas accessible to persons with severe mobility impairment to be provided with accessible means of egress.

(20) **Smokeproof Enclosure.** See 3.3.239.

### 7.1.3 Separation of Means of Egress.

See also Section 8.2.

**7.1.3.1 Exit Access Corridors.** Corridors used as exit access and serving an area having an occupant load exceeding 30 shall be separated from other parts of the building by walls having not less than a 1-hour fire resistance rating in accordance with Section 8.3, unless otherwise permitted by the following:

(1) This requirement shall not apply to existing buildings, provided that the occupancy classification does not change.
(2) This requirement shall not apply where otherwise provided in Chapters 11 through 43.

Paragraph 7.1.3.1 requires protection via fire-rated corridor walls of exit access corridors serving more than 30 occupants. Note that the requirement for the corridor walls to be fire resistance rated, which is not a requirement for the floor/ceiling or roof/ceiling assemblies forming the top and bottom of the corridor compartment, provides separation only between the corridor and other spaces on the same floor. To provide the 1-hour separation between the corridor and the remainder of the floor, as required by 7.1.3.1, the fire barriers forming the corridor walls must extend above any ceiling membranes so as to be sealed tightly against the floor or roof above.

To learn if any separation between the corridor and spaces on floors above or below is required, one has to rely on, for example, the provisions of 8.6.1(1) to ensure that the floor is constructed as a smoke barrier — or the provisions of subsection __.1.6 of an occupancy chapter that require fire resistance–rated floor construction.

Paragraph 7.1.3.1(1) exempts existing corridors, provided that the occupancy classification does not change. Therefore, if the occupancy classification of an existing building does change, the 1-hour corridor wall requirement applies, unless the specific occupancy involved has different requirements. Most of the occupancy chapters establish new exit access corridor wall requirements that supersede the requirements of 7.1.3.1. Also, some of the occupancy chapters establish corridor wall requirements for existing buildings. Such provisions usually appear in subsection __.3.6. For example, 14.3.6 addresses special requirements for corridor walls in new educational occupancies and 15.3.6 addresses special requirements for corridor walls in existing educational occupancies. If no special requirements appear in an occupancy chapter, the provisions of 7.1.3.1 prevail.

Paragraph 7.1.3.1 does not require corridors; however, it does require that, where corridors do exist and where they serve an area having an occupant load of more than 30 persons, they must be separated from other (i.e., noncorridor) spaces on that floor by corridor walls. Section 8.3 regulates the construction of the fire barrier forming the corridor walls and the opening protection. Wall segments that serve both as a corridor wall and as part of an exit enclosure must meet the more stringent provisions required for the enclosure of exits. Similarly, wall segments that serve both as a corridor wall and enclosure protection of hazardous contents areas must meet the more stringent of the applicable provisions. In some cases, the provisions for corridor walls and those for hazardous area protection require a minimum 1-hour fire resistance rating. Yet, the minimum required fire protection rating of door assemblies in such walls might vary, with a minimum 45-minute rating required for the hazardous area protection and only a 20-minute rating for the corridor wall. Determining which set of requirements is more stringent involves comparing all related requirements, not only the fire resistance rating of the wall.

Exhibit 7.4 is an example of the protection of exit access corridors required by 7.1.3.1. Note the difference in the required protection for the corridor wall segments serving also as enclosure protection from the hazardous contents area (see Section 8.7) and as part of the enclosure of an exit (see 7.1.3.2).

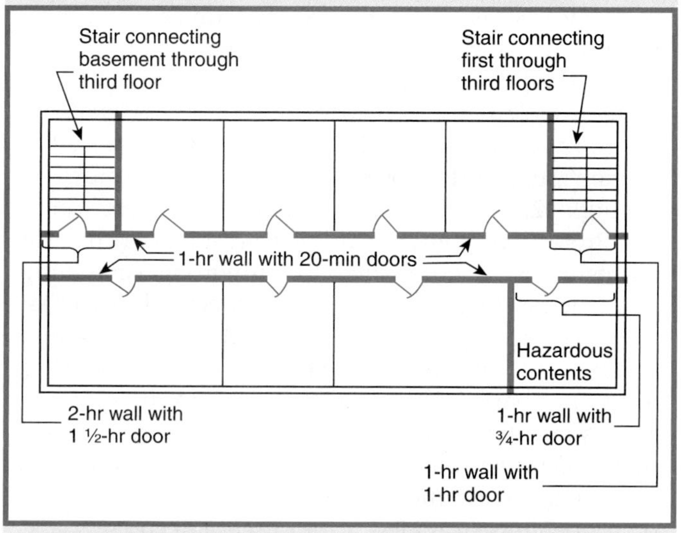


***Exhibit 7.4*** *Protection of exit access corridors.*

**7.1.3.2 Exits.**

**7.1.3.2.1** Where this *Code* requires an exit to be separated from other parts of the building, the separating construction shall meet the requirements of Section 8.2 and the following:

(1)* The separation shall have a minimum 1-hour fire resistance rating where the exit connects three or fewer stories.

**A.7.1.3.2.1(1)** In existing buildings, existing walls in good repair and consisting of lath and plaster, gypsum wallboard, or masonry units can usually provide satisfactory protection for the purposes of this requirement where a 1-hour fire resistance rating is required. Further evaluation might be needed where a 2-hour fire resistance rating is required. Additional guidelines can be found in Appendix D of NFPA 914, *Code for Fire Protection of Historic Structures*, and in the *SFPE Handbook of Fire Protection Engineering*.

(2)* The separation shall have a minimum 2-hour fire resistance rating where the exit connects four or more stories, unless one of the following conditions exists:

(a) In existing non-high-rise buildings, existing exit stair enclosures shall have a minimum 1-hour fire resistance rating.

(b) In existing buildings protected throughout by an approved, supervised automatic sprinkler system in accordance with Section 9.7, existing exit stair enclosures shall have a minimum 1-hour fire resistance rating.

(c) The minimum 1-hour enclosures in accordance with 28.2.2.1.2, 29.2.2.1.2, 30.2.2.1.2, and 31.2.2.1.2 shall be permitted as an alternative to the requirement of 7.1.3.2.1(2).

**A.7.1.3.2.1(2)** In existing buildings, existing walls in good repair and consisting of lath and plaster, gypsum wallboard, or masonry units can usually provide satisfactory protection for the purposes of this requirement where a 1-hour fire resistance rating is required. Further evaluation might be needed where a 2-hour fire resistance rating is required. Additional guidelines can be found in Appendix O of NFPA 914, *Code for Fire Protection of Historic Structures*, and in the *SFPE Handbook of Fire Protection Engineering*.

(3) **Reserved.**

(4) The minimum 2-hour fire resistance–rated separation required by 7.1.3.2.1(2) shall be constructed of an assembly of noncombustible or limited-combustible materials and shall be supported by construction having a minimum 2-hour fire resistance rating, unless otherwise permitted by 7.1.3.2.1(6).

(5)* Structural elements, or portions thereof, that support exit components and either penetrate into a fire resistance–rated assembly or are installed within a fire resistance–rated wall assembly shall be protected, as a minimum to the fire resistance rating required by 7.1.3.2.1(1) or (2).

**A.7.1.3.2.1(5)** It is not the intent to require the structural elements supporting outside stairs, or structural elements that penetrate within exterior walls or any other wall not required to have a fire resistance rating, to be protected by fire resistance–rated construction.

(6) In Type III, Type IV, and Type V construction, as defined in NFPA 220, *Standard on Types of Building Construction (see 8.2.1.2)*, fire-retardant-treated wood enclosed in noncombustible or limited-combustible materials shall be permitted.

(7) Openings in the separation shall be protected by fire door assemblies equipped with door closers complying with 7.2.1.8.

(8)* Openings in exit enclosures shall be limited to door assemblies from normally occupied spaces and corridors and door assemblies for egress from the enclosure, unless one of the following conditions exists:

(a) Openings in exit passageways in mall buildings as provided in Chapters 36 and 37 shall be permitted.

(b) In buildings of Type I or Type II construction, as defined in NFPA 220, *Standard on Types of Building Construction (see 8.2.1.2)*, existing fire protection–rated door assemblies to interstitial spaces shall be permitted, provided that such spaces meet all of the following criteria:

i. The space is used solely for distribution of pipes, ducts, and conduits.
ii. The space contains no storage.
iii. The space is separated from the exit enclosure in accordance with Section 8.3.

(c) Existing openings to mechanical equipment spaces protected by approved existing fire protection–rated door assemblies shall be permitted, provided that the following criteria are met:

i. The space is used solely for non-fuel-fired mechanical equipment.
ii. The space contains no storage of combustible materials.
iii. The building is protected throughout by an approved, supervised automatic sprinkler system in accordance with Section 9.7.

**A.7.1.3.2.1(8)** Means of egress from the level of exit discharge is permitted to pass through an exit stair enclosure or exit passageway serving other floors. Doors for convenience purposes and unrelated to egress also are permitted to provide access to and from exit stair enclosures and exit passageways, provided that such doors are from corridors or normally occupied spaces. It is also the intent of this provision to prohibit exit enclosure windows, other than approved vision panels in doors, that are not mounted in an exterior wall.

(9) Penetrations into, and openings through, an exit enclosure assembly shall be limited to the following:

(a) Door assemblies permitted by 7.1.3.2.1(8)
(b)*Electrical conduit serving the exit enclosure

**A.7.1.3.2.1(9)(b)** Penetrations for electrical wiring are permitted where the wiring serves equipment permitted by the authority having jurisdiction to be located within the exit enclosure, such as security systems, public address systems, and fire department emergency communications devices.

(c) Required exit door openings
(d) Ductwork and equipment necessary for independent stair pressurization
(e) Water or steam piping necessary for the heating or cooling of the exit enclosure
(f) Sprinkler piping
(g) Standpipes
(h) Existing penetrations protected in accordance with 8.3.5
(i) Penetrations for fire alarm circuits, where the circuits are installed in metal conduit and the penetrations are protected in accordance with 8.3.5

(10) Penetrations or communicating openings shall be prohibited between adjacent exit enclosures.

Exits must provide protection from fire originating inside or outside the exit. Protection from fire originating within the enclosure is accomplished by prohibiting use of the enclosure for any purpose that could possibly interfere with the exit functioning as a protected path of travel (see 7.1.3.2.3) and by limiting the combustibility of interior wall, ceiling, and floor finish materials within exit enclosures (see 7.1.4). Details on interior wall, ceiling, and floor finish are contained in Section 10.2 and subsection __.3.3 of Chapters 12 through 42.

Protection from fire originating outside the exit enclosure is accomplished by providing separating construction having the required specified degree of fire resistance and by careful control of openings into the exit enclosure itself. The only openings permitted in the fire barriers between the exit and the building spaces are those for entering the exit from any normally occupied space or corridor and those for leaving the exit to reach the exit discharge. In other words, only openings provided for an occupant to enter and leave the exit enclosure are permitted.

Exhibit 7.5 depicts an egress arrangement on the ground floor of a building where occupants of that floor can enter the two exit stair enclosures, although such door assemblies are not required, because the

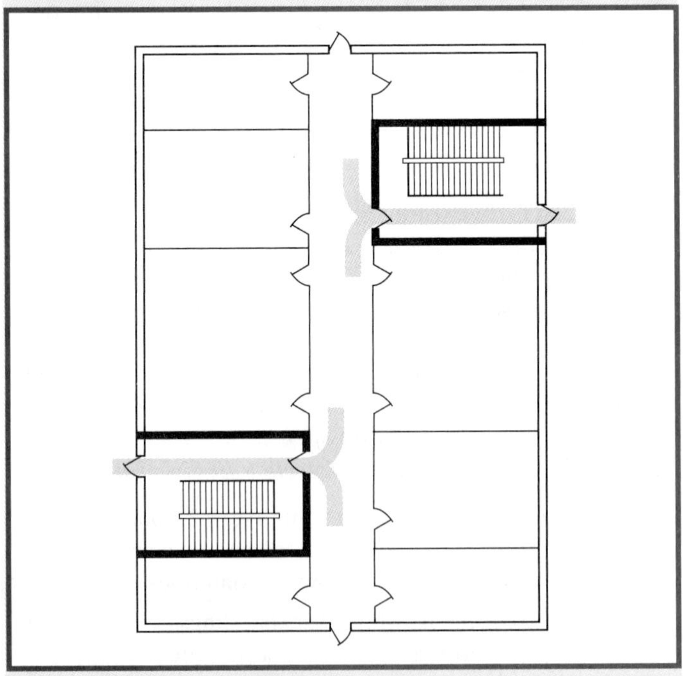

***Exhibit 7.5*** *Convenience door assemblies permitted from ground floor into exit enclosure.*

door assemblies at the end of the corridor that discharge directly outside provide the required means of egress for the ground floor occupants. Earlier editions of the *Code* limited door assemblies into exit stair enclosures to those *necessary* for access to the enclosure. Some authorities having jurisdiction (AHJ) interpreted that limitation as prohibiting the convenience door assembly from the ground floor to the exit stair enclosure. The *Code* was revised to delete the concept of necessity for openings and now states that openings in exit enclosures are limited to door assemblies from normally occupied spaces and corridors and door assemblies for egress from the enclosure. Thus, the arrangement depicted in Exhibit 7.5, with the convenience door assemblies into the stair enclosures on the ground floor, is permitted.

The required degree of fire resistance–rated separation for the exit enclosure depends on the number of stories or floor levels the exit connects, not the height of the building. It is possible to have stairs in a high-rise building connecting only three or fewer stories. In such a case, the enclosing construction is not required to be more than 1-hour fire resistance rated. See Exhibit 7.6. Where connecting four stories or more, exit stairs must be separated from other spaces within the building by 2-hour fire resistance–rated noncombustible, limited-combustible, or fire-retardant-treated wood construction. Where connecting three or fewer stories, the separation is permitted to be reduced to a minimum 1-hour rating. Via 7.1.3.2.1(2)(a) and 7.1.3.2.1(2)(b), existing exit stair enclosures in existing non-high-rise buildings or in existing sprinklered buildings — regardless of height — are permitted a 1-hour fire resistance rating. As indicated by 7.1.3.2.1(2)(c), some occupancy chapters reduce the 2-hour fire resistance–rated construction requirement to 1 hour — even for new construction — if the building is protected throughout by an approved, supervised automatic sprinkler system. An example can be found in 28.2.2.1.2, applicable to new hotels.

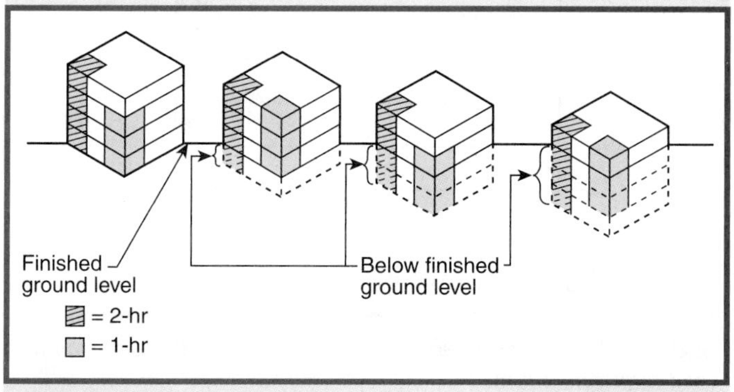


***Exhibit 7.6*** *Required separating construction for exit stairs.*

The door assemblies in walls of exit enclosures are to be 1-hour fire protection–rated door assemblies where used in 1-hour fire resistance–rated enclosures, and $1\frac{1}{2}$-hour fire protection–rated door assemblies where used in 2-hour fire resistance–rated enclosures. See Table 8.3.4.2. Paragraph 8.3.4.3 modifies the provisions of Table 8.3.4.2 by permitting existing $\frac{3}{4}$-hour fire protection–rated door assemblies to continue in use in lieu of the minimum 1-hour fire protection rating required by the table.

If a pair of fire door leaves opening in the same direction without a center mullion post between the door leaf panels is to be used in an opening in an exit enclosure, it would be prudent to choose a pair of door leaves listed for use without an overlapping astragal plate. Pairs of door leaves with an astragal must be arranged to close in a particular sequence to ensure full closure. A coordinator is required to accomplish the sequential closing, and the record of coordinators functioning properly is poor. However, a pair of door leaves without an astragal could pass considerable smoke through any gap between the meeting edges of the leaves and into the exit; therefore, the use of pairs of fire door leaves opening in the same direction into an exit enclosure, without a center mullion post, should be discouraged.

The provisions of 7.1.3.2.1(4) and (6) work together to limit the combustibility of the minimum 2-hour fire resistance–rated separating construction required by 7.1.3.2.1(2). Additionally, such 2-hour separating construction must be supported by construction having a minimum 2-hour fire resistance rating. The effect of this requirement is that, in a building with floor/ceiling assemblies of less than a 2-hour fire resistance rating, the exit stair enclosure fire barrier walls are not permitted to be supported by the building floors. Rather, the exit stair enclosure needs to be a self-supporting shaft system.

The provision of 7.1.3.2.1(5) is new to the 2009 edition of the *Code*. It supplements the requirement of 7.1.3.2.1(4) to help ensure that structural elements that support exit stair components are protected to the same level as required for the exit enclosure. The new provision will prevent the early failure of exit enclosures and related egress elements. For example, a hanger rod supporting a stair landing must not be installed within a wall cavity, as the cavity and outer wall membrane do not provide the required minimum fire resistance rating that the entire wall assembly provides (i.e., the fire resistance rating achieved by the combination of the outer wall membrane, cavity, and inner wall membrane). The text of A.7.1.3.2.1(5) clarifies that outside walls that are not required to be fire rated to complete the separation of the exit stair from the remainder of the floor are permitted to be penetrated by structural elements, such as the stair landing hanger rod referenced earlier in this paragraph.

In accordance with 7.1.3.2.1(8), the only openings permitted in the exit enclosure are for door assemblies providing access into the enclosure from normally occupied spaces and corridors and for door assemblies providing egress from the enclosure into the exit discharge. These door assemblies are required to be self-closing fire door assemblies as described in 7.2.1.8. No opening through the exit enclosure walls — including a door opening — is permitted from storage rooms, closets, boiler rooms, equipment spaces, utility rooms, electrical vaults, or similar spaces that are not normally occupied. Access panels to access building spaces cannot be installed in the walls or ceilings of exit enclosures, regardless of whether the access panels have a fire resistance rating.

Paragraph 7.1.3.2.1(8)(a) permits openings from normally unoccupied spaces within the exit enclosures created by exit passageways in mall buildings, as detailed in Chapters 36 and 37. By consulting the provisions of 36.4.4.6.2 and 37.4.4.6.2, one finds that rooms housing building service equipment, service elevators, and janitor closets — spaces not normally occupied — are permitted to open directly onto mall building exit passageways. For an explanation of this deviation from the requirement of 7.1.3.2.1(8), see the commentary following 36/37.4.4.

Paragraph 7.1.3.2.1(8)(b) recognizes that, in some existing buildings, it is safe to permit unoccupied rooms to open directly onto an exit stair enclosure. For example, in some existing hospitals, it is common to have interstitial spaces above the ceiling of each floor for purposes of running pipes, ducts, and conduits. The interstitial spaces appear much like separate floors. For example, in an elevation view of a four-story hospital, it would appear that there are eight stories. Patients would occupy every other floor, and the alternating "floors" created by the interstitial spaces would house the service pipes, ducts, and conduits. This arrangement is depicted in Exhibit 7.7. Access to the patient floors and to the interstitial space "floors" would be by means of fire protection rated–door assemblies from the stair enclosure. See 7.1.3.2.1(8)(b) for the other criteria necessary to permit the existing situation to be continued in use.

Exit enclosure penetrations generally are prohibited for new construction.

Penetrations for ductwork for pressurization of smokeproof enclosures might be permitted (see 7.2.3), but penetration by other ductwork is prohibited. Penetrations are permitted by 7.1.3.2.1(9) for the following:

1. Water and steam piping necessary for the heating and cooling of the exit enclosure
2. Electrical conduit serving the exit enclosure
3. Fire alarm system circuit wiring installed in metallic conduit and serving the building
4. Standpipe and sprinkler piping serving the building

The technical committee carefully compiled the list of penetrations permitted by 7.1.3.2.1(9) to be a complete list rather than a partial list of examples. Given that fire alarm system circuit wiring installed in metallic conduit is permitted, some designers and contractors have attempted to justify placing control panels within the exit enclosure. It was not the committee's intent to permit fire alarm system controls and associated components, other than circuit wiring in metallic conduit, to be installed within the exit enclosure.

Openings to the exterior of the building are not regulated, provided that there is no potential fire exposure from an adjacent source. Such openings need not be protected with fire protection–rated assemblies, because they are not separating the exit from other parts of the building. However, where the exterior wall of the exit stair enclosure is not fire resistance rated, such stair is subject to the provisions of 7.2.2.5.2. See Figure A.7.2.2.5.2(c) for an example of the fire-rated separating construction needed for an exterior

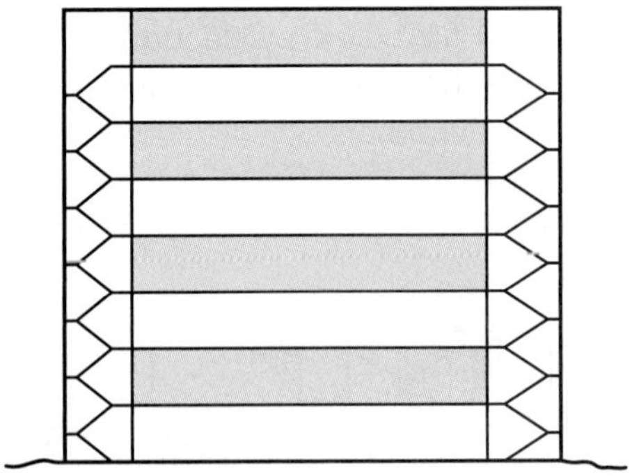


***Exhibit 7.7** Unoccupied interstitial spaces with openings to exit stair enclosure.*

wall segment adjacent to, and exposing, the nonrated exterior wall of an exit stair enclosure at an angle of less than 180 degrees.

**7.1.3.2.2** An exit enclosure shall provide a continuous protected path of travel to an exit discharge.

Paragraph 7.1.3.2.2 emphasizes that exit enclosures, and the protection they afford the occupants, must be continuous. It is a fundamental premise that, once an occupant has been provided the level of protection afforded by an exit, that level of protection must be maintained to the exit discharge.

Paragraph 7.1.3.2.2 prohibits an exit stair or exit ramp arrangement that requires a person to leave the exit enclosure, become exposed to conditions on a floor, and then re-enter the exit enclosure to continue moving to the exit discharge. Exhibit 7.8 shows an unacceptable arrangement. The discontinuity of leaving the stair enclosure, and then re-entering the stair enclosure to continue moving to the level of exit discharge, creates too great a potential for exposing occupants to danger and blocking their egress route.

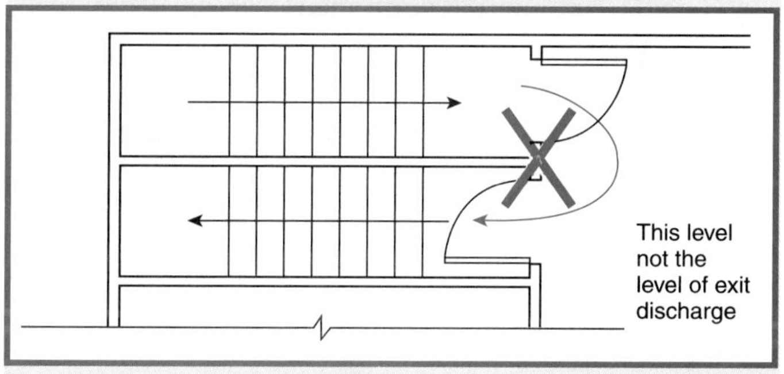


***Exhibit 7.8*** *Unacceptable arrangement for enclosing a stair serving as a required exit.*

**7.1.3.2.3*** An exit enclosure shall not be used for any purpose that has the potential to interfere with its use as an exit and, if so designated, as an area of refuge. *(See also 7.2.2.5.3.)*

**A.7.1.3.2.3** This provision prohibits the use of exit enclosures for storage or for installation of equipment not necessary for safety. Occupancy is prohibited other than for egress, refuge, and access. The intent is that the exit enclosure essentially be "sterile" with respect to fire safety hazards.

Paragraph 7.1.3.2.3 prohibits the use of an exit enclosure for any purpose that could potentially interfere with its use as an exit or as an area of refuge. For example, use of an enclosed exit stair to house vending machines, copying machines, or storage, or to run electrical distribution wires and cables to areas of the building, is prohibited. Standpipes and emergency lighting that are part of the life safety features are permitted only if their arrangement does not interfere with the passage of people. This limitation covers more than mechanical obstruction of the egress path; it includes any use that could interfere with the use of the exit. See also 7.1.10.1 and 7.2.2.5.3.

The prohibitions of the previous paragraph also apply to exit passageways, because they also are exit enclosures.

### 7.1.4 Interior Finish in Exit Enclosures.

**7.1.4.1* Interior Wall and Ceiling Finish in Exit Enclosures.** Interior wall and ceiling finish shall be in accordance with Section 10.2. In exit enclosures, interior wall and ceiling finish materials complying with Section 10.2 shall be Class A or Class B.

**A.7.1.4.1** See Chapters 12 through 42 for further limitations on interior wall and ceiling finish.

**7.1.4.2* Interior Floor Finish in Exit Enclosures.** New interior floor finish in exit enclosures, including stair treads and risers, shall be not less than Class II in accordance with Section 10.2.

**A.7.1.4.2** See Chapters 12 through 42 for further limitations on interior floor finish.

Paragraph 7.1.4.1 regulates interior wall and ceiling finish within exit enclosures, such as enclosed exit stairs. The intent is to minimize the possibility of fire spreading into and within the exit enclosure. Except as modified by occupancy Chapters 12 through 42, the interior wall and ceiling finish in exit enclosures is required to be either Class A or Class B, as detailed in Section 10.2. Because 7.1.4.1 does not prohibit the use of the provisions of 10.2.8.1, Class C interior wall and ceiling finish would be permitted within an exit enclosure if automatic sprinklers protected the enclosure and adjacent areas of the building.

As explained in the commentary following 4.4.2.3, the occupancy chapters can modify the requirements of Chapters 1 through 4 and Chapters 6 through 10. In some cases, the modification results in a more stringent requirement. In others, the result is a relaxation of a base chapter requirement. Interior finish is addressed in detail in Section 10.2, with specific limitations in subsection __.3.3 of the occupancy chapters. For example, for new interior wall and ceiling finish materials in health care occupancies, the requirements of 18.3.3 result in more stringent criteria for wall and ceiling finish within exit enclosures than are required by 7.1.4. Where new interior wall finish is installed in a nonsprinklered health care occupancy, the requirement is for Class A — not Class B — materials. If the enclosure and adjacent smoke compartments of the building are sprinklered, the requirement is for Class B — not Class C — materials. In this case, the occupancy chapter, considering the needs of its typical occupant group (i.e., persons incapable of self-preservation for whom a defend-in-place strategy is employed), tailors its provisions to help achieve the intended minimum level of life safety.

### 7.1.5* Headroom.

**A.7.1.5** For the purpose of this requirement, projections include devices such as lighting equipment, emergency signaling equipment, environmental controls and equipment, security devices, signs, and decorations that are typically limited in area.

**7.1.5.1** Means of egress shall be designed and maintained to provide headroom in accordance with other sections of this *Code*, and such headroom shall be not less than 7 ft 6 in. (2285 mm), with projections from the ceiling not less than 6 ft 8 in. (2030 mm) with a tolerance of $-\frac{3}{4}$ in. (−19 mm), above the finished floor, unless otherwise specified by the following:

(1) In existing buildings, the ceiling height shall be not less than 7 ft (2135 mm) from the floor, with projections from the ceiling not less than 6 ft 8 in. (2030 mm) nominal above the floor.
(2) Headroom in industrial equipment access areas as provided in 40.2.5.2 shall be permitted.

**7.1.5.2** The minimum ceiling height shall be maintained for not less than two-thirds of the ceiling area of any room or space, provided that the ceiling height of the remaining ceiling area is not less than 6 ft 8 in. (2030 mm).

**7.1.5.3** Headroom on stairs shall be not less than 6 ft 8 in. (2030 mm) and shall be measured vertically above a plane parallel to, and tangent with, the most forward projection of the stair tread.

The minimum 7 ft 6 in. (2285 mm) ceiling height and the minimum 6 ft 8 in. (2030 mm) clearance below any projections descending from the minimum ceiling height is expressed with a tolerance of $-\frac{3}{4}$ in. (−19 mm) rather than as an absolute minimum height. Thus, it is the intent of 7.1.5.1 to recognize the clearance provided in passing through the door frame opening associated with a standard 6 ft 8 in. (2030 mm) door leaf where the door stop built into the door frame at the top of the door opening encroaches on the height of the opening. Paragraph 7.1.5.3 and the dimensional criteria of 7.2.2.2.1 also permit the 6 ft 8 in. (2030 mm) minimum headroom height on stairways. Paragraph 7.1.5.3 explains how to measure the headroom on stairs. Headroom measurement is illustrated in Exhibit 7.9. The dimension 6 ft 8 in. (2030 mm) is permitted for projections descending from the ceiling and for stairs.

Earlier editions of the *Code* left unanswered the question of how many 6 ft 8 in. (2030 mm) projections are too many, so as to leave too little area with at least 7 ft 6 in. (2285 mm) of headroom height. Since the 2000 edition, 7.1.5.2 has required the 7 ft 6 in. (2285 mm) minimum headroom to be maintained for at least two-thirds of the ceiling area of any room or space.

For industrial occupancies, 40.2.5.2 extends the use of the minimum 6 ft 8 in. (2030 mm) headroom allowance to industrial equipment access walkways, platforms, ramps, and stairs that serve as a component of the means of egress for not more than 20 people.

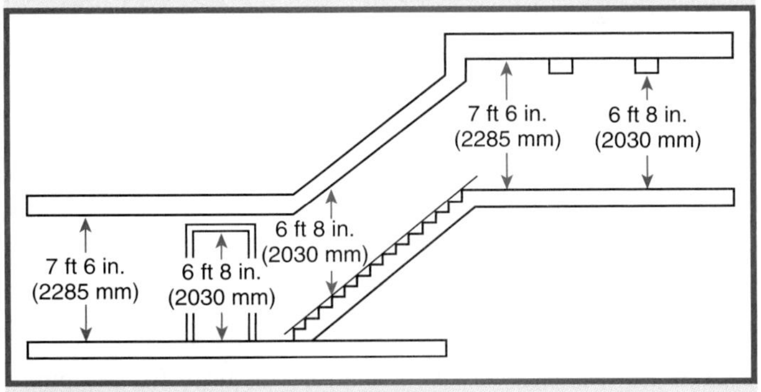


*Exhibit 7.9 Headroom measurement.*

### 7.1.6 Walking Surfaces in the Means of Egress.

**7.1.6.1 General.**

**7.1.6.1.1** Walking surfaces in the means of egress shall comply with 7.1.6.2 through 7.1.6.4.

**7.1.6.1.2** Approved existing walking surfaces shall be permitted.

The vast majority of a building occupant's egress travel time is spent on walking surfaces, rather than passing through door assemblies or traversing other egress components detailed in Section 7.2. Yet, editions of the *Code* prior to 2000 remained silent on the needed characteristics of walking surfaces.

The current provisions applicable to walking surfaces are minimal. They address elevation changes that might cause tripping hazards, maximum slope, and slip resistance that relates to safe use. By addressing, for example, slip resistance in the generalized paragraph applicable to walking surfaces (see 7.1.6.4), it is no longer necessary to repeat similar provisions for the applicable components of means of egress, such as ramps, stair treads, and landing surfaces. It is expected that the provisions of 7.1.6 will be further expanded, such as by codifying measurable slip-resistance criteria, for future editions of the *Code*. The technology has not yet evolved to the degree needed to achieve technical committee consensus on which provisions need to be mandated and which equipment is to be used to take measurements for judging compliance with the criteria mandated.

**7.1.6.2 Changes in Elevation.** Abrupt changes in elevation of walking surfaces shall not exceed $^1/_4$ in. (6.3 mm). Changes in elevation exceeding $^1/_4$ in. (6.3 mm), but not exceeding $^1/_2$ in. (13 mm), shall be beveled with a slope of 1 in 2. Changes in elevation exceeding $^1/_2$ in. (13 mm) shall be considered a change in level and shall be subject to the requirements of 7.1.7.

**7.1.6.3 Level.** Walking surfaces shall comply with the following:

(1) Walking surfaces shall be nominally level.
(2) The slope of a walking surface in the direction of travel shall not exceed 1 in 20, unless the ramp requirements of 7.2.5 are met.
(3) The slope perpendicular to the direction of travel shall not exceed 1 in 48.

**7.1.6.4* Slip Resistance.** Walking surfaces shall be slip resistant under foreseeable conditions. The walking surface of each element in the means of egress shall be uniformly slip resistant along the natural path of travel.

**A.7.1.6.4** The foreseeable slip conditions are those that are likely to be present at the location of the walking surface during the use of the building or area. A foreseeable condition of a swimming pool deck is that it is likely to be wet.

Regarding the slip resistance of treads, it should be recognized that, when walking up or down stairs, a person's foot exerts a smaller horizontal force against treads than is exerted when walking on level floors. Therefore, materials used for floors that are acceptable as slip resistant (as described by ASTM F 1637, *Standard Practice for Safe Walking Surfaces*) provide adequate slip resistance where used for stair treads. Such slip resistance includes the important leading edges of treads, the part of the tread that the foot first contacts during descent, which is the most critical direction of travel. If stair treads are wet, there is an increased danger of slipping, just as there is an increased danger of slipping on wet floors of similar materials. A small wash or drainage slope on exterior stair treads is, therefore, recommended to shed water. *(See Templer, J. A., The Staircase: Studies of Hazards, Falls, and Safer Design, Cambridge, MA: MIT Press, 1992.)*

### 7.1.7 Changes in Level in Means of Egress.

**7.1.7.1** Changes in level in means of egress shall be achieved by an approved means of egress where the elevation difference exceeds 21 in. (535 mm).

**7.1.7.2*** Changes in level in means of egress not in excess of 21 in. (535 mm) shall be achieved either by a ramp complying with the requirements of 7.2.5 or by a stair complying with the requirements of 7.2.2.

**A.7.1.7.2** Aside from the problems created for persons who are mobility impaired, small changes of elevations in floors are best avoided because of the increased occurrence of missteps where the presence of single steps, a series of steps, or a ramp is not readily apparent. Although small changes of elevation pose significant fall risks in the case of individual movement, they are even more undesirable where crowds traverse the area.

A contrasting marking stripe on each stepping surface can be helpful at the nosing or leading edge so that the location of each step is readily apparent, especially when viewed in descent. Such stripes should be not less than 1 in. (25 mm), but should not exceed 2 in. (51 mm), in width. Other methods could include a relatively higher level of lighting, contrasting colors, contrasting textures, highly prominent handrails, warning signs, a combination thereof, or other similar means. The construction or application of marking stripes should be such that slip resistance is consistent over the walking surface and no tripping hazard is created *(see also A.7.2.2.3.3.2)*. Depending on the distractions of the surroundings, the familiarity of users with a particular small change of level, and especially the number of people that might be in a group traversing the change of level (thereby reducing visibility of the level changes), a strong argument can be made for the elimination of steps and ramps that might pose a risk of missteps.

**7.1.7.2.1** Where a ramp is used, the presence and location of ramped portions of walkways shall be readily apparent.

**7.1.7.2.2** Where a stair is used, the tread depth of such stair shall be not less than 13 in. (330 mm).

**7.1.7.2.3** Tread depth in industrial equipment access areas as provided in 40.2.5.2 shall be permitted.

**7.1.7.2.4** The presence and location of each step shall be readily apparent.

Prior to 1988, the *Code* prohibited stairs where changes of elevation were less than 21 in. (535 mm), because steps spanning such small elevation differences often go unnoticed and create conditions conducive to missteps. The minimum 13 in. (330 mm) tread depth and the requirement to make the presence and location of each step readily apparent were established to help reduce missteps. The text of A.7.1.7.2 provides additional details on stair arrangement to help reduce the problem.

Exhibit 7.10 illustrates an arrangement intended to meet the requirements of 7.1.7. In the exhibit, tread depth has been increased over the usual minimum 11 in. (280 mm) to a minimum of 13 in. (330 mm). The leading edge of each tread has been marked to make its presence and location readily apparent.

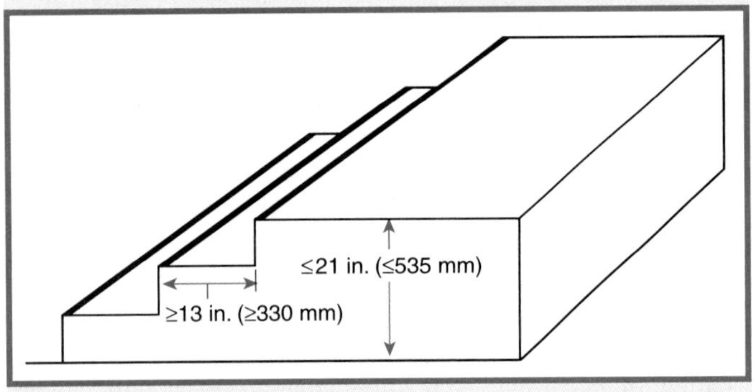


***Exhibit 7.10** Special features for stairs involving changes in elevation of 21 in. (535 mm) or less.*

Small elevation differences connected by ramps might also go unnoticed and create conditions conducive to missteps. Paragraph 7.1.7.2.1 covers the hazards of trips and other missteps on ramps where such hazards are not clear to persons walking in an area where a small change of elevation is otherwise not evident. Although the consequences of a misstep are usually not as severe on ramps as on stairs, hazard mitigation is needed.

Single risers and other combinations of a few risers are considered stairs and must meet all the requirements for stairs. Because such risers are considered stairs, handrails are needed along the natural path of egress travel.

### 7.1.8* Guards.

Guards in accordance with 7.2.2.4 shall be provided at the open sides of means of egress that exceed 30 in. (760 mm) above the floor or the finished ground level below.

**A.7.1.8** Elements of the means of egress that might require protection with guards include stairs, landings, escalators, moving walks, balconies, corridors, passageways, floor or roof openings, ramps, aisles, porches, and mezzanines.

Escalators and moving walks, other than previously approved existing escalators and moving walks, are prohibited from serving as components of the required means of egress. Building occupants using the escalator at the time of fire or similar emergency must traverse some portion of the escalator to gain access to a required egress route. For those building occupants using the escalator, such travel along the escalator is part of their means of egress. The requirement that guards be provided at the open side of means of egress that exceed 30 in. (760 mm) above the floor or grade below is meant to be applied to escalators and moving walks.

The text of A.7.1.8 reminds the user that guards need to be located at more than the open sides of stairs. Because guards have applicability to a range of locations within a building [i.e., wherever there is a vertical drop of more than 30 in. (760 mm)], the requirement for guards is located in the general provisions of Section 7.1. The detailed provisions for guards are found in 7.2.2 for stairs but apply for all guards, regardless of where the guards are located.

### 7.1.9 Impediments to Egress.

Any device or alarm installed to restrict the improper use of a means of egress shall be designed and installed so that it cannot, even in case of failure, impede or prevent emergency use of such means of egress, unless otherwise provided in 7.2.1.6 and Chapters 18, 19, 22, and 23.

### 7.1.10 Means of Egress Reliability.

**7.1.10.1* General.** Means of egress shall be continuously maintained free of all obstructions or impediments to full instant use in the case of fire or other emergency.

**A.7.1.10.1** A proper means of egress allows unobstructed travel at all times. Any type of barrier including, but not limited to, the accumulations of snow and ice in those climates subject to such accumulations is an impediment to free movement in the means of egress.

For a given occupancy, the combination of requirements contained in Chapters 7 and 8 and in the corresponding occupancy chapter provides for an adequately sized and protected means of egress system. The provision in 7.1.10.1 emphasizes the importance of keeping the egress system usable at all times. In the case of a Class A mercantile occupancy, for example, the minimum 60 in. (1525 mm) exit access aisle width required by 36.2.5.6 and 37.2.5.6 must not, subsequent to receipt of the store's occupancy permit, be filled with mid-aisle displays that reduce the aisle width. Similarly, in a business occupancy with a new exit stair of the minimum 44 in. (1120 mm) width required by Table 7.2.2.2.1.2(B), the stair width must not be reduced by the introduction of a mechanized chairlift that is installed, for example, to comply with legislation mandating accessibility for persons with mobility impairments. [For additional guidance on the installation of stair descent devices, see A.7.2.12.2.3(2).] In an apartment building complex, the required width of the outside exit discharge sidewalk that runs along the side of the building must not be reduced by the presence of a trash dumpster on either a temporary or permanent basis.

Paragraph 7.1.10.1 does not designate responsibility for keeping the means of egress (i.e., exit accesses, exits, and exit discharges) free and clear of obstructions. The individuals responsible for each facility — whether managers, owners, or operators — must make certain that the required egress components are maintained in usable condition. The authority having jurisdiction has the power to enforce this requirement.

Shortly after the 2006 edition of the *Code* was published, NFPA staff received inquiries from authorities having jurisdiction looking for requirements they could use in their enforcement efforts to ban the introduction of artificial smoke into a building upon activation of an intrusion alarm. The intent behind the introduction of the artificial smoke was to disorient intruders and make it difficult for them to travel through the building. Emergency responders called to the building were similarly disoriented, making it dangerous to enter the building. Paragraph 7.1.10.1, by requiring that the means of egress be continuously maintained free of all obstructions and impediments to full instant use in case of fire or other emergency, provides authorities having jurisdiction with a tangible requirement that they can enforce to prohibit intrusion alarms from discharging smoke to obscure the egress path. Also see 4.6.1.2, which gives the AHJ the authority to determine any requirements that are essential for the safety of building occupants and that are not specifically provided for by the *Code*.

**7.1.10.2 Furnishings and Decorations in Means of Egress.**

Paragraphs 7.1.10.2.1 through 7.1.10.2.3 provide guidance for the interior decoration and maintenance of buildings that serve, for example, as restaurants and theaters, where mirrored wall surfaces and excessive decoration can camouflage and, in some cases, obstruct exits. For such occupancies, care must be taken to ensure that the required, standard, well-marked exit access that leads to an unobstructed exit is not obscured in the pursuit of period or style authenticity. For example, a restaurant that is heavily decorated with red wall coverings might use green exit signs to help meet the requirements of these paragraphs, despite the fact that Chapter 7 does not specify exit sign color.

**7.1.10.2.1** No furnishings, decorations, or other objects shall obstruct exits or their access thereto, egress therefrom, or visibility thereof.

**7.1.10.2.2** No obstruction by railings, barriers, or gates shall divide the means of egress into sections appurtenant to individual rooms, apartments, or other occupied spaces. Where the authority having jurisdiction finds the required path of travel to be obstructed by furniture or other movable objects, the authority shall be permitted to require that such objects be secured out of the way or shall be permitted to require that railings or other permanent barriers be installed to protect the path of travel against encroachment.

Paragraph 7.1.10.2.2 relates to the arrangement of furniture, as well as to the arrangement of railings, gates, or barriers found in lobbies, foyers, waiting spaces, or staging areas of businesses, hospitals, health care clinics, hotels, and apartments. Because these large spaces are often subdivided by furniture (e.g., chairs, tables, and plants) or by railings and gates, furnishings must be prevented from blocking access to exits.

Paragraph 7.1.10.2.2 recommends fastening furnishings so that they are clear of access to exits or placing railings around furnishings to ensure that they are held within a fixed area and cannot be easily moved or rearranged. The *Code* recognizes the problem created by storage that is placed within the exit access aisles of storage rooms in mercantile occupancies, which is a violation of *Code* requirements. Both Chapters 36 and 37, in accordance with the provisions of 36.2.5.11(4) and 37.2.5.11(4), require an unobstructed egress path to be maintained as a specific condition for permitting egress to pass through storerooms.

**7.1.10.2.3** Mirrors shall not be placed on exit door leaves. Mirrors shall not be placed in or adjacent to any exit in such a manner as to confuse the direction of egress.

### 7.1.11 Sprinkler System Installation.

Where another provision of this chapter requires an automatic sprinkler system, the sprinkler system shall be installed in accordance with the subparts of 9.7.1.1 permitted by the applicable occupancy chapters.

Paragraph 9.7.1.1 lists the three NFPA sprinkler installation standards as options for other sections of the *Code* to reference where the installation of automatic sprinklers is required. Some provisions of Chapter 7 mandate the installation of sprinklers as a condition for using a particular feature. For example, the delayed-egress locking provisions of 7.2.1.6.1 require that the building be protected by either a fire detection system or an automatic sprinkler system. Yet, Chapter 7 is a core chapter that might apply to any occupancy. Thus, the requirement of 7.1.11 leaves the choice of an applicable sprinkler system installation standard to the appropriate occupancy chapter.

## 7.2 Means of Egress Components

Many different components of a building or structure are encountered while traversing a means of egress. These components comprise the means of egress and include such items as door assemblies, including necessary hardware; stairs and ramps, including handrails and guards; horizontal exits; exit passageways; and areas of refuge. The composition, properties, use, limits, and function of such components have an effect on the usability of the means of egress system.

Portable ladders, rope ladders, and similar devices are not recognized by the *Code* as providing any portion of the required capacity of a means of egress. In addition, they should not be considered in any way as an upgrade of an inadequate existing means of egress. Although such devices might be used to provide additional safety under emergency conditions, they are unreliable and can lead to a false sense of security. Such devices are often unusable by small children, older people, persons with disabilities, or those who simply have not been trained in their use.

Changing technology and product development are responsible for the availability of supplemental evacuation equipment with features more desirable than those inherent in portable ladders, rope ladders, and similar traditional escape devices. Supplemental evacuation equipment (e.g., exterior platforms, accessed by building occupants via windows in outside walls, that travel vertically against the building walls by a cable and hoist system to carry occupants to ground level) receives no credit as satisfying any of the *Code*-mandated means of egress provisions. However, if a building owner voluntarily installs such a system, the *Code* user should implement additional safeguards to help ensure that the supplemental evacuation equipment does not interfere with use of the normal egress components, create a dangerous situation for users, or impart a false sense of security that could lead to a delay in building egress. Such safeguards are detailed in new Annex C, Supplemental Evacuation Equipment.

The components of a means of egress are required to meet certain standards, be built in a prescribed manner, and perform at a level specified by the *Code*. Depending on whether the component is part of the access to an exit, is itself the exit, or is part of the exit discharge, the applicable requirements might differ. In most instances, the requirements applicable to a given component are the same, regardless of where it is used within the means of egress system. For example, for new stair construction, the riser height must not exceed 7 in. (180 mm), the tread depth must be at least 11 in. (280 mm), and the handrails must be installed at both sides — regardless of where the stairs are placed within the means of egress (unenclosed exit access stairs, enclosed exit stairs, or outside exit discharge stairs).

### 7.2.1 Door Openings.

**7.2.1.1 General.**

Door assemblies serve multiple purposes that relate to the comfort and safety of building occupants and provide protection from the following:

1. Weather, drafts, noise, and disturbance from adjoining areas
2. Trespass by unauthorized persons
3. Fire and smoke, with which this *Code* is concerned

The three broad categories of door asemblies, each providing varying degrees of protection from fire and smoke, follow.

**1.** *Non-fire-rated door assembly.* A non-fire-rated door assembly is a door assembly such as is used in one- and two-family dwelling construction or a door assembly to a small coat closet in an office building. Although not fire rated, such door assemblies do provide a limited degree of protection, especially from smoke, if closed.

**2.** *Fire-rated door assembly.* A fire protection–rated door assembly is referred to as a *fire door assembly.* It has passed the standard fire test for door assemblies, as prescribed by NFPA 252, *Standard Methods of Fire Tests of Door Assemblies.*[4] During such fire testing, a fire door assembly withstands a severe fire and hose stream exposure for a given time period, which can be specified by a *Code* requirement. The fire protection rating required by the *Code* for a given application varies, depending on the uses and occupancy type involved.

**3.** *Smoke-resisting door assembly.* A smoke-resisting door assembly might or might not have a fire protection rating. Its function is to provide a temporary barrier against the passage of heat, smoke, and gases. Some smoke-resisting door assemblies required by the *Code* must meet performance and installation criteria specified in NFPA 105, *Standard for the Installation of Smoke Door Assemblies and Other Opening Protectives.*[5]

None of the door assemblies discussed in this commentary will perform satisfactorily if left open during a fire, thus allowing the entry of fire and combustion products into what should be a safer area than the fire area. The history of fires is full of tragic examples of those who died because of an open door assembly. There are also many examples of people saved because a door leaf was closed. Less frequent, but nonetheless tragic, are those situations in which door openings needed for escape were blocked or locked, resulting in dire consequences. Numerous *Code* requirements, particularly those contained in 7.2.1, address these concerns.

Some types of door assemblies that are designed to prevent the spread of fire through wall openings for property protection purposes might be unsuitable for use in means of egress. Certain door assemblies pose the potential for entrapment if they cannot be operated or for personal injury if they are used; examples include various rolling-shutter and sliding door assemblies. However, under limited conditions, certain horizontal-sliding door assemblies are permitted to be within the exit access path. For example, 7.2.1.4.1(7) is used by 39.2.2.2.8, 40.2.2.2.4, and 42.2.2.2.4 to permit existing sliding door assemblies to be positioned within the exit access path of existing business, industrial, and storage occupancies if additional criteria are met. The provisions help to ensure that the door leaf will be open when conditions in the door opening's vicinity are tenable for people movement and closed once it is no longer safe for people to seek egress via that exit access path.

See also 7.2.1.14 for a specialized form of sliding door assembly that has desirable life safety features.

**7.2.1.1.1** A door assembly in a means of egress shall conform to the general requirements of Section 7.1 and to the special requirements of 7.2.1.

Wherever the *Code* refers to a fire protection–rated door assembly or fire door assembly, it is referring to the entire assembly. If any single component is not properly provided, installed, and functioning, the assembly is not a fire protection–rated assembly. For example, if a listed fire door leaf and frame are installed with positive latch and hinges but the required self-closing device is omitted, the assembly cannot be considered a fire door assembly and is not considered to have any particular fire protection rating.

**7.2.1.1.2** Every door opening and every principal entrance that is required to serve as an exit shall be designed and constructed so that the path of egress travel is obvious and direct. Windows that, because of their physical configuration or design and the materials used in their construction, have the potential to be mistaken for door openings shall be made inaccessible to the occupants by barriers or railings.

The purpose of the barriers or railings required by 7.2.1.1.2 is to prevent an occupant from walking through a window. Such barriers are not required to comply with the requirements of 7.2.2.4 applicable to guards. For example, intermediate rails or balusters spaced to meet the 4 in. (100 mm) diameter sphere requirement of 7.2.2.4.5.3 are not needed. A simple barrier rail, without ornamental grille-like fill or closely spaced balusters, will adequately warn occupants to avoid walking into a glass wall or large windowpane.

**7.2.1.1.3 Occupied Building.**

**7.2.1.1.3.1** For the purposes of Section 7.2, a building shall be considered to be occupied at any time it meets any of the following criteria:

(1) It is open for general occupancy.
(2) It is open to the public.
(3) It is occupied by more than 10 persons.

**7.2.1.1.3.2** Where means of egress doors are locked in a building that is not considered occupied, occupants shall not be locked beyond their control in buildings or building spaces, except for lockups in accordance with 22.4.5 and 23.4.5, detention and correctional occupancies, and health care occupancies.

Many industrial, storage, and business occupancy buildings are never open to or accessible to the public; the only occupants are employees and authorized visitors. Therefore, the term *occupied* in 7.2.1.1.3.1 also includes the condition of being *open for general occupancy*. That is, the facility is *operating* or *functioning*.

The intent of permitting a building with 10 or fewer occupants to be considered unoccupied — if it is not open for general occupancy and not open to the public — is to allow small security details or small cleaning crews inside a building without applying all the *Code* requirements. This will allow door assemblies to be locked and lights to be turned off without violating the *Code*. The limited number of occupants will use lights as they need them and then turn them off. In the case of security personnel, they will carry their own lights and keys. For example, see the criterion of 7.2.1.5.4.1(4) for making a key available to occupants, which is applicable to a special type of key-operated dead bolt lock.

The wording of 7.2.1.1.3.2 reiterates that it is not the intent to allow people, no matter how few the number, to be locked in a building without a ready means of egress. Even in detention and correctional facilities, where locked door assemblies are permitted, 24-hour staffing must be provided in sufficient numbers to start the release of locks necessary for emergency evacuation or rescue and initiate other necessary emergency actions within 2 minutes of alarm. See 22.7.1.1(2) and 23.7.1.1(2).

**7.2.1.2 Door Leaf Width.**

The title of 7.2.1.2 is Door Leaf Width, but, for other than the atypical case where door leaf width is specified [see 7.2.1.2.3.1 and, for example, 7.2.1.2.3.2(4)], the provisions of 7.2.1.2 address clear width of the door opening and egress capacity width of the door opening.

Door width measurements might be used in calculating egress capacity or in determining if a minimum door width requirement is met. Depending on the purpose for which the door width measurement is used, the allowable encroachments on opening width vary. See the commentary following 7.2.1.2.1.1(6) and 7.2.1.2.2.2.

**7.2.1.2.1* Measurement of Clear Width.**

The method of measuring door width required by 7.2.1.2.1.1 and 7.2.1.2.1.2 is for meeting minimum door-opening, clear width requirements specified elsewhere in the *Code*, not for determining the egress capacity of the door opening. For example, 7.2.1.2.3.2 requires new door openings in means of egress to be not less than 32 in. (810 mm) in clear width, based on the need for an occupant traveling in a wheelchair to be able to move the wheelchair through the door opening, with allowance for the wheelchair user's arms and hands to guide the wheels.

**A.7.2.1.2.1** Figure A.7.2.1.2.1(a) and Figure A.7.2.1.2.1(b) illustrate the method of measuring clear width for doors.

In cases where a chapter requires a door width, for example, of not less than 36 in. (915 mm), this requirement can be met by a door leaf of the minimum specified width if the term *clear width* does not appear as part of the minimum width requirement. A pair of cross-corridor doors subject to such a requirement would be judged under the following criteria:

(1) Each door leaf is required to be not less than 36 in. (915 mm) in width.
(2) The pair of doors is required to provide sufficient, clear, unobstructed width (which will be less than the door leaf width measurement) to handle its assigned occupant load, based on a calculation using the appropriate egress capacity factor in Table 7.3.3.1.

Where swinging doors do not open at least 90 degrees, the clear width of the doorway should be measured between the face of the door and the stop.

It is not the intent to regulate projections above the 6 ft 8 in. (2030 mm) height.

**7.2.1.2.1.1 Swinging Door Assemblies.** For swinging door assemblies, clear width shall be measured as follows:

(1) The measurement shall be taken at the narrowest point in the door opening.
(2) The measurement shall be taken between the face of the door leaf and the stop of the frame.

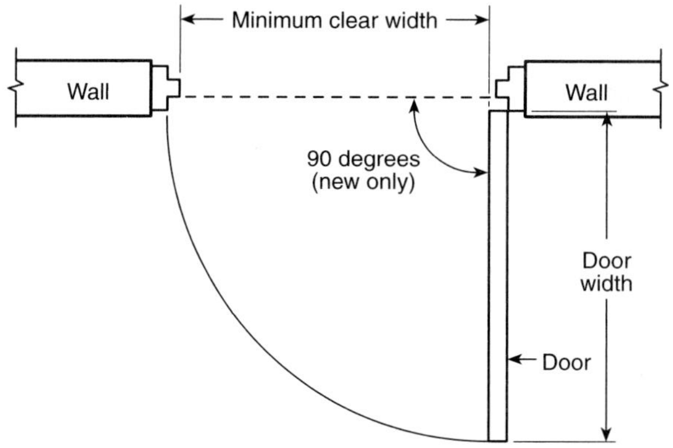


*Figure A.7.2.1.2.1(a) Minimum Clear Width.*

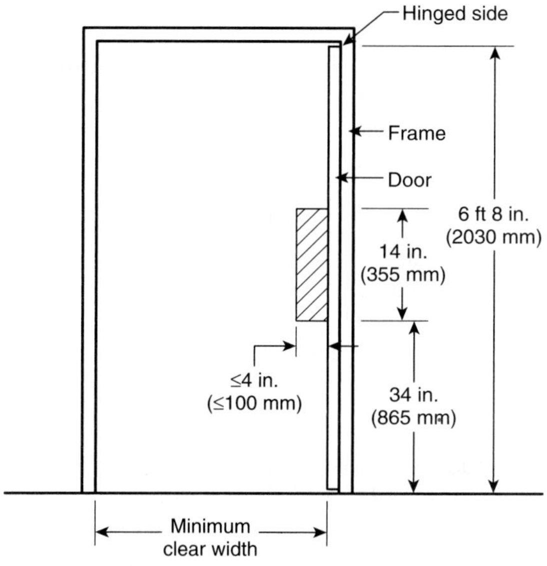


*Figure A.7.2.1.2.1(b) Minimum Clear Width with Permitted Obstructions.*

(3) For new swinging door assemblies, the measurement shall be taken with the door leaf open 90 degrees.
(4) For any existing door assembly, the measurement shall be taken with the door leaf in the fully open position.
(5) Projections of not more than 4 in. (100 mm) into the door opening width on the hinge side shall not be considered reductions in clear width, provided that such projections are for purposes of accommodating panic hardware or fire exit hardware and are located not less than 34 in. (865 mm), and not more than 48 in. (1220 mm), above the floor.
(6) Projections exceeding 6 ft 8 in. (2030 mm) above the floor shall not be considered reductions in clear width.

Where clear width is used to judge whether a *Code* provision for minimum door width is met, no projections into the clear width within 34 in. (865 mm) of the floor are permitted, as addressed in 7.2.1.2.1.1(5). Thus, where 7.2.1.2.3.2 requires door openings to be at least 32 in. (810 mm) in clear width, full clear width must be available near the floor to accommodate, for example, the width and height of a wheelchair and the wheelchair user's arms and hands.

At heights above 34 in. (865 mm), encroachment on clear width is permitted only on the hinge side of the door opening, and then only if the projection into the clear width does not exceed 4 in. (100 mm). Further, such projection is only for purposes of permitting panic hardware or fire exit hardware — installed in accordance with 7.2.1.7.1(2) at the minimum 34 in. (865 mm) mounting height set for new installations and the maximum mounting height of 48 in. (1220 mm) for new and existing installations — to encroach on clear width. Note, however, that projections above the floor of more than 6 ft 8 in. (2030 mm) are permitted by 7.2.1.2.1.1(6). Thus, for many door assemblies that exceed the minimum nominal height of 6 ft 8 in. (2030 mm), the projection created by a magnetic lock or hydraulic door leaf closer attached beneath the top member of the door frame is not an encroachment on door width. For door assemblies utilizing a minimum 6 ft 8 in. (2030 mm) height door frame, magnetic locks or hydraulic door leaf closers attached beneath the top member of the door frame will encroach on the space within the 6 ft 8 in. (2030 mm) vertical distance of the floor and constitute a reduction in clear width. In this case, where the minimum 6 ft 8 in. (2030 mm) height door frame is used, the concerns of the AHJ with excessive encroachment by the hydraulic leaf closer have often been allayed where the closer is mounted to the door leaf, and not suspended beneath the top member of the door frame, so as to move out of the door opening when the door leaf swings open.

Figure A.7.2.1.2.1(b) shows a 14 in. (355 mm) vertical range for mounting the panic hardware or fire exit hardware permitted by 7.2.1.2.1.1(5), to encroach a maximum of 4 in. (100 mm) into the clear width without penalty. The 14 in. (355 mm) range is the difference between the 34 in. (865 mm) and 48 in. (1220 mm) criteria specified in 7.2.1.2.1.1(5), which are extracted from the minimum and maximum mounting heights for new panic hardware and new fire exit hardware per 7.2.1.7.1(2)(a).

The concepts described in this commentary are illustrated in Figure A.7.2.1.2.1(a) and Figure A.7.2.1.2.1(b).

**7.2.1.2.1.2 Other than Swinging Door Assemblies.** For other than swinging door assemblies, clear width shall be measured as follows:

(1) The measurement shall be taken at the narrowest point in the door opening.
(2) The measurement shall be taken as the door opening width when the door leaf is in the fully open position.
(3) Projections exceeding 6 ft 8 in. (2030 mm) above the floor shall not be considered reductions in clear width.

**7.2.1.2.2* Measurement of Egress Capacity Width.**

**A.7.2.1.2.2** Figure A.7.2.1.2.2(a) and Figure A.7.2.1.2.2(b) illustrate the method of measuring egress capacity width for purposes of calculating door egress capacity.

**7.2.1.2.2.1 Swinging Door Assemblies.** For swinging door assemblies, egress capacity width shall be measured as follows:

(1) The measurement shall be taken at the narrowest point in the door opening.

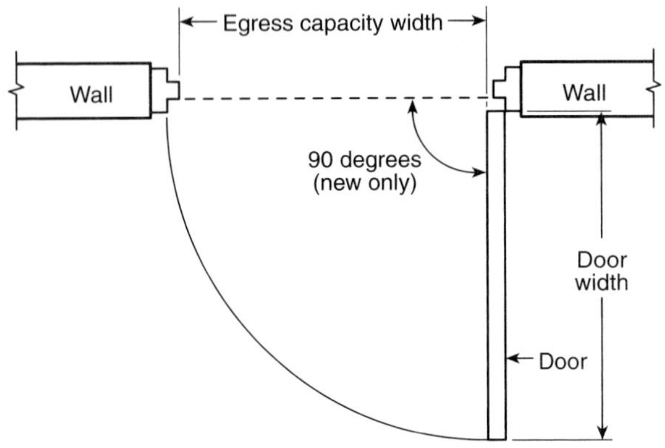


*Figure A.7.2.1.2.2(a) Door Width — Egress Capacity.*

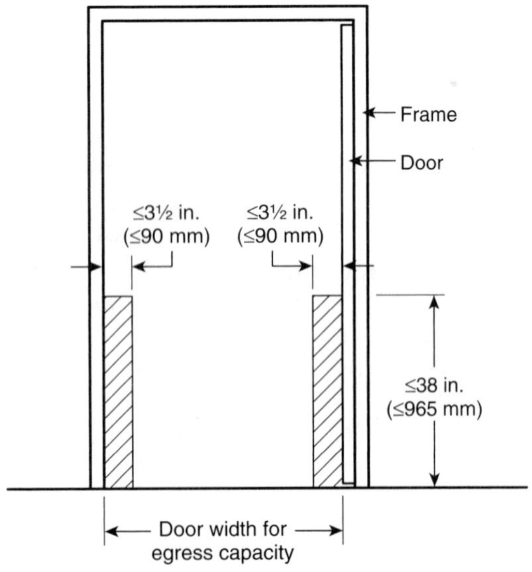


*Figure A.7.2.1.2.2(b) Door Width — Egress Capacity with Permitted Obstructions.*

(2) The measurement shall be taken between the face of the door leaf and the stop of the frame.
(3) For new swinging doors assemblies, the measurement shall be taken with the door leaf open 90 degrees.
(4) For any existing door assembly, the measurement shall be taken with the door leaf in the fully open position.
(5) Projections not more than $3\frac{1}{2}$ in. (90 mm) at each side of the door openings at a height of not more than 38 in. (965 mm) shall not be considered reductions in egress capacity width.
(6) Projections exceeding 6 ft 8 in. (2030 mm) above the floor shall not be considered reductions in egress capacity width.

**7.2.1.2.2.2 Other than Swinging Door Assemblies.** For other than swinging door assemblies, egress capacity width shall be measured as follows:

(1) The measurement shall be taken at the narrowest point in the door opening.
(2) The measurement shall be taken as the door opening width when the door leaf is in the fully open position.
(3) Projections not more than $3\frac{1}{2}$ in. (90 mm) at each side of the door openings at a height of not more than 38 in. (965 mm) shall not be considered reductions in egress capacity width.
(4) Projections exceeding 6 ft 8 in. (2030 mm) above the floor shall not be considered reductions in egress capacity width.

The method of measuring door width required by 7.2.1.2.2.1 and 7.2.1.2.2.2 is to determine the egress capacity of the door assembly, not to meet minimum door size requirements specified elsewhere in the *Code*. The method of measuring door width required by 7.2.1.2.1 is for meeting minimum door-opening, clear width requirements specified elsewhere in the *Code*, not for determining the egress capacity of the door assembly.

The egress capacity width will be less than the door leaf width, because deductions in width are made for the stops built into the door frame and for the encroachment created by the thickness of the door leaf where its stile edge, to which the hinges are secured, extends into the door opening.

The width measurement for new door assemblies that can be opened at least 90 degrees is to be made with the door leaf open 90 degrees. Door leaves that open more than 90 degrees — permitting the stile edge of the door leaf to move out of the door opening — receive no additional width credit, based on the inability of most people to push a door leaf open more than 90 degrees prior to moving through the door opening, especially a door assembly with a self-closing device.

Paragraph 7.2.1.2.2.1(4) exempts existing door assemblies from the 90-degree requirement. Rather, the egress capacity width measurement for existing door assemblies is made with the door leaf in the fully open position — regardless of whether that position is less than or more than 90 degrees.

Exhibit 7.11 depicts a new door assembly. It also might apply to an existing door assembly that opens exactly 90 degrees. The 44 in. (1120 mm) width door leaf provides approximately 40½ in. (1030 mm) of egress capacity width, measured in accordance with 7.2.1.2.2.1 (1), (2), and (3). Note the reduction in egress width, as compared to the door leaf width, caused by the stop in the door frame at the left of the exhibit and the stile edge of the door leaf at the right of the exhibit.

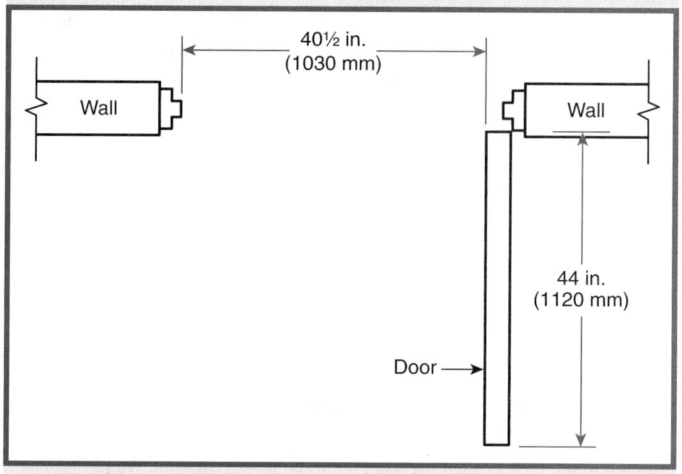


***Exhibit 7.11*** *Egress capacity width for new door leaf open 90 degrees and for existing door leaf that opens 90 degrees.*

Exhibit 7.12 depicts an existing door assembly for which the door leaf can be opened more than 90 degrees so that the stile edge of the door leaf moves out of the framed door opening. The 44 in. (1120 mm) width door leaf provides approximately 42 in. (1065 mm) of egress capacity width, measured in accordance with 7.2.1.2.2.1 (1), (2), and (4). Note the reduction in egress width, as compared to the door leaf width, caused by the stops at each side of the door frame.

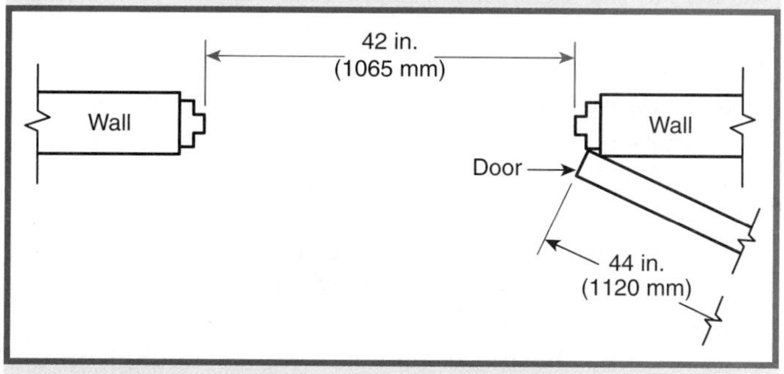


***Exhibit 7.12*** *Egress capacity width for existing door assembly with door leaf that opens more than 90 degrees.*

Exhibit 7.13 depicts an existing door assembly for which the door leaf can be opened less than 90 degrees due to the presence of a pipe column that prevents the door leaf from opening any further. The 44 in. (1120 mm) width door leaf provides approximately 38 in. (965 mm) of egress capacity width, measured in accordance with 7.2.1.2.2.1 (1), (2), and (4). Note the reduction in egress width, as compared to the door leaf width, caused by the stop at the left of the exhibit and the door leaf itself as it extends into the door opening at the right of the exhibit due to the obstruction caused by the pipe column. The 38 in. (965 mm) dimension is measured in accordance with 7.2.1.2.2.1(2) to the face of the door leaf at a point where the intersection with the door leaf creates a right angle, thus ensuring that the minimum width is measured.

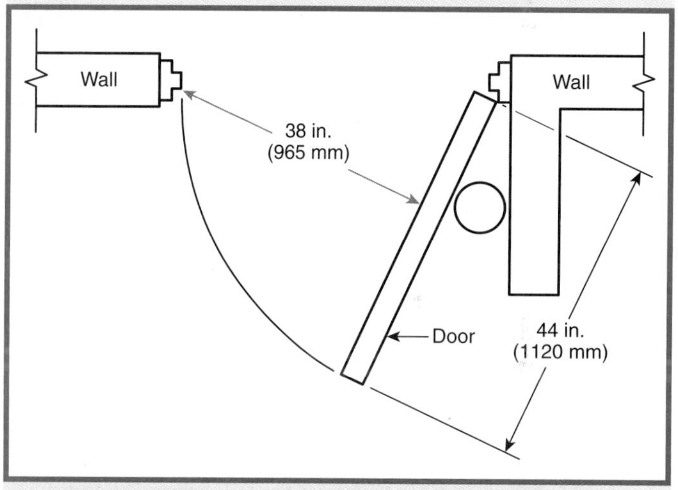


***Exhibit 7.13*** *Egress capacity width for existing door assembly with door leaf that opens less than 90 degrees.*

The wording of 7.2.1.2.2.1(5) permits projections of not more than 3½ in. (90 mm) at each side of the door opening, provided that such projections do not extend above 38 in. (965 mm) in height. For example, for a 40 in. (1015 mm) capacity width door opening, although there might be only 33 in. (840 mm) of *true* opening width between the projections near floor level, capacity calculations are permitted that assume an available capacity width of 40 in. (1015 mm).

The concepts described in this commentary are illustrated in Figure A.7.2.1.2.2(a) and Figure A.7.2.1.2.2(b).

**7.2.1.2.3 Minimum Door Leaf Width.**

**7.2.1.2.3.1** For purposes of determining minimum door opening width, the clear width in accordance with 7.2.1.2.1 shall be used, unless door leaf width is specified.

**7.2.1.2.3.2** Door openings in means of egress shall be not less than 32 in. (810 mm) in clear width, unless one of the following conditions exists:

(1) Where a pair of door leaves is provided, one door leaf shall provide not less than a 32 in. (810 mm) clear width opening.
(2) Exit access door assemblies serving a room not exceeding 70 $ft^2$ (6.5 $m^2$) and not required to be accessible to persons with severe mobility impairments shall be not less than 24 in. (610 mm) in door leaf width.
(3) Door openings serving a building or portion thereof not required to be accessible to persons with severe mobility impairments shall be permitted to be 28 in. (710 mm) in door leaf width.
(4) In existing buildings, the existing door leaf width shall be not less than 28 in. (710 mm).
(5) Door openings in detention and correctional occupancies, as otherwise provided in Chapters 22 and 23, shall not be required to comply with 7.2.1.2.3.
(6) Interior door openings in dwelling units as otherwise provided in Chapter 24 shall not be required to comply with 7.2.1.2.3.
(7) A power-operated door leaf located within a two-leaf opening shall be exempt from the minimum 32 in. (810 mm) single-leaf requirement in accordance with 7.2.1.9.1.5.
(8) Revolving door assemblies, as provided in 7.2.1.10, shall be exempt from the minimum 32 in. (810 mm) width requirement.
(9)* Where a single door opening is provided for discharge from a stairway required to be a minimum of 56 in. (1420 mm) wide in accordance with 7.2.2.2.1.2(B), and such door assembly serves as the sole means of exit discharge from such stairway, the clear width of the door opening, measured in accordance with 7.2.1.2.2, shall be not less than two-thirds the required width of the stairway.

**A.7.2.1.2.3.2(9)** The relative egress carrying capacity of door openings and stairs is based on the two-to-three ratio used in Table 7.3.3.1 to help balance the capacity of various egress elements and ensure that downstream egress facilities do not form a bottleneck or constriction to flow. For example, a stairway with a nominal width of 56 in. (1420 mm) should be served by an exit discharge door with a minimum width opening of 37 in. (940 mm) if only one discharge door is provided. It might be advantageous for two discharge doors to serve such a stairway, each with a more typical clear opening width of 32 in. (810 mm). This would facilitate access, into the exit, of fire fighters and other emergency responders without causing undue interference to evacuees attempting to transition from the stair to the exit discharge door.

Generally, various door assemblies are encountered as one travels the means of egress route. Each door opening must provide sufficient egress capacity width to accommodate the number of people expected to pass through that door opening during emergency egress as required by Section 7.3 and must meet any clear widths specified by other provisions of the *Code*. The egress capacity door width necessary to accommodate a specified number of persons is calculated from the occupant load served and the capacity factors applicable to level egress components, as provided in Table 7.3.3.1. Regardless of the occupant load served and the corresponding calculated minimum egress capacity width required, new door openings generally are not permitted to be less than 32 in. (810 mm) in clear width, as specified by the base requirement of 7.2.1.2.3.2.

Note that a clear width of 32 in. (810 mm) permits the passage of wheelchairs; however, it might not be adequate for the normal use of the door opening for purposes other than emergency egress. Thus, door widths in excess of those required by the *Code* are often provided voluntarily for purposes of day-to-day function. Door widths in excess of the minimum specified in 7.2.1.2.3.2 often are provided where a bank of doors are needed to serve a large occupant load and the number of door assemblies is to be minimized. For example, a bank of four door assemblies, each with a 48 in. (1220 mm) door leaf, providing 15 ft (4570 mm) of clear width and capacity for 900 persons might be used in place of a bank of six door assemblies, each with a 34 in. (865 mm) door leaf, providing 15 ft (4570 mm) of clear width and capacity for 900 persons.

If a door assembly in a new business occupancy is to serve 120 occupants, for example, the minimum egress capacity door width calculated from the perspective of occupant load served would be 24 in. (610 mm) [i.e., calculated as 120 persons × 0.2 in./person (120 persons × 5 mm/person) — see 7.3.3.1]. However, a door opening providing only 24 in. (610 mm) of egress capacity width would not satisfy 7.2.1.2.3.2, which requires that, as a minimum, the door opening must provide 32 in. (810 mm) of clear width. Because more than one requirement affects door width, a comparison must be made between the calculated minimum width for egress capacity purposes and the more arbitrary minimum width requirement of 7.2.1.2.3.2.

Having performed the comparison, the greater width — in this case, 32 in. (810 mm) — must be used.

Where another *Code* section specifies a minimum door width greater than 32 in. (810 mm), the greater width must be provided. Generally, the greater width is specified in terms of clear width. For example, in new health care occupancies, the minimum width for patient room door openings and cross-corridor door openings is 41½ in. (1055 mm) in clear width [see 18.2.3.6(1)]. The 41½ in. (1055 mm) minimum clear width requirement unintentionally connotes a precision and accuracy that one might expect resulted from a detailed research program; in reality, it represents an attempt to quantify the clear width realized when a typical 44 in. (1120 mm) wide door leaf is swung to its 90-degree open position. For many editions of the *Code*, new health care occupancies specified the required minimum as 44 in. (1120 mm) of door leaf width, not of clear opening.

The exemptions of 7.2.1.2.3.2(1) through (8) modify the minimum 32 in. (810 mm) clear width requirement so as to recognize smaller door opening widths for the specific situations they address. The provision addressed by 7.2.1.2.3.2(9) is not an exemption to the 32 in. (810 mm) clear width criterion but is an additional requirement. Commentary on this provision follows.

Paragraph 7.2.1.2.3.2(1) exempts one of the door leaves used in a pair of door leaves from the 32 in. (810 mm) clear width criterion, because the minimum 32 in. (810 mm) clear width opening provided by the other door leaf can serve to accommodate a wheelchair user.

Paragraph 7.2.1.2.3.2(2) permits a small room, likely occupied by only a couple of people and not required to be accessible to people with severe mobility impairments, to use a 24 in. (610 mm) width door assembly. This exemption does not specify clear width, so a minimum 24 in. (610 mm) wide door leaf would be sufficient.

Paragraph 7.2.1.2.3.2(3) also addresses door assemblies serving spaces not required to be accessible to people with severe mobility impairments. In lieu of a room size, the exemption can be applied, regardless of occupant load, but the door leaf width must be at least 28 in. (710 mm).

Earlier editions of the *Code* specified that no single door leaf in a door opening was permitted to be less than 28 in. (710 mm) wide. To prevent automatically creating a situation of noncompliance where there had previously been compliance, 7.2.1.2.3.2(4) exempts existing buildings from the minimum 32 in. (810 mm) clear width requirement if the door width, that is, the leaf width, is at least 28 in. (710 mm).

For security and operations purposes, 7.2.1.2.3.2(5) permits detention and correctional facilities to have door assemblies of smaller width. See Chapters 22 and 23.

Chapter 24 establishes that door assemblies within dwelling units are within the means of escape and not the means of egress. Paragraphs 24.2.4.1 and 24.2.4.2 permit such door assemblies, whether new or existing, to be a minimum of 28 in. (710 mm) in leaf width and, in some cases, 24 in. (610 mm). Paragraph 7.2.1.2.3.2(6) recognizes this permission.

The provision of 7.2.1.2.3.2(9) relates to minimum stair criteria in 7.2.2. The stair provisions of 7.2.2.2.1.2 require extra stair width for buildings, such as high-rise buildings, where it is expected that occupants will still be in the process of egressing the building when emergency responders, such as fire fighters, arrive. The extra stair width helps to facilitate counterflow — the downward movement of building occupants that occurs while emergency responders are simultaneously moving up the same stairs — and allows faster stair travel by building occupants.

The provision of 7.2.1.2.3.2(9) requires the single door assembly from the stair enclosure to the exit discharge to be sized so that occupants do not need to queue on the stairs while waiting for their turn to move through the door opening. The two-to-three ratio of door-opening width to stair width is consistent with the capacity factors of Table 7.3.3.1, that is, 0.2 in. (5 mm) per person for level travel, such as that through door openings, and 0.3 in. (7.6 mm) per person for stair travel. The two-to-three ratio is further explained in A.7.2.1.2.3.2(9).

It is the intent of the *Code* that a door opening not create a bottleneck in the means of egress. At times, another component of the means of egress might be larger than required, creating the illusion of a bottleneck at an appropriately sized door opening. However, a door opening with a width that is adequate for the occupant load served and with at least a 32 in. (810 mm) clear width is sufficient for other than the special case addressed by 7.2.1.2.3.2(9). A door opening serving a hallway often is not as wide as the hallway. This is illustrated in Exhibit 7.14. Because operational features of the occupancy, in addition to the occupant load, are considered in determining needed corridor width, the corridor might be wider than the exit door opening serving the corridor. In Exhibit 7.14, which depicts a new school, the corridor is required by 14.2.3.2 to be 6 ft (1830 mm) wide, as a minimum, and wider only if that section of corridor serves more than 360 persons [i.e., based on a calculation using the capacity factor of 0.2 in. (5 mm) per person for level travel from Table

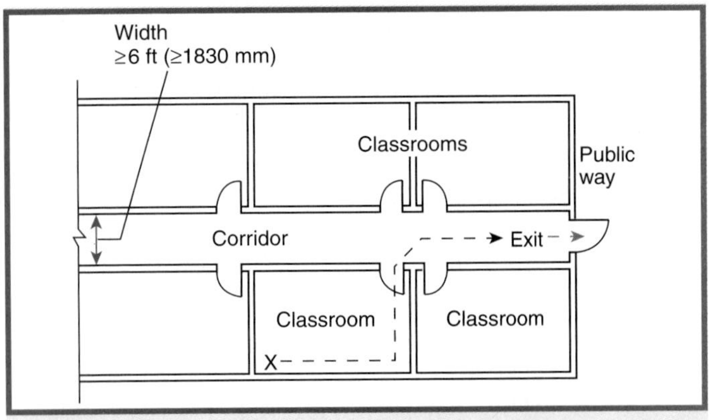


*Exhibit 7.14 Exit door-opening width and corridor width relationship.*

7.3.3.1]. The exit door opening is required by 7.2.1.2.3.2 to be 32 in. (810 mm) wide, as a minimum, and wider only if it serves more than 160 persons (again, based on a calculation using the capacity factor for level travel).

In a health care occupancy, the corridor and door opening widths are usually much wider than the occupant load dictates. In this instance, the sizes of the corridor and door openings are governed by the necessity to move patients on gurneys. Patients are often connected to medical equipment that must be moved with the patients along the means of egress route.

Note that, since the 1997 edition, the *Code* no longer restricts door leaf width to a maximum of 48 in. (1220 mm). Provided that the door leaf and its hardware are maintained in good working order, there is insufficient reason to limit the maximum width of a door leaf.

**7.2.1.3 Floor Level.**

**7.2.1.3.1** The elevation of the floor surfaces on both sides of a door opening shall not vary by more than $^1/_2$ in. (13 mm), unless otherwise permitted by 7.2.1.3.5 or 7.2.1.3.6.

**7.2.1.3.2** The elevation of the floor surfaces required by 7.2.1.3.1 shall be maintained on both sides of the door openings for a distance not less than the width of the widest leaf.

**7.2.1.3.3** Thresholds at door openings shall not exceed $^1/_2$ in. (13 mm) in height.

**7.2.1.3.4** Raised thresholds and floor level changes in excess of $^1/_4$ in. (6.3 mm) at door openings shall be beveled with a slope not steeper than 1 in 2.

**7.2.1.3.5** In existing buildings, where the door opening discharges to the outside or to an exterior balcony or exterior exit access, the floor level outside the door opening shall be permitted to be one step lower than that of the inside, but shall be not more than 8 in. (205 mm) lower.

**7.2.1.3.6** In existing buildings, a door assembly at the top of a stair shall be permitted to open directly at a stair, provided that the door leaf does not swing over the stair and that the door opening serves an area with an occupant load of fewer than 50 persons.

The detailed dimensional tolerances specified for thresholds at door openings are intended to permit persons in wheelchairs, persons using assistive mobility devices like walkers, and those with difficulty lifting their feet to move easily through those openings. Arrangements meeting the criteria useful to persons with disabilities provide for the safe use of door assemblies by other occupants.

In earlier editions, the *Code* permitted the floor level outside exterior door assemblies to be one step — up to 8 in. (205 mm) — lower than the floor level inside the door opening. This was permitted to avoid blocking the outward swing of the door leaf by a buildup of snow or ice. The requirements of 7.2.1.3.1 are practical for new construction because of the importance of avoiding tripping hazards, and because other provisions of the *Code* require that the means of egress be maintained free of obstructions and protected from the weather, thus providing for the removal of snow or ice accumulations. Existing buildings continue to be permitted to use one exterior step. See 7.2.1.3.5.

Paragraph 7.2.1.3.6 recognizes an existing situation in which the door leaf of a door assembly at the top of a stair opens directly at the stair without providing a level landing on the stair side of the door opening. In this case, however, the door leaf swings away from the stair, rather than swinging over the stair. See Exhibit 7.15. This situation is permitted in ex-

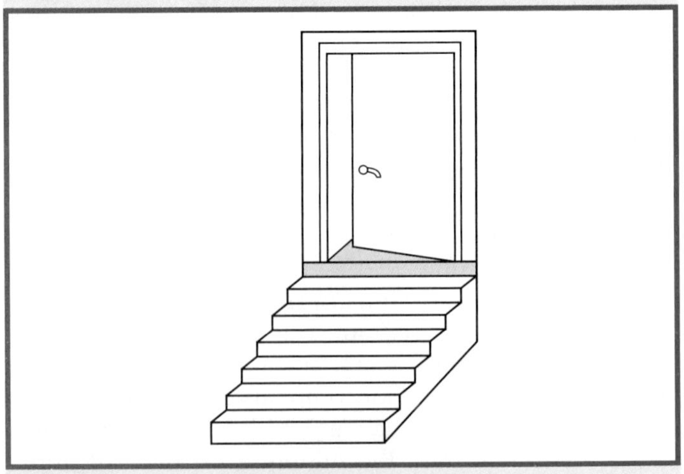

*Exhibit 7.15 Door leaf opening directly at the top of a stair, but not swinging over the stair.*

isting buildings where the area served by the door assembly has an occupant load of fewer than 50 persons. Paragraph 7.2.2.3.2.5 permits this situation as an exemption to the requirement of 7.2.2.3.2 that there be a level landing on each side of the door opening that is at least as deep in the direction of stair run as the door leaf is wide. The wording of 7.2.1.3.6 and 7.2.2.3.2.5 are identical. The dual placement of the exemption is helpful to *Code* users. One user might see the issue as being related to doors and seek guidance via the provisions of 7.2.1, while another user might see the issue as being related to stairs and seek guidance via the provisions of 7.2.2.

The exemption permitted by 7.2.1.3.6 does not permit the dangerous practice of swinging the door leaf out over the stair, because it would force a person climbing the stairs to reach for the doorknob and back away by descending to a tread located a riser or two lower in order to pull the door leaf open while attempting to maintain stability on the stair. Neither does the exemption permit another dangerous practice of opening a door leaf directly at the bottom of a stair without providing a level landing on the stair side of the door opening. Such an action would force a person descending the stair to lean forward and downward to reach the latch release and then push the door leaf open while standing on a tread located one or more risers above the base of the door opening while attempting to maintain stability on the stair.

**7.2.1.4 Swing and Force to Open.**

**7.2.1.4.1* Swinging-Type Door Assembly Requirement.** Any door assembly in a means of egress shall be of the side-hinged or pivoted-swinging type, and shall be installed to be capable of swinging from any position to the full required width of the opening in which it is installed, unless otherwise specified as follows:

(1) Door assemblies in dwelling units, as provided in Chapter 24, shall be permitted.
(2) Door assemblies in residential board and care occupancies, as provided in Chapters 32 and 33, shall be permitted.
(3) Where permitted in Chapters 11 through 43, horizontal-sliding or vertical-rolling security grilles or door assemblies that are part of the required means of egress shall be permitted, provided that they meet the following criteria:

    (a) Such grilles or door assemblies shall remain secured in the fully open position during the period of occupancy by the general public.
    (b) On or adjacent to the grille or door opening, there shall be a readily visible, durable sign in letters not less than 1 in. (25 mm) high on a contrasting background that reads as follows: THIS DOOR TO REMAIN OPEN WHEN THE BUILDING IS OCCUPIED.
    (c) Door leaves or grilles shall not be brought to the closed position when the space is occupied.
    (d) Door leaves or grilles shall be operable from within the space without the use of any special knowledge or effort.
    (e) Where two or more means of egress are required, not more than half of the means of egress shall be equipped with horizontal-sliding or vertical-rolling grilles or door assemblies.

(4) Horizontal-sliding door assemblies shall be permitted under any of the following conditions:

    (a) Horizontal-sliding door assemblies in detention and correctional occupancies, as provided in Chapters 22 and 23, shall be permitted.
    (b) Horizontal-sliding door assemblies complying with 7.2.1.14 shall be permitted.
    (c) Unless prohibited by Chapters 11 through 43, horizontal-sliding door assemblies serving a room or area with an occupant load of fewer than 10 shall be permitted, provided that all of the following criteria are met:

        i. The area served by the door assembly has no high hazard contents.
        ii. The door assembly is readily operable from either side without special knowledge or effort.
        iii. The force required to operate the door assembly in the direction of door leaf travel is not more than 30 lbf (133 N) to set the door leaf in motion and is not more than 15 lbf (67 N) to close the door assembly or open it to the minimum required width.
        iv. The door assembly complies with any required fire protection rating, and, where rated, is self-closing or automatic-closing by means of smoke detection in accordance with 7.2.1.8 and is installed in accordance with NFPA 80, *Standard for Fire Doors and Other Opening Protectives.*
        v. Corridor door assemblies required to be self-latching shall have a latch or other mechanism that ensures that the door leaf will not rebound into a partially open position if forcefully closed.

    (d) Where private garages, business areas, industrial areas, and storage areas with an occupant load not exceeding 10 contain only low or ordinary hazard contents, door openings to such areas and private garages shall be permitted to be horizontal-sliding door assemblies.

(5) Where private garages, business areas, industrial areas, and storage areas with an occupant load not exceeding 10 contain only low or ordinary hazard contents, door openings to such areas and private garages shall be permitted to be vertical-rolling door assemblies.

(6) Revolving door assemblies complying with 7.2.1.10 shall be permitted.

(7) Existing fusible link–operated horizontal-sliding or vertical-rolling fire door assemblies shall be permitted to be used as provided in Chapters 39, 40, and 42.

Paragraph 7.2.1.4.1 requires that door assemblies within the means of egress be of the side-hinged or pivoted-swinging type. These types of door assemblies are most familiar to the general public, and their operation is readily understood.

Furthermore, 7.2.1.4.1 requires that the door leaf be capable of swinging to the full required width of the opening. The required width is determined by two width considerations. The first consideration involves the width required for egress capacity purposes. For example, if a door assembly in a business occupancy needs to accommodate 180 persons, the applicable capacity factor from Table 7.3.3.1 dictates that the door opening provide a 36 in. (915 mm) egress capacity width [i.e., calculated as 180 persons × 0.2 in./person (180 persons × 5 mm/person)]. The second consideration involves the minimum clear width required, regardless of occupant load served. For the same business occupancy, the minimum clear width is specified in 7.2.1.2.3.2 as 32 in. (810 mm). The required width is the larger of the two widths — in this example, the 36 in. (915 mm) calculated from the egress capacity consideration.

Paragraph 7.2.1.4.1 (1) and (2) recognize that some occupancy chapters provide exemptions to the requirement that door assemblies be of the side-hinged or pivoted-swinging type. Chapters 24, 32, and 33, which apply to one- and two-family dwellings and residential board and care occupancies, do not require that door leaves be swinging. These exemptions recognize the smaller numbers of persons using door assemblies within dwellings and the familiarity those occupants have with the operation of other door assembly types, such as sliding door assemblies.

Paragraph 7.2.1.4.1(3) permits horizontal-sliding or vertical-rolling security grilles or door assemblies to be used in lieu of side-hinged- or pivoted-swinging-type door assemblies, provided that the exemption is specifically permitted by the applicable occupancy chapter. This exemption permits the type of security door assemblies and grilles normally found in mall buildings.

Note that there is a difference between 7.2.1.4.1(3)(a) and 7.2.1.4.1(3)(c). Paragraph 7.2.1.4.1(3)(a) requires that the door assembly be fully open when the public occupies the space, while 7.2.1.4.1(3)(c) states that the grille or door leaf cannot be closed when the space is occupied. This allows the common practice of leaving the grille or door leaf partially closed at closing time and other times when restricting entry to the general public is desired. See the explanation of the term *occupied* in 7.2.1.1.3 and its commentary.

The following occupancies permit the use of horizontal-sliding or vertical-rolling door assemblies complying with 7.2.1.4.1(3). See the referenced paragraphs for additional restrictions, if any, imposed by the occupancy chapter:

1. Assembly occupancies (12.2.2.2.2, 13.2.2.2.2)
2. Mercantile occupancies (36.2.2.2.7, 37.2.2.2.7)
3. Business occupancies (38.2.2.2.7, 39.2.2.2.7)

As referenced in 7.2.1.4.1(4)(a), detention and correctional occupancies permit certain sliding door assemblies, because swinging door leaves can become readily accessible weapons for use by residents against staff.

Paragraph 7.2.1.4.1(4)(b) recognizes the use of a special form of horizontal-sliding door assembly under detailed conditions. One of the characteristic features of this door assembly is its operability in the direction of door leaf travel when a specified force is applied in the direction of occupant travel. See also 7.2.1.14.

Paragraph 7.2.1.4.1(4)(c) is new to the 2009 edition of the *Code* and is an expansion of a provision that was new to the 2006 edition and applied only to horizontal-sliding door assemblies in health care occupancies. The new provision recognizes horizontal-sliding door assemblies serving fewer than 10 persons in any occupancy, unless an occupancy chapter specifically prohibits use of the provision. See the detailed criteria in 7.2.1.4.1(4)(c) i. through 7.2.1.4.1(4)(c) v.

Paragraphs 7.2.1.4.1(4)(d) and 7.2.1.4.1(5) recognize that many private garages, small businesses, and industrial and storage buildings typically have only vertical-rolling or horizontal-sliding door assembly and no side-hinged door assemblies. Provided that the maximum 10-person occupant load is not exceeded and there are no high hazard contents, such door assemblies are permitted to substitute for side-hinged or pivoted-swinging door assemblies.

Paragraph 7.2.1.4.1(6) cross-references the provisions of 7.2.1.10, which apply to revolving door assemblies. If 7.2.1.4.1(6) did not exist, it might be assumed, incorrectly, that revolving door assemblies violate the requirement for door assemblies to be side-hinged or pivoted-swinging.

Paragraph 7.2.1.4.1(7) legitimizes the provisions of 39.2.2.2.8, 40.2.2.2.4, and 42.2.2.2.4 that permit existing fusible link-operated sliding door assemblies to be positioned within the exit access of existing business, industrial, and storage occupancies if additional criteria are met. These provisions help to ensure that the door leaf is open when conditions in the door opening's vicinity are tenable for occupant movement and that it is closed once it is no longer safe for persons to seek egress via that exit access path.

**A.7.2.1.4.1** Where doors are subject to two-way traffic, or where their opening can interfere with pedestrian traffic, an appropriately located vision panel can reduce the chance of accidents.

Swinging doors in horizontal- or vertical-rolling partitions should be permitted in a means of egress where the following criteria are met:

(1) The door or doors comply with 7.2.1.4.
(2) The partition in which the doors are mounted complies with the applicable fire protection rating and closes upon smoke detection or power failure at a speed not exceeding 9 in./s (230 mm/s) and not less than 6 in./s (150 mm/s).
(3) The doors mounted in the partition are self-closing or automatic-closing in accordance with 7.2.1.8.

**7.2.1.4.2 Door Leaf Swing Direction.** Door leaves required to be of the side-hinged or pivoted-swinging type shall swing in the direction of egress travel under any of the following conditions:

(1) Where serving a room or area with an occupant load of 50 or more, except under the following conditions:
  (a) Door leaves in horizontal exits shall not be required to swing in the direction of egress travel where permitted by 7.2.4.3.8.1 or 7.2.4.3.8.2.
  (b) Door leaves in smoke barriers shall not be required to swing in the direction of egress travel in existing health care occupancies, as provided in Chapter 19.
(2) Where the door assembly is used in an exit enclosure, unless the door opening serves an individual living unit that opens directly into an exit enclosure
(3) Where the door opening serves a high hazard contents area

The provisions regulating the direction of door leaf swing appear in 7.2.1.4.2 and 7.2.4.3.8(1).

Paragraph 7.2.1.4.2(1) requires all door leaves serving in the means of egress from a room or area with an occupant load of 50 or more persons to swing in the direction of egress travel. For example, if the occupant load of a room with two exit access door assemblies is 80 persons, the door leaves of both door assemblies are required to swing in the direction of egress travel. The 50-person criterion is not related to the number of persons expected to use a given door opening but, rather, to the total occupant load of the room. Therefore, it would be incorrect in the case of this 80-person example to claim that 40 persons will move to each of the two door openings, that the 40-person number is fewer than the 50-person threshold, and that neither door leaf needs to swing in the direction of egress travel. The fact that the total occupant load of the room is more than 50 persons is sufficient condition to require the exit access door leaves to swing in the direction of egress travel.

Paragraph 7.2.1.4.2(2) requires a door leaf used in an exit enclosure to swing in the direction of egress travel. An example of a door leaf used in an exit enclosure is the door leaf in the opening between an exit access corridor and an enclosed exit stair. The main entrance and exit door leaf from an office building lobby to the outside is not a door leaf used in an exit enclosure, although it is an exit door. Door leaf swing direction for such a door would be regulated by the 50-person criterion of 7.2.1.4.2(1).

Paragraph 7.2.1.4.2(3) requires a door leaf serving a high hazard contents area to swing in the direction of egress travel. Persons leaving high hazard contents spaces under fire or similar emergency must not be impeded, as would occur if they had to stop and pull a door toward them before egressing the space.

Paragraph 7.2.4.3.8(1) requires a swinging fire door assembly used in a horizontal exit to swing in the direction of egress travel.

If none of the requirements of 7.2.1.4.2 (1) through (3), or 7.2.4.3.8(1) applies, a door leaf is permitted to swing against the direction of egress travel.

Ideally, all door leaves in a means of egress would swing in the direction of egress travel. However, because of operational concerns, there are cases where door leaf swing in the direction of egress travel is not desirable. For example, a classroom door leaf that swings into a corridor serving as an exit access for several classrooms might open against another door leaf or against the flow of people and possibly restrict the width available as corridor exit access. The *Code* recognizes this danger and permits the classroom/corridor door leaf from a room with an occupant load of fewer than 50 persons to swing against the direction of egress travel. This provision limits the number of people using a door opening whose door leaf swings against egress travel to that which is safe. The *Code* also recognizes similar constraints with regard to an exterior exit door assembly; although such a door assembly is considered an exit but not within an exit enclosure, the *Code* does not require that it swing in the direction of egress travel, unless it serves 50 or more occupants.

Exhibit 7.16 illustrates considerations involved in evaluating door leaf swing direction as addressed in 7.2.1.4.2. Door assembly C is permitted to swing back into the room if the room has an occupant load of fewer than 50 persons and does not have high hazard contents [see 7.2.1.4.2 (1) and (3)]. Door assembly D must swing in the direction of egress travel if the room has an occupant load of 50 or more [see 7.2.1.4.2 (1)]. Door assembly E, although it is an exit door assembly, is not used in an exit enclosure [see 7.2.1.4.2(2)], so its door leaf is permitted to swing back into the room if the occupant load is fewer than 50 and the room does not have high hazard contents. Door assemblies A and B are related to the encroachment-related provisions of 7.2.1.4.3. They open into the corridor directly opposite each other. Although this does not violate any *Code* provision, it is preferable that door leaves do not swing in a direction that blocks the use of the corridor when both are open.

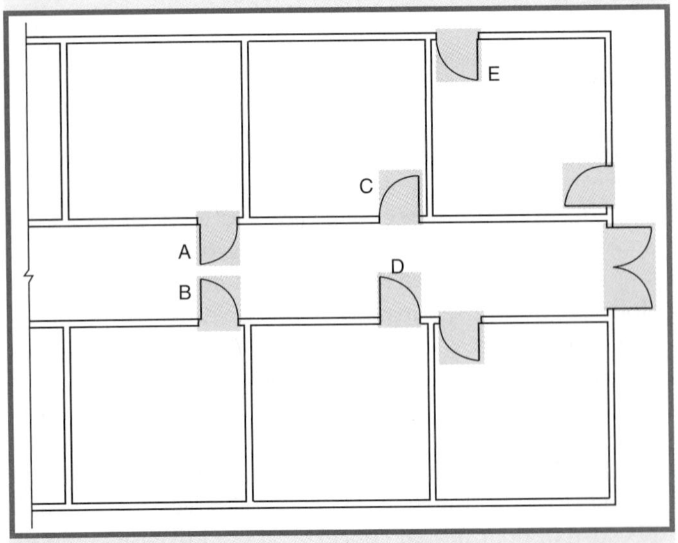


**Exhibit 7.16** *Door leaf swing direction considerations.*

Paragraph 7.2.1.4.2(1)(a) recognizes that the provisions of 7.2.4.3.8.1 exempt door leaves in horizontal exits from having to swing in the direction of egress travel in accordance with specific allowances and conditions for existing health care occupancies and existing detention and correctional occupancies. For these occupancies, staff is expected to be able to control occupant movement at horizontal exit door assemblies to prevent a crowd from pushing against a door leaf that is arranged to open only by swinging back toward the occupants. See 7.2.4.3.8.1. Also see 7.2.4.3.8.2 for an exemption with applicability to any occupancy that recognizes the impracticality of replacing an existing horizontal exit door leaf with a pair of door leaves where the corridor does not have sufficient width to accommodate the pair.

Paragraph 7.2.1.4.2(1)(b) exempts smoke barrier door assemblies from having to swing in the direction of egress travel in existing health care facilities. Such door assemblies usually span the width of a corridor. Because existing health care occupancies are permitted to have corridors as narrow as 48 in. (1220 mm), it might be impractical to install a pair of door leaves swinging in opposite directions. The single door leaf recognized by the exception swings in the correct direction for occupants on one side and swings against the direction of egress travel for occupants on the other side. Because staff directs the egress or relocation movement necessary during an emergency, the direction of door leaf swing problem is alleviated.

The exemption offered by 7.2.1.4.2(2) addresses the common design in apartment buildings in which door assemblies from the exit enclosure into apartment units normally swing into the apartment units. This design is common in a three-story, single-exit garden apartment. The swing of the door leaf in this arrangement is not a significant concern. The exemption also addresses another situation common to hotels where guest room door assemblies frequently open directly into an exit enclosure created to enclose a formerly open stair. Because it is often necessary to use part of the corridor to create a stair landing for the newly enclosed exit stair, the exemption offers some relief without compromising safety.

Per 7.2.1.4.2(3), door leaves to hazardous contents areas must swing in the direction of egress travel. A conflict sometimes arises between this requirement and the desire of those responsible for explosion control — who prefer that door leaves to areas subject to explosion be required to swing inward to impede spreading the effects of a blast to adjacent rooms and spaces. In new construction, this conflict can usually be resolved if the hazardous contents area can be located along an outside wall of the main building; the required egress door assemblies then open directly to the outside — which is desirable for life safety. This arrangement is also favorable for explosion relief, because it easily allows the door leaves to swing outward. In existing situations, or where the hazardous area must be located internal to a building and away from exterior walls, the conflict is not easily resolved. The AHJ needs to work with the building owner, insurer, and other involved parties to determine how best to reduce the exposure hazard while adequately providing needed life safety to those who work in the hazardous area. See also Section 7.11.

**7.2.1.4.3 Door Leaf Encroachment.**

**7.2.1.4.3.1*** During its swing, any door leaf in a means of egress shall leave not less than one-half of the required width of an aisle, a corridor, a passageway, or a landing unobstructed and shall project not more than 7 in. (180 mm) into the required width of an aisle, a corridor, a passageway, or a landing, when fully open, unless both of the following conditions are met:

(1) The door opening provides access to a stair in an existing building.
(2) The door opening meets the requirement that limits projection to not more than 7 in. (180 mm) into the required width of the stair landing when the door leaf is fully open.

**A.7.2.1.4.3.1** The requirements of 7.2.1.4.3 are not intended to apply to the swing of cross-corridor doors, such as smoke barrier doors and horizontal exits.

Door leaves capable of swinging a full 180 degrees, so that they rest nearly flat against the wall in which the door opening is installed, have a greater utility than doors leaves capable of swinging only 90 degrees. The 180-degree-swinging door leaf can be fully opened into a corridor without significant intrusion on corridor width. The 90-degree-swinging door leaf, however, might have to open into an unusually wide corridor, be set into an alcove, or otherwise be recessed so as not to exceed the maximum encroachment permitted by 7.2.1.4.3.1.

Note that 7.2.1.4.3.1 requires that, during its swing, a door leaf must leave unobstructed at least one-half of the required width of a corridor. Note that this requirement is concerned with the required corridor width, which is not necessarily the same as the actual width. For example, in a corridor that is required to be 44 in. (1120 mm) wide but that is voluntarily constructed to be 56 in. (1420 mm) wide, a 34 in. (865 mm) wide door leaf — a door leaf that provides the minimum 32 in. (810 mm) clear width required by 7.2.1.2.3 — would swing to encroach on 34 in. (865 mm) of the corridor width. Although this encroachment is more than one-half of the *actual* corridor width, it does leave one-half of the *required* corridor width [22 in. (560 mm)] unobstructed. Such an arrangement meets the requirement of 7.2.1.4.3.1.

Door leaves that swing within a recessed pocket of the corridor, so as not to protrude into the required corridor width, provide the best arrangement for clear passage through an exit access corridor. Door leaves that swing 180 degrees so that they come to rest against a wall and do not extend into more than 7 in. (180 mm) of required corridor width provide an acceptable arrangement. A door leaf that swings 90 degrees so that it comes to rest in the path of travel is considered not to encroach excessively on the exit access corridor width if not more than 7 in. (180 mm) of the required width of the corridor remains obstructed. Additionally, any door leaf swinging into the corridor must leave at least one-half of the required corridor width unobstructed during its entire swing. See Exhibit 7.17.

Door leaves of door assemblies serving as an entrance into an enclosed stair must not unduly block the stair landing or the stairs. Ideally, the door leaf should not reduce the required width either during its

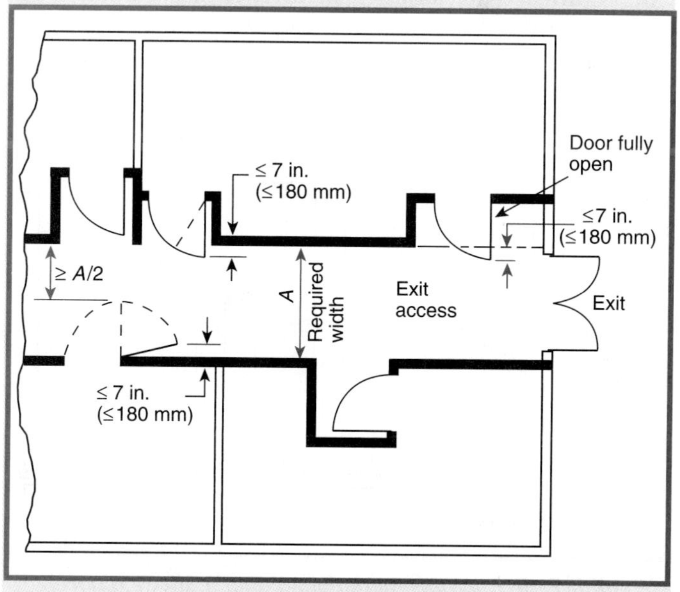


***Exhibit 7.17*** *Door leaf swing into a corridor.*

swing or while at rest. However, the *Code* does permit encroachment on the stair landing, as shown in Exhibit 7.18. For most stairs, Table 7.2.2.2.1.2(B) requires a 44 in. (1120 mm) clear width. In cases such as these, the $B \geq A/2$ rule shown in Exhibit 7.18 requires that the clearance between the leading edge of the opening door leaf and stair newel post be at least 22 in. (560 mm). However, where the total occupant load of all floors served by the stair is fewer than 50 persons, 7.2.2.2.1.2(A) permits a 36 in. (915 mm) wide stair; in this case, the $B \geq A/2$ rule requires that the clearance between the leading edge of the opening door leaf and stair newel post be at least 18 in. (455 mm).

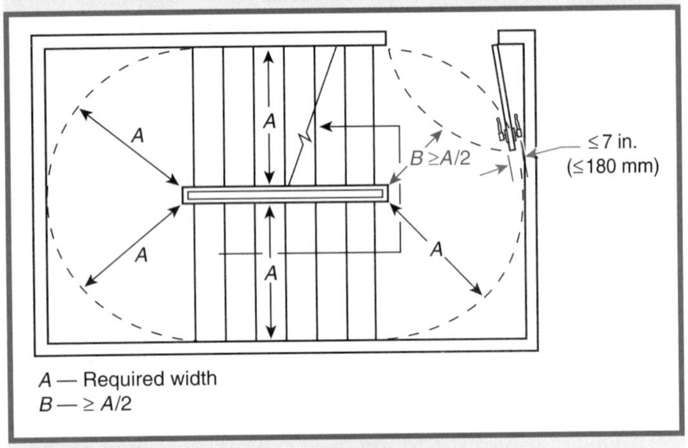


***Exhibit 7.18*** *Minimum required unobstructed clearance with door leaf encroaching on landing in new buildings.*

An acceptable arrangement for a door leaf opening onto a stair landing in an existing building is shown in Exhibit 7.19. In lieu of a $B \geq A/2$ rule, existing stairs are not required to maintain a specified clearance between the leading edge of the opening door leaf and stair newel post. However, the maximum 7 in. (180 mm) encroachment when the door leaf is fully open still applies.

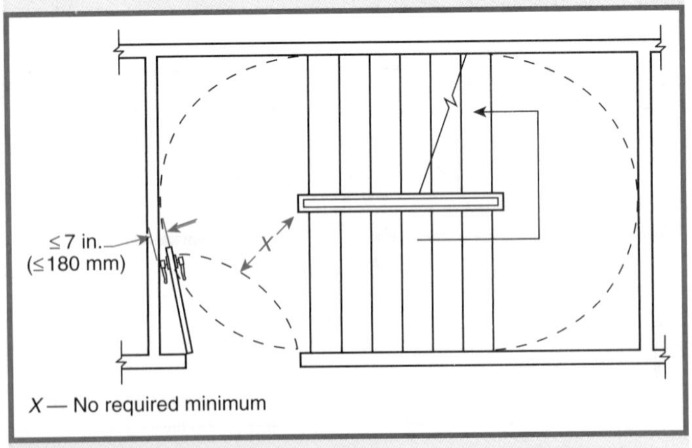


***Exhibit 7.19*** *Encroachment during door leaf swing not limited in existing buildings.*

**7.2.1.4.3.2** Surface-mounted latch release hardware on the door leaf shall be exempt from being included in the maximum 7 in. (180 mm) projection requirement of 7.2.1.4.3.1, provided that both of the following criteria are met:

(1) The hardware is mounted to the side of the door leaf that faces the aisle, corridor, passageway, or landing when the door leaf is in the open position.
(2) The hardware is mounted not less than 34 in. (865 mm), and not more than 48 in. (1220 mm), above the floor.

The provision of 7.2.1.4.3.2 is new to the 2009 edition of the *Code* and specifies that latch release hardware that is surface mounted to the side of the door leaf that faces the aisle, corridor, passageway, or landing when the door leaf is in the open position is exempted from inclusion in the maximum 7 in. (180 mm) projection specified in 7.2.1.4.3.1, provided that such hardware is mounted 34 in. to 48 in. (865 mm to 1220 mm) above the floor. The application of the requirement is illustrated in Exhibit 7.18 and Exhibit 7.19. Note in the exhibits that the hardware on the back side of the door leaf is counted in the maximum 7 in. (180 mm) projection, but the hardware on the side of the door leaf that faces the landing is not. The new provision is consistent with the door-opening clear width encroachment criteria of 7.2.1.2.1.1(5) as depicted in Figure A.7.2.1.2.1(b). It will help to alleviate the problem where the AHJ cites the door leaf encroachment as excessive because of the latch release hardware that protrudes into the egress path. Wheelchair users are able to travel past the door without being encumbered, as the hardware must be at least 34 in. (865 mm) off the floor.

**7.2.1.4.4 Screen Door Assemblies and Storm Door Assemblies.** Screen door assemblies and storm door assemblies used in a means of egress shall be subject to the requirements for direction of swing that are applicable to other door assemblies used in a means of egress.

Various functional arrangements of screen or storm door assemblies can be provided without allowing a door leaf to swing against the direction of egress travel. A screen or storm door assembly might be permitted to be used in proximity to a door opening with an ordinary door assembly by providing a vestibule of sufficient size to allow the inner door leaf to swing outward without interfering with the operation of the door leaf at the outer end of the vestibule. See Exhibit 7.20.

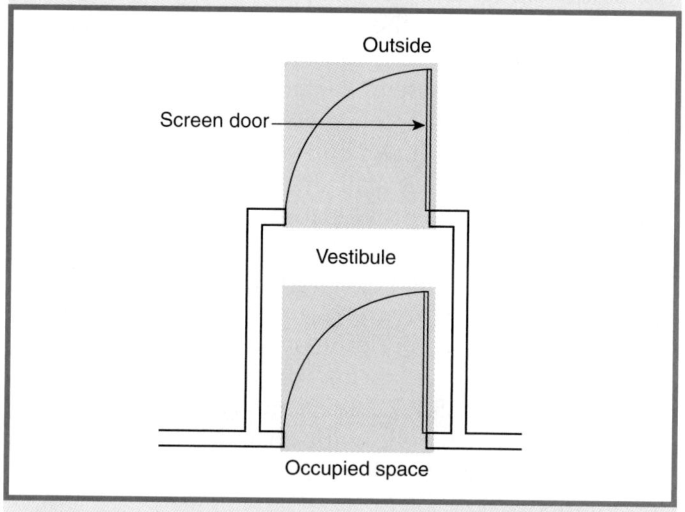


***Exhibit 7.20** Arrangement of vestibule leading to screen door assembly complying with 7.2.1.4.4.*

**7.2.1.4.5 Door Leaf Operating Forces.** The forces required to fully open any door leaf manually in a means of egress shall not exceed 15 lbf (67 N) to release the latch, 30 lbf (133 N) to set the leaf in motion, and 15 lbf (67 N) to open the leaf to the minimum required width, unless otherwise specified as follows:

(1) The forces specified in 7.2.1.4.5 shall be applied to the latch stile.
(2) The opening forces for interior side-hinged or pivoted-swinging door leaves without closers shall not exceed 5 lbf (22 N).
(3) The opening forces for existing door leaves in existing buildings shall not exceed 50 lbf (222 N) applied to the latch stile.
(4) The opening forces for horizontal-sliding door leaves in detention and correctional occupancies shall be as provided in Chapters 22 and 23.
(5) The opening forces for power-operated door leaves shall be as provided in 7.2.1.9.

The *Code* recognizes that several movements are necessary to move a door leaf from its closed to its fully open position. Paragraph 7.2.1.4.5 identifies each of those movements and limits the force needed to accomplish each. The force required to unlatch the door assembly is limited to 15 lbf (67 N); the force necessary to start the door leaf in motion, or to overcome its inertia, is limited to not more than 30 lbf (133 N); and the force necessary to move the door leaf to its required open position is limited to not more than 15 lbf (67 N).

Care must be taken to ensure that the 30 lbf (133 N) needed to overcome the inertia of a door leaf in a means of egress is not exceeded for door assemblies opening into pressurized stairs. The pressure necessary to protect the stair often might be such that 30 lbf (133 N) is insufficient to open the door leaf. The use of barometric relief dampers or other pressure-regulating methods might be required. See NFPA 92A, *Standard for Smoke-Control Systems Utilizing Barriers and Pressure Differences*.[6]

A person with severe mobility impairment, such as someone who uses a wheelchair, might find it difficult or impossible to exert even the 15 lbf (67 N) specified by 7.2.1.4.5. Specification of a lower operating force for self-closing door assemblies might adversely affect the door assembly closer's ability to perform its intended function of returning an open door leaf to the fully closed and latched position. For interior side-hinged or pivoted-swinging door assemblies without closers, no conflict exists between the needs of a closer and those of a person with physical disabilities. Therefore, 7.2.1.4.5(2) specifies that such door assemblies be operable when not more than 5 lbf (22 N) is applied at the latch stile.

Circumstances such as wet floors, smooth-soled shoes, and light body weight can render many people incapable of exerting 50 lbf (222 N) horizontally. Therefore, the maximum 50 lbf (222 N) operating requirement of earlier editions of the *Code* remains applicable only to existing door assemblies via the provisions of 7.2.1.4.5(3).

Paragraphs 7.2.1.4.5(4) and (5) address special situations where the operating force requirements of 7.2.1.4.5 cannot be applied. For horizontal-sliding door assemblies in detention and correctional occupancies, see 22.2.11.6 and 23.2.11.6. For requirements specific to power-operated door assemblies, see 7.2.1.9.

**7.2.1.5 Locks, Latches, and Alarm Devices.**

An increase in thefts, muggings, and similar crimes has led to the practice of providing extra security on door assemblies within the means of egress. Such a practice, particularly where door assemblies to exit stairs and exit discharges are involved, is an open invitation to tragedy in the event of fire or other emergency. The provisions of 7.2.1.5 are aimed at preventing locked door assemblies in means of egress or any other unnecessary interference with the orderly movement of people through door openings in the event of fire. The *Code* has attempted to accomplish this objective while maintaining features that are essential to security within the building.

A study of structural fires reported to U.S. fire departments between 1981 and 1985 found that an average of 117 fire deaths a year involved locks or gates that prevented escape.[7] Most of these deaths occurred in fires in residential occupancies. The report also described a number of incidents, including those that follow.

In a Texas dwelling fire, seven people died when a space heater ignited a sofa. Two of the adults who died were overcome while they struggled to unlock the dead bolt lock on the front door assembly and the security bars.

In another Texas dwelling fire, three people died when a bedridden woman accidentally ignited her bedding with a cigarette. The other two victims died while trying to escape past burglar bars, double-cylinder dead bolt locks, and a security bar on a sliding glass door assembly.

The report also found that makeshift security arrangements, such as windows that had been nailed shut, were factors in more multiple-fatality fires than in cases where more expensive security devices, such as security bars and gates, were used. The conflict between some security provisions and sound fire safety practices takes many forms.

The requirement that door assemblies be easily openable from the egress side is consistent with the concept that all components in the means of egress must be under the control of the occupants. This requirement prohibits the use of key locks or hard-to-use devices, such as door handles or latches covered with glass that has to be broken. Where panic hardware or fire exit hardware is used, no device that might interfere with its operation can be used; however, this does not prevent the use of alarm connections that indicate that the door assembly is in use.

Requirements for door assemblies leading to exits also apply to door assemblies that open to roofs, where — for example — exit stairs from a high-rise portion of the building discharge to the roof of the low-rise portion of the building, and to exit discharge door assemblies leading to the street or other public way.

**7.2.1.5.1** Door leaves shall be arranged to be opened readily from the egress side whenever the building is occupied.

**7.2.1.5.2** Locks, if provided, shall not require the use of a key, a tool, or special knowledge or effort for operation from the egress side.

Paragraph 7.2.1.5.1 establishes the principle that, when a building is occupied, door assemblies must be able to be opened easily from the side from which egress is to be made. Paragraph 7.2.1.5.2 prohibits the installation of locks that require the use of a key, tool, or special knowledge or effort to open the door leaf from the egress side. Door assemblies are generally permitted to be locked from the nonegress side, so as to prevent unauthorized entry into a building. However, door assemblies from an exit stair enclosure to the building floors might have to provide for re-entry as detailed in 7.2.1.5.7.

See the commentary following 7.2.1.5.5, which explains the concept whereby a door assembly with a magnetic lock, with building access via a card reader, can be considered a normal door assembly in compliance with 7.2.1.5.1, 7.2.1.5.2, and 7.2.1.5.9 if the door leaf has a lever handle with an integral switch that releases the lock to allow free egress by building occupants.

**7.2.1.5.3** The requirements of 7.2.1.5.1 and 7.2.1.5.2 shall not apply where otherwise provided in Chapters 18 through 23.

Paragraph 7.2.1.5.3 cross-references the provisions applicable to health care occupancies and detention and correctional occupancies where door assemblies locked against egress by building occupants are permitted under specific conditions. For examples, see 18.1.1.1.5, 18.2.2.2.2, 18.2.2.2.4, 18.2.2.2.5, and similar provisions in Chapter 19. Also see 22.2.11.2 and 22.2.11.7 through 22.2.11.10 and similar provisions in Chapter 23.

**7.2.1.5.4 Key-Operated Locks.**

**7.2.1.5.4.1** Exterior door assemblies shall be permitted to have key-operated locks from the egress side, provided that the following criteria are met:

(1) This alternative is permitted in Chapters 11 through 43 for the specific occupancy.
(2) A readily visible, durable sign in letters not less than 1 in. (25 mm) high on a contrasting background that reads as follows is located on or adjacent to the door leaf: THIS DOOR TO REMAIN UNLOCKED WHEN THE BUILDING IS OCCUPIED.
(3) The locking device is of a type that is readily distinguishable as locked.
(4) A key is immediately available to any occupant inside the building when it is locked.

**7.2.1.5.4.2** The alternative provisions of 7.2.1.5.4.1 shall be permitted to be revoked by the authority having jurisdiction for cause.

The provisions of 7.2.1.5.4 address key-operated locks that must meet four conditions — one of which is that the appropriate occupancy chapter must specifically permit use of the exemption. Compliance with 7.2.1.5.4.1(3), which requires that the locking device be of a type readily distinguishable as locked, is to be judged by the authority having jurisdiction. Locks specifically designed to meet this requirement often have an indicating window mechanism that displays the word "open" when the device is in the unlocked position and displays the word "locked" when the device is in the locked position.

In permitting up to 10 persons in a locked building (i.e., an *unoccupied* building, as addressed in 7.2.1.1.3), the *Code* does not dismiss such occupants as unimportant. The *Code* recognizes that there are instances where a building must be occupied by security personnel or by janitorial crews when it is locked. Such persons are generally familiar with the premises, and the *Code* requires that they have keys available for egress when necessary. Also see the commentary following 7.2.1.1.3.2.

The occupancies in the list that follows permit the use of the key-operated lock addressed by 7.2.1.5.4. Additional restrictions that might be imposed by the occupancy chapter are contained in the paragraphs referenced within parentheses in the list. For example, in new assembly occupancies, use of a key-operated lock is restricted to the main exit of a building with an occupant load of not more than 500 persons. In addition, the main exit of the assembly occupancy is required to consist of a single door leaf or single pair of door leaves, and any latch on the door leaf or leaves is required to be released by panic hardware.

The occupancies permitting the use of the key-operated lock addressed in 7.2.1.5.4 are as follows:

1. Assembly occupancies (12.2.2.2.4, 13.2.2.2.4)
2. Mercantile occupancies (36.2.2.2.2, 37.2.2.2.2)
3. Business occupancies (38.2.2.2.2, 39.2.2.2.2)

**7.2.1.5.5 Electrically Controlled Egress Door Assemblies.** Door assemblies in the means of egress shall be permitted to be electrically locked if equipped with approved, listed hardware that incorporates a built-in switch, provided that the following conditions are met:

(1) The hardware for occupant release of the lock is affixed to the door leaf.
(2) The hardware has an obvious method of operation that is readily operated in the direction of egress.
(3) The hardware is capable of being operated with one hand in the direction of egress.
(4) Operation of the hardware interrupts the power supply directly to the electric lock and unlocks the door assembly in the direction of egress.
(5) Loss of power to the hardware automatically unlocks the door assembly in the direction of egress.

The provisions of 7.2.1.5.5 are new to the 2009 edition of the *Code* and address electrically controlled egress door assemblies as a normal door assembly and not as a special locking arrangement. Note that the new provisions are positioned within 7.2.1.5, related to traditional locks and latches, and not within 7.2.1.6, which addresses specialized, nontraditional locking arrangements like delayed-egress locking systems and access-controlled egress door assemblies.

The door assemblies addressed by 7.2.1.5.5 typically take the form of a door leaf that is held locked to its frame via an electromagnet. Authorities having jurisdiction, in enforcing the provisions of earlier editions of the *Code*, often required any door assembly with an electromagnetic lock to comply with one of the sets of provisions of 7.2.1.6 for special locking arrangements, regardless of how the lock was operated. The new text has the effect of equating the electrically controlled lock to a traditional, mechanically latched or locked door.

The criteria detailed in 7.2.1.5.5 (1) through (5) ensure that the electrically controlled egress door assembly meets the requirements of 7.2.1.5.1, 7.2.1.5.2, and 7.2.1.5.9, as well as additional safeguards imposed, because the lock is electrically controlled. See also the third sentence of A.7.2.1.5.9.

**7.2.1.5.6** Where permitted in Chapters 11 through 43, key operation shall be permitted, provided that the key cannot be removed when the door leaf is locked from the side from which egress is to be made.

Paragraph 7.2.1.5.6 permits the "captive key" hardware, as is permitted in lodging and rooming houses via the provisions of 26.2.3.6. The captive key lock has the potential for misuse and must be used carefully. The design of the lock is such that an occupant could unlock the door assembly from the inside, thus freeing the key; move through the door opening, taking the key to the outside; lock the door assembly from the outside; and leave the property — potentially leaving others locked in the building. Thus, this lock is permitted limited use within the occupancy chapters.

**7.2.1.5.7*** Every door assembly in a stair enclosure serving more than four stories, unless permitted by 7.2.1.5.7.2, shall meet one of the following conditions:

(1) Re-entry from the stair enclosure to the interior of the building shall be provided.
(2) An automatic release that is actuated with the initiation of the building fire alarm system shall be provided to unlock all stair enclosure door assemblies to allow re-entry.
(3) Selected re-entry shall be provided in accordance with 7.2.1.5.7.1.

**A.7.2.1.5.7** It is intended that the re-entry provisions apply only to enclosed exit stairs, not to outside stairs. This arrangement makes it possible to leave the stairway at such floor if the fire renders the lower part of the stair unusable during egress or if the occupants seek refuge on another floor.

Every door assembly in a stair enclosure serving more than four stories in a new building [see 7.2.1.5.7.2 (1) and (2)] must be arranged to permit re-entry into the building. However, the *Code* recognizes the need for varying degrees of security and does specify some equivalent alternatives. Stairway door assemblies are permitted to be locked to the stairwell side if arranged to unlock automatically upon initiation of the fire alarm system. Selected re-entry is addressed in the commentary associated with 7.2.1.5.7.1.

**7.2.1.5.7.1** Door assemblies on stair enclosures shall be permitted to be equipped with hardware that prevents re-entry into the interior of the building, provided that the following criteria are met:

(1) There shall be not less than two levels where it is possible to leave the stair enclosure to access another exit.
(2) There shall be not more than four stories intervening between stories where it is possible to leave the stair enclosure to access another exit.
(3) Re-entry shall be possible on the top story or next-to-top story served by the stair enclosure, and such story shall allow access to another exit.
(4) Door assemblies allowing re-entry shall be identified as such on the stair side of the door leaf.
(5) Door assemblies not allowing re-entry shall be provided with a sign on the stair side indicating the location of the nearest door opening, in each direction of travel, that allows re-entry or exit.

Paragraph 7.2.1.5.7.1 permits some stair enclosure door assemblies, regardless of occupancy, to be locked to prevent re-entry on selected floors. In such instances, there must be at least two levels with unlocked door assemblies providing a way out of the stairway, one of which must be the top floor or the next to top floor; the other is usually the door assembly at the level of exit discharge. Because the *Code* prohibits more than four floors between floors that provide a way out of the stairway, stair enclosures serving more than six or seven stories must have more than two unlocked re-entry points. This arrangement provides flexibility in buildings that, perhaps for security reasons, need to prevent re-entry on certain floors, while at the same time ensuring that one can re-enter the building without having to travel up or down too many flights of stairs. See Exhibit 7.21. Any door assembly providing a way out of the stair enclosure must be identified as such on the stairwell side.

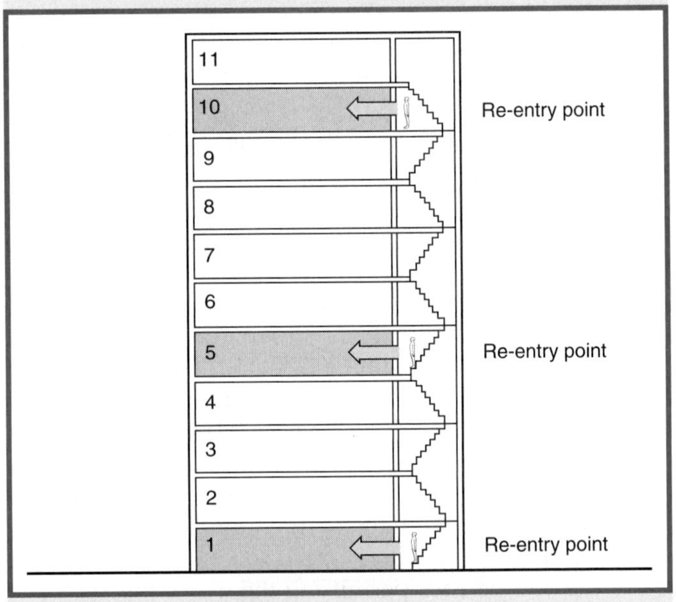


***Exhibit 7.21*** *Stairway re-entry option.*

**7.2.1.5.7.2** The requirements of 7.2.1.5.7, except as provided in 7.2.1.5.7.3, shall not apply to the following:

(1) Existing installations in buildings that are not high-rise buildings as permitted in Chapters 11 through 43
(2) Existing installations in high-rise buildings as permitted in Chapters 11 through 43 where the occupancy is within a building protected throughout by an approved, supervised automatic sprinkler system in accordance with 9.7.1
(3) Existing approved stairwell re-entry installations as permitted by Chapters 11 through 43

(4) Stair enclosures serving a building permitted to have a single exit in accordance with Chapters 11 through 43
(5) Stair enclosures in health care occupancies where otherwise provided in Chapter 18
(6) Stair enclosures in detention and correctional occupancies where otherwise provided in Chapter 22

**7.2.1.5.7.3** When the provisions of 7.2.1.5.7.2 are used, signage on the stair door leaves shall be required as follows;

(1) Door assemblies allowing re-entry shall be identified as such on the stair side of the door leaf.
(2) Door assemblies not allowing re-entry shall be provided with a sign on the stair side indicating the location of the nearest door opening, in each direction of travel, that allows re-entry or exit.

In editions of the *Code* prior to 2009, the re-entry provisions were exempted for any existing stair installation where the applicable occupancy chapter specifically provided an exemption. The provisions of 7.2.1.5.7.2 (2) and (3) are new to the 2009 edition. Existing stair installations in a high-rise building are permitted to be exempted by the applicable occupancy chapter only if the building is fully sprinklered. Where the existing high-rise building is not sprinklered, re-entry in accordance with 7.2.1.5.7 is required.

Where an existing stairwell re-entry installation does not meet all the criteria of 7.2.1.5.7, the provision of 7.2.1.5.7.2(3) establishes that the existing installation can be continued in use if approved. The term *approved* means acceptable to the AHJ, and its definition appears in 3.2.1.

Paragraph 7.2.1.5.7.2(4) recognizes that re-entry in buildings permitted to have a single exit is not necessary. In most single-exit buildings, the door assemblies from the stairway open directly into the occupant space. Most of the single-exit buildings recognized by the occupancy chapters are not more than four stories in height and are exempt from the stairwell re-entry provisions via the base paragraph of 7.2.1.5.7.

Paragraphs 7.2.1.5.7.2(5) and (6) specify, for correlation with the occupancy chapters, that health care occupancies and detention and correctional occupancies are exempt from the stair enclosure re-entry provisions. The exemption is based on the level of protection provided via a defend-in-place approach that minimizes the need for vertical evacuation by stairs or, where such movement is needed, relies heavily on staff with access to keys to direct the evacuation or relocation.

The provisions of 7.2.1.5.7.3 are new to the 2009 edition of the *Code* and require signage in each exit stair enclosure serving more than four stories and not providing re-entry in accordance with the criteria of 7.2.1.5.7 (1), (2), or (3). The signage must be installed on the stair side of each door leaf. The provisions of 7.2.1.5.7.3 are illustrated by the example that follows.

An existing business occupancy building is six stories in height above grade plane. Egress from all floors above floor 1 is provided by two remote exit stair enclosures that are accessed by a corridor on each floor. On floors 2 through 6, all door leaves from the corridor to the exit stair enclosures are locked from the stairwell side so as to prevent re-entry as permitted by 39.2.2.2.4(1) and 7.2.1.5.7.2(1). On floor 1, the door from the corridor to each stair enclosure is left unlocked so as to permit re-entry onto the floor. In accordance with 7.2.1.5.7.3(2), the exit stair enclosure door leaves on floors 2 through 6 must be provided with signage, on the stair side, indicating that re-entry is provided at floor 1.

**7.2.1.5.8** If a stair enclosure allows access to the roof of the building, the door assembly to the roof either shall be kept locked or shall allow re-entry from the roof.

Paragraph 7.2.1.5.8 was written to prevent building occupants from being trapped on a roof by a locked door assembly that does not permit re-entry into the building. If security concerns, for example, dictate that rooftop door assemblies are to be locked against entry from the outside, then the door assemblies also need to be locked from the inside to prevent unauthorized building occupants from going to the roof and becoming trapped. Note that there is no requirement that stair enclosure door assemblies provide rooftop access. Heroic helicopter rescues from rooftops of burning buildings are Hollywood movie illusions that seldom happen in real life.

**7.2.1.5.9*** A latch or other fastening device on a door leaf shall be provided with a releasing device that has an obvious method of operation and that is readily operated under all lighting conditions.

**A.7.2.1.5.9** Examples of devices that might be arranged to release latches include knobs, levers, and bars. This requirement is permitted to be satisfied by the use of conventional types of hardware, whereby the door is released by turning a lever, knob, or handle or by pushing against a bar, but not by unfamiliar methods of operation, such as a blow to break glass. It is also within the intent of this requirement that switches integral to traditional doorknobs, lever handles, or bars, and that interrupt the power supply to an electromagnetic lock, be permitted, provided that they are affixed to the door leaf. The operating devices should be capable of being operated with one hand and should not require tight grasping, tight pinching, or twisting of the wrist to operate.

Paragraph 7.2.1.5.9 requires that, where a latch or other similar device is provided, the method of operation of its releasing device must be obvious, even in the dark. The intention of this requirement is that the method of release be one that is familiar to the average person. Generally, a two-step release, such as a knob and an independent slide bolt, is not permitted. In most occupancies, it is important that a single action unlatch the door assembly. See the commentary following 7.2.1.5.9.5 for an explanation of night latches permitted as a device in addition to the main latch/lock on residential occupancy dwelling unit door assemblies.

See the commentary following 7.2.1.5.5, which explains the concept whereby a door assembly with a electrically controlled lock can be considered a normal door assembly in compliance with 7.2.1.5.1, 7.2.1.5.2, and 7.2.1.5.9 if the door assembly meets the criteria detailed in 7.2.1.5.5 (1) through (5), which include an arrangement where the locked door leaf is provided with a lever handle with an integral switch that releases the lock to allow free egress by building occupants.

**7.2.1.5.9.1** The releasing mechanism for any latch, other than for existing installations, shall be located not less than 34 in. (865 mm), and not more than 48 in. (1220 mm), above the finished floor.

**7.2.1.5.9.2** The releasing mechanism shall open the door leaf with not more than one releasing operation, unless otherwise specified in 7.2.1.5.9.3 and 7.2.1.5.9.4.

**7.2.1.5.9.3*** Egress door assemblies from individual living units and guest rooms of residential occupancies shall be permitted to be provided with devices, including automatic latching devices, that require not more than one additional releasing operation, provided that such device is operable from the inside without the use of a key or tool and is mounted at a height not exceeding 48 in. (1220 mm) above the finished floor.

**A.7.2.1.5.9.3** Examples of devices that, when used with a latch, can be arranged to require not more than one additional releasing operation include night latches, dead bolts, and security chains.

**7.2.1.5.9.4** Existing security devices permitted by 7.2.1.5.9.3 shall be permitted to have two additional releasing operations.

**7.2.1.5.9.5** Existing security devices permitted by 7.2.1.5.9.3, other than automatic latching devices, shall be located not more than 60 in. (1525 mm) above the finished floor.

Paragraph 7.2.1.5.9.1 specifies that the latch release mechanism be located at least 34 in. (865 mm) and not more than 48 in. (1220 mm) above the floor, so that the latch release is located in a position that is neither too low nor too high to be reached by persons in wheelchairs. The maximum mounting height for the latch release also helps to ensure that children can reach the latch. Note that 7.2.1.5.9.1 does not clearly reflect intent with respect to existing installations. In editions of the *Code* through 2000, exemptions were formatted as self-contained exceptions. The applicable exception clearly stated that only the 34 in. (865 mm) minimum mounting height was not applicable to existing installations. The exception did not exempt existing installations from the 48 in. (1220 mm) maximum mounting height. The editorial reformatting that was done in preparation of the 2003 edition of the *Code* unintentionally confused the issue. The lack of clarity on the subject was noted while reviewing the commentary for the 2009 edition of this handbook. The technical committee responsible for Chapter 7 will be asked to fix the text during the next revision cycle.

Paragraphs 7.2.1.5.9.3 and 7.2.1.5.9.4 provide an exemption to the requirement for a single releasing mechanism. The exemption recognizes the use, in residential living units and hotel guest rooms, of one additional device requiring release in new construction and two additional devices requiring release in existing installations. It permits an existing condition to continue where a hotel room door assembly, for example, has hardware arranged such that one operation releases the security chain or bar (i.e., night latch), another operation releases the dead bolt (usually via a thumb turn-type knob), and a third operation releases the door latch, usually by turning the doorknob or operating the door lever. However, in new installations, if a night latch or security device is installed, one operation would release the security device and a second operation, such as turning the doorknob or operating the door lever, would have to release both the dead bolt and normal door latch.

Also, the *Code* prohibits supplemental automatic latching security devices from being located more than 48 in. (1220 mm) above the floor, even in existing buildings (see 7.2.1.5.9.3). This prohibition is intended to prevent children and wheelchair users from being trapped in a space when an automatic latching device that is located above reach range engages, locking the door assembly. Existing security devices that must be physically engaged are permitted in locations not more than 60 in. (1525 mm) above the floor (see 7.2.1.5.9.5), based on the assumption that the person engaging such a device is present to disengage it when needed.

**7.2.1.5.10** Where pairs of door leaves are required in a means of egress, one of the following criteria shall be met:

(1) Each leaf of the pair shall be provided with a releasing device that does not depend on the release of one leaf before the other.
(2) Approved automatic flush bolts shall be used and arranged such that the following criteria are met:
    (a) The door leaf equipped with the automatic flush bolts shall have no doorknob or surface-mounted hardware.
    (b) Unlatching of any leaf shall not require more than one operation.

The requirement of 7.2.1.5.10(1) for independent releasing hardware applies only to pairs of door leaves in a common door opening where both door leaves are required for means of egress. If a second leaf is provided for a reason other than required egress, that leaf can have a releasing mechanism that requires the egress leaf to be released first. However, in such a case, the leaf not used for egress must be arranged so as not to be mistaken for the egress door leaf.

Paragraph 7.2.1.5.10(2) permits a pair of door leaves — both a part of the required means of egress — to be placed within a common frame, whereby one leaf has no visible releasing hardware but has approved automatic flush bolts that release that leaf when the other leaf, which has visible hardware, is released. Therefore, the user is directed to the leaf with releasing hardware and disengages the latch on that leaf, and the other leaf automatically unlatches to allow its use if pushed in the direction of door leaf travel.

**7.2.1.5.11*** Devices shall not be installed in connection with any door assembly on which panic hardware or fire exit hardware is required where such devices prevent or are intended to prevent the free use of the leaf for purposes of egress, unless otherwise provided in 7.2.1.6.

**A.7.2.1.5.11** Examples of devices prohibited by this requirement include locks, padlocks, hasps, bars, chains, or combinations thereof.

It is not the intent of 7.2.1.5.11 to require panic hardware or fire exit hardware; that requirement is specified by the various occupancy chapters. Rather, 7.2.1.5.11 requires that, where panic hardware or fire exit hardware is installed, no device or arrangement is to interfere with its intended function. The intended function is the release of the latch when pressure — such as that exerted by persons pushing up against the door leaf — is applied to the bar or pad extending across the majority of the door leaf width [see 7.2.1.7.1(1)].

**7.2.1.6* Special Locking Arrangements.**

The special locking arrangements described in 7.2.1.6 include delayed-egress locking systems and access-controlled egress door assemblies. Each of these terms has a specific, but limited, meaning for purposes of applying the *Code*. For example, a building operator installs a magnetic lock on an outside door assembly and provides a card reader outside the building that releases the door assembly lock, so that only authorized persons are allowed entry to the building. Further, a lever handle is mounted on the inside surface of the door leaf and has an integral switch that releases the magnetic lock whenever a building occupant operates the lever. The building operator refers to this system as an access-controlled egress door assembly, but it is not the access-controlled egress door assembly addressed in 7.2.1.6.2, and it is not subject to those requirements. Rather, the door assembly locking system described is an electrically controlled egress door assembly subject to the provisions of 7.2.1.5.5. Such door assemblies in accordance with 7.2.1.5.5 comply with 7.2.1.5.1, 7.2.1.5.2, and 7.2.1.5.9 so as not to be special locking arrangements. The concept is further explained by A.7.2.1.6.2 and the third sentence of A.7.2.1.5.9.

NFPA staff answers *Code* questions from NFPA members and authorities having jurisdiction under a program referred to internally as Advisory Services. In 2005, a safety officer for a pharmaceutical manufacturer called. He explained that some of the pharmaceutical manufacturing facility exit door assemblies had magnetic locks released by card readers for both entry and exit. A consultant's report suggested to the safety officer that panic bar or push-pad releases be added to the door assemblies to directly release the lock for use in emergencies and that the facility continue to have employees use their pass cards for normal (i.e., nonemergency) entry/exit. Thus, the door assemblies would be treated as normal, manually released door assemblies not subject to any special provisions, such as those for access-controlled egress door assemblies. The safety officer could not understand that he should not refer to the access-controlled egress door assembly provisions of the *Code* and that the door assemblies in question were not termed *access-controlled* by NFPA *101*. He thought that the facility door assemblies were required to be tied into the fire alarm panel because of the access-controlled egress door assembly provisions. It took further explanation and reference to the text of A.7.2.1.5.9 and A.7.2.1.6.2 to assuage his concerns. With the 2009 edition, the issue is further clarified by the introduction of the new provisions on electrically controlled egress door assemblies as detailed in 7.2.1.5.5.

**A.7.2.1.6** None of the special locking arrangements addressed in 7.2.1.6 are intended to allow *credentialed egress, request to exit*, or similar provisions, where an occupant cannot leave the building without swiping a card through a reader. Where such an arrangement is desired to keep track of occupants, the swiping of cards needs to be procedural but not necessary for releasing the door lock or latch. Free egress needs to be available at all times. Another option to free egress is the use of a delayed-egress locking system.

**7.2.1.6.1 Delayed-Egress Locking Systems.** Approved, listed, delayed-egress locking systems shall be permitted to be installed on door assemblies serving low and ordinary hazard contents in buildings protected throughout by an approved, supervised automatic fire detection system in accordance with Section 9.6 or an approved, supervised automatic sprinkler system in accordance with Section 9.7, and where permitted in Chapters 11 through 43, provided that the following criteria are met:

(1) The provisions of 7.2.1.6.2 for access-controlled egress door assemblies shall not apply to door assemblies with delayed-egress locking systems.
(2) The door leaves shall unlock upon actuation of one of the following:
   (a) Approved, supervised automatic sprinkler system in accordance with Section 9.7
   (b) Not more than one heat detector of an approved, supervised automatic fire detection system in accordance with Section 9.6
   (c) Not more than two smoke detectors of an approved, supervised automatic fire detection system in accordance with Section 9.6
(3) The door leaves shall unlock upon loss of power controlling the lock or locking mechanism.
(4)* An irreversible process shall release the lock within 15 seconds, or 30 seconds where approved by the authority having jurisdiction, upon application of a force to the release device required in 7.2.1.5.9 under the following conditions:
   (a) The force shall not be required to exceed 15 lbf (67 N).
   (b) The force shall not be required to be continuously applied for more than 3 seconds.
   (c) The initiation of the release process shall activate an audible signal in the vicinity of the door opening.
   (d) Once the lock has been released by the application of force to the releasing device, relocking shall be by manual means only.

**A.7.2.1.6.1(4)** It is not the intent to require a direct physical or electrical connection between the door release device and the lock. It is the intent to allow door movement initiated by operating the door release device required in 7.2.1.5.9 as one option to initiate the irreversible process.

Several factors need to be considered in approving an increase in delay time from 15 seconds to 30 seconds. Some of the factors include occupancy, occupant density, ceiling height, fire hazards present, fire protection features provided, and the location of the delayed-egress locks. An example of a location where the increase in delay time might not be approved is at an exit stair discharge door.

(5)* A readily visible, durable sign in letters not less than 1 in. (25 mm) high and not less than ⅛ in. (3.2 mm) in stroke width on a contrasting background that reads as follows shall be located on the door leaf adjacent to the release device:

PUSH UNTIL ALARM SOUNDS

DOOR CAN BE OPENED IN 15 SECONDS

**A.7.2.1.6.1(5)** In the event that the authority having jurisdiction has permitted increased operation time, the sign should reflect the appropriate time.

Delayed-egress locking systems prevent a door leaf from being opened for 15 seconds or 30 seconds under either nonemergency conditions or those encountered very early in a fire or similar emergency. Delayed-egress locking systems are to be used only where specifically permitted by the appropriate occupancy chapter. Their use is further limited to buildings protected throughout by either an approved, supervised automatic fire detection system or an approved, supervised automatic sprinkler system.

Paragraph 7.2.1.6.1(1) serves mainly as a reminder that delayed-egress locking systems and access-controlled egress door assembly locking are two different features that are not to be intermixed. In the case of the delayed-egress locking systems, the releasing mechanism is mounted on the door leaf, and the system delays occupants from initially opening the door leaf. Access-controlled egress door assembly locking involves a door assembly that is not provided with an occupant-activated releasing mechanism on the door leaf and, therefore, relies on a motion detector to sense the approaching occupant, with the door leaf unlocking as the occupant reaches the door leaf.

Paragraph 7.2.1.6.1(2) requires that the locking devices unlock upon activation of the corresponding detection or sprinkler system. The required detection system provides early warning; the alternately required sprinkler system provides early control of the fire — with each system performing to the degree necessary to make tolerable the delay experienced in waiting for the door leaf to be unlocked.

Paragraph 7.2.1.6.1(3) provides a fail-safe feature where, upon loss of the electrical power that controls the lock, immediate unlocking occurs. Note that, where the door leaf is unlocked, it is not required to be unlatched. Building occupants might need to operate the actuating bar or push pad to release the latch before opening the door. See the commentary three paragraphs below this paragraph.

Paragraph 7.2.1.6.1(4) requires that, once the release device is manually activated, the door leaf must unlock within 15 seconds, or 30 seconds with specific permission of the authority having jurisdiction. This action must be irreversible and cannot require the user to maintain pressure on the release device for more than 3 seconds. To provide occupants attempting egress with cues to indicate that the system is functioning, a signal is sounded in the vicinity of the door opening. Additionally, the signage required by 7.2.1.6.1(5) provides useful, reassuring information.

After the door leaf is unlatched and physically opened (i.e., swung on its hinges away from the door frame), it is permitted to be relocked by manual means only. Relocking generally involves returning the door leaf to its closed and latched position and then resetting the system to engage the lock. Relatching is not prohibited, provided that the releasing mechanism (i.e., the push pad or actuating bar), when operated, unlatches the door leaf without any delay.

Note that the unlocking required by 7.2.1.6.1(2), (3), and (4) need not automatically open the door leaf. Rather, the door leaf is permitted to remain latched. The unlocking allows the user to open the door leaf immediately by operating the releasing mechanism on the door leaf. Security is not sacrificed. Of course, any exterior exit door assembly is permitted to be locked against building entry at any time.

The occupancies in the list that follows permit the use of delayed-egress locking systems in accordance with 7.2.1.6.1. Additional restrictions that might be imposed by the occupancy chapter are contained in the paragraphs referenced within parentheses in the list. For example, lodging and rooming houses, hotels and dormitories, and apartment buildings permit delayed-egress locking systems if all the conditions of 7.2.1.6.1 are met and only one such lock is encountered along any natural path of egress travel.

The occupancies permitting delayed-egress locking systems are as follows:

1. Assembly occupancies (12.2.2.2.5, 13.2.2.2.5)
2. Educational occupancies (14.2.2.2.3, 15.2.2.2.3)
3. Day-care occupancies (16.2.2.2.3, 17.2.2.2.3)
4. Health care occupancies [18.2.2.2.4(2), 19.2.2.2.4(2)]
5. Ambulatory health care occupancies (20.2.2.2, 21.2.2.2)
6. Lodging or rooming houses (26.2.3.5.2)
7. Hotels and dormitories (28.2.2.2.2.2, 29.2.2.2.2.2)
8. Apartment buildings (30.2.2.2.2.2, 31.2.2.2.2.2)
9. Residential board and care occupancies [32.2.2.5.5.1, 32.3.2.2.2(4), 33.2.2.5.5.1, 33.3.2.2.2(4)]
10. Mercantile occupancies (36.2.2.2.5, 37.2.2.2.5)
11. Business occupancies (38.2.2.2.5, 39.2.2.2.5)
12. Industrial occupancies (40.2.2.2.2)
13. Storage occupancies (42.2.2.2.2, 42.8.2.2.2.2)

**7.2.1.6.2* Access-Controlled Egress Door Assemblies.** Where permitted in Chapters 11 through 43, door assemblies in the means of egress shall be permitted to be equipped with an approved entrance and egress access control system, provided that all the following criteria are met:

(1) A sensor shall be provided on the egress side, arranged to detect an occupant approaching door leaves that are arranged to unlock in the direction of egress upon detection of an approaching occupant or loss of power to the sensor.
(2) Loss of power to the part of the access control system that locks the door leaves shall automatically unlock the door leaves in the direction of egress.
(3) Door leaves shall be arranged to unlock in the direction of egress from a manual release device located 40 in. to 48 in. (1015 mm to 1220 mm ) vertically above the floor and within 60 in. (1525 mm) of the secured door openings.
(4) The manual release device specified in 7.2.1.6.2(3) shall be readily accessible and clearly identified by a sign that reads as follows: PUSH TO EXIT.
(5) When operated, the manual release device shall result in direct interruption of power to the lock —

independent of the access control system electronics — and the door leaves shall remain unlocked for not less than 30 seconds.

(6) Activation of the building fire-protective signaling system, if provided, shall automatically unlock the door leaves in the direction of egress, and they shall remain unlocked until the fire-protective signaling system has been manually reset.

(7) The activation of manual fire alarm boxes that activate the building fire-protective signaling system specified in 7.2.1.6.2(6) shall not be required to unlock the door leaves.

(8) Activation of the building automatic sprinkler or fire detection system, if provided, shall automatically unlock the door leaves in the direction of egress, and they shall remain unlocked until the fire-protective signaling system has been manually reset.

**A.7.2.1.6.2** It is not the intent to require doors that restrict access but comply with 7.2.1.5.9 to comply with the access-controlled egress door provisions of 7.2.1.6.2.

The access-controlled egress door assemblies addressed by 7.2.1.6.2 are intended to be locked against access from the outside of the building and require a magnetic card or similar instrument for authorized entry. However, such door assemblies must be arranged for free egress use whenever the building is occupied. The *Code* addresses these door assemblies under the subject of special locking arrangements because such door assemblies generally do not have the leaf-mounted manual latch/lock release typically installed on egress door assemblies. The absence of the door leaf-mounted manual latch/lock release prevents a person on the outside from inserting a wire hanger or other tool between the gaps at the door leaf edges to reach the release. Use of access-controlled egress door assemblies requires specific occupancy chapter permission.

See the commentary following 7.2.1.6, which explains the concept whereby a door assembly with a magnetic lock, with building access via a card reader, can be considered a normal door assembly in accordance with 7.2.1.5.5 if the door leaf has a lever handle with an integral switch that releases the lock to allow free egress by building occupants.

The occupancies in the list that follows permit the use of access-controlled egress door assemblies in accordance with 7.2.1.6.2. Additional restrictions that might be imposed by the occupancy chapter are contained in the paragraphs referenced within parentheses in the list. For example, the provisions of 36.2.2.2.6 and 37.2.2.2.6, which apply to mercantile occupancies, permit access-controlled egress door assemblies if all conditions of 7.2.1.6.2 are met and the building is protected throughout by an approved, supervised fire detection system or an approved automatic sprinkler system. The provisions of 12.2.2.2.6 and 13.2.2.2.6, which apply to assembly occupancies, permit access-controlled egress door assemblies if all conditions of 7.2.1.6.2 are met and such doors are not locked from the egress side when the assembly occupancy is occupied — in other words, the access control locking system is permitted to be engaged only in the hours when the assembly occupancy is not occupied.

The occupancies permitting access-controlled egress door assemblies are as follows:

1. Assembly occupancies (12.2.2.2.6, 13.2.2.2.6)
2. Educational occupancies (14.2.2.2.3, 15.2.2.2.3)
3. Day-care occupancies (16.2.2.2.3, 17.2.2.2.3)
4. Health care occupancies [18.2.2.2.4(3), 19.2.2.2.4(3)]
5. Ambulatory health care occupancies (20.2.2.2, 21.2.2.2)
6. Hotels and dormitories (28.2.2.2.2.3, 29.2.2.2.2.3)
7. Apartment buildings (30.2.2.2.2.3, 31.2.2.2.2.3)
8. Residential board and care occupancies [32.2.2.5.5.2, 32.3.2.2.2(5), 33.2.2.5.5.2, 33.3.2.2.2(5)]
9. Mercantile occupancies (36.2.2.2.6, 37.2.2.2.6)
10. Business occupancies (38.2.2.2.6, 39.2.2.2.6)
11. Industrial occupancies (40.2.2.2.3)
12. Storage occupancies (42.2.2.2.3, 42.8.2.2.2.2)

Paragraph 7.2.1.6.2(1) provides for the door leaf to unlock when a sensor detects an occupant approaching the door opening. This method is the normal primary means of releasing the lock to allow occupants to leave the building. If the sensor and the release system fail, the requirements of 7.2.1.6.2(3) through (5) provide a backup system consisting of a manual lock release mounted at a usable height in the immediate vicinity of the door opening. The *Code* permits the manual release to be installed as much as 60 in. (1525 mm) from the secured door assembly, recognizing that the glass sidelights featured on many of these door assemblies are an impractical place to install a manual release device.

Additionally, 7.2.1.6.2(2) requires a fail-safe feature to unlock the door leaf immediately upon loss of the electrical power that controls the lock.

Paragraphs 7.2.1.6.2(1) through (5) work together to help ensure that the door opening is usable at all times, before and during a fire emergency. Paragraphs 7.2.1.6.2(6) and (8) provide added assurance that the door opening is usable under fire emergency conditions. If the building has a fire alarm system, initiation of that system (by devices other than manual fire alarm boxes) must unlock the door leaf. If the building has either a fire detection system or a sprinkler system, activation of such system must unlock the door leaf.

Paragraph 7.2.1.6.2(7) clarifies that, if the building fire alarm system is initiated by a manual fire alarm box (formerly called a pull station), the door assembly is not required to unlock. This provision prevents an occupant who is intent on circumventing the security provided by such a door assembly from pulling the manual fire alarm box lever, which would initiate the alarm system and unlock the door assembly. Such an alarm initiation would readily defeat the purpose of the access-controlled egress door assembly locking provisions, which were developed to address security needs. The life safety features of the provisions of 7.2.1.6.2 are sufficient so as not to require an alarm initiation via a manual fire alarm box to unlock the door assembly.

Provided that the applicable occupancy chapter permits access-controlled egress door assemblies, and such occupancy chapter does not add an additional requirement limiting location, the provisions of 7.2.1.6.2 are meant to permit access-controlled egress door assemblies to be installed and used anywhere in the egress path; and there can be multiple such devices encountered along any egress path. Unlike the delayed-egress lock, there is no waiting period before the door leaf is usable, other than having to push a release button in the not-so-common situation where the electronics controlling the access-controlled device (such as the motion detector) fail.

**7.2.1.6.3 Elevator Lobby Exit Access Door Assemblies Locking.** Where permitted in Chapters 11 through 43, door assemblies separating the elevator lobby from the exit access required by 7.4.1.6.1 shall be permitted to be electronically locked, provided that all the following criteria are met:

(1) The electronic switch for releasing the lock is listed in accordance with UL 294, *Standard for Access Control System Units*
(2) The building is protected throughout by a fire alarm system in accordance with Section 9.6.
(3) The building is protected throughout by an approved, supervised automatic sprinkler system in accordance with Section 9.7.
(4) Waterflow in the sprinkler system required by 7.2.1.6.3(3) is arranged to initiate the building fire alarm system.
(5) The elevator lobby is protected by an approved, supervised smoke detection system in accordance with Section 9.6.
(6) Detection of smoke by the detection system required by 7.2.1.6.3(5) is arranged to initiate the building fire alarm system.
(7) Initiation of the building fire alarm system by other than manual fire alarm boxes unlocks the elevator lobby door assembly.
(8) Loss of power to the elevator lobby electronic lock system unlocks the elevator lobby door assemblies.
(9) The elevator lobby electronic lock system is not supplied with emergency or standby electrical power.
(10) Once unlocked, the elevator lobby door assemblies remain unlocked until the building fire alarm system has been manually reset.
(11) Where the elevator lobby door assemblies remain latched after being unlocked, latch-releasing hardware in accordance with 7.2.1.5.9 is affixed to the door leaves.
(12) A two-way communication system is provided for communication between the elevator lobby and a central control point that is constantly staffed.
(13) The central control point staff required by 7.2.1.6.3(12) is capable, trained, and authorized to provide emergency assistance.
(14) The provisions of 7.2.1.6.1 for delayed-egress locking systems are not applied to the elevator lobby door assemblies.
(15)* The provisions of 7.2.1.6.2 for access-controlled egress door assemblies are not applied to the elevator lobby door assemblies.

**A.7.2.1.6.3(15)** It is not the intent to prohibit elevator lobby doors from being equipped with card access systems for gaining access, for example, to tenant spaces. It is the access-controlled egress door system described in 7.2.1.6.2 that is prohibited from being installed on the same door as the lock addressed by 7.2.1.6.3.

The provisions of 7.2.1.6.3 are new to the 2009 edition of the *Code* and provide the technical details supporting the exemption offered by 7.4.1.6.3 to the requirements of 7.4.1.6.1 and 7.4.1.6.2 for unencumbered access to at least one exit from each elevator landing and lobby.

The provisions of 7.2.1.6.3 for the locking of elevator lobby access door assemblies are permitted to be used only where another portion of the *Code*, typically an occupancy chapter, specifically permits their use. Many of the occupancy chapters were revised concurrently with the development of 7.2.1.6.3 to permit its use.

The occupancies permitting the locking of elevator lobby access door assemblies are as follows:

1. Assembly occupancies (12.2.2.2.7, 13.2.2.2.7)
2. Educational occupancies (14.2.2.2.4, 15.2.2.2.4)

3. Day-care occupancies (16.2.2.2.4, 17.2.2.2.4)
4. Health care occupancies [18.2.2.2.4(4), 19.2.2.2.4(4)]
5. Ambulatory health care occupancies (20.2.2.3, 21.2.2.3)
6. Hotels and dormitories (28.2.2.2.2.4, 29.2.2.2.2.4)
8. Apartment buildings (30.2.2.2.2.4, 31.2.2.2.2.4)
9. Mercantile occupancies (36.2.2.2.3, 37.2.2.2.3)
10. Business occupancies (38.2.2.2.3, 39.2.2.2.3)

Where the provisions of 7.2.1.6.3 are used, all the criteria detailed in 7.2.1.6.3(1) through (15) must be met. When the criteria of all 15 items are met, the locked door between the elevator lobby or landing and the exit should present a minimal, but tolerable, obstruction to speedy egress. The criteria blend a host of provisions for fire detection and alarm systems, sprinkler systems, occupant and staff two-way communication systems, and automatic lock release systems.

**7.2.1.7 Panic Hardware and Fire Exit Hardware.**

The difference between panic hardware and fire exit hardware is that fire exit hardware is tested and listed for use on fire-rated door assemblies; panic hardware is not (see 7.2.1.7.2). As the terms imply, *panic hardware* and *fire exit hardware* are designed for ease of use and functional reliability under conditions that range from an orderly evacuation to that of hurried egress that might accompany a fast-spreading fire. See 3.3.124.1 and 3.3.124.2 for definitions of *fire exit hardware* and *panic hardware*, respectively.

The provisions of 7.2.1.7 do not require panic hardware; they do, however, set the requirements for such hardware if another portion of the *Code*, typically the applicable occupancy chapter, requires it.

The occupancies in the list that follows require the use of panic hardware or fire exit hardware. Additional restrictions that might be imposed by the occupancy chapter are contained in the paragraphs referenced within parentheses in the list.

The occupancies that require the use of panic hardware or fire exit hardware are as follows:

1. Assembly occupancies (12.2.2.2.3, 13.2.2.2.3)
2. Educational occupancies (14.2.2.2.2, 15.2.2.2.2)
3. Day-care occupancies (16.2.2.2.2, 17.2.2.2.2)

Although not required for occupancies other than assembly, educational, and day-care, panic hardware or fire exit hardware is often used in other occupancies, either because an assembly occupancy is located within the multiple occupancy or because it is used as a means of complying with 7.2.1.5.9. Additionally, 7.11.6, which applies to high hazard contents areas, permits door assemblies from spaces with occupant loads of more than five persons to be provided with a latch or lock only if panic hardware or fire exit hardware is installed to release the latch or lock.

**7.2.1.7.1** Where a door assembly is required to be equipped with panic or fire exit hardware, such hardware shall meet the following criteria:

(1) It shall consist of a cross bar or a push pad, the actuating portion of which extends across not less than one-half of the width of the door leaf.
(2) It shall be mounted as follows:
   (a) New installations shall be not less than 34 in. (865 mm), and not more than 48 in. (1220 mm), above the floor.
   (b) Existing installations shall be not less than 30 in. (760 mm), and not more than 48 in. (1220 mm), above the floor.
(3) It shall be constructed so that a horizontal force not to exceed 15 lbf (66 N) actuates the cross bar or push pad and latches.

Panic hardware and fire exit hardware are required to be instantly and easily released. New panic hardware and fire exit hardware installations are to be located 34 in. to 48 in. (865 mm to 1220 mm) above the floor [for existing installations — 30 in. to 48 in. (760 mm to 1220 mm)]. The actuating member or bar (see 3.3.4) is required to extend at least one-half the width of the door leaf, so as to create a target width sufficient to ensure that it will be engaged by the bodies of occupants pushing up against the door leaf. Such hardware, where mounted to a door leaf surface, might reduce the usable, clear width of a door opening. Provided that the hardware is installed at least 34 in. (865 mm) above the floor, the provisions of 7.2.1.2.1.1(5) permit a 4 in. (100 mm) encroachment on clear width without forcing a reduction in reported clear width. This is depicted in Figure A.7.2.1.2.1(b). Installed below 34 in. (865 mm), the panic hardware or fire exit hardware might create a reduction in clear width sufficient to obstruct wheelchair passage through the opening associated with a 34 in. (865 mm) width door leaf. Where panic hardware is installed below 34 in. (865 mm), such as at the 30 in. (760 mm) height permitted for existing hardware by 7.2.1.7.1(2)(b), the clear width measurement is reduced by the amount of the panic hardware encroachment.

The maximum force that the panic hardware or fire exit hardware actuating bar or member can require for operation is 15 lbf (66 N). Note that this is the force needed to release the latching device only. The force needed to open the door leaf itself is governed by 7.2.1.4.5.

**7.2.1.7.2** Only approved panic hardware shall be used on door assemblies that are not fire-rated door assemblies. Only approved fire exit hardware shall be used on fire-rated door assemblies.

It is not the intent of 7.2.1.7.2 to require the use of panic hardware or fire exit hardware. The two requirements of this paragraph are as follows:

1. Only approved hardware is to be used, which means such hardware must be acceptable to the authority having jurisdiction (AHJ), which generally relies on laboratory listing of the hardware. See the definition of *approved* in 3.2.1.
2. Where such hardware is used on a fire-rated door assembly, it must be that special form of panic hardware termed *fire exit hardware* (see 3.3.124.1), which ensures that it has been tested for use on fire-rated door assemblies (with the AHJ generally making approval conditional on the device being listed; see 3.2.5).

Fire exit hardware is tested for use on fire-rated door assemblies; panic hardware is not.

**7.2.1.7.3** Required panic hardware and fire exit hardware, in other than detention and correctional occupancies as otherwise provided in Chapters 22 and 23, shall not be equipped with any locking device, set screw, or other arrangement that prevents the release of the latch when pressure is applied to the releasing device.

**7.2.1.7.4** Devices that hold the latch in the retracted position shall be prohibited on fire exit hardware, unless such devices are listed and approved for such a purpose.

It is the intent of the *Code* to permit the use of the delayed-egress lock described by 7.2.1.6.1 where panic hardware is required if the applicable occupancy chapter specifically permits use of the delayed-egress lock. In these cases, the actuating member or bar, which 7.2.1.7.1(1) requires to extend across at least half the door leaf width, serves as the device that initiates the irreversible process that results in the door leaf unlocking within the 15 seconds or 30 seconds specified.

Panic hardware, which is prohibited from being used on fire-rated door assemblies, often features the ability to "dog" the bar in the down position, so as to hold the door leaf latch in the retracted position. This latch-retracting feature is not available on fire exit hardware, because it would violate the listing of the rated fire door assembly. Rated door assemblies must self-latch upon being brought to the closed position by the required closing device. A latch helps to keep the door leaf closed under the pressures generated by a fire.

**7.2.1.8 Self-Closing Devices.**

**7.2.1.8.1*** A door leaf normally required to be kept closed shall not be secured in the open position at any time and shall be self-closing or automatic-closing in accordance with 7.2.1.8.2, unless otherwise permitted by 7.2.1.8.3.

**A.7.2.1.8.1** Examples of doors designed to normally be kept closed include those to a stair enclosure or horizontal exit.

**7.2.1.8.2** In any building of low or ordinary hazard contents, as defined in 6.2.2.2 and 6.2.2.3, or where approved by the authority having jurisdiction, door leaves shall be permitted to be automatic-closing, provided that the following criteria are met:

(1) Upon release of the hold-open mechanism, the leaf becomes self-closing.
(2) The release device is designed so that the leaf instantly releases manually and, upon release, becomes self-closing, or the leaf can be readily closed.
(3) The automatic releasing mechanism or medium is activated by the operation of approved smoke detectors installed in accordance with the requirements for smoke detectors for door leaf release service in *NFPA 72, National Fire Alarm Code*.
(4) Upon loss of power to the hold-open device, the hold-open mechanism is released and the door leaf becomes self-closing.
(5) The release by means of smoke detection of one door leaf in a stair enclosure results in closing all door leaves serving that stair.

**7.2.1.8.3** The elevator car doors, and the associated hoistway enclosure doors, at the floor level designated for recall in accordance with the requirements of 9.4.3 shall be permitted to remain open during Phase I Emergency Recall Operation.

Fire door assemblies in a means of egress route should be kept in the closed position, particularly those serving as entrances to a stair enclosure or positioned in a horizontal exit; however, it is in these two locations that door assemblies so often are held open by some type of door leaf stopping chock to aid in the free flow of normal traffic. This practice establishes conditions conducive to the rapid spread of fire, smoke, and heat to other sections of the building — the very situation that the stringent compartmentation requirements for the exit enclosure intend to prevent.

Recognizing that tampering with the self-closing feature might occur — and in an effort to encourage the use of effective positive measures, rather than ineffective prohibitions that often go ignored — the *Code* presents criteria for holding door leaves in the open position. It permits door leaves to be held open in buildings that house low or ordinary hazard contents or where the authority having jurisdiction gives approval.

Specific requirements found elsewhere in the *Code* mandate the use of automatic-closing devices rather than making their use an option. For example, 7.2.4.3.10 requires that horizontal exit door assemblies that span a corridor be automatic-closing in accordance with 7.2.1.8. The requirement of 7.2.4.3.10 recognizes that cross-corridor door assemblies without an automatic release feature are often wedged open to facilitate normal pedestrian movement. Such wedges compromise the safety intended to be provided by the horizontal exit door assembly.

The provisions of 7.2.1.8.2 permit door leaves to be held open by an automatic releasing device. The triggering of the automatic release is done through the operation of smoke detectors installed in accordance with the requirements for smoke detectors for door release service as specified in *NFPA 72*®, *National Fire Alarm Code*®.[8] Fusible links are not an acceptable trigger in this system, because untenable smoke conditions could easily render an exit enclosure or adjoining fire compartment unusable long before the temperature in the vicinity of the door opening has risen enough to operate the fusible link.

Additionally, loss of power to the device providing the hold-open feature must cause immediate automatic release. A manual method of release is also required. The manual method might involve tugging on the door leaf to cause its release. Therefore, magnetic devices with significant holding forces that are not easily overcome by a deliberate tug on the door leaf cannot be used. Once the hold-open device is released, the self-closing device installed on the door leaf swings the door leaf to its closed position. On a fire protection–rated door assembly, the required door latch then engages.

The door leaves held open in accordance with the provisions of 7.2.1.8.2 can be arranged to close simultaneously throughout the building or only in the affected zones. Zoning is generally better, because it permits door assemblies in areas unaffected by the emergency to remain open to accommodate normal use. If protecting a room, that room might be considered a zone. If protecting a stair enclosure, the entire stair enclosure is considered a zone, and the signal to close one door leaf in the enclosing walls must close all door leaves in that stair enclosure.

With the exception of certain hazardous areas where flash fires or explosions could occur, the use of automatic closers in accordance with these provisions is permitted. Use of automatic-closing equipment should be encouraged to prevent door leaves from being secured open by other means. Wedges, for example, need to be removed manually before the self-closer installed on the door leaf can move the door leaf to its closed position.

Paragraph 7.2.1.8.3 helps to coordinate the door leaf closing requirements of 7.2.1.8 with the provisions of 9.4.3 for elevator recall. The Fire Fighters' Emergency Operations requirements for elevators, as mandated by 9.4.3 and detailed in ASME A17.1/CSA B44, *Safety Code for Elevators and Escalators*,[9] mandate that an elevator — once recalled — to remain at the designated recall floor with the elevator shaft and elevator car door leaves held in the open position. The open door leaves allow responding fire service personnel to ensure the elevator has been recalled. Paragraph 7.2.1.8.3 legitimizes a feature that would otherwise be prohibited by 7.2.1.8.1.

**7.2.1.9* Powered Door Leaf Operation.**

**A.7.2.1.9** Horizontal-sliding doors installed in accordance with 7.2.1.14 should not be considered powered doors subject to the provisions of 7.2.1.9.

Powered doors are divided into two categories — power assisted and power operated. Power-assisted doors that conform to ANSI/BHMA A156.19, *American National Standard for Power Assist and Low Energy Power Operated Doors*, use limited power to operate the door. They require fewer safeguards as compared to full power–operated doors. These door operators are for swinging doors only. Power-operated doors that conform to ANSI/BHMA A156.10, *American National Standard for Power Operated Pedestrian Doors*, require more power to operate the door and require additional safeguards to provide protection against personal injury. Power-operated doors can be swinging, sliding, or folding doors.

**7.2.1.9.1* General.** Where means of egress door leaves are operated by power upon the approach of a person or are provided with power-assisted manual operation, the design shall be such that, in the event of power failure, the leaves open manually to allow egress travel or close when necessary to safeguard the means of egress.

**A.7.2.1.9.1** An example of the type of door addressed by 7.2.1.9.1 is one actuated by a motion-sensing device upon the approach of a person.

**7.2.1.9.1.1** The forces required to manually open the door leaves specified in 7.2.1.9.1 shall not exceed those required in 7.2.1.4.5, except that the force required to set the leaf in motion shall not exceed 50 lbf (222 N).

**7.2.1.9.1.2** The door assembly shall be designed and installed so that, when a force is applied to the door leaf on the side from which egress is made, it shall be capable of swinging from any position to provide full use of the required width of the opening in which it is installed. *(See 7.2.1.4.)*

**7.2.1.9.1.3** A readily visible, durable sign in letters not less than 1 in. (25 mm) high on a contrasting background that reads as follows shall be located on the egress side of each door opening:

IN EMERGENCY, PUSH TO OPEN

Power-operated sliding door assemblies activated by an automatic mechanism are permitted, provided that their movement can be manually overpowered and the door leaf can be made to swing in the direction of egress travel while still providing the required egress capacity. The feature for manual operation must work at all times, even when other features of the door assembly's mechanism (such as the treadle, the electric eye, or the sliding rail) have failed. Such a door leaf must be arranged so it can be made to swing manually from any position, whether fully or partially closed. Care must be taken to ensure that the enclosing construction of any door leaf pocket does not defeat its ability to swing. Note that the breakaway feature cannot require a force in excess of 50 lbf (222 N).

The sign advising that the door leaf can be pushed open in an emergency provides the user with information that might not be intuitively obvious. Typically, the user sees the door operate under power, which involves the door leaf sliding to the side of the opening. The emergency manual mode of operation often relies on a breakaway feature that allows the door assembly to become side-hinged and swinging when pushed in the direction of egress travel.

**7.2.1.9.1.4** Sliding, power-operated door assemblies in an exit access serving an occupant load of fewer than 50 that manually open in the direction of door leaf travel, with forces not exceeding those required in 7.2.1.4.5, shall not be required to have the swing-out feature required by 7.2.1.9.1.2. The required sign shall be in letters not less than 1 in. (25 mm) high on a contrasting background and shall read as follows:

IN EMERGENCY, SLIDE TO OPEN

Recall that swinging door leaves, other than those in exit enclosures, serving an occupant load of fewer than 50 persons are permitted to swing against the direction of egress travel. Paragraph 7.2.1.9.1.4 considers a sliding door leaf that can be manually opened with forces not exceeding those required of swinging door leaves to be equivalent to a door leaf that swings against the direction of egress travel. Paragraph 7.2.1.9.1.4 then exempts the breakaway feature described in the commentary that follows 7.2.1.9.1.3.

Again, because the door leaf is power-operated during normal use, a sign must be provided advising the user that force can be used to slide the door leaf to its open position in an emergency mode — that is, on loss of power or equipment malfunction.

**7.2.1.9.1.5*** In the emergency breakout mode, a door leaf located within a two-leaf opening shall be exempt from the minimum 32 in. (810 mm) single-leaf requirement of 7.2.1.2.3.2(1), provided that the clear width of the single leaf is not less than 30 in. (760 mm).

**A.7.2.1.9.1.5** Although a single power-operated door leaf located within a two-leaf opening might alone not provide more than 30 in. (760 mm) of clear width in the emergency breakout mode, where both leaves are broken out to become side hinged, the required egress width is permitted to be provided by the width of the entire opening.

**7.2.1.9.1.6** For a biparting sliding door assembly in the emergency breakout mode, a door leaf located within a multiple-leaf opening shall be exempt from the minimum 32 in. (810 mm) single-leaf requirement of 7.2.1.2.3.2(1) if a clear opening of not less than 32 in. (810 mm) is provided by all leafs broken out.

Paragraphs 7.2.1.9.1.5 and 7.2.1.9.1.6 recognize a design limitation of power-operated door assemblies currently manufactured and widely in use. Power-operated door assemblies that are capable of providing the minimum 32 in. (810 mm) clear width for a single leaf, as required by 7.2.1.2.3.2, generally are not capable of providing the same minimum 32 in. (810 mm) clear width in the emergency breakout mode. As long as there are multiple leaves within a single opening and each is provided with the breakout feature, the 32 in. (810 mm) single-leaf requirement is relaxed, because the minimum required width can be provided by the entire opening with multiple door leaves broken out.

**7.2.1.9.1.7** Door assemblies complying with 7.2.1.14 shall be permitted to be used.

**7.2.1.9.1.8** The requirements of 7.2.1.9.1 through 7.2.1.9.1.7 shall not apply in detention and correctional occupancies where otherwise provided in Chapters 22 and 23.

**7.2.1.9.2 Self-Closing or Self-Latching Door Leaf Operation.** Where door leaves are required to be self-closing or self-latching and are operated by power upon the approach of a person, or are provided with power-assisted manual operation, they shall be permitted in the means of egress where they meet the following criteria:

(1) The door leaves can be opened manually in accordance with 7.2.1.9.1 to allow egress travel in the event of power failure.
(2) New door leaves remain in the closed position, unless actuated or opened manually.
(3) When actuated, new door leaves remain open for not more than 30 seconds.
(4) Door leaves held open for any period of time close — and the power-assist mechanism ceases to function — upon operation of approved smoke detectors installed in such a way as to detect smoke on either side of the door opening in accordance with the provisions of *NFPA 72, National Fire Alarm Code.*
(5) Door leaves required to be self-latching are either self-latching or become self-latching upon operation of approved smoke detectors per 7.2.1.9.2(4).
(6) New power-assisted swinging door assemblies comply with BHMA/ANSI A156.19, *American National Standard for Power Assist and Low Energy Power Operated Doors.*

If a door assembly that is required to be self-closing or self-latching by a provision of the *Code* is a powered door assembly, the possibility of competing functions creating conflict exists. The intent of the self-closing or self-latching requirement is to keep the door leaf in its closed position, except when someone is moving through the door opening; the intent of a powered door assembly is either to cause the door leaf to open automatically upon approach of a person or to open via power assist when a limited force is applied against the door leaf. Under fire conditions, boxes falling from shelving, for example, might cause either the approach-actuated powered door assembly or force-actuated power-assist door assembly to open. The provisions of 7.2.1.9.2(4) require that, upon detection of smoke, the door leaf closes and the power-assist mechanism ceases to function. This requirement emphasizes that the need for the door leaf to be in its closed position is paramount compared to the need to open the door leaf easily under fire conditions.

**7.2.1.10 Revolving Door Assemblies.**

Note that 7.2.1.10.1 applies to all revolving door assemblies, whether they are in the means of egress or not. Paragraph 7.2.1.10.2 applies to revolving door assemblies within required means of egress. Paragraphs 7.2.1.10.3 and 7.2.1.10.4 apply specifically to those revolving door assemblies that are not within the required means of egress.

**7.2.1.10.1** Revolving door assemblies, whether used or not used in the means of egress, shall comply with the following:

(1) Revolving door wings shall be capable of being collapsed into a book-fold position, unless they are existing revolving doors approved by the authority having jurisdiction.
(2) When revolving door wings are collapsed into the book-fold position, the parallel egress paths formed shall provide an aggregate width of 36 in. (915 mm), unless they are approved existing revolving door assemblies.
(3) Revolving door assemblies shall not be used within 10 ft (3050 mm) of the foot or the top of stairs or escalators.
(4) A dispersal area acceptable to the authority having jurisdiction shall be located between stairs or escalators and the revolving door assembly.
(5) The revolutions per minute (rpm) of revolving door wings shall not exceed the values in Table 7.2.1.10.1.
(6) Each revolving door assembly shall have a conforming side-hinged swinging door assembly in the same wall as the revolving door within 10 ft (3050 mm) of the revolving door, unless one of the following conditions applies:

***Table 7.2.1.10.1 Revolving Door Assembly Maximum Speed***

| Inside Diameter | | Power-Driven Speed Control (rpm) | Manual Speed Control (rpm) |
|---|---|---|---|
| ft/in. | mm | | |
| 6 ft 6 in. | 1980 | 11 | 12 |
| 7 ft | 2135 | 10 | 11 |
| 7 ft 6 in. | 2285 | 9 | 11 |
| 8 ft | 2440 | 9 | 10 |
| 8 ft 6 in. | 2590 | 8 | 9 |
| 9 ft | 2745 | 8 | 9 |
| 9 ft 6 in. | 2895 | 7 | 8 |
| 10 ft | 3050 | 7 | 8 |

(a) Revolving door assemblies shall be permitted without adjacent swinging door assemblies, as required by 7.2.1.10.1(6), in street floor elevator lobbies, provided that no stairways or door openings from other parts of the building discharge through the lobby and the lobby has no occupancy other than as a means of travel between the elevators and street.

(b) The requirement of 7.2.1.10.1(6) shall not apply to existing revolving door assemblies where the number of revolving door assemblies does not exceed the number of swinging door assemblies within 20 ft (6100 mm) of the revolving door assembly.

The provisions of 7.2.1.10.1, which apply to revolving door assemblies, address collapsibility, width of egress path, location, speed of rotation, and supplementary swinging door assemblies. Paragraphs 7.2.1.10.1(1) and (2) require collapsibility to provide egress paths, albeit narrow paths, to each side of the center column with attached book-fold position door leaves. Paragraph 7.2.1.10.1(3), which requires that revolving door assemblies not be used within 10 ft (3050 mm) of the foot or top of stairs or escalators, is meant to prevent the crushing accumulation of occupants if egress travel is slowed at the door opening. Paragraph 7.2.1.10.1(6) provides redundant egress via a nearby side-hinged swinging door leaf if the revolving door assembly prevents egress upon failure of its emergency features. Paragraph 7.2.1.10.1(6)(a) specifies a safe arrangement under which the additional swinging door assembly is not needed.

**7.2.1.10.2** Where permitted in Chapters 11 through 43, revolving door assemblies shall be permitted as a component in a means of egress, provided that the following criteria are met:

(1) Revolving door openings shall not be given credit for more than 50 percent of the required egress capacity.
(2) Each revolving door opening shall not be credited with more than a 50-person capacity or, if of not less than a 9 ft (2745 mm) diameter, a revolving door assembly shall be permitted egress capacity based on the clear opening width provided when collapsed into a book-fold position.
(3) Revolving door wings shall be capable of being collapsed into a book-fold position when a force not exceeding 130 lbf (580 N) is applied to the wings within 3 in. (75 mm) of the outer edge.

The occupancies in the list that follows permit the use of a revolving door assembly in a means of egress. Additional restrictions that might be imposed by the occupancy chapter are contained in the paragraphs referenced in parentheses in the list.

The occupancies permitting a revolving door assembly within the means of egress are as follows:

1. Assembly occupancies (12.2.2.2.8, 13.2.2.2.8)
2. Hotels and dormitories (28.2.2.2.3, 29.2.2.2.3)
3. Apartment buildings (30.2.2.2.3, 31.2.2.2.3)
4. Existing residential board and care facilities [33.3.2.2.2(6)]
5. Mercantile occupancies (36.2.2.2.9, 37.2.2.2.9)
6. Business occupancies (38.2.2.2.9, 39.2.2.2.9)

Revolving door assemblies present the potential for problems when too many people try to use them in too short a period of time. The congestion created by such a situation is one reason why their use is prohibited at the foot or top of stairs. This potential danger is also why they are not permitted to provide more than 50 percent of the required egress capacity. Where revolving door assemblies are used, they each receive credit for a maximum of 50 persons, regardless of the width of the revolving panel.

**7.2.1.10.3** Revolving door assemblies not used as a component of a means of egress shall have a collapsing force not exceeding 180 lbf (800 N).

**7.2.1.10.4** The requirement of 7.2.1.10.3 shall not apply to revolving door assemblies, provided that the collapsing force is reduced to a force not to exceed 130 lbf (580 N) under the following conditions:

(1) Power failure, or removal of power to the device holding the wings in position
(2) Actuation of the automatic sprinkler system, where such a system is provided
(3) Actuation of a smoke detection system that is installed to provide coverage in all areas within the building that are within 75 ft (23 m) of the revolving door assemblies
(4) Actuation of a clearly identified manual control switch in an approved location that reduces the holding force to a force not to exceed 130 lbf (580 N)

Note that the provisions of 7.2.1.10.3 apply if the door assembly is not within the required means of egress. Note that 7.2.1.10.4 permits revolving door assemblies not used as a component of a means of egress to have a collapsing force in excess of the 180 lbf (800 N) specified in 7.2.1.10.3 provided that the criteria of 7.2.1.10.4(1) through (4) are met. Thus, the criteria contained in 7.2.1.10.4 need to be satisfied only if the collapsing force is in excess of 180 lbf (800 N) under normal operating conditions.

**7.2.1.11 Turnstiles.**

The intent of 7.2.1.11 is to provide guidance on how best to place turnstiles in a building, to describe the circumstances under which they are permitted, and to reduce the chances of their improper use during an emergency.

**7.2.1.11.1** Turnstiles or similar devices that restrict travel to one direction or are used to collect fares or admission charges shall not be placed so as to obstruct any required means of egress, unless otherwise specified in 7.2.1.11.1.1 and 7.2.1.11.1.2.

**7.2.1.11.1.1** Approved turnstiles not exceeding 39 in. (990 mm) in height that turn freely in the direction of egress travel shall be permitted where revolving door assemblies are permitted in Chapters 11 through 43.

**7.2.1.11.1.2** Where turnstiles are approved by the authority having jurisdiction and permitted in Chapters 11 through 43, each turnstile shall be credited for a capacity of 50 persons, provided that such turnstiles meet the following criteria:

(1) They freewheel in the egress direction when primary power is lost, and freewheel in the direction of egress travel upon manual release by an employee assigned in the area.
(2) They are not given credit for more than 50 percent of the required egress width.
(3) They are not in excess of 39 in. (990 mm) in height and have a clear width of not less than $16\frac{1}{2}$ in. (420 mm).

**7.2.1.11.2** Turnstiles exceeding 39 in. (990 mm) in height shall meet the requirements for revolving door assemblies in 7.2.1.10.

**7.2.1.11.3** Turnstiles located in, or furnishing access to, required exits shall provide not less than $16\frac{1}{2}$ in. (420 mm) clear width at and below a height of 39 in. (990 mm) and at least 22 in. (560 mm) clear width at heights above 39 in. (990 mm).

Generally, turnstiles are installed to prevent or control entry. As such, they are not always suitable for installation in a means of egress. Turnstiles are permitted in means of egress locations where revolving door assemblies are permitted, unless an occupancy chapter specifically prohibits recognition of the turnstile; see the commentary following 7.2.1.10.2(3) for a list of occupancies that permit revolving door assemblies within the means of egress. Although assembly occupancies appear in the list as recognizing the use of revolving door assemblies, 12.2.2.2.9 and 13.2.2.2.9 prohibit turnstiles from serving within the means of egress.

The reference in 7.2.1.11.1.1 to revolving door assemblies is not meant to imply that there is a relationship between their purpose and that of turnstiles. The revolving door assembly is not meant to restrict traffic in either direction, while the turnstile is often used to do just that, with the restriction or obstruction to traffic movement usually in the direction of building entry. Yet, if a turnstile does not restrict egress, it might be assumed to be the equivalent of a revolving door assembly. At heights not exceeding 39 in. (990 mm), a freewheeling turnstile is not required to provide the collapsibility features required of a revolving door assembly; turnstiles with heights exceeding 39 in. (990 mm) must be provided with all the features applicable to revolving door assemblies.

Some turnstiles do not turn in the direction of entry until coin-operated. Others require no coin for operation and are used simply to count numbers of people. Perhaps the most dangerous are those that do not bar entry but specifically bar egress. This situation might occur in large mercantile occupancies where turnstiles turn freely on entering but do not turn in the direction of egress, thereby causing patrons to reroute their egress through checkout stands. It is possible that the patrons of locations using one-way turnstiles are quite aware of this limitation and know the correct path to take for emergency egress; however, this knowledge cannot be relied on, especially if the turnstiles are placed near the exit door assemblies. In emergencies, occupants might head for what appears to be the shortest route to the outside, only to find it blocked by a turnstile preventing movement in that direction.

Some occupancy chapters, via their recognition of revolving doors (see 7.2.1.11.1.1), permit turnstiles to provide a portion of the required egress capacity, provided that they are in strict compliance with the dimensional criteria and performance requirements of 7.2.1.11.1.2. Turnstiles are not permitted to provide more than 50 percent of the required egress capacity, and no single turnstile can be given egress capacity for more than 50 persons.

**7.2.1.12 Door Openings in Folding Partitions.** Where permanently mounted folding or movable partitions divide a room into smaller spaces, a swinging door leaf or open doorway shall be provided as an exit access from each such space, unless otherwise specified in 7.2.1.12.1 and 7.2.1.12.2.

**7.2.1.12.1** A door leaf or opening in the folding partition shall not be required, provided that all of the following criteria are met:

(1) The subdivided space is not used by more than 20 persons at any time.
(2) The use of the space is under adult supervision.
(3) The partitions are arranged so that they do not extend across any aisle or corridor used as an exit access to the required exits from the story.
(4) The partitions conform to the interior finish and other requirements of this *Code*.
(5) The partitions are of an approved type, have a simple method of release, and are capable of being opened quickly and easily by experienced persons in case of emergency.

**7.2.1.12.2** Where a subdivided space is provided with not less than two means of egress, the swinging door leaf in the folding partition specified in 7.2.1.12 shall not be required, and one such means of egress shall be permitted to be equipped with a horizontal-sliding door assembly complying with 7.2.1.14.

Although 7.2.1.12.1(3) might appear to be so stringent as to make the exemption offered by 7.2.1.12.1 unworkable, it prohibits the extension of the partition across the exit access for the rest of the floor, not the extension of the partition across the exit access for the small space created by closing the partition.

**7.2.1.13 Balanced Door Assemblies.** If panic hardware is installed on balanced door leaves, the panic hardware shall be of the push-pad type, and the pad shall not extend more than approximately one-half the width of the door leaf, measured from the latch stile. *[See 7.2.1.7.1(1).]*

Balanced door assemblies do not have side hinges; instead, they have a pivot point that is offset from the stile edge of the door leaf. This arrangement helps reduce the force needed to open the door leaf. With balanced door assemblies, where the hinge or pivot point is set in from the edge of the door leaf, care must be taken to position the panic hardware actuating bar on the latch side of the pivot point; otherwise, pushing on the actuating bar might actually help to hold the door leaf closed. This arrangement might be effectively accomplished using push-pad panic hardware, which more readily instructs the user where to push.

Exhibit 7.22 depicts a balanced door assembly; Exhibit 7.23 illustrates the difference between panic hardware with an actuating bar and panic hardware with a push pad serving as the actuating member.

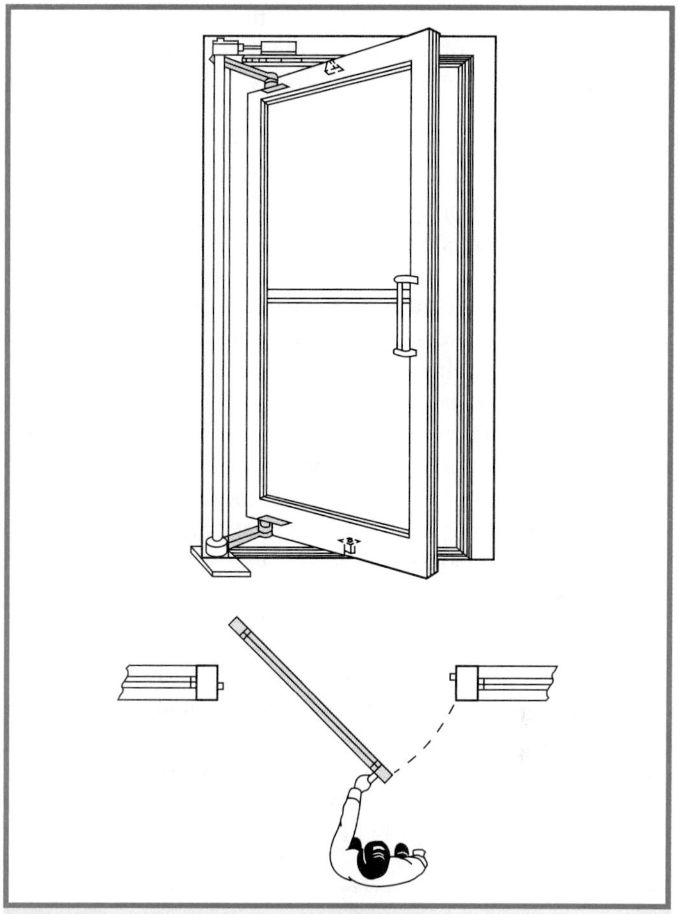

***Exhibit 7.22*** *Balanced door assembly.*

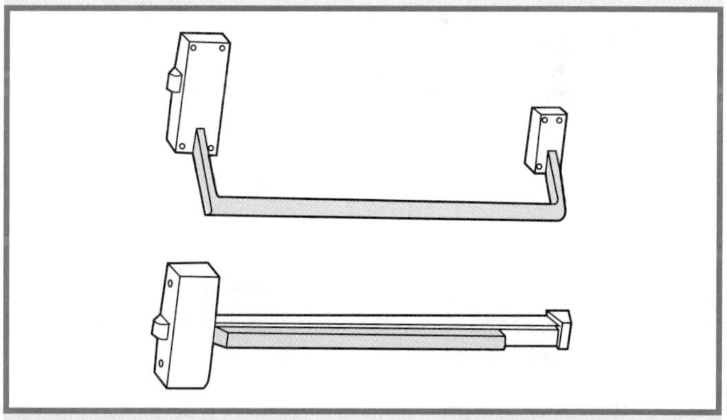

***Exhibit 7.23*** *Panic hardware with actuating bar (top) and panic hardware with push-pad actuating member (bottom).*

**7.2.1.14 Horizontal-Sliding Door Assemblies.** Horizontal-sliding door assemblies shall be permitted in means of egress, provided that the following criteria are met:

(1) The door leaf is readily operable from either side without special knowledge or effort.

(2) The force that, when applied to the operating device in the direction of egress, is required to operate the door leaf is not more than 15 lbf (67 N).
(3) The force required to operate the door leaf in the direction of travel is not more than 30 lbf (133 N) to set the leaf in motion and is not more than 15 lbf (67 N) to close the leaf or open it to the minimum required width.
(4) The door leaf is operable using a force of not more than 50 lbf (222 N) when a force of 250 lbf (1100 N) is applied perpendicularly to the leaf adjacent to the operating device, unless the door opening is an existing horizontal-sliding exit access door assembly serving an area with an occupant load of fewer than 50.
(5) The door assembly complies with the fire protection rating, if required, and, where rated, is self-closing or automatic-closing by means of smoke detection in accordance with 7.2.1.8 and is installed in accordance with NFPA 80, *Standard for Fire Doors and Other Opening Protectives*.

The special type of horizontal-sliding door assembly addressed by 7.2.1.14 is different from a traditional horizontal-sliding door assembly. When force is applied in the direction of egress travel to the door actuator, the door leaf must slide to the side to allow passage. This concept is illustrated in Exhibit 7.24.

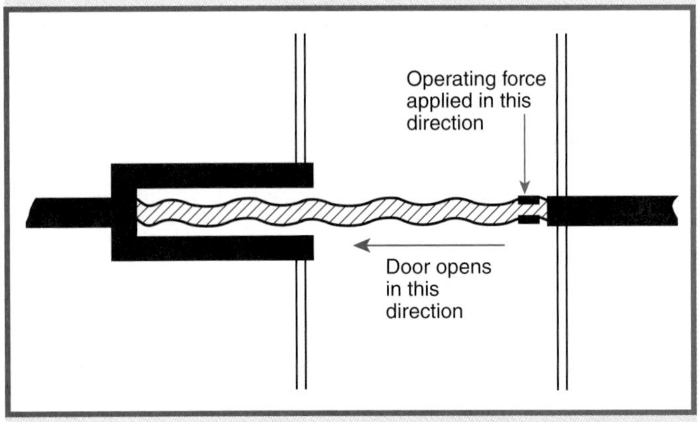


***Exhibit 7.24*** *Horizontal-sliding door assembly operation.*

Although the provisions of 7.2.1.14 do not require specific occupancy chapter permission for use of horizontal-sliding door assemblies, some occupancy chapters impose additional restrictions. For example, 28.2.2.2.4 prohibits the installation of these door assemblies across a corridor in a new hotel or dormitory.

The requirements for the installation of horizontal-sliding door assemblies address the following:

1. Simple method of operation from either side without special knowledge or effort
2. Force necessary to operate the door assembly
3. Fire protection rating applicable to door assembly location and purpose
4. Automatic-closing means by smoke detection or means for self-closing

The force requirements of 7.2.1.14(3) and (4) help to ensure that the door assembly can be operated if the usual method of operation required by 7.2.1.14(2) fails.

It is important that sliding door assemblies, other than those addressed by 7.2.1.4.1(4)(c), be evaluated for compliance with all the requirements of 7.2.1.14. Traditional sliding door assemblies do not comply with these requirements; an example of a type of door assembly that does comply is shown in Exhibit 7.25.

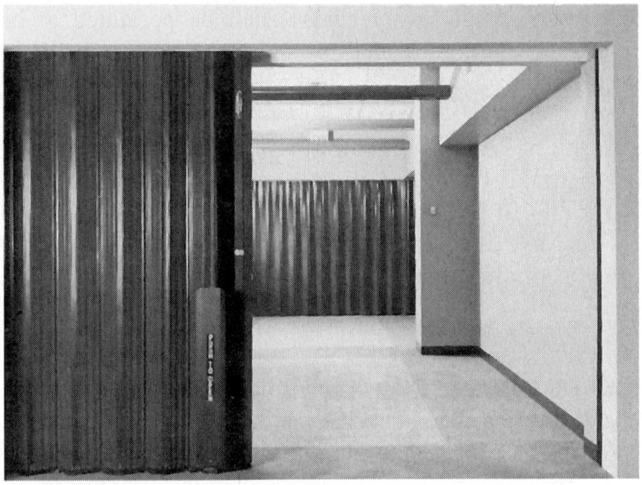

***Exhibit 7.25*** *Horizontal-sliding door assembly addressed by 7.2.1.14. (Photo courtesy of Won-Door Corp.)*

**7.2.1.15 Inspection of Door Openings.**

**7.2.1.15.1** Where required by Chapters 11 through 43, door assemblies for which the door leaf is required to swing in the direction of egress travel shall be inspected and tested not less than annually in accordance with 7.2.1.15.2 through 7.2.1.15.8.

The provisions of 7.2.1.15 are new to the 2009 edition of the *Code* and address the inspection and testing of door openings. The criteria for the inspection and testing of door openings apply only where specifically required by another portion of the *Code*, typically an occupancy chapter.

The occupancies requiring inspection of door openings are as follows:

1. Assembly occupancies (12.7.1.3, 13.7.1.3)
2. Educational occupancies (14.7.3.3, 15.7.3.3)
3. Day-care occupancies (16.7.3.4, 17.7.3.4)
4. Residential board and care occupancies (32.7.7, 33.7.7)

The annual inspection and testing requirements of 7.2.1.15, where required by another portion of the *Code*, have applicability, for other than fire-rated door assemblies (see 7.2.1.15.2), to only those door leaves that are required to swing in the direction of egress travel. Door leaves that are required to swing in the direction of egress travel include those from spaces with an occupant load of 50 or more persons [see 7.2.1.4.2(1)] and those used in an exit enclosure [see 7.2.1.4.2(2)]. This application threshold was chosen to help ensure that the egress doors used most frequently on a normal day-to-day basis and those designed to accommodate larger numbers of occupants under emergency egress or relocation are inspected and tested. Door leaves that get used frequently are more apt to experience wear that adversely affects operability and leads to failure. Door leaves that are infrequently used, like those into exit stair enclosures in high-rise buildings, might be misaligned within their frames so as to be difficult to open within the operating forces requirements of 7.2.1.4.5. The door inspection and testing criteria of 7.2.15 are intended to help identify problems with door openings and ensure that such problems are remedied.

**7.2.1.15.2** Fire-rated door assemblies shall be inspected and tested in accordance with NFPA 80, *Standard for Fire Doors and Other Opening Protectives.*

Fire-rated door assemblies are required by 8.3.3.1 to be in accordance with the requirements of NFPA 80, *Standard for Fire Doors and Other Opening Protectives.*[10] NFPA 80 requires fire-rated door assemblies to be inspected and tested in accordance with the criteria contained in that document. The requirement of 7.2.1.15.2 is redundant in that it applies even if it were not included as part of the provisions of 7.2.1.15. It is helpful to the *Code* user to have the road map to the complete package of inspection and testing criteria for door openings presented in one place.

Following the publication of the 2007 edition of NFPA 80, the Door and Hardware Institute (DHI) released, through its Foundation for the Advancement of Life Safety and Security, guides on the annual safety inspection required by NFPA 80 for swinging fire doors with builders hardware. The guides are targeted to three audiences — the inspector, the AHJ, and the owner. The three guides are titled as follows:

1. *Inspector's Guide: Swinging Fire Doors with Builders Hardware — Annual Safety Inspections*[11]
2. *AHJ's Guide: Swinging Fire Doors with Builders Hardware — Annual Safety Inspections*[12]
3. *Owner's Guide: Swinging Fire Doors with Builders Hardware — Annual Safety Inspections*[13]

Additional information on the DHI educational program can be accessed at *www.lifesafetyandsecurity.org and www.dhi.org.*

**7.2.1.15.3** The inspection and testing interval for fire-rated and nonrated door assemblies shall be permitted to exceed 12 months under a written performance-based program in accordance with 5.2.2 of NFPA 80, *Standard for Fire Doors and Other Opening Protectives.*

The introductory requirements of 7.2.1.15.1 set the inspection and testing interval as once per year. Paragraph 7.2.1.15.3 provides an exemption so that the inspection interval can exceed 12 months where a written performance-based program in accordance with NFPA 80 is implemented. Subsection 5.2.2 of NFPA 80 addresses the performance-based option for extending the inspection and testing interval. As explained in Annex J of NFPA 80, the concept of a performance-based inspection and testing frequency program is to establish the type and frequency of inspection needed to demonstrate that the door assemblies are operational. The goal is to balance the inspection frequency with proven reliability of the door assemblies; thus, the performance-based option is required to include historical data acceptable to the AHJ. The goal of a performance-based inspection program is also to adjust test and inspection frequencies commensurate with historical, documented equipment performance and desired reliability. Program attributes that should be considered in the adjustment of test and inspection frequencies include maintenance programs, usage frequencies, history of repairs, building condition, and consequence of failure of the door assemblies.

**7.2.1.15.4** A written record of the inspections and testing shall be signed and kept for inspection by the authority having jurisdiction.

The required written record of the inspection and testing must be signed, preferably by the individual who performed the inspection and testing.

**7.2.1.15.5** Functional testing of door assemblies shall be performed by individuals who can demonstrate knowledge and understanding of the operating components of the type of door being subjected to testing.

The functional testing of door assemblies is not required to be performed by a licensed or certified individual. Rather, the person performing the functional testing must be able to demonstrate knowledge and understanding of the operating components of the type of door assemblies required to be inspected at the facility. See the commentary following 7.2.1.15.2 relative to the educational program developed by the Door and Hardware Institute for the inspection of swinging fire doors.

**7.2.1.15.6** Door assemblies shall be visually inspected from both sides of the opening to assess the overall condition of the assembly.

The overall condition of the door assembly can be visually evaluated only if inspected from both sides of the door opening. Some features are evident from only the pull side of the door opening, as the stops in the frame prevent viewing the feature; other features, like the door closer, are evident only from the push side of the door opening.

**7.2.1.15.7** As a minimum, the following items shall be verified:

(1) Floor space on both sides of the openings is clear of obstructions, and door leaves open fully and close freely.
(2) Forces required to set door leaves in motion and move to the fully open position do not exceed the requirements in 7.2.1.4.5.
(3) Latching and locking devices comply with 7.2.1.5.
(4) Releasing hardware devices are installed in accordance with 7.2.1.5.9.1.
(5) Door leaves of paired openings are installed in accordance with 7.2.1.5.10.
(6) Door closers are adjusted properly to control the closing speed of door leaves in accordance with accessibility requirements.
(7) Projection of door leaves into the path of egress does not exceed the encroachment permitted by 7.2.1.4.3.
(8) Powered door openings operate in accordance with 7.2.1.9.
(9) Signage required by 7.2.1.4.1(3), 7.2.1.5.4, 7.2.1.6, and 7.2.1.9 is intact and legible.
(10) Door openings with special locking arrangements function in accordance with 7.2.1.6
(11) Security devices that impede egress are not installed on openings, as required by 7.2.1.5.11.

The criteria required to be verified in 7.2.1.15.7(1) through (11) were developed to evaluate post-installation operating performance where the installation was made to comply with door assembly criteria of 7.2.1. Fire-rated door assemblies must also meet additional criteria as detailed in Section 5.2 of NFPA 80 (see the commentary following 7.2.1.15.2).

**7.2.1.15.8** Door openings not in proper operating condition shall be repaired or replaced without delay.

The purpose of the inspection and testing program is to identify problems with door assemblies. Paragraph 7.2.1.15.8 completes the process by requiring that problems be corrected without delay. The correction of the problem is part of the overall inspection and testing program and needs to be documented in the written record required by 7.2.1.15.4.

### 7.2.2 Stairs.

Stairs, whether interior or exterior to a building, serve multiple functions, including allowing normal occupant movement among the floors of a building, providing emergency egress in case of fire, and facilitating rescue and fire control operations conducted by fire fighters.

Stairs are used within any of the three components of a means of egress system; that is, the exit access, the exit, and the exit discharge. The *Code* focuses much attention on stairs to help ensure their effective use during emergency egress. These requirements for emergency egress use help to ensure that stairs are also safe to use on a regular basis. As one of the most commonly used building elements on a day-to-day, nonemergency basis, stairs are one of the most common scenes of trips and falls.

Earlier editions of the *Code* addressed monumental stairs, but only to require that such stairs follow all the provisions applicable to standard stairs. The *Code* does not define the term *monumental stair*. A monumental stair is simply a regular stair that has been embellished for visual effect. The paragraph on monumental stairs was deleted because it added nothing to the *Code*, in that monumental stairs were required to meet all the usual stair criteria. A monumental stair is not a subset of stairs that have special features — it is a regular stair that might have extra width or substantial architectural detail. Contrast this description with a spiral stair (as addressed in 7.2.2.2.3), which cannot meet the usual stair criteria and, therefore, must meet its own set of requirements if it is to be recognized within the means of egress.

**7.2.2.1 General.**

**7.2.2.1.1** Stairs used as a component in the means of egress shall conform to the general requirements of Section 7.1 and to the special requirements of 7.2.2, unless otherwise specified in 7.2.2.1.2.

**7.2.2.1.2** The requirement of 7.2.2.1.1 shall not apply to the following:

(1) Aisle stairs in assembly occupancies, as provided in Chapters 12 and 13
(2) Approved existing noncomplying stairs

Assembly occupancy aisle stairs (i.e., stepped aisles) are detailed in 12.2.5.6 and 13.2.5.6.

Although stairs can serve within any of the three components of the means of egress, they are most often located within an exit. To be considered an exit, interior stairs must be separated from the other spaces on the floor in accordance with 7.1.3.2. Unenclosed interior stairs might serve as exit access but are not exits. Where an interior stair connects two or more stories, it creates a vertical opening and must meet the requirements applicable to such, regardless of whether it is an exit. See the vertical opening protection provisions of Section 8.6.

It is sometimes more difficult to determine whether outside stairs are part of the exit access, the exit, or the exit discharge. To be considered an exit, outside stairs need to be separated from the interior of the building by fire-rated construction in accordance with 7.2.2.6.3. Outside stairs adjacent to the building that are unprotected would normally be considered part of the exit access where serving occupants of upper stories, with the user reaching the exit and exit discharge simultaneously at the base of the last stair flight. Where stairs occur in a sidewalk that connects an exit door assembly to a public way, the stairs are part of the exit discharge.

**7.2.2.2 Dimensional Criteria.**

**7.2.2.2.1 Standard Stairs.**

**7.2.2.2.1.1** Stairs shall meet the following criteria:

(1) New stairs shall be in accordance with Table 7.2.2.2.1.1(a) and 7.2.2.2.1.2.
(2)* Existing stairs shall be permitted to remain in use, provided that they meet the requirements for existing stairs shown in Table 7.2.2.2.1.1(b).

**A.7.2.2.2.1.1(2)** It is the intent of 7.2.2.2.1.1(2) to permit the use of Table 7.2.2.2.1.1(b) in existing buildings, even where there is a change in occupancy per 4.6.12. Safety improvements should be made that are reasonable and feasible at minimal cost. Improvements include removal, repair, or replacement of step coverings, as described in A.7.2.2.3.5, particularly Figure A.7.2.2.3.5(e), and addition of functional handrails and guardrails in place of, or in conjunction with, other rails, as described in 7.2.2.4.

*Table 7.2.2.2.1.1(a) New Stairs*

| | Dimensional Criteria | |
|---|---|---|
| Feature | ft/in. | mm |
| Minimum width | See 7.2.2.2.1.2. | |
| Maximum height of risers | 7 in. | 180 |
| Minimum height of risers | 4 in. | 100 |
| Minimum tread depth | 11 in. | 280 |
| Minimum headroom | 6 ft 8 in. | 2030 |
| Maximum height between landings | 12 ft | 3660 |
| Landing | See 7.2.1.3, 7.2.1.4.3.1, and 7.2.2.3.2. | |

*Table 7.2.2.2.1.1(b) Existing Stairs*

| | Dimensional Criteria | |
|---|---|---|
| Feature | ft/in. | mm |
| Minimum width clear of all obstructions, except projections not more than $4\frac{1}{2}$ in. (114 mm) at or below handrail height on each side | 36 in. | 915 |
| Maximum height of risers | 8 in. | 205 |
| Minimum tread depth | 9 in. | 230 |
| Minimum headroom | 6 ft 8 in. | 2030 |
| Maximum height between landings | 12 ft | 3660 |
| Landing | See 7.2.1.3 and 7.2.1.4.3.1. | |

(3) Approved existing stairs shall be permitted to be rebuilt in accordance with the following:
   (a) Dimensional criteria of Table 7.2.2.2.1.1(b)
   (b) Other stair requirements of 7.2.2

(4) The requirements for new and existing stairs shall not apply to stairs located in industrial equipment access areas where otherwise provided in 40.2.5.2.

Editions of the *Code* prior to 1981 required that the height of every riser and the width of every tread be so proportioned that the sum of two risers and a tread, exclusive of the tread nosing or projection, was not less than 24 in. (610 mm) nor more than 25 in. (635 mm). This requirement was deleted because it was based on a 300-year-old French formula in which the inch was a slightly larger unit of measure than it is today. Moreover, people's feet and stride length — the basis for the formula — were somewhat smaller at that time. Also, the requirement was originally intended only for stairs of moderate steepness or pitch. These reasons, as well as information gathered by researchers on people movement, explain why the requirement was replaced by requirements that ensure good step geometry.

Because of the hardship and impracticality of rebuilding all existing stairs to the newer requirements, the *Code* permits existing stairs in existing buildings to comply with previous requirements. It also permits existing stairs to be rebuilt to the previous dimensional criteria, because a new stair might not fit in an existing stair enclosure. However, the rebuilt stair utilizing the older geometry must meet all other requirements of 7.2.2, including those relating to handrails. The text of A.7.2.2.2.1.1(2) provides guidance for judging the improvements that are reasonable.

The provisions applicable to the width of new stairs were changed for the 2006 edition of the *Code*. See the commentary that follows 7.2.2.2.1.2(F).

Prior to the 2006 edition of the *Code*, existing stairs were classified as either Class A or Class B, depending on their tread depth and riser height. The Class A stair was a safer stair than Class B because it was limited to a maximum riser height of 7½ in. (190 mm) instead of the 8 in. (205 mm) permitted for Class B stairs; and it was required to have a minimum tread depth of 10 in. (255 mm) instead of the 9 in. (230 mm) permitted for Class B stairs. The last two occupancies that required existing stairs to be Class A dropped the requirement — it had applied to existing stairs used for student access in educational occupancies and existing stairs used for client access in day-care occupancies. Therefore, Table 7.2.2.2.1.1(b) was revised to reflect that the criteria associated with what had been Class B stairs have become the minimum recognized by all the occupancy chapters. As such, there was no longer a need to differentiate existing stairs as being Class A or Class B — they currently are referred to simply as existing stairs.

See 7.1.7 for special requirements where stairs provide a total elevation change of not more than 21 in. (535 mm).

**7.2.2.2.1.2 Minimum New Stair Width.**

**(A)** Where the total occupant load of all stories served by the stair is fewer than 50, the minimum width clear of all obstructions, except projections not more than 4½ in. (114 mm) at or below handrail height on each side, shall be 36 in. (915 mm).

**(B)*** Where stairs serve occupant loads exceeding that permitted by 7.2.2.2.1.2(A), the minimum width clear of all obstructions, except projections not more than 4½ in. (114 mm) at or below handrail height on each side, shall be in accordance with Table 7.2.2.2.1.2(B) and the requirements of 7.2.2.2.1.2(C), (D), (E), and (F).

*Table 7.2.2.2.1.2(B) New Stair Width*

| Total Cumulative Occupant Load Assigned to the Stair | Width |
|---|---|
| <2000 persons | 44 in. (1120 mm) |
| ≥2000 persons | 56 in. (1420 mm) |

**A.7.2.2.2.1.2(B)** The stair width requirement of 7.2.2.2.1.2(B) is based on accumulating the occupant load on each story the stair serves.

The accumulating of occupant load is done for the purposes of the requirements of 7.2.2.2.1.2 only. The egress capacity requirements of Section 7.3 are NOT cumulative on a story-by-story basis.

If additional exits provide egress capacity, the occupant load served by such additional exits, up to the limit permitted for the egress capacity of such additional exits, is not added to the total occupant load considered for the minimum stair width requirements of 7.2.2.2.1.2.

If horizontal exits are provided on any of the stories, the total occupant load of all compartments on the story with the horizontal exits is used in the calculation of the minimum stair width requirements of 7.2.2.2.1.2. The number of stairs permitted through application of horizontal exit requirements in 7.2.4 is not affected by the minimum stair width requirements of 7.2.2.2.1.2.

The examples that follow illustrate applications of the minimum stair width requirement.

A stair in a building two stories in height above grade plane that has 2000 persons on the second story, among 10 equally sized stairs that serve the second story, would be considered to have an occupant load of 200 persons for the purposes of applying Table 7.2.2.2.1.2(B). The minimum width of such a stair would be 44 in. (1120 mm).

For a building with a relatively large floor area, a typical 44 in. (1120 mm) stair would not be required to be increased in width until it serves a building approximately 14 stories in height above grade plane, calculated as follows:

$$\frac{2000 \text{ persons}}{147 \text{ persons per floor for a 44 in. (1120 mm) width stair}} \approx 14 \text{ stories}$$

For egress in the descending direction, only the stair width below the 14 stories with the total occupant load of 2000 persons per stair, or 4000 persons if served by two equally sized stairs, would need to be increased to 56 in. (1420 mm). If the building is 20 stories in height above grade plane, only the stairs on the lowest 7 stories would be required to have the 56 in. (1420 mm) width.

For a building 41 stories in height above grade plane with 200 persons on each story (or 8000 persons overall, not including the level of exit discharge), with two equally sized stairs, each stair would be considered to have an occupant load of 4000 persons for the purposes of applying Table 7.2.2.2.1.2(B). Only the portion of the stair serving 2000 persons would be required to have the wider width. If each story provides the same floor area for occupancy, the upper 20 stories would have 44 in. (1120 mm) stairs, and the lowest 20 stories would have the 56 in. (1420 mm) stairs, as a minimum.

**(C)** The total cumulative occupant load assigned to a particular stair shall be that stair's prorated share of the total occupant load, as stipulated in 7.2.2.2.1.2(D) and (E), calculated in proportion to the stair width.

**(D)** For downward egress travel, stair width shall be based on the total number of occupants from stories above the level where the width is measured.

**(E)** For upward egress travel, stair width shall be based on the total number of occupants from stories below the level where the width is measured.

**(F)** The clear width of door openings discharging from stairways required to be a minimum of 56 in. (1420 mm) wide in accordance with 7.2.2.2.1.2(B) shall be in accordance with 7.2.1.2.3.2(9).

The provisions of 7.2.2.2.1.2 apply to the minimum required width of new stairs as mandated by 7.2.2.2.1.1(1).

Paragraph 7.2.2.2.1.2(A) permits a new stair to have a 36 in. (915 mm) minimum width if the total occupant load of all stories served by the stair is fewer than 50. This is an exemption to the 44 in. (1120 mm) minimum width criterion of Table 7.2.2.2.1.2(B). It recognizes that the small total number of persons who will use the stair will do so in little time compared to larger groups where persons avoid each other by staggering their entry onto the stair and by locating themselves so as to leave space between users.

Table 7.2.2.2.1.2(B) requires stairs serving large total cumulative occupant loads, such as those common to high-rise buildings, to be a minimum of 56 in. (1420 mm) in width. The increased width helps to facilitate counterflow on the stairs as might be experienced where building occupants have not completed their evacuation via stairs at the time emergency responders, such as fire fighters, arrive at the building. The minimum 56 in. (1420 mm) stair width lessens the challenges to stair use where occupant egress travel in one direction on the stairs (typically downward) occurs simultaneously with emergency responders use of the stairs in the opposite direction (typically upward) for ingress.

Paragraph 7.2.2.2.1.2(C) provides guidance on determining the total cumulative occupant load. Paragraph 7.2.2.2.1.2(D) provides that the width increase is not required to be applied to the upper stories where the total cumulative occupant load using that portion of the stairs is less than the 2000-person threshold. The Examples that follow illustrate these provisions.

***Example 1: Determining Stair Width, 14-Story Building***

Exhibit 7.26 depicts a 14-story building with a 300-person occupant load per floor. Floors 2 through 14 use the two exit stairs for egress. The occupants of

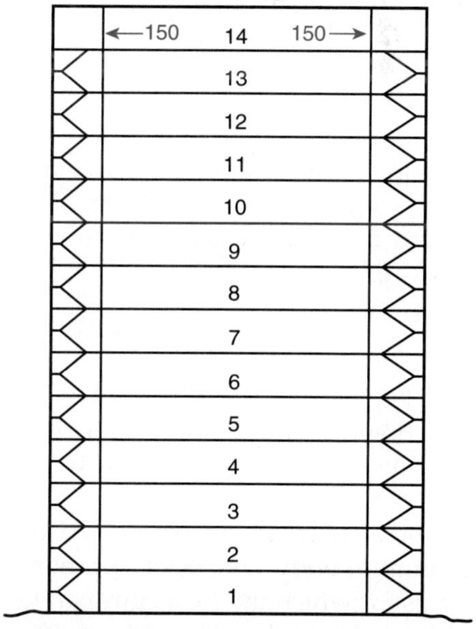


***Exhibit 7.26*** *Building where total cumulative occupant load does not require a 56 in. (1420 mm) minimum stair width.*

the first floor use door assemblies directly to the outside (not shown) for egress. The means of egress system is designed for half of the occupant load of floors 2 through 14 to use the stair at the left of the exhibit, and for the other half to use the stair at the right of the exhibit. The sum of the 150 persons from each of floors 2 through 14 is considered the total cumulative occupant load assigned to each of the two stairs for purposes of applying 7.2.2.2.1.2(B). The total cumulative occupant load assigned to each of the two stairs is calculated as follows:

$$\frac{13 \text{ floors} \times 150 \text{ persons}}{\text{per floor per stair}} = 1950 \text{ persons per stair}$$

Thus, the 2000-person threshold of Table 7.2.2.2.1.2(B) is not reached. No part of either stair is required to be increased to a minimum width of 56 in. (1420 mm). The stairs must be at least 44 in. (1120 mm) wide [per Table 7.2.2.2.1.2(B)], and wider if needed from a capacity consideration. In this case, the stairs must be 45 in. (1140 mm) wide, based on the following capacity calculation, which does not accumulate the occupant load from floor to floor in accordance with 7.3.1.4:

150 persons × 0.3 in. per person = 45 in.
(150 persons × 7.6 mm per person = 1140 mm)

***Example 2: Determining Stair Width, 28-Story Building***

Exhibit 7.27 depicts a 28-story building (i.e., the 14-story building from Exhibit 7.26 with 14 more stories added). See Example 1 for a description of the means of egress and occupant load for each floor. The sum of the 150 persons per stair from each of floors 2 through 28 is considered the total cumulative occupant load assigned to each of the two stairs for purposes of applying 7.2.2.2.1.2(B). The total cumulative occupant load assigned to each of the two stairs is calculated as follows:

$$\frac{27 \text{ floors} \times 150 \text{ persons}}{\text{per floor per stair}} = 4050 \text{ persons per stair}$$

Thus, the 2000-person threshold of Table 7.2.2.2.1.2(B) is exceeded. Some part of each of the two stairs is required to be increased to a minimum width of 56 in. (1420 mm).

Paragraph 7.2.2.2.1.2(D) exempts, from the increased minimum width, the upper portion of each of the two stairs for which the total cumulative occupant load assigned is fewer than 2000 persons. In this case, the transition point between the 45 in. (1140 mm) width required of the stair from a capacity consideration and the 56 in. (1420 mm) minimum width that facilitates counterflow occurs at the fifteenth story, calculated as follows:

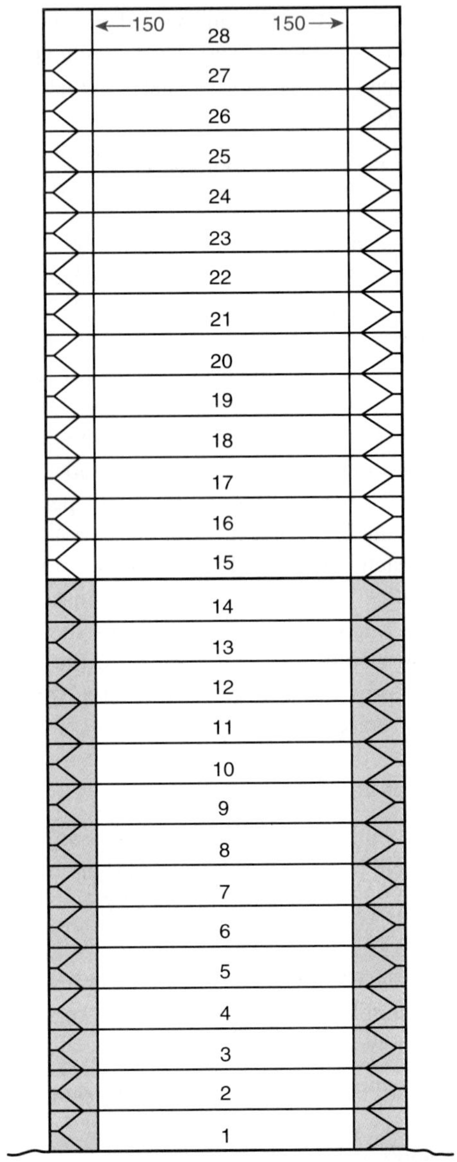


***Exhibit 7.27*** *Building where total cumulative occupant load requires a 56 in. (1420 mm) minimum stair width for the lower portion of the building.*

$$\frac{2000 \text{ persons}}{150 \text{ persons per floor}} = 13.3 \text{ floors}$$

$$28 \text{ stories} - 13 \text{ upper stories} = \text{fifteenth story}$$

The stairs below the fifteenth story must provide the minimum 56 in. (1420 mm) width required by Table 7.2.2.2.1.2(B). This is shown in the shaded, lower portion of the stair enclosures in Exhibit 7.27.

***Example 3: Determining Stair Width, Three-Story Mall Building***

Exhibit 7.28 depicts the third story of a new three-story mall building that utilizes horizontal exits for half of the required egress capacity, as permitted by 7.2.4.1.2 and 36.2.2.5. The occupant load of the third story is 6000 persons, of which the 20 exit stairs accommodate 3000 and the horizontal exits accommodate the other 3000. The second story is arranged and occupied the same as the third story. Occupants of the first floor are provided with adequate egress not involving use of the stairs.

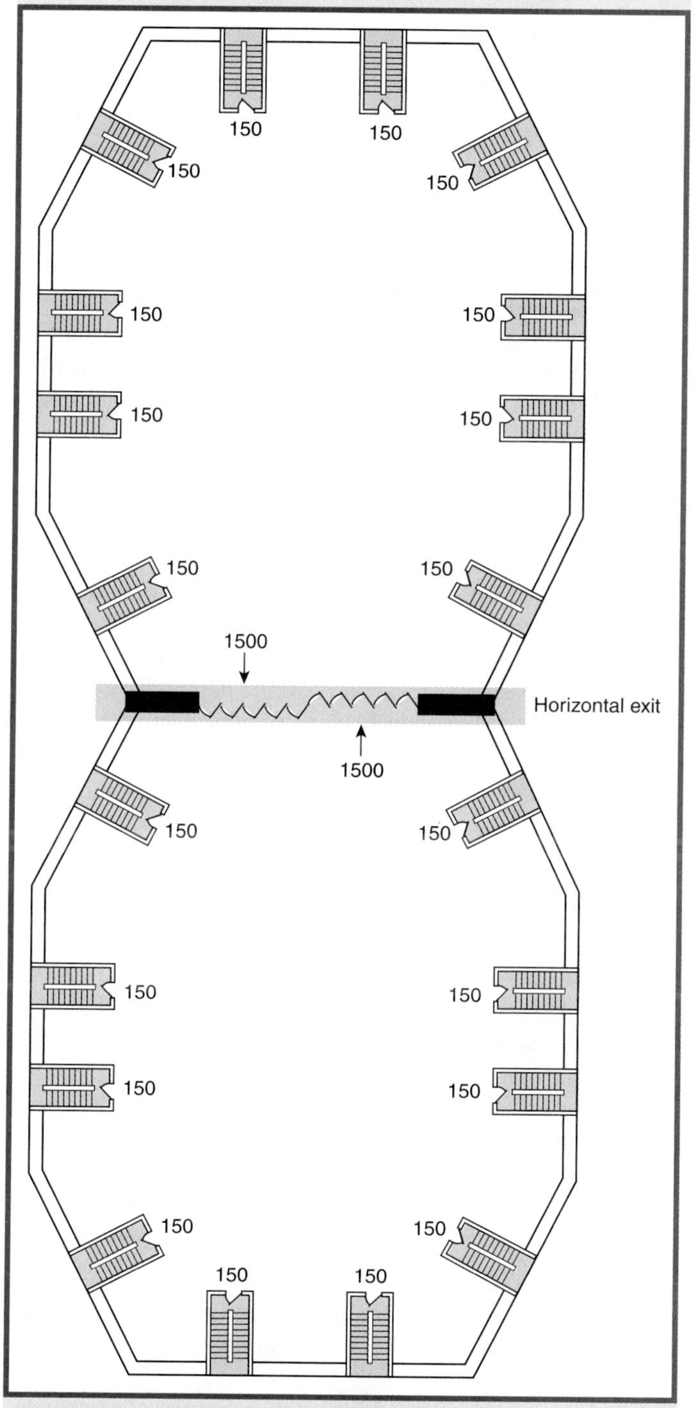


***Exhibit 7.28*** *Horizontal exits excluded in calculating total cumulative occupant load assigned to each stair.*

The fourth paragraph of A.7.2.2.2.1.2(B) describes how to calculate the total cumulative occupant load assigned to each stair where horizontal exits exist. All occupants are to be assigned only to the stairs, without any consideration given to the horizontal exits, although the horizontal exits do count toward satisfying the required egress capacity and the required number of exits. The reasoning behind excluding the horizontal exits from consideration is that persons using them have to wait on the safe side of the horizontal exit for their chance to use the exit stairs, which were not sized to handle the total occupant load of the floor. Therefore, for any of the stairs having a total cumulative occupant load of 2000 or more, it can be expected that the occupants will not have completed their evacuation stair travel when emergency responders arrive — and counterflow will occur on the stairs.

The total cumulative occupant load assigned to each of the 20 stairs is the sum of the occupant loads of floors 2 and 3 divided by the number of stairs, because, in this case, the stairs are all evenly sized. The calculation is as follows:

$$\frac{12{,}000 \text{ persons}}{20 \text{ stairs}} = 600 \text{ persons}$$

Thus, the 2000-person threshold of Table 7.2.2.2.1.2(B) is not reached. The stairs are not required to be increased to a minimum width of 56 in. (1420 mm). For the arrangement shown in Exhibit 7.28, the building would need to be at least eight stories high before any stair would be assigned a 2000-person or greater total cumulative occupant load so as to require a 56 in. (1420 mm) minimum stair width. A more realistic egress system design that would accommodate the 3000 persons per floor apportioned in Example 3 to the 20 stairs (i.e., the half of the floor's occupant load not apportioned to the horizontal exits) would typically involve fewer, but wider, stairs than the 45 in. (1140 mm) width used in this example, so as to make the 56 in. (1420 mm) criterion a nonissue.

Paragraph 7.2.2.2.1.2(F) serves as a reference to remind the user that related door width criteria are located in 7.2.1.2.3.2(9). The requirement of 7.2.1.2.3.2(9) ensures that, where a single door assembly serves as the discharge for stairs required to meet the 56 in. (1420 mm) minimum width criterion of Table 7.2.2.2.1.2(B), the door assembly is sized in proper proportion to the stair capacity so as not to create a bottleneck at the door opening. See the commentary on 7.2.1.2.3.2(9).

**7.2.2.2.2 Curved Stairs.**

**7.2.2.2.2.1** New curved stairs shall be permitted as a component in a means of egress, provided that the depth of tread is not less than 11 in. (280 mm) at a point 12 in. (305 mm) from the narrower end of the tread and the smallest radius is not less than twice the stair width.

**7.2.2.2.2.2** Existing curved stairs shall be permitted as a component in a means of egress, provided that the depth of tread is not less than 10 in. (255 mm) at a point 12 in. (305 mm) from the narrower end of the tread and the smallest radius is not less than twice the stair width.

Paragraph 7.2.2.2.2.1 relates the degree of curvature to the width of the curved stair, as shown in Exhibit 7.29. Dimension *B* must be at least twice dimension *A*. Dimension *C*, the tread depth, is measured at the so-called inner walking line (where the stair users' feet land when walking on the inner part of the stair); tread depth must be at least 11 in. (280 mm). This relationship of smallest radius to stair width should be based on the actual width of the stair, rather than on the required width. Otherwise, unsafe conditions toward the outside of wide-curved stairs could be created.

The measurement method for curved stairs that is specified by the *Code* is based on how such stairs are used, with reference to a minimum 11 in. (280 mm) tread depth at the inner walking line. This concept has been used in the *Code's* requirement for winders for some time (see 7.2.2.2.4). With the minimum tread depth stated as a dimension similar to that applicable to other stairs permitted in the required means of egress, it is more evident that curved stairs are an acceptable egress component for any occupancy.

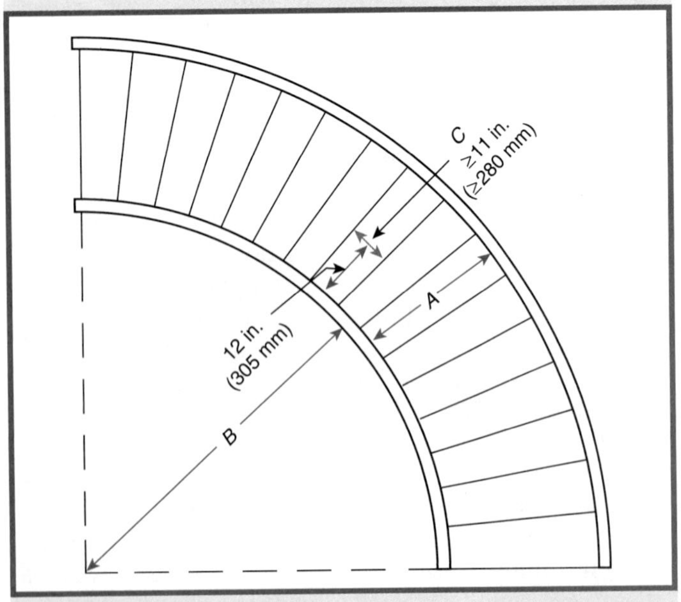


***Exhibit 7.29*** *Curved stairs.*

**7.2.2.2.3 Spiral Stairs.**

**7.2.2.2.3.1** Where specifically permitted for individual occupancies by Chapters 11 through 43, spiral stairs shall be permitted as a component in a means of egress in accordance with 7.2.2.2.3.2 through 7.2.2.2.3.4.

**7.2.2.2.3.2** Spiral stairs shall be permitted, provided that the following criteria are met:

(1) Riser heights shall not exceed 7 in. (180 mm).
(2) The stairway shall have a tread depth of not less than 11 in. (280 mm) for a portion of the stairway width sufficient to provide egress capacity for the occupant load served in accordance with 7.3.3.1.
(3) At the outer side of the stairway, an additional 10½ in. (265 mm) of width shall be provided clear to the other handrail, and this width shall not be included as part of the required egress capacity.
(4) Handrails complying with 7.2.2.4 shall be provided on both sides of the spiral stairway.
(5) The inner handrail shall be located within 24 in. (610 mm), measured horizontally, of the point where a tread depth of not less than 11 in. (280 mm) is provided.
(6) The turn of the stairway shall be such that the outer handrail is at the right side of descending users.

**7.2.2.2.3.3** Where the occupant load served does not exceed three, spiral stairs shall be permitted, provided that the following criteria are met:

(1) The clear width of the stairs shall be not less than 26 in. (660 mm).
(2) The height of risers shall not exceed 9½ in. (240 mm).
(3) The headroom shall be not less than 6 ft 6 in. (1980 mm).
(4) Treads shall have a depth not less than 7½ in. (190 mm) at a point 12 in. (305 mm) from the narrower edge.
(5) All treads shall be identical.
(6) Handrails shall be provided on both sides of the stairway.

**7.2.2.2.3.4** Where the occupant load served does not exceed five, existing spiral stairs shall be permitted, provided that the requirements of 7.2.2.2.3.3(1) through (5) are met.

Spiral stairs can be used only where expressly permitted by the appropriate occupancy chapter. Some occupancy chapters establish additional limitations. For example, in assembly occupancies, spiral stairs are permitted only from lighting and access catwalks, galleries, and gridirons. In apartment buildings, spiral stairs are permitted only within a dwelling unit, not within the common spaces and egress paths serving multiple dwelling units.

The occupancies that permit spiral stairs are as follows:

1. Assembly occupancies (12.2.2.3.2.2, 13.2.2.3.2.2)
2. Detention and correctional occupancies (22.2.2.3.2, 23.2.2.3.2)
3. One- and two-family dwellings (24.2.5.5)
4. Apartment buildings (30.2.2.3.3, 31.2.2.3.3)
5. Mercantile occupancies (36.2.2.3.2, 37.2.2.3.2)
6. Business occupancies (38.2.2.3.2, 39.2.2.3.2)
7. Industrial occupancies (40.2.2.3.2)
8. Storage occupancies (42.2.2.3.2)

The requirement of 7.2.2.2.3.2 is significant in that it includes a spiral stair geometry that can be used without a prespecified maximum occupant limit. The number of occupants permitted to use a spiral stair depends on how much egress width is provided. The term *egress width* has a specific meaning in this instance. It excludes the narrow part of the tapered tread that has less than 11 in. (280 mm) of tread depth. It also excludes the outer 10½ in. (265 mm) of tread width. Note that handrails are required at both sides. Also, the turn of the stairway must be such that the outer handrail is available to descending users at their right side. These criteria are depicted in Exhibit 7.30. An additional criterion is that the riser height not exceed 7 in. (180 mm), as is required for traditional stairs in accordance with Table 7.2.2.2.1.1(a).

The requirement of 7.2.2.2.3.3 retains the dimensional criteria for spiral stairs from earlier editions of the *Code* but changes the maximum number of occupants served by the stair from five to three and requires that handrails be provided at both sides of the stair.

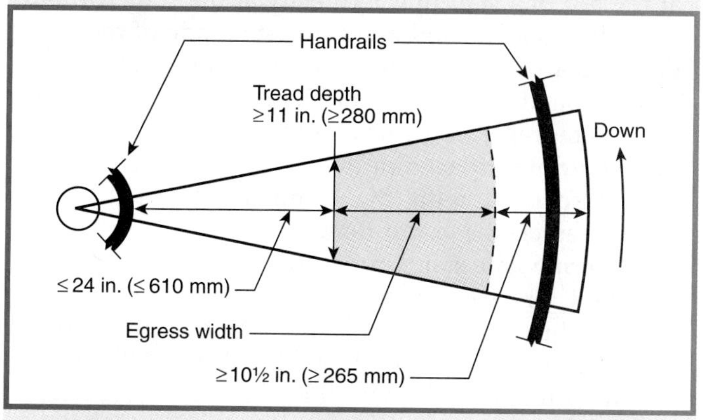


***Exhibit 7.30** Spiral stair tread dimensional criteria reflecting the requirements of 7.2.2.2.3.2.*

The requirement of 7.2.2.2.3.4 applies to existing spiral stairs. The traditional five-person limit and the requirement that a handrail be at the open side have been retained.

**7.2.2.2.4* Winders.**

**A.7.2.2.2.4** If properly designed and constructed, stairs with winders are not necessarily more dangerous than other stairs. Attention to the following factors helps to make winders generally more effective for egress and safety. Handrails should be continuous, without breaks at newel posts, from story to story. Handrails located at a greater than normal distance from the inner turn of winders can improve safety by constraining stair users to walk on the portion of the treads providing deeper treads, which should have not less than 11 in. (280 mm) of depth. Combinations of straight flights and winders are best arranged with winders located only below the straight flight. This arrangement is best because the winders provide larger tread dimensions over much of their width than do typical treads on straight flights. A descending person will, thus, be unlikely to experience a reduction of tread depth during descent, a condition of nonuniformity that is best avoided.

**7.2.2.2.4.1** Where specified in Chapters 11 through 43, winders shall be permitted in stairs, provided that they meet the requirements of 7.2.2.2.4.2 and 7.2.2.2.4.3.

**7.2.2.2.4.2** New winders shall have a tread depth of not less than 6 in. (150 mm) and a tread depth of not less than 11 in. (280 mm) at a point 12 in. (305 mm) from the narrowest edge.

**7.2.2.2.4.3** Existing winders shall be permitted to be continued in use, provided that they have a tread depth of not less than 6 in. (150 mm) and a tread depth of not less than 9 in. (230 mm) at a point 12 in. (305 mm) from the narrowest edge.

A winder is a tapered tread used to change the direction the stair runs. Because winders introduce a variation in the stair geometry and their effective tread depths are less than 11 in. (280 mm), they are suited to limited applications. At one time, the *Code* prohibited winders. Chapter 7 now sets applicable criteria for winders if the appropriate occupancy chapter specifically permits their use. Other than within dwelling units, the *Code* limits winders to existing installations. Exhibit 7.31 illustrates the dimensional criteria required.

Some occupancy chapters include additional limitations in addition to the criteria of 7.2.2.2.4. For

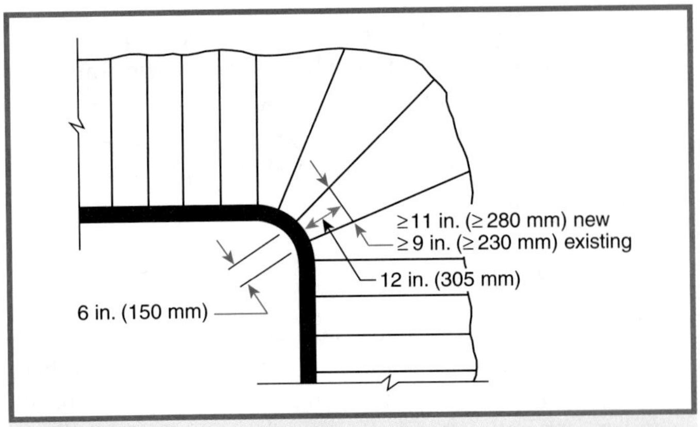


***Exhibit 7.31*** *Acceptable winders.*

example, in new apartment buildings, winders are permitted to serve only within a living unit and not within the common spaces, such as corridors and lobbies.

The occupancies that permit winders are as follows:

1. One- and two-family dwellings (24.2.5.5)
2. Lodging or rooming houses (26.2.2.4)
3. Apartment buildings (30.2.2.3.4, 31.2.2.3.4)
4. Residential board and care occupancies (32.2.2.6.2, 33.2.2.6.2)
5. Existing mercantile occupancies (37.2.2.3.3)
6. Existing business occupancies (39.2.2.3.3)
7. Existing industrial occupancies (40.2.2.3.3)
8. Existing storage occupancies (42.2.2.3.3, 42.8.2.2.3.3)

**7.2.2.3 Stair Details.**

**7.2.2.3.1 Construction.**

**7.2.2.3.1.1** All stairs serving as required means of egress shall be of permanent fixed construction, unless they are stairs serving seating that is designed to be repositioned in accordance with Chapters 12 and 13.

The requirement of 7.2.2.3.1.1 recognizes the functional requirement in theaters, for example, where seating sections are added, removed, or repositioned, depending on the specific theatrical production. It is impractical for stairs associated with such seating sections to be of fixed, permanent construction.

**7.2.2.3.1.2** Each stair, platform, and landing, not including handrails and existing stairs, in buildings required in this *Code* to be of Type I or Type II construction shall be of noncombustible material throughout.

The requirement of 7.2.2.3.1.2 covers the combustibility of materials used to construct new stairs. Stairs are permitted to be of combustible construction if the building is not required, by the __1.6 subsection of the applicable occupancy chapter, to be of Type I or Type II construction as defined in NFPA 220, *Standard on Types of Building Construction*.[14] For example, the occupancy chapter might not have any requirements related to minimum building construction type, or the occupancy chapter might permit Type III, Type IV, or Type V construction. If the building is required to be of Type I or Type II construction, the materials used for new stair construction (i.e., stairs, platforms, and landings) must be noncombustible.

**7.2.2.3.2 Landings.**

**7.2.2.3.2.1** Stairs shall have landings at door openings, except as permitted in 7.2.2.3.2.5.

**7.2.2.3.2.2** Stairs and intermediate landings shall continue with no decrease in width along the direction of egress travel.

**7.2.2.3.2.3** In new buildings, every landing shall have a dimension, measured in the direction of travel, that is not less than the width of the stair.

**7.2.2.3.2.4** Landings shall not be required to exceed 48 in. (1220 mm) in the direction of travel, provided that the stair has a straight run.

**7.2.2.3.2.5** In existing buildings, a door assembly at the top of a stair shall be permitted to open directly to the stair, provided that the door leaf does not swing over the stair and the door opening serves an area with an occupant load of fewer than 50 persons.

Stairs must have landings at door openings. It is unsafe to move through a door opening and immediately begin vertical travel on a stair. Paragraph 7.2.2.3.2.5 permits an existing situation in which a door assembly at the top of a stair opens directly at the stair without providing a level landing on the stair side of the door opening. In this case, however, the door leaf swings away from the stair, rather than swinging over the stair. Paragraph 7.2.1.3.6 recognizes the same concept of a step-down at exterior door assemblies. See Exhibit 7.15, associated with the commentary on 7.2.1.3.6, which depicts the exemption.

Intermediate stair landings of the minimum depth specified for new construction by 7.2.2.3.2.3 serve as effective breaks in runs of stairs, which allow persons who slip or trip to halt their fall. Exhibit 7.32 illustrates the minimum landing width addressed by 7.2.2.3.2.2 and the minimum landing depth addressed by 7.2.2.3.2.3 and 7.2.2.3.2.4.

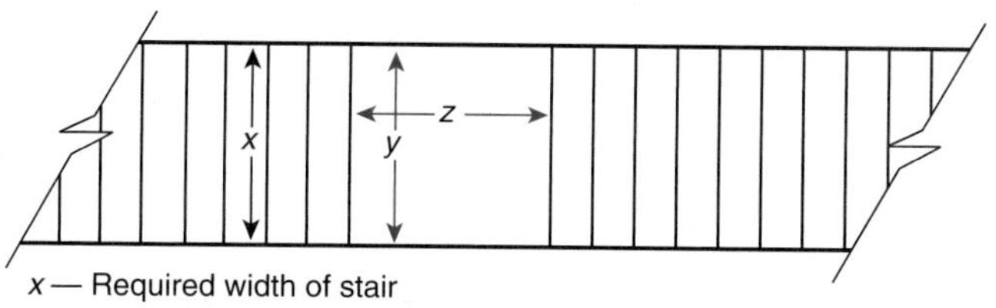


***Exhibit 7.32*** *Required width of intermediate landings; required depth of new intermediate landings.*

**7.2.2.3.3 Tread and Landing Surfaces.**

**7.2.2.3.3.1** Stair treads and landings shall be solid, without perforations, unless otherwise permitted in 7.2.2.3.3.4.

**7.2.2.3.3.2*** Stair treads and landings shall be free of projections or lips that could trip stair users.

**A.7.2.2.3.3.2** The tripping hazard referred to in 7.2.2.3.3.2 occurs especially during descent, where the tread walking surface has projections such as strips of high-friction materials or lips from metal pan stairs that are not completely filled with concrete or other material. Tread nosings that project over adjacent treads can also be a tripping hazard. ICC/ANSI A117.1, *American National Standard for Accessible and Usable Buildings and Facilities,* illustrates projecting nosing configurations that minimize the hazard.

Where environmental conditions (such as illumination levels and directionality or a complex visual field that draws a person's attention away from stair treads) lead to a hazardous reduction in one's ability to perceive stair treads, they should be made of a material that allows ready discrimination of the number and position of treads. In all cases, the leading edges of all treads should be readily visible during both ascent and descent. A major factor in injury-producing stair accidents, and in the ability to use stairs efficiently in conditions such as egress, is the clarity of the stair treads as separate stepping surfaces.

**7.2.2.3.3.3** If not vertical, risers on other than existing stairs shall be permitted to slope under the tread at an angle not to exceed 30 degrees from vertical, provided that the projection of the nosing does not exceed 1½ in. (38 mm).

**7.2.2.3.3.4** The requirement of 7.2.2.3.3.1 shall not apply to noncombustible grated stair treads and landings in the following occupancies:

(1) Assembly occupancies as otherwise provided in Chapters 12 and 13
(2) Detention and correctional occupancies as otherwise provided in Chapters 22 and 23
(3) Industrial occupancies as otherwise provided in Chapter 40
(4) Storage occupancies as otherwise provided in Chapter 42

Solid treads and solid landing floors provide a visual barrier that shields the user's view of the vertical drop beneath the stair. Persons with a fear of high places are more comfortable using such stairs. Grated and expanded metal treads and landings might catch a user's heel and present a tripping hazard. Noncombustible, grated stair treads are permitted in areas not accessed by the general public, such as catwalks and gridirons in theaters, resident housing areas in prisons, factories and other industrial occupancies, and storage occupancies.

The *Code* does not directly mandate solid risers on stairs. Rather, the requirement of 7.2.2.3.3.2 for treads to be free of projections or lips that could trip stair users is a performance-based provision that indirectly mandates solid risers on egress stairs used in the upward direction. Given that a riser is provided, the maximum slope specified by 7.2.2.3.3.3 — established as 30 degrees from the vertical with not more than a 1½ in. (38 mm) nosing projection — is intended to keep the toes of ascending users from becoming caught under the tread if users have a disability that prevents them from pulling their foot backwards to clear the lip created by the stair tread. The provision of 7.2.2.3.3.3 does not apply to existing stairs.

**7.2.2.3.4* Tread and Landing Slope.** The tread and landing slope shall not exceed ¼ in./ft (21 mm/m) (a slope of 1 in 48).

**A.7.2.2.3.4** A small drainage slope for stair treads subject to wetting can improve tread slip resistance *(see also A.7.2.2.3.3.2)*. A consistent slope to a side of the stair, where drainage is possible, might be preferable to a front-to-back slope of the treads. Providing a pitch of ⅛ in./ft to ¼ in./ft (10 mm/m to 21 mm/m) aids the shedding of water from a nominally horizontal surface.

Sloping treads and landings are intentionally used to avoid water accumulation on stairs. They might also be unintentionally created where treads and landings erode unevenly through usage or where differential settlement occurs, affecting the treads or landings. The limitation in slope is intended to reduce the dimensional nonuniformity of the effective riser heights and to reduce the chance of occupants slipping.

**7.2.2.3.5* Riser Height and Tread Depth.** Riser height shall be measured as the vertical distance between tread nosings. Tread depth shall be measured horizontally, between the vertical planes of the foremost projection of adjacent treads and at a right angle to the tread's leading edge, but shall not include beveled or rounded tread surfaces that slope more than 20 degrees (a slope of 1 in 2.75). At tread nosings, such beveling or rounding shall not exceed ½ in. (13 mm) in horizontal dimension.

**A.7.2.2.3.5** Figure A.7.2.2.3.5(a), Figure A.7.2.2.3.5(b), Figure A.7.2.2.3.5(c), and Figure A.7.2.2.3.5(d) illustrate the method for measuring riser height and tread depth. Stairs that are covered with resilient floor coverings might need additional tread depth beyond the minimum specified in the

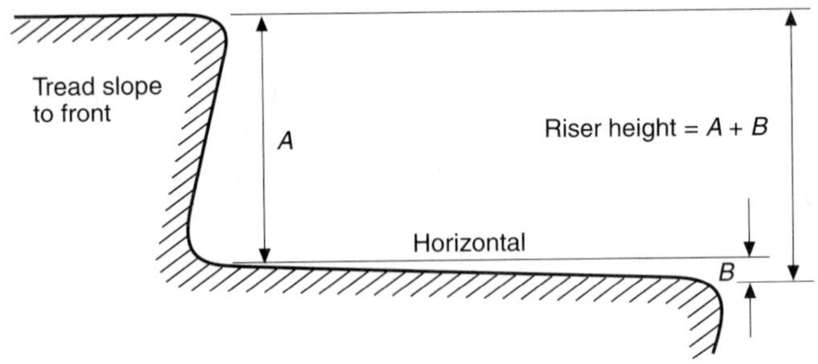


***Figure A.7.2.2.3.5(a)*** *Riser Measurement with Tread Slope to Front.*

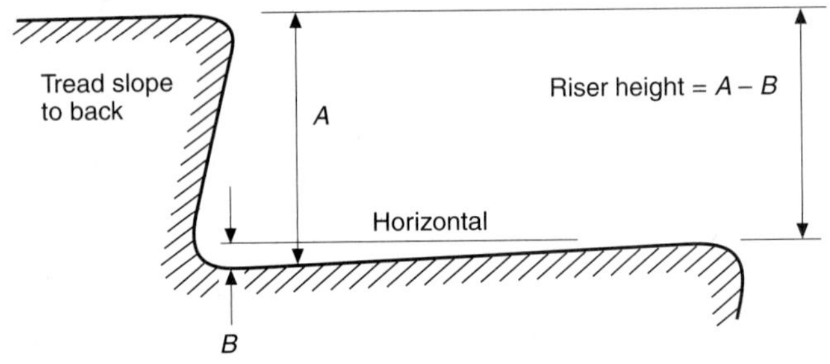


***Figure A.7.2.2.3.5(b)*** *Riser Measurement with Tread Slope to Back.*

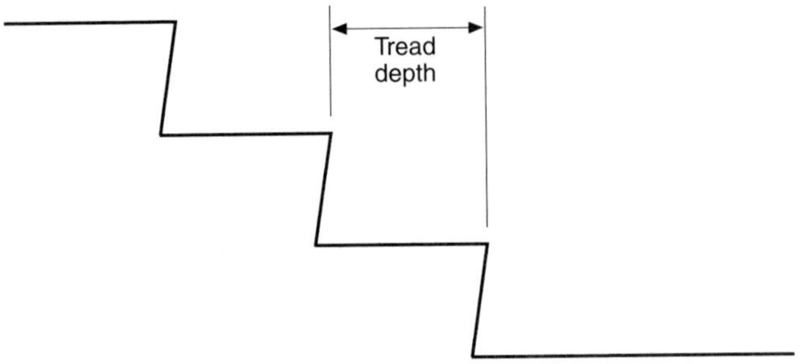


***Figure A.7.2.2.3.5(c)*** *Tread Depth.*

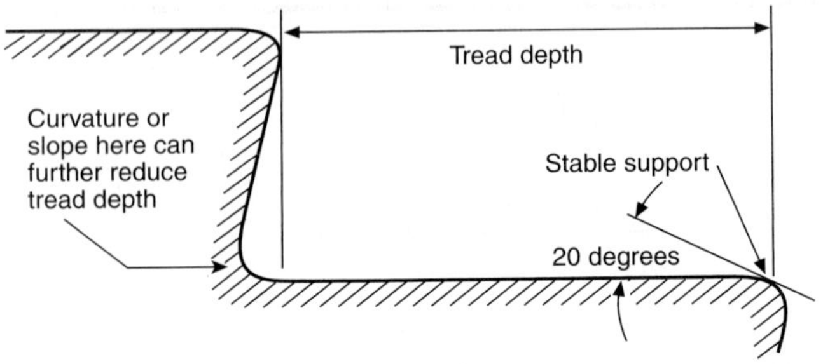


***Figure A.7.2.2.3.5(d)*** *Tread Measurement with Stable Support at Leading Edge.*

*Code*. Any horizontal projection of resilient covering materials beyond the tread nosing and riser, such as carpet and underlayment, can interfere with users' feet and thereby reduce usable tread depth. At the tread nosing, such resilient covering materials might not be capable of providing stable support for users' feet. Generally, effective tread depth is reduced by the uncompressed thickness of such resilient coverings and might be further reduced over time if coverings are not well secured and consequently might move forward at the nosings. *[See Figure A.7.2.2.3.5(e).]*

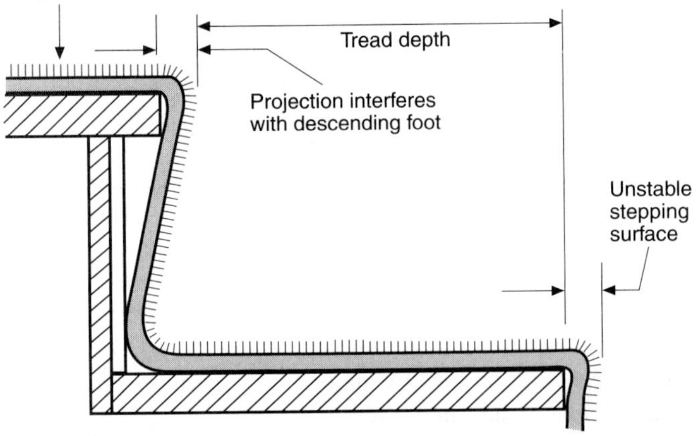


***Figure A.7.2.2.3.5(e)*** *Tread Measurement with Unstable Stepping Surface at Leading Edge.*

Measurement of riser and tread dimensions needs to represent the actual heights and depths experienced by those using the stairs. Therefore, the tread dimension is not to include any part of the tread that is not functional for normal foot placement, especially where the tread slopes more than 20 degrees from the horizontal. Normal placement of the foot onto the step nosings results in an initial contact angle of less than 20 degrees. Therefore, any part of the nosing sloping more than an angle of 20 degrees is ineffective and might create a tripping hazard. The limitation of a ½ in. (13 mm) horizontal dimension for beveling or rounding of the step nosings is also related to tripping hazards. This beveling or rounding also reduces the chance of a slip occurring when the foot initially contacts the nosing during descent of the stair. By following this rule, the designer also achieves acceptable step dimensions, while keeping the space used for the stair to a minimum.

Stair designers should keep in mind the possibility that a stair that was originally installed without floor coverings or with a resilient covering like sheet vinyl might someday be carpeted, thereby possibly reducing significantly the effective tread depth of the steps. Designing such stairs to provide slightly more than the minimum required tread depth is especially prudent in these cases. In addition, those responsible for maintaining stairs should keep in mind that the addition of resilient coverings might reduce step tread dimensions to below the standard, and the dimensions will be further reduced if the coverings are not installed and maintained tight against the underlying steps.

**7.2.2.3.6 Dimensional Uniformity.**

**7.2.2.3.6.1** Variation in excess of $^3/_{16}$ in. (4.8 mm) in the depth of adjacent treads or in the height of adjacent risers shall be prohibited, unless otherwise permitted in 7.2.2.3.6.3.

**7.2.2.3.6.2** The tolerance between the largest and smallest riser or between the largest and smallest tread shall not exceed $^3/_8$ in. (9.5 mm) in any flight.

Many accidents have resulted from irregularities in stair geometry from one step to an adjacent step or over an entire run of stairs. There should be no design irregularities. Variations due to construction are permitted, provided that the variation between adjacent treads or adjacent risers does not exceed $^3/_{16}$ in. (4.8 mm) and that the difference between the largest and smallest riser, as well as the difference between the largest and smallest tread, in any flight of stairs does not exceed $^3/_8$ in. (9.5 mm).

Exhibit 7.33 illustrates a stair that has various nonuniformities or irregularities. Note that the treads are not all uniformly horizontal, and the risers are not all vertical. This situation, which illustrates construction errors, is sometimes encountered with cast-in-place concrete stairs. Exhibit 7.33 shows unacceptable nonuniformities of the dimensions measured in accordance with 7.2.2.3.6.1 and 7.2.2.3.6.2. The nonuniformities measured at the backs of the treads and along the risers might be greater or smaller, depending on how the treads and risers slope.

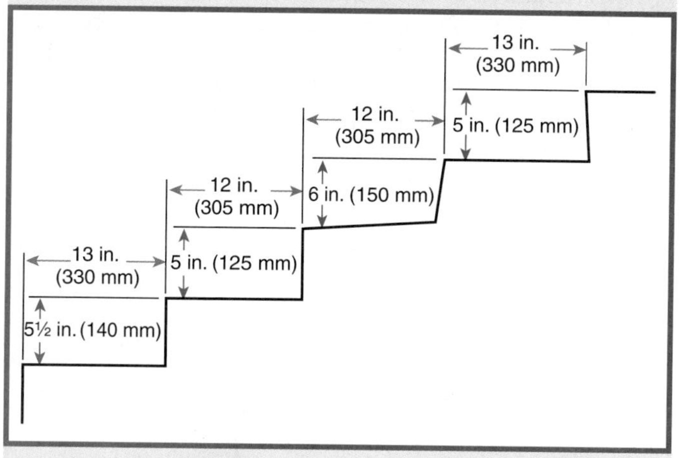


***Exhibit 7.33*** *Variations in tread and riser dimensions.*

**7.2.2.3.6.3** Where the bottom or top riser adjoins a sloping public way, walk, or driveway having an established finished ground level and serves as a landing, the bottom or top riser shall be permitted to have a variation in height of not more than 1 in. in every 12 in. (25 mm in every 305 mm) of stairway width.

**7.2.2.3.6.4*** All tread nosings of stairs utilizing the provision of 7.2.2.3.6.3 shall be marked in accordance with 7.2.2.5.4.3. Those portions of the marking stripe at locations where the riser height below the nosing is inconsistent by more than $^3/_{16}$ in. (4.8 mm), relative to other risers in the stair flight, shall be distinctively colored or patterned, incorporating safety yellow, to warn descending users of the inconsistent geometry relative to other steps in the flight.

**A.7.2.2.3.6.4** "Safety yellow" is the widely used, standard color (described in ANSI/NEMA Z535.1, *Standard for Safety Colors*) to be used for a "caution" function, as a solid color or in alternating, angled yellow-black bars or other geometric combination that draws attention beyond merely designating a nosing. Other nosings, not located above nonuniform risers, need only contrast with the remainder of the step and can be of any color providing contrast relative to the remainder of the tread. Note that similar specification of distinctive and contrasting nosing markings is called for in assembly seating aisle stairs *(See, respectively, 12.2.5.6.6(7) and 12.2.5.6.9.1.)* The safety problems of exterior stairs in assembly aisles and adjacent to a sloping public way are similar, as each individual step has to be visually detected in a reliable fashion. In addition, the presence and location of steps with unavoidably nonuniform risers must be effectively communicated, especially when viewed in the descent direction. Widely varying light conditions further heighten the need for such markings.

Where the riser at the base of a stair abuts sloping public property, such as a public sidewalk, the building owner usually has no right to alter the grade of the public property. Therefore, 7.2.2.3.6.3 accepts a certain minimum across-the-stair slope not in excess of 1 in 12, as shown in Exhibit 7.34. A similar across-the-stair slope is permitted along the top riser.

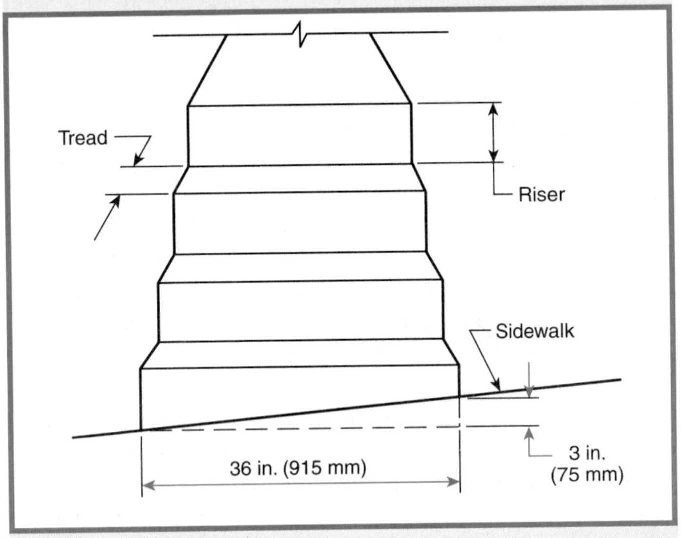


***Exhibit 7.34*** *Permissible across-the-stair slope.*

The provision of 7.2.2.3.6.4 is new to the 2009 edition of the *Code*. It requires that all the tread nosings (not just the top or bottom nosing) in a flight of stairs utilizing the across-the-stair slope allowance of 7.2.2.3.6.3 be provided with marking stripes. The text of A.7.2.2.3.6.4 explains the rationale for such requirement. Exhibit 7.35 depicts the required marking stripes, which are visible by stair users in ascending and descending the stairs.

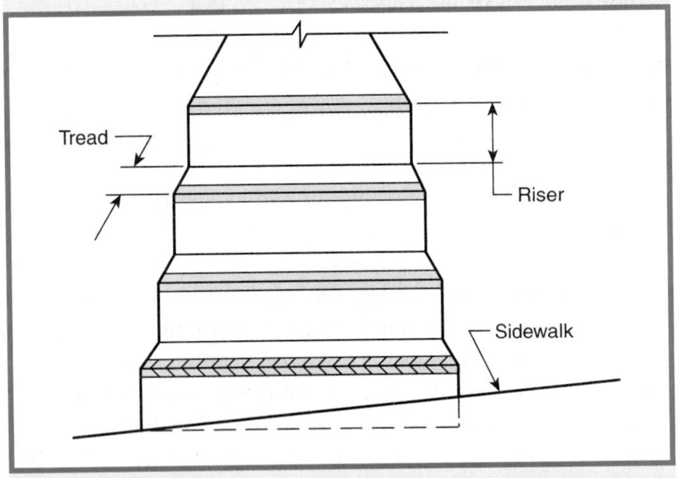


***Exhibit 7.35*** *Marking stripes to caution stair user of across-the-stair slope.*

**7.2.2.4 Guards and Handrails.**

Subsection 7.1.8 requires guards along the open sides of means of egress paths where there is a vertical drop of at least 30 in. (760 mm). This requirement is positioned in the general requirements of Section 7.1, because the open sides of means of egress paths occur in places other than just stairs. If the requirement of 7.1.8 to provide guards had instead been positioned within the provisions of 7.2.2 for stairs, it might go unnoticed by *Code* users concerned with egress components other than stairs. Thus, the actual requirement to provide guards appears in 7.1.8, and the details on how to provide guards are positioned within the provisions of 7.2.2.

The requirement for guards at open sides of means of egress has a particular impact on stairs that historically have required only handrails. Guards must be provided on open sides of the stair — including those that "switch back" between adjacent stair flights, regardless of the horizontal distance between those flights. The minimum 42 in. (1065 mm) high guard, as contrasted with the minimum 34 in. (865 mm) handrail, is needed to prevent a ninety-fifth percentile male from falling over the rail upon striking the side of a stair. On switch-back flights of stairs, the required guard is intended to keep a person from falling to the adjacent stair flight. See 7.2.2.4.5 for guard details — especially 7.2.2.4.5.2(3), which permits existing guards on existing stairs to be a minimum of 30 in. (760 mm) high.

Where the *Code* permits guards to be omitted, specific language is provided. For example, in 12.2.11.1.6, which applies to new assembly occupancies, guards are exempted on the audience side of stages; raised platforms; and other raised floor areas, such as runways, ramps, and side stages used for entertainment or presentations. Similarly, permanent guards are not required at vertical openings in the performance area of stages. Nor are guards required in assembly occupancies where the side of an elevated walking surface is required to be open for the normal functioning of special lighting or for the access and use of other special equipment.

NFPA staff members are often asked whether guards can be omitted at the open edge of loading docks. Given that the *Code* provides no specific exemption for loading docks, it is the intent that the general provisions for guards apply. However, Chapter 4 gives the authority having jurisdiction (AHJ) great latitude in making judgment calls where protection equivalent to that required by the *Code* is provided. Examples of judgment calls made by the AHJ are presented in the three scenarios that follow.

*Scenario 1.* A loading dock is 30 ft (9.1 m) deep [i.e., the building wall is set back 30 ft (9.1 m) from the open edge of the dock]. At the open edge of the dock, there is more than 30 in. (760 mm) of vertical drop to the ground below. The egress system relies on passage along the width of the loading dock as part of the exit discharge leading to the public way. A 44 in. (1120 mm) wide aisle has been stenciled on the floor running parallel to, and adjacent to, the building wall. Building management strictly enforces a policy that keeps the aisle clear at all times. The authority having jurisdiction judges that, in traveling along the designated path, the building occupants never come close to the open edge of the dock and, thus, guards are not required.

*Scenario 2.* The same physical arrangement exists as in scenario 1, but the AHJ inspects the facility and finds stacked materials in the designated aisle and across the depth of the loading dock. During emergency egress, the building occupants would need to travel close to the open edge of the dock to get around the stacked materials. The AHJ judges that, in this case, the guard provisions need to be followed.

*Scenario 3.* The loading dock is only 10 ft (3050 mm) deep. Materials are placed in a haphazard fashion on the dock. There is no designated egress path and, thus, building occupants can be expected to have to travel near the open edge of the dock. The AHJ judges that guards are needed.

**7.2.2.4.1 Handrails.**

**7.2.2.4.1.1** Stairs and ramps shall have handrails on both sides, unless otherwise permitted in 7.2.2.4.1.5 or 7.2.2.4.1.6.

**7.2.2.4.1.2** In addition to the handrails required at the sides of stairs by 7.2.2.4.1.1, the following provisions shall apply:

(1) For new stairs, handrails shall be provided within 30 in. (760 mm) of all portions of the required egress width.
(2) For existing stairs, handrails shall meet the following criteria:
  (a) They shall be provided within 44 in. (1120 mm) of all portions of the required egress width.
  (b) Such stairs shall not have their egress capacity adjusted to a higher occupant load than permitted by the capacity factor in Table 7.3.3.1 if the stair's clear width between handrails exceeds 60 in. (1525 mm).

**7.2.2.4.1.3** Where new intermediate handrails are provided in accordance with 7.2.2.4.1.2, the minimum clear width between handrails shall be 20 in. (510 mm).

**7.2.2.4.1.4*** The required egress width shall be provided along the natural path of travel.

**A.7.2.2.4.1.4** The intent of this provision is to place handrails for the required egress width only, regardless of the actual width. The required egress width is provided along the natural path of travel to and from the building. Examples of this requirement are shown in Figure A.7.2.2.4.1.4. The reduced intermediate handrail spacing of 60 in. (1525 mm), along with a handrail height within the permissible height limits, allows users to reach and grasp one handrail. Except as noted in 7.2.2.4.2 and 7.2.2.4.4, handrails are not required on stair landings.

**7.2.2.4.1.5** If a single step or a ramp is part of a curb that separates a sidewalk from a vehicular way, it shall not be required to have a handrail.

**7.2.2.4.1.6** Existing stairs, existing ramps, stairs within dwelling units and within guest rooms, and ramps within dwelling units and guest rooms shall be permitted to have a handrail on one side only.

Handrails are required on each side of new stairs and ramps, but they are not required on landings, except as noted in 7.2.2.4.2 at inside turns on stairs and in 7.2.2.4.4.10 as a short horizontal extension of the stair handrail. Handrails are also required on at least one side of existing stairs. The handrails provide support for people using stairs, act as a feature that stair users can grab to arrest a fall, and can serve as a guide for users if smoke enters the stairway in a quantity sufficient to obscure vision or if the stair lighting system fails.

For handrails to be effective, they must be within reach of each file of people using the stair. Paragraph 7.2.2.4.1.2(1) requires intermediate handrails for new stairs such that no portion of the stair is more than 30 in. (760 mm) horizontal distance from a handrail. Paragraph 7.2.2.4.1.2(2)(a) requires intermediate handrails for existing stairs only where the absence of such an intermediate handrail creates a portion of the stair that is more than 44 in. (1120 mm) horizontal distance from a handrail. The maximum 30 in. (760 mm) distance from a point on a new stair to the nearer handrail is based on the fact that people can only reach approximately 24 in. (610 mm) to the side to grasp a handrail and that a person's arms extend from the side of the body, not from the centerline. Exhibit 7.36 depicts people movement on a stair, seen in overhead plan view. The staggered filling of the stair surfaces is typical of that observed during building evacuation where movement, speed, density, and flow are near optimum for safe, comfortable crowd movement.

Because 7.2.2.2.1.2(A), 7.2.2.2.1.2(B), and 7.3.2.2 permit new handrails to project as much as $4\frac{1}{2}$ in. (114 mm) into the stair clear width at each side of the stair,

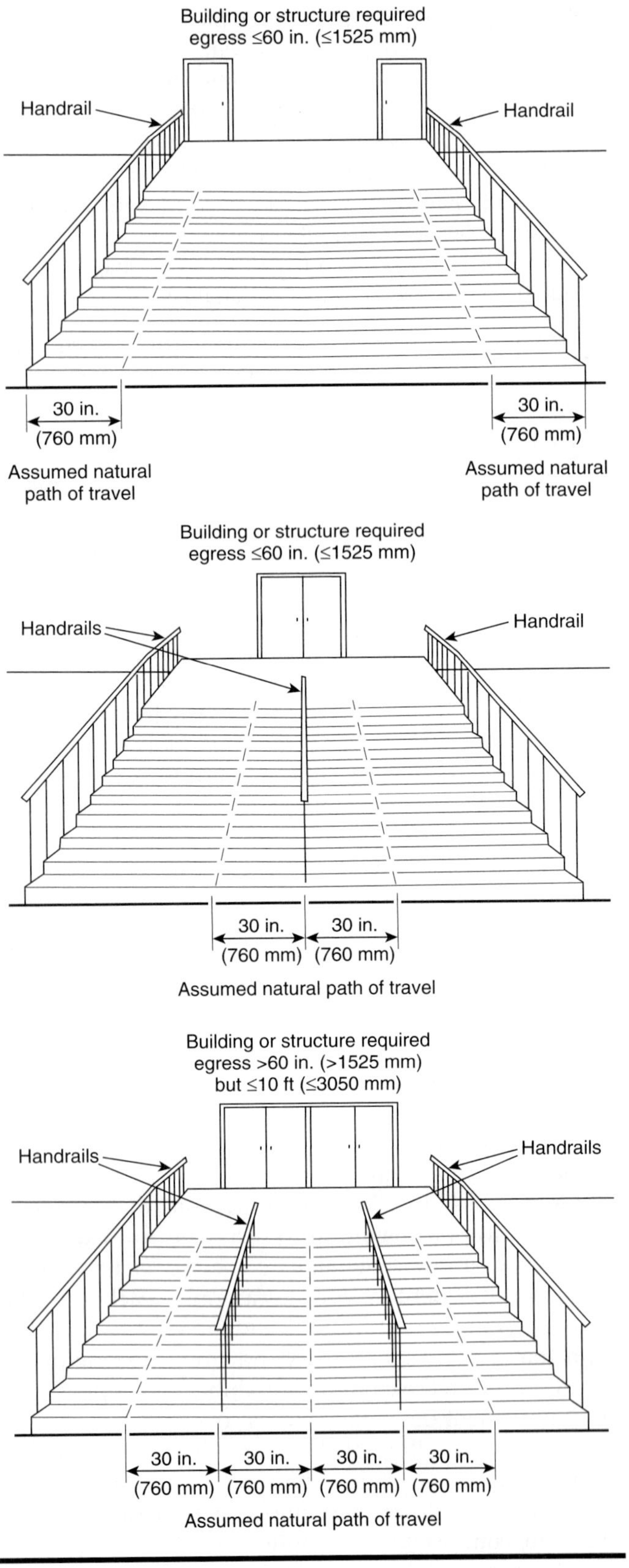


***Figure A.7.2.2.4.1.4*** *Assumed Natural Paths of Travel on Monumental Stairs with Various Handrail Locations.*

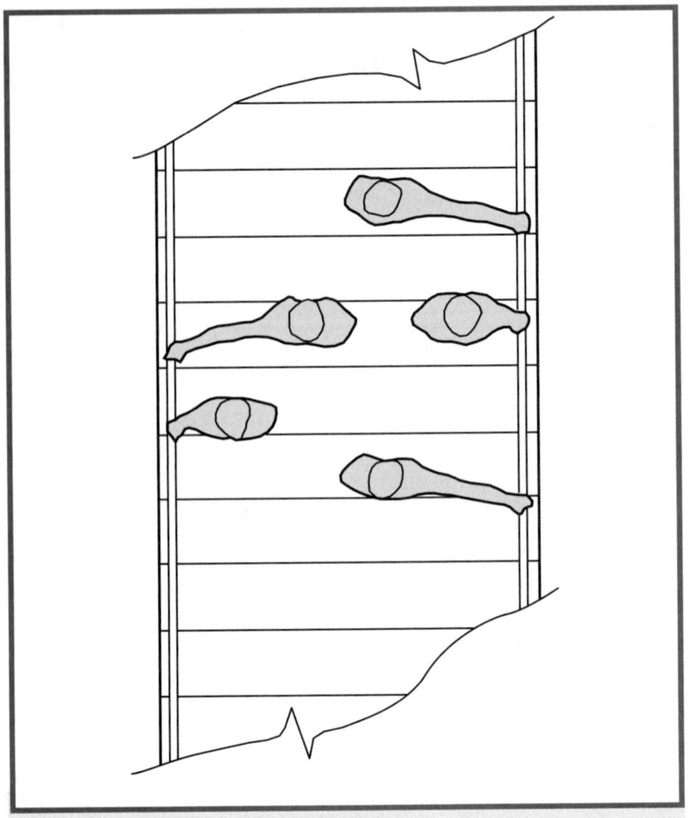

***Exhibit 7.36*** *Overhead plan view of stair with handrails within maximum 30 in. (760 mm) reach.*

center handrails are needed on new stairs more than, approximately, 5 ft 9 in. (1750 mm) wide, or $4\frac{1}{2}$ in. + 30 in. + 30 in. + $4\frac{1}{2}$ in. (114 mm + 760 mm + 760 mm + 114 mm), as illustrated in Exhibit 7.37.

Because Table 7.2.2.2.1.1(b) and 7.3.2.2 permit existing handrails to project as much as $4\frac{1}{2}$ in. (114 mm) into the stair clear width at each side of the stair, center handrails are needed on existing stairs more than, approximately, 8 ft 1 in. (2470 mm) wide, or $4\frac{1}{2}$ in. + 44 in. + 44 in. + $4\frac{1}{2}$ in. (114 mm + 1120 mm + 1120 mm + 114 mm), as illustrated in Exhibit 7.38.

Paragraph 7.2.2.4.1.2(2)(b) is new to the 2009 edition of the *Code*. It prohibits existing stairways with a clear width between handrails in excess of 60 in. (1525 mm) from using the capacity factor adjustment offered in 7.3.3.2 to stairways wider than 44 in. (1120 mm). The normal stair capacity factor of 0.3 in. (7.6 mm) per person is especially needed where a stair user is more than 30 in. (760 mm) from a handrail, which might have the effect of slowing people movement on the stair.

On monumental stairs, which are characterized by their extreme widths, the required handrails should be located along the normal path of travel to and from the

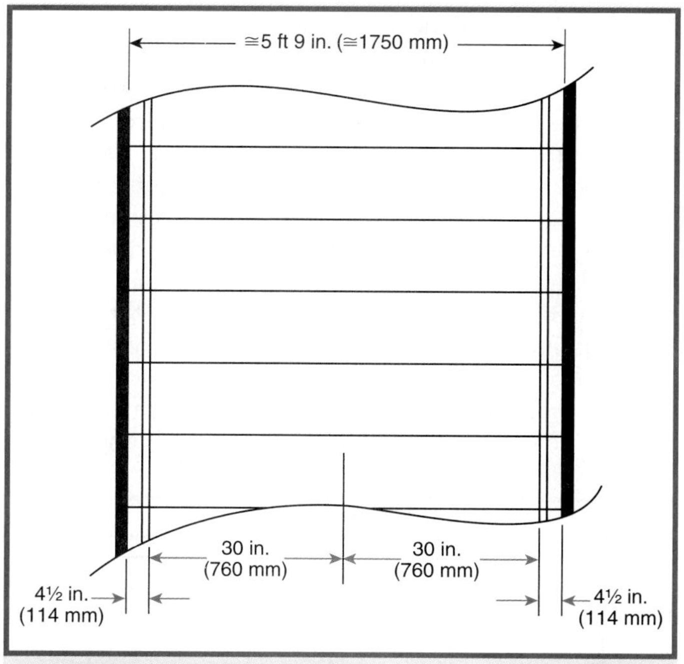


**Exhibit 7.37** *Maximum required width permitted without center handrail on new stair.*

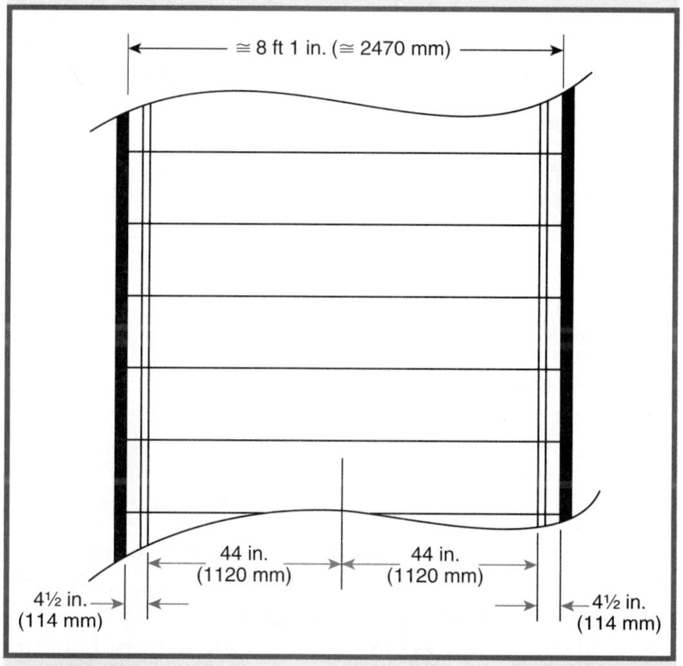


**Exhibit 7.38** *Maximum required width permitted without center handrail on existing stair.*

building. Figure A.7.2.2.4.1.4 illustrates the placement of handrails required on stairs that provide more width than required for egress. Handrails are provided along the natural paths of travel from the associated door assemblies.

**7.2.2.4.2 Continuity.** Required guards and handrails shall continue for the full length of each flight of stairs. At turns of new stairs, inside handrails shall be continuous between flights at landings.

It is not the intent of this *Code* to require handrails on stair landings. However, new handrails on the inside turn of switchback stairs (stairs that change direction at a landing) must be continuous. See the turn detailed in the plan view of Figure A.7.2.2.4.4.

The commentary following 7.2.2.4 explains the need for guards on open sides of stairs where there is at least a 30 in. (760 mm) vertical drop. The 30 in. (760 mm) criterion — considered alone — would seem to exempt the guard from running alongside the last couple of risers at the base of each stair flight; however, this criterion must be considered in conjunction with 7.2.2.4.2, which mandates that the required guard is to continue for the full length of each flight of stairs.

**7.2.2.4.3 Projections.** The design of guards and handrails and the hardware for attaching handrails to guards, balusters, or walls shall be such that there are no projections that might engage loose clothing. Openings in guards shall be designed to prevent loose clothing from becoming wedged in such openings.

**7.2.2.4.4* Handrail Details.**

**A.7.2.2.4.4** Figure A.7.2.2.4.4 illustrates some of the requirements of 7.2.2.4.4.

See 12.2.5.6.8 and 13.2.5.6.8 for requirements for handrails on aisle stairs in assembly occupancies.

**7.2.2.4.4.1** New handrails on stairs shall be not less than 34 in. (865 mm), and not more than 38 in. (965 mm), above the surface of the tread, measured vertically to the top of the rail from the leading edge of the tread.

**7.2.2.4.4.2** Existing required handrails shall be not less than 30 in. (760 mm), and not more than 38 in. (965 mm), above the surface of the tread, measured vertically to the top of the rail from the leading edge of the tread.

**7.2.2.4.4.3** The height of required handrails that form part of a guard shall be permitted to exceed 38 in. (965 mm), but shall not exceed 42 in. (1065 mm), measured vertically to the top of the rail from the leading edge of the tread.

**7.2.2.4.4.4*** Additional handrails that are lower or higher than the main handrail shall be permitted.

**A.7.2.2.4.4.4** Additional handrails, beyond those required by the *Code*, are permitted at heights other than those

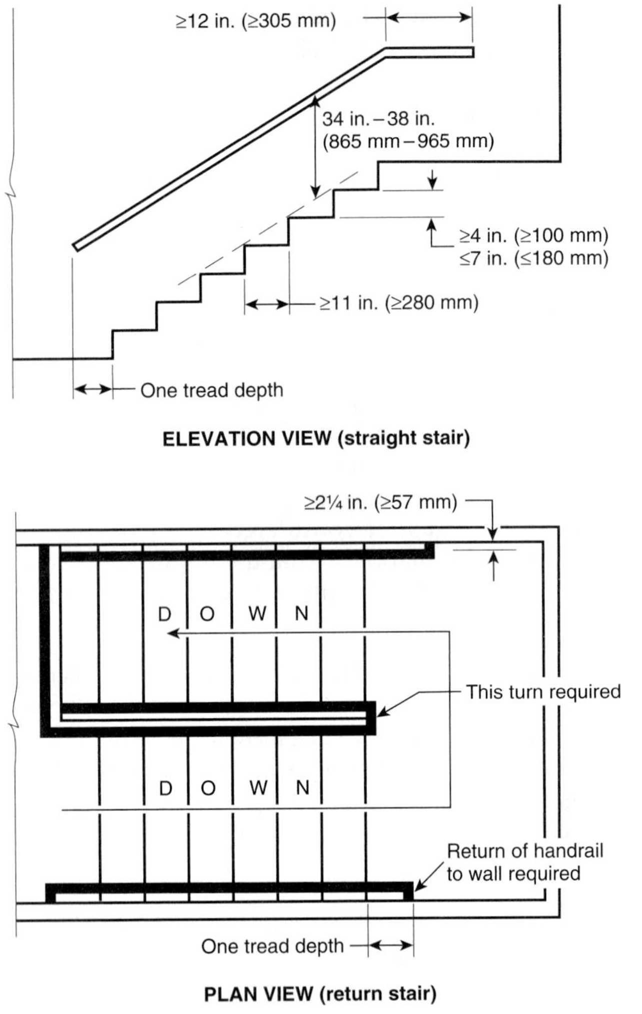


***Figure A.7.2.2.4.4*** *Handrail Details.*

stipulated. For example, where children under the age of five are major users of a facility, an additional handrail at a height in the range of 28 in. to 32 in. (710 mm to 810 mm) might be useful. Generally, children prefer to use, and can effectively use, handrails that are located at shoulder to head height due to their developmental characteristics and their less developed balance and walking abilities. At age 3, head height ranges from 35 in. to 40 in. (890 mm to 1015 mm); shoulder height averages 29 in. (735 mm). At age 5, head height ranges from 39 in. to 46 in. (990 mm to 1170 mm); shoulder height ranges from 31 in. to 37 in. (785 mm to 940 mm).

Handrail height was the subject of extensive research by the National Research Council Canada.

Very high handrails have been tested in field and laboratory conditions. Heights up to about 42 in. (1065 mm) are very effective in helping people stabilize themselves to arrest a fall. Therefore, a guard-height railing that also meets the graspability criteria for handrails (see 7.2.2.4.4.6) serves well as a handrail also. This dual function is the reason 7.2.2.4.4.3 permits the rail at the top of a 42 in. (1065 mm) high guard to serve as a handrail if it meets the graspability criteria. Three different types of studies of handrail height for stairs all concluded that the handrail heights previously required by the *Code* were inadequate. The studies included anthropometric analyses, such as the analysis illustrated in Exhibit 7.39, field studies of the use of various handrails, and laboratory studies where the functional capability of users to grasp a handrail — as if arresting a fall — were able to be accurately measured and compared for a range of handrail conditions.

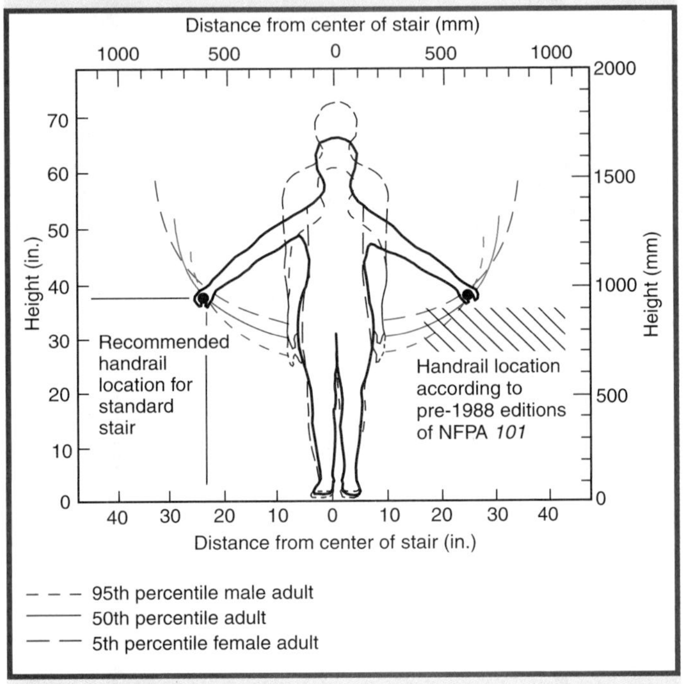


***Exhibit 7.39*** *Anthropometric analysis of reach.*

One of the studies leading to the requirement for higher handrails and closer lateral spacing included the anthropometric analysis of user capability to reach a handrail positioned to the side, as shown in Exhibit 7.39. The left side of the exhibit shows the recommended height and spacing of handrails; on the right is the location of handrails permitted by pre-1988 editions of the *Code*. People in the middle of a wide stair are unable to reach the lower, more distant handrails; therefore, this condition is not desirable when a stair is crowded, as during emergency egress.

The studies included a wide range of ages and sizes of people, from young children to those in their

70s. Most functional heights — even for elderly persons tested — were in the range of 36 in. to 38 in. (915 mm to 965 mm), and the average height most preferred by elderly persons tested was about 37 in. (940 mm). These studies were reported in "Review of Stair-Safety Research with an Emphasis on Canadian Studies" by Jake Pauls.[15] The recommendation for lower handrails for young children is particularly important for family dwellings and for child day-care facilities.

Exhibit 7.40 is a frame from the documentary film, *The Stair Event*. It shows field testing of an adjustable-height handrail in an aisle stair in Canada's Edmonton Commonwealth Stadium. Evidence from such field testing, from anthropometric analyses, and from laboratory testing with a range of younger and older adults led to the higher handrail heights first introduced in the 1988 edition of the *Code*. The upper handrail is located 37 in. (940 mm) above tread nosings, which, in the laboratory testing, was the average preferred height for elderly people and an especially effective height for arresting a fall that occurs while descending a stair. The lower railing, provided for children, is approximately 24 in. (610 mm) above the tread nosings. Note that, even in this case of ascent, one of the children has chosen to use the higher railing, located at about his shoulder height, in preference to the lower one. A moment after this frame was taken, the smaller of the two boys also chose to use the upper handrail, which was located at about the height of his head. This behavior has been observed in other studies of children; that is, when given a choice of handrail heights, they often select one between shoulder and head height.

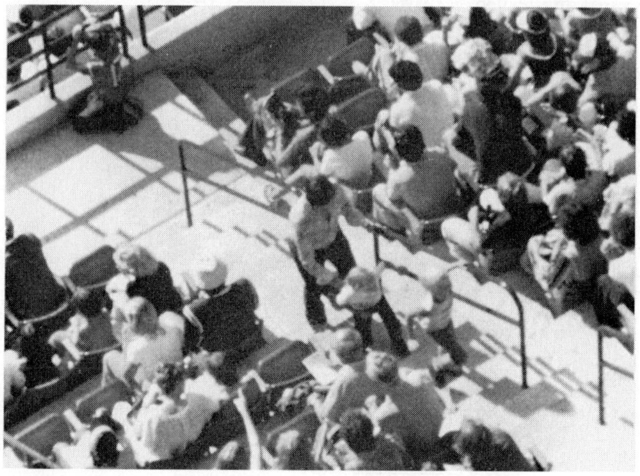

***Exhibit 7.40*** *Field testing of handrail height. (Photo courtesy of Jake Pauls.)*

**7.2.2.4.4.5** New handrails shall be installed to provide a clearance of not less than 2¼ in. (57 mm) between the handrail and the wall to which it is fastened.

**7.2.2.4.4.6** Handrails shall include one of the following features:

(1) Circular cross section with an outside diameter of not less than 1¼ in. (32 mm) and not more than 2 in. (51 mm)

(2)* Shape that is other than circular with a perimeter dimension of not less than 4 in. (100 mm), but not more than 6¼ in. (160 mm), and with the largest cross-sectional dimension not more than 2¼ in. (57 mm), provided that graspable edges are rounded so as to provide a radius of not less than ⅛ in. (3.2 mm)

**A.7.2.2.4.4.6(2)** Handrails should be designed so they can be grasped firmly with a comfortable grip and so the hand can be slid along the rail without encountering obstructions. The profile of the rail should comfortably match the hand grips. For example, a round profile, such as is provided by the simplest round tubing or pipe having an outside diameter of 1½ in. to 2 in. (38 mm to 51 mm), provides good graspability for adults. Factors such as the use of a handrail by small children and the wall-fixing details should be taken into account in assessing handrail graspability. The most functional, as well as the most preferred, handrail shape and size is circular with a 1½ in. (38 mm) outside diameter (according to research conducted using adults). Handrails used predominantly by children should be designed at the lower end of the permitted dimensional range.

Handrails are one of the most important components of a stair; therefore, design excesses such as oversized wood handrail sections should be avoided, unless there is a readily perceived and easily grasped handhold provided. In handrail design, it is useful to remember at all times the effectiveness of a simple round profile that allows some locking action by fingers as they curl around the handrail.

Perimeter dimension, referred to in 7.2.2.4.4.6(2), is the length of the shortest loop that wraps completely around the railing.

**7.2.2.4.4.7** New handrails shall be continuously graspable along their entire length.

In earlier editions of the *Code*, a minimum 1½ in. (38 mm) clearance was required between a new handrail and the wall to which it was fastened. The current provision, as detailed in 7.2.2.4.4.5, increases the required minimum clearance to 2¼ in. (57 mm) for new handrails in recognition of the fact that 1½ in. (38 mm) is an inadequate clearance for both a normal grasp and an emergency grasp of the handrail.

Paragraph 7.2.2.4.4.6 introduces a subtle but important requirement for handrails — graspability. People are incapable of exerting sufficient finger pressure to grasp a handrail adequately where using only a *pinch grip;* a *power grip,* where fingers curl around and under a properly shaped and sized railing, is much more effective. Exhibit 7.41 shows examples of acceptable and unacceptable handrails. Example 1 shows a handrail with a shape and an offset from the wall that provides graspability. Example 2 shows a handrail of a size and shape that are unacceptable from a graspability standpoint.

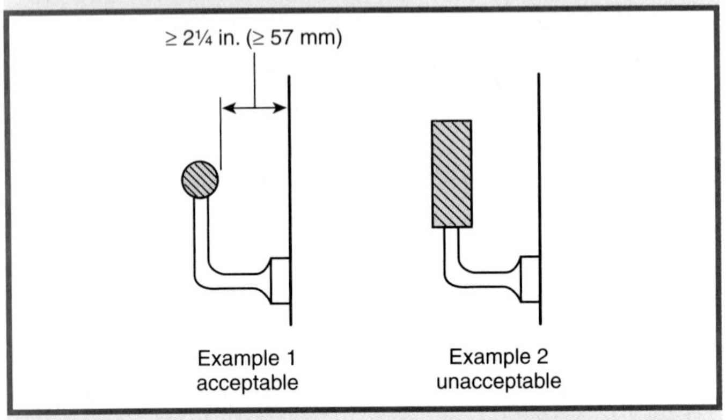


***Exhibit 7.41** Handrail graspability features.*

Exhibit 7.42 illustrates acceptable, unacceptable, and marginal handrail shapes and sizes, based on a Canadian study that used younger and older adults and tested functional capability as well as user preference. The traditional residential handrail, shown at the bottom center, did not perform well in the functional testing; it was not a comfortable shape to grasp in comparison with other shapes. A key difference between the acceptable and unacceptable handrail shapes is the ability to wrap the fingers around the handrail completely to achieve a power grip. Unacceptable shapes allow only a pinch grip, which is ineffective in arresting a fall, even for people with ordinary hand dexterity and strength.

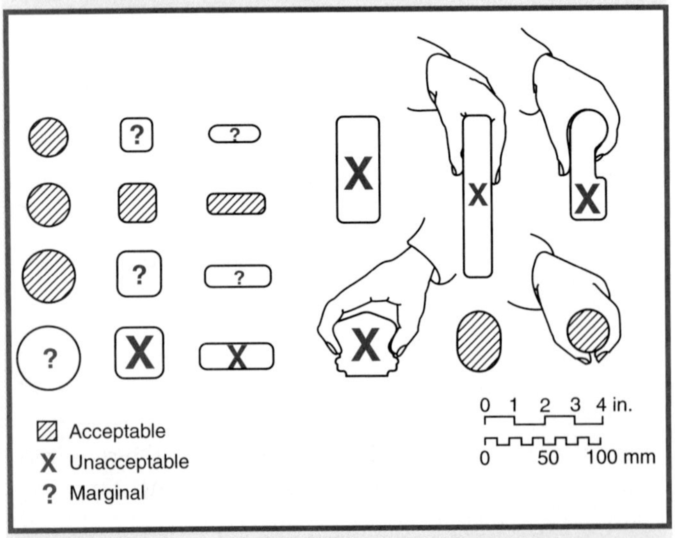


***Exhibit 7.42** Acceptable, unacceptable, and marginal handrail shapes.*

**7.2.2.4.4.8** Handrail brackets or balusters attached to the bottom surface of the handrail shall not be considered to be obstructions to graspability, provided that the following criteria are met:

(1) They do not project horizontally beyond the sides of the handrail within $1\frac{1}{2}$ in. (38 mm) of the bottom of the handrail and provided that, for each additional $\frac{1}{2}$ in. (13 mm) of handrail perimeter dimension greater than 4 in. (100 mm), the vertical clearance dimension of $1\frac{1}{2}$ in. (38 mm) is reduced by $\frac{1}{8}$ in. (3.2 mm).
(2) They have edges with a radius of not less than 0.01 in. (0.25 mm).

Paragraph 7.2.2.4.4.8 recognizes that handrail brackets and other forms of support are necessary but need to be designed to allow the hand to slide along the handrail without encountering obstructions that would force the release of the hand's grip. Exhibit 7.43 shows a handrail that has been positioned above the horizontal extension of the supporting bracket by the required minimum $1\frac{1}{2}$ in. (38 mm). Note how the fingers of the hand have sufficient space to point downward in a natural grasping position without encountering the handrail bracket.

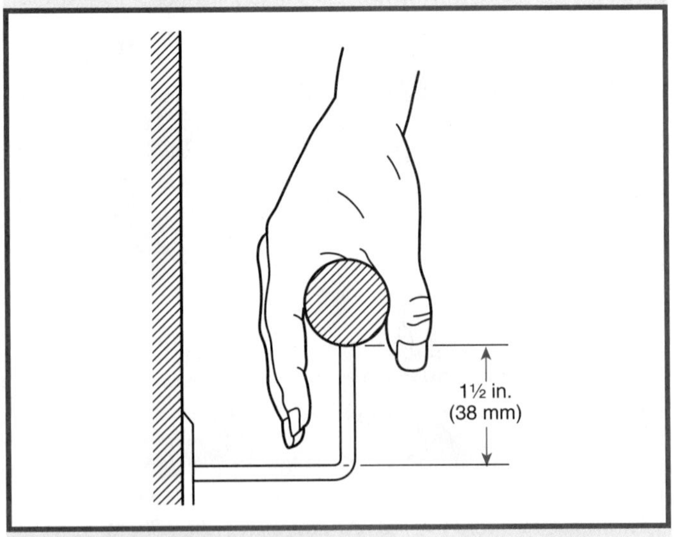


***Exhibit 7.43** Minimum clearance to handrail brackets.*

**7.2.2.4.4.9** New handrail ends shall be returned to the wall or floor or shall terminate at newel posts.

**7.2.2.4.4.10** In other than dwelling units, new handrails that are not continuous between flights shall extend horizontally, at the required height, not less than 12 in. (305 mm) beyond the top riser and continue to slope for a depth of one tread beyond the bottom riser.

**7.2.2.4.4.11** Within dwelling units, handrails shall extend, at the required height, to at least those points that are directly above the top and bottom risers.

The handrail extensions required by 7.2.2.4.4.10 are depicted in Figure A.7.2.2.4.4. At the top of the stair, the handrail extends horizontally for at least 12 in. (305 mm) past the top riser; at the bottom of the stair, the handrail continues past the bottom riser but does so at the same sloped angle as the remainder of the handrail positioned over the stair treads. The handrail extensions allow the stair users, who want to hold the handrail continuously while traveling along the stair, to grasp the handrail at their side — rather than ahead — before beginning to move vertically on the stair, and to continue to grasp the handrail at their side until vertical movement on the stair has been completed.

Paragraph 7.2.2.4.4.11 recognizes that the handrail extensions required by 7.2.2.4.4.10 need space at the top and bottom of stair flights that is typically not provided within dwelling units (e.g., hotel guest suites, apartment units, and single-family homes). It also recognizes that fewer occupants are expected to use a stair within a dwelling unit than a stair in the common space of a building (e.g., an enclosed exit stair serving the upper floors of a large apartment building). The provision permits handrails on stairs within dwelling units to end at points directly above the top and bottom risers. Where the stair users want to hold the handrail continuously while traveling along the stair, the users will need to reach forward to grasp the handrail before beginning to move vertically and will end their travel with their arm extended behind the plane of their backs.

**7.2.2.4.5 Guard Details.** See 7.1.8 for guard requirements.

**7.2.2.4.5.1** The height of guards required in 7.1.8 shall be measured vertically to the top of the guard from the surface adjacent thereto.

**7.2.2.4.5.2** Guards shall be not less than 42 in. (1065 mm) high, except as permitted by one of the following:

(1) Existing guards within dwelling units shall be permitted to be not less than 36 in. (915 mm) high.
(2) The requirement of 7.2.2.4.5.2 shall not apply in assembly occupancies where otherwise provided in Chapters 12 and 13.
(3)* Existing guards on existing stairs shall be permitted to be not less than 30 in. (760 mm) high.

**A.7.2.2.4.5.2(3)** This reduction in required height applies only to the stair, not to the landings.

**7.2.2.4.5.3*** Open guards, other than approved existing open guards, shall have intermediate rails or an ornamental pattern such that a sphere 4 in. (100 mm) in diameter is not able to pass through any opening up to a height of 34 in. (865 mm), and the following also shall apply:

(1) The triangular openings formed by the riser, tread, and bottom element of a guardrail at the open side of a stair shall be of such size that a sphere 6 in. (150 mm) in diameter is not able to pass through the triangular opening.
(2) In detention and correctional occupancies, in industrial occupancies, and in storage occupancies, the clear distance between intermediate rails, measured at right angles to the rails, shall not exceed 21 in. (535 mm).

**A.7.2.2.4.5.3** Vertical intermediate rails are preferred to reduce climbability.

The criterion for a 6 in. (150 mm) diameter sphere was changed to a 4 in. (100 mm) diameter sphere for the 1991 edition of the *Code*. This change was made based on the submission of a proposal that received the backing of the American Academy of Pediatrics. Approximately 950 out of 1000 children under age 10 can pass through a 6 in. (150 mm) wide opening. To prevent small children from falling through guards or being caught in openings, the configuration and construction of a guard must meet certain minimum requirements. Rather than requiring detailed specifications to be met for intermediate rails, the *Code* sets a performance criterion that permits alternative solutions.

The 4 in. (100 mm) diameter sphere criterion applies only to the portion of the guard that extends from the walking surface to a height of 34 in. (865 mm), even though the top rail of the guard must extend to a minimum height of 42 in. (1065 mm). See Exhibit 7.44.

Paragraph 7.2.2.4.5.3 exempts approved existing open guards from the maximum 4 in. (100 mm) diameter sphere criterion. Note that the phrase "approved existing open guards" has a different meaning than the phrase "previously approved open guards." See 3.3.73.1 and 3.3.198. In evaluating whether existing guards that do not meet the maximum 4 in. (100 mm) diameter sphere criterion are to be permitted to continue in use, it does not matter whether such guards received prior approval from the authority having

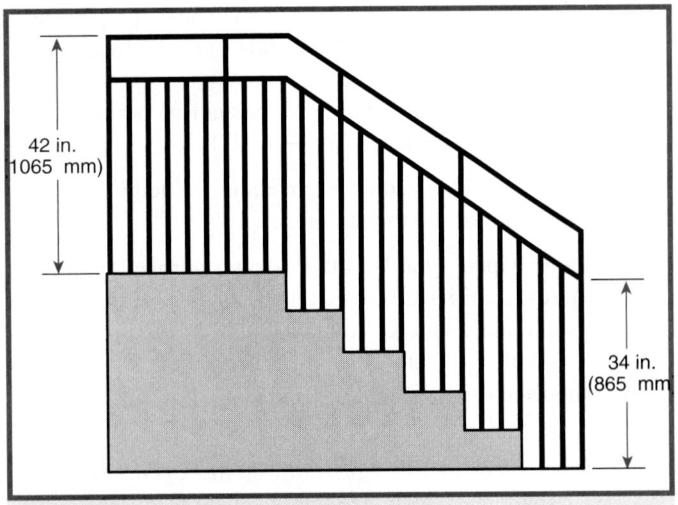


***Exhibit 7.44*** *Height extension for application of 4 in. (100 mm) diameter sphere criterion for guards.*

jurisdiction (AHJ). Instead, approval by the current AHJ is needed. Consider the following three examples:

1. The AHJ examines the existing open guards and finds that they meet a 6 in. (150 mm) diameter sphere criterion. The AHJ knows that older editions of the *Code* mandated a maximum 6 in. (150 mm) spacing and, therefore, approves the existing installation for continued use.
2. The AHJ examines the existing open guards and finds that they meet a 20 in. (510 mm) diameter sphere criterion. The AHJ knows that older editions of the *Code* did not permit anything larger than 6 in. (150 mm) spacing and, therefore, does not approve the existing installation for continued use.
3. The AHJ examines the existing open guards and finds that they meet an 8 in. (205 mm) diameter sphere criterion. The AHJ knows that older editions of the *Code* did not permit anything larger than 6 in. (150 mm) spacing and makes a judgment call on whether to approve the existing installation for continued use.

**7.2.2.5 Enclosure and Protection of Stairs.**

**7.2.2.5.1 Enclosures.**

**7.2.2.5.1.1** All inside stairs serving as an exit or exit component shall be enclosed in accordance with 7.1.3.2.

**7.2.2.5.1.2** Inside stairs, other than those serving as an exit or exit component, shall be protected in accordance with Section 8.6.

**7.2.2.5.1.3** In existing buildings, where a two-story exit enclosure connects the story of exit discharge with an adjacent story, the exit shall be permitted to be enclosed only on the story of exit discharge, provided that not less than 50 percent of the number and capacity of exits on the story of exit discharge are independent of such enclosures.

Paragraphs 7.2.2.5.1.1 and 7.2.2.5.1.2 emphasize that enclosure protection for stairs depends on whether they serve within an exit or involve a vertical opening between floors. Stairs that are not used as exits but that involve vertical openings are not subject to the requirements of 7.1.3.2; they must be protected in accordance with Section 8.6. Many interior stairs serve as exits and are vertical openings — they must, therefore, meet the requirements of 7.1.3.2 for exits as well as those of Section 8.6. Compliance with Section 8.6 does not ensure compliance with 7.1.3.2. Stairs that are neither within an exit nor part of vertical openings, such as stairs to a platform or stage, or those running between two different floor levels on the same story, do not have to comply with either 7.1.3.2 or Section 8.6.

The provisions of 7.2.2.5.1.3 recognize existing two-story stairs that, rather than being fully enclosed by a fire-rated shaft at both the top and bottom, are separated only from the level of exit discharge. Be-

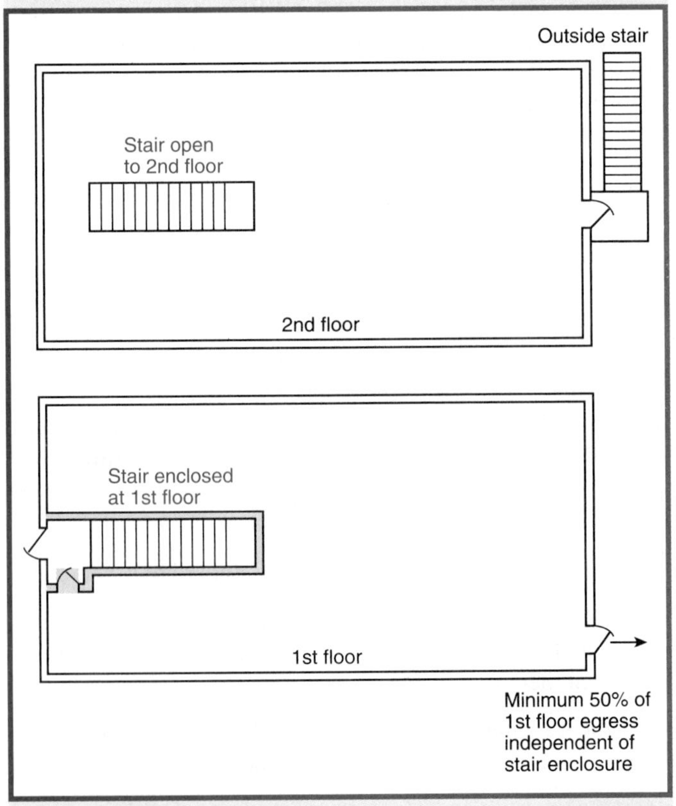


***Exhibit 7.45*** *Partial enclosure of existing stair.*

cause such stairs are open to another floor, they might compromise the use of the stair enclosure for egress purposes by occupants of the level of exit discharge. The *Code* requires that at least half of the egress for the level of exit discharge be independent of the stair enclosure. This requirement limits the effect of occupants who are forced to travel into an enclosure that is smoke-filled due to a fire on another floor that is open to the stair. See Exhibit 7.45. In Exhibit 7.45, the existing stair connecting the first and second floors, although separated from the first floor, is open to the second floor. This arrangement is permitted because a minimum of 50 percent of the first floor egress can be satisfied independently from use of the stair enclosure via the door assembly that opens directly to the outside at grade level at the right of the exhibit.

**7.2.2.5.2* Exposures.**

**A.7.2.2.5.2** The purpose of this provision is to protect the exterior wall of a stairway from fires in other portions of the building. If the exterior wall of the stair is flush with the building exterior wall, the fire would need to travel around 180 degrees in order to impact the stair. This has not been a problem in existing buildings, so no protection is required. However, if the angle of exposure is less than 180 degrees, protection of either the stair wall or building wall is required.

Figure A.7.2.2.5.2(a), Figure A.7.2.2.5.2(b), and Figure A.7.2.2.5.2(c) illustrate the requirement, assuming nonrated glass on the exterior wall of the stair is used.

**7.2.2.5.2.1** Where nonrated walls or unprotected openings enclose the exterior of a stairway, other than an existing stairway, and the walls or openings are exposed by other parts of the building at an angle of less than 180 degrees, the building enclosure walls within 10 ft (3050 mm) horizontally of the nonrated wall or unprotected opening shall be constructed as required for stairway enclosures, including opening protectives.

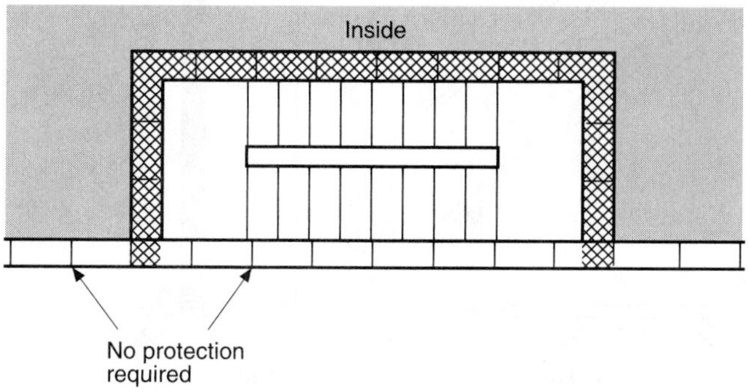


***Figure A.7.2.2.5.2(a)*** *Stairway with Nonrated Exterior Wall in Same Plane as Building Exterior Wall.*

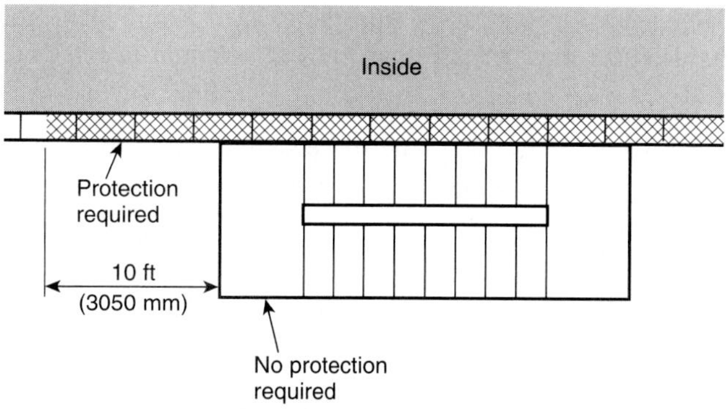


***Figure A.7.2.2.5.2(b)*** *Stairway with Unprotected Exterior Perimeter Protruding Past Building Exterior Wall.*

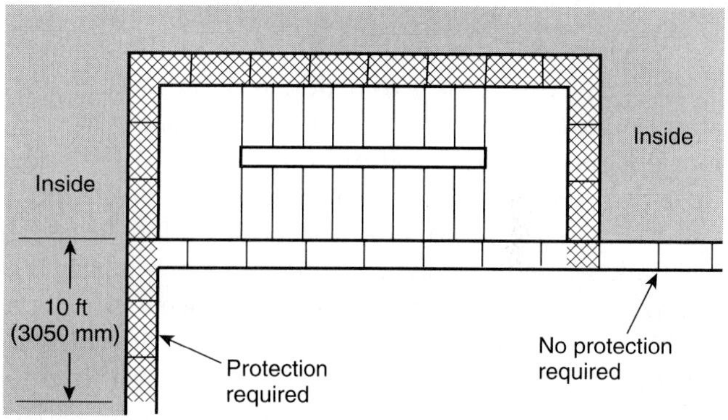


***Figure A.7.2.2.5.2(c)*** *Stairway with Nonrated Exterior Wall Exposed by Adjacent Exterior Wall of Building.*

**7.2.2.5.2.2** Construction shall extend vertically from the finished ground level to a point 10 ft (3050 mm) above the topmost landing of the stairs or to the roofline, whichever is lower.

**7.2.2.5.2.3** The fire resistance rating of the separation extending 10 ft (3050 mm) from% the stairs shall not be required to exceed 1 hour where openings have a minimum $\frac{3}{4}$-hour fire protection rating.

The provisions of 7.2.2.5.2.1 through 7.2.2.5.2.3 are well explained by A.7.2.2.5.2, including Figure A.7.2.2.5.2(a), Figure A.7.2.2.5.2(b), and Figure A.7.2.2.5.2(c).

**7.2.2.5.3* Usable Space.** Enclosed, usable spaces within exit enclosures shall be prohibited, including under stairs, unless otherwise permitted by 7.2.2.5.3.2.

**A.7.2.2.5.3** An example of a use with the potential to interfere with egress is storage.

**7.2.2.5.3.1** Open space within the exit enclosure shall not be used for any purpose that has the potential to interfere with egress.

**7.2.2.5.3.2** Enclosed, usable space shall be permitted under stairs, provided that the following criteria are met:

(1) The space shall be separated from the stair enclosure by the same fire resistance as the exit enclosure.
(2) Entrance to the enclosed, usable space shall not be from within the stair enclosure. *(See also 7.1.3.2.3.)*

Paragraphs 7.2.2.5.3 and 7.2.2.5.3.1 state that, within an exit enclosure, no enclosed, usable space is permitted, nor is any open space permitted to be used for any purpose that could interfere with the use of the exit enclosure. Per 7.2.2.5.3.2, an enclosed, usable space under a stair is permitted to be considered outside the exit enclosure if the walls and soffits of the enclosed space meet the same protection requirements as the stair enclosure, thereby separating the space from the exit enclosure, and if the door assembly to the space does not open into the exit enclosure. The provision of 7.2.2.5.3.2 is depicted in Exhibit 7.46. Note that fire resistance–rated construction isolates the space beneath the last run of stair so that the space is no longer within the exit enclosure. Note also that a door assembly that is outside the exit enclosure is used to enter the space, as a door communicating between the space and the exit enclosure would violate the provision of 7.1.3.2.1(8).

**7.2.2.5.4* Stairway Identification.**

**A.7.2.2.5.4** Figure A.7.2.2.5.4 shows an example of a stairway marking sign.

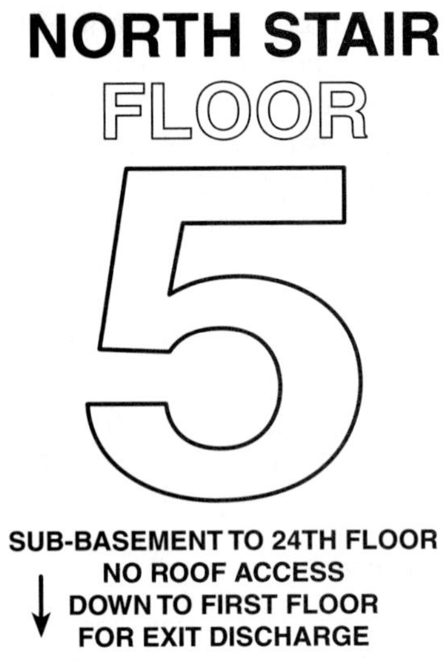


*Figure A.7.2.2.5.4 Example of a Stairway Marking Sign.*

**7.2.2.5.4.1** New enclosed stairs serving three or more stories and existing enclosed stairs serving five or more stories shall comply with 7.2.2.5.4.1(A) through (M).

**(A)** The stairs shall be provided with special signage within the enclosure at each floor landing.

**(B)** The signage shall indicate the floor level.

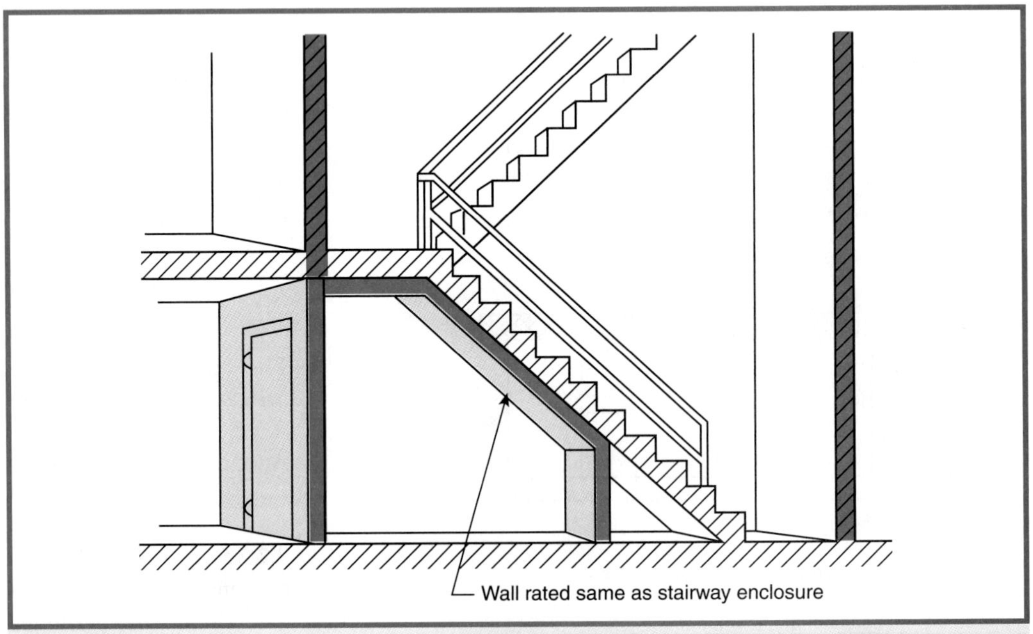


***Exhibit 7.46** Enclosed, usable space under flight of stairs.*

**(C)** The signage shall indicate the terminus of the top and bottom of the stair enclosure.

**(D)** The signage shall indicate the identification of the stair enclosure.

**(E)** The signage shall indicate the floor level of, and the direction to, exit discharge.

**(F)** The signage shall be located inside the enclosure approximately 60 in. (1525 mm) above the floor landing in a position that is visible when the door is in the open or closed position.

**(G)** The signage shall comply with 7.10.8.1 and 7.10.8.2 of this *Code*.

**(H)** The floor level designation shall also be tactile in accordance with ICC/ANSI A117.1, *American National Standard for Accessible and Usable Buildings and Facilities*.

**(I)** The signage shall be painted or stenciled on the wall or on a separate sign securely attached to the wall.

**(J)** The stairway identification letter shall be located at the top of the sign in minimum 1 in. (25 mm) high lettering and shall be in accordance with 7.10.8.2.

**(K)*** Signage that reads NO ROOF ACCESS and is located under the stairway identification letter shall designate stairways that do not provide roof access. Lettering shall be a minimum of 1 in. (25 mm) high and shall be in accordance with 7.10.8.2.

**A.7.2.2.5.4.1(K)** It is not the intent to require a sign that reads ROOF ACCESS, as such message might be misinterpreted by building occupants as an alternative egress route. However signs that read ROOF ACCESS are not prohibited, as many such signs have been installed in existing buildings so as to make a requirement for removal impractical. Historically, the ROOF ACCESS sign has provided information for the fire department. Where there is no roof access, such information will be posted via a NO ROOF ACCESS sign. The absence of the NO ROOF ACCESS sign should be understood by the fire department to mean that roof access is possible.

**(L)** The floor level number shall be located in the middle of the sign in minimum 5 in. (125 mm) high numbers and shall be in accordance with 7.10.8.2. Mezzanine levels shall have the letter "M" or other appropriate identification letter preceding the floor number, while basement levels shall have the letter "B" or other appropriate identification letter preceding the floor level number.

**(M)** Identification of the lower and upper terminus of the stairway shall be located at the bottom of the sign in minimum 1 in. (25 mm) high letters or numbers and shall be in accordance with 7.10.8.2.

**7.2.2.5.4.2** Wherever an enclosed stair requires travel in an upward direction to reach the level of exit discharge, special signs with directional indicators showing the direction to the level of exit discharge shall be provided at each floor level landing from which upward direction of travel is required, unless otherwise provided in 7.2.2.5.4.2(A) and 7.2.2.5.4.2(B), and the following also shall apply:

(1) Such signage shall comply with 7.10.8.1 and 7.10.8.2.
(2) Such signage shall be visible when the door leaf is in the open or closed position.

**(A)** The requirement of 7.2.2.5.4.2 shall not apply where signs required by 7.2.2.5.4.1 are provided.

**(B)** The requirement of 7.2.2.5.4.2 shall not apply to stairs extending not more than one story below the level of exit discharge where the exit discharge is clearly obvious.

**7.2.2.5.4.3* Stairway Tread Marking.** Where new contrasting marking is applied to stairs, such marking shall comply with the following:

(1) The marking shall include a continuous strip as a coating on, or as a material integral with, the full width of the leading edge of each tread.
(2) The marking shall include a continuous strip as a coating on, or as a material integral with, the full width of the leading edge of each landing nosing.
(3) The marking strip width, measured horizontally from the leading vertical edge of the nosing, shall be consistent at all nosings.
(4) The marking strip width shall be 1 in. to 2 in. (25 mm to 51 mm).

**A.7.2.2.5.4.3** For stair nosing marking, surface-applied material, such as adhesive-backed tape and magnetic strips, should not be used, as it is not durable under the scuffing from users' feet and, in coming loose, it creates a tripping hazard. While a carefully applied and consistently maintained coating is acceptable, contrasting color or photoluminescent material integral with the nosings is preferable because of its permanence. See also 7.1.6.4 and 7.2.2.3.6 for slip resistance uniformity requirements, as well as prohibition of projections on the treads.

Guidance on the use of photoluminescent marking is provided by ASTM E 2030, *Guide for Recommended Uses of Photoluminesent (Phosphorescent) Safety Markings*. Additional marking, for example, at the side boundaries of the stair, should be applied in accordance with the guidance provided therein.

**7.2.2.5.4.4*** Where new contrast marking is provided for stairway handrails, it shall be applied to, or be part of, at least the upper surface of the handrail; have a minimum width of $\frac{1}{2}$ in. (13 mm); and extend the full length of each handrail. After marking, the handrail shall comply with 7.2.2.4.4.

**A.7.2.2.5.4.4** Coatings and other applied markings, if used, should be durable for the expected usage, especially at end terminations of the marking and at changes in stair direction where usage is more extensive and hand forces are larger.

The provisions of 7.2.2.5.4 require the posting of important information at each floor landing in each stairwell if a new stair serves three or more stories or an existing stair serves five or more stories. The information is for fire-fightin%g personnel and building occupants in an emergency. The term *signage* is used to signify that the required information might appear on multiple signs mounted adjacent to each other. The information most helpful to fire fighters can be put on one sign, and the information most useful to occupants on another. See Figure A.7.2.2.5.4.

The signage must identify the stair, indicate the floor level of the landing [this information additionally must be tactile per 7.2.2.5.4.1(H)] and where the stairwell terminates at the top and bottom, and identify and show the direction to the exit discharge. Exhibit 7.47 illustrates the placement required to ensure that the sign is readily visible, whether the door leaf is open or closed.

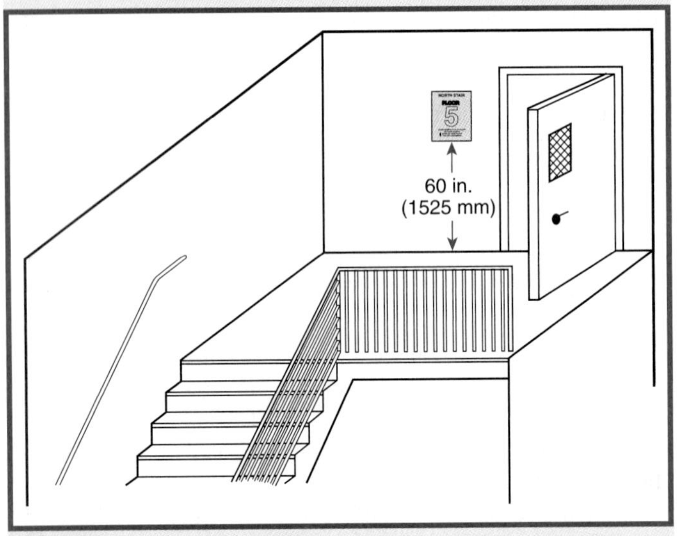


***Exhibit 7.47** Stair sign placement.*

The indication of the direction to the level of exit discharge can be extremely useful to occupants of a building, especially if they are located below the level of exit discharge. The natural tendency of occupants is to attempt egress by traveling downward in a stair; this is counterproductive where the exit discharge is located on an upper level. Also, many buildings have multiple levels of entrance, which create confusion with respect to travel direction in a given stair.

The requirements of 7.2.2.5.4 are not exempted for existing buildings, because it is feasible and cost-effective to install signs providing the required information. Because stair enclosures are usually not as aesthetically well finished as occupied portions of a building, the requirement for the signage (other than for the tactile floor level designator) is often met by stenciling the information directly onto the walls.

The provision of 7.2.2.5.4.1(K) was revised for the 2009 edition of the *Code*. In prior editions, roof access or lack of roof access was required to be designated by a sign. In many cases, roof access was provided for emergency responders only, and a sign reading "Roof Access" was misleading to building occupants. The current provision requires that only the lack of roof access be designated by a sign.

The provisions of 7.2.2.5.4.4 do not mandate that contrasting marking be applied to stair handrails. Where such contrast marking is provided for handrails, it regulates such installation so that the markings are useful and not misleading. For example, it requires that the marking stripe extend the full length of each handrail so the stair user can assess the extent of the stair flight before beginning any vertical movement on the stair. Marking stripes, where applied, will usually take the form of a photoluminescent or glow-in-the-dark material. See 7.2.2.5.5.10.

The criteria of 7.2.2.5.4.3(1) through (4) are needed to prevent the marking strips from providing misleading cues to stair users that might make use of the stair less safe or more confusing than if the marking strips were not installed. For example, 7.2.2.5.4.3(4) limits the marking strip to a maximum width of 2 in. (51 mm) to ensure that all but the leading edge of the tread is left unmarked, so a person using the stair in the downward direction sees individual tread edges and not one continuously marked sloping plane. The undesired continuously marked sloping plane would create a ramp effect, with no indication of the location of the leading edge of each tread.

**7.2.2.5.5 Exit Stair Path Markings.** Where exit stair path markings are required in Chapters 11 through 43, such markings shall be installed in accordance with 7.2.2.5.5.1 through 7.2.2.5.5.11.

**7.2.2.5.5.1 Exit Stair Treads.** Exit stair treads shall incorporate a marking stripe that is applied as a paint/coating or be a material that is integral with the nosing of each step. The marking stripe shall be installed along the horizontal leading edge of the step and shall extend the full width of the step. The marking stripe shall also meet the following requirements:

(1) The marking stripe shall be not more than $^1/_2$ in. (13 mm) from the leading edge of each step and shall not overlap the leading edge of the step by more than $^1/_2$ in. (13 mm) down the vertical face of the step.
(2) The marking stripe shall have a minimum horizontal width of 1 in. (25 mm) and a maximum width of 2 in. (51 mm).
(3) The dimensions and placement of the marking stripe shall be uniform and consistent on each step throughout the exit enclosure.
(4) Surface-applied marking stripes using adhesive-backed tapes shall not be used.

**7.2.2.5.5.2 Exit Stair Landings.** The leading edge of exit stair landings shall be marked with a solid and continuous marking stripe consistent with the dimensional requirements for stair treads and shall be the same length as, and consistent with, the stripes on the steps.

**7.2.2.5.5.3 Exit Stair Handrails.** All handrails and handrail extensions shall be marked with a solid and continuous marking stripe and meet the following requirements:

(1) The marking stripe shall be applied to the upper surface of the handrail or be a material integral with the upper surface of the handrail for the entire length of the handrail, including extensions.
(2) The marking stripe shall have a minimum horizontal width of 1 in. (25 mm).
(3) The dimensions and placement of the marking stripe shall be uniform and consistent on each handrail throughout the exit enclosure.

**7.2.2.5.5.4 Perimeter Demarcation Marking.** Stair landings, exit passageways, and other parts of the floor areas within the exit enclosure shall be provided with a solid and continuous perimeter demarcation marking stripe on the floor. The marking stripe shall also meet the following requirements:

(1) The marking stripe shall have a minimum horizontal width of 1 in. (25 mm) and a maximum width of 2 in. (51 mm), with interruptions not exceeding 4 in. (100 mm).
(2) The marking stripe shall be applied within 2 in. (51 mm) of the wall.
(3) The marking stripe shall continue in front of all door openings swinging into the exit enclosure. However, the marking stripe shall not be applied in front of door openings discharging from the exit enclosure.
(4) The dimensions and placement of the perimeter demarcation marking stripe shall be uniform and consistent throughout the exit enclosure.
(5) Surface-applied marking stripes using adhesive-backed tapes shall not be used.

**7.2.2.5.5.5* Obstacles.** Obstacles that are in the exit enclosure at or below 6 ft 6 in. (1980 mm) in height, and that project more than 4 in. (100 mm) into the egress path, shall be identified with markings not less than 1 in. (25 mm) in horizontal width comprised of a pattern of alternating equal bands of luminescent material and black; and with the alternating bands not more than 2 in. (51 mm) in horizontal width and angled at 45 degrees.

**A.7.2.2.5.5.5** Examples of obstacles addressed by 7.2.2.5.5.5 are standpipes, hose cabinets, and wall projections.

**7.2.2.5.5.6 Doors Serving Exit Enclosure.** All doors serving the exit enclosure that swing out from the enclosure in the direction of egress travel shall be provided with a marking stripe on the top and sides of the door(s) frame(s). The marking stripe shall also meet the following requirements:

(1) The marking stripe shall have a minimum horizontal width of 1 in. (25 mm) and a maximum width of 2 in. (51 mm).
(2) Gaps shall be permitted in the continuity of door frame markings where a line is fitted into a corner or bend, but shall be as small as practicable, and in no case shall gaps be greater than 1 in. (25 mm).
(3) Where the door molding does not provide enough flat surface on which to locate the marking stripe, the marking stripe shall be located on the wall surrounding the frame.
(4) The dimensions and placement of the marking stripe shall be uniform and consistent on all doors in the exit enclosure.

**7.2.2.5.5.7 Door Hardware Marking.** The door hardware for the doors serving the exit enclosure that swing out from the enclosure in the direction of egress travel shall be provided with a marking stripe. The marking stripe shall also meet the following requirements:

(1) The door hardware necessary to release the latch shall be outlined with a marking stripe having a minimum horizontal width of 1 in. (25 mm).
(2) Where panic hardware is installed, the following criteria shall be met:
    (a) The marking stripe shall have a minimum horizontal width of 1 in. (25 mm) and be applied to the entire length of the actuating bar or touch pad.
    (b) The placement of the marking stripe shall not interfere with viewing of any instructions on the actuating bar or touch pad.

**7.2.2.5.5.8 Emergency Exit Symbol.** An emergency exit symbol with a luminescent background shall be applied on all doors serving the exit enclosure that swing out from the enclosure in the direction of egress travel. The emergency exit symbol shall also meet the following requirements:

(1) The emergency exit symbol shall meet the requirements of NFPA 170, *Standard for Fire Safety and Emergency Symbols*.
(2) The emergency exit symbol applied on the door shall be not higher than 18 in. (455 mm) above the finished floor.

**7.2.2.5.5.9 Uniformity.** Placement and dimensions of the marking stripes shall be consistent and uniform throughout the same exit enclosure.

**7.2.2.5.5.10 Materials.** Exit stair path markings shall be made of any material, including paint, provided that an electrical charge is not required to maintain the required luminescence. Such materials shall include, but shall not be limited to, self-luminous materials and photoluminescent materials. Materials shall comply with one of the following:

(1) ASTM E 2073, *Standard Test Method for Photopic Luminance of Photoluminescent (Phosphorescent) Markings*, except that the charging source shall be 1 ft-candle (10.8 lux) of fluorescent illumination for 60 minutes, and the minimum luminance shall be 5 milli-candelas per square meter after 90 minutes
(2) UL 1994, *Standard for Luminous Egress Path Marking Systems*
(3) An alternate standard deemed equivalent and approved by the authority having jurisdiction

**7.2.2.5.5.11 Exit Stair Illumination.** Exit enclosures where photoluminescent materials are installed shall be continuously illuminated for at least 60 minutes prior to periods when the building is occupied. Lighting control devices that automatically turn exit enclosure lighting on and off, based on occupancy, shall not be installed.

The provisions of 7.2.2.5.5 on exit stair path markings were significantly expanded for the 2009 edition of the *Code*. The provisions were assembled from a variety of sources including General Services Administration standards and the New York City requirements applicable to high-rise buildings. Detailed criteria are presented as a set of requirements that run from the base paragraph of 7.2.2.5.5 through 7.2.2.5.5.11. The provisions are formatted so as to provide the "how-to" details where exit stair path markings are required by some other section of the *Code*, typically the occupancy chapters, although there is potential that exit stair path marking might be mandated in future editions by other provisions of the core chapters. For example, exit path markings might be used to enhance the high-rise building protection provisions detailed in Section 11.8.

No provision of the 2009 edition of the *Code* mandates the use of 7.2.2.5.5. Users of the *Code* should view the requirements of 7.2.2.5.5 as guidance that should be followed where exit stair path markings are provided voluntarily, as such markings, if not properly installed, might have the effect of making the stair less usable than a stair with no markings. Dr. Guyléne Proulx and colleagues at the National Research Council Canada's Institute for Research in Construction have actively evaluated photoluminescent markings in stairwells. Some of their work is summarized in the following research reports:

1. *Evaluation of the Effectiveness of Different Photoluminescent Stairwell Installations for the Evacuation of Office Building Occupants*[16]
2. *Evaluation and Comparison of Different Installations of Photoluminescent Marking in Stairwells of a High-rise Building*[17]

The criteria of 7.2.2.5.5 help to prevent the marking stripes from providing misleading cues to stair users that might make use of the stair less safe or more confusing than if the marking stripes were not installed. For example, 7.2.2.5.5.1(2) limits the marking stripe that extends across the full width of the leading edge of the stair tread to a maximum width of 2 in. (51 mm) to ensure that all but the leading edge of the tread is left unmarked, so a person using the stair in the downward direction sees individual tread edges, and not one continuously marked sloping plane. The undesired continuously marked sloping plane would create a ramp effect, with no indication of the location of the leading edge of each tread.

For future editions, the provisions of 7.2.2.5.5 and those of Section 7.10 for photoluminescent (PL) exit signs will need to be correlated. For example, 7.2.2.5.5.11 requires that, where exit stair path marking is installed using PL materials, the materials must be continuously illuminated for at least 60 minutes prior to periods when the building is occupied. Before a photoluminescent material can release electromagnetic radiation in the form of visible light, it must store incident electromagnetic radiation that typically reaches the material in the form of visible light. The illumination requirement of 7.2.2.5.5.11 is inconsistent with the philosophy applied to PL exit signs in Section 7.10. Photoluminescent exit signs are required by 7.10.7.1 to be listed in accordance with ANSI/UL 924, *Standard for Emergency Lighting and Power Equipment*.[18] ANSI/UL 924 requires that the sign be marked with a caution note that external illumination is required at all times that the building is occupied, but does not require any mention of providing a charging illumination prior to building occupancy. Further, 7.10.7.2 specifies that the face of the PL sign must be continuously illuminated while the building is occupied, so as to charge the PL material, but says nothing about providing illumination prior to building occupancy.

**7.2.2.6 Special Provisions for Outside Stairs.**

**7.2.2.6.1 Access.** Where approved by the authority having jurisdiction, outside stairs shall be permitted to lead to roofs of other sections of a building or an adjoining building where the construction is fire resistive and there is a continuous and safe means of egress from the roof. *(See also 7.7.6.)*

**7.2.2.6.2* Visual Protection.** Outside stairs shall be arranged to avoid any impediments to their use by persons having a fear of high places. Outside stairs more than 36 ft (11 m) above the finished ground level, other than previously approved existing stairs, shall be provided with an opaque visual obstruction not less than 48. in. (1220 mm) in height.

**A.7.2.2.6.2** The guards that are required by 7.1.8 and detailed in 7.2.2.4.5 will usually meet this requirement where the stair is not more than 36 ft (11 m) above the finished ground level. Special architectural treatment, including application of such devices as metal or masonry screens and grilles, will usually be necessary to comply with the intent of this requirement for stairs over 36 ft (11 m) above the finished ground level.

Outside stairs frequently have an open side. Required rails and guards help to prevent falls but do nothing to shield the user's view of the vertical drop. The fear of using such stairs, and the resultant decrease in the effectiveness of the stair as an egress component, justify the requirement for an opaque visual obstruction. The opaque visual barrier, required for stairs more than 36 ft (11 m) above the finished ground level, is required to be a minimum of 48 in. (1220 mm) high — a height that exceeds the 42 in. (1065 mm) criterion for guards at the open edge.

**7.2.2.6.3 Separation and Protection of Outside Stairs.**

**7.2.2.6.3.1** Outside stairs shall be separated from the interior of the building by construction with the fire resistance rating required for enclosed stairs with fixed or self-closing opening protectives, except as follows:

(1) Outside stairs serving an exterior exit access balcony that has two remote outside stairways or ramps shall be permitted to be unprotected.
(2) Outside stairs serving two or fewer adjacent stories, including the story where the exit discharges, shall be permitted to be unprotected where there is a remotely located second exit.
(3) In existing buildings, existing outside stairs serving three or fewer adjacent stories, including the story where the exit discharges, shall be permitted to be unprotected where there is a remotely located second exit.
(4) The fire resistance rating of a separation extending 10 ft (3050 mm) from the stairs shall not be required to exceed 1 hour where openings have a minimum $\frac{3}{4}$-hour fire protection rating.
(5) Outside stairs in existing buildings protected throughout by an approved, supervised automatic sprinkler system in accordance with Section 9.7 shall be permitted to be unprotected.

**7.2.2.6.3.2** Wall construction required by 7.2.2.6.3.1 shall extend as follows:

(1) Vertically from the finished ground level to a point 10 ft (3050 mm) above the topmost landing of the stairs or to the roofline, whichever is lower
(2) Horizontally for not less than 10 ft (3050 mm)

**7.2.2.6.3.3** Roof construction required by 7.2.2.6.3.1 shall meet the following criteria:

(1) It shall provide protection beneath the stairs.
(2) It shall extend horizontally to each side of the stair for not less than 10 ft (3050 mm).

The provisions of 7.2.2.6.3 address the proximity of outside stairs to openings in the building wall through which fire emerging from the building could render the stairs useless as a means of egress. Protection against such an occurrence is achieved as follows:

1. Protection from openings by separation distances
2. Protection of openings by fire-rated door assemblies and fire-rated windows, which is required if the openings are positioned such that the separation distances are less than are required

The arrangement typical of old fire escapes, where a window access is positioned immediately below a fire escape landing, creates the potential for fire exposure of the fire escape and is not permitted for outside stairs. The separation and protection provisions in 7.2.2.6.3 for outside stairs are illustrated in Exhibit 7.48 through Exhibit 7.50.

In Exhibit 7.48, if openings are within 10 ft (3050 mm) of the outside stairs, they must be protected (see 7.2.2.6.3.2). However, the fire resistance ratings in the 10 ft (3050 mm) extension need not exceed 1 hour, and the fire protection rating for the opening need not exceed $\frac{3}{4}$ hour.

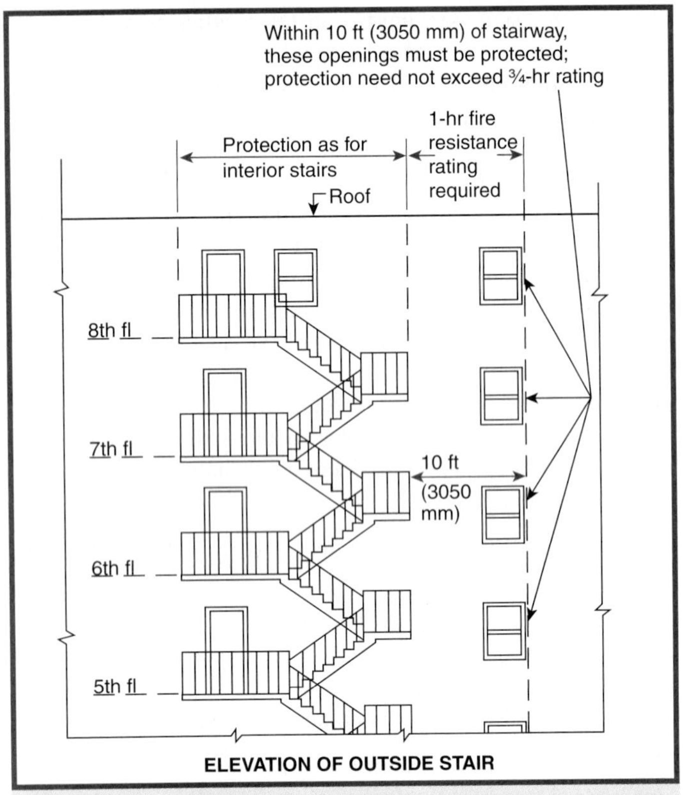


***Exhibit 7.48*** *Protection of openings for outside stairs — Example 1.*

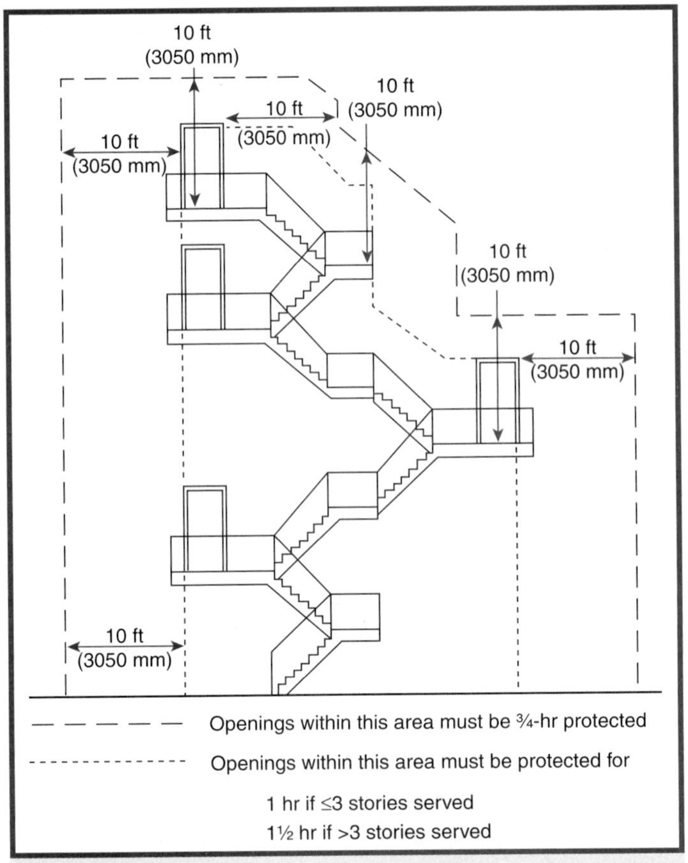


***Exhibit 7.49*** *Protection of openings for outside stairs — Example 2.*

In Exhibit 7.49, the fire resistance rating for the walls of the 10 ft (3050 mm) extension is a minimum of 1 hour. The fire resistance rating required for the walls within the short dashed lines is based on the number of stories served by the outside stair — the same as for interior stairs — as addressed in 7.1.3.2.1.

In Exhibit 7.50, the exemption permitted by 7.2.2.6.3.1(1) is illustrated in Part (a) of Exhibit 7.50. The exemption permitted by 7.2.2.6.3.1(2), which is restricted to stairways serving not more than two adjacent stories, is illustrated in Part (b) of Exhibit 7.50. Part (b) also illustrates the exemption permitted by 7.2.2.6.3.1(3), though that exemption permits stairways to serve up to three adjacent stories and is restricted to use in existing buildings.

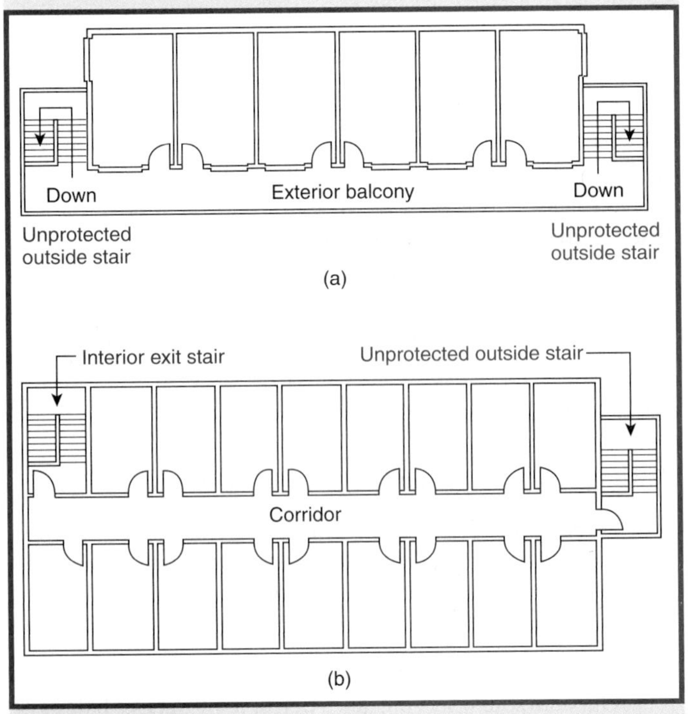


***Exhibit 7.50*** *Protection of openings for outside stairs — Example 3 and Example 4.*

**7.2.2.6.4 Protection of Openings.** All openings below an outside stair shall be protected with an assembly having a minimum ¾-hour fire protection rating as follows:

(1) Where located in an enclosed court *(see 3.3.46.1)*, the smallest dimension of which does not exceed one-third its height

(2) Where located in an alcove having a width that does not exceed one-third its height and a depth that does not exceed one-fourth its height

Exhibit 7.51 illustrates the provisions of 7.2.2.6.4(2). All openings along the alcove walls and located at an elevation less than the outside stairs are required to be protected if *D* (depth) is less than or equal to one-fourth of *H* (height) and *W* (width) is less than or equal to one-third of *H*.

*Example*

$H$ = 60 ft (18.3 m)

$D$ = 15 ft (4570 mm)

$W$ = 20 ft (6100 mm)

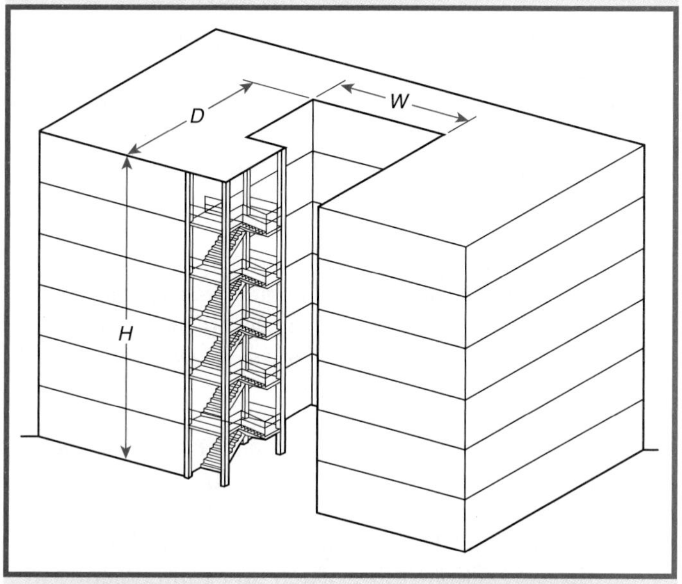


***Exhibit 7.51*** *Bases for required protection of openings below open, outside stairs discharging to an alcove.*

Therefore, in this example, all openings along the alcove walls and located at an elevation less than the outside stairs must be protected by opening protectives (e.g., fire windows) with a minimum fire protection rating of $^3/_4$ hour.

Note that the alcove depicted in Exhibit 7.51 is considered an alcove because it is open on one side. Paragraph 7.2.2.6.4(1) addresses an enclosed court, as defined in 3.3.46.1. It requires that if either *D* or *W* is one-third or less of *H*, all openings along the enclosed court walls and located at an elevation less than the outside stairs must be protected by opening protectives (e.g., fire windows) with a minimum fire protection rating of $^3/_4$ hour.

**7.2.2.6.5* Water Accumulation.** Outside stairs and landings, other than existing outside stairs and landings, shall be designed to minimize water accumulation on their surfaces.

**A.7.2.2.6.5** See A.7.2.2.3.4.

**7.2.2.6.6 Openness.** Outside stairs, other than existing outside stairs, shall be not less than 50 percent open on one side. Outside stairs shall be arranged to restrict the accumulation of smoke.

Paragraph 7.2.2.6.6 does not specify that the longer side of the new outside stair must be the side that is arranged to be at least 50 percent open. The shorter side of the stair can be arranged to be at least 50 percent open, if such arrangement complies with the performance-based requirement imposed by the second sentence of 7.2.2.6.6.

### 7.2.3 Smokeproof Enclosures.

**7.2.3.1 General.** Where smokeproof enclosures are required in other sections of this *Code,* they shall comply with 7.2.3, unless they are approved existing smokeproof enclosures.

A smokeproof enclosure has traditionally taken the form of an exit stair enclosure provided with additional features that limit the infiltration of heat, smoke, and fire gases from a fire in any part of a building. A pressurized stair enclosure is an example of this form of smokeproof enclosure. Smokeproof enclosures, other than exit stair enclosures, include pressurized elevator hoistway shafts. A smokeproof enclosure improves protection against the products of combustion entering the enclosure. The *Code* requires the use of smokeproof enclosures in 31.2.11.1 for existing, nonsprinklered, high-rise apartment building stairs. The provisions for smokeproof enclosures also are mandated for hoistway shaft systems for elevators providing access from an area of refuge to a public way in accordance with 7.2.12.2.4(3).

**7.2.3.2 Performance Design.** An appropriate design method shall be used to provide a system that meets the definition of *smokeproof enclosure (see 3.3.239).* The smokeproof enclosure shall be permitted to be created by using natural ventilation, by using mechanical ventilation incorporating a vestibule, or by pressurizing the stair enclosure.

Paragraph 7.2.3.2 requires that smokeproof enclosures meet the performance criterion contained in the definition of *smokeproof enclosure* in 3.3.239. Paragraph 7.2.3.2 also specifies three different means of creating smokeproof enclosures, as follows:

1. By use of natural ventilation as detailed in 7.2.3.7

2. By mechanical ventilation in accordance with 7.2.3.8
3. By pressurizing the enclosure as outlined in 7.2.3.9

However, the *Code* does not restrict the design to one of the three methods detailed in the previous paragraph if the design meets the performance requirements and is acceptable to the authority having jurisdiction. This alternative is especially important for existing smokeproof enclosures, because they often do not meet all the prescriptive-based specifications that follow.

Exhibit 7.52 illustrates four variations of exit stair enclosure smokeproof enclosures that meet the specific *Code* criteria contained in 7.2.3.4 through 7.2.3.8. Plan A utilizes an open-air vestibule. Plan B shows entrance to the smokeproof enclosure by way of an outside balcony. Plan C provides a stair enclosure entrance common to two building areas. In Plan D, smoke and gases entering the vestibule are exhausted by mechanical ventilation. In each case, a double entrance to the stair enclosure with at least one side open or vented is characteristic of the type of construction. Pressurization of the stair enclosure in the event of fire provides an attractive alternative and is a means of eliminating the need for an entrance vestibule.

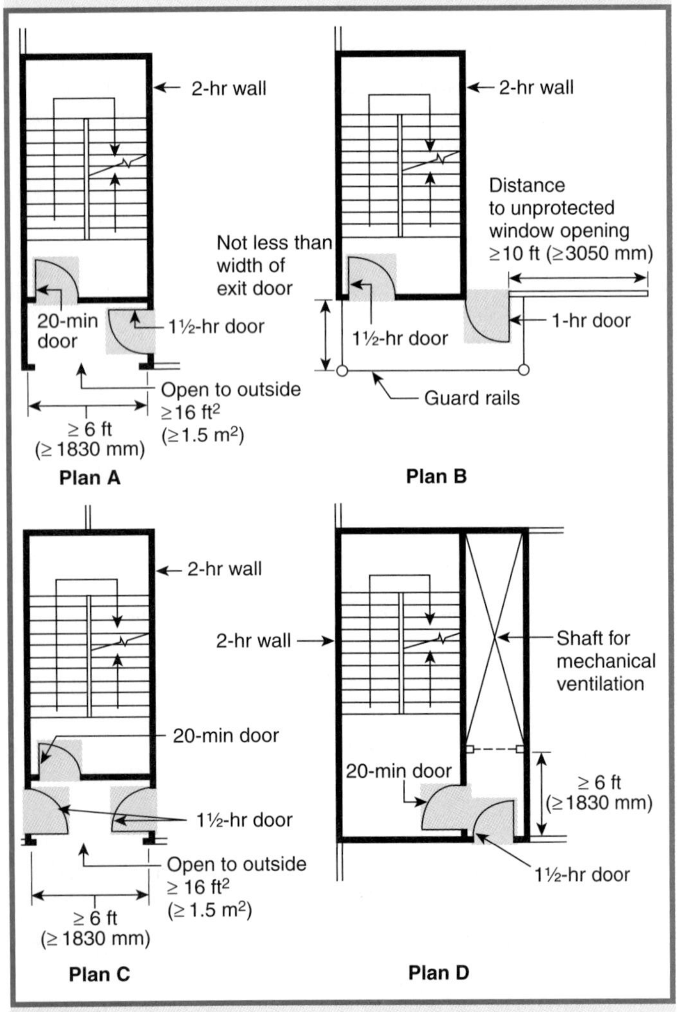


***Exhibit 7.52*** *Four variations of smokeproof enclosures.*

**7.2.3.3 Enclosure.** A smokeproof enclosure shall be enclosed from the highest point to the lowest point by barriers having 2-hour fire resistance ratings. Where a vestibule is used, it shall be within the 2-hour-rated enclosure and shall be considered part of the smokeproof enclosure.

**7.2.3.4 Vestibule.** Where a vestibule is provided, the door opening into the vestibule shall be protected with an approved fire door assembly having a minimum 1½-hour fire protection rating, and the fire door assembly from the vestibule to the smokeproof enclosure shall have a minimum 20-minute fire protection rating. Door leaves shall be designed to minimize air leakage and shall be self-closing or shall be automatic-closing by actuation of a smoke detector within 10 ft (3050 mm) of the vestibule door opening. New door assemblies shall be installed in accordance with NFPA 105, *Standard for the Installation of Smoke Door Assemblies and Other Opening Protectives.*

Paragraph 7.2.3.3 requires that the smokeproof enclosure and all of its components be within the required 2-hour fire resistance–rated enclosure, with openings therein protected by a door assembly having a 1½-hour fire protection rating. Such an arrangement protects the smokeproof enclosure from the direct attack of fire. However, per 7.2.3.4, the assembly from the vestibule (within the 2-hour-rated enclosure) into the actual stairway requires only a 20-minute fire protection rating, because the purpose of this door assembly is to minimize air or smoke leakage. Such door assemblies, other than in existing installations, are required to be smoke leakage–rated door assemblies installed in accordance with NFPA 105, *Standard for the Installation of Smoke Door Assemblies and Other Opening Protectives.* The AHJ is to qualitatively evaluate existing door assemblies with respect to their ability to restrict smoke movement through the gaps between the door leaf and the door frame.

**7.2.3.5 Discharge.** Every smokeproof enclosure shall discharge into a public way, into a yard or court having direct access to a public way, or into an exit passageway. Such exit passageways shall be without openings, other than the entrance to the smokeproof enclosure and the door opening to the outside yard, court, or public way. The exit passageway shall be separated from the remainder of the building by a 2-hour fire resistance rating.

Note that 7.2.3.5 prohibits smokeproof enclosures from discharging through the level of exit discharge. Thus, the provisions of 7.7.2, which otherwise permit up to 50 percent of the exit stair enclosures to discharge through areas on the level of exit discharge, do not apply to exit stair enclosures that are smokeproof enclosures. The requirement of 7.2.3.5 emphasizes the need for continuity to a public way, the exit discharge that leads to a public way, or an exit passageway that leads to an exit discharge that leads to a public way. Because an exit passageway is an exit, it is permitted to have only those openings necessary for building occupant egress and to support the life safety features required within the exit passageway; for example, penetrations for electrical conduit serving the lighting within the exit passageway.

**7.2.3.6 Access.** For smokeproof enclosures other than those consisting of a pressurized enclosure complying with 7.2.3.9, access to the smokeproof enclosure shall be by way of a vestibule or by way of an exterior balcony.

**7.2.3.7 Natural Ventilation.** Smokeproof enclosures using natural ventilation shall comply with 7.2.3.3 and the following:

(1) Where access to the enclosure is by means of an open exterior balcony, the door assembly to the enclosure shall have a minimum $1\frac{1}{2}$-hour fire protection rating and shall be self-closing or shall be automatic-closing by actuation of a smoke detector.
(2) Openings adjacent to the exterior balcony specified in 7.2.3.7(1) shall be protected in accordance with 7.2.2.6.4.
(3) Every vestibule shall have a net area of not less than 16 $ft^2$ (1.5 $m^2$) of opening in an exterior wall facing an exterior court, yard, or public space not less than 20 ft (6100 mm) in width.
(4) Every vestibule shall have a minimum dimension of not less than the required width of the corridor leading to it and a dimension of not less than 6 ft (1830 mm) in the direction of travel.

**7.2.3.8 Mechanical Ventilation.** Smokeproof enclosures using mechanical ventilation shall comply with 7.2.3.3 and the requirements of 7.2.3.8.1 through 7.2.3.8.4.

**7.2.3.8.1** Vestibules shall have a dimension of not less than 44 in. (1120 mm) in width and not less than 6 ft (1830 mm) in the direction of travel.

**7.2.3.8.2** The vestibule shall be provided with not less than one air change per minute, and the exhaust shall be 150 percent of the supply. Supply air shall enter and exhaust air shall discharge from the vestibule through separate tightly constructed ducts used only for such purposes. Supply air shall enter the vestibule within 6 in. (150 mm) of the floor level. The top of the exhaust register shall be located not more than 6 in. (150 mm) below the top of the trap and shall be entirely within the smoke trap area. Door leaves, when in the open position, shall not obstruct duct openings. Controlling dampers shall be permitted in duct openings if needed to meet the design requirements.

**7.2.3.8.3** To serve as a smoke and heat trap and to provide an upward-moving air column, the vestibule ceiling shall be not less than 20 in. (510 mm) higher than the door opening into the vestibule. The height shall be permitted to be decreased where justified by engineering design and field testing.

**7.2.3.8.4** The stair shall be provided with a dampered relief opening at the top and supplied mechanically with sufficient air to discharge at least 2500 $ft^3$/min (70.8 $m^3$/min) through the relief opening while maintaining a positive pressure of not less than 0.10 in. water column (25 $N/m^2$) in the stair, relative to the vestibule with all door leaves closed.

Exhibit 7.53 illustrates an elevation view of a smokeproof enclosure vestibule that uses mechanical ventilation. The minimum height of the door opening, specified as 6 ft 8 in. (2030 mm) in Exhibit 7.53, is mandated by 7.1.5.1, not by 7.2.3.8.

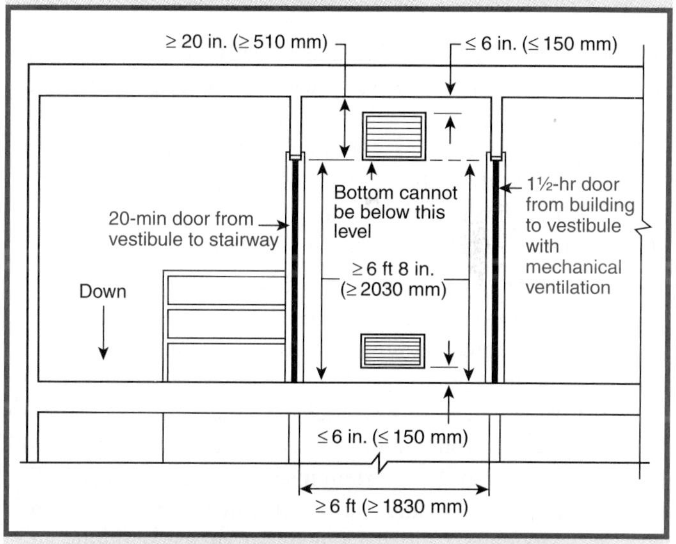


***Exhibit 7.53** Mechanical ventilation form of smokeproof enclosure.*

**7.2.3.9 Enclosure Pressurization.**

**7.2.3.9.1*** Smokeproof enclosures using pressurization shall use an approved engineered system with a design pressure difference across the barrier of not less than 0.05 in. water column (12.5 $N/m^2$) in sprinklered buildings, or 0.10 in. water column (25 $N/m^2$) in nonsprinklered buildings, and shall be capable of maintaining these pressure differences under likely conditions of stack effect or wind. The pressure difference across door openings shall not exceed that which allows the door leaves to begin to be opened by a force of 30 lbf (133 N) in accordance with 7.2.1.4.5.

**A.7.2.3.9.1** The design pressure differences required by 7.2.3.9.1 are based on specific gas temperatures and ceiling heights. The system is required to be approved, because anticipated conditions might be different from those on which the design pressure differences were calculated and, thus, different design pressure differences might be needed. For additional information on necessary minimum design pressure differences, including calculational techniques, or maximum pressure differences across doors to ensure reasonable operating forces, see NFPA 92A, *Standard for Smoke-Control Systems Utilizing Barriers and Pressure Differences.*

Pressurized stairs are permitted to be used as smokeproof enclosures in either nonsprinklered or sprinklered buildings. However, the design pressure difference across the barrier in a nonsprinklered building is required to be twice that required in a sprinklered building.

**7.2.3.9.2** Equipment and ductwork for pressurization shall be located in accordance with one of the following specifications:

(1) Exterior to the building and directly connected to the enclosure by ductwork enclosed in noncombustible construction
(2) Within the enclosure with intake and exhaust air vented directly to the outside or through ductwork enclosed by a 2-hour fire-resistive rating
(3) Within the building under the following conditions:
  (a) Where the equipment and ductwork are separated from the remainder of the building, including other mechanical equipment, by a 2-hour fire-resistive rating
  (b) Where the building, including the enclosure, is protected throughout by an approved, supervised automatic sprinkler system installed in accordance with Section 9.7, and the equipment and ductwork are separated from the remainder of the building, including other mechanical equipment, by not less than a 1-hour fire-resistive rating

**7.2.3.9.3** In all cases specified by 7.2.3.9.2(1) through (3), openings into the required fire resistance–rated construction shall be limited to those needed for maintenance and operation and shall be protected by self-closing fire protection–rated devices in accordance with 8.3.4.

Exhibit 7.54, Exhibit 7.55, and Exhibit 7.56 illustrate arrangements that comply with 7.2.3.9.2. In Exhibit

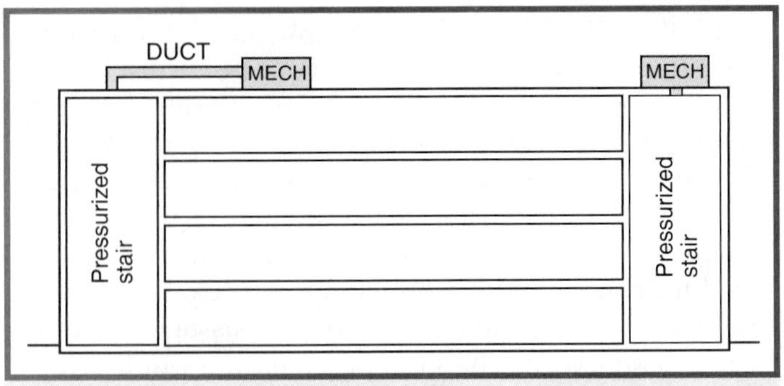


***Exhibit 7.54** Mechanical equipment and ductwork complying with 7.2.3.9.2(1).*

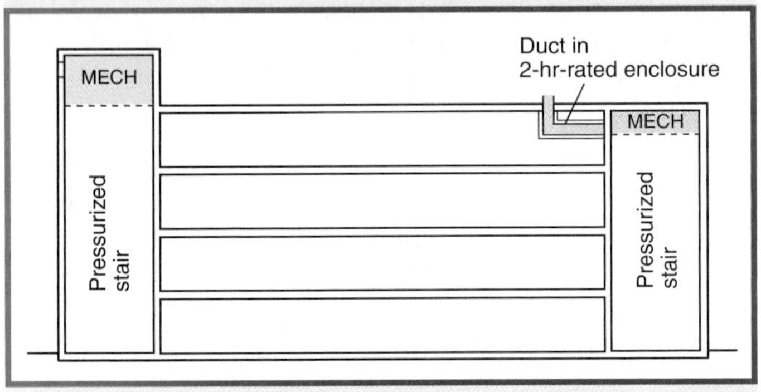


***Exhibit 7.55** Mechanical equipment and ductwork complying with 7.2.3.9.2(2).*

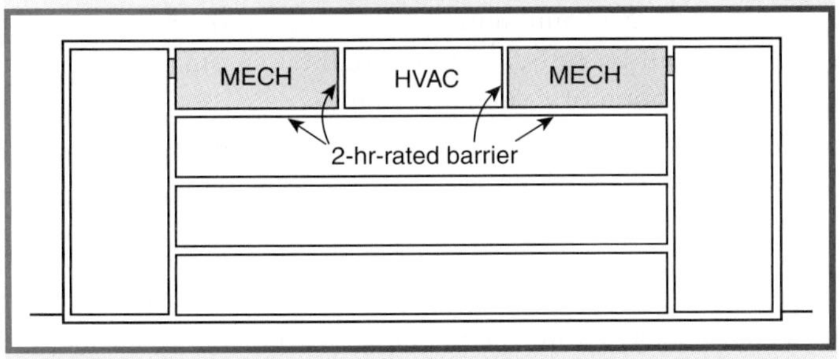


***Exhibit 7.56** Mechanical equipment and ductwork complying with 7.2.3.9.2(3).*

7.56, the required fire-rated separation is permitted to be reduced from 2 hours to 1 hour where the building, including the stairway enclosure, is protected throughout by an approved, supervised automatic sprinkler system.

**7.2.3.10 Activation of Mechanical Ventilation and Pressurized Enclosure Systems.**

**7.2.3.10.1** For both mechanical ventilation and pressurized enclosure systems, the activation of the systems shall be initiated by a smoke detector installed in an approved location within 10 ft (3050 mm) of each entrance to the smokeproof enclosure.

Paragraph 7.2.3.10.1 was revised for the 2009 edition of the *Code* to clarify that a smoke detector for activation of the ventilation system must be positioned at each entrance to the smokeproof enclosure. In prior editions, the requirement was for a smoke detector to be positioned at the entrance. Each entrance must be monitored for smoke.

**7.2.3.10.2** The required mechanical system shall operate upon the activation of the smoke detectors specified in 7.2.3.10.1 and by manual controls accessible to the fire department. The required system also shall be initiated by the following, if provided:

(1) Waterflow signal from a complete automatic sprinkler system
(2) General evacuation alarm signal *(see 9.6.3.6)*

**7.2.3.11 Door Leaf Closers.** The activation of an automatic-closing device on any door leaf in the smokeproof enclosure shall activate all other automatic-closing devices on door leaves in the smokeproof enclosure.

**7.2.3.12 Emergency Power Supply System (EPSS).** Power shall be provided as follows:

(1) A Type 60, Class 2, Level 2 EPSS for new mechanical ventilation equipment shall be provided in accordance with NFPA 110, *Standard for Emergency and Standby Power Systems.*
(2) A previously approved existing standby power generator installation with a fuel supply adequate to operate the equipment for 2 hours shall be permitted in lieu of 7.2.3.12(1).
(3) The generator shall be located in a room separated from the remainder of the building by fire barriers having a minimum 1-hour fire resistance rating.

A Type 60 emergency power supply system (EPSS) must restore power within 60 seconds of the failure of the primary power source. A Class 2 EPSS must be capable of operating at its rated load without being refueled for a minimum of 2 hours. Level 2 performance is specified based on the technical committee's judgment that failure of the EPSS is less critical to human life and safety.

For an example where Level 1 performance, for EPSS critical to human life and safety, is specified in the *Code*, see 7.9.2.2, which is related to new emergency power systems for emergency lighting. See also NFPA 110, *Standard for Emergency and Standby Power Systems.*[19]

**7.2.3.13 Testing.** Before the mechanical equipment is accepted by the authority having jurisdiction, it shall be tested to confirm that it is operating in compliance with the requirements of 7.2.3. All operating parts of the system shall be tested semiannually by approved personnel, and a log shall be kept of the results.

## 7.2.4 Horizontal Exits.

### 7.2.4.1 General.

**7.2.4.1.1** Where horizontal exits are used in the means of egress, they shall conform to the general requirements of Section 7.1 and the special requirements of 7.2.4.

**7.2.4.1.2*** Horizontal exits shall be permitted to be substituted for other exits where the total egress capacity and the total number of the other exits (stairs, ramps, door openings leading outside the building) is not less than half that required for the entire area of the building or connected buildings, and provided that none of the other exits is a horizontal exit, unless otherwise permitted by 7.2.4.1.3.

**A.7.2.4.1.2** An example of one way to provide the required egress capacity from the upper floor of a department store building measuring 350 ft × 200 ft (107 m × 61 m), with an occupant load of 1166 per floor, would be to furnish eight 1120 mm (44 in.) stairs. *[See Figure A.7.2.4.1.2(a).]*

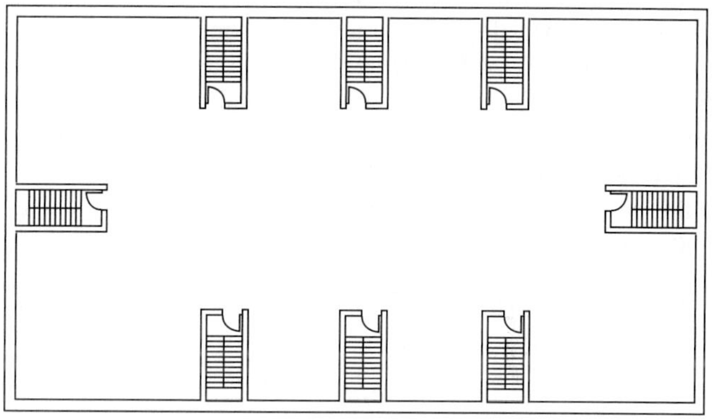

***Figure A.7.2.4.1.2(a)*** *Eight Exits, Required to Provide Necessary Egress Capacity, with None via Horizontal Exit.*

The building is assumed to be divided into two sections by a fire barrier meeting the requirements for a horizontal exit, one 130 ft × 200 ft (40 m × 61 m), and the other 220 ft × 200 ft (67 m × 61 m), with two pairs of 46 in. (1170 mm) double egress doors, with each door providing 44 in. (1120 mm) of clear egress width. *[See Figure A.7.2.4.1.2(b).]* The smaller section, considered separately, will require the equivalent of three 44 in. (1120 mm) exit stairs, and the larger section will require five such exits. The horizontal exits will serve as one of the three exits required for the smaller section, and two of the five exits required for the larger section. Therefore, only two 44 in. (1120 mm) exit stairs from the smaller section and three 44 in. (1120 mm) exit stairs from the larger section will be required if the exits

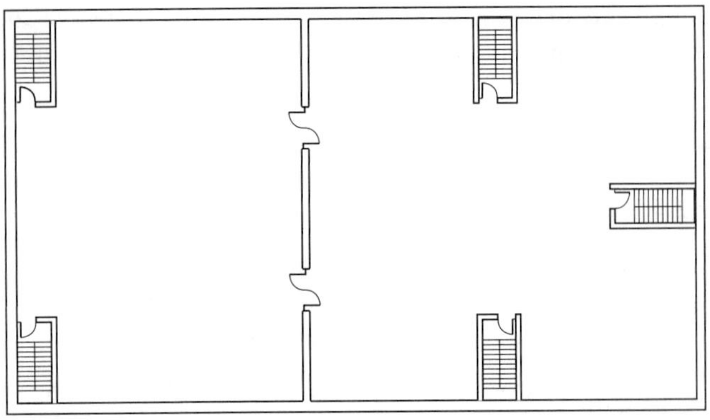

*Figure A.7.2.4.1.2(b) Number of Stairs Reduced by Three Through Use of Two Horizontal Exits; Egress Capacity Not Reduced.*

can be arranged to meet the requirements for the 150 ft (46 m) travel distance permitted from any point in a nonsprinklered building. Thus, the total number of exit stairs required for the building will be five, as compared to eight if no horizontal exit had been provided.

Another option would be the use of two 56 in. (1420 mm) exit stairs from the larger section, which would reduce the total number of stairways required from the floor to four *[see Figure A.7.2.4.1.2(c)]*. However, if the building were further subdivided by a second fire wall meeting the requirements for a horizontal exit, no further reduction in stairways would be permitted in order to comply with the requirement that horizontal exits provide a maximum of one-half of egress capacity.

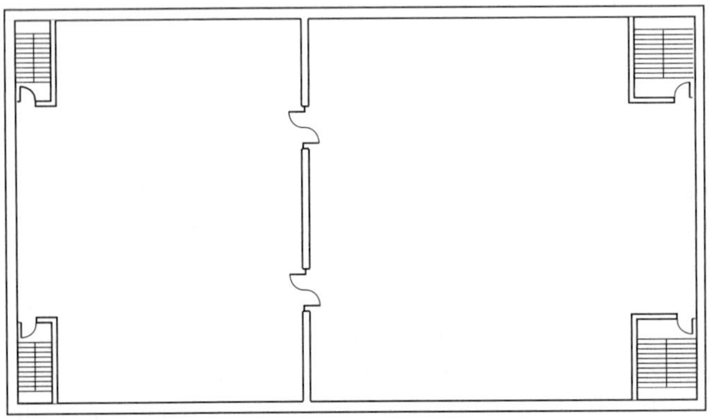

*Figure A.7.2.4.1.2(c) Number of Stairs Further Reduced by Widening Stairs in Larger Compartment, But Not to Less than One-Half the Required Number and Capacity of Exits from That Compartment.*

**7.2.4.1.3** The requirement of 7.2.4.1.2 shall not apply to the following:

(1) Health care occupancies as otherwise provided in Chapters 18 and 19

(2) Detention and correctional occupancies as otherwise provided in Chapters 22 and 23

A horizontal exit is a combination of fire-rated walls with fire-rated door assemblies providing passage from one building area into another building area; each area is a fire compartment independent of the other compartment. A horizontal exit, however, need not be confined to one building. It can be used as a bridge from one building to another. Just as with other types of exits, the horizontal exit has components consisting of door assemblies and enclosure walls. Structural features, such as bridges and balconies, are sometimes used in the passage from one area to the other. Horizontal exits typically do not include stairs or ramps, because they are usually located on the same level as the area from which escape is desired. See the definition of *horizontal exit* in 3.3.75.1, which includes the words "passage through . . . a fire barrier to an area of refuge on approximately the same level . . ."

Horizontal exits are internal exits that might be located some distance from a door assembly leading to the outside at the level of exit discharge or to an exit stair enclosure on a floor above the level of exit discharge, so the *Code* permits them to provide not more than one-half the required number of exits and not more than one-half of the egress capacity of the building or buildings that they connect. However, in health care occupancies and detention and correctional occupancies, special exemptions apply to permit additional reliance on horizontal exits as part of a defend-in-place protection strategy, as noted in 7.2.4.1.3.

Before any space can be used as an occupant accumulation area on either side of a horizontal exit, it must satisfy certain criteria. Such a space, although separated with 2-hour fire barriers (see 7.2.4.3 for details on the fire barrier), cannot be used as a horizontal exit unless there is at least one standard type of exit (not an additional horizontal exit) leading from the space to ensure occupants are not trapped within a fire compartment with no other way out. Additionally, the compartment must be large enough to provide occupant accumulation space for the occupants of both the fire compartment containing the fire and the non-fire compartment, allowing 3 $ft^2$ (0.28 $m^2$) of floor space per person. The accumulation space permits occupants of the refuge compartment to wait in safety until the standard type of exits from the compartment (which are not required to be sized to accommodate the total accumulated number of occupants) can accommodate everyone.

The required accumulation space per person is increased in health care occupancies, because occupants might be on gurneys and stretchers; the accumulation space is also increased in detention and correctional occupancies, where the residents are normally held in the non-fire compartment for a considerable time, rather than being released to the outside, because crowded conditions might lead to behavioral problems among the residents. The nature of a horizontal exit is such that it provides psychological comfort. Being held in an area or building that is away from the fire reassures occupants and prevents disorderly movement.

Exhibit 7.57 illustrates how to apply the requirement of 7.2.4.1.2 when substituting horizontal exits for other exits. Note that the door assemblies in the horizontal exits (circled) substitute for exit stair enclosures. For example, the two horizontal exit door leaves that swing into Compartment A are permitted to be substituted for the exit stair enclosures in Compartment B that are designated as numbers 1 and 3 [see 7.2.4.3.8(1)]. The two horizontal exit door leaves that swing into Compartment B might provide sufficient egress width to be substituted for two of the exit stair enclosures in Compartment A, but to do so would violate the limitation of 7.2.4.1.2 that horizontal exits not comprise more than one-half of the required number of exits for a compartment, so only one exit stair enclosure, designated as number 2, is rendered unnecessary in Compartment A via the creation of the horizontal exits.

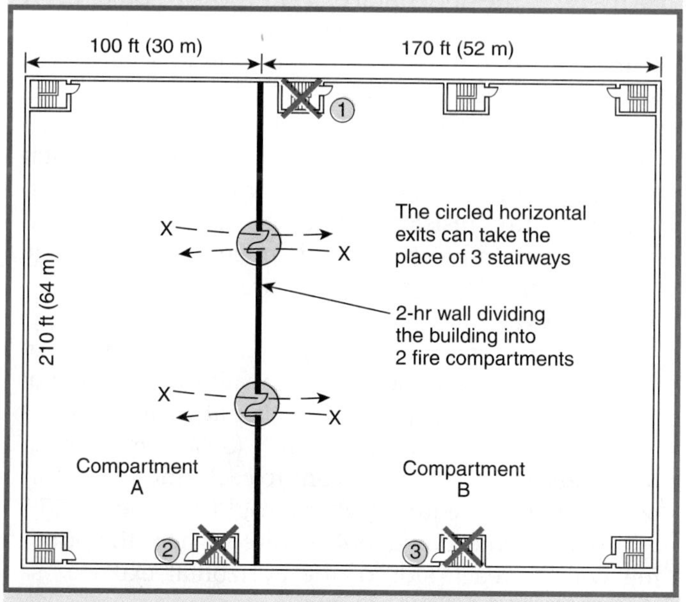


***Exhibit 7.57*** *Example of substituting horizontal exits for other exits.*

**7.2.4.2 Fire Compartments.**

**7.2.4.2.1** Every fire compartment for which credit is permitted in connection with a horizontal exit(s) also shall have at least one additional exit, but not less than 50 percent of the required number and capacity of exits, that is not a horizontal exit, unless otherwise provided in 7.2.4.2.1.2.

**7.2.4.2.1.1** Any fire compartment not having an exit leading outside shall be considered as part of an adjoining compartment with an exit leading to the outside.

**7.2.4.2.1.2** The requirement of 7.2.4.2.1 shall not apply to the following:

(1) Health care occupancies as otherwise provided in Chapters 18 and 19
(2) Detention and correctional occupancies as otherwise provided in Chapters 22 and 23

**7.2.4.2.2** Every horizontal exit for which credit is permitted shall be arranged so that there are continuously available paths of travel leading from each side of the exit to stairways or other means of egress leading to outside the building.

**7.2.4.2.3** Wherever either side of a horizontal exit is occupied, the door leaves used in connection with the horizontal exit shall be unlocked from the egress side, unless otherwise permitted for the following:

(1) Health care occupancies as provided in Chapters 18 and 19
(2) Detention and correctional occupancies as provided in Chapters 22 and 23

**7.2.4.2.4** The floor area on either side of a horizontal exit shall be sufficient to hold the occupants of both floor areas and shall provide at least 3 $ft^2$ (0.28 $m^2$) clear floor area per person, unless otherwise permitted for the following:

(1) Health care occupancies as provided in Chapters 18 and 19
(2) Detention and correctional occupancies as provided in Chapters 22 and 23

The design of a horizontal exit and the incorporation of a horizontal exit into a building are not complicated. For proper arrangement of the total means of egress system, it is simply a matter of designing each separated portion, or compartment, as if it were a completely separate building. The point of passage through the door assembly in the horizontal exit is treated as if it were passage through an exterior exit door assembly. Egress capacity for each compartment is calculated to accommodate the occupant load of the compartment before anyone leaves and before anyone from an adjacent compartment arrives.

Although each compartment must contain sufficient available floor area [at least 3 $ft^2$ (0.28 $m^2$) per person for the total occupant load of both the compartment in question and the number of occupants from the adjacent compartment that are credited with traveling through the doors in the horizontal exit], such floor area is intended to serve as temporary refuge, as occupants are not expected to remain in the safe compartment indefinitely. Egress from the safe compartment continues through its other exits, such as enclosed exit stairs or door assemblies to the outside. The 2-hour fire resistance–rated barrier separating the safe compartment from the compartment of fire origin provides the additional time needed for all occupants to egress the building. Egress through other exits might be relatively slow, because such exits are typically sized for some portion of the initial occupant load of that safe compartment alone, not the combined load that includes occupants from other compartments.

**7.2.4.3 Fire Barriers.**

**7.2.4.3.1** Fire barriers separating buildings or areas between which there are horizontal exits shall have a minimum 2-hour fire resistance rating, unless otherwise provided in 7.2.4.4.1, and shall provide a separation that is continuous to the finished ground level. *(See also Section 8.3.)*

**7.2.4.3.2 Reserved.**

**7.2.4.3.3** Where a fire barrier provides a horizontal exit in any story of a building, such fire barrier shall not be required on other stories, provided that the following criteria are met:

(1) The stories on which the fire barrier is omitted are separated from the story with the horizontal exit by construction having a fire resistance rating at least equal to that of the horizontal exit fire barrier.
(2) Vertical openings between the story with the horizontal exit and the open fire area story are enclosed with construction having a fire resistance rating at least equal to that of the horizontal exit fire barrier.
(3) All required exits, other than horizontal exits, discharge directly to the outside.

Exhibit 7.58 illustrates how the exemption detailed in 7.2.4.3.3 can be used to avoid extending the 2-hour fire resistance–rated barrier vertically through all floors. Horizontal exits occur on floors 5 and 6 only. Fire-rated floor/ceiling assemblies and associated supporting construction (beams, girders, columns) provide the needed separation between the floors with horizontal exits and those without them.

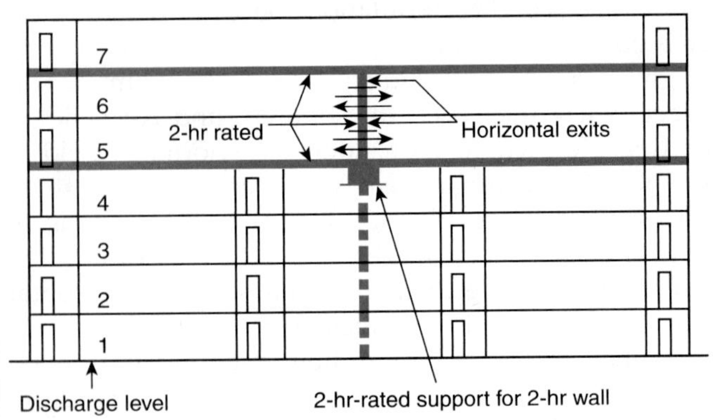


***Exhibit 7.58** Building with horizontal exits on certain floors only.*

**7.2.4.3.4** Where fire barriers serving horizontal exits, other than existing horizontal exits, terminate at outside walls, and the outside walls are at an angle of less than 180 degrees for a distance of 10 ft (3050 mm) on each side of the horizontal exit, the outside walls shall have a minimum 1-hour fire resistance rating, with opening protectives having a minimum $^3/_4$-hour fire protection rating, for a distance of 10 ft (3050 mm) on each side of the horizontal exit.

Paragraph 7.2.4.3.4 requires additional protection where the horizontal exit wall joins the building's exterior wall if there is potential at that location for fire to spread to the adjoining fire compartment. Such potential is judged to exist where the building walls on each side of the horizontal exit expose each other at an angle of less than 180 degrees. The intent is the same as in 7.2.2.6.3 for the protection of exterior walls associated with outside stairs.

The required 10 ft (3050 mm) extensions to each side of the 2-hour fire resistance–rated horizontal exit only need to have a 1-hour fire resistance rating. One-hour fire resistance–rated walls are permitted $^3/_4$-hour fire protection–rated opening protectives; therefore, the rated extensions are permitted to use fire windows.

The concept of the 180-degree rule is illustrated in Exhibit 7.59. Where the building walls on each side of the horizontal exit expose each other at an angle of less than 180 degrees, additional 10 ft (3050 mm), 1-hour fire protection–rated extensions to each side of the horizontal exit are required. At the right of Exhibit 7.59, additional protection is not required where the building walls at each side of the horizontal exit expose each other at a full 180 degrees.

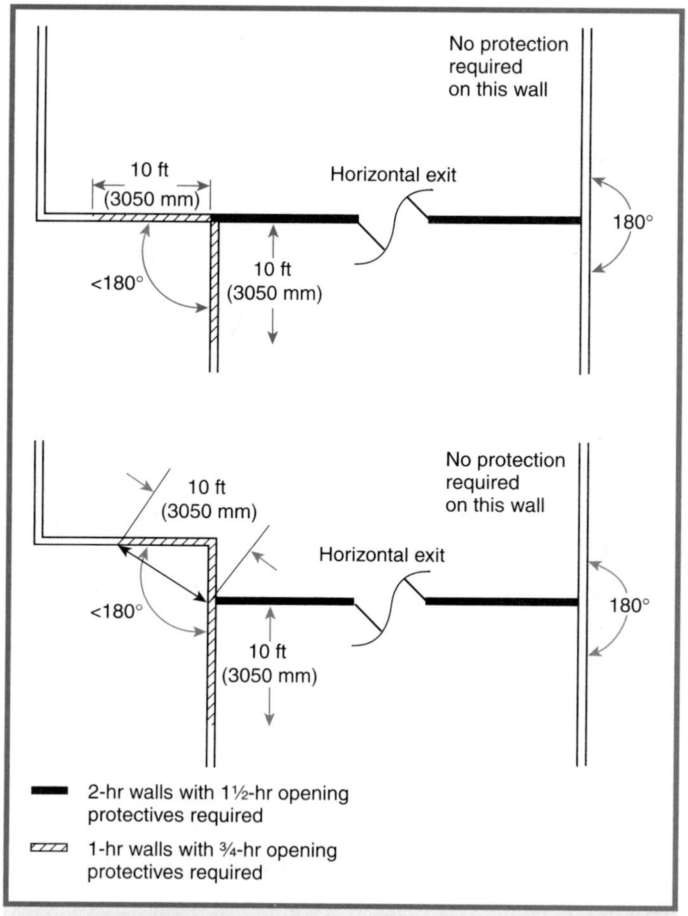


***Exhibit 7.59** Protection of building exterior walls abutting a horizontal exit.*

**7.2.4.3.5** Fire barriers forming horizontal exits shall not be penetrated by ducts, unless one of the following criteria is met:

(1) The ducts are existing penetrations protected by approved and listed fire dampers.
(2) The building is protected throughout by an approved, supervised automatic sprinkler system in accordance with Section 9.7.
(3) The duct penetrations are those permitted in detention and correctional occupancies as otherwise provided in Chapters 22 and 23 and are protected by combination fire dampers/smoke leakage–rated dampers that meet the smoke damper actuation requirements of 8.5.5.

Paragraph 7.2.4.3.5 addresses horizontal exit barrier penetrations other than those provided for door assemblies used for accessing the adjacent fire compartments. Because horizontal exit barriers usually subdivide floor spaces, any prohibition on penetrations by ductwork complicates the design and installation of the heating, ventilating, and air-conditioning system.

Paragraph 7.2.4.3.5(1) recognizes existing ductwork penetrations only if the penetrations are protected by listed fire dampers that are also approved by the authority having jurisdiction.

Paragraph 7.2.4.3.5(2) provides for an acceptable level of safety and permits duct penetrations. Such penetrations are permitted if sprinklers protect the building throughout. The penetrating duct also requires an approved fire damper, because the horizontal exit is a 2-hour fire-rated barrier.

Paragraph 7.2.4.3.5(3) recognizes that local policy prohibits some detention and correctional occupancies from having automatic sprinkler protection. Nonsprinklered buildings are not permitted to use 7.2.4.3.5(2), yet horizontal exits are desirable means of egress features in this defend-in-place occupancy. Duct penetrations, therefore, are permitted if protected by combination fire/smoke leakage–rated dampers that meet the smoke damper actuation requirements of 8.5.5.

**7.2.4.3.6** Any opening in the fire barriers specified in 7.2.4.3.5 shall be protected as provided in 8.3.4.

**7.2.4.3.7** Door assemblies in horizontal exits shall comply with 7.2.1.4, unless they are sliding door assemblies in industrial or storage occupancies as otherwise provided in Chapters 40 and 42.

An exemption for industrial occupancies in Chapter 40 and an exemption for storage occupancies in Chapter 42 permit a fire-rated sliding door assembly in addition to a swinging door assembly in a door opening in a horizontal exit. Such a door assembly might be installed for property protection, insurance-related reasons, or building code compliance. See 40.2.2.5.2 and 42.2.2.5.2.

**7.2.4.3.8** Unless otherwise specified in 7.2.4.3.8.1 and 7.2.4.3.8.2, swinging fire door assemblies shall be permitted in horizontal exits, provided that the criteria of both 7.2.4.3.8(1) and (2), or the criteria of both 7.2.4.3.8(1) and (3), are met as follows:

(1) The door leaves shall swing in the direction of egress travel.
(2) In other than sleeping room areas in detention and correctional occupancies, where a horizontal exit serves areas on both sides of a fire barrier, adjacent openings

with swinging door leaves that open in opposite directions shall be provided, with signs on each side of the fire barrier identifying the door leaf that swings with the travel from that side.

(3) The door assemblies shall be of any other approved arrangement, provided that the door leaves always swing with any possible egress travel.

**7.2.4.3.8.1** The requirements of 7.2.4.3.8 shall not apply to horizontal exit door leaf swing as provided in Chapters 19 and 23.

**7.2.4.3.8.2** The requirements of 7.2.4.3.8 shall not apply to horizontal exit door assemblies in corridors not more than 6 ft (1830 mm) wide in existing buildings.

Paragraph 7.2.4.3.8.2 recognizes the impracticality and hardship of installing a pair of door leaves that meets the minimum width requirements of 7.2.1.2.3.2 in an opening across an existing corridor that is 6 ft (1830 mm) or less in width.

**7.2.4.3.9** Door leaves in horizontal exits shall be designed and installed to minimize air leakage. New door assemblies in horizontal exits shall be installed in accordance with NFPA 105, *Standard for the Installation of Smoke Door Assemblies and Other Opening Protectives.*

Note that new door assemblies in horizontal exits are required to meet performance-based smoke leakage criteria contained in NFPA 105, *Standard for the Installation of Smoke Door Assemblies,* as well as the criterion of the first sentence of 7.2.4.3.9 related to minimization of air leakage. Existing door assemblies are evaluated qualitatively against the air leakage minimization criterion only.

**7.2.4.3.10*** All fire door assemblies in horizontal exits shall be self-closing or automatic-closing in accordance with 7.2.1.8.

**A.7.2.4.3.10** Fusible link–actuated automatic-closing doors do not qualify for use in horizontal exits under these provisions, because smoke might pass through the opening before there is sufficient heat to release the hold-open device. Such doors are also objectionable because, once closed, they are difficult to open and would inhibit orderly egress.

**7.2.4.3.11** Horizontal exit door assemblies located across a corridor, other than approved existing door assemblies, shall be automatic-closing in accordance with 7.2.1.8.2.

Because cross-corridor door assemblies are so commonly wedged open in violation of *Code* requirements, 7.2.4.3.11 does not offer the option of using self-closing door assemblies but mandates the use of automatic-closing door assemblies in these horizontal exit, cross-corridor locations. Because the authority having jurisdiction can observe if the wedging open of door leaves has been a problem in existing installations, 7.2.4.3.11 gives the enforcer the authority to permit existing self-closing door assemblies to continue to be used.

**7.2.4.4 Bridges Serving Horizontal Exits Between Buildings.** The provisions of 7.2.4.4 shall apply to bridges serving horizontal exits between buildings and to the associated horizontal exit fire barrier.

**7.2.4.4.1** The minimum 2-hour fire resistance–rated barrier required by 7.2.4.3.1 shall extend as follows:

(1) Vertically from the ground to a point 10 ft (3050 mm) above the bridge or to the roofline, whichever is lower
(2) Horizontally for not less than 10 ft (3050 mm) to each side of the bridge

**7.2.4.4.2** Any opening in the fire barrier addressed in 7.2.4.4.1 shall be protected with fire door assemblies or fixed fire window assemblies having a $^3/_4$-hour fire protection rating, unless otherwise provided in 7.2.4.4.3.

**7.2.4.4.3** The requirement of 7.2.4.4.2 shall not apply to approved existing bridges.

**7.2.4.4.4** Where the bridge serves as a horizontal exit in one direction, the horizontal exit door leaf shall be required to swing only in the direction of egress travel, unless the door leaf complies with the swing requirements for the following:

(1) Existing health care occupancies in Chapter 19
(2) Existing detention and correctional occupancies in Chapter 23

**7.2.4.4.5** Where the bridge serves as a horizontal exit in both directions, door leaves shall be provided in pairs that swing in opposite directions, with only the door leaf swinging in the direction of egress travel included when determining egress capacity, unless otherwise provided in 7.2.4.4.5.1 through 7.2.4.4.5.3.

**7.2.4.4.5.1** Approved existing door assemblies on both ends of the bridge shall be permitted to swing out from the building.

**7.2.4.4.5.2** The requirement of 7.2.4.4.5 shall not apply to existing bridges if the bridge has sufficient floor area to accommodate the occupant load of either connected building or fire area based on 3 ft$^2$ (0.28 m$^2$) per person.

**7.2.4.4.5.3** The requirement of 7.2.4.4.5 shall not apply to horizontal exit door leaf swing as provided for the following:

(1) Existing health care occupancies in Chapter 19
(2) Existing detention and correctional occupancies in Chapter 23

**7.2.4.4.6** Every bridge shall be not less than the width of the door opening to which it leads and shall be not less than 44 in. (1120 mm) wide for new construction.

**7.2.4.4.7** In climates subject to the accumulation of snow and ice, the bridge floor shall be protected to prevent the accumulation of snow and ice.

**7.2.4.4.8** In existing buildings, one step not exceeding 8 in. (205 mm) shall be permitted below the level of the inside floor.

### 7.2.5 Ramps.

Ramps are permitted as a part of a means of egress and are preferred over stairs under some circumstances. To quote from a 1974 publication:

> One can consider ramps and steps simply as prosthetic devices for assisting the human organism in climbing from floor to floor . . . When one must consider the energy cost of both horizontal and vertical movement, one finds that a ramp with a gradient of less than about eight degrees is more economical than any stairway that is likely to be encountered in normal activity.[20]

A study by the National Bureau of Standards, now the National Institute of Standards and Technology (NIST), states, in part:

> For certain occupancies, such as schools and institutions, they [ramps] are believed to be more satisfactory and their use in these buildings is recommended . . . Ramps have a rate of discharge between that of stairways and level passageways.[21]

**7.2.5.1 General.** Every ramp used as a component in a means of egress shall conform to the general requirements of Section 7.1 and to the special requirements of 7.2.5.

**7.2.5.2 Dimensional Criteria.** The following dimensional criteria shall apply to ramps:

(1) New ramps shall be in accordance with Table 7.2.5.2(a), unless otherwise permitted by the following:

(a) Table 7.2.5.2(a) shall not apply to industrial equipment access areas as provided in 40.2.5.2.

*Table 7.2.5.2(a) New Ramps*

| Feature | Dimensional Criteria | |
|---|---|---|
| | in. | mm |
| Minimum width clear of all obstructions, except projections not more than $4\frac{1}{2}$ in. (114 mm) at or below handrail height on each side | 44 | 1120 |
| Maximum slope | 1 in 12 | |
| Maximum cross slope | 1 in 48 | |
| Maximum rise for a single ramp run | 30 | 760 |

(b) The maximum slope requirement shall not apply to ramps in assembly occupancies as provided in Chapter 12.
(c) The maximum slope or maximum rise for a single ramp run shall not apply to ramps providing access to vehicles, vessels, mobile structures, and aircraft.

(2) Existing ramps shall be permitted to remain in use or be rebuilt, provided that they meet the requirements shown in Table 7.2.5.2(b), unless otherwise permitted by the following:

(a) The requirements of Table 7.2.5.2(b) shall not apply to industrial equipment access areas as provided in 40.2.5.2.
(b) The maximum slope or maximum height between landings for a single ramp run shall not apply to ramps providing access to vehicles, vessels, mobile structures, and aircraft.
(c) Approved existing ramps with slopes not steeper than 1 in 6 shall be permitted to remain in use.
(d) Existing ramps with slopes not steeper than 1 in 10 shall not be required to be provided with landings.

*Table 7.2.5.2(b) Existing Ramps*

| Feature | Dimensional Criteria | |
|---|---|---|
| | ft/in. | mm |
| Minimum width | 30 in. | 760 |
| Maximum slope | 1 in 8 | |
| Maximum height between landings | 12 ft | 3660 |

The dimensional criteria and other details applicable to ramps were extensively rewritten for the 1994 edition of the *Code*. In the 1994 and 1997 editions, the maximum allowed slope of a new ramp varied with the total vertical rise provided by the ramp. In each subsequent edition, the slope of new ramps has been limited to a maximum of 1 in 12. Such ramps are particularly useful for persons with severe mobility impairment. See ICC/ANSI A117.1, *American National Standard for Accessible and Usable Buildings and Facilities.* Paragraph 7.2.5.2(2) continues to recognize existing ramps and the rebuilding of existing ramps to the former criteria.

Paragraphs 7.2.5.2(1)(c) and 7.2.5.2(2)(b) recognize that ramps providing access to vehicles, vessels, mobile structures, and aircraft must be able to accommodate the variety of conditions encountered. For example, not all ships have entrances mounted at the same height, and, due to tidal influences, the water level rises and falls with respect to a stationary pier. Because ships are regulated under special rules, have their own exiting programs, and usually provide staff assistance during the disembarkation process, ramps to ships are exempt from the maximum ramp slope requirements of Table 7.2.5.2(a) and Table 7.2.5.2(b).

**7.2.5.3 Ramp Details.**

**7.2.5.3.1 Construction.** Ramp construction shall be as follows:

(1) All ramps serving as required means of egress shall be of permanent fixed construction.
(2) Each ramp in buildings required by this *Code* to be of Type I or Type II construction shall be any combination of noncombustible or limited-combustible material or fire-retardant-treated wood.
(3) Ramps constructed with fire-retardant-treated wood shall be not more than 30 in. (760 mm) high, shall have an area of not more than 3000 $ft^2$ (277 $m^2$), and shall not occupy more than 50 percent of the room area.
(4) The ramp floor and landings shall be solid and without perforations.

**7.2.5.3.2 Landings.** Ramp landings shall be as follows:

(1) Ramps shall have landings located at the top, at the bottom, and at door leaves opening onto the ramp.
(2) The slope of the landing shall be not steeper than 1 in 48.
(3) Every landing shall have a width not less than the width of the ramp.
(4) Every landing, except as otherwise provided in 7.2.5.3.2(5), shall be not less than 60 in. (1525 mm) long in the direction of travel, unless the landing is an approved existing landing.
(5) Where the ramp is not part of an accessible route, the ramp landings shall not be required to exceed 48 in. (1220 mm) in the direction of travel, provided that the ramp has a straight run.
(6) Any changes in travel direction shall be made only at landings, unless the ramp is an existing ramp.
(7) Ramps and intermediate landings shall continue with no decrease in width along the direction of egress travel.

Landings are required to be nearly horizontal to provide transition areas to and from ramps that are usable to persons with severe mobility impairments (see 3.3.228). Landings at door openings allow for movement through the door opening without the burden of dealing with a sloping floor section. The requirement for intermediate landings on ramps is similar to that part of 7.2.2.3.2 applicable to landings on stairs.

The minimum 60 in. (1525 mm) landing depth, measured in the direction of travel, is intended to accommodate a person in a wheelchair. Thus, 7.2.5.3.2(5) permits the landing depth on straight run portions of the ramp to be decreased to 48 in. (1220 mm) where the ramp is not part of an accessible route (see 3.3.3).

The effect of 7.2.5.3.2(6) is to prohibit curved ramps. With a curved ramp, the travel direction changes continually. The change in direction is accomplished by introducing a cross slope that might make use of the ramp by persons with severe mobility impairments overly burdensome. Thus, the *Code* requires that any changes in travel direction occur only at level landings.

**7.2.5.3.3 Drop-Offs.** Ramps and landings with drop-offs shall have curbs, walls, railings, or projecting surfaces that prevent people from traveling off the edge of the ramp. Curbs or barriers shall be not less than 4 in. (100 mm) in height.

**7.2.5.4 Guards and Handrails.**

**7.2.5.4.1** Guards complying with 7.2.2.4 shall be provided for ramps, unless otherwise provided in 7.2.5.4.4.

**7.2.5.4.2** Handrails complying with 7.2.2.4 shall be provided along both sides of a ramp run with a rise greater than 6 in. (150 mm), unless otherwise provided in 7.2.5.4.4.

**7.2.5.4.3** The height of handrails and guards shall be measured vertically to the top of the guard or rail from the walking surface adjacent thereto.

**7.2.5.4.4** The requirements of 7.2.5.4.1 and 7.2.5.4.2 shall not apply to guards and handrails provided for ramped aisles in assembly occupancies as otherwise provided in Chapters 12 and 13.

Ramps are subject to the guard and handrail requirements of 7.2.2.4. However, per 7.2.5.4.2, the handrail requirements apply only to ramps with a rise of more than 6 in. (150 mm).

**7.2.5.5 Enclosure and Protection of Ramps.** Ramps in a required means of egress shall be enclosed or protected as a stair in accordance with 7.2.2.5 and 7.2.2.6.

**7.2.5.6 Special Provisions for Outside Ramps.**

Outside ramps are permitted to serve as part of a means of egress, subject to the applicable criteria governing exit access, exits, and exit discharge.

**7.2.5.6.1* Visual Protection.** Outside ramps shall be arranged to avoid any impediments to their use by persons having a fear of high places. Outside ramps more than 36 ft (11 m) above the finished ground level shall be provided with an opaque visual obstruction not less than 48. in. (1220 mm) in height.

**A.7.2.5.6.1** The guards required by 7.1.8 and detailed in 7.2.2.4.5 for the unenclosed sides of ramps will usually meet this requirement where the ramp is not more than 36 ft (11 m) above the finished ground level. Special architectural treatment, including application of such devices as metal or masonry screens and grilles, will usually be necessary to comply with the intent of the requirements for ramps over 36 ft (11 m) above the finished ground level.

**7.2.5.6.2* Water Accumulation.** Outside ramps and landings shall be designed to minimize water accumulation on their surfaces.

**A.7.2.5.6.2** Providing a pitch of $\frac{1}{8}$ in./ft to $\frac{1}{4}$ in./ft (10 mm/m to 21 mm/m) will aid the shedding of water from a nominally horizontal surface.

### 7.2.6* Exit Passageways.

**A.7.2.6** An exit passageway serves as a horizontal means of exit travel that is protected from fire in a manner similar to an enclosed interior exit stair. Where it is desired to offset exit stairs in a multistory building, an exit passageway can be used to preserve the continuity of the protected exit by connecting the bottom of one stair to the top of the stair that continues to the street floor. Probably the most important use of an exit passageway is to satisfy the requirement that at least 50 percent of the exit stairs discharge directly outside from multistory buildings *(see 7.7.2)*. Thus, if it is impractical to locate the stair on an exterior wall, an exit passageway can be connected to the bottom of the stair to convey the occupants safely to an outside exit door. In buildings of extremely large area, such as shopping malls and some factories, the exit passageway can be used to advantage where the travel distance to reach an exit would otherwise be excessive.

The word *exit*, used in the term *exit passageway*, helps to distinguish between an exit passageway and an ordinary passageway or corridor that serves as exit access. An exit passageway is an exit; it provides a path of travel offering the same level of protection and safety that is required of an enclosed exit stair. An exit passageway is a versatile feature, because it can be used to extend an exit, or, as is done in many cases, it can be used to bring an exit closer to where the occupants are located.

In Exhibit 7.60, an exit passageway is used to continue the exit to the outside from one of the two enclosed interior exit stairs. This arrangement might be used to help comply with the requirements of 7.7.2, which mandate that at least one-half of the egress capacity and at least one-half of the number of exits must discharge directly to the outside at the level of exit discharge.

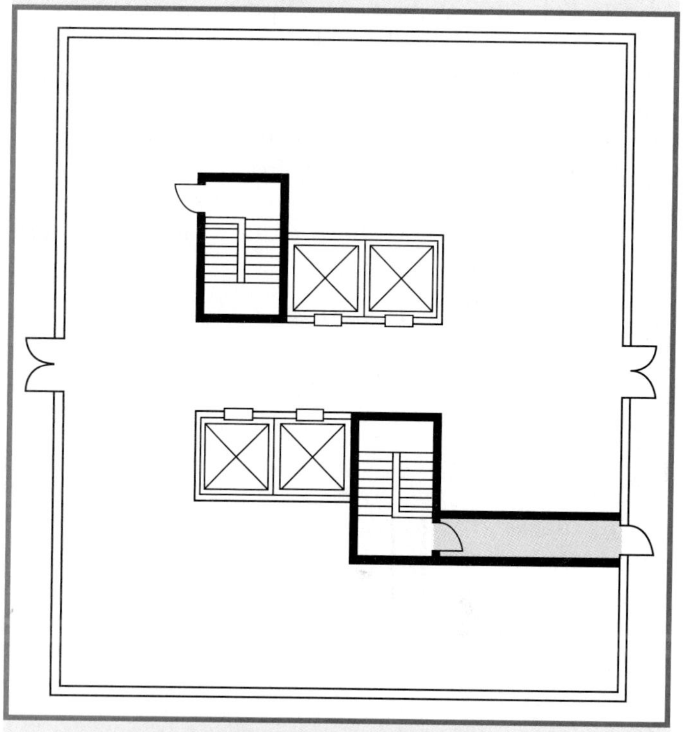

***Exhibit 7.60*** *Exit passageway used to connect exit stair with exterior of building.*

Extending the exit stair's required enclosure to include a portion of the corridor creates an exit passageway that brings the exit closer to the occupants, as is demonstrated in Exhibit 7.61. Travel distance measurement ends at entrance E1 to the exit passageway. The distance from X to E2 exceeds the allowed travel distance. The distance from X to E1 is within the allowed travel distance. Extension of an exit stair's enclosure is often used where travel distance to the exit enclosure would otherwise be in excess of *Code* allowance. Because it is an exit, an exit passageway qualifies as the point at which travel distance measurement ends in accordance with Section 7.6.

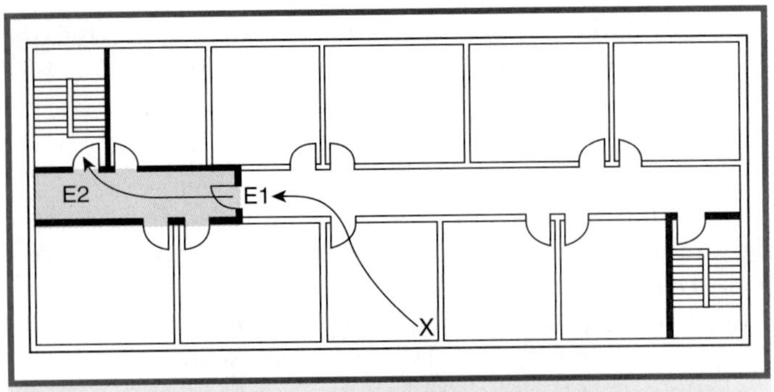


*Exhibit 7.61* Exit passageway used to keep travel distance from becoming excessive.

In Exhibit 7.62, the two exit passageways marked A bring exits within allowable travel distances for the occupants in the mall (similar to the exit passageway illustrated in Exhibit 7.61). The exit passageway marked B allows occupants of multiple stores in the mall to enter the exit directly from the rear of each store. This arrangement is often used to limit, for security purposes, the number of door assemblies that open directly to the outside.

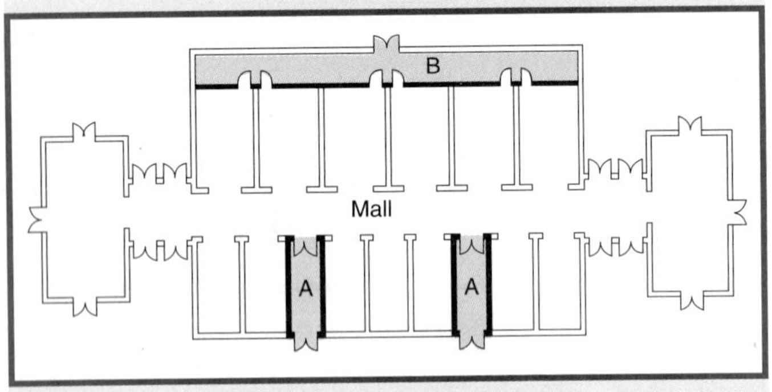


*Exhibit 7.62* Exit passageways used for multiple purposes in mall building.

**7.2.6.1* General.** Exit passageways used as exit components shall conform to the general requirements of Section 7.1 and to the special requirements of 7.2.6.

**A.7.2.6.1** Examples of building elements that might be arranged as exit passageways include hallways, corridors, passages, tunnels, underfloor passageways, or overhead passageways.

**7.2.6.2 Enclosure.** An exit passageway shall be separated from other parts of the building as specified in 7.1.3.2, and the following alternatives shall be permitted:

(1) Fire windows in accordance with 8.3.3 shall be permitted to be installed in the separation in a building protected throughout by an approved, supervised automatic sprinkler system in accordance with Section 9.7.

(2) Existing fixed wired glass panels in steel sash shall be permitted to be continued in use in the separation in buildings protected throughout by an approved, supervised automatic sprinkler system in accordance with Section 9.7.

**7.2.6.3 Stair Discharge.** An exit passageway that serves as a discharge from a stair enclosure shall have not less than the same fire resistance rating and opening protective fire protection rating as those required for the stair enclosure.

Paragraph 7.2.6.2 requires exit passageways to have walls with the hourly fire resistance ratings and door assemblies with the fire protection ratings required of exit stair enclosures, as detailed in 7.1.3.2.1(1) or (2) and 8.3.4.2. The requirement also limits door openings into, and penetrations through, the exit enclosure created by the exit passageway, as detailed in 7.1.3.2.1(8) and (9). In Exhibit 7.63, new exit passageway A on the first floor — the level of exit discharge — opens at one end to a five-story exit stair enclosure and, at the other end, to a door assembly to the outside. This exit passageway also serves as a horizontal continuation of,

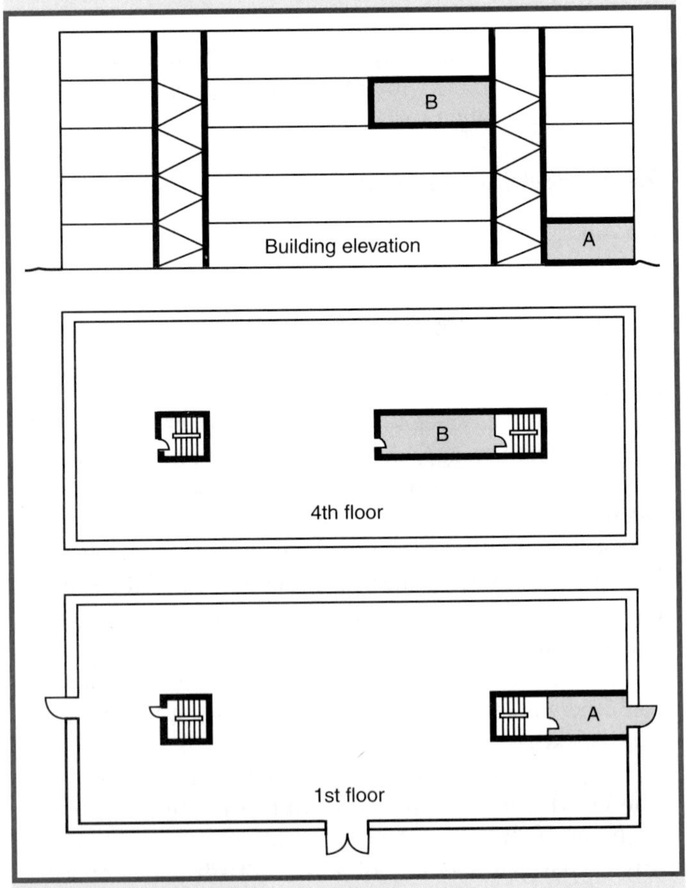


*Exhibit 7.63* Exit passageways with fire resistance–rated enclosures and fire protection–rated door assemblies.

and discharge for, the stair enclosure. In serving as a discharge for the exit stair, the exit passageway must provide the same degree of protection required of the stair enclosure. Given that the exit stair must be enclosed by 2-hour fire resistance–rated construction because it is new and serves four or more stories, the exit passageway must also be enclosed by 2-hour fire resistance–rated construction. This protection is addressed in 7.2.6.3.

In Exhibit 7.63, exit passageway B, on the fourth floor, is used to provide the safety of an exit to occupants traveling to the exit stair enclosure. This exit passageway might have been built to meet the travel distance limitation. If a fire-rated wall and door assembly separate exit passageway B from the new 2-hour exit stair enclosure, the required rating of exit passageway B is only 1 hour, because the exit passageway serves only the occupants of the fourth floor. A similar 1-hour fire resistance–rated enclosure requirement applies, for example, to a horizontal exit serving a single story of a shopping mall building. Contrast this configuration with exit passageway A on the first floor, which potentially serves occupants of the second through fifth floors and must provide a continuation of the 2-hour separation required of the new stair enclosure.

For the same reasons that the exit stair enclosure cannot have door assemblies opening directly onto it from normally unoccupied spaces, a storage room, for example, is prohibited from opening directly onto exit passageways A and B and the exit stair enclosures. Penetrations through the enclosing walls are limited to those necessary for the functioning of life safety systems, such as lighting powered by electrical cables that enter the exit enclosure via properly sealed conduit penetrations. Ductwork for climate control is prohibited from penetrating enclosing walls. Thus, the exit passageways and the exit stair enclosures must receive their heating and cooling by systems independent of those serving the remainder of the building. Ductwork serving other parts of the floor must be routed around the outside of, not through, the exit passageway enclosures.

**7.2.6.4 Width.**

**7.2.6.4.1** The width of an exit passageway shall be sized to accommodate the aggregate required capacity of all exits that discharge through it, unless one of the following conditions applies:

(1)* Where an exit passageway serves occupants of the level of exit discharge as well as other stories, the capacity shall not be required to be aggregated.

**A.7.2.6.4.1(1)** Where an exit passageway serves occupants on the level of exit discharge as well as other floors, it should not be required that the occupant loads be added, thus increasing the width of the exit passageway. The situation is the same as that in which occupants from the level of exit discharge join occupants from upper floors for a few feet of horizontal travel through a stair enclosure.

(2) As provided in Chapters 36 and 37, an exit passageway in a mall building shall be permitted to accommodate occupant loads independently from the mall and the tenant spaces. *(See 36.2.2.7.2 and 37.2.2.7.2.)*

The text in A.7.2.6.4(1) explains the exemption to aggregating the capacity of exit passageways where accommodating occupant loads from various floors. See A.36.2.2.7.2 and the commentary associated with 36.2.2.7.2 (which is positioned within a block of commentary after 36/37.2.2.12.2) for a detailed explanation of the situation permitted in mall buildings by 7.2.6.4(2).

**7.2.6.4.2** In new construction, the minimum width of any exit passageway into which an exit stair discharges, or that serves as a horizontal transfer within an exit stair system, shall meet the following criteria:

(1) The minimum width of the exit passageway shall be not less than two-thirds of the width of the exit stair.
(2) Where stairs are credited with egress capacity in accordance with 7.3.3.2, the exit passageway width shall be sized to accommodate the same capacity as the stair, with such capacity determined by use of the capacity factors in Table 7.3.3.1.

Level travel through exit passageways is typically calculated using a capacity factor of 0.2 in. (5 mm) per person and stair travel width is typically calculated using a capacity factor of 0.3 in. (7.6 mm) per person in accordance with Table 7.3.3.1. The provision of 7.2.6.4.2(1) maintains the 2:3 ratio derived from comparing the two capacity factors and might seem redundant with the requirements of 7.3.3.1. It is presented as part of 7.2.6.4.2 to provide a foundation on which the provision of 7.2.6.4.2(2) builds. The provision of 7.2.6.4.2(2) provides guidance on how to size the exit passageway that serves a stair that utilizes the enhanced capacity provisions of 7.3.3.2. See the commentary that follows A.7.3.3.2.

**7.2.6.5 Floor.** The floor shall be solid and without perforations.

### 7.2.7 Escalators and Moving Walks.

Escalators and moving walks shall not constitute a part of the required means of egress, unless they are previously approved existing escalators and moving walks.

Older editions of the *Code* permitted some egress capacity credit for escalators. However, because riser/tread sections of escalators and standing surfaces of moving walks are removed for maintenance, it cannot be ensured that occupants will be able to walk on these devices when emergency egress is needed. Therefore, new escalators and moving walks receive no credit within the required means of egress. Existing, previously approved escalators and moving walks are permitted to continue to be used as part of the means of egress if permitted by the appropriate occupancy chapter. Although not permitted as part of the required means of egress in new construction, new escalators and moving walks, where installed, must comply with ASME A17.1/CSA B44, *Safety Code for Elevators and Escalators*, and existing escalators and moving walks must comply with ASME A17.3, *Safety Code for Existing Elevators and Escalators.*[22] See 9.4.2.1 and 9.4.2.2.

Escalators are acceptable as an egress component in existing buildings only in the following occupancies:

1. Existing assembly occupancies (13.2.2.8)
2. Existing hotels and dormitories (29.2.2.8)
3. Existing apartment buildings (31.2.2.8)
4. Existing mercantile occupancies (37.2.2.8)
5. Existing business occupancies (39.2.2.8)
6. Existing industrial occupancies (40.2.2.8)

When evaluating existing escalators for occupant egress, the factors that follow should be considered.

**1.** The escalator should comply with the applicable requirements for stairs in 7.2.2. It is assumed that, where escalators serve as required means of egress, they will continue to operate in case of fire. However, if they stop due to electric current failure or other cause, they can be used as ordinary stairs.

**2.** Escalators constituting a means of egress should operate only in the direction of egress. Usually escalators are provided in pairs, with one stairway moving up and another moving down; however, if the electric power fails and both stop, two stairs would be available for movement in the egress direction. In this situation, one might propose that both stairways be accepted as constituting a means of egress, since the power could be turned off intentionally. The problem is that, in an emergency, the power might not be turned off, and one stairway would continue to move against traffic. For this reason, only those escalators moving in the direction of egress should be permitted to be part of a means of egress.

**3.** Escalators should be of the horizontal-tread type and, with the exception of step tread surfaces, handrails, and step wheels, should be of noncombustible construction throughout.

**4.** A single escalator that is 32 in. (810 mm) wide should be given credit for 75 people. An escalator that is 48 in. (1220 mm) wide should be given credit for 150 people. Even though a person does not have to exert any energy or do any moving while on an operating escalator, there are many people who are frightened by escalators and many who are extremely cautious in approaching them. These are factors that could contribute to a bottleneck as user movement is impeded. Thus, it is recognized that an escalator would have to be wider than a stair to accommodate the same number of people.

**5.** There should be unobstructed spaces of at least 4 in. (100 mm) outside the handrail and above the handrail for the full length of the escalator.

**6.** No single escalator should travel uninterrupted for more than one story.

The guidelines of 1 through 6 in this commentary were taken from older editions of the *Code* and were required in those years when escalators were given egress credit in new construction and are offered here as guidance for existing escalator installations credited with serving within the means of egress.

Even in an existing building, an escalator cannot be counted as an exit unless it is enclosed as an exit in accordance with 7.1.3.2. Such an arrangement is rare. Typically, an existing escalator is not enclosed and might, at most, serve as exit access or exit discharge.

Most of the same principles that apply to the design and operation of escalators also apply when evaluating existing moving walkways. The major difference is that a moving walkway that moves in the direction of egress travel can be evaluated in terms of the usual egress width and associated capacity rather than the larger dimensions specified for escalators in item 4 of this commentary.

### 7.2.8 Fire Escape Stairs.

Fire escape stairs and ladders have fallen into disfavor for a variety of reasons, including the following:

1. Unsightly appearance
2. Possible icing in winter weather

3. Expense of maintenance (i.e., the metal is subject to corrosion)
4. Possibility of users being trapped by a fire issuing from unprotected openings at a lower level
5. Fear of height and, therefore, objection to using fire escape stairs and ladders

On the other hand, well-maintained fire escape stairs can and have saved many lives when smoke-filled stairs have become impassable. A classic example is the June 5, 1946, fire in the 22-story LaSalle Hotel in Chicago. Hundreds of people made their escape from the building on outside fire escape stairs.[23]

In the past, fire fighters have found outside fire escape stairs advantageous. However, instances can be cited where corroded fire escapes have collapsed, or where people have been fatally burned because fire broke out of windows or door assemblies at a lower level as they were descending on a fire escape. The *Code* requires proper means of egress using interior or outside stairs and the gradual phasing out of fire escape stairs as new buildings replace existing buildings.

Fire escape stairs can, however, help correct serious means of egress deficiencies in existing buildings and are helpful to fire department rescue and fire-fighting efforts. If fire escape stairs are part of an existing building, or must be included on a building (perhaps due to insufficient space for an outside stair in accordance with 7.2.2), they must adhere to the provisions of the *Code* to provide an acceptable level of life safety.

**7.2.8.1 General.**

**7.2.8.1.1** Fire escape stairs shall comply with the provisions of 7.2.8, unless they are approved existing fire escape stairs.

Fire escape stairs, as specified in 7.2.8 of the *Code*, should not be confused with the outside stairs covered in 7.2.2. Neither should the fire escape stairs specified by 7.2.8 of the *Code* be confused with the inferior fire escapes that are commonly found on old buildings. Such steep, inadequate, and flimsy fire escapes, unshielded against fire in the structure to which they are attached, might give an occupant a false sense of security. Such escape stairs are not recognized by this *Code*.

Even the fire escape stairs constructed in accordance with this *Code* have limitations that might prevent their effective use during a fire. Even where window protection is provided, conditions might be such that fire, or the smoke from fire, on lower floors might render the stairs impassable before the occupants of the upper floors have had time to use them. Fire escape stairs might be blocked by snow or ice when they are most needed. People are likely to be timid about descending fire escape stairs from a considerable height, so their downward travel is much slower than for travel on inside stairs. Slower travel is a factor even where *Code*-specified solid-tread stairs without perforations are used in place of ordinary slatted-tread construction. Fire escape stairs are not the usual means of egress. Occupants of buildings will not use them as readily in the case of fire as they will an inside stair, which is the more common egress component. Because fire escape stairs are an emergency device and are not ordinarily used, their proper upkeep is often neglected.

**7.2.8.1.2** Fire escape stairs shall not constitute any of the required means of egress, unless otherwise provided in 7.2.8.1.2.1 and 7.2.8.1.2.2.

**7.2.8.1.2.1** Fire escape stairs shall be permitted on existing buildings as provided in Chapters 11 through 43 but shall not constitute more than 50 percent of the required means of egress.

**7.2.8.1.2.2** New fire escape stairs shall be permitted to be erected on existing buildings only where the authority having jurisdiction has determined that outside stairs are impractical. *(See 7.2.2.)*

**7.2.8.1.2.3** New fire escape stairs permitted by 7.2.8.1.2.2 shall not incorporate ladders or access windows, regardless of occupancy classification or occupant load served.

No recognition of any kind is given by the *Code* to the use of fire escape stairs in new buildings for any of the three parts of a means of egress. A token recognition of 50 percent of egress capacity is given for their use in existing buildings, simply because the fire escape stairs have already been installed or because such stairs might be the only feasible way in which to upgrade a means of egress in an existing building.

In most cases, outside stairs complying with 7.2.2 must be used rather than fire escape stairs. However, the *Code* recognizes that, in the case of some existing buildings, there are situations in which modifying stairs to comply with 7.2.2 would be impractical. For example, the space between the building and the property line might be too narrow to accommodate a *Code*-conforming stair, or it might be necessary to have the stair located over a sidewalk, alley, or similar space that cannot be permanently blocked by stair construction.

Fire escape stairs are regarded as an expedient remedy for deficiencies in means of egress of existing buildings, where it might not be feasible to provide outside stairs or properly enclosed, additional inside stairways required by the *Code*.

Because effective use of fire escape stairs might be seriously impaired by conditions such as snow and ice, the authorities having jurisdiction might wish to impose additional requirements because of climate. In such a case, egress capacity credit for the fire escape stairs might be reduced.

**7.2.8.1.3** Fire escape stairs of the return-platform type with superimposed runs, or of the straight-run type with a platform that continues in the same direction, shall be permitted. Either type shall be permitted to be parallel to, or at right angles to, buildings. Either type shall be permitted to be attached to buildings or erected independently of buildings and connected by walkways.

**7.2.8.2 Protection of Openings.** Fire escape stairs shall be exposed to the smallest possible number of window and door openings, and each opening shall be protected with approved fire door or fire window assemblies where the opening or any portion of the opening is located as follows:

(1) Horizontally, within 15 ft (4570 mm) of any balcony, platform, or stairway constituting a component of the fire escape stair
(2) Below, within three stories or 36 ft (11 m) of any balcony, platform, walkway, or stairway constituting a component of the fire escape stair, or within two stories or 24 ft (7320 mm) of a platform or walkway leading from any story to the fire escape stair
(3) Above, within 10 ft (3050 mm) of any balcony, platform, or walkway, as measured vertically, or within 10 ft (3050 mm) of any stair tread surface, as measured vertically
(4) Facing a court served by a fire escape stair, where the least dimension of the court does not exceed one-third of the height to the uppermost platform of the fire escape stair, measured from the finished ground level
(5) Facing an alcove served by a fire escape stair, where the width of the alcove does not exceed one-third, or the depth of the alcove does not exceed one-fourth, of the height to the uppermost platform of the fire escape stair, measured from the finished ground level

**7.2.8.2.1** The requirements of 7.2.8.2 shall not apply to openings located on the top story where stairs do not lead to the roof.

**7.2.8.2.2** The requirements of 7.2.8.2 shall be permitted to be modified by the authority having jurisdiction where automatic sprinkler protection is provided, where the occupancy is limited to low hazard contents, or where other special conditions exist.

**7.2.8.2.3** The requirements of 7.2.8.2 for the protection of window openings shall not apply where such window openings are necessary for access to existing fire escape stairs.

**7.2.8.3 Access.**

**7.2.8.3.1** Access to fire escape stairs shall be in accordance with 7.2.8.4 and 7.5.1.1.1 through 7.5.1.2.2.

Exhibit 7.64 illustrates the minimum opening dimensions for windows that open onto fire escape stairs serving more than 10 occupants. The exhibit also depicts the maximum interior measurements from the floor to the windowsill. See Table 7.2.8.4.1(a) and Table 7.2.8.4.1(b).

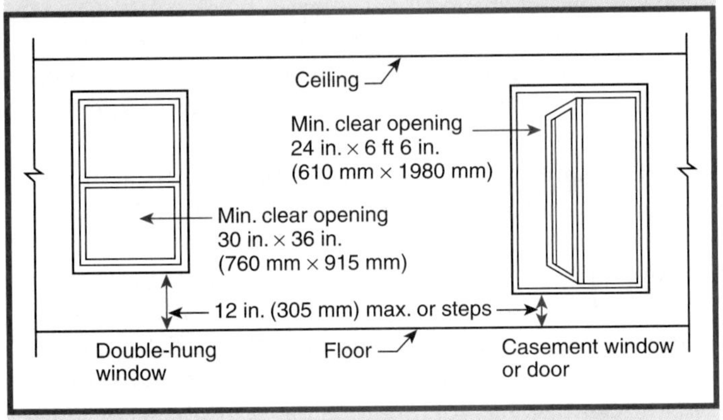


***Exhibit 7.64*** *Window openings for access to fire escape stairs.*

**7.2.8.3.2** Where access is permitted by way of windows, the windows shall be arranged and maintained so as to be easily opened. Screening or storm windows that restrict free access to the fire escape stair shall be prohibited.

**7.2.8.3.3** Fire escape stairs shall extend to the roof in all cases where the roof is subject to occupancy or provides an area of safe refuge, unless otherwise provided in 7.2.8.3.4.

**7.2.8.3.4** Where a roof has a pitch that does not exceed 1 to 6, fire escape ladders in accordance with 7.2.9 or alternating tread devices in accordance with 7.2.11 shall be permitted to provide access to the roof.

**7.2.8.3.5** Access to a fire escape stair shall be directly to a balcony, landing, or platform; shall not exceed the floor or windowsill level; and shall not be more than 8 in. (205 mm) below the floor level or 18 in. (455 mm) below the windowsill level.

The height requirements of 7.2.8.3.5 establish the maximum distance, on the outside of the building, down to the balcony, landing, or platform of the fire escape stair, measured from the windowsill level or from the floor level.

**7.2.8.4 Stair Details.**

Generally, the requirements for fire escape stairs are similar to those specified for outside stairs. The major difference between the two types of stairs is the dimensions in Commentary Table 7.1, which details the differences between the generally accepted fire escape stair of existing buildings and the lighter fire escape stair considered acceptable for small existing buildings serving 10 or fewer occupants.

The existing fire escape stair with a minimum width of 22 in. (560 mm) is a type that is permitted for buildings of small or moderate size, depending on the specific features of an installation.

The existing fire escape stair with a minimum width of 18 in. (455 mm) represents the absolute minimum that is permitted. Because of access over windowsills, steep pitch, and a narrow width, travel down such stairs will be necessarily slow and possibly dangerous. Even worse are stairs with spiral stair treads or stairs that terminate at a balcony above ground level with a fixed or movable ladder extending downward from the balcony. Such stairs are suitable only in situations that involve a very small number of occupants.

**7.2.8.4.1 General.** Fire escape stairs shall comply with the requirements of Table 7.2.8.4.1(a). Replacement of fire escape stairs shall comply with the requirements of Table 7.2.8.4.1(b).

**7.2.8.4.2 Slip Resistance.** Stair treads and landings of new or replacement fire escape stairs shall have slip-resistant surfaces.

**7.2.8.5 Guards, Handrails, and Visual Enclosures.**

**7.2.8.5.1** All fire escape stairs shall have walls or guards and handrails on both sides in accordance with 7.2.2.4.

**7.2.8.5.2** Replacement fire escape stairs in occupancies serving more than 10 occupants shall have visual enclosures to avoid any impediments to their use by persons having a fear of high places. Fire escape stairs more than 36 ft (11 m) above the finished ground level shall be provided with an opaque visual obstruction not less than 48 in. (1220 mm) in height.

**7.2.8.6 Materials and Strength.**

**7.2.8.6.1** Noncombustible materials shall be used for the construction of all components of fire escape stairs.

**7.2.8.6.2** The authority having jurisdiction shall be permitted to approve any existing fire escape stair that has been shown by load test or other satisfactory evidence to have adequate strength.

**7.2.8.7* Swinging Stairs.**

**A.7.2.8.7** Swinging stairs, although superior to fire escape ladders, are generally unsatisfactory, even for emergency use. Although such stairs are permitted by this *Code*, they should not be used where it is reasonably possible to terminate the fire escape stair at the finished ground level.

***Commentary Table 7.1 Differences Between Outside Stairs and Fire Escape Stairs***

| Design Factor | New Outside Stair | Existing Outside Stair | Fire Escape Stair: Standard | Fire Escape Stair: Small Buildings |
|---|---|---|---|---|
| Accepted as means of egress | Yes | Yes | Existing buildings | Existing buildings |
| Width | 44 in. (1120 mm)† | 44 in. (1120 mm)† | 22 in. (560 mm) | 18 in. (455 mm) |
| Maximum rise | 7 in. (180 mm) | 8 in. (205 mm) | 9 in. (230 mm) | 12 in. (305 mm) |
| Minimum tread | 11 in. (280 mm) | 9 in. (230 mm) | 9 in. (230 mm) | 6 in. (150 mm) |
| Tread construction | Solid | Solid | Solid, with perforations permitted | Metal bars |
| Access by windows | No | No | Yes | Yes |
| Swinging stair accepted | No | No | Yes | Yes |
| Ladder accepted | No | No | No | Yes |

Note: The capacity of normal fire escape stairs is 45 persons if accessed by door assemblies, and 20 persons if accessed by windows where it is necessary to climb over a sill. On small buildings, the capacity is 10 persons; 5 persons if winders or a ladder from bottom landing; 1 person if both winders and a ladder from bottom landing.

†36 in. (915 mm) where serving occupant load of fewer than 50.

*Table 7.2.8.4.1(a) Fire Escape Stairs*

| Feature | Serving More Than 10 Occupants | Serving 10 or Fewer Occupants |
|---|---|---|
| Minimum widths | 22 in. (560 mm) clear between rails | 18 in. (455 mm) clear between rails |
| Minimum horizontal dimension of any landing or platform | 22 in. (560 mm) clear | 18 in. (455 mm) clear |
| Maximum riser height | 9 in. (230 mm) | 12 in. (305 mm) |
| Minimum tread, exclusive of nosing | 9 in. (230 mm) | 6 in. (150 mm) |
| Minimum nosing or projection | 1 in. (25 mm) | No requirement |
| Tread construction | Solid 1/2 in. (13 mm) diameter perforations permitted | Flat metal bars on edge or square bars secured against turning, spaced 1 1/4 in. (32 mm) maximum on centers |
| Winders | None | Permitted subject to capacity penalty |
| Risers | None | No requirement |
| Spiral | None | Permitted subject to capacity penalty |
| Maximum height between landings | 12 ft (3660 mm) | No requirement |
| Headroom, minimum | 6 ft 8 in. (2030 mm) | 6 ft 8 in. (2030 mm) |
| Access to escape | Door or casement windows, 24 in. × 6 ft 8 in. (610 mm × 1980 mm); or double-hung windows, 30 in. × 36 in. (760 mm × 915 mm) clear opening | Windows providing a clear opening of at least 20 in. (510 mm) in width, 24 in. (610 mm) in height, and 5.7 $ft^2$ (0.53 $m^2$) in area |
| Level of access opening | Not over 12 in. (305 mm) above floor; steps if higher | Not over 12 in. (305 mm) above floor; steps if higher |
| Discharge to the finished ground level | Swinging stair section permitted if approved by authority having jurisdiction | Swinging stair, or ladder if approved by authority having jurisdiction |
| Capacity | 1/2 in. (13 mm) per person, if access by door; 1 in. (25 mm) per person, if access by climbing over windowsill | 10 persons; if winders or ladder from bottom balcony, 5 persons; if both, 1 person |

In cases where the use of a fire escape stair would block a sidewalk or other public way or provide ready access for intruders, the following solution is offered:

1. The discharge can be counterweighted.
2. The unlocked swinging stair can be designed so that a 150 lb (68 kg) weight applied at one quarter of the length of the stair from the pivot point causes the stair to drop into the usable position. See 7.2.8.7.7.

**7.2.8.7.1** A single swinging stair section shall be permitted to terminate fire escape stairs over sidewalks, alleys, or driveways where it is impractical to make the termination with fire escape stairs.

**7.2.8.7.2** Swinging stair sections shall not be located over doors, over the path of travel from any other exit, or in any locations where there are likely to be obstructions.

**7.2.8.7.3** The width of swinging stair sections shall be at least that of the fire escape stairs above.

**7.2.8.7.4** The pitch of swinging stair sections shall not exceed the pitch of the fire escape stairs above.

**7.2.8.7.5** Guards and handrails shall be provided in accordance with 7.2.2.4 and shall be similar in height and construction to those used with the fire escape stairs above. Guards and handrails shall be designed to prevent any possibility of injury to persons where stairs swing downward. The clearance between moving sections and any other portion of the stair system where hands have the potential to be caught shall be not less than 4 in. (100 mm).

**7.2.8.7.6** If the distance from the lowest platform to the finished ground level is not less than 12 ft (3660 mm), an intermediate balcony not more than 12 ft (3660 mm) from the finished ground level and not less than 7 ft (2135 mm) in the clear underneath shall be provided, with width not less than that of the stairs and length not less than 48 in. (1220 mm).

*Table 7.2.8.4.1(b) Replacement Fire Escape Stairs*

| Feature | Serving More Than 10 Occupants | Serving 10 or Fewer Occupants |
|---|---|---|
| Minimum widths | 22 in. (560 mm) clear between rails | 22 in. (560 mm) clear between rails |
| Minimum horizontal dimension of any landing or platform | 22 in. (560 mm) | 22 in. (560 mm) |
| Maximum riser height | 9 in. (230 mm) | 9 in. (230 mm) |
| Minimum tread, exclusive of nosing | 10 in. (255 mm) | 10 in. (255 mm) |
| Tread construction | Solid, ½ in. (13 mm) diameter perforations permitted | Solid, ½ in. (13 mm) diameter perforations permitted |
| Winders | None | Permitted subject to 7.2.2.2.4 |
| Spiral | None | Permitted subject to 7.2.2.2.3 |
| Risers | None | None |
| Maximum height between landings | 12 ft (3660 mm) | 12 ft (3660 mm) |
| Headroom, minimum | 6 ft 8 in. (2030 mm) | 6 ft 8 in. (2030 mm) |
| Access to escape | Door or casement windows, 24 in. × 6 ft 8 in. (610 mm × 1980 mm); or double-hung windows, 30 in. × 36 in. (760 mm × 915 mm) clear opening | Windows providing a clear opening of at least 20 in. (510 mm) in width, 24 in. (610 mm) in height, and 5.7 $ft^2$ (0.53 $m^2$) in area |
| Level of access opening | Not over 12 in. (305 mm) above floor; steps if higher | Not over 12 in. (305 mm) above floor; steps if higher |
| Discharge to the finished ground level | Swinging stair section permitted if approved by authority having jurisdiction | Swinging stair section permitted if approved by authority having jurisdiction |
| Capacity | ½ in. (13 mm) per person, if access by door; 1 in. (25 mm) per person, if access by climbing over windowsill | 10 persons |

**7.2.8.7.7** Swinging stairs shall be counterbalanced about a pivot, and cables shall not be used. A weight of 150 lb (68 kg) located one step from the pivot shall not cause the stairs to swing downward, and a weight of 150 lb (68 kg) located one-quarter of the length of the swinging stairs from the pivot shall cause the stairs to swing down.

**7.2.8.7.8** The pivot for swinging stairs shall be of a corrosion-resistant assembly or shall have clearances to prevent sticking due to corrosion.

**7.2.8.7.9*** Devices shall not be installed to lock a swinging stair section in the up position.

**A.7.2.8.7.9** A latch is desirable for holding swinging stairs down after they have swung to the finished ground level.

**7.2.8.8 Intervening Spaces.**

**7.2.8.8.1** Where approved by the authority having jurisdiction, fire escape stairs shall be permitted to lead to an adjoining roof that is crossed before continuing downward travel. The direction of travel shall be clearly marked, and walkways with guards and handrails complying with 7.2.2.4 shall be provided.

**7.2.8.8.2** Where approved by the authority having jurisdiction, fire escape stairs shall be permitted to be used in combination with inside or outside stairs complying with 7.2.2, provided that a continuous safe path of travel is maintained.

### 7.2.9 Fire Escape Ladders.

**7.2.9.1 General.** Fire escape ladders complying with 7.2.9.2 and 7.2.9.3 shall be permitted in the means of egress only where providing one of the following:

(1) Access to unoccupied roof spaces as permitted in 7.2.8.3.4
(2) Second means of egress from storage elevators as permitted in Chapter 42
(3) Means of egress from towers and elevated platforms around machinery or similar spaces subject to occu-

pancy not to exceed three persons who are all capable of using the ladder

(4) Secondary means of egress from boiler rooms or similar spaces subject to occupancy not to exceed three persons who are all capable of using the ladder

(5) Access to the finished ground level from the lowest balcony or landing of a fire escape stair for small buildings as permitted in 7.2.8.4 where approved by the authority having jurisdiction

The *Code* does not intend to encourage the use of ladders but intends to provide access to an exit from any regularly occupied area. The *Code* contains provisions for fire escape ladders only because these ladders are sometimes one of the only practical means of moving from one space to another along what might be a path of escape from spaces not normally occupied. The *Code* does specify requirements for ladder construction and installation to ensure structural integrity and ease of use if ladders must be used. The provisions of 7.2.9.1 constitute the minimal recognition given fire escape ladders by this *Code*. Subsection 7.2.11 also addresses alternating tread devices for use under conditions similar to those specified for fire escape ladders.

**7.2.9.2 Construction and Installation.**

**7.2.9.2.1** Fire escape ladders shall comply with ANSI A14.3, *Safety Requirements for Fixed Ladders*, unless one of the following criteria is met:

(1) Approved existing ladders complying with the edition of this *Code* that was in effect when the ladders were installed shall be permitted.

(2) Industrial stairs complying with the minimum requirements for fixed stairs of ANSI/ASSE A1264.1, *Safety Requirements for Workplace Floor and Wall Openings, Stairs and Railing Systems*, shall be permitted where fire escape ladders are permitted in accordance with Chapter 40.

Fixed industrial stairs can have dimensional criteria that are comparable to ladders or that are nearly comparable to existing means of egress stairs in accordance with 7.2.2. Paragraph 7.2.9.2.1(2) recognizes that some industrial stairs are safer to use than ladders and permits such stairs to be used at locations where fire escape ladders are permitted in industrial occupancies.

**7.2.9.2.2** Ladders shall be installed with a pitch that exceeds 75 degrees.

**7.2.9.3 Access.** The lowest rung of any ladder shall not be more than 12 in. (305 mm) above the level of the surface beneath it.

### 7.2.10 Slide Escapes.

**7.2.10.1 General.**

**7.2.10.1.1** A slide escape shall be permitted as a component in a means of egress where permitted in Chapters 11 through 43.

Slide escapes are permitted in means of egress only in high hazard industrial occupancies and existing storage occupancies. See 40.2.2.11 and 42.2.2.10.

Ordinarily, an occupant enters a slide escape through a window or special opening in an exterior wall. From that point on, the slide escape functions as an exit discharge. If the slide escape is entered from within the building, it is considered an exit and must be protected by enclosure as required by 7.1.3.2.

Where provided, slide escapes should be used regularly in practice drills or for normal egress so that occupants are familiar with their use.

A slide pole of the type found in fire stations is not considered a slide escape.

**7.2.10.1.2** Each slide escape shall be of an approved type.

**7.2.10.2 Capacity.**

**7.2.10.2.1** Slide escapes, where permitted as a required means of egress, shall be rated at a capacity of 60 persons.

**7.2.10.2.2** Slide escapes shall not constitute more than 25 percent of the required egress capacity from any building or structure or any individual story thereof, unless otherwise provided for industrial occupancies in Chapter 40.

The 25 percent limitation on slide escapes as required means of egress emphasizes that other, more common egress components must comprise the majority of the egress capacity.

### 7.2.11* Alternating Tread Devices.

**A.7.2.11** Special consideration should be given prior to the application of such devices where children, the elderly, or physically disabled persons use such devices. These devices present obstacles in ascent and descent that differ from those for stairs and ladders.

**7.2.11.1** Alternating tread devices complying with 7.2.11.2 shall be permitted in the means of egress only where providing one of the following:

(1) Access to unoccupied roof spaces as permitted in 7.2.8.3.4
(2) Second means of egress from storage elevators as permitted in Chapter 42
(3) Means of egress from towers and elevated platforms around machinery or similar spaces subject to occupancy not to exceed three persons who are all capable of using the alternating tread device
(4) Secondary means of egress from boiler rooms or similar spaces subject to occupancy not to exceed three persons who are all capable of using the alternating tread device

**7.2.11.2** Alternating tread devices shall comply with the following:

(1) Handrails shall be provided on both sides of alternating tread devices in accordance with 7.2.2.4.4, except as provided in 7.2.11.3.
(2) The clear width between handrails shall be not less than 17 in. (430 mm) and not more than 24 in. (610 mm).
(3) Headroom shall be not less than 6 ft 8 in. (2030 mm).
(4) The angle of the device shall be between 50 degrees and 68 degrees to horizontal.
(5) The height of the riser shall not exceed 9½ in. (240 mm).
(6) Treads shall have a projected tread depth of not less than 5⅘ in. (145 mm), measured in accordance with 7.2.2, with each tread providing 9½ in. (240 mm) of depth, including tread overlap.
(7) A distance of not less than 6 in. (150 mm) shall be provided between the alternating tread device handrail and any other object.
(8) The initial tread of the alternating tread device shall begin at the same elevation as the platform, landing, or floor surface.
(9) The alternating treads shall not be laterally separated by a distance of more than 2 in. (51 mm).
(10) The occupant load served shall not exceed three.

**7.2.11.3** Handrails of alternating tread devices shall comply with the following:

(1) The handrail height of alternating tread devices, measured above tread nosings, shall be uniform, not less than 30 in. (760 mm), and not more than 34 in. (865 mm).
(2) Handrails for alternating tread devices shall be permitted to terminate at a location vertically above the top and bottom risers.
(3) Handrails for alternating tread devices shall not be required to be continuous between flights or to extend beyond the top or bottom risers.
(4) Alternating tread device guards, with a top rail that also serves as a handrail, shall have a height of not less than 30 in. (760 mm), and not more than 34 in. (865 mm), measured vertically from the leading edge of the device tread nosing.
(5) Open guards of alternating tread devices shall have rails such that a sphere 21 in. (535 mm) in diameter is not able to pass through any opening.

As used in the *Code*, an alternating tread device is an intermediate form of climbing implement that is a cross between a ladder and a stair. It consists of a steep succession of treads that alternate from the left side to the right side at intervals of one riser height. A person using the device is forced to place the correct foot on each tread. This alternating tread design, now generally manufactured as a series of treads supported by a central spine, permits stairlike half-treads to be used with ladderlike slopes. The use of such devices, which might be awkward due to unfamiliarity or infrequent use, might be acceptable for some occupancies and locations where the alternative means of changing levels are ladders or ships' ladders, devices that generally have pitches of 50 degrees to 75 degrees. Such pitches are approximately twice those permitted for stairs by the *Code*.

An advantage of alternating tread devices is that one can descend with one's back to the device — unlike a ladder where one can only descend safely while facing the ladder because of the more limited surface area and depth of ladder rungs. A further benefit of the device is that objects can be carried more easily while ascending or descending, because the handrails provide support under the arms, which are left free.

The *Code* limits the use of alternating tread devices to those situations where a ladder is acceptable. Exhibit 7.65 is a photograph of an alternating tread device.

The provisions of 7.2.11.3 for handrails on alternating tread devices are new to the 2009 edition of the *Code*. In earlier editions, 7.2.11.2(1) required that the handrails provided on both sides of the alternating tread device be in accordance with the handrail provisions of 7.2.2.4.4. Paragraph 7.2.11.2(1) was revised to permit the handrails to be in accordance with 7.2.11.3. Due to the steepness of the alternating tread device, a handrail height in the range of 30 in. to 34 in. (760 mm to 865 mm) is best suited ergonomically for the majority of users. The 17 in. to 24 in. (430 mm to 610 mm) width between handrails positions the user very near

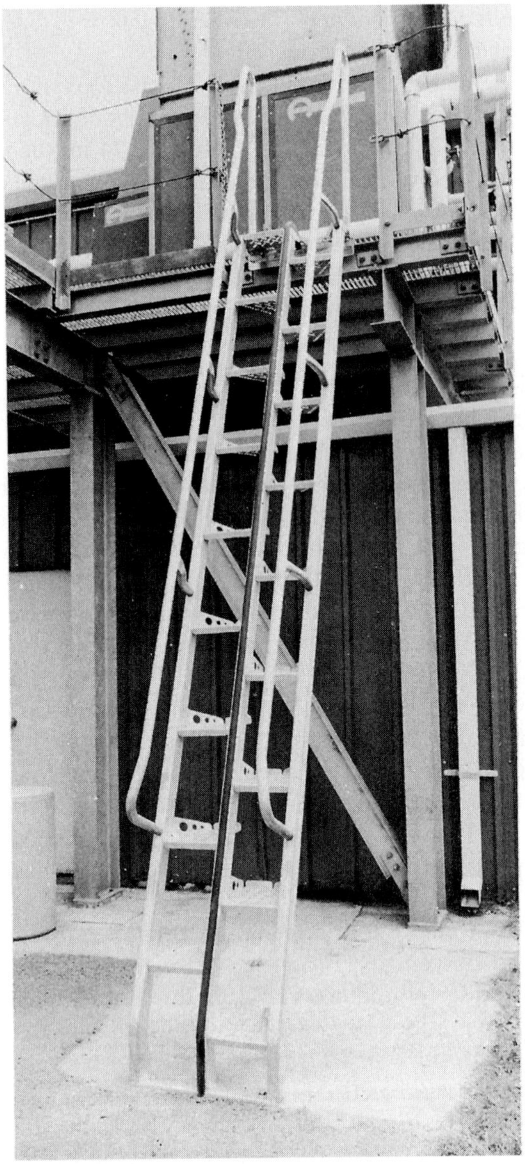

*Exhibit 7.65 Alternating tread device.*

the sides of the device, so that the handrails restrict lateral movement and provide support under the arms. A handrail with height in excess of 34 in. (865 mm) begins to encroach on the user's armpit, and, at some height above 34 in. (865 mm), the user's arm can no longer be extended over the handrail.

### 7.2.12 Areas of Refuge.

Subsection 7.2.12 presents the detailed criteria applicable to an area of refuge. The term *area of refuge* and the related terms *accessible area of refuge* and *accessible means of egress* are defined in 3.3.20, 3.3.20.1, and 3.3.161.1, respectively.

Subsection 7.5.4 requires accessible means of egress in new construction in areas accessible to persons with severe mobility impairment. Because an accessible means of egress must be usable by a person with severe mobility impairment, the components most commonly used in such means of egress are ramps and areas of refuge. Areas of refuge are extensively used from the upper stories of multistory buildings where it might not be feasible to install ramp systems.

The criteria of 7.2.12 were written to bring the *Code* into substantial agreement with the *Americans with Disabilities Act Accessibility Guidelines for Buildings and Facilities* (ADAAG); its successor, the *ADA and ABA Accessibility Guidelines for Buildings and Facilities* (ADA-ABA-AG); and ICC/ANSI A117.1, *American National Standard for Accessible and Usable Buildings and Facilities.* Inclusion in this 2009 edition of the expanded requirements of 7.2.12.1.1 for a two-way communication system, even in a building that is protected throughout by automatic sprinklers, moves the *Code* ahead of ADAAG, ADA-ABA-AG, and ICC/ANSI A117.1 in providing persons with severe mobility impairments with an egress system that approaches that provided to occupants who can use stairs.

#### 7.2.12.1 General.

**7.2.12.1.1** An area of refuge used as part of a required accessible means of egress in accordance with 7.5.4; consisting of a story in a building that is protected throughout by an approved, supervised automatic sprinkler system in accordance with Section 9.7; and having an accessible story that is one or more stories above or below a story of exit discharge shall meet the following criteria:

(1) Each elevator landing shall be provided with a two-way communication system for communication between the elevator landing and the fire command center or a central control point approved by the authority having jurisdiction.
(2) Directions for the use of the two-way communication system, instructions for summoning assistance via the two-way communication system, and written identification of the location shall be posted adjacent to the two-way communication system.
(3) The two-way communication system shall include both audible and visible signals.

**7.2.12.1.2** An area of refuge used as part of a required accessible means of egress in accordance with 7.5.4 in other than a building that is protected throughout by an approved, supervised automatic sprinkler system in accordance with Section 9.7 shall meet the following criteria:

(1) The area of refuge shall meet the general requirements of Section 7.1.
(2) The area of refuge shall meet the requirements of 7.2.12.2 and 7.2.12.3.

The provisions of 7.2.12.1.1 and 7.2.12.1.2 and the definition of *area of refuge* in 3.3.20 are interrelated. Their combined effect is to permit three forms of area of refuge to serve as part of an accessible means of egress, as outlined in paragraphs 1 through 3, which follow.

**1.** On a floor of a building not protected throughout by an approved, supervised automatic sprinkler system, the area of refuge serving as part of an accessible means of egress must meet the special requirements of 7.2.12.2 and 7.2.12.3, as well as the general requirements of Section 7.1.

**2.** On a floor of a building protected throughout by an approved, supervised automatic sprinkler system — and involving an occupancy that is not exempt from the minimum two accessible rooms provision of the definition of *area of refuge* — an area of refuge serving as part of an accessible means of egress is exempt from the special requirements of 7.2.12.2 and 7.2.12.3. However, the area of refuge must meet the general requirements of Section 7.1, consist of at least two accessible rooms or spaces separated from each other by smoke-resisting partitions, and meet the criteria of 7.2.12.1.1 (1) through (3) related to a two-way communication system. The following occupancies are not exempt from the minimum two accessible rooms provision of the definition of *area of refuge*:

1. Assembly occupancies
2. Educational occupancies
3. Day-care occupancies
4. Health care occupancies (which are exempt from accessible means of egress criteria because of the level of life safety provided by the protect-in-place strategy employed by Chapter 18)
5. Detention and correctional occupancies
6. Residential board and care occupancies
7. Industrial occupancies
8. Storage occupancies

**3.** On a floor of a building protected throughout by an approved, supervised automatic sprinkler system — and involving an occupancy that is exempt from the minimum two accessible rooms provision of the definition of *area of refuge* — an area of refuge serving as part of an accessible means of egress is exempt from the special requirements of 7.2.12.2 and 7.2.12.3 and is also exempt from having to provide the two accessible rooms or spaces separated from each other by smoke-resisting partitions. However, the area of refuge must meet the general requirements of Section 7.1 and meet the criteria of 7.2.12.1.1 (1) through (3) related to a two-way communication system. The following occupancies are exempt from the minimum two accessible rooms provision of the definition of *area of refuge*:

1. Hotels and dormitories (28.2.2.12.2, 29.2.2.12.2)
2. Apartment buildings (30.2.2.12.2, 31.2.2.12.2)
3. Mercantile occupancies (36.2.2.12.2, 37.2.2.12.2)
4. Business occupancies (38.2.2.12.2, 39.2.2.12.2)

**7.2.12.2 Accessibility.**

**7.2.12.2.1** Required portions of an area of refuge shall be accessible from the space they serve by an accessible means of egress.

To help ensure that persons with mobility impairments can access the area of refuge, 7.2.12.2.1 requires such accessibility via an accessible means of egress. Thus, a person attempting to reach the area of refuge must be provided with either level floor travel or ramp travel, not stairs. Similarly, the door assembly to the area of refuge must provide sufficient clear width, typically the 32 in. (810 mm) minimum specified by 7.2.1.2.3.2, to allow a person in a wheelchair to move through the door opening. See the definition of *accessible means of egress* in 3.3.161.1.

**7.2.12.2.2** Required portions of an area of refuge shall have access to a public way via an exit or an elevator without requiring return to the building spaces through which travel to the area of refuge occurred.

An area of refuge is intended to provide only a temporary point of safety to allow delayed-egress travel from any level. Therefore, an area of refuge cannot be a room or space whose only access to the building spaces is via the room or space through which the user arrived. Such an arrangement might trap a person within the area of refuge, since no egress has been provided other than that which requires travel back through the space where the fire is located. Rather, the area of refuge must provide access to a public way via either an elevator or an exit, such as an enclosed exit stair.

**7.2.12.2.3*** Where the exit providing egress from an area of refuge to a public way that is in accordance with 7.2.12.2.2 includes stairs, the clear width of landings and stair flights, measured between handrails and at all points below handrail height, shall be not less than 48 in. (1220 mm), unless otherwise permitted by the following:

(1) The minimum 48 in. (1220 mm) clear width shall not be required where the area of refuge is separated from the remainder of the story by a horizontal exit meeting the requirements of 7.2.4. *(See also 7.2.12.3.4.)*

(2)* For stairs where egress is in the descending direction, a clear width of not less than 37 in. (940 mm), measured at and below handrail height, shall be permitted where all of the following are met:

(a) An approved stair descent device is provided on each floor served by the stair.

(b) Additional approved stair descent devices are provided on floors with an occupant load exceeding 200 at the ratio of one device per 200 occupants.

(c) The required approved stair descent devices are provided in an approved location on the floor.

(3) Existing stairs and landings that provide a clear width of not less than 37 in. (940 mm), measured at and below handrail height, shall be permitted.

**A.7.2.12.2.3** The clear width of not less than 48 in. (1220 mm) is needed for a three-person carry of an occupied wheelchair up or down a stair. This procedure, as well as the more difficult two-person wheelchair carry or roll, requires training and experience. Safer, alternative stair descent measures for transporting a person who normally requires a wheelchair include evacuation chairs and self-braking stair descent devices. In addition to having such devices available where needed, and having persons trained and experienced in their use, it is important to have people trained and experienced in wheelchair transfer techniques.

In view of the logistical difficulties as well as the dangers inherent in carrying occupied wheelchairs or otherwise transporting their occupants on stairs, the preferred means of egress from an area of refuge consists of facilities normally employed for ingress and egress by people using wheelchairs. Foremost among these options are elevators meeting the fire fighters' emergency operations requirements of ASME A17.1/CSA B44, *Safety Code for Elevators and Escalators.*

**A.7.2.12.2.3(2)** Stair descent devices using stair-bearing belted tracks, for example, provide a safer, more effective evacuation option than carrying an occupied wheelchair or other carried device down the stairs and on landings. The use of stair descent devices is recommended.

The design, manufacture, selection, maintenance, and operation of stairway descent devices should take into account the following recommendations and general guidance information:

(1) The minimum carrying capacity of the device should be 350 lb (159 kg) and should be rated for the maximum permitted slope of the stair served.

(2) For existing stairs with 8 in. (205 mm) riser height and 9 in. (230 mm) tread depth, the 350 lb (159 kg) carrying capacity specified in A.7.2.12.2.3(2)(1) should be maintained at a slope or pitch of 42 degrees or 1.0 unit vertical for 1.1 units horizontal.

(3) The rated maximum carrying capacity and maximum stair pitch should be labeled on the device, and the device should only be operated within the labeled limits of load and stair slope or pitch.

(4) The maximum descent speed should be capable of being controlled during operation, without undue restraint by the operator(s), to 30 in./s (760 mm/s), measured along the slope of the stair.

(5) When operated according to the manufacturer's instructions and loaded to its maximum stated capacity, the device should come reliably to a complete stop within a distance of 12 in. (305 mm), measured along the landing or stair slope, on a stair with a slope or pitch within the device's maximum stated capability, and the following also should apply:

(a) The device should have a break.

(b) On walking surfaces other than stairs, the device should maintain a parked position, without rolling, so that the operator can attend to other activities, including assisting the passenger to transfer from or to other mobility devices.

(6) Minimum stairway width and landing depth requirements, especially at landings where turns occur, should be disclosed by the manufacturer, and only devices appropriate to the building's stairways should be provided in the building.

(7) Slowing or delays when transitioning between stairway landings and stair flights should cause no more than minimal delay to the movement of pedestrians using the stairway in the vicinity of the device and, generally, should not significantly reduce the flow of evacuees using the stairway system.

(8) When descending stairs, the device should be easily operable by one person who is trained on its use, and the following also should apply:

(a) Above average weight or strength should not be required for proper operation.

(b) Lifting or carrying of the device, when occupied, should normally not be required.

(9) Unless designed specifically for use on stairs with nonrectangular treads (e.g., winder treads), with operators trained for such use, the device should be operated only on stairways with straight flights having rectangular treads.

(10) On straight flights, the device should be designed to have supporting contact with at least two treads, except during the transition between landings and stair flights.

(11) The device should be equipped with restraining straps that securely hold the passenger, including the chest, waist, thighs, knees, ankles, and arms to prevent injury, and the length and quantity of straps should be designed to accommodate a range of passenger sizes and weights up to the maximum capacity of the device.
(12) The seat or seat sling should have open sides and be positioned at an appropriate height to allow transfer with minimal operator assistance, and the specific procedure used for a particular transfer should be determined through discussion between the passenger and the operator(s).
(13) Setup of the device should be described in procedures posted on the device, should require no other tools or expertise beyond that of available operators, and should take approximately 10 seconds to set up from storage condition to readiness for transfer.
(14) In addition to descending stairs, the device should be able to travel across ramped or horizontal surfaces, such as stair landings and hallways, so that it can follow an entire egress route to the exterior of the building.
(15) The device's seating system should provide adequate support of the passenger to minimize the potential for discomfort or injury, recognizing that people with physical disabilities, who will be the main occupants of the device, are often unusually susceptible to pressure-related injuries and spasm, while being unable to perceive the warning signs of pain.
(16) If cabinets or storage covers are provided, they should include signage or labeling that clearly identifies the device and its use, and the device should be readily retrievable from storage without use of a key or special tool.
(17) The building evacuation plan should include the location of the devices, a process for verifying the availability of trained operators, and other critical information as is required for the building.
(18) The manufacturer of the device should provide comprehensive training materials with each device, and the following also should apply:

(a) All designated operators should be trained in accordance with these instructions.
(b) Evacuation drills that involve actual use of the device by the designated operators, including transfer and transport of building occupants with disabilities, should occur at least quarterly.

(19) The device should be inspected and tested annually in accordance with the manufacturer's recommendations, and preventive maintenance should be performed in accordance with the manufacturer's recommendations.
(20) Device capabilities differing significantly from those spelled out in the foregoing recommendations (e.g., carrying capacity, higher normal speed, and fail-safe braking systems) should be disclosed by the manufacturer in a manner readily known to operators whose training should take such differences into account.
(21) Limitations of the device based on stair nosing geometry and nature of stairway covering should be disclosed by the manufacturer in specifications, operating instructions, and labeling.
(22) Carrying handles, if installed on the device, should provide secure gripping surfaces and adequate structural and geometric design to facilitate carrying by two or more operators, and the following also should be considered:

(a) Carrying might be necessitated by damaged or otherwise irregular walking surfaces that do not facilitate rolling with the device's wheels or tracks.
(b) Carrying might also be necessitated by the existence of an ascending stair along the means of egress (e.g., in the exit discharge path.)

(23) Unless specialized operator training is undertaken, use of a stairway descent device on stairways with unusually large treads and on escalators should be attempted only under the following conditions:

(a) The device is designed for extra-long distance between the tread nosings [e.g., about 16 in. (405 mm) on escalators, as opposed to about 12 in. to 13 in. (305 mm to 330 mm) on typical exit stairways].
(b) Such specialized training might entail maintaining a downward force on the device operating handle.

The *Code* requires 48 in. (1220 mm) of clear width between handrails on exit stairs that provide the required access from the area of refuge to the exit discharge. The 48 in. (1220 mm) clear width requirement is wider than the minimum 44 in. (1120 mm) stair width required by Table 7.2.2.2.1.2(B), which might provide as little as 35 in. (890 mm) of clear width between handrails. [A $4\frac{1}{2}$ in. (114 mm) encroachment is currently permitted at each side of the stair by 7.2.2.2.1.2(A), Table 7.2.2.2.1.1(b), and 7.3.2.2. Prior to the 2003 edition of the *Code*, the permitted encroachment was $3\frac{1}{2}$ in. (90 mm).] The extra width is required to facilitate the carrying of persons in wheelchairs, as explained in A.7.2.12.2.3. The minimum 48 in. (1220 mm) stair width is a clear width dimension, measured between handrails. The allowances of 7.2.2.2.1.2(A), Table 7.2.2.2.1.1(b), and 7.3.2.2 that permit handrails to encroach as much as $4\frac{1}{2}$ in. (114 mm) on each side of a stair without considering the reduced clear width do not apply. For a stair with normal handrails to provide the required 48 in. (1220 mm) clear width, the stair needs to be approximately 57 in. (1445 mm) wide.

Paragraph 7.2.12.2.3(1) exempts areas of refuge created by horizontal exits from the extra-wide stair requirement. Horizontal exits in accordance with 7.2.4 consist of barriers with a minimum 2-hour fire resistance rating. The 2-hour rating increases the time for which the area of refuge can maintain tenable conditions. It is believed that this increase in time allows a slower evacuation on a narrower, typical stair to be effectively accomplished.

Paragraph 7.2.12.2.3(2) recognizes a 44 in. (1120 mm) stair with handrails encroaching up to $3\frac{1}{2}$ in. (90 mm), as permitted by earlier editions of the *Code*, so as to provide a minimum 37 in. (940 mm) of clear width. However, egress must be in the descending direction, which is easier than climbing stairs and lifting persons with disabilities. Also, special stair descent devices must be provided on each floor served by the stair, so that occupied wheelchairs do not need to be carried on stairs. Special controlled-descent boards, chairs, and other devices, which are operable by one able-bodied person, are available. Such devices, typically using stair-bearing belted tracks, can be effectively used with the 37 in. (940 mm) of clear width afforded by some 44 in. (1120 mm) width stairs.

Significant guidance on the stair descent devices addressed in 7.2.12.2.3(2) is provided in A.7.2.12.2.3(2)(1) through A.7.2.12.2.3(2)(23). The detailed criteria serve as a de facto product standard, in that the industry that manufactures stair descent devices has no recognized product standard. The intent of A.7.2.12.2.3(2) is to influence the manufacturers to provide equipment that complies with the criteria in order to receive the approval of the AHJ as required by 7.2.12.2.3(2)(a). Exhibit 7.66 through Exhibit 7.68 depict a stair descent device.

Paragraph 7.2.12.2.3(3) recognizes that areas of refuge might be created in existing buildings with existing 44 in. (1120 mm) stairs that provide only 37 in. (940 mm) of clear width because of the $3\frac{1}{2}$ in. (90 mm) handrail encroachment permitted by earlier editions of the *Code*. To require the stairs in such buildings to be widened retroactively would create a severe hardship.

**7.2.12.2.4*** Where an elevator provides access from an area of refuge to a public way that is in accordance with 7.2.12.2.2, the following criteria shall be met:

(1) The elevator shall be approved for fire fighters' emergency operations as provided in ASME A17.1/CSA B44, *Safety Code for Elevators and Escalators*.

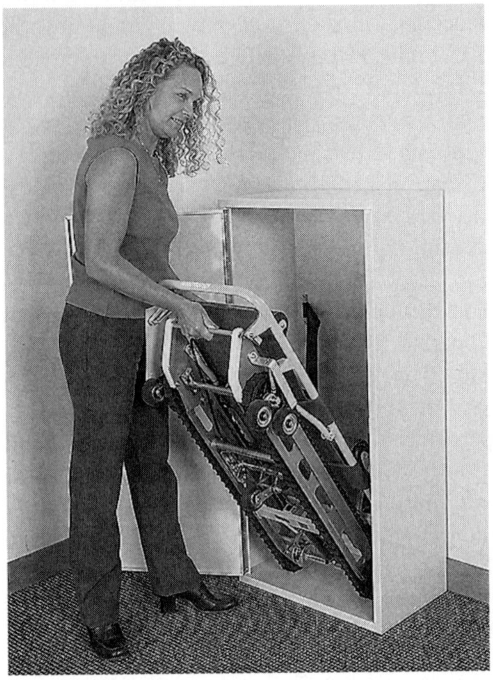

***Exhibit 7.66*** *Stair descent device readily accessed in vicinity of exit stair. (Photo courtesy of Garaventa Lift)*

(2) The power supply shall be protected against interruption from fire occurring within the building but outside the area of refuge.

(3) The elevator shall be located in a shaft system meeting the requirements for smokeproof enclosures in accordance with 7.2.3, unless otherwise provided in 7.2.12.2.4.1 and 7.2.12.2.4.2.

**A.7.2.12.2.4** The use of elevators for egress, especially during an emergency such as a fire, is not an approach to be taken without considerable planning, ongoing effort, and a high degree of understanding by everyone involved with the evacuation of persons with mobility impairments. Due in part to the limited capacity of elevators, as well as to the conflicting demands for elevator use for fire-fighting activities, even elevators in accordance with 7.2.12.2.4 cannot be considered as satisfying any of the *Code's* requirements for egress capacity, number of means of egress, or travel distance to an exit.

**7.2.12.2.4.1** The smokeproof enclosure specified in 7.2.12.2.4(3) shall not be required for areas of refuge that are more than 1000 ft² (93 m²) and that are created by a horizontal exit meeting the requirements of 7.2.4.

**7.2.12.2.4.2** The smokeproof enclosure specified in 7.2.12.2.4(3) shall not be required for elevators complying with 7.2.13.

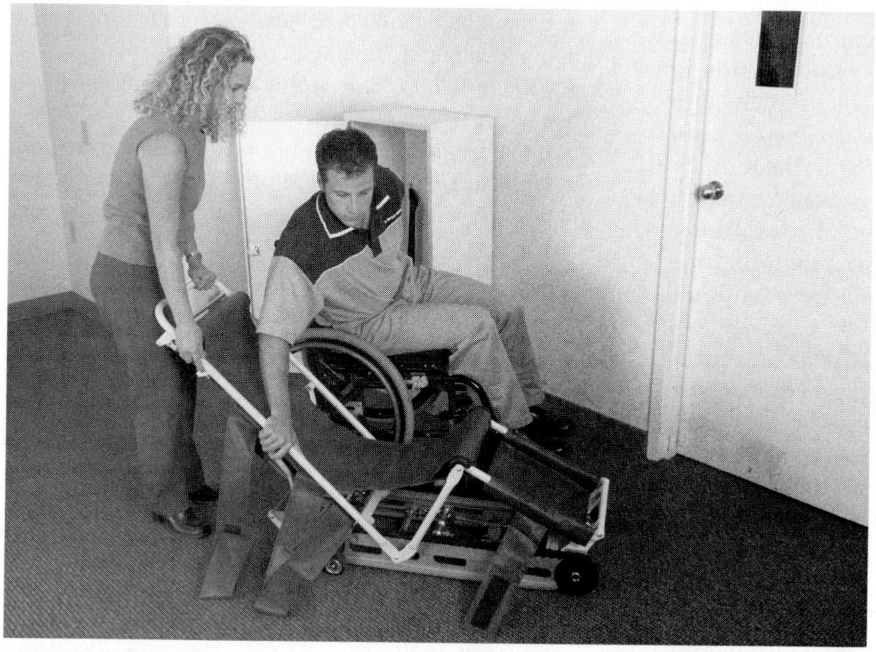

**Exhibit 7.67** *Person transferring from wheelchair to stair descent device. (Photo courtesy of Garaventa Lift)*

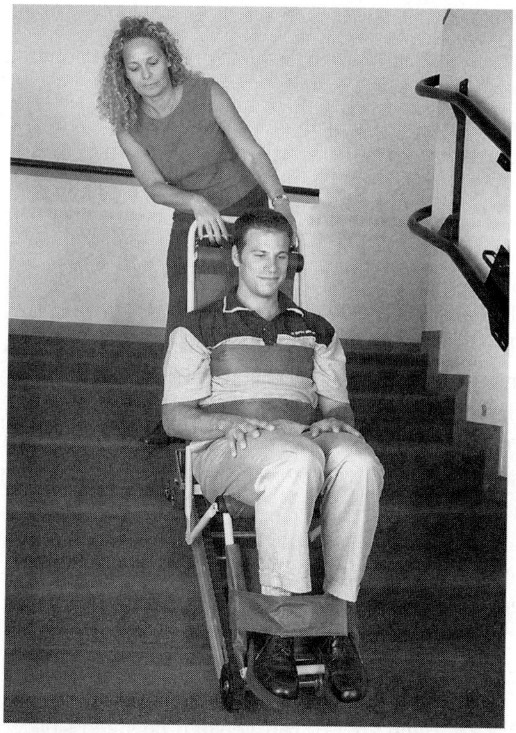

**Exhibit 7.68** *Stair descent device in use. (Photo courtesy of Garaventa Lift)*

An elevator used to provide the required access from the area of refuge to the exit discharge must be safe to operate in a building with a fire. The *Code* requires such an elevator to have the Fire Fighters' Emergency Operations features required by ASME A17.1/CSA B44, *Safety Code for Elevators and Escalators*. One of these features is elevator recall, whereby the elevator is taken out of service if smoke is detected in the elevator machine room or any elevator lobby the elevator serves. Fire service personnel or other trained persons can put the elevator back into service for manual operation by the trained personnel.

Also, the power supply for the elevator must be protected against interruption caused by fire occurring within the building but outside the area of refuge. The electrical wiring would require enclosure within protecting construction — both for the horizontal runs across any floor and the vertical runs from floor to floor — wherever such wiring is outside the area of refuge. The *Code's* intent is to ensure that, if it is safe to operate an elevator within a portion of the building, a fire in some other area will not adversely affect the power to the elevator. If the fire is in the same area as the elevator, it will not be safe to operate. Therefore, the electrical wiring in the same area as the elevator is not required to be protected.

For an elevator to pass a fire floor safely, its shaft must be kept free of smoke. The elevator must be located in a shaft system meeting the requirements of 7.2.3 for smokeproof enclosures. To achieve such compliance, it will probably be necessary for the elevator landing on each floor to be separated from the remainder of the floor via the creation of an enclosed elevator lobby. The requirement for smokeproof enclosure is a performance-based, rather than prescriptive, requirement for elevator vestibules. See 7.2.3 for additional details on smokeproof enclosures.

Paragraph 7.2.12.2.4.1 exempts the smokeproof enclosure for elevators in areas of refuge where those areas of refuge are more than 1000 $ft^2$ (93 $m^2$) and are created by horizontal exits. Horizontal exits in accordance with 7.2.4 consist of barriers with a minimum 2-hour fire resistance rating. The 2-hour rating increases the time for which the area of refuge can maintain tenable conditions. The minimum area criterion helps to ensure that small amounts of smoke entering the area of refuge do not smoke-log the area, so as to make it unusable.

**7.2.12.2.5** The area of refuge shall be provided with a two-way communication system for communication between the area of refuge and a central control point. The door opening to the stair enclosure or the elevator door and the associated portion of the area of refuge that the stair enclosure door opening or elevator door serves shall be identified by signage. *(See 7.2.12.3.5.)*

**7.2.12.2.6*** Instructions for summoning assistance, via the two-way communication system, and written identification of the area of refuge location shall be posted adjacent to the two-way communication system.

**A.7.2.12.2.6** The instructions should include the following:

(1) Directions to find other means of egress
(2) Advice that persons able to use exit stairs do so as soon as possible, unless they are assisting others
(3) Information on planned availability of assistance in the use of stairs or supervised operation of elevators and how to summon such assistance
(4) Directions for use of the emergency communications system

To facilitate an adequate degree of understanding of the use of areas of refuge and of the associated assisted egress procedures, information should be provided to those using the facilities. The exact content of the information, its organization (e.g., as a set of instructions), and its format (e.g., either posted instructions in the area of refuge or information otherwise transmitted to facility users) should be determined on a case-by-case basis. The information should be tailored to the specific facility, its emergency plan, the intended audience, and the intended presentation format. Suggested information content addressing two situations follows.

*Refuge with Elevator Use.* An area of refuge provided in the elevator lobby serves as a staging area for persons unable to use stairs and needing assistance for their evacuation during an emergency. The elevator(s) will be taken out of automatic service and operated by emergency service personnel. Persons unable to evacuate down the exit stairs without assistance and needing transportation by elevator should make certain the elevator lobby doors are closed while they wait in the elevator lobby for assistance. The two-way communication system should be used if there is a delay of more than several minutes in the arrival of an elevator that will provide transportation to the level of exit discharge. Alternatively, another refuge area, and assistance with evacuation, is available in the designated exit stair.

*Refuge with Stair Use.* An area of refuge within the designated exit stair serves as a staging area for persons needing assistance for their evacuation during an emergency. Persons unable to use the stairs unassisted, or who wish to move down the stairs at a slower pace, should wait on the stair landing. The two-way communication system should be used if assistance is needed.

The provisions of 7.2.12.2.5 for a two-way communication system are reached via the roadmap provided in 7.2.12.1.2, meaning that the building in question is not protected throughout by an approved, supervised automatic sprinkler system. For sprinklered buildings, the two-way communication provisions of 7.2.12.1.1 apply. In a nonsprinklered building, either an elevator or a stair is provided as access from the area of refuge to a public way; however, persons with mobility impairments might not be able to use the elevator or stair without assistance. For example, an elevator might have been called out of service because smoke was detected in one of the elevator lobbies serving that elevator or in the elevator machine room. A person in a wheelchair would need to call for help. Therefore, the *Code* requires a two-way communication system between the area of refuge and a central control point; the communication system is used to summon assistance. Additionally, signage and instructions are required to help complete the package of features for use by persons with disabilities.

**7.2.12.3 Details.**

**7.2.12.3.1*** Each area of refuge shall be sized to accommodate one wheelchair space of 30 in. × 48 in. (760 mm × 1220 mm) for every 200 occupants, or portion thereof, based on the occupant load served by the area of refuge. Such wheelchair spaces shall maintain the width of a means of egress to not less than that required for the occupant load served and to not less than 36 in. (915 mm).

**A.7.2.12.3.1** Figure A.7.2.12.3.1 illustrates the application of the minimum space requirement to an area of refuge located within an exit stair enclosure. Note that each of the two required spaces is sufficient to allow the parking of a standard wheelchair. Preferably, such spaces should be provided adjacent to each other in a location where the presence of people taking temporary shelter in an area of refuge will be immediately apparent to rescue personnel and other evacuees.

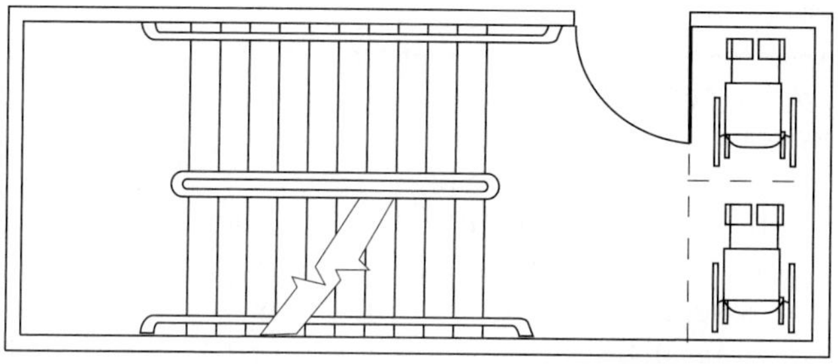

***Figure A.7.2.12.3.1*** *Exit Stair Used as an Area of Refuge.*

**7.2.12.3.2*** For any area of refuge that does not exceed 1000 ft$^2$ (93 m$^2$), it shall be demonstrated by calculation or test that tenable conditions are maintained within the area of refuge for a period of 15 minutes when the exposing space on the other side of the separation creating the area of refuge is subjected to the maximum expected fire conditions.

Areas of refuge of less than 1000 ft$^2$ (93 m$^2$) might be more easily affected than larger areas by the products of combustion from a fire in the area on the other side of the separating barrier. Thus, tenability must be demonstrated by calculation or test. An area of refuge within an exit stair enclosure, as shown in Figure A.7.2.12.3.1, would be required to demonstrate tenability. However, an area of refuge consisting of half of a 2200 ft$^2$ (205 m$^2$) floor would not be required to do so.

**A.7.2.12.3.2** The method of meeting the tenability performance criteria required of an area of refuge of less than 1000 ft$^2$ (93 m$^2$) can involve controlling the exposing fire (e.g., via automatic sprinkler protection), installing smoke-resisting doors in the smoke-resisting barriers *(see* NFPA 105, *Standard for the Installation of Smoke Door Assemblies and Other Opening Protectives),* providing smoke control to prevent or limit smoke migration through cracks or other leakage paths *(see* NFPA 92A, *Standard for Smoke-Control Systems Utilizing Barriers and Pressure Differences),* or providing other means or a combination of these means.

Calculations, if used, need to be based on established engineering relationships and equations. Such calculational procedures are described in NFPA 92A, and the *SFPE Handbook of Fire Protection Engineering*. Tenable conditions are those that maintain the temperature of any smoke in the area of refuge at less than 200°F (93°C) if the smoke is more than 60 in. (1525 mm) above the floor, and at less than 120°F (49°C) if the smoke descends below the 60 in. (1525 mm) level in the area of refuge. Also, if the smoke descends below the 60 in. (1525 mm) level, tenable conditions require not less than 16 percent oxygen and not more than 30,000 ppm/min exposure to carbon monoxide. The exposing conditions used in the calculations should be in accordance with the following:

(1) The exposing space is sprinkler protected, and the following conditions also exist:
   (a) The temperature of the exposing smoke is 200°F (93°C).
   (b) The smoke layer extends to the floor.
   (c) The oxygen content is 16 percent.
   (d) The carbon monoxide concentration is 2000 ppm (0.2 percent).
(2) The exposing space is a nonsprinklered corridor finished with Class A interior wall and ceiling finish, and the following conditions also exist:
   (a) The temperature of the exposing smoke is 600°F (316°C).
   (b) The smoke layer extends to a level 24 in. (610 mm) above the floor.
   (c) The oxygen content is 3 percent.
   (d) The carbon monoxide concentration is 50,000 ppm (5 percent).
(3) The exposing space is either not a corridor or, if a corridor, the corridor is not finished with a Class A interior wall and ceiling finish, and the following conditions also exist:
   (a) The temperature of the exposing smoke is 1500°F (815°C).
   (b) The smoke layer extends to a level 24 in. (610 mm) above the floor.
   (c) The oxygen content is 3 percent.
   (d) The carbon monoxide concentration is 50,000 ppm (5 percent).

**7.2.12.3.3** Access to any designated wheelchair space in an area of refuge shall not pass through more than one adjoining wheelchair space.

**7.2.12.3.4*** Each area of refuge shall be separated from the remainder of the story by a barrier having a minimum 1-hour fire resistance rating, unless one of the following criteria applies:

(1) A greater rating is required in other provisions of this *Code*.

(2) The barrier is an existing barrier with a minimum 30-minute fire resistance rating.

**A.7.2.12.3.4** Requirements for fire resistance ratings in excess of 1 hour, fire protection ratings in excess of 20 minutes, and prohibitions on duct penetrations appear in other *Code* sections. For example, if the barrier creating the area of refuge is also part of an exit stair enclosure that connects two or more stories, or is a horizontal exit, a minimum 2-hour fire resistance rating for the barrier and a minimum $1^1/_2$-hour fire protection rating for opening protectives, such as doors, would be required for most occupancies.

For further information on door openings in smoke-resisting barriers, see NFPA 105, *Standard for the Installation of Smoke Door Assemblies and Other Opening Protectives.*

Generally, by providing one barrier that subdivides a floor area, two areas of refuge can be created. This subdivision method and the possibility of creating areas of refuge within compartmented elevator lobbies or on enlarged stair landings of exit stair enclosures make less onerous any requirement for a story to have more than one accessible means of egress.

**7.2.12.3.4.1** New fire door assemblies serving an area of refuge shall be smoke leakage–rated in accordance with 8.2.2.5.

**7.2.12.3.4.2** The barriers specified in 7.2.12.3.4, and any openings in them, shall minimize air leakage and resist the passage of smoke.

**7.2.12.3.4.3** Door assemblies in the barriers specified in 7.2.12.3.4 shall have not less than a 20-minute fire protection rating, unless a greater rating is required in other provisions of this *Code*, and shall be either self-closing or automatic-closing in accordance with 7.2.1.8.

**7.2.12.3.4.4** Ducts shall be permitted to penetrate the barrier specified in 7.2.12.3.4, unless prohibited in other provisions of this *Code*, and shall be provided with smoke-actuated dampers or other approved means to resist the transfer of smoke into the area of refuge.

As explained in the commentary following 7.2.12.1.2, these requirements for fire resistance–rated separating barriers and fire protection–rated separating door assemblies are not required for areas of refuge in buildings protected throughout by approved, supervised automatic sprinkler systems per 7.2.12.1.2.

Exhibit 7.69 through Exhibit 7.73 illustrate various arrangements of areas of refuge.

Exhibit 7.69 illustrates an area of refuge in a new sprinklered business occupancy. The area of refuge is used to meet the requirements for accessible means of egress, because persons with severe mobility impairment are able to access the floor via the elevator. Paragraph 38.2.2.12.2 exempts the floor that serves as an area of refuge from having to provide two rooms or spaces separated from each other by smoke-resistant partitions if the new business occupancy building is protected throughout by an approved, supervised automatic sprinkler system. The open floor area depicted therefore meets the requirements for an area of refuge, provided that the two-way communication system (as noted by the accessible phone symbol) is installed in accordance with 7.2.12.1.1. The accessible phone symbol is detailed in NFPA 170, *Standard for Fire Safety and Emergency Symbols.*[24]

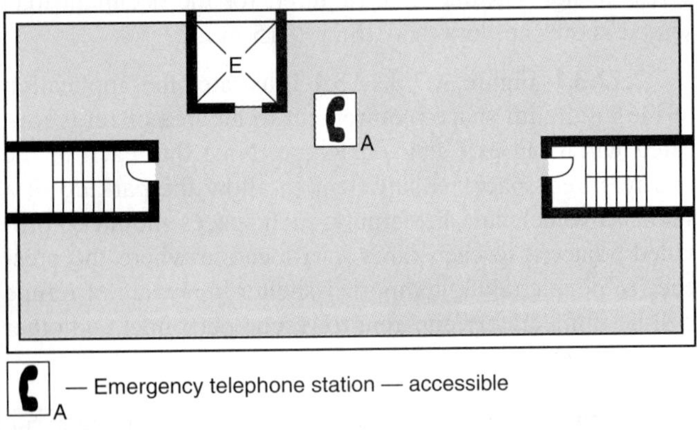


**Exhibit 7.69** *Area of refuge in new sprinklered business occupancy.*

Exhibit 7.70 depicts an area of refuge in a new sprinklered industrial occupancy. The area of refuge is used to meet the requirements for accessible means of egress, because persons with severe mobility impairment are able to access the floor via the elevator. Industrial occupancies are not exempt from the area of refuge provision for two rooms or spaces separated from each other by smoke-resistant partitions. Thus, in

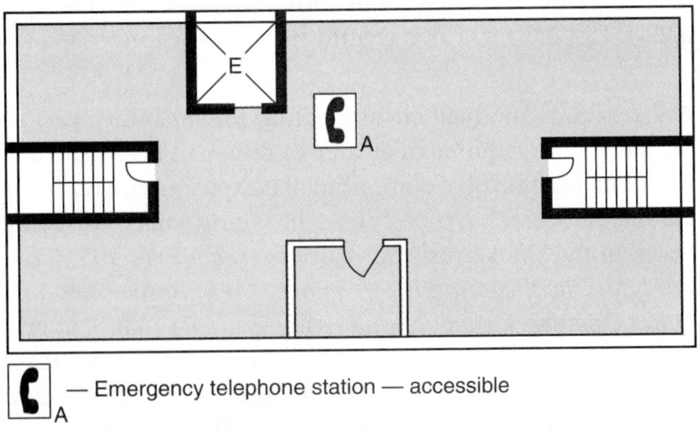


**Exhibit 7.70** *Area of refuge in new sprinklered industrial occupancy.*

this building, which is protected throughout by an approved, supervised automatic sprinkler system, a second room is provided on this floor. Note that the second room can be anywhere on the floor; it doesn't have to be adjacent to or in an exit stair enclosure. Although the separating barriers and door assembly are not required to be fire rated, they must be smoke resistant as addressed in the definition of *area of refuge* in 3.3.20. With this arrangement, the floor meets the requirements for an area of refuge, provided that the two-way communication system (as noted by the NFPA 170 accessible phone symbol) is installed in accordance with 7.2.12.1.1.

Exhibit 7.71 depicts areas of refuge in nonsprinklered new construction. The area of refuge is used to meet the requirements for accessible means of egress, because persons with severe mobility impairment are able to access the floor via the elevator. The barrier dividing the floor into two areas of refuge has a 1-hour fire resistance rating; the door assembly has a 20-minute fire protection rating. Each area is more than 1000 ft² (93 m²), and no tenability calculations are required. In the area of refuge at the left, the elevator is provided with the special features detailed in 7.2.12.2.4 and serves as access to the public way; the stair in this compartment is permitted to have the usual 44 in. (1120 mm) width. In the area of refuge at the right, the stair serves as access to the public way and must be approximately 57 in. (1455 mm) wide to provide the required 48 in. (1220 mm) clear width between handrails. Two-way communication capability (as noted by the NFPA 170 accessible phone symbol), signage, and posted instructions are required in each area of refuge in accordance with 7.2.12.2.5 and 7.2.12.2.6.

Exhibit 7.72 depicts areas of refuge created by a horizontal exit in nonsprinklered new construction.

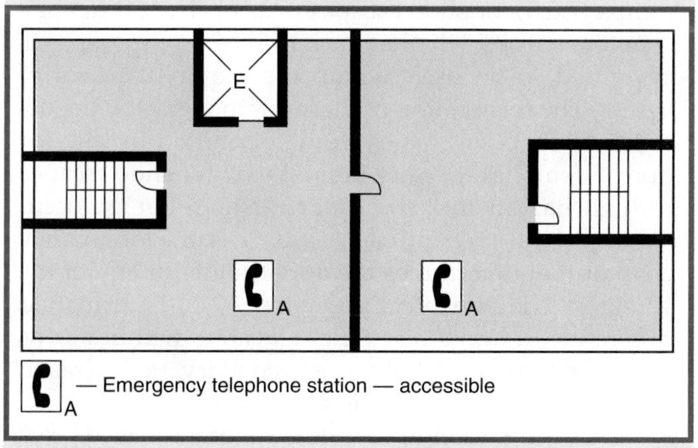


***Exhibit 7.71** Areas of refuge in nonsprinklered new construction.*

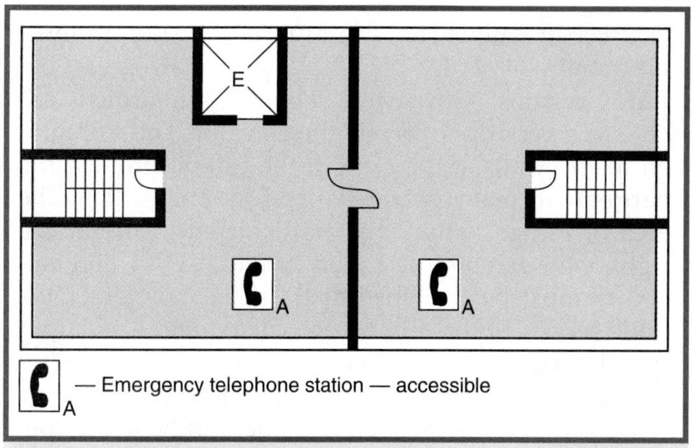


***Exhibit 7.72** Areas of refuge created by horizontal exit in nonsprinklered new construction.*

The area of refuge is used to meet the requirements for accessible means of egress, because persons with severe mobility impairment are able to access the floor via the elevator. The barrier dividing the floor into two areas of refuge is a horizontal exit with a 2-hour fire resistance rating; the door assemblies have a 1½-hour fire protection rating. Each area is more than 1000 ft² (93 m²), so no tenability calculations are required. Because the separating barrier is a horizontal exit, the stairs are permitted to be typical 44 in. (1120 mm) width stairs that might provide only 35 in. (890 mm) of clear width between handrails, and the elevator is not required to have the special features detailed in 7.2.12.2.4. Two-way communication capability (as noted by the NFPA 170 accessible phone symbol), signage, and posted instructions are required in each area of refuge in accordance with 7.2.12.2.5 and 7.2.12.2.6.

Exhibit 7.73 depicts an area of refuge that uses space within the exit stair enclosure in nonsprinklered

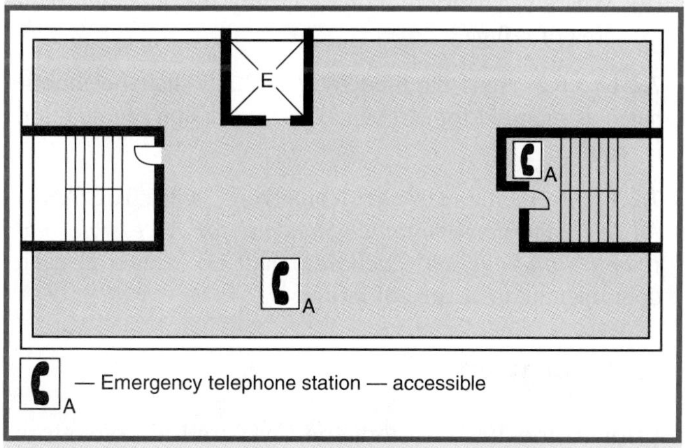


***Exhibit 7.73** Two areas of refuge — one using space within an exit stair enclosure — in nonsprinklered new construction.*

new construction. The area of refuge is used to meet the requirements for accessible means of egress, because persons with severe mobility impairment are able to access the floor via the elevator. The exit stair enclosure walls at the right of the exhibit provide the barrier that creates two areas of refuge on the floor. The area of refuge within that exit stair enclosure at the right of the exhibit is less than 1000 $ft^2$ (93 $m^2$), and tenability must be demonstrated. The remainder of the floor serves as the second area of refuge; it is larger than 1000 $ft^2$ (93 $m^2$), and no tenability calculation is required. Stairs provide access from each area of refuge to a public way, as the elevator does not have the special features detailed in 7.2.12.2.4. The stairs must be approximately 57 in. (1455 mm) wide to provide the required 48 in. (1220 mm) clear width between handrails. Two-way communication capability (as noted by the NFPA 170 accessible phone symbol), signage, and posted instructions are required in each area of refuge in accordance with 7.2.12.2.5 and 7.2.12.2.6.

**7.2.12.3.5** Each area of refuge shall be identified by a sign that reads as the follows:

AREA OF REFUGE

**7.2.12.3.5.1** The sign required by 7.2.12.3.5 shall conform to the requirements of ICC/ANSI A117.1, *American National Standard for Accessible and Usable Buildings and Facilities*, for such signage and shall display the international symbol of accessibility. Signs also shall be located as follows:

(1) At each door opening providing access to the area of refuge
(2) At all exits not providing an accessible means of egress, as defined in 3.3.161.1
(3) Where necessary to indicate clearly the direction to an area of refuge

**7.2.12.3.5.2** Signs required by 7.2.12.3.5 shall be illuminated as required for exit signs where exit sign illumination is required.

**7.2.12.3.6** Tactile signage complying with ICC/ANSI A117.1, *American National Standard for Accessible and Usable Buildings and Facilities*, shall be located at each door opening to an area of refuge.

### 7.2.13 Elevators.

Prior to the 1997 edition, the *Code* credited elevators only as a means of moving persons with mobility impairment from an area of refuge to the exit discharge (see 7.2.12). Elevators were not recognized as a component of typical means of egress. The concept of elevators as a component of the means of egress, which is addressed in 7.2.13, was new to the 1997 edition of the *Code*.

**7.2.13.1* General.** An elevator complying with the requirements of Section 9.4 and 7.2.13 shall be permitted to be used as a second means of egress from a tower, as defined in 3.3.262, provided that the following criteria are met:

(1) The tower and any attached structure shall be protected throughout by an approved, supervised automatic sprinkler system in accordance with Section 9.7.
(2) The tower shall be subject to occupancy not to exceed 90 persons.
(3) Primary egress discharges shall be directly to the outside.
(4) No high hazard content areas shall exist in the tower or attached structure.
(5) One hundred percent of the egress capacity shall be provided independent of the elevators.
(6) An evacuation plan that specifically includes the elevator shall be implemented, and staff personnel shall be trained in operations and procedures for elevator emergency use in normal operating mode prior to fire fighter recall.
(7) The tower shall not be used by the general public.

**A.7.2.13.1** It is the intent of 7.2.13.1 that elevators serving as a means of egress serve only independent towers or the tower portion of any integral structure. For elevators that are used as a component in the means of egress, the elevator lobbies, elevator shaft, and machine room need to be protected from the effects of fire.

Subsections 7.2.1 through 7.2.12 are formatted to describe one of 12 potential components of means of egress, such as door assemblies (7.2.1), stairs (7.2.2), ramps (7.2.5), or slide escapes (7.2.10). The occupancy chapters specify whether each of these components is permitted to be used within the required means of egress. The recognition of these components by the occupancy chapters ranges from "permitted by all" for door assemblies to "very limited use" for slide escapes in high hazard industrial and existing storage occupancies. However, in each case, it is the occupancy chapter that determines the applicability of any of the 12 egress components. Subsection 7.2.13 is formatted differently. It limits the use of elevators within means of egress to serving only as a secondary, not primary, means of egress from towers.

The recognition of elevators for emergency egress is limited to towers not used by the general public [see 7.2.13.1(7)]. The occupants will generally be employees, who are familiar with the structure because of repeated occupancy. Although members of the public have likely been taught not to use elevators during fire or similar emergency, the tower's employees can be trained to use elevators effectively for egress.

Note that 7.2.13.1(1) requires the tower to be sprinklered to keep conditions tenable while the elevator is being used. Paragraph 7.2.13.1(2) limits occupancy in the tower to a maximum of 90 persons. Paragraph 7.2.13.1(5) requires that 100 percent of the egress capacity be provided without considering the capacity provided by the elevator. Thus, the elevator helps to satisfy the requirement for a redundant, second egress route, but the primary route (typically a stair) must be sized to accommodate the entire occupant load.

The restrictions imposed on the use of elevator evacuation systems as part of the required means of egress resulted from the consensus process by which the *Code* is revised. One faction favored recognition of elevator evacuation systems in the means of egress for any occupancy. The other faction did not want elevators to be recognized at all for purposes of satisfying any egress requirements.

In March 2004, ASME (the developer of ASME A17.1/CSA B44, *Safety Code for Elevators and Escalators*) sponsored a symposium, cosponsored by NFPA, on the use of elevators in fire emergencies for egress and for fire service use. Recommendations from the symposium were distributed to a host of code-making bodies, including NFPA, to promote concurrent development of provisions to support such elevator use. At the time this commentary was being updated for this edition of the *Code*, two ASME task groups — one on the use of elevators by building occupants during emergencies and one on the use of elevators by emergency responders during emergencies — had nearly completed their detailed hazard analyses required by the ASME procedures for the development of code requirements in new subject areas. NFPA staff is participating in the ASME task groups.

Preliminary work by the task groups indicates that it should be feasible to develop code criteria to permit occupants to use elevators safely after activation of the building fire alarm system and up until the time that a smoke detector in an elevator lobby or associated elevator machine room recalls the elevator. At that time, the elevator will remain locked-out from use until emergency responders place the elevator back into service. Emergency responders (typically fire service personnel) can then use some of the building elevators to ferry occupants to safe discharge levels, while other elevators are used to carry fire fighters and their equipment to floors in the vicinity of the fire floor.

In anticipation that a completed ASME hazard analysis bears out the feasibility of using elevators for evacuation, the NFPA Technical Committee on Means of Egress developed new Annex B on elevators for occupant-controlled evacuation prior to phase I emergency recall operations for the 2009 edition of the *Code*. The new annex uses existing elevator technology and enhanced building construction and occupant information systems. It does not permit the evacuation elevator to receive any credit within the required means of egress system. It is a first step toward recognizing evacuation elevators as part of the required means of egress — a recognition that might be possible for a future edition. In the meantime, elevators continue to receive credit toward satisfying area of refuge criteria applied to an accessible means of egress, via the provisions of 7.2.12 and 7.5.4, and as a second means of egress from a tower in accordance with the provisions of 7.2.13.

**7.2.13.2 Elevator Evacuation System Capacity.**

**7.2.13.2.1** The elevator car shall have a capacity of not less than eight persons.

**7.2.13.2.2** The elevator lobby shall have a capacity of not less than 50 percent of the occupant load of the area served by the lobby. The capacity shall be calculated based on 3 $ft^2$ (0.28 $m^2$) per person and shall also include one wheelchair space of 30 in. × 48 in. (760 mm × 1220 mm) for every 50 persons, or portion thereof, of the total occupant load served by that lobby.

**7.2.13.3 Elevator Lobby.** Every floor served by the elevator shall have an elevator lobby. Barriers forming the elevator lobby shall have a minimum 1-hour fire resistance rating and shall be arranged as a smoke barrier in accordance with Section 8.5.

**7.2.13.4 Elevator Lobby Door Assemblies.** Elevator lobby door assemblies shall have a minimum 1-hour fire protection rating. The transmitted temperature end point shall not exceed 450°F Δ (250°C Δ) above ambient at the end of 30 minutes of the fire exposure specified in the test method referenced in 8.3.3.2. Elevator lobby door leaves shall be self-closing or automatic-closing in accordance with 7.2.1.8.

**7.2.13.5 Door Leaf Activation.** The elevator lobby door leaves shall close in response to a signal from a smoke detector located directly outside the elevator lobby adjacent to or on each door opening. Elevator lobby door leaves shall be permitted to close in response to a signal from the building fire alarm system. Where one elevator lobby door leaf closes by means of a smoke detector or a signal from the building fire alarm system, all elevator lobby door leaves serving that elevator evacuation system shall close.

**7.2.13.6* Water Protection.** Building elements shall be used to restrict water exposure of elevator equipment.

**A.7.2.13.6** One or more of the following approaches can be used to restrict exposure of elevator equipment to water:

(1) A combination of sealed elevator lobby doors, sloped floors, floor drains, and sealed elevator shaft walls is used.
(2) The elevator is mounted on the building exterior that normally operates in the elements, and seals are used on the elevator lobby doors.
(3) The elevator shaft is separated from the building at each floor by an exterior elevator lobby designed to prevent water entry into the elevator shaft.

Information gained from ongoing research concerning waterflow and elevators could lead to the development of water-resistive or water-protected elevator equipment specifically for fire applications. Such equipment should be used only with the building elements (e.g., sealed elevator lobby doors, sloped floors, floor drains) for which it is developed. Further information is available from the NIST publication, *Feasibility of Fire Evacuation by Elevators at FAA Control Towers*.

**7.2.13.7* Power and Control Wiring.** Elevator equipment, elevator communications, elevator machine room cooling, and elevator controller cooling shall be supplied by both normal and standby power. Wiring for power and control shall be located and properly protected to ensure a minimum 1 hour of operation in the event of a fire.

**A.7.2.13.7** Cooling equipment dedicated to the elevator machine room can be used to minimize requirements for standby power.

**7.2.13.8* Communications.** Two-way communication systems shall be provided between elevator lobbies and a central control point and between elevator cars and a central control point. Communications wiring shall be protected to ensure a minimum 1 hour of operation in the event of fire.

**A.7.2.13.8** Communication between elevator lobbies and a central control point can be by telephone or intercom. Auditory alarms should be designed so that they do not interfere with people talking on communications systems.

**7.2.13.9* Elevator Operation.** Elevators shall be provided with fire fighters' emergency operations in accordance with ASME A17.1/CSA B44, *Safety Code for Elevators and Escalators*.

**A.7.2.13.9** Smoke detection in the elevator lobby will result in a Phase I recall of the elevators. The elevators will then be automatically taken out of normal service and will be available to be operated by emergency service personnel.

**7.2.13.10 Maintenance.** Where an elevator lobby is served by only one elevator car, the elevator evacuation system shall have a program of scheduled maintenance during times of building shutdown or low building activity. Repairs shall be performed within 24 hours of breakdown.

**7.2.13.11 Earthquake Protection.** Elevators shall have the capability of orderly shutdowns during earthquakes at locations where such shutdowns are an option of ASME A17.1/CSA B44, *Safety Code for Elevators and Escalators*.

**7.2.13.12 Signage.** Signage shall comply with 7.10.8.4.

## 7.3 Capacity of Means of Egress

### 7.3.1 Occupant Load.

**7.3.1.1 Sufficient Capacity.**

**7.3.1.1.1** The total capacity of the means of egress for any story, balcony, tier, or other occupied space shall be sufficient for the occupant load thereof.

**7.3.1.1.2** For other than existing means of egress, where more than one means of egress is required, the means of egress shall be of such width and capacity that the loss of any one means of egress leaves available not less than 50 percent of the required capacity.

It is a basic concept of the *Code* that the means of egress system be sized to accommodate all people occupying a building. Sizing is accomplished via a code-specified method of matching the occupant load of a floor against the calculated egress capacity of the egress components serving the floor. The sizing criteria do not ensure that all occupants can leave immediately, but they do provide for sufficient quick movement without unacceptable queuing; that is, occupants might have to wait in line to pass through an exit stair enclosure door assembly to begin moving down the stairs, especially where occupants of upper floors who have already entered the stair enclosure are simultaneously using the stairs for egress travel in the downward direction.

The geometry of a building, its occupancy and related occupant load, and the travel distance to exits dictate, in large measure, the location of exits, the number of exits, and the capacity of exits and access thereto. As a consequence, the exits themselves influence the plan and layout of the entire means of egress system. The number of people that the means of egress system can accommodate is determined not solely by the capacity of the exits but also by the number of persons each component within the exit access and exit discharge can accommodate. Very wide corridors that lead to very wide exit stair enclosure door assemblies that then lead to much narrower stairs provide a system comparable to average-width corridors that lead to average-width exit stair enclosure door assemblies that then lead to average-width stairs. A means of egress system is only as good as its most constricting component.

The number of people or occupant load for which the means of egress system must provide egress capacity is calculated or otherwise determined. The occupant load is to reflect the maximum number of people anticipated to occupy the building rooms or spaces at any given time and under all probable situations. The occupant load must not be based only on normal occupancy.

The provision of 7.3.1.1.2 is new to the 2009 edition of the *Code*. It has the effect of requiring that new egress systems employing two means of egress be balanced in size, so that each egress route accommodates at least half of the occupant load of the floor. It also has the effect of requiring that new egress systems employing more than two means of egress be sized so that no one egress route is credited with accommodating more than half of the occupant load of the floor. The requirement is aimed at preventing a situation where the loss of any one egress route reduces the remaining egress capacity to less than half of that needed to accommodate the occupant load of the floor. Application of the provision of 7.3.1.1.2 is demonstrated in the examples that follow.

*Example 1*

The occupant load of a floor in a new building is 350 persons. Two means of egress are provided. Egress route 1 is of sufficient width to accommodate 200 persons, and egress route 2 accommodates 150. The two egress routes, together, exactly accommodate the 350 person occupant load of the floor. If fire or similar emergency were to render egress route 1 unusable, the performance-based criterion of 7.3.1.1.2 would not be met, as less than half the required egress capacity remains usable [i.e., 150 < 350/2]. The designer chooses to resize both egress routes so that each accommodates 175 persons. Following the redesign, the arrangement is again evaluated against the criterion of 7.3.1.1.2. The loss of any one of the two egress routes leaves available not less than 50 percent of the required egress capacity of the floor as required by 7.3.1.1.2.

*Example 2*

The occupant load of a floor in a new building is 350 persons. Two means of egress are provided. Egress route 1 is of sufficient width to accommodate 200 persons, and egress route 2 accommodates 175. The two egress routes, together, accommodate 375 persons, which is 25 persons more than required to be accommodated for the 350 person occupant load of the floor. If fire or similar emergency were to render egress route 1 unusable, the performance-based criterion of 7.3.1.1.2 would be met, as at least half the required egress capacity (i.e., 350/2 = 175) remains usable as required by 7.3.1.1.2.

*Example 3*

The occupant load of a floor in a new building is 640 persons. Three means of egress are provided in accordance with 7.4.1.2. Egress route 1 is of sufficient width to accommodate 340 persons, and egress route 2 and egress route 3 each accommodate 150 persons. The three egress routes, together, exactly accommodate the 640-person occupant load of the floor. If a fire or similar emergency were to render egress route 1 unusable, the performance-based criterion of 7.3.1.1.2 would not be met, as less than half the required egress capacity remains usable via the combination of egress route 2 and egress route 3 [i.e., 150 + 150 = 300; 300 < 640/2]. The designer chooses to resize all three egress routes so that egress route 1 accommodates 320 persons and egress route 2 and egress route 3 each accommodate 160 persons. Following the redesign, the arrangement is again evaluated against the criterion of 7.3.1.1.2. The loss of egress route 1 leaves available not less than 50 percent of the required egress capacity of the floor as required by 7.3.1.1.2.

**7.3.1.2* Occupant Load Factor.** The occupant load in any building or portion thereof shall be not less than the number of persons determined by dividing the floor area assigned to that use by the occupant load factor for that use as specified in Table 7.3.1.2, Figure 7.3.1.2(a), and Figure 7.3.1.2(b). Where both gross and net area figures are given for the same occupancy, calculations shall be made by applying the gross area figure to the gross area of the portion of the building devoted to the use for which the gross area figure is specified and by applying the net area figure to the net area of the portion of the building devoted to the use for which the net area figure is specified.

*Table 7.3.1.2 Occupant Load Factor*

| Use | ($ft^2$ per person)[a] | ($m^2$ per person)[a] |
|---|---|---|
| **Assembly Use** | | |
| Concentrated use, without fixed seating | 7 net | 0.65 net |
| Less concentrated use, without fixed seating | 15 net | 1.4 net |
| Bench-type seating | 1 person/18 linear in. | 1 person/455 linear mm |
| Fixed seating | Number of fixed seats | Number of fixed seats |
| Waiting spaces | See 12.1.7.2 and 13.1.7.2. | See 12.1.7.2 and 13.1.7.2. |
| Kitchens | 100 | 9.3 |
| Library stack areas | 100 | 9.3 |
| Library reading rooms | 50 net | 4.6 net |
| Swimming pools | 50 (water surface) | 4.6 (water surface) |
| Swimming pool decks | 30 | 2.8 |
| Exercise rooms with equipment | 50 | 4.6 |
| Exercise rooms without equipment | 15 | 1.4 |
| Stages | 15 net | 1.4 net |
| Lighting and access catwalks, galleries, gridirons | 100 net | 9.3 net |
| Casinos and similar gaming areas | 11 | 1 |
| Skating rinks | 50 | 4.6 |
| **Educational Use** | | |
| Classrooms | 20 net | 1.9 net |
| Shops, laboratories, vocational rooms | 50 net | 4.6 net |
| **Day-Care Use** | 35 net | 3.3 net |
| **Health Care Use** | | |
| Inpatient treatment departments | 240 | 22.3 |
| Sleeping departments | 120 | 11.1 |
| Ambulatory health care | 100 | 9.3 |
| **Detention and Correctional Use** | 120 | 11.1 |
| **Residential Use** | | |
| Hotels and dormitories | 200 | 18.6 |
| Apartment buildings | 200 | 18.6 |
| Board and care, large | 200 | 18.6 |
| **Industrial Use** | | |
| General and high hazard industrial | 100 | 9.3 |
| Special-purpose industrial | NA | NA |
| **Business Use (other than below)** | 100 | 9.3 |
| Air traffic control tower observation levels | 40 | 3.7 |
| **Storage Use** | | |
| In storage occupancies | NA | NA |
| In mercantile occupancies | 300 | 27.9 |
| In other than storage and mercantile occupancies | 500 | 46.5 |
| **Mercantile Use** | | |
| Sales area on street floor[b,c] | 30 | 2.8 |
| Sales area on two or more street floors[c] | 40 | 3.7 |
| Sales area on floor below street floor[c] | 30 | 2.8 |
| Sales area on floors above street floor[c] | 60 | 5.6 |
| Floors or portions of floors used only for offices | See business use. | See business use. |
| Floors or portions of floors used only for storage, receiving, and shipping, and not open to general public | 300 | 27.9 |
| Mall buildings[d] | Per factors applicable to use of space[e] | |

NA: Not applicable. The occupant load is the maximum probable number of occupants present at any time.

[a]All factors are expressed in gross area unless marked "net."

[b]For the purpose of determining occupant load in mercantile occupancies where, due to differences in the finished ground level of streets on different sides, two or more floors directly accessible from streets (not including alleys or similar back streets) exist, each such floor is permitted to be considered a street floor. The occupant load factor is one person for each 40 $ft^2$ (3.7 $m^2$) of gross floor area of sales space.

[c]For the purpose of determining occupant load in mercantile occupancies with no street floor, as defined in 3.3.253, but with access directly from the street by stairs or escalators, the floor at the point of entrance to the mercantile occupancy is considered the street floor.

[d]For any food court or other assembly use areas located in the mall that are not included as a portion of the gross leasable area of the mall building, the occupant load is calculated based on the occupant load factor for that use as specified in Table 7.3.1.2. The remaining mall area is not required to be assigned an occupant load.

[e]The portions of the mall that are considered a pedestrian way and not used as gross leasable area are not required to be assessed an occupant load based on Table 7.3.1.2. However, means of egress from a mall pedestrian way are required to be provided for an occupant load determined by dividing the gross leasable area of the mall building (not including anchor stores) by the appropriate lowest whole number occupant load factor from Figure 7.3.1.2(a) or Figure 7.3.1.2(b).

Each individual tenant space is required to have means of egress to the outside or to the mall based on occupant loads calculated by using the appropriate occupant load factor from Table 7.3.1.2.

Each individual anchor store is required to have means of egress independent of the mall.

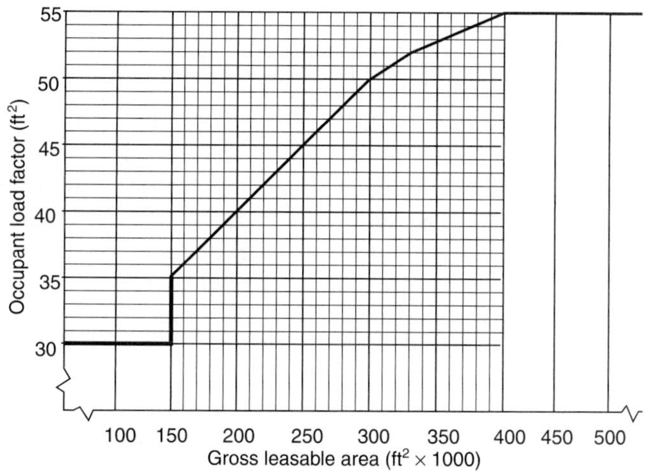


***Figure 7.3.1.2(a)*** *Mall Building Occupant Load Factors (U.S. Customary Units).*

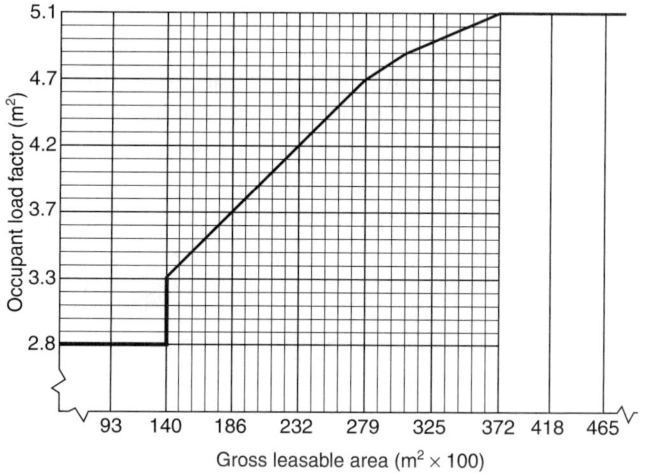


***Figure 7.3.1.2(b)*** *Mall Building Occupant Load Factors (SI Units).*

**A.7.3.1.2** The normal occupant load is not necessarily a suitable criterion, because the greatest hazard can occur when an unusually large crowd is present, which is a condition often difficult for authorities having jurisdiction to control by regulatory measures. The principle of this *Code* is to provide means of egress for the maximum probable number of occupants, rather than to attempt to limit occupants to a number commensurate with available means of egress. However, limits of occupancy are specified in certain special cases for other reasons.

Suggested occupant load factors for components of large airport terminal buildings are given in Table A.7.3.1.2. However, the authority having jurisdiction might elect to use different occupant load factors, provided that egress requirements are satisfied.

***Table A.7.3.1.2 Airport Terminal Occupant Load Factors***

| Airport Terminal Area | ft² (gross) | m² (gross) |
|---|---|---|
| Concourse | 100 | 9.3 |
| Waiting areas | 15 | 1.4 |
| Baggage claim | 20 | 1.9 |
| Baggage handling | 300 | 27.9 |

The figure used in determining the occupancy load for mall shopping centers of varying sizes was arrived at empirically by surveying over 270 mall shopping centers, by studying mercantile occupancy parking requirements, and by observing the number of occupants per vehicle during peak seasons.

These studies show that, with an increase in shopping center size, there is a decrease in the number of occupants per square foot of gross leasable area.

This phenomenon is explained when one considers that, above a certain shopping center gross leasable area [approximately 600,000 ft² (56,000 m²)], there exists a multiplicity of the same types of stores. The purpose of duplicate types of stores is to increase the choices available to a customer for any given type of merchandise. Therefore, when shopping center size increases, the occupant load increases as well, but at a declining rate. In using Figure 7.3.1.2(a) or Figure 7.3.1.2(b), the occupant load factor is applied only to the gross leasable area that uses the mall as a means of egress.

Occupant load is determined by the nature of the use of a building or space and the amount of space available for that use. Since different generic uses are characterized by different occupant densities, Table 7.3.1.2 has established occupant load factors for each use. The first column of the table is deliberately headed "use" rather than "occupancy," because the use of an area might differ from its occupancy classification. For example, a meeting room for fewer than 50 people in an office building is not an assembly occupancy; it is a business occupancy [see 6.1.14.1.3(2)], but its occupant load is based on an assembly use. The same concept applies to a classroom in a university, which, although classified as a business occupancy, has an occupant load based on educational use (for traditional classroom style) or assembly use (for lecture style with theater-type seating).

The occupant load factor, as a density factor, assumes the presence of at least one person for each specified unit of area. Note that some values are for net area, while others are based on gross area. The gross area figure applies to the building as a whole (the area within the confining perimeter walls of the building, including areas that are occupied by shafts and other elements that people do not occupy); the net area figure applies to actual occupied spaces, such as classroom spaces, and does not include the corridors, the area occupied by walls, or other unoccupied areas.

Cases of mixed use might exist where, for example, an assembly use space having an occupant load based on net floor area might be located in a building that is primarily a business occupancy, a classification for which the occupant load is based on gross area. In such instances, the net area calculations should be performed for those specific areas that use occupant load factors based on net area; the remaining floor area can then be used to calculate the occupant load for the uses employing gross floor area. This is illustrated in Exhibit 7.74.

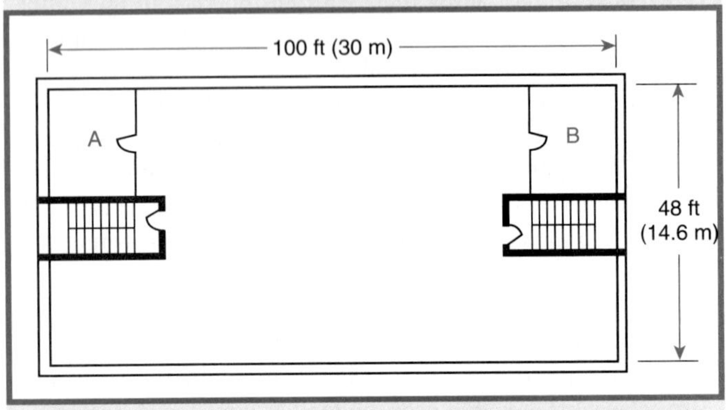


***Exhibit 7.74*** *Floor area for occupant load considerations.*

In Exhibit 7.74, the majority of the 4800 ft² (446 m²) gross floor area [i.e., 100 ft × 48 ft (30 m × 14.6 m)] is used for business purposes and is occupied by desks, chairs, file cabinets, office machines, and associated office personnel. Rooms A and B are conference rooms with tables and chairs used on a regular basis, primarily by company personnel from other floors in the building. These rooms can be expected to be occupied simultaneously with the remainder of the floor. Each conference room provides 320 ft² (30 m²) of net usable area. Because neither conference room can accommodate 50 or more persons, an assembly occupancy is not created. Rather, the floor is a business occupancy with some incidental assembly use [again, see 6.1.14.1.3(2)].

Because occupant load is calculated based on use of the space (not occupancy classification), the occupant load of the floor shown in Exhibit 7.74 is calculated using occupant load factors for both an assembly use, which is based on net area, and a business use, which is based on gross area. The occupant load of the assembly use spaces (conference rooms A and B) is calculated first. Using Table 7.3.1.2, a net area factor of 15 ft² (1.4 m²) per person for assembly, "less concentrated use," is chosen. [Note that the concept of "less concentrated use" refers to the possible concentration of occupants where, because of the presence of tables and chairs, there are fewer occupants than would be possible without the tables and chairs, which is an example of "concentrated use."] The two conference rooms must be assumed to have a combined occupant load of at least 43 persons, according to the following calculation:

$$\frac{640\ \text{ft}^2}{15\ \text{ft}^2\ \text{per person}} = 43\ \text{persons}$$

$$\frac{60\ \text{m}^2}{1.4\ \text{m}^2\ \text{per person}} = 43\ \text{persons}$$

Next, the occupant load of the remainder of the floor must be calculated. The use is business, so a gross area factor of 100 ft² (9.3 m²) per person is chosen per Table 7.3.1.2. Because the net area usable as conference rooms has already been assigned an occupant load, that area can be subtracted from the gross floor area, and the remaining business use area is then assigned an occupant load as follows:

$$(4800\ \text{ft}^2\ \text{gross area}) - (640\ \text{ft}^2\ \text{net assembly use area}) = 4160\ \text{ft}^2$$

$$[(446\ \text{m}^2\ \text{gross area}) - (60\ \text{m}^2\ \text{net assembly use area}) = 386\ \text{m}^2]$$

$$\frac{4160\ \text{ft}^2\ \text{gross business use area}}{100\ \text{ft}^2\ \text{per person}} = 42\ \text{persons}$$

$$\left[\frac{386\ \text{m}^2\ \text{gross business use area}}{9.3\ \text{m}^2\ \text{per person}} = 42\ \text{persons}\right]$$

Adding together the assembly use occupant load (43) and the business use occupant load (42) results in a minimum occupant load of 85 persons for the floor. See the paragraph that follows for an explanation of conditions under which the occupant load might be a number greater than that calculated using the floor area and occupant load factor calculation. However, the occupant load is not permitted to be a number smaller than that calculated, even where the building operator plans to limit the number of occupants.

Egress capacity must be provided for at least the occupant load (expressed in number of persons) determined by dividing each area of the space by the appropriate occupant load factor. This calculated occupant load must serve as the minimum starting point for egress sizing, regardless of whether the building operator claims that the occupant load will never reach the occupant load determined by calculation. However, if the building operator plans to have more occupants present than the number determined by calculation using occupant load factors, the means of egress system must be sized to accommodate that larger number. In return for providing the larger egress system, the building operator is permitted to claim the larger number of persons as the occupant load. This concept is further explained in the commentary following 7.3.1.3.2.

Table 7.3.1.2 provides an occupant load factor for ambulatory health care use. The entry clarifies that, in the same way that the provisions for ambulatory health care occupancies build on those for business occupancies, the 100 $ft^2$ (9.3 $m^2$) per person characteristic of a business use is appropriate for ambulatory health care use.

Note that the occupant load for storage use classified as a storage occupancy (e.g., a warehouse) is determined not by calculation, but through negotiation between the designer or owner and the AHJ, based on actual use and population (see 42.1.7). There is no occupant load factor for storage use in a storage occupancy in Table 7.3.1.2. However, Table 7.3.1.2 provides occupant load factors for storage use in occupancies other than a storage occupancy (e.g., a central storage room in a hospital) to allow occupant load to be aggregated via calculations for each use area on a building floor.

**7.3.1.3 Occupant Load Increases.**

**7.3.1.3.1** The occupant load in any building or portion thereof shall be permitted to be increased from the occupant load established for the given use in accordance with 7.3.1.2 where all other requirements of this *Code* are also met, based on such increased occupant load.

**7.3.1.3.2** The authority having jurisdiction shall be permitted to require an approved aisle, seating, or fixed equipment diagram to substantiate any increase in occupant load and shall be permitted to require that such a diagram be posted in an approved location.

The *Code*'s intent for other than assembly occupancies is not to restrict the occupant load of a building based on the floor area of the building. Nor is the *Code* specifying the minimum area needed by each occupant for efficient use of the space. An occupant load is established for use in sizing the means of egress system and in determining thresholds at which additional provisions, such as mandatory sprinklers, become applicable. If *Code* provisions can be met for a larger number of persons than the calculation determines, the larger number of occupants is permitted to be present, provided that the AHJ is satisfied that the egress system (including corridors, aisles, stairs, and other means of egress components) can accommodate the larger occupant load.

For example, an office of 20,000 $ft^2$ (1860 $m^2$) gross area would be assigned an occupant load of 200 persons if the typical 100 $ft^2$ (9.3 $m^2$) per person occupant load factor were used. However, the occupant load would be permitted to be increased (e.g., to 400 persons to accommodate the occupant load of a telemarketing call center where staff occupy tiny cubicles) if all *Code* provisions dependent on numbers of persons were met for the increased load.

Assembly occupancies have special but similar provisions for increasing occupant load. Densities greater than one person for each 5 $ft^2$ (0.46 $m^2$) are prohibited, because movement speeds are reduced to a crawl where the density exceeds one person for each 3 $ft^2$ (0.28 $m^2$) density. This density is approaching the jam point at which movement stops, as addressed in the commentary following 12/13.1.7.4.

**7.3.1.4 Exits Serving More than One Story.** Where an exit serves more than one story, only the occupant load of each story considered individually shall be used in computing the required capacity of the exit at that story, provided that the required egress capacity of the exit is not decreased in the direction of egress travel.

Paragraph 7.3.1.4 provides that, once a maximum required egress capacity is determined, such required capacity must be maintained — in the direction of egress travel — for the remainder of the egress system.

Required stair width is determined by the required egress capacity of each floor the stair serves, considered independently. It is not necessary to accumulate occupant loads from floor to floor to determine stair width. Each story or floor level is considered separately when calculating the occupant load to be served by the means of egress from that floor. The size or width of the stair need only accommodate the portion of the floor's occupant load assigned to that stair. However, in a multistory building, the floor requiring the greatest egress capacity dictates the minimum stair width from that floor to the level of exit discharge in the direction of egress travel. It is not permissible to reduce such stair width along the remainder of the stair runs encountered in traveling to the level of exit discharge; that is, stairs encountered in the direction of egress travel. Exits serving floors above the floor of greatest egress capacity are permitted to use egress components sized to handle the largest demand created by any floor served by that section of stair run.

Exhibit 7.75 illustrates the intent of 7.3.1.4. It is not necessary to accumulate required egress capacity from floor to floor; no decrease in egress capacity is permitted in the direction of egress travel.

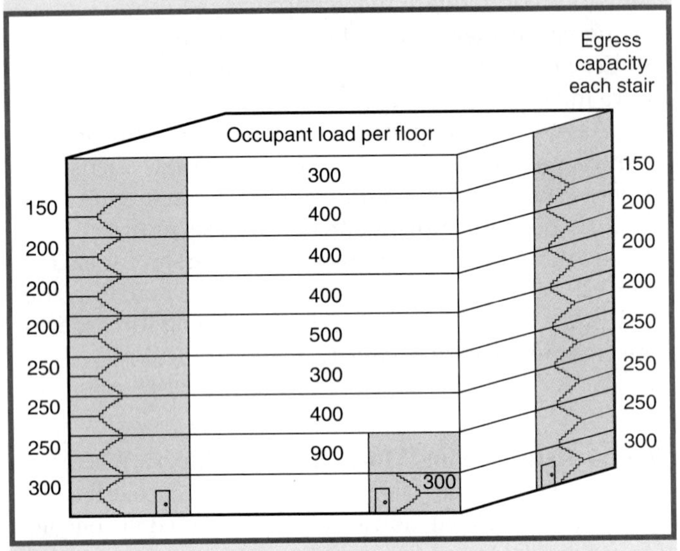


***Exhibit 7.75*** *Capacity of exit stairs serving multiple floors.*

**7.3.1.5 Capacity from a Point of Convergence.** Where means of egress from a story above and a story below converge at an intermediate story, the capacity of the means of egress from the point of convergence shall be not less than the sum of the capacity of the two means of egress.

Exhibit 7.76 illustrates the intent of 7.3.1.5. Convergence from floors above and below requires the accumulation of required egress capacity. Note that occupants of the second floor move down the stairs and converge with occupants of the basement, who are traveling up the stairs. From the merge point (i.e., the ground level stair landing) to the public way, the egress path must accommodate the 300-person combined occupant load represented as the sum of those persons moving downward and upward on the stair.

The occupants of the first floor (X) experience level travel through the stair enclosure; they are not considered to have merged from above or below; and egress capacity for the first floor occupants is not added to that of the second floor and basement.

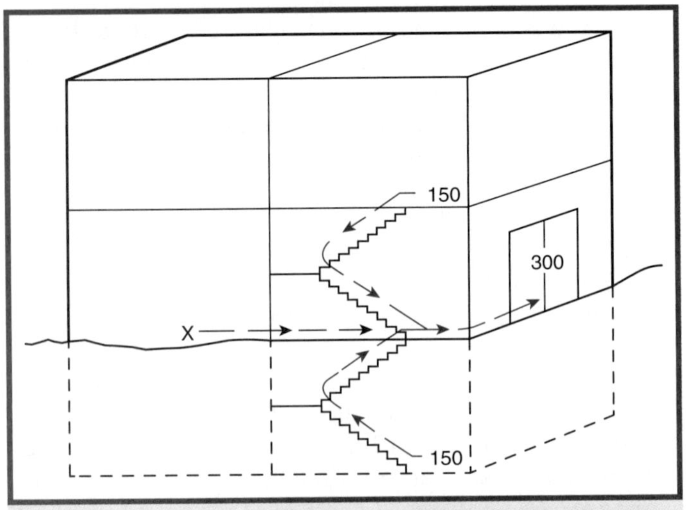


***Exhibit 7.76*** *Capacity of egress system from point on stairs where occupants from floors above and below converge.*

**7.3.1.6 Egress Capacity from Balconies and Mezzanines.** Where any required egress capacity from a balcony or mezzanine passes through the room below, that required capacity shall be added to the required egress capacity of the room below.

Mezzanines and balconies are considered as part of the room in which they are located. Occupants of mezzanines and balconies experience the effects of a fire in the room to which such spaces are open as readily as do the occupants of those spaces. Thus, mezzanines and balconies must have their occupant load added to that of the room or space in which they are located if their egress passes through that room or space.

An example is depicted in Exhibit 7.77. There is no direct access to the enclosed exit stair from the mezzanine; therefore, egress from the mezzanine is down the open stair and through the main floor. Thus, the street floor egress capacity must accommodate the occupant load of the street floor and that of the mezzanine. If the main floor has an occupant load of 200 persons and the mezzanine has an occupant load of 50 persons, the egress capacity for the main floor must accommodate at least 250 persons.

### 7.3.2 Measurement of Means of Egress.

**7.3.2.1** The width of means of egress shall be measured in the clear at the narrowest point of the egress component under consideration, unless otherwise provided in 7.3.2.2 or 7.3.2.3.

**7.3.2.2** Projections within the means of egress of not more than 4½ in. (114 mm) on each side shall be permitted at a

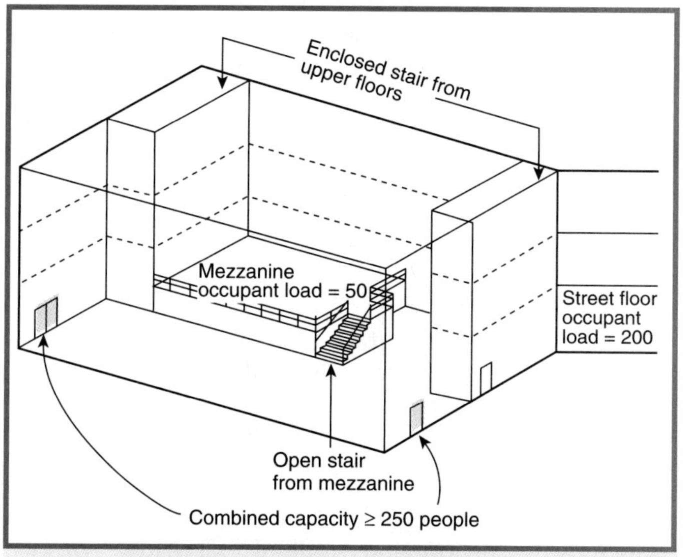


***Exhibit 7.77*** *Capacity of main floor with mezzanine egress through that floor.*

height of 38 in. (965 mm) and below. In the case of stair and landing handrails forming part of a guard, in accordance with 7.2.2.4.4.3, such projections shall be permitted at a height of 42 in. (1065 mm) and below.

**7.3.2.3** In health care and ambulatory health care occupancies, projections shall be permitted in corridors in accordance with Chapters 18 through 21.

Paragraph 7.3.2.2 permits maximum 4½ in. (114 mm) projections at each side of an egress component for purposes of determining width for use in egress capacity calculations, provided that such projections occur at a height of not more than 38 in. (965 mm), which is the maximum mounting height for handrails. Note that such encroachments are not limited to items such as handrails that are required by the *Code*. The encroachment might be the result of wainscoting applied to the lower portion of a wall, or it might be caused by the metal stringers to which metal pan stair treads and risers are welded.

A 4½ in. (114 mm) encroachment is permitted by 7.3.2.2 along stairs, corridors, passageways, and other components of the means of egress (other than door openings) for purposes of calculating egress capacity. The egress capacity of door openings is regulated by 7.2.1.2.2.1, which substitutes a maximum 3½ in. (90 mm) projection at each side of the door opening in place of the 4½ in. (114 mm) projection permitted by 7.3.2.2. Figure A.7.2.1.2.2(b) depicts the allowable encroachment at each side of a door opening.

For purposes of determining whether a door opening provides the minimum required width (such as that needed for a person in a wheelchair to pass through a door opening), see 7.2.1.2.1.1, Figure A.7.2.1.2.1.1(a), and Figure A.7.2.1.2.1.1(b). Similarly, the minimum 48 in. (1220 mm) clear width between handrails, as required by 7.2.12.2.3 for stairs serving areas of refuge, does not allow for encroachments, based on the need to provide sufficient clear width to carry a person in a wheelchair on the stair.

Projections at or below 38 in. (965 mm) (i.e., handrail height), and not exceeding 4½ in. (114 mm), do not adversely restrict the effective egress width of stairs or corridors, because the human body is normally widest at shoulder level. Also, the body sway associated with walking, particularly on stairs, is greater at shoulder height than it is at waist height. Other projections, however, might constitute obstructions and cause impediments to the free flow of pedestrian travel. The *Code*, therefore, bases the measurements of widths of means of egress used for egress capacity calculation purposes on the clear, net, usable, unobstructed width. Only those projections specified are permitted to encroach on the required width without having to subtract the encroaching space from the overall width before performing the egress width calculation.

Paragraph 7.3.2.3 serves as a reminder that the provisions of 7.3.2 are modified to permit encroachments in health care and ambulatory health care occupancy corridors where the corridor width is at least 6 ft (1830 mm) — a width far greater than the 36 in. (915 mm) minimum established for egress components by 7.3.4.1. See, for example, 18.2.3.4(2) and (3) and 18.2.3.5(2) and (3).

### 7.3.3* Egress Capacity.

**A.7.3.3** In egress capacity calculations, standard rounding should be used.

**7.3.3.1** Egress capacity for approved components of means of egress shall be based on the capacity factors shown in Table 7.3.3.1, unless otherwise provided in 7.3.3.2 .

A significant change in egress capacity calculations was introduced in the 1988 edition of the *Code*. The unit of exit width formerly used as a measure of egress capacity was replaced by a system of smaller increments of egress width and capacity. For egress widths that were close to, and no smaller than, the previously used units [22 in. (560 mm)] and half units [12 in. (305 mm)], there is little difference in the egress capacities

*Table 7.3.3.1 Capacity Factors*

| Area | Stairways (width per person) | | Level Components and Ramps (width per person) | |
|---|---|---|---|---|
| | in. | mm | in. | mm |
| Board and care | 0.4 | 10 | 0.2 | 5 |
| Health care, sprinklered | 0.3 | 7.6 | 0.2 | 5 |
| Health care, nonsprinklered | 0.6 | 15 | 0.5 | 13 |
| High hazard contents | 0.7 | 18 | 0.4 | 10 |
| All others | 0.3 | 7.6 | 0.2 | 5 |

calculated by the two methods. For other widths, such as for door assemblies and nonstandard stairs, the new method of using smaller increments (approximating a linear formula) provides increased egress capacity. This concept is demonstrated in the examples that follow.

*Example 1*

The common combination of a 34 in. (865 mm) clear width door opening that provides access to a stair 44 in. (1120 mm) wide with a 34 in. (865 mm) clear width discharge door opening has a capacity based on the capacity of its least efficient element. The individual capacities of the elements are calculated by dividing the widths by the appropriate capacity factor from Table 7.3.3.1. The door openings have a capacity of 34 in. (865 mm) divided by 0.2 in. (5 mm) per person, or 170 persons. The stair has a capacity of 44 in. (1120 mm) divided by 0.3 in. (7.6 mm) per person, or 147 persons. The capacity of the exit is 147, the smaller of the two capacities. Under the use of the pre-1988 unit of exit width method, the capacities were 150 for the $1\frac{1}{2}$-unit door assemblies [those 34 in. (865 mm) or more in width] and 150 for the 2-unit stair.

*Example 2*

If the entry door opening provides 32 in. (810 mm) in clear width, the stair is 54 in. (1370 mm) wide, and the discharge door opening provides 36 in. (915 mm) in clear width, the individual capacities are, respectively, as follows:

1. 32 in. (810 mm) divided by 0.2 in. (5 mm) per person, or 160 persons, for the entry door opening
2. 54 in. (1370 mm) divided by 0.3 in. (7.6 mm) per person, or 180 persons, for the stair
3. 36 in. (915 mm) divided by 0.2 in. (5 mm) per person, or 180 persons, for the discharge door opening

Therefore, the capacity of the overall combination is the smallest of the three capacities — 160 persons, as provided by the entry door opening. Under the previous unit of exit width method, the capacities would have been, respectively, as follows:

1. 1 unit for the entry door opening multiplied by 100 persons per unit, or 100 persons
2. 2 units for the stair multiplied by 75 persons per unit, or 150 persons
3. 1.5 units for the discharge door opening multiplied by 100 persons per unit, or 150 persons

Therefore, the capacity for the combination, as calculated using the previous unit of exit width, would have been only 100 persons, based on the entry door opening. The unit of exit width procedure unfairly penalized the door opening because it was 2 in. (51 mm) short of the width needed to be credited with $1\frac{1}{2}$ units of exit width, or a 150-person capacity.

The width per person figures specified in Table 7.3.3.1 are based on previously used values credited for full units. The chief difference is that small increments are now considered to add to the capacity. Although Canadian research studies of egress movement in tall office buildings and in larger assembly occupancy buildings have demonstrated the validity of the small increment approach, there was evidence for this approach even in some significant early studies of egress and exit design. Two early, influential reports are of interest. One dates from 1935 in the United States,[25] the other was published in 1958 in Great Britain.[26] Both reports are provided in a discussion of the issue of exit unit size that was published in 1984 in *Fire Technology*.[27] The reports clearly show that the small increment approach was an unsettled issue, even in those reports that were thought to support only the unit width method. More recent evidence has related egress facility width and crowd flow capacity. Clear documentation shows that crowds do not move in regular files or lanes, especially on stairs where side-to-side body sway almost prevents people from walking shoulder to shoulder. The combination of the recent evidence and documentation has led to the change to the more linear small increment method.

The capacity factors found in Table 7.3.3.1 are simply derived from previously used combinations of egress component width and capacity, such as 75 persons per 22 in. unit of exit width for stairs (22 divided by 75 is 0.293, which, when rounded to the closest single digit, is 0.3). Similarly, for level and ramped components, the derivation is simply 22 divided by 100, which is rounded to 0.2.

The differences in the width factors specified in Table 7.3.3.1 arise from the following:

1. Stairs entail a totally different type of movement, by both individuals and crowds, than do level and ramped components.
2. For stairs, there are differences in biomechanics, as well as a difficulty in the ability to see (or otherwise detect) the next stepping surface in order to avoid misstepping and suffering a fall and resulting injury.
3. The approximate ratio of 3 to 2, relating the required widths for vertical travel on stairs and level travel on floors, is based on previous ratios and on empirical observations.

The greater range of width requirements for different occupancies reflects the following two factors:

1. The need for a much more rapid egress time in the case of high hazard occupancies
2. The slower movement and greater need for assistance from others during evacuations in nonsprinklered health care and related institutional and semi-institutional occupancies

In summary, given the designer's knowledge of the occupancy, the occupant load of the floor level, and the type of egress component, the required minimum width for each component can be determined by simple multiplication (i.e., multiply the occupant load by the appropriate width-per-person factor found in Table 7.3.3.1 to obtain the minimum width of the component under consideration). If the width of the component under consideration is known, divide that width by the appropriate width-per-person factor to obtain the number of persons the component can accommodate over the entire evacuation. These calculated minimum widths are then considered along with other *Code* requirements, including minimum widths based on other factors, to design a system in which performance will be closely matched from one part of the system to another.

**7.3.3.2*** For stairways wider than 44 in. (1120 mm) and subject to the 0.3 in. (7.6 mm) width per person capacity factor, the capacity shall be permitted to be increased using the following equation:

$$C = 146.7 + \left(\frac{Wn - 44}{0.218}\right)$$

where:

$C$ = capacity, in persons, rounded to the nearest integer

$Wn$ = nominal width of the stair as permitted by 7.3.2.2 (in.)

**A.7.3.3.2** The effective capacity of stairways has been shown by research to be proportional to the effective width of the stairway, which is the nominal width minus 12 in. (305 mm). This phenomenon, and the supporting research, were described in the chapter, "Movement of People," in the first, second, and third editions of the *SFPE Handbook of Fire Protection Engineering* and was also addressed in Appendix D of the 1985 edition of NFPA *101*, among several other publications. In 1988, this appendix was moved to form Chapter 2 of the 1988 edition of NFPA 101M, *Alternative Approaches to Life Safety*. (This document was later designated as NFPA 101A, *Guide on Alternative Approaches to Life Safety*, and this chapter remained in the document through the 1998 edition.) In essence, the effective width phenomenon recognizes that there is an edge or boundary effect at the sides of a circulation path. It has been best examined in relation to stairway width, where the edge effect was estimated to be 6 in. (150 mm) on each side, but a similar phenomenon occurs with other paths, such as corridors and doors, although quantitative estimates of their edge effect are not as well established as they have been for stairways, at least those stairways studied in Canada during the late 1960s through the 1970s in office building evacuation drills and in crowd movement in a variety of buildings with assembly occupancy.

More recent studies have not been performed to determine how the edge effect might be changing (or has changed) with demographic changes to larger, heavier occupants moving more slowly, and thus swaying laterally, to maintain balance when walking. The impact of such demographic changes, which are significant and influential for evacuation flow and speed of movement on stairs, for example, has the effect of increasing the time of evacuation in a way that affects all stair widths, but will be most pronounced for nominal widths less than 56 in. (1422 mm).

Without taking into account occupant demographic changes in the last few decades that affect evacuation performance, especially on stairs, the formula for enhanced capacity of stairways wider than 44 in. (1120 mm) assumes that any portion of the nominal width greater than 44 in. (1120 mm) is as effective proportionally as the effective width of a nominal 44 in. (1120 mm) stair, that is, 32 in. (810 mm). Thus, the denominator (0.218) in the equation is simply the effective width of 32 in. (810 mm) divided by the capacity of 147 persons that is credited, by the 0.3 in. (7.6 mm) capacity factor in Table 7.3.3.1, to the corresponding nominal width, 44 in. (1120 mm).

The resulting permitted stairway capacities, based on occupant load of single stories (in accordance with 7.3.1.4), for several stairway widths are shown in Table A.7.3.3.2.

*Table A.7.3.3.2 Stairway Capacities*

| Permitted Capacity (no. of persons) | Nominal Width | | Clear Width Between Handrails[a] | | Effective Width | |
|---|---|---|---|---|---|---|
| | in. | mm | in. | mm | in. | mm |
| 120[b] | 36 | 915 | 28 | 710 | 24 | 610 |
| 147 | 44 | 1120 | 36 | 915 | 32 | 810 |
| 202 | 56 | 1420 | 48 | 1220 | 44 | 1120 |
| 257 | 68 | 1725 | 60 | 1525[c] | 56 | 1420 |

[a]A reasonable handrail incursion of only 4 in. (100 mm), into the nominal width, is assumed on each side of the stair, although 7.3.3.2 permits a maximum incursion of 4½ in. (114 mm) on each side.

[b]Other *Code* sections limit the occupant load for such stairs more severely (e.g., 50 persons in 7.2.2.2.1.2). Such lower limits are partly justified by the relatively small effective width of such stairs, which, if taken into account by Table 7.3.3.1, would result in a correspondingly low effective capacity of only 110 persons (24 divided by 0.218), or a more realistic capacity factor of 0.327, applicable to nominal width.

[c] A clear width of 60 in. (1525 mm) is the maximum permitted by the handrail reachability criteria of 7.2.2.4.1.2. Although some prior editions of the *Code* permitted wider portions of stairs [up to 88 in. (2240 mm), between handrails], such wider portions are less effective for reasonably safe crowd flow and generally should not be used for major crowd movement. To achieve the maximum possible, reasonably safe egress capacity for such stairs, retrofit of an intermediate — not necessarily central — handrail is recommended; for example, with an intermediate handrail located 36 in. (915 mm) from the closest side handrail. In this case, the effective capacity would be 358 persons for the formerly permitted, now retrofitted, stair. This is based on a retrofitted, effective width of about 78 in. (1980 mm) [subtracting 2 in. (51 mm) from each usable side of a handrail and assuming a 2 in. (51 mm) wide, retrofitted intermediate handrail].

The enhanced capacity provision of 7.3.3.2 is new to the 2009 edition of the *Code*. It permits stairs that are wider than 44 in. (1120 mm) for which the 0.3 in. (7.6 mm) per person capacity factor from the last row (i.e., the entry for "all others") of Table 7.3.3.1 is applied to be credited with more capacity than results from the standard calculation performed by dividing the clear width of the stair by the 0.3 in (7.6 mm) per person capacity factor. The rationale for the enhanced capacity allowance is detailed in the extensive commentary of A.7.3.3.2.

The equation in 7.3.3.2 is presented only in inch-pound units. Where SI units are used, the equation for calculating capacity, C, is as follows:

$$C = 146.7 + \left[\frac{(Wn - 1120)}{5.45}\right]$$

where the nominal stair width is expressed in mm.

An example of use of the enhanced capacity permitted by 7.3.3.2 follows. A 56 in. (1420 mm) stair has encroachments at handrail height and below that do not exceed the 4½ in. (114 mm) permitted at each side by 7.3.2.2. The stair exceeds the 44 in. (1120 mm) width specified in 7.3.3.2 and is in a business occupancy, so as to be subject to the 0.3 in. (7.6 mm) per person capacity factor from the last row of Table 7.3.3.1. The traditional capacity calculation involves taking the 56 in. (1420 mm) clear width and dividing it by 0.3 in. (7.6 mm) per person, which results in a traditional capacity of 187 persons. The nominal width of the stair, for purposes of performing the enhanced capacity calculation permitted by 7.3.3.2, is the full 56 in. (1420 mm) clear width, and the calculation is performed as follows:

$$\text{Enhanced capacity, } C = 146.7 + \left[\frac{(56 \text{ in.} - 44 \text{ in.})}{0.218}\right]$$

$$C = 146.7 + \left[\frac{12}{0.218}\right]$$

$$C = 146.7 + 55$$

$$C = 202$$

In SI units:

$$\text{Enhanced capacity, } C = 146.7 + \left[\frac{(1420 \text{ mm} - 1120 \text{ mm})}{5.45}\right]$$

$$C = 146.7 + \left[\frac{300}{5.45}\right]$$

$$C = 146.7 + 55$$

$$C = 202$$

Note that 7.2.2.4.1.2(2)(b) prohibits the enhanced capacity option of 7.3.3.2 from being applied to existing stairs where portions of the stair are more than 30 in. (760 mm) from a handrail as permitted by 7.2.2.4.1.2(2)(a).

**7.3.3.3** The required capacity of a corridor shall be the occupant load that utilizes the corridor for exit access divided by the required number of exits to which the corridor connects, but the corridor capacity shall be not less than the required capacity of the exit to which the corridor leads.

An example of the provisions of 7.3.3.2 is shown in Exhibit 7.78. A corridor system serves a floor with a 660-person occupant load and three means of egress. The corridor must be wide enough to accommodate the portion of the floor's occupant load that it serves. Typical design practice is to divide the floor occupant load by the number of means of egress provided. In this three-exit example, no portion of the corridor needs capacity for more than one-third of the floor's occu-

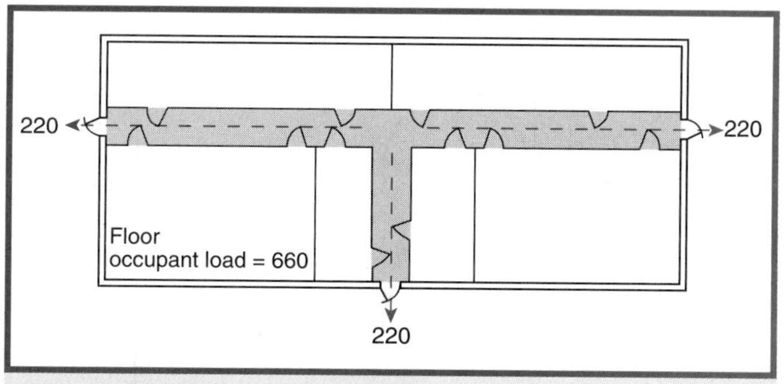


***Exhibit 7.78*** *Corridor capacity.*

pant load, which by calculation (660 ÷ 3) is 220 persons. The required corridor width is determined to be 44 in. (1120 mm) wide [220 persons × 0.2 in. (5 mm) per person]. Some occupancies, such as health care occupancies, require wider minimum corridor widths than the 44 in. (1120 mm) width calculated.

The *Code* states that the required corridor capacity cannot be less than the required capacity of the exit to which it leads. In other words, the corridor is not permitted to create a bottleneck that is too narrow and impedes the flow of occupants to the exit door opening.

### 7.3.4 Minimum Width.

**7.3.4.1** The width of any means of egress, unless otherwise provided in 7.3.4.1.1 through 7.3.4.1.3, shall be as follows:

(1) Not less than that required for a given egress component in this chapter or Chapters 11 through 43
(2) Not less than 36 in. (915 mm)

**7.3.4.1.1*** The width of exit access that is formed by furniture and movable partitions, that serves not more than six people, and that has a length not exceeding 50 ft (15 m) shall meet both of the following criteria:

(1) The width shall be not less than 18 in. (455 mm), at and below a height of 38 in. (965 mm), and not less than 28 in. (710 mm) above a height of 38 in. (965 mm).
(2) A width of not less than 36 in. (915 mm) for new exit access, and not less than 28 in. (710 mm) for existing exit access, shall be capable of being provided without moving permanent walls.

**A.7.3.4.1.1** The criteria of 7.3.4.1.1 provide for minimum widths for small spaces such as individual offices. The intent is that these reductions in required width apply to spaces formed by furniture and movable walls, so that accommodations can easily be made for mobility-impaired individuals. One side of a path could be a fixed wall, provided that the other side is movable. This does not exempt the door widths or widths of fixed-wall corridors, regardless of the number of people or length.

Figure A.7.3.4.1.1(a) and Figure A.7.3.4.1.1(b) present selected anthropometric data for adults. The male and female figures depicted in the figures are average, 50th percentile, in size. Some dimensions apply to very large, 97.5 percentile, adults (noted as 97.5 P).

Paragraph 7.3.4.1.1 and the associated annex material explain the intent behind permitting spaces, such as individual offices or workstations, an exemption from the 36 in. (915 mm) minimum width requirement of 7.3.4.1(2) for new construction. If any one path (e.g., a "miniaisle") requires a maximum of six people to travel not more than 50 ft (15 m) to reach a minimum 36 in. (915 mm) wide egress path (e.g., a major aisle), the path is permitted to be as narrow as 28 in. (710 mm). The width of the path is permitted to be reduced further to 18 in. (455 mm) near the floor, but not at points more than 38 in. (965 mm) above the floor, as might be characteristic of a small floor-mounted bookcase.

Other paths within the same room are permitted the same reduction in required width, provided that each individually meets the six-person and 50 ft (15 m)

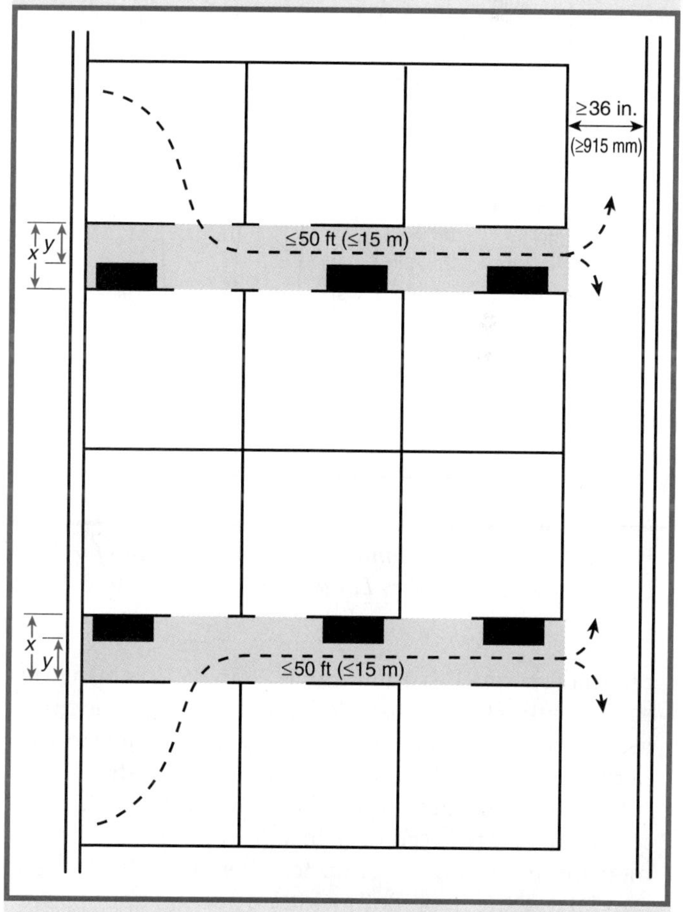


***Exhibit 7.79*** *Minimum exit access width created by movable furniture and partitions.*

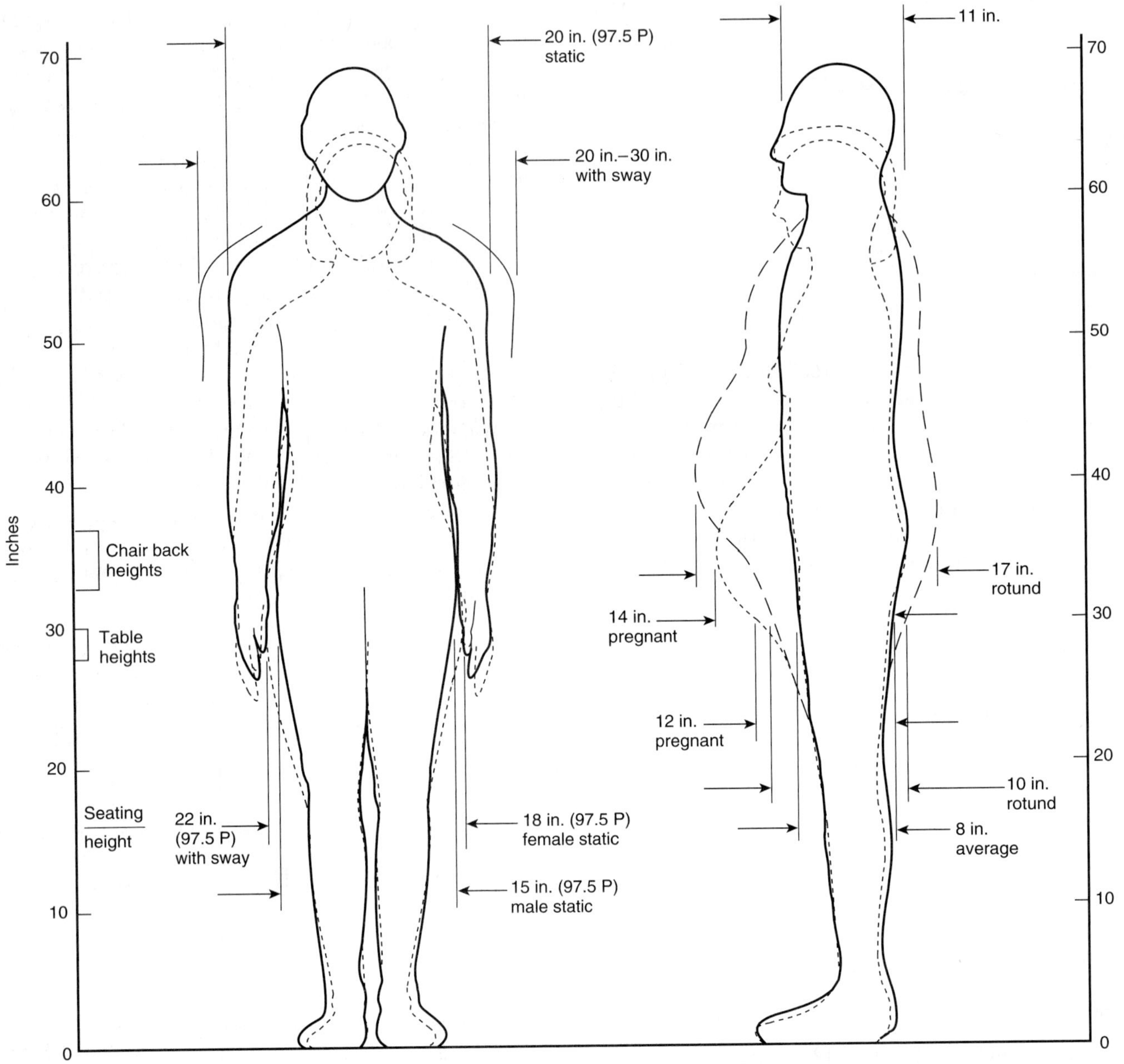


***Figure A.7.3.4.1.1(a)*** *Anthropometric Data (in in.) for Adults; Males and Females of Average, 50th Percentile, Size; Some Dimensions Apply to Very Large, 97.5 Percentile (97.5 P), Adults.*

criteria for travel to a minimum 36 in. (915 mm) wide egress path. This is illustrated in Exhibit 7.79. The minimum 28 in. (710 mm) width (shown as dimension *x*) permitted by 7.3.4.1.1(1) is a relaxation of the 36 in. (915 mm) minimum required by 7.3.4.1(2). This width can be further reduced to 18 in. (455 mm) (shown as dimension *y*) at floor level up to a height of 38 in. (965 mm) above the floor. Both width reduction options are conditional on a maximum of six people traveling not more than 50 ft (15 m) along a resultant miniaisle to reach a minimum 36 in. (915 mm) wide exit access component, such as an aisle.

Use of 7.3.4.1.1 is not limited to business occupancies. The same provisions could be applied to factory workstations in an industrial occupancy or to library study carrels in an assembly occupancy.

The provision of 7.3.4.1.1(2), related to the ability to increase the available width to 36 in. (915 mm) without moving permanent walls, is intended to keep the overall width exemption from denying accessibility to

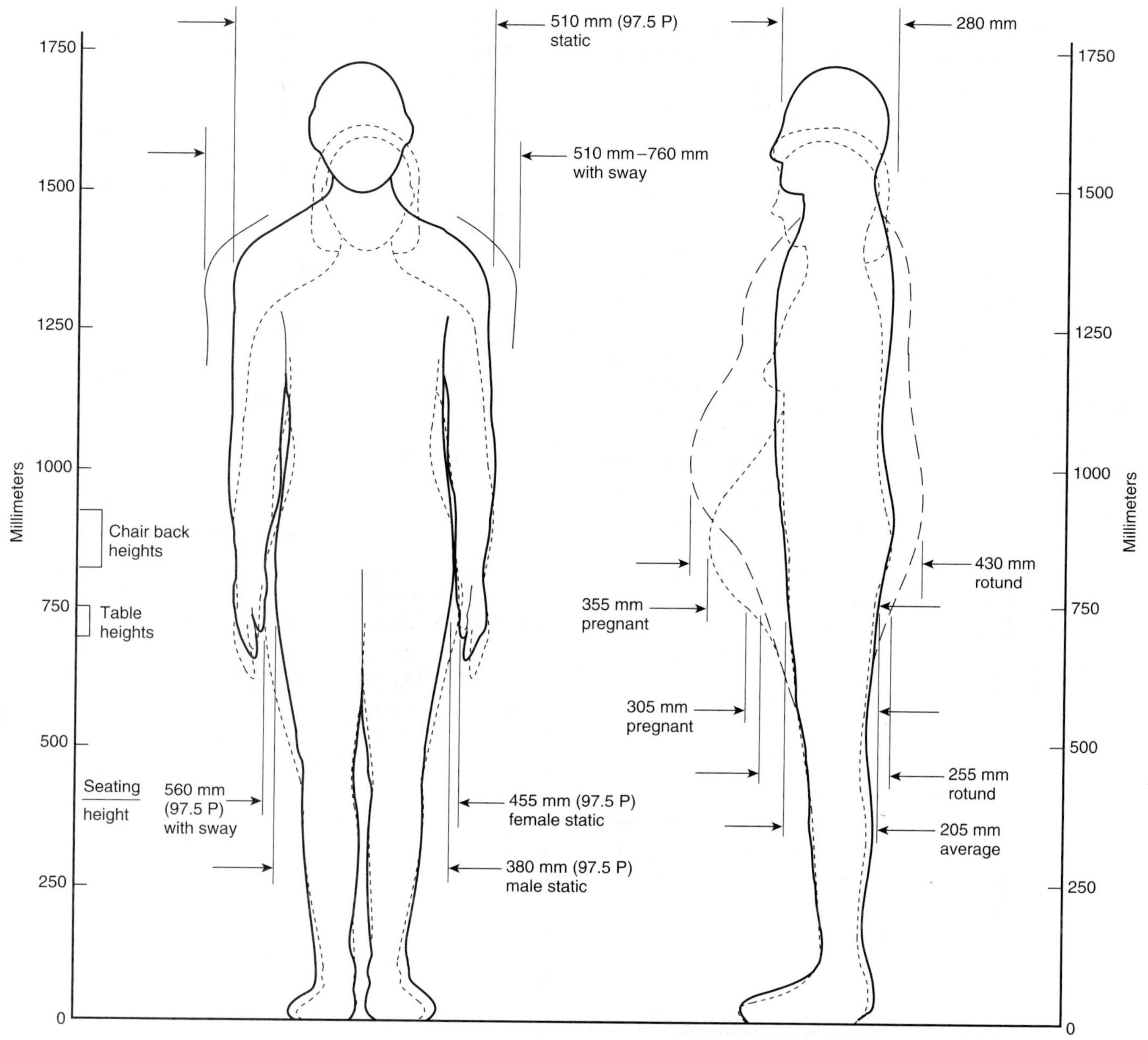


***Figure A.7.3.4.1.1(b)*** *Anthropometric Data (in mm) for Adults; Males and Females of Average, 50th Percentile, Size; Some Dimensions Apply to Very Large, 97.5 Percentile (97.5 P), Adults.*

persons with severe mobility impairment. For example, if a person who uses a wheelchair has seniority to claim the prime workstation with a window to the outside, but such workstation is currently arranged so that it is accessed by a miniaisle only 28 in. (710 mm) wide, the building maintenance engineer must be able to detach from the floor, reposition, and reattach cubicle partitions to increase the miniaisle to a 36 in. (915 mm) width.

**7.3.4.1.2** In existing buildings, the width of exit access shall be permitted to be not less than 28 in. (710 mm).

**7.3.4.1.3** The requirement of 7.3.4.1 shall not apply to the following:

(1) Doors as otherwise provided for in 7.2.1.2
(2) Aisles and aisle accessways in assembly occupancies as otherwise provided in Chapters 12 and 13
(3) Industrial equipment access as otherwise provided in 40.2.5.2

The minimum width required in any egress path is dependent on the occupancy and is thus specified in Chapters 12 through 42 for individual occupancies. The widths are based on experience and on observations of the manner in which people move along paths used for egress purposes. The minimum width permitted for any new egress component, other than a door opening, is 36 in. (915 mm), but most occupancies require additional width for specific components. Educational occupancies require a corridor width of not less than 6 ft (1830 mm). New health care occupancies require a corridor width of not less than 8 ft (2440 mm), which reflects the need to move bedridden patients and multiple lines of people along the path to an exit. Hotels, apartment buildings, and business occupancies generally require 44 in. (1120 mm) minimum width corridors. Some occupancies rely wholly on the provisions of 7.3.4.1, so as not to specify their own minimum widths.

**7.3.4.2** Where a single exit access leads to an exit, its capacity in terms of width shall be not less than the required capacity of the exit to which it leads.

**7.3.4.3** Where more than one exit access leads to an exit, each shall have a width adequate for the number of persons it accommodates.

The intent of 7.3.4.2 and 7.3.4.3 is to balance the flow of persons from the exit access to the exit to avoid a bottleneck and to ensure that the occupants being served by the exit can, in fact, reach it. The design and sizing of egress paths involve apportioning part of the overall occupant load to the various available paths. Where there are multiple paths, no one path needs to accommodate all of the occupants by itself.

## 7.4 Number of Means of Egress

### 7.4.1 General.

**7.4.1.1** The number of means of egress from any balcony, mezzanine, story, or portion thereof shall be not less than two, except under one of the following conditions:

(1) A single means of egress shall be permitted where permitted in Chapters 11 through 43.
(2) A single means of egress shall be permitted for a mezzanine or balcony where the common path of travel limitations of Chapters 11 through 43 are met.

Most of the occupancy chapters provide redundancy with respect to the number of means of egress by requiring at least two means of egress. Some occupancies identify specific arrangements under which only a single means of egress is permitted. Where large numbers of occupants are to be present on any floor or portion of a floor in new construction, more than two means of egress must be provided as required by 7.4.1.2.

Mezzanines are required to have the same number of means of egress as any story of the building, unless an occupant can reach either the single exit or a point (at or past the bottom of a single open stair) where access to two exits becomes available within the allowable common path of travel permitted for the applicable occupancy.

Exhibit 7.80 illustrates the mezzanine provisions of 7.4.1.1 and 7.4.1.1(2), which are not intended to override the provisions for openness of mezzanines imposed by 8.6.9.3. In Exhibit 7.80, Part (a) illustrates the requirement for a minimum of two means of egress per 7.4.1.1. One means of egress is an open stair to the floor below, and the other is an enclosed exit stair. Both could be open stairs to the floor below, unless the openness requirements of 8.6.9.3 are not met. If the mezzanine were enclosed, such that the enclosed area

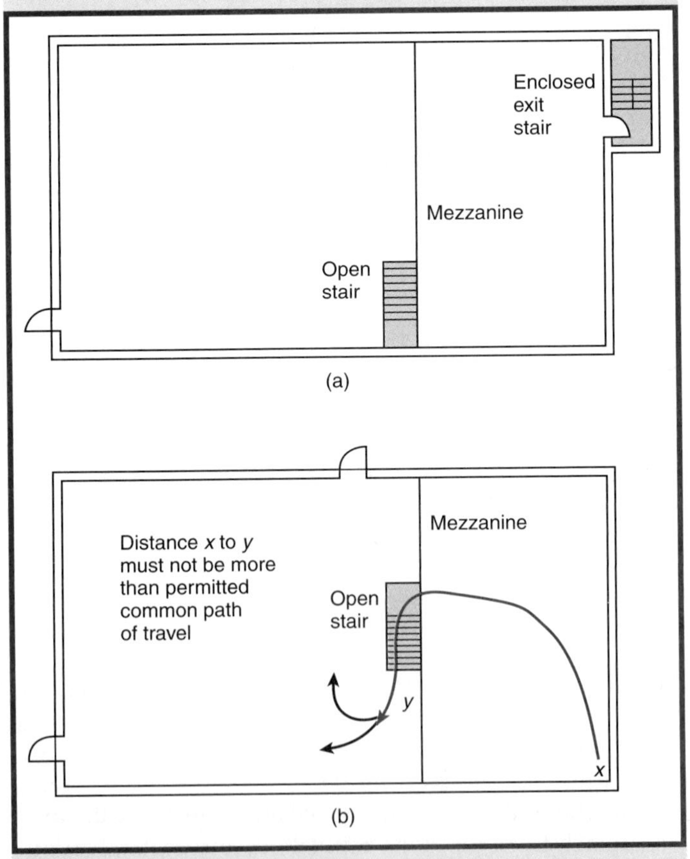


***Exhibit 7.80** Number of means of egress from mezzanines.*

had an occupant load of more than 10 persons, 8.6.9.3 would require a second means of egress [similar to the enclosed exit stair in Part (a)] that provides direct access from the enclosed area to an exit at the mezzanine level. In Part (b) of Exhibit 7.80, a single means of egress is permitted in accordance with 7.4.1.1(2), because the common path of travel is within the limits specified for the occupancy involved.

See also Section 7.5 with respect to remoteness of exits and common paths of travel; 7.6.4 with respect to measuring travel distance in the plane of the tread nosings on open stairs; and 8.6.9 on mezzanines.

**7.4.1.2** The number of means of egress from any story or portion thereof, other than for existing buildings as permitted in Chapters 11 through 43, shall be as follows:

(1) Occupant load more than 500 but not more than 1000 — not less than 3
(2) Occupant load more than 1000 — not less than 4

Chapter 7 requires a minimum number of means of egress, unless otherwise specified by the occupancy chapters. Several occupancies establish not only the minimum number of means of egress but also the minimum number of actual exits that must be provided on each floor. For example, for new educational occupancies, 14.2.4 requires access to two exits and further requires that both of the exits be provided on the floor. In contrast, for industrial occupancies, 40.2.4.1.1 requires access to two exits and further requires that at least one of the exits is to be located on the floor. Access to the other exit can involve traveling to another floor via an egress component such as an open stair, provided that such open stair is permitted by the provisions for protection of vertical openings.

In most occupancies, meeting the requirements for egress capacities and travel distances means the required minimum number of means of egress will automatically be met. However, in occupancies characterized by high occupant loads, such as assembly and mercantile occupancies, compliance with requirements for more than two exits per floor might require specific attention.

**7.4.1.3** Accessible means of egress in accordance with 7.5.4 that do not utilize elevators shall be permitted to serve as any or all of the required minimum number of means of egress.

Because an accessible means of egress can effectively serve the needs of persons with mobility impairments, the same accessible means of egress should effectively serve the needs of persons without disabilities. Therefore, the *Code* permits accessible means of egress to fulfill any requirements for means of egress. However, this permission does not apply to elevators because of the small number of occupants accommodated during each run of the elevator and concerns that the elevator might be automatically called out of service upon the detection of smoke in the elevator machine room or an elevator lobby or landing on any floor served by the elevator.

**7.4.1.4** The occupant load of each story considered individually shall be required to be used in computing the number of means of egress at each story, provided that the required number of means of egress is not decreased in the direction of egress travel.

Similar to the procedures for determining required egress capacity (see 7.3.1.4), the number of required means of egress is based on a floor-by-floor consideration, rather than the accumulation of the occupant loads of all floors. For example, see Exhibit 7.81, where the fourth floor of the building has an occupant load of 700 persons and would require three means of egress. The third floor of the same building has an occupant load of 400 persons and would require two means of egress; regardless of the fact that the two floors together have an occupant load in excess of 1000 persons, four means of egress are not required. However, the number of means of egress cannot decrease as an occupant proceeds along the egress path. The three exits required from the fourth floor in this example

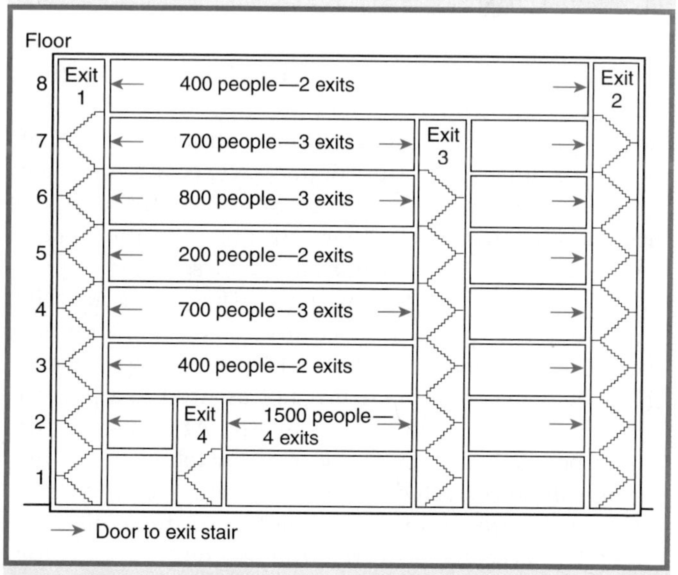


***Exhibit 7.81*** *Minimum number of required means of egress for new construction.*

cannot be merged into two exits on the third floor, even though the third floor requires only two exits. On any floor requiring only two exits, one of the three exits could be left inaccessible (blind) on that floor, as shown at Exit 3 in Exhibit 7.81 on the third and fifth floors. The second floor, with an occupant load of 1500 persons, requires a fourth means of egress.

**7.4.1.5** Doors other than the hoistway door; the elevator car door; and doors that are readily openable from the car side without a key, a tool, special knowledge, or special effort shall be prohibited at the point of access to an elevator car.

Paragraph 7.4.1.5 prohibits the installation of a door assembly at the entrance to an elevator, unless that door leaf is readily operable by those in the elevator. This prohibition prevents entrapment between the elevator and the door assembly. The primary concern is the potential for an occupant to enter this small space and become trapped during a fire.

**7.4.1.6 Elevator Landing and Lobby Exit Access.**

**7.4.1.6.1** Each elevator landing and lobby shall have access to at least one exit.

**7.4.1.6.2** The elevator landing and lobby exit access required by 7.4.1.6.1 shall not require the use of a key, a tool, special knowledge, or special effort, unless permitted by 7.4.1.6.3.

**7.4.1.6.3** Doors separating the elevator lobby from the exit access required by 7.4.1.6.1 shall be permitted to be electronically locked in accordance with 7.2.1.6.3.

The purpose of 7.4.1.6.1 and 7.4.1.6.2 is to ensure that an occupant who has gained access to an elevator lobby can get out of the lobby without the use of a tool or key. It is not uncommon, especially in office buildings where a tenant occupies an entire floor, for the elevator lobby door assemblies to the tenant space to be locked after normal business hours to prevent entry into the tenant space. This problem is illustrated in Exhibit 7.82. Because the door assemblies between the elevator lobby and the tenant spaces can be locked, access to an exit is not assured to a person who arrives at the floor via elevator. At least one exit must be accessible from the elevator lobby. The situation can be corrected by repositioning one of the exit stair enclosures depicted at the top of the exhibit so that it is accessed directly from within the elevator lobby.

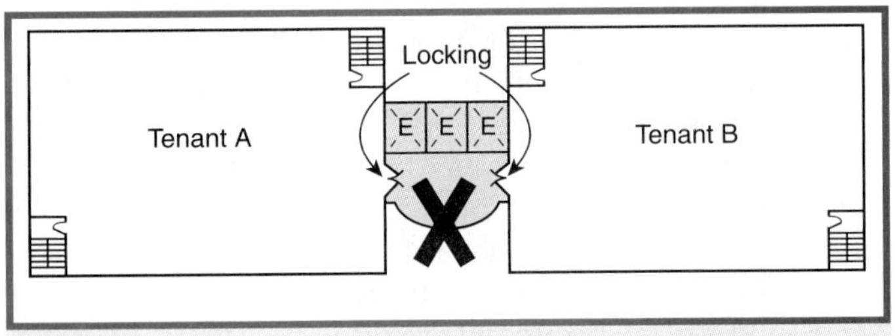


***Exhibit 7.82** Exit access from an elevator lobby.*

The provision of 7.4.1.6.3 is new to the 2009 edition of the *Code* and, rather than providing the detailed criteria required of locked elevator lobby exit access door assemblies, references the criteria of 7.2.1.6.3 as an exemption to the requirements of 7.4.1.6.1 and 7.4.1.6.2. The provisions of 7.2.1.6.3 for elevator lobby exit access door assemblies locking are correctly positioned within the 7.2.1 subsection on door openings and, more importantly, within 7.2.1.6, special locking arrangements provisions, as locked elevator lobby exit access doors are a special form of permitted door assembly locking. See the commentary following A.7.2.1.6.3(15).

### 7.4.2 Spaces About Electrical Equipment.

**7.4.2.1 600 Volts, Nominal, or Less.** The minimum number of means of egress for working space about electrical equipment, other than existing electrical equipment, shall be in accordance with *NFPA 70, National Electrical Code*, Article 110.26(C).

**7.4.2.2 Over 600 Volts, Nominal.** The minimum number of means of egress for working space about electrical equipment, other than existing electrical equipment, shall be in accordance with *NFPA 70, National Electrical Code*, Article 110.33(A).

The provisions of 7.4.2 are new to the 2009 edition of the *Code* and are intended to serve as a reminder that *NFPA 70®, National Electrical Code®*,[28] has criteria for ingress and egress for working space around electrical equipment that are more specific, and potentially more stringent, than those of this *Code*. Users had complained that, after designing an egress system in accordance with this *Code*, they were cited for not complying with *NFPA 70*.

## 7.5 Arrangement of Means of Egress

### 7.5.1 General.

**7.5.1.1** Exits shall be located and exit access shall be arranged so that exits are readily accessible at all times.

**7.5.1.1.1*** Where exits are not immediately accessible from an open floor area, continuous passageways, aisles, or corridors leading directly to every exit shall be maintained and shall be arranged to provide access for each occupant to not less than two exits by separate ways of travel, unless otherwise provided in 7.5.1.1.3 and 7.5.1.1.4.

**A.7.5.1.1.1** See A.7.5.1.5.

**7.5.1.1.2** Exit access corridors shall provide access to not less than two approved exits, unless otherwise provided in 7.5.1.1.3 and 7.5.1.1.4.

**7.5.1.1.3** The requirements of 7.5.1.1.1 and 7.5.1.1.2 shall not apply where a single exit is permitted in Chapters 11 through 43

**7.5.1.1.4** Where common paths of travel are permitted for an occupancy in Chapters 11 through 43, such common paths of travel shall be permitted but shall not exceed the limit specified.

Paragraphs 7.5.1.1.1 and 7.5.1.1.2 reinforce the desirability of always being able to move in different directions from any location, so as to allow different paths of travel to different exits. However, typical floor layouts and furnishing arrangements often create spaces where travel in a single direction is necessary for a limited distance before it becomes possible to travel in different directions.

Paragraph 7.5.1.1.3 recognizes that a single exit creates a condition under which travel is possible in only one direction. The conditions under which an occupancy chapter permits a single exit usually produce a situation that is as safe as, or safer than, a building that is provided with two exits but that includes substantial common path of travel before access to both exits is possible.

Paragraph 7.5.1.1.4 recognizes common paths of travel within the limits set by the individual occupancy chapters. For additional information on common paths of travel, see A.7.5.1.5.

**7.5.1.2** Corridors shall provide exit access without passing through any intervening rooms other than corridors, lobbies, and other spaces permitted to be open to the corridor, unless otherwise provided in 7.5.1.2.1 and 7.5.1.2.2.

**7.5.1.2.1** Approved existing corridors that require passage through a room to access an exit shall be permitted to continue to be used, provided that the following criteria are met:

(1) The path of travel is marked in accordance with Section 7.10.
(2) Doors to such rooms comply with 7.2.1.
(3) Such arrangement is not prohibited by the applicable occupancy chapter.

The requirement of 7.5.1.2, which mandates that corridors provide access to at least two exits without passing through intervening rooms (other than corridors and lobbies), was new to the 1997 edition of the *Code*, though a similar requirement had been in effect for health care occupancies for many years.

The exit access arrangement illustrated in Exhibit 7.83 is deficient. Occupants reaching the corridor have access only to exit B without leaving the protection afforded by the corridor. Paragraph 7.5.1.2 requires access to both exit A and exit B without leaving the corridor and traveling within another use area. One possible solution to this problem would be to extend the corridor walls to the far left of the floor so as to connect directly with exit stair enclosure A.

Paragraph 7.5.1.2.1 recognizes the continued use of existing corridors that force occupants to travel through a room to access an exit where such existing corridors are approved. Per the definition of 3.2.1, the term *approved* means acceptable to the authority having jurisdiction, so it is the current AHJ who must approve the existing corridor arrangement in order for it to be continued in use. If the exemption were not permitted, existing arrangements that were in compliance with earlier editions of the *Code* might suddenly be considered noncompliant.

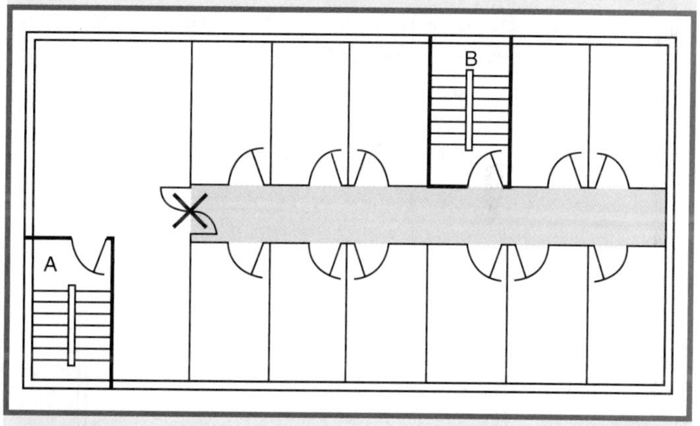


***Exhibit 7.83** Deficient corridor exit access.*

**7.5.1.2.2** Corridors that are not required to be fire resistance rated shall be permitted to discharge into open floor plan areas.

**7.5.1.3** Remoteness shall be provided in accordance with 7.5.1.3.1 through 7.5.1.3.7.

The provisions of 7.5.1.3.1 through 7.5.1.3.7 were revised for the 2009 edition of the *Code* to expand the applicability of the remoteness criteria from what had been only the remoteness of exits to include the remoteness of exit accesses, the remoteness of exits, and the remoteness of exit discharges.

The concept of remoteness of exit accesses is illustrated in Exhibit 7.84 [which is an adaptation of Figure A.7.5.1.3.2(c)]. For purposes of this illustration, the building is new construction and is not sprinklered, so as to be subject to both the qualitative remoteness criterion of 7.5.1.3.1 and the quantitative, one-half diagonal measurement remoteness criterion of 7.5.1.3.2. By the requirements of editions of the *Code* prior to 2009, Exit 1 and Exit 2, which are about as remotely located from each other as physically possible, easily comply with the one-half diagonal separation distance criterion of 7.5.1.3.2 for exits. Yet, the L-shaped partition around which occupants must travel to reach Exit 1 has the effect of making the exit accesses less remotely located from each other than the exits, as all occupants are drawn toward Exit 2 before reaching point A, where access to Exit 1 becomes possible. The distance from point A to point B designates the separation distance between exit accesses that the requirements of 7.5.1.3.1 and 7.5.1.3.2 are intended to regulate. Without having to resort to measuring with a scale, it is apparent that the exit accesses do not meet the minimum one-half diagonal ($\frac{1}{2}$ *D*) requirement of 7.5.1.3.2. It is not obvious whether the distance from point A to point B provides sufficient separation between exit accesses to meet the qualitative provision of 7.5.1.3.1, which requires that the exit accesses be remotely located from each other to minimize the possibility that more than one of the exit accesses has the potential to be blocked by any one fire or other emergency condition. Such judgment is left to the authority having jurisdiction, which might be influenced by the fact that the diagonal measurement criterion of 7.5.1.3.2 was not met. If the building were sprinklered, the provision of 7.5.1.3.3 would be applied in lieu of that of 7.5.1.3.2, so as to decrease the required separation distance from one-half the diagonal to one-third the diagonal. Again, although less obvious than before, the remoteness test for the exit accesses would fail, as the distance from point A to point B is less than one-third the diagonal ($\frac{1}{3}$ *D*).

The provisions of 7.5.1.3.1 through 7.5.1.3.3, in addition to regulating the remoteness of exit accesses and the remoteness of exits, require that exit discharges be remotely located from each other. The concept of remoteness of exit discharges is illustrated in Exhibit 7.85. The shaded paths outside the nonsprinklered building are exit discharges. One provides the exit discharge path from Exit 1 to the public way, and the other provides the exit discharge path from Exit 2 to the public way. The proximity of the two exit discharge paths, measured as the distance between point A and point B, is insufficient to meet the one-half diagonal ($\frac{1}{2}$ *D*) requirement of 7.5.1.3.2. Although Exit 1 is sufficiently remote from Exit 2 to comply with 7.5.1.3.2, the exit discharges are not, and the situation

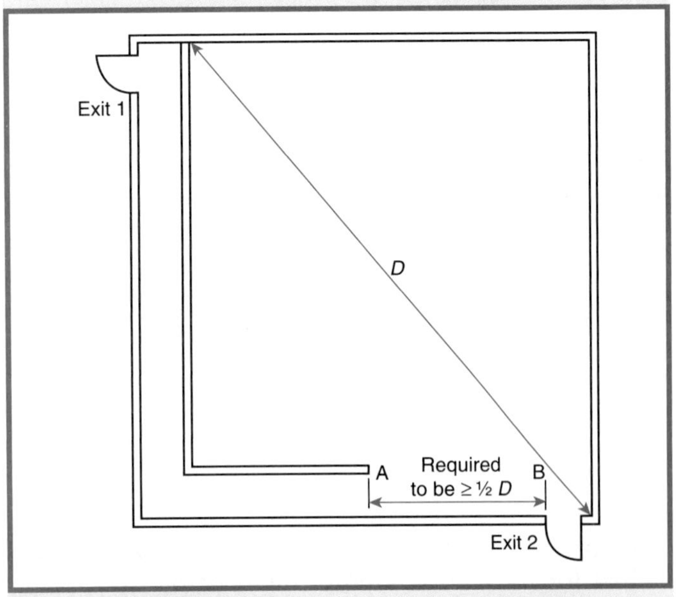


**Exhibit 7.84** *Testing the remoteness of exit accesses.*

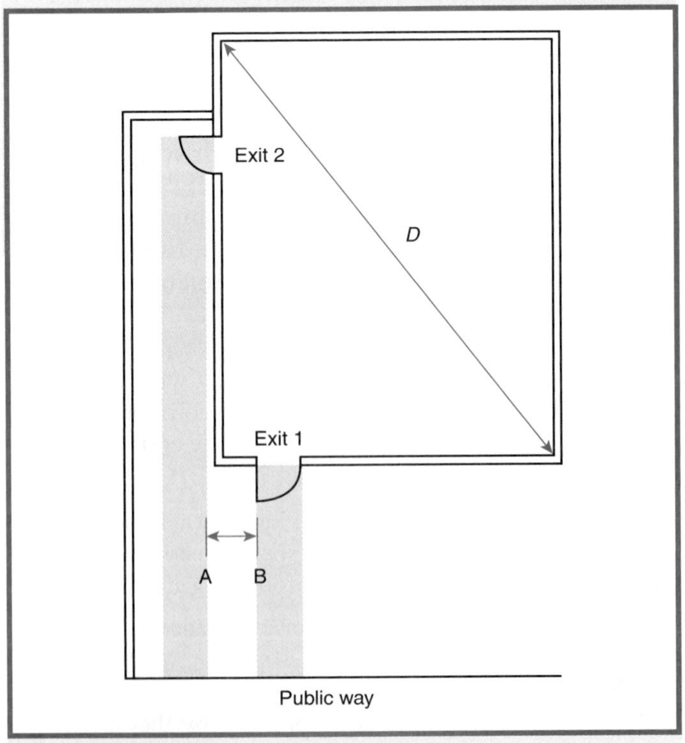


**Exhibit 7.85** *Testing the remoteness of exit discharges.*

must be remedied. One possible solution might be to move Exit 1 to the far right end of the building exterior wall in which it is currently positioned.

Exhibit 7.86 addresses the case of testing the remoteness of exit discharges where three exits are provided. The provision of 7.5.1.3.6 requires that at least two of the required exit discharges be remote from each other. The provision of 7.5.1.3.7 requires that any additional required exit discharges be located so that, if one of the required exit discharges becomes blocked, the others are available. Assume that the single-story, nonsprinklered building depicted has an occupant load of more than 500 persons, so as to require three means of egress in accordance with 7.4.1.2. The separation distance between the exit discharges from Exit 1 and Exit 3, measured as the distance from point C to point E, is sufficient to meet the one-half diagonal ($^1/_2 D$) requirement of 7.5.1.3.2. Thus, two of the three required exit discharges are remote from each other as required by 7.5.1.3.6. It is left to the authority having jurisdiction to decide whether the loss of the exit discharge serving Exit 1 leaves the exit discharge serving Exit 2 available as required by 7.5.1.3.7. The *Code* provides no further guidance on what the term *available* means, other than to connote that an exit discharge can be judged as being available without being remote from its nearest neighbor, as defined by the criteria of 7.5.1.3.1, 7.5.1.3.2, or 7.5.1.3.3.

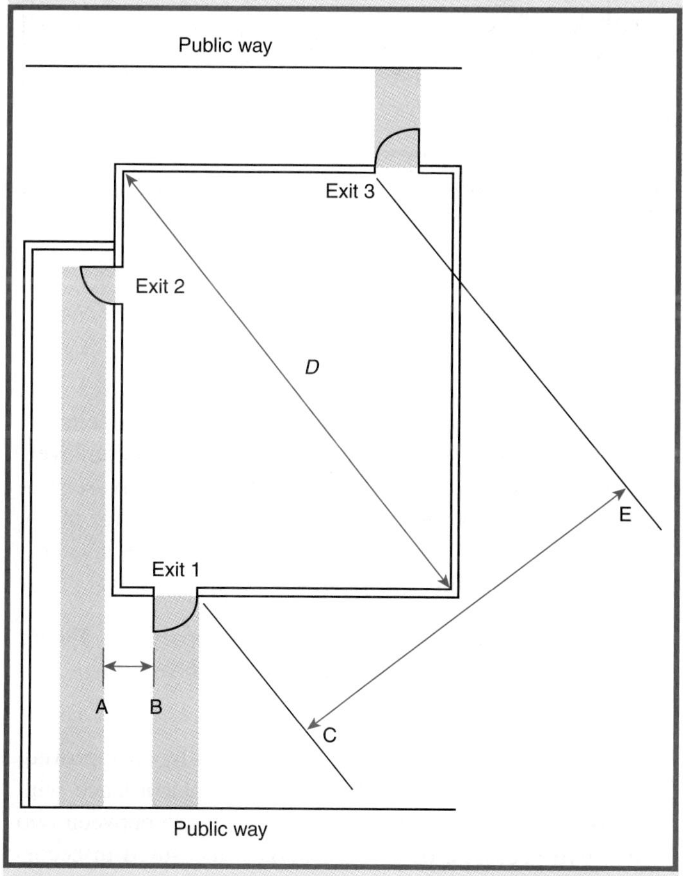


***Exhibit 7.86*** *Testing the remoteness of exit discharges with three exits.*

**7.5.1.3.1** Where more than one exit, exit access, or exit discharge is required from a building or portion thereof, such exits, exit accesses, or exit discharges shall be remotely located from each other and be arranged to minimize the possibility that more than one has the potential to be blocked by any one fire or other emergency condition.

It is a precept of life safety in buildings, repeated many times in the *Code*, that if multiple exits are required, they need to be not only separate, but also remote, from one another. Although the objective of this requirement is clear (if one exit is blocked by smoke or fire, the other needs to be maintained available), the term *remote* cannot always be clearly defined.

Where exits are located at each end of a long corridor or at each end or side of a building, they qualify as remotely located exits. However, core-type buildings with elevators, service shafts, and stairs in one central or side core introduce some challenging problems with respect to exit remoteness. Exhibit 7.87 shows two core-type buildings that illustrate this problem.

Exhibit 7.87 (top view) shows a plan approximating that of the Rault Center Building in New Orleans, where five women were trapped by fire on the fifteenth floor. Travel to both exit stairs was blocked by fire, and the women eventually jumped to the roof of an adjacent eight-story building. Four of the five died.[29]

Exhibit 7.87 (bottom view) shows the plan of the twentieth floor of a New York City office building. An incendiary device was set off somewhere near the lobby reception area. One of 15 people on the floor at the time made it to the stair exit, but the other 14 were trapped and rescued by fire fighters. One of the 14 died.[30]

With more attention given to life safety during the design stage, a much better solution might have been devised for these buildings. In the upper plan view of Exhibit 7.88, the exit stairs are not as remote from each other as practicable. They are both located on the same end of the core, a detriment when tenants, current and future, lay out their own partition arrangements to suit their needs. By removing the elevator lobby from the core, as shown in the lower plan of Exhibit 7.88, and adding a minimum 1-hour fire resistance–rated corridor around three sides of the

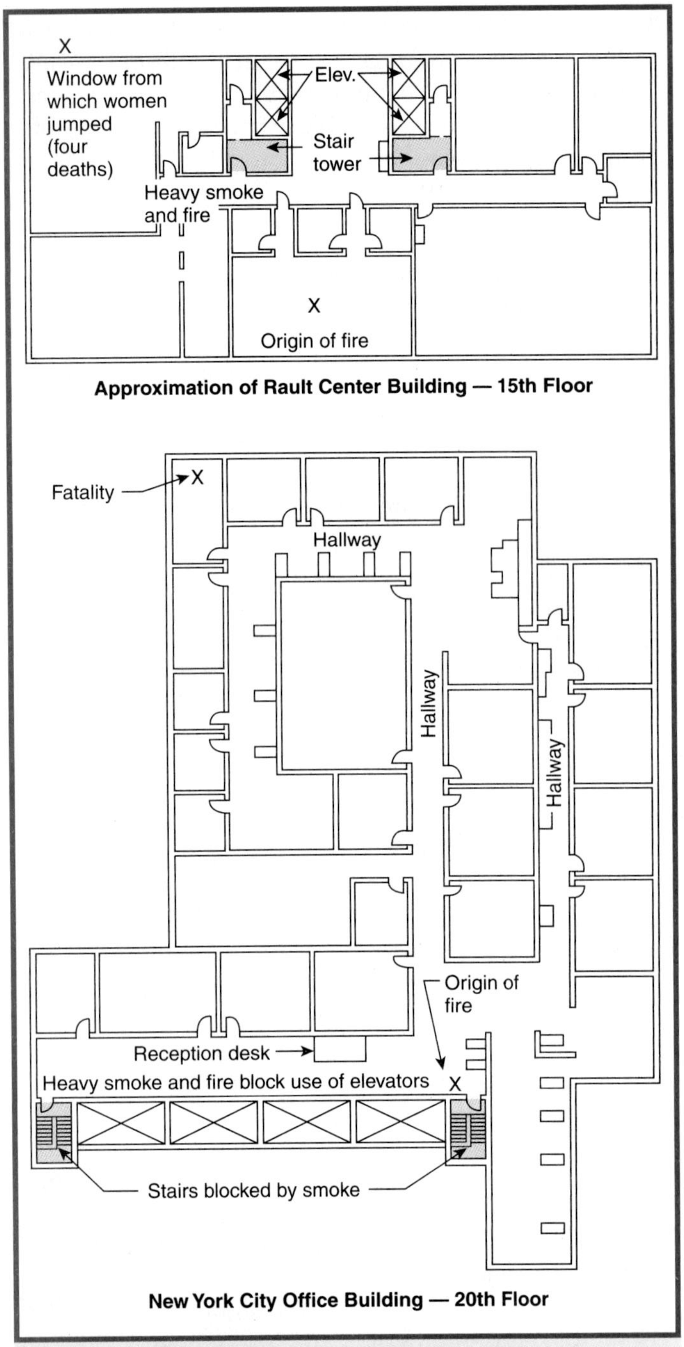


*Exhibit 7.87 Plan views of upper floors of two core-type high-rise buildings where fires occurred.*

core, the designer can ensure that tenants will have viable access to two exits (and that the exits are sufficiently remote to meet the minimum one-half diagonal requirement of 7.5.1.3.2 where the separation distance is measured along the corridor as permitted by 7.5.1.3.4). The exhibit illustrates how, with thought, imagination, and little, if any, added expense, a poor design can be greatly improved.

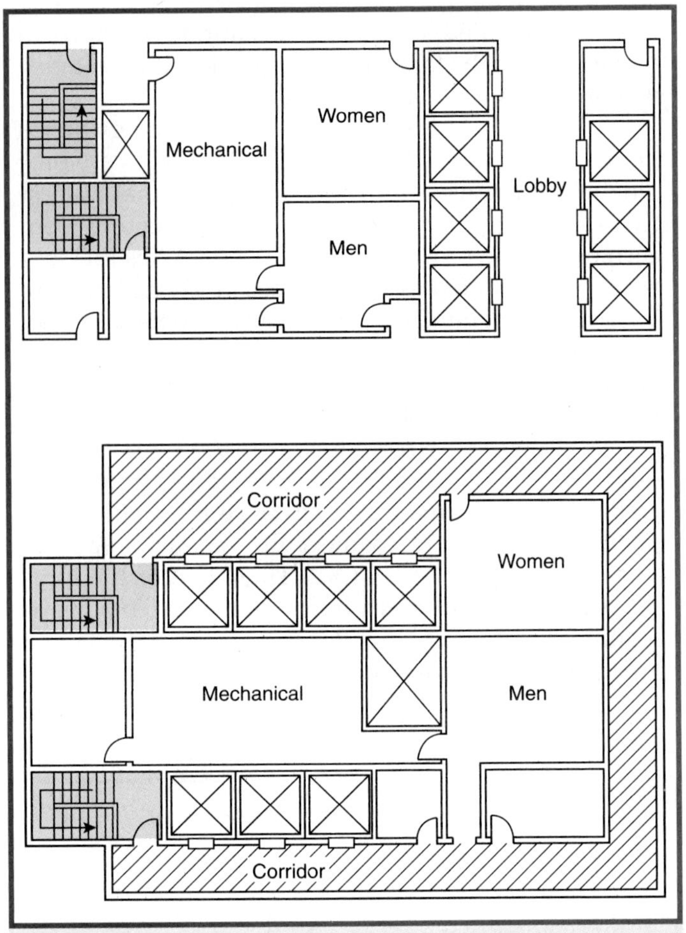


*Exhibit 7.88 Access to exits in core-type multitenant buildings.*

Also see the commentary following 7.5.1.3.7.

**7.5.1.3.2*** Where two exits, exit accesses, or exit discharges are required, they shall be located at a distance from one another not less than one-half the length of the maximum overall diagonal dimension of the building or area to be served, measured in a straight line between the nearest edge of the exits, exit accesses, or exit discharges, unless otherwise provided in 7.5.1.3.3 through 7.5.1.3.5.

**A.7.5.1.3.2** Figure A.7.5.1.3.2(a) through Figure A.7.5.1.3.2(e) illustrate the method of measurement intended by 7.5.1.3.2.

**7.5.1.3.3** In buildings protected throughout by an approved, supervised automatic sprinkler system in accordance with Section 9.7, the minimum separation distance between two exits, exit accesses, or exit discharges, measured in accordance with 7.5.1.3.2, shall be not less than one-third the length of the maximum overall diagonal dimension of the building or area to be served.

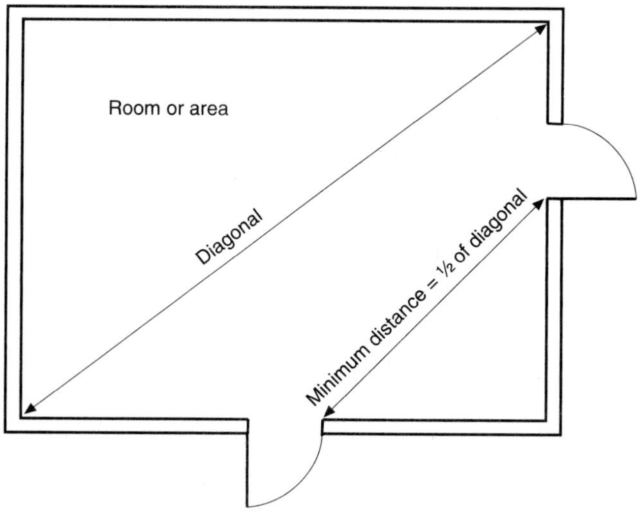


*Figure A.7.5.1.3.2(a)* *Diagonal Rule for Exit Remoteness.*

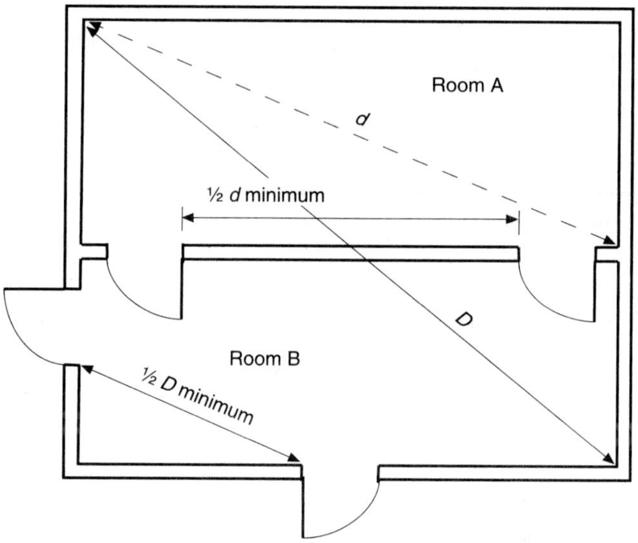


*Figure A.7.5.1.3.2(b)* *Diagonal Rule for Exit and Exit Access Door Remoteness.*

**7.5.1.3.4*** In other than high-rise buildings, where exit enclosures are provided as the required exits specified in 7.5.1.3.2 or 7.5.1.3.3 and are interconnected by not less than a 1-hour fire resistance–rated corridor, exit separation shall be measured along the shortest line of travel within the corridor.

**A.7.5.1.3.4** Figure A.7.5.1.3.4 illustrates the method of measuring exit separation distance along the line of travel within a minimum 1-hour fire resistance–rated corridor.

**7.5.1.3.5** In existing buildings, where more than one exit, exit access, or exit discharge is required, such exits, exit ac-

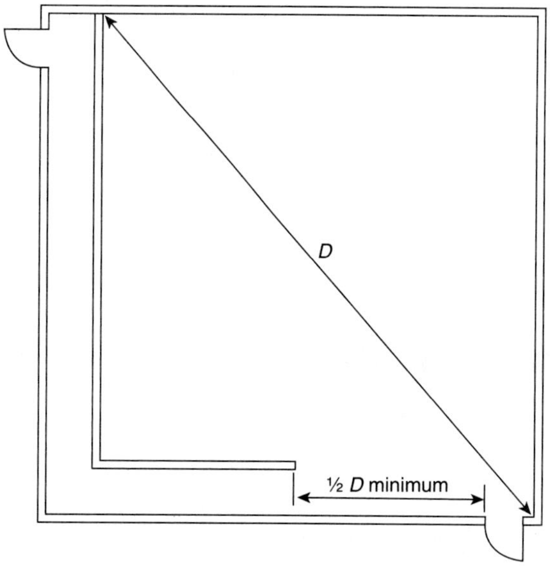


*Figure A.7.5.1.3.2(c)* *Diagonal Rule for Exit and Access Remoteness.*

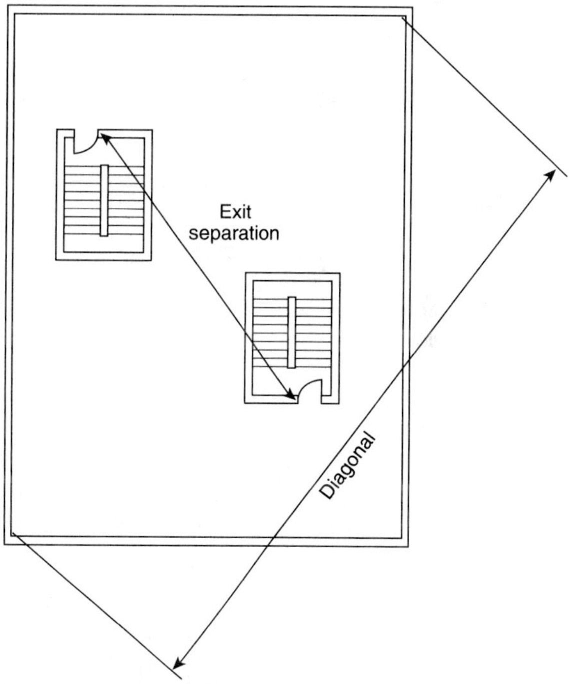


*Figure A.7.5.1.3.2(d)* *Exit Separation and Diagonal Measurement of Area Served.*

cesses, or exit discharges shall be exempt from the diagonal measurement separation distance criteria of 7.5.1.3.2 and 7.5.1.3.3, provided that such exits, exit accesses, or exit discharges are remotely located in accordance with 7.5.1.3.1.

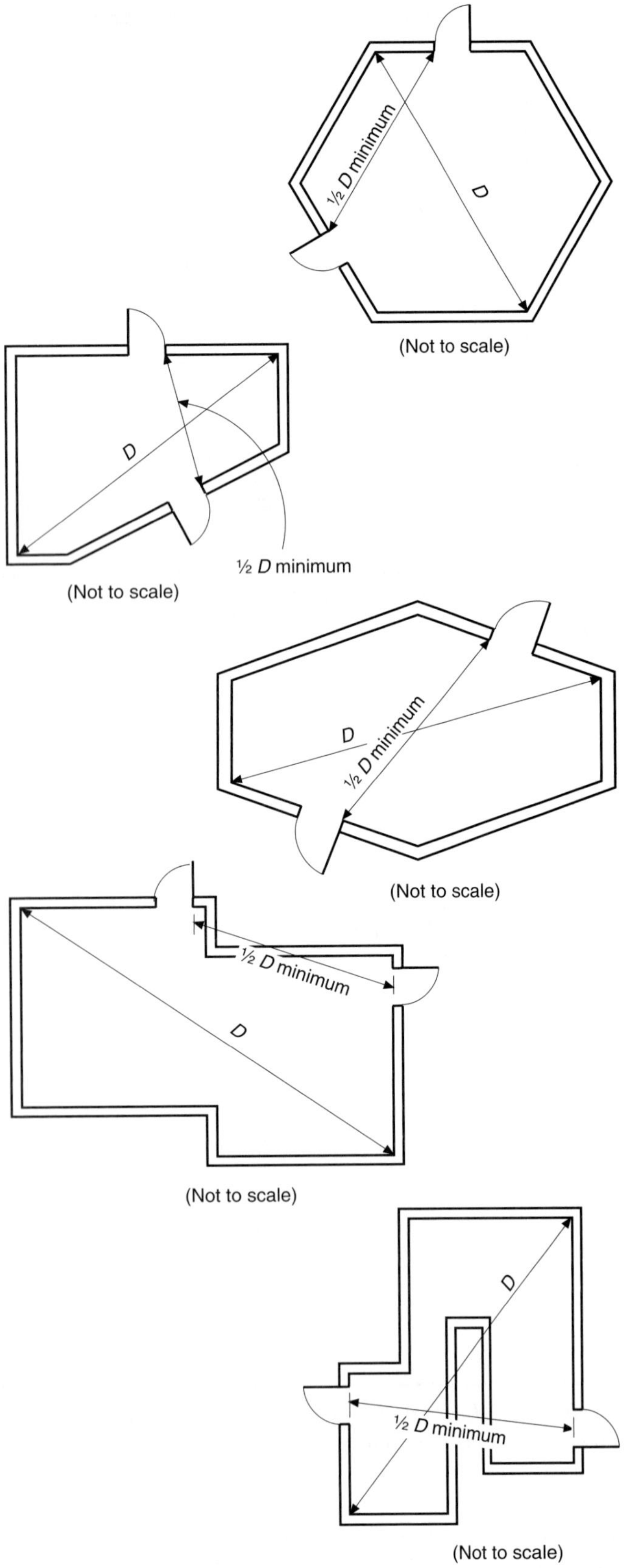


*Figure A.7.5.1.3.2(e)* *Diagonal Measurement for Unusually Shaped Areas.*

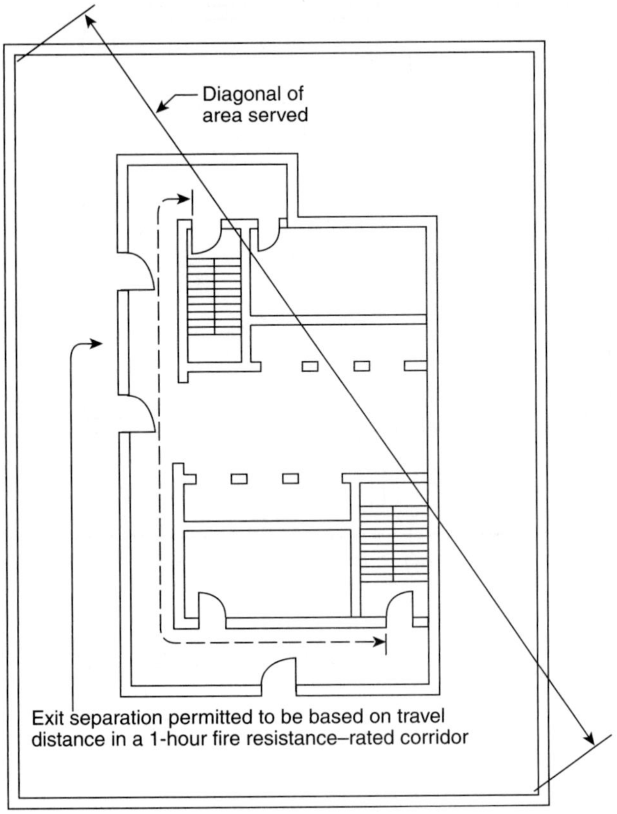


*Figure A.7.5.1.3.4* *Exit Separation Measured Along Corridor Path.*

**7.5.1.3.6** In other than existing buildings, where more than two exits, exit accesses, or exit discharges are required, at least two of the required exits, exit accesses, or exit discharges shall be arranged to comply with the minimum separation distance requirement.

**7.5.1.3.7** The balance of the exits, exit accesses, or exit discharges specified in 7.5.1.3.6 shall be located so that, if one becomes blocked, the others are available.

Since 1988, the *Code* has contained a remoteness formula referred to as the "one-half diagonal rule." This basic rule is stated in 7.5.1.3.2. Figure A.7.5.1.3.2(a) through Figure A.7.5.1.3.2(e) detail the application of the rule. The *Code* uses the one-half diagonal rule to quantify remoteness and to make certain that exit accesses, exits, and exit discharges are sufficiently remote to ensure, with reasonable certainty, that the same fire will not obstruct multiple egress routes. The exit separation is permitted by 7.5.1.3.3 to be reduced to one-third of the maximum overall diagonal measurement in fully sprinklered buildings, because the sprinkler system is expected to control the fire so that the use of multiple egress paths will not be lost.

Although existing buildings are exempted by the provision of 7.5.1.3.5 from the diagonal rule of 7.5.1.3.2 and 7.5.1.3.3, they must meet the remoteness requirement via the performance requirement of 7.5.1.3.1. Therefore, in existing buildings, remoteness is not required to be judged via the diagonal rule; it must be met via the provision of 7.5.1.3.1.

Exhibit 7.89 illustrates the provision of 7.5.1.3.4, which permits the distance between exit enclosures to be measured along a minimum 1-hour fire resistance–rated corridor with appropriate fire protection–rated door assemblies. Although the exit enclosures are physically closer to each other than the dimension measured along the corridor, the exits will behave, under fire conditions, as if they were the corridor length apart.

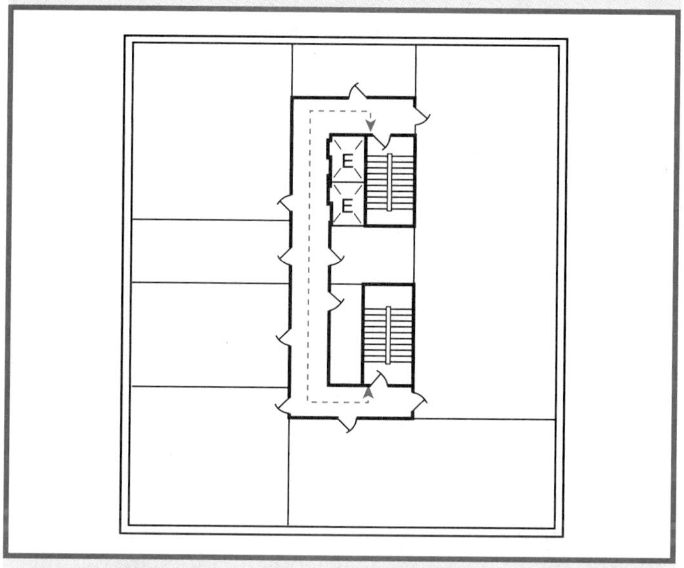


***Exhibit 7.89*** *Exit remoteness measured along 1-hour-rated corridor.*

**7.5.1.4** Interlocking or scissor stairs shall comply with 7.5.1.4.1 and 7.5.1.4.2.

**7.5.1.4.1** New interlocking or scissor stairs shall be permitted to be considered only as a single exit.

**7.5.1.4.2*** Existing interlocking or scissor stairs shall be permitted to be considered separate exits, provided that they meet the following criteria:

(1) They are enclosed in accordance with 7.1.3.2.
(2) They are separated from each other by 2-hour fire resistance–rated noncombustible construction.
(3) No protected or unprotected penetrations or communicating openings exist between the stair enclosures.

**A.7.5.1.4.2** It is difficult in actual practice to construct scissor stairs so that products of combustion that have entered one stairway do not penetrate into the other. Their use as separate required exits is discouraged. The term *limited-combustible* is intentionally not included in 7.5.1.4.2. The user's attention is directed to the definitions of limited-combustible and noncombustible in 3.3.160.2 and 3.3.160.3, respectively.

New scissors stairs are restricted by 7.5.1.4.1 to serving only as a single exit, because it is nearly impossible to ensure that the fire-rated and smoke-resisting separations provided between the two entwined stairs are complete and will stay complete over the life of the building. For example, standpipes are run vertically through the scissor stairs so as to create openings that connect the two stairs.

For existing installations, scissors stairs are regulated by 7.5.1.4.2 to ensure that they will perform similarly to two more widely separated exit stairs under fire conditions. Some design professionals believe scissors stairs are hazardous and should not be permitted; others believe just the opposite. Generally, the principal objection is that scissors stairs cannot be reliably built to create an absolute barrier to the passage of fire, smoke, and toxic gases between the stairs. Even if such a barrier is created, there is still concern that settling of the building or exposure to fire conditions might result in the cracking of the separating walls, landings, and stair runs, which could allow fire, smoke, and gases to pass from one exit stair into its entwined neighbor. On the other hand, those who do not believe that scissors stairs present such problems point to their advantages in reducing construction costs and saving space.

Paragraph 7.5.1.4.2(2) requires existing scissors stairs to have noncombustible, 2-hour fire resistance–rated separating construction. Some form of masonry or poured concrete wall, landing, or stair run is normally used to meet the definition of *noncombustible (material)* (see 3.3.160.3). Although scissors stairs can be located with their entrances remote from one another and their discharges also remotely placed, the remoteness requirements are applicable to scissors stairs only if they are to be considered as separate exits. Where not sufficiently separated or not remote from each other — or in new construction — scissors stairs cannot be used as separate exits but can be considered as a single exit, with their combined egress width providing increased capacity over that of a single stair. These points are illustrated in Exhibit 7.90 and Exhibit 7.91.

In Exhibit 7.90, the two existing entwined stairways sharing the same enclosing walls are called scissors stairs. To be considered separate exits, the existing stairs must be completely separated from each other. In effect, each stair enclosure must consist of a fire resistance–rated tube entwined around the other stair in a form similar to a helix. This arrangement results in

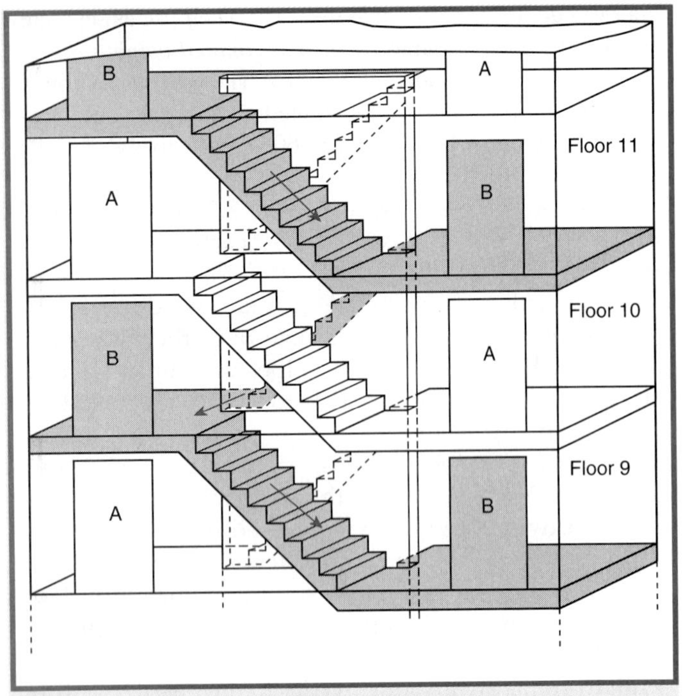


***Exhibit 7.90*** *Scissors stairs.*

space and cost savings by permitting the stairs to share the common enclosing walls that separate them from the remainder of the building. With this arrangement, two independent escape paths are created, similar to those provided by two independent stair enclosures positioned at a distance from each other. The continuity of all walls provides a complete separation at all points. The arrows designate the direction of egress travel in stair B.

Exhibit 7.91 illustrates some of the advantages of scissors stairs versus conventional exit stairs. The two stairs, positioned at the center of the exhibit and highlighted by placement within the oval, are entwined to create a set of scissors stairs. They provide the same degree of remoteness as the separate and independent stairs shown by the dashed lines at the sides of the exhibit and encircled. Travel distance to either the scissors stairs or the independent stairs is equal, even if the independent exit stairs are located at the opposite corners (X).

**7.5.1.5*** Exit access shall be arranged so that there are no dead ends in corridors, unless permitted by, and limited to the lengths specified in, Chapters 11 through 43.

A dead end exists in a corridor where the corridor continues past an exit and creates a pocket into which an occupant might travel. The occupant then recognizes there is no exit at that end of the pocket and is forced

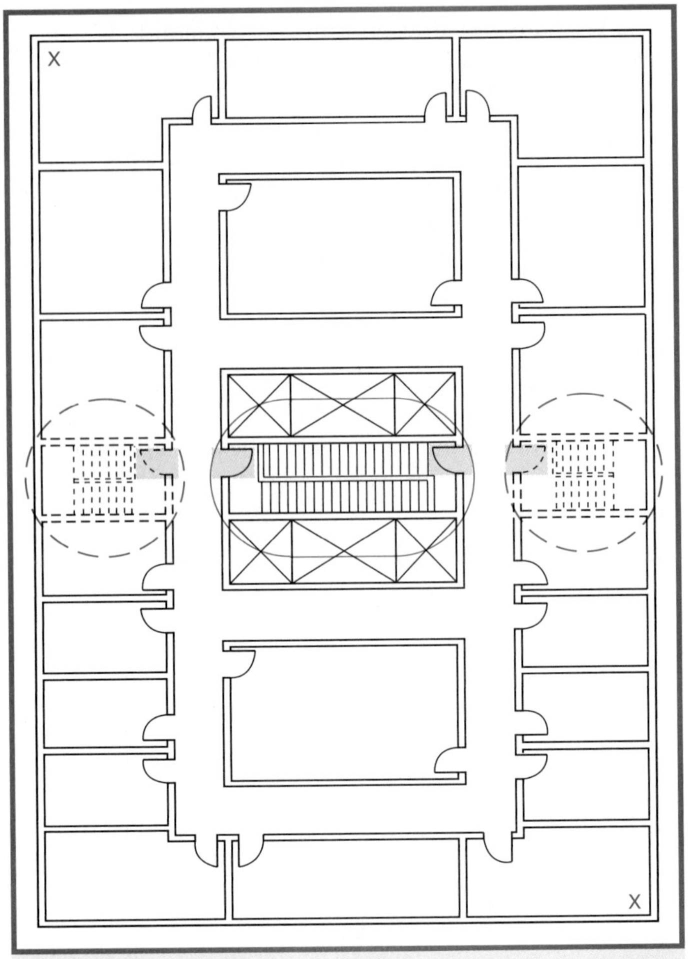


***Exhibit 7.91*** *Scissors stairs contrasted with conventional exit stairs.*

into retracing the original path to reach the exit. Although relatively short dead-end corridors are permitted for all occupancies by the chapter applicable to that occupancy, it is a better practice to avoid them; dead-end corridors increase the danger of people becoming trapped during a fire. Note that compliance with the limits on dead-end corridors does not necessarily mean that the requirements for remoteness of exits are met. Requirements for remoteness are especially difficult to meet in small buildings or buildings with short public corridors.

Exhibit 7.92 illustrates examples of two common types of dead-end corridors. In moving toward exits, occupants from building spaces other than the rooms served by the dead-end portion of the corridor could mistakenly travel into the dead end. Similarly, any occupant of the floor might mistakenly travel into the dead end created by the elevator lobby, which is connected to the corridor so as not to be discerned by the occupants as being anything other than a corri-

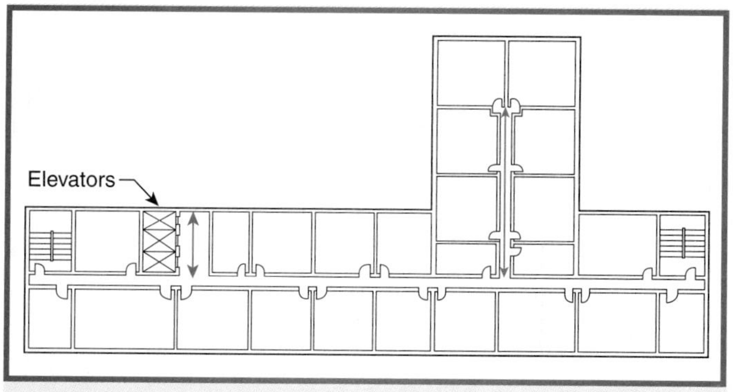


***Exhibit 7.92*** *Examples of common types of dead-end corridors.*

dor. Neither of the dead-end corridor pockets leads to an exit.

For persons occupying the two rooms located at the very end of the dead-end corridor section at the top of Exhibit 7.92, the travel from those rooms through this portion of the corridor system involves the concept of common path of travel, not dead-end corridors. Because the concepts of dead-end corridors and common path of travel are often confused, dead-end corridors have been blamed for fire deaths more correctly attributable to common path of travel problems. For example, the report on a 1977 Rhode Island dormitory fire in which 10 people died reads:

> Dead-end corridors approximately 61 feet long existed at each end of the dormitory. These dead ends were allowed by the Rhode Island building code in effect at the time when the building renovations were made in 1972. . . . A factor contributing to four of the . . . deaths and several of the injuries was the long, dead-end corridor. Residents who left their rooms in this dead end were . . . [kept from reaching] their only exit.[31]

For the occupants of the other five rooms with door assemblies opening into the dead-end corridor section at the top of Exhibit 7.92, the concepts of both dead-end corridors and common path of travel are applicable. Although occupants must travel in one direction to reach an exit, they also might mistakenly turn the wrong way when leaving their rooms and travel into the remainder of the dead-end corridor pocket, only to have to reverse direction and retrace their steps to reach an exit.

**A.7.5.1.5** The terms *dead end* and *common path of travel* are commonly used interchangeably. Although the concepts of each are similar in practice, they are two different concepts.

A common path of travel exists where a space is

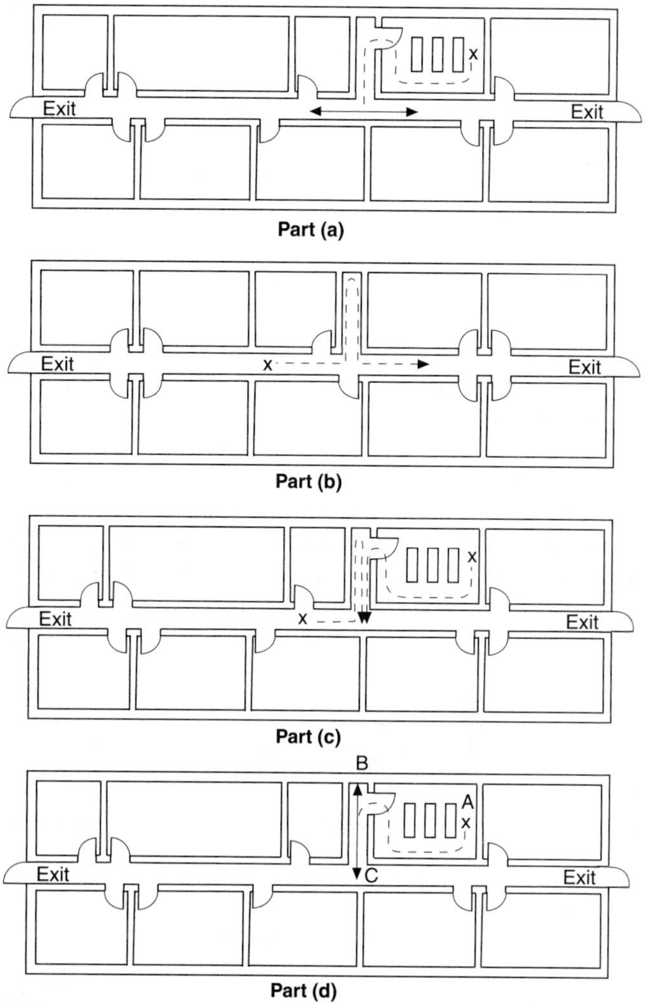


***Figure A.7.5.1.5*** *Common Paths of Travel and Dead-End Corridors.*

arranged so that occupants within that space are able to travel in only one direction to reach any of the exits or to reach the point at which the occupants have the choice of two paths of travel to remote exits. Part (a) of Figure A.7.5.1.5 is an example of a common path of travel.

While a dead end is similar to a common path of travel, a dead end can exist where there is no path of travel from an occupied space but can also exist where an occupant enters a corridor thinking there is an exit at the end and, finding none, is forced to retrace his or her path to reach a choice of exits. Part (b) of Figure A.7.5.1.5 is an example of such a dead-end arrangement.

Combining the two concepts, part (c) of Figure A.7.5.1.5 is an example of a combined dead-end/common path of travel problem.

Common paths of travel and dead-end travel are measured using the same principles used to measure travel distance as described in Section 7.6. Starting in the room shown in part (d) of Figure A.7.5.1.5, measurement is made from the most remote point in the room, A, along the natural path of travel and through the doorway along the centerline of the corridor to point C, located at the centerline of the corridor, which then provides the choice of two different paths to remote exits; this is common path of travel. The space between point B and point C is a dead end. *(See 3.3.42 for the definition of common path of travel.)*

Common paths of travel are explained in A.7.5.1.5. The portion of the exit access travel to which an occupant is steered in one direction only without the option of traveling in another independent direction toward an exit is common path of travel (see definition in 3.3.42). Exhibit 7.93 shows examples of common paths of travel (illustrated by the dashed lines). In each case illustrated, an occupant is steered in only one direction before reaching a point at which travel in independent directions becomes possible. Common path of travel might exist only within rooms and occupied spaces, or it might exist within the combination of room space and corridors.

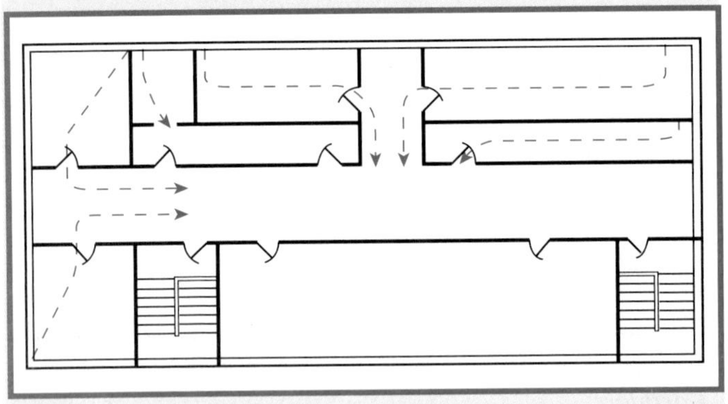

***Exhibit 7.93** Common paths of travel.*

Exhibit 7.94 depicts an approximation of the Rault Center Building shown in the top view of Exhibit 7.87 under the discussion of exit remoteness following 7.5.1.3.1. In Part (a), the dashed lines indicate the extent of the three dead-end corridor pockets. In Part (b), the dashed lines illustrate the numerous common paths of travel.

Note that the paths shown by the dashed lines are meant to include travel around all obstacles, such as furniture. Where furniture placement is not known, common path and travel distance are typically evaluated assuming an occupant has to traverse a distance equal to the length plus the width of the room in order to reach the door opening. Common path of travel measurement shares some common5% guidelines with travel distance measurement. See the commentary following A.7.6.1.

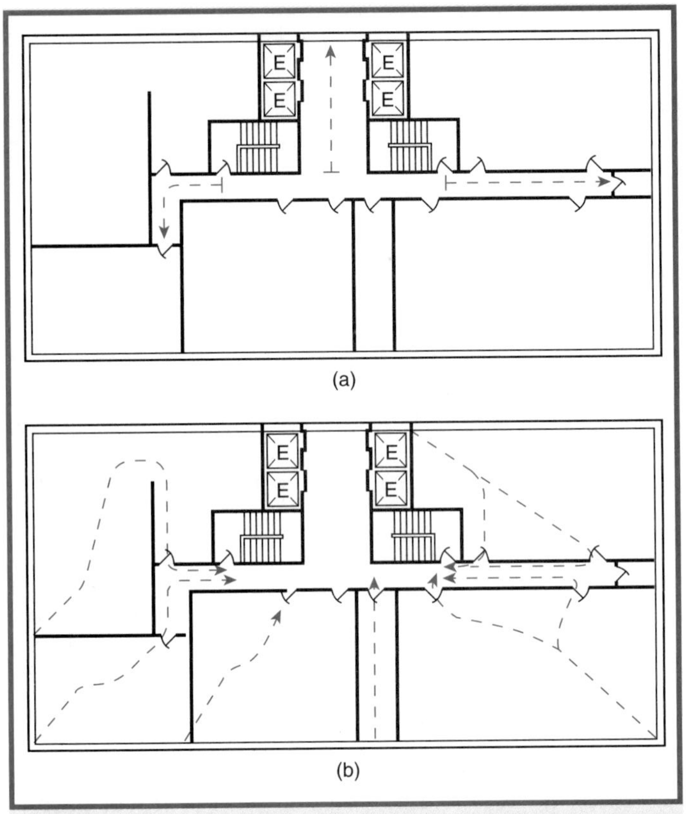


***Exhibit 7.94** Dead-end corridors and common paths of travel.*

**7.5.1.6** Exit access from rooms or spaces shall be permitted to be through adjoining or intervening rooms or areas, provided that such rooms or areas are accessory to the area served. Foyers, lobbies, and reception rooms constructed as required for corridors shall not be construed as intervening rooms. Exit access shall be arranged so that it is not necessary to pass through any area identified under Protection from Hazards in Chapters 11 through 43.

Paragraph 7.5.1.6 permits exit access travel through adjoining spaces if such spaces are accessory to the area served and such travel is not through any area identified under protection from hazards in an occupancy chapter (generally subsection __.3.2). Exhibit 7.95 illustrates exit access travel through intervening spaces that are under the control of the tenant and are not hazardous. Even though the hazardous contents storage room is under the control of the occupants of tenant space A, the hazard makes passage through the room unsafe. Passage from tenant space A into tenant space B is not permitted, because there is no assurance that the door assembly into tenant space B will be left unlocked, unblocked, and usable to occupants of tenant space A.

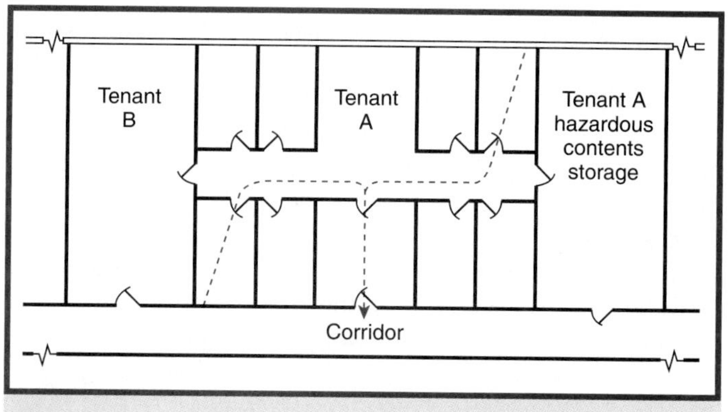


*Exhibit 7.95* Exit access through adjoining rooms.

### 7.5.2 Impediments to Egress.

See also 7.1.9 and 7.2.1.5.

**7.5.2.1*** Access to an exit shall not be through kitchens, storerooms other than as provided in Chapters 36 and 37, restrooms, workrooms, closets, bedrooms or similar spaces, or other rooms or spaces subject to locking, unless passage through such rooms or spaces is permitted for the occupancy by Chapter 18, 19, 22, or 23.

**A.7.5.2.1** It is not the intent that an area with equipment such as a beverage brewpot, microwave oven, and a toaster be considered a kitchen.

Paragraph 7.5.2.1, in combination with 7.5.1.6, prevents exit access from passing through certain rooms either due to increased relative hazard or potential blockage or locking. The text of A.7.5.2.1 clarifies that the presence of beverage brewpots, microwave ovens, and toasters, commonly found in employee break areas that often are located in spaces not separated from the remainder of an open floor plan, do not cause such spaces to be classified as kitchens through which 7.5.1.6 and 7.5.2.1 restrict exit access.

**7.5.2.2*** Exit access and exit doors shall be designed and arranged to be clearly recognizable.

**A.7.5.2.2** Doors that lead through wall paneling, and that harmonize in appearance with the rest of the wall to avoid detracting from some desired aesthetic or decorative effect, are not acceptable, because casual occupants might not be aware of such means of egress even though it is visible.

**7.5.2.2.1** Hangings or draperies shall not be placed over exit doors or located so that they conceal or obscure any exit, unless otherwise provided in 7.5.2.2.2.

**7.5.2.2.2** Curtains shall be permitted across means of egress openings in tent walls, provided that the following criteria are met:

(1) They are distinctly marked in contrast to the tent wall so as to be recognizable as means of egress.
(2) They are installed across an opening that is at least 6 ft (1830 mm) in width.
(3) They are hung from slide rings or equivalent hardware so as to be readily moved to the side to create an unobstructed opening in the tent wall that is of the minimum width required for door openings.

See the commentary following A.7.1.10.1 for more information on maintaining means of egress free of obstructions or impediments.

### 7.5.3 Exterior Ways of Exit Access.

The provisions of 7.5.3 apply to exit access in the typical motel arrangement where exit access from the guest rooms is provided by door openings to an open-air exit access balcony to an open stair. This arrangement is also common in apartment buildings and office buildings in warm climates. An understanding of these provisions is important, because many of the exemptions from the mandatory sprinkler requirements for the various residential occupancies conditionally apply where exterior exit access is provided.

**7.5.3.1** Exit access shall be permitted to be by means of any exterior balcony, porch, gallery, or roof that conforms to the requirements of this chapter.

**7.5.3.2** The long side of the balcony, porch, gallery, or similar space shall be at least 50 percent open and shall be arranged to restrict the accumulation of smoke.

Exterior ways of exit access need significant openings to the exterior so as not to become smoke-logged and unusable. Paragraph 7.5.3.2 establishes that at least 50 percent of the long side of the balcony, porch, gallery, or similar space is required to be open.

**7.5.3.3** Exterior exit access balconies shall be separated from the interior of the building by walls and opening protectives as required for corridors, unless the exterior exit access balcony is served by at least two remote stairs that can be accessed without any occupant traveling past an unprotected opening to reach one of the stairs, or unless dead ends on the exterior exit access do not exceed 20 ft (6100 mm).

Paragraph 7.5.3.3 requires the exterior exit access to be protected by separating construction from the interior of the building via the same rules that are applicable to corridors. However, this requirement does not apply to exit access served by at least two remote stairs, as detailed. Such an arrangement is used more often than the rated construction required by 7.5.3.3. To use this arrangement, access must be possible to both of the required remote stairs, one of which must be reachable without traveling past an unprotected opening.

Exhibit 7.96 illustrates four arrangements permitted by 7.5.3.3. In Part (a) and Part (b), it is possible for occupants of all rooms to reach one of the stairs without having to travel past any opening from which fire might issue; thus, fire-rated walls and door assemblies are not required. In Part (c), the occupants of rooms at the ends of the building must travel past other rooms to reach a stair; thus, fire resistance–rated walls and fire protection–rated opening protectives, such as windows and door assemblies, are required in the areas indicated.

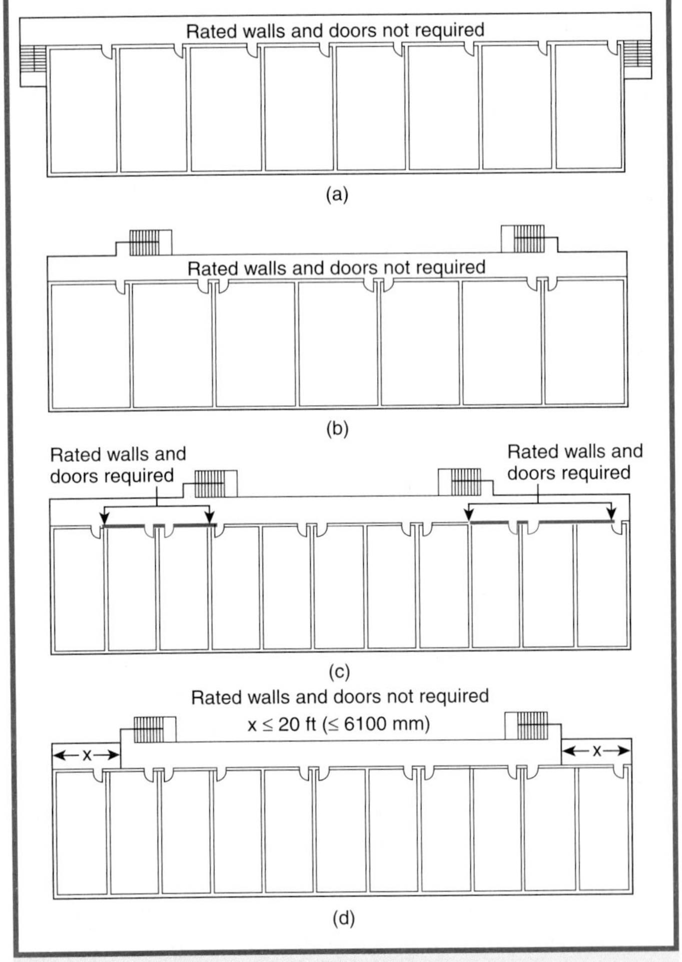


***Exhibit 7.96*** *Exterior ways of exit access.*

In Part (d), the alternative of 7.5.3.3, related to limiting the length of the exit access balcony dead end, is used to exempt the fire-rated wall construction and fire-rated opening protectives along the exterior exit access path. Provided that the exit access balcony dead end, denoted by the distance X, does not exceed 20 ft (6100 mm), the occupant using the exterior exit access will not be exposed to an excessive number of unprotected openings.

**7.5.3.4** Exterior exit access shall be arranged so that there are no dead ends in excess of those permitted for dead-end corridors in Chapters 11 through 43.

Because 7.5.3.3 permits unrated construction along a maximum 20 ft (6100 mm) dead-end exterior exit access path, it seems logical to recognize longer dead ends, as permitted by some of the occupancy chapters, where the exterior exit access path is protected by rated walls and rated opening protectives.

### 7.5.4 Accessible Means of Egress.

**7.5.4.1*** Areas accessible to people with severe mobility impairment, other than in existing buildings, shall have not less than two accessible means of egress, unless otherwise provided in 7.5.4.1.2 through 7.5.4.1.4.

**A.7.5.4.1** An accessible means of egress should comply with the accessible route requirements of ICC/ANSI A117.1, *American National Standard for Accessible and Usable Buildings and Facilities.*

**7.5.4.1.1** Access within the allowable travel distance shall be provided to not less than one accessible area of refuge or one accessible exit providing an accessible route to an exit discharge.

**7.5.4.1.2** A single accessible means of egress shall be permitted from buildings or areas of buildings permitted to have a single exit.

**7.5.4.1.3** Accessible means of egress shall not be required in health care occupancies protected throughout by an approved, supervised automatic sprinkler system in accordance with Section 9.7.

**7.5.4.1.4** Exit access travel along the accessible means of egress shall be permitted to be common for the distances permitted as common paths of travel.

Paragraph 7.5.4.1 requires that, in other than existing buildings, accessible means of egress be provided for all areas accessible to persons with severe mobility impairment. The term *accessible means of egress* is defined in 3.3.161.1 as "a means of egress that provides an accessible route to an area of refuge, a horizontal exit, or a public way." The term *severe mobility impairment* is defined in 3.3.228 as "the ability to move to stairs but without the ability to use the stairs."

For a single-story building with typical exit door assemblies to the exterior at finished ground level (grade), the requirement for accessible means of egress is normally met without having to provide any additional features. For a multistory building involving vertical travel to ground, the requirement for accessible means of egress from the upper floors might be met by providing ramps. Because ramp systems use considerable space, the requirement for accessible means of egress from the upper floors will most often be met by providing areas of refuge meeting the requirements of 7.2.12.

Exhibit 7.97 illustrates arrangements providing accessible means of egress. In Part (a) and Part (b), accessible means of egress are provided via finished ground level door assemblies or ramps from the second story.

In Part (c), areas of refuge with rated barrier and extra-width stairs in accordance with 7.2.12 provide accessible means of egress. In Part (d), the floor of a fully sprinklered building with a second accessible room on the floor creates an area of refuge via the definition in 3.3.20, thus providing one accessible means of egress.

The *Code* does not require areas of refuge; it requires accessible means of egress. The easiest way to meet the requirements for accessible means of egress in multistory buildings is by providing areas of refuge. See 7.2.12 and its associated commentary.

Paragraph 7.5.4.1 clarifies that the requirement for accessible means of egress is not retrospectively required in existing buildings, unless specifically required by the applicable occupancy chapter.

Note that Paragraph 7.5.4.1 requires a minimum of two accessible means of egress, unless one of the exceptions of 7.5.4.1.2 or 7.5.4.1.3 is met. Assume that the buildings depicted in Exhibit 7.97 are classified as other than health care occupancies, so that the exemption offered by 7.5.4.1.3 does not apply. Assume also that the __.2.4 subsection of the applicable occupancy chapter does not permit a single means of egress and, therefore, the exemption offered by 7.5.4.1.2 does not apply. Part (a), Part (b), and Part (c) depict floors with two accessible means of egress.

Part (d) depicts a single area of refuge with access to two exits. The intent of 7.2.12.1 is that the sprinklering of the building and the presence of two exits create the equivalent of two accessible means of egress. Persons with severe mobility impairment are able to await rescue assistance in tenable conditions until emergency responders arrive. The two exit stair enclosures, although not of the minimum width addressed in 7.2.12.2.3, provide sufficient width for emergency responders to carry the occupant on the stair to finished grade level, albeit at a slow pace. The

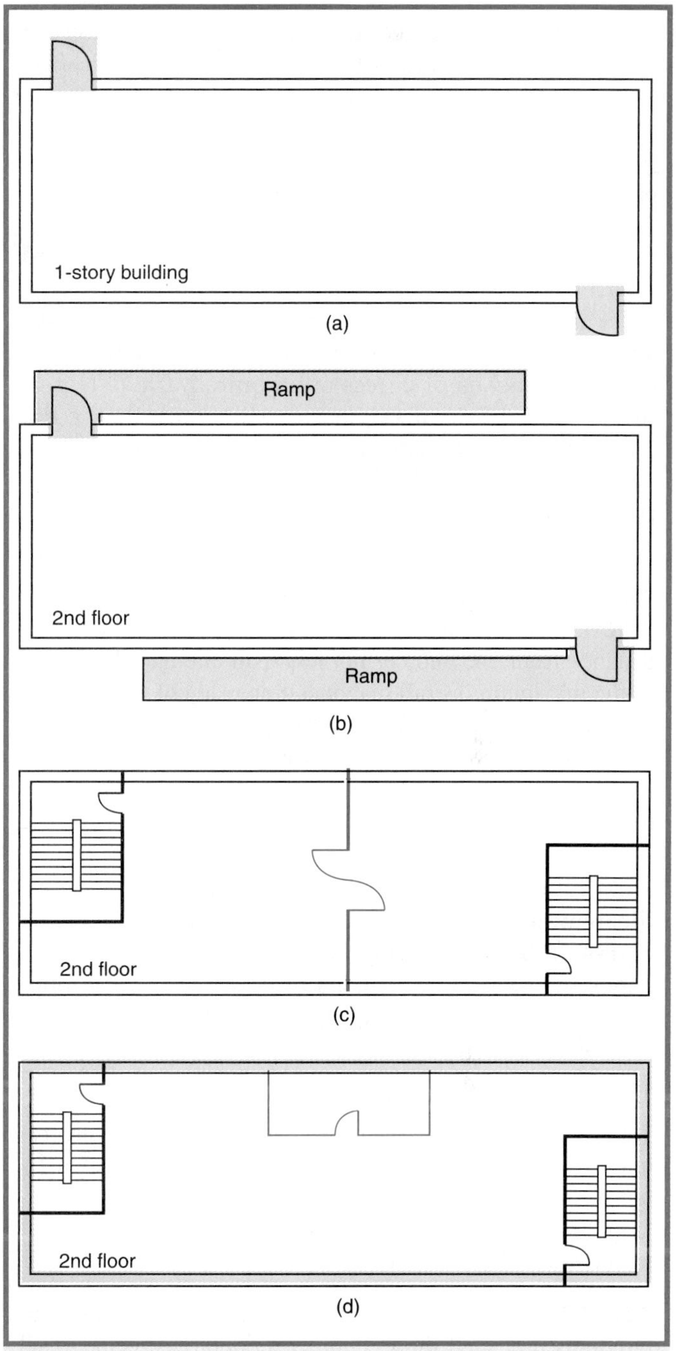


***Exhibit 7.97** Accessible means of egress.*

sprinklers are expected to control the fire to permit the exit stair enclosures to be used well into the fire. If one of the exit stair enclosures is not usable, the other provides an alternative route. Taken together, the features provided in the sprinklered building (including the communication system required by 7.2.12.1.1) serve to provide the equivalent of two accessible means of egress. The *Code* text of 7.5.4 and 7.2.12 does not clearly explain this concept.

Paragraph 7.5.4.1.4 does not permit a single accessible means of egress; rather, it permits that, where two accessible means of egress are required, travel is permitted to be along a single accessible path that is not longer than the distance permitted as common path of travel before travel along two separate accessible paths must become available.

**7.5.4.2** Where two accessible means of egress are required, the exits serving such means of egress shall be located at a distance from one another not less than one-half the length of the maximum overall diagonal dimension of the building or area to be served. This distance shall be measured in a straight line between the nearest edge of the exit doors or exit access doors, unless otherwise provided in 7.5.4.2.1 through 7.5.4.2.3.

Paragraph 7.5.4.2 establishes criteria for judging the remoteness of exits serving accessible means of egress paths. It is analogous to 7.5.1.3.2, which establishes remoteness for means of egress using the one-half diagonal rule in nonsprinklered buildings. See A.7.5.1.3.2.

**7.5.4.2.1** Where exit enclosures are provided as the required exits specified in 7.5.4.2 and are interconnected by not less than a 1-hour fire resistance–rated corridor, exit separation shall be permitted to be measured along the line of travel within the corridor.

**7.5.4.2.2** The requirement of 7.5.4.2 shall not apply to buildings protected throughout by an approved, supervised automatic sprinkler system in accordance with Section 9.7.

**7.5.4.2.3** The requirement of 7.5.4.2 shall not apply where the physical arrangement of means of egress prevents the possibility that access to both accessible means of egress will be blocked by any one fire or other emergency condition as approved by the authority having jurisdiction.

**7.5.4.3** Each required accessible means of egress shall be continuous from each accessible occupied area to a public way or area of refuge in accordance with 7.2.12.2.2.

**7.5.4.4** Where an exit stair is used in an accessible means of egress, it shall comply with 7.2.12.2.3 and either shall incorporate an area of refuge within an enlarged story-level landing or shall be accessed from an area of refuge.

**7.5.4.5** To be considered part of an accessible means of egress, an elevator shall be in accordance with 7.2.12.2.4.

**7.5.4.6** To be considered part of an accessible means of egress, a smoke barrier in accordance with Section 8.5 with not less than a 1-hour fire resistance rating, or a horizontal exit in accordance with 7.2.4, shall discharge to an area of refuge in accordance with 7.2.12.

**7.5.4.7** Accessible stories that are four or more stories above or below a story of exit discharge shall have not less than one elevator complying with 7.5.4.5, except as modified in 7.5.4.8.

**7.5.4.8** Where elevators are required by 7.5.4.7, the smokeproof enclosure required by 7.2.12.2.4 shall not be required in buildings protected throughout by an approved, supervised automatic sprinkler system in accordance with 9.7.1.1(1).

**7.5.4.9** An area of refuge used as part of a required accessible means of egress shall be in accordance with 7.2.12.

Where it might be necessary to carry persons and their wheelchairs on stairs for four or more stories to the ground level, the *Code* requires at least one elevator complying with 7.5.4.5, which imposes special elevator features and protection in accordance with 7.2.12.2.4. However, if automatic sprinklers protect the building throughout, the elevator shaft system is exempted from the smokeproof enclosure requirement of 7.2.12.2.4(3). This is consistent with the premise that sprinklers control fires so as to limit smoke production.

Paragraph 7.5.4.9 completes the package by requiring areas of refuge used as part of accessible means of egress to follow the detailed criteria for areas of refuge presented in 7.2.12.

## 7.6* Measurement of Travel Distance to Exits

**A.7.6** Table A.7.6 is a compilation of the requirements of the individual occupancy chapters (Chapters 12 through 42) for permissible length of common path of travel, dead-end corridors, and travel distance to not less than one of the required exits.

A dead end exists where an occupant enters a corridor thinking there is an exit at the end and, finding none, is

*Table A.7.6 Common Path, Dead-End, and Travel Distance Limits (by occupancy)*

| | Common Path Limit | | | | Dead-End Limit | | | | Travel Distance Limit | | | |
|---|---|---|---|---|---|---|---|---|---|---|---|---|
| | Unsprinklered | | Sprinklered | | Unsprinklered | | Sprinklered | | Unsprinklered | | Sprinklered | |
| **Type of Occupancy** | ft | m | ft | m | ft | m | ft | m | ft | m | ft | m |
| **Assembly** | | | | | | | | | | | | |
| New | 20/75 | 6.1/23[a] | 20/75 | 6.1/23[a] | 20 | 6.1[b] | 20 | 6.1[b] | 200 | 61[c] | 250 | 76[c] |
| Existing | 20/75 | 6.1/23[a] | 20/75 | 6.1/23[a] | 20 | 6.1[b] | 20 | 6.1[b] | 200 | 61[c] | 250 | 76[c] |
| **Educational** | | | | | | | | | | | | |
| New | 75 | 23 | 100 | 30 | 20 | 6.1 | 50 | 15 | 150 | 45 | 200 | 61 |
| Existing | 75 | 23 | 100 | 30 | 20 | 6.1 | 50 | 15 | 150 | 45 | 200 | 61 |
| **Day Care** | | | | | | | | | | | | |
| New | 75 | 23 | 100 | 30 | 20 | 6.1 | 50 | 15 | 150 | 45[d] | 200 | 61[d] |
| Existing | 75 | 23 | 100 | 30 | 20 | 6.1 | 50 | 15 | 150 | 45[d] | 200 | 61[d] |
| **Health Care** | | | | | | | | | | | | |
| New | NR | NR | NR | NR | 30 | 9.1 | 30 | 9.1 | NA | NA | 200 | 61[d] |
| Existing | NR | NR | NR | NR | NR | NR | NR | NR | 150 | 45[d] | 200 | 61[d] |
| **Ambulatory Health Care** | | | | | | | | | | | | |
| New | 75 | 23[e] | 100 | 30[e] | 20 | 6.1 | 50 | 15 | 150 | 45[d] | 200 | 61[d] |
| Existing | 75 | 23[e] | 100 | 30[e] | 50 | 15 | 50 | 15 | 150 | 45[d] | 200 | 61[d] |
| **Detention and Correctional** | | | | | | | | | | | | |
| New — Use Condition II, III, IV | 50 | 15 | 100 | 30 | 50 | 15 | 50 | 15 | 150 | 45[d] | 200 | 61[d] |
| New — Use Condition V | 50 | 15 | 100 | 30 | 20 | 6.1 | 20 | 6.1 | 150 | 45[d] | 200 | 61[d] |
| Existing — Use Condition II, III, IV, V | 50 | 15[f] | 100 | 30[f] | NR | NR | NR | NR | 150 | 45[d] | 200 | 61[d] |
| **Residential** | | | | | | | | | | | | |
| One- and two-family dwellings | NR | NR | NR | NR | NR | NR | NR | NR | NR | NR | NR | NR |
| Lodging or rooming houses | NR | NR | NR | NR | NR | NR | NR | NR | NR | NR | NR | NR |
| Hotels and dormitories | | | | | | | | | | | | |
| New | 35 | 10.7[g,h] | 50 | 15[g,h] | 35 | 10.7 | 50 | 15 | 175 | 53[d,i] | 325 | 99[d,i] |
| Existing | 35 | 10.7[g] | 50 | 15[g] | 50 | 15 | 50 | 15 | 175 | 53[d,h] | 325 | 99[d,h] |
| Apartments | | | | | | | | | | | | |
| New | 35 | 10.7[g] | 50 | 15[g] | 35 | 10.7 | 50 | 15 | 175 | 53[d,i] | 325 | 99[d,i] |
| Existing | 35 | 10.7[g] | 50 | 15[g] | 50 | 15 | 50 | 15 | 175 | 53[d,i] | 325 | 99[d,i] |
| Board and care | | | | | | | | | | | | |
| Small, new and existing | NR | NR | NR | NR | NR | NR | NR | NR | NR | NR | NR | NR |
| Large, new | NA | NA | 125 | 38[h] | NA | NA | 30 | 9.1 | NA | NA | 325 | 99[d,i] |
| Large, existing | 110 | 33 | 160 | 49 | 50 | 15 | 50 | 15 | 175 | 53[d,i] | 325 | 99[d,i] |
| **Mercantile** | | | | | | | | | | | | |
| Class A, B, C | | | | | | | | | | | | |
| New | 75 | 23 | 100 | 30 | 20 | 6.1 | 50 | 15 | 150 | 45 | 250 | 76 |
| Existing | 75 | 23 | 100 | 30 | 50 | 15 | 50 | 15 | 150 | 45 | 250 | 76 |
| Open air | NR | NR | NR | NR | 0 | 0 | 0 | 0 | NR | NR | NR | NR |
| Mall | | | | | | | | | | | | |
| New | 75 | 23 | 100 | 30 | 20 | 6.1 | 50 | 15 | 150 | 45 | 400 | 120[j] |
| Existing | 75 | 23 | 100 | 30 | 50 | 15 | 50 | 15 | 150 | 45 | 400 | 120[j] |
| **Business** | | | | | | | | | | | | |
| New | 75 | 23[k] | 100 | 30[k] | 20 | 6.1 | 50 | 15 | 200 | 61 | 300 | 91 |
| Existing | 75 | 23[k] | 100 | 30[k] | 50 | 15 | 50 | 15 | 200 | 61 | 300 | 91 |

*(continues)*

*Table A.7.6 Continued*

| | Common Path Limit | | | | Dead-End Limit | | | | Travel Distance Limit | | | |
|---|---|---|---|---|---|---|---|---|---|---|---|---|
| | Unsprinklered | | Sprinklered | | Unsprinklered | | Sprinklered | | Unsprinklered | | Sprinklered | |
| **Type of Occupancy** | **ft** | **m** | **ft** | **m** | **ft** | **m** | **ft** | **m** | **ft** | **m** | **ft** | **m** |
| **Industrial** | | | | | | | | | | | | |
| General | 50 | 15 | 100 | 30 | 50 | 15 | 50 | 15 | 200 | 61[l] | 250 | 75[m] |
| Special purpose | 50 | 15 | 100 | 30 | 50 | 15 | 50 | 15 | 300 | 91 | 400 | 122 |
| High hazard | 0 | 0 | 0 | 0 | 0 | 0 | 0 | 0 | 0 | 0 | 75 | 23 |
| Aircraft servicing hangars, finished ground level floor | 50 | 15[n] | 100 | 30[n] | 50 | 15[n] | 50 | 15[n] | note l | note l | note l | note l |
| Aircraft servicing hangars, mezzanine floor | 50 | 15[n] | 75 | 23[n] | 50 | 15[n] | 50 | 15[n] | 75 | 23 | 75 | 23 |
| **Storage** | | | | | | | | | | | | |
| Low hazard | NR | NR | NR | NR | NR | NR | NR | NR | NR | NR | NR | NR |
| Ordinary hazard | 50 | 15 | 100 | 30 | 50 | 15 | 100 | 30 | 200 | 61 | 400 | 122 |
| High hazard | 0 | 0 | 0 | 0 | 0 | 0 | 0 | 0 | 75 | 23 | 100 | 30 |
| Parking structures, open[o] | 50 | 15 | 50 | 15 | 50 | 15 | 50 | 15 | 300 | 91 | 400 | 122 |
| Parking structures, enclosed | 50 | 15 | 50 | 15 | 50 | 15 | 50 | 15 | 150 | 45 | 200 | 60 |
| Aircraft storage hangars, finished ground level floor | 50 | 15[n] | 100 | 30[n] | 50 | 15[n] | 50 | 15[n] | note l | note l | note l | note l |
| Aircraft servicing hangars, mezzanine floor | 50 | 15[n] | 75 | 23[n] | 50 | 15[n] | 50 | 15[n] | 75 | 23 | 75 | 23 |
| Underground spaces in grain elevators | 50 | 15[n] | 100 | 30[n] | 50 | 15[n] | 100 | 30[n] | 200 | 61 | 400 | 122 |

NR: No requirement. NA: Not applicable.

[a]For common path serving >50 persons, 20 ft (6.1 m); for common path serving ≤50 persons, 75 ft (23 m).

[b]Dead-end corridors of 20 ft (6.1 m) permitted; dead-end aisles of 20 ft (6.1 m) permitted.

[c]See Chapters 12 and 13 for special considerations for smoke-protected assembly seating in arenas and stadia.

[d]This dimension is for the total travel distance, assuming incremental portions have fully utilized their permitted maximums. For travel distance within the room, and from the room exit access door to the exit, see the appropriate occupancy chapter.

[e]See business occupancies, Chapters 38 and 39.

[f]See Chapter 23 for special considerations for existing common paths.

[g]This dimension is from the room/corridor or suite/corridor exit access door to the exit; thus, it applies to corridor common path.

[h]See the appropriate occupancy chapter for requirements for second exit access based on room area.

[i]See the appropriate occupancy chapter for special travel distance considerations for exterior ways of exit access.

[j]See 36.4.4 and 37.4.4 for special travel distance considerations in covered malls considered to be pedestrian ways.

[k]See Chapters 38 and 39 for special common path considerations for single-tenant spaces.

[l]See Chapters 40 and 42 for special requirements on spacing of doors in aircraft hangars.

[m]See Chapter 40 for industrial occupancy special travel distance considerations.

[n]See Chapters 40 and 42 for special requirements if high hazard conditions exist.

[o]See 42.8.2.6.2 for special travel distance considerations in open parking structures.

forced to retrace the path traveled to reach a choice of egress travel paths. Although relatively short dead ends are permitted by this *Code*, it is better practice to eliminate them wherever possible, as they increase the danger of persons being trapped in case of fire. Compliance with the dead-end limits does not necessarily mean that the requirements for remoteness of exits have been met. Such lack of compliance is particularly true in small buildings or buildings with short public hallways. Adequate remoteness can be obtained in such cases by further reducing the length of dead ends. *(See also A.7.5.1.5.)*

The *Code* specifies the maximum distance that occupants are permitted to travel from their position in a building to the nearest exit. There is no formula by which this distance can be established.

Maximum allowed travel distances are based on factors that include the following:

1. Number, age, and physical condition of building occupants and the rate at which they can be expected to move
2. Type and number of obstructions (e.g., display cases, seating, heavy machinery) around which occupants must travel
3. Number of people in any room or space and the distance from the farthest point in that room to the door opening
4. Amount and nature of combustibles expected in a particular occupancy
5. Rapidity with which fire might spread (a function of type of construction, materials used, degree of compartmentation, and presence or absence of automatic fire detection and extinguishing systems)

Allowable travel distances will vary with the type and size of occupancy and the degree of hazard present. Table A.7.6 is an aggregation of the maximum travel distance allowances specified elsewhere in the *Code*, typically from the __.2.6 subsection of each occupancy chapter. As shown in Table A.7.6, maximum travel distances can vary from 75 ft (23 m) in nonsprinklered high hazard storage occupancies to 400 ft (120 m) in sprinklered mall buildings or sprinklered special-purpose industrial occupancies meeting additional criteria. For most occupancies, the allowable travel distance is permitted to be increased if the building is protected throughout by automatic sprinkler systems.

Where the occupant has been provided with at least two paths of travel to an exit, it becomes important that the time needed to travel the shorter of the two paths is not so great as to place the occupant in further danger. There are no formulae or exact criteria for determining maximum permitted travel distances. Many factors have been considered and weighed in establishing these distances; they are the result of observing people who are in motion, consensus judgment, and many years of studying the results of fires in which the pre-fire conditions of a building were known.

Excessive travel distances can be a factor in large losses of life in fires, because they increase the time required to reach the safety of an exit, whether the exit is a door assembly directly to the outside or into a properly enclosed exit stair on an upper floor of a building. There is evidence that excessive travel distances played a role in a number of the fatalities on the casino floor at the MGM Grand Hotel fire in Las Vegas in 1980.[32] Of the 85 fatalities, 18 victims were located on the casino level, and some apparently were overrun by the flame front.

**7.6.1*** The travel distance to an exit shall be measured on the floor or other walking surface as follows:

(1) Along the centerline of the natural path of travel, starting from the most remote point subject to occupancy
(2) Curving around any corners or obstructions, with a 12 in. (305 mm) clearance therefrom
(3) Terminating at one of the following:
    (a) Center of the doorway
    (b) Other point at which the exit begins
    (c) Smoke barrier in an existing detention and correctional occupancy as provided in Chapter 23

**A.7.6.1** The natural exit access (path of travel) is influenced by the contents and occupancy of the building. Furniture, fixtures, machinery, or storage can serve to increase the length of travel. It is good practice in building design to recognize the influence of contents and occupancy by spacing exits for a completely open floor area at closer intervals than are required, thus reducing the hazard of excessive travel distances due to the introduction of furniture, fixtures, machinery, or storage and minimizing the possibility of violating the travel distance requirements of this *Code*.

Exhibit 7.98 illustrates the path along which travel distance to an exit is measured. In Part (a), the stair is not appropriately enclosed to qualify as an exit; second-floor travel distance measurement continues to the first floor at the exit door opening to the outside. In Part (b), the stair is properly enclosed and constitutes an exit; travel distance measurement ends on the second floor at the entrance door opening to the exit stair enclosure. The travel paths marked as 1 through 6 show that travel distance is measured as follows:

1. Starting at the most remote point subject to occupancy
2. On the floor or other walking surface
3. Along the centerline of the natural path of travel
4. Around corners and obstructions with a clearance of 12 in. (305 mm)
5. Over open exit access ramps and open exit access stairs in the plane of tread nosings
6. Ending where the exit begins

Travel distance is that length of travel to an exterior exit door opening [as shown in Exhibit 7.98, Part (a)], an enclosed exit stair [as shown in Exhibit 7.98, Part (b)], an exit passageway, or a horizontal exit. It includes

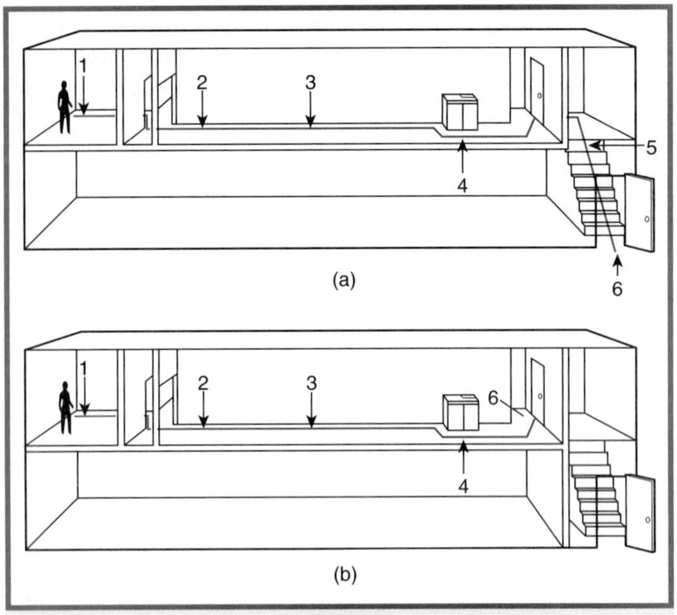


**Exhibit 7.98** *Measuring travel distance to an exit.*

all travel within the occupied space until an occupant reaches that level of protection afforded by the nearest exit. Therefore, where stairs form part of an exit access rather than an exit, the travel over such stairs is included in the travel distance measurement [as shown in Exhibit 7.98, Part (a)].

The measurement of travel distance along stairs, as detailed in 7.6.4, is to be made in the plane of the tread nosings, not along each riser and tread. This measurement is illustrated in Exhibit 7.99.

In reviewing plans for compliance with the travel distance limitations established for any occupancy, it is important to know the natural path of travel and the obstacles that are present. In Exhibit 7.100, Part (a) and Part (b) depict the same building. In Part (a), points X and Y are located at the same physical distance from the nearest exit door opening. Without further information related to the layout of furniture and partitions, it isn't clear whether the occupant will be able to travel in a straight line, as shown from point Y to the exit door opening, or will need to follow a longer travel path that zigzags around obstacles, as shown from point X to the exit door opening. A prudent designer, with lack of knowledge about the actual placement of furniture and partitions, will not assume that travel distance is a straight-line measurement. Rather, the prudent designer would estimate the travel distance to be at least the distance calculated by adding travel path segments L1 and L2.

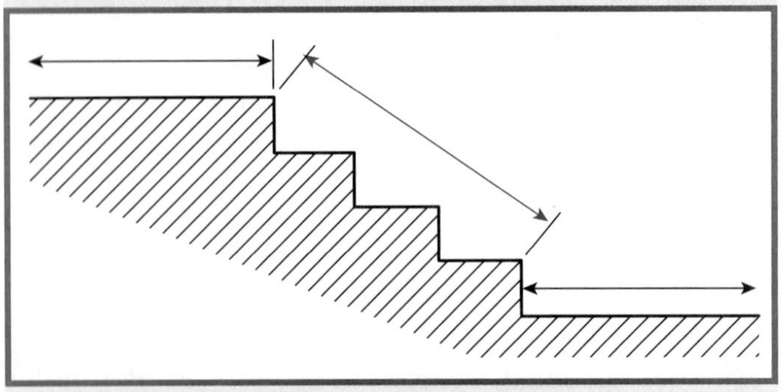

**Exhibit 7.99** *Measuring travel distance on stairs.*

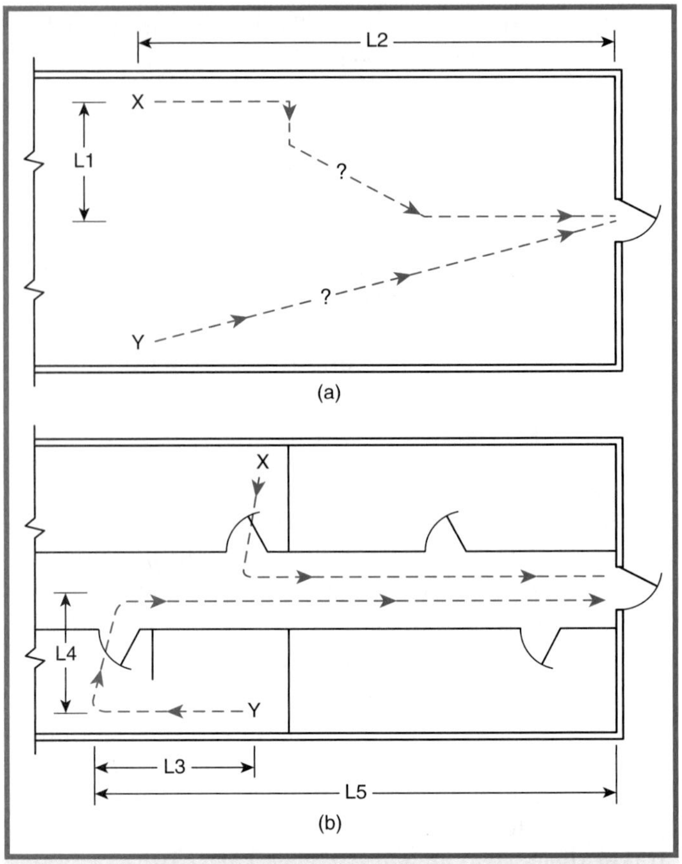


**Exhibit 7.100** *Measuring travel distance along the natural path of travel.*

In Exhibit 7.100, Part (b), the placement of partitions appears on the plan. An occupant is unable to travel in a straight "beeline" path to the exit door opening from either point X or point Y; the partitions preclude this. Further, the occupant at point Y must first move in a direction opposite from that of the building's exit door opening to reach the room door opening before turning and traveling in a direction toward the exit door opening. In this case, the travel distance is calculated by adding together travel path segments L3, L4, and L5.

**7.6.2*** Where open stairways or ramps are permitted as a path of travel to required exits, the distance shall include the travel on the stairway or ramp and the travel from the end of the stairway or ramp to an outside door or other exit in addition to the distance traveled to reach the stairway or ramp.

**A.7.6.2** Examples of locations where open stairways might exist include between mezzanines or balconies and the floor below.

**7.6.3** Where any part of an exterior exit is within 10 ft (3050 mm) of horizontal distance of any unprotected building opening, as permitted by 7.2.2.6.3 for outside stairs, the travel distance to the exit shall include the length of travel to the finished ground level.

The intent of 7.6.3 is to clarify that, if the exterior stair is exposed to unprotected building openings within 10 ft (3050 mm) horizontal distance, it is not considered an exit but is considered exit access; the travel distance, therefore, includes the measurement along the stair. The concept is illustrated in Exhibit 7.101. The openings in the wall that separates the rooms from the exit access balcony are not required to be fire rated in accordance with 7.5.3.3 (see the commentary that follows 7.5.3.3). Exterior Stair 1 is less than 10 ft (3050 mm) from the unprotected building openings (dimension d1). It cannot be considered an exit stair but, rather, an exit access stair in accordance with 7.6.3. The travel distance from point x must be measured to the bottom of the stair. Exterior Stair 2 is positioned 10 ft (3050 mm) from the unprotected building openings (dimension d2). It can be considered an exit in accordance with 7.6.3. The travel distance from point y needs to be measured only to the point on the stair landing that is 10 ft (3050 mm) from the unprotected exterior wall.

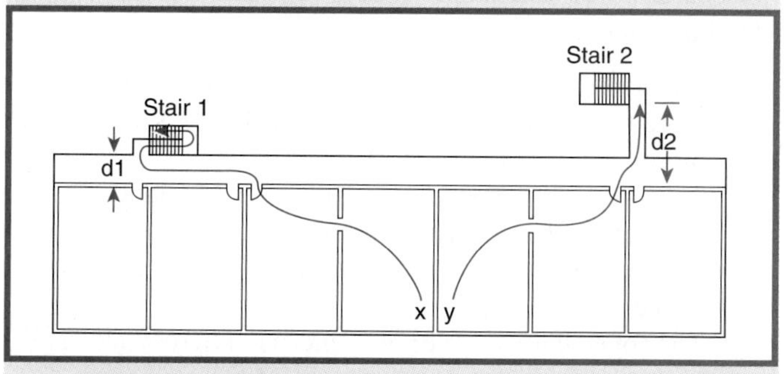


***Exhibit 7.101** Measuring travel distance with egress paths that include exterior stairs.*

**7.6.4** Where measurement includes stairs, the measurement shall be taken in the plane of the tread nosing.

**7.6.5** The travel distance in any occupied space to not less than one exit, measured in accordance with 7.6.1 through 7.6.4, shall not exceed the limits specified in this *Code*. *(See 7.6.6.)*

The maximum permitted travel distance is that length of travel path that must not be exceeded to reach the nearest exit. Although more than one exit might be required, the travel distance to exits other than the closest exit is not regulated.

**7.6.6** Travel distance limitations shall be as provided in Chapters 11 through 43 and, for high hazard areas, shall be in accordance with Section 7.11.

Although Section 7.6 establishes the method for measuring travel distance, it does not set the maximum travel distance permitted for a specific occupancy. Travel distance limitations are contained in other sections of the *Code*, typically the __.2.6 subsection of Chapters 12 through 42. Travel distance limitations might be found in portions of the *Code* that are not occupancy chapters — for example, see 7.11.1 for special travel distance provisions applicable to areas with high hazard contents. The travel distance limitations specified in the occupancy chapters are summarized in Table A.7.6.

In the 1988 edition of the *Code*, the maximum permitted travel distances were increased in most occupancies to maintain the status quo, because an exemption was deleted that permitted the travel within small rooms or spaces to be excluded from the overall measurement of travel distance. This former provision exempted rooms that contained six or fewer people, and that had a travel distance within them of less than 50 ft (15 m), from being included in the overall travel distance measurement.

## 7.7 Discharge from Exits

### 7.7.1* Exit Termination.

Exits shall terminate directly, at a public way or at an exterior exit discharge, unless otherwise provided in 7.7.1.2 through 7.7.1.4.

**A.7.7.1** An exit from the upper stories in which the direction of egress travel is generally downward should not be arranged so that it is necessary to change to travel in an upward direction at any point before discharging to the outside. A similar prohibition of reversal of the vertical component of travel should be applied to exits from stories below the floor of exit discharge. However, an exception is permitted in the case of stairs used in connection with overhead or underfloor exit passageways that serve the street floor only.

It is important that ample roadways be available from buildings in which there are large numbers of occupants so that exits will not be blocked by persons already outside. Two or more avenues of departure should be available for all but very small places. Location of a larger theater — for example, on a narrow dead-end street — might be prohibited by the authority having jurisdiction under this rule, unless some alternate way of travel to another street is available.

Exterior walking surfaces within the exit discharge are not required to be paved and often are provided by grass or similar surfaces. Where discharging exits into yards, across lawns, or onto similar surfaces, in addition to providing the required width to allow all occupants safe access to a public way, such access also is required to meet the following:

(1) Provisions of 7.1.7 with respect to changes in elevation
(2) Provisions of 7.2.2 for stairs, as applicable
(3) Provisions of 7.2.5 for ramps, as applicable
(4) Provisions of 7.1.10 with respect to maintaining the means of egress free of obstructions that would prevent its use, such as snow and the need for its removal in some climates

**7.7.1.1** Yards, courts, open spaces, or other portions of the exit discharge shall be of the required width and size to provide all occupants with a safe access to a public way.

**7.7.1.2** The requirement of 7.7.1 shall not apply to interior exit discharge as otherwise provided in 7.7.2.

**7.7.1.3** The requirement of 7.7.1 shall not apply to rooftop exit discharge as otherwise provided in 7.7.6.

**7.7.1.4** Means of egress shall be permitted to terminate in an exterior area of refuge for detention and correctional occupancies as otherwise provided in Chapters 22 and 23.

The principle addressed in 7.7.1 is that, once a building occupant reaches an exit (the protected portion of the means of egress), the level of protection afforded by that exit cannot be reduced or eliminated. Therefore, except as noted, all exits must be continuous to a public way or other safe place or to an exit discharge that must, in turn, be continuous to the public way.

It is not sufficient to allow the egress system to terminate at the outside of a building, because there might not be enough space to provide safe movement away from the building. Also, the terminus of the egress system cannot be located at the outside in a closed court from which travel back through the building might be necessary to get away from the building. In such a case, an exit passageway at least as wide as the exit itself, and constructed as specified for exits, is required to provide travel from the courtyard to the safe place.

### 7.7.2 Discharge Through Areas on Level of Exit Discharge.

Not more than 50 percent of the required number of exits, and not more than 50 percent of the required egress capacity, shall discharge through areas on the level of exit discharge, unless otherwise permitted in 7.7.2.1 and 7.7.2.2 and provided that the criteria of 7.7.2.3 through 7.7.2.7 also are met.

**7.7.2.1** One hundred percent of the exits shall be permitted to discharge through areas on the level of exit discharge in detention and correctional occupancies as otherwise provided in Chapters 22 and 23.

**7.7.2.2** In existing buildings, the 50 percent limit on egress capacity shall not apply if the 50 percent limit on the required number of exits is met.

**7.7.2.3** The discharge specified in 7.7.2 shall lead to a free and unobstructed way to the exterior of the building, and such way shall be readily visible and identifiable from the point of discharge from the exit.

**7.7.2.4** The level of discharge shall be protected throughout by an approved automatic sprinkler system in accordance with Section 9.7, or the portion of the level of discharge used for discharge shall be protected by an approved automatic sprinkler system in accordance with Section 9.7 and shall be separated from the nonsprinklered portion of the floor by a fire resistance rating meeting the requirements for the enclosure of exits. *(See 7.1.3.2.1.)*

**7.7.2.5** The requirement of 7.7.2.4 shall not apply where the discharge area is a vestibule or foyer that meets all of the following criteria:

(1) The depth from the exterior of the building shall be not more than 10 ft (3050 mm), and the length shall be not more than 30 ft (9140 mm).
(2) The foyer shall be separated from the remainder of the level of discharge by construction providing protection not less than the equivalent of wired glass in steel frames.
(3) The foyer shall serve only as means of egress and shall include an exit directly to the outside.

**7.7.2.6** The entire area on the level of discharge shall be separated from areas below by construction having a fire resistance rating not less than that required for the exit enclosure, unless otherwise provided in 7.7.2.7.

**7.7.2.7** Levels below the level of discharge in an atrium shall be permitted to be open to the level of discharge where such level of discharge is protected in accordance with 8.6.7.

The provisions of 7.7.2 permit a portion of the exit discharge from exits from floors above and below the level of exit discharge (LED) to pass through portions of the LED rather than discharge directly to the outside. Compliance with the criteria of 7.7.2 provides users of an exit stair enclosure that discharges through the level of exit discharge with approximately the same level of protection offered to users of exit enclosures that discharge directly to the outside.

Note that, where an exit from floors above or below the LED is a smokeproof enclosure, the provisions of 7.2.3.5 require the smokeproof enclosure to discharge directly outside. In cases where more than one *Code* requirement applies to a situation, the more stringent requirement takes priority, unless a specific exemption is provided. The provisions of 7.7.2 do not specifically exempt the requirement of 7.2.3.5; were not written with the intent of providing such an exemption; and are not permitted to be used to discharge occupants through the LED.

Among the questions most often asked regarding the *Code* are those that concern the requirements of 7.7.2.4 related to providing sprinkler protection on the LED. The intent of 7.7.2.4 is to require sprinkler protection in the portion of the LED that is used as exit discharge and to provide that portion of the LED with fire-rated separation from all other portions of the LED that are not sprinklered. The requirement of 7.7.2.4 can be met by either of the following means:

**1.** Protecting the entire LED by automatic sprinklers; and separating the LED from any floor below by fire-rated construction with the minimum fire rating required for the exit that discharges occupants though the LED (see 7.1.3.2.1)

**2.** Providing automatic sprinkler protection in only the portion of the LED used for exit discharge travel from the exit stair enclosure door opening to the door opening to the outside; separating the sprinklered portion of the LED from the rest of the LED by construction as required for the exit that discharges occupants though the LED; and separating the LED from any floor below by fire-rated construction with the minimum fire rating required for the exit that discharges occupants though the LED

An exemption to the sprinkler requirement of 7.7.2.4 is offered by 7.7.2.5 and involves providing a maximum 10 ft × 30 ft (3050 mm × 9140 mm) wired-glass foyer, which can be used only for egress and, thus, has no occupancy of its own.

Use of the 50 percent rule of 7.7.2 for discharge through the level of exit discharge is not dependent on occupancy permission; thus, it can be used in all occupancies. However, detention and correctional occupancies (see 22/23.2.7.3 and 22/23.2.7.4) permit 100 percent of the exits and 100 percent of the egress capacity to discharge through the level of exit discharge. Hotels and dormitories establish additional requirements limiting the distance occupants are permitted to travel within their exit discharge through the LED to the opening to the outside (see 28.2.7.3 and 29.2.7.3).

Exhibit 7.102 illustrates exit discharge arrangements meeting the requirements of 7.7.2. The equally sized stairs provide four required exits from the upper floors. Exit stair A discharges directly outside. Exit stair B is also considered to discharge directly outside, because its attached exit passageway affords protected passage to the door opening to the outside without leaving the protection offered by an exit. The other two exit stairs, C and D, are permitted to discharge across the first floor (the LED), because they do not constitute more than 50 percent of the number of exits from an

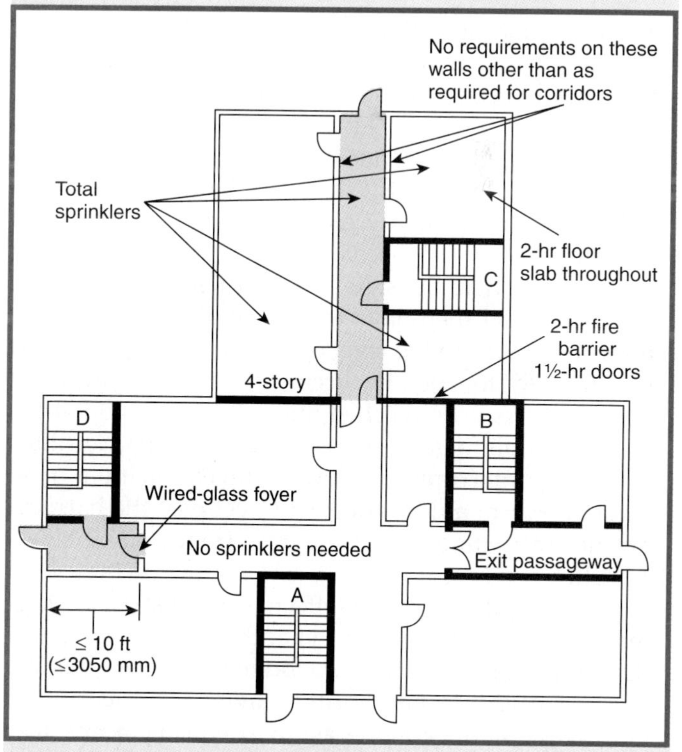


***Exhibit 7.102*** *Exit discharge.*

upper floor or more than 50 percent of the egress capacity of any upper floor. Exit stair C discharges into an area on the discharge level that is sprinklered and separated from the remainder of the floor and the basement, which are not sprinklered. The hourly fire resistance rating of the floor slab and the separating fire barrier are the same as required for the enclosure of exit stair C [e.g., a 2-hour rating if the stair is new and serves four or more stories in accordance with 7.1.3.2.1(2)]. Exit stair D discharges into a wired-glass foyer in the nonsprinklered portion of the floor in accordance with 7.7.2.5.

### 7.7.3 Arrangement and Marking of Exit Discharge.

**7.7.3.1** Where more than one exit discharge is required, exit discharges shall be arranged to meet the remoteness criteria of 7.5.1.3.

**7.7.3.2** The exit discharge shall be arranged and marked to make clear the direction of egress to a public way. Stairs shall be arranged so as to make clear the direction of egress to a public way. Stairs that continue more than one-half story beyond the level of exit discharge shall be interrupted at the level of exit discharge by partitions, doors, or other effective means.

The provision of 7.7.3.1 is new to the 2009 edition of the *Code*. It serves as a reminder that exit discharges, like exits and exit accesses, are required to be remote as addressed in 7.5.1.3.

Exhibit 7.103 illustrates a stair design intended to minimize the possibility that occupants traveling on stairs will inadvertently continue their stair descent past the level of exit discharge (LED), stop at the basement level where the stair ends but where there is no discharge, and then have to reverse direction and retrace their steps to the level of exit discharge. The barrier needed to cue the occupant that the level of discharge has been reached might be a partition with door assembly, a gate, or another physical barrier that effectively interrupts the flow of travel, forcing a person to perform a deliberate act to get past the barrier, but not restricting required egress from floors below the LED.

The words "or other effective means" open the realm of possibilities that the authority having jurisdiction (AHJ) is permitted to judge as meeting the intent of 7.7.3.2. Most authorities having jurisdiction do not accept signage alone as an adequate means for capturing the stair users' attention, as it was the failure of such signage that led to the development of the re-

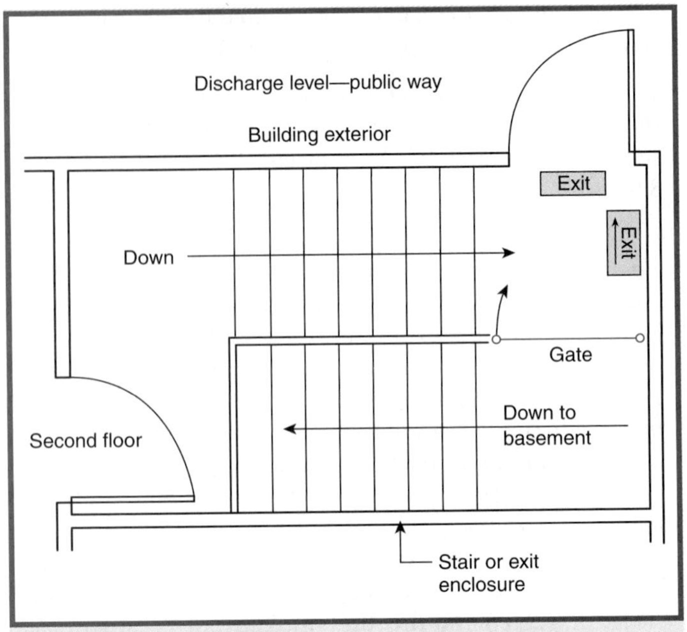


***Exhibit 7.103*** *Interruption of exit stair at LED.*

quirement. As explained in the previous paragraph, it typically takes a physical barrier to have the effect of interrupting the flow of travel past the LED.

### 7.7.4 Components of Exit Discharge.

Doors, stairs, ramps, corridors, exit passageways, bridges, balconies, escalators, moving walks, and other components of an exit discharge shall comply with the detailed requirements of this chapter for such components.

### 7.7.5 Signs.

See 7.2.2.5.4.

### 7.7.6 Discharge to Roofs.

Where approved by the authority having jurisdiction, exits shall be permitted to discharge to roofs or other sections of the building or an adjoining building where the following criteria are met:

(1) The roof/ceiling assembly construction has a fire resistance rating not less than that required for the exit enclosure.
(2) A continuous and safe means of egress from the roof is available.

An exit discharge to a roof is not acceptable, unless there is another continuous and safe means of egress from the roof and the roof construction affords protection against fire that is at least equivalent to that of the exit enclosure (e.g., the exit stair) that discharged occupants to the roof. Helicopter rescue from roofs is not dependable enough to be given credit as an exit; many factors in such a rescue are too unpredictable for this method to be a consideration.

Outside stairs leading to the roofs of other sections of the building or onto the roofs of adjoining buildings are acceptable as part of the means of egress, but only with the approval of the AHJ. The conditions and settings of such paths of travel are likely to be so varied that it is virtually impossible to cover them by written provisions. Ideally the AHJ judges each situation individually.

## 7.8 Illumination of Means of Egress

When fire occurs in a building, the degree of visibility in aisles, corridors, stairs, and exit passageways might mean the difference between orderly evacuation and chaos and, possibly, the difference between life and death. A brief glance at the history of fires reveals several noteworthy fires in which the failure of normal or emergency lighting was a major factor in the casualties incurred. The following is a list of some of these fires:

| | |
|---|---|
| Iroquois Theater, Chicago, 1903 | 602 deaths[33] |
| Cocoanut Grove Night Club, Boston, 1942 | 492 deaths[34] |
| Baltimore Oyster Roast, Baltimore, 1956 | 11 deaths[35] |
| Apartment house, Boston, 1971 | 8 deaths[36] |
| Summerland amusement complex, Isle of Man, 1973 | 50 deaths[37] |
| Psychiatric hospital, Mississippi, 1978 | 15 deaths[38] |

The report on the 1971 Massachusetts apartment fire where eight people died stated "Among the conditions contributing to the . . . loss of life were . . . the lack of emergency lighting and the lack of illuminated exit signs."

The report on the 1973 fire in the amusement complex on the Isle of Man in Great Britain, where 50 people died, stated "The problems with the evacuation are . . . (5) An insufficient number of exit signs and directional signs . . . (7) The emergency lighting did not come on when the main power was shut off by a staff member in an act of misguided zeal."

The report on the 1978 mental hospital fire in Mississippi, where 15 people died, stated:

> Heat and flame . . . impinged directly on the emergency lighting conduit, causing . . . a short circuit to occur. The short tripped the circuit breaker . . . leaving the north end of the building without emergency lighting. However, in this fire, the emergency lighting circuits on the first floor were not used. The dual-function lighting circuits were switched in the "off" position in both wards. The attendant entering Ward 1 to evacuate the residents did not turn the lights on. In Ward 2, the attendants could not reach the switch, and the circuit shorted out soon after the discovery of the fire. The darkness contributed to the difficulty in evacuating both wards.[39]

A lack of illuminated exit signs in several key places was also noted in the report.

### 7.8.1 General.

**7.8.1.1*** Illumination of means of egress shall be provided in accordance with Section 7.8 for every building and structure where required in Chapters 11 through 43. For the purposes of this requirement, exit access shall include only designated stairs, aisles, corridors, ramps, escalators, and passageways leading to an exit. For the purposes of this requirement, exit discharge shall include only designated stairs, aisles, corridors, ramps, escalators, walkways, and exit passageways leading to a public way.

**A.7.8.1.1** Illumination provided outside the building should be to either a public way or a distance away from the building that is considered safe, whichever is closest to the building being evacuated.

The means of egress (i.e., exit access, exit, and exit discharge) encompasses practically all spaces where persons can be present. The subject addressed by Section 7.8 is illumination of means of egress. It would seem that the title of Section 7.8 indicates that such illumination needs to be provided throughout all portions of the exit access, the exit, and the exit discharge, but this is not so. Illumination is required throughout the exit (e.g., an enclosed exit stair or exit passageway). Yet, 7.8.1.1 clarifies that, for the purposes of applying the requirements of Section 7.8, the portions of the exit access and exit discharge requiring illumination are only the "designated" egress paths, such as aisles, corridors, stairs, and ramps. "Designated" is meant to indicate designation by the authority having jurisdiction (AHJ). For example, most authorities having jurisdiction do not designate the space within an individual's work cubicle as a portion of the exit access required to be illuminated, but the aisles serving multiple cubicles are typically designated as requiring illumination.

Illumination of means of egress is not required unless specifically called for in the appropriate occupancy chapter. However, all occupancy chapters do require illumination, but there are a few exemptions. For example, in new assembly occupancies, 12.2.8 exempts private-party tents not larger than 1200 ft$^2$ (112 m$^2$) from the illumination requirement. Subsection __.2.8 (e.g., 36.2.8 for new mercantile occupancies) of each occupancy chapter provides illumination requirements.

**7.8.1.2** Illumination of means of egress shall be continuous during the time that the conditions of occupancy require that the means of egress be available for use, unless otherwise provided in 7.8.1.2.2.

**7.8.1.2.1** Artificial lighting shall be employed at such locations and for such periods of time as are necessary to maintain the illumination to the minimum criteria values herein specified.

**7.8.1.2.2** Automatic, motion sensor–type lighting switches shall be permitted within the means of egress, provided that the switch controllers are equipped for fail-safe operation, the illumination timers are set for a minimum 15-minute duration, and the motion sensor is activated by any occupant movement in the area served by the lighting units.

**7.8.1.3*** The floors and other walking surfaces within an exit and within the portions of the exit access and exit discharge designated in 7.8.1.1 shall be illuminated as follows:

(1) During conditions of stair use, the minimum illumination for new stairs shall be at least 10 ft-candle (108 lux), measured at the walking surfaces.
(2) The minimum illumination for floors and walking surfaces, other than new stairs during conditions of stair use, shall be to values of at least 1 ft-candle (10.8 lux), measured at the floor.
(3) In assembly occupancies, the illumination of the walking surfaces of exit access shall be at least 0.2 ft-candle (2.2 lux) during periods of performances or projections involving directed light.
(4)* The minimum illumination requirements shall not apply where operations or processes require low lighting levels.

**A.7.8.1.3(4)** Some processes, such as manufacturing or handling of photosensitive materials, cannot be performed in areas provided with the minimum specified lighting levels. The use of spaces with lighting levels below 1 ft-candle (10.8 lux) might necessitate additional safety measures, such as written emergency plans, training of new employees in emergency evacuation procedures, and periodic fire drills.

**A.7.8.1.3** A desirable form of means of egress lighting is by lights recessed in walls about 12 in. (305 mm) above the floor. Such lights are not likely to be obscured by smoke.

The *Code* requires that there be at least 1 ft-candle (10.8 lux) of illumination at floor level.

Paragraph 7.8.1.3(1), requiring at least 10 ft-candle (108 lux) for new stairs during conditions of stair use, was added for the 2003 edition of the *Code*. Note that, during conditions where the stair is not being used but the building is occupied, there must be at least 1 ft-candle (10.8 lux) of illumination on the stair walking surfaces in compliance with 7.8.1.3(2). An arrangement that might be used to comply with 7.8.1.3(1) and (2) would include illuminating the stair to a minimum of 1 ft-candle (10.8 lux) during periods that the building is occupied and using motion detectors to sense occupant presence in any portion of the stair enclosure that, upon activation, would increase the illumination level to the minimum 10 ft-candle (108 lux) requirement.

When motion pictures, slides, and the like are being shown in theaters, auditoriums, and other assembly occupancies, 7.8.1.3(3) permits the level of illumination to be reduced to 0.2 ft-candle (2.2 lux).

Paragraph 7.8.1.3(4) recognizes that some operations (e.g., photographic film manufacturing) require low lighting levels. Special precautions can be taken for occupant life safety so as not to have to require a minimum illumination level.

**7.8.1.4*** Required illumination shall be arranged so that the failure of any single lighting unit does not result in an illumination level of less than 0.2 ft-candle (2.2 lux) in any designated area.

**A.7.8.1.4** An example of the failure of any single lighting unit is the burning out of an electric bulb.

All lights, circuits, or auxiliary power must be arranged to ensure continuity of egress lighting, although the performance level is permitted to decline from 1 ft-candle (10.8 lux) to 0.2 ft-candle (2.2 lux) if a system element fails. Continuity of egress lighting can be accomplished by means such as use of duplicate light bulbs in fixtures or overlapping light patterns from neighboring fixtures.

**7.8.1.5** The equipment or units installed to meet the requirements of Section 7.10 also shall be permitted to serve the function of illumination of means of egress, provided that all requirements of Section 7.8 for such illumination are met.

### 7.8.2 Sources of Illumination.

**7.8.2.1*** Illumination of means of egress shall be from a source considered reliable by the authority having jurisdiction.

**A.7.8.2.1** An example of a power source with reasonably ensured reliability is a public utility electric service.

**7.8.2.2** Battery-operated electric lights and other types of portable lamps or lanterns shall not be used for primary illumination of means of egress. Battery-operated electric lights shall be permitted to be used as an emergency source to the extent permitted under Section 7.9.

## 7.9 Emergency Lighting

### 7.9.1 General.

**7.9.1.1*** Emergency lighting facilities for means of egress shall be provided in accordance with Section 7.9 for the following:

(1) Buildings or structures where required in Chapters 11 through 43
(2) Underground and limited access structures as addressed in Section 11.7
(3) High-rise buildings as required by other sections of this *Code*
(4) Doors equipped with delayed-egress locks
(5) Stair shaft and vestibule of smokeproof enclosures, for which the following also apply:
   (a) The stair shaft and vestibule shall be permitted to include a standby generator that is installed for the smokeproof enclosure mechanical ventilation equipment.
   (b) The standby generator shall be permitted to be used for the stair shaft and vestibule emergency lighting power supply.
(6) New access-controlled egress doors in accordance with 7.2.1.6.2.

**A.7.9.1.1** Emergency lighting outside the building should provide illumination to either a public way or a distance away from the building that is considered safe, whichever is closest to the building being evacuated.

Emergency lighting is not required unless specifically called for in the appropriate occupancy chapter or by a provision of 7.9.1.1. Most occupancy chapters require emergency lighting in medium to large buildings. Subsection __.2.9 of each occupancy chapter (e.g., 12.2.9 and 36.2.9 for new assembly and new mercantile occupancies, respectively) provides emergency lighting requirements.

**7.9.1.2** For the purposes of 7.9.1.1, exit access shall include only designated stairs, aisles, corridors, ramps, escalators, and passageways leading to an exit. For the purposes of 7.9.1.1, exit discharge shall include only designated stairs, ramps, aisles, walkways, and escalators leading to a public way.

The means of egress (i.e., exit access, exit, and exit discharge) encompasses practically all spaces where persons can be present. The subject addressed by Section 7.9 is emergency lighting of means of egress. It would seem that the title of Section 7.9 indicates that such emergency lighting needs to be provided throughout all portions of the exit access, the exit, and the exit discharge, but this is not so. Emergency lighting is required throughout the exit (e.g., in an enclosed exit stair or exit passageway). Yet, 7.9.1.2 clarifies that, for the purposes of applying the requirements of Section 7.9, the portions of the exit access and exit discharge requiring emergency lighting are only the "designated" egress paths, such as aisles, corridors, stairs, and ramps. "Designated" is meant to indicate designation by the AHJ. For example, most authorities having jurisdiction do not designate the space within an individual's work cubicle as a portion of the exit access required to be provided with emergency lighting, but the aisles serving multiple cubicles are typically designated as requiring emergency lighting.

**7.9.1.3** Where maintenance of illumination depends on changing from one energy source to another, a delay of not more than 10 seconds shall be permitted.

An on-site generator driven by a prime mover must be automatically started and capable of picking up the emergency lighting load within 10 seconds. If the generator is not able to supply power within this time frame, an auxiliary power source must be provided. For example, unit lighting packs with their integral batteries might be used to provide emergency lighting immediately upon loss of normal power, with a switchover to other lighting fixtures supplied by power from the generator at a later point in the incident during which normal power was lost.

Some turbine-driven emergency generators take longer than 10 seconds to reach operating speed. A backup battery pack, such as an uninterruptible power supply (UPS), capable of delivering emergency power for a few minutes might be used in conjunction with any on-site generator that cannot meet the 10-second requirement. As another alternative, unit lighting packs with their integral batteries might be used to provide emergency lighting immediately upon loss of normal power, with a switchover to other lighting fixtures supplied by power from the generator at a later point in the incident during which normal power was lost.

*NFPA 70, National Electrical Code*, permits use of an emergency generator for load shedding and peak load shaving, provided that these loads can be disconnected when normal power to the emergency lighting system is lost.

Although not required by *NFPA 70*, the use of bypass-isolation transfer switches might be considered. See Exhibit 7.104. These devices allow maintenance and repair of the transfer switch mechanism without interruption of power to the emergency loads. Bypass switches are interlocked to prevent simultaneous interconnection of the two power sources, and isolation of the transfer switch is usually accomplished by operation of a drawout handle. This type of construction might be used where continuity of electrical service to the emergency system is essential.

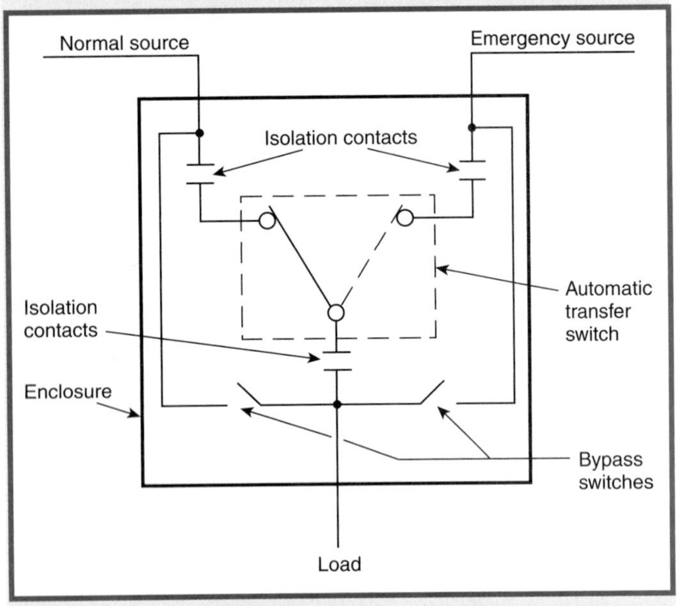


***Exhibit 7.104** Schematic of bypass-isolation transfer switch.*

### 7.9.2 Performance of System.

**7.9.2.1*** Emergency illumination shall be provided for a minimum of $1\frac{1}{2}$ hours in the event of failure of normal lighting. Emergency lighting facilities shall be arranged to provide initial illumination that is not less than an average of 1 ft-candle (10.8 lux) and, at any point, not less than 0.1 ft-candle (1.1 lux), measured along the path of egress at floor level. Illumination levels shall be permitted to decline to not less than an average of 0.6 ft-candle (6.5 lux) and, at any point, not less than 0.06 ft-candle (0.65 lux) at the end of $1\frac{1}{2}$ hours. A maximum-to-minimum illumination uniformity ratio of 40 to 1 shall not be exceeded.

**A.7.9.2.1** The illumination uniformity ratio is determined by the following formula:

$$\frac{\text{Maximum illumination at any point}}{\text{Minimum illumination at any point}}$$

The *Code* requires a 1 ft-candle (10.8 lux) average and establishes a 0.1 ft-candle (1.1 lux) minimum, with a uniformity ratio maximum of 40 to 1 to prevent excessively bright and dark spots.

**7.9.2.2** New emergency power systems for emergency lighting shall be at least Type 10, Class 1.5, Level 1, in accordance with NFPA 110, *Standard for Emergency and Standby Power Systems.*

A Type 10 emergency power supply system (EPSS) must restore power within 10 seconds of the failure of the primary power source. A Class 1.5 EPSS must be capable of operating at its rated load without being refueled for a minimum of $1\frac{1}{2}$ hours. Level 1 performance is specified based on the technical committee's judgment that failure of the EPSS is critical to human life and safety. For an example where Level 2 performance, for EPSS less critical to human life and safety, is specified in the *Code*, see 7.2.3.12 related to powering mechanical ventilation equipment for smokeproof enclosures. See also NFPA 110, *Standard for Emergency and Standby Power Systems.*

**7.9.2.3*** The emergency lighting system shall be arranged to provide the required illumination automatically in the event of any interruption of normal lighting due to any of the following:

(1) Failure of a public utility or other outside electrical power supply
(2) Opening of a circuit breaker or fuse
(3) Manual act(s), including accidental opening of a switch controlling normal lighting facilities

**A.7.9.2.3** Where approved by the authority having jurisdiction, this requirement is permitted to be met by means such as the following.

(1) Two separate electric lighting systems with independent wiring, each adequate alone to provide the specified lighting, as follows:
   (a) One such system is permitted to be supplied from an outside source, such as a public utility service, and the other from an electric generator on the premises driven by an independent source of power.
   (b) Both sources of illumination should be in regular

simultaneous operation whenever the building is occupied during periods of darkness.

(2) An electric circuit, or circuits, used only for means of egress illumination, with two independent electric sources arranged so that, on the failure of one, the other will automatically and immediately operate, as follows:

(a) One such source is permitted to be a connection from a public utility, or similar outside power source, and the other an approved storage battery with suitable provision to keep it automatically charged.

(b) The battery should be provided with automatic controls that, after operation of the battery due to failure of the primary power source or operation for the purpose of turning off the primary electric source for the lights, will shut off the battery after its specified period of operation and will automatically recharge and ready the battery for further service when the primary current source is turned on again.

(3) Electric battery–operated emergency lighting systems complying with the provisions of 7.9.2.3 and operating on a separate circuit and at a voltage different from that of the primary light can be used where permitted. *(See NFPA 70, National Electrical Code.)*

These requirements are not intended to prohibit the connection of a feeder serving exit lighting and similar emergency functions ahead of the service disconnecting means, but such provision does not constitute an acceptable alternate source of power. Such a connection furnishes only supplementary protection for emergency electrical functions, particularly where intended to allow the fire department to open the main disconnect without hampering exit activities. Provision should be made to alert the fire department that certain power and lighting is fed by an emergency generator and will continue operation after the service disconnect is opened.

Where emergency lighting is provided by automatic transfer between normal power service and an emergency generator, it is the intent to prohibit the installation, for any reason, of a single switch that can interrupt both energy sources.

The emergency lighting provisions of 7.9.2.3 are more stringent than those in *NFPA 70, National Electrical Code*. Compliance with the criterion of 7.9.2.3(2), related to interruption of normal lighting due to the opening of a circuit breaker or fuse, requires careful design and installation. The requirement can be met by providing a minimum of two lighting circuits in a room. If the breaker controlling one of the two lighting circuits is opened, there is still illumination in the room, so that there is no interruption of normal lighting and no resulting requirement to switch over to emergency lighting.

The second breaker serving the lighting circuits in the room should be installed on a subpanel separate from the subpanel serving the first breaker. If a common subpanel were used for both lighting circuits, the opening of the main breaker in that subpanel would interrupt normal lighting in the room so as to trigger the need to provide emergency lighting. The common subpanels would introduce the need to monitor those subpanels for the purpose of automatically switching over to emergency lighting — a complication that would be unacceptable to most building operators.

The wiring for the independent lighting subpanels needs to come together somewhere in order to provide them with power, and that typically occurs at the main service entrance/panel. The main breaker can be monitored in the same way that the incoming public power is monitored, so as to automatically provide emergency lighting upon interruption of power.

Six methods of providing emergency power are recognized in *NFPA 70*; however, some of these sources do not meet the requirements for emergency lighting under the *Life Safety Code*.

Storage batteries are an acceptable emergency source and are permitted to be used to supply continuous, required emergency lighting. For this arrangement, two separate lighting systems with independent wiring are employed. One system is permitted to be supplied from a public utility, and the other from storage batteries. Each supply source must have sufficient capacity, and emergency lighting must be designed so that adequate light is available for a specified time if one system fails.

Instead of installing two separate wiring systems, a single emergency system connected to an automatic transfer switch is often used. The two sources of power, normal and emergency, are connected to the transfer switch, which automatically switches the emergency lighting load from the normal source to the emergency source upon loss of normal power. When normal power is restored, the emergency load is transferred back to the normal source.

Batteries that are used for the emergency source must be suitable for the application. Automotive-type batteries are not acceptable.

Where an on-site generator is the emergency power source, it is generally controlled by a transfer switch. Upon loss of normal emergency power, a signal is sent to start the generator. When the generator is running at rated speed and its output voltage is correct, the emergency load is connected to this source by operation of the automatic transfer switch. This transfer must take place in 10 seconds or less. See Exhibit 7.105.

Exhibit 7.106 shows two methods of obtaining an emergency power supply by connection ahead of the service disconnecting means. Although not prohibited by *NFPA 70*, this method does not comply with the requirements for emergency lighting of the *Life Safety Code* and might not be acceptable to the authority having jurisdiction (AHJ). Before considering this method to supply emergency power for other than emergency lighting, the reliability of the utility system in the area must be evaluated, and the risk to building occupants must be carefully considered. This arrangement only provides protection from electrical failures in the occupancy, such as blown fuses, tripped circuit breakers, or a localized fire at such locations as the electrical service or distribution panels. In such instances, the availability of the emergency source is dependent on the reliability of the public utility.

The advantage of connecting the emergency lighting circuit to the main power line on the live side of the main disconnect is service continuity if employees or fire fighters throw the main switch as a precautionary measure. The *Code* does not prohibit this practice; however, this method does not meet the requirements for emergency lighting.

Two separate services, one for normal power and the other for emergency power, are also recognized by *NFPA 70*, subject to approval by the AHJ but, again, not accepted by the *Life Safety Code* for emergency lighting. Usually, this method provides a higher degree of reliability than the connection ahead of the service disconnecting means but does not satisfy the requirements of 7.9.2.3. However, underground loop systems in downtown areas of large cities are quite

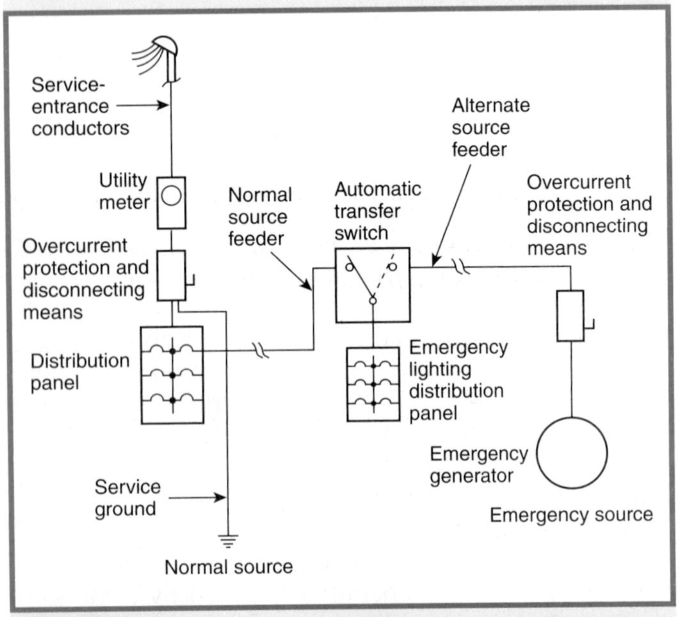


**Exhibit 7.105** *Arrangement of normal and alternate sources where emergency power is supplied from on-site generator.*

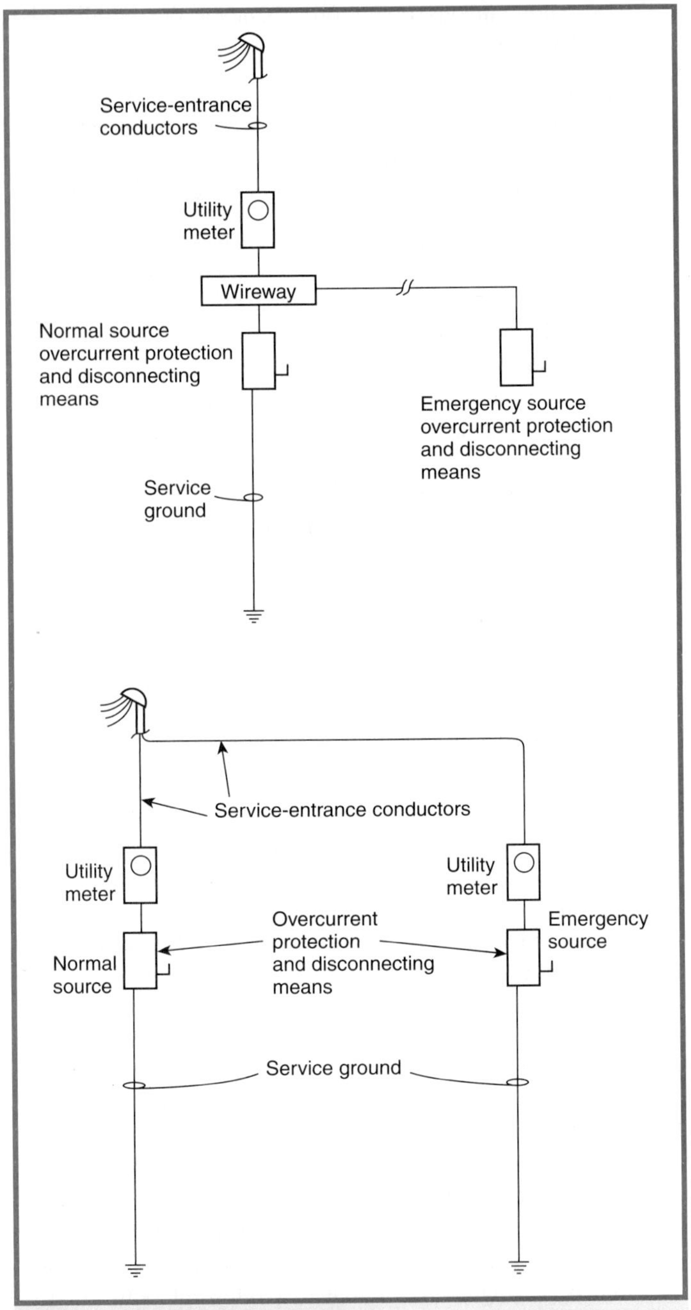


**Exhibit 7.106** *Two methods (not Life Safety Code–compliant) of obtaining an emergency source by connection ahead of service disconnecting means.*

reliable. Many public utilities have not experienced an outage on their loop systems for many years, but there is no protection from any electrical failures that might occur outside of the occupancy. One way to reduce the possibility of simultaneous loss of both power sources is to use different voltages for the normal and emergency systems, taking power for each system from separate manholes or employing other schemes that provide both electrical and physical separation between the normal and emergency sources. See Exhibit 7.107.

Individual battery-operated lights can also be used for emergency lighting. Specific rules in *NFPA 70* govern the installation of these products, referred to in *NFPA 70* as "unit equipment."

To qualify for emergency lighting, each piece of unit equipment must have a rechargeable battery, a battery-charging means, provisions for one or more lamps, and a relay to energize the lamps automatically upon failure of the normal supply. Unit equipment must be connected to the same branch circuit that supplies normal lighting to the area in which the unit equipment is located. Connection to this branch circuit must be ahead of, or on the line side of, any switches controlling the normal lighting. An exception in *NFPA 70* permits connection of unit equipment directly to a branch circuit from a panel board that also supplies a minimum of three normal lighting circuits to the area in which the unit equipment is installed. The overcurrent device protecting this unit equipment circuit must be provided with a lock-on feature that will prevent accidental disconnection.

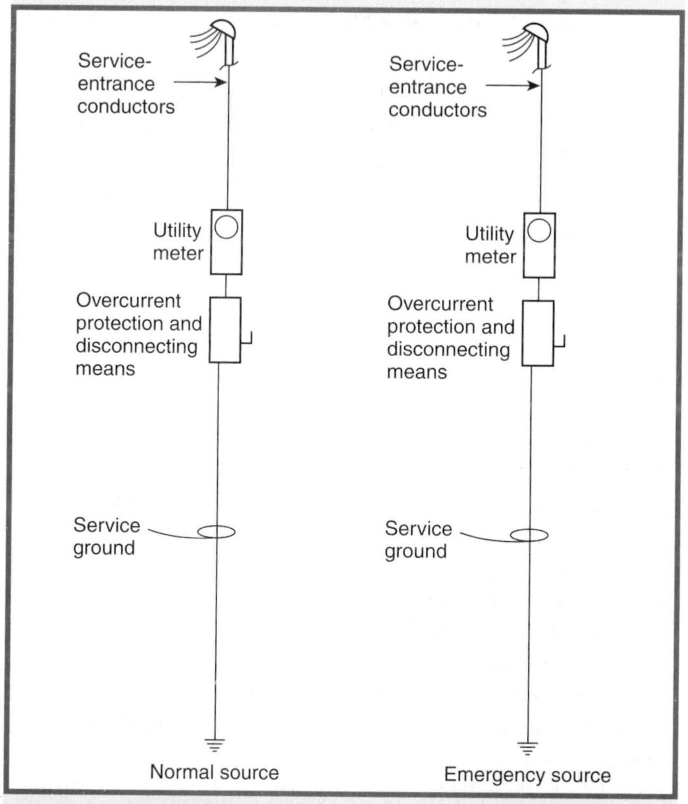


***Exhibit 7.107** Two separate services to the same building permitted by NFPA 70, National Electrical Code, but not recognized by the Life Safety Code for emergency lighting.*

**7.9.2.4** Emergency generators providing power to emergency lighting systems shall be installed, tested, and maintained in accordance with NFPA 110, *Standard for Emergency and Standby Power Systems*. Stored electrical energy systems, where required in this *Code*, other than battery systems for emergency luminaires in accordance with 7.9.2.5, shall be installed and tested in accordance with NFPA 111, *Standard on Stored Electrical Energy Emergency and Standby Power Systems*.

The provision of 7.9.2.4 was revised for the 2009 edition of the *Code* to clarify that battery systems for emergency luminaires are to comply with 7.9.2.5, which requires listing per ANSI/UL 924, *Standard for Emergency Lighting and Power Equipment*.

**7.9.2.5** Unit equipment and battery systems for emergency luminaires shall be listed to ANSI/UL 924, *Standard for Emergency Lighting and Power Equipment*.

**7.9.2.6*** Existing battery-operated emergency lights shall use only reliable types of rechargeable batteries provided with suitable facilities for maintaining them in properly charged condition. Batteries used in such lights or units shall be approved for their intended use and shall comply with *NFPA 70, National Electrical Code*.

**A.7.9.2.6** Automobile-type lead storage batteries are not suitable by reason of their relatively short life when not subject to frequent discharge and recharge as occurs in automobile operation.

For proper selection and maintenance of appropriate batteries, see *NFPA 70, National Electrical Code*.

**7.9.2.7** The emergency lighting system shall be either continuously in operation or shall be capable of repeated automatic operation without manual intervention.

### 7.9.3 Periodic Testing of Emergency Lighting Equipment.

**7.9.3.1** Required emergency lighting systems shall be tested in accordance with one of the three options offered by 7.9.3.1.1, 7.9.3.1.2, or 7.9.3.1.3.

**7.9.3.1.1** Testing of required emergency lighting systems shall be permitted to be conducted as follows:

(1) Functional testing shall be conducted monthly with a minimum of 3 weeks and a maximum of 5 weeks between tests, for not less than 30 seconds, except as otherwise permitted by 7.9.3.1.1(2).
(2)* The test interval shall be permitted to be extended beyond 30 days with the approval of the authority having jurisdiction.
(3) Functional testing shall be conducted annually for a minimum of $1\frac{1}{2}$ hours if the emergency lighting system is battery powered.
(4) The emergency lighting equipment shall be fully operational for the duration of the tests required by 7.9.3.1.1(1) and (3).
(5) Written records of visual inspections and tests shall be kept by the owner for inspection by the authority having jurisdiction.

**A.7.9.3.1.1(2)** Technical justification for extending test intervals past 30 days should be based on recorded event history (data) and should include evaluation of the following criteria:

(1) Number of egress lighting units
(2) Number of 30-second tests for analysis
(3) Re-evaluation period (confirm or adjust intervals)
(4) Number of fixtures found obstructed
(5) Number of fixtures found misaligned
(6) Fixtures found to be missing
(7) Fixtures found damaged
(8) Battery design
(9) Type of light source
(10) Fixture design (manufacturer)
(11) Number of light fixtures per exit path
(12) Existence of fire, smoke, and thermal barriers
(13) Evacuation capability
(14) Maximum egress time
(15) Hours of occupancy
(16) Number of recorded bulb failures
(17) Number of recorded fixture failures
(18) Single fixture reliability
(19) Repairs — mean time to repair
(20) Lighted egress path probability of success or failure — monthly upper tolerance limit
(21) Lighted egress path probability of success or failure — quarterly upper tolerance limit (estimated)

**7.9.3.1.2** Testing of required emergency lighting systems shall be permitted to be conducted as follows:

(1) Self-testing/self-diagnostic battery-operated emergency lighting equipment shall be provided.
(2) Not less than once every 30 days, self-testing/self-diagnostic battery-operated emergency lighting equipment shall automatically perform a test with a duration of a minimum of 30 seconds and a diagnostic routine.
(3) Self-testing/self-diagnostic battery-operated emergency lighting equipment shall indicate failures by a status indicator.
(4) A visual inspection shall be performed at intervals not exceeding 30 days.
(5) Functional testing shall be conducted annually for a minimum of $1\frac{1}{2}$ hours.
(6) Self-testing/self-diagnostic battery-operated emergency lighting equipment shall be fully operational for the duration of the $1\frac{1}{2}$ hour test.
(7) Written records of visual inspections and tests shall be kept by the owner for inspection by the authority having jurisdiction.

**7.9.3.1.3** Testing of required emergency lighting systems shall be permitted to be conducted as follows:

(1) Computer-based, self-testing/self-diagnostic battery-operated emergency lighting equipment shall be provided.
(2) Not less than once every 30 days, emergency lighting equipment shall automatically perform a test with a duration of a minimum of 30 seconds and a diagnostic routine.
(3) The emergency lighting equipment shall automatically perform annually a test for a minimum of $1\frac{1}{2}$ hours.
(4) The emergency lighting equipment shall be fully operational for the duration of the tests required by 7.9.3.1.3(2) and (3).
(5) The computer-based system shall be capable of providing a report of the history of tests and failures at all times.

Periodic testing of emergency lighting equipment is needed to help ensure such equipment will perform as needed upon failure of normal power. The functional test, required to be conducted by 7.9.3.1.1(1), 7.9.3.1.2(2), and 7.9.3.1.3(2), ensures that the bulbs and other equipment work. Additionally, for battery-powered equipment, the 30-second performance criterion for the functional test demonstrates that batteries have more than a residual charge. The $1\frac{1}{2}$-hour performance criterion required yearly for battery-powered equipment ensures sufficient battery life to provide emergency lighting for the $1\frac{1}{2}$ hours required by 7.9.2.1.

The self-testing/self-diagnostic systems permitted by 7.9.3.1.2 and 7.9.3.1.3 use newer technologies and equipment to automate the testing, thereby reducing the manual labor needed to keep the emergency lighting systems in proper operating condition.

Note that 7.9.3.1.1(1) was revised and 7.9.3.1.1(2) is new to the 2009 edition of the *Code*. In prior editions, the functional test, which must be performed manually (as contrasted with the functional testing that is conducted automatically by the self-testing/self-diagnostic systems addressed in 7.9.3.1.2 and 7.9.3.1.3), was required to be conducted at 30-day intervals. Where that requirement was followed exactly, testing performed on January 31 would be performed again the following year on January 25 due to the forward creep caused by 31-day months. The former requirement also offered no leniency for scheduling the testing to avoid weekends when the person responsible for conducting the testing might not normally be present. The new language of 7.9.3.1.1(1) offers flexibility without permitting someone to test, for example, on January 31 and again the next day, February 1, and claim compliance with having tested once in each of those months.

The provision of 7.9.3.1.1(2) offers further flexibility by allowing the AHJ to extend the testing frequency. The text of A.7.9.3.1.1(2) provides guidance on the nature of the technical justification needed to qualify for such an extension.

## 7.10 Marking of Means of Egress

In the fatal Westchase Hilton Hotel fire, which occurred in Houston, Texas, in March of 1982, "several people were confused by the exit markings or the similarity of exit doors and adjacent storage room doors. The directional exit signs within the exit foyers at the ends of the hotel corridors indicated that the exit path from this point would be perpendicular to the exit access corridor. Some of the occupants moved toward the locked storage room doors and away from the exits."[40]

### 7.10.1 General.

**7.10.1.1 Where Required.** Means of egress shall be marked in accordance with Section 7.10 where required in Chapters 11 through 43.

Marking of means of egress is not required unless specifically called for by the applicable occupancy chapter. Subsection __.2.10 of each occupancy chapter (e.g., 12.2.10 for new assembly occupancies) details where exit signs and directional exit signs are required.

**7.10.1.2 Exits.**

**7.10.1.2.1*** Exits, other than main exterior exit doors that obviously and clearly are identifiable as exits, shall be marked by an approved sign that is readily visible from any direction of exit access.

**A.7.10.1.2.1** Where a main entrance also serves as an exit, it will usually be sufficiently obvious to occupants so that no exit sign is needed.

The character of the occupancy has a practical effect on the need for signs. In any assembly occupancy, hotel, department store, or other building subject to transient occupancy, the need for signs will be greater than in a building subject to permanent or semipermanent occupancy by the same people, such as an apartment house where the residents are presumed to be familiar with exit facilities by reason of regular use thereof. Even in a permanent residence-type building, however, there is a need for signs to identify exit facilities such as outside stairs that are not subject to regular use during the normal occupancy of the building.

There are many types of situations where the actual need for signs is debatable. In cases of doubt, however, it is desirable to be on the safe side by providing signs, particularly because posting signs does not ordinarily involve any material expense or inconvenience.

The requirement for the locations of exit signs visible from any direction of exit access is illustrated in Figure A.7.10.1.2.1.

**7.10.1.2.2*** Horizontal components of the egress path within an exit enclosure shall be marked by approved exit or directional exit signs where the continuation of the egress path is not obvious.

The provision of 7.10.1.2.2 is new to the 2009 edition of the *Code*. Some exit stair enclosures, particularly in high-rise buildings where the upper portion of the tower presents a smaller footprint than the base of the building, include horizontal components (much like exit passageways) at floors where the stair enclosure that serves the next group of floors immediately below shifts horizontally in position. Although exit and directional exit signs are not normally needed within an exit stair enclosure that is stacked vertically without offsets because occupants simply move downward from floor to floor, the presence of the horizontal passageway might confound the egress path. Where the continuation of the egress path is not obvious, 7.10.1.2.2 requires additional exit or directional exit signs.

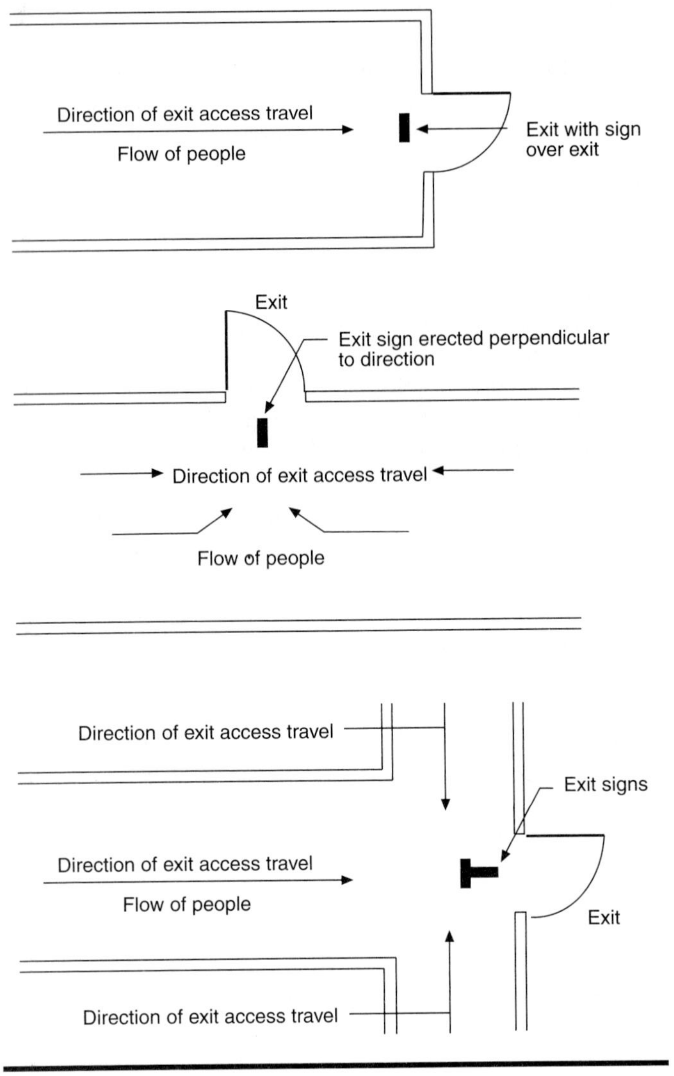


*Figure A.7.10.1.2.1 Location of Exit Signs.*

**A.7.10.1.2.2** The direction of travel to the exit discharge within a stair enclosure with horizontal components in excess of the typical landings might need additional signage to be readily visible or obvious. Exit signs should be installed above doors through which the egress path leads. Directional exit signs should be installed where the horizontal egress path changes directions. The stairway marking signs required by 7.2.2.5.4, provided within the stair enclosure at each floor landing, indicate the vertical direction to exit discharge.

**7.10.1.3 Exit Door Tactile Signage.** Tactile signage shall be provided to meet the following criteria, unless otherwise provided in 7.10.1.4:

(1) Tactile signage shall be located at each exit door requiring an exit sign.
(2) Tactile signage shall read as follows: EXIT.
(3) Tactile signage shall comply with ICC/ANSI A117.1, *American National Standard for Accessible and Usable Buildings and Facilities.*

**7.10.1.4 Existing Exemption.** The requirements of 7.10.1.3 shall not apply to existing buildings, provided that the occupancy classification does not change.

All exit door assemblies required to have an exit sign are also required to have tactile signage, unless the exit door assembly is in an existing building and the occupancy classification does not change. The required tactile signage allows persons with vision impairment to identify the door assembly as an exit. For the same reasons that the requirements of 7.5.4 on accessible means of egress are not required for existing buildings, tactile signage is not required in existing buildings, unless the occupancy classification changes.

**7.10.1.5 Exit Access.**

**7.10.1.5.1** Access to exits shall be marked by approved, readily visible signs in all cases where the exit or way to reach the exit is not readily apparent to the occupants.

**7.10.1.5.2*** New sign placement shall be such that no point in an exit access corridor is in excess of the rated viewing distance or 100 ft (30 m), whichever is less, from the nearest sign.

**A.7.10.1.5.2** For externally illuminated signs in accordance with 7.10.6 and internally illuminated signs listed without a viewing distance, the rated viewing distance should be considered to be 100 ft (30 m). However, placing signs to meet the 100 ft (30 m) viewing distance in other than exit access corridors might create operating difficulties or encourage placement of a sign above the line of sight. To resolve the viewing distance versus placement issue, consideration should be given to proportionally increasing the level of illumination and the size of the exit legend to the viewing distance, if signs are placed at greater distances.

The placement distance requirement in 7.10.1.5.2 applies only to new exit sign installations in corridors. Internally illuminated signs are required by 7.10.7.1 to be listed in accordance with ANSI/UL 924, *Standard for Emergency Lighting and Power Equipment.* The testing procedures of ANSI/UL 924 determine a distance rating for the listed sign. Externally illuminated signs are not required to be listed and do not have a distance rating associated with them; however, they are subject to the maximum 100 ft (30 m) placement distance requirement.

The requirement by 7.10.1.5.2 to position internally illuminated signs based on their listed distance rating is another step toward promoting performance-based design in lieu of the traditional prescription-based approach [i.e., use of the maximum 100 ft (30 m) distance]. Listed exit signs are required to be marked with a distance rating only if the rating is other than the 100 ft (30 m) default value.

**7.10.1.6* Floor Proximity Exit Signs.** Where floor proximity exit signs are required in Chapters 11 through 43, such signs shall comply with 7.10.3, 7.10.4, 7.10.5, and 7.10.6 for externally illuminated signs and 7.10.7 for internally illuminated signs. Such signs shall be located near the floor level in addition to those signs required for doors or corridors. The bottom of the sign shall be not less than 6 in. (150 mm), but not more than 18 in. (455 mm), above the floor. For exit doors, the sign shall be mounted on the door or adjacent to the door, with the nearest edge of the sign within 4 in. (100 mm) of the door frame.

**A.7.10.1.6** See A.7.10.3.

Because locations near the ceiling might be the first to become obstructed by smoke, the provision of 7.10.1.6 makes it possible for the occupancy chapters to specify floor proximity signs to supplement the regular exit signs that are usually placed above the exit door opening or near the ceiling in corridors. Such signs are not intended to replace standard exit signs but are designed as an extra asset to a building occupant seeking egress in a smoke-filled environment. Because the signs are positioned near the floor, they will be among the last signs to become obscured by the descending smoke layer.

The provisions of 7.10.1.6 can be used as guidance on the placement and installation of floor proximity signs, even though they might not be required.

The only occupancies currently mandating floor proximity exit signs are assembly occupancies, where they are required in special amusement buildings in accordance with the provisions of 12.4.7.7.2 and 13.4.7.7.2.

**7.10.1.7* Floor Proximity Egress Path Marking.** Where floor proximity egress path marking is required in Chapters 11 through 43, an approved floor proximity egress path marking system that is internally illuminated shall be installed within 18 in. (455 mm) of the floor. Floor proximity egress path marking systems shall be listed in accordance with ANSI/UL 1994, *Standard for Luminous Egress Path Marking Systems*. The system shall provide a visible delineation of the path of travel along the designated exit access and shall be essentially continuous, except as interrupted by doorways, hallways, corridors, or other such architectural features. The system shall operate continuously or at any time the building fire alarm system is activated. The activation, duration, and continuity of operation of the system shall be in accordance with 7.9.2. The system shall be maintained in accordance with the product manufacturing listing.

**A.7.10.1.7** See 3.3.135.2 for the definition of the term *internally illuminated.*

Paragraph 7.10.1.7 provides a standard for floor proximity egress path marking for mandatory use by the occupancy chapters or for voluntary use by any party. This type of marking has been mandatory on aircraft for several years. It is not mandatory for any occupancy under the *Code*. However, it could be used as part of the directional exit marking required for special amusement buildings by the provisions of 12.4.7.7.3 and 13.4.7.7.3. Such systems are required by 7.10.1.7 to be listed (see 3.2.5 for the definition of the term *listed*).

The provisions of 7.10.1.7 require that floor proximity egress path marking systems be internally illuminated. Photoluminescent egress path markers (like photoluminescent exit signs addressed in 7.10.7.2) are internally illuminated. The photoluminescent material stores incident electromagnetic radiation, typically from ambient light sources, and releases it in the form of visible light. The intensity and duration of the ambient light used for charging the photoluminescent material varies by product and manufacturer. Thus, 7.10.1.7 requires that the system be maintained in accordance with the product manufacturing listing.

Exhibit 7.108 depicts photoluminescent egress path marking in an exit stair enclosure during normal lighting and during a blackout.

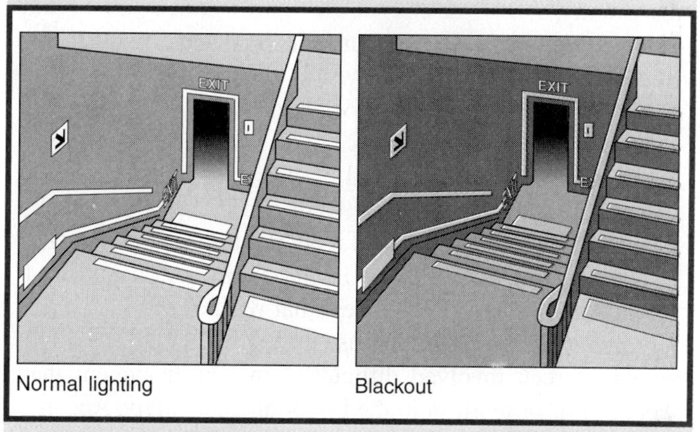


***Exhibit 7.108** Photoluminescent egress path marking in an exit stair enclosure.*

**7.10.1.8* Visibility.** Every sign required in Section 7.10 shall be located and of such size, distinctive color, and design that it is readily visible and shall provide contrast with decorations, interior finish, or other signs. No decorations, furnishings, or equipment that impairs visibility of a sign shall be permitted. No brightly illuminated sign (for other than exit purposes), display, or object in or near the line of vision of the required exit sign that could detract attention from the exit sign shall be permitted.

In some locations, an otherwise adequate exit sign or directional exit sign might be rendered inconspicuous by a high-intensity illuminated advertising sign in the immediate vicinity. For this reason, such signs are not permitted in the line of vision of any required sign addressed by Section 7.10.

The maximum mounting height for directional exit signs not associated with an egress opening is not specified, and the minimum mounting height for exit signs and directional exit signs is not specified (see 7.10.1.9). Usually they are placed above exit door openings and above head height. There are those who argue, with reason, that smoke builds up more rapidly at higher levels, and signs positioned near the floor would be visible for a much longer time during a fire. However, when several people are moving toward an exit, those in the rear might not be able to see signs located near the floor because of the obstruction created by those ahead of them. Also, in the absence of careful housekeeping, such signs might be damaged or blocked. Thus, 7.10.1.8 treats the subject as a visibility issue and requires that the signs be located to be readily visible and to provide contrast with their surroundings. See also 7.10.1.9 and its related commentary.

**A.7.10.1.8** In stores, for example, an otherwise adequate exit sign could be rendered inconspicuous by a high-intensity illuminated advertising sign located in the immediate vicinity.

Red is the traditional color for exit signs and is required by law in many places. However, at an early stage in the development of the *Code*, a provision made green the color for exit signs, following the concept of traffic lights in which green indicates safety and red is the signal to stop. During the period when green signs were specified by the *Code*, many such signs were installed, but the traditional red signs also remained. In 1949, the Fire Marshals Association of North America voted to request that red be restored as the required exit sign color, because it was found that the provision for green involved difficulties in law enactment that were out of proportion to the importance of safety. Accordingly, the 10th edition of the *Code* specified red where not otherwise required by law. The present text avoids any specific requirement for color, based on the assumption that either red or green will be used in most cases and that there are some situations in which a color other than red or green could actually provide better visibility.

As indicated in A.7.10.1.8, the issue of sign color has been the subject of considerable debate. The predecessor to this *Code*, the *Building Exits Code* (see the commentary following 1.1.1) required, from its first edition in 1927 through 1947, that exit signs use white letters on a green field, unless such color was contrary to local law. The text in A.7.10.1.8 describes the development of events since 1949. Currently, color is not specified.

**7.10.1.9 Mounting Location.** The bottom of new egress markings shall be located at a vertical distance of not more than 6 ft 8 in. (2030 mm) above the top edge of the egress opening intended for designation by that marking. Egress markings shall be located at a horizontal distance of not more than the required width of the egress opening, as measured from the edge of the egress opening intended for designation by that marking to the nearest edge of the marking.

Paragraph 7.10.1.9 addresses the mounting location of exit signs associated with an egress opening such as a door opening, an archway, or a portal. Its provisions are meant to keep the sign from being located too high above the egress opening and too far to the side of the egress opening, at which point the sign would be less effective in designating the opening as the egress route.

Exhibit 7.109 illustrates the maximum distance at which the nearest sign edge is permitted to be positioned above and to the side of the egress opening,

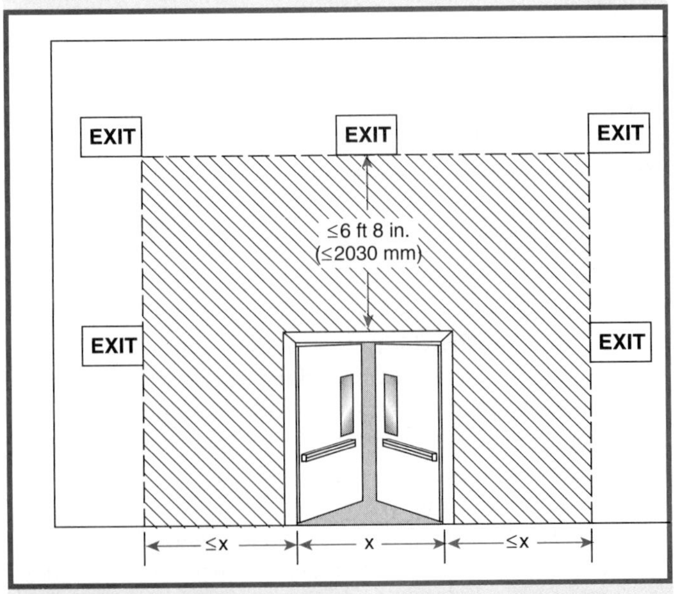


***Exhibit 7.109** Maximum permitted distance of sign edge above and to the side of egress opening.*

which, in this illustration, is a pair of door leaves. Measurement *x*, shown below the door leaves, is the required width of the egress opening.

### 7.10.2 Directional Signs.

**7.10.2.1*** A sign complying with 7.10.3 with a directional indicator showing the direction of travel shall be placed in every location where the direction of travel to reach the nearest exit is not apparent.

**A.7.10.2.1** A sign complying with 7.10.2 and indicating the direction of the nearest approved exit should be placed at the point of entrance to any escalator or moving walk. *(See A.7.10.3.)*

The provision of 7.10.2.1 mandates that a directional sign be placed where the direction of travel to reach the nearest exit is not apparent. The directional sign uses an exit sign to which one or two directional indicators are added. For externally illuminated signs, which are not required to be laboratory listed, the detailed criteria for the directional indicator appear in 7.10.6.2. Internally illuminated signs, which are required to be tested and listed in accordance with ANSI/UL 924, *Standard for Emergency Lighting and Power Equipment*, have their directional indicators evaluated by the performance criteria of the ANSI/UL 924 test procedure; they are exempt from the specification-based criteria of 7.10.6.2.

The requirement of 7.10.2.1 is somewhat performance-based in that it adds another directional exit sign wherever the direction of travel to reach the nearest exit is not apparent. The enforcement of this provision will typically be somewhat subjective, because a judgment call must be made as to whether the direction of travel to reach the nearest exit is apparent. A strict reading and application of the requirement, especially with respect to the word "nearest," could conceivably lead to the installation of many more signs than are practically needed.

Exhibit 7.110 depicts a warehouse with storage racks and aisles. The racks are of sufficient height and construction to prevent an occupant located within almost any aisle from seeing either of the exit door assemblies from the building. The designer is charged with specifying exit sign and directional sign placement that meets the provisions of Section 7.10. An occupant standing at point X within an aisle has a choice of many possible paths for travel to the two exit door assemblies; there are no dead-end aisles in which to become trapped. The criterion test for exit sign placement is 7.10.2.1, which requires that a directional sign be placed in every location where the direction of travel to reach the "nearest" exit is not apparent. Exit

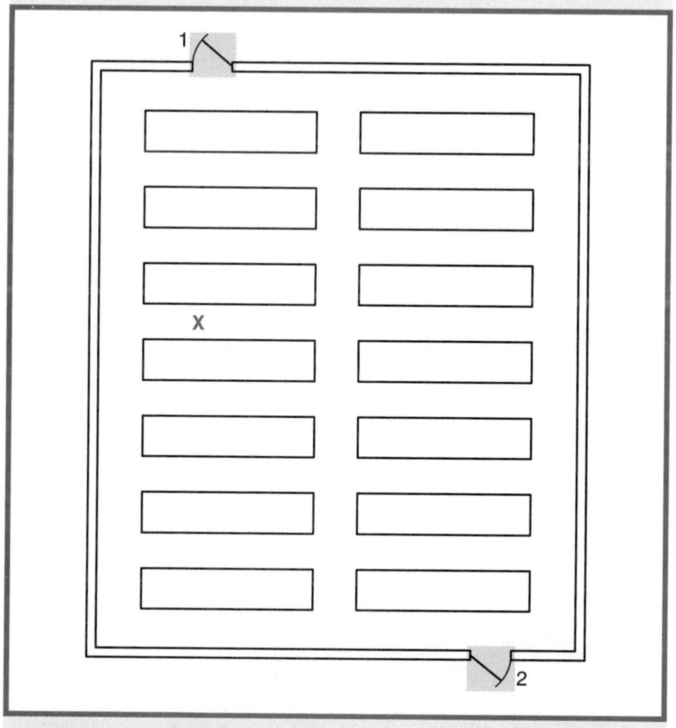


***Exhibit 7.110** Warehouse exit sign and directional sign placement to be determined.*

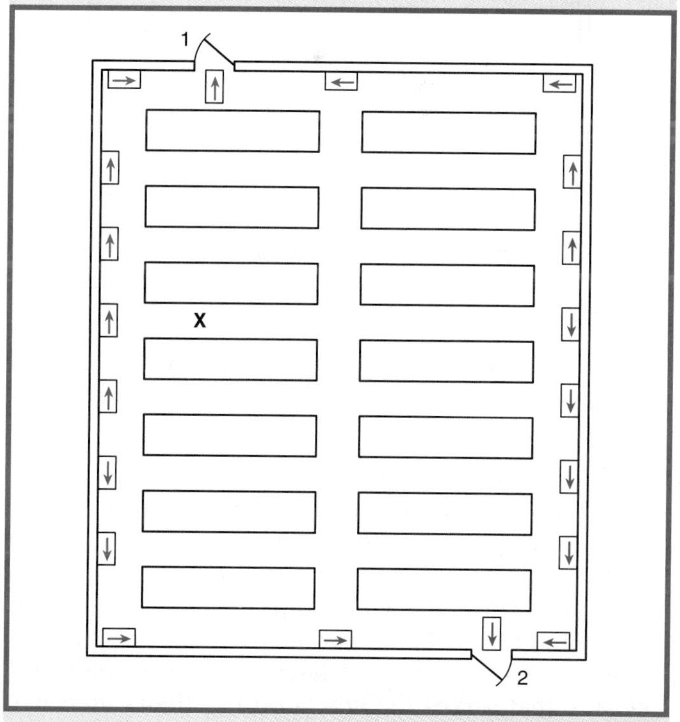


***Exhibit 7.111** Excessive placement of directional signs.*

door assembly 1 is the nearest exit, but neither exit door assembly 1 nor exit door assembly 2 can be seen from within the aisle or from within any of the three cross-aisles. A strict interpretation of 7.10.2.1, coupled with the requirement of 7.10.1.2.1 that the exit door assemblies themselves be provided with exit signs, could lead to the installation of 20 signs, as shown in Exhibit 7.111. A reasonable person would argue that it is neither unreasonable nor unsafe to reduce the number of signs so as to require the occupant to travel to either of the two nearest cross-aisles in order to see a directional sign that leads to an exit. A check for reasonableness could lead to the placement of eight signs, as shown in Exhibit 7.112.

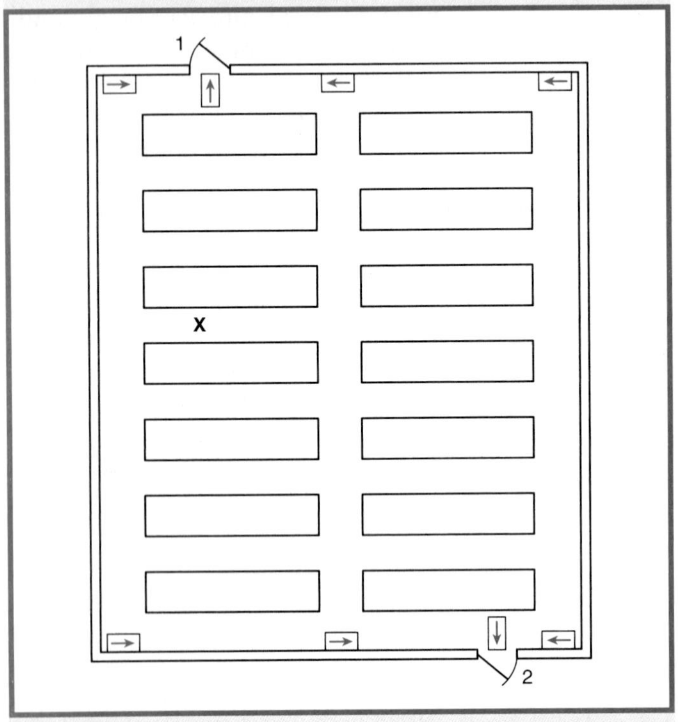


***Exhibit 7.112** Reasonable placement of directional signs.*

**7.10.2.2** Directional exit signs shall be provided within horizontal components of the egress path within exit enclosures as required by 7.10.1.2.2.

The provisions of 7.10.2.2 are new to the 2009 edition of the *Code*. Some exit stair enclosures, particularly in high-rise buildings where the upper portion of the tower presents a smaller footprint than the base of the building, include horizontal components (much like exit passageways) at floors where the stair enclosure that serves the next group of floors immediately below shifts horizontally in position. Although directional exit signs are not normally needed within an exit stair enclosure that is stacked vertically without offsets because occupants simply move downward from floor to floor, the presence of the horizontal passageway might confound the egress path. Where the continuation of the egress path is not obvious, 7.10.1.2.2 requires additional exit signs or directional exit signs.

### 7.10.3* Sign Legend.

**A.7.10.3** Where graphics are used, the symbols provided in NFPA 170, *Standard for Fire Safety and Emergency Symbols*, should be used. Such signs need to provide equal visibility and illumination and are to comply with the other requirements of Section 7.10.

**7.10.3.1** Signs required by 7.10.1 and 7.10.2 shall read as follows in plainly legible letters, or other appropriate wording shall be used:

EXIT

**7.10.3.2*** Where approved by the authority having jurisdiction, pictograms in compliance with NFPA 170, *Standard for Fire Safety and Emergency Symbols*, shall be permitted.

**A.7.10.3.2** Pictograms are permitted to be used in lieu of, or in addition to, signs with text.

Paragraph 7.10.3.1 permits other wording in lieu of the word EXIT where the alternative wording is appropriate. In countries where Spanish is the predominant language, one might find the word SALIDA. In Canada, where signage appears in both French and English, exit signs have been increased in size to accommodate the words EXIT and SORTIE.

Although 7.10.3.1 refers to wording "in plainly legible letters," it is evident from the language of 7.10.3.2 that graphics, or pictograms, in lieu of words are permitted with the approval of the AHJ. Graphics have the advantage of being nonspecific to a written language. Paragraph 7.10.3.2 specifies that the pictograms comply with NFPA 170, *Standard for Fire Safety and Emergency Symbols*. NFPA 170 provides a symbol for an emergency exit that should be considered the equivalent of the *Life Safety Code*'s exit sign. NFPA 170 also provides two symbols that — when used together — designate an emergency exit route. This diptych uses the emergency exit symbol and an arrow symbol and should be considered the equivalent of the *Code*'s directional exit sign. See Exhibit 7.113 and Exhibit 7.114.

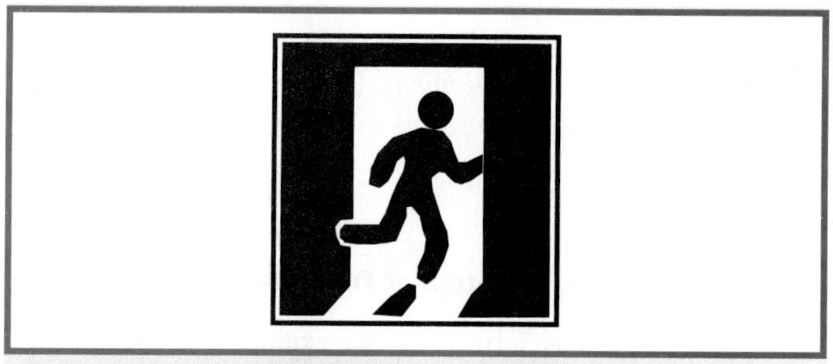

*Exhibit 7.113 NFPA 170 symbol for emergency exit.*

*Exhibit 7.114 NFPA 170 symbols for emergency exit route.*

### 7.10.4* Power Source.

Where emergency lighting facilities are required by the applicable provisions of Chapters 11 through 43 for individual occupancies, the signs, other than approved self-luminous signs and listed photoluminescent signs in accordance with 7.10.7.2, shall be illuminated by the emergency lighting facilities. The level of illumination of the signs shall be in accordance with 7.10.6.3 or 7.10.7 for the required emergency lighting duration as specified in 7.9.2.1. However, the level of illumination shall be permitted to decline to 60 percent at the end of the emergency lighting duration.

**A.7.10.4** It is not the intent of this paragraph to require emergency lighting but only to have the sign illuminated by emergency lighting if emergency lighting is required and provided.

It is not the intent to require that the entire stroke width and entire stroke height of all letters comprising the word EXIT be visible per the requirements of 7.10.6.3 under normal or emergency lighting operation, provided that the sign is visible and legible at a 100 ft (30 m) distance under all room illumination conditions.

The text of A.7.10.4 explains that it is not the intent of 7.10.4 to require an emergency power source for the illumination of exit signs. Rather, it is the intent that the required exit signs are provided with emergency power if the occupancy is required to have emergency lighting. For example, there are business occupancies that are small enough to be exempt from the emergency lighting requirement of 38.2.9.1 and 39.2.9.1. Yet, business occupancies are required to have exit signs in accordance with Section 7.10. Such exit signs are required to be illuminated per 7.10.5.1. In a small business occupancy that is exempt from emergency lighting, if a power failure occurs, the exit signs are permitted to go dark. The business occupancy example can be contrasted with an assembly occupancy. Assembly occupancies are required to have emergency lighting and exit signs. The exit signs must be illuminated in accordance with 7.10.5.1 when the building's normal power is available; the illumination must also be maintained in accordance with 7.10.4 upon failure of the normal power service.

### 7.10.5 Illumination of Signs.

**7.10.5.1* General.** Every sign required by 7.10.1.2, 7.10.1.5, or 7.10.8.1, other than where operations or processes require low lighting levels, shall be suitably illuminated by a reliable light source. Externally and internally illuminated signs shall be legible in both the normal and emergency lighting mode.

**A.7.10.5.1** See A.7.8.1.3(4).

Internally illuminated signs are particularly useful in occupancies where reduction of normal illumination is permitted, such as in movie theaters. However, the intent of 7.10.5.1 is to treat externally illuminated and internally illuminated signs equally, with no preference shown to one or the other. Subsequent subsections then treat each type of sign via a specialized package of requirements, such as 7.10.6 for externally illuminated signs and 7.10.7 for internally illuminated signs. This format is provided because externally illuminated signs are not required to be tested and listed by a laboratory. Due to the lack of testing, it is necessary for the *Code* to specify detailed criteria, such as the letter height and stroke width addressed in 7.10.6.1.1 and illumination levels as addressed in 7.10.6.3. Because internally illuminated signs must be laboratory tested and listed, the *Code* can rely on the listing to ensure that necessary criteria are met.

**7.10.5.2* Continuous Illumination.**

**A.7.10.5.2** It is the intent to prohibit the use of a freely accessible light switch to control the illumination of either an internally or externally illuminated exit sign.

**7.10.5.2.1** Every sign required to be illuminated by 7.10.6.3, 7.10.7, and 7.10.8.1 shall be continuously illuminated as required under the provisions of Section 7.8, unless otherwise provided in 7.10.5.2.2.

**7.10.5.2.2*** Illumination for signs shall be permitted to flash on and off upon activation of the fire alarm system.

**A.7.10.5.2.2** The flashing repetition rate should be approximately one cycle per second, and the duration of the off-time should not exceed $\frac{1}{4}$ second per cycle. During on-time, the illumination levels need to be provided in accordance with 7.10.6.3. Flashing signs, when activated with the fire alarm system, might be of assistance.

### 7.10.6 Externally Illuminated Signs.

**7.10.6.1* Size of Signs.**

**A.7.10.6.1** Experience has shown that the word EXIT, or other appropriate wording, is plainly legible at 100 ft (30 m) if the letters are as large as specified in 7.10.6.1.

**7.10.6.1.1** Externally illuminated signs required by 7.10.1 and 7.10.2, other than approved existing signs, unless otherwise provided in 7.10.6.1.2, shall read EXIT or shall use other appropriate wording in plainly legible letters sized as follows:

(1) For new signs, the letters shall be not less than 6 in. (150 mm) high, with the principal strokes of letters not less than $\frac{3}{4}$ in. (19 mm) wide.
(2) For existing signs, the required wording shall be permitted to be in plainly legible letters not less than 4 in. (100 mm) high.
(3) The word EXIT shall be in letters of a width not less than 2 in. (51 mm), except the letter I, and the minimum spacing between letters shall be not less than $\frac{3}{8}$ in. (9.5 mm).
(4) Sign legend elements larger than the minimum established in 7.10.6.1.1(1) through (3) shall use letter widths, strokes, and spacing in proportion to their height.

**7.10.6.1.2** The requirements of 7.10.6.1.1 shall not apply to marking required by 7.10.1.3 and 7.10.1.7.

Traditionally, the letters in an exit sign have been required to be 6 in. (150 mm) in height, with the principal strokes not less than $\frac{3}{4}$ in. (19 mm) wide. In an effort to increase visibility, the *Code* requires that the letters, other than *I*, be at least 2 in. (51 mm) wide and have a minimum spacing between letters of $\frac{3}{8}$ in. (9.5 mm). These dimensional criteria have been maintained, but they apply only to externally illuminated signs. Internally illuminated signs are exempt from these criteria, because they must be tested and listed in accordance with ANSI/UL 924, *Standard for Emergency Lighting and Power Equipment*. The ANSI/UL 924 test procedures include assessing the readability of a sign's letters.

**7.10.6.2* Size and Location of Directional Indicator.**

**A.7.10.6.2** Figure A.7.10.6.2 shows examples of acceptable locations of directional indicators with regard to left and right orientation. Directional indicators are permitted to be placed under the horizontal stroke of the letter T, provided that spacing of not less than $\frac{3}{8}$ in. (10 mm) is maintained from the horizontal and vertical strokes of the letter T.

EXIT>
<EXIT
<EXIT>

*Figure A.7.10.6.2 Directional Indicators.*

**7.10.6.2.1** Directional indicators, unless otherwise provided in 7.10.6.2.2, shall comply with the following:

(1) The directional indicator shall be located outside of the EXIT legend, not less than $\frac{3}{8}$ in. (9.5 mm) from any letter.
(2) The directional indicator shall be of a chevron type, as shown in Figure 7.10.6.2.1.

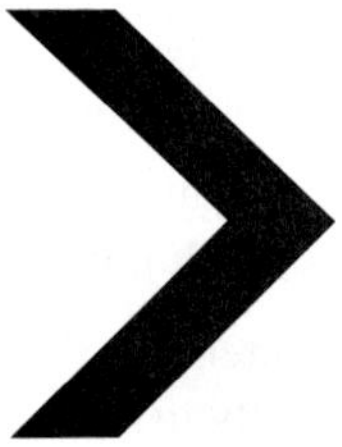

*Figure 7.10.6.2.1 Chevron-Type Indicator.*

(3) The directional indicator shall be identifiable as a directional indicator at a distance of 40 ft (12 m).
(4) A directional indicator larger than the minimum established for compliance with 7.10.6.2.1(3) shall be proportionately increased in height, width, and stroke.
(5) The directional indicator shall be located at the end of the sign for the direction indicated.

**7.10.6.2.2** The requirements of 7.10.6.2.1 shall not apply to approved existing signs.

To improve the effectiveness of directional indicators on directional exit signs, the requirements have been changed over the past several years. The directional indicator cannot be positioned between the letters in the word EXIT. The directional indicator, which formerly was an arrow, must be a chevron. Research showed that a chevron indicator was more effective than an arrow. Performance criteria are specified to ensure that the chevron is of adequate size, contrast, and illumination. A specific size is not required, because size depends on factors such as color, contrast, and illumination. However, the directional indicator must be identifiable as a directional indicator at a minimum distance of 40 ft (12 m), which is another performance-based requirement.

**7.10.6.3* Level of Illumination.** Externally illuminated signs shall be illuminated by not less than 5 ft-candles (54 lux) at the illuminated surface and shall have a contrast ratio of not less than 0.5.

**A.7.10.6.3** Colors providing a good contrast are red or green letters on matte white background. Glossy background and glossy letter colors should be avoided.

The average luminance of the letters and background is measured in footlamberts or candela per square meter. The contrast ratio is computed from these measurements by the following formula:

$$\text{Contrast} = \frac{L_g - L_e}{L_g}$$

Where $L_g$ is the greater luminance and $L_e$ is the lesser luminance, either the variable $L_g$ or $L_e$ is permitted to represent the letters, and the remaining variable will represent the background. The average luminance of the letters and background can be computed by measuring the luminance at the positions indicated in Figure A.7.10.6.3 by numbered circles.

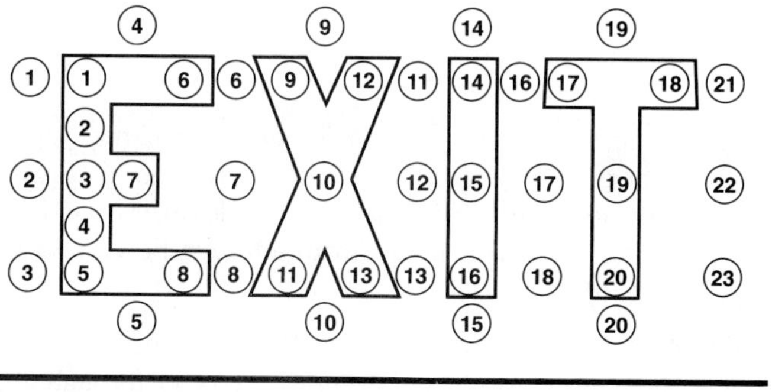

*Figure A.7.10.6.3 Measurement of Exit Sign Luminance.*

## 7.10.7 Internally Illuminated Signs.

**7.10.7.1 Listing.** Internally illuminated signs shall be listed in accordance with ANSI/UL 924, *Standard for Emergency Lighting and Power Equipment*, unless they meet one of the following criteria:

(1) They are approved existing signs.
(2) They are existing signs having the required wording in legible letters not less than 4 in. (100 mm) high.
(3) They are signs that are in accordance with 7.10.1.3 and 7.10.1.6.

Internally illuminated signs must be laboratory tested and listed in accordance with ANSI/UL 924, *Standard for Emergency Lighting and Power Equipment*. Reliance is placed on the laboratory having conducted a comprehensive examination. By relying on the laboratory listing, the *Code* does not need to address the detailed criteria that it requires of externally illuminated signs, which are not required to be listed.

**7.10.7.2* Photoluminescent Signs.** The face of a photoluminescent sign shall be continually illuminated while the building is occupied. The illumination levels on the face of the photoluminescent sign shall be in accordance with its listing. The charging illumination shall be a reliable light source, as determined by the authority having jurisdiction. The charging light source, shall be of a type specified in the product markings.

**A.7.10.7.2** Photoluminescent signs need a specific minimum level of light on the face of the sign to ensure that the sign is charged for emergency operation and legibility in both the normal and emergency modes. Additionally, the type of light source (for example, incandescent, fluorescent, halogen, metal halide) is important. Each light source produces different types of visible and invisible light (for example, UV) that might affect the ability of some photoluminescent signs to charge and might also affect the amount of light output available during emergency mode. This type of sign would not be suitable where the illumination levels are permitted to decline. The charging light source should not be connected to automatic timers, because continuous illumination of the sign is needed; otherwise, the sign illumination would not be available, because it would be discharged.

A photoluminescent sign absorbs light from an activation light source in order to emit light (i.e., luminesce). The sign continues to emit light for a time after the activation light source has been removed. The requirements of 7.10.7.2 for photoluminescent signs were new to the 2000 edition of the *Code*. Note that these requirements are contained as a subset of the internally illuminated sign requirements of 7.10.7. A photoluminescent sign is an internally illuminated sign. Photoluminescent exit signs are permitted, provided that they are listed in accordance with ANSI/UL 924, *Standard for Emergency Lighting and Power Equipment*, and meet the criteria of 7.10.7.2. The criteria of 7.10.7.2 are meant to highlight some of the special considerations needed to use photoluminescent exit signs effectively for life safety.

**7.10.8 Special Signs.**

**7.10.8.1 Sign Illumination.**

**7.10.8.1.1** Where required by other provisions of this *Code*, special signs shall be illuminated in accordance with 7.10.5, 7.10.6.3, and 7.10.7.

**7.10.8.1.2** Where emergency lighting facilities are required by the applicable provisions of Chapters 11 through 43, the required illumination of special signs shall additionally be provided under emergency lighting conditions.

**7.10.8.2 Characters.** Special signs, where required by other provisions of this *Code*, shall comply with the visual character requirements of ICC/ANSI A117.1, *American National Standard for Accessible and Usable Buildings and Facilities*.

**7.10.8.3* No Exit.**

**A.7.10.8.3** The likelihood of occupants mistaking passageways or stairways that lead to dead-end spaces for exit doors and becoming trapped governs the need for exit signs. Thus, such areas should be marked with a sign that reads as follows:

NO EXIT

Supplementary identification indicating the character of the area, such as TO BASEMENT, STOREROOM, LINEN CLOSET, or the like, is permitted to be provided.

**7.10.8.3.1** Any door, passage, or stairway that is neither an exit nor a way of exit access and that is located or arranged so that it is likely to be mistaken for an exit shall be identified by a sign that reads as follows:

# NO

EXIT

**7.10.8.3.2** The NO EXIT sign shall have the word NO in letters 2 in. (51 mm) high, with a stroke width of $^3/_8$ in. (9.5 mm), and the word EXIT in letters 1 in. (25 mm) high, with the word EXIT below the word NO, unless such sign is an approved existing sign.

**7.10.8.4 Elevator Signs.** Elevators that are a part of a means of egress *(see 7.2.13.1)* shall have the following signs with a minimum letter height of $^5/_8$ in. (16 mm) posted in every elevator lobby:

(1)* Signs that indicate that the elevator can be used for egress, including any restrictions on use

**A.7.10.8.4(1)** These signs are to be used in place of signs that indicate that elevators are not to be used during fires. Examples of these signs include the following:

In the Event of Fire, This Elevator Will Be Used
by the Fire Department for Evacuation of People.

PROTECTED ELEVATOR —
USABLE IN EMERGENCIES

(2)* Signs that indicate the operational status of elevators

**A.7.10.8.4(2)** The wording of these signs should reflect human behavior in fires and the control specifics of the elevator system. Subparagraph 7.10.8.4 addresses signs, but provisions for notification of the vision impaired need to be considered. For information about human behavior with respect to elevator evacuation, see Groner and Levin, "Human Factor Considerations in the Potential for Using Elevators in Building Emergency Evacuation Plans"; Levin and Groner, "Human Behavior Aspects of Staging Areas for Fire Safety in GSA Buildings"; and Levin and Groner, "Human Factor Considerations for the Potential Use of Elevators for Fire Evacuation of FAA Air Traffic Control Towers." Some examples of messages on signs that could be displayed are shown in Table A.7.10.8.4(2).

***Table A.7.10.8.4(2) Elevator Status Messages***

| Elevator Status | Message |
|---|---|
| Normal use | Elevator in Service |
| Elevators recalled and waiting for fire service | Please Wait for Fire Department or Use Stairs |
| Elevator out of service | Elevator Out of Service |

The requirements in 7.10.8.4 for elevator signs apply only where the elevator is part of the means of egress. The only current application is for elevators used as the second means of egress from a tower. See 7.2.13.1.

**7.10.8.5* Evacuation Diagram.** Where a posted floor evacuation diagram is required in Chapters 11 through 43, floor evacuation diagrams reflecting the actual floor arrangement and exit locations shall be posted and oriented in a location and manner acceptable to the authority having jurisdiction.

**A.7.10.8.5** Egress paths with multiple turns can often be confusing with respect to which exit route will lead to the closest exit door. Floor evacuation diagrams can eliminate the guesswork by giving the occupant a point of reference by the YOU ARE HERE symbol. The entire floor plan should be shown with the primary and secondary exit routes, exit stairs, and elevators clearly identified. For further information, see ASTM E 2238, *Standard Guide for Evacuation Route Diagrams*.

The provision of 7.10.8.5 is new to the 2009 edition of the *Code* and is formatted such that it applies only where a posted floor evacuation diagram is required by another provision of the *Code*. A floor diagram, reflecting the actual floor arrangement and exit locations, is required for hotels and dormitories by 28.7.4.1 and 29.7.4.1. It is important that the floor evacuation diagram be oriented so that, if an exit is shown at the right of the diagram, the exit is actually located to the right of the person facing the sign. In a hotel with guest rooms located at both sides of the corridor, the floor diagram for the rooms at one side of the corridor will need to be the mirror image of the floor diagram for the rooms at the other side of the corridor.

### 7.10.9 Testing and Maintenance.

**7.10.9.1 Inspection.** Exit signs shall be visually inspected for operation of the illumination sources at intervals not to exceed 30 days or shall be periodically monitored in accordance with 7.9.3.1.3.

**7.10.9.2 Testing.** Exit signs connected to, or provided with, a battery-operated emergency illumination source, where required in 7.10.4, shall be tested and maintained in accordance with 7.9.3.

## 7.11 Special Provisions for Occupancies with High Hazard Contents

See Section 6.2.

The wording associated with the classification of high hazard contents in 6.2.2.4 states that "high hazard contents shall be classified as those that are likely to burn with extreme rapidity or from which explosions are likely."

**7.11.1*** Where the contents are classified as high hazard, exits shall be provided and arranged to allow all occupants to escape from the building or structure, or from the hazardous area thereof, to the outside or to a place of safety with a travel distance of not more than 75 ft (23 m), measured as required in 7.6.1, unless otherwise provided in 7.11.2.

**A.7.11.1** Seventy-five feet (23 m) can be traversed in approximately 10 seconds to 15 seconds, even when allowing for a momentary delay to decide which way to go, during which it can be assumed that the average individual can hold his or her breath.

Subsection 7.11.1 does not limit occupants to a 75 ft (23 m) travel distance but requires escape from the hazardous area itself with not more than 75 ft (23 m) of travel. The place of safety outside the hazardous area is permitted to be within the building's exit access; additional travel might be necessary to reach an exit.

**7.11.2** The requirement of 7.11.1 shall not apply to storage occupancies as otherwise provided in Chapter 42.

**7.11.3** Egress capacity for high hazard contents areas shall be based on 0.7 in./person (18 mm/person) for stairs or 0.4 in./person (10 mm/person) for level components and ramps in accordance with 7.3.3.1.

**7.11.4** Not less than two means of egress shall be provided from each building or hazardous area thereof, unless all of the following criteria are met:

(1) Rooms or spaces do not exceed 200 ft$^2$ (18.6 m$^2$).
(2) Rooms or spaces have an occupant load not exceeding three persons.
(3) Rooms or spaces have a travel distance to the room door not exceeding 25 ft (7620 mm).

Subsection 7.11.4 recognizes that it is not always necessary or feasible to provide two ways out of very small high hazard contents spaces. Provided that all three conditional features — limited room area, occupant load, and travel distance to room door opening — can be met, a single means of egress is permitted.

**7.11.5** Means of egress, for rooms or spaces other than those that meet the criteria of 7.11.4(1) through (3), shall be arranged so that there are no dead ends in corridors.

**7.11.6** Doors serving high hazard contents areas with occupant loads in excess of five shall be permitted to be provided with a latch or lock only if the latch or lock is panic hardware or fire exit hardware complying with 7.2.1.7.

It is not the intent of the *Code* to apply the provisions of Section 7.11 to the hazardous contents areas addressed by subsection __.3.2 of each occupancy chapter. Those hazardous contents areas are generally rooms or spaces with contents that make them somewhat more hazardous than the rooms or spaces normally associated with a given occupancy. For example, soiled linen storage rooms in a health care occupancy create contents that are more hazardous than those within a patient room, but they don't create a hazard that warrants protection as high hazard contents by Section 7.11. The decision as to when an area is sufficiently hazardous to warrant protection as high hazard contents by the requirements of Section 7.11 is left to the authority having jurisdiction via use of the classification criteria in 6.2.2.4.

## 7.12 Mechanical Equipment Rooms, Boiler Rooms, and Furnace Rooms

Section 7.12 applies to mechanical equipment rooms, boiler rooms, and furnace rooms in all buildings, regardless of occupancy. The number of exits and common path of travel limitations in these spaces are addressed independently of the occupancy in which they are located. The presence of these rooms does not result in a facility being designated a multiple occupancy.

**7.12.1** Mechanical equipment rooms, boiler rooms, furnace rooms, and similar spaces shall be arranged to limit common path of travel to a distance not exceeding 50 ft (15 m), unless otherwise permitted by the following:

(1) A common path of travel not exceeding 100 ft (30 m) shall be permitted in the following locations:
   (a) In buildings protected throughout by an approved, supervised automatic sprinkler system in accordance with Section 9.7
   (b) In mechanical equipment rooms with no fuel-fired equipment
   (c) In existing buildings

(2) In an existing building, a common path of travel not exceeding 150 ft (46 m) shall be permitted, provided that all of the following criteria are met:
   (a) The building is protected throughout by an approved, supervised automatic sprinkler system installed in accordance with Section 9.7.
   (b) No fuel-fired equipment is within the space.
   (c) The egress path is readily identifiable.

(3) The requirement of 7.12.1 shall not apply to rooms or spaces in existing health care occupancies complying with the arrangement of means of egress provisions of 19.2.5 and the travel distance limits of 19.2.6.

**7.12.2** Stories used exclusively for mechanical equipment, furnaces, or boilers shall be permitted to have a single means of egress where the travel distance to an exit on that story is not in excess of the common path of travel limitations of 7.12.1.

Paragraph 7.12.2 is especially useful in equipment penthouses and for basement furnace and boiler rooms. As long as the common path of travel specified by 7.12.1 is not exceeded, a story used exclusively for mechanical equipment, boilers, or furnaces is permitted to be served by a single exit.

### References Cited in Commentary


1. ICC/ANSI A117.1, 2003 edition, *American National Standard for Accessible and Usable Buildings and Facilities*, American National Standards Institute Inc., 25 West 43rd Street, 4th floor, New York, NY 10036.
2. *Americans with Disabilities Act Accessibility Guidelines for Buildings and Facilities* (ADAAG), U.S. Architectural and Transportation Barriers Compliance Board, Washington, DC, 1992.
3. *ADA and ABA Accessibility Guidelines for Buildings and Facilities* (ADA-ABA-AG), U.S. Architectural and Transportation Barriers Compliance Board, Washington, DC, 2004.
4. NFPA 252, *Standard Methods of Fire Tests of Door Assemblies*, 2008 edition, National Fire Protection Association, Quincy, MA.
5. NFPA 105, *Standard for the Installation of Smoke Door Assemblies and Other Opening Protectives*, 2007 edition, National Fire Protection Association, Quincy, MA.
6. NFPA 92A, *Standard for Smoke-Control Systems Utilizing Barriers and Pressure Differences*, 2009 edition, National Fire Protection Association, Quincy, MA.
7. Norton, A., "When Security Provisions Threaten Fire Safety," *Fire Journal®* 82, no. 6 (November/December 1988): 40, 42, 45, 76–77.
8. *NFPA 72®, National Fire Alarm Code®*, 2007 edition, National Fire Protection Association, Quincy, MA.
9. ASME A17.1/CSA B44, *Safety Code for Elevators and Escalators*, 2007 edition, American Society of Mechanical Engineers, Three Park Avenue, New York, NY 10016-5590.
10. NFPA 80, *Standard for Fire Doors and Other Opening Protectives*, 2007 edition, National Fire Protection Association, Quincy, MA.
11. *Inspector's Guide: Swinging Fire Doors with Builders Hardware — Annual Safety Inspections*, 2007 edition,

Door and Hardware Institute, 14150 Newbrook Drive, Chantilly, VA 20151-2232.

12. *AHJ's Guide: Swinging Fire Doors with Builders Hardware — Annual Safety Inspections*, 2007 edition, Door and Hardware Institute, 14150 Newbrook Drive, Chantilly, VA 20151-2232.
13. *Owner's Guide: Swinging Fire Doors with Builders Hardware — Annual Safety Inspections*, 2007 edition, Door and Hardware Institute, 14150 Newbrook Drive, Chantilly, VA 20151-2232.
14. NFPA 220, *Standard on Types of Building Construction*, 2009 edition, National Fire Protection Association, Quincy, MA.
15. Pauls, J., "Review of Stair-Safety Research with an Emphasis on Canadian Studies," *Ergonomics* 28, no. 7 (1985): 999–1010.
16. Proulx, G., et al., *Evaluation of the Effectiveness of Different Photoluminescent Stairwell Installations for the Evacuation of Office Building Occupants*, IRC-RR-232, National Research Council Canada, Ottawa, Ontario, 2007.
17. Bénichou, N. and Proulx, G., *Evaluation and Comparison of Different Installations of Photoluminescent Marking in Stairwells of a Highrise Building*, NRCC-49230, National Research Council Canada, Ottawa, Ontario, 2008.
18. ANSI/UL 924, *Standard for Emergency Lighting and Power Equipment*, 2006 edition, Underwriters Laboratories Inc., 333 Pfingsten Road, Northbrook, IL 60062-2096.
19. NFPA 110, *Standard for Emergency and Standby Power Systems*, 2005 edition, National Fire Protection Association, Quincy, MA.
20. Fitch, Templar, Corcoran, "The Dimensions of Stairs," *Scientific American* (October 1974).
21. *Design and Construction of Building Exits*, Miscellaneous Publication M 51, October 10, 1935, National Bureau of Standards, Washington, DC (out of print).
22. ASME A17.3, *Safety Code for Existing Elevators and Escalators*, 2005 edition, American Society of Mechanical Engineers, Three Park Avenue, New York, NY 10016-5590.
23. Lyons, P. R., *Fire in America*, NFPA SPP-33, National Fire Protection Association, Quincy, MA, 1976, p. 190.
24. NFPA 170, *Standard for Fire Safety and Emergency Symbols*, 2006 edition, National Fire Protection Association, Quincy, MA.
25. *Design and Construction of Building Exits*, Miscellaneous Publication M 51, October 10, 1935, National Bureau of Standards, Washington, DC (out of print).
26. Research Report No. 95, August 1958, "Second Report of the Operational Research Team on the Capacity of Footways," London: London Transit Board Research.
27. Pauls, J., "Development of Knowledge about Means of Egress," *Fire Technology* 20, no. 2 (May 1984): 28–40.
28. *NFPA 70®, National Electrical Code®*, 2008 edition, National Fire Protection Association, Quincy, MA.
29. Watrous, L. D., "High-Rise Fire in New Orleans," *Fire Journal®* 67, no. 3 (May 1973): 6–9.
30. Mendes, R. F., *Fighting High-Rise Building Fires — Tactics and Logistics*, NFPA FSP-44, National Fire Protection Association, Quincy, MA, 1975.
31. Demers, D. P., "Ten Students Die in Providence College Dormitory Fire," *Fire Journal®* 72, no. 4 (July 1978): 59–63, 103.
32. NFPA LS-4, 1982, "Investigation Report on the MGM Grand Hotel Fire, Las Vegas, NV, Nov. 21, 1980."
33. Moulton, R. S., "Emergency Lighting for Fire Safety," *NFPA Quarterly* 50, no. 2 (October 1956): 93–96.
34. See note 33.
35. See note 33.
36. Willey, A. E., "Unsafe Existing Conditions! Apartment House Fire, Boston, Massachusetts," *Fire Journal®* 65, no. 4 (July 1971): 16–23.
37. Lathrop, J. K., "The Summerland Fire: 50 Die on Isle of Man," *Fire Journal®* 69, no. 2 (March 1975): 5–12.
38. Bell, J., "Fifteen Residents Die in Mental Hospital Fire," *Fire Journal®* 73, no. 4 (July 1979): 68–76.
39. See note 38.
40. NFPA Investigation Report, "Westchase Hilton Hotel Fire, Houston, Texas, March 6, 1982, 12 Fatalities."

CHAPTER 8

# Features of Fire Protection

Chapter 8 establishes minimum requirements for features of fire protection, which include the following:

1. Construction
2. Compartmentation through use of fire barriers
3. Protection of vertical openings
4. Protection of concealed spaces
5. Subdivision of building spaces through use of smoke barriers and smoke partitions
6. Protection from hazards

This chapter specifies a menu of protection options that are mandated to varying degrees by specific occupancy chapters. Some of the provisions apply as requirements to all occupancies.

While the title suggests that the chapter encompasses any and all subject matter dealing with fire protection and fire safety, Chapter 8 focuses on a number of passive building features that contribute to minimizing the impact of a fire on the building occupants. The bulk of this protection scheme is associated with a series of methods and techniques that are used to control the construction and compartmentation features of a building.

Managing the spread of a fire from the room of origin, or between floors in a building, is an important consideration. Managing the spread of fire through the construction of barriers designed to limit the transfer of heat, smoke, and, in some cases, both, is achieved by compartmentation. Chapter 8 contains the minimum requirements for the construction of fire barriers, smoke barriers, and smoke partitions. These barriers are frequently used to enclose means of egress components, such as exit stairs, corridors, and exit passageways. For exit enclosures, the requirements of Chapter 8 are applied in conjunction with those of Chapter 7, which imposes additional restrictions, since exits are considered "safe havens" within a building. The *Code* mandates that openings through or into separated areas be protected with appropriately rated doors, windows, or other devices that will prevent or minimize the spread of heat and other products of combustion into or through these areas.

Recognizing that there are acceptable, safe methods for permitting building spaces to be open to each other, Chapter 8 addresses openings between floors, such as atria and mezzanines that communicate among multiple floor levels of a building.

A building's structural integrity during a fire is directly related to the fire resistance of its structural components. The *Code* regulates building construction in those occupancies where it is expected that evacuation will take an extended period of time (such as in assembly occupancies), or where occupants will be defended in place (such as in health care occupancies), by specifying minimum types of construction for those occupancies in accordance with Section 8.2.

## 8.1 General

### 8.1.1 Application.

The features of fire protection set forth in this chapter shall apply to both new construction and existing buildings.

Lack of compartmentation and rapid fire development have been significant factors in numerous multiple-fatality fires, especially in residential occupancies. Smoke spread throughout a floor not subdivided by smoke barriers has been identified as a factor contributing to loss of life in fires reported in health care occupancies. Unprotected vertical openings have repeatedly provided the route for fire spread in various occupancies. The ongoing role played by these factors in fires demonstrates the need to apply Chapter 8 requirements to both new construction and existing buildings.

### 8.1.2 Automatic Sprinkler Systems.

Where another provision of this chapter requires an automatic sprinkler system, the automatic sprinkler system shall be installed in accordance with the subparts of 9.7.1.1, as permitted by the applicable occupancy chapter.

## 8.2 Construction and Compartmentation

The general requirements in Section 8.2 aid in limiting the spread of smoke and fire and protect exit access corridors, exits, and other areas of the building from fire in adjoining areas and on other floors. Construction and compartmentation requirements vary by occupancy and are specified in Chapters 12 through 42 of the *Code*.

To preserve the integrity of a fire or smoke compartment, all openings and penetrations for doors, ducts, and building services (e.g., electric power, telephone, water supply, and waste lines) must also be effectively closed or fitted with automatic closures. Equally important, and sometimes overlooked, are concealed spaces, particularly those above suspended ceilings, that frequently have been the means of spreading fire into otherwise protected areas.[1] In some instances, these interstitial spaces might be 8 ft (2440 mm) or more in height; in others, they might serve as supply- or return-air plenums for heating, ventilating, and air-conditioning systems. Proper protection of concealed spaces can include firestopping, draftstopping, installation of automatic sprinklers, area limitations, and other limitations on the combustibility of contents, interior finishes, and construction materials. For specific concealed space protection details, see 8.6.10.

In Section 8.2, and throughout the *Code*, a distinction is made between smoke partitions, smoke barriers, and fire barriers. The function of a smoke partition and a smoke barrier is to restrict or minimize the passage of smoke, including fire gases. Fire barriers need to be reasonably airtight under increased air pressure on the fire side due to heated air expansion and must prevent the passage of heat and flame for a designated time. Fire barriers also must be capable of withstanding direct impingement by the fire, as determined by large-scale tests conducted in accordance with one of the following:

1. NFPA 251, *Standard Methods of Tests of Fire Resistance of Building Construction and Materials*[2]
2. ASTM E 119, *Standard Test Methods for Fire Tests of Building Construction and Materials*[3]
3. ANSI/UL 263, *Standard for Fire Tests of Building Construction and Materials*[4]

In addition, doors in fire barriers must be capable of withstanding the effects of fire, as determined by large-scale tests in accordance with one of the following:

1. NFPA 252, *Standard Methods of Fire Tests of Door Assemblies*[5]
2. ASTM E 2074, *Standard Test Method for Fire Tests of Door Assemblies, Including Positive Pressure Testing of Side-Hinged and Pivoted Swinging Door Assemblies*[6]
3. ANSI/UL 10B, *Standard for Fire Tests of Door Assemblies*[7]
4. ANSI/UL 10C, *Standard for Positive Pressure Fire Tests of Door Assemblies*[8]

Prior to the 2006 edition of the *Code*, only NFPA 251 and NFPA 252 were referenced. In subsequent editions, comparable ASTM and ANSI/UL standards are also referenced, as they are deemed to be equivalent to the NFPA standards.

### 8.2.1 Construction.

**8.2.1.1** Buildings or structures occupied or used in accordance with the individual occupancy chapters, Chapters 11 through 43 shall meet the minimum construction requirements of those chapters.

**8.2.1.2*** NFPA 220, *Standard on Types of Building Construction*, shall be used to determine the requirements for the construction classification.

**A.8.2.1.2** Table A.8.2.1.2 is from *NFPA 5000, Building Construction and Safety Code*, and is reproduced in this annex for the convenience of users of this *Code*.

The *Code* is not a building code. However, in certain occupancies, minimum construction requirements are established to help maintain structural integrity for the time needed for evacuation. In the case of health care occupancies, significant time is needed to ensure the

*Table A.8.2.1.2 Fire Resistance Ratings for Type I Through Type V Construction (hours)*

| | Type I | | Type II | | | Type III | | Type IV | Type V | |
|---|---|---|---|---|---|---|---|---|---|---|
| | 442 | 332 | 222 | 111 | 000 | 211 | 200 | 2HH | 111 | 000 |
| **Exterior Bearing Walls**[a] | | | | | | | | | | |
| Supporting more than one floor, columns, or other bearing walls | 4 | 3 | 2 | 1 | 0[b] | 2 | 2 | 2 | 1 | 0[b] |
| Supporting one floor only | 4 | 3 | 2 | 1 | 0[b] | 2 | 2 | 2 | 1 | 0[b] |
| Supporting a roof only | 4 | 3 | 1 | 1 | 0[b] | 2 | 2 | 2 | 1 | 0[b] |
| **Interior Bearing Walls** | | | | | | | | | | |
| Supporting more than one floor, columns, or other bearing walls | 4 | 3 | 2 | 1 | 0 | 1 | 0 | 2 | 1 | 0 |
| Supporting one floor only | 3 | 2 | 2 | 1 | 0 | 1 | 0 | 1 | 1 | 0 |
| Supporting roofs only | 3 | 2 | 1 | 1 | 0 | 1 | 0 | 1 | 1 | 0 |
| **Columns** | | | | | | | | | | |
| Supporting more than one floor, columns, or other bearing walls | 4 | 3 | 2 | 1 | 0 | 1 | 0 | H | 1 | 0 |
| Supporting one floor only | 3 | 2 | 2 | 1 | 0 | 1 | 0 | H | 1 | 0 |
| Supporting roofs only | 3 | 2 | 1 | 1 | 0 | 1 | 0 | H | 1 | 0 |
| **Beams, Girders, Trusses, and Arches** | | | | | | | | | | |
| Supporting more than one floor, columns, or other bearing walls | 4 | 3 | 2 | 1 | 0 | 1 | 0 | H | 1 | 0 |
| Supporting one floor only | 2 | 2 | 2 | 1 | 0 | 1 | 0 | H | 1 | 0 |
| Supporting roofs only | 2 | 2 | 1 | 1 | 0 | 1 | 0 | H | 1 | 0 |
| **Floor-Ceiling Assemblies** | 2 | 2 | 2 | 1 | 0 | 1 | 0 | H | 1 | 0 |
| **Roof-Ceiling Assemblies** | 2 | 1½ | 1 | 1 | 0 | 1 | 0 | H | 1 | 0 |
| **Interior Nonbearing Walls** | 0 | 0 | 0 | 0 | 0 | 0 | 0 | 0 | 0 | 0 |
| **Exterior Nonbearing Walls**[c] | 0[b] | 0[b] | 0[b] | 0[b] | 0[b] | 0[b] | 0[b] | 0[b] | 0[b] | 0[b] |

H: Heavy timber members *(see NFPA 5000 for requirements).*

[a]See 7.3.2.1 of *NFPA 5000.*

[b]See Section 7.3 of *NFPA 5000.*

[c]See 7.2.3.2.12, 7.2.4.2.3, and 7.2.5.6.8 of *NFPA 5000.* [***5000:*** Table 7.2.1.1]

safety of nonambulatory occupants; a safe fire and smoke compartment needs to be established within the building but away from the compartment or zone of fire origin.

Minimum construction requirements are not mandated by 8.2.1; however, the detailed classification criteria of NFPA 220, *Standard on Types of Building Construction,* are referenced.[9] Therefore, construction types specified in other sections of the *Code* (particularly in Chapters 12 through 42 — the occupancy chapters) can use a shorthand notation, such as Type I(332), without additional, expansive detail. The user then refers to NFPA 220 for the necessary details.

**8.2.1.3** Where the building or facility includes additions or connected structures of different construction types, the rating and classification of the structure shall be based on one of the following:

(1) Separate buildings, if a 2-hour or greater vertically aligned fire barrier wall in accordance with NFPA 221, *Standard for High Challenge Fire Walls, Fire Walls, and Fire Barrier Walls,* exists between the portions of the building

(2) Separate buildings, if provided with previously approved separations

(3) Least fire-resistive construction type of the connected portions, if separation as specified in 8.2.1.3(1) or (2) is not provided

Some buildings are composed of sections and wings of differing construction types. For example, the portion of the building first constructed might be of Type III(200) (sometimes referred to as "ordinary") construction; an addition might be of Type II(111) (noncombustible-protected) construction; and the most current section of the building might be of Type V(000) (combustible-unprotected) construction (see Exhibit 8.1). Prior to the 2000 edition of the *Code*, it was left to the user and the authority having jurisdiction (AHJ) to determine the construction type classification assigned to a building with multiple construction types. The minimum fire resistance rating required of a vertically aligned fire barrier to create the equivalent of separate buildings, each of one construction type, is now specified by 8.2.1.3.

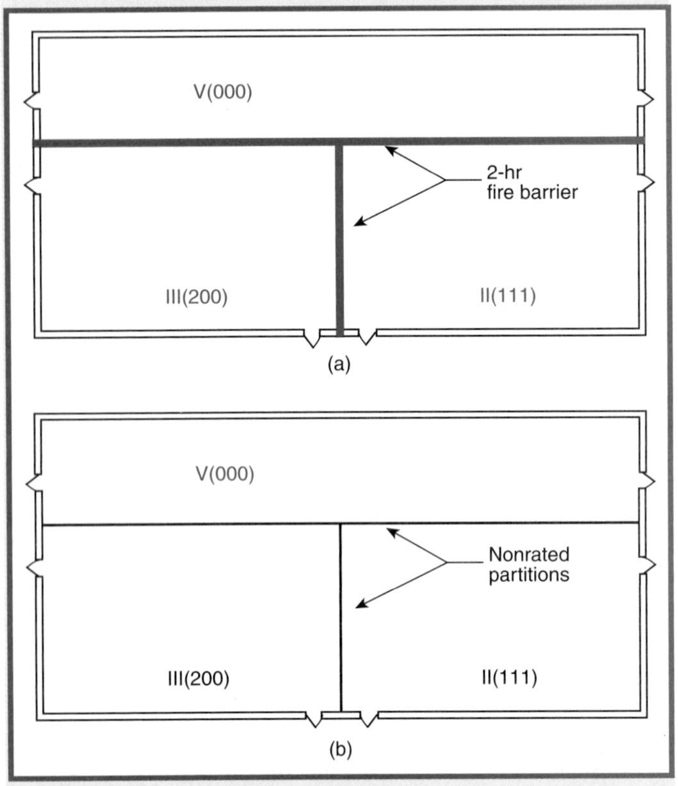


***Exhibit 8.1*** *Building composed of sections with varying construction types.*

In Exhibit 8.1, Part (a), the minimum 2-hour fire resistance–rated, vertically aligned fire barrier (i.e., a wall, not a floor) is provided between the three portions of the building with differing construction types. For purposes of applying the minimum construction requirements, each section is permitted to be treated as a separate building; one building is of Type III(200) construction, a second building is of Type II(111) construction, and a third is of Type V(000) construction. In Exhibit 8.1, Part (b), the nonrated partitions separating the portions of the building do not provide a minimum 2-hour fire resistance rating, so the building is classified as one building having the least fire resistance offered by any of the three construction types. Thus, the building construction is classified as Type V(000).

Table A.8.2.1.2 provides the *Code* user with a reprint of the key table from NFPA 220, which is extracted from *NFPA 5000®, Building Construction and Safety Code®*. The table summarizes portions of NFPA 220 and *NFPA 5000*. Note that the shorthand notation, such as Type I(332), provides the minimum hourly fire resistance ratings required to meet the definition of that construction type for only three components of the building — exterior bearing walls, structural frame/columns/girders, and floor construction. To meet the definition fully, other building components, such as roof construction and interior bearing walls, need to have certain minimum fire resistance ratings. Thus, the shorthand notation alone does not provide all the needed information. NFPA 220 should be consulted as necessary.

The minimum construction requirements of other sections of the *Code* might establish criteria, in addition to those of NFPA 220, for use in judging compliance with the definition of a specific building construction type. Chapter 18, which is applicable to new health care occupancies, recognizes that an overall life safety package is necessary for a population that is incapable of self-preservation and, thus, is difficult to protect. Therefore, 18.1.6.4 requires that, for a building to be classified as either Type I or Type II construction, it must meet the requirements of NFPA 220 and have noncombustible or limited-combustible interior nonbearing walls. NFPA 220 does not address interior nonbearing walls.

Commentary Table 8.1 matches the various NFPA 220 and *NFPA 5000, Building Construction and Safety Code*,[10] construction types with their approximate equivalent construction types, as contained in the following model building codes used throughout the United States:

1. Uniform Building Code (UBC)[11]
2. BOCA *National Building Code* (BNBC)[12]
3. *Standard Building Code* (SBC)[13]
4. *International Building Code* (IBC)[14]

For example, a building that is classified by NFPA 220 and *NFPA 5000* as Type II(111) is classified by the UBC as Type II 1-hour, by the BNBC as Type 2B, by the SBC as Type IV 1-hour, and by the IBC as Type IIA.

***Commentary Table 8.1 Cross-Reference of Building Construction Types***

| NFPA 220/NFPA 5000 | I(442) | I(332) | II(222) | II(111) | II(000) | III(211) | III(200) | IV(2HH) | V(111) | V(000) |
|---|---|---|---|---|---|---|---|---|---|---|
| UBC | — | I FR | II FR | II 1 hr | II N | III 1 hr | III N | IV HT | V 1 hr | V N |
| B/NBC | 1A | 1B | 2A | 2B | 2C | 3A | 3B | 4 | 5A | 5B |
| SBC | I | II | — | IV 1 hr | IV UNP | V 1 hr | V UNP | III | VI 1 hr | VI UNP |
| IBC | — | IA | IB | IIA | IIB | IIIA | IIIB | IV HT | VA | VB |

UBC — Uniform Building Code.
B/NBC — National Buillding Code.
SBC — Standard Building Code.
UNP — Unprotected.
IBC — International Building Code.

When using the *Life Safety Code* in conjunction with one of these building codes, the authority having jurisdiction might consider using Commentary Table 8.1 to establish (per Section 1.4) corresponding construction classifications.

## 8.2.2 General.

**8.2.2.1** Where required by other chapters of this *Code*, every building shall be divided into compartments to limit the spread of fire and restrict the movement of smoke.

**8.2.2.2** Fire compartments shall be formed with fire barriers that comply with Section 8.3.

**8.2.2.3*** Fire compartments shall be formed by fire barriers complying with one of the following:

(1) The fire barriers are continuous from outside wall to outside wall or from one fire barrier to another, or a combination thereof, including continuity through all concealed spaces, such as those found above a ceiling, including interstitial spaces.
(2) The fire barriers are continuous from outside wall to outside wall or from one fire barrier to another, or from the floor to the bottom of the interstitial space, provided that the construction assembly forming the bottom of the interstitial space has a fire resistance rating not less than that of the fire barrier.

**A.8.2.2.3** To ensure that a fire barrier is continuous, it is necessary to seal completely all openings where the fire barrier abuts other fire barriers, the exterior walls, the floor below, and the floor or ceiling above. In 8.2.2.3(2), the fire resistance rating of the bottom of the interstitial space is provided by that membrane alone. Ceilings of rated floor/ceiling and roof/ceiling assemblies do not necessarily provide the required fire resistance.

In Exhibit 8.2, the bold, solid lines designate a variety of fire barriers that meet the requirement of horizontal continuity to prevent a fire from spreading around the end of the barrier into the adjoining fire compartment.

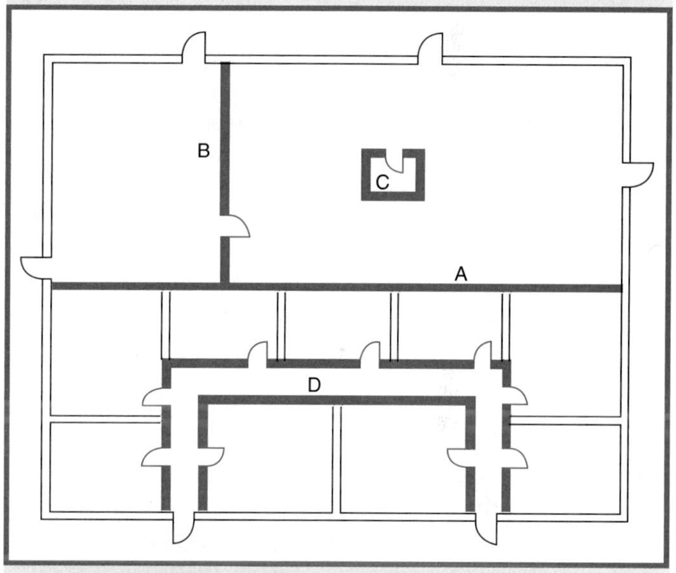


***Exhibit 8.2** Typical fire barriers.*

Fire barrier A divides the building into two distinct fire compartments by running continuously from an outside wall to an outside wall. This barrier could have, but does not have, door openings that would be protected by fire protection–rated door assemblies meeting the requirements of 8.3.4. Fire barrier B further subdivides the building into a third fire compartment and achieves its required continuity by running from an outside wall to a fire barrier (barrier A). The door opening is permitted if protected by an appropriately rated fire door assembly.

The fire barriers surrounding room C meet the horizontal continuity requirement by running from one fire barrier to another fire barrier to another; they envelop the room. This arrangement is commonly used to isolate a room and, thus, meet the protection requirements associated with protecting a hazardous area, such as a storage room or mechanical equipment room, as specified by the applicable occupancy chapter.

Fire barriers are often used to meet the protection and isolation requirements associated with corridors. Corridor D is protected by fire barriers that run from an outside wall to a fire barrier, to another fire barrier, to an outside wall. They isolate the corridor from other spaces on the floor and meet the horizontal continuity requirements.

In addition to horizontal continuity, fire barriers are required to be vertically continuous through all interstitial spaces, as described in 8.2.2.3(1).

In some cases, interstitial spaces above ceilings and between floors contain a considerable fuel load and are readily accessible. The possibility that an interstitial space will be used for storage should not be overlooked. These factors must be considered to determine whether an interstitial space is, in fact, another floor. See Exhibit 7.7, which illustrates an exit enclosure and egress provision of Chapter 7 but also shows interstitial spaces that constitute the equivalent of separate floors.

In lieu of a fire barrier being vertically continuous through the interstitial spaces to the underside of the floor or roof above, 8.2.2.3(2) permits it to terminate at the ceiling, but only where the ceiling membrane, by itself, provides a fire resistance rating equivalent to that required for the fire barrier. It is the intent of 8.2.2.3(2) to require both horizontal and vertical continuity where this option is utilized.

Normally, ceilings are tested as part of a floor/ceiling or roof/ceiling assembly rather than being tested alone. The test does not indicate the performance of the ceiling by itself but, rather, the performance of the total assembly. For example, the ceiling of a 1-hour floor/ceiling assembly might experience failure in a fire in less than 20 minutes, but the overall assembly might pass the 1-hour test. A designer or contractor might refer to a 1-hour or 2-hour ceiling and request permission to terminate a fire barrier at the ceiling, but, in reality, the ceiling is part of a 1-hour or 2-hour floor/ceiling or roof/ceiling assembly. Because the ceiling itself does not provide the appropriately rated fire barrier against which the wall assembly can be terminated, the fire barrier must run through and above the ceiling; it must extend from the floor to the underside of the floor or roof above.

Tests reported by the Gypsum Association in the *Fire Resistance Design Manual* indicate that two layers of ⅝ in. (16 mm), fire-rated, Type X gypsum wallboard, applied at right angles to the underside of 2 in. × 10 in. nominal (38 mm × 254 mm actual) wood joists and spaced 24 in. (610 mm) on centers, with the face layer of the gypsum board offset by 24 in. (610 mm) from the base layer joints, will provide 1-hour fire resistance protection for the wood framing.[15] Using this information, the authority having jurisdiction could judge that such a ceiling meets the intent of 8.2.2.3(2) and could permit a 1-hour fire resistance–rated wall assembly to terminate tightly against the underside of such a ceiling.

Part (a) of Exhibit 8.3 shows a 1-hour fire resistance–rated wall assembly continuing up through the ceiling and void space of a 1-hour fire resistance–rated floor/ceiling assembly, so as to terminate tightly against the underside of the floor slab to achieve the required vertical continuity. (Although, in this example, the floor/ceiling assembly has a 1-hour fire resistance rating, such a rating is not necessarily required.) In Exhibit 8.3, Part (b), 8.2.2.3(2) is used to permit the 1-hour-rated wall assembly to terminate at a ceiling that provides the required 1-hour fire resistance rating by itself.

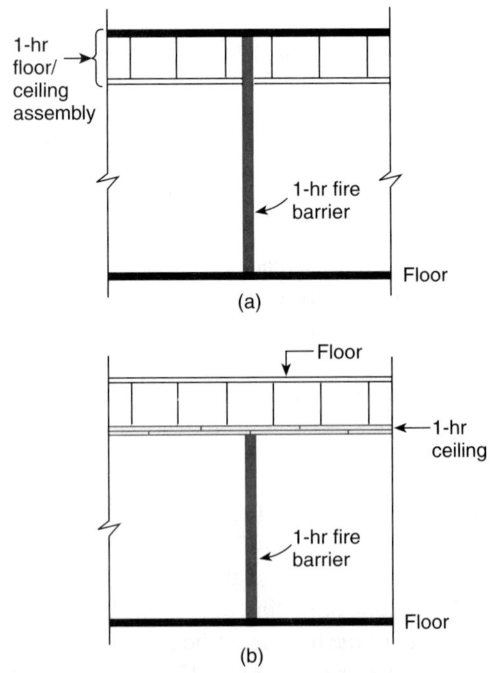


***Exhibit 8.3*** *Fire barrier vertical continuity.*

**8.2.2.4** Walls used as fire barriers shall comply with Chapter 7 of NFPA 221, *Standard for High Challenge Fire Walls, Fire Walls, and Fire Barrier Walls*. The NFPA 221 limitation on percentage width of openings shall not apply.

The requirement in 8.2.2.4 that fire barrier walls must meet NFPA 221, *Standard for High Challenge Fire Walls, Fire Walls, and Fire Barrier Walls*,[16] recognizes that the NFPA technical committee responsible for the development of NFPA 221 has specialized expertise in this area. The detailed provisions of NFPA 221 for fire barrier walls include requirements that are outside the scope of this *Code* but that are necessary to ensure the anticipated level of protection.

**8.2.2.5** Where door assemblies are required elsewhere in this *Code* to be smoke leakage–rated in accordance with 8.2.2.5, door assemblies shall comply with the following:

(1) They shall be tested in accordance with ANSI/UL 1784, *Standard for Air Leakage Tests for Door Assemblies*.
(2) The maximum air leakage rate of the door assembly shall be 3.0 $ft^3/min/ft^2$ (0.9 $m^3/min/m^2$) of door opening at 0.10 in. water column (25 $N/m^2$) for both the ambient and elevated temperature tests.
(3) Door assemblies shall be installed in accordance with NFPA 105, *Standard for the Installation of Smoke Door Assemblies and Other Opening Protectives*.

Minimum criteria for air leakage rates of door assemblies are specified by 8.2.2.5 to provide a smoke-tight assembly. However, the criteria in 8.2.2.5 are mandatory only when referenced by another section of the *Code* — such as in Chapters 12 through 42. Currently, only new fire doors serving areas of refuge are required to meet the 8.2.2.5 air-leakage rate criteria (see 7.2.12.3.4.1).

### 8.2.3 Fire Resistance–Rated Construction.

**8.2.3.1*** The fire resistance of structural elements and building assemblies shall be determined in accordance with test procedures set forth in NFPA 251, *Standard Methods of Tests of Fire Resistance of Building Construction and Materials*; ASTM E 119, *Standard Test Methods for Fire Tests of Building Construction and Materials*; or ANSI/UL 263, *Standard for Fire Tests of Building Construction and Materials*, or other approved test methods, or analytical methods approved by the authority having jurisdiction. Materials used to construct fire resistance–rated elements and assemblies shall be limited to those permitted in this *Code*.

**A.8.2.3.1** NFPA 251, *Standard Methods of Tests of Fire Resistance of Building Construction and Materials*; ANSI/UL 263, *Standard for Fire Tests of Building Construction and Materials*; and ASTM E 119, *Standard Test Methods for Fire Tests of Building Construction and Materials*, are considered nationally recognized methods of determining fire resistance and have been found to yield equivalent test methods.

**8.2.3.2** Fire resistance–rated floor and roof assemblies shall be classified as restrained or unrestrained in accordance with NFPA 251, *Standard Methods of Tests of Fire Resistance of Building Construction and Materials*; ASTM E 119, *Standard Test Methods for Fire Tests of Building Construction and Materials*; or UL 263, *Standard for Fire Tests of Building Construction and Materials*; or other approved test methods. The construction shall be considered restrained only where a registered design professional has furnished the authority having jurisdiction with satisfactory documentation verifying that the construction is restrained. The classification of fire resistance–rated floor and roof construction shall be identified on the plans as restrained or unrestrained.

The fire resistance of a fire barrier is determined by the test method described in NFPA 251, *Standard Methods of Tests of Fire Resistance of Building Construction and Materials*; ASTM E 119, *Standard Test Methods for Fire Tests of Building Construction and Materials*; and ANSI/UL 263, *Standard for Fire Tests of Building Construction and Materials*. The NFPA 251/ASTM E 119/ANSI/UL 263 test standard provides for the rating of the construction of the particular assembly and the actual testing of the assembly in the test furnace. The test is conducted under very rigid conditions, so that test results on the same assembly are reproducible and tests of different assemblies are comparable. During the test, the assembly being tested is loaded the same way it would be expected to be loaded where installed in a building. Temperatures in the furnace are generated in strict accordance with the standard time–temperature curve and reach levels of 1000°F (538°C), 1300°F (704°C), 1550°F (843°C), 1700°F (927°C), 1850°F (1010°C), and 2000°F (1093°C) at intervals of 5, 10, 30, 60, 120, and 240 minutes into the test, respectively. Temperatures both in the furnace and on the unexposed side of the assembly being tested are monitored, and results are recorded at specified intervals and locations. During the course of the test, cotton waste is placed against the unexposed surface and observed for flaming.

The following are acceptance criteria for a successfully completed fire test on an assembly for a specified time period:

1. Cotton waste on unexposed side does not ignite.
2. Temperature rise on unexposed side does not exceed 325°F (180°C) at any point or an average of 250°F (139°C).
3. Assembly continues to support design loads.

The criteria in items 1 through 3 apply to floor, roof, wall, and partition assemblies. In addition, wall and partition assemblies that are to be rated at 1 hour or more are subjected to the hose stream test. A duplicate specimen of the assembly to be rated is tested in the furnace for one-half the time specified as the fire resistance rating in the fire endurance test. This specimen is then removed from the furnace and immediately subjected to the hose stream test. If there is any projection of water beyond the unexposed surface, the assembly is considered to have failed.

Testing laboratories commonly perform the NFPA 251/ASTM E 119/ANSI/UL 263 testing. The laboratories normally issue a report of the test and then list or approve the assembly. Listings of tested fire resistance–rated assemblies are found in publications and on websites of laboratories that conduct fire testing, such as the following:

1. *UL Fire Resistance Directory*[17]
2. FM Global *Approval Guide*[18]
3. *Intertek Directory of Listed Products* [contains all listings for ETL, Warnock Hersey (WHI), and Omega Point Laboratories (OPL)[19]]

It is important that the assembly constructed is the same as that listed or approved. For example, if a floor/ceiling assembly calls for clips on the ceiling tiles, the clips must be installed and maintained. Another example is the special treatment often required for lights or air ducts in suspended ceilings. A common problem in walls is the installation of an untested material between the wallboard and the studs or the installation of recessed wall fixtures, which requires the removal of wallboard.

**8.2.3.3** Structural elements that support fire barriers shall be permitted to have only the fire resistance rating required for the construction classification of the building, provided that both of the following criteria are met:

(1) Such structural elements support nonbearing wall or partition assemblies that have a required 1-hour fire resistance rating or less.
(2) Such structural elements do not serve as exit enclosures or protection for vertical openings.

If 8.2.3.3 were not included in the *Code*, a two-story building, for example, used for an occupancy that (1) permits Type II(000) construction to be occupied and (2) requires the presence of 1-hour fire resistance–rated corridor walls, would be required to upgrade all construction supporting the nonbearing second-floor corridor walls (i.e., the columns, beams, and girders supporting the second floor) to a 1-hour fire resistance rating. Because the purpose of 1-hour-rated corridor walls is not to provide structural integrity but to provide barriers that create fire compartments on the floor on which they are installed, 8.2.3.3 permits the unprotected, noncombustible Type II(000) building to be occupied in accordance with subsection ___.1.6 of the applicable occupancy chapter.

Exhibit 8.4 further illustrates the use of 8.2.3.3. The floor shown in Part (a) is the second floor of a two-story building that, given its occupancy, is permitted to be in a building of Type II(000) construction, as defined by NFPA 220, *Standard on Types of Building Construction* (see A.8.2.1.2 and its associated commentary). In addition, the occupancy in question requires

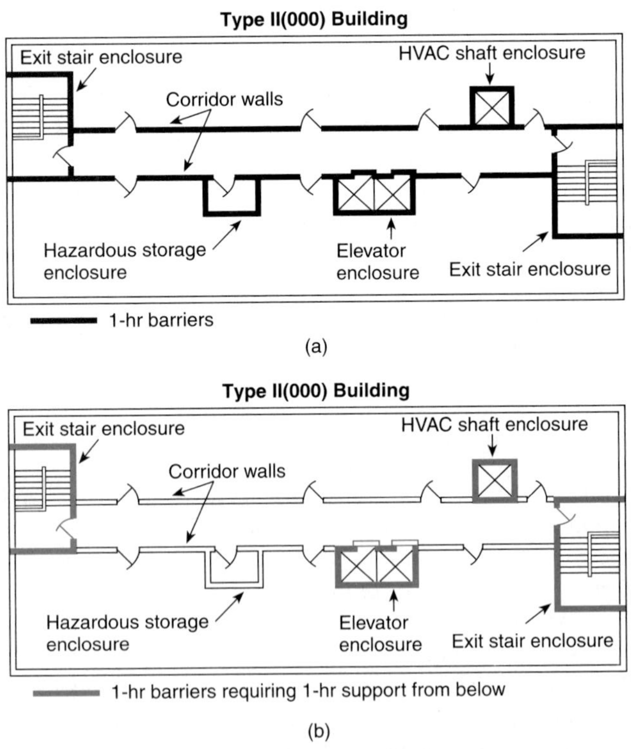


***Exhibit 8.4*** *Fire barriers and rated structural supports.*

(1) corridor walls with a 1-hour fire resistance rating and (2) enclosure of hazardous area rooms, interior exit stairs, and vertical openings, such as elevator and ventilating (HVAC) shafts, by 1-hour fire resistance–rated barriers. As shown in Part (b) of Exhibit 8.4, 8.2.3.3 permits the building construction that supports the second-floor corridor walls and the walls enclosing the hazardous storage room to remain unprotected, but such construction is to be noncombustible, as specified by building construction Type II(000). However, the second-floor 1-hour-rated fire barriers enclosing the exit stairs, and the elevator shaft and the HVAC shaft, must be supported by 1-hour fire resistance–rated construction. In Part (b), only those fire barriers depicted by bold, solid lines are required to be supported by 1-hour-rated construction from below.

**8.2.3.4** The requirement of 8.2.3.3 shall not apply to health care occupancy structural elements supporting floor assemblies in accordance with the provisions of 18.1.6 and 19.1.6.

### 8.2.4 Analytical Methods.

**8.2.4.1** Analytical methods utilized to determine the fire resistance of building assemblies shall comply with 8.2.4.2 or 8.2.4.3.

**8.2.4.2*** Where calculations are used to establish the fire resistance rating of structural elements or assemblies, they shall be permitted to be performed in accordance with ASCE/SFPE 29, *Standard Calculation Methods for Structural Fire Protection*. Where calculations are used to establish the fire resistance rating of concrete or masonry elements or assemblies, the provisions of ACI 216.1/TMS 0216.1, *Standard Method for Determining Fire Resistance of Concrete and Masonry Construction Assemblies*, shall be permitted to be used.

**A.8.2.4.2** The intent of this provision is to allow the provisions of either ASCE/SFPE 29, *Standard Calculation Methods for Structural Fire Protection*, or ACI 216.1/TMS 0216.1, *Standard Method for Determining Fire Resistance of Concrete and Masonry Assemblies*, for the calculation for fire resistance of concrete or masonry elements or assemblies.

**8.2.4.3** Except for the methods specified in 8.2.4.2, analytical methods used to calculate the fire resistance of building assemblies or structural elements shall be approved. Where an approved analytical method is utilized to establish the fire resistance rating of a structural element or building assembly, the calculations shall be based upon the fire exposure and acceptance criteria specified in NFPA 251, *Standard Methods of Tests of Fire Resistance of Building Construction and Materials*; ASTM E 119, *Standard Test Methods for Fire Tests of Building Construction and Materials*; or UL 263, *Standard for Fire Tests of Building Construction and Materials*.

Analytical methods are alternate methods of determining the fire resistance ratings of construction assemblies in lieu of the large-scale test in accordance with NFPA 251/ASTM E 119/ANSI/UL 263, as specified in 8.2.3.1. For example, a designer who wants to provide a 2-hour fire resistance rating for a W14 × 233 steel column by boxing the column with gypsum wallboard cannot find such an assembly in the *UL Fire Resistance Directory*. Design No. X520 and design No. X521 come very close to providing the needed information but deal with W14 × 228 steel columns; the designs show that, with one layer of ½ in. (13 mm) thick gypsum wallboard, the assembly will provide a 2-hour fire resistance rating. The *UL Fire Resistance Directory* further explains that most structural steel producers began rolling a new series of structural shapes in accordance with ASTM A 6/A6M, *Standard Specification for General Requirements for Rolled Structural Steel Bars, Plates, Shapes, and Sheet Piling*,[20] in 1978 and that some of the column sizes specified for individual designs might have been discontinued. Instead of making a judgment call as to whether the W14 × 233 column will provide the same rating as the discontinued W14 × 228 shape by comparing flange and web thickness, the designer calculates the fire resistance rating of a W14 × 233 steel column with a single layer of ½ in. (13 mm) gypsum wallboard built around the column in a box profile using criteria from ASCE/SFPE 29, *Standard Calculation Methods for Structural Fire Protection*,[21] as referenced in 8.2.4.2.

Based on results from accumulated fire test data, ASCE/SFPE 29 presents the following formula for calculating the fire endurance of steel columns protected by gypsum wallboard:

$$R = 2.17\left[\frac{h\left(\frac{W'}{D}\right)}{2}\right]^{0.75}$$

where

$R$ = fire resistance (hr)
$h$ = thickness of gypsum wallboard (in.)
$W'$ = weight of steel column and gypsum wallboard protection (lb/ft)
$D$ = heated perimeter of steel column (in.) [for box profile, inside perimeter of gypsum wallboard material, calculated as $D = 2(a + b)$ per Exhibit 8.5]

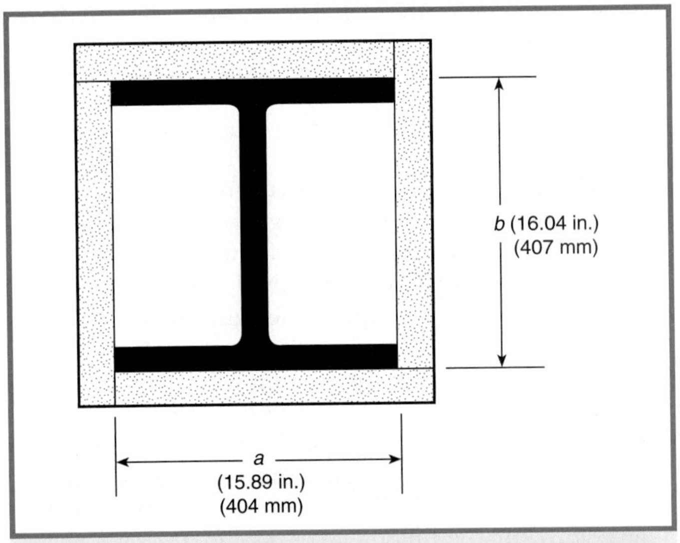


**Exhibit 8.5** *Box profile of gypsum wallboard around steel column for which fire resistance rating of assembly can be calculated.*

The total weight ($W'$) of both the column and its gypsum wallboard protection is calculated using the following formula:

$$W' = \frac{W + 50(h)(D)}{144}$$

where W = weight of steel column (lb/ft)

Performing the calculations yields the following:

$$D = 2(a + b)$$
$$= 2(15.89 + 16.04)$$
$$= 63.86 \text{ in.}$$
$$W' = \frac{W + 50(h)(D)}{144}$$
$$= 233 + \frac{50(0.5)(63.86)}{144}$$
$$= 244.09 \text{ lb/ft}$$
$$\frac{W'}{D} = \frac{244.09}{63.86} = 3.82$$
$$R = 2.17\left[\frac{h\left(\frac{W'}{D}\right)}{2}\right]^{0.75}$$
$$= 2.17\left[\frac{(0.50)(3.82)}{2}\right]^{0.75}$$
$$= 2.1 \text{ hr}$$

Based on the calculation for fire endurance, the designer specifies, with a degree of comfort, that the 2-hour fire resistance rating for the assembly consisting of the W14 × 233 steel column and gypsum wallboard box profile enclosure be achieved using a single layer of ½ in. (13 mm) gypsum wallboard.

In addition to calculation methods for determining the fire resistance of structural steel construction, ASCE/SFPE 29 includes calculation methods for plain and reinforced concrete construction, timber and wood structural elements, and masonry construction. Alternatively, the designer is permitted to use the American Concrete Institute standard ACI 216.1/TMS 0216.1, *Standard Method for Determining Fire Resistance of Concrete and Masonry Construction Assemblies*, to calculate the fire resistance of concrete and masonry construction assemblies.[22] The authority having jurisdiction must approve calculation methods other than those described in the ASCE and ACI standards, as specified in 8.2.4.3.

## 8.3 Fire Barriers

### 8.3.1 General.

Fire barriers used to provide enclosure, subdivision, or protection under this *Code* shall be classified in accordance with one of the following fire resistance ratings:

(1) 3-hour fire resistance rating
(2) 2-hour fire resistance rating
(3) 1-hour fire resistance rating
(4)* ½-hour fire resistance rating

**A.8.3.1(4)** Walls in good condition with lath and plaster, or gypsum board of not less than ½ in. (13 mm) on each side, can be considered as providing a minimum ½-hour fire resistance rating. Additional information on archaic material assemblies can be found in Appendix I of NFPA 914, *Code for Fire Protection of Historic Structures*.

Fire resistance testing of building construction per NFPA 251/ASTM E 119/ANSI/UL 263 permits assemblies to be assigned fire resistance ratings up through the category of "8 hours and over." Ratings of more than 2 hours are used primarily in protecting property; however, some occupancy separations require 3-hour fire barriers per Table 6.1.14.4.1(b). The *Code* requires not more than a 2-hour fire resistance rating for building construction, even in the health care and detention and correctional occupancy chapters. These chapters promote a defend-in-place strategy, because such a strategy emphasizes life safety over property protection. Thus, in the ___.1.6 subsections in the health care and detention and correctional occupancy chapters, construction Types I(442), I(332), and II(222) are grouped to be treated as equivalent. A design professional can specify that material assemblies with 3-hour or 4-hour fire resistance ratings be used. However, no reduction in requirements is permitted, other than those permitted for construction with a 2-hour fire resistance rating.

Prior to the 1997 edition, the *Code* included ¾-hour and ⅓-hour fire resistance rating classifications in addition to the current ½ hour classification. The range of fractional-hour ratings mistakenly implied a degree of accuracy and precision. The range was revised so that the only fire resistance rating of less than 1 hour is the ½-hour classification. Because some occupancies, such as existing health care occupancies, previously permitted a fire resistance rating of ⅓ hour but now require a rating of ½ hour, A.8.3.1(4) provides guidance on evaluating existing fire barriers. The change from the ⅓-hour to the ½-hour classification was not intended to create a condition of noncompliance where existing fire barriers had previously complied with *Code* requirements. A previously approved ⅓-hour fire resistance–rated barrier should be considered as complying with the requirement for a ½-hour fire barrier.

### 8.3.2 Walls.

**8.3.2.1** The fire-resistive materials, assemblies, and systems used shall be limited to those permitted in this *Code* and this chapter.

**8.3.2.1.1*** Fire resistance–rated glazing tested in accordance with NFPA 251, *Standard Methods of Tests of Fire Resistance of Building Construction and Materials*, shall be permitted.

**A.8.3.2.1.1** Fire resistance–rated glazing complying with 8.3.2, where not installed in a door, is considered a wall, not an opening protective.

**8.3.2.1.2** New fire resistance–rated glazing shall bear the identifier "W-XXX" where "XXX" is the fire resistance rating in minutes. Such identification shall be permanently affixed.

The provisions of 8.3.2.1.1 and 8.3.2.1.2 recognize that glazing material that has been tested as a wall assembly in accordance with NFPA 251 is permitted to be used in fire barrier walls with no limitations, other than those imposed by the product's listing. New glazing material tested and used as such must be appropriately labeled as specified in 8.3.2.1.2.

**8.3.2.2** The construction materials and details for fire-resistive assemblies and systems for walls described shall comply with all other provisions of this *Code*, except as modified herein.

**8.3.2.3** Interior walls and partitions of nonsymmetrical construction shall be evaluated from both directions and assigned a fire resistance rating based on the shorter duration obtained in accordance with NFPA 251, *Standard Methods of Tests of Fire Resistance of Building Construction and Materials*; ASTM E 119, *Standard Test Methods for Fire Tests of Building Construction and Materials*; or ANSI/UL 263, *Standard for Fire Tests of Building Construction and Materials*. When the wall is tested with the least fire-resistive side exposed to the furnace, the wall shall not be required to be subjected to tests from the opposite side.

### 8.3.3 Fire Doors and Windows.

**8.3.3.1** Openings required to have a fire protection rating by Table 8.3.4.2 shall be protected by approved, listed, labeled fire door assemblies and fire window assemblies and their accompanying hardware, including all frames, closing devices, anchorage, and sills in accordance with the requirements of NFPA 80, *Standard for Fire Doors and Other Opening Protectives*, except as otherwise specified in this *Code*.

**8.3.3.2*** Fire protection ratings for products required to comply with 8.3.3 shall be as determined and reported by a nationally recognized testing agency in accordance with NFPA 252, *Standard Methods of Fire Tests of Door Assemblies*; ASTM E 2074, *Standard Test Method for Fire Tests of Door Assemblies, Including Positive Pressure Testing of Side-Hinged and Pivoted Swinging Door Assemblies*; ANSI/UL 10B, *Standard for Fire Tests of Door Assemblies*; or ANSI/UL 10C, *Standard for Positive Pressure Fire Tests of Door Assemblies*; or NFPA 257, *Standard on Fire Test for Window and Glass Block Assemblies*; ASTM E 2010, *Standard Test Method for Positive Pressure Fire Tests of Window Assemblies*; or ANSI/UL 9, *Standard for Fire Tests of Window Assemblies*.

**A.8.3.3.2** Some door assemblies have been tested to meet the conditions of acceptance of NFPA 251, *Standard Methods of Tests of Fire Resistance of Building Construction and Materials*; ASTM E 119, *Standard Test Methods for Fire Tests of Building Construction and Materials*; or ANSI/UL 263, *Standard for Fire Tests of Building Construction and Materials*. Where such assemblies are used, the provisions of 8.3.2 should be applied instead of those of 8.3.3.2.

**8.3.3.2.1** Fire protection–rated glazing shall be evaluated under positive pressure in accordance with NFPA 257, *Standard on Fire Test for Window and Glass Block Assemblies*.

**8.3.3.2.2** All products required to comply with 8.3.3.2 shall bear an approved label.

**8.3.3.2.3*** Labels on fire door assemblies shall be maintained in a legible condition.

**A.8.3.3.2.3** In existing installations, it is important to be able to determine the fire protection rating of the fire door. However, steel door frames that are well set in the wall might be judged as acceptable even if the frame label is not legible.

**8.3.3.3** Unless otherwise specified, fire doors shall be self-closing or automatic-closing in accordance with 7.2.1.8.

Fire protection–rated door assemblies are tested in accordance with NFPA 252, *Standard Methods of Fire Tests of Door Assemblies,* also commonly known as ASTM E 2074, *Standard Test Method for Fire Tests of Door Assemblies, Including Positive Pressure Testing of Side-Hinged and Pivoted Swinging Door Assemblies.*[23] Such assemblies must be installed in accordance with the requirements of NFPA 80, *Standard for Fire Doors and Other Opening Protectives.*[24] Where the *Code* uses the term *door,* it includes not only the door leaf or slab but also the doorway, frame, and necessary hardware, including hinges. Where describing a fire door, the applicable standards similarly define a fire protection–rated assembly as including all these components as well as a listed door closer and positive latching.

If they are to be effective, fire doors must be not only closed but also held closed. Building fires are capable of generating pressures sufficient to force fire doors open if they are not held closed with positive latching, thereby rendering the doors incapable of protecting the opening in which they are installed.

The acceptance criteria for fire protection–rated assemblies, such as fire doors, differ from those for fire resistance–rated construction, such as a wall or floor/ceiling assembly. The limitation of temperature rise through the fire door is not normally a measure of acceptance, although it is a measure of acceptance for a fire resistance–rated assembly such as a wall. In addition, during the course of the fire test, fire doors will expand on the exposed side and, as a result, will warp — sometimes expanding through the door opening at the top of the door. This expansion and warping can result in some flaming through the top of the door openings. The test standards recognize this phenomenon, and a certain amount of such flaming is permitted under the acceptance criteria. This does not adversely affect safety, given that fire protection–rated assemblies are intended to protect relatively small openings in larger fire resistance–rated barriers. Also, to maintain the door as usable, combustible materials are not typically stored in front of the door opening.

**8.3.3.4** Floor fire door assemblies shall be tested in accordance with NFPA 288, *Standard Methods of Fire Tests of Floor Fire Door Assemblies Installed Horizontally in Fire Resistance–Rated Floor Systems*, and shall achieve a fire resistance rating not less than the assembly being penetrated. Floor fire door assemblies shall be listed and labeled.

**8.3.3.5** Fire protection–rated glazing shall be permitted in fire barriers having a required fire resistance rating of 1 hour or less and shall be of an approved type with the appropriate fire protection rating for the location in which the barriers are installed.

**8.3.3.6*** Glazing in fire window assemblies, other than in existing fire window installations of wired glass and other fire-rated glazing material, shall be of a design that has been tested to meet the conditions of acceptance of NFPA 257, *Standard on Fire Test for Window and Glass Block Assemblies*; ASTM E 2010, *Standard Test Method for Positive Pressure Fire Tests of Window Assemblies*; or ANSI/UL 9, *Standard for Fire Tests of Window Assemblies.* Fire protection–rated glazing in fire door assemblies, other than in existing fire-rated door assemblies, shall be of a design that has been tested to meet the conditions of acceptance of NFPA 252, *Standard Methods of Fire Tests of Door Assemblies*; ASTM E 2074, *Standard Test Method for Fire Tests of Door Assemblies, Including Positive Pressure Testing of Side-Hinged and Pivoted Swinging Door Assemblies*; ANSI/UL 10B, *Standard for Fire Tests of Door Assemblies*; or ANSI/UL 10C, *Standard for Positive Pressure Fire Tests of Door Assemblies.*

**A.8.3.3.6** Some window assemblies have been tested to meet the conditions of acceptance of NFPA 251, *Standard Methods of Tests of Fire Resistance of Building Construction and Materials*; ASTM E 119, *Standard Test Methods for Fire Tests of Building Construction and Materials*; or ANSI/UL 263, *Standard for Fire Tests of Building Construction and Materials.* Where such assemblies are used, the provisions of 8.3.2 should be applied instead of those of 8.3.3.6.

**8.3.3.7** Fire resistance–rated glazing complying with 8.3.2.1.1 shall be permitted in fire doors and fire window assemblies in accordance with their listings.

**8.3.3.8** Wired glass of $^1/_4$ in. (6 mm) thickness and labeled for fire protection purposes shall be permitted to be used in approved opening protectives, provided that the maximum size specified by the listing is not exceeded. Other glazing materials that have been tested and labeled to indicate the type of opening to be protected for fire protection purposes shall be permitted to be used in approved opening protectives in accordance with their listing, with the maximum sizes tested.

**8.3.3.9** Nonsymmetrical fire protection–rated glazing systems shall be tested with each face exposed to the furnace, and the assigned fire protection rating shall be that of the shortest duration obtained from the two tests conducted in compliance with NFPA 257, *Standard on Fire Test for Window and Glass Block Assemblies*; ASTM E 2010, *Standard Test Method for Positive Pressure Fire Tests of Window Assemblies*; or ANSI/UL 9, *Standard for Fire Tests of Window Assemblies*.

**8.3.3.10** The total combined area of glazing in fire-rated window assemblies and fire-rated door assemblies used in fire barriers shall not exceed 25 percent of the area of the fire barrier that is common with any room, unless the installation meets one of the following criteria:

(1) The installation is an existing fire window installation of wired glass and other fire-rated glazing material in approved metal frames.
(2) The installation is an existing fire window installation of wired glass and other fire-rated glazing materials in approved frames.
(3) The fire protection–rated glazing material is installed in approved existing frames.

**8.3.3.11** Fire protection–rated glazing shall bear identification as described in 8.3.3.11.1 or 8.3.3.11.2 and shall be permanently affixed.

**8.3.3.11.1** Fire protection–rated glazing used in doors shall bear a four-part identification in the form of D — H (or NH) — T (or NT) — XXX, with the component parts defined as follows:

(1) D, which indicates that the glazing is to be used in fire door assemblies and that the glazing meets the fire protection requirements of NFPA 252, *Standard Methods of Fire Tests of Door Assemblies*
(2) H, which indicates that the glazing meets the hose stream requirements of the test standard
(3) NH, which indicates that the glazing does not meet the hose stream requirements of the test standard
(4) T, which indicates that the glazing has a maximum transmitted temperature endpoint of not more than 450°F (250°C) above ambient at the end of 30 minutes of standard fire test exposure
(5) NT, which indicates that the glazing does not have a temperature rise rating
(6) XXX, which is the placeholder that specifies the fire protection rating period, in minutes

**8.3.3.11.2** Fire protection–rated glazing used in fire resistance–rated walls and partitions shall bear the identification OH-XXX, which is defined as follows:

(1) OH indicates that the glazing meets both the fire protection and the hose stream requirements of NFPA 257, *Standard on Fire Test for Window and Glass Block Assemblies*; ASTM E 2010, *Standard Test Method for Positive Pressure Fire Tests of Window Assemblies*; or ANSI/UL 9, *Standard for Fire Tests of Window Assemblies*; and is permitted to be used in openings.
(2) XXX indicates the fire protection rating period, in minutes, that was tested.

The requirements of 8.3.3.5 through 8.3.3.11.2 provide specifications for fire window assemblies that parallel those covered by 8.3.3.1 through 8.3.3.4 for fire door assemblies. New glazing for use in fire barriers and fire doors is regulated by performance-oriented criteria, which refer to fire-rated glazing, in lieu of the more traditional but prescriptive requirements previously applicable to wired glass. The requirements limit the installation of fire windows used in fire barriers to not more than 25 percent of the area of the fire barrier that is common with any room; however, 8.3.3.10 continues to recognize the current practice of using greater percentages of wired glass for existing fire windows and vision panels in fire doors subject to the stated limitations.

The marking requirements for fire protection–rated glazing in 8.3.3.11 first appeared in the 2006 edition of the *Code*. The markings vary, depending on whether the glazing is installed in a door (8.3.3.11.1) or a wall (8.3.3.11.2), and provide details on the test criteria at a glance. The prescribed marking scheme is consistent with the requirements of *NFPA 5000, Building Construction and Safety Code*, and other model building codes used throughout the United States.

### 8.3.4 Opening Protectives.

**8.3.4.1** Every opening in a fire barrier shall be protected to limit the spread of fire and restrict the movement of smoke from one side of the fire barrier to the other.

**8.3.4.2*** The fire protection rating for opening protectives in fire barriers, fire-rated smoke barriers, and fire-rated smoke partitions shall be in accordance with Table 8.3.4.2, except as otherwise permitted in 8.3.4.3 or 8.3.4.4.

**A.8.3.4.2** Longer ratings might be required where opening protectives are provided for property protection as well as life safety. NFPA 80, *Standard for Fire Doors and Other Opening Protectives*, should be consulted for standard practice in the selection and installation of fire door assemblies and fire window assemblies.

**Table 8.3.4.2.** A vision panel in a fire door is not a fire window, and, thus, it is not the intent of the"NP" notations

***Table 8.3.4.2 Minimum Fire Protection Ratings for Opening Protectives in Fire Resistance–Rated Assemblies***

| Component | Walls and Partitions (hr) | Fire Door Assemblies (hr) | Fire Window Assemblies (hr) |
|---|---|---|---|
| Elevator hoistways | 2 | 1½ | NP |
| | 1 | 1 | NP |
| Vertical shafts (including stairways, exits, and refuse chutes) | 2 | 1½ | NP |
| | 1 | 1 | NP |
| | ½ | ⅓ | NP |
| Fire barriers | 3 | 3 | NP |
| | 2 | 1½ | NP |
| | 1 | ¾ | ¾ |
| | ½ | ⅓* | ⅓ |
| Horizontal exits | 2 | 1½ | NP |
| Horizontal exits served by bridges between buildings | 2 | ¾ | ¾ |
| Exit access corridors† | 1 | ⅓ | ¾ |
| | ½ | ⅓ | ⅓ |
| Smoke barriers† | 1 | ⅓ | ¾ |
| Smoke partitions†, ‡ | ½ | ⅓ | ⅓ |

NP: Not permitted.

† Fire doors are not required to have a hose stream test per NFPA 252, *Standard Methods of Fire Tests of Door Assemblies*; ASTM E 2074, *Standard Test Method for Fire Tests of Door Assemblies, Including Positive Pressure Testing of Side-Hinged and Pivoted Swinging Door Assemblies*; ANSI/UL 10B, *Standard for Fire Tests of Door Assemblies*; or ANSI/UL 10C, *Standard for Positive Pressure Fire Tests of Door Assemblies*.

‡ For residential board and care, see 32.2.3.1 and 33.2.3.1.

in the "Fire Window Assemblies" column of Table 8.3.4.2 to prohibit vision panels in fire doors.

Note that Table 8.3.4.2 does not mandate fire resistance ratings for the components listed; rather, it specifies the fire protection rating needed for openings where the listed components are required to be rated by another section of the *Code*. For example, not all exit access corridors are required to be rated. However, where corridor walls are required by another section of the *Code* to have a 1-hour rating, the doors therein must have a ⅓-hour (or 20-minute) fire protection rating.

**8.3.4.3** Existing fire door assemblies having a minimum ¾-hour fire protection rating shall be permitted to continue to be used in vertical openings and in exit enclosures in lieu of the minimum 1-hour fire protection rating required by Table 8.3.4.2.

**8.3.4.4** Where a 20-minute fire protection–rated door is required in existing buildings, an existing 1¾ in. (44 mm) solid-bonded wood-core door, an existing steel-clad (tin-clad) wood door, or an existing solid-core steel door with positive latch and closer shall be permitted, unless otherwise specified by Chapters 11 through 43.

Fire barriers have fire *resistance* ratings, as addressed in 8.3.1; opening protectives, such as fire doors, have fire *protection* ratings, as discussed in 8.3.3. For a better understanding of the difference in test methods used for rating fire barriers and fire doors, compare the commentary following 8.2.3.2 and 8.3.3.3.

In general, 1-hour fire barriers for the protection of vertical openings (e.g., the shafts enclosing maximum three-story exit stairs) require doors with a 1-hour fire protection rating. One-hour fire barriers for other than vertical opening protection, such as those used to isolate a hazardous contents room, require doors with a ¾-hour fire protection rating.

The provisions of 8.3.3.1 permit Chapter 7 and the occupancy chapters to alter the general rule specified in the previous paragraph. However, for the most part, such alteration is usually done only with regard to the requirement that corridor walls be of a 1-hour fire resistance rating. Table 8.3.4.2 permits a 1-hour or ½-hour fire resistance–rated corridor wall or 1-hour fire resistance–rated smoke barrier to have a door with a 20-minute fire protection rating.

Health care and ambulatory health care occupancies, for example, permit the omission of the self-closing devices on patient room doors installed in corridor walls. In this case, the special requirements recognize the functional needs for open doors in these facilities, and a true fire protection–rated patient room door assembly is not required.

The fire protection ratings of the opening protectives are sometimes permitted to be of a lower rating than the fire resistance rating of the fire barrier openings to be protected. For example, a 2-hour fire resistance–rated fire barrier is permitted to have its openings protected by 1½-hour fire protection–rated door assemblies. The perceived mismatch of ratings actually accomplishes a reasonable, practical match — as explained in the paragraphs that follow.

The test procedures on which the ratings are based, that is, NFPA 251/ASTM E 119/ANSI/UL 263 for fire barriers and NFPA 252/ASTM E 2074 (see commentary following 8.3.3.3) for fire doors, are different.

Although combustibles placed against a fire resistance–rated wall expose the wall to a considerable fire challenge, a fire protection–rated door assembly does not usually have combustibles placed against it, because the opening must be clear to use the door. Such a scenario suggests that, if a door — for example, a second door to a storage room that is no longer needed — is not to be used and combustible storage is to be placed at the door opening, the door should be removed and the opening filled with material to restore the wall to its required fire resistance rating.

### 8.3.5 Penetrations.

The provisions of 8.3.5 shall govern the materials and methods of construction used to protect through-penetrations and membrane penetrations in fire walls, fire barrier walls, and fire resistance–rated horizontal assemblies. The provisions of 8.3.5 shall not apply to approved existing materials and methods of construction used to protect existing through-penetrations and existing membrane penetrations in fire walls, fire barrier walls, or fire resistance–rated horizontal assemblies, unless otherwise required by Chapters 11through 43.

**8.3.5.1* Firestop Systems and Devices Required.** Penetrations for cables, cable trays, conduits, pipes, tubes, combustion vents and exhaust vents, wires, and similar items to accommodate electrical, mechanical, plumbing, and communications systems that pass through a wall, floor, or floor/ceiling assembly constructed as a fire barrier shall be protected by a firestop system or device. The firestop system or device shall be tested in accordance with ASTM E 814, *Standard Test Method for Fire Tests of Through Penetration Fire Stops*, or ANSI/UL 1479, *Standard for Fire Tests of Through-Penetration Firestops*, at a minimum positive pressure differential of 0.01 in. water column (2.5 N/m$^2$) between the exposed and the unexposed surface of the test assembly.

**A.8.3.5.1** ASTM E 2174, *Standard Practice for On-Site Inspection of Installed Fire Stops*, provides guidance for the inspection of through-penetration fire stop systems tested in accordance with ASTM E 814, *Standard Test Method for Fire Tests of Through-Penetration Fire Stops*, and ANSI/UL 1479, *Standard for Fire Tests of Through-Penetration Firestops*.

One source of information on tested materials, devices, and systems for protecting through-penetrations of fire resistance–rated barriers is Volume 2 of the *UL Fire Resistance Directory*, published by Underwriters Laboratories.[25] Such devices and systems are designed to resist the spread of fire through openings in fire resistance–rated floor or wall barriers that accommodate penetrating items, such as electrical cables, cable trays, conduits, and pipes. Underwriters Laboratories classifies such devices and systems with respect to installation in a wall only, installation in a floor only, or installation in a wall or floor. The basic standard used by UL to investigate products in this category is ANSI/UL 1479, *Standard for Fire Tests of Through-Penetration Firestops*,[26] which is similar to ASTM E 814, *Standard Test Method for Fire Tests of Through-Penetration Fire Stops*.[27] A sampling of the currently classified devices includes the use of the following:

1. Ceramic fibers
2. Foamed silicones
3. Mineral wool batts
4. Intumescent sheets
5. Sealing blankets and plugs
6. Fittings and couplings
7. Various caulks, putties, and mastics
8. Spring-loaded guillotine blades

Over the life of a building, it is important to maintain the integrity of barriers to protect against fire penetration. Renovations or any changes to building utilities will tend to violate the compartmentation provided when a building is first occupied.

Exhibit 8.6 illustrates some of the typical fire barrier penetrations, which are addressed by 8.3.5.

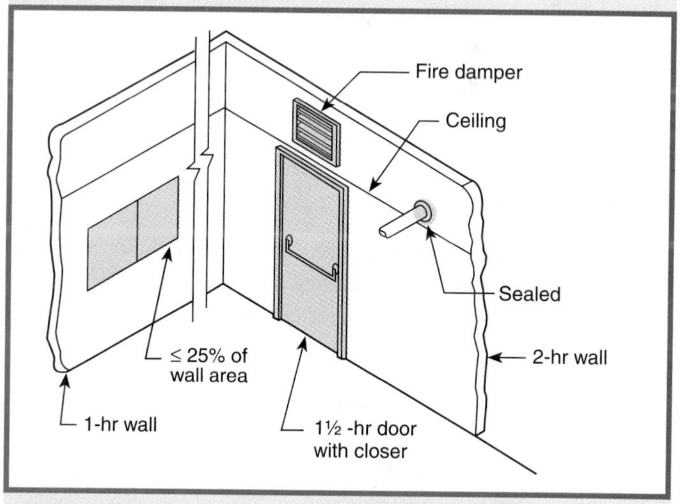


***Exhibit 8.6** Typical penetrations of a fire barrier.*

**8.3.5.1.1** The requirements of 8.3.5.1 shall not apply where otherwise permitted by any one of the following:

(1) Where penetrations are tested and installed as part of an assembly tested and rated in accordance with NFPA

251, *Standard Methods of Tests of Fire Resistance of Building Construction and Materials*; ASTM E 119, *Standard Test Methods for Fire Tests of Building Construction and Materials*; or ANSI/UL 263, *Standard for Fire Tests of Building Construction and Materials*

(2) Where penetrations through floors are enclosed in a shaft enclosure designed as a fire barrier

(3) Where concrete, grout, or mortar has been used to fill the annular spaces around cast-iron, copper, or steel piping that penetrates one or more concrete or masonry fire resistance–rated assemblies and both of the following criteria are also met:

  (a) The nominal diameter of each penetrating item shall not exceed 6 in. (150 mm), and the opening size shall not exceed 1 $ft^2$ (0.09 $m^2$).

  (b) The thickness of the concrete, grout, or mortar shall be the full thickness of the assembly.

(4) Where firestopping materials are used with the following penetrating items, the penetration is limited to one floor, and the firestopping material is capable of preventing the passage of flame and hot gases sufficient to ignite cotton waste when subjected to the time—temperature fire conditions of NFPA 251 under a minimum positive pressure differential of 0.01 in. water column (2.5 Pa) at the location of the penetration for the time period equivalent to the required fire resistance rating of the assembly penetrated:

  (a) Steel, ferrous, or copper cables
  (b) Cable or wire with steel jackets
  (c) Cast-iron, steel, or copper pipes
  (d) Steel conduit or tubing

**8.3.5.1.2** The maximum nominal diameter of the penetrating item, as indicated in 8.3.5.1.1(4)(a) through (d), shall not be greater than 4 in. (100 mm) and shall not exceed an aggregate 100 $in.^2$ (64,520 $mm^2$) opening in any 100 $ft^2$ (9.3 $m^2$) of floor or wall area.

**8.3.5.1.3** Firestop systems and devices shall have a minimum 1-hour F rating, but not less than the required fire resistance rating of the fire barrier penetrated.

**8.3.5.1.4** Penetrations in fire-rated horizontal assemblies shall have a minimum 1-hour T rating, but not less than the fire resistance rating of the horizontal assembly. Rated penetrations shall not be required for the following:

(1) Floor penetrations contained within the cavity of a wall assembly
(2) Penetrations through floors or floor assemblies where the penetration is not in direct contact with combustible material

**8.3.5.2 Sleeves.** Where the penetrating item uses a sleeve to penetrate the wall or floor, the sleeve shall be securely set in the wall or floor, and the space between the item and the sleeve shall be filled with a material that complies with 8.3.5.1.

**8.3.5.3 Insulation and Coverings.** Insulation and coverings for penetrating items shall not pass through the wall or floor unless the insulation or covering has been tested as part of the firestop system or device.

**8.3.5.4 Transmission of Vibrations.** Where designs take transmission of vibrations into consideration, any vibration isolation shall meet one of the following conditions:

(1) It shall be provided on either side of the wall or floor.
(2) It shall be designed for the specific purpose.

**8.3.5.5 Transitions.**

**8.3.5.5.1** Where piping penetrates a fire resistance–rated wall or floor assembly, combustible piping shall not connect to noncombustible piping within 36 in. (915 mm) of the firestop system or device without demonstration that the transition will not reduce the fire resistance rating, except in the case of previously approved installations.

**8.3.5.5.2** Unshielded couplings shall not be used to connect noncombustible piping to combustible piping unless it can be demonstrated that the transition complies with the fire-resistive requirements of 8.3.5.1.

**8.3.5.6 Membrane Penetrations.**

The term *membrane penetration* refers to openings for penetrations made through one side only of a fire resistance–rated assembly, as defined in *NFPA 5000, Building Construction and Safety Code*. The provisions of 8.3.5.6 address such penetrations, which, if not properly protected, would compromise the fire-resistive integrity of the barrier. The term *through-penetration*, on the other hand, refers to openings for penetrations that pass through both sides of a fire barrier.

**8.3.5.6.1** Membrane penetrations for cables, cable trays, conduits, pipes, tubes, combustion vents and exhaust vents, wires, and similar items to accommodate electrical, mechanical, plumbing, and communications systems that pass through a membrane of a wall, floor, or floor/ceiling assembly constructed as a fire barrier shall be protected by a firestop system or device and shall comply with 8.3.5.1 through 8.3.5.5.2.

**8.3.5.6.2** The firestop system or device shall be tested in accordance with ASTM E 814, *Standard Test Method for Fire Tests of Through Penetration Fire Stops*, or ANSI/UL 1479, *Standard for Fire Tests of Through-Penetration Firestops*, at a minimum positive pressure differential of 0.01 in. water column (2.5 $N/m^2$) between the exposed and the unexposed surface of the test assembly, unless one of the following applies:

(1) Membrane penetrations of ceilings that are not an integral part of a fire resistance–rated floor/ceiling or roof/ceiling assembly shall be permitted.
(2) Membrane penetrations of steel, ferrous, or copper conduits, and pipes, tubes, or combustion vents or exhaust vents, shall be permitted where the annular space is protected with an approved material and the aggregate area of the openings does not exceed 0.7 $ft^2$ (0.06 $m^2$) in any 100 $ft^2$ (9.3 $m^2$) of ceiling area.
(3) Electrical outlet boxes and fittings shall be permitted, provided that such devices are listed for use in fire resistance–rated assemblies and are installed in accordance with their listing.
(4) The annular space created by the membrane penetration of a fire sprinkler shall be permitted, provided that the space is covered by a metal escutcheon plate.

**8.3.5.6.3** Where walls or partitions are required to have a minimum 1-hour fire resistance rating, recessed fixtures shall be installed in the wall or partition in such a manner that the required fire resistance is not reduced, unless one of the following is met:

(1) Any steel electrical box not exceeding 0.1 $ft^2$ (0.01 $m^2$) shall be permitted where the aggregate area of the openings provided for the boxes does not exceed 0.7 $ft^2$ (0.06 $m^2$) in any 100 $ft^2$ (9.3 $m^2$) of wall area, and, where outlet boxes are installed on opposite sides of the wall, the boxes shall be separated by one of the following:
   (a) Horizontal distance of not less than 24 in. (610 mm)
   (b) Horizontal distance of not less than the depth of the wall cavity, where the wall cavity is filled with cellulose loose-fill, rock wool, or slag wool insulation
   (c)* Solid fireblocking

**A.8.3.5.6.3(1)(c)** Criteria associated with fireblocking can be found in 8.14.2 of *NFPA 5000, Building Construction and Safety Code*.

   (d) Other listed materials and methods
(2) Membrane penetrations for any listed electrical outlet box made of any material shall be permitted, provided that such boxes have been tested for use in fire resistance–rated assemblies and are installed in accordance with the instructions included in the listing.
(3) The annular space created by the membrane penetration of a fire sprinkler shall be permitted, provided that the space is covered by a metal escutcheon plate.

**8.3.5.7 Openings for Air-Handling Ductwork.** Openings in fire barriers for air-handling ductwork or air movement shall be protected in accordance with 9.2.1.

In referencing 9.2.1 for the protection of openings in fire barriers for air-handling ductwork or air movement, 8.3.5.7 mandates that the requirements of NFPA 90A, *Standard for the Installation of Air-Conditioning and Ventilating Systems*,[28] and not the usual *Life Safety Code* requirements for opening protectives (contained in 8.3.4), apply to heating, ventilating, and air-conditioning (HVAC) system penetrations of fire barriers. NFPA 90A requires that approved fire dampers be provided in all air-transfer openings in barriers that are required to have a fire resistance rating. It also requires that approved fire dampers be provided where ducts penetrate barriers that are required to have a fire resistance rating of 2 hours or more. Thus, although any air-transfer opening would have to be provided with a fire damper in a required fire barrier of any rating, penetrations by ducts would not have to be provided with fire dampers if the required rating of the fire barrier were less than 2 hours. These requirements are depicted in Exhibit 8.7.

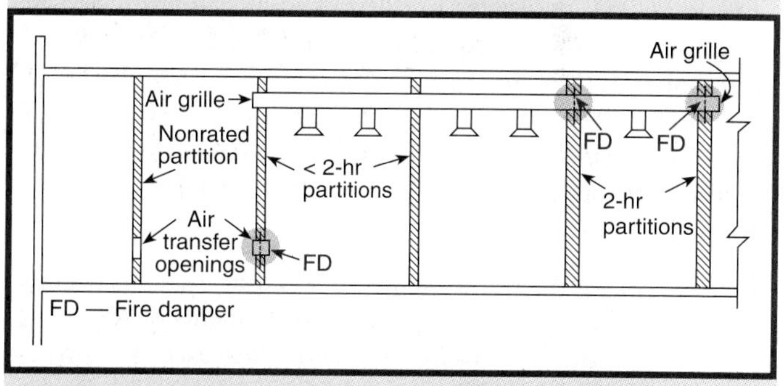


***Exhibit 8.7** Fire damper requirements of NFPA 90A for HVAC penetrations of fire barriers.*

## 8.3.6 Joints.

**8.3.6.1** The provisions of 8.3.6 shall govern the materials and methods of construction used to protect joints in between and at the perimeter of fire barriers or, where fire barriers meet other fire barriers, the floor or roof deck above, or the outside walls. The provisions of 8.3.6 shall not apply to approved existing materials and methods of construction used to protect existing joints in fire barriers, unless otherwise required by Chapters 11 through 43.

**8.3.6.2** Joints made within or at the perimeter of fire barriers shall be protected with a joint system that is capable of limiting the transfer of smoke.

**8.3.6.3** Joints made within or between fire barriers shall be protected with a smoke-tight joint system that is capable of limiting the transfer of smoke.

**8.3.6.4** Testing of the joint system in a fire barrier shall be representative of the actual installation suitable for the required engineering demand without compromising the fire resistance rating of the assembly or the structural integrity of the assembly.

**8.3.6.5*** Joints made within or between fire resistance–rated assemblies shall be protected with a joint system that is designed and tested to prevent the spread of fire for a time period equal to that of the assembly in which the joint is located. Such materials, systems, or devices shall be tested as part of the assembly in accordance with the requirements of ASTM E 1966, *Standard Test Method for Fire-Resistive Joint Systems*, or ANSI/UL 2079, *Standard for Tests for Fire Resistance of Building Joint Systems*.

**A.8.3.6.5** On-site inspection of firestopping is important in maintaining the integrity of any vertical or horizontal fire barrier. Two standard practice documents were developed with the ASTM process to allow inspections of through-penetration firestops, joints, and perimeter fire barrier systems. ASTM E 2393, *Standard Practice for On-Site Inspection of Installed Fire Resistive Joint Systems and Perimeter Fire Barriers*, provides guidance for the inspection of fire-resistive joints and perimeter fire barrier joint systems tested in accordance with the requirements of ASTM E 1966, *Standard Test Method for Fire-Resistive Joint Systems*, or with ANSI/UL 2079, *Standard for Tests for Fire Resistance of Building Joint Systems*. ASTM E 2393 contains a standardized report format, which would lead to greater consistency for inspections.

**8.3.6.6** All joint systems shall be tested at their maximum joint width in accordance with the requirements of ASTM E 1966, *Standard Test Method for Fire-Resistive Joint Systems*, or ANSI/UL 2079, *Standard for Tests for Fire Resistance of Building Joint Systems*, under a minimum positive pressure differential of 0.01 in. water column (2.5 N/m$^2$) for a time period equal to that of the assembly. All test specimens shall comply with the minimum height or length required by the standard. Wall assemblies shall be subjected to a hose stream test in accordance with NFPA 251, *Standard Methods of Tests of Fire Resistance of Building Construction and Materials*; ASTM E 119, *Standard Test Methods for Fire Tests of Building Construction and Materials*; or ANSI/UL 263, *Standard for Fire Tests of Building Construction and Materials*.

**8.3.6.7* Exterior Curtain Walls and Perimeter Joints.**

**A.8.3.6.7** The provisions of 8.3.6.7 are intended to restrict the interior vertical passage of flame and hot gases from one floor to another at the location where the floor intersects the exterior wall assembly. The requirements of 8.3.6.7 mandate sealing the opening between a floor and an exterior wall assembly to provide the same fire performance as that required for the floor. ASTM E 2307, *Standard Test Method for Determining Fire Resistance of Perimeter Fire Barrier Systems Using Intermediate-Scale, Multi-Story Test Apparatus*, is a test method for evaluating the performance of perimeter fire barrier systems. Some laboratories have tested and listed perimeter fire barrier systems essentially in accordance with the ASTM method. The ASTM test method evaluates the performance of perimeter fire barrier systems in terms of heat transfer and fire spread inside a building through the floor/exterior wall intersection. The current test method does not assess the ability of perimeter fire barrier systems to prevent the spread of fire from story to story via the exterior. However, some laboratories have included additional temperature measurement criteria in their evaluation of the exterior wall, and also evaluate vision glass breakage as additional pass/fail criteria in an attempt to at least partially address this leapfrog effect.

**8.3.6.7.1** Voids created between the fire resistance–rated floor assembly and the exterior curtain wall shall be protected with a perimeter joint system that is designed and tested in accordance with ASTM E 2307, *Standard Test Method for Fire Resistance of Perimeter Fire Barriers Using Intermediate-Scale, Multi-story Apparatus*.

**8.3.6.7.2** The perimeter joint system shall have an F rating equal to the fire resistance rating of the floor assembly.

It is important that joints between and within fire barriers be protected by materials tested to ensure the integrity of the barrier. Like a weak link in a chain, an improperly protected joint in a fire barrier is likely to be the point of failure when exposed to fire.

## 8.4 Smoke Partitions

The concept of the smoke partition is intended to serve as another menulike item that can be referenced by other parts of the *Code*, especially the occupancy chapters, instead of repeating detailed criteria in many chapters. For an example of a mandate for the use of the smoke partition provisions of Section 8.4 in large residential board and care occupancies, see 32.3.3.6.3 and 33.3.3.6.3.2.

The smoke partition provisions offer options not available prior to the 2000 edition of the *Code* under the provisions for fire barriers and smoke barriers. For example, a smoke partition is not always required to have a fire resistance rating, but a fire barrier must have a rating. Also, a smoke partition is not required to have a smoke damper where ductwork penetrates the partition, but a duct penetration of a smoke barrier typically is required to do so.

### 8.4.1* General.

Where required elsewhere in this *Code*, smoke partitions shall be provided to limit the transfer of smoke.

**A.8.4.1** Although a smoke partition is intended to limit the free movement of smoke, it is not intended to provide an area that would be free of smoke.

Chapter 8 does not require the installation of smoke partitions but provides detailed criteria for smoke partitions where required by other sections of the *Code*. A smoke partition is a continuous membrane designed to form a barrier to limit the transfer of smoke.

### 8.4.2 Continuity.

The following shall apply to smoke partitions:

(1) They shall extend from the floor to the underside of the floor or roof deck above, through any concealed spaces, such as those above suspended ceilings, and through interstitial structural and mechanical spaces.

(2)* They shall be permitted to extend from the floor to the underside of a monolithic or suspended ceiling system where the following conditions are met:

  (a) The ceiling system forms a continuous membrane.
  (b) A smoke-tight joint is provided between the top of the smoke partition and the bottom of the suspended ceiling.
  (c) The space above the ceiling is not used as a plenum.

(3) Smoke partitions enclosing hazardous areas shall be permitted to terminate at the underside of a monolithic or suspended ceiling system where the following conditions are met:

  (a) The ceiling system forms a continuous membrane.
  (b) A smoke-tight joint is provided between the top of the smoke partition and the bottom of the suspended ceiling.
  (c) Where the space above the ceiling is used as a plenum, return grilles from the hazardous area into the plenums are not permitted.

**A.8.4.2(2)** An architectural, exposed, suspended-grid acoustical tile ceiling with penetrations for sprinklers, ducted HVAC supply and return-air diffusers, speakers, and recessed light fixtures is capable of limiting the transfer of smoke.

A smoke partition should be thought of as a barrier that reasonably limits, but does not necessarily prevent, smoke transfer. As such, there are suspended ceiling systems and monolithic surfaced ceilings that provide resistance to smoke transfer that is approximately equal to that of the traditional, nonrated corridor wall or partition. Smoke partitions are permitted to terminate tightly against the underside of such ceilings in accordance with 8.4.2(2). The concept is further described in A.8.4.2(2). The list of acceptable penetrating items (e.g., speakers, recessed light fixtures, and ducted HVAC air diffusers) makes it clear that a smoke partition is not intended to prevent all smoke transfer; rather, it limits the transfer of smoke to an acceptable level to provide for occupant life safety.

### 8.4.3 Opening Protectives.

**8.4.3.1** Doors in smoke partitions shall comply with 8.4.3.2 through 8.4.3.5.

**8.4.3.2** Doors shall comply with the provisions of 7.2.1.

**8.4.3.3** Doors shall not include louvers.

**8.4.3.4*** Door clearances shall be in accordance with NFPA 80, *Standard for Fire Doors and Other Opening Protectives*.

**A.8.4.3.4** Gasketing of doors should not be necessary, as the clearances in NFPA 80, *Standard for Fire Doors and Other Opening Protectives*, effectively achieve resistance to the passage of smoke if the door is relatively tight-fitting.

For swinging doors with builder's hardware, NFPA 80, *Standard for Fire Doors and Other Opening Protectives*, permits clearances of not more than $\frac{1}{8}$ in. (3.2 mm) [$\pm \frac{1}{16}$ in. (1.6 mm) for steel doors] between the door frame and the top and sides of the door. The clearance under the bottom of a fire door is permitted to be not more than $\frac{3}{4}$ in. (19 mm).

With the permitted clearances, some smoke will pass to the opposite side of a closed door. It is important to remember that the intent of the smoke partition is not to prevent all smoke transfer but, rather, to limit the transfer of smoke to an acceptable level.

**8.4.3.5** Doors shall be self-closing or automatic-closing in accordance with 7.2.1.8.

The five provisions applicable to doors in smoke partitions are individually addressed in 8.4.3.1 through 8.4.3.5 to allow each to be singled out in the references made by other sections of the *Code* that require smoke partitions. For example, 33.3.3.6.3.2 exempts existing large residential board and care occupancies in sprinklered buildings from the self-closing requirement of 8.4.3.5 but retains the other door provisions.

### 8.4.4 Penetrations.

The provisions of 8.4.4 shall govern the materials and methods of construction used to protect through-penetrations and membrane penetrations of smoke partitions.

**8.4.4.1** Penetrations for cables, cable trays, conduits, pipes, tubes, vents, wires, and similar items to accommodate electrical, mechanical, plumbing, and communications systems that pass through a smoke partition shall be protected by a system or material that is capable of limiting the transfer of smoke.

**8.4.4.2** Where designs take transmission of vibrations into consideration, any vibration isolation shall meet one of the following conditions:

(1) It shall be provided on either side of the smoke partition.
(2) It shall be designed for the specific purpose.

### 8.4.5 Joints.

**8.4.5.1** The provisions of 8.4.5 shall govern the materials and methods of construction used to protect joints in between and at the perimeter of smoke partitions or, where smoke partitions meet other smoke partitions, the floor or roof deck above, or the outside walls. The provisions of 8.4.5 shall not apply to approved existing materials and methods of construction used to protect existing joints in smoke partitions, unless otherwise required by Chapters 11 through 43.

**8.4.5.2** Joints made within or at the perimeter of smoke partitions shall be protected with a joint system that is capable of limiting the transfer of smoke.

### 8.4.6 Air-Transfer Openings.

**8.4.6.1 General.** The provisions of 8.4.6 shall govern the materials and methods of construction used to protect air-transfer openings in smoke partitions.

**8.4.6.2* Smoke Dampers.** Air-transfer openings in smoke partitions shall be provided with approved smoke dampers designed and tested in accordance with the requirements of ANSI/UL 555S, *Standard for Smoke Dampers*, to limit the transfer of smoke.

**A.8.4.6.2** An air-transfer opening, as defined in NFPA 90A, *Standard for the Installation of Air-Conditioning and Ventilating Systems*, is an opening designed to allow the movement of environmental air between two contiguous spaces.

**8.4.6.3 Smoke Damper Ratings.** Smoke damper leakage ratings shall be not less than Class II. Elevated temperature ratings shall be not less than 250°F (140°C).

**8.4.6.4 Smoke Detectors.** Dampers in air-transfer openings shall close upon detection of smoke by approved smoke detectors installed in accordance with *NFPA 72, National Fire Alarm Code*.

If ductwork runs to a smoke partition, pierces the partition, and continues its run on the other side of the partition, no transfer opening exists. Given that no transfer opening is present, there is no requirement for a smoke damper. If such ducted HVAC systems without dampers are to spread smoke, such smoke spread will occur due to the buoyant forces of the hot fire gases, because the provisions of NFPA 90A, *Standard for the Installation of Air-Conditioning and Ventilating Systems*, require the automatic shutdown of most of the fans that would otherwise circulate smoke through the ductwork.

## 8.5 Smoke Barriers

### 8.5.1* General.

Where required by Chapters 11 through 43, smoke barriers shall be provided to subdivide building spaces for the purpose of restricting the movement of smoke.

**A.8.5.1** Wherever smoke barriers and doors therein require a degree of fire resistance, as specified by requirements in the various occupancy chapters (Chapters 12 through 42), the construction should be a fire barrier that has been specified to limit the spread of fire and restrict the movement of smoke.

Although a smoke barrier is intended to restrict the movement of smoke, it might not result in tenability throughout the adjacent smoke compartment. The adjacent smoke compartment should be safer than the area on the fire side, thus allowing building occupants to move to that area. Eventually, evacuation from the adjacent smoke compartment might be required.

It is imprecise to refer to a "1-hour smoke barrier." It is more accurate to refer to a "smoke barrier that additionally has a 1-hour fire resistance rating." A barrier with only a fire resistance rating does not necessarily make an effective smoke barrier. For example, a fire barrier, if rated at less than 2 hours, would not be required to have either a fire damper or a smoke damper where ductwork penetrates the barrier. A smoke barrier, in accordance with Section 8.5, would have ducted penetrations protected by smoke dampers per 8.5.5.2. For additional information on fire barrier testing, rating, and installation, see the commentary following 8.2.3.2 and 8.3.5.7.

**8.5.2* Continuity.**

**A.8.5.2** To ensure that a smoke barrier is continuous, it is necessary to seal completely all openings where the smoke barrier abuts other smoke barriers, fire barriers, exterior walls, the floor below, and the floor or ceiling above. It is not the intent to prohibit a smoke barrier from stopping at a fire barrier if the fire barrier meets the requirements of a smoke barrier (i.e., the fire barrier is a combination smoke barrier/fire barrier).

**8.5.2.1** Smoke barriers required by this *Code* shall be continuous from an outside wall to an outside wall, from a floor to a floor, or from a smoke barrier to a smoke barrier, or by use of a combination thereof.

**8.5.2.2** Smoke barriers shall be continuous through all concealed spaces, such as those found above a ceiling, including interstitial spaces.

**8.5.2.3** A smoke barrier required for an occupied space below an interstitial space shall not be required to extend through the interstitial space, provided that the construction assembly forming the bottom of the interstitial space provides resistance to the passage of smoke equal to that provided by the smoke barrier.

In occupancies where evacuation is a last resort or is expected to be otherwise delayed, smoke barriers and doors will require a degree of fire resistance, as specified by the requirements found in the *Code*'s occupancy chapters (Chapters 12 through 42).

Other openings in smoke and fire barriers must be protected as well. HVAC ducts provide a ready path for smoke and fire to travel from one area to another unless carefully protected. Penetrations in walls and ceiling construction for utility lines and other building services must be firestopped to prevent fire spread. The hidden spaces above suspended ceilings and attic spaces are out of sight and easily overlooked.

The provision of 8.5.2.3 must be used with care. Several chapters require the smoke barrier to be fire resistance rated and, therefore, the smoke barrier would be permitted to terminate at the ceiling only if the ceiling were of the same rating (see commentary following A.8.2.2.3). Also, even if no fire resistance rating were required, it is difficult to ensure that a ceiling is smoke-tight, unless it is of monolithic construction without air-handling penetrations. This kind of construction is often found in apartment buildings, hotels, and dormitories; consequently, the provision of 8.5.2.3 can be useful.

**8.5.3 Fire Barrier Used as Smoke Barrier.**

A fire barrier shall be permitted to be used as a smoke barrier, provided that it meets the requirements of Section 8.5.

**8.5.4 Opening Protectives.**

**8.5.4.1*** Doors in smoke barriers shall close the opening, leaving only the minimum clearance necessary for proper operation, and shall be without undercuts, louvers, or grilles.

**A.8.5.4.1** The clearance for proper operation of smoke doors is defined as $\frac{1}{8}$ in. (3.2 mm). For additional information on the installation of smoke control door assemblies, see NFPA 105, *Standard for the Installation of Smoke Door Assemblies and Other Opening Protectives.*

NFPA 105, *Standard for the Installation of Smoke Door Assemblies and Other Opening Protectives,*[29] acknowledges that no nationally recognized test for the measurement of smoke leakage exists. However, NFPA 105 notes that ANSI/UL 1784, *Standard for Air Leakage Tests of Door Assemblies,*[30] can be used to measure ambient and warm air leakage rates of door assemblies.

ANSI/UL 1784, which is also referenced in 8.2.2.5, should determine satisfactory performance if recognized design features are also taken into account, such as close-fitting assemblies, limited deflections, and the use of gasketing and sealing materials. The document then provides performance criteria for determining maximum air leakage rates expressed in air volume per time per area of door opening.

**8.5.4.2** Where required by Chapters 11 through 43, doors in smoke barriers shall comply with the requirements of 8.2.2.5.

**8.5.4.3** Latching hardware shall not be required on doors in smoke barriers where permitted by Chapters 11 through 43.

**8.5.4.4*** Doors in smoke barriers shall be self-closing or automatic-closing in accordance with 7.2.1.8 and shall comply with the provisions of 7.2.1.

**A.8.5.4.4** Where, because of operational necessity, it is desired to have smoke barrier doors that are usually open, such doors should be provided with hold-open devices that are activated to close the doors by means of the operation of smoke detectors and other alarm functions.

Doors in smoke barriers are not generally required to have a fire protection rating, unless the occupancy chapter requires the smoke barrier itself to have a fire resistance rating. Therefore, any door that resists the passage of smoke, even a hollow-core wood door or glass door, is acceptable, provided that it is tight-fitting. Stops at the head and sides of the door help resist the passage of smoke. Where a pair of doors is used, it is recommended (and required for cross-corridor door assemblies in new health care occupancies) that they open in opposite directions from each other so that rabbets, bevels, or astragals can be provided at the meeting edges without the use of coordinators. See also 18.3.7.11.

Doors in smoke barriers, although not the equivalent of fire doors and not completely smoke-tight, are effective in restricting the spread of smoke and reducing drafts, which might otherwise spread fire rapidly. Where an occupancy chapter requires the smoke barrier to have a fire resistance rating, a 20-minute fire protection–rated door assembly in a smoke partition should be accepted as a reasonable barrier. It has been shown through tests that the commonly used $1\frac{3}{4}$ in. (44 mm) thick solid-bonded wood-core door assembly can be expected to fail in fire tests in 22 minutes to 24 minutes, but it has performed well in actual fires when closed.[31]

Doors in a fire separation, horizontal exit, or smoke barrier should be closed at all times to impede the spread of smoke and fire gases. Functionally, however, keeping the doors closed decreases efficiency. In a health care occupancy, for example, closed doors limit patient observation by staff. To accommodate such situations, it is practical to presume that the door will be kept open, even with the use of wood chocks or other makeshift devices. Where operational necessity dictates that smoke barrier doors normally are to be kept open, such doors should be provided with hold-open devices that are triggered to close the doors by the operation of smoke detectors (see Exhibit 8.8). See 7.2.1.8.2 for details on hold-open devices with automatic release mechanisms. For additional information on the use of smoke detectors for releasing service, see the commentary to A.9.6.3.2.3.

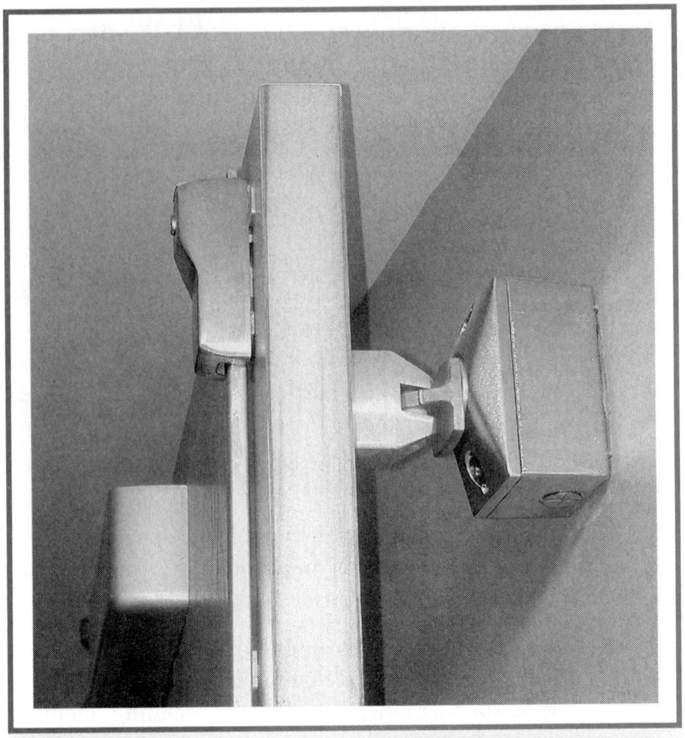

***Exhibit 8.8*** *Hold-open mechanism on automatic-closing door.*

**8.5.4.5** Fire window assemblies shall comply with 8.3.3.

## 8.5.5 Ducts and Air-Transfer Openings.

**8.5.5.1 General.** The provisions of 8.5.5 shall govern the materials and methods of construction used to protect ducts and air-transfer openings in smoke barriers.

**8.5.5.2 Smoke Dampers.** Where a smoke barrier is penetrated by a duct or air-transfer opening, a smoke damper designed and tested in accordance with the requirements of ANSI/UL 555S, *Standard for Smoke Dampers*, shall be installed. Where a smoke barrier is also constructed as a fire barrier, a combination fire/smoke damper designed and tested in accordance with the requirements of ANSI/UL 555, *Standard for Fire Dampers*, and ANSI/UL 555S shall be installed.

**8.5.5.3 Smoke Damper Exemptions.** Smoke dampers shall not be required under any of the following conditions:

(1) Where specifically exempted by provisions in Chapters 11 through 43
(2) Where ducts or air-transfer openings are part of an engineered smoke control system
(3) Where the air in ducts continues to move and the air-handling system installed is arranged to prevent recirculation of exhaust or return air under fire emergency conditions

Paragraph 8.5.5.3(2) addresses the omission of dampers in ducts that must remain open so that an engineered smoke control system can operate. The provision of 8.5.5.3(3) applies only in very limited cases. It can be used only on small ventilation systems, because NFPA 90A, *Standard for the Installation of Air-Conditioning and Ventilating Systems*, requires that systems over

15,000 ft$^3$/min (7080 L/s) that are not part of a smoke control system shut down upon detection of smoke.

Even without the restriction of NFPA 90A, it is difficult to ensure that the air-handling system will be in continuous operation. Because of increased awareness of energy conservation, many systems are cycled or shut down during parts of the day. The cycling or shutdown feature might be added later without recognizing its potential detriment to building life safety. However, the provisions of 8.5.5.3(3) can be useful for ductwork for small ventilation systems, such as those for toilet rooms or small suites.

(4) Where the air inlet or outlet openings in ducts are limited to a single smoke compartment

Paragraph 8.5.5.3(4) addresses situations where an "express" duct has no openings other than in a single smoke compartment. This provision can reasonably be extended to situations illustrated in Exhibit 8.9. Per the requirements of NFPA 90A, *Standard for the Installation of Air-Conditioning and Ventilating Systems*, only a single floor can be penetrated by ductwork not enclosed within a rated shaft system, and such an installation requires a fire damper at the plane of the floor where the penetration is located. Ducts penetrating more than one floor must be enclosed within an appropriately fire-rated shaft. Thus, where a smoke damper is exempted by 8.5.5.3(5), the resulting openings can potentially act as a minor route for smoke migration from one floor to another before the actuation of a fire damper. The floor, as a whole, serves as an adequate smoke barrier in accordance with the requirements of 8.6.1.

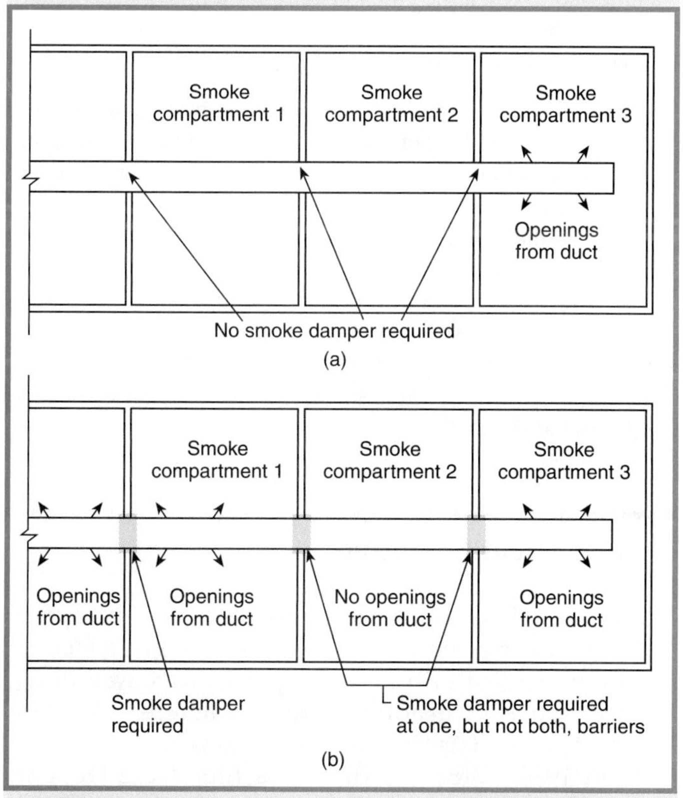


***Exhibit 8.9** Position of smoke dampers in air-handling ductwork.*

(5) Where ducts penetrate floors that serve as smoke barriers

(6) Where ducts penetrate smoke barriers forming a communicating space separation in accordance with 8.6.6(4)(a).

**8.5.5.4 Installation, Testing, and Maintenance.**

**8.5.5.4.1** Air-conditioning, heating, ventilating ductwork, and related equipment, including smoke dampers and combination fire and smoke dampers, shall be installed in accordance with NFPA 90A, *Standard for the Installation of Air-Conditioning and Ventilating Systems*, and NFPA 105, *Standard for the Installation of Smoke Door Assemblies and Other Opening Protectives*.

**8.5.5.4.2** Smoke dampers and combination fire and smoke dampers shall be inspected, tested, and maintained in accordance with NFPA 105, *Standard for the Installation of Smoke Door Assemblies and Other Opening Protectives*.

**8.5.5.4.3** The equipment specified in 8.5.5.4.1 shall be installed in accordance with the requirements of 8.5.5, the manufacturer's installation instructions, and the equipment listing.

**8.5.5.5 Access and Identification.** Access to the dampers shall be provided for inspection, testing, and maintenance. The access openings shall not reduce the fire resistance rating of the fire barrier assembly.

**8.5.5.6 Smoke Damper Ratings.** Smoke damper leakage ratings shall be not less than Class II. Elevated temperature ratings shall be not less than 250°F (140°C).

**8.5.5.7 Smoke Detectors.**

**8.5.5.7.1** Required smoke dampers in ducts penetrating smoke barriers shall close upon detection of smoke by approved smoke detectors in accordance with *NFPA 72, National Fire Alarm Code*, unless one of the following conditions exists:

(1) The ducts penetrate smoke barriers above the smoke barrier doors, and the door release detector actuates the damper.

(2) Approved smoke detector installations are located within the ducts in existing installations.

**8.5.5.7.2** Where a duct is provided on one side of the smoke barrier, the smoke detectors on the duct side shall be in accordance with 8.5.5.7.1.

**8.5.5.7.3** Required smoke dampers in air-transfer openings shall close upon detection of smoke by approved smoke detectors in accordance with *NFPA 72, National Fire Alarm Code*.

*NFPA 72®, National Fire Alarm Code®*,[32] provides information on the installation of smoke detectors that close smoke dampers. The damper is permitted to be closed by the same detector that closes the door in a smoke barrier if the duct penetrates the wall above the door. Existing installations of detectors installed within ducts, which might not be in total compliance with *NFPA 72*, continue to be recognized.

### 8.5.6 Penetrations.

**8.5.6.1** The provisions of 8.5.6 shall govern the materials and methods of construction used to protect through-penetrations and membrane penetrations of smoke barriers.

**8.5.6.2** Penetrations for cables, cable trays, conduits, pipes, tubes, vents, wires, and similar items to accommodate electrical, mechanical, plumbing, and communications systems that pass through a wall, floor, or floor/ceiling assembly constructed as a smoke barrier, or through the ceiling membrane of the roof/ceiling of a smoke barrier assembly, shall be protected by a system or material capable of restricting the transfer of smoke.

**8.5.6.3** Where a smoke barrier is also constructed as a fire barrier, the penetrations shall be protected in accordance with the requirements of 8.3.5 to limit the spread of fire for a time period equal to the fire resistance rating of the assembly and 8.5.6 to restrict the transfer of smoke, unless the requirements of 8.5.6.4 are met.

**8.5.6.4** Where sprinklers penetrate a single membrane of a fire resistance–rated assembly in buildings equipped throughout with an approved automatic fire sprinkler system, noncombustible escutcheon plates shall be permitted, provided that the space around each sprinkler penetration does not exceed $\frac{1}{2}$ in. (13 mm), measured between the edge of the membrane and the sprinkler.

**8.5.6.5** Where the penetrating item uses a sleeve to penetrate the smoke barrier, the sleeve shall be securely set in the smoke barrier, and the space between the item and the sleeve shall be filled with a material capable of restricting the transfer of smoke.

**8.5.6.6** Where designs take transmission of vibrations into consideration, any vibration isolation shall meet one of the following conditions:

(1) It shall be provided on either side of the smoke barrier.
(2) It shall be designed for the specific purpose.

### 8.5.7 Joints.

**8.5.7.1** The provisions of 8.5.7 shall govern the materials and methods of construction used to protect joints in between and at the perimeter of smoke barriers or, where smoke barriers meet other smoke barriers, the floor or roof deck above, or the outside walls. The provisions of 8.5.7 shall not apply to approved existing materials and methods of construction used to protect existing joints in smoke barriers, unless otherwise required by Chapters 11 through 43.

**8.5.7.2** Joints made within or at the perimeter of smoke barriers shall be protected with a joint system that is capable of limiting the transfer of smoke.

**8.5.7.3** Joints made within or between smoke barriers shall be protected with a smoke-tight joint system that is capable of limiting the transfer of smoke.

**8.5.7.4** Smoke barriers that are also constructed as fire barriers shall be protected with a joint system that is designed and tested to resist the spread of fire for a time period equal to the required fire resistance rating of the assembly and restrict the transfer of smoke.

**8.5.7.5** Testing of the joint system in a smoke barrier that also serves as fire barrier shall be representative of the actual installation suitable for the required engineering demand without compromising the fire resistance rating of the assembly or the structural integrity of the assembly.

As in the case of fire barriers, it is important to maintain the integrity of smoke barriers over the life of a building. Exhibit 8.10 illustrates some of the key items regarding smoke barrier penetrations discussed in 8.5.3 through 8.5.7.

## 8.6 Vertical Openings

Unprotected or improperly protected vertical openings have consistently been major contributing factors in multiple-death fires. This is particularly well illustrated by the two deadliest hotel fires in recent decades in the United States and its possessions.[33]

In 1986, 97 people died in a fire at the Dupont Plaza Hotel in San Juan, Puerto Rico. The unprotected vertical opening between the ballroom level, where

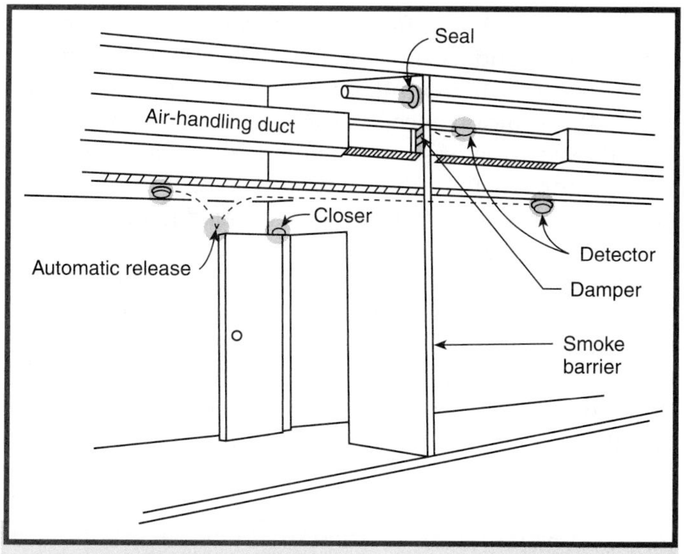


**Exhibit 8.10** *Typical penetrations of a smoke barrier.*

the fire originated, and the casino level, where nearly all the deaths occurred, would not be permitted by the *Code*, given the lack of other fire protection design features of that area.[34]

In the 1980 MGM Grand Hotel fire in Las Vegas, Nevada, where 85 people died, smoke spread via unprotected vertical openings (concealed spaces, elevator shafts) and insufficiently protected exit stair enclosures.[35] Many factors contributed to the vertical smoke spread, including the following:

1. Unprotected seismic joint shafts and elevator hoistways
2. Insufficiently fire resistance–rated construction used in interior stair enclosures
3. Exposure of exit stair and exit passageway spaces to casino level plenum air
4. Heating, ventilating, and air-conditioning systems with fire dampers that did not operate

Most of the hotel and motel fires of recent decades that have resulted in 10 or more fatalities have involved unprotected vertical openings, typically unenclosed interior stairs.

### 8.6.1 Floor Smoke Barriers.

Every floor that separates stories in a building shall meet the following criteria:

(1) It shall be constructed as a smoke barrier in accordance with Section 8.5.
(2) It shall be permitted to have openings as described by 8.6.6, 8.6.7, 8.6.8, or Chapters 11 through 43

Prior to the 2006 edition of the *Code*, floors were required to provide a basic degree of smoke compartmentation, consistent with the definition of the term *smoke barrier* in 3.3.27.2, without meeting the detailed requirements of Section 8.5. In the 2006 edition, a reference to Section 8.5 in 8.6.1(1) was added to require all floors to meet the detailed requirements for true smoke barriers. Note that duct penetrations through a floor are exempt from the requirement for a smoke damper at the penetration by 8.5.5.3(5).

Paragraph 8.6.1(2) emphasizes that the communicating space, atrium, and convenience opening concepts addressed in 8.6.6, 8.6.7, and 8.6.8, respectively, continue to be permitted, along with other unprotected vertical openings where permitted by the occupancy chapters. The use of such openings between floors should not be deemed to be in conflict with the requirements of Section 8.5 or 8.6.1(1).

### 8.6.2* Continuity.

Openings through floors shall be enclosed with fire barrier walls, shall be continuous from floor to floor, or floor to roof, and shall be protected as appropriate for the fire resistance rating of the barrier.

**A.8.6.2** Openings might include items such as stairways; hoistways for elevators, dumbwaiters, and inclined and vertical conveyors; shaftways used for light, ventilation, or building services; or expansion joints and seismic joints used to allow structural movements.

### 8.6.3 Continuity Exemptions.

The requirements of 8.6.2 shall not apply where otherwise permitted by the following:

(1) Where pneumatic tube conveyors are protected in accordance with 8.3.5.1
(2) Where specified by 8.6.6, 8.6.7, 8.6.8.1, 8.6.8.2, or Chapters 11 through 43
(3) Where escalators and moving walks are protected in accordance with 8.6.8.5 or 8.6.8.6
(4) Where expansion or seismic joints are designed to prevent the penetration of fire and are shown to have a fire resistance rating of not less than that required for the floor when tested in accordance with ANSI/UL 2079, *Standard for Tests for Fire Resistance of Building Joint Systems*
(5) Where existing mail chutes meet one of the following criteria:
    (a) The cross-sectional area does not exceed 0.1 $ft^2$ (0.01 $m^2$).
    (b) The building is protected throughout by an approved automatic sprinkler system in accordance with Section 9.7.

It is important to note that 8.6.1 and 8.6.2 apply to all occupancies, unless a specific occupancy chapter provides an alternative option. Protection of vertical openings is normally covered in the ___.3.1 subsection of each occupancy chapter (e.g., 12.3.1 for new assembly occupancies or 18.3.1 for new health care occupancies).

Protection of vertical openings is extremely important in reducing fire casualties. In report after report of fires involving fatalities, unprotected vertical openings were a major factor contributing to loss of life.

Vertical fire spread is also a major factor contributing to the extensive property damage that is characteristic of large-loss building fires; thus, a correlation frequently exists between loss of life from fire and monetary loss from fire. Vertical fire spread relates directly to the lack of protection for vertical openings, because the principal structural weakness responsible for the vertical spread of fire is the absence of the fire cutoffs at openings between floors.

Exhibit 8.11 illustrates some typical floor openings in buildings. If the exit stairs at each end of the building are not properly enclosed per the requirements of 7.1.3.2, they do not qualify as exits. If the exit stairs do not comply with the requirements of Section 8.6 and the ___.3.1 subsection of the appropriate occupancy chapter, they create unprotected vertical openings. The other floor openings illustrated in Exhibit 8.11 are not affected by the requirements applicable to exits, but do, if not properly enclosed, create unprotected vertical openings.

Based on lessons learned from the Las Vegas MGM Grand Hotel fire, the 1988 edition of the *Code* expanded the list of floor openings to include expansion joints and seismic joints that allow structural movement. In lieu of full enclosure from floor to floor, 8.6.3(4) specifically recognizes the use of fire protection–rated expansion or seismic joints with a minimum rating of not less than the required fire resistance rating of the floor. Without appropriately rated joints, the enclosure requirements might be satisfied by an arrangement of walls and doors as shown in Exhibit 8.12. Back-to-back fire resistance–rated barriers and cross-corridor fire protection–rated door assemblies accomplish the enclosure of the seismic joint running horizontally across the building and vertically through all floors.

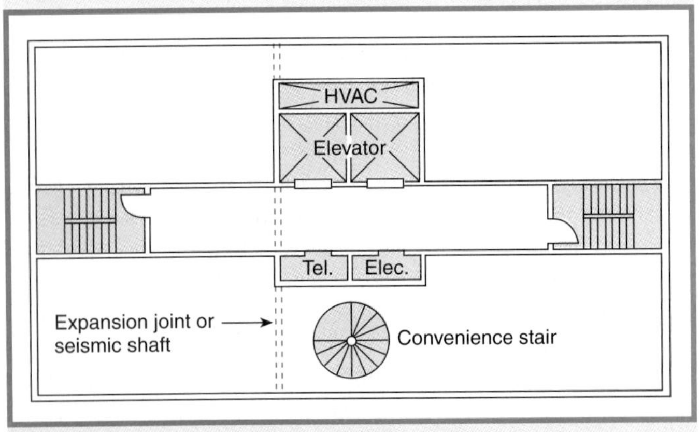


***Exhibit 8.11*** *Typical floor openings that, if not properly enclosed, might spread the effects of a fire from floor to floor.*

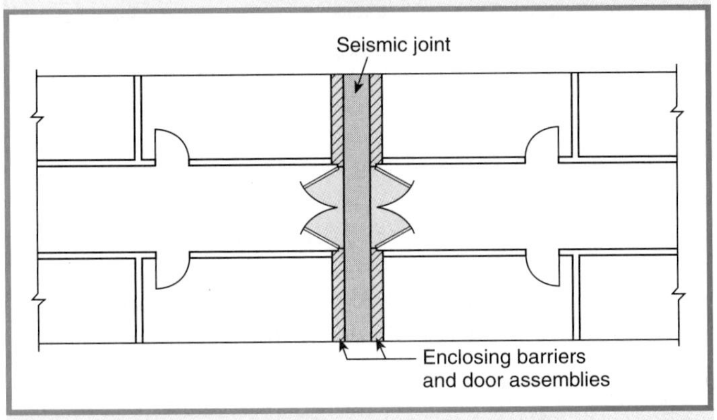


***Exhibit 8.12*** *Enclosure of seismic joint.*

## 8.6.4 Shafts.

Shafts that do not extend to the bottom or the top of the building or structure shall comply with either 8.6.4.1, 8.6.4.2, or 8.6.4.3.

**8.6.4.1** Shafts shall be enclosed at the lowest or highest level of the shaft, respectively, with construction in accordance with 8.6.5.

**8.6.4.2** Shafts shall be permitted to terminate in a room or space having a use related to the purpose of the shaft, provided that the room or space is separated from the remainder of the building by construction having a fire resistance rating and opening protectives in accordance with 8.6.5 and 8.3.4.

**8.6.4.3** Shafts that do not extend to the bottom or top of the building or structure shall be permitted to be protected by approved fire dampers installed in accordance with their listing at the lowest or highest floor level, as applicable, within the shaft enclosure.

Some shafts commonly found in buildings do not extend through the entire height of the building. For example, in a high-rise building, a percentage of the overall number of elevator shafts will service only the lower-rise portion of the building. Such shafts might run from the street level through the twentieth floor of a 40-story building. In a typical hotel that devotes the first couple of stories to assembly occupancy uses and locates guest rooms above in the hotel occupancy tower, the shafts associated with guest room bathroom exhaust might begin at the third floor and continue to the roof. In such cases, although the shaft walls are constructed of fire resistance–rated assemblies, an unprotected shaft ceiling/top or unprotected shaft floor/bottom would allow fire and other products of combustion to travel vertically to some other part of the building. Because of this concern, 8.6.4.1 requires that those shaft ceilings or shaft floors be protected by construction as required for the shaft walls.

Exhibit 8.13 illustrates various shaft arrangements. Shafts that do not run the full height of a building must be capped by floors or ceilings of fire resistance–rated construction at least equal to the required rating of the shaft-enclosing walls. Shaft A runs vertically for the full height of the building and requires only vertical fire barriers to separate the shaft from the remainder of the building interior. Because neither shaft B nor shaft C extends the full height of the building, horizontal fire barriers (a floor for shaft B and a ceiling for shaft C) must be provided to complete the shaft envelope. Shaft D, which is used for heating, ventilating, and air-conditioning (HVAC), extends vertically from the second floor to the roof; 8.6.4.2 makes it unnecessary to install a rated floor barrier between shaft D and the mechanical equipment room, E. In this case, the ceiling and walls of the mechanical equipment room, used for purposes related to the use of the HVAC shaft, must be constructed of material of at least the same hourly rating as required for shaft D. The room enclosure thus becomes an extension of the shaft. Access to room E from within the building would be gained through appropriately rated fire door assemblies.

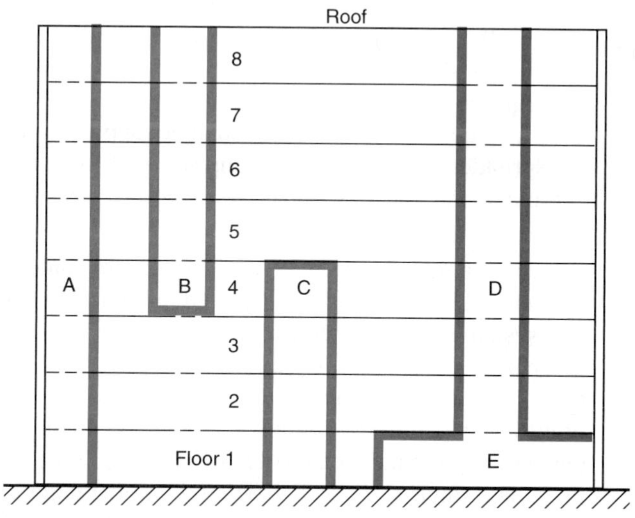


**Exhibit 8.13** *Shaft enclosures.*

### 8.6.5* Required Fire Resistance Rating.

The minimum fire resistance rating for the enclosure of floor openings shall be as follows *(see 7.1.3.2.1 for enclosure of exits)*:

(1) Enclosures connecting four or more stories in new construction — 2-hour fire barriers
(2) Other enclosures in new construction — 1-hour fire barriers
(3) Existing enclosures in existing buildings — ½-hour fire barriers
(4) Enclosures for lodging and rooming houses — as specified in Chapter 26
(5) Enclosures for new hotels — as specified in Chapter 28
(6) Enclosures for new apartment buildings — as specified in Chapter 30

**A.8.6.5** The application of the 2-hour rule in buildings not divided into stories is permitted to be based on the number of levels of platforms or walkways served by the stairs.

Where addressing vertical openings, the *Code* does not use the height of buildings or a designated number of floors above ground as the basis for its rated enclosure requirements. Rather, such requirements are based on the total number of floors connected by the vertical opening. For example, if there is a vertical opening between the second, third, and fourth stories of an eight-story building, the opening connects fewer than four floors and the enclosure must be of 1-hour, rather than 2-hour, fire resistance–rated construction.

Where a vertical opening in new construction connects four stories or more, the enclosure protection afforded must have at least a 2-hour fire resistance rating. This requirement applies whether the stories are above the exit discharge level, below the exit discharge level, or any combination thereof. Where a vertical opening in new construction connects three or fewer stories, the enclosure rating must be at least 1 hour. Existing vertical openings, regardless of the number of stories they connect, require protection by ½-hour fire resistance–rated enclosures.

See Exhibit 8.14 for illustrations of the vertical opening protection requirements for new construction. Although Exhibit 8.14 depicts vertical openings that resemble exit stair enclosures, the same requirements apply to any type of vertical opening, including exit access stairs and elevator, electrical, HVAC, and seismic shafts.

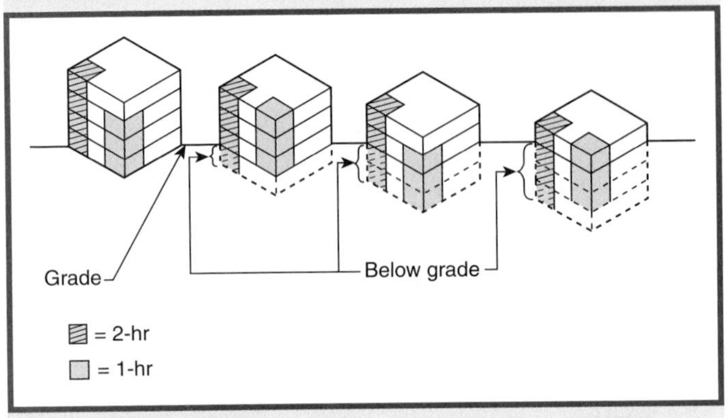


***Exhibit 8.14*** *Vertical opening protection requirements.*

Experience shows that, under some circumstances, each of the 1-hour and 2-hour rating levels provides a comfortable period of time for the occupants of a building to evacuate. On the other hand, there are times when the integrity of the construction will be taxed to its limit (e.g., during a fire that has gone undetected for a long period). This type of fire can generate heavy smoke and toxic gases that complicate evacuation by blocking the exit access.

An interior exit stair (see definition of *exit* in 3.3.75) must be enclosed to be separated from other building spaces and to provide a protected way of travel to the exit discharge. If not properly enclosed, the exit not only fails to meet the definition of an exit but also creates an unprotected vertical opening. Thus, an exit stair must meet the requirements for enclosure of an exit (see 7.1.3.2), as well as those for protection of vertical openings in accordance with 8.6.5, as modified by the applicable occupancy chapter. Because the requirements for exit enclosures are more stringent than the requirements for protection of vertical openings, once the more stringent requirements have been met, the other requirements are usually met automatically.

The provisions of 8.6.5(4) through (6) reference the lodging or rooming, hotel, and apartment occupancy chapters, which permit modifications to the requirements of 8.6.5 under certain conditions. Some of the provisions permit 1-hour-rated enclosures, regardless of the number of stories connected, if the building is protected throughout by automatic sprinklers and it is not a high-rise building. Although these occupancy chapters use such modifications to temper the basic Chapter 8 requirements with respect to the enclosure of vertical openings, it is possible for a specific occupancy chapter to be more stringent. For example, see 19.3.1.1, which requires 1-hour enclosures in existing health care occupancies rather than the ½-hour enclosures that would otherwise be permitted by 8.6.5(3).

### 8.6.6 Communicating Space.

Unless prohibited by Chapters 11 through 43, unenclosed floor openings forming a communicating space between floor levels shall be permitted, provided that the following conditions are met:

(1) The communicating space does not connect more than three contiguous stories.

(2) The lowest or next-to-lowest story within the communicating space is a street floor.

(3) The entire floor area of the communicating space is open and unobstructed, such that a fire in any part of the space will be readily obvious to the occupants of the space prior to the time it becomes an occupant hazard.

(4) The communicating space is separated from the remainder of the building by fire barriers with not less than a 1-hour fire resistance rating, unless one of the following is met:

  (a) In buildings protected throughout by an approved automatic sprinkler system in accordance with Section 9.7, a smoke barrier in accordance with Section 8.5 shall be permitted to serve as the separation required by 8.6.6(4).

  (b) The requirement of 8.6.6(4) shall not apply to fully sprinklered residential housing units of detention and correctional occupancies in accordance with 22.3.1(2) and 23.3.1.1(2).

(5) The communicating space has ordinary hazard contents protected throughout by an approved automatic sprinkler system in accordance with Section 9.7 or has only low hazard contents. *(See 6.2.2.)*

(6) Egress capacity is sufficient to allow all the occupants of all levels within the communicating space to simultaneously egress the communicating space by considering it as a single floor area in determining the required egress capacity.

(7)* Each occupant within the communicating space has access to not less than one exit without having to traverse another story within the communicating space.

**A.8.6.6(7)** Given that a mezzanine meeting the maximum one-third area criterion of 8.6.9.2.1 is not considered a story, it is permitted, therefore, to have 100 percent of its exit access within the communicating area run back through the story below.

(8) Each occupant not in the communicating space has access to not less than one exit without having to enter the communicating space.

Subsection 8.6.6 recognizes a vertical opening that is exempt from the normal enclosure requirements of 8.6.5 under the following two conditions:

1. The pertinent occupancy chapter for the occupancy type in question does not specifically prohibit use of the provision.
2. All the alternative protection provisions of 8.6.6(1) through (8) are met.

The provisions of 8.6.6 are often referred to as the "mini-atrium" requirements. Because they are limited to a maximum three-story vertical opening, the requirements are not as stringent as those of 8.6.7, which apply to atria that can involve vertical openings that communicate among any number of stories. A two- or three-story communicating space can be adequately protected by the requirements of 8.6.6 without having to apply the more stringent requirements of 8.6.7. The fact that a two- or three-story space is labeled as an "atrium" on building plans does not necessarily mean that it must be protected by the requirements of 8.6.7. A two- or three-story vertical opening, irrespective of what it is called, is permitted to be protected per the requirements of 8.6.6, provided that doing so is not prohibited by the occupancy chapter(s) involved and the requirements of 8.6.6(1) through (8) are met.

Paragraphs 1 through 8, which follow, explain and illustrate the provisions of 8.6.6(1) through (8).

**1.** The vertical space cannot connect or communicate among more than three stories, and all connected stories are required to be contiguous to each other. However, the building housing the vertical opening in question is permitted to be more than three stories in height. For example, the vertical opening might communicate among floors 1 through 3 of a six-story building, as shown in Exhibit 8.15.

**2.** The lowest of the maximum three communicating floor levels must be at, or not more than one level below, the street level. In other words, the vertical opening can communicate among only the first, second, and third floors or among the basement and first and second floors. See the space labeled *A* in Exhibit 8.15. As previously mentioned, additional building floor levels might be present either above or below the floors involving the vertical opening, but these additional floors cannot be left open to the vertical opening. The more stringent set of provisions for atria per 8.6.7 should be considered where it is necessary or desirable either to have more than three levels open or to locate the communicating levels such that the lowest level does not meet the placement requirement with respect to street level.

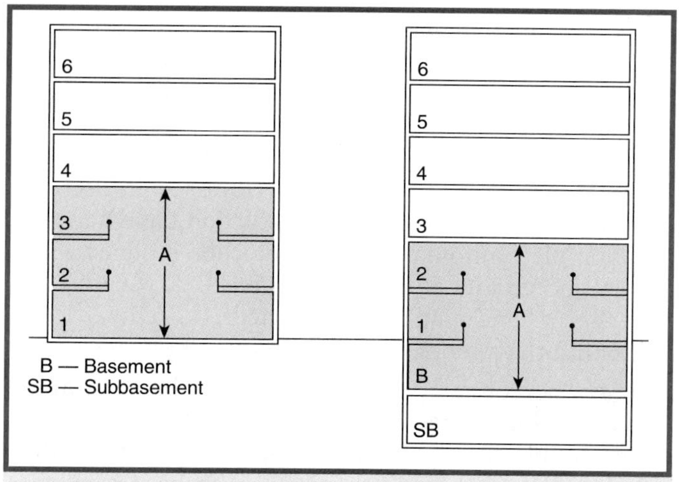


***Exhibit 8.15*** *Permitted location of three-story vertical opening.*

**3.** The communicating space includes all of the areas within the vertical opening itself and all of the adjoining areas left open to the vertical opening, as well as those areas not separated by minimum 1-hour fire resistance–rated barriers. The communicating space must be open and unobstructed, so that occupants of the space will be aware of fire and smoke conditions emanating from any part of the communicating space prior to the time that such conditions become a hazard.

The provisions of 8.6.6 were originally written to recognize typical mercantile occupancy construction practices, which left partial, mezzanine-like floors open to the main street-level shopping floor below. These arrangements were sufficiently open so that, where coupled with the other provisions, they allowed sufficient time for the necessary awareness of emergency conditions and for occupants to use the egress system. These provisions were not intended to be used for an unenclosed stair. The size of the small opening created by an unenclosed stair is insufficient to provide occupants on all levels connected by the stair with the needed degree of awareness.

Between the two extremes of vast amounts of openness (as in the case of the mezzanine-like floors described in the previous paragraph) and little or no openness (as depicted by the unenclosed stair), judging sufficient openness can be difficult. Through the use of the equivalency concept addressed in Section 1.4, some authorities having jurisdiction have permitted complete automatic smoke detection systems with proper occupant notification features to be substituted for the openness and unobstructedness required by 8.6.6(3) for awareness and early warning purposes.

**4.** The communicating space must be separated from the remainder of the building by fire barriers with a minimum 1-hour fire resistance rating. Once the boundaries of the communicating space are established, based on determining how much area is open enough [per the requirement of 8.6.6(3) referenced in the previous paragraph] to allow awareness and early warning, then areas outside these boundaries must be separated from the communicating space associated with the vertical opening by barriers with a minimum 1-hour fire resistance rating. If the building is fully sprinklered, the barriers are permitted to be nonrated but must resist the passage of smoke and meet the other smoke barrier requirements of Section 8.5. It is assumed that the sprinkler system will control the fire and make fire resistance–rated barriers unnecessary. The smoke barriers will control the limited smoke, under sprinklered conditions, and help maintain a tenable means of egress route.

For example, consider a hotel building with fingerlike guest room wings fanning out from the vertical opening. It can be assumed that the guest room wing corridors will need separation from the vertical opening, because occupants in the corridor on the second or third floor will not be readily aware of a fire on the first floor before it becomes a hazard to their safety. The required 1-hour separation can be provided, while maintaining the perception of openness, by isolating the guest room wings from the vertical opening through the use of pairs of cross-corridor doors held open with automatic release devices. See Exhibit 8.16.

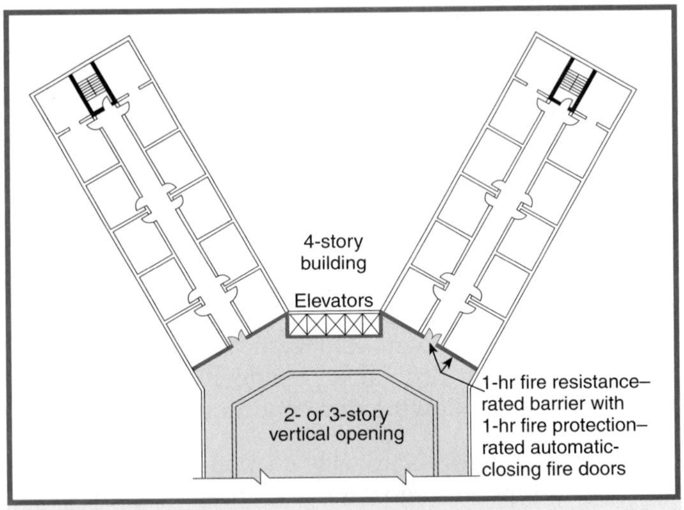


***Exhibit 8.16*** *Separation of two- or three-story communicating space from remainder of building.*

**5.** If the communicating space (the vertical opening itself and all adjoining areas open to it, as described in the first paragraph of item 3) contains *ordinary hazard contents* (as specified in Section 6.2 of this *Code*, as opposed to *ordinary hazard occupancies* as defined in NFPA 13, *Standard for the Installation of Sprinkler Systems*)[36], all areas within the confines of the communicating space must be sprinklered. If the contents are *low hazard contents* (as specified in Section 6.2 of this *Code*, rather than *light hazard occupancies* as defined in NFPA 13), no sprinkler system is required by 8.6.6. However, as intended by Section 6.2, most occupancies contain ordinary hazard contents. Because only low hazard and ordinary hazard contents are addressed in 8.6.6(5), high hazard contents are prohibited from any communicating spaces recognized by 8.6.6.

Although sprinkler system protection is required with ordinary hazard contents, only the communicating space (as previously defined) needs to be sprinklered, as specified by 8.6.6. The sprinkler system should cover all areas within the boundaries established by the 1-hour fire barriers that are required by 8.6.6(4). See Exhibit 8.16.

In Exhibit 8.16, the cross-corridor fire doors are held open by automatic release devices so that the corridor appears to be open to the communicating area of the vertical opening. Yet, because there are doors and a barrier at that location, they demarcate the boundary between the communicating space and the floor area outside the communicating space. Sprinkler protection must be provided for the vertical opening and the shaded adjoining areas up to the 1-hour barriers.

**6.** Because all occupants within the communicating area might be exposed within a short time to the effects of a fire within the area, simultaneous evacuation capability needs to be provided. Thus, the combined occupant load for all spaces, on all levels, within the boundaries of the communicating area needs to be included when sizing the means of egress for the communicating area. This requirement is more stringent than the provision of 7.3.1.4, which does not require the accumulation of occupant loads from various floors when determining the required egress capacity for exit stairs.

**7.** Per the requirements of 8.6.6(3) and (4), the communicating space is that space that is sufficiently open to the vertical opening to allow ready awareness of fire conditions on that and other levels within the communicating space. Areas that are remote enough from the vertical opening to lose the requisite awareness must be located on the other side of 1-hour fire resistance–rated fire barriers and are considered to be outside the communicating space. Thus, in a typical office building making use of the provisions of 8.6.6, for example, some occupants work and are normally stationed within the communicating space, while others work and are stationed outside the communicating space. This arrangement is shown in Exhibit 8.17.

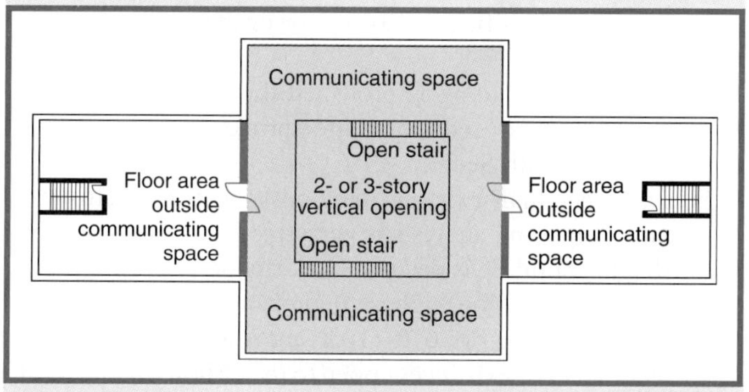


***Exhibit 8.17** Exit access arrangement for building using the two- or three-story vertical opening provision.*

Occupants located within the communicating space must have access to at least one exit without having to traverse another story within the communicating space per 8.6.6(7). The communicating space shown in Exhibit 8.17 would meet this requirement by allowing occupants to travel horizontally across the communicating space, pass through the fire doors in the fire-rated barrier into one of the building wings designated as "floor area outside communicating space," and continue to that wing's enclosed exit stair. In other words, the occupants of the communicating space are not permitted to use the open stairs exclusively to travel to another level of the communicating space to reach the required exits.

In the example illustrated in Exhibit 8.17, assume that some occupants of the communicating space are farther from either of the enclosed exit stairs, which are located at each end of the building, than the travel distance permitted by other *Code* requirements. Further, assume that those same occupants of the communicating space can travel down the open stair and across the bottom floor of the vertical opening to an exterior exit door within the permitted travel distance limitation. The open stair, although it is not an exit, could be considered as exit access, and the door to the outside at the lowest level of the vertical opening could then be regarded as the nearest *Code*-complying exit for those occupants. Either of the enclosed exit stairs at the end of the building could then serve as the second exit for those occupants of the communicating space. The enclosed exit stairs would then serve the following three purposes, none of which would be as the primary exit for those occupants of the communicating space:

**a.** The stairs would satisfy the business occupancy chapters' requirements that the minimum two required exits be located on the floor.
**b.** Either stair would satisfy the requirement of 8.6.6(7) that the occupants of the communicating space have access to at least one exit without having to traverse another story within the communicating space.
**c.** Each stair would satisfy the requirement of 8.6.6(8), discussed in the commentary that follows in paragraph 8, which mandates that each occupant not located within the communicating space is to have access to at least one exit without entering the communicating space.

**8.** Although all occupants must have access to two separate exits, the occupants who are located on any of the maximum of three floors that are permitted to communicate with the vertical opening, but who are not within the communicating space (as illustrated in Exhibit 8.17 by the wings located at each end of the building), must be able to reach one of the two required exits without entering the communicating space. Locating an enclosed exit stair within each of the floor areas outside the communicating space satisfies this requirement.

The provisions of 8.6.6 are permitted, unless prohibited by an occupancy chapter. For an example of an occupancy that prohibits the two- or three-story vertical opening, see 18.3.1.5 and 19.3.1.5, which apply to new and existing health care occupancies, respectively. For an example of an occupancy that provides requirements in addition to those of 8.6.6(1) through (8), see 14.3.1.2 and 15.3.1.2, which apply to new and existing educational occupancies, respectively. Chapters 14 and 15 require that the entire building, rather than only the communicating space, be protected by a supervised automatic sprinkler system.

### 8.6.7* Atriums.

**A.8.6.7** Where atriums are used, there is an added degree of safety to occupants because of the large volume of space into which smoke can be dissipated. However, there is a need to ensure that dangerous concentrations of smoke are promptly removed from the atrium, and the exhaust system needs careful design. For information about systems that can be used to provide smoke protection in these spaces, see the following:

(1) NFPA 92B, *Standard for Smoke Management Systems in Malls, Atria, and Large Spaces*
(2) *Principles of Smoke Management*

Unless prohibited by Chapters 11 through 43, an atrium shall be permitted, provided that the following conditions are met:

(1) The atrium is separated from the adjacent spaces by fire barriers with not less than a 1-hour fire resistance rating with opening protectives for corridor walls, unless one of the following is met:
   (a) The requirement of 8.6.7(1) shall not apply to existing, previously approved atriums.
   (b) Any number of levels of the building shall be permitted to open directly to the atrium without enclosure based on the results of the engineering analysis required in 8.6.7(5).
   (c)* Glass walls and inoperable windows shall be permitted in lieu of the fire barriers where all the following are met:
      i. Automatic sprinklers are spaced along both sides of the glass wall and the inoperable windows at intervals not to exceed 6 ft (1830 mm).
      ii. The automatic sprinklers specified in 8.6.7(1)(c)(i) are located at a distance from the glass wall not to exceed 12 in. (305 mm) and arranged so that the entire surface of the glass is wet upon operation of the sprinklers.
      iii. The glass wall is of tempered, wired, or laminated glass held in place by a gasket system that allows the glass framing system to deflect without breaking (loading) the glass before the sprinklers operate.
      iv. The automatic sprinklers required by 8.6.7(1)(c)(i) are not required on the atrium side of the glass wall and the inoperable window where there is no walkway or other floor area on the atrium side above the main floor level.
      v. Doors in the glass walls are of glass or other material that resists the passage of smoke.
      vi. Doors in the glass walls are self-closing or automatic-closing upon detection of smoke.
      vii. The glass is continuous vertically, without horizontal mullions, window treatments, or other obstructions that would interfere with the wetting of the entire glass surface.

**A.8.6.7(1)(c)** The intent of the requirement for closely spaced sprinklers is to wet the atrium glass wall to ensure that the surface of the glass is wet upon operation of the sprinklers, with a maximum spacing of sprinklers of 6 ft (1830 mm) on centers. Provided that it can be shown that the glass can be wet by the sprinklers using a given discharge rate, and that the 6 ft (1830 mm) spacing is not exceeded, the intent of the requirement is met. It is important that the entire glass area surface is wet. Due consideration should be given to the height of the glass panels and any horizontal members that might interfere with sprinkler wetting action.

(2) Access to exits is permitted to be within the atrium, and exit discharge in accordance with 7.7.2 is permitted to be within the atrium.
(3) The occupancy within the atrium meets the specifications for classification as low or ordinary hazard contents. *(See 6.2.2.)*
(4) The entire building is protected throughout by an approved, supervised automatic sprinkler system in accordance with Section 9.7.
(5)* For other than existing, previously approved atriums, an engineering analysis is performed that demonstrates that the building is designed to keep the smoke layer interface above the highest unprotected opening to adjoining spaces, or 6 ft (1830 mm) above the highest floor level of exit access open to the atrium, for a period equal to 1.5 times the calculated egress time or 20 minutes, whichever is greater.

**A.8.6.7(5)** See NFPA 92B, *Standard for Smoke Management Systems in Malls, Atria, and Large Spaces*. The engineering analysis should include the following elements:

(1) Fire dynamics, including the following:
   (a) Fire size and location
   (b) Materials likely to be burning
   (c) Fire plume geometry
   (d) Fire plume or smoke layer impact on means of egress
   (e) Tenability conditions during the period of occupant egress
(2) Response and performance of building systems, including passive barriers, automatic detection and extinguishing, and smoke control
(3) Response time required for building occupants to reach building exits, including any time required to exit through the atrium as permitted by 8.6.7(2)

(6)* In other than existing, previously approved atriums, where an engineered smoke control system is installed to meet the requirements of 8.6.7(5), the system is independently activated by each of the following:

(a) Required automatic sprinkler system
(b) Manual controls that are readily accessible to the fire department

**A.8.6.7(6)** Activation of the ventilation system by manual fire alarms, extinguishing systems, and detection systems can cause unwanted operation of the system, and it is suggested that consideration be given to zoning of the activation functions so the ventilation system operates only when actually needed.

Atria are permitted in accordance with 8.6.7, unless prohibited by an occupancy chapter. Although no occupancy chapter currently prohibits atria, some impose additional limitations. For example, health care occupancies prohibit the open floors addressed by 8.6.7(1)(b) from involving patient sleeping and treatment rooms. Thus, there would need to be, at a minimum, a smoke-resisting membrane, such as a glass window, between the patient room and the atrium space.

Exhibit 8.18 and Exhibit 8.19 illustrate a typical atrium.

The provisions of 8.6.7 address a vertical opening that communicates among more than the three floors addressed by the communicating space, or "mini-atrium," provisions of 8.6.6. Although the atrium provisions are not prohibited from being used for two- or three-story, atrium-like vertical openings, the provisions of 8.6.6 should adequately protect a two- or three-story "mini-atrium." The design professional should be permitted to protect such areas in accordance with the less stringent provisions of 8.6.6, provided that the occupancy chapter in question does not prohibit doing so. For example, the ___.3.1 subsections of Chapters 18 and 19, which address the protection of vertical openings in health care occupancies, prohibit the use of the mini-atrium provisions of 8.6.6. Thus, in health care occupancies, a two- or three-story atrium-like vertical opening is permitted only if it meets all

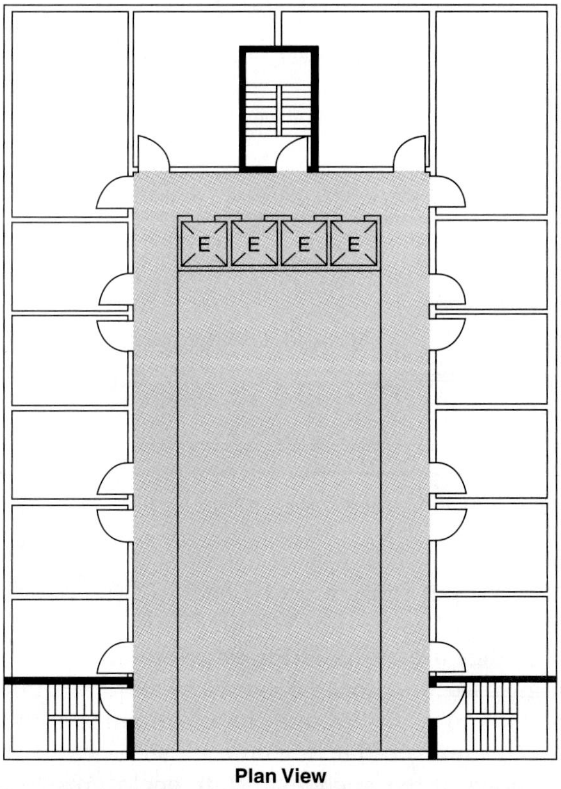


***Exhibit 8.18*** *Plan view of a typical atrium.*

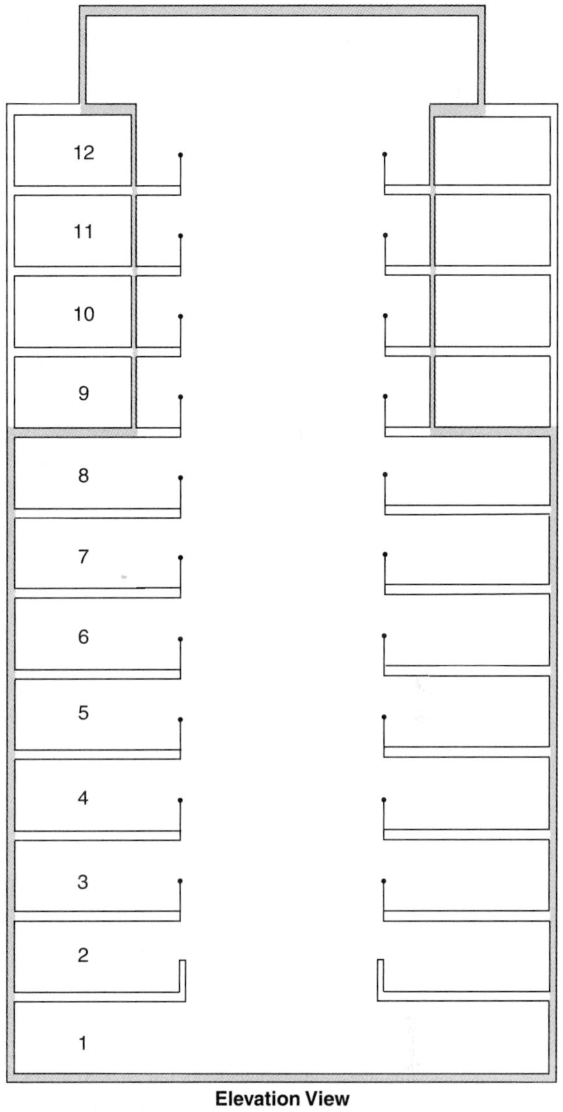


***Exhibit 8.19*** *Elevation view of a typical atrium.*

criteria of 8.6.7 applicable to atria. For certain designs, 8.6.6 is not desirable due to its restriction on exit access within the vertical opening. For example, a three-story hotel would prefer to use the more stringent provisions of 8.6.7, because they would permit the guest rooms to have exit access through the atrium, whereas 8.6.6 would not permit exit access to be solely through the communicating space.

The protection provisions of 8.6.7(1) through (6) are explained and illustrated in paragraphs 1 through 6, which follow.

**1.** In accordance with the requirements of 8.6.5(1), a vertical opening of four or more stories in new construction generally must be separated from the rest of the building by an enclosure of 2-hour fire resistance–rated construction. However, the atrium provisions work together as an overall package in permitting the construction that separates other areas of the building from the atrium to be reduced to a 1-hour fire resistance rating. Further, the doors in the 1-hour atrium fire barrier are permitted to be 20-minute fire protection–rated assemblies, as permitted for corridor doors. Thus, the intent of the 1-hour separation requirement is mainly to provide a carefully constructed smoke-resistant barrier.

Per 8.6.7(1)(b), any number of levels is permitted to be left open to the atrium, based on the engineering analysis required in 8.6.7(5). In Exhibit 8.20, floors 2 through 5 have been left open to the atrium. (In Exhibit 8.19, the open levels occur on floors 1 through 8.) Some occupancy chapters modify the atrium requirements as needed to afford the users of those occupancies the level of life safety needed. For example, for health care occupancies, Chapters 18 and 19 limit the location of the open levels permitted by 8.6.7(1)(b) so that patient treatment and sleeping rooms are not left open to the atrium.

To allow visual contact between the atrium and floors that have not been proven by engineering analysis to warrant openness, 8.6.7(1)(c) exempts the 1-hour-rated separation if a smoke-resisting separation is provided. The use of glass walls, vision panels, and windows in lieu of 1-hour-rated fire barriers is recognized by 8.6.7(1)(c). The intent of the requirement for directing closely spaced sprinklers at the glass walls is explained in A.8.6.7(1)(c).

The concept of wetting the glass that is exposed to a fire, without specifying a water application rate, is similar to boiling water in a Pyrex® container over an open flame. As long as there is some water present to absorb the heat, the glass itself does not reach excessive temperatures that would cause failure. To ensure that water will reach the surface of the glass, window blinds and draperies must not be placed between the line of closely spaced sprinklers and the glass. Careful design will allow for the sprinklers to be placed close enough to the glass so that blinds and draperies can be installed using normal installation practice.

The permission to omit lines of closely spaced sprinklers on the atrium side of glass walls, which are to be used in lieu of 1-hour fire resistance–rated barriers, is intended to apply to the floor levels above the atrium main floor level. In other words, if glass walls are used on the main floor level in lieu of a 1-hour fire barrier, sprinklers must be installed on both sides of the glass at that level, because combustibles might be placed on the floor on the atrium side of the glass. A similar condition occurs on floors 6, 7, and 8, where combustibles could be placed on the balcony floor adjacent to the glass. See Exhibit 8.20.

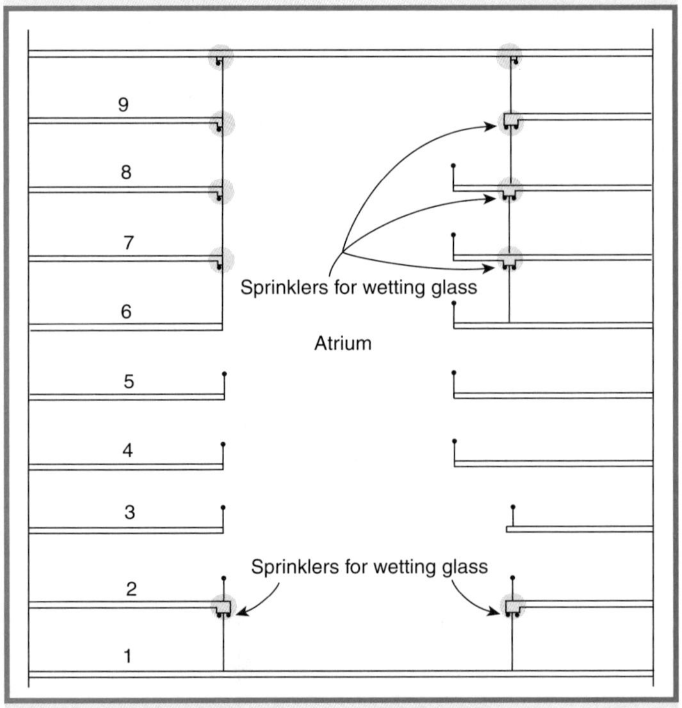


***Exhibit 8.20*** *Floor levels open to atrium.*

**2.** The exit stairs must be enclosed in accordance with the exit enclosure requirements of 7.1.3.2, although they are permitted to be within the communicating space and located so as to require building occupants to walk through the communicating space of the atrium in order to gain access to them. Exhibit 8.18 shows three such exit stair enclosures located within the communicating space, with all occupants of the floor required to walk within the communicating space across the interior exit access balcony of that floor in order to gain access to the stairs. Up to 50 percent of those three exits — that is, one exit in the given example — is permitted to discharge occupants from upper or lower floors through the level of exit discharge in accordance with 7.7.2, thus forcing some occupants to walk across the floor of the atrium to reach a door to the outside. The stringent requirements of 8.6.7(1) through (6) ensure an adequate overall life safety package, allowing the exit access and as much as half of the exit discharge to be within the atrium.

**3.** The occupancy within the atrium [the vertical opening and all floor areas left open to the vertical opening, such as balcony-like walking surfaces and the levels permitted to be left completely open via the provisions of 8.6.7(1)(b)] is limited to low hazard or ordinary hazard contents, as addressed in 6.2.2. High hazard contents are thus prohibited from being placed within the atrium but could be within hazardous area rooms surrounded by fire barriers in accordance with the provisions of Section 8.7. Because the provisions of 8.6.7(4) require that the building be completely protected by an approved, supervised automatic sprinkler system, the presence of only low hazard contents within the communicating space does not exempt the space from the sprinkler requirement. However, under the communicating space, or "mini-atrium" provisions of 8.6.6, such an exemption is permitted.

**4.** The entire building, not only the communicating space involving the atrium opening, must be protected by an approved, supervised automatic sprinkler system meeting the requirements of Section 9.7. Assuming that the atrium is located in a hotel building of five or more stories, for example, the provisions of Section 9.7 require the use of NFPA 13, *Standard for the Installation of Sprinkler Systems*.

A question that frequently arises is whether sprinklers are required, or whether they will be effective, at the ceilings of atria, which can be very high relative to the floor level. Prior to the 1997 edition of the *Code*, an exception allowed the authority having jurisdiction to permit the omission of sprinklers at the tops of atria where the ceiling height was greater than 55 ft (17 m) above the floor. This exception was removed for the 1997 and subsequent editions because there is no scientific evidence to suggest that sprinklers are ineffective at such heights. In fact, data submitted to the technical committee responsible for these provisions indicates that sprinklers can effectively extinguish or control fires at heights on the order of 100 ft (30 m) above the floor. Neither this *Code* nor NFPA 13 permits the omission of sprinklers from the ceilings of atria.

**5.** An engineered smoke control or smoke removal system acceptable to the authority having jurisdiction has been required since the atrium provisions were first introduced into the *Life Safety Code* in the 1981 edition. As advisory, but nonmandatory, information, the appendix of earlier editions suggested that, depending on atrium height and volume, either four or six air changes per hour could provide the smoke exhaust rate needed to meet the tenability conditions intended by the requirement for atrium smoke control.

The guideline for six air changes per hour came to be considered law by many authorities having jurisdiction and was thus accepted as the norm by many system designers. Authorities having jurisdiction then subjected such systems to acceptance testing using smoke bombs that produce cold smoke, which does not have the heat, buoyancy, and entrainment of air from a real fire. The acceptance criteria were further complicated by those who mistakenly believed that the intent of the smoke control requirement was, for example, that no smoke be visible within the atrium at the end of a 10-minute test. Designers found that, to ensure that the acceptance test could be passed, the system should provide approximately 10 to 12 air changes per hour. In effect, atria smoke control systems were typically designed to pass the acceptance test with no consideration or assurance of effective smoke control under fire conditions. NFPA 92B, *Standard for Smoke Management Systems in Malls, Atria, and Large Spaces*, warns that a system designed in accordance with NFPA 92B and capable of providing the intended smoke management might not pass smoke bomb tests.[37] Conversely, it is possible for a system that is incapable of providing the intended smoke management to pass smoke bomb tests. Because of the impracticality of conducting real fire tests within an atrium, the acceptance tests described in NFPA 92B are directed at those aspects of smoke management systems that can be verified through direct measurement.

Using performance-based criteria, 8.6.7(5) requires that an engineering analysis be performed to demonstrate that smoke will be managed for the time needed to evacuate the building. To accomplish this, 8.6.7(5) requires the analysis to prove that the smoke layer interface will be maintained above the highest unprotected opening to adjoining spaces, or 6 ft (1830 mm) above the highest floor level of exit access open to the atrium for a time equal to 1½ times the calculated egress time or 20 minutes, whichever is greater. For a protect-in-place occupancy, such as health care, the evacuation time is considered to be infinite, which means that the smoke control performance criteria must be maintained indefinitely.

In Exhibit 8.19, floors 1 through 8 are open to the atrium and floors 9 through 12 use the atrium balconies for exit access. An engineering analysis will most likely determine that a high-capacity smoke management system will be needed to meet the performance-based criteria for maintaining the smoke layer interface 6 ft (1830 mm) above the walking surface of the twelfth-floor exit access balcony (the highest floor level with exit access in the atrium). The smoke control system will need to begin removing smoke early in the fire, because there is little accumulation capacity in the space above the twelfth floor and beneath the ceiling of the atrium. Contrast this situation with that shown in Exhibit 8.21, in which floors 10 through 12 do not use the atrium for exit access. Although a smoke control system will be needed to meet the performance-based smoke control criteria, the system might be of a less aggressive design, given that the smoke can bank down from the ceiling of the atrium to below the tenth floor before affecting occupant egress.

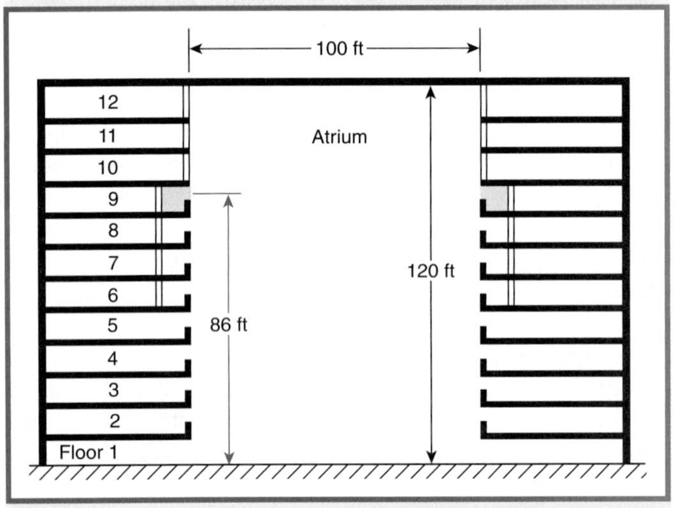


***Exhibit 8.21*** *Twelve-story atrium for which smoke control is to be provided.*

NFPA 92B, *Standard for Smoke Management Systems in Malls, Atria, and Large Spaces*, quantifies the physics associated with atrium smoke control and presents methodologies for system design in an understandable and useful format. The requirements of NFPA 92B allow the system designer to design a system and prepare the associated documentation for the AHJ to assess for adequacy in meeting the performance criteria of 8.6.7(5). For example, the designer and the AHJ agree that an acceptable design must provide for the level of smoke filling to be maintained at least 6 ft (1830 mm) above the highest floor level open to the atrium and the highest floor level used for exit access within the atrium for a minimum of 20 minutes after actuation of the fire alarm system.

The following example, which is illustrated in Exhibit 8.21, makes use of the provisions of NFPA 92B in designing a smoke management system that meets the smoke-filling criterion agreed to by the designer and the AHJ.

The proposed atrium building is to be 12 stories in height, with the fifth floor as the highest level open to the atrium and the ninth floor as the highest walking level within the atrium. Further, the atrium ceiling is to be 120 ft (36.6 m) above the floor; the atrium opening is to be rectangular with horizontal dimensions of 100 ft × 200 ft (30.5 m × 61 m); and the atrium is to be furnished with upholstered furniture and wood and plastic tables characteristic of the fire loading typically associated with a business occupancy.

Note that the following example and analysis use the formulae from those portions of NFPA 92B that use the conventional U.S. Customary units (e.g., feet, square feet, Btu per second, pounds per cubic foot, cubic feet per minute). Although it is standard practice within this handbook to provide metric or SI units, SI equivalents are not provided in the calculations that follow. Rather, the reader is referred to NFPA 92B, where SI unit forms of all 22 equations used in the standard are available.

If the designer prefers to install spot smoke detectors for activation of the smoke control system and initiation of the building fire alarm at the top of the atrium only, the designer would need to determine if smoke will reach the ceiling or stratify at a given distance below the ceiling in the case of the selected design fire. Stratification occurs when the temperature of the rising plume equals the temperature of the surrounding air and the fire has insufficient energy to "push" the smoke layer any higher.

Computational methods, which are beyond the scope of this analysis, are available for determining the potential for stratification below the atrium ceiling. For example, in an atrium that is known to have a discrete ambient temperature change at a given elevation above the floor level (perhaps due to solar loading), the designer can determine the height at which the fire plume centerline temperature equals the ambient temperature. Stratification can be assumed to occur at that height. See Annex H of NFPA 92B for additional discussion on stratification.

To further compound the issue, detection of smoke by spot-type detectors at ceiling heights greater than 30 ft requires its own engineering analysis, which is also beyond the scope of this example. For such analyses, consult Schifiliti and Pucci's "Fire Detection Modeling, State of the Art."[38]

Stratification is not a concern after the smoke management system activates, because the natural buoyancy of the smoke (or lack thereof) will be negligible compared to the pressure differences and air movement created by the system. Stratification can, however, have a significant adverse effect on the time to system initiation from the start of the fire. The designer might wish to design the detection system for activation of the smoke management system in a manner that ensures prompt detection, regardless of the ambient conditions in the atrium at the time of the fire. Projected-beam smoke detectors, which are capable of measuring the light obscuration caused by smoke particles, can be arranged to quickly detect either a developing smoke layer or the rising smoke plume. In either case, a series of beam detectors is to be installed at strategic points within the atrium. Projected-beam smoke detectors can be arranged to provide a highly reliable means of detecting a fire within the atrium in its early stages. In all cases, the requirements of *NFPA 72, National Fire Alarm Code*, and the detector manufacturer's installation guidelines should be followed.

For the remainder of this exercise, it is assumed that the atrium is provided with projected-beam smoke detectors arranged to activate the smoke management system and initiate the building fire alarm relatively quickly following the onset of fire, and before the smoke level descends to within 6 ft of the highest level of exit access open to the atrium.

Having equated the furniture arrangement as typical of the combustible loading associated with a business occupancy, the designer feels comfortable assuming a typical heat release rate per unit floor area of 20 Btu/ft$^2$-s, which realistically translates to a design fire heat release rate, $Q$, from steady fire of 5000 Btu/s. The convective portion of the heat release rate, $Q_c$, can be estimated as 70 percent of the heat release rate, $Q$.

The designer next calculates the volumetric exhaust rate required to keep smoke 86 ft above the atrium floor (i.e., 6 ft above the highest walking level in the atrium, which, in this case, is the ninth floor balcony whose floor is at the 80 ft elevation). From the provisions of NFPA 92B, the designer locates the design fire in the center of the floor of the atrium so as to keep the fire away from the walls and, thus, create the worst-case condition. With the fire at the center of the atrium floor, an axisymmetric fire plume is expected for which air is entrained from all sides and along the entire height of the plume, until the plume becomes submerged in the smoke layer (see Exhibit 8.22). This leads the designer to the use of equation 6.2.1.1a of NFPA 92B to determine the flame height, as follows:

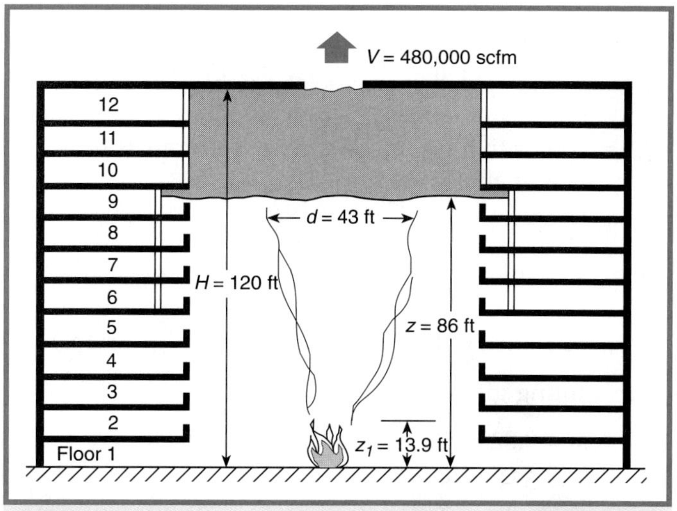


***Exhibit 8.22*** *Axisymmetric fire plume and associated smoke interface.*

$$z_l = 0.533Q_c^{2/5}$$

where:

$z_l$ = limiting elevation (ft)
$Q_c$ = convective portion of heat release rate (Btu/s), established previously as 70 percent of the heat release rate, $Q$

In this case,

$$Q_c = 0.7(5000 \text{ Btu/s}) = 3500 \text{ Btu/s}$$

Substituting gives

$$z_l = 0.533(3500)^{2/5} = 13.9 \text{ ft}$$

With the design interface of the smoke layer at 86 ft above the floor level, the flame height is less than the design smoke layer height. Thus, equation 6.2.1.1b of NFPA 92B can be used to determine the smoke production rate at the height of the smoke layer interface as follows:

$$m = [0.022Q_c^{1/3} z^{5/3}] + 0.0042Q_c \text{ (for } z > z_l)$$

where:

$m$ = smoke production rate at height of smoke layer interface (lb/s)
$Q_c$ = convective portion of heat release rate (Btu/s)
$z$ = height above the fuel (ft)

In this case,

$Q_c$ = 3500 Btu/s, as developed in previous calculations
$z$ = 86 ft (i.e., 6 ft above the 80 ft walking surface)

Substituting gives

$$m = 0.022(3500)^{1/3}(86)^{5/3} + 0.0042(3500)$$
$$= 574 \text{ lb/s}$$

If the smoke exhaust rate is equal to the smoke production rate, the smoke layer depth will be stabilized at the design height (i.e., the 86 ft elevation) and, thus, all balconies and areas open to the atrium will remain tenable as the fire continues to burn.

Before converting the smoke production rate to a volumetric flow rate, it is necessary to determine the temperature rise above ambient of the smoke at time of venting in order to establish the density of the smoke during the vented stage. As explained by the last note in Table G.1.3 of NFPA 92B, the maximum temperature rise will occur if the total heat loss factor is equal to zero. Use the vented stage temperature rise formula from Table G.1.3, simplified by setting the total heat loss factor equal to zero, to determine $\Delta T$ as follows:

$$\Delta T = \frac{60\ Q_c}{(\rho c V)}$$

which, as shown in equation 6.2.5 of NFPA 92B, can be reduced to

$$\Delta T = \frac{Q_c}{mc}$$

where:

$\Delta T$ = temperature rise above ambient of smoke at time of venting (°F)
$Q_c$ = 3500 Btu/s, as developed in previous calculations
$m$ = 574 lb/s, as developed in previous calculations
$c$ = 0.24 Btu/lb-°F, specific heat of smoke, assuming smoke equals air

Substituting gives

$$\Delta T = \frac{3500}{574(0.24)}$$
$$= 25°\text{F}$$

Assuming ambient temperature of 68°F, the temperature of smoke is $T_s$ = 25 + 68 = 93°F.

Using equation A.6.4 of NFPA 92B, the density of smoke at 93°F can be calculated as follows:

$$\rho = \frac{144P_{atm}}{R(T + 460)}$$

where:

$\rho$ = density of heated smoke (lb/ft$^3$)
$P_{atm}$ = atmospheric pressure (lb/in.$^2$) (for this example, use standard atmospheric pressure: 14.7 lb/in.$^2$)
$R$ = gas constant (53.34)
$T$ = temperature of smoke (°F)

Substituting gives

$$\rho = \frac{[144(14.7)]}{[53.34(93 + 460)]}$$
$$= 0.0717 \text{ lb/ft}^3$$

The smoke production rate can be converted to a volumetric flow rate using equation 6.4 of NFPA 92B as follows:

$$V = 60\,\frac{m}{\rho}$$

where:

$V$ = volumetric flow rate (scfm)
$m$ = smoke production rate, 574 lb/sec as previously calculated
$\rho$ = density of heated smoke, 0.0717 lb/ft$^3$ as previously calculated

Substituting gives

$$V = 60\left[\frac{574}{0.0717}\right]$$
$$= 480{,}335 \text{ scfm}$$

The preceding calculations assume that the smoke plume has not widened to contact the walls of the atrium prior to reaching the design interface height of 86 ft above the atrium floor in this example. As a plume rises, it also widens. If the plume were to contact all of the walls of the atrium prior to reaching the ceiling, the smoke interface would be considered as occurring at the height of contact with all of the surrounding walls. No additional smoke generation can be assumed to occur above that height, because additional air entrainment into the plume is considered to be negligible above the point of contact. To check if the widening plume has contacted the walls of the atrium, equation 6.2.4 of NFPA 92B can be used to predict the total plume diameter, at the interface height, as follows:

$$d = 0.5z$$
$$= 0.5(86)$$
$$= 43 \text{ ft}$$

where:

$d$ = plume diameter (ft)
$z$ = interface height (ft)

Thus, in this 100 ft × 200 ft atrium area, the smoke does not contact the walls prior to reaching the design interface height of 86 ft. Mechanical systems capable of extracting approximately 480,000 scfm are then designed. The substantiation package is submitted to the authority having jurisdiction for approval.

Acceptance testing of the system then involves verifying the function of the system components in the intended sequence for varying initiation scenarios. In addition, the system should be evaluated by measuring the following:

1. Total volumetric flow rate
2. Airflow velocities
3. Airflow direction
4. Door-opening forces (forces permitted by the *Code* must not be exceeded when the smoke management system is operating)
5. Pressure differences
6. Ambient indoor and outdoor temperatures
7. Wind speed and direction

If the measurements are within the previously agreed upon system design specifications, the system should be deemed as passing. Note again that no reference is made to the use of subjective test criteria, such as cold smoke bombs. The measurements are obtained objectively and can be performed by professional mechanical, HVAC, or fire protection engineers. NFPA 92A, *Standard for Smoke-Control Systems Utilizing Barriers and Pressure Differences*,[39] and NFPA 92B, *Standard for Smoke Management Systems in Malls, Atria, and Large Spaces*, offer detailed provisions on the equipment needed and procedures for conducting acceptance tests on engineered smoke management systems.

**6.** The provisions of 8.6.7(6) address the activation of mechanical systems that might be designed to meet the performance-based smoke management requirements of 8.6.7(5). In some buildings that have large atrium openings but no upper floors open to the atrium, and no exit access on those upper floors through the atrium, and that are used by ambulatory occupants, it might be possible to meet smoke control criteria without any mechanical systems by allowing the large atrium to accumulate smoke above the heads of all atrium occupants. The purpose of the engineering analysis required by 8.6.7(5) is to determine which type of mechanical smoke control, if any, is needed. Alternatively, tenability of the means of egress might be able to be maintained through passive ventilation of the atrium. The required engineering analysis should evaluate several protection scenarios.

As addressed by A.8.6.7(6), automatic activation of the atrium smoke management system, especially upon initiation of the building alarm system via operation of a manual fire alarm box, could result in the activation of the smoke management system in the incorrect mode. For example, a building occupant walking along the sixth-floor exit access balcony within the atrium might see flames and smoke on the third floor, which is open to the atrium. The occupant might walk to the exit stair enclosure on the sixth floor and operate the manual fire alarm box. The building fire alarm system might incorrectly assume that the fire is on the sixth level. The third floor, which is the actual fire floor, might incorrectly be identified as a non-fire floor. The smoke management system might positively pressurize the third floor and move large volumes of air across the third-floor opening into the atrium in an effort to keep smoke from entering the third-floor communicating space. In reality, the smoke management system would accomplish exactly the opposite of that which it was designed to do; it would spread the smoke and other products of combustion from the third-floor fire into the atrium. The sixth floor would mistakenly be negatively pressurized (exhausted) and would pull in the smoke and gases from the third-floor fire via the atrium. For this reason, NFPA 92A and NFPA 92B require smoke management systems to activate only via automatic initiating devices, such as smoke detectors and automatic sprinklers. However, controls for manual operation of the system by the fire department are required by 8.6.7(6)(b). Smoke management systems should not be arranged to activate via manual fire alarm boxes that are accessible to building occupants.

The manual controls required by 8.6.7(6)(b) must be readily accessible to the responding fire department personnel, so that the smoke management system's mode of operation can be overridden and tailored to the specific needs of the emergency responders. These and other concepts on effective smoke management are covered in NFPA 92A and NFPA 92B.

### 8.6.8 Convenience Openings.

**8.6.8.1** A vertical opening serving as other than an exit enclosure, connecting only two adjacent stories and piercing only one floor, shall be permitted to be open to one of the two stories.

Paragraph 8.6.8.1 recognizes a maximum two-story stair that is separated from one of the two floors, but not both. The separating barrier keeps the effects of a fire on one of the two levels from spreading to the other floor. Because the stair is not an exit, this arrangement does not violate the requirements of 7.1.3.2 pertaining to exit enclosures. Exhibit 8.23 illustrates this provision. As an alternative, the stair could be separated from floor 3 and open to floor 2. A stair meeting 8.6.8.1 might be permitted to be used for exit access, but it is not permitted to be considered an exit because it is not enclosed on all levels.

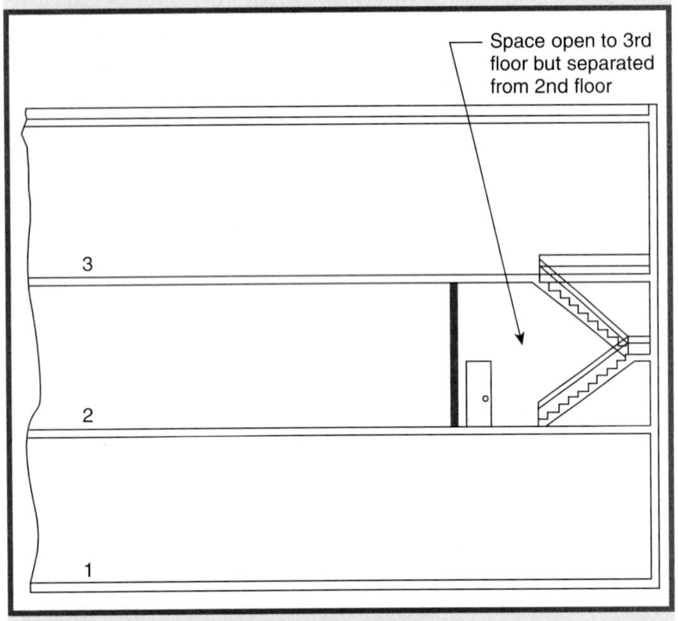


*Exhibit 8.23 Verticial opening protection by fire barrier at one floor level only.*

**8.6.8.2** Where permitted by Chapters 11 through 43, unenclosed vertical openings not concealed within the building construction shall be permitted as follows:

(1) Such openings shall connect not more than two adjacent stories (one floor pierced only).
(2) Such openings shall be separated from unprotected vertical openings serving other floors by a barrier complying with 8.6.5.
(3) Such openings shall be separated from corridors.
(4) In new construction, the convenience opening shall be separated from the corridor referenced in 8.6.8.2(3) by a smoke partition, unless Chapters 11 through 43 require the corridor to have a fire resistance rating.
(5)* Such openings shall not serve as a required means of egress.

**A.8.6.8.2(5)** This requirement prohibits means of egress down or up the convenience opening. It does not prohibit means of escape from running down or up the convenience opening within residential dwelling units.

The provisions of 8.6.8.2 address a convenience opening, often taking the form of a convenience stair, which many of the occupancy chapters have recognized for many years. Prior to the 1997 edition of the *Code*, occupancy chapters specified the detailed criteria contained in 8.6.8.2(1) through (4). The provisions now appear in 8.6.8.2 with the conditional statement "where permitted by Chapters 11 through 43." Therefore, any occupancy chapter can reference the provisions of 8.6.8.2 without having to repeat the detailed criteria. For example, in 38.3.1.1, which applies to new business occupancies, the detailed criteria have been dropped and 38.3.1.1(1) permits "unenclosed vertical openings in accordance with 8.6.8.2." This permits, for example, a two-level office or reference library in an office building to have an unenclosed convenience stair.

The application of 38.3.1.1(1) is restricted by 8.6.8.2(1) to two adjacent levels only. The opening must be separated from other vertical openings serving other floors per 8.6.8.2(2); this requirement prevents the linking of individual openings that would otherwise create a means for spreading the effects of fire among multiple floors. The areas connected by the opening must be separated from corridors per 8.6.8.2(3). Where the applicable occupancy chapter does not require corridor protection, the spaces containing the convenience opening must be separated from corridors by smoke partitions per 8.6.8.2(4). The convenience opening is not permitted to be part of the means of egress per 8.6.8.2(5). The space would be required to have access to exits on both levels so occupants would not have to rely on an open stair as part of the required means of egress. One possible application of these provisions is shown in Exhibit 8.24.

**8.6.8.3** For other than existing hoistways in existing buildings, elevator cars located within a building shall be enclosed as follows:

(1) Where there are three or fewer elevator cars in the building, they shall be permitted to be located within the same hoistway enclosure.

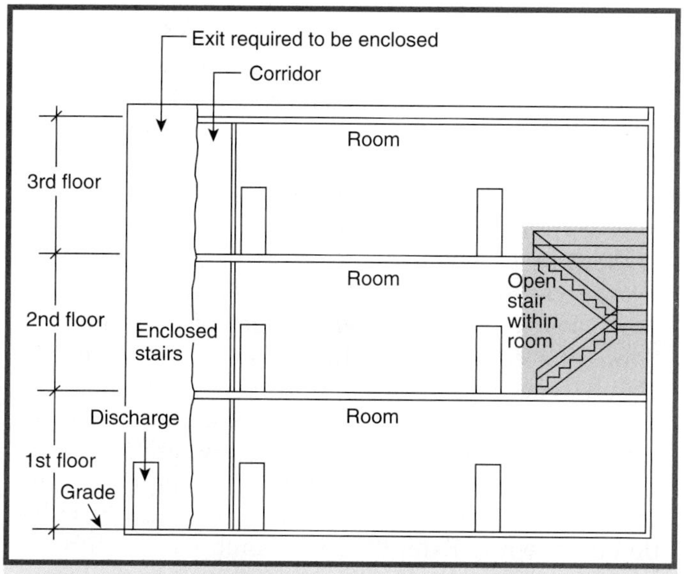


***Exhibit 8.24*** *Elevation view of unenclosed two-story stair serving as a convenience opening.*

(2) Where there are four elevator cars in the building, they shall be divided in such a manner that not less than two separate hoistway enclosures are provided.

(3) Where there are more than four elevator cars in the building, the number of elevator cars located within a single hoistway enclosure shall not exceed four.

The requirements addressed by 8.6.8.3 help to ensure that smoke and fire in an elevator hoistway will not prevent the use of all elevators in any building that has 4 or more elevators. If a building has 4 elevators, a maximum of 3 elevators is permitted within the same elevator hoistway or shaft. If the building has more than 4 elevators, not more than 4 elevators can be in one shaft. If smoke and fire prevent the use of the elevators within one hoistway, an elevator in another hoistway might be usable. Because of the maximum limit of 4 elevators per hoistway, a building with 9 to 12 elevators must have a minimum of three hoistways.

The requirements of 8.6.8.3 mesh well with the high-rise building requirements of 11.8.5.2, which apply to standby power. The required standby power system must be connected to at least one elevator serving all floors of the building. Additionally, elevator standby power must be transferable to any elevator. If the hoistway containing the elevator initially powered by the standby power system becomes untenable, the switching requirement will allow for an elevator in a different hoistway to be placed back into service.

**8.6.8.4** Service openings for conveyors, elevators, and dumbwaiters, where required to be open on more than one story at the same time for purposes of operation, shall be provided with closing devices in accordance with 7.2.1.8.

**8.6.8.5** Any escalators and moving walks serving as a required exit in existing buildings shall be enclosed in the same manner as exit stairways. *(See 7.1.3.2.)*

Where used as an exit, an escalator must be completely enclosed with fire-rated construction, including entrance and discharge doors. It is rare to find an escalator enclosed in such a manner. Escalators located within the required means of egress in existing buildings that maintain compliance with the *Code* usually make use of one of the provisions of 8.6.8.6 to avoid creating an unprotected vertical opening. By doing so, they are classified as exit access. Note that 7.2.7 prohibits escalators from constituting any part of the required means of egress in new buildings. Thus, in new construction, an escalator can be installed but is not recognized as satisfying the requirements for exit access, exit, or exit discharge.

**8.6.8.6** Any escalators and moving walks not constituting an exit shall have their floor openings enclosed or protected as required for other vertical openings, unless otherwise permitted by the following:

(1) The requirement of 8.6.8.6 shall not apply to escalators in large open areas, such as atriums and enclosed shopping malls.

(2)* In buildings protected throughout by an approved automatic sprinkler system in accordance with Section 9.7, escalator and moving walk openings shall be permitted to be protected in accordance with the method detailed in NFPA 13, *Standard for the Installation of Sprinkler Systems*, or in accordance with a method approved by the authority having jurisdiction.

**A.8.6.8.6(2)** The intent is to place a limitation on the size of the opening to which the protection applies. The total floor opening should not exceed twice the projected area of the escalator or moving walk at the floor. Also, the arrangement of the opening is not intended to circumvent the requirements of 8.6.7.

As with any opening through a floor, the openings around the outer perimeter of the escalators should be considered as vertical openings.

(3) In buildings protected throughout by an approved automatic sprinkler system in accordance with Section 9.7, escalator and moving walk openings shall be permitted to be protected by rolling steel shutters appropriate for the fire resistance rating of the vertical opening as follows:

(a) The shutters shall close automatically and independently of each other upon smoke detection and sprinkler operation.
(b) A manual means of operating and testing the operation of the shutters shall be provided.
(c) The shutters shall be operated not less than once a week to ensure that they remain in proper operating condition.
(d) The shutters shall operate at a speed not to exceed 30 ft/min (0.15 m/s) and shall be equipped with a sensitive leading edge.
(e) The leading edge shall arrest the progress of a moving shutter and cause it to retract a distance of approximately 6 in. (150 mm) upon the application of a force not exceeding 20 lbf (90 N) applied to the surface of the leading edge.
(f) The shutter, following the retraction specified in 8.6.8.6(3)(e), shall continue to close.
(g) The operating mechanism for the rolling shutter shall be provided with standby power complying with the provisions of *NFPA 70, National Electrical Code*.

The provisions of 8.6.8.6 provide that new escalators (which cannot be part of the means of egress) and existing escalators not serving as exits (see 8.6.8.5) need not be enclosed if certain provisions are met.

The sprinkler–draft curtain method is detailed in NFPA 13, *Standard for the Installation of Sprinkler Systems*. It consists of surrounding the escalator opening, in an otherwise fully sprinklered building, with an 18 in. (455 mm) deep draft stop located on the underside of the floor to which the escalator ascends. This draft stop serves to delay the heat, smoke, and combustion gases developed in the early stages of a fire on that floor from entering into the escalator well. A row of closely spaced automatic sprinklers located outside of the draft stop also surrounds the escalator well. As sprinklers along this surrounding row are individually activated by heat, their water discharge patterns combine to create a water curtain. A typical installation is shown in Exhibit 8.25. In combination with the sprinkler system in the building, this system should delay fire spread effectively and allow time for evacuation.

Prior editions of the *Code* detailed several methods that permitted the use of unenclosed escalators in completely sprinklered buildings where the escalators were not used as exits. In addition to the sprinkler–draft curtain or rolling shutter methods, the authority

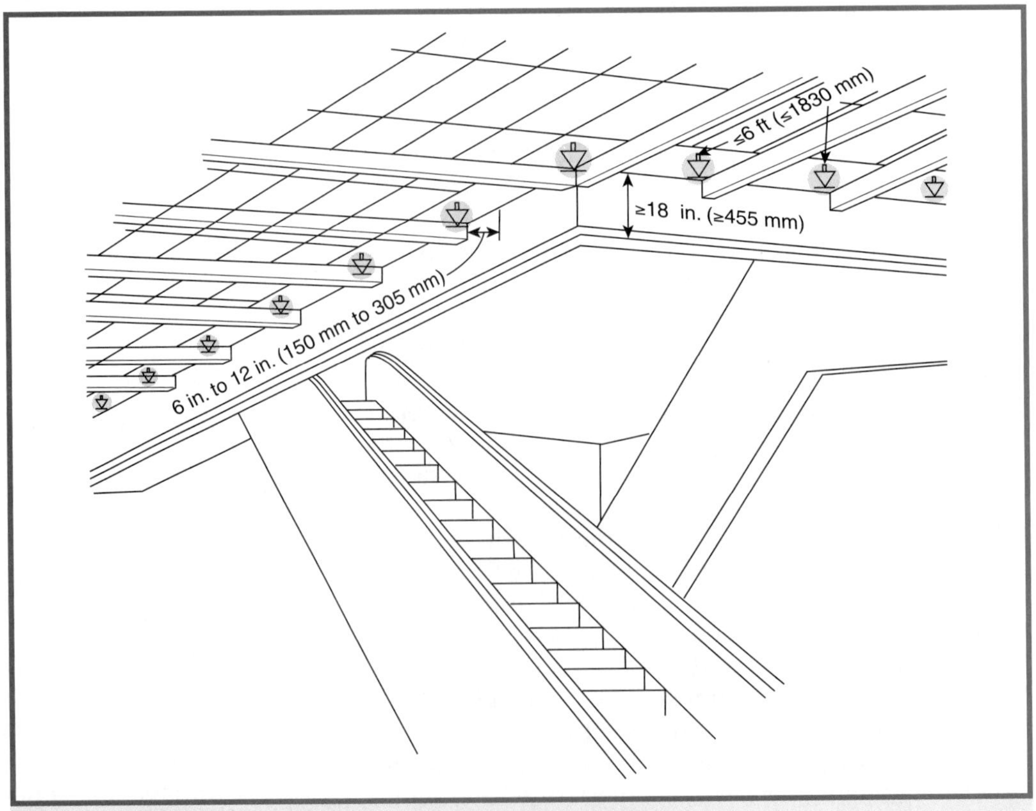


***Exhibit 8.25*** *Sprinklers around an escalator opening.*

having jurisdiction might consider one of the following when evaluating existing buildings:

1. Sprinkler-vent method
2. Spray nozzle method
3. Partial enclosure method

These three methods are detailed in the paragraphs that follow.

**Sprinkler-Vent Method.** Under the conditions specified, escalator or moving walk openings are permitted to be protected by the sprinkler-vent method, which consists of a combination of an automatic fire or smoke detection system, an automatic exhaust system, and an automatic water curtain. This combination of fire protection and system design is required to meet the criteria of paragraphs 1 through 8, which follow, and to be approved by the authority having jurisdiction.

**1.** The exhaust system should be capable of creating a downdraft through the escalator or moving walk floor opening. The downdraft should have an average velocity of not less than 300 ft/min (1.5 m/s) under normal conditions for a period of not less than 30 minutes. This requirement can be met by providing an air intake from the outside of the building above the floor opening. The test of the system under "normal" conditions requires that the velocity of the downdraft be developed when windows or doors on the several stories normally used for ventilation are open. The size of the exhaust fan and exhaust ducts must be sufficient to meet such ventilation conditions. Experience indicates that fan capacity should be based on a rating of not less than 500 $ft^3/min/ft^2$ ($8.3\ m^3/s/m^2$) of moving stairway opening to obtain the 300 ft/min (1.5 m/s) velocity required. If the building is provided with an air-conditioning system arranged to be automatically shut down in the event of fire, the test condition should be met with the air-conditioning system shut down. The 300 ft/min (1.5 m/s) downdraft through the opening provides for the testing of the exhaust system without requiring the expansion of air that would be present under actual fire conditions.

**2.** Operation of the exhaust system for any floor opening should be initiated by an approved device on the involved story and should use one of the following means, in addition to a manual means, for operating and testing the system:

**a.** Heat detectors (fixed-temperature, rate-of-rise, or a combination of both)
**b.** Waterflow in the sprinkler system
**c.** Approved supervised smoke detection located so that the presence of smoke is detected before it enters the stairway

**3.** Electric power supply to all parts of the exhaust system and its control devices should be designed and installed for maximum reliability. The electric power supply provision of NFPA 20, *Standard for the Installation of Stationary Pumps for Fire Protection*,[40] can be used as a guide to design and installation features that help to ensure maximum reliability.

**4.** Any fan or duct used in connection with an automatic exhaust system should be of the approved type and should be installed in accordance with the applicable standards in Chapter 2 and Annex D.

**5.** Periodic tests should be made of the automatic exhaust system, at least quarterly, to maintain the system and the control devices in good working condition.

**6.** The water curtain should be formed by open sprinklers or by spray nozzles located and spaced to form a complete and continuous barrier along all exposed sides of the floor opening and to reach from the ceiling to the floor. Water discharge for the water curtain should be not less than approximately 3 gal/min/lineal ft (0.6 L/s/lineal m) of water curtain, measured horizontally around the opening.

**7.** The water curtain should operate automatically from thermal-response elements of a fixed-temperature type. These elements should be located with respect to the ceiling/floor opening so that the water curtain actuates upon the advance of heat toward the escalator or moving walk opening.

**8.** Every automatic exhaust system (including all motors, controls, and automatic water curtain system) should be electrically supervised in an approved manner that is similar to that specified for automatic sprinkler system supervision.

**Spray Nozzle Method.** Under the conditions specified, escalator openings are permitted to be protected by the spray nozzle method, which consists of a combination of an automatic fire or smoke detection system and a system of high-velocity water spray nozzles. This combination of fire protection and system design should meet the criteria of paragraphs 1 through 8, which follow, and be approved by the authority having jurisdiction.

**1.** Spray nozzles should be of the open type and should have a solid conical spray pattern with discharge angles between 45 degrees and 90 degrees. The number of nozzles, their discharge angles, and their location should be such that the escalator or moving walk opening between the top of the wellway housing and the treadway will be completely filled with dense spray on operation of the system.

**2.** The number and size of nozzles and water supply should be sufficient to deliver a discharge of 2 gal of water/ft$^2$/min (1.4 L of water/m$^2$/s) through the wellway, with the area to be figured perpendicularly to the treadway. See Exhibit 8.26.

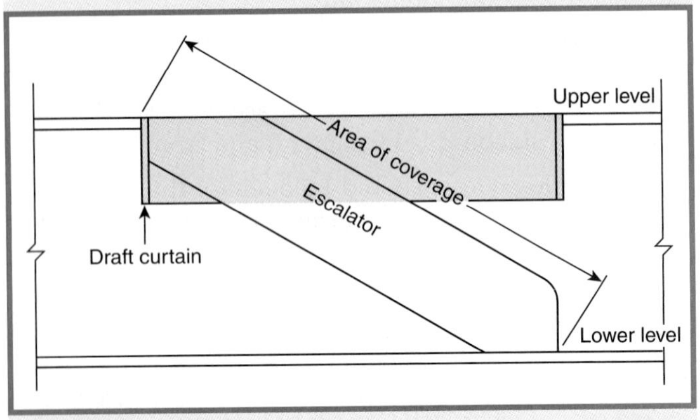


***Exhibit 8.26*** *Area of coverage for spray nozzle method of protecting escalator openings.*

**3.** Spray nozzles should be located to take full advantage of the cooling and counterdraft effect. They should be positioned so that the centerline of spray discharge is as closely in line as possible with the slope of the escalator or moving walk, not more than an angle of 30 degrees with the top slope of the wellway housing. Nozzles should also be positioned so that the centerline of discharge is at an angle of not more than 30 degrees from the vertical sides of the wellway housing.

**4.** Spray nozzles should discharge at a minimum pressure of 25 lb/in.$^2$ (172 kPa). Water supply piping is permitted to be taken from the sprinkler system, provided that an adequate supply of water is available for the spray nozzles and that the water pressure at the sprinkler farthest from the supply riser is not reduced beyond the required minimum. Water supply taken from the sprinkler system is designed to provide protection from life hazards to the wellway opening during the exit period but is not to be relied on to provide an effective floor cutoff.

**5.** Control valves should be readily accessible to minimize water damage.

**6.** A noncombustible or limited-combustible draft curtain should be provided that extends at least 20 in. (510 mm) below and around the opening, and a solid noncombustible wellway housing at least 60 in. (1525 mm) long, measured parallel to the handrail and extending from the top of the handrail enclosure to the soffit of the stairway or ceiling above, should also be provided at each escalator floor opening. Where necessary, spray nozzles should be protected against mechanical damage or tampering that might interfere with proper discharge. See Exhibit 8.27.

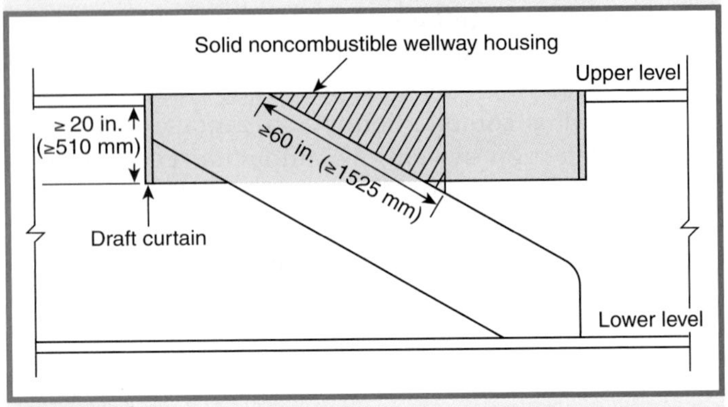


***Exhibit 8.27*** *The draft curtain and wellway housing method of protecting vertical openings.*

**7.** The spray nozzle system should operate automatically from thermal-response elements of the fixed-temperature type and be located with respect to the ceiling/floor opening so that the spray nozzle system actuates upon the advance of heat toward the escalator opening. Supervised smoke detection located in or near the escalator opening is permitted to be used to sound an alarm. The spray nozzle system should also be provided with manual means of operation. It is not desirable to have smoke detectors activate the spray nozzles; safeguards against accidental discharge must be provided to prevent both panic and property damage.

**8.** Control valves for the spray nozzle system and approved smoke detection or thermostatic devices should be electrically supervised in accordance with the applicable provisions of 9.7.2.

**Partial Enclosure Method.** Under the conditions specified, escalator or moving walk openings are permitted to be protected by a partial enclosure, or so-called kiosk, designed to provide an effective barrier to the spread of smoke from floor to floor. This method of fire protection should meet the criteria of paragraphs 1 and 2, which follow, and be approved by the AHJ.

**1.** Partial enclosure construction should provide fire resistance equivalent to that specified for stairway enclosures in the same building, with openings therein protected by approved, self-closing fire doors. The openings also are permitted to be of approved wired-glass and metal frame construction with wired-glass panel doors.

**2.** Fire doors are permitted to be equipped with an electric opening mechanism, which opens the door automatically upon the approach of a person. The mechanism should return the door to its closed position upon any interruption of electric current supply, and it should be adjusted so that the pressures generated by a fire will not cause the door to open.

### 8.6.9 Mezzanines.

**8.6.9.1 General.** Multilevel residential housing areas in detention and correctional occupancies in accordance with Chapters 22 and 23 shall be exempt from the provisions of 8.6.9.2 and 8.6.9.3.

**8.6.9.2 Area Limitations.**

**8.6.9.2.1** The aggregate area of mezzanines located within a room, other than those located in special-purpose industrial occupancies, shall not exceed one-third the open area of the room in which the mezzanines are located. Enclosed space shall not be included in a determination of the size of the room in which the mezzanine is located.

**8.6.9.2.2** No limit on the number of mezzanines in a room shall be required.

**8.6.9.2.3** For purposes of determining the allowable mezzanine area, the aggregate area of the mezzanines shall not be included in the area of the room.

**8.6.9.3 Openness.** The openness of mezzanines shall be in accordance with 8.6.9.3.1 or 8.6.9.3.2.

**8.6.9.3.1** All portions of a mezzanine, other than walls not more than 42 in. (1065 mm) high, columns, and posts, shall be open to and unobstructed from the room in which the mezzanine is located, unless the occupant load of the aggregate area of the enclosed space does not exceed 10.

**8.6.9.3.2** A mezzanine having two or more means of egress shall not be required to open into the room in which it is located if not less than one of the means of egress provides direct access from the enclosed area to an exit at the mezzanine level.

The mezzanine provisions of 8.6.9 were developed for the 1991 edition of the *Code*. They are based on a report prepared by the Board for the Coordination of the Model Codes (BCMC) in an attempt to standardize the treatment of mezzanines among three former U.S. regional building code officials' organizations and NFPA.

The aggregate area of a mezzanine within a room must not exceed one-third the open area (the unenclosed space) of the room in which the mezzanine is located. The area of the mezzanine is not considered to be part of the total open area of the room for the purposes of this calculation. For other purposes, the area of the mezzanine is considered part of the area of the room. Because a mezzanine is limited to such size, it is exempted from being counted as a building story — thus affecting the applicability of *Code* requirements based on the number of building stories or floors.

Exhibit 8.28 illustrates the use of the one-third area rule for determining whether a level is a mezzanine. A 1000 $ft^2$ (93 $m^2$) partial level is positioned above a 3000 $ft^2$ (279 $m^2$) main room. This is depicted in the plan view at the top of the figure. Because the one-third area rule compares the area of the upper level to the *open* area of the room in which the partial floor level is located, only the unenclosed space of the room is used in the calculation. In Elevation A in Exhibit 8.28, the space below the partial floor level is enclosed. The enclosed area beneath the partial upper level is not counted in the area of the main floor. In this case, the area of the upper level is approximately half the area

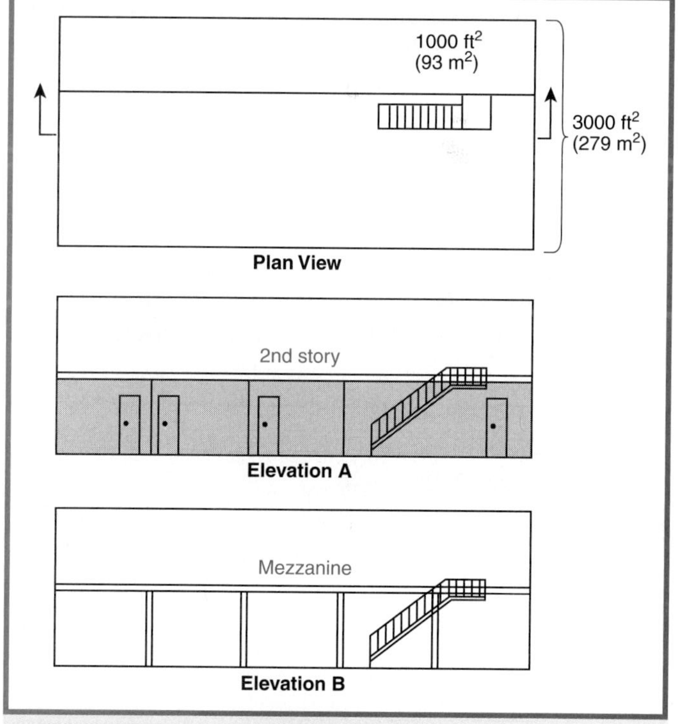


***Exhibit 8.28** Determining whether partial upper level meets one-third area rule to qualify as a mezzanine.*

of the open space on the main room below. The size of this area exceeds the one-third allowance, which means that the partial upper level is considered a floor and not a mezzanine. Contrast this arrangement with the arrangement shown in Elevation B in Exhibit 8.28. In this case, the space below the partial floor level is open to the main room. The 1000 $ft^2$ (93 $m^2$) area of the partial floor level is compared to the full 3000 $ft^2$ (279 $m^2$) area of the room below. The one-third area rule is met, and the upper level is considered a mezzanine, provided that the other provisions of 8.6.9 are met.

The openness requirements of 8.6.9.3 are intended to provide the mezzanine occupants with a degree of awareness of fire conditions on the floor below that is equivalent to the awareness of the occupants of the fire floor. Because the mezzanine sits above the floor of which it is considered a part, untenable smoke concentrations and the associated loss of visibility due to smoke obscuration might affect the mezzanine level before similarly affecting the floor below. In the same way that openness and awareness are required via the mini-atrium provisions of 8.6.6(3), the occupants of the mezzanine should be alerted to a fire in any part of the two-level space before the fire becomes a hazard to their safety.

In recognition of such openness, the *Code* treats the mezzanine no differently than an area or room on the level below the mezzanine. If the mezzanine depicted in Exhibit 8.29 were located in a business occupancy, for example, it would be required to follow the same exit access arrangement rules of any other room on the floor below. Thus, if all occupants could travel across the mezzanine, down the open stair to the room below, and as far across the floor of that room as necessary to reach a point where they had access to two different egress paths, and if that total distance did not exceed the allowable common path of travel [i.e., 75 ft (23 m), or 100 ft (30 m) if sprinklered per 38.2.5.3, for the new business occupancy in this example], a single exit access from the mezzanine to the floor below would be permitted. If the allowable common path of travel were exceeded, the mezzanine would require a second, remote exit access.

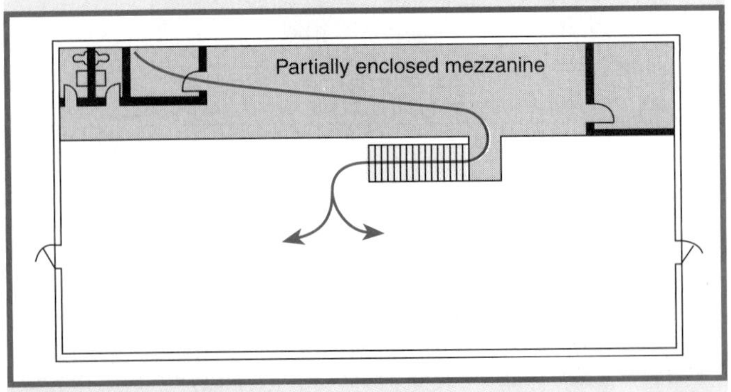


***Exhibit 8.29*** *Open mezzanine.*

Paragraph 8.6.9.3.1 recognizes that walls not more than 42 in. (1065 mm) high can serve as guards to prevent falls over the open side of a mezzanine but are low enough to achieve the openness requirement. See 7.2.2.4 for guard requirements.

A limited amount of enclosed space on the mezzanine is also permitted by 8.6.9.3.1 to allow for toilet rooms, limited storage, small offices, and similar areas normally separated from the open area of the mezzanine. In Exhibit 8.29, the mezzanine is partially enclosed such that the total occupant load of all enclosed rooms does not exceed 10 persons. This permits a partially enclosed mezzanine to use all the benefits available to a fully open mezzanine.

Paragraph 8.6.9.3.2 exempts a mezzanine from being open to the room in which it is located if the occupants of the mezzanine are provided with at least two means of egress and if one of those means of egress provides direct access to an exit at the mezzanine level. This provision permits the mezzanine in Exhibit 8.30 to be enclosed, because one of its two means of egress provides access from the mezzanine directly into an exit stair enclosure that discharges to the outside. Occupants of the mezzanine are then judged as being adequately safe from a fire on the level below because, even if they learn about that fire later than they would have if the mezzanine were open, one of their means of egress does not require them to return through the room below.

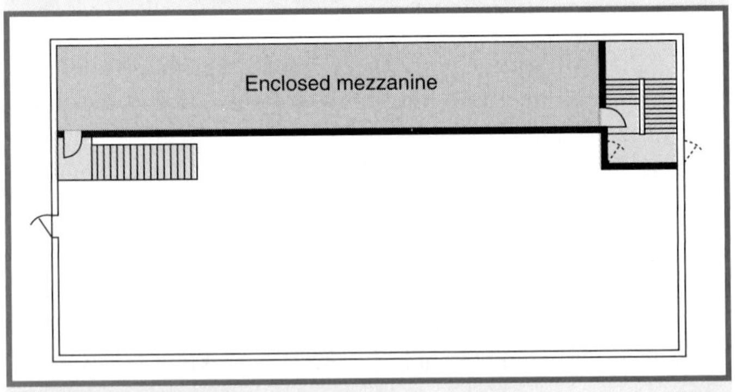


***Exhibit 8.30*** *Enclosed mezzanine.*

### 8.6.10 Concealed Spaces and Draftstops.

**8.6.10.1** Any concealed combustible space in which building materials having a flame spread index greater than Class A are exposed shall be draftstopped as follows:

(1) Every exterior and interior wall and partition shall be firestopped at each floor level, at the top story ceiling level, and at the level of support for roofs.
(2) Every unoccupied attic space shall be subdivided by draftstops into areas not to exceed 3000 $ft^2$ (280 $m^2$).
(3) Any concealed space between the ceiling and the floor or roof above shall be draftstopped for the full depth of the space along the line of support for the floor or roof structural members and, if necessary, at other locations to form areas not to exceed 1000 $ft^2$ (93 $m^2$) for any space between the ceiling and floor, and 3000 $ft^2$ (280 $m^2$) for any space between the ceiling and roof.

**8.6.10.2** The requirements of 8.6.10.1 shall not apply where any of the following conditions are met:

(1) Where the space is protected throughout by an approved automatic sprinkler system in accordance with Section 9.7
(2)* Where concealed spaces serve as plenums

**A.8.6.10.2(2)** See NFPA 90A, *Standard for the Installation of Air-Conditioning and Ventilating Systems.*

(3) Where the installation is an existing installation

**8.6.10.3** Draftstopping materials shall be not less than $\frac{1}{2}$ in. (13 mm) thick gypsum board, $\frac{15}{32}$ in. (12 mm) thick plywood, or other approved materials that are adequately supported.

**8.6.10.4** The integrity of all draftstops shall be maintained.

The vertical spread of fire through shafts, chases, and hollow wall construction and the horizontal spread of fire through plenums and open attics are phenomena common to many serious fires. Where such spaces are protected with automatic sprinklers, the risk of unseen fires is minimized. Certain additional precautions are required where automatic sprinkler protection is not installed in new buildings, and where the materials used have a flame spread rating of more than 25 (i.e., other than Class A interior finish).

Draftstopping of attic spaces is particularly important in shopping centers composed of one story and an attic and in two-story apartment buildings or row houses. Experience has shown that fire starting in one of these occupancy units frequently breaks into the attic space, spreads through the attic, and travels down into adjoining units.

Numerous fires in garden-type apartments have demonstrated two common weaknesses that relate to the lack of adequate firestopping and draftstopping. The following two areas are frequently not firestopped:

1. Between the underside of the roof deck and the top of fire barriers that do not extend through the roofline
2. Inside the pipe chase that contains the plumbing vent stack

The vent stack is of particular concern, because it frequently is located between two mirror-image apartment units and interconnects all the floors of the apartment building. A fire that travels into this concealed space can spread to the attic and soon involve the entire structure.

The term *draft stop* is defined in 3.3.60 as "a continuous membrane used to subdivide a concealed space to resist the passage of smoke and heat."

**8.6.10.5** In existing buildings, firestopping and draftstopping shall be provided as required by Chapters 11 through 43.

An example of an occupancy chapter requirement for firestopping is found in 19.1.6.7, which requires firestopping between the basement and first floor in existing health care occupancies.

## 8.7 Special Hazard Protection

### 8.7.1 General.

**8.7.1.1*** Protection from any area having a degree of hazard greater than that normal to the general occupancy of the building or structure shall be provided by one of the following means:

(1) Enclosing the area with a fire barrier without windows that has a 1-hour fire resistance rating in accordance with Section 8.3
(2) Protecting the area with automatic extinguishing systems in accordance with Section 9.7
(3) Applying both 8.7.1.1(1) and (2) where the hazard is severe or where otherwise specified by Chapters 11 through 43

**A.8.7.1.1** Areas requiring special hazard protection include, but are not limited to, areas such as those used for storage of combustibles or flammables, areas housing heat-producing appliances, or areas used for maintenance purposes.

The effects of fire originating in hazardous areas are minimized by isolating those areas that have a high potential for fire or a high fuel load in accordance with 8.7.1.1. The occupancy chapters identify the particular hazards against which protection is to be provided and generally address them in the ___.3.2 subsection of each occupancy chapter. For example, see Table 22.3.2.1, which is applicable to hazardous areas in new detention and correctional occupancies. This subsection addresses the fundamental fire protection concept of either protecting against known hazards via automatic extinguishment systems or isolating known hazards by means of fire-rated construction. The authority having jurisdiction is responsible for determining the criteria that define a hazardous area.

**8.7.1.2** In new construction, where protection is provided with automatic extinguishing systems without fire-resistive separation, the space protected shall be enclosed with smoke partitions in accordance with Section 8.4, unless otherwise permitted by one of the following conditions:

(1) Where mercantile occupancy general storage areas and stockrooms are protected by automatic sprinklers in accordance with Section 9.7
(2) Where hazardous areas in industrial occupancies are protected by automatic extinguishing systems in accordance with 40.3.2
(3) Where hazardous areas in detention and correctional occupancies are protected by automatic sprinklers in accordance with 22.3.2

The provisions of 8.7.1.2 require a smoke-resisting enclosure, which includes both surrounding wall barriers and opening protectives such as self-closing doors, where the allowance of 8.7.1.1(2) is used, to protect the hazardous area with automatic sprinklers in lieu of a fire barrier enclosure. The smoke-resisting enclosure, although it lacks a mandated fire resistance rating, will help to contain the smoke generated prior to sprinkler activation and subsequent to fire control. This concept is illustrated in Exhibit 8.31. Paragraph 8.7.1.2(1) permits omission of the additional smoke-resisting enclosure or separation for general storage areas in mercantile occupancies that are protected by automatic sprinklers. For example, in a shoe store, a sprinklered shoe storage area could be left open to the sales area. The clerk might go behind a partial-height partition without going through a door opening to get shoes. Another example is a department store, which usually positions its general storage rooms behind floor-to-ceiling wall barriers at the rear of the store along exterior walls. In this case, double-acting doors (i.e., those that can swing both into and out of the storage room) that might not adequately resist the passage of smoke as required by 8.7.1.2 could be used if the storage area were sprinklered.

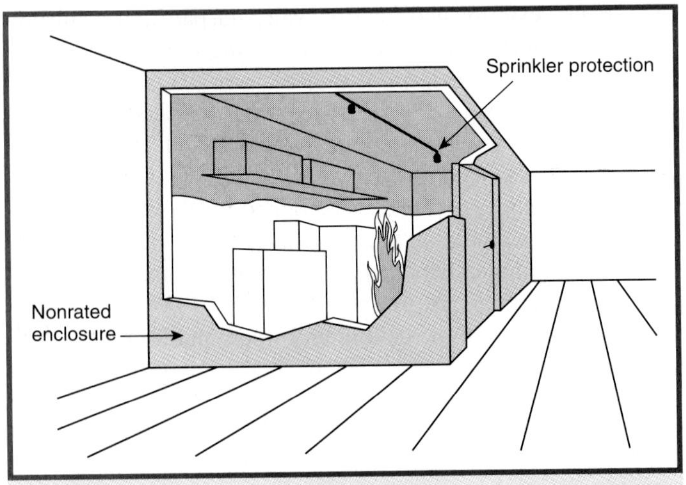


***Exhibit 8.31*** *Sprinkler-protected hazardous contents area.*

The provision of 8.7.1.2(2) exempts hazardous areas in industrial occupancies from the additional smoke-resisting enclosure requirement if those areas are protected by automatic extinguishing systems. The nonhazardous areas might not be sprinklered, but the protected hazardous areas can be left open to the nonhazardous areas.

**8.7.1.3** Doors in barriers required to have a fire resistance rating shall have a minimum $^{3}/_{4}$-hour fire protection rating and shall be self-closing or automatic-closing in accordance with 7.2.1.8.

## 8.7.2* Explosion Protection.

Where hazardous processes or storage is of such a character as to introduce an explosion potential, an explosion venting system or an explosion suppression system specifically designed for the hazard involved shall be provided.

**A.8.7.2** For details, see NFPA 68, *Standard on Explosion Protection by Deflagration Venting*.

If a potential hazard is of an explosive nature, explosion venting or an explosion suppression system is required. NFPA 68, *Standard on Explosion Protection by Deflagration Venting*,[41] contains details of acceptable venting systems; NFPA 69, *Standard on Explosion Prevention Systems*,[42] covers suppression systems. NFPA 654, *Standard for the Prevention of Fire and Dust Explosions from the Manufacturing, Processing, and Handling of Combustible Particulate Solids*,[43] is useful where explosive dusts are encountered.

### 8.7.3 Flammable Liquids and Gases.

**8.7.3.1** The storage and handling of flammable liquids or gases shall be in accordance with the following applicable standards:

(1) NFPA 30, *Flammable and Combustible Liquids Code*
(2) NFPA 54, *National Fuel Gas Code*
(3) NFPA 58, *Liquefied Petroleum Gas Code*

**8.7.3.2*** No storage or handling of flammable liquids or gases shall be permitted in any location where such storage would jeopardize egress from the structure, unless otherwise permitted by 8.7.3.1.

**A.8.7.3.2** NFPA 58, *Liquefied Petroleum Gas Code*, permits portable butane-fueled appliances in restaurants and in attended commercial food catering operations where fueled by not in excess of two 10 oz (0.28 kg) LP-Gas capacity, nonrefillable butane containers having a water capacity not in excess of 1.08 lb (0.4 kg) per container. Containers are required to be directly connected to the appliance, and manifolding of containers is not permitted. Storage of cylinders is also limited to 24 containers, with an additional 24 permitted where protected by a 2-hour fire resistance–rated barrier.

### 8.7.4 Laboratories.

**8.7.4.1** Laboratories that use chemicals shall comply with NFPA 45, *Standard on Fire Protection for Laboratories Using Chemicals*, unless otherwise modified by other provisions of this *Code*.

**8.7.4.2** Laboratories in health care occupancies and medical and dental offices shall comply with NFPA 99, *Standard for Health Care Facilities*.

### 8.7.5* Hyperbaric Facilities.

All occupancies containing hyperbaric facilities shall comply with NFPA 99, *Standard for Health Care Facilities*, Chapter 20, unless otherwise modified by other provisions of this *Code*.

**A.8.7.5** While the scope of NFPA 99, *Standard for Health Care Facilities*, is limited to health care occupancies, it is the intent that this requirement be applied to hyperbaric facilities used in all occupancies.

Hyperbaric facilities can be found in a variety of occupancies, in addition to health care occupancies. For example, hyperbaric chambers have been installed in amusement centers and physical fitness centers and have been promoted as health-enhancing aids. Paragraph 8.7.5 extends the use of the provisions of NFPA 99, *Standard for Health Care Facilities*,[44] to hyperbaric facilities, regardless of occupancy classification.

## References Cited in Commentary


1. NFPA SPP-24, *Designing Buildings for Fire Safety*, National Fire Protection Association, Boston, 1975, pp. 72-74.
2. NFPA 251, *Standard Methods of Tests of Fire Resistance of Building Construction and Materials*, 2006 edition, National Fire Protection Association, Quincy, MA.
3. ASTM E 119, *Standard Test Methods for Fire Tests of Building Construction and Materials*, 2007a edition, ASTM International, 100 Barr Harbor Drive, P. O. Box C700, West Conshohocken, PA 19428-2959.
4. ANSI/UL 263, *Standard for Fire Tests of Building Construction and Materials*, Underwriters Laboratories Inc., 333 Pfingsten Road, Northbrook, IL 60062-2096.
5. NFPA 252, *Standard Methods of Fire Tests of Door Assemblies*, 2008 edition, National Fire Protection Association, Quincy, MA.
6. ASTM E 2074, *Standard Test Method for Fire Tests of Door Assemblies, Including Positive Pressure Testing of Side-Hinged and Pivoted Swinging Door Assemblies*, 2000e edition, ASTM International, 100 Barr Harbor Drive, P.O. Box C700, West Conshohocken, PA 19428-2959.
7. ANSI/UL 10B, *Standard for Fire Tests of Door Assemblies*, 1997 edition, Revised 2001, Underwriters Laboratories Inc., 333 Pfingsten Road, Northbrook, IL 60062-2096.
8. ANSI/UL 10C, *Standard for Positive Pressure Fire Tests of Door Assemblies*, 1998 edition, Revised 2001, Underwriters Laboratories Inc., 333 Pfingsten Road, Northbrook, IL 60062-2096.
9. NFPA 220, *Standard on Types of Building Construction*, 2009 edition, National Fire Protection Association, Quincy, MA.
10. *NFPA 5000®, Building Construction and Safety Code®*, 2009 edition, National Fire Protection Association, Quincy, MA.
11. *Uniform Building Code*, International Conference of Building Officials, Whittier, CA.
12. BOCA *National Building Code*, Building Officials and Code Administrators International, Inc., Country Club Hills, IL.
13. *Standard Building Code*, Southern Building Code Congress International, Inc., Birmingham, AL.
14. *International Building Code*, International Code Council, Inc., 5203 Leesburg Pike, Suite 600, Falls Church, VA 22041.
15. *Fire Resistance Design Manual*, Gypsum Association, 810 First Street, NE, Suite 510, Washington, DC 20002.
16. NFPA 221, *Standard for High Challenge Fire Walls,*

*Fire Walls, and Fire Barrier Walls*, 2009 edition, National Fire Protection Association, Quincy, MA.
17. *UL Fire Resistance Directory*, 2007 edition, Underwriters Laboratories Inc., 333 Pfingsten Road, Northbrook, IL 60062-2096.
18. *2008 Approval Guide*, FM Global Research, FM Global, 1301 Atwood Avenue, P.O. Box 7500, Johnston, RI 02919.
19. *Intertek Directory of Listed Products*, Intertek, 165 Main Street, Cortland, NY 13045.
20. ASTM A 6/A6M, *Standard Specification for General Requirements for Rolled Structural Steel Bars, Plates, Shapes, and Sheet Piling*, 2008 edition, ASTM International, 100 Barr Harbor Drive, P.O. Box C700, West Conshohocken, PA 19428-2959.
21. ASCE/SFPE 29, *Standard Calculation Methods for Structural Fire Protection*, 1999 edition, American Society of Civil Engineers, 1801 Alexander Bell Drive, Reston, VA 20191-4400.
22. ACI 216.1/TMS 0216.1 *Standard Method for Determining Fire Resistance of Concrete and Masonry Construction Assemblies*, 1997 edition, American Concrete Institute, P.O. Box 9094, Farmington Hills, MI 48333.
23. ASTM E 2074, *Standard Test Method for Fire Tests of Door Assemblies, Including Positive Pressure Testing of Side-Hinged and Pivoted Swinging Door Assemblies*, 2000e edition, ASTM International, 100 Barr Harbor Drive, P.O. Box C700, West Conshohocken, PA 19428-2959.
24. NFPA 80, *Standard for Fire Doors and Other Opening Protectives*, 2007 edition, National Fire Protection Association, Quincy, MA.
25. Vol. 2, *UL Fire Resistance Directory*, Underwriters Laboratories Inc., 333 Pfingsten Road, Northbrook, IL 60062-2096.
26. ANSI/UL 1479, *Standard for Fire Tests of Through-Penetration Firestops*, 2003 edition, Revised 2007, Underwriters Laboratories Inc., 333 Pfingsten Road, Northbrook, IL 60062-2096.
27. ASTM E 814, *Standard Test Method for Fire Tests of Through-Penetration Fire Stops*, 2002 edition, ASTM International, 100 Barr Harbor Drive, P.O. Box C700, West Conshohocken, PA 19428-2959.
28. NFPA 90A, *Standard for the Installation of Air-Conditioning and Ventilating Systems*, 2009 edition, National Fire Protection Association, Quincy, MA.
29. NFPA 105, *Standard for the Installation of Smoke Door Assemblies and Other Opening Protectives*, 2007 edition, National Fire Protection Association, Quincy, MA.
30. ANSI/UL 1784, *Standard for Air Leakage Tests of Door Assemblies*, 2001 edition, Revised 2004, Underwriters Laboratories Inc., 333 Pfingsten Road, Northbrook, IL 60062-2096.
31. Degenkolb, J., "The 20-Minute Door and Other Considerations," *Building Standards*, XLV, no. 1 (January/February 1976).
32. *NFPA 72®, National Fire Alarm Code®*, 2007 edition, National Fire Protection Association, Quincy, MA.
33. Hall, Jr., J., "Report Prepared for the House Subcommittee on Science, Research, and Technology on H.R. 94, The Hotel and Motel Fire Safety Act of 1989," NFPA Fire Analysis and Research Division, National Fire Protection Association, Quincy, MA, March 2, 1989.
34. Klem, T., "Investigation Report on the Dupont Plaza Hotel Fire," National Fire Protection Association, Quincy, MA, 1987.
35. Best, R. and Demers, D., "Investigation Report on the MGM Grand Hotel Fire," National Fire Protection Association, Quincy, MA, 1980.
36. NFPA 13, *Standard for the Installation of Sprinkler Systems*, 2007 edition, National Fire Protection Association, Quincy, MA.
37. NFPA 92B, *Standard for Smoke Management Systems in Malls, Atria, and Large Spaces*, 2005 edition, National Fire Protection Association, Quincy, MA.
38. Schifiliti, R. and Pucci, W., "Fire Detection Modeling, State of the Art," Fire Detection Institute, Bloomfield, CT, 1996.
39. NFPA 92A, *Standard for Smoke-Control Systems Utilizing Barriers and Pressure Differences*, 2009 edition, National Fire Protection Association, Quincy, MA.
40. NFPA 20, *Standard for the Installation of Stationary Pumps for Fire Protection*, 2007 edition, National Fire Protection Association, Quincy, MA.
41. NFPA 68, *Standard on Explosion Protection by Deflagration Venting* , 2007 edition, National Fire Protection Association, Quincy, MA.
42. NFPA 69, *Standard on Explosion Prevention Systems*, 2008 edition, National Fire Protection Association, Quincy, MA.
43. NFPA 654, *Standard for the Prevention of Fire and Dust Explosions from the Manufacturing, Processing, and Handling of Combustible Particulate Solids*, 2006 edition, National Fire Protection Association, Quincy, MA.
44. NFPA 99, *Standard for Health Care Facilities*, 2005 edition, National Fire Protection Association, Quincy, MA.

CHAPTER 9

# Building Service and Fire Protection Equipment

As the title indicates, Chapter 9 divides the types of equipment commonly found in buildings into two categories: building service and fire protection. For the most part, the requirements for building service equipment are handled by direct reference to another code or standard, with little or no modification or additional requirements in the occupancy chapters. The result is that compliance with the referenced document is required in order for the building to achieve overall compliance with the *Life Safety Code.* Fire protection systems, particularly fire alarm and automatic sprinkler systems, are handled quite differently. For these systems, the *Code* presents a menu of general provisions that are used in conjunction with the installation standards. To apply these provisions, a specific requirement from another section of the *Code* must require their use. For example, 9.6.2.1 addresses fire alarm system signal initiation and 12.3.4.2 mandates the use of those provisions for fire alarm systems in new assembly occupancies.

The features that maintain a building safe from fire are varied and work in combination to provide protection for the occupants under a range of potentially adverse conditions. This chapter addresses those systems that help either to maintain a safe environment or to keep the occupants safe from the effects of a fire.

Section 9.6 identifies types of fire alarm initiating and notification systems. The fire alarm system plays an important role in notifying the building occupants of a fire, as well as in summoning help from outside sources, such as the fire department.

Section 9.7 applies to systems or features used to provide an active method for controlling the effects of a fire. These systems and features include automatic systems (such as sprinkler systems) as well as manual systems (such as standpipes and portable fire extinguishers).

Note that the occupancy chapters mandate the type of system required and the conditions under which that system is required.

## 9.1 Utilities

### 9.1.1 Gas.

Equipment using gas and related gas piping shall be in accordance with NFPA 54, *National Fuel Gas Code*, or NFPA 58, *Liquefied Petroleum Gas Code*, unless such installations are approved existing installations, which shall be permitted to be continued in service.

Although the referenced documents do not specify whether gas piping is permitted to pass through an exit enclosure, such as an enclosed stair, other provisions of the *Life Safety Code* apply. For example, see the provisions of 7.1.3.2.1(8) and (9) and the commentary following 7.1.3.2.1(10). These provisions stress that the only openings permitted in the enclosure walls between an exit and other building spaces are those needed to provide access into the exit from any normally occupied space and those needed to provide access out of the exit at the level of exit discharge. In other words, only those openings used by an occupant to enter and leave the exit enclosure are permitted. Gas piping is not permitted to pass through exit enclosure walls. Conversely, the *Code* does not prohibit the installation of gas piping in elevator shafts, dumbwaiters, or chutes. However, these areas are clearly prohibited from containing gas piping by NFPA 54, *National Fuel Gas Code.*[1] Thus, the *Code* and the reference document are used together to address installation safety and life safety.

### 9.1.2 Electrical Systems.

Electrical wiring and equipment shall be in accordance with *NFPA 70, National Electrical Code*, unless such installations are approved existing installations, which shall be permitted to be continued in service.

Because electrical wiring might require a complicated system or array involving many specifications and design details, the *Code* does not repeat them; rather, it references *NFPA 70®, National Electrical Code®*,[2] for design and installation guidance.

The *Life Safety Code* requirements for emergency lighting addressed by Section 7.9 and, in particular, by 7.9.2.3, with respect to independence of the emergency lighting source and distribution network, exceed the more general guidelines of *NFPA 70*. See the commentary throughout Section 7.9.

### 9.1.3 Emergency Generators and Standby Power Systems.

Where required for compliance with this *Code*, emergency generators and standby power systems shall comply with 9.1.3.1 and 9.1.3.2.

**9.1.3.1** Emergency generators and standby power systems shall be installed, tested, and maintained in accordance with NFPA 110, *Standard for Emergency and Standby Power Systems*.

**9.1.3.2** New generator controllers shall be monitored by the fire alarm system, where provided, or at an attended location, for the following conditions:

(1) Generator running
(2) Generator fault
(3) Generator switch in nonautomatic position

### 9.1.4 Stored Electrical Energy Systems.

Stored electrical energy systems shall be installed, tested, and maintained in accordance with NFPA 111, *Standard on Stored Electrical Energy Emergency and Standby Power Systems*.

## 9.2 Heating, Ventilating, and Air-Conditioning

### 9.2.1 Air-Conditioning, Heating, Ventilating Ductwork, and Related Equipment.

Air-conditioning, heating, ventilating ductwork, and related equipment shall be in accordance with NFPA 90A, *Standard for the Installation of Air-Conditioning and Ventilating Systems*, or NFPA 90B, *Standard for the Installation of Warm Air Heating and Air-Conditioning Systems*, as applicable, unless such installations are approved existing installations, which shall be permitted to be continued in service.

For the proper installation of HVAC systems, 9.2.1 refers the *Code* user to NFPA 90A, *Standard for the Installation of Air-Conditioning and Ventilating Systems*.[3] For occupancies with small overall volumes, such as one- and two-family dwellings, the *Code* refers the user to NFPA 90B, *Standard for the Installation of Warm Air Heating and Air-Conditioning Systems*.[4]

For example, NFPA 90A addresses fire damper requirements for both ductwork and air-transfer grilles that penetrate fire resistance–rated barriers. NFPA 90A also prohibits means of egress corridors in health care, detention and correctional, and residential occupancies from being used as a portion of a supply-, return-, or exhaust-air system serving adjoining areas. Exhibit 9.1 identifies some of the areas where fire dampers and smoke dampers would be required by NFPA 90A.

### 9.2.2 Ventilating or Heat-Producing Equipment.

Ventilating or heat-producing equipment shall be in accordance with NFPA 91, *Standard for Exhaust Systems for Air Conveying of Vapors, Gases, Mists, and Noncombustible Particulate Solids*; NFPA 211, *Standard for Chimneys, Fireplaces, Vents, and Solid Fuel–Burning Appliances*; NFPA 31, *Standard for the Installation of Oil-Burning Equipment*; NFPA 54, *National Fuel Gas Code*; or *NFPA 70, National Electrical Code*, as applicable, unless such installations are approved existing installations, which shall be permitted to be continued in service.

### 9.2.3 Commercial Cooking Equipment.

Commercial cooking equipment shall be in accordance with NFPA 96, *Standard for Ventilation Control and Fire Protection of Commercial Cooking Operations*, unless such installations are approved existing installations, which shall be permitted to be continued in service.

The occupancy chapters that address the protection of commercial cooking equipment do so in the provisions for the protection of hazards. To understand the intent of the *Code*, close attention must be paid to the manner in which the protection is addressed.

For example, for health care occupancies, 18.3.2.5.2 states that domestic cooking equipment used for food warming or limited cooking is not required to be protected; nor must the space be segregated from the rest of the building. For day-care occupancies, a

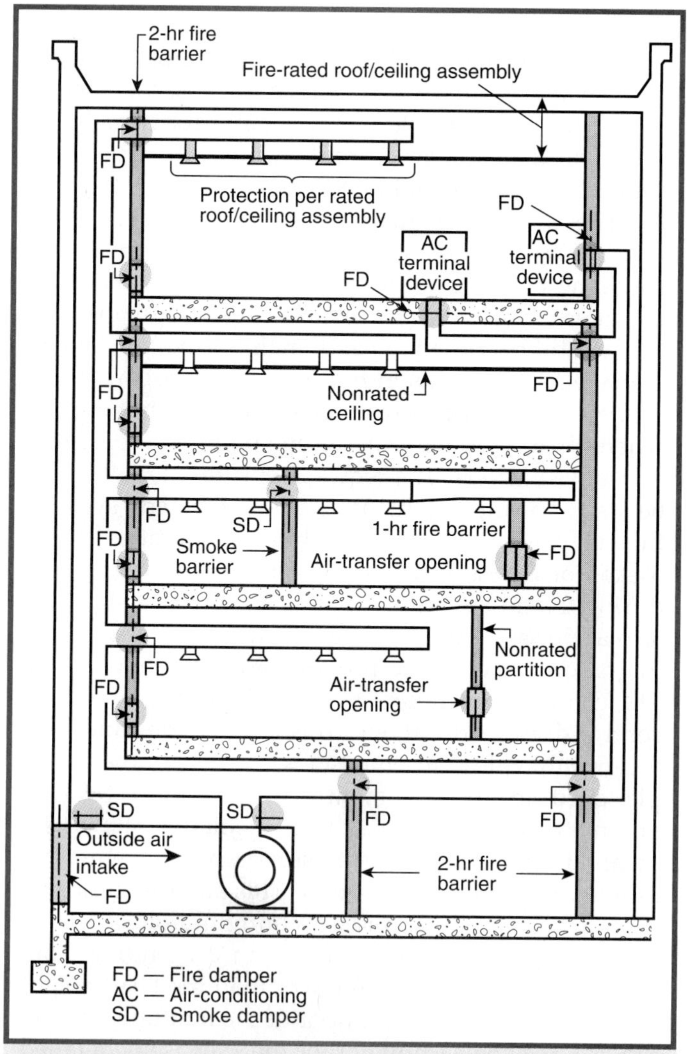


**Exhibit 9.1** *Partition and fire barrier penetration protection.*

similar provision appears in 16.3.2.5; however, this provision requires the approval of the authority having jurisdiction (AHJ) to exempt protection and segregation of domestic cooking equipment (the term *approved* is defined in 3.2.1 as "acceptable to the authority having jurisdiction"). Paragraphs 12.3.2.2 and 13.3.2.2, which apply to assembly occupancies, and 22.3.2.4 and 23.3.2.4, which apply to detention and correctional occupancies, permit a kitchen to be open to the rest of a building only if the cooking equipment is protected in accordance with 9.2.3.

In occupancy chapters that do not refer to the protection of cooking equipment, NFPA 96, *Standard for Ventilation Control and Fire Protection of Commercial Cooking Operations,*[5] needs to be consulted to determine the criteria that define commercial cooking equipment and its appropriate required protection.

### 9.2.4 Ventilating Systems in Laboratories Using Chemicals.

Ventilating systems in laboratories using chemicals shall be in accordance with NFPA 45, *Standard on Fire Protection for Laboratories Using Chemicals*, or NFPA 99, *Standard for Health Care Facilities*, as appropriate.

NFPA 45, *Standard on Fire Protection for Laboratories Using Chemicals,*[6] contains requirements for construction, ventilation, and fire protection in laboratory buildings, as well as for units and work areas in all buildings. Additional requirements for laboratories in health care occupancies are found in NFPA 99, *Standard for Health Care Facilities.*[7] The requirements of both documents are to be applied to laboratories in health care facilities.

## 9.3 Smoke Control

**9.3.1** Where required by the provisions of another section of this *Code*, smoke control systems shall be installed, inspected, tested, and maintained in accordance with NFPA 92A, *Standard for Smoke-Control Systems Utilizing Barriers and Pressure Differences*; NFPA 92B, *Standard for Smoke Management Systems in Malls, Atria, and Large Spaces*; NFPA 204, *Standard for Smoke and Heat Venting*; or nationally recognized standards, engineering guides, or recommended practices, as approved by the authority having jurisdiction.

The provision of 9.3.1 does not itself require smoke control systems; it mandates that, if such systems are installed for *Code* compliance, they must be installed, inspected, tested, and maintained in accordance with NFPA 92A, *Standard for Smoke-Control Systems Utilizing Barriers and Pressure Differences,*[8] NFPA 92B, *Standard for Smoke Management Systems in Malls, Atria, and Large Spaces,*[9] or NFPA 204, *Standard for Smoke and Heat Venting,* as applicable. Prior to this edition of the *Code*, no smoke control system standards existed. Rather, the noted NFPA documents were guides and recommended practices. As such, they could not be referenced in the body of the *Code* as mandatory requirements. Subsequent to the publication of the 2006 edition of this *Code*, the noted documents were revised as standards and are now referenced herein as mandatory requirements.

NFPA 92A addresses smoke control systems that use barriers, airflows, and pressure differences to confine the smoke of a fire to the zone of fire origin and, thus, maintain a tenable environment in other zones. The requirements of NFPA 92A can be used to create a smokeproof enclosure using the stair pressurization method described in 7.2.3.9. The standard also covers smoke control for elevator hoistways by employing the following methods, either singly or in combination:

1. Fire floor exhaust
2. Elevator lobby pressurization
3. Smoke-tight elevator lobby construction
4. Elevator hoistway pressurization

NFPA 92A also addresses, in detail, zoned smoke control under which a building can be divided into a number of smoke control zones. Each zone is separated from the others by partitions, floors, and doors that can be closed to inhibit the movement of smoke. A smoke control zone can consist of one or more floors, or a floor can consist of more than one smoke control zone. Some arrangements of smoke control zones are depicted in Exhibit 9.2. The smoke zones are indicated by minus signs — negative pressurization or exhaust — and positively pressurized spaces are indicated by plus signs. All nonsmoke zones might be pressurized, as in Part (a) and Part (c), or only those nonsmoke zones that are adjacent to the smoke zone might be pressurized, as in Part (b) and Part (d). In Part (e), the smoke zone has been limited to a portion of a floor.

The subject of maintaining tenable conditions within large zones of fire origin (such as atria and shopping malls) is addressed by NFPA 92B. NFPA 92B provides technical data relevant to the design, installation, testing, operation, and maintenance of smoke management systems in buildings with large-volume spaces. These systems manage smoke within the space where the fire exists or between spaces not separated by smoke barriers. The requirements of NFPA 92B can be used to implement smoke management systems that help to maintain a tenable environment in the means of egress from large-volume building spaces during the time required for evacuation. The standard also addresses the control and reduction of the smoke migration between the fire area and adjacent spaces. The commentary following A.8.6.7 on atrium smoke control draws extensively from the theories and protection strategies presented in NFPA 92B. In the example cited in the commentary following A.8.6.7, a volumetric exhaust rate, *V*, was calculated following a detailed analysis of the physics associated with fire growth and smoke generation. This analysis concerns a particular atrium building configuration in which the exhaust rate keeps smoke from descending from the ceiling level to a level lower than the head height of persons on the highest floor of the building open to the atrium. The summation of the exercise is detailed in Exhibit 8.22 and is generalized in Exhibit 9.3.

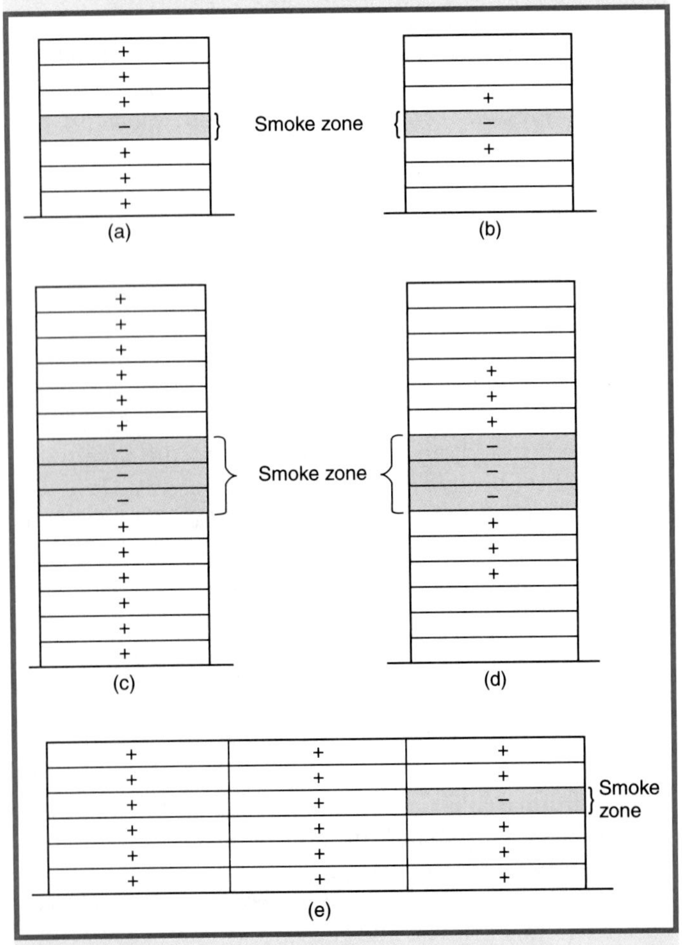


***Exhibit 9.2** Smoke control zone arrangement.*

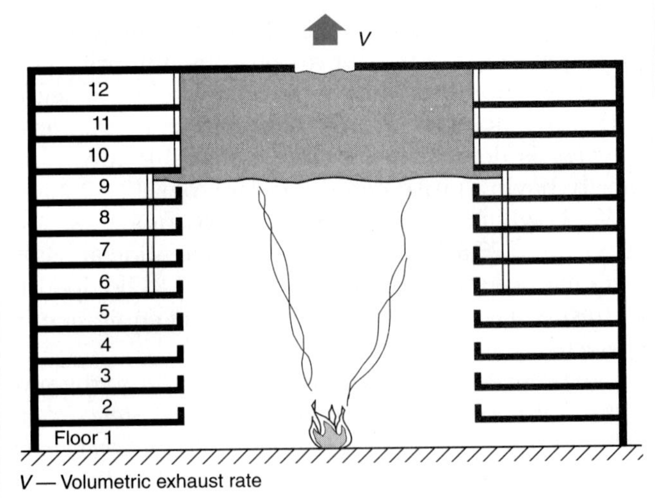


***Exhibit 9.3** Control of smoke layer.*

An approved maintenance and testing program must be provided to ensure the operational integrity of smoke control systems. A combination public address system and emergency occupant notification system is used routinely, and any problems with the system will be readily apparent; a smoke control system dedicated to emergency use only is not subject to daily use. Therefore, maintenance and testing of smoke control systems are necessary.

**9.3.2** The engineer of record shall clearly identify the intent of the system, the design method used, the appropriateness of the method used, and the required means of inspecting, testing, and maintaining the system.

**9.3.3** Acceptance testing shall be performed by a special inspector in accordance with Section 9.8.

### 9.3.4 Smoke Control System Operation.

**9.3.4.1** Floor- or zone-dependent smoke control systems shall be automatically activated by sprinkler waterflow or smoke detection systems.

**9.3.4.2** Means for manual operation of smoke control systems shall be provided at an approved location.

## 9.4 Elevators, Escalators, and Conveyors

### 9.4.1* General.

An elevator, other than an elevator in accordance with 7.2.13, shall not be considered a component in a required means of egress but shall be permitted as a component in an accessible means of egress.

**A.9.4.1** Under certain conditions, elevators are recognized as means of egress.

The use of elevators for emergency evacuation purposes, where operated by trained emergency service personnel (e.g., building personnel, fire personnel), should be incorporated into the building evacuation program. Elevators are normally capable of manual, in-car fire fighter operation (Phase II) after elevator recall (Phase I). In addition, there usually are two or more shafts wherever there are more than three elevators, which further enhances the possibilities for elevator use during an emergency evacuation where operated by trained personnel.

In high-rise buildings, in towers, or in deep underground spaces where travel over considerable vertical distance on stairs can cause persons incapable of such physical effort to collapse before they reach the street exit, stairways are permitted to be used for initial escape from the immediate area of danger, and elevators are permitted to be used to complete the travel to the street.

It can be reasonably assumed that, in all buildings of sufficient height to indicate the need for elevators, elevators will be provided for normal use; for this reason, no requirements for mandatory installation of elevators are included in the *Code*.

For additional information on elevators, see ASME A17.1/CSA B44,, *Safety Code for Elevators and Escalators*, and ASME A17.3, *Safety Code for Existing Elevators and Escalators*.

In much earlier *Code* editions, the egress capacity of elevators was calculated based on the assumption that three average elevators were roughly equivalent to the formerly used single unit of stairway exit width. Because of this assumption, elevators were accepted as required egress components under certain limited conditions. No such credit has been given since 1956 because of some inherent characteristics that might make elevators unsuitable for emergency exit use. These characteristics are accentuated in modern automatic elevators where no operator is available to exercise judgment in the control of the elevator in case of fire or other emergency. The reasons that elevators are not credited as part of the required means of egress are summarized in paragraphs 1 through 4, which follow.

**1.** People seeking to escape from a fire by using an elevator might have to wait at the elevator door for some time; during that time, they might be exposed to fire or smoke, or they might panic.

**2.** Automatic elevators travel to floors by responding to call buttons, both in the elevator car and in elevator lobbies. Because this operation cannot be canceled once a button is pressed, it is possible for an elevator descending from floors above a fire to stop automatically at the floor of the fire. The doors will open automatically, thus exposing occupants to fire and smoke.

A further consideration is that an elevator shaft will act as a "chimney" in a multistory building. Unless positively pressurized with respect to the fire floor, the shaft can carry heat and smoke from a fire and expose passengers to hazardous levels of both — even if the elevator does not stop at the fire floor and continues to function. An elevator moving within its shaft enclosure might act as a piston within a cylinder and push the smoke and fire gases to floors not initially involved.

**3.** Modern elevators will not operate until the doors are fully closed. In an emergency, a large number of people might try to crowd into an elevator, preventing the doors from closing and preventing the elevator from operating.

**4.** Any power failure, such as the burnout of electric supply cables during a fire, might render the elevators inoperative or might cause people to become trapped in elevators stopped between floors. Under fire conditions, there might not be enough time to rescue the trapped occupants through emergency escape hatches or doors.

Exhibit 9.4 is an example of an appropriate elevator placard used to notify occupants that an elevator is unsuitable for emergency egress use.

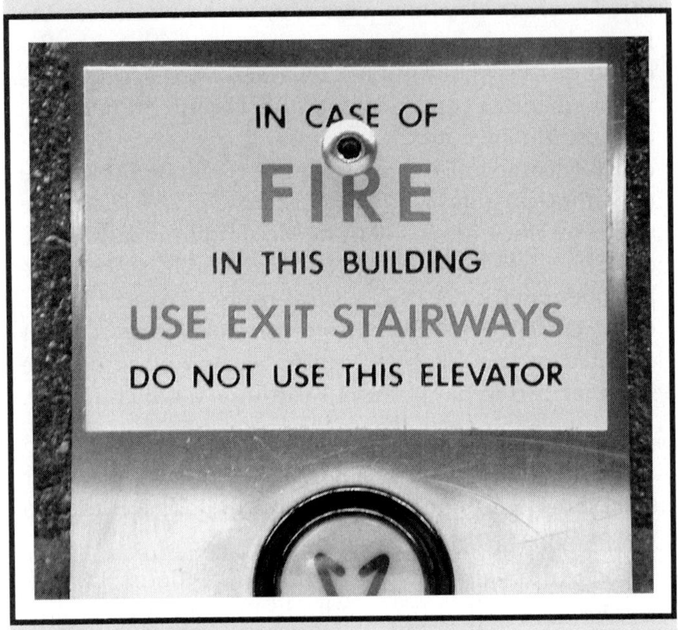


***Exhibit 9.4*** *Elevator placard.*

Recognizing the viability of elevators to facilitate the movement of people, the *Code* has, in recent editions, added guidelines addressing their use in limited circumstances. The four circumstances under which an elevator can be part of a building's evacuation plan are described in paragraphs 1 through 4, which follow.

**1.** An elevator can be used in a high-rise building for assisting in a staged evacuation. Though it cannot be used as a component of the means of egress, an elevator can be a useful tool in the evacuation of a high-rise building.

**2.** An elevator can be used as a means of evacuating people from an area of refuge. Elevators are an effective means of transporting people with severe mobility impairments. The criteria for the use of elevators for evacuation from an area of refuge are established in 7.2.12.2.4. Also see the commentary on 7.2.12.

**3.** In underground assembly occupancies, the *Code* might require an elevator or escalator for the purpose of assisting in an emergency evacuation in an upward direction. An example of the *Code* requiring an elevator to be used under emergency conditions can be found in 12.4.3.3, which requires each level of a new assembly occupancy with a floor level more than 30 ft (91 m) below the level of exit discharge to be divided into at least two smoke compartments. Per 12.4.3.3.2, each compartment must be provided with a mechanical means of moving people vertically, such as an elevator or escalator. These requirements are in addition to those of Section 11.7, which addresses underground and limited access structures. In Exhibit 9.5, an escalator is used in smoke zone A and an elevator is used in smoke zone B to meet the requirements of 12.4.3.3.2.

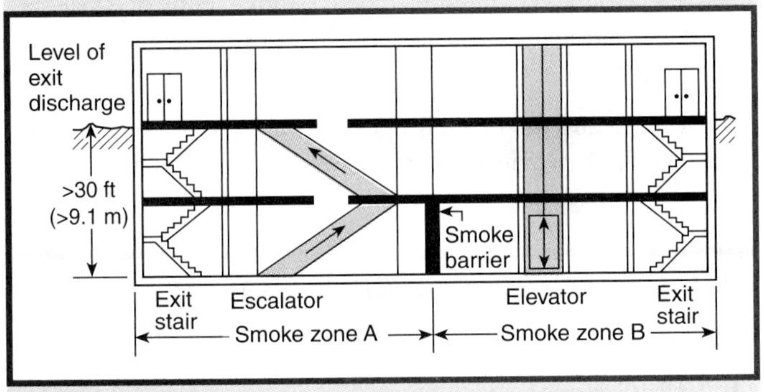


***Exhibit 9.5*** *Elevator and escalator use in underground assembly occupancy.*

**4.** In special types of towers (typically air traffic control towers), the *Code* recognizes the use of an elevator as a secondary means of egress. See the commentary on 7.2.13.

### 9.4.2 Code Compliance.

For elevator installations, the *Code* requires compliance with either of the following:

1. ASME A17.1/CSA B44, *Safety Code for Elevators and Escalators*[11]
2. ASME A17.3, *Safety Code for Existing Elevators and Escalators*[12]

The *Code* additionally requires that a sprinkler system, if installed, meet the requirements of NFPA 13,

*Standard for the Installation of Sprinkler Systems.*[13] ASME A17.1/CSA B44 permits sprinklers in elevator hoistways and machine rooms in accordance with NFPA 13, subject to the following provisions:

1. All risers and returns are to be located outside these spaces.
2. Branch lines in the hoistway are to supply only the sprinklers on that level.
3. A means for disconnecting the main line power supply to the affected elevator automatically upon, or prior to, the application of water from sprinklers located in the machine room or hoistway is to be provided as follows:
   a. The means must be independent of the elevator control and cannot be self-resetting.
   b. The activation of sprinklers outside the hoistway or machine room is not to disconnect the main line power supply.
   c. Smoke detectors are not to be used to activate sprinklers in these spaces or to disconnect the main line power supply.

ASME A17.1/CSA B44 and ASME A17.3 are also referenced because the *Code* recognizes the use of elevators and escalators under limited conditions and because fire fighters might need to use elevators during fire suppression operations. Compliance with these documents makes it possible to recall elevators to the ground floor or other designated floor during a fire, thus taking the elevators out of service. The provisions also permit fire fighters to manually override the controls and use the elevators as necessary.

Where elevators are to be used for occupant evacuation, the *Code* provides additional requirements by way of an adoptable annex— see Annex B, Elevators for Occupant-Controlled Evacuation Prior to Phase I Emergency Recall Operations. Annex B, while not part of the body of the *Code*, is written in mandatory language so that it can be separately adopted by authorities having jurisdiction. Its requirements augment those of ASME A17.1/CSA B44 and Section 9.4 of this *Code*.

**9.4.2.1** Except as modified herein, new elevators, escalators, dumbwaiters, and moving walks shall be in accordance with the requirements of ASME A17.1/CSA B44, *Safety Code for Elevators and Escalators*.

**9.4.2.2** Except as modified herein, existing elevators, escalators, dumbwaiters, and moving walks shall conform to the requirements of ASME A17.3, *Safety Code for Existing Elevators and Escalators*.

### 9.4.3 Fire Fighters' Emergency Operations.

**9.4.3.1** All new elevators shall conform to the Fire Fighters' Emergency Operations requirements of ASME A17.1/CSA B44, *Safety Code for Elevators and Escalators*.

**9.4.3.2** All existing elevators having a travel distance of 25 ft (7620 mm) or more above or below the level that best serves the needs of emergency personnel for fire-fighting or rescue purposes shall conform to the Fire Fighters' Emergency Operations requirements of ASME A17.3, *Safety Code for Existing Elevators and Escalators*.

Because an elevator stopping at a fire floor (intentionally or unintentionally) is an extreme hazard, the *Code* mandates compliance with the Fire Fighters' Emergency Operations requirements of ASME A17.1/CSA B44 and ASME A17.3 in both new and existing buildings. The Fire Fighters' Emergency Operations requirements establish elevator recall activated by smoke detection in each elevator lobby and in associated elevator machine rooms. A three-position, key-operated switch, normally located in the main lobby at the elevator, controls the recall function. The requirements mandate specific functions for the "on," "off," and "bypass" positions of this switch. The requirements also provide for *emergency in-car operations*, or what is often referred to as *fire fighters' service*. Fire fighters' service requires a three-position, key-operated switch in each elevator car. The functions of the "on," "off," and "hold" positions are specified in the elevator code. For specific details, refer to ASME A17.1/CSA B44. Explanatory material on these rules can be found in the ASME A17.1/CSA B44 *Handbook on Safety Code for Elevators and Escalators*.[14]

Supplement 2 of this *Life Safety Code Handbook* contains extracts from ASME A17.1/CSA B44 regarding this issue, as well as commentary from the ASME A17.1/CSA B44 *Handbook on Safety Code for Elevators and Escalators*.

### 9.4.4 Number of Cars.

The number of elevator cars permitted in a hoistway shall be in accordance with 8.6.8.3.

### 9.4.5* Elevator Machine Rooms.

Elevator machine rooms that contain solid-state equipment for elevators, other than existing elevators, having a travel distance exceeding 50 ft (15 m) above the level of exit discharge, or exceeding 30 ft (9.1 m) below the level of exit discharge, shall be provided with independent ventilation or air-conditioning systems to maintain temperature during fire fighters' emergency operations for elevator operation *(see 9.4.3)*. The operating temperature shall be established by the elevator equipment manufacturer's specifications. When standby power is connected to the elevator, the machine room ventilation or air-conditioning shall be connected to standby power.

**A.9.4.5** Continued operation of solid-state elevator equipment is contingent on maintaining the ambient temperature in the range specified by the elevator manufacturer. If the machine room ventilation/air-conditioning is connected to the general building system, and that system is shut down during a fire, the fire department might lose the use of elevators due to excessive heat in the elevator machine room.

The intent of the requirement for a ventilation or an air-conditioning system to help keep the elevator controls operable is explained in 9.4.5 and A.9.4.5. For many typical installations, this requirement can be met by installing an independent through-the-wall air-conditioning unit. Regardless of shutdown of the building's HVAC system, the independent unit will continue to run, provided that its power supply is not interrupted.

### 9.4.6 Elevator Testing.

Because emergency responders might use elevators to move personnel and equipment, and potentially to assist in the evacuation of mobility-impaired occupants, it is important to provide an appropriate level of elevator testing to help ensure that elevators can be used when needed under fire and other emergency conditions.

**9.4.6.1** Elevators shall be subject to periodic inspections and tests as specified in ASME A17.1/CSA B44, *Safety Code for Elevators and Escalators*.

**9.4.6.2** All elevators equipped with fire fighters' emergency operations in accordance with 9.4.3 shall be subject to a monthly operation with a written record of the findings made and kept on the premises as required by ASME A17.1/CSA B44, *Safety Code for Elevators and Escalators*.

**9.4.6.3** The elevator inspections and tests required by 9.4.6.1 shall be performed at frequencies complying with one of the following:

(1) Inspection and test frequencies specified in Appendix N of ASME A17.1/CSA B44, *Safety Code for Elevators and Escalators*
(2) Inspection and test frequencies specified by the authority having jurisdiction

### 9.4.7 Openings to Exit Enclosures.

Conveyors, elevators, dumbwaiters, and pneumatic conveyors serving various stories of a building shall not open to an exit enclosure.

Openings in exit enclosures are strictly limited by the provisions of 7.1.3.2.1(8) to doors that provide access to the exit from normally occupied spaces or corridors and means to leave the exit enclosure. Elevators and other conveyors are not considered normally occupied areas. Additionally, an elevator, with its associated cables, controls, and mechanical equipment, would introduce combustibles into an exit enclosure, which conflicts with the objective of making the exit enclosure a safe place free of combustibles.

## 9.5 Rubbish Chutes, Incinerators, and Laundry Chutes

### 9.5.1 Enclosure.

**9.5.1.1** Rubbish chutes and laundry chutes shall be separately enclosed by walls or partitions in accordance with the provisions of Section 8.3.

**9.5.1.2** Inlet openings serving chutes shall be protected in accordance with Section 8.3.

**9.5.1.3** The doors of chutes specified in 9.5.1.2 shall open only to a room that is designed and used exclusively for accessing the chute opening.

**9.5.1.4** The room used for accessing the chute opening shall be separated from other spaces in accordance with Section 8.7.

**9.5.1.5** The requirements of 9.5.1.1 through 9.5.1.4 shall not apply where otherwise permitted by the following:

(1) Existing installations having properly enclosed service chutes and properly installed and maintained service openings shall be permitted to have inlets open to a corridor or normally occupied space.
(2) Rubbish chutes and laundry chutes shall be permitted to open into rooms not exceeding 400 ft$^2$ (37 m$^2$) that are used for storage, provided that the room is protected by automatic sprinklers.

Laundry chutes are often associated with a laundry/storage room. The provision of 9.5.1.5(2) permits chutes to open into such rooms, provided that the area of the room does not exceed 400 ft$^2$ (37 m$^2$). Without this provision, the user might interpret the words "used exclusively" (see 9.5.1.3) as limiting the use of that room to serving the chute only.

### 9.5.2 Installation and Maintenance.

Rubbish chutes, laundry chutes, and incinerators shall be installed and maintained in accordance with NFPA 82, *Standard on Incinerators and Waste and Linen Handling Systems and Equipment*, unless such installations are approved existing installations, which shall be permitted to be continued in service.

Shafts containing waste and linen chutes must be enclosed according to the requirements for the protection of vertical openings found in Section 8.6. The installation of the chute itself must meet the requirements of NFPA 82, *Standard on Incinerators and Waste and Linen Handling Systems and Equipment.*[15]

Additional concerns regarding chutes opening to other parts of the building need to be addressed. For convenience, service openings for loading are usually located to be accessible from corridors on the upper floors of the building. However, these corridors also serve as exit access, and a fire in the chute with an open loading door could result in the obstruction of the corridor by smoke and other products of combustion. To address this hazard, the *Code* and NFPA 82 require the construction of service opening rooms to form a buffer between the chute and the building space. The special hazard protection provisions in Section 8.7 for the separation of the service opening are referenced in 9.5.1.4. The result is a room that is separated from the rest of the building by construction with a 1-hour fire resistance rating or protected with an automatic extinguishing system. The door to this room is required to have a $^3/_4$-hour fire protection rating. Exhibit 9.6 illustrates the protection arrangement required for waste and linen chutes by NFPA 82.

Additionally, NFPA 82 requires the service opening room to be sized to maintain a minimum 6 in. (150 mm) clearance between the closed chute loading door and the closed room door. Exhibit 9.7 illustrates the measurement of this clearance.

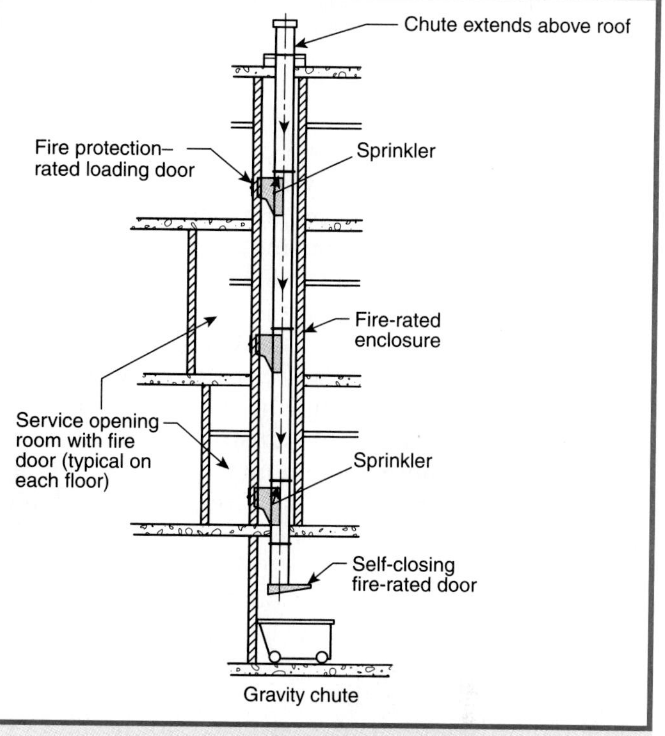


***Exhibit 9.6*** *Protection of waste and linen chutes.*

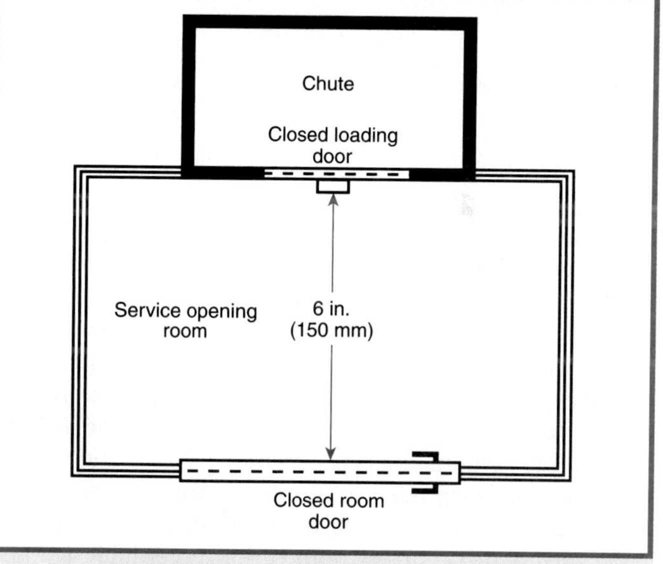


***Exhibit 9.7*** *Clearance in service opening room.*

## 9.6 Fire Detection, Alarm, and Communications Systems

### 9.6.1* General.

**A.9.6.1** The provisions of Section 9.6 cover the basic functions of a complete fire alarm system, including fire detection, alarm, and communications. These systems are primarily intended to provide the indication and warning of abnormal conditions, the summoning of appropriate aid, and the control of occupancy facilities to enhance protection of life.

Some of the provisions of Section 9.6 originated with *NFPA 72, National Fire Alarm Code*. For purposes of this

*Code*, some provisions of Section 9.6 are more stringent than those of *NFPA 72*, which should be consulted for additional details.

The provision for early warning of fire accompanied by notification of emergency responders is a key element of a fire protection program. If people are involved, then protective signaling carries even greater importance. The intent of A.9.6.1 is to provide guidance on establishing objectives for the performance of the fire alarm system and to allow individual system designs to address occupancy-specific variables.

Certain occupancies might not be required to have a fire alarm system at all. In industrial and storage occupancies, for example, the number of occupants in the facility or the hazard classification of the contents of the building determines whether an alarm system is required. In educational, mercantile, and business occupancies, there are usually enough people present (at least during a part of the day) to discover an incipient fire. For these occupancies, the *Code* imposes less rigid requirements for fire alarm systems than it does for certain other occupancies. Conversely, for health care occupancies, the provisions for fire alarm systems are quite detailed with respect to notification and emergency functions, such as the automatic closure of smoke barrier doors.

**9.6.1.1** The provisions of Section 9.6 shall apply only where specifically required by another section of this *Code*.

Section 9.6 applies only where specifically referenced by another section of the *Code*. Primarily, such references appear in the occupancy chapters. Careful attention to the provisions in the occupancy chapters is necessary, as they might contain references to specific paragraphs in Section 9.6. For example, 12.3.4.1.1 for new assembly occupancies contains a general reference to all the requirements of 9.6.1; however, 12.3.4.3.5 contains a provision that permits the omission of visible signals in assembly seating areas where the occupant load exceeds 1000 and an alternative visible means of occupant notification acceptable to the AHJ, such as an electronic message board, is provided as indicated in 9.6.3.5.7.

**9.6.1.2** Fire detection, alarm, and communications systems installed to make use of an alternative permitted by this *Code* shall be considered required systems and shall meet the provisions of this *Code* applicable to required systems.

The provisions of 9.6.1.2 remind the user that a fire detection, an alarm, or an associated communications system that is installed to take advantage of a *Code* alternative becomes a required system and is subject to the same requirements as any other required system, including maintenance. An example of this provision is a new business occupancy that is not required to have a fire alarm system on the basis of the thresholds established in 38.3.4.1. If, for security reasons, delayed-egress locks were to be installed, they would have to meet the provisions of 7.2.1.6.1. Paragraph 7.2.1.6.1(2) requires that the locks automatically release upon the activation of an approved, supervised automatic sprinkler system in accordance with Section 9.7; activation of any heat detector; or activation of not more than two smoke detectors of an approved, supervised automatic fire detection system installed in accordance with Section 9.6. If a fire alarm system is utilized to automatically release a delayed-egress lock, it becomes a required system and must be installed and maintained in accordance with Section 9.6.

**9.6.1.3** A fire alarm system required for life safety shall be installed, tested, and maintained in accordance with the applicable requirements of *NFPA 70, National Electrical Code*, and *NFPA 72, National Fire Alarm Code*, unless it is an approved existing installation, which shall be permitted to be continued in use.

**9.6.1.4** All systems and components shall be approved for the purpose for which they are installed.

Approval of both the system as a whole and its individual components is required. The authority having jurisdiction grants such approval (see the definition of *approved* in 3.2.1). Substantiating data could be provided in the form of test reports, approvals or listings issued by organizations such as FM Global or Underwriters Laboratories Inc., or testing or evaluation by another recognized source.

**9.6.1.5*** To ensure operational integrity, the fire alarm system shall have an approved maintenance and testing program complying with the applicable requirements of *NFPA 70, National Electrical Code*, and *NFPA 72, National Fire Alarm Code*.

**A.9.6.1.5** Records of conducted maintenance and testing and a copy of the certificate of compliance should be maintained.

The operational integrity of a fire alarm system cannot be ensured without proper maintenance and testing. Thus, the *Code* requires that an approved — that is, acceptable to the authority having jurisdiction — maintenance and testing program be operational on an ongoing basis. An important part of the program is retention of system acceptance records and subsequent operational test records, so that comparisons can be made to initial system specifications.

**9.6.1.6*** Where a required fire alarm system is out of service for more than 4 hours in a 24-hour period, the authority having jurisdiction shall be notified, and the building shall be evacuated, or an approved fire watch shall be provided for all parties left unprotected by the shutdown, until the fire alarm system has been returned to service.

**A.9.6.1.6** A fire watch should at least involve some special action beyond normal staffing, such as assigning an additional security guard(s) to walk the areas affected. Such individuals should be specially trained in fire prevention and in occupant and fire department notification techniques, and they should understand the particular fire safety situation for public education purposes. *(Also see* NFPA 601, *Standard for Security Services in Fire Loss Prevention.)*

The term *out of service* in 9.6.1.6 is intended to imply that a significant portion of the fire alarm system is not in operation, such as an entire initiating device, signaling line, or notification appliance circuit. It is not the intent of the *Code* to require notification of the authority having jurisdiction, or evacuation of the portion of the building affected, for a single nonoperating device or appliance.

A fire alarm system might be shut down for any number of reasons during the life of a building. Some shutdowns are preplanned, controlled, and of short duration, such as during periodic testing and maintenance. Others might be preplanned and of longer duration, such as during times of building or system rehabilitation. Emergency shutdown of the system can be the result of power failure, fire, or other physical damage and might result in a short or lengthy shutdown to repair the system. Advance planning should help ensure that the system, or most of the system, can be restored to service despite the scope of the renovation or the extent of an unexpected impairment. If the alarm system is required by the *Code*, or if it was installed to make use of one of the alternatives offered by the *Code*, it must be in operable condition for the building to be considered *Code* compliant.

Instead of designating a building with an inoperative alarm system as noncompliant and prohibiting occupancy under all conditions in accordance with the provisions of 4.6.10.1, 9.6.1.6 differentiates between those alarm system impairments that last less than 4 hours within a 24-hour period and those that last longer. Continued occupancy of a building that has an alarm system impairment of more than 4 hours cumulative within any 24-hour period can be tolerated only if a fire watch acceptable to the authority having jurisdiction is provided. Such lengthy impairments generally indicate a situation that involves a problem more serious in nature than typical system maintenance or testing.

It is the intent of the *Code* that the fire watch result in a heightened awareness of the building's operations and environment. Individuals assigned to the fire watch should be able to recognize fire hazards and understand the procedures for occupant and fire department notification and occupant evacuation in an emergency.

When developing a plan to address system shutdown, it is important to consider the nature of the shutdown, the location, the increased hazards that are involved, and the actions necessary to mitigate the hazards. The authority having jurisdiction should be involved in the development of such a plan.

A parallel requirement in 9.7.6 addresses sprinkler system shutdown.

**9.6.1.7** For the purposes of this *Code*, a complete fire alarm system shall provide functions for initiation, notification, and control, which shall perform as follows:

(1) The initiation function provides the input signal to the system.
(2) The notification function is the means by which the system advises that human action is required in response to a particular condition.
(3) The control function provides outputs to control building equipment to enhance protection of life.

**9.6.1.8 Protection of Fire Alarm System.**

**9.6.1.8.1*** In areas that are not continuously occupied, and unless otherwise permitted by 9.6.1.8.1.1, 9.6.1.8.1.2, or 9.6.1.8.1.3, automatic smoke detection shall be installed to provide notification of fire at the following locations:

(1) Each fire alarm control unit
(2) Notification appliance circuit power extenders
(3) Supervising station transmitting equipment

**A.9.6.1.8.1** The *Code* intends that only one smoke detector is required to be installed at the fire alarm control unit, the notification circuit power extenders, and the supervising station transmitting equipment, even when the area of the room would require more than one smoke detector if installed according to the spacing rules in *NFPA 72, National Fire Alarm Code*, Chapter 5.

**9.6.1.8.1.1** The provisions of 9.6.1.8.1(2) and 9.6.1.8.1(3) shall not apply to existing alarm systems.

**9.6.1.8.1.2** Where ambient conditions prohibit installation of a smoke detector, a heat detector shall be used.

**9.6.1.8.1.3** Automatic smoke detection shall not be required where buildings are protected throughout by an approved, supervised automatic sprinkler system in accordance with Section 9.7 and the area containing the fire alarm control unit is sprinklered.

The provisions of 9.6.1.8 are intended to provide early notification of a fire that might adversely affect components of the fire alarm system and prevent it from operating properly. Note that smoke detectors are not required to provide such early notification where the building is protected throughout by an approved, supervised automatic sprinkler system per 9.6.1.8.1.3. Further note, however, that the occupancy chapters can further modify these provisions. For example, see 30.3.4.6, which requires a smoke detector to protect the fire alarm control unit in new apartment buildings, regardless of the presence of automatic sprinklers, because sufficient smoke can be produced to damage the control unit prior to the activation of sprinklers.

### 9.6.2 Signal Initiation.

**9.6.2.1** Where required by other sections of this *Code*, actuation of the complete fire alarm system shall be initiated by, but shall not be limited to, any or all of the following means:

(1) Manual fire alarm initiation
(2) Automatic detection
(3) Extinguishing system operation

The capability for manual fire alarm initiation is a requirement common to all occupancies that require the installation of a fire alarm system. Initiation by automatic detection or extinguishing system operation is permitted to serve in lieu of manual initiation for some occupancies. In some cases, an occupancy chapter might require initiation by automatic detection or extinguishing system operation. For example, new educational occupancies are not generally required to have an automatic sprinkler system; however, if such a system is installed, 14.3.4.2.2 requires automatic alarm system initiation by operation of the sprinkler system in addition to the manual means. In new health care occupancies, automatic sprinklers are required, and 18.3.4.2.1 states that initiation of the alarm system is to be by manual means and by sprinkler system waterflow alarms. In new Class A mercantile occupancies, a fire alarm system and an automatic sprinkler system are required. However, 36.3.4.2(1) only requires alarm initiation by manual means. Alarm initiation by means of sprinkler system activation is permitted by 36.3.4.2(3) to serve in lieu of manual initiation, but it is not required.

Where both manual and automatic means for alarm system initiation are used, they should be complementary. If one system becomes inoperative — for example, failure of the manual initiation circuit — the second should continue to function properly and initiate the alarm upon automatic detection of fire or smoke.

**9.6.2.2** Manual fire alarm boxes shall be used only for fire-protective signaling purposes. Combination fire alarm and guard's tour stations shall be acceptable.

**9.6.2.3** A manual fire alarm box shall be provided as follows, unless modified by another section of this *Code*:

(1) For new alarm system installations, the manual fire alarm box shall be located within 5 ft (1.5 m) of exit doorways.
(2) For existing alarm system installations, the manual fire alarm box either shall be provided in the natural exit access path near each required exit or within 5 ft (1.5 m) of exit doorways.

**9.6.2.4** Manual fire alarm boxes shall be mounted on both sides of grouped openings over 40 ft (12.2 m) in width, and within 5 ft (1.5 m) of each side of the opening.

The provisions of 9.6.2.3 and 9.6.2.4, which are new to the 2009 edition of the *Code*, are intended to correlate with the requirements of *NFPA 72®, National Fire Alarm Code®*,[16] for the placement of manual fire alarm boxes. Previous editions of the *Code* only required manual fire alarm boxes to be located near each required exit in the natural exit access path; such arrangement is still permitted by 9.6.2.3(2) for existing installations. For new installations, manual fire alarm boxes must be located within 5 ft (1.5 m) of exit doors, which include doors directly to the outside and doors to exit stair enclosures. See Exhibit 9.8 for an example of the application of 9.6.2.4 to manual fire alarm boxes at grouped openings.

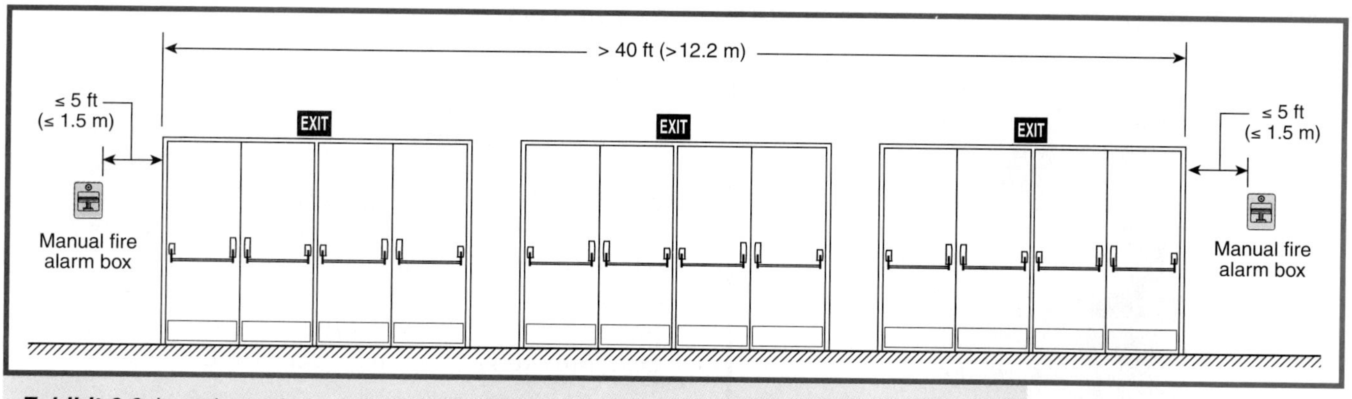


***Exhibit 9.8*** *Locations of manual fire alarm boxes at grouped openings.*

**9.6.2.5*** Additional manual fire alarm boxes shall be located so that, on any given floor in any part of the building, no horizontal distance on that floor exceeding 200 ft (60 m) shall need to be traversed to reach a manual fire alarm box.

**A.9.6.2.5** It is not the intent of 9.6.2.5 to require manual fire alarm boxes to be attached to movable partitions or to equipment, nor is it the intent to require the installation of permanent structures for mounting purposes only.

In a large open area, such as a convention hall, it would be impractical to require the installation of manual fire alarm boxes on mounting posts in the middle of the floor. However, it would be reasonable to apply the maximum spacing requirements to boxes located on the perimeter wall of the space.

**9.6.2.6*** For fire alarm systems using automatic fire detection or waterflow detection devices to initiate the fire alarm system in accordance with Chapters 11through 43, not less than one manual fire alarm box shall be provided to initiate a fire alarm signal. The manual fire alarm box shall be located where required by the authority having jurisdiction.

**A.9.6.2.6** The manual fire alarm box required by 9.6.2.6 is intended to provide a means to manually activate the fire alarm system when the automatic fire detection system or waterflow devices are out of service due to maintenance or testing, or where human discovery of the fire precedes automatic sprinkler system or automatic detection system activation. Where the fire alarm system is connected to a monitoring facility, the manual fire alarm box required by 9.6.2.6 should be connected to a separate circuit that is not placed "on test" when the detection or sprinkler system is placed on test. The manual fire alarm box should be located in an area that is accessible to occupants of the building and should not be locked.

**9.6.2.7*** Each manual fire alarm box on a system shall be accessible, unobstructed, and visible.

**A.9.6.2.7** Manual fire alarm boxes can include those with key-operated locks for detention areas or psychiatric hospitals, manual fire alarm boxes in areas where explosive vapors or dusts might be a hazard, or manual fire alarm boxes in areas with corrosive atmospheres. The appearance of manual fire alarm boxes for special uses often differs from those used in areas of normal occupancy. Manual fire alarm boxes, such as those with locks, that are located in areas where the general public has limited access might need to have signage advising persons to seek assistance from staff in the event a fire is noted.

Paragraphs 9.6.2.3 through 9.6.2.7 establish the criteria for the placement of manual fire alarm boxes. The intent is to provide maximum visibility and easy access to increase the probability that building occupants will initiate an alarm as they exit the building. If alarm boxes are not located conveniently or are obstructed from view, it is unlikely that an occupant will look for one. A typical manual fire alarm box is shown in Exhibit 9.9.

The requirement of 9.6.2.6 is also found in *NFPA 72, National Fire Alarm Code*, and is restated in the *Life Safety Code* for additional emphasis. This requirement affects initiation arrangement for occupancies that permit alarm initiation by automatic detection or extinguishing system operation in lieu of manual initiation. For example, a business occupancy using either 38.3.4.2(2) or (3) for alarm initiation would still be required to have one manual fire alarm box in the building in a location approved by the authority having jurisdiction. The single required fire alarm box is intended to be utilized to initiate the required fire alarm to provide occupant notification in the event the automatic initiation circuit is out of service for testing, maintenance, or repair. It is not necessarily intended to be accessible to the general public, although it might be if so required by the authority having jurisdiction.

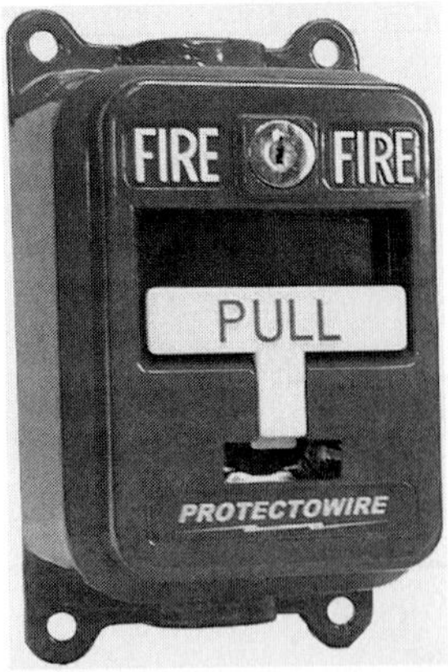


*Exhibit 9.9 Typical manual fire alarm box. (Source: Protectowire; photo courtesy of Mammoth Fire Alarms, Inc., Lowell, MA)*

**9.6.2.8** Where a sprinkler system provides automatic detection and alarm system initiation, it shall be provided with an approved alarm initiation device that operates when the flow of water is equal to or greater than that from a single automatic sprinkler.

**9.6.2.9** Where a total (complete) coverage smoke detection system is required by another section of this *Code*, automatic detection of smoke in accordance with *NFPA 72, National Fire Alarm Code*, shall be provided in all occupiable areas in environments that are suitable for proper smoke detector operation.

Paragraph 9.6.2.9 specifies the locations for smoke detectors where a total (complete) coverage smoke detection system is required to be installed throughout an occupancy by another section of the *Code*. Smoke detection systems are not required by the *Code* in every occupancy where a fire alarm system is required. Many occupancies require neither a smoke detection system nor smoke alarms. For example, in business occupancies that are large enough to mandate the fire alarm requirement, the occupants are assumed to be awake and alert when the building is occupied, so the *Code* relies on the occupants to initiate the alarm via manual fire alarm boxes (see 38.3.4.2 and 39.3.4.2).

Other occupancies require smoke detection systems to be installed in selected areas. For example, in new nursing homes, smoke detection systems are generally required in the corridors (see 18.3.4.5.3). Where such limited coverage systems are required by the occupancy chapters, it is not necessary to meet the complete (total) coverage requirements of 9.6.2.9.

**9.6.2.10 Smoke Alarms.**

Smoke alarms need to be positioned correctly. If they are too close to a wall/ceiling intersection, particularly over a door, air currents might cause heat and smoke to bypass the unit completely. Likewise, their location with respect to a dropped beam or other construction can have a similar nullifying effect. Problems can arise where partitions are moved without regard to the location of existing detectors. These problems are illustrated in Exhibit 9.10. *NFPA 72, National Fire Alarm Code*, provides extensive guidance in this area.

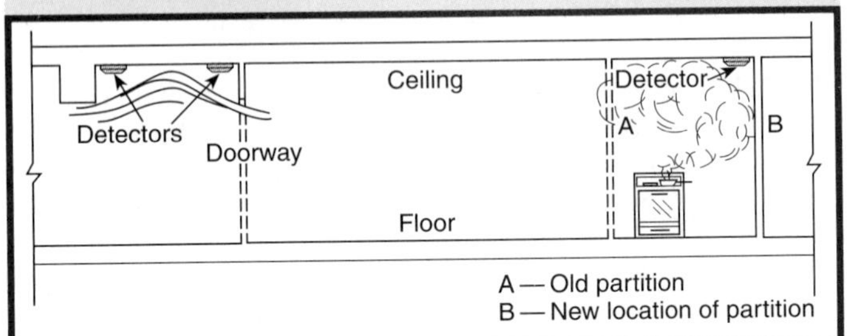


*Exhibit 9.10 Detector location problems to be avoided.*

**9.6.2.10.1 General.**

The provisions of 9.6.2.10.1 reference the use of *NFPA 72* where single-station and multiple-station smoke alarms that are not part of a fire alarm system are used. See the commentary following 9.6.2.10.2 through 9.6.2.10.4.

The terms *smoke alarm* and *smoke detector* are frequently, and incorrectly, used interchangeably. A smoke alarm is a device that, upon the presence of smoke, sounds an integral alarm. Smoke alarms are typically powered by the building electrical system and might be provided with battery backup; in some cases, such as in existing one- and two-family dwellings, they are permitted to be powered solely by batteries. Smoke alarms are typically found within dwelling units and within sleeping rooms of lodging or rooming houses and hotels and dormitories.

Smoke alarms can be either the single-station type or the multiple-station type. *Single station* means that, when a smoke alarm senses smoke, only that device sounds its integral sounding alarm. The term *multiple-station* refers to smoke alarms that are interconnected such that, when one alarm senses smoke, all the interconnected devices sound their integral alarms. Interconnected multiple-station smoke alarms are typically used within individual dwelling units to alert sleeping occupants located in different rooms to a fire in the dwelling.

A smoke detector is a component of a fire alarm system. In the presence of smoke, a smoke detector sends an electronic signal to the fire alarm control panel, which, in turn, initiates a predetermined action (such as activating the building evacuation alarm). Smoke detectors usually receive their power from the fire alarm system and contain no integral sounding devices.

In an occupancy such as a hotel, it might be desirable to protect the guest rooms with system smoke detectors rather than single-station smoke alarms. The *Code*, however, prohibits the guest room smoke detectors from sounding the general building evacuation alarm (see 9.6.2.10.4). Provided that the system smoke detectors are arranged to function like single- or multiple-station smoke alarms by sounding an alarm only within the protected guest room or suite, and perhaps annunciate a supervisory signal at the front desk, 9.6.2.10.1.4 permits system smoke detectors to be used in the guest rooms in lieu of single- or multiple-station smoke alarms. The use of such system smoke detectors might provide an enhanced level of reliability, since the wiring connecting the detectors to the fire alarm control panel will be supervised for integrity in accordance with *NFPA 72*.

**9.6.2.10.1.1** Where required by another section of this *Code*, single-station and multiple-station smoke alarms shall be in accordance with *NFPA 72, National Fire Alarm Code*, unless otherwise provided in 9.6.2.10.1.2, 9.6.2.10.1.3, or 9.6.2.10.1.4.

**9.6.2.10.1.2** The installation of smoke alarms in sleeping rooms shall be required where required by Chapters 11 through 43.

**9.6.2.10.1.3*** The interconnection of smoke alarms shall apply only to new construction as provided in 9.6.2.10.3.

**A.9.6.2.10.1.3** *NFPA 72, National Fire Alarm Code*, mandates smoke alarms in all sleeping rooms, and interconnection of smoke alarms is required for both new and existing installations. Per, 9.6.2.10.1.2, the residential occupancy chapters determine whether smoke alarms are needed within sleeping rooms. Paragraph 9.6.2.10.1.3 limits the requirement for interconnection of smoke alarms to those in new construction. This *Code* does not intend to require compliant, existing smoke alarm installations to be interconnected. This *Code* is periodically revised to add retrospective requirements only where the need is clearly substantiated.

**9.6.2.10.1.4** System smoke detectors in accordance with *NFPA 72, National Fire Alarm Code*, and arranged to function in the same manner as single-station or multiple-station smoke alarms shall be permitted in lieu of smoke alarms.

**9.6.2.10.2** Smoke alarms, other than existing battery-operated smoke alarms as permitted by other sections of this *Code*, shall be powered in accordance with the requirements of *NFPA 72, National Fire Alarm Code*.

Single-station and multiple-station smoke alarms, unless exempted by 9.6.2.10.2, must be powered as required by *NFPA 72, National Fire Alarm Code*. In general, they must be powered by the building electrical system; they must not rely solely on battery power. This provision is based on the experience that battery-operated detectors do not provide the reliability with respect to uninterrupted power supply that building electrical system power provides. Batteries are often removed to avoid nuisance alarms caused by kitchen or bathroom vapors or for use in other devices, such as radios and electronic toys; dead batteries are often not replaced. However, 9.6.2.10.2 allows the occupancy chapters to permit battery-operated, single-station smoke alarms. Such exemptions recognize battery-operated alarms in existing one- and two-family dwellings; in existing lodging or rooming houses; and, under certain conditions, in existing board and care facilities.

It is not the intent of 9.6.2.10.2 to prohibit low-power wireless technology, in which a battery-operated alarm reports by radio transmission to an alarm panel, if such a device complies with *NFPA 72, National Fire Alarm Code*. In turn, *NFPA 72* requires such systems to indicate a missing battery or low battery power condition at the remotely located alarm system panel. Compliance with the provisions of *NFPA 72* applicable to low-power wireless systems increases the power source reliability to a level comparable to that provided by connection to the building electrical service.

**9.6.2.10.3*** In new construction, where two or more smoke alarms are required within a dwelling unit, suite of rooms, or similar area, they shall be arranged so that operation of any smoke alarm shall cause the alarm in all smoke alarms within the dwelling unit, suite of rooms, or similar area to sound, unless otherwise permitted by the following:

(1) The requirement of 9.6.2.10.3 shall not apply where permitted by another section of this *Code*.
(2) The requirement of 9.6.2.10.3 shall not apply to configurations that provide equivalent distribution of the alarm signal.

**A.9.6.2.10.3** A dwelling unit is that structure, area, room, or combination of rooms, including hotel rooms/suites, in which a family or individual lives. A dwelling unit includes living areas only and not common usage areas in multifamily buildings, such as corridors, lobbies, and basements.

Audibility over background noises, such as running water, home appliances, and audio systems, with intervening doors closed between the occupants and the detector sounding device, is of key importance. In multistory or large-area living units, multiple smoke alarms should be interconnected, so that the sensing of smoke by one sounds the alarms of all devices within that living unit.

*NFPA 72* specifies the audibility requirements for alarm signals in sleeping areas. Audible appliances must have a sound level that is at least 15 dB above the average ambient sound level, 5 dB above the maximum sound level having a duration of at least 60 seconds, or a sound level of at least 75 dBA, whichever is greater. The sound level is measured at the pillow level in the sleeping room, with any doors between the sleeping room and the audible appliance in the closed position.

**9.6.2.10.4** The alarms shall sound only within an individual dwelling unit, suite of rooms, or similar area and shall not actuate the building fire alarm system, unless otherwise permitted by the authority having jurisdiction. Remote annunciation shall be permitted.

The intent behind requiring smoke detection within an individual living unit without requiring connection to the overall building alarm system is to provide notification of a smoke condition within a guest room, guest suite, or dwelling unit to its occupants. Once the occupants escape from their unit to the building's common areas, they can use the manual fire alarm boxes to sound the building alarm to notify the remaining building occupants of the emergency.

Interconnection of dwelling unit smoke alarms to the building alarm system can result in numerous nuisance alarms due to the detection of cooking vapors or steam from showers. Nuisance alarms can lead to complacency, or worse, the deliberate disablement of the system and the resulting lack of early warning. Thus, where a complete fire detection (versus smoke detection) system is required, it usually includes system smoke detection within building common areas and system heat detection within individual dwelling units. Single- or multiple-station smoke alarms are then still necessary within each dwelling unit to afford the occupants of each unit early warning of smoke conditions within their unit.

**9.6.2.11** Where required by Chapters 11 through 43, an automatic fire detection system shall be provided in hazardous areas for initiation of the signaling system.

### 9.6.3 Occupant Notification.

**9.6.3.1** Occupant notification shall be provided to alert occupants of a fire or other emergency where required by other sections of this *Code*.

**9.6.3.2** Occupant notification shall be in accordance with 9.6.3.3 through 9.6.3.10.2, unless otherwise provided in 9.6.3.2.1 through 9.6.3.2.4.

Note that 9.6.3.5 requires that occupant notification be provided by audible and visible signals. Thus, where an occupancy chapter requires an alarm system that provides occupant notification in accordance with Section 9.6, visible signals (as well as the traditional audible signals) must be provided. See also the modifications to the visible signal requirement in 9.6.3.5.1 through 9.6.3.5.8. For example, existing alarm systems are exempt from the requirement for visible signals per 9.6.3.5.3.

**9.6.3.2.1*** Elevator lobby, hoistway, and associated machine room smoke detectors used solely for elevator recall, and heat detectors used solely for elevator power shutdown, shall not be required to activate the building evacuation alarm if the power supply and installation wiring to such detectors are monitored by the building fire alarm system, and if the activation of such detectors initiates a supervisory signal at a constantly attended location.

**A.9.6.3.2.1** Elevator lobbies have been considered areas subject to unwanted alarms due to factors such as low ceilings and smoking. In the past several years, new features have become available to reduce this problem. These features are, however, not necessarily included in any specific installation.

**9.6.3.2.2*** Smoke detectors used solely for closing dampers or heating, ventilating, and air-conditioning system shutdown shall not be required to activate the building evacuation alarm, provided that the power supply and installation wiring to the detectors are monitored by the building fire alarm system, and the activation of the detectors initiates a supervisory signal at a constantly attended location.

**A.9.6.3.2.2** The concept addressed is that detectors used for releasing service, such as door or damper closing and fan shutdown, are not required to sound the building alarm.

**9.6.3.2.3*** Smoke detectors located at doors for the exclusive operation of automatic door release shall not be required to activate the building evacuation alarm, provided that the power supply and installation wiring to the detectors are monitored by the building fire alarm system, and the activation of the detectors initiates a supervisory signal at a constantly attended location.

**A.9.6.3.2.3** The concept addressed is that detectors used for releasing service, such as door or damper closing and fan shutdown, are not required to sound the building alarm.

The provisions of 9.6.3.2.2 and 9.6.3.2.3 reaffirm that not all detectors are required to sound the building alarm simply because they are installed on the premises. Detectors used for releasing service, such as for the release of an automatic door hold-open device that allows a door to be self-closing in the presence of smoke, need only perform their intended function as long as the detector wiring is monitored and a supervisory signal is annunciated at a constantly attended location when the detectors activate. In areas where smoke detection — complete with occupant notification via the building alarm system — is needed to provide the intended level of life safety, the *Code* specifically requires either a complete or partial smoke detection system. Interconnection with the building alarm should not be mandated in the hope of receiving additional detection coverage; such a detector might have been installed for another purpose, such as releasing service.

New health care occupancies, via 18.3.4.3.1, prohibit the use of 9.6.3.2.3. Thus, if a smoke detector is installed as part of an automatic door release (see 7.2.1.8.2), the activation of the detector must result in occupant notification through the building fire alarm system.

**9.6.3.2.4** Detectors in accordance with 22.3.4.3.1(2) and 23.3.4.3.1(2) shall not be required to activate the building evacuation alarm.

**9.6.3.3** Where permitted by Chapters 11 through 43, a presignal system shall be permitted where the initial fire alarm signal is automatically transmitted without delay to a municipal fire department, to a fire brigade (if provided), and to an on-site staff person trained to respond to a fire emergency.

Instead of immediately and automatically sounding a general alarm throughout the building, a presignal system delays the general alarm by sounding an alarm only at an approved and constantly attended area. This area could be, for example, a fire brigade station, guard station, or similar location with staff trained to investigate the signal's origin and subsequently activate a general alarm if necessary.

A delay in sounding the general alarm is inherent in a presignal system, but the delay might do more harm than good in those occupancies with populations that are difficult to evacuate or protect. Therefore, the *Code* requires an occupancy chapter to specifically recognize a presignal system to permit its use. No new occupancy chapter permits presignal systems, but they are permitted in some existing occupancies. For example, 40.3.4.3.3 permits an existing presignal system in an industrial occupancy.

A presignal system used in accordance with the provisions of 9.6.3.3 is permitted to delay only the general occupant notification and must, at time of initiation, achieve immediate and automatic notification of emergency forces.

**9.6.3.4** Where permitted by Chapters 11 through 43, a positive alarm sequence shall be permitted, provided that it is in accordance with *NFPA 72, National Fire Alarm Code*.

Given that smoke detector sensitivity should result in alarm system initiation sooner than that achieved by either heat detection or manual discovery and use of a pull station, 9.6.3.4 addresses positive alarm sequence, which has detailed requirements in *NFPA 72, National Fire Alarm Code*. Positive alarm sequence offers relief from nuisance alarms in buildings equipped with detection technology by permitting a delay in occupant notification. The detector senses smoke, automatically and without delay, sending an alarm signal to a constantly attended location, so that trained staff can investigate the origin of the signal. Positive alarm sequence includes all of the following features:

1. The signal received at the attended location must be acknowledged within 15 seconds, or immediate occupant notification (and emergency forces notification, if required) must occur.
2. Trained personnel have up to 180 seconds during the alarm investigation phase to evaluate the fire condition and reset the system; if the system is not reset within 180 seconds, immediate occupant notification (and emergency forces notification, if required) must occur.
3. If a second automatic fire detector is actuated during the investigation phase, immediate occupant notification (and emergency forces notification, if required) must occur.

4. If any other initiating device, such as a manual pull station, is actuated during the investigation phase, immediate occupant notification (and emergency forces notification, if required) must occur.
5. The system must provide a means to bypass the positive alarm sequence.

Positive alarm sequence is permitted only if an occupancy chapter specifically allows it by direct reference to 9.6.3.4. The only occupancies that do not permit occupant notification by positive alarm sequence are new and existing residential board and care occupancies.

**9.6.3.5** Unless otherwise provided in 9.6.3.5.1 through 9.6.3.5.8, notification signals for occupants to evacuate shall be audible and visible signals in accordance with *NFPA 72, National Fire Alarm Code*, and ICC/ANSI A117.1, *American National Standard for Accessible and Usable Buildings and Facilities*, or other means of notification acceptable to the authority having jurisdiction shall be provided.

**9.6.3.5.1** Areas not subject to occupancy by persons who are hearing impaired shall not be required to comply with the provisions for visible signals.

Visible alarm devices, in addition to the audible alarms, are needed in buildings occupied by persons who are hearing impaired. The provision of 9.6.3.5.1 recognizes that not all buildings are subject to occupancy by those who are hearing impaired. For example, in a high hazard industrial occupancy where, due to employee safety concerns, an adequate hearing level has been judged to be a legitimate condition of employment, there should be no life safety need for visible signals in addition to the audible signals. As the provisions of the *Americans with Disabilities Act and Architectural Barriers Act Accessibility Guidelines for Buildings and Facilities*,[17] discussed in the commentary associated with 7.2.12, receive wider implementation or are expanded in scope, few locations will exist where it is certain that persons with hearing impairments will not be present.

**9.6.3.5.2** Visible-only signals shall be provided where specifically permitted in health care occupancies in accordance with the provisions of Chapters 18 and 19.

**9.6.3.5.3** Existing alarm systems shall not be required to comply with the provision for visible signals.

**9.6.3.5.4** Visible signals shall not be required in lodging or rooming houses in accordance with the provisions of Chapter 26.

**9.6.3.5.5** Visible signals shall not be required in exit stair enclosures.

**9.6.3.5.6** Visible signals shall not be required in elevator cars.

Visible occupant notification appliances are not required to be installed in exit stairs or elevator cars as noted in 9.6.3.5.5 and 9.6.3.5.6, respectively. These provisions recognize that, upon entering an exit stair, occupants have reached a safe location and are in the process of egressing the building. Notification appliances in exit stair enclosures can create confusion and slow down the evacuation process. Likewise, if an occupant is in an elevator and the building alarm activates, occupants will become aware of the alarm condition when the doors open and proceed to egress the building. See also 9.6.3.6.4 and 9.6.3.6.5 for parallel provisions addressing audible notification appliances.

**9.6.3.5.7*** Public mode visual notification appliances in accordance with *NFPA 72* shall not be required in designated areas as permitted by Chapters 11 through 43, provided that they are replaced with approved alternative visible means.

**A.9.6.3.5.7** Visual notification appliances installed in large volume spaces, such as arenas, stadiums, malls and atriums, can be alternative devices which are not listed as visible notification appliances for fire alarm systems provided that the notification objective of the visual signal is reasonably achieved. Examples of alternative devices include, but are not limited to, scoreboards, message boards, and other electronic devices that meet the performance objectives of visible fire alarm appliances in large volume spaces.

It is the intent to permit the omission of visible notification appliances as identified in 9.6.3.5.7 provided that the adjacent areas that have not been specifically designated as exempt are provided with visible notification as required by 9.6.3.5.

**9.6.3.5.8*** Where visible signals are not required, as permitted by 9.6.3.5.7, documentation of such omission shall be maintained in accordance with 9.7.7.

**A.9.6.3.5.8** Documentation should be maintained with the as-built drawings so that inspection and testing personnel understand that the visible appliances have been exempted from certain areas and, therefore, can note the deviation on the acceptance test documentation and ongoing inspection reports. This will provide inspection and testing personnel with necessary details regarding the omission of visible notification appliances.

In large-volume spaces, such as stadiums, standard visual alarm notification appliances (strobes) might not prove to be effective for hearing-impaired occupants. The provisions of 9.6.3.5.7 and 9.6.3.5.8, which are new to the 2009 edition of the *Code,* permit alternative means of visual notification, provided that permission is granted by the applicable occupancy chapter (only new assembly occupancies with an occupant load of more than 1000 are currently permitted to utilize the provision of 9.6.3.5.7 via 12.3.4.3.5). Such alternative means of visual notification might be provided by electronic signage or video displays strategically located throughout the space or by the electronic scoreboards provided within a stadium or arena. It is anticipated that, in such occupancies, hearing-impaired occupants will not only see the messages, but they will also take cues from other occupants responding to the audible alarm notification.

**9.6.3.6** The general evacuation alarm signal shall operate in accordance with one of the methods prescribed by 9.6.3.6.1 through 9.6.3.6.3.

**9.6.3.6.1** The general evacuation alarm signal shall operate throughout the entire building.

**9.6.3.6.2*** Where total evacuation of occupants is impractical due to building configuration, only the occupants in the affected zones shall be notified initially. Provisions shall be made to selectively notify occupants in other zones to afford orderly evacuation of the entire building.

**A.9.6.3.6.2** To approve an evacuation plan to selectively notify building occupants, the authority having jurisdiction should consider several building parameters, including building compartmentation, detection and suppression system zones, occupant loads, and the number and arrangement of the means of egress.

In high-rise buildings, it is typical to evacuate the fire floor, the floor(s) above, and the floor immediately below. Other areas are then evacuated as the fire develops.

The provision of 9.6.3.6.2 normally applies to high-rise buildings. It provides for zoned, staged evacuation. This provision anticipates that the portions of the building that do not receive the initial alarm are separated from the areas of immediate emergency by adequate fire resistance-rated construction, such as the 2-hour fire separation that is usually provided between floors of high-rise buildings.

The use of staged evacuation requires occupants to be regularly trained and to have a basic understanding of the building's life safety systems and features. After witnessing the collapse of the World Trade Center on September 11, 2001, many building occupants might not be comfortable remaining in a high-rise building under any fire condition. By conducting routine training, their comfort level can be increased by raising their awareness of how buildings are designed to limit the spread of fire from the area of origin through compartmentation and the installation of automatic sprinkler systems. This training becomes very important, since the exit stairs in most existing high-rise buildings are not designed to accommodate the evacuation of the entire building population all at once. See 7.2.2.2.1.2 for increased width requirements for stairs serving 2000 occupants or more that were new to the 2006 edition of the *Code*.

**9.6.3.6.3** Where occupants are incapable of evacuating themselves because of age, physical or mental disabilities, or physical restraint, the private operating mode, as described in *NFPA 72, National Fire Alarm Code*, shall be permitted to be used. Only the attendants and other personnel required to evacuate occupants from a zone, area, floor, or building shall be required to be notified. The notification shall include means to readily identify the zone, area, floor, or building in need of evacuation.

The provisions of 9.6.3.6.3, which address the private operating mode for occupant notification, commonly apply to health care occupancies and detention and correctional occupancies. It is common in these occupancies to use coded messages or a similar method to announce the location of a fire emergency throughout the facility. This allows all members of the emergency response team, regardless of current location within a potentially sprawling facility, to respond to their assigned emergency duties. For example, despite the fact that the facility engineer might be in a building remote from that having the emergency when the coded alarm sounds throughout the facility, the engineer will receive the proper notification to carry out the previously assigned task of checking the fire pump to ensure that it is ready to operate, if needed.

Likewise, *NFPA 72* modifies the requirements for the placement of visible notification appliances where the private operating mode is utilized. For example, it might not be necessary to locate visible notification appliances in the patient rooms of a hospital or nursing home, since notification is intended to be provided via a coded message to staff, who will initiate the emergency plan. In such a case, visible signals might be limited to those areas subject to occupancy by the general public (such as lobbies, corridors, cafeterias, public restrooms). The authority having jurisdiction ultimately determines where visible notification appliances must be located.

**9.6.3.6.4** The general evacuation signal shall not be required in exit stair enclosures.

**9.6.3.6.5** The general evacuation signal shall not be required in elevator cars.

**9.6.3.7** Audible alarm notification appliances shall be of such character and so distributed as to be effectively heard above the average ambient sound level that exists under normal conditions of occupancy.

The authority having jurisdiction should review carefully the types and locations of fire alarm notification appliances. Given that audibility above ambient sound level is of primary importance and that each additional sounding device adds cost to a system, a balance should be maintained so that excessive costs are not incurred, while the installation of sufficient devices for adequate audibility is ensured. The provision of sufficient devices is extremely important in hotels and apartment buildings. Sounding devices located in corridors might not be audible within living units or guest rooms, especially in newer construction, due to the increased use of acoustical insulation for sound isolation.

In newer hotels, it has become common to install alarm notification appliances within each guest room to meet the audibility requirements of *NFPA 72*. With water running in the bathroom, the television operating on high volume, and the air-conditioning system in use, the horn or speaker within the room achieves the required occupant notification, whereas a similar device located in the corridor alone might not. Additionally, the alarm device often used is a speaker that can produce an alarm tone or deliver a specific voice message. A speaker device is particularly useful in a high-rise building; although it is important to get an initial message to all rooms, different messages might also need to be sent to different parts of the building as part of a zoned or staged evacuation plan. See the commentary following A.9.6.3.6.2 for additional information on staged evacuation.

**9.6.3.8** Audible alarm notification appliances shall produce signals that are distinctive from audible signals used for other purposes in a given building.

Where the provisions of Chapters 11 through 43 require an evacuation alarm signal, the standard fire alarm evacuation signal described in *NFPA 72, National Fire Alarm Code*, should be used. The standard fire alarm evacuation signal is a three-pulse temporal pattern using any appropriate sound. This signal is illustrated in Exhibit 9.11. The pattern consists of an "on" phase (1) lasting 0.5 second followed by an "off" phase (2) lasting 0.5 second, for three successive "on" periods; these are followed by an "off" phase (3) lasting 1.5 seconds. The signal should be repeated for a period appropriate for the purposes of evacuation of the building, but for not less than 180 seconds. A single-stroke bell or chime sounded at "on" intervals lasting 1 second, with a 2-second "off" interval after each third "on" stroke, is permitted.

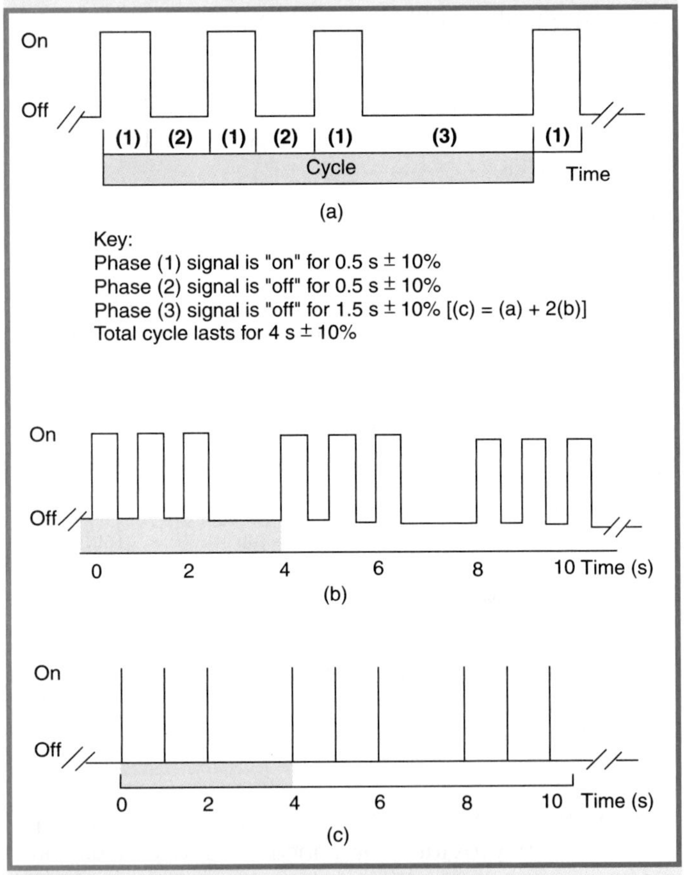


***Exhibit 9.11*** *Standard fire alarm evacuation signal.*

The manner of sounding alarms should be standardized to obtain uniformity throughout as large a geographic area as practicable, so that people moving from one location to another will not be misled and confused by differences in the manner of sounding alarms.

Two multiple-fatality fires in hotel occupancies that occurred in late 1978 and 1979 illustrate the need for standardized fire alarm signals with adequate audibility. In both incidents, which occurred in the middle of the night, many survivors reported not hearing any alarm device or mistaking the alarm for telephones or alarm clocks. An additional multiple-fatality fire in a hotel in 1978 illustrated the special problems with alarm notification where occupants are hearing impaired. In this fire, several elderly occupants removed hearing aids before going to bed, thus challenging the adequacy of the alarm's audibility.

**9.6.3.9** Automatically transmitted or live voice evacuation or relocation instructions shall be permitted to be used to notify occupants and shall comply with either 9.6.3.9.1 or 9.6.3.9.2.

Where occupant notification is provided by voice announcements, the notification means must comply with either: (1) *NFPA 72, National Fire Alarm Code,* as referenced in 9.6.3.9.1; or (2) where permitted by Chapters 11 through 43, the alternative criteria specified in 9.6.3.9.2.

**9.6.3.9.1** Automatically transmitted or live voice evacuation or relocation instructions shall be in accordance with *NFPA 72, National Fire Alarm Code*.

**9.6.3.9.2*** Where permitted by Chapters 11 through 43, automatically transmitted or live voice announcements shall be permitted to be made via a voice communication or public address system that complies with the following:

(1) Occupant notification, either live or recorded, shall be initiated at a constantly attended receiving station by personnel trained to respond to an emergency.
(2) An approved secondary power supply shall be provided for other than existing, previously approved systems.
(3) The system shall be audible above the expected ambient noise level.
(4) Emergency announcements shall take precedence over any other use.

**A.9.6.3.9.2** The provisions of 9.6.3.9.2 offer an alternative to the emergency voice alarm and communications system provisions (live voice or recorded voice announcements) of *NFPA 72, National Fire Alarm Code*. Occupancies, such as large-venue assembly occupancies and mercantile mall buildings, are occupancies in which the physical configuration (e.g., large-volume spaces), function, and human behavior (including elevated levels of occupant-generated noise) present challenges with respect to effective occupant notification by standard means in accordance with *NFPA 72*. Because the routine operation of these occupancies demands highly reliant, acoustically capable, and sufficiently audible public address systems, properly trained staff can be relied on to use these public address systems to effect occupant evacuation, relocation, or both.

As 9.6.3.9.2 specifically permits an alternative means of notification to that prescribed by *NFPA 72*, it does not mandate that the secondary power supply and the intelligibility and audibility facets of the public address system comply with *NFPA 72* or suggest that equivalency with the related provisions of *NFPA 72* is required. However, it is anticipated that, when approving the secondary power and audibility capabilities of public address systems, authorities having jurisdiction will ensure that these systems are conceptually comparable to the emergency voice alarm and communications system provisions of *NFPA 72*, such that a reliable and effective occupant notification system is provided.

The voice announcement occupant notification criteria in 9.6.3.9.2 provides an alterative arrangement to that specified by *NFPA 72, National Fire Alarm Code,* where specifically permitted by Chapters 11 through 43. These criteria permit the use of a public address system that is not part of an approved fire alarm system, provided that it has a secondary power supply and its audibility characteristics are such that announcements will be heard over the anticipated ambient noise in the occupancy. In addition, provisions must be made such that any emergency announcements will override the system's "normal" applications (for example, music or paging announcements). These criteria are new to Chapter 9 for the 2009 edition of the *Code*, but they are based on criteria previously found in the assembly, mercantile, and business occupancy chapters. The provisions of 9.6.3.9.2 consolidate the criteria and make them available to be referenced by any occupancy chapter.

It is the *Code's* intent that these alternative voice announcement occupant notification criteria are to be used in occupancies where the public address system is used routinely in the venue and, as a result, has an inherent high degree of reliability. An example of such a venue might be a sports arena in which the public address system is used to make announcements pertinent to the contest, and which has been designed to be heard over the expected crowd noise. The occupancies that currently permit the arrangement described in 9.6.3.9.2 are the following:

1. Assembly occupancies (12.3.4.3.6, 13.3.4.3.6)
2. Mall buildings (36.4.4.4.3.1, 37.4.4.4.3.1)
3. Existing mercantile occupancies (37.3.4.3.1)
4. Existing bulk merchandising retail buildings (37.4.5.4.3)
5. Existing business occupancies (39.3.4.3)

**9.6.3.10** Unless otherwise permitted by another section of this *Code*, audible and visible fire alarm notification appliances shall comply with either 9.6.3.10.1 or 9.6.3.10.2.

An example of a use permitted by another section of the *Code*, as specified in 9.6.3.10, appears in 14.3.4.3.1.3 for educational occupancies; the fire alarm system is permitted to be used to designate class change, provided that the fire alarm signal is distinctively different from the class change signal and overrides all other use and provided that such arrangement is acceptable to the authority having jurisdiction (see 9.6.3.10.2).

**9.6.3.10.1** Audible and visible fire alarm notification appliances shall be used only for fire alarm system or other emergency purposes.

**9.6.3.10.2** Emergency voice/alarm communication systems shall be permitted to be used for other purposes, subject to the approval of the authority having jurisdiction, if the fire alarm system takes precedence over all other signals, with the exception of mass notification inputs.

The provision of 9.6.3.10.2 requires the approval of the authority having jurisdiction to permit a voice communication system to be used for some other purpose. The system designer or building operator and the authority having jurisdiction should determine how susceptible the system is to deliberate tampering. For example, in a business occupancy where a combination emergency voice communication and daily background music system is installed with a speaker located in the ceiling directly over an employee's desk, it should be predicted that the constant background music might irritate the employee to the point that the speaker will be muffled or otherwise disabled. Therefore, the requirement that the fire alarm system take precedence over all other signals becomes futile; a disabled speaker cannot deliver the required emergency message.

### 9.6.4 Emergency Forces Notification.

**9.6.4.1** Where required by another section of this *Code*, emergency forces notification shall be provided to alert the municipal fire department and fire brigade (if provided) of fire or other emergency.

**9.6.4.2** Where fire department notification is required by another section of this *Code*, the fire alarm system shall be arranged to transmit the alarm automatically via any of the following means acceptable to the authority having jurisdiction and shall be in accordance with *NFPA 72, National Fire Alarm Code*:

(1) Auxiliary fire alarm system
(2) Central station fire alarm system
(3) Proprietary supervising station fire alarm system
(4) Remote supervising station fire alarm system

Paragraphs 1 through 4, which follow, help differentiate among the four alarm transmission methods for fire department notification in 9.6.4.2.

**1.** *Auxiliary fire alarm system.* An auxiliary fire alarm system is a system connected to a municipal fire alarm system for transmitting an alarm of fire to the public fire service communication center. Fire alarms from an auxiliary alarm system are received at the public fire service communication center on the same equipment and by the same methods as alarms transmitted manually from municipal fire alarm boxes located on streets.

**2.** *Central station fire alarm system.* A central station fire alarm system is a system or group of systems in which the operations of circuits and devices are signaled automatically to, recorded in, maintained by, and supervised from a listed central station staffed by competent and experienced servers and operators. Upon receipt of a signal, the staff takes such action as is required. Such service is controlled and operated by a person or firm whose business is the furnishing, maintaining, and monitoring of supervised fire alarm systems.

**3.** *Proprietary supervising station fire alarm system.* A proprietary supervising station fire alarm system is an installation of fire alarm systems that serves contiguous or noncontiguous properties under one ownership from a proprietary supervising station located at the protected property, where trained, competent personnel are in constant attendance. This system includes the proprietary supervising station; power supplies; signal initiating devices; initiating device circuits; signal notification appliances; equipment for the automatic, permanent, visual recording of signals; and equipment for initiating the operation of emergency building control services.

**4.** *Remote supervising station fire alarm system.* A remote supervising station fire alarm system is a system installed to transmit alarm, supervisory, and trouble signals from one or more protected premises to a remote supervising station location at which appropriate action is taken.

**9.6.4.3** For existing installations where none of the means of notification specified in 9.6.4.2(1) through (4) are available, an approved plan for notification of the municipal fire department shall be permitted.

The extensive availability of reliable communications systems has limited the necessity for the provision of 9.6.4.3 (formerly permitted for all occupancies) to existing installations only.

## 9.6.5 Fire Safety Functions.

**9.6.5.1** Fire safety functions shall be installed in accordance with the requirements of *NFPA 72, National Fire Alarm Code*.

**9.6.5.2** Where required by another section of this *Code*, the following functions shall be actuated:

(1) Release of hold-open devices for doors or other opening protectives

Doors are permitted by 7.2.1.8.2 to be automatic-closing if (among other requirements) the detection of smoke automatically releases the device holding the door open, thus allowing the door to become self-closing. The provisions of 7.2.1.8.2 do not require the building alarm system to release the doors. The health care occupancy chapters are more stringent on the subject and require that the automatic closing of doors must also occur upon initiation of the building's required fire alarm system (see 18.2.2.2.7 and 19.2.2.2.7). This is an example of an occupancy chapter mandating 9.6.5.2(1) as a requirement that is needed in addition to the provisions of 7.2.1.8.2.

(2) Stairwell or elevator shaft pressurization
(3) Smoke management or smoke control systems

Manual fire alarm boxes generally should not be used to activate smoke control systems, other than stair tower pressurization systems, due to the likelihood of a person signaling an alarm from a location outside the smoke zone of fire origin. Such alarm initiation could put the smoke management system in an undesirable mode of operation and cause it to spread smoke from one zone to another, rather than restrict it. The installation of smoke control systems is addressed by NFPA 92A, *Standard for Smoke-Control Systems Utilizing Barriers and Pressure Differences*, and NFPA 92B, *Standard for Smoke Management Systems in Malls, Atria, and Large Spaces*.

(4) Unlocking of doors

For an example of a *Code* requirement for the activation of the alarm system to unlock a door, see the provisions for delayed-egress door locking addressed by 7.2.1.6.1.

(5) Elevator recall and shutdown

ASME A17.1/CSA B44, *Safety Code for Elevators and Escalators*, and ASME A17.3, *Safety Code for Existing Elevators and Escalators* (which are referenced mandatorily by Section 9.4), prohibit the recall of elevators by detectors, other than those installed in elevator lobbies, hoistways, and associated elevator machine rooms. Recall by other detectors can lead to numerous nuisance recalls under conditions where it would be safe to operate elevators. To avoid taking elevators out of service every time any building smoke detector activates, the recall feature is sometimes deliberately disabled. ASME A17.1/CSA B44 and ASME A17.3 impose the recall restriction to keep the recall feature operational. The elevator lobby, hoistway, and machine room detectors are permitted to be part of the building fire alarm system, provided that only the activation of those detectors initiates elevator recall.

In addition to the items listed in 9.6.5.2(1) though (5), fire alarm systems can be used to perform other fire safety control functions. For example, new special amusement buildings are addressed in 12.4.7. Those that operate in reduced lighting levels (e.g., a haunted house amusement) must, upon actuation of the required automatic smoke detection system or the required automatic sprinkler system, increase illumination in the means of egress to at least the minimum level required by Section 7.8. The requirements applicable to special amusement buildings augment the concept of using the alarm system to initiate an emergency control function by mandating that conflicting or confusing sounds and visual effects stop upon actuation of the required automatic smoke detection system or the required automatic sprinkler system. Thus, in a haunted house amusement, all audible and visual special effects would cease upon alarm, so as not to confuse the patrons. A fire alarm horn or strobe might not be recognized if forced to compete with the background special effects common to such an occupancy.

## 9.6.6 Location of Controls.

Operator controls, alarm indicators, and manual communications capability shall be installed at a convenient location acceptable to the authority having jurisdiction.

At times it is not practical, either physically or from a security standpoint, to locate fire alarm system controls adjacent to an entrance. For example, controls for proprietary fire alarm systems designed in accordance with *NFPA 72, National Fire Alarm Code*, for reasons of security, often need to be located away from public areas. Thus, the *Code* does not require that controls be located adjacent to an entrance. However, because the controls are intended to be used by the fire department, they need to be located as approved by the authority having jurisdiction (AHJ). Where the fire department does not serve as the AHJ, it should be consulted to determine an acceptable location.

### 9.6.7 Annunciation.

Subsection 9.6.7 establishes provisions for fire alarm annunciation, which are then referenced by other sections of the *Code* as part of the overall life safety package needed for specific occupancies. Alarm annunciation allows trained individuals — such as building engineers, security and safety officers, and responding fire service personnel — to read the indicator lamps or alphanumeric displays of an annunciator panel to identify circuits, associated building locations, and conditions that warrant attention or investigation.

**9.6.7.1** Where alarm annunciation is required by another section of this *Code*, it shall comply with 9.6.7.2 through 9.6.7.7.

**9.6.7.2** Alarm annunciation at the control center shall be by means of audible and visible indicators.

Alarm annunciation at the control center, as specified in 9.6.7.2, must be by means of audible as well as visible indicators to capture the attention of the trained attendant, who might have numerous job functions within or near the control center that might distract attention from the annunciator panel. Where a control center is not required or otherwise provided, the annunciator panel should be located in or near a public space, such as an entrance lobby, so that trouble and supervisory signals will get the attention of a passerby, who can then notify the building's maintenance staff.

**9.6.7.3** For the purposes of alarm annunciation, each floor of the building, other than floors of existing buildings, shall be considered as not less than one zone, unless otherwise permitted by 9.6.7.4.3, 9.6.7.4.4, 9.6.7.4.5, or by another section of this *Code*.

**9.6.7.4** If a floor area exceeds 22,500 ft$^2$ (2090 m$^2$), additional fire alarm zoning shall be provided, and the length of any single fire alarm zone shall not exceed 300 ft (91 m) in any direction, except as provided in 9.6.7.4.1 through 9.6.7.4.5 or as otherwise modified by another section of this *Code*.

**9.6.7.4.1** Where permitted by another section of this *Code*, fire alarm zones shall be permitted to exceed 22,500 ft$^2$ (2090 m$^2$), and the length of a zone shall be permitted to exceed 300 ft (91 m) in any direction.

**9.6.7.4.2** Where the building is protected by an automatic sprinkler system in accordance with 9.7.1.1(1), the area of the fire alarm zone shall be permitted to coincide with the allowable area of the sprinkler system.

**9.6.7.4.3** Unless otherwise prohibited elsewhere in this *Code*, where a building not exceeding four stories in height is protected by an automatic sprinkler system in accordance with 9.7.1.1(1), the sprinkler system shall be permitted to be annunciated on the fire alarm system as a single zone.

The provision of 9.6.7.4.3, which is new to the 2009 edition of the *Code*, permits the waterflow from a sprinkler system that meets NFPA 13, *Standard for the Installation of Sprinkler Systems*, to be annunciated as a single zone in buildings up to four stories in height, unless the occupancy chapters prohibit such arrangement. Lacking this provision, sprinkler systems would have to be arranged so that every floor would be provided with a waterflow switch to permit each floor to be annunciated separately. Such a requirement would limit the sprinkler system design flexibility and would prohibit the use of the so-called "birdcage" design in which multiple vertical risers act as loops for hydraulic efficiency. The only occupancy chapter that prohibits this arrangement is new health care (see 18.3.4.3.3.3).

**9.6.7.4.4** Where the building is protected by an automatic sprinkler system in accordance with 9.7.1.1(2), the sprinkler system shall be permitted to be annunciated on the fire alarm system as a single zone.

**9.6.7.4.5** Where the building is protected by an automatic sprinkler system in accordance with 9.7.1.1(3), the sprinkler system shall be permitted to be annunciated on the fire alarm system as a single zone.

Paragraphs 9.6.7.4.1 through 9.6.7.4.5 provide a choice of zone locations and zone sizes for meaningful annunciation. In a new multiple-story building required to have alarm annunciation by another section of the *Code*, 9.6.7.3 would not permit two or more floors to be considered as a single zone, unless the building were a residential occupancy sprinklered in accordance with NFPA 13R, *Standard for the Installation of Sprinkler Systems in Residential Occupancies up to and Including Four Stories in Height,*[18] NFPA 13D, *Standard for the Installation of Sprinkler Systems in One-and Two-Family Dwellings and Manufactured Homes,*[19] or as otherwise permitted by 9.6.7.4.3, in which case the sprinkler system would be permitted to be annunciated as a single zone. In buildings other than those sprinklered in accordance with NFPA 13 (up to four stories, other than new health care), NFPA 13R, or NFPA 13D, floors must be annunciated separately; otherwise an alarm condition would be annunciated as originating in a zone that includes multiple floors and, thus, would not identify the specific location of the fire. Such a situation might delay the investigation and associated emergency response effort. Existing alarm annunciation systems are exempted from the requirement of 9.6.7.3, so as not to unfairly render existing *Code*-complying installations abruptly noncompliant, thereby avoiding the need for major alterations or a complete replacement of the alarm system.

Residential sprinkler systems in accordance with NFPA 13R and NFPA 13D commonly utilize a so-called "birdcage" piping configuration in which the sprinkler branch lines are run vertically through the building, rather than horizontally, providing an economical design alternative. (The resulting piping network resembles a birdcage, thus the name.) With such a configuration, however, it is not practical to provide waterflow devices for every floor, since each branch line typically serves multiple floors. Therefore, a single waterflow device is provided on the supply piping ahead of the branch lines, resulting in the sprinkler system being annunciated as a single zone. Although such an arrangement might increase the time required for emergency responders to locate the fire, it is considered a reasonable alternative for residential occupancies not exceeding four stories in height utilizing sprinkler systems compliant with NFPA 13R or NFPA 13D.

It is further specified in 9.6.7.4 that no one zone, for alarm annunciation purposes, even if located entirely on one floor of the building, is permitted to be so large that it delays identification of the location from which the alarm was initiated. The permitted zone size, 22,500 ft$^2$ (2090 m$^2$), is intended to coordinate with the maximum permitted smoke compartment size in health care and detention and correctional occupancies. The maximum zone area and zone dimensional criteria are modified by 9.6.7.4.2 for fully sprinklered buildings, allowing the alarm system zoning to coincide with the area of the sprinkler system zone. Depending on the sprinkler system's design, this might result in a zone as large as 52,000 ft$^2$ (4831 m$^2$). This requirement helps to achieve consistency in reporting alarms from signaling system devices and from sprinkler system waterflow to the alarm annunciator. Although a sprinkler system might be designed and installed by parties other than those who design and install fire alarm systems, the coordination of these two systems is needed during the design phase to ensure that they complement each other.

**9.6.7.5** A system trouble signal shall be annunciated at the control center by means of audible and visible indicators.

**9.6.7.6** A system supervisory signal shall be annunciated at the control center by means of audible and visible indicators.

Alarm system trouble signals and supervisory signals must be annunciated by both audible and visible indicators in accordance with 9.6.7.5 and 9.6.7.6 to help ensure that personnel will respond to the indication. Trouble signals indicate such conditions as a circuit break or ground occurring in the fire alarm system wiring. Supervisory signals indicate a problem with the supervision of sprinkler systems, such as a closed valve. Supervisory signals can also be associated with the supervision of other extinguishing systems and equipment or the maintenance features of other fire protection systems.

**9.6.7.7** Where the system serves more than one building, each building shall be annunciated separately.

## 9.7 Automatic Sprinklers and Other Extinguishing Equipment

### 9.7.1 Automatic Sprinklers.

**9.7.1.1*** Each automatic sprinkler system required by another section of this *Code* shall be in accordance with one of the following:

(1) NFPA 13, *Standard for the Installation of Sprinkler Systems*
(2) NFPA 13D, *Standard for the Installation of Sprinkler Systems in One- and Two-Family Dwellings and Manufactured Homes*
(3) NFPA 13R, *Standard for the Installation of Sprinkler Systems in Residential Occupancies up to and Including Four Stories in Height*

**A.9.7.1.1** For a discussion of the effectiveness of automatic sprinklers, as well as a general discussion of automatic sprinklers, see the NFPA *Fire Protection Handbook*. Where partial sprinkler protection is permitted by another section of this *Code*, the limited area systems provisions of NFPA 13, *Standard for the Installation of Sprinkler Systems*, should apply.

The *Code* requirements for automatic sprinklers are based on the sprinkler experience record, which shows that, where installed properly, a sprinkler system is the most effective tool for protecting and safeguarding against loss of life and property. Occupants of a building who are aware of the presence of sprinkler protection can feel secure that any fire will be detected and extinguished or controlled at its origin.

Numerous myths exist regarding the operation of automatic sprinklers. Some are reinforced by misrepresentations in the news media or the entertainment industry. The following facts should serve to debunk these myths:

1. Sprinkler systems do not operate when smoke detectors operate.
2. All sprinklers in the building do not operate simultaneously, unless specifically designed to do so (such as in the case of a deluge system protecting an unusual hazard).
3. Sprinklers do not spray water that has been superheated by the fire, resulting in the scalding of building occupants.
4. Sprinkler system operation does not cause drowning or electrocution of building occupants.
5. Sprinkler system operation does not increase the amount of smoke generated by the fire; rather, it dramatically reduces the generation of smoke and other hazardous products of combustion.

Automatic sprinkler systems remain the single most effective means of controlling fire spread for the widest range of buildings and areas. It is for this reason that the *Code* permits the relaxation of many of its requirements based on the presence of sprinklers.

NFPA 13, *Standard for the Installation of Sprinkler Systems*, covers installation details for standard automatic sprinkler systems. In the interest of both life safety from fire and the protection of property, it will generally be beneficial to provide a complete standard automatic sprinkler installation to protect the entire property. Sprinklers prove beneficial even in situations where the *Code* requires sprinklers only for the isolation and protection of hazardous contents areas.

NFPA 13 is the authoritative source for sprinkler systems with respect to design, installation, and character and adequacy of water supply. Even though there are usually some areas in a building where fires are more likely to start than others, it is impossible to predict with absolute certainty where a fire might start and protect only those areas. Thus, where sprinklers are installed, they should be installed throughout a building. The basic requirements of NFPA 13 for spacing, locating, and positioning sprinklers are based on principles that include sprinkler installation throughout the building — including combustible concealed spaces. The *Life Safety Code*, however, in an effort to promote the use of sprinkler systems by reducing the costs, permits sprinklers to be omitted from small closets and bathrooms in various residential occupancies but considers those occupancies to be fully sprinklered. For an example, see 29.3.5.5, which applies to existing hotels and dormitories.

NFPA 13D, *Standard for the Installation of Sprinkler Systems in One- and Two-Family Dwellings and Manufactured Homes*, was developed after extensive research that included full-scale fire tests. NFPA 13D introduced the concept of a quick-response residential sprinkler. Unlike its standard spray sprinkler counterpart, a quick-response residential sprinkler operates very quickly once its rated temperature is reached. It begins controlling a fire early in its growth. In addition to being quick to respond, residential sprinklers (as mandated by NFPA 13D) have a specifically designed spray pattern that delivers water to nearly the full height of the walls of small rooms that are characteristic of residential occupancies.

NFPA 13R, *Standard for the Installation of Sprinkler Systems in Residential Occupancies up to and Including Four Stories in Height*, was first published in 1989. NFPA 13R extends the technological and economic benefits of an NFPA 13D-type system to larger residential buildings, while mandating additional requirements that are commensurate with increased building size. The requirements help to ensure improved protection against injury and life loss to building occupants, including those within the room of fire origin.

NFPA 25, *Standard for the Inspection, Testing, and Maintenance of Water-Based Fire Protection Systems*,[20] provides information on required maintenance procedures for automatic sprinkler systems.

**9.7.1.2** Sprinkler piping serving not more than six sprinklers for any isolated hazardous area shall be permitted to be connected directly to a domestic water supply system having a capacity sufficient to provide 0.15 gpm/ft$^2$ (6.1 mm/min) throughout the entire enclosed area. An indicating shutoff valve, supervised in accordance with 9.7.2 or NFPA 13, *Standard for the Installation of Sprinkler Systems*, shall be installed in an accessible, visible location between the sprinklers and the connection to the domestic water supply.

The general provisions of Section 8.7 for special hazard protection — in combination with the specific requirements of the ___3.2 subsection of each occupancy chapter — make extensive use of sprinklering hazardous contents rooms in otherwise nonsprinklered buildings. Such sprinklers are permitted by 9.7.1.2 to be supplied by the domestic water supply and its associated distribution piping. The domestic water supply must provide a sufficient volume of water at the appropriate pressure to deliver a sprinkler discharge density of 0.15 gpm/ft$^2$ (6.1 mm/min) within the hazardous contents room. For a 100 ft$^2$ (9.3 m$^2$) room, the water supply would have to provide at least 15 gpm (57 L/min) at the pressure appropriate to such a discharge from a specific size and model of sprinkler. Additionally, the provisions of 9.7.1.2 can be used (in lieu of a devoted sprinkler system piping network and water supply) only if any given room requires six or fewer sprinklers for adequate protection, based on the spacing and location rules of the applicable installation standards referenced in 9.7.1.1. Another hazardous contents room on the same floor, or in some other part of the building, can obtain its protection by repeating a similar maximum six-sprinkler installation in accordance with 9.7.1.2.

**9.7.1.3*** In areas protected by automatic sprinklers, automatic heat-detection devices required by other sections of this *Code* shall not be required.

**A.9.7.1.3** Properly designed automatic sprinkler systems provide the dual function of both automatic alarms and automatic extinguishment. Dual function is not provided in those cases where early detection of incipient fire and early notification of occupants are needed to initiate actions in behalf of life safety earlier than can be expected from heat-sensitive fire detectors.

Because the operation of an automatic sprinkler system is initiated by a heat-sensing element and works on the same principle as an automatic heat detection and alarm system, a sprinkler system is judged to be capable of serving the same purpose. Even though some sprinkler systems do not sound an alarm on activation, many do. Furthermore, although a particular sprinkler system might not sound an alarm, it does immediately initiate extinguishment; this is a feature that is at least as valuable, if not more so, than a system that sounds an alarm only.

Detection of smoke, on the other hand, can be accomplished at the incipient stages of a fire and can give rise to an earlier warning than that provided by heat detection, so smoke detection is considered in a somewhat different light. One school of thought is that a system that starts suppression of a fire immediately upon detection is better than one that simply detects the fire and sounds an alarm, even though the latter is quicker to initiate an alarm signal. Others believe, however, that an early alarm is more advantageous. The first group is concerned with the immediate suppression or containment of fire; it might take considerable time for fire fighters to arrive. The second group stresses immediate notification of occupants. The *Code* recognizes the value of both strategies, and strives for a balanced approach to occupant protection by requiring, in some occupancies, both early warning and automatic suppression systems, depending on the characteristics of the occupants. The extent of protection provided should be commensurate with the ability of the occupants, as a group, to evacuate or relocate to a safe location within the building before the egress routes become unusable from the effects of a fire.

**9.7.1.4** Automatic sprinkler systems installed to make use of an alternative permitted by this *Code* shall be considered required systems and shall meet the provisions of this *Code* that apply to required systems.

The provisions of 9.7.1.4 remind the user that an automatic sprinkler system voluntarily installed as a *Code* alternative is considered a required system; therefore, it is subject to the same requirements (including maintenance) that apply to a sprinkler system specifically mandated by the *Code*. For example, if an occupancy that does not require a sprinkler system permits the use of the delayed-egress door lock addressed by 7.2.1.6.1, and if the designer or building operator meets one of the unlocking provisions of 7.2.1.6.1 via the installation of an approved, supervised automatic sprinkler system, the sprinkler system is considered a required system. Therefore, the system must meet all requirements that apply to a similar system installed to comply with the *Code* in addition to those of the alternative system, such as delayed-egress door locking.

### 9.7.2 Supervision.

Sprinkler system supervision is not required by 9.7.2. The requirements of 9.7.2 apply where a supervised automatic sprinkler system is specified by the *Code*. Most of the occupancy chapters that require an automatic sprinkler system for life safety purposes also require the system to be supervised in accordance with 9.7.2.

**9.7.2.1* Supervisory Signals.** Where supervised automatic sprinkler systems are required by another section of this *Code*, supervisory attachments shall be installed and monitored for integrity in accordance with *NFPA 72, National Fire Alarm Code*, and a distinctive supervisory signal shall be provided to indicate a condition that would impair the satisfactory operation of the sprinkler system. System components and parameters that are required to be monitored shall include, but shall not be limited to, control valves, fire pump power supplies and running conditions, water tank levels and temperatures, tank pressure, and air pressure on dry-pipe valves. Supervisory signals shall sound and shall be displayed either at a location within the protected building that is constantly attended by qualified personnel or at an approved, remotely located receiving facility.

**A.9.7.2.1** *NFPA 72, National Fire Alarm Code*, provides details of standard practice in sprinkler supervision. Subject to the approval of the authority having jurisdiction, sprinkler supervision is also permitted to be provided by direct connection to municipal fire departments or, in the case of very large establishments, to a private headquarters providing similar functions. *NFPA 72* covers such matters.

Where municipal fire alarm systems are involved, reference should also be made to NFPA 1221, *Standard for the Installation, Maintenance, and Use of Emergency Services Communications Systems*.

One reason why the automatic sprinkler system has attained a high level of satisfactory performance and response to fire conditions is that, through supervision, it can be kept in operative condition. Of course, keeping the system operative depends on routine maintenance and the owner's willingness to repair the system when there are indications of impairment. Features of the system, such as the following, can be automatically monitored:

1. Opening and closing of water control valves
2. Power supplies for required fire pumps
3. Water tank level

If an undesirable situation develops, a signal is annunciated in the protected building or relayed to a monitoring facility.

A supervisory system will also indicate or activate a waterflow alarm. In addition to being transmitted to an alarm-monitoring agency, the waterflow alarm can be transmitted directly to the fire department. The signals for electrical and mechanical problems need not burden the fire department unnecessarily, yet those indicating a fire can be received directly.

**9.7.2.2 Alarm Signal Transmission.** Where supervision of automatic sprinkler systems is provided in accordance with another provision of this *Code*, waterflow alarms shall be transmitted to an approved, proprietary alarm-receiving facility, a remote station, a central station, or the fire department. Such connection shall be in accordance with 9.6.1.3.

## 9.7.3 Other Automatic Extinguishing Equipment.

**9.7.3.1** In any occupancy where the character of the fuel for fire is such that extinguishment or control of fire is accomplished by a type of automatic extinguishing system in lieu of an automatic sprinkler system, such system shall be installed in accordance with the appropriate standard, as determined in accordance with Table 9.7.3.1.

***Table 9.7.3.1 Fire Suppression System Installation Standards***

| Fire Suppression System | Installation Standard |
|---|---|
| Low-, medium-, and high-expansion foam systems | NFPA 11, *Standard for Low-, Medium-, and High-Expansion Foam* |
| Carbon dioxide systems | NFPA 12, *Standard on Carbon Dioxide Extinguishing Systems* |
| Halon 1301 systems | NFPA 12A, *Standard on Halon 1301 Fire Extinguishing Systems* |
| Water spray fixed systems | NFPA 15, *Standard for Water Spray Fixed Systems for Fire Protection* |
| Deluge foam-water sprinkler systems | NFPA 16, *Standard for the Installation of Foam-Water Sprinkler and Foam-Water Spray Systems* |
| Dry chemical systems | NFPA 17, *Standard for Dry Chemical Extinguishing Systems* |
| Wet chemical systems | NFPA 17A, *Standard for Wet Chemical Extinguishing Systems* |
| Water mist systems | NFPA 750, *Standard on Water Mist Fire Protection Systems* |
| Clean agent extinguishing systems | NFPA 2001, *Standard on Clean Agent Fire Extinguishing Systems* |

Use of special types of extinguishing systems is a matter of engineering judgment on the part of the designer, working in collaboration with the owner and the authority having jurisdiction. For example, it might be undesirable to install automatic sprinklers in a portion of a facility used for storage of water-reactive materials, such as magnesium. The application of water to such materials can significantly exacerbate a fire problem.

It is not the intent of 9.7.3.1 to permit a required sprinkler system to be replaced by a gaseous suppression system in a portion of a building where the application of water might be harmful to the building contents or equipment (e.g., computer or telecommunications equipment). To be effective, such systems typically depend on a limited quantity of extinguishing agent, and the protected room must be essentially airtight to allow the extinguishing agent concentration to remain sufficiently high for the time necessary to extinguish the fire. If the room enclosure is penetrated and not properly sealed, or if a door is propped open, the extinguishing system might not function as intended, and once the system discharges its extinguishing agent, there is typically no backup agent. Where a sprinkler system is required and there is concern about the application of water to the contents or equipment for reasons other than the ability of water to control or extinguish a fire involving such contents, an area could be protected by both a gaseous extinguishing system and an automatic sprinkler system; the special system will serve as a first line of defense in the event of a fire, and, if it fails to extinguish the fire for whatever reason, the sprinkler system will activate. If there is concern about accidental activation of a sprinkler system, a pre-action system can be installed whereby the sprinkler piping is dry until an automatic detection system senses smoke or fire in the room. Even then, water will not be discharged from the system unless a sprinkler reaches its design discharge temperature.

The NFPA standards listed in Table 9.7.3.1 provide mandatory requirements for the installation and maintenance of such special types of extinguishing systems.

**9.7.3.2** If the extinguishing system is installed in lieu of a required, supervised automatic sprinkler system, the activation of the extinguishing system shall activate the building fire alarm system, where provided. The actuation of an extinguishing system that is not installed in lieu of a required, supervised automatic sprinkler system shall be indicated at the building fire alarm system, where provided.

The activation of a special extinguishing system — installed in lieu of a required supervised automatic sprinkler system — must activate the building fire alarm system where provided per 9.7.3.2. This system provides early warning to building occupants so that necessary action, probably evacuation, can occur. If the special extinguishing system is not serving as a substitute for the required supervised automatic sprinkler system, its activation need only be indicated at the fire alarm control panel or remote annunciator.

A kitchen exhaust hood and duct extinguishing system is an example of a special extinguishing system not serving as a substitute for a required supervised automatic sprinkler system. The operation of a kitchen exhaust hood and duct extinguishing system would have to be indicated at the fire alarm panel, but would not have to result in the activation of audible and visible occupant notification signals.

### 9.7.4 Manual Extinguishing Equipment.

**9.7.4.1*** Where required by the provisions of another section of this *Code*, portable fire extinguishers shall be installed, inspected, and maintained in accordance with NFPA 10, *Standard for Portable Fire Extinguishers*.

**A.9.7.4.1** For a description of standard types of extinguishers and their installation, maintenance, and use, see NFPA 10, *Standard for Portable Fire Extinguishers*. The labels of recognized testing laboratories on extinguishers provide evidence of tests indicating the reliability and suitability of the extinguisher for its intended use. Many unlabeled extinguishers are offered for sale that are substandard by reason of insufficient extinguishing capacity, questionable reliability, or ineffective extinguishing agents for fires in ordinary combustible materials or because they pose a personal hazard to the user.

Portable fire extinguishers are required throughout health care, ambulatory health care, detention and correctional, new large board and care, mercantile, and business occupancies, but only in the hazardous areas of nonsprinklered hotels and dormitories, nonsprinklered apartment buildings, and existing large board and care occupancies. Where the *Code* requires portable extinguishers, the number, types, and locations required can be found in NFPA 10, *Standard for Portable Fire Extinguishers*.[21]

**9.7.4.2** Where required by the provisions of another section of this *Code*, standpipe and hose systems shall be provided in accordance with NFPA 14, *Standard for the Installation of Standpipe and Hose Systems*. Where standpipe and hose systems are installed in combination with automatic sprinkler systems, installation shall be in accordance with the appropriate provisions established by NFPA 13, *Standard for the Installation of Sprinkler Systems*, and NFPA 14, *Standard for the Installation of Standpipe and Hose Systems*.

The *Code* requires standpipes only in certain occupancy chapters. For example, standpipes are required on stages of assembly occupancies and in detention and correctional occupancies. Standpipe provisions also appear as part of the Section 11.8 menu of provisions applicable to high-rise buildings (see 11.8.2.2). The following occupancy chapters mandatorily reference Section 11.8 and, thus, require fire department–use standpipes for high-rise buildings:

1. New assembly occupancies (12.4.4)
2. New educational occupancies (14.4.2)
3. New day-care occupancies (16.4.2)
4. Existing day-care occupancies (17.4.2)
5. New health care occupancies (18.4.2)
6. New detention and correctional occupancies (22.4.3)
7. New hotels and dormitories (28.4.1.1)
8. New apartment buildings (30.4.1.1)
9. New large residential board and care occupancies (32.3.4)
10. New business occupancies (38.4.2)

### 9.7.5 Maintenance and Testing.

All automatic sprinkler and standpipe systems required by this *Code* shall be inspected, tested, and maintained in accordance with NFPA 25, *Standard for the Inspection, Testing, and Maintenance of Water-Based Fire Protection Systems.*

### 9.7.6* Sprinkler System Shutdown.

**A.9.7.6** A fire watch should at least involve some special action beyond normal staffing, such as assigning an additional security guard(s) to walk the areas affected. Such individuals should be specially trained in fire prevention and in the use of fire extinguishers and occupant hose lines, in notifying the fire department, in sounding the building fire alarm, and in understanding the particular fire safety situation for public education purposes. Some authorities having jurisdiction require fire fighters to be assigned to the area, with direct radio communication to the local fire department. *(Also see* NFPA 601, *Standard for Security Services in Fire Loss Prevention.)*

**9.7.6.1** Where a required automatic sprinkler system is out of service for more than 4 hours in a 24-hour period, the authority having jurisdiction shall be notified, and the building shall be evacuated or an approved fire watch shall be provided for all parties left unprotected by the shutdown until the sprinkler system has been returned to service.

**9.7.6.2** Sprinkler impairment procedures shall comply with NFPA 25, *Standard for the Inspection, Testing, and Maintenance of Water-Based Fire Protection Systems.*

A sprinkler system might be shut down for any number of reasons during the life of a building. Some shutdowns are preplanned, controlled, and of short duration, such as those during periodic testing and maintenance. Others might be preplanned and of longer duration, such as shutdowns during times of building or system renovation. Emergency shutdown of the system can be the result of fire or other physical damage and might result in a short or lengthy shutdown to repair the system. Advance planning should help ensure that the system, or most of the system, can be restored to service, despite the scope of the renovation or the extent of an unexpected impairment. If the sprinkler system is required by the *Code,* or if it was installed to make use of one of the alternatives offered by the *Code,* it must be in operable condition for the building to be considered *Code* compliant.

Instead of designating a building with an inoperative sprinkler system as noncompliant and prohibiting occupancy under all conditions in accordance with the provisions of 4.6.10.1, 9.7.6.1 differentiates between those sprinkler system impairments that last less than 4 hours within a 24-hour period and those that last longer. Continued occupancy of a building that has a sprinkler system impairment of more than 4 hours cumulative within any 24-hour period can be tolerated only if a fire watch acceptable to the authority having jurisdiction is provided. Such lengthy impairments generally indicate a situation that involves a problem more serious in nature than typical system maintenance or testing.

It is the intent of the *Code* that the fire watch result in a heightened awareness of the building's operations and environment. Individuals assigned to the fire watch should be able to recognize fire hazards and understand the procedures for occupant and fire department notification and occupant evacuation in an emergency.

When developing a plan to address system shutdown, it is important to consider the nature of the shutdown, the location, the increased hazards that are involved, and the actions necessary to mitigate the hazards. The authority having jurisdiction should be involved in the development of these plans.

A parallel requirement in 9.6.1.6 addresses fire alarm system impairments.

### 9.7.7 Documentation.

All required documentation regarding the design of the fire protection system and the procedures for maintenance, inspection, and testing of the fire protection system shall be maintained at an approved, secured location for the life of the fire protection system.

### 9.7.8 Record Keeping.

Testing and maintenance records required by NFPA 25, *Standard for the Inspection, Testing, and Maintenance of Water-Based Fire Protection Systems*, shall be maintained at an approved, secured location.

## 9.8 Special Inspections and Tests

**9.8.1** Where required by another section of this *Code*, special inspections and tests shall be performed to verify the operation of the fire protection system in its final condition for acceptance by the authority having jurisdiction.

**9.8.2** The special inspector's relevant experience in the design, installation, and testing of the fire protection systems being tested shall be documented.

**9.8.3** The design documents shall provide the procedures and methods to be used and items subject to special inspections and tests.

**9.8.4** The special inspector shall submit an inspection and test report to the authority having jurisdiction and registered design professional in responsible charge.

Section 9.8 recognizes the complex nature of certain life safety systems in buildings. Where required by another section of the *Code*, special inspections must be performed, and design and test documentation must be provided to the authority having jurisdiction to ensure the system will perform as intended during a fire. Currently, only engineered smoke management systems must be submitted to special inspections and tests, as required by 9.3.3, to ensure all relevant parties (building owner's representative, design professional, and AHJ) understand the goals and objectives of the system (e.g., to maintain the means of egress tenable for a given time period to facilitate evacuation) and the required performance criteria needed to achieve the stated goals (e.g., the pressure differences needed between smoke zones and other performance criteria). See NFPA 92A, *Standard for Smoke-Control Systems Utilizing Barriers and Pressure Differences*, and NFPA 92B, *Standard for Smoke Management Systems in Malls, Atria, and Large Spaces*, for additional details on smoke control system design.

### References Cited in Commentary


1. NFPA 54, *National Fuel Gas Code*, 2009 edition, National Fire Protection Association, Quincy, MA.
2. *NFPA 70®*, *National Electrical Code®*, 2008 edition, National Fire Protection Association, Quincy, MA.
3. NFPA 90A, *Standard for the Installation of Air-Conditioning and Ventilating Systems*, 2009 edition, National Fire Protection Association, Quincy, MA.
4. NFPA 90B, *Standard for the Installation of Warm Air Heating and Air-Conditioning Systems*, 2009 edition, National Fire Protection Association, Quincy, MA.
5. NFPA 96, *Standard for Ventilation Control and Fire Protection of Commercial Cooking Operations*, 2008 edition, National Fire Protection Association, Quincy, MA.
6. NFPA 45, *Standard on Fire Protection for Laboratories Using Chemicals*, 2004 edition, National Fire Protection Association, Quincy, MA.
7. NFPA 99, *Standard for Health Care Facilities*, 2005 edition, National Fire Protection Association, Quincy, MA.
8. NFPA 92A, *Standard for Smoke-Control Systems Utilizing Barriers and Pressure Differences*, 2009 edition, National Fire Protection Association, Quincy, MA.
9. NFPA 92B, *Standard for Smoke Management Systems in Malls, Atria, and Large Spaces*, 2009 edition, National Fire Protection Association, Quincy, MA.
10. NFPA 204, *Standard for Smoke and Heat Venting*, 2007 edition, National Fire Protection Association, Quincy, MA.
11. ASME A17.1/CSA B44, *Safety Code for Elevators and Escalators*, 2007 edition, American Society of Mechanical Engineers, Three Park Avenue, New York, NY 10016-5990.
12. ASME A17.3, *Safety Code for Existing Elevators and* Escalators, 2005 edition, American Society of Mechanical Engineers, Three Park Avenue, New York, NY 10016-5990.
13. NFPA 13, *Standard for the Installation of Sprinkler Systems*, 2007 edition, National Fire Protection Association, Quincy, MA.
14. ASME *Handbook* A17.1, 2007 edition, American Society of Mechanical Engineers, Three Park Avenue, New York, NY 10016-5990.
15. NFPA 82, *Standard on Incinerators and Waste and Linen Handling Systems and Equipment*, 2004 edition, National Fire Protection Association, Quincy, MA.
16. *NFPA 72®*, *National Fire Alarm Code®*, 2007 edition, National Fire Protection Association, Quincy, MA.
17. *Americans with Disabilities Act and Architectural Barriers Act Accessibility Guidelines for Buildings and*

*Facilities*, 2004 edition, U.S. Architectural and Transportation Barriers Compliance Board, 1331 F Street, NW, Suite 100, Washington, DC.

18. NFPA 13R, *Standard for the Installation of Sprinkler Systems in Residential Occupancies up to and Including Four Stories in Height*, 2007 edition, National Fire Protection Association, Quincy, MA.
19. NFPA 13D, *Standard for the Installation of Sprinkler Systems in One- and Two-Family Dwellings and Manufactured Homes*, 2007 edition, National Fire Protection Association, Quincy, MA.
20. NFPA 25, *Standard for the Inspection, Testing, and Maintenance of Water-Based Fire Protection Systems*, 2008 edition, National Fire Protection Association, Quincy, MA.
21. NFPA 10, *Standard for Portable Fire Extinguishers*, 2007 edition, National Fire Protection Association, Quincy, MA.

CHAPTER 10

# Interior Finish, Contents, and Furnishings

Historically, many fire fatalities have been attributed to the quick spread of fire. Often the fire spread occurs along the expanses of exposed wall and ceiling coverings and via the contents of the building. Such was the case with The Station nightclub fire in West Warwick, Rhode Island, in February 2003. In that fire, pyrotechnics ignited acoustical foam wall and ceiling surfaces, resulting in a rapidly developing fire and the death of 100 people.

Chapter 10 establishes basic requirements for interior wall, ceiling, and floor finish and for furnishings and contents. This chapter specifies a menu of protection options, which are mandated to varying degrees by specific occupancy chapters. However, some of the requirements of this chapter apply to all occupancies.

Section 10.2 provides requirements for interior finish, which includes wall, ceiling, and floor finishes. The concept behind the requirements is to slow the flame spread across these finish surfaces to allow additional time for occupants to relocate within, or evacuate from, a building. The fire characteristics of interior finish can play a dramatic role in life safety when a fire occurs.

Section 10.3 addresses the contents and furnishings in a building. Very few occupancy chapters mandate the use of the provisions of this section. Where provisions of this section are formatted so as to apply to any occupancy unless specifically exempted, many occupancy chapters provide such exemptions. The occupancies for which the regulation of furnishings and contents is part of the overall life safety scheme involve occupants who are nonambulatory, who are otherwise restrained or detained, or who are asleep. Contrast this application with the provisions for interior finish that are mandated by all of the occupancy chapters.

## 10.1 General

Interior finish has been a significant factor in rapid flame spread in many of the deadliest U.S. fires of recent decades. The paragraphs that follow describe a few examples of such fires.

In June 1989, five people died on the floor of origin of an "intense, rapidly developing fire on the sixth floor of an office building" in Atlanta, Georgia.[1] In this fire, ". . . the fire spread was so fast that the blaze in the corridor had burned itself out by the time fire fighters entered the sixth floor about seven minutes after the initial alarm . . . This is not the first time that multiple layers of wall coverings have been identified as a contributing factor in a fire . . . It is evident that this condition existed in the Atlanta building, that the materials in those layers contributed to the total load in the corridor, and that it is likely they contributed to the rate of fire spread."

Regarding the 1986 Dupont Plaza Hotel fire (see Exhibit 10.1) in which 96 people died: "Under the NFPA *Life Safety Code*, interior finish in all ballrooms, including the room of origin, should have been Class A or Class B. The wall finish of the room of origin contributed to the rapid fire growth."[2]

In the 1981 Las Vegas Hilton Hotel fire, combustible carpeting on the walls and ceilings of elevator lobbies contributed to horizontal fire spread on the floor of origin and vertical spread involving 22 floors. Eight people died.[3]

In a 1978 Holiday Inn fire that killed 10 people, "lightweight plywood paneling in stairway did not meet *Life Safety Code*, was involved early in fire, and produced rapid growth and spread." In a 1979 Holiday Inn fire that also killed 10 people, "carpeting and some wall covering in corridors had excessively high flame-spread properties."[4]

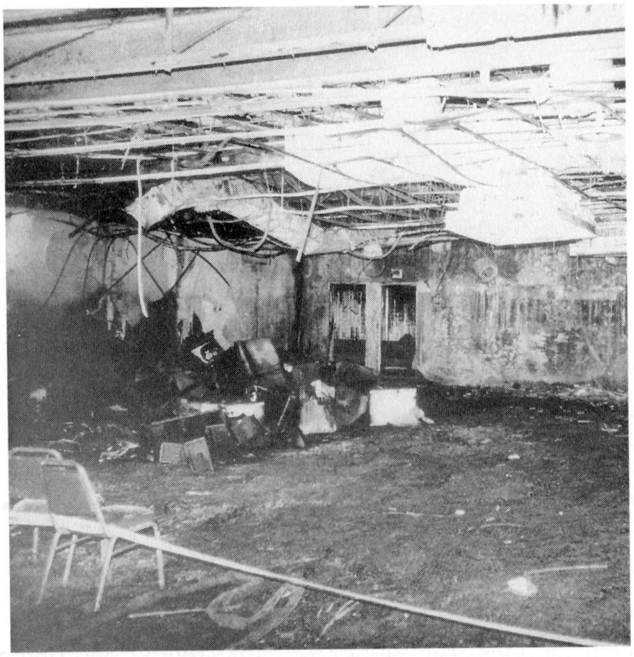

*Exhibit 10.1 Dupont Plaza Hotel Fire, in which rapid fire growth was, in part, due to wall finish in room of origin.*

In a 1972 Springfield, Illinois, convalescent nursing home fire that killed 10 of the 41 patients, "the wood-panel finish accelerated fire spread . . . Combustible interior finish — especially interior finish such as the wood paneling in this facility — should not be allowed where infirm people are housed . . . The paneling on the stairway had completely burned away, permitting fire spread into the first floor through holes in the plaster."[5]

Regarding the 1970 Pioneer International Hotel fire where 28 died:

> Under the NFPA *Life Safety Code*, interior finish in all ballrooms, including the room of origin, corridors and stairs were carpeted (100 percent acrylic), with two layers of padding under carpet in corridors and carpeting extending 22 inches up the walls. Above the carpeted areas of the wall were sections of wood, wallpaper, and plastic-laminated plywood. Interior finish contributed to fire.[6]

### 10.1.1 Application.

The interior finish, contents, and furnishings provisions set forth in this chapter shall apply to new construction and existing buildings.

Highly combustible interior wall and ceiling finishes and easily ignited contents and furnishings are repeatedly reported as factors in fire spread in various occupancies. The repeated contribution of these factors to fire spread demonstrates the need to apply Chapter 10 requirements to both new and existing installations.

### 10.1.2 Automatic Sprinkler Systems.

Where another provision of this chapter requires an automatic sprinkler system, the automatic sprinkler system shall be installed in accordance with the subparagraph of 9.7.1.1 as permitted by the applicable occupancy chapter.

The protection provided by automatic sprinklers, especially with respect to preventing flashover (see 3.3.104), is recognized via certain exemptions in Chapter 10. For example, in locations protected by automatic sprinklers, 10.2.8.1 permits the use of Class C interior wall and ceiling finish materials where Class B would otherwise be required. It is important that the sprinkler system be designed and installed in accordance with the proper standard. Paragraph 10.1.2 relegates the appropriate sprinkler system installation standard to the applicable occupancy chapter. For example, sprinkler systems required for new health care occupancies must be installed per NFPA 13, *Standard for the Installation of Sprinkler Systems*,[7] because 18.3.5.4 references 9.7.1.1(1); yet, for hotels and dormitories, 28.3.5.3 recognizes sprinkler systems installed per NFPA 13R, *Standard for the Installation of Sprinkler Systems in Residential Occupancies up to and Including Four Stories in Height*,[8] if the hotel or dormitory is not more than four stories in height; otherwise the sprinkler system must be installed per NFPA 13.

### 10.1.3 Special Definitions.

A list of special terms used in this chapter follows:

(1) **Contents and Furnishings.** See 3.3.45.

The term *contents and furnishings* is defined in 3.3.45 as "any movable objects in a building for functional, operational, or decorative reasons, excluding parts of the building structure, building service equipment, and items meeting the definition of interior finish." Application of the definition of *interior finish* in 3.3.84.2 and the provisions of 10.2.1.3 will result in some items commonly considered by building occupants as contents or furnishings being classified and treated under the stricter provisions applicable to interior finish.

(2) **Flashover.** See 3.3.104.

The term *flashover* is defined in 3.3.104 as "a transition phase in the development of a compartment fire in which surfaces exposed to thermal radiation reach ignition temperature more or less simultaneously and fire spreads rapidly throughout the space." The space in which flashover occurs is not tenable for human occupancy, and tenability is not ensured in adjacent spaces not adequately separated from the fire compartment. The provisions of Section 10.2, and the associated interior finish limitations imposed by the occupancy chapters, are directed at preventing a fire involving the interior finish materials alone from resulting in flashover.

(3) **Interior Finish.** See 3.3.84.2.

The term *interior finish* is defined in 3.3.84.2 as "the exposed surfaces of walls, ceilings, and floors within buildings."

The faster a fire develops, the greater the threat it represents to the occupants of a building, and the more difficult it will be to control. Wall and ceiling surfaces of a building have a major influence on how fast a fire develops. In establishing restrictions for the use of interior finish materials, the *Code*'s intention is to limit the spread of fire across the interior surfaces of a building.

Any large fire within a building represents a threat to occupants. A successful fire protection strategy attempts to limit the size of fires. Any interior finish that acts as a "fuse" to spread flame and involve objects remote from the point of origin, or that contributes fuel to the early growth of a fire and causes a large fire, is undesirable. The restrictions found in the *Code* for wall and ceiling finishes vary, depending on the occupancy characteristics. Where occupants are immobile or where security measures restrict freedom of movement (as in health care facilities or detention and correctional facilities), conservative interior finish limits are set. In contrast, more relaxed limits are permitted in industrial or storage occupancies where occupants are assumed to be alert and mobile.

Interior finishes are the interior surfaces of a building that are generally secured in place. Thus, wall, ceiling, and column coverings are considered interior wall and ceiling finishes. The surfaces of movable walls or folding partitions are also to be treated as interior finishes (see 10.2.1.3). However, the *Code* permits the authority having jurisdiction (AHJ) to exercise judgment in determining the criteria that constitute interior finish. For example, a loosely hanging tapestry placed against a wall would not normally be considered interior finish. However, a large tapestry that is secured to and covers a major portion of a wall could promote the rapid growth of fire and might be judged as constituting interior finish.

Furnishings (including high-backed, plastic-upholstered restaurant booths) are not normally considered as interior finish, even in cases where the furnishings are fixed in place. However, some furnishings are considered interior finish, as detailed in 10.2.1.3. See the definition of *contents and furnishings* in 3.3.45 and in the commentary following 10.1.3(1).

(4) **Interior Ceiling Finish.** See 3.3.84.1.

The term *interior ceiling finish* is defined in 3.3.84.1 as "the interior finish of ceilings." Flame spread typically occurs from burning furnishings located at floor level, moving upward vertically along wall surfaces to the ceiling, and spreading across the ceiling surface. Where ceiling materials are not controlled as interior finish, the spread of fire across the ceiling surface might outpace that of the building occupants moving toward exits.

(5) **Interior Floor Finish.** See 3.3.84.3.

The term *interior floor finish* is defined in 3.3.84.3 as "the interior finish of floors, ramps, stair treads and risers, and other walking surfaces." Interior floor finish includes both exposed surfaces of structural floor systems and decorative floor treatments, such as wood flooring, carpet, or other resilient flooring materials. Coverings on stair risers and treads are regulated as interior floor finish, even though risers involve vertical applications. This regulation recognizes that floor coverings on stair risers and treads will perform similarly to other floor surfaces during a fire.

(6) **Interior Wall Finish.** See 3.3.84.4.

The term *interior wall finish* is defined in 3.3.84.4 as "the interior finish of columns, fixed or movable walls, and fixed or movable partitions." Wall surfaces serve as the medium for spreading flame from burning furnishings, located at floor level, upward vertically to the ceiling. The likelihood of flashover is greatly reduced if flame can be stopped from reaching the ceiling.

Many of the provisions of Section 10.2 are focused at slowing the flame spread on wall surfaces.

## 10.2* Interior Finish

**A.10.2** The requirements pertaining to interior finish are intended to restrict the spread of fire over the continuous surface forming the interior portions of a building.

Table A.10.2 shows the fire test methods and classification criteria that apply to different interior finish materials.

### 10.2.1* General.

**A.10.2.1** The presence of multiple paint layers has the potential for paint delamination and bubbling or blistering of paint. Testing (NFPA *Fire Technology*, August 1974, "Fire Tests of Building Interior Covering Systems," David Waksman and John Ferguson, Institute for Applied Technology,

***Table A.10.2 Fire Testing of Interior Finish Materials***

| Material | Test Method | Acceptance Criterion | Application Requirement | Section |
|---|---|---|---|---|
| Interior wall and ceiling finish materials, except as shown in this table | ASTM E 84 or ANSI/UL 723 | Class A, in accordance with 10.2.3.4 (1) | As required by relevant sections | 10.2.3 |
| | ASTM E 84 or ANSI/UL 723 | Class B, in accordance with 10.2.3.4 (2) | As required by relevant sections | 10.2.3 |
| | ASTM E 84 or ANSI/UL 723 | Class C, in accordance with 10.2.3.4 (3) | As required by relevant sections | 10.2.3 |
| | NFPA 286 | In accordance with 10.2.3.7.2 | Permitted where Class A, B, or C is required by relevant sections | 10.2.3.2 |
| Materials having thickness <$^1/_{28}$ in. (0.90 mm) applied directly to the surface of walls or ceilings | No testing required | | | 10.2.1.2 |
| Exposed portions of structural members complying with requirements for buildings of Type IV (2HH) construction in accordance with NFPA 220 | No testing required | | | 10.2.3.1 |
| Cellular or foamed plastics (exposed foamed plastics and foamed plastics used in conjunction with textile or vinyl facing or cover) | NFPA 286 | In accordance with 10.2.3.7.2 | Permitted where Class A, B, or C is required by relevant sections | 10.2.4.3.1.1(1) |
| | ANSI/UL 1715 | Pass | Permitted where Class A, B, or C is required by relevant sections | 10.2.4.3.1.1(2) |
| | ANSI/UL 1040 | Pass | Permitted where Class A, B, or C is required by relevant sections | 10.2.4.3.1.1(3) |
| | FM 4880 | Pass | Permitted where Class A, B, or C is required by relevant sections | 10.2.4.3.1.1(4) |
| | Suitable large-scale fire test that substantiates combustibility characteristics for use intended under actual fire conditions | Pass | Permitted where Class A, B, or C is required by relevant sections | 10.2.4.3.1 |

*Table A.10.2 Continued*

| Material | Test Method | Acceptance Criterion | Application Requirement | Section |
|---|---|---|---|---|
| Textile wall coverings | NFPA 286 | In accordance with 10.2.3.7.2 | Permitted where Class A, B, or C is required by relevant sections | 10.2.4.1(6) |
| | NFPA 265, Method B | In accordance with 10.2.3.7.1 | Permitted on walls and partitions | 10.2.4.1(5) |
| | ASTM E 84 or ANSI/UL 723 | Class A, in accordance with 10.2.3.4 (1) | Permitted on walls, but also requires sprinklers per Section 9.7 | 10.2.4.1(1) |
| | ASTM E 84 or ANSI/UL 723 | Class A, in accordance with 10.2.3.4 (1) | Permitted on partitions not exceeding three-quarters of the floor-to-ceiling height or not exceeding 8 ft (2440 mm) in height, whichever is less | 10.2.4.1(2) |
| | ASTM E 84 or ANSI/UL 723 | Class A, in accordance with 10.2.3.4 (1) | Permitted to extend not more than 48 in. (1220 mm) above finished floor on ceiling-height walls and ceiling-height partitions | 10.2.4.1(3) |
| | ASTM E 84 or ANSI/UL 723 | Class A, in accordance with 10.2.3.4 (1) | Previously approved existing installations of textile material having a Class A rating permitted to be continued to be used | 10.2.4.1(4) |
| Expanded vinyl wall coverings | NFPA 286 | In accordance with 10.2.3.7.2 | Permitted where Class A, B, or C is required by relevant sections | 10.2.4.2(6) |
| | NFPA 265, Method B | In accordance with 10.2.3.7.1 | Permitted on walls and partitions | 10.2.4.2(5) |
| | ASTM E 84 or ANSI/UL 723 | Class A, in accordance with 10.2.3.4 (1) | Permitted on walls, but also requires sprinklers per Section 9.7 | 10.2.4.2(1) |
| | ASTM E 84 or ANSI/UL 723 | Class A, in accordance with 10.2.3.4 (1) | Permitted on partitions not exceeding three-quarters of the floor-to-ceiling height or not exceeding 8 ft (2440 mm) in height, whichever is less | 10.2.4.2(2) |
| | ASTM E 84 or ANSI/UL 723 | Class A, in accordance with 10.2.3.4 (1) | Permitted to extend not more than 48 in. (1220 mm) above finished floor on ceiling-height walls and ceiling-height partitions | 10.2.4.2(3) |
| | ASTM E 84 or ANSI/UL 723 | Class A, B, or C, in accordance with 10.2.3.4 | Existing installations of materials with appropriate wall finish classification for occupancy involved, and with classification in accordance with the provisions of 10.2.3.4 | 10.2.4.2(4) |

*(continues)*

*Table A.10.2 Continued*

| Material | Test Method | Acceptance Criterion | Application Requirement | Section |
|---|---|---|---|---|
| Textile ceiling coverings | NFPA 286 | In accordance with 10.2.3.7.2 | Permitted where Class A, B, or C is required by relevant sections | 10.2.4.1(6) |
| | ASTM E 84 or ANSI/UL 723 | Class A, in accordance with 10.2.3.4 (1) | Permitted on walls, but also requires sprinklers per Section 9.7 | 10.2.4.1(1) |
| | ASTM E 84 or ANSI/UL 723 | Class A, in accordance with 10.2.3.4 (1) | Previously approved existing installations of textile material having a Class A rating permitted to be continued to be used | 10.2.4.1(4) |
| Expanded vinyl ceiling coverings | NFPA 286 | In accordance with 10.2.3.7.2 | Permitted where Class A, B, or C is required by relevant sections | 10.2.4.2(6) |
| | ASTM E 84 or ANSI/UL 723 | Class A, in accordance with 10.2.3.4 (1) | Permitted on walls, but also requires sprinklers per Section 9.7 | 10.2.4.2(1) |
| | ASTM E 84 or ANSI/UL 723 | Class A, B, or C, in accordance with 10.2.3.4 | Existing installations of materials with appropriate wall finish classification for occupancy involved, and with classification in accordance with the provisions of 10.2.3.4 | 10.2.4.2(4) |
| Interior trim, other than foamed plastic and other than wall base | ASTM E 84 or ANSI/UL 723 | Class C, in accordance with 10.2.3.4 | Interior wall and ceiling trim and incidental finish, other than wall base not in excess of 10 percent of the aggregate wall and ceiling areas of any room or space where interior wall and ceiling finish of Class A or Class B is required | 10.2.5.1 |
| | NFPA 286 | In accordance with 10.2.3.7.2 | Permitted where Class A, B, or C is required by relevant sections | 10.2.3.2 |
| Foamed plastic used as interior trim | ASTM E 84 or ANSI/UL 723 | Flame spread index ≤ 75 | (1) Minimum density of interior trim required to be 20 lb/ft$^3$ (320 kg/m$^3$) | 10.2.4.3.2 |
| | | | (2) Maximum thickness of interior trim required to be ½ in. (13 mm), and maximum width required to be 4 in. (100 mm) | 10.2.4.3.2 |
| | | | (3) Interior trim not permitted to constitute more than 10 percent of the wall or ceiling area of a room or space | 10.2.4.3.2 |
| | NFPA 286 | In accordance with 10.2.3.7.2 | Permitted where Class A, B, or C is required by relevant sections | 10.2.3.2 |

*Table A.10.2 Continued*

| Material | Test Method | Acceptance Criterion | Application Requirement | Section |
|---|---|---|---|---|
| Fire-retardant coatings | NFPA 703 | Class A, B, or C, when tested by ASTM E 84 or ANSI/UL 723, in accordance with 10.2.3.4 | Required flame spread or smoke development classification of existing surfaces of walls, partitions, columns, and ceilings permitted to be secured by applying approved fire-retardant coatings to surfaces having higher flame spread ratings than permitted; such treatments required to be tested, or listed and labeled for application to material to which they are applied | 10.2.6.1 |
| Carpet and carpetlike interior floor finishes | ASTM D 2859 | Pass | All areas | 10.2.7.1 |
| Floor coverings, other than carpet, judged to represent an unusual hazard (excluding traditional finish floors and floor coverings, such as wood flooring and resilient floor coverings) | NFPA 253 | Critical radiant flux ≥ 0.1 W/cm$^2$ | All areas | 10.2.7.2 |
| Interior floor finish, other than carpet and carpetlike materials | NFPA 253 | Class I: Critical radiant flux ≥ 0.45 W/cm$^2$, in accordance with 10.2.7.4 | As required by relevant sections | 10.2.7.3 |
| | NFPA 253 | Class II: Critical radiant flux ≥ 0.22 W/cm$^2$, in accordance with 10.2.7.4 | As required by relevant sections | 10.2.7.3 |
| Wall base [interior floor trim material used at junction of wall and floor to provide a functional or decorative border, and not exceeding 6 in. (150 mm) in height] | NFPA 253 | Class II: Critical radiant flux ≥ 0.22 W/cm$^2$, in accordance with 10.2.7.4 | All areas | 10.2.5.2 |
| | NFPA 253 | Class I: Critical radiant flux ≥ 0.45 W/cm$^2$, in accordance with 10.2.7.4 | If interior floor finish is required to meet Class I critical radiant flux | 10.2.5.2 |
| Floor finish of traditional type, such as wood flooring and resilient floor coverings | No testing required | | | 10.2.2.2 |

National Bureau of Standards) has shown that adding up to two layers of paint with a dry film thickness of about 0.007 in. (0.18 mm) will not change the fire properties of surface-covering systems. Testing has shown that the fire properties of the surface-covering systems are highly substrate dependent and that thin coatings generally take on the characteristics of the substrate. When exposed to fire, the delamination, bubbling, and blistering of paint can result in an accelerated rate of flame spread.

**10.2.1.1** Classification of interior finish materials shall be in accordance with tests made under conditions simulating actual installations, provided that the authority having jurisdiction shall be permitted to establish the classification of any material on which a rating by standard test is not available, unless otherwise provided in 10.2.1.2.

Paragraph 10.2.1.1 presents two concepts.

First, for interior finish materials to be classified properly based on performance under a standardized test, such test needs to be indicative of the conditions under which the material will actually be installed. For example, thin wood paneling applied directly to wall framing studs can be expected to spread flame differently than thin wood paneling applied to gypsum wallboard. This concept is explained, in part, in A.10.2.1. See also the commentary following A.10.2.3.4.

Second, the authority having jurisdiction (AHJ) is responsible for classifying interior finish materials for which standardized test data is not available. The AHJ is free to use whatever tools are available (such as experience, intuition, comparative field testing) and will generally take the conservative approach of banning the use of suspect materials for which there is no corroborating data. The regulation of interior finish materials is an important part of the total package of life safety offered by compliance with the *Code*.

**10.2.1.2** Materials applied directly to the surface of walls and ceilings in a total thickness of less than $^{1}/_{28}$ in. (0.9 mm) shall not be considered interior finish and shall be exempt from tests simulating actual installation if they meet the requirements of Class A interior wall or ceiling finish when tested in accordance with 10.2.3 using fiber cement board as the substrate material.

Paragraph 10.2.1.2 addresses the issue of thin coverings, which was covered in earlier editions of the *Code* by a simply worded, performance-based criterion that was difficult to use and enforce. The *Code* recognized that thin coverings [those less than $^{1}/_{28}$ in. (0.9 mm) in thickness] with surface-burning characteristics not greater than that of paper would not significantly affect the fire performance of the basic wall or ceiling material. If assurance were provided that such a thin covering had surface-burning characteristics not greater than those of paper, the thin material would not be subject to regulation as an interior finish. Therefore, the material's flame spread rating wasn't needed, which, in turn, meant that no fire testing was required. The problem was that, without running fire tests, it was impossible to determine whether a thin material had surface-burning characteristics that were greater than those of paper.

The wording of 10.2.1.2 does not exempt thin materials from testing, but it does exempt thin materials from testing with the actual substrate or backing material that will be used in the final installed state. If there were no exemption, thin materials, such as paint (whose liquid suspension state dries to become a thin layer of material) and wallpaper, would be required to be fire tested in combination with numerous backing materials. A complete set of test results, representative of the many forms of substrates in common use, would be prohibitively expensive to collect. Paragraph 10.2.1.2 permits the material to be tested only with fiber cement board as the substrate material. If the material, where tested in that configuration, meets the requirements for Class A interior finish [see 10.2.3.4(1)], it is not considered as interior finish, and further regulation by Section 10.2 is exempted.

Thermally thin coverings, such as paint and wallpaper coverings, where secured to a noncombustible substrate such as fiber cement board, will not significantly alter the performance of the substrate during a fire. However, thicker coverings, such as multiple layers of wallpaper, can and have contributed to rapid fire growth. For example, multiple layers of wall coverings contributed to rapid fire growth in the multiple-death fire in the Holiday Inn in Cambridge, Ohio, which occurred on July 31, 1979.[9]

The provision of 10.2.1.2 has the effect of requiring any wall or ceiling covering (or multiple layers of such covering) of more than $^{1}/_{28}$ in. (0.9 mm) in thickness to undergo the full test series required of other interior finish materials so as to be representative of actual installations.

Painted surfaces might be evaluated using the steps that follow:

1. Determine the classification of the interior finish material (e.g., wood wainscoting) in its unpainted configuration, and verify that it complies with the applicable limits (e.g., 38.3.3, if the occupancy is new business, and 7.1.4 for exit enclosures).

2. Obtain a paint product for which the manufacturer has documented that it achieves a Class A rating when applied to a substrate of cement fiber board and tested in accordance with ASTM E 84, *Standard Test Method for Surface Burning Characteristics of Building Materials,* or ANSI/UL 723, *Standard for Test for Surface Burning Characteristics of Building Materials.*
3. Apply the paint to the substrate described in step 1 above such that the thickness is less than $\frac{1}{28}$ in. (0.9 mm).
4. Where the above steps 1 through 3 are followed, the paint is exempt from being tested on the substrate on which it is actually installed.

Where the thickness of an interior finish material is $\frac{1}{28}$ in. (0.9 mm) or greater, it must be tested as it will actually be installed. For example, the performance of thermally thin coverings is altered by the nature of the substrate over which they are installed.[10] Adhesives might also be an important factor in performance. In the case of composites (such as textile wall coverings over gypsum board), the adhesive should be sufficient to maintain a bond between the "finish" and the substrate. However, excess adhesive might contribute to a fire. Tests of textile wall coverings have shown that changing adhesives, or simply changing the application rate for the same adhesive, might significantly alter product performance.[11] Tests to qualify assemblies should use adhesives and application rates similar to actual installations.

Similarly, a product that undergoes testing in intimate contact with a mineral board should be installed in contact with a mineral board or similar substrate. Also, where products are tested in intimate contact with a substrate, results might be altered if the product is installed with air space behind the covering.

**10.2.1.3*** Fixed or movable walls and partitions, paneling, wall pads, and crash pads applied structurally or for decoration, acoustical correction, surface insulation, or other purposes shall be considered interior finish and shall not be considered decorations or furnishings.

**A.10.2.1.3** Such partitions are intended to include washroom water closet partitions.

Prior to the 2006 edition of the *Code*, there was significant confusion among users on how to address materials placed on walls after construction and occupancy of the building. Often when materials were brought into an occupied building and attached to the walls, the authority having jurisdiction (AHJ) was petitioned to treat such materials as decorations or furnishings. If the AHJ agreed to classifying such materials as decorations or furnishings, then the materials might go unregulated or, at best, would be tested per NFPA 701, *Standard Methods of Fire Tests for Flame Propagation of Textiles and Films*[12] (see 10.3.1), which is not the appropriate test for interior finish materials. The criteria in 10.2.1.3, which was new to the 2006 edition of the *Code*, provides the needed clarification.

Pads are often attached to walls in school gymnasiums to cushion the blow if a student crashes into the wall. Such pads applied to, or placed against, walls need to be treated as interior wall finish. Similar pads placed on the floor should be considered as contents and furnishings.

### 10.2.2* Use of Interior Finishes.

**A.10.2.2** Table A.10.2.2 provides a compilation of the interior finish requirements of the occupancy chapters (Chapters 12 through 42).

***Table A.10.2.2 Interior Finish Classification Limitations***

| Occupancy | Exits | Exit Access Corridors | Other Spaces |
|---|---|---|---|
| Assembly — New | | | |
| >300 occupant load | A | A or B | A or B |
| | I or II | I or II | NA |
| ≤300 occupant load | A | A or B | A, B, or C |
| | I or II | I or II | NA |
| Assembly — Existing | | | |
| >300 occupant load | A | A or B | A or B |
| ≤300 occupant load | A | A or B | A, B, or C |
| Educational — New | A | A or B | A or B; C on low partitions† |
| | I or II | I or II | NA |
| Educational — Existing | A | A or B | A, B, or C |
| Day-Care Centers — New | A | A | A or B |
| | I or II | I or II | NA |

*(continues)*

*Table A.10.2.2* ***Continued***

| Occupancy | Exits | Exit Access Corridors | Other Spaces |
|---|---|---|---|
| Day-Care Centers — Existing | A or B | A or B | A or B |
| Day-Care Homes — New | A or B | A or B | A, B, or C |
| | I or II | | NA |
| Day-Care Homes — Existing | A or B | A, B, or C | A, B, or C |
| Health Care — New | A | A | A |
| | NA | B on lower portion of corridor wall† | B in small individual rooms† |
| | I or II | I or II | NA |
| Health Care — Existing | A or B | A or B | A or B |
| Detention and Correctional — New (sprinklers mandatory) | A or B | A or B | A, B, or C |
| | I or II | I or II | NA |
| Detention and Correctional — Existing | A or B | A or B | A, B, or C |
| | I or II | I or II | NA |
| One- and Two-Family Dwellings and Lodging or Rooming Houses | A, B, or C | A, B, or C | A, B, or C |
| Hotels and Dormitories — New | A | A or B | A, B, or C |
| | I or II | I or II | NA |
| Hotels and Dormitories — Existing | A or B | A or B | A, B, or C |
| | I or II† | I or II† | NA |
| Apartment Buildings — New | A | A or B | A, B, or C |
| | I or II | I or II | NA |
| Apartment Buildings — Existing | A or B | A or B | A, B, or C |
| | I or II† | I or II† | NA |
| Residential Board and Care — *(See Chapters 32 and 33.)* | | | |
| Mercantile — New | A or B | A or B | A or B |
| | I or II | | NA |
| Mercantile — Existing | | | |
| Class A or Class B stores | A or B | A or B | Ceilings — A or B; walls — A, B, or C |
| Class C stores | A, B, or C | A, B, or C | A, B, or C |
| Business and Ambulatory Health Care — New | A or B | A or B | A, B, or C |
| | I or II | | NA |
| Business and Ambulatory Health Care — Existing | A or B | A or B | A, B, or C |
| Industrial | A or B | A, B, or C | A, B, or C |
| | I or II | I or II | NA |
| Storage | A or B | A, B, or C | A, B, or C |
| | I or II | | NA |

NA: Not applicable.

Notes:

(1) Class A interior wall and ceiling finish — flame spread, 0–25 (new applications), smoke developed, 0–450.

(2) Class B interior wall and ceiling finish — flame spread, 26–75 (new applications), smoke developed, 0–450.

(3) Class C interior wall and ceiling finish — flame spread, 76–200 (new applications), smoke developed, 0–450.

(4) Class I interior floor finish — critical radiant flux, not less than 0.45 W/cm$^2$.

(5) Class II interior floor finish — critical radiant flux, not more than 0.22 W/cm$^2$, but less than 0.45 W/cm$^2$.

(6) Automatic sprinklers — where a complete standard system of automatic sprinklers is installed, interior wall and ceiling finish with a flame spread rating not exceeding Class C is permitted to be used in any location where Class B is required and with a rating of Class B in any location where Class A is required; similarly, Class II interior floor finish is permitted to be used in any location where Class I is required, and no critical radiant flux rating is required where Class II is required. These provisions do not apply to new detention and correctional occupancies.

(7) Exposed portions of structural members complying with the requirements for heavy timber construction are permitted.

†See corresponding chapters for details.

Traditional floor coverings, such as wood flooring and resilient tile, do not contribute to the early growth of fire. Paragraph 10.2.2.2 has the effect of exempting traditional floor coverings from the restrictions that would otherwise be applicable. However, the authority having jurisdiction (AHJ) can require substantiation of the performance of any unfamiliar floor covering. For example, imitation wood floors made of plastic, artificial turf, artificial surfaces of athletic fields, and certain types of carpeting are products that might merit substantiation. If the AHJ judges that a floor covering warrants testing and substantiation, or if an occupancy chapter imposes restrictions, then the floor covering would be treated as interior floor finish. It would, therefore, be regulated on the basis of tests conducted in accordance with the flooring radiant panel test required in 10.2.7.

**10.2.2.1** Requirements for interior wall and ceiling finish shall apply as follows:

(1) Where specified elsewhere in this *Code* for specific occupancies *(see Chapter 7 and Chapters 11 through 43)*
(2) As specified in 10.2.4

**10.2.2.2*** Requirements for interior floor finish shall apply under any of the following conditions:

(1) Where floor finish requirements are specified elsewhere in the *Code*
(2)* Where carpet or carpetlike material not meeting the requirements of ASTM D 2859, *Standard Test Method for Ignition Characteristics of Finished Textile Floor Covering Materials*, is used

**A.10.2.2.2(2)** Compliance with 16 CFR 1630, *Standard for the Surface Flammability of Carpets and Rugs* (FFI-70), is considered equivalent to compliance with ASTM D 2859, *Standard Test Method for Ignition Characteristics of Finished Textile Floor Covering Materials.*

(3) Where the fire performance of the floor finish cannot be demonstrated to be equivalent to floor finishes with a critical radiant flux of at least 0.1 W/cm$^2$
(4) Where the fire performance of the floor finish is unknown

**A.10.2.2.2** This paragraph recognizes that traditional finish floors and floor coverings, such as wood flooring and resilient floor coverings, have not proved to present an unusual hazard.

## 10.2.3* Interior Wall or Ceiling Finish Testing and Classification.

Interior wall or ceiling finish that is required elsewhere in this *Code* to be Class A, Class B, or Class C shall be classified based on test results from ASTM E 84, *Standard Test Method for Surface Burning Characteristics of Building Materials*, or ANSI/UL 723, *Standard for Test for Surface Burning Characteristics of Building Materials*, except as indicated in 10.2.3.1 or 10.2.3.2.

**A.10.2.3** See A.10.2.4.1.

Flame spread and smoke development are both recorded in the results of a test conducted in accordance with ASTM E 84, *Standard Test Method for Surface Burning Characteristics of Building Materials*,[13] or ANSI/UL 723, *Standard for Test of Surface Burning Characteristics of Building Materials*.[14] The test is also referred to as the "Steiner tunnel test" (named after its inventor) and, generically, as the "room tunnel test." See also Supplement 3, Fire Tests for *Life Safety Code* Users, of this handbook.

**10.2.3.1** Exposed portions of structural members complying with the requirements for Type IV(2HH) construction in accordance with NFPA 220, *Standard on Types of Building Construction*, or with 7.2.5 of *NFPA 5000*, *Building Construction and Safety Code*, shall be exempt from testing and classification in accordance with ASTM E 84, *Standard Test Method for Surface Burning Characteristics of Building Materials*, or ANSI/UL 723, *Standard for Test for Surface Burning Characteristics of Building Materials*.

Type IV(2HH) construction has traditionally been called "heavy timber construction." Exposed surfaces of the structural members, such as wood columns, beams, and girders, meet the definition of interior wall and ceiling finish. All heavy timber structural members are required to be of substantial thickness, as detailed in NFPA 220, *Standard on Types of Building Construction*,[15] and *NFPA 5000®*, *Building Construction and Safety Code®*.[16] Thus, none are thermally thin, so they do not present the concerns addressed in the commentary that follows 10.2.1.2.

Paragraph 10.2.3.1 recognizes that exposed surfaces of heavy timber structural members can be safely used where Class A, Class B, or Class C interior finish is required. Such wood members often have flame spread ratings in the range of 76 to 200 and, therefore, are classified as Class C interior finish. The exemption is based on the fact that the structural members are located at intervals and do not constitute a continuous surface that allows flame to spread, for example, across a ceiling.

**10.2.3.2** Interior wall and ceiling finish tested in accordance with NFPA 286, *Standard Methods of Fire Tests for*

*Evaluating Contribution of Wall and Ceiling Interior Finish to Room Fire Growth*, and meeting the conditions of 10.2.3.7.2 shall be permitted to be used where interior wall and ceiling finish is required to be Class A in accordance with ASTM E 84, *Standard Test Method for Surface Burning Characteristics of Building Materials*, or ANSI/UL 723, *Standard for Test for Surface Burning Characteristics of Building Materials*.

Paragraph 10.2.3.2 permits materials that meet the criteria specified in 10.2.3.7.2, where tested in accordance with NFPA 286, *Standard Methods of Fire Tests for Evaluating Contribution of Wall and Ceiling Interior Finish to Room Fire Growth*,[17] to be used as both interior wall finish and interior ceiling finish, even where other *Code* provisions require interior wall and ceiling finish to be Class A in accordance with 10.2.3.4(1). Testing per NFPA 286, combined with performance as required by 10.2.3.7.2, represents an improvement over testing in accordance with ASTM E 84 or ANSI/UL 723 and classification in accordance with 10.2.3.4. ASTM E 84 and ANSI/UL 723 test a sample that is mounted in a horizontal orientation to cover the 18 in. (455 mm) wide by 24 ft (7.3 m) long ceiling of the test tunnel. NFPA 286 tests a sample that fully covers three walls of the 8 ft (2440 mm) wide by 12 ft (3660 mm) long by 8 ft (2440 mm) high test chamber — and the ceiling as well if the results are to be applied to interior ceiling finish. See the commentary following 10.2.3.7.2.

Note that 10.2.3.2 does not require testing per NFPA 286; rather, it offers this test procedure as an alternative to that of meeting the Class A classification criteria of 10.2.3.4(1), based on results from the more traditional ASTM E 84 or ANSI/UL 723 test protocol.

**10.2.3.3** For fire-retardant coatings, see 10.2.6.

**10.2.3.4*** Products required to be tested in accordance with ASTM E 84, *Standard Test Method for Surface Burning Characteristics of Building Materials*, or ANSI/UL 723, *Standard for Test for Surface Burning Characteristics of Building Materials*, shall be classified as follows in accordance with their flame spread and smoke development, except as indicated in 10.2.3.4(4):

(1) Class A interior wall and ceiling finish shall be characterized by the following:
  (a) Flame spread index, 0–25
  (b) Smoke developed index, 0–450
(2) Class B interior wall and ceiling finish shall be characterized by the following:
  (a) Flame spread index, 26–75
  (b) Smoke developed index, 0–450
(3) Class C interior wall and ceiling finish shall be characterized by the following:
  (a) Flame spread index, 76–200
  (b) Smoke developed index, 0–450
(4) Existing interior finish shall be exempt from the smoke development criteria of 10.2.3.4(1)(b), (2)(b), and (3)(b).

**A.10.2.3.4** It has been shown that the method of mounting interior finish materials might affect actual performance. Where materials are tested in intimate contact with a substrate to determine a classification, such materials should be installed in intimate contact with a similar substrate. Such details are especially important for "thermally thin" materials. For further information, see ASTM E 84, *Standard Test Method for Surface Burning Characteristics of Building Materials*.

Some interior wall and ceiling finish materials, such as fabrics not applied to a solid backing, do not lend themselves to a test made in accordance with ASTM E 84. In such cases, the large-scale test outlined in NFPA 701, *Standard Methods of Fire Tests for Flame Propagation of Textiles and Films*, is permitted to be used.

Prior to 1978, the test report described by ASTM E 84 included an evaluation of the fuel contribution as well as the flame spread rating and the smoke development value. However, it is now recognized that the measurement on which the fuel contribution is based does not provide a valid measure. Therefore, although the data are recorded during the test, the information is no longer normally reported. Classification of interior wall and ceiling finish thus relies only on flame spread index and smoke development value.

The 450 smoke development value limit is based solely on obscuration. *(See A.10.2.4.1.)*

Samples are tested in accordance with ASTM E 84 or ANSI/UL 723, as mandated by 10.2.3.4, using a noncombustible, fiber cement board backing. Specimens are tested with adhesives and joints and under other conditions that simulate the actual installation of a product in a building. These fire test standards provide a general indication of product performance only if the product is installed in a fashion similar to that which has been tested. Available data demonstrate that the performance of interior finish materials varies, depending on mounting conditions.[18] For example, a product installed over a combustible substrate tends to propagate fire more readily than would be typical of the same product installed over a noncombustible substrate.

Further, a wall covering installed with air space behind the covering tends to spread flame more readily than one installed in contact with a noncombustible substrate. Therefore, mounting techniques must be carefully considered in the evaluation of probable product performance.

Exhibit 10.2 illustrates the ASTM E 84 room tunnel test apparatus. The same apparatus is required for testing per ANSI/UL 723.

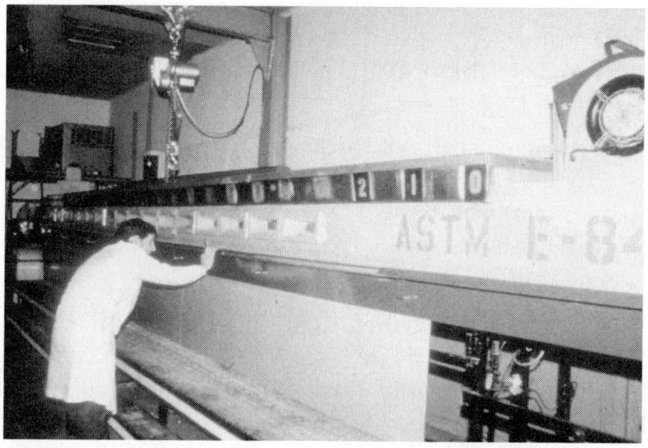


***Exhibit 10.2*** *ASTM E 84 room tunnel test apparatus. (Photo courtesy of Hughes Associates, Inc.)*

Interior wall and ceiling finish classifications in accordance with 10.2.3.4 are based mainly on flame spread ratings, with an additional requirement that smoke development not exceed a common value of 450, regardless of the class into which the material falls based on flame spread. Flame spread ratings offer a general indication of the speed with which fire might spread across the surface of a material. In assessing the hazard posed by a material on the basis of flame spread, it is assumed that a person might be close to the fire and would be directly exposed to the energy associated with the actual flames. By contrast, the purpose of smoke development ratings is to address visual obscuration of the egress path by smoke. Thus, an interior wall and ceiling finish material with a low smoke development value should provide better visibility in a given egress route than a material with a high smoke development value. Given that the smoke development value is a cumulative measurement over the prescribed test duration, it is based on both quantity and rate of smoke liberation.

The *Code* requires the use of specific classes of interior wall and ceiling finish materials, which are differentiated by their allowable flame spread rating, based on consideration of their installed location within the building, the building's egress paths, and the occupancy in question. Different classes of interior finish materials are specified for an office area, for example, as opposed to an exit stair enclosure or exit access corridor. The different classes recognize that, when escaping a building, people must move away from the flames while traveling through the means of egress toward an exit. The classes of interior finishes that are considered acceptable within an open office, therefore, are different from those that are required for exit enclosures. Similarly, occupancies used by those who are mobility impaired have stricter interior finish requirements than occupancies used by fully ambulatory occupants. For example, although both hospitals and hotels provide sleeping accommodations, interior finish requirements for hospitals are more stringent, because hospital patients are less capable of self-preservation.

The same smoke development limit is used for all three flame spread classifications. This limit recognizes that smoke generated during a fire might affect visibility both in the vicinity of, and remote from, the fire. Large buildings can be quickly filled with smoke as a result of a fire. An upper limit has been established, therefore, that applies to new interior finish materials, regardless of their location.

Per 10.2.3.4(4), existing buildings are exempted from the smoke development limitation. In existing buildings, existing interior finish materials are restricted only on the basis of flame spread. Prior to the 1976 edition, the *Code* did not regulate interior finish materials based on smoke development. As a general rule, the replacement of existing materials only because they were previously approved exclusively on the basis of flame spread is not warranted.

The smoke development limit of 450 was determined on the basis of research conducted by Underwriters Laboratories Inc. A 5000 $ft^3$ (140 $m^3$) room was filled with smoke from the tunnel test chamber. The room was equipped with illuminated exit signs. The time required to reach various stages of exit sign obscuration was recorded and compared to the smoke development rating for the different materials involved. The report states that "materials having smoke developed ratings above 325 showed 'good' to 'marginal' visibility — scale readings of 3 to 4.8 — in a few cases; other materials produced conditions of 'marginal' to obscuration in the six-minute period."[19]

Considering both time and smoke levels, the limit of 450 on smoke ratings as used in the *Code* has been judged to be reasonable. There is no direct relationship between flame spread and smoke development. For example, in the report referenced in the previous paragraph, one material had a flame spread index of 490 and a smoke developed index of 57, while another had a flame spread index of 44 and a smoke developed index of 1387.

The smoke development limit of 450 is based solely on the level of visual obscuration. Although not addressed by the requirements for interior finishes, other important factors used in evaluating materials on the basis of smoke generation are the effects of irritability and toxicity caused by gases. Smoke might also act as an irritant, further reducing visibility, and might, in addition, have a debilitating physiological effect on people attempting to escape from a building. Such effects are not evaluated by the current smoke development limit. Previous editions of the *Code* permitted the authority having jurisdiction to regulate products presenting an "unreasonable life hazard due to the character of the products of decomposition." This provision was deleted in the 1988 edition of the *Code* due to its unenforceable nature. The adverse physiological effects on the human body caused by exposure to heat and the effects of inhaling hot gases should also be considered as part of an overall hazard risk assessment and should be considered separately from the interior finish requirements of Section 10.2.

**10.2.3.5** The classification of interior finish specified in 10.2.3.4 shall be that of the basic material used by itself or in combination with other materials.

**10.2.3.6** Wherever the use of Class C interior wall and ceiling finish is required, Class A or Class B shall be permitted. Where Class B interior wall and ceiling finish is required, Class A shall be permitted.

Paragraph 10.2.3.6 recognizes that the *Code* sets minimum criteria. An interior finish material that performs better than that specifically prescribed by the *Code* is always permitted.

**10.2.3.7*** Products tested in accordance with NFPA 265, *Standard Methods of Fire Tests for Evaluating Room Fire Growth Contribution of Textile Coverings on Full Height Panels and Walls*, shall comply with the criteria of 10.2.3.7.1. Products tested in accordance with NFPA 286, *Standard Methods of Fire Tests for Evaluating Contribution of Wall and Ceiling Interior Finish to Room Fire Growth*, shall comply with the criteria of 10.2.3.7.2.

**A.10.2.3.7** The methodology specified in NFPA 265, *Standard Methods of Fire Tests for Evaluating Room Fire Growth Contribution of Textile Coverings on Full Height Panels and Walls*, includes provisions for measuring smoke obscuration. Such measurement is considered desirable, but the basis for specific recommended values is not currently available. *(See A.10.2.4.1.)*

**10.2.3.7.1** Products shall be tested using Method B of the test protocol of NFPA 265, *Standard Methods of Fire Tests for Evaluating Room Fire Growth Contribution of Textile Coverings on Full Height Panels and Walls*. The following conditions shall be met:

(1) Flame shall not spread to the ceiling during the 40 kW exposure.
(2) During the 150 kW exposure, the following criteria shall be met:
    (a) Flame shall not spread to the outer extremities of the sample on the 8 ft × 12 ft (2440 mm × 3660 mm) wall.
    (b) Flashover shall not occur.

The *Code* recognizes the use of Method B of NFPA 265, *Standard Methods of Fire Tests for Evaluating Room Fire Growth Contribution of Textile Coverings on Full Height Panels and Walls*,[20] but not Method A. Method B is the more rigorous test and requires that the test specimens be mounted to cover fully both 8 ft × 12 ft (2440 mm × 3660 mm) walls and the 8 ft × 8 ft (2440 mm × 2440 mm) rear wall. Method A is a screening test for which the test specimen is mounted as 24 in. (610 mm) wide strips at the intersection of two adjacent walls and along the top of those two walls where they meet the ceiling. See also Supplement 3, Fire Tests for *Life Safety Code* Users.

The NFPA 265 test compartment is depicted in Exhibit 10.3.

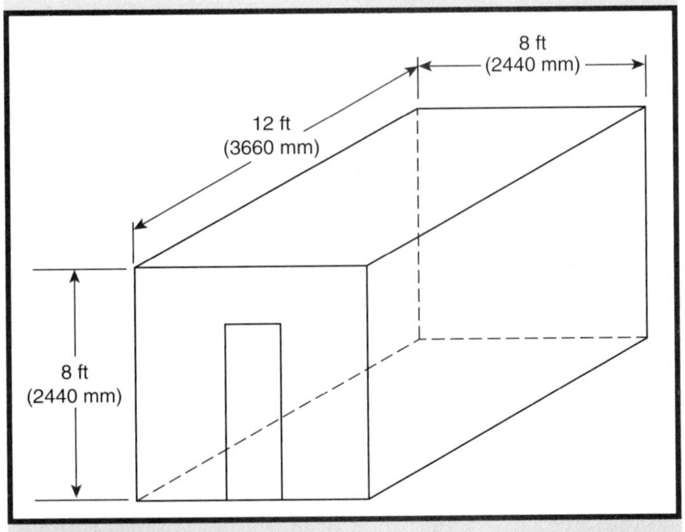


***Exhibit 10.3*** *Test compartment required by NFPA 265.*

**10.2.3.7.2** The following conditions shall be met when using the test protocol of NFPA 286, *Standard Methods of Fire Tests for Evaluating Contribution of Wall and Ceiling Interior Finish to Room Fire Growth*:

(1) Flames shall not spread to the ceiling during the 40 kW exposure.
(2) During the 160 kW exposure, the following criteria shall be met:
  (a) Flame shall not spread to the outer extremities of the sample on the 8 ft × 12 ft (2440 mm × 3660 mm) wall.
  (b) Flashover shall not occur.
(3) The peak heat release rate throughout the test shall not exceed 800 kW.
(4) For new installations, the total smoke released throughout the test shall not exceed 1000 $m^2$.

NFPA 286, *Standard Methods of Fire Tests for Evaluating Contribution of Wall and Ceiling Interior Finish to Room Fire Growth,* was developed specifically to measure the following:

1. Extent of flame spread and burning relative to the realistically sized and mounted sample
2. Whether flashover occurs
3. Peak rate of heat release
4. Total smoke released throughout the test

The peak heat release rate of 800 kW, as specified by 10.2.3.7.2(3), was new to the 2006 edition of the *Code*. It was added because 10.2.3.2 permits materials that meet the criteria specified in 10.2.3.7.2, where tested in accordance with NFPA 286, to be used as both interior wall finish and interior ceiling finish, even where other *Code* provisions require interior wall and ceiling finish to be Class A in accordance with 10.2.3.4(1). Some interior finish materials can be produced less expensively, so as to be somewhat less fire safe if they need to meet only the criteria of 10.2.3.7.2 (based on testing per NFPA 286) without a peak heat release rate criterion, instead of having to pass the flame spread criteria for Class A required by 10.2.3.4(1) (based on testing per ASTM E 84 or ANSI/UL 723). The peak heat release rate criterion associated with testing per NFPA 286 helps equalize the anomaly in the test methods. See also Supplement 3, Fire Tests for *Life Safety Code* Users.

Materials that meet the criteria for Class A interior finish when tested per ASTM E 84 or ANSI/UL 723, and that do not flash over the test room when tested per NFPA 286, typically have a peak heat release rate of less than 400 kW. The 800 kW peak heat release rate criterion of 10.2.3.7.2(3) was chosen to help ensure that materials that have already been tested are not unnecessarily penalized.

The test room used for NFPA 286 testing is the same size as that used for NFPA 265 testing and is shown in Exhibit 10.3. If the test results are to be applied only to interior wall finish, then the test specimens are mounted to cover fully both 8 ft × 12 ft (2440 mm × 3660 mm) walls and the 8 ft × 8 ft (2440 mm × 2440 mm) rear wall. If the test results are to be applied both to interior wall finish and interior ceiling finish, then, in addition, the test specimen is mounted to cover the ceiling. If the test results are to be applied only to interior ceiling finish, then the test specimen is mounted to cover the ceiling only.

## 10.2.4* Specific Materials.

**A.10.2.4** Surface nonmetallic raceway products, as permitted by *NFPA 70, National Electrical Code*, are not interior finishes.

**10.2.4.1* Textile Wall and Textile Ceiling Materials.** The use of textile materials on walls or ceilings shall comply with one of the following conditions:

(1) Textile materials having a Class A rating *(see 10.2.3.4)* shall be permitted on the walls or ceilings of rooms or areas protected by an approved automatic sprinkler system.
(2) Textile materials having a Class A rating *(see 10.2.3.4)* shall be permitted on partitions that do not exceed three-quarters of the floor-to-ceiling height or do not exceed 8 ft (2440 mm) in height, whichever is less.
(3) Textile materials having a Class A rating *(see 10.2.3.4)* shall be permitted to extend not more than 48 in. (1220 mm) above the finished floor on ceiling-height walls and ceiling-height partitions.
(4) Previously approved existing installations of textile material having a Class A rating *(see 10.2.3.4)* shall be permitted to be continued to be used.
(5) Textile materials shall be permitted on walls and partitions where tested in accordance with NFPA 265, *Standard Methods of Fire Tests for Evaluating Room Fire Growth Contribution of Textile Coverings on Full Height Panels and Walls. (See 10.2.3.7.)*
(6) Textile materials shall be permitted on walls, partitions, and ceilings where tested in accordance with NFPA 286, *Standard Methods of Fire Tests for Evaluating Contribution of Wall and Ceiling Interior Finish to Room Fire Growth. (See 10.2.3.7.)*

Textile materials are permitted to be used as interior wall or ceiling finish only where such materials meet any one of the provisions of 10.2.4.1(1) through (6). The language in the *Code* prior to the 2006 edition did not clearly explain this.

Prior to the 1988 edition of the *Code*, the danger of carpetlike textile coverings used on walls and ceilings was recognized and regulated by a requirement that only Class A tufted or napped carpetlike materials be used, even in a sprinklered building. In 1981, eight people died at the nonsprinklered Las Vegas Hilton Hotel when a fire began in an elevator lobby and was fueled by carpetlike textile wall and ceiling finishes that did not meet the qualifications for Class A interior finish.[21] Other than the textile wall and ceiling finish materials, sheer sunscreen material at the window, and a cushioned seat pad on a metal bench, there was little combustible material to fuel the fire in the elevator lobby. See Exhibit 10.4. Yet, the elevator lobby went to flashover, the fire broke out the windows and extended to a nearly identical elevator lobby on the floor above, and the events repeated themselves in a leapfrog fashion, burning out the elevator lobbies from the eighth floor through the twenty-fourth floor. See Exhibit 10.5.

Research sponsored by the American Textile Manufacturers Institute (ATMI) and conducted by the Fire Research Laboratory of the University of California at Berkeley between March 1985 and January 1986 was described in the report "Room Fire Experiments of Textile Wall Coverings."[22] This research demonstrated that consideration of only the flame spread rating, as measured by ASTM E 84 or ANSI/UL 723, might not reliably predict the fire behavior of textile wall and ceiling coverings. Test results indicate that not all Class A textile wall coverings are alike with respect to their potential for producing room flashover; some are capable of producing room flashover when subjected to an ignition source scenario that models a small fuel item (such as a wastebasket) igniting a chair or similar furnishing, while others are not. Simply requiring textile wall coverings to be classified as Class A interior wall and ceiling finishes does not ensure the level of life safety intended by the *Code*.

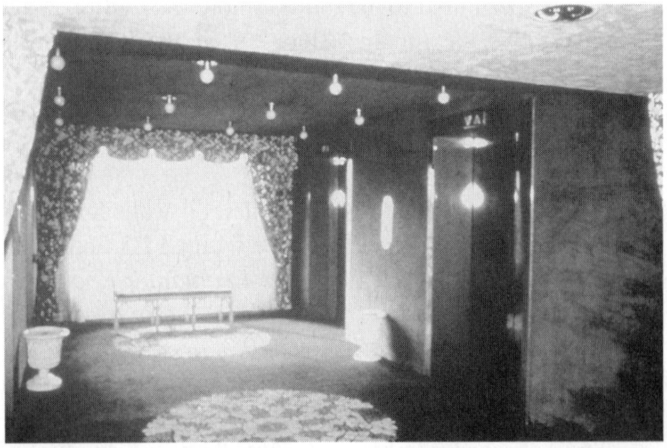

**Exhibit 10.4** *Elevator lobby with carpetlike textile wall and ceiling finish material.*

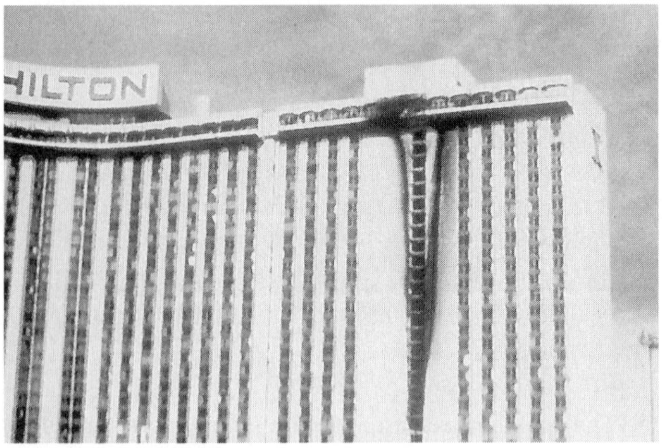


**Exhibit 10.5** *Resulting fire spread involving elevator lobbies on eighth through twenty-fourth floors.*

The testing at the University of California was conducted in an 8 ft × 12 ft × 8 ft (2440 mm × 3660 mm × 2440 mm) high room using a gas diffusion burner as an ignition source. Products undergoing evaluation — various textile wall coverings — were applied to the walls; the gas diffusion burner and ignition source were placed in the corner of the room. Two of the 16 products tested — one a tufted wall covering, the other a woven wall covering — were known to have flame spread ratings of 25 or less when tested in accordance with ASTM E 84 or ANSI/UL 723. When tested using the room-corner procedure, these two products readily spread flame and caused the fire in the test room to grow quickly to a large size, causing full room involvement — that is, flashover. Concerns about the performance of these low flame spread textile wall coverings led to the requirement of 10.2.4.1(5) for full-scale room-corner testing to qualify products for use in nonsprinklered buildings.

The tests revealed that the method of mounting, including adhesive and application rate, can be critically important to product fire performance. Changing the application rate of the same adhesive or changing the adhesive can cause a product that is assumed to be safe to exhibit unsatisfactory performance.

Caution should be exercised when using combinations of textile wall and ceiling coverings. Experience has shown that combinations of textile wall and ceiling coverings might result in intense burning. The University of California testing included only wall coverings; research conducted at the Illinois Institute of Technology Research Institute indicates that flame spread is more likely to occur with combinations of combustible wall and ceiling coverings than in those situations involving only combustible wall coverings or only combustible ceiling coverings.[23] Therefore, full-scale room-corner testing, using an appropriately sized ignition source, is necessary to substantiate the performance of textile wall and ceiling coverings.

With the publication of NFPA 265, *Standard Methods of Fire Tests for Evaluating Room Fire Growth Contribution of Textile Coverings on Full Height Panels and Walls*, a nationally recognized room-corner fire test to be used specifically for textile wall coverings became available. Its use is addressed in 10.2.3.7, 10.2.3.7.1, and 10.2.4.1(5).

Paragraph 10.2.4.1(6) expands the options for specialized fire tests representative of an actual installation by recognizing the use of NFPA 286, *Standard Methods of Fire Tests for Evaluating Contribution of Wall and Ceiling Interior Finish to Room Fire Growth.* See the commentary that follows 10.2.3.7.2(4).

Paragraphs 10.2.4.1(1) through (4) address other conditions under which textile wall coverings are permitted to be used.

**A.10.2.4.1** Previous editions of the *Code* have regulated textile materials on walls and ceilings using ASTM E 84, *Standard Test Method for Surface Burning Characteristics of Building Materials*, or ANSI/UL 723, *Standard for Test for Surface Burning Characteristics of Building Materials.* Full-scale room/corner fire test research has shown that flame spread indices produced by ASTM E 84 or ANSI/UL 723 might not reliably predict all aspects of the fire behavior of textile wall and ceiling coverings.

NFPA 265, *Standard Methods of Fire Tests for Evaluating Room Fire Growth Contribution of Textile Coverings on Full Height Panels and Walls*, and NFPA 286, *Standard Methods of Fire Tests for Evaluating Contribution of Wall and Ceiling Interior Finish to Room Fire Growth*, both known as room/corner tests, were developed for assessing the fire and smoke obscuration performance of textile wall coverings and interior wall and ceiling finish materials, respectively. As long as an interior wall or ceiling finish material is tested by NFPA 265 or NFPA 286, as appropriate, using a mounting system, substrate, and adhesive (if appropriate) that are representative of actual use, the room/corner test provides an adequate evaluation of a product's flammability and smoke obscuration behavior. Manufacturers, installers, and specifiers should be encouraged to use NFPA 265 or NFPA 286, as appropriate — but not both — because each of these standard fire tests has the ability to characterize actual product behavior, as opposed to data generated by tests using ASTM E 84 or ANSI/UL 723, which only allow comparisons of one product's performance with another. If a manufacturer or installer chooses to test a wall finish in accordance with NFPA 286, additional testing in accordance with ASTM E 84 or ANSI/UL 723 is not necessary.

The test results from ASTM E 84 or ANSI/UL 723 are suitable for classification purposes but should not be used as input into fire models, because they are not generated in units suitable for engineering calculations. Actual test results for heat, smoke, and combustion product release from NFPA 265, and from NFPA 286, are suitable for use as input into fire models for performance-based design.

**10.2.4.2* Expanded Vinyl Wall and Expanded Vinyl Ceiling Materials.** The use of expanded vinyl wall or expanded vinyl ceiling materials shall comply with one of the following conditions:

(1) Materials having a Class A rating *(see 10.2.3.4)* shall be permitted on the walls or ceilings of rooms or areas protected by an approved automatic sprinkler system.
(2) Materials having a Class A rating *(see 10.2.3.4)* shall be permitted on partitions that do not exceed three-quarters of the floor-to-ceiling height or do not exceed 8 ft (2440 mm) in height, whichever is less.
(3) Materials having a Class A rating *(see 10.2.3.4)* shall be permitted to extend not more than 48 in. (1220 mm) above the finished floor on ceiling-height walls and ceiling-height partitions.
(4) Existing installations of materials with the appropriate wall finish classification for the occupancy involved, and with classification in accordance with the provisions in 10.2.3.4, shall be permitted to be continued to be used.
(5) Materials shall be permitted on walls and partitions where tested in accordance with NFPA 265, *Standard Methods of Fire Tests for Evaluating Room Fire Growth Contribution of Textile Coverings on Full Height Panels and Walls. (See 10.2.3.7.)*
(6) Textile materials shall be permitted on walls, partitions, and ceilings where tested in accordance with NFPA 286, *Standard Methods of Fire Tests for Evaluating Contribution of Wall and Ceiling Interior Finish to Room Fire Growth. (See 10.2.3.7.)*

**A.10.2.4.2** Expanded vinyl wall covering consists of a woven textile backing, an expanded vinyl base coat layer, and a nonexpanded vinyl skin coat. The expanded base coat layer is a homogeneous vinyl layer that contains a blowing agent. During processing, the blowing agent decomposes, which causes this layer to expand by forming closed cells. The total thickness of the wall covering is approximately 0.055 in. to 0.070 in. (1.4 mm to 1.8 mm).

The provisions of 10.2.4.2, which address expanded vinyl wall coverings and expanded vinyl ceiling coverings (described in A.10.2.4.2), are similar to those of 10.2.4.1, which are applicable to textile wall coverings.

**10.2.4.3 Cellular or Foamed Plastic.** Cellular or foamed plastic materials shall not be used as interior wall and ceiling finish unless specifically permitted by 10.2.4.3.1 or 10.2.4.3.2. The requirements of 10.2.4.3 through 10.2.4.3.2 shall apply both to exposed foamed plastics and to foamed plastics used in conjunction with a textile or vinyl facing or cover.

**10.2.4.3.1*** Cellular or foamed plastic materials shall be permitted where subjected to large-scale fire tests that substantiate their combustibility and smoke release characteristics for the use intended under actual fire conditions. The tests shall be performed on a finished foamed plastic assembly related to the actual end-use configuration, including any cover or facing, and at the maximum thickness intended for use. Suitable large-scale fire tests shall include those shown in 10.2.4.3.1.1.

**A.10.2.4.3.1** Both NFPA 286, *Standard Methods of Fire Tests for Evaluating Contribution of Wall and Ceiling Interior Finish to Room Fire Growth*, and ANSI/UL 1715, *Standard for Fire Test of Interior Finish Material*, contain smoke obscuration criteria. ANSI/UL 1040, *Standard for Fire Test of Insulated Wall Construction*, and FM 4880, *Approval Standard for Class I Insulated Wall or Wall and Roof/Ceiling Panels; Plastic Interior Finish Materials; Plastic Exterior Building Panels; Wall/Ceiling Coating Systems; Interior or Exterior Finish Systems*, do not include smoke obscuration criteria. Smoke obscuration is an important component of the fire performance of cellular or foamed plastic materials.

**10.2.4.3.1.1** The following are suitable fire tests for assessing the combustibility of cellular or foamed plastic materials as interior finish:

(1) NFPA 286, *Standard Methods of Fire Tests for Evaluating Contribution of Wall and Ceiling Interior Finish to Room Fire Growth*, with the acceptance criteria of 10.2.3.7.2
(2) ANSI/UL 1715, *Standard for Fire Test of Interior Finish Material*
(3) ANSI/UL 1040, *Standard for Fire Test of Insulated Wall Construction*
(4) FM 4880, *Approval Standard for Class 1 Insulated Wall or Wall and Roof/Ceiling Panels; Plastic Interior Finish Materials; Plastic Exterior Building Panels; Wall/Ceiling Coating Systems; Interior or Exterior Finish Systems*

**10.2.4.3.1.2** New installations of cellular or foamed plastic materials tested in accordance with ANSI/UL 1040, *Standard for Fire Test of Insulated Wall Construction*, or FM 4880, *Approval Standard for Class 1 Insulated Wall or Wall and Roof/Ceiling Panels; Plastic Interior Finish Materials; Plastic Exterior Building Panels; Wall/Ceiling Coating Systems; Interior or Exterior Finish Systems*, shall also be tested for smoke release. Suitable smoke release tests include the following:

(1) Additional measurements of smoke release into the duct that demonstrate that the total smoke released throughout the test does not exceed 1000 $m^2$
(2) NFPA 286, *Standard Methods of Fire Tests for Evaluating Contribution of Wall and Ceiling Interior Finish to Room Fire Growth*, with the acceptance criterion of 10.2.3.7.2(4)
(3) ASTM E 84, *Standard Test Method for Surface Burning Characteristics of Building Materials*; or ANSI/UL 723, *Standard for Test for Surface Burning Characteristics for Building Materials*; with a smoke developed index not exceeding 450

**10.2.4.3.2** Cellular or foamed plastic shall be permitted for trim not in excess of 10 percent of the wall or ceiling area, provided that it is not less than 20 lb/ft$^3$ (320 kg/m$^3$) in density, is limited to $\frac{1}{2}$ in. (13 mm) in thickness and 4 in. (100 mm) in width, and complies with the requirements for Class A or Class B interior wall and ceiling finish as described in 10.2.3.4; however, the smoke developed index shall not be limited.

The prohibition of 10.2.4.3 on the use of foamed plastics within buildings is based on actual fire experience in which foamed plastics have contributed to very rapid fire development.[24] It also acknowledges that tunnel testing per ASTM E 84 or ANSI/UL 723 (see 10.2.3.4) might not accurately assess the potential hazard of plastics in general. Therefore, if cellular or foamed plastics are to be used within a building, their use needs to be substantiated on the basis of large-scale fire tests that simulate conditions of actual use. Four such tests are offered in 10.2.4.3.1.1(1) through (4). In addition, smoke release criteria new to the 2009 edition of the *Code* are specified in 10.2.4.3.1.2.

Note that the provisions of 10.2.4.3 through 10.2.4.3.2 apply not only to exposed foamed plastics but also to foamed plastics used as backings for textile or vinyl facings or cover materials. An assembly comprised of foamed plastic backings in conjunction with a textile or vinyl facing or cover is expected to behave differently under fire tests than if just the textile or vinyl facing were tested alone.

Paragraph 10.2.4.3.2 permits the limited use of cellular or foamed plastics as a substitute for traditional wood trim, assuming their performance under fire exposure will be comparable to that of wood. To control the mass of the material that can be used, limits have been established on width and thickness. The intent in establishing a minimum density of 20 $lb/ft^3$ (320 $kg/m^3$) is to prohibit the use of lightweight [1 $lb/ft^3$ to 3 $lb/ft^3$ (16 $kg/m^3$ to 48 $kg/m^3$)], readily available, foamed plastics as trim.

Limiting plastic trim to Class A or Class B materials, in combination with the 10 percent area limit for walls and ceilings, imposes a greater restriction than that which applies to wood. This limitation ensures that the performance of the plastic trim will be equivalent or superior to that of more traditional materials.

In establishing the 10 percent limit, it is intended that the trim will be used around doors and windows or at the junction of walls and ceilings. Therefore, the trim will be somewhat uniformly distributed throughout the room. There would be a significant difference in the probable performance of wall and ceiling finish if the 10 percent limit were concentrated in one area.

**10.2.4.4* Light-Transmitting Plastics.** Light-transmitting plastics shall be permitted to be used as interior wall and ceiling finish if approved by the authority having jurisdiction.

**A.10.2.4.4** Light-transmitting plastics are used for a variety of purposes, including light diffusers, exterior wall panels, skylights, canopies, glazing, and the like. Previous editions of the *Code* have not addressed the use of light-transmitting plastics. Light-transmitting plastics will not normally be used in applications representative of interior finishes. Accordingly, ASTM E 84, *Standard Test Method for Surface Burning Characteristics of Building Materials*, or ANSI/UL 723, *Standard for Test for Surface Burning Characteristics of Building Materials,* can produce test results that might or might not apply.

Light-transmitting plastics are regulated by model building codes such as *NFPA 5000, Building Construction and Safety Code*. Model building codes provide adequate regulation for most applications of light-transmitting plastics. Where an authority having jurisdiction determines that a use is contemplated that differs from uses regulated by model building codes, light-transmitting plastics in such applications can be substantiated by fire tests that demonstrate the combustibility characteristics of the light-transmitting plastics for the use intended under actual fire conditions.

Building code provisions typically regulate light-transmitting plastics. Paragraph 10.2.4.4 gives the authority having jurisdiction the ability to regulate light-transmitting plastics; A.10.2.4.4 offers guidance for such regulation. See Chapter 48, Plastics, of *NFPA 5000, Building Construction and Safety Code,* for additional guidance.

**10.2.4.5 Decorations and Furnishings.** Decorations and furnishings that do not meet the definition of interior finish, as defined in 3.3.84.2, shall be regulated by the provisions of Section 10.3.

**10.2.4.6 Metal Ceiling and Wall Panels.** Listed factory finished Class A metal ceiling and wall panels shall be permitted to be finished with one additional application of paint. Such painted panels shall be permitted for use in areas where Class A interior finishes are required. The total paint thickness shall not exceed $\frac{1}{28}$ in. (0.9 mm).

Metal-based ceiling and wall panels are used extensively in custom-designed acoustical ceiling and wall systems. Often the customer desires a special custom color to meet aesthetic requirements. Although the manufacturer can certify the performance of the factory finish, it is not possible to test and certify all the custom colors that are requested. These finishes are applied post-production, using a process where thickness of paint application is controlled. The $\frac{1}{28}$ in. (0.9 mm) thickness criterion used in 10.2.4.6 is taken from 10.2.1.2 as a safe thickness for which the exemption does not sacrifice safety.

### 10.2.5 Trim and Incidental Finish.

**10.2.5.1 General.** Interior wall and ceiling trim and incidental finish, other than wall base in accordance with 10.2.5.2 and bulletin boards, posters, and paper in accordance with 10.2.5.3, not in excess of 10 percent of the aggregate wall and ceiling areas of any room or space shall be permitted to be Class C materials in occupancies where interior wall and ceiling finish of Class A or Class B is required.

**10.2.5.2 Wall Base.** Interior floor trim material used at the junction of the wall and the floor to provide a functional or decorative border, and not exceeding 6 in. (150 mm) in height, shall meet the requirements for interior wall finish for its location or the requirements for Class II interior floor finish as described in 10.2.7.4 using the test described in 10.2.7.3. If a Class I floor finish is required, the interior floor trim shall be Class I.

**10.2.5.3 Bulletin Boards, Posters, and Paper.**

**10.2.5.3.1** Bulletin boards, posters, and paper attached directly to the wall shall not exceed 20 percent of the aggregate wall area to which they are applied.

**10.2.5.3.2** The provision of 10.2.5.3.1 shall not apply to artwork and teaching materials in sprinklered educational or day-care occupancies in accordance with 14.7.4.3(2), 15.7.4.3(2), 16.7.4.3(2), or 17.7.4.3(2).

Subsection 10.2.5 is intended to permit the use of wood trim around doors and windows as a decoration or as functional molding (such as for chair rails). Wood trim must meet the criteria for Class C materials. See 10.2.4.3.2 for restrictions applicable to plastic trim. Where such trim is used in rooms or spaces requiring the use of Class A or Class B materials, the trim is permitted to constitute not more than 10 percent of the aggregate wall or ceiling area to ensure that the trim will be more or less uniformly distributed throughout the room or space. If the trim is concentrated in a single, sizable, continuous pattern (e.g., on one wall of a room), the materials could contribute to rapid fire growth.

The provisions of 10.2.5.2 for wall base and 10.2.5.3 for bulletin boards, posters, and paper were new for the 2006 edition of the *Code*. The wall base provisions of 10.2.5.2 regulate the common practice of running flooring up onto the lowest portion of a wall where it meets the floor. The 6 in. (150 mm) maximum height criterion recognizes the limitations of judging an interior wall finish material based on a test method developed to evaluate flame spread for interior floor finish materials exposed to a flaming radiant heat source. Note that, even where the interior floor finish of a room or space is not required to be Class I or Class II in accordance with 10.2.7.4, the flooring material wrapped up onto the wall is required to be tested and classified per 10.2.7.3 and 10.2.7.4.

The educational and day-care occupancy chapters have regulated artwork and teaching materials that are attached directly to walls for many editions of the *Code* — see 14.7.4.3, 15.7.4.3, 16.7.4.3, and 17.7.4.3. The provisions of 10.2.5.3 codify the subject for all occupancies. Bulletin boards, posters, and paper attached directly to a wall serve as de facto interior finish materials with the potential for spreading flame. The 20 percent maximum aggregate wall area criterion of 10.2.5.3.1 helps ensure that there are not sufficient expanses of such materials, for which classification per 10.2.3.4 is unfeasible and unenforceable, that could spread flame more quickly than would occur with wall finish materials complying with applicable interior finish requirements based on testing per ASTM E 84 or ANSI/UL 723.

## 10.2.6* Fire-Retardant Coatings.

**A.10.2.6** Fire-retardant coatings need to be applied to surfaces properly prepared for the material, and application needs to be consistent with the product listing. Deterioration of coatings applied to interior finishes can occur due to repeated cleaning of the surface or painting over applied coatings.

**10.2.6.1*** The required flame spread or smoke development classification of existing surfaces of walls, partitions, columns, and ceilings shall be permitted to be secured by applying approved fire-retardant coatings to surfaces having higher flame spread ratings than permitted. Such treatments shall be tested, or shall be listed and labeled for application to the material to which they are applied, and shall comply with the requirements of NFPA 703, *Standard for Fire Retardant–Treated Wood and Fire-Retardant Coatings for Building Materials*.

**A.10.2.6.1** It is the intent of the *Code* to mandate interior wall and ceiling finish materials that obtain their fire performance and smoke developed characteristics in their original form. However, in renovations, particularly those involving historic buildings, and in changes of occupancy, the required fire performance or smoke developed characteristics of existing surfaces of walls, partitions, columns, and ceilings might have to be secured by applying approved fire-retardant coatings to surfaces having higher flame spread ratings than permitted. Such treatments should comply with the requirements of NFPA 703, *Standard for Fire Retardant–Treated Wood and Fire-Retardant Coatings for Building Materials*. When fire-retardant coatings are used, they need to be applied to surfaces properly prepared for the material, and application needs to be consistent with the product listing. Deterioration of coatings applied to interior finishes can occur due to repeated cleaning of the surface or painting over applied coatings, but permanency must be assured in some appropriate fashion. Fire-retardant coatings must possess the desired degree of permanency and be maintained so as to retain the effectiveness of the treatment under the service conditions encountered in actual use.

**10.2.6.2** Fire-retardant coatings shall possess the desired degree of permanency and shall be maintained so as to retain the effectiveness of the treatment under the service conditions encountered in actual use.

Fire-retardant paints, coatings, and penetrants are sometimes used to improve the flame spread ratings of materials or assemblies used as interior finishes within buildings. Fire-retardant treatments are permitted to be used to satisfy the flame spread requirements only for existing interior finish materials within existing buildings.

Fire retardants are generally surface treatments that — through intumescence or other chemical reaction — will delay the ignition and slow the flame spread of a material. The nature of the material to which the treatment has been applied is not changed. Fire exposures of sufficient duration or intensity can ultimately cause a treated material to burn. Therefore, as a rule, materials with favorable intrinsic performance characteristics are preferred over those that achieve a satisfactory level of performance through the use of externally applied treatments. However, external treatments, where properly applied and maintained, can be effective in achieving reasonable fire performance.

Note that 10.2.6.1 permits fire-retardant coatings to be either tested or listed, as the product might have been tested with adequate results but not yet listed when being considered for application. Additionally, such products must comply with NFPA 703, *Standard for Fire Retardant–Treated Wood and Fire-Retardant Coatings for Building Materials,*[25] which contains criteria related to testing.

Fire-retardant paints, coatings, and penetrants must be applied in strict accordance with the manufacturer's instructions. Most fire-retardant coatings require an application rate that is three-to-four times greater than that of ordinary paints. Application is usually done by brush, spray, immersion, or pressure treatment. The treatment should be reapplied or renewed at regular intervals. Treatments that might be removed by regular maintenance, washing, or cleaning procedures will require periodic examination and reapplication to maintain the required level of performance.

The use of fire retardants can improve the performance of some materials from Class C to Class B; similarly, Class B materials can, in some cases, be upgraded to Class A. Likewise, materials having flame spread ratings in excess of 200 can sometimes be upgraded to Class C.

In approving fire-retardant treatments, the authority having jurisdiction should take into consideration that, in reducing flame spread, some fire-retardant treatments increase a material's capacity for smoke generation.

### 10.2.7 Interior Floor Finish Testing and Classification.

**10.2.7.1** Carpet and carpetlike interior floor finishes shall comply with ASTM D 2859, *Standard Test Method for Ignition Characteristics of Finished Textile Floor Covering Materials.*

**10.2.7.2*** Floor coverings, other than carpet for which 10.2.2.2 establishes requirements for fire performance, shall have a minimum critical radiant flux of 0.1 W/cm$^2$.

**A.10.2.7.2** The fire performance of some floor finishes has been tested, and traditional finish floors and floor coverings, such as wood flooring and resilient floor coverings, have not proved to present an unusual hazard.

**10.2.7.3*** Interior floor finishes shall be classified in accordance with 10.2.7.4, based on test results from NFPA 253, *Standard Method of Test for Critical Radiant Flux of Floor Covering Systems Using a Radiant Heat Energy Source*, or ASTM E 648, *Standard Test Method for Critical Radiant Flux of Floor Covering Systems Using a Radiant Heat Energy Source.*

**A.10.2.7.3** The flooring radiant panel provides a measure of a floor covering's tendency to spread flames where located in a corridor and exposed to the flame and hot gases from a room fire. The flooring radiant panel test method is to be used as a basis for estimating the fire performance of a floor covering installed in the building corridor. Floor coverings in open building spaces and in rooms within buildings merit no further regulation, provided that it can be shown that the floor covering is at least as resistant to spread of flame as a material that meets the U.S. federal flammability standard 16 CFR 1630, *Standard for the Surface Flammability of Carpets and Rugs* (FF 1-70). All carpeting sold in the U.S. since 1971 is required to meet this standard and, therefore, is not likely to become involved in a fire until a room reaches or approaches flashover. Therefore, no further regulations are necessary for carpet other than carpet in exitways and corridors.

It has not been found necessary or practical to regulate interior floor finishes on the basis of smoke development.

Full-scale fire tests and fire experience have shown floor coverings in open building spaces merit no regulation beyond the United States federally mandated DOC FF 1-70 "pill test." This is because floor coverings meeting the FF 1-70 regulation will not spread flame significantly until a room fire approaches flashover. At flashover, the spread of flame across a floor covering will have minimal impact on the already existing hazard. The minimum critical radiant flux of a floor covering that will pass the FF 1-70 regulation has been determined to be approximately 0.04 W/cm$^2$ *(see Annex B, Tu, King-Mon and Davis, Sanford, "Flame Spread of Carpet Systems Involved in Room Fires")*. The flooring radiant panel is only able to determine critical radiant flux values to 0.1 W/cm$^2$. This provision will prevent use of a noncomplying material, which might create a problem, especially when the *Code* is used outside the United States, where federal regulation FF 1-70 is not mandated.

Experience and full-scale fire test data have shown that floor coverings of modest resistance to flame spread are unlikely to become involved in the early growth of a fire. The testing of flooring materials in accordance with 10.2.7.1 and 10.2.7.2 is relatively easy to accomplish. The testing helps to identify floor finish materials that have a modest resistance to flame spread.

Where floor coverings are regulated by the occupancy chapters, the evaluation is based on tests conducted in accordance with NFPA 253, *Standard Method of Test for Critical Radiant Flux of Floor Covering Systems Using a Radiant Heat Energy Source,*[26] also known as ASTM E 648, *Standard Test Method for Critical Radiant Flux of Floor Covering Systems Using a Radiant Heat Energy Source.*[27] The flooring radiant panel test was specifically developed to evaluate the tendency of a floor covering to propagate flame. See also Supplement 3, Fire Tests for *Life Safety Code* Users, of this handbook.

Fire tests conducted by the National Bureau of Standards (now the National Institute of Standards and Technology) demonstrate that carpet that passes the federal flammability standard 16 CFR 1630, "Standard for the Surface Flammability of Carpets and Rugs"[28] (also known as FF 1-70 or the pill test), is not likely to become involved in a fire until a room reaches or approaches flashover.[29] Since all carpet manufactured for sale in the United States has been required since April 1971 to meet the pill test, no further regulation is necessary for carpet located within rooms.

On the other hand, it has been shown that floor coverings might propagate flame under the influence of a sizable exposure fire. For example, it has been shown that carpet located in a corridor might spread flame when subjected to the energy emanating from the doorway of a room fully developed in fire. The fire discharges flame and hot gases into the corridor, causing a radiant heat energy exposure to the floor. It has been shown that the level of energy radiating onto the floor is a significant factor in determining whether progressive flaming will occur. NFPA 253 and ASTM E 648 measure the minimum energy required on the floor covering to sustain flame, measured in W/cm². This minimum value is the *critical radiant flux*. The flooring radiant panel test, therefore, measures a floor covering's tendency to spread flames where located in a corridor and exposed to flame and hot gases from a room fire.

Interior floor finishes must be tested as proposed for use. For example, if a carpet is to be used with a separate underlayment, the carpet must be tested as such. The flooring radiant panel test specifies that a carpet is permitted to be tested using either the standard underlayment specified in NFPA 253, ASTM E 648, or the actual underlayment proposed for use. Data generated using the standard underlayment is intended to permit the tested carpet to be used over any other underlayment. Where assembly tests are conducted with other than the standard underlayment, the results of such tests are valid only for the specific combination tested.

Floor coverings are not regulated on the basis of smoke generation. Smoke development limits are not believed to be practical or necessary, because floor coverings generally will not contribute to a fire until the fire has grown to large proportions. The minimal benefits achieved by imposing smoke development limits do not usually warrant such regulation. In addition, it is not considered practical to regulate on the basis of smoke development, because no regulatory test method that exists has been shown to be capable of producing data that correlates with the performance of products in actual fires.

**10.2.7.4** Interior floor finishes shall be classified as follows in accordance with the critical radiant flux ratings:

(1) Class I interior floor finish shall be characterized by a critical radiant flux not less than 0.45 W/cm², as determined by the test described in 10.2.7.3.
(2) Class II interior floor finish shall be characterized by a critical radiant flux not less than 0.22 W/cm² but less than 0.45 W/cm², as determined by the test described in 10.2.7.3.

The greater its critical radiant flux value, the greater the resistance of a floor finish to flame propagation. Thus, a Class I interior floor finish with a critical radiant flux of 0.45 W/cm² or greater should perform better under fire conditions than a Class II interior floor finish material with its lesser critical radiant flux value range of 0.22 W/cm² to less than 0.45 W/cm². Contrast this classification with that of interior wall and ceiling interior finish materials in 10.2.3.4, in which higher flame spread ratings generally denote poorer performance under fire conditions.

**10.2.7.5** Wherever the use of Class II interior floor finish is required, Class I interior floor finish shall be permitted.

### 10.2.8 Automatic Sprinklers.

**10.2.8.1** Unless specifically prohibited elsewhere in this *Code*, where an approved automatic sprinkler system is in accordance with Section 9.7, Class C interior wall and ceiling finish materials shall be permitted in any location where Class B is required, and Class B interior wall and ceiling finish materials shall be permitted in any location where Class A is required.

**10.2.8.2** Unless specifically prohibited elsewhere in this *Code*, where an approved automatic sprinkler system is in accordance with Section 9.7, Class II interior floor finish shall be permitted in any location where Class I interior floor finish is required, and where Class II is required, no critical radiant flux rating shall be required.

Fire testing and actual fire experience have shown that automatic sprinklers prevent flame spread across the surface of a wall, ceiling, or floor covering so as to prevent flashover [see commentary following 10.1.3(2)]. Flame spread limits (applicable to interior wall and ceiling finishes) and critical radiant flux limits (applicable to interior floor finishes) are more lenient in areas protected by an automatic sprinkler system. However, there is a value beyond which the potential for flame spread becomes unacceptably high. For example, in occupancies with the most lenient interior finish requirements, which include fully sprinklered buildings, interior wall and ceiling finishes must meet the criteria for Class C materials.

Note that the provisions of 10.2.8.1 and 10.2.8.2 are formatted so as to apply, unless specifically prohibited elsewhere in the *Code*. For examples of an occupancy chapter prohibiting the interior finish requirements from being further relaxed based on sprinkler protection, see 22.3.3.2 and 22.3.3.3.2, applicable to new detention and correctional occupancies. All new detention and correctional occupancies are required to be sprinklered (see 22.3.5.2). The interior finish limitations established in 22.3.3.2 and 22.3.3.3.2 are based on the presence of sprinklers. The prohibition on use of 10.2.8.1 and 10.2.8.2 keeps the user from taking a second, unjustified credit for the sprinklers.

## 10.3 Contents and Furnishings

Section 10.3 provides a detailed menu of provisions that apply to contents and furnishings (e.g., draperies, upholstered furniture, and mattresses) that can be adopted singly, in various combinations, or in their entirety in accordance with an occupancy's individual operating features requirements. These requirements typically appear in Section ___.7 of an occupancy chapter. For example, the provisions for detention and correctional occupancies (22.7.4 and 23.7.4) make extensive, mandatory use of all provisions outlined in the Section 10.3 menu. Provisions for residential board and care occupancies (32.7.5, 33.7.5, A.32.7.5, and A.33.7.5) make mandatory and advisory use of various menu items contained in Section 10.3.

**10.3.1*** Where required by the applicable provisions of this *Code*, draperies, curtains, and other similar loosely hanging furnishings and decorations shall meet the flame propagation performance criteria contained in NFPA 701, *Standard Methods of Fire Tests for Flame Propagation of Textiles and Films*.

**A.10.3.1** Testing per NFPA 701, *Standard Methods of Fire Tests for Flame Propagation of Textiles and Films*, applies to textiles and films used in a hanging configuration. If the textiles are to be applied to surfaces of buildings or backing materials as interior finishes for use in buildings, they should be treated as interior wall and ceiling finishes in accordance with Section 10.2 of this *Code*, and they should then be tested for flame spread index and smoke developed index values in accordance with ASTM E 84, *Standard Test Method for Surface Burning Characteristics of Building Materials*, or ANSI/UL 723, *Standard for Test for Surface Burning Characteristics of Building Materials*, or for flame spread and flashover in accordance with NFPA 265, *Standard Methods of Fire Tests for Evaluating Room Fire Growth Contribution of Textile Coverings on Full Height Panels and Walls*. Films and other materials used as interior finish applied to surfaces of buildings should be tested for flame spread index and smoke developed index values in accordance with ASTM E 84 or ANSI/UL 723 or for heat and smoke release and flashover in accordance with NFPA 286, *Standard Methods of Fire Tests for Evaluating Contribution of Wall and Ceiling Interior Finish to Room Fire Growth*.

The test results from NFPA 701 are suitable for classification purposes but should not be used as input into fire models, because they are not generated in units suitable for engineering calculations.

The testing requirements of NFPA 701, *Standard Methods of Fire Tests for Flame Propagation of Textiles and Films*, measure the level of hazard posed by draperies and other loosely hanging fabrics and films. NFPA 701 describes procedures for an intermediate-scale test (referred to as Test Method 1) and a large-scale test (referred to as Test Method 2). The applicable test method is determined, in part, by the weight of the material per unit area (i.e., areal density). Both tests involve applying a flame to a vertically positioned sample for a specified time. Upon removal of the flame-producing burner, the sample must self-extinguish and must not have charred beyond a specified distance in order to pass the test. Additionally, with the intermediate-scale test, a specified maximum percent weight loss cannot be exceeded.

Exhibit 10.6 illustrates a representative setup for a folded test sample for the large-scale (Test Method 2) test from NFPA 701. The hanging textile sample is approximately 47 in. (1200 mm) long. See also Supplement 3, Fire Tests for *Life Safety Code* Users, of this handbook.

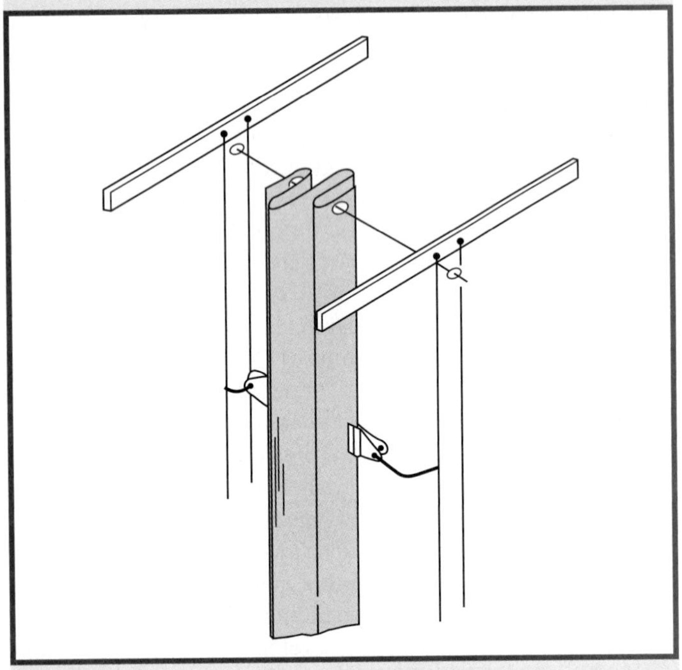

***Exhibit 10.6*** *NFPA 701 test sample in folds.*

## 10.3.2 Smoldering Ignition of Upholstered Furniture and Mattresses.

**10.3.2.1* Upholstered Furniture.** Newly introduced upholstered furniture, except as otherwise permitted by Chapters 11 through 43, shall be resistant to a cigarette ignition (i.e., smoldering) in accordance with one of the following:

(1) The components of the upholstered furniture shall meet the requirements for Class I when tested in accordance with NFPA 260, *Standard Methods of Tests and Classification System for Cigarette Ignition Resistance of Components of Upholstered Furniture*, or with ASTM E 1353, *Standard Test Methods for Cigarette Ignition Resistance of Components of Upholstered Furniture*.

(2) Mocked-up composites of the upholstered furniture shall have a char length not exceeding $1\frac{1}{2}$ in. (38 mm) when tested in accordance with NFPA 261, *Standard Method of Test for Determining Resistance of Mock-Up Upholstered Furniture Material Assemblies to Ignition by Smoldering Cigarettes*, or with ASTM E 1352 *Standard Test Method for Cigarette Ignition Resistance of Mock-Up Upholstered Furniture Assemblies*.

**A.10.3.2.1** The Class I requirement associated with testing in accordance with NFPA 260, *Standard Methods of Tests and Classification System for Cigarette Ignition Resistance of Components of Upholstered Furniture*, or with ASTM E 1353, *Standard Test Methods for Cigarette Ignition Resistance of Components of Upholstered Furniture*, and the char length of not more than $1\frac{1}{2}$ in. (38 mm) required with testing in accordance with NFPA 261, *Standard Method of Test for Determining Resistance of Mock-Up Upholstered Furniture Material Assemblies to Ignition by Smoldering Cigarettes*, or with ASTM E 1352, *Standard Test Method for Cigarette Ignition Resistance of Mock-Up Upholstered Furniture Assemblies*, are indicators that the furniture item or mattress is resistant to a cigarette ignition. A fire that smolders for an excessive period of time without flaming can reduce the tenability within the room or area of fire origin without developing the temperatures necessary to operate automatic sprinklers.

The test results from NFPA 260, or from ASTM E 1353, and from NFPA 261, or from ASTM E 1352, are suitable for classification purposes but should not be used as input into fire models, because they are not generated in units suitable for engineering calculations.

**10.3.2.2* Mattresses.** Newly introduced mattresses, except as otherwise permitted by Chapters 11 through 43, shall have a char length not exceeding 2 in. (51 mm) when tested in accordance with 16 CFR 1632, "Standard for the Flammability of Mattresses and Mattress Pads" (FF 4-72).

**A.10.3.2.2** The char length of not more than 2 in. (51 mm) required in 16 CFR 1632, *Standard for the Flammability of Mattresses and Mattress Pads* (FF 4-72), is an indicator that the mattress is resistant to a cigarette ignition. United States federal regulations require mattresses in this country to comply with 16 CFR 1632.

The provisions of 10.3.2 address ignition by cigarettes or other smoldering sources in an attempt to reduce the incidence of fires involving upholstered furniture and mattresses. Such ignition sources can smolder for considerable periods before producing flaming ignition.

Note that the formatting of 10.3.2.1 and 10.3.2.2 changed for the 2006 edition of the *Code* to require cigarette ignition testing of newly introduced upholstered furniture and newly introduced mattresses for all occupancies unless "otherwise permitted by Chapters 11 through 43." In earlier editions, the provisions were formatted to apply only where the occupancy chapter required such compliance. The cigarette ignition testing of upholstered furniture and mattresses is exempted for the following occupancies:

1. Day-care homes (16.7.4.4, 17.7.4.4)
2. Health care, if sprinklered (18.7.5.2, 18.7.5.4, 19.7.5.2, 19.7.5.4)
3. One- and two-family dwellings (24.3.3.4)
4. Lodging or rooming houses (26.7.1.1)
5. Apartment buildings (30.7.2.1, 31.7.2.1)
6. Residential board and care, with smoke alarm in sleeping room (32.7.5.2, 32.7.5.3, 33.7.5.2, 33.7.5.3)
7. Mercantile (36.7.5, 37.7.5)
8. Business (38.7.5, 39.7.5)
9. Industrial (Section 40.7)
10. Storage (Section 42.9)

The following fire test methods address the cigarette ignition resistance of upholstered furniture:

1. NFPA 260, *Standard Methods of Tests and Classification System for Cigarette Ignition Resistance of Components of Upholstered Furniture,*[30] and ASTM E 1353, *Standard Test Methods for Cigarette Ignition Resistance of Components of Upholstered Furniture*[31]
2. NFPA 261, *Standard Method of Test for Determining Resistance of Mock-Up Upholstered Furniture Material Assemblies to Ignition by Smoldering Cigarettes,*[32] and ASTM E 1352, *Standard Test Method for Cigarette Ignition Resistance of Mock-Up Upholstered Furniture Assemblies*[33]

One federal test method that is specified for judging the cigarette ignition resistance of mattresses is 16 CFR 1632, "Standard for the Flammability of Mattresses and Mattress Pads."[34] When purchasing upholstered furniture, consumers should check for flammability labeling. See Exhibit 10.7 and Exhibit 10.8 for a representative flammability hangtag found on upholstered furniture. The hangtag is produced by the Upholstered Furniture Action Council (UFAC), a voluntary furniture manufacturing industry association. The UFAC hangtag program, developed in 1982, was designed to help reduce the number of cigarette-ignited fires in upholstered furniture. Manufacturers that participate in the program — and use the UFAC hangtags — agree to meet the construction criteria outlined by the program (which essentially is testing for compliance with NFPA 260 or ASTM E 1353). The hangtag, which is applied by the manufacturer to the finished piece of furniture at the factory, indicates to the consumer that the furniture meets the specified ignition resistance criteria.

NFPA 260 and ASTM E 1353 test individual components of upholstered furniture, such as cover fabric, interior fabric, welt cord, filling/padding, decking materials, and barrier materials. Specimens of the component to be tested are assembled with specimens of standardized materials to create a miniature horizontal base panel and vertical panel tester, a mocked-up arrangement that simulates the junction and sur-

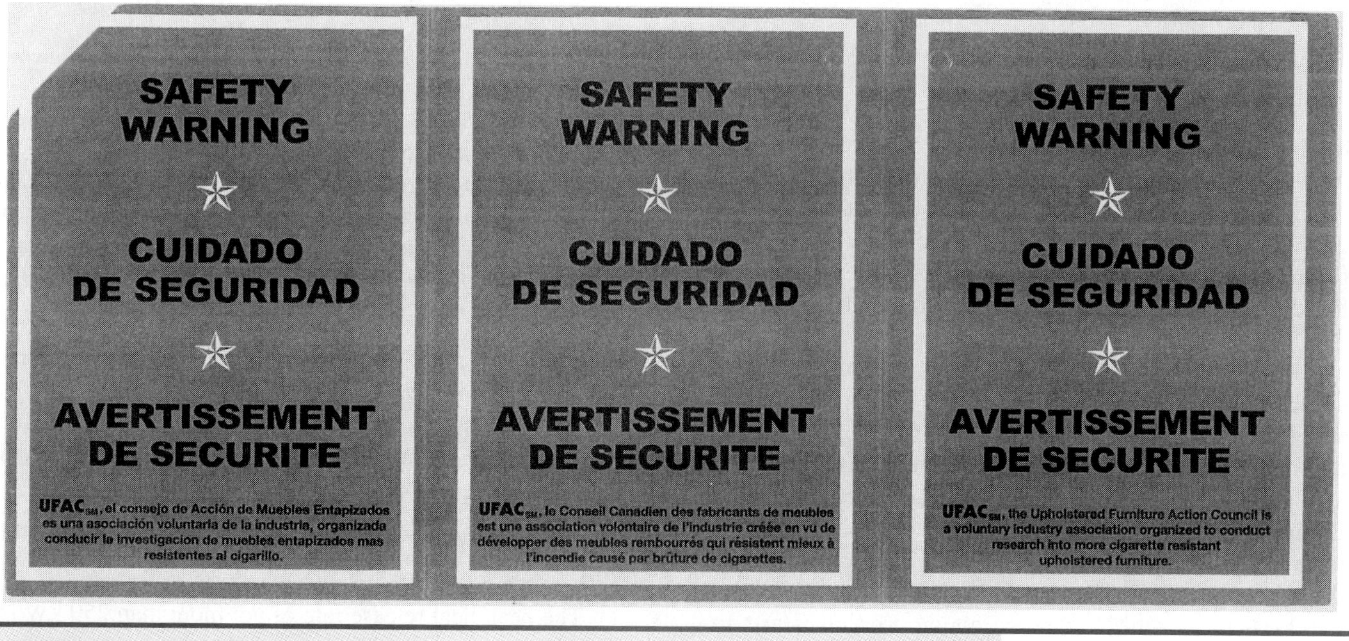


***Exhibit 10.7** Upholstered furniture flammability hangtag — front. (Courtesy of the Upholstered Furniture Action Council)*

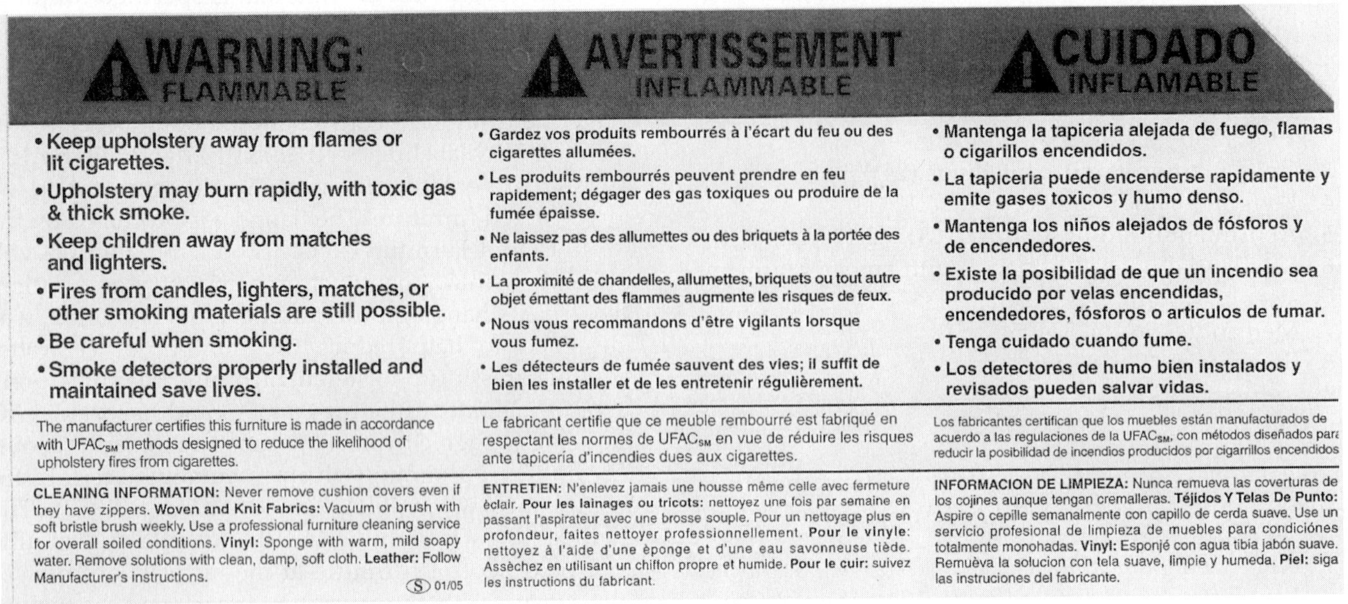


***Exhibit 10.8*** *Upholstered furniture flammability hangtag — back. (Courtesy of the Upholstered Furniture Action Council)*

rounding area of a seat cushion and back cushion in a piece of upholstered furniture. Standardizing all the components of the mocked-up tester, except the component being tested, allows the test to measure the ignition resistance of the test component. Components that meet the test criteria are designated as Class I materials. Components that do not meet the test criteria are designated as Class II materials. Upholstered furniture constructed from components that individually received a Class I designation is judged to be resistant to cigarette ignition without testing the actual combination of materials. Cigarette ignition–resistant upholstered furniture can also be constructed using Class II cover fabric materials over conventional polyurethane foam cushions if a Class I barrier material is used between the Class II fabric and the conventional foam cushion.

NFPA 261 and ASTM E 1352 test a mocked-up assembly consisting of all the actual components that will be used to construct the piece of upholstered furniture, rather than testing the components individually. The test procedure specifies that a char length is to be measured and reported. There are no pass/fail criteria within the document, so 10.3.2.1(2) specifies that the char length not exceed 1½ in. (38 mm) if the mocked-up assembly is to be considered resistant to cigarette ignition.

NFPA 260, ASTM E 1353, NFPA 261, and ASTM E 1352 address the cigarette ignition resistance of upholstered furniture; 16 CFR 1632 addresses the cigarette ignition resistance of mattresses. For this test method, 10.3.2.2 establishes that a char length not exceeding 2 in. (51 mm) qualifies the mattress as resistant to cigarette ignition.

See also Supplement 3, Fire Tests for *Life Safety Code* Users, of this handbook.

**10.3.3*** Where required by the applicable provisions of this *Code*, upholstered furniture, unless the furniture is located in a building protected throughout by an approved automatic sprinkler system, shall have limited rates of heat release when tested in accordance with ASTM E 1537, *Standard Test Method for Fire Testing of Upholstered Furniture*, as follows:

(1) The peak rate of heat release for the single upholstered furniture item shall not exceed 80 kW.
(2) The total energy released by the single upholstered furniture item during the first 10 minutes of the test shall not exceed 25 MJ.

**A.10.3.3** The intent of the provisions of 10.3.3 is as follows:

(1) The peak heat release rate of not more than 250 kW by a single upholstered furniture item was chosen based on maintaining a tenable environment within the room of fire origin, and the sprinkler exception was developed

because the sprinkler system helps to maintain tenable conditions, even if the single upholstered furniture item were to have a peak rate of heat release in excess of 250 kW.

(2) The total energy release of not more than 40 MJ by the single upholstered furniture item during the first 5 minutes of the test was established as an additional safeguard to protect against the adverse conditions that would be created by an upholstered furniture item that released its heat in other than the usual measured scenario, and the following should also be noted:
   (a) During the test for measurement of rate of heat release, the instantaneous heat release value usually peaks quickly and then quickly falls off, so as to create a triangle-shaped curve.
   (b) In the atypical case, if the heat release were to peak and remain steady at that elevated level, as opposed to quickly falling off, the 250 kW limit would not ensure safety.
   (c) Only a sprinkler exception is permitted in lieu of the test because of the ability of the sprinkler system to control the fire.

Actual test results for heat, smoke, and combustion product release from ASTM E 1537, *Standard Test Method for Fire Testing of Upholstered Furniture*, might be suitable for use as input into fire models for performance-based design.

The provisions of 10.3.2 address only one important property of upholstered furniture and mattresses — their resistance to cigarette ignition. The provisions of 10.3.3 and 10.3.4 supplement those provisions by addressing rates of heat release. Different combustible materials vary in their potential to produce heat. Some plastic materials, for example, have twice as much potential heat per weight of material as wood. However, if a material with twice the potential heat were to burn only half as fast as a material with lower potential, the two materials would liberate about the same amount of heat during any given period and create approximately equivalent hazards. If one material with a heat potential approximately equal to another material were to burn twice as fast as the other, it would liberate about twice as much heat during any given period and, thus, create a greater hazard than the slower burning material. Therefore, the property of a material or group of materials expressed by a rate of heat release is important in regulating the combustibility of upholstered furniture and mattresses for use in nonsprinklered areas.

It is noted that the values in A.10.3.3 differ from those in the actual *Code* requirement of 10.3.3. The *Code* values were revised for the 2009 edition to correspond with the values found in California Technical Bulletin 133[35]; the associated annex text was inadvertently overlooked. The values will be corrected for a future edition of the *Code*. Although the values in A.10.3.3 are incorrect, A.10.3.3 adequately describes the intent of the rates of heat release provisions, which is to prevent any single furniture item from causing room flashover. The material in A.10.3.3 also explains how automatic sprinklers, in certain cases, can serve in lieu of a low rate of heat release.

**10.3.4*** Where required by the applicable provisions of this *Code*, mattresses, unless the mattress is located in a building protected throughout by an approved automatic sprinkler system, shall have limited rates of heat release when tested in accordance with ASTM E 1590, *Standard Test Method for Fire Testing of Mattresses*, as follows:

(1) The peak rate of heat release for the mattress shall not exceed 100 kW.
(2) The total energy released by the mattress during the first 10 minutes of the test shall not exceed 25 MJ.

**A.10.3.4** The intent of the provisions of 10.3.4 is as follows:

(1) The peak heat release rate of not more than 250 kW by a single mattress was chosen based on maintaining a tenable environment within the room of fire origin, and the sprinkler exception was developed because the sprinkler system helps to maintain tenable conditions, even if the single mattress were to have a peak rate of heat release in excess of 250 kW.
(2) The total energy release of not more than 40 MJ by the single mattress during the first 5 minutes of the test was established as an additional safeguard to protect against the adverse conditions that would be created by a mattress that released its heat in other than the usual measured scenario, and the following should also be noted:
   (a) During the test for measurement of rate of heat release, the instantaneous heat release value usually peaks quickly and then quickly falls off, so as to create a triangle-shaped curve.
   (b) In the atypical case, if the heat release were to peak and remain steady at that elevated level, as opposed to quickly falling off, the 250 kW limit would not ensure safety.
   (c) Only a sprinkler exception is permitted in lieu of the test because of the ability of the sprinkler system to control the fire.

Actual test results for heat, smoke, and combustion product release from ASTM E 1590, *Standard Test Method for Fire Testing of Mattresses*, might be suitable for use as input into fire models for performance-based design.

See the commentary following A.10.3.3.

It is noted that the values in A.10.3.4 differ from those in the actual *Code* requirement of 10.3.4. The *Code* values were revised for the 2009 edition to correspond with the values found in California Technical Bulletin 129[36]; the associated annex text was inadvertently overlooked. The values will be corrected for a future edition of the *Code.* Although the values in A.10.3.4 are incorrect, A.10.3.4 adequately describes the intent of the rates of heat release provisions, which is to prevent any single furniture item from causing room flashover. The material in A.10.3.4 also explains how automatic sprinklers, in certain cases, can serve in lieu of a low rate of heat release.

**10.3.5*** Furnishings or decorations of an explosive or highly flammable character shall not be used.

**A.10.3.5** Christmas trees that are not effectively flame-retardant treated, ordinary crepe paper decorations, and pyroxylin plastic decorations might be classified as highly flammable.

The *Code* relies on the authority having jurisdiction to exercise judgment in determining whether materials are of an explosive or highly flammable nature.

**10.3.6** Fire-retardant coatings shall be maintained to retain the effectiveness of the treatment under service conditions encountered in actual use.

See NFPA 703, *Standard for Fire Retardant–Treated Wood and Fire-Retardant Coatings for Building Materials.*

**10.3.7*** Where required by the applicable provisions of this *Code*, furnishings and contents made with foamed plastic materials that are unprotected from ignition shall have a heat release rate not exceeding 100 kW when tested in accordance with UL 1975, *Standard for Fire Tests for Foamed Plastics Used for Decorative Purposes.*

**A.10.3.7** ANSI/UL 1975, *Standard for Fire Tests for Foamed Plastics Used for Decorative Purposes*, is not intended for evaluating interior wall and ceiling finish materials.

Actual test results for heat, smoke, and combustion product release from ANSI/UL 1975 might be suitable for use as input into fire models intended for performance-based design.

## References Cited in Commentary

1. Isner, M., "Five Die in High-Rise Office Building Fire," *Fire Journal®* 84, no. 4 (July/August 1990): 50–57, 59.
2. Klem, T., "Investigation Report on the Dupont Plaza Hotel Fire," National Fire Protection Association, Quincy, MA, 1987.
3. National Fire Protection Association, "Investigation Report on the Las Vegas Hilton Hotel Fire," *Fire Journal®* 76, no. 1 (January 1982): 52–63.
4. Hall, Jr., J., "Report Prepared for the House Subcommittee on Science, Research, and Technology on H.R. 94, The Hotel and Motel Fire Safety Act of 1989," NFPA Fire Analysis and Research Division, National Fire Protection Association, Quincy, MA, March 2, 1989.
5. Watrous, L., "Ten Die in Convalescent Home Fire," *Fire Journal®* 66, no. 5 (September 1972): 16–20.
6. Hall, Jr., J., "Report Prepared for the House Subcommittee on Science, Research, and Technology on H.R. 94, The Hotel and Motel Fire Safety Act of 1989," NFPA Fire Analysis and Research Division, National Fire Protection Association, Quincy, MA, March 2, 1989.
7. NFPA 13, *Standard for the Installation of Sprinkler Systems*, 2007 edition, National Fire Protection Association, Quincy, MA.
8. NFPA 13R, *Standard for the Installation of Sprinkler Systems in Residential Occupancies up to and Including Four Stories in Height,* 2007 edition, National Fire Protection Association, Quincy, MA.
9. Demers, D., "Familiar Problems Cause 10 Deaths in Hotel Fire," *Fire Journal®* 74, no. 1 (January 1980): 52–56.
10. Waksman, D. and Ferguson, J. B., "Fire Tests of Building Interior Covering Systems," *Fire Technology* 10, no. 3 (August 1974): 211–220.
11. Fisher F. et al., "Room Fire Experiments of Textile Wall Coverings," Fire Research Laboratory, University of California, Berkeley, March 1986.
12. NFPA 701, *Standard Methods of Fire Tests for Flame Propagation of Textiles and Films*, 2004 edition, National Fire Protection Association, Quincy, MA.
13. ASTM E 84, *Standard Test Method for Surface Burning Characteristics of Building Materials*, 2004 edition, ASTM International, 100 Barr Harbor Drive, P.O. Box C700, West Conshohocken, PA 19428-2959.
14. ANSI/UL 723, *Standard for Test of Surface Burning Characteristics of Building Materials*, 2003 edition, Revised 2005, Underwriters Laboratories Inc., 333 Pfingsten Road, Northbrook, IL 60062-2096.

15. NFPA 220, *Standard on Types of Building Construction*, 2009 edition, National Fire Protection Association, Quincy, MA.
16. *NFPA 5000®, Building Construction and Safety Code®*, 2009 edition, National Fire Protection Association, Quincy, MA.
17. NFPA 286, *Standard Methods of Fire Tests for Evaluating Contribution of Wall and Ceiling Interior Finish to Room Fire Growth,* 2006 edition, National Fire Protection Association, Quincy, MA.
18. Waksman, D. and Ferguson, J. B., "Fire Tests of Building Interior Covering Systems," *Fire Technology* 10, no. 3(August 1974): 211–220.
19. "Study of Smoke Ratings Developed in Standard Fire Tests in Relation to Visual Observations," Bulletin of Research, No. 56, April 1965, Underwriters Laboratories Inc., 333 Pfingsten Road, Northbrook, IL 60062-2096.
20. NFPA 265, *Standard Methods of Fire Tests for Evaluating Room Fire Growth Contribution of Textile Coverings on Full Height Panels and Walls,* 2007 edition, National Fire Protection Association, Quincy, MA.
21. National Fire Protection Association, "Investigation Report on the Las Vegas Hilton Hotel Fire," *Fire Journal®* 76, no. 1 (January 1982): 52–63.
22. Fisher F. et al., "Room Fire Experiments of Textile Wall Coverings," Fire Research Laboratory, University of California, Berkeley, March 1986.
23. Christian, W. J. and Waterman, T. E., "Flame Spread in Corridors: Effects of Location and Area of Wall Finish," *Fire Journal®* 65, no. 4 (July 1971): 25–32.
24. Sharry, J., "Foamed Plastic Fire: Fire Spreads 430 Feet in Eight Minutes," *Fire Journal®* 69, no. 1 (January 1975): 5–6, 56.
25. NFPA 703, *Standard for Fire Retardant–Treated Wood and Fire-Retardant Coatings for Building Materials,* 2009 edition, National Fire Protection Association, Quincy, MA.
26. NFPA 253, *Standard Method of Test for Critical Radiant Flux of Floor Covering Systems Using a Radiant Heat Energy Source,* 2006 edition, National Fire Protection Association, Quincy, MA.
27. ASTM E 648, *Standard Test Method for Critical Radiant Flux of Floor-Covering Systems Using a Radiant Heat Energy Source*, 2006 edition, ASTM International, 100 Barr Harbor Drive, P.O. Box C700, West Conshohocken, PA 19428-2959.
28. Title 16, *Code of Federal Regulations*, Part 1630, "Standard for the Surface Flammability of Carpets and Rugs" (FF 1-70), U.S. Government Printing Office, Washington, DC 20402, published annually.
29. King-Mon, T. and Davis, S., "Flame Spread of Carpet Systems Involved in Room Fires," NBSIR 76-1013, June 1976, National Bureau of Standards (currently National Institute of Standards and Technology, Gaithersburg, MD 20899-1070.
30. NFPA 260, *Standard Methods of Tests and Classification System for Cigarette Ignition Resistance of Components of Upholstered Furniture,* 2009 edition, National Fire Protection Association, Quincy, MA.
31. ASTM E 1353, *Standard Test Methods for Cigarette Ignition Resistance of Components of Upholstered Furniture,* 2002 edition, ASTM International, 100 Barr Harbor Drive, P.O. Box C700, West Conshohocken, PA 19428-2959.
32. NFPA 261, *Standard Method of Test for Determining Resistance of Mock-Up Upholstered Furniture Material Assemblies to Ignition by Smoldering Cigarettes,* 2009 edition, National Fire Protection Association, Quincy, MA.
33. ASTM E 1352, *Standard Test Method for Cigarette Ignition Resistance of Mock-Up Upholstered Furniture Assemblies*, 2002 edition, ASTM International, 100 Barr Harbor Drive, P.O. Box C700, West Conshohocken, PA 19428-2959.
34. Title 16, *Code of Federal Regulations*, Part 1632, "Standard for the Flammability of Mattresses and Mattress Pads" (FF 4-72), U.S. Government Printing Office, Washington, DC 20402, published annually.
35. Technical Bulletin 133, *Flammability Test Procedure for Seating Furniture for Use in Public Occupancies,* 1991 edition, State of California, Department of Consumer Affairs, Bureau of Home Furnishings and Thermal Insulation, 3485 Orange Grove Avenue, North Highlands, CA 95660-5595.
36. Technical Bulletin 129, *Flammability Test Procedure for Mattresses for Use in Public Buildings,* 1992 edition, State of California, Department of Consumer Affairs, Bureau of Home Furnishings and Thermal Insulation, 3485 Orange Grove Avenue, North Highlands, CA 95660-5595.

# CHAPTER 11

# Special Structures and High-Rise Buildings

Chapter 11 is formatted differently from the other chapters of the *Code*. It is the last of the core chapters that precedes the occupancy chapters. Its scope is potentially applicable to all occupancies. Each subsection is targeted to specific special structures or *unusual* surroundings within which a *usual* occupancy might exist. The facilities to which Chapter 11 provisions might be applied range from a refinery petroleum-cracking plant to an air traffic control tower. While the life safety and functional use considerations of these properties might, at times, seem to conflict, Chapter 11 provides the necessary guidance to make them safe as well as functional.

Examples of usual occupancies housed in unusual surroundings or special structures include a large convention center located on a pier, so that the facility is surrounded by water on three sides, and a moderately sized restaurant located on an upper level of an air traffic control tower. Exhibit 11.1 is an example of a usual occupancy in an unusual surrounding.

An authority having jurisdiction (AHJ) should ensure that any engineered solutions to the special structure's inherent egress deficiencies provide an overall level of life safety equivalent to that specified by the requirements of the occupancy chapter that applies to the structure's use. In some cases, a structure might be so unusual that the only practical option is a complete performance-based design in accordance with Chapter 5.

Chapter 11 also regulates water-surrounded structures, vehicles and vessels, and limited access (referred to as *windowless* prior to the 2003 edition of the *Code*) and underground structures. These provisions apply, regardless of the occupancy classification. For example, a permanently moored ship that is used as a hotel with restaurants and other entertainment facilities must comply with Chapter 12 or Chapter 13 for assembly occupancies, and Chapter 28 or Chapter 29 for hotels and dormitories, as appropriate, by virtue of the language in 11.6.2. The Queen Mary, which has been permanently moored in Long Beach, California, since 1967 is an example of such an occupancy. See Exhibit 11.2.

Section 11.8 presents a series of unique provisions applicable to high-rise buildings. The various occupancy chapters might mandate the use of some, all, or none of those provisions. It is important to note that Section 11.8 applies only where referenced by another section of the *Code*.

Sections 11.9 through 11.11 provide a series of requirements applicable to membrane structures and tents. Similar requirements were originally contained in NFPA 102, *Standard for Grandstands, Folding and Telescopic Seating, Tents, and Membrane Structures*.[1] However, the requirements for such seating are now within the scope of this *Code* (and that of *NFPA 5000*®, *Building Construction and Safety Code*®[2]). As such, NFPA 102 is now extracted, in its entirety, from NFPA *101* and *NFPA 5000*.

## 11.1 General Requirements

### 11.1.1 Application.

The requirements of Sections 11.1 through 11.11 shall apply to occupancies regulated by Chapters 12 through 42 that are in a special structure. The applicable provisions of Chapters 12 through 42 shall apply, except as modified by this chapter. Section 11.8 shall apply to high-rise buildings only where specifically required by Chapters 12 through 42.

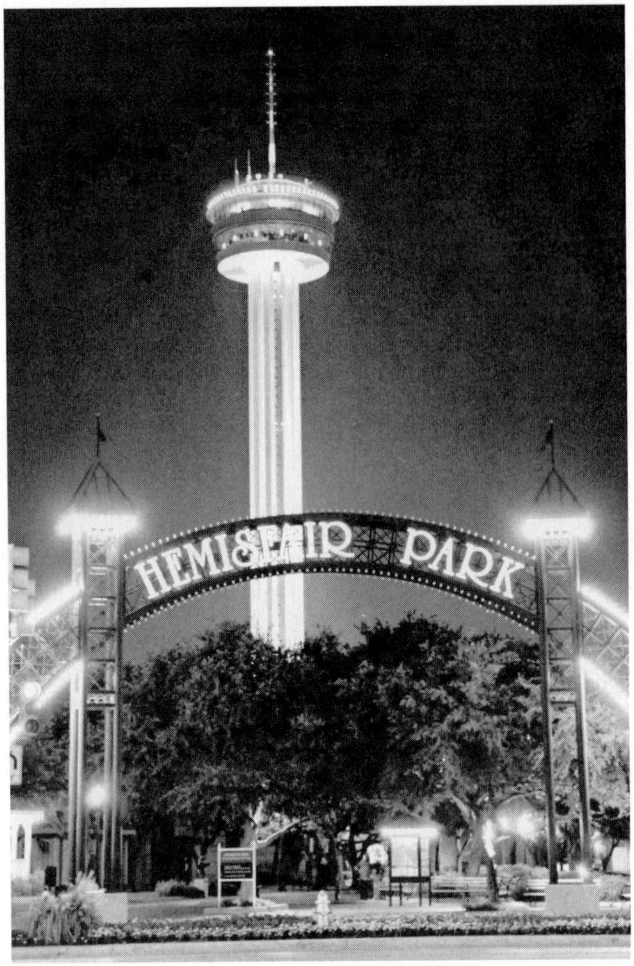


***Exhibit 11.1*** *Tower of the Americas in San Antonio, TX. (Photo courtesy of Landry's Restaurants, Inc.)*

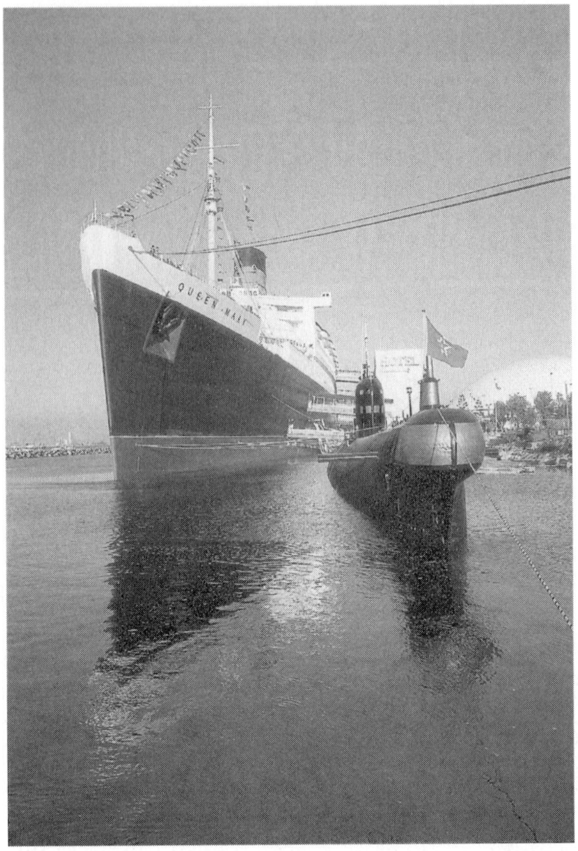


***Exhibit 11.2*** *The Queen Mary in Long Beach, CA. (Photo courtesy of the Queen Mary, Long Beach, CA)*

Occupancies in special structures can pose a challenge to life safety. Sections 11.1 through 11.6 are intended to supplement the requirements of the occupancy chapters (Chapters 12 through 42); their provisions might serve as requirements that must be satisfied in addition to those found in the applicable occupancy chapter. For example, 11.5.2.2 contains additional provisions that apply to a pier used for other than cargo handling or storage. Therefore, in the case of an amusement pier, the requirements of Chapter 12 or Chapter 13 for assembly occupancies would apply as well as those of 11.5.2.2.

The provisions of Chapter 11 also might take the form of a modification of a requirement that is permitted to be used for an occupancy in a special structure but that would not be permitted in a usual structure housing the same occupancy. For example, if a business occupancy is housed in a tower, 11.3.2.4.1 permits a single exit from the tower under a strict set of conditions. However, if a similar business occupancy is located on an upper floor of a multistory building that is not a tower, Chapter 38 or Chapter 39 would require that two exits be provided on the floor housing the business occupancy. In other words, Chapter 11 might offer an exemption based on the inherent difficulty of providing two remote exits from a tower. Yet, the exemption isn't a waiver that ignores life safety; rather, the exemption provides criteria and limitations that ensure a safe means of tolerating a single exit.

In addition to the provisions applicable to an occupancy via its appropriate occupancy chapter (Chapters 12 through 42), occupancies housed in underground and limited access structures must comply with the provisions of Section 11.7, which include the following:

1. Complete automatic sprinkler protection, unless certain criteria are met (see 11.7.3.4)
2. Emergency lighting (see 11.7.3.5)
3. Smoke venting (in underground structures only; see 11.7.4.4)

4. Directional signage for egress paths (in underground structures only; see 11.7.4.5)

An occupancy in a high-rise building must comply with the requirements of Section 11.8 only to the degree specified by the applicable occupancy chapter. For example, for new hotels, 28.4.1 requires compliance with the full package of high-rise building provisions of Section 11.8; for new mercantile occupancies, 36.4.2 requires only sprinkler systems in accordance with 11.8.3.1, rather than the complete high-rise package. For most existing buildings, the applicable occupancy chapter does not make mandatory use of any of the provisions of Section 11.8, although some require existing high-rise buildings to be sprinklered in accordance with Section 9.7 rather than 11.8.3.

Although the *Code* provisions present an essentially complete package of requirements for life safety, the provision of adequate means of egress from many special structures requires unique solutions. In many instances, engineered solutions will supplement the minimum provisions of Chapter 11 and the applicable occupancy chapter. However, the unique character of a structure should not become an excuse for reducing safety to life. The *Code* user is cautioned to exercise careful judgment when determining the egress requirements for special structures.

### 11.1.2 Multiple Occupancies.

See 6.1.14.

### 11.1.3 Special Definitions.

Special terms used in this chapter are located within each special structure section.

### 11.1.4 Classification of Occupancy.

Occupancies regulated by Chapters 12 through 42 that are in special structures shall meet the requirements of those chapters, except as modified by this chapter.

### 11.1.5 Classification of Hazard of Contents.

Classification of hazard of contents shall be in accordance with Section 6.2.

### 11.1.6 Minimum Construction Requirements.

Minimum construction requirements shall be in accordance with the applicable occupancy chapter.

### 11.1.7 Occupant Load.

The occupant load of special structures shall be based on the use of the structure as regulated by Chapters 12 through 42.

### 11.1.8 Automatic Sprinkler Systems.

Where another provision of this chapter requires an automatic sprinkler system, the automatic sprinkler system shall be installed in accordance with the subparts of 9.7.1.1 as permitted by the applicable occupancy chapter.

## 11.2 Open Structures

### 11.2.1 Application.

**11.2.1.1 General.** The provisions of Section 11.1 shall apply.

**11.2.1.2 Definition — Open Structure.** See 3.3.254.7.

### 11.2.2* Means of Egress.

**A.11.2.2** Escape chutes, controlled descent devices, and elevators are permitted to provide escape routes in special structures; however, they should not be substituted for the provisions of this *Code*.

**11.2.2.1 General.** The means of egress provisions of the applicable occupancy, Chapters 12 through 42, shall apply, except as modified by 11.2.2.2 through 11.2.2.10.

**11.2.2.2 Means of Egress Components.**

**11.2.2.2.1 Fire Escape Ladders.** Open structures that are designed for occupancy by not more than three persons shall be permitted to be served by fire escape ladders complying with 7.2.9.

**11.2.2.2.2 Reserved.**

**11.2.2.3 Capacity of Means of Egress.** Open structures shall be exempt from the requirements for capacity of means of egress.

Paragraph 11.2.2.3 recognizes the multiple means of egress paths available from open structures, such as those found in petrochemical and process industries. An open structure is actually an access platform to the equipment it surrounds or supports. Normal occupancy is very limited in number and occasional in frequency. If a fire blocks one means of egress, a number of alternate means of egress remain available. An escape route is provided by the fixed means of egress, and rescue is possible from any portion of the structure by use of the emergency procedures of fire-fighting personnel. The potential for exposure of portions of the structure not involved in a fire is minimal, because, in open platforms, flames, heat, and smoke are safely dispersed directly into the atmosphere and not into the uninvolved portions of the structure.

**11.2.2.4 Number of Means of Egress.**

**11.2.2.4.1*** Open structures at the finished ground level are exempt from the requirements for number of means of egress.

**A.11.2.2.4.1** The grade level of open structures, which by their very nature contain an infinite number of means of egress, are exempt from the requirements for number of means of egress.

**11.2.2.4.2** Open structures occupied by not more than three persons, with travel distance of not more than 200 ft (61 m), shall be permitted to have a single exit.

**11.2.2.5 Arrangement of Means of Egress.** (No modifications.)

**11.2.2.6 Travel Distance to Exits.** Open structures shall be exempt from travel distance limitations.

**11.2.2.7 Discharge from Exits.** Open structures permitted to have a single exit per 11.2.2.4 shall be permitted to have 100 percent of the exit discharge through areas on the level of exit discharge.

**11.2.2.8 Illumination of Means of Egress.** Open structures shall be exempt from illumination of means of egress requirements.

**11.2.2.9 Emergency Lighting.** Open structures shall be exempt from emergency lighting requirements.

**11.2.2.10 Marking of Means of Egress.** Open structures shall be exempt from marking of means of egress requirements.

### 11.2.3 Protection.

**11.2.3.1 Protection of Vertical Openings.** Open structures shall be exempt from protection of vertical opening requirements.

**11.2.3.2 Protection from Hazards.** Every open structure, other than those structures with only occasional occupancy, shall have automatic, manual, or other protection that is appropriate to the particular hazard and that is designed to minimize danger to occupants in case of fire or other emergency before they have time to use the means of egress.

**11.2.3.3 Interior Finish.** (No modifications.)

**11.2.3.4 Detection, Alarm, and Communications Systems.** Open structures shall be exempt from requirements for detection, alarm, and communications systems.

**11.2.3.5 Extinguishing Requirements.** (No modifications.)

## 11.3 Towers

### 11.3.1 Application.

**11.3.1.1 General.** The provisions of Section 11.1 shall apply.

**11.3.1.2 Definition — Tower.** See 3.3.262.

**11.3.1.3 Use of Accessory Levels.**

**11.3.1.3.1 Sprinklered Towers.** In towers protected throughout by an automatic sprinkler system in accordance with Section 9.7, the levels located below the observation level shall be permitted to be occupied only for the following uses that support tower operations:

(1) Use as electrical and mechanical equipment rooms, including emergency power, radar, communications, and electronics rooms
(2)* Incidental accessory uses

**A.11.3.1.3.1(2)** The incidental accessory uses are intended to apply to small office spaces or lounge areas and similar uses that are used by tower employees.

**11.3.1.3.2 Nonsprinklered Towers.** The levels located within a tower below the observation level and the equipment room for that level in nonsprinklered towers shall not be occupied.

### 11.3.2 Means of Egress.

**11.3.2.1 General.** The means of egress provisions of the applicable occupancy chapter, Chapters 12 through 42, shall apply, except as modified by 11.3.2.2 through 11.3.2.10.

**11.3.2.2 Means of Egress Components.**

**11.3.2.2.1 Fire Escape Ladders.** Towers, such as forest fire observation or railroad signal towers, that are designed for occupancy by not more than three persons shall be permitted to be served by fire escape ladders complying with 7.2.9.

**11.3.2.2.2 Elevators.** Towers subject to occupancy by not more than 90 persons shall be permitted to use elevators in the means of egress in accordance with 7.2.13.

**11.3.2.3 Capacity of Means of Egress.**

**11.3.2.3.1** Means of egress for towers shall be provided for the number of persons expected to occupy the space.

**11.3.2.3.2** Spaces not subject to human occupancy because of machinery or equipment shall be excluded from consideration.

**11.3.2.4* Number of Means of Egress.**

**A.11.3.2.4** The Washington Monument in Washington, DC, is an example of a tower where it would be impracticable to provide a second stairway.

**11.3.2.4.1** Towers shall be permitted to have a single exit, provided that the following conditions are met:

(1) The tower shall be subject to occupancy by fewer than 25 persons.
(2) The tower shall not be used for living or sleeping purposes.
(3) The tower shall be of Type I, Type II, or Type IV construction. *(See 8.2.1.)*
(4) The tower interior wall and ceiling finish shall be Class A or Class B.
(5) No combustible materials shall be located within the tower, under the tower, or within the immediate vicinity of the tower, except necessary furniture.
(6) No high hazard occupancies shall be located within the tower or within its immediate vicinity.
(7) Where the tower is located above a building, the single exit from the tower shall be provided by one of the following:
    (a) Exit enclosure separated from the building with no door openings to or from the building
    (b) Exit enclosure leading directly to an exit enclosure serving the building, with walls and door separating the exit enclosures from each other, and another door allowing access to the top floor of the building that provides access to a second exit serving that floor

Paragraph 11.3.2.4.1 permits a single means of egress from a tower if additional criteria are met. Determination of the total occupant load of a tower should be based on the actual number of people expected to occupy the facility [see 11.3.2.4.1(1)]. Limitations on the combustibility and interior finish of the structure are established, so that the potential exposure of the tower occupants to fire is minimal. Types I, II, and IV construction [see 11.3.2.4.1(3)] are defined in *NFPA 5000, Building Construction and Safety Code,* and NFPA 220, *Standard on Types of Building Construction.*[3]

One difficulty associated with the requirements for exits in towers is the accurate determination of the level of exposure of the tower to combustible materials under, or in the immediate vicinity of, the structure. The authority having jurisdiction (AHJ) and other *Code* users should use careful judgment to ensure that arbitrary limitations are not established that excessively restrict the use of the tower. For example, a forest fire tower is usually located in a clearing in a large forest. The proximity of trees to the tower could be interpreted as constituting combustible materials in the immediate vicinity of the tower. Reasonable clearances between the tower and forest — such as a clear space of 50 ft to 100 ft (15 m to 30 m) — could be considered adequate separation for the life safety of the tower's occupants. Similar judgment is required where evaluating the clearance between high hazard occupancies and towers.

The provisions of 11.3.2.4.1(7) are illustrated in Exhibit 11.3. Where the tower is located above a building, special precautions must be taken to prevent use of the tower's single means of egress from being compromised by a fire in the building below. In Exhibit 11.3, Part (a), the single exit stair enclosure for the tower is separated from the building by rated construction in accordance with 7.1.3.2. Additionally, the single exit

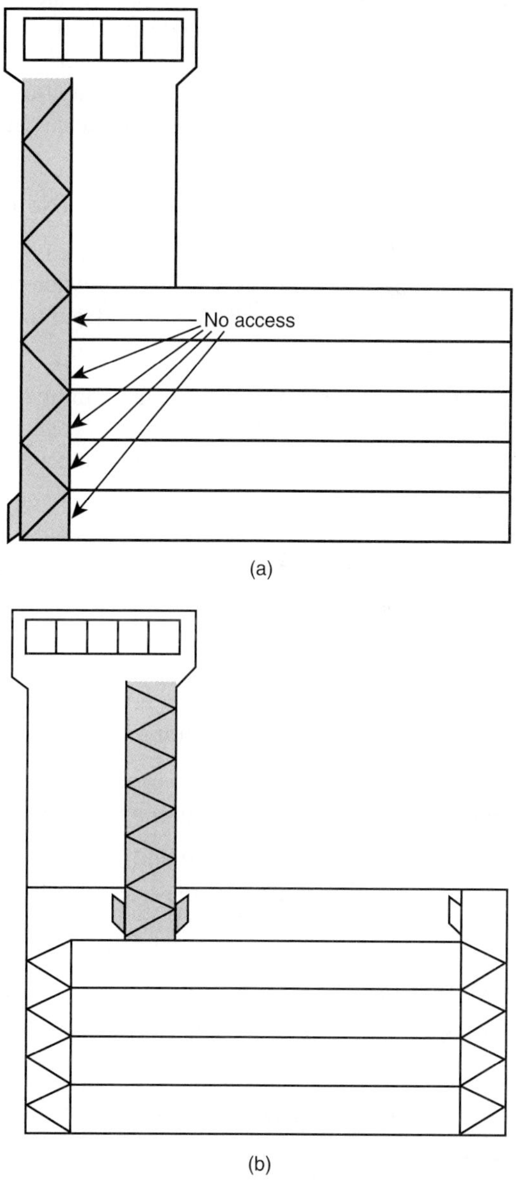


***Exhibit 11.3*** *Single exit from a tower.*

stair enclosure for the tower has no openings to the floors of the building above which the tower is positioned, thus preventing a fire on the building floors from entering the enclosure.

In Exhibit 11.3, Part (b), the single exit stair positioned above the building serves the tower. It provides direct access to the exit stair enclosure on the left, which also serves the building floors. If a fire prevents the use of the exit stair enclosure on the left, the tower stair allows tower occupants to traverse the top floor of the building and access a second exit stair enclosure on the right.

**11.3.2.4.2** Towers with 360-degree line-of-sight requirements shall be permitted to have a single means of egress for a distance of travel not exceeding 75 ft (23 m), or 100 ft (30 m) if the tower is protected throughout by an approved, supervised automatic sprinkler system in accordance with Section 9.7.

**11.3.2.5 Arrangement of Means of Egress.** (No modifications.)

**11.3.2.6 Travel Distance to Exits.** Towers where ladders are permitted by 11.3.2.2.1 shall be exempt from travel distance limitations.

**11.3.2.7 Discharge from Exits.** Towers permitted to have a single exit per 11.3.2.4 shall be permitted to have 100 percent of the exit discharge through areas on the level of exit discharge.

**11.3.2.8 Illumination of Means of Egress.** Towers where ladders are permitted by 11.3.2.2.1 shall be exempt from illumination of means of egress requirements.

**11.3.2.9 Emergency Lighting.**

**11.3.2.9.1** Towers where ladders are permitted by 11.3.2.2.1 shall be exempt from emergency lighting requirements.

**11.3.2.9.2** Locations not routinely inhabited by humans shall be exempt from emergency lighting requirements.

**11.3.2.9.3** Structures occupied only during daylight hours, with windows arranged to provide the required level of illumination of all portions of the means of egress during such hours, shall be exempt from emergency lighting requirements where approved by the authority having jurisdiction.

**11.3.2.10 Marking of Means of Egress.**

**11.3.2.10.1** Towers where ladders are permitted by 11.3.2.2.1 shall be exempt from marking of means of egress requirements.

**11.3.2.10.2** Locations not routinely inhabited by humans shall be exempt from marking of means of egress requirements.

### 11.3.3 Protection.

**11.3.3.1 Protection of Vertical Openings.**

**11.3.3.1.1** Towers where ladders are permitted by 11.3.2.2.1 shall be exempt from protection of vertical opening requirements.

**11.3.3.1.2** In towers where the support structure is open and there is no occupancy below the top floor level, stairs shall be permitted to be open with no enclosure required, or fire escape stairs shall be permitted.

**11.3.3.2 Protection from Hazards.** Every tower, other than structures with only occasional occupancy, shall have automatic, manual, or other protection that is appropriate to the particular hazard and that is designed to minimize danger to occupants in case of fire or other emergency before they have time to use the means of egress.

**11.3.3.3 Interior Finish.** (No modifications.)

**11.3.3.4 Detection, Alarm, and Communications Systems.** Towers designed for occupancy by not more than three persons shall be exempt from requirements for detection, alarm, and communications systems.

**11.3.3.5 Extinguishing Requirements.** (No modifications.)

**11.3.3.6 Corridors.** (No modifications.)

### 11.3.4 Additional Requirements for Air Traffic Control Towers.

The provisions of 11.3.4, which are new to the 2009 edition of the *Code*, provide additional requirements for an air traffic control tower (ATCT), which is defined in 3.3.262.1 as "an enclosed structure or building at airports with elevated levels for support of equipment and occupied for observation, control, operation, and signaling of aircraft in flight and on the ground." These criteria are intended to supplement the general tower provisions of Section 11.3, as well as the applicable occupancy chapter provisions (typically Chapters 38 and 39 for business occupancies); they recognize that conditions at ATCTs include critical public safety functions and unique occupancy conditions, such as the potential for delayed evacuation and limited occupant loads. The criteria for single-exit ATCTs in 11.3.4.4.1 are based on those agreed upon by the U.S. Department of Transportation — Federal Aviation Administration (FAA) and the U.S. Department of Labor — Occupational Safety & Health Administration (OSHA). The level of protection afforded by life safety features, such as fire-resistive or noncombustible construction (11.3.4.3), smokeproof enclosures (11.3.4.4.5), fire alarm and detection systems (11.3.4.5.1), and automatic sprinklers (11.3.4.5.2), is deemed to be sufficient to accommodate the unique operational requirements for ATCTs that might otherwise compromise occupant life safety from fire.

**11.3.4.1 Definition — Air Traffic Control Tower.** See 3.3.262.1.

**11.3.4.2 Use of Accessory Levels.** The levels located below the observation level shall be permitted to be occupied only for the following uses that support tower operations:

(1) Use as electrical and mechanical equipment rooms, including emergency and standby power, radar, communications, and electronics rooms
(2)* Incidental accessory uses

**A.11.3.4.2(2)** The incidental accessory uses are intended to apply to small office spaces or lounge areas and similar uses that are used by tower employees.

**11.3.4.3 Minimum Construction Requirements.** New air traffic control towers shall be of Type I or Type II construction. *(See 8.2.1.)*

**11.3.4.4 Means of Egress.**

**11.3.4.4.1 Number of Means of Egress.** Air traffic control towers shall be permitted to have a single exit, provided that the following conditions are met in addition to the requirements of 11.3.2.4:

(1) Each level of new air traffic control towers, served by a single exit, shall be subject to a calculated occupant load of 15 or fewer persons.
(2) The requirements of 11.3.2.4.1(1) shall not apply to existing air traffic control towers.
(3) Smoke detection shall be provided throughout air traffic control towers to meet the requirements of partial coverage, as defined in 5.5.2.2 of *NFPA 72, National Fire Alarm Code,* and shall include coverage of all of the following:
    (a) Occupiable areas
    (b) Common areas
    (c) Work spaces
    (d) Equipment areas
    (e) Means of egress
    (f) Accessible utility shafts
(4) The requirements of 11.3.2.4.1(5) shall not apply.
(5) Rooms or spaces used for the storage, processing, or use of combustible supplies shall be permitted in quantities deemed acceptable by the authority having jurisdiction.

**11.3.4.4.2 Egress for Occupant Load.** Means of egress for air traffic control towers shall be provided for the occupant load, as determined in accordance with 7.3.1.

**11.3.4.4.3 Areas Excluded from Occupant Load.** Shafts, stairs, and spaces and floors not subject to human occupancy shall be excluded from consideration in determining the total calculated occupant load of the tower as required by 11.3.2.4.1(1) and 11.3.4.4.1(3).

**11.3.4.4.4 Single Means of Egress.** A single means of egress shall be permitted from the observation level of an air traffic control tower, as permitted by 11.3.2.4.2.

**11.3.4.4.5 Smokeproof Enclosures.** For other than existing, previously approved air traffic control towers, smokeproof exit enclosures complying with 7.2.3 shall be provided for all air traffic control tower exit stair enclosures.

**11.3.4.4.6 Discharge from Exits.** Air traffic control towers shall comply with the requirements of 7.7.2.

**11.3.4.5 Protection.**

**11.3.4.5.1 Detection, Alarm, and Communications Systems.** For other than existing, previously approved air traffic control towers, air traffic control towers shall be provided with a fire alarm system in accordance with Section 9.6. Smoke detection shall be provided throughout the air traffic control tower to meet the requirements for selective coverage, as defined in 5.5.2.2 of *NFPA 72, National Fire Alarm Code*, and shall include coverage of all of the following:

(1) Equipment areas
(2) Outside each opening into exit enclosures
(3) Along the single means of egress permitted from observation levels in 11.3.2.4.2
(4) Outside each opening into the single means of egress permitted from observation levels in 11.3.2.4.2

**11.3.4.5.2 Extinguishing Requirements.** New air traffic control towers shall be protected throughout by an approved, supervised automatic sprinkler system in accordance with Section 9.7.

**11.3.4.6 Contents and Furnishings.** Contents and furnishings in air traffic control towers shall comply with 10.3.1, 10.3.2, 10.3.6, and 10.3.7.

**11.3.4.7 Uses.** Sleeping areas shall be prohibited in air traffic control towers.

## 11.4 Water-Surrounded Structures

### 11.4.1 Application.

**11.4.1.1 General.** The provisions of Sections 11.1 and 11.4 shall apply to those structures that are not under the jurisdiction of the U.S. Coast Guard and not designed and arranged in accordance with U.S. Coast Guard regulations.

**11.4.1.2 Definition — Water-Surrounded Structure.** See 3.3.254.12.

### 11.4.2 Means of Egress.

**11.4.2.1 General.** The means of egress provisions of the applicable occupancy chapter, Chapters 12 through 42, shall apply, except as modified by 11.4.2.2 through 11.4.2.10.

**11.4.2.2 Means of Egress Components.** (No modifications.)

**11.4.2.3 Capacity of Means of Egress.** Spaces in water-surrounded structures that are not subject to human occupancy because of machinery or equipment shall be exempt from the requirements for capacity of means of egress.

**11.4.2.4 Number of Means of Egress.** (No modifications.)

**11.4.2.5 Arrangement of Means of Egress.** (No modifications.)

**11.4.2.6 Travel Distance to Exits.** (No modifications.)

**11.4.2.7 Discharge from Exits.** Structures permitted to have a single exit per the applicable occupancy chapter shall be permitted to have 100 percent of the exit discharge through areas on the level of exit discharge.

**11.4.2.8 Illumination of Means of Egress.** (No modifications.)

**11.4.2.9 Emergency Lighting.**

**11.4.2.9.1** Locations not routinely inhabited by humans are exempt from emergency lighting requirements.

**11.4.2.9.2** Structures occupied only during daylight hours, with windows arranged to provide the required level of illumination of all portions of the means of egress during such hours, shall be exempt from emergency lighting requirements where approved by the authority having jurisdiction.

**11.4.2.10 Marking of Means of Egress.** Locations not routinely inhabited by humans shall be exempt from marking of means of egress requirements.

### 11.4.3 Protection.

**11.4.3.1 Protection of Vertical Openings.** (No modifications.)

**11.4.3.2 Protection from Hazards.** Every water-surrounded structure, other than structures with only occasional occupancy, shall have automatic, manual, or other protection that is appropriate to the particular hazard and that is designed to minimize danger to occupants in case of fire or other emergency before they have time to use the means of egress.

**11.4.3.3 Interior Finish.** (No modifications.)

**11.4.3.4 Detection, Alarm, and Communications Systems.** (No modifications.)

**11.4.3.5 Extinguishing Requirements.** (No modifications.)

**11.4.3.6 Corridors.** (No modifications.)

## 11.5* Piers

**A.11.5** For further information on pier fire protection, see NFPA 307, *Standard for the Construction and Fire Protection of Marine Terminals, Piers, and Wharves.*

### 11.5.1 Application.

The provisions of Section 11.1 shall apply.

### 11.5.2 Number of Means of Egress.

The intent of 11.5.2 is to recognize the open nature of a pier and to equate a pier with a public way for purposes of egress arrangement. Note that 11.5.2.1 applies to cargo and storage piers, which are occupied by a limited number of people, the majority of whom are accustomed to the arrangement of piers. The risk to life safety is considered minimal under these conditions, and one means of egress is acceptable. The provisions of 11.5.2.2 apply to buildings on piers that are not used exclusively to moor cargo vessels and store materials.

**11.5.2.1** Piers used exclusively to moor cargo vessels and to store material shall be exempt from number of means of egress requirements where provided with proper means of egress from structures thereon to the pier and a single means of access to the mainland, as appropriate to the pier's arrangement.

**11.5.2.2** Buildings on piers not meeting the requirements of 11.5.2.1 and occupied for other than cargo handling and storage shall be in accordance with both of the following:

(1) Means of egress shall be arranged in accordance with Chapters 12 through 43
(2) One of the following measures shall be provided on piers extending over 150 ft (46 m) from shore to minimize the possibility that fire under or on the pier blocks the escape of occupants to shore:
   (a) The pier shall be arranged to provide two separate ways to travel to shore, such as by two well-separated walkways or independent structures.
   (b) The pier deck shall be open, fire resistive, and set on noncombustible supports.

(c) The pier shall be open, unobstructed, and not less than 50 ft (15 m) in width if less than 500 ft (150 m) long, or its width shall be not less than 10 percent of its length if more than 500 ft (150 m) long.
(d) The pier deck shall be provided with an approved automatic sprinkler system in accordance with Section 9.7 for combustible substructures and all superstructures.
(e) The sprinkler system specified in 11.5.2.2(2)(d) shall be supervised where required by the applicable occupancy chapter, Chapters 12 through 42.

The provisions of 11.5.2.2 apply to pier structures other than those structures exempted by 11.5.2.1. Note that these provisions must be applied in addition to those contained in Chapters 12 through 42. For piers that extend more than 150 ft (46 m) from shore, the provisions of 11.5.2.2(2)(a) through (d) are not required to be applied in total; in other words, the pier is required to comply with only one of the four subparts [subpart (e) is applied in conjunction with subpart (d)].

## 11.6* Vehicles and Vessels

**A.11.6** Fire safety information for manufactured home parks is found in NFPA 501A, *Standard for Fire Safety Criteria for Manufactured Home Installations, Sites, and Communities*.

### 11.6.1 Vehicles.

Where immobile, attached to a building, or permanently fixed to a foundation, and where subject to human occupancy, the following vehicles shall comply with the requirements of this *Code* that are appropriate to buildings of similar occupancy:

(1) Trailers
(2) Railroad cars
(3) Streetcars
(4) Buses
(5) Conveyances similar to those in 11.6.1(1) through (4)

### 11.6.2 Vessels.

Any ship, barge, or other vessel permanently fixed to a foundation or mooring, or unable to get underway by means of its own power, and occupied for purposes other than navigation shall be subject to the requirements of this *Code* that apply to buildings of similar occupancy.

## 11.7 Underground and Limited Access Structures

### 11.7.1 Application.

The provisions of Section 11.1 shall apply.

### 11.7.2 Special Definitions.

A list of special terms used in Section 11.7 follows:

(1) **Limited Access Structure.** See 3.3.254.3.
(2) **Underground Structure.** See 3.3.254.11.

### 11.7.3 Special Provisions for Underground and Limited Access Structures.

**11.7.3.1** A structure or portion of a structure that does not have openings in compliance with 11.7.3.1.1 and 11.7.3.1.2 shall be designated as a limited access structure and shall comply with 11.7.3.4 and 11.7.3.5.

**11.7.3.1.1 One-Story Structures.** One-story structures shall have finished ground level doors or emergency access openings in accordance with 11.7.3.2 on two sides of the building, spaced not more than 125 ft (38 m) apart on the exterior walls.

**11.7.3.1.2 Multiple-Story Structures.** Multiple-story structures shall comply with the following:

(1) The story at the finished ground level shall comply with 11.7.3.1.1.
(2) Other stories shall be provided with emergency access openings in accordance with 11.7.3.2 on two sides of the building, spaced not more than 30 ft (9140 mm) apart.

**11.7.3.2*** Emergency access openings shall consist of a window, panel, or similar opening that complies with all of the following:

(1) The opening shall have dimensions of not less than 22 in. (560 mm) in width and 24 in. (610 mm) in height and shall be unobstructed to allow for ventilation and rescue operations from the exterior.
(2) The bottom of the opening shall be not more than 44 in. (1120 mm) above the floor.
(3) The opening shall be readily identifiable from both the exterior and interior.
(4) The opening shall be readily openable from both the exterior and interior.

**A.11.7.3.2** It is not the intent that emergency access openings be readily openable from the exterior by the public but that they can easily be opened with normal fire department equipment.

The provision of emergency access openings for ventilation and rescue exempts stories below the level of exit discharge from classification as underground structures. In Exhibit 11.4, the basement is not considered to be underground if the following conditions apply:

1. Openings are provided on at least two sides.
2. Openings are located entirely above the adjoining grade level.
3. Openings comprise a minimum of 20 $ft^2$ per 50 lineal ft (1.9 $m^2$ per 15 lineal m) of walls.
4. X = minimum width of 22 in. (560 mm) of unobstructed opening.
   Y = minimum height of 24 in. (610 mm) of unobstructed opening.
   Z = maximum of 44 in. (1120 mm) from floor to bottom of opening.
5. Openings are readily identifiable.
6. Openings are readily openable.

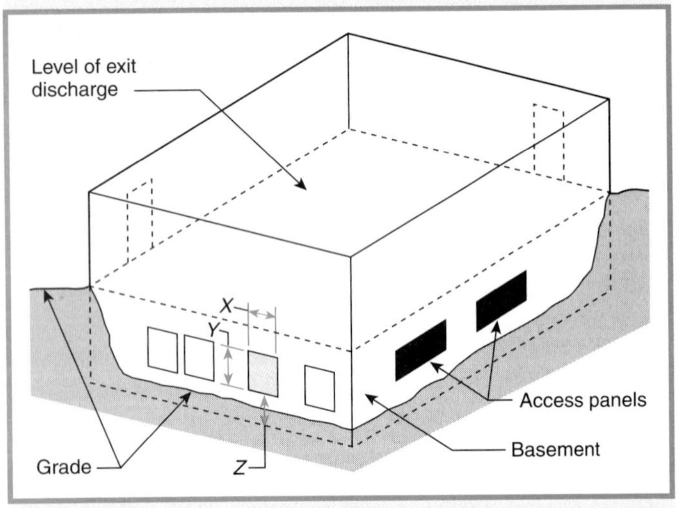


***Exhibit 11.4*** *Emergency access openings.*

As explained in A.11.7.3.2, it is not required that the public be able to readily open access openings from the exterior. Rather, such openings need to be opened easily from the outside by the fire department, using equipment normally carried on fire apparatus. Building occupants should also be able to open them easily from the interior.

Openings are permitted in the form of a window, a door, or an access panel.

Note that a structure is not considered to be a limited access structure if certain provisions are made for emergency access openings for ventilation and rescue. The provisions are more stringent for multistory structures than for single-story structures.

**11.7.3.3** A structure or portion of a structure shall not be considered an underground structure if the story is provided, on not less than two sides, with not less than 20 $ft^2$ (1.9 $m^2$) of emergency access opening located entirely above the adjoining finished ground level in each 50 lineal ft (15 lineal m) of exterior enclosing wall area.

**11.7.3.4** Underground and limited access structures, and all areas and floor levels traversed in traveling to the exit discharge, shall be protected by an approved, supervised automatic sprinkler system in accordance with Section 9.7, unless such structures meet one of the following criteria:

(1) They have an occupant load of 50 or fewer persons in new underground or limited access portions of the structure.
(2) They have an occupant load of 100 or fewer persons in existing underground or limited access portions of the structure.
(3) The structure is a one-story underground or limited access structure that is permitted to have a single exit per Chapters 12 through 43, with a common path of travel not greater than 50 ft (15 m).

**11.7.3.5** Underground or limited access portions of structures and all areas traversed in traveling to the exit discharge, other than in one- and two-family dwellings, shall be provided with emergency lighting in accordance with Section 7.9.

## 11.7.4 Additional Provisions for Underground Structures.

**11.7.4.1** A structure or portion of a structure shall not be considered an underground structure if the story is provided, on not less than two sides, with not less than 20 $ft^2$ (1.9 $m^2$) of emergency access opening located entirely above the adjoining finished ground level in each 50 lineal ft (15 lineal m) of exterior enclosing wall area.

**11.7.4.2** The requirements of 11.7.3 shall apply.

**11.7.4.3** Exits from underground structures with an occupant load of more than 100 persons in the underground portions of the structure and having a floor used for human occupancy located more than 30 ft (9140 mm) below the lowest level of exit discharge, or having more than one level located below the lowest level of exit discharge, shall be provided with outside smoke-venting facilities or other means to prevent the exits from becoming charged with smoke from any fire in the areas served by the exits.

**11.7.4.4** The underground portions of an underground structure, other than an existing underground structure, shall be provided with approved automatic smoke venting in accordance with Section 9.3 where the underground structure has the following features:

(1) Occupant load of more than 100 persons in the underground portions of the structure
(2) Floor level used for human occupancy located more than 30 ft (9140 mm) below the lowest level of exit discharge, or more than one level located below the lowest level of exit discharge
(3) Combustible contents, combustible interior finish, or combustible construction

**11.7.4.5** Exit stair enclosures in underground structures having a floor level used for human occupancy located more than 30 ft (9140 mm) below the lowest level of exit discharge, or having more than one level located below the lowest level of exit discharge, shall be provided with signage in accordance with 7.2.2.5.4 at each floor level landing traversed in traveling to the exit discharge. The signs shall include a chevron-shaped indicator to show direction to the exit discharge.

The provisions contained in 11.7.1 through 11.7.4.5 that regulate life safety in underground and limited access structures are minimal. The intent of the provisions is to supplement, not to provide a means of circumventing, the life safety provisions contained in other chapters of the *Code*. If the building under consideration is a limited access structure or located underground and — due to its occupancy classification — subject to stricter requirements than those contained in Section 11.7, the stricter provisions of the *Code* must be applied. For example, the provisions of 12.4.3 — which apply to new assembly occupancies located in limited access or underground structures or portions thereof — require that each level more than 30 ft (9140 mm) below the level of exit discharge be equipped with a mechanical means of moving occupants vertically, such as an elevator or escalator. Section 11.7 has no such requirement.

Limited access and underground structures pose enhanced risks to life safety, because the buildings cannot be easily vented of products of combustion. In an area from which there is no direct access to the outside and where there are no windows to allow outside fire department rescue operations and ventilation, fire or smoke might cause occupants to panic. Therefore, additional corrective measures, such as complete automatic sprinkler protection and automatic smoke-venting systems, must be provided where necessary to ensure an adequate level of life safety.

The provisions of 11.7.4.5 address the need for cues to guide occupants toward the exit and level of exit discharge. Traveling upward in an exit stair might appear illogical, because most egress from buildings involves downward travel within an exit stair enclosure. However, the direction of travel chosen by an occupant can depend on how the occupant entered the building. Paragraph 11.7.4.5 requires signs to be provided within the exit stair enclosure to direct occupants to the exit discharge. The directional indicator must be of the same chevron design as required by 7.10.6.2.

Although it is not referenced directly by the *Code*, NFPA 520, *Standard on Subterranean Spaces*,[4] offers guidance on protecting occupants in these variations of underground or limited access structures. A subterranean space is defined as a cavern resulting from the extraction of subsurface-located material from underground areas in a manner that does not disturb the surface area of the property, except in the vicinity of the entrances and ventilation openings.

The headquarters for the North American Aerospace Defense Command (NORAD), housed in Cheyenne Mountain, Colorado Springs, Colorado, is an example of a subterranean space. Such spaces are also commonly used as storage occupancies due to their relatively constant climates. These spaces can be massive in size, complete with roadways and rails for transporting goods in and out, and some contain buildings within the spaces. NFPA 520 includes requirements on construction features, such as compartmentation and smoke control; means of egress; fire alarm, detection, and suppression systems; emergency preparedness; and fire department provisions, such as communications systems, preplanning, and access.

## 11.8 High-Rise Buildings

Section 11.8 does not itself require that any special provisions be applied to high-rise buildings. Instead, it provides a menu of options for high-rise buildings that can be wholly or partially mandated by other *Code* sections. For example, Chapters 12, 14, 16, 17, 18, 28, 30, 32, and 38 (which apply to new assembly occupancies, new educational occupancies, new and existing daycare occupancies, new health care occupancies, new hotels and dormitories, new apartment buildings, new large residential board and care facilities, and new business occupancies, respectively) require high-rise buildings to comply with the entire package of requirements contained in Section 11.8. Chapter 22 (which applies to new detention and correctional occupancies) requires high-rise buildings to comply with the provisions of 11.8.3, which require sprinklers and standpipes. Chapters 15, 36, 40, and 42 (for existing educational occupancies, new mercantile occupancies, industrial occupancies, and storage occupancies, respectively) require that new high-rise buildings be sprinklered in accordance with 11.8.3.1.

Exhibit 11.5 illustrates the criteria under which a building is classified as high-rise, as specified by the definition of *high-rise building* in 3.3.32.7. Measurement of the vertical distance criterion begins at ground level on the lowest side of the building that provides fire department vehicle access and ends at the floor of the highest occupiable story. If the vertical distance measurement made in this manner exceeds 75 ft (23 m), the building is considered to be a high-rise building.

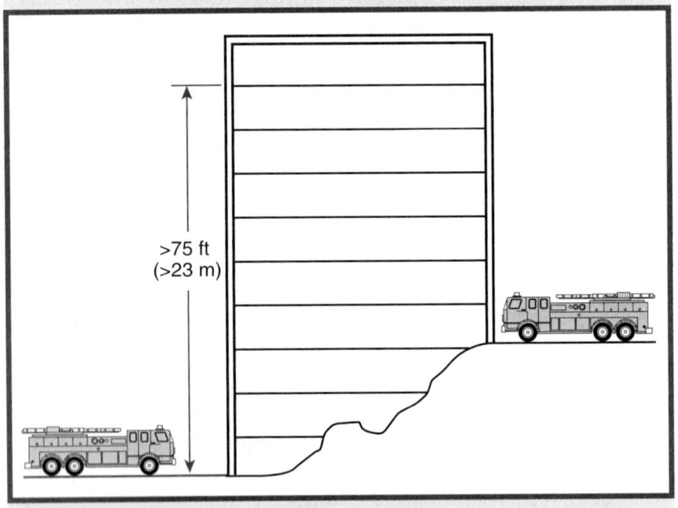


***Exhibit 11.5*** *Determining if building is high-rise in accordance with the 75 ft (23 m) criterion.*

The 75 ft (23 m) criterion used for defining a high-rise building was first added to the 1988 edition of the *Code*. Previously, individual occupancy chapters set their own criteria. Business and health care occupancies used provisions similar to the 75 ft (23 m) criterion, while residential occupancies used a six-story criterion. The current method establishes consistency for use throughout the *Code*. The current criteria have been accepted fairly well throughout the United States, but some local jurisdictions set a lower height at which high-rise building provisions apply. Although the definition does not include buildings less than 75 ft (23 m) in height, such buildings can experience the same challenges as true high-rise buildings, because they are set back over a larger one-story section, out of reach of fire department ladders. Although the definition does not address the subject completely, it provides a generally acceptable method for determining whether a building is a high-rise building.

High-rise buildings pose several problems, as follows:

1. Potential for wide distribution of smoke to all floors due to significant stack effect (i.e., natural draft) within stair towers and other tall shafts
2. Difficulty in evacuation
3. Difficulty experienced by fire service personnel in reaching the fire

### 11.8.1 General.

**11.8.1.1** Where required by Chapters 12 through 43, the provisions of Section 11.8 shall apply to high-rise buildings, as defined in 3.3.32.7.

**11.8.1.2** In addition to the requirements of Section 11.8, compliance with all other applicable provisions of this *Code* shall be required.

### 11.8.2 Means of Egress Requirements.

**11.8.2.1 Reserved.**

**11.8.2.2 Elevator Lobby Exit Access Door Locking.** In other than newly constructed high-rise buildings, locks in accordance with 7.2.1.6.3 shall be permitted.

### 11.8.3 Extinguishing Requirements.

**11.8.3.1*** High-rise buildings shall be protected throughout by an approved, supervised automatic sprinkler system in accordance with Section 9.7. A sprinkler control valve and a waterflow device shall be provided for each floor.

**A.11.8.3.1** Where an occupancy chapter (Chapters 12 through 42) permits the omission of sprinklers in specific spaces, such as small bathrooms and closets in residential occupancies, the building is still considered to be protected throughout for the purposes of 11.8.3.1.

**11.8.3.2** High-rise buildings shall be protected throughout by a Class I standpipe system in accordance with Section 9.7.

Paragraph 11.8.3.2 expands the menu of provisions that can be mandated for high-rise buildings — in accordance with the various occupancy chapters — to include standpipes. Exhibit 11.6 is an example of a typical standpipe.

Although the *Life Safety Code* has traditionally considered standpipes mainly as property protection devices, limited mandatory standpipe requirements for life safety purposes have been included for many editions of the *Code*. Standpipes are required on stages in assembly occupancies and in detention and correctional occupancies (see 12.4.5.12, 13.4.5.12, 22.3.5.5,

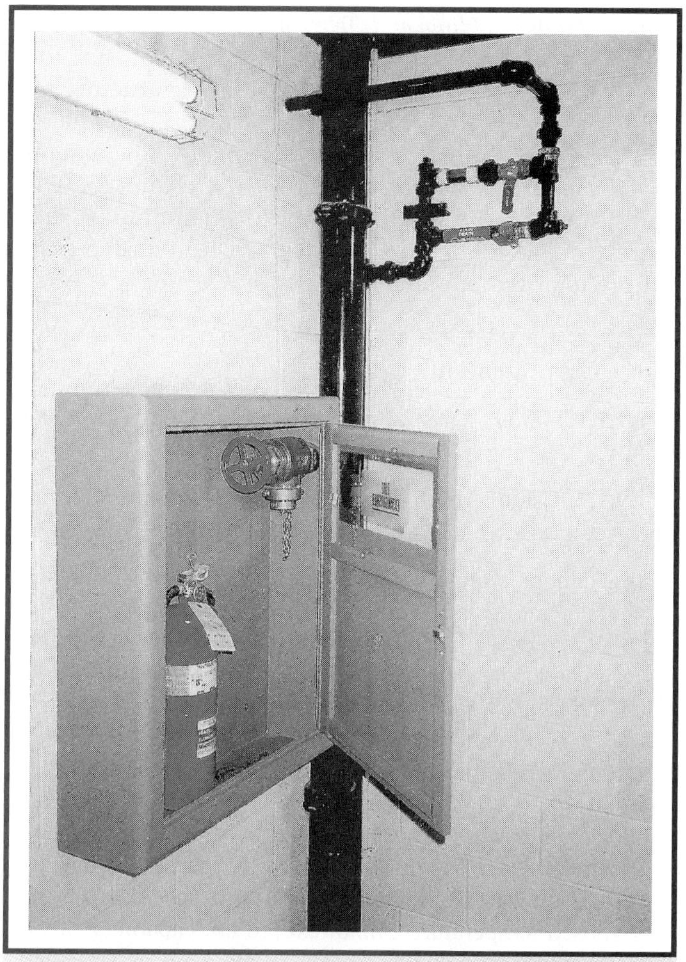

***Exhibit 11.6*** *Typical combination sprinkler/standpipe system with a $2\frac{1}{2}$ in. (64 mm) fire department valve.*

and 23.3.5.5). These requirements are based on the following:

1. Occupants will not be able to leave the fire area immediately, either due to the presence of large numbers of people, as is characteristic of an assembly occupancy, or because doors to the outside will be locked, as might be expected in a detention and correctional occupancy.
2. Trained personnel will be present early in the fire development to make effective use of the standpipe and hose.

Standpipes in high-rise buildings can serve to increase life safety, as well as property protection, because of the lengthy evacuation times associated with tall buildings. In many cases, fire emergency plans advise occupants who are not in immediate danger of exposure to fire to remain within the building to allow responding fire service personnel better access to the standpipes within the exit stair enclosures (staged evacuation). Use of standpipes at that time supplements the operation of the required automatic sprinkler system. See the commentary following A.9.6.3.6.2 for additional information on staged evacuation.

### 11.8.4 Detection, Alarm, and Communications Systems.

**11.8.4.1*** A fire alarm system using an approved emergency voice/alarm communication system shall be installed in accordance with Section 9.6.

**A.11.8.4.1** The need for voice communication can be based on a decision regarding staged or partial evacuation versus total evacuation of all floors. The determination of need is a function of occupancy classification and building height.

**11.8.4.2** Two-way telephone service shall be in accordance with 11.8.4.2.1 and 11.8.4.2.2.

**11.8.4.2.1** Two-way telephone communication service shall be provided for fire department use. This system shall be in accordance with *NFPA 72, National Fire Alarm Code*. The communications system shall operate between the emergency command center and every elevator car, every elevator lobby, and each floor level of exit stairs.

**11.8.4.2.2** The requirement of 11.8.4.2.1 shall not apply where the fire department radio system is approved as an equivalent system.

### 11.8.5 Emergency Lighting and Standby Power.

**11.8.5.1** Emergency lighting in accordance with Section 7.9 shall be provided.

**11.8.5.2** Requirements for standby power shall be as specified in 11.8.5.2.1 through 11.8.5.2.4.

**11.8.5.2.1** Type 60, Class 1, Level 1, standby power in accordance with Article 701 of *NFPA 70, National Electrical Code*, and NFPA 110, *Standard for Emergency and Standby Power Systems*, shall be provided.

**11.8.5.2.2** The standby power system shall have a capacity and rating sufficient to supply all equipment required to be connected by 11.8.5.2.4.

**11.8.5.2.3** Selective load pickup and load shedding shall be permitted in accordance with *NFPA 70, National Electrical Code*.

**11.8.5.2.4** The standby power system shall be connected to the following:

(1) Electric fire pump
(2) Emergency command center equipment and lighting

(3) Not less than one elevator serving all floors, with standby power transferable to any elevator
(4) Mechanical equipment for smokeproof enclosures
(5) Mechanical equipment required to conform with the requirements of Section 9.3

**11.8.5.3** Power for detection, alarm, and communications systems shall be in accordance with *NFPA 72, National Fire Alarm Code*.

### 11.8.6* Emergency Command Center.

**A.11.8.6** It is not the intent of the paragraph to require any of the equipment in the list, other than the telephone for fire department use, but only to provide the controls, panels, annunciators, and similar equipment at this location if the equipment is provided or required by another section of the *Code*.

**11.8.6.1** An emergency command center shall be provided in a location approved by the fire department.

**11.8.6.2** The emergency command center shall contain the following:

(1) Voice fire alarm system panels and controls
(2) Fire department two-way telephone communication service panels and controls where required by another section of this *Code*
(3) Fire detection and fire alarm system annunciation panels
(4) Elevator floor location and operation annunciators
(5) Elevator fire recall switch in accordance with ASME A17.1/CSA B44, *Safety Code for Elevators and Escalators*
(6) Elevator emergency power selector switch(es) where provided in accordance with ASME A17.1/CSA B44.
(7) Sprinkler valve and waterflow annunciators
(8) Emergency generator status indicators
(9) Controls for any automatic stairway door unlocking system
(10) Fire pump status indicators
(11) Telephone for fire department use with controlled access to the public telephone system

### 11.8.7 Emergency Plans.

Emergency plans shall be provided in accordance with 4.8.2.

## 11.9 Permanent Membrane Structures

The material in Section 11.9 was transferred into the 2000 edition of the *Code* from NFPA 102, *Standard for Grandstands, Folding and Telescopic Seating, Tents, and Membrane Structures*, so that all the provisions for life safety needed for a permanent membrane structure reside in this *Code*. Other material from NFPA 102 that is specific to assembly seating was moved to the assembly occupancy chapters — Chapters 12 and 13. The provisions applicable to permanent membrane structures are included in Chapter 11 because they can apply to any occupancy.

### 11.9.1 Application.

**11.9.1.1 General.** The provisions of Section 11.1 shall apply.

**11.9.1.2 Use of Membrane Roofs.** Membrane roofs shall be used in accordance with the following:

(1) Membrane materials shall not be used where fire resistance ratings are required for walls or roofs.
(2) Where every part of the roof, including the roof membrane, is not less than 20 ft (6100 mm) above any floor, balcony, or gallery, a noncombustible or limited-combustible membrane shall be permitted to be used as the roof in any construction type.
(3) With approval of the authority having jurisdiction, membrane materials shall be permitted to be used where every part of the roof membrane is sufficiently above every significant fire potential, such that the imposed temperature cannot exceed the capability of the membrane, including seams, to maintain its structural integrity.

**11.9.1.3 Testing.** Testing of membrane materials for compliance with the requirements of Section 11.9 for use of the categories of noncombustible and limited-combustible materials shall be performed on weathered-membrane material, as defined in 3.3.160.4.

**11.9.1.4 Flame Spread Index.** The flame spread index of all membrane materials exposed within the structure shall be Class A in accordance with Section 10.2.

**11.9.1.5 Roof Covering Classification.** Roof membranes shall have a roof covering classification, as required by the applicable building codes, when tested in accordance with NFPA 256, *Standard Methods of Fire Tests of Roof Coverings*, ASTM E 108, *Standard Test Methods for Fire Tests of Roof Coverings*; or ANSI/UL 790, *Test Methods for Fire Tests of Roof Coverings*.

**11.9.1.6 Flame Propagation Performance.**

**11.9.1.6.1** All membrane structure fabric shall meet the flame propagation performance criteria contained in NFPA 701, *Standard Methods of Fire Tests for Flame Propagation of Textiles and Films*.

**11.9.1.6.2** One of the following shall serve as evidence that the fabric materials have the required flame propagation performance:

(1) The authority having jurisdiction shall require a certificate or other evidence of acceptance by an organization acceptable to the authority having jurisdiction.
(2) The authority having jurisdiction shall require a report of tests made by other inspection authorities or organizations acceptable to the authority having jurisdiction.

**11.9.1.6.3** Where required by the authority having jurisdiction, confirmatory field tests shall be conducted using test specimens from the original material, which shall have been affixed at the time of manufacture to the exterior of the structure.

### 11.9.2 Tensioned-Membrane Structures.

One well-known tensioned-membrane structure is the main terminal building at Denver International Airport, as shown in Exhibit 11.7.

**11.9.2.1** The design, materials, and construction of the building shall be based on plans and specifications prepared by a licensed architect or engineer knowledgeable in tensioned-membrane construction.

**11.9.2.2** Material loads and strength shall be based on physical properties of the materials verified and certified by an approved testing laboratory.

**11.9.2.3** The membrane roof for structures in climates subject to freezing temperatures and ice buildup shall be composed of two layers separated by an air space through which heated air can be moved to guard against ice accumulation. As an alternative to the two layers, other approved methods that protect against ice accumulation shall be permitted.

**11.9.2.4** Roof drains shall be equipped with electrical elements to protect against ice buildup that can prevent the drains from functioning. Such heating elements shall be served by on-site standby electrical power in addition to the normal public service. As an alternative to such electrical elements, other approved methods that protect against ice accumulation shall be permitted.

### 11.9.3 Air-Supported and Air-Inflated Structures.

**11.9.3.1 General.** In addition to the general provisions of 11.9.1, the requirements of 11.9.3 shall apply to air-supported and air-inflated structures.

**11.9.3.2 Pressurization (Inflation) System.** The pressurization system shall consist of one or more operating blower units. The system shall include automatic control of

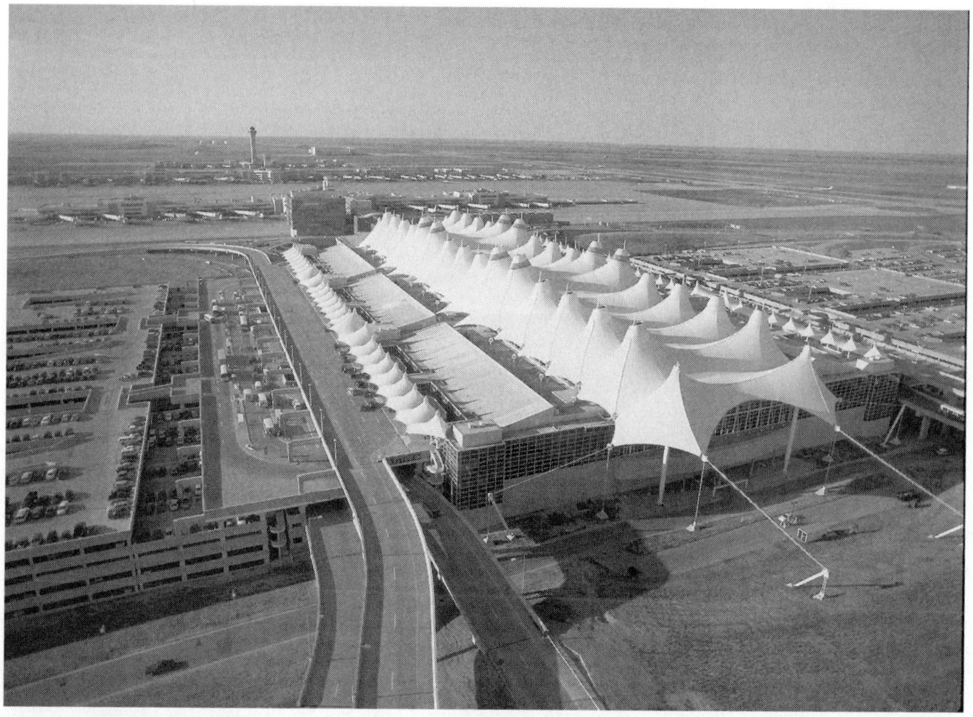

***Exhibit 11.7*** *Example of a tensioned-membrane structure: Denver International Airport. (Photo courtesy of the Denver International Airport)*

auxiliary blower units to maintain the required operating pressure. Such equipment shall meet the following requirements:

(1) Blowers shall be powered by continuous-rated motors at the maximum power required.
(2) Blowers shall have personnel protection, such as inlet screens and belt guards.
(3) Blower systems shall be weather protected.
(4) Blower systems shall be equipped with backdraft check dampers.
(5) Not less than two blower units shall be provided, each of which has capacity to maintain full inflation pressure with normal leakage.
(6) The blowers shall be designed to be incapable of overpressurization.
(7) The auxiliary blower unit(s) shall operate automatically if there is any loss of internal pressure or if an operating blower unit becomes inoperative.
(8) The design inflation pressure and the capacity of each blower system shall be certified by a professional engineer.

**11.9.3.3 Standby Power System.**

**11.9.3.3.1*** A fully automatic standby power system shall be provided. The system shall be either an auxiliary engine generator set capable of running the blower system or a supplementary blower unit that is sized for 1 times the normal operating capacity and is powered by an internal combustion engine.

**A.11.9.3.3.1** The requirements of this paragraph can be considered as a Class 4, Type 60, system per NFPA 110, *Standard for Emergency and Standby Power Systems.*

**11.9.3.3.2** The standby power system shall be fully automatic to ensure continuous inflation in the event of any failure of the primary power. The system shall be capable of operating continuously for a minimum of 4 hours.

**11.9.3.3.3** The sizing and capacity of the standby power system shall be certified by a professional engineer.

The indoor sports facility pictured in Exhibit 11.8 is an example of an air-supported structure. Because it houses an assembly occupancy, it must also meet the requirements of Chapter 12 or Chapter 13, as applicable. For such an occupancy, special attention should be paid to the crowd manager requirements of 12/13.7.6.

The "sports dome" pictured in Exhibit 11.8 was destroyed by a blizzard in 2005. Fortunately, it was unoccupied when it collapsed.

### 11.9.4 Maintenance and Operation.

**11.9.4.1** Instructions in both operation and maintenance shall be transmitted to the owner by the manufacturer of the tensioned-membrane, air-supported, or air-inflated structure.

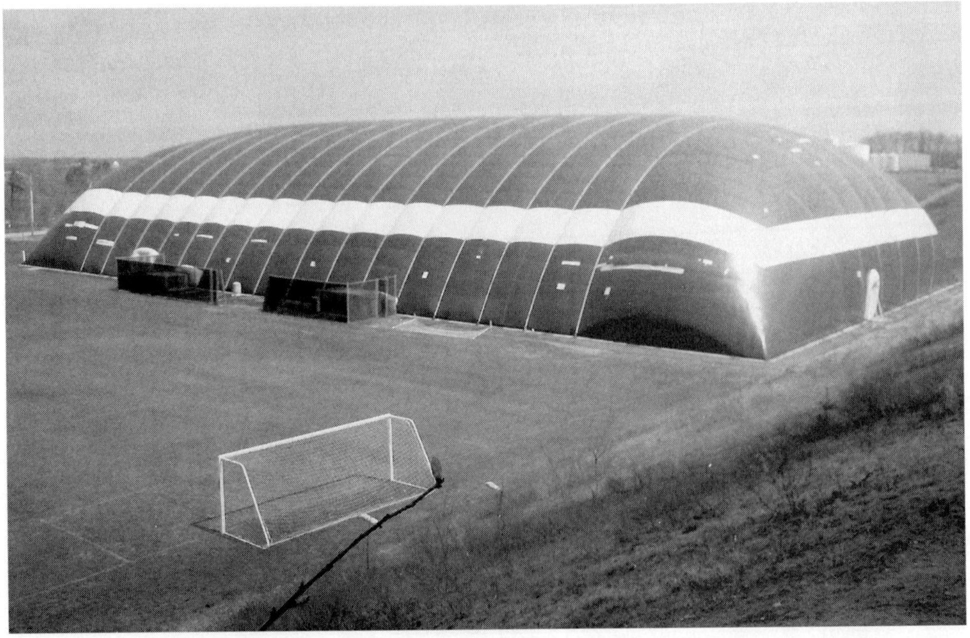

***Exhibit 11.8*** *An air-supported structure housing sporting fields.*

**11.9.4.2** Annual inspection and required maintenance of each structure shall be performed to ensure safety conditions. At least biennially, the inspection shall be performed by a professional engineer, registered architect, or individual certified by the manufacturer.

### 11.9.5 Services.

**11.9.5.1 Fired Heaters.**

**11.9.5.1.1** Only labeled heating devices shall be used.

**11.9.5.1.2** Fuel-fired heaters and their installation shall be approved by the authority having jurisdiction.

**11.9.5.1.3** Containers for liquefied petroleum gases shall be installed not less than 60 in. (1525 mm) from any temporary membrane structure and shall be in accordance with the provisions of NFPA 58, *Liquefied Petroleum Gas Code*.

**11.9.5.1.4** Tanks shall be secured in the upright position and protected from vehicular traffic.

**11.9.5.2 Electric Heaters.**

**11.9.5.2.1** Only labeled heaters shall be permitted.

**11.9.5.2.2** Electric heaters, their placement, and their installation shall be approved by the authority having jurisdiction.

**11.9.5.2.3** Heaters shall be connected to electricity by electric cable that is suitable for outside use and is of sufficient size to handle the electrical load.

## 11.10 Temporary Membrane Structures

The material in Section 11.10 was transferred into the 2000 edition of the *Code* from NFPA 102, *Standard for Grandstands, Folding and Telescopic Seating, Tents, and Membrane Structures*, so that all the provisions for life safety needed for a temporary membrane structure reside in this *Code*. Other material from NFPA 102 that is specific to assembly seating was moved to the assembly occupancy chapters — Chapters 12 and 13. The provisions applicable to temporary membrane structures are included in Chapter 11 because they can apply to any occupancy.

### 11.10.1 Application.

**11.10.1.1 General.** The provisions of Section 11.1 shall apply.

**11.10.1.2 Required Approval.** Membrane structures designed to meet all the requirements of Section 11.10 shall be permitted to be used as temporary buildings subject to the approval of the authority having jurisdiction.

**11.10.1.3 Alternative Requirements.** Temporary tensioned-membrane structures shall be permitted to comply with Section 11.11 instead of Section 11.10.

**11.10.1.4 Roof Covering Classification.** Roof membranes shall have a roof covering classification, as required by the applicable building codes, when tested in accordance with NFPA 256, *Standard Methods of Fire Tests of Roof Coverings*; ASTM E 108, *Standard Test Methods for Fire Tests of Roof Coverings*; or ANSI/UL 790, *Test Methods for Fire Tests of Roof Coverings*.

**11.10.1.5 Flame Propagation Performance.**

**11.10.1.5.1** All membrane structure fabric shall meet the flame propagation performance criteria contained in NFPA 701, *Standard Methods of Fire Tests for Flame Propagation of Textiles and Films*.

**11.10.1.5.2** One of the following shall serve as evidence that the fabric materials have the required flame propagation performance:

(1) The authority having jurisdiction shall require a certificate or other evidence of acceptance by an organization acceptable to the authority having jurisdiction.
(2) The authority having jurisdiction shall require a report of tests made by other inspection authorities or organizations acceptable to the authority having jurisdiction.

**11.10.1.5.3** Where required by the authority having jurisdiction, confirmatory field tests shall be conducted using test specimens from the original material, which shall have been affixed at the time of manufacture to the exterior of the structure.

### 11.10.2 Fire Hazards.

**11.10.2.1** The finished ground level enclosed by any temporary membrane structure, and the finished ground level for a reasonable distance but for not less than 10 ft (3050 mm) outside of such a structure, shall be cleared of all flammable or combustible material or vegetation that is not used for necessary support equipment. The clearing work shall be accomplished to the satisfaction of the authority having jurisdiction prior to the erection of such a structure. The premises shall be kept free from such flammable or combustible materials during the period for which the premises are used by the public.

**11.10.2.2** Where prohibited by the authority having jurisdiction, smoking shall not be permitted in any temporary membrane structure.

### 11.10.3 Fire-Extinguishing Equipment.

Portable fire-extinguishing equipment of approved types shall be furnished and maintained in temporary membrane structures in such quantity and in such locations as directed by the authority having jurisdiction.

### 11.10.4 Tensioned-Membrane Structures.

**11.10.4.1** The design, materials, and construction of the building shall be based on plans and specifications prepared by a licensed architect or engineer knowledgeable in tensioned-membrane construction.

**11.10.4.2** Material loads and strength shall be based on physical properties of the materials verified and certified by an approved testing laboratory.

**11.10.4.3** The membrane roof for structures in climates subject to freezing temperatures and ice buildup shall be composed of two layers separated by an air space through which heated air can be moved to guard against ice accumulation. As an alternative to the two layers, other approved methods that protect against ice accumulation shall be permitted.

**11.10.4.4** Roof drains shall be equipped with electrical elements to protect against ice buildup that can prevent the drains from functioning. Such heating elements shall be served by on-site standby electrical power in addition to the normal public service. As an alternative to such electrical elements, other approved methods that protect against ice accumulation shall be permitted.

### 11.10.5 Air-Supported and Air-Inflated Structures.

**11.10.5.1 General.** In addition to the general provisions of 11.10.1, the requirements of 11.10.5 shall apply to air-supported and air-inflated structures.

**11.10.5.2 Pressurization (Inflation) System.** The pressurization system shall consist of one or more operating blower units. The system shall include automatic control of auxiliary blower units to maintain the required operating pressure. Such equipment shall meet the following requirements:

(1) Blowers shall be powered by continuous-rated motors at the maximum power required.
(2) Blowers shall have personnel protection, such as inlet screens and belt guards.
(3) Blower systems shall be weather protected.
(4) Blower systems shall be equipped with backdraft check dampers.
(5) Not less than two blower units shall be provided, each of which has capacity to maintain full inflation pressure with normal leakage.
(6) Blowers shall be designed to be incapable of overpressurization.
(7) The auxiliary blower unit(s) shall operate automatically if there is any loss of internal pressure or if an operating blower unit becomes inoperative.
(8) The design inflation pressure and the capacity of each blower system shall be certified by a professional engineer.

**11.10.5.3 Standby Power System.**

**11.10.5.3.1** A fully automatic standby power system shall be provided. The system shall be either an auxiliary engine generator set capable of running the blower system or a supplementary blower unit that is sized for 1 times the normal operating capacity and is powered by an internal combustion engine.

**11.10.5.3.2** The standby power system shall be fully automatic to ensure continuous inflation in the event of any failure of the primary power. The system shall be capable of operating continuously for a minimum of 4 hours.

**11.10.5.3.3** The sizing and capacity of the standby power system shall be certified by a professional engineer.

### 11.10.6 Maintenance and Operation.

**11.10.6.1** Instructions in both operation and maintenance shall be transmitted to the owner by the manufacturer of the tensioned-membrane, air-supported, or air-inflated structure.

**11.10.6.2** Annual inspection and required maintenance of each structure shall be performed to ensure safety conditions. At least biennially, the inspection shall be performed by a professional engineer, registered architect, or individual certified by the manufacturer.

### 11.10.7 Services.

**11.10.7.1 Fired Heaters.**

**11.10.7.1.1** Only labeled heating devices shall be used.

**11.10.7.1.2** Fuel-fired heaters and their installation shall be approved by the authority having jurisdiction.

**11.10.7.1.3** Containers for liquefied petroleum gases shall be installed not less than 60 in. (1525 mm) from any temporary membrane structure and shall be in accordance with the provisions of NFPA 58, *Liquefied Petroleum Gas Code*.

**11.10.7.1.4** Tanks shall be secured in the upright position and protected from vehicular traffic.

**11.10.7.2 Electric Heaters.**

**11.10.7.2.1** Only labeled heaters shall be permitted.

**11.10.7.2.2** Heaters used inside a temporary membrane structure shall be approved.

**11.10.7.2.3** Heaters shall be connected to electricity by electric cable that is suitable for outside use and is of sufficient size to handle the electrical load.

## 11.11 Tents

The material in Section 11.11 was transferred into the *Code* from NFPA 102, *Standard for Grandstands, Folding and Telescopic Seating, Tents, and Membrane Structures,* so that all the provisions for life safety needed for a tent reside in this *Code*. Other material from NFPA 102 that is specific to assembly seating was moved to the assembly occupancy chapters — Chapters 12 and 13. The provisions applicable to tents are included in Chapter 11 because they can apply to any occupancy.

### 11.11.1 General.

**11.11.1.1** The provisions of Section 11.1 shall apply.

**11.11.1.2** Tents shall be permitted only on a temporary basis.

**11.11.1.3** Tents shall be erected to cover not more than 75 percent of the premises, unless otherwise approved by the authority having jurisdiction.

### 11.11.2 Flame Propagation Performance.

**11.11.2.1** All tent fabric shall meet the flame propagation performance criteria contained in NFPA 701, *Standard Methods of Fire Tests for Flame Propagation of Textiles and Films.*

**11.11.2.2** One of the following shall serve as evidence that the tent fabric materials have the required flame propagation performance:

(1) The authority having jurisdiction shall require a certificate or other evidence of acceptance by an organization acceptable to the authority having jurisdiction.
(2) The authority having jurisdiction shall require a report of tests made by other inspection authorities or organizations acceptable to the authority having jurisdiction.

**11.11.2.3** Where required by the authority having jurisdiction, confirmatory field tests shall be conducted using test specimens from the original material, which shall have been affixed at the time of manufacture to the exterior of the tent.

### 11.11.3 Location and Spacing.

**11.11.3.1** There shall be a minimum of 10 ft (3050 mm) between stake lines.

**11.11.3.2** Adjacent tents shall be spaced to provide an area to be used as a means of emergency egress. Where 10 ft (3050 mm) between stake lines does not meet the requirements for means of egress, the distance necessary for means of egress shall govern.

**11.11.3.3** Tents not occupied by the public and not used for the storage of combustible material shall be permitted to be erected less than 10 ft (3050 mm) from other structures where the authority having jurisdiction deems such close spacing to be safe from hazard to the public.

**11.11.3.4** Tents, each not exceeding 1200 $ft^2$ (112 $m^2$) in finished ground level area and located in fairgrounds or similar open spaces, shall not be required to be separated from each other, provided that safety precautions meet the approval of the authority having jurisdiction.

**11.11.3.5** The placement of tents relative to other structures shall be at the discretion of the authority having jurisdiction, with consideration given to occupancy, use, opening, exposure, and other similar factors.

### 11.11.4 Fire Hazards.

**11.11.4.1** The finished ground level enclosed by any tent, and the finished ground level for a reasonable distance, but for not less than 10 ft (3050 mm) outside of such a tent, shall be cleared of all flammable or combustible material or vegetation that is not used for necessary support equipment. The clearing work shall be accomplished to the satisfaction of the authority having jurisdiction prior to the erection of such a tent. The premises shall be kept free from such flammable or combustible materials during the period for which the premises are used by the public.

**11.11.4.2** Where prohibited by the authority having jurisdiction, smoking shall not be permitted in any tent.

### 11.11.5 Fire-Extinguishing Equipment.

Portable fire-extinguishing equipment of approved types shall be furnished and maintained in tents in such quantity and in such locations as directed by the authority having jurisdiction.

### 11.11.6 Services.

**11.11.6.1 Fired Heaters.**

**11.11.6.1.1** Only labeled heating devices shall be used.

**11.11.6.1.2** Fuel-fired heaters and their installation shall be approved by the authority having jurisdiction.

**11.11.6.1.3** Containers for liquefied petroleum gases shall be installed not less than 60 in. (1525 mm) from any tent and shall be in accordance with the provisions of NFPA 58, *Liquefied Petroleum Gas Code.*

**11.11.6.1.4** Tanks shall be secured in the upright position and protected from vehicular traffic.

**11.11.6.2 Electric Heaters.**

**11.11.6.2.1** Only labeled heaters shall be permitted.

**11.11.6.2.2** Heaters used inside a tent shall be approved.

**11.11.6.2.3** Heaters shall be connected to electricity by electric cable that is suitable for outside use and is of sufficient size to handle the electrical load.

## References Cited in Commentary

1. NFPA 102, *Standard for Grandstands, Folding and Telescopic Seating, Tents, and Membrane Structures*, 2006 edition, National Fire Protection Association, Quincy, MA.
2. *NFPA 5000®, Building Construction and Safety Code®*, 2009 edition, National Fire Protection Association, Quincy, MA.
3. NFPA 220, *Standard on Types of Building Construction*, 2009 edition, National Fire Protection Association, Quincy, MA.
4. NFPA 520, *Standard on Subterranean Spaces*, 2005 edition, National Fire Protection Association, Quincy, MA.

CHAPTERS 12 AND 13

# New and Existing Assembly Occupancies

Chapters 12 and 13 are the first of the numerous occupancy chapters that address a specific building use based on the occupancy classification system developed in Chapter 6. The occupancy chapters of the *Code* work together with the core chapters to implement the fundamental requirements of the core chapters, as appropriate to a specific use. The occupancy chapters provide a complete road map to all applicable provisions in the core chapters via the mandatory references and specific permissions contained in the occupancy chapters.

The requirements for assembly occupancies are based on protecting concentrations of occupants in a building or area.

The occupant load factors for assembly uses (see Table 7.3.1.2) accurately reflect the large numbers of occupants in a given area that are characteristic of such use. Large numbers of occupants present unique challenges, such as arranging and designing the egress facilities to move the occupants efficiently and quickly. In addition, there are issues that must be balanced, such as sloping the floor to achieve line of sight for audience spectators (e.g., during theater performances, sporting events, or concerts) without creating stepped aisles that are too steep to use effectively.

The level of life safety mandated by Chapters 12 and 13 addresses many conditions that are often taken for granted by the public. The exit access from occupant seating areas to aisles in a movie theater, for example, is regulated by these chapters, as is the arrangement of tables and chairs in a restaurant (see 12/13.2.5.7). This regulation provides a reasonable egress path if a fire occurs.

Section 12/13.4 addresses special provisions and contains a series of specific and unique rules for assembly occupancies. The concept of smoke-protected assembly seating (see 12/13.4.2) is intended to provide a realistic egress capacity for an assembly occupancy that performs under fire conditions as if it were outdoors. This concept departs somewhat from the prescriptive rules usually imposed on an occupancy. The use of smoke-protected assembly seating, however, requires a life safety evaluation in accordance with 12/13.4.1 that addresses many aspects associated with the potential threat to a large number of occupants.

Other special subjects addressed in Section 12/13.4 include stages and platforms (12/13.4.5), projection rooms (12/13.4.6), special amusement buildings (12/13.4.7), grandstands (12/13.4.8), folding and telescopic seating (12/13.4.9), and airport loading walkways (12/13.4.10).

Assembly occupancies include, but are not limited to, buildings or portions of buildings used for gatherings of 50 or more people for such purposes as deliberation, worship, entertainment, eating, drinking, amusement, or awaiting transportation. Assembly occupancies also include special amusement buildings (such as a fun house attraction at an amusement park or a multilevel play structure in a fast-food restaurant), regardless of occupant load (see item 2 of 6.1.2.1 and 12/13.4.7).

For other than special amusement buildings, the criteria for assembly occupancy classification include the 50-person threshold addressed in the previous paragraph and consideration of the activities in which those persons are involved. The activities that lead to the classification of an occupancy as an assembly occupancy include those detailed in item 1 of 6.1.2.1 — deliberation, worship, entertainment, drinking, amusement, awaiting transportation, or similar uses. For example, working at a desk in a large open-plan office area is not an assembly use, so the presence of 50 or more persons in the office space constitutes a business occupancy, not an assembly occupancy. Examples of assembly occupancies include the following, if they have an occupant load of at least 50 persons:

1. Armories
2. Assembly halls
3. Auditoriums
4. Bowling establishments
5. Churches
6. Club rooms
7. Conference rooms
8. Courtrooms
9. Dance halls
10. Discotheques
11. Drinking establishments
12. Exposition halls
13. Gymnasiums
14. Libraries
15. Mortuary chapels
16. Motion picture theaters
17. Multilevel play structures (regardless of occupant load)
18. Museums
19. Nightclubs
20. Pool rooms
21. Recreation piers
22. Restaurants
23. Skating rinks
24. Theaters

Passenger stations and terminals of air, surface, underground, and marine public transportation facilities are also considered assembly occupancies. If the jurisdiction enforcing the *Code* has adopted NFPA 130, *Standard for Fixed Guideway Transit and Passenger Rail Systems*,[1] requirements for transit stations might fall under NFPA 130 rather than this *Code*. See NFPA 130 for additional details.

Assembly occupancies with an occupant load of fewer than 50 persons (except for special amusement buildings) are considered incidental to the predominant occupancy in which they are located. For example, a conference room with fewer than a 50-person occupant load (see 7.3.1.2) that is located in an office area is considered part of the overall business occupancy. A freestanding diner with an occupant load of fewer than 50 persons is normally assigned a mercantile occupancy classification. Regardless of occupancy classification, the occupant load for areas of assembly use needs to be calculated based on the use of the space, not the occupancy classification, using the occupant load factors of Table 7.3.1.2 for assembly uses.

## 12.1 General Requirements

### 12.1.1 Application.

The requirements of this chapter shall apply to new buildings or portions thereof used as an assembly occupancy. *(See 1.3.1.)*

## 13.1 General Requirements

### 13.1.1 Application.

**13.1.1.1** The requirements of this chapter shall apply to existing buildings or portions thereof currently occupied as assembly occupancies, unless otherwise specified by 13.1.1.2. *(See 3.3.178.2 for definition of assembly occupancy.)*

**13.1.1.2** An existing building housing an assembly occupancy established prior to the effective date of this *Code* shall be permitted to be approved for continued use if it conforms to, or is made to conform to, the provisions of this *Code* to the extent that, in the opinion of the authority having jurisdiction, reasonable life safety against the hazards of fire, explosion, and panic is provided and maintained.

**13.1.1.3** Additions to existing buildings shall conform to the requirements of 4.6.8.

**13.1.1.4** Existing portions of buildings shall be upgraded if the addition results in an increase in the required minimum number of separate means of egress in accordance with 7.4.1.2.

**13.1.1.5** Existing portions of the structure shall not be required to be modified, provided that both of the following criteria are met:

(1) The new construction has not diminished the fire safety features of the facility.
(2) The addition does not result in an increase in the required minimum number of separate means of egress in accordance with 7.4.1.2.

**13.1.1.6** An assembly occupancy in which an occupant load increase results in an increase in the required minimum number of separate means of egress, in accordance with 7.4.1.2, shall meet the requirements for new construction.

The provisions for new assembly occupancies are addressed in Chapter 12; the provisions for existing assembly occupancies (i.e., existing conditions in assembly occupancies) are addressed in Chapter 13.

In editions of the *Code* prior to 2006, renovations, additions, and changes of occupancy were required to comply with the requirements for new construction. For assembly occupancies, such renovations, additions, and changes of occupancy were required to meet the provisions of Chapter 12, while existing conditions were subject to the provisions of Chapter 13. The subject is now addressed by Chapter 43, Building Rehabilitation. The chapter was written to promote the adaptive reuse of existing buildings without sacrificing the needed level of life safety. The provisions of Chapter 43 blend the requirements for new construction with those for existing conditions so as to require additional life safety features as the rehabilitation work category increases in complexity. The rehabilitation work categories are repair, renovation, modification, reconstruction, change of use, change of occupancy classification, and addition. See 4.6.8, 4.6.12, and Chapter 43.

Paragraph 13.1.1.3 mandates that additions to existing assembly occupancies meet the requirements of 4.6.8, which mandates the use of Chapter 43. Per 43.8.1.1(1), the addition must comply with the requirements for new construction (i.e., Chapter 12 for assembly occupancies). The provisions of 43.8.1.1(2) require that the existing portion of the building comply with the requirements for existing conditions (i.e., Chapter 13 for existing assembly occupancies), but 13.1.1.4 adds a requirement. Per 13.1.1.4, if construction of an addition causes the occupant load to increase to the point that 7.4.1.2 would require an increase in the required minimum number of means of egress, then the existing portion of the building must be upgraded to meet the requirements for new construction.

For example, prior to the addition, the floor area of an existing assembly occupancy might be such that the occupant load is 900 persons, which, per 7.4.1.2 (and 13.2.4.3), requires the assembly occupancy to be provided with three means of egress. After the addition, the increased floor area accommodates an occupant load of 1100 persons, which, per 7.4.1.2, requires four means of egress. The increase in required minimum number of means of egress — from three to four — results in the existing assembly occupancy being subject to the provisions of Chapter 12 for new assembly occupancies.

The provisions of 13.1.1.6 are similar to those of 13.1.1.4 in that, if the occupant load increases so that an increase in the required minimum number of separate means of egress is mandated by 7.4.1.2, the existing building must be modified to comply with the requirements of Chapter 12 for new assembly occupancies. Paragraph 13.1.1.4 addresses such changes occurring as a result of an addition; 13.1.1.6 encompasses such situations as renovation of an existing building or a higher occupant load being granted by the authority having jurisdiction (AHJ) under the provisions of 7.3.1.3.

For example, large dining tables might be replaced by small cocktail tables, permitting a larger occupant load even though the building size has not increased. The occupant load prior to the change in table size was 550 persons, which, per 13.2.4.2, requires the assembly occupancy to be provided with two means of egress. After the new tables are installed, the occupant load is increased to 650 persons, which, per 13.2.4.3, requires three means of egress. The increase in required minimum number of means of egress — from two to three — results in the existing assembly occupancy being subject to the provisions of Chapter 12 for new assembly occupancies.

CHAPTER 12 • New

### 12.1.2 Multiple Occupancies.

**12.1.2.1 General.** Multiple occupancies shall be in accordance with 6.1.14.

**12.1.2.2* Simultaneous Occupancy.** Exits shall be sufficient for simultaneous occupancy of both the assembly occupancy and other parts of the building, except where the authority having jurisdiction determines that the conditions are such that simultaneous occupancy will not occur.

**A.12.1.2.2** For example, an assembly room for the residents of a detention occupancy will not normally be subject to simultaneous occupancy.

CHAPTER 13 • Existing

### 13.1.2 Multiple Occupancies.

**13.1.2.1 General.** Multiple occupancies shall be in accordance with 6.1.14.

**13.1.2.2* Simultaneous Occupancy.** Exits shall be sufficient for simultaneous occupancy of both the assembly occupancy and other parts of the building, except where the authority having jurisdiction determines that the conditions are such that simultaneous occupancy will not occur.

**A.13.1.2.2** For example, an assembly room for the residents of a detention occupancy will not normally be subject to simultaneous occupancy.

The provision of 12/13.1.2.2 that exempts exits from the simultaneous occupancy requirement should be used judiciously, with all possible uses being considered before it is judged whether simultaneous occupancy will occur. For example, a school gymnasium might normally be used only by the school occupants; however, it might be used by an outside group during school hours, such as occurs when school gymnasiums function as polling locations on election day. See Exhibit 12/13.1. A means of egress system sized to accommodate simultaneous occupancy provides maximum flexibility in the use of the building.

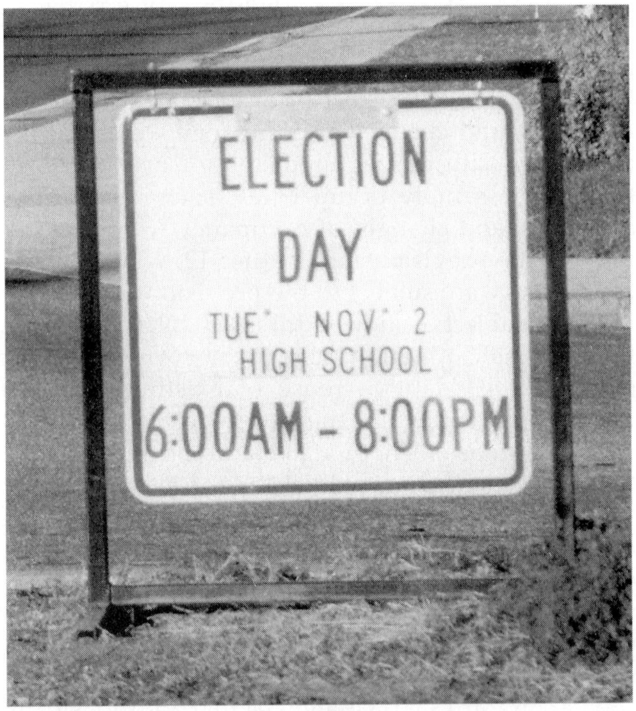


***Exhibit 12/13.1*** *Use of school building for simultaneous mixed occupancy purposes.*

CHAPTER 12 • New

**12.1.2.3 Assembly and Mercantile Occupancies in Mall Buildings.**

**12.1.2.3.1** The provisions of Chapter 12 shall apply to the assembly occupancy tenant space.

**12.1.2.3.2** The provisions of 36.4.4 shall be permitted to be used outside the assembly occupancy tenant space.

CHAPTER 13 • Existing

**13.1.2.3 Assembly and Mercantile Occupancies in Mall Buildings.**

**13.1.2.3.1** The provisions of Chapter 13 shall apply to the assembly occupancy tenant space.

**13.1.2.3.2** The provisions of 37.4.4 shall be permitted to be used outside the assembly occupancy tenant space.

CHAPTER 12 • New

Paragraph 12/13.1.2.3 addresses the common situation in which mall buildings include assembly occupancies in addition to mercantile and other occupancies. The assembly occupancies are required to comply with the requirements of Chapters 12 and 13 up to the point in the egress system at which the occupants reach the mall. The remainder of the egress path — which passes through the mall and discharges to the public way — is addressed in the mercantile occupancy chapters in the specialized mall building provisions of 36/37.4.4. Subsection 36/37.4.4 requires that egress from the mall be sufficient for an occupant load based on the gross leasable area of the overall mall building, not a calculation directly related to the area of only the mall (i.e., the covered pedestrian way that connects the various stores and assembly areas). Although this calculation method does not take into consideration the actual number of persons sent into the mall from the assembly occupancy, it is reliable. The concept is addressed in the commentary following 36/37.4.4.10.2.

### 12.1.3* Special Definitions.

A list of special terms used in this chapter follows:

(1) **Aisle Accessway.** See 3.3.11.
(2) **Exhibit.** See 3.3.71.
(3) **Exhibitor.** See 3.3.72.
(4) **Exposition.** See 3.3.78.
(5) **Exposition Facility.** See 3.3.82.1.
(6) **Festival Seating.** See 3.3.221.1.
(7) **Flow Time.** See 3.3.107.
(8) **Fly Gallery.** See 3.3.108.
(9) **Gridiron.** See 3.3.117.
(10) **Legitimate Stage.** See 3.3.246.1.
(11) **Life Safety Evaluation.** See 3.3.148.
(12) **Multilevel Play Structure.** See 3.3.254.5.
(13) **Multipurpose Assembly Occupancy.** See 3.3.178.2.1.
(14) **Pinrail.** See 3.3.194.
(15) **Platform.** See 3.3.195.
(16) **Proscenium Wall.** See 3.3.268.2.
(17) **Regular Stage.** See 3.3.246.2.
(18) **Smoke-Protected Assembly Seating.** See 3.3.221.4.
(19) **Special Amusement Building.** See 3.3.32.10.
(20) **Stage.** See 3.3.246.
(21) **Temporary Platform.** See 3.3.195.1.

**A.12.1.3** An understanding of the term *accessory room* might be useful to the enforcer of the *Code*, although the term is not used within the *Code*. An accessory room includes a dressing room, the property master's work and storage rooms, the carpenter's room, or similar rooms necessary for legitimate stage operations.

CHAPTER 13 • Existing

### 13.1.3* Special Definitions.

A list of special terms used in this chapter follows:

(1) **Aisle Accessway.** See 3.3.11.
(2) **Exhibit.** See 3.3.71.
(3) **Exhibitor.** See 3.3.72.
(4) **Exposition.** See 3.3.78.
(5) **Exposition Facility.** See 3.3.82.1.
(6) **Festival Seating.** See 3.3.221.1.
(7) **Flow Time.** See 3.3.107.
(8) **Fly Gallery.** See 3.3.108.
(9) **Gridiron.** See 3.3.117.
(10) **Legitimate Stage.** See 3.3.246.1.
(11) **Life Safety Evaluation.** See 3.3.148.
(12) **Multilevel Play Structure.** See 3.3.254.5.
(13) **Pinrail.** See 3.3.194.
(14) **Platform.** See 3.3.195.
(15) **Proscenium Wall.** See 3.3.268.2.
(16) **Regular Stage.** See 3.3.246.2.
(17) **Smoke-Protected Assembly Seating.** See 3.3.221.4.
(18) **Special Amusement Building.** See 3.3.32.10.
(19) **Stage.** See 3.3.246.
(20) **Temporary Platform.** See 3.3.195.1.

**A.13.1.3** An understanding of the term *accessory room* might be useful to the enforcer of the *Code*, although the term is not used within the *Code*. An accessory room includes a dressing room, the property master's work and storage rooms, the carpenter's room, or similar rooms necessary for legitimate stage operations.

The terms in 12/13.1.3 have special meanings with respect to assembly occupancies. The commentary that follows addresses some of the terms. For definitions of all these terms, see Chapter 3.

The term *aisle accessway* is that part of the exit access (typically the row space occupied by one's legs and feet) located between where an occupant is seated and an aisle. For seating at tables (e.g., classroom style), the aisle accessway is typically the space located between the back of an occupant's chair and the table immediately behind. See 12/13.2.5.5 and 12/13.2.5.7.

The definitions of the terms *exhibit*, *exhibitor*, *exposition*, and *exposition facility* relate to the provisions in 12/13.7.5. The terms are consistent with terms used by the exposition industry.

The term *festival seating* is addressed in 12/13.2.5.4.1.

The term *flow time* is used in the technical literature on egress and is important to understand in relation to the *Code*'s requirements for the capacity of means of egress. Flow time is the time taken by a crowd to pass, for example, through a doorway during group egress. Flow time contributes to the total time needed to evacuate an area after an emergency is detected and an alarm is sounded. In the case of large assembly buildings, flow time is often the largest component of total evacuation time, which also includes the time taken to respond to an alarm before egress begins and to travel the length of an egress route. Although Chapters 12 and 13 of the *Code* do not specifically require that flow time be used, the term is provided to help improve understanding of the nominal performance expected in complying with particular egress capacity requirements.

The term *life safety evaluation* is used in 12/13.1.7.3, 12/13.2.5.4.1(2), 12/13.4.1, and 12/13.4.2.2. See A.12/13.4.1.1 and A.12/13.4.1.3 in particular. A life safety evaluation addresses more than fire safety. A life safety evaluation considers all life safety hazards that could endanger occupants and require rapid egress or other measures to maintain occupant safety. For example, fire might not be the most likely hazard in some large assembly facilities. Injuries and deaths might result from the actions of a large number of people occupying a limited space during normal occupancy conditions, such as when spectators become especially enthusiastic during an event. A sudden change in weather at an outdoor facility or a partial structural collapse might cause occupants to attempt to escape an area. Such situations must be taken into account during a life safety evaluation. In some cases, special expertise will be required to assess, design, or manage social and behavioral factors in addition to fire and structural safety considerations. In general, the life safety evaluation requires a comprehensive understanding of occupant characteristics, especially if densely crowded conditions exist.

*Multilevel play structures* have become commonplace. Some are entities unto themselves and draw patrons strictly because of the amusement offered. Others are operated in conjunction with some other business, such as the play structures attached to fast-food restaurants. Multilevel play structures are considered special amusement buildings. Special amusement buildings are assembly occupancies, regardless of occupant load. See 6.1.2.1 and 12/13.4.7.

The term *multipurpose assembly occupancy* is synonymous with the term *multipurpose room*, as used in 12.3.5.3(1). Multipurpose rooms are often part of a school, office building, fellowship hall, or other occupancy.

The definition of the term *special amusement building* (see 3.3.32.10), which has application in the provisions of 12/13.4.7, addresses both the structure of such buildings and their use. The structure might be a permanent building or a semitrailer truck or other similar enclosure that is semipermanent or mobile. Special amusement buildings are not open-air structures. Structures that are not fully enclosed (e.g., a merry-go-round with a roof and no side walls) are not special amusement buildings as explained in A.3.3.32.10. The definition also includes special amusement buildings within larger structures, such as an amusement building within a shopping mall. Theaters, movie houses, or similar assembly occupancies used for amusement or entertainment are not defined as special amusement buildings.

The terms *platform* and *stage* are defined so as to differentiate between the two. The definition of stage should be examined in conjunction with the definition of platform. The critical features in defining a stage are hanging curtains, drops, and scenery. An arrangement without these features is most likely a platform. The intent is to include nontheatrical stages, such as those in many grade schools, under the definition of platform. However, many school stages are actually regular stages, because they use scenery. Hanging curtains commonly used on platforms are normally used to conceal lighting or to provide a more aesthetic appearance. A potential problem is the arrangement commonly known as theater-in-the-round. For *Code*-application purposes, if a theater-in-the-round uses scenery, leg drops, or curtains suspended on or above it, it is considered a stage; if it uses only lighting with a valance to hide the electrical fixtures, it is a platform.

CHAPTER 12 • New

### 12.1.4* Classification of Occupancy.

See 6.1.2.

**A.12.1.4** Assembly occupancy requirements should be determined on a room-by-room basis, a floor-by-floor basis, and a total building basis. The requirements for each room should be based on the occupant load of that room, and the requirements for each floor should be based on the occupant load of that floor, but the requirements for the assembly building overall should be based on the total occupant load. Therefore, it is quite feasible to have several assembly occupancies with occupant loads of 300 or less grouped together in a single building. Such a building would be an assembly occupancy with an occupant load of over 1000.

CHAPTER 13 • Existing

### 13.1.4* Classification of Occupancy.

See 6.1.2.

**A.13.1.4** Assembly occupancy requirements should be determined on a room-by-room basis, a floor-by-floor basis, and a total building basis. The requirements for each room should be based on the occupant load of that room, and the requirements for each floor should be based on the occupant load of that floor, but the requirements for the assembly building overall should be based on the total occupant load. Therefore, it is quite feasible to have several assembly occupancies with occupant loads of 300 or less grouped together in a single building. Such a building would be an assembly occupancy with an occupant load of over 1000.

The 1994 edition of the *Code* was the last to subclassify assembly occupancies as Class A, Class B, or Class C. The subclassification scheme was based on the number of occupants and permitted requirements to be written for application to one or more of the subclasses. In subsequent editions of the *Code*, different requirements apply to different assembly occupancies with different occupant loads. Such requirements explicitly state the occupant load threshold at which the particular requirement becomes applicable. For example, see the minimum construction requirements in Table 12/13.1.6 that apply, for a given construction type and given floor elevation level, to occupant loads of 300 or 1000.

Exhibit 12/13.2 can be used to illustrate when occupant loads of assembly use spaces are to be aggregated for purposes of assembly occupancy classification and application of the provisions of Chapters 12 and 13. Part (a) of Exhibit 12/13.2 depicts six meeting rooms used by adults for training in a wing of an office building. Each room has an occupant load of 49 persons, calculated using the assembly use occupant load factor for less concentrated use, without fixed seating, from Table 7.3.1.2. Each room is considered individually for purposes of testing its occupant load against the 50-person assembly occupancy threshold of 6.1.2.1. None of the six rooms meets the 50-person criterion, so there is no assembly occupancy. Per 6.1.14.1.3(2), the assembly use meeting rooms are classified as business occupancies, based on their being incidental to the predominant business occupancy. The meeting rooms are exempt from the aggregation of occupant load on a floor-by-floor basis as detailed in A.12/13.1.4, because, as business occupancies, they are not subject to the

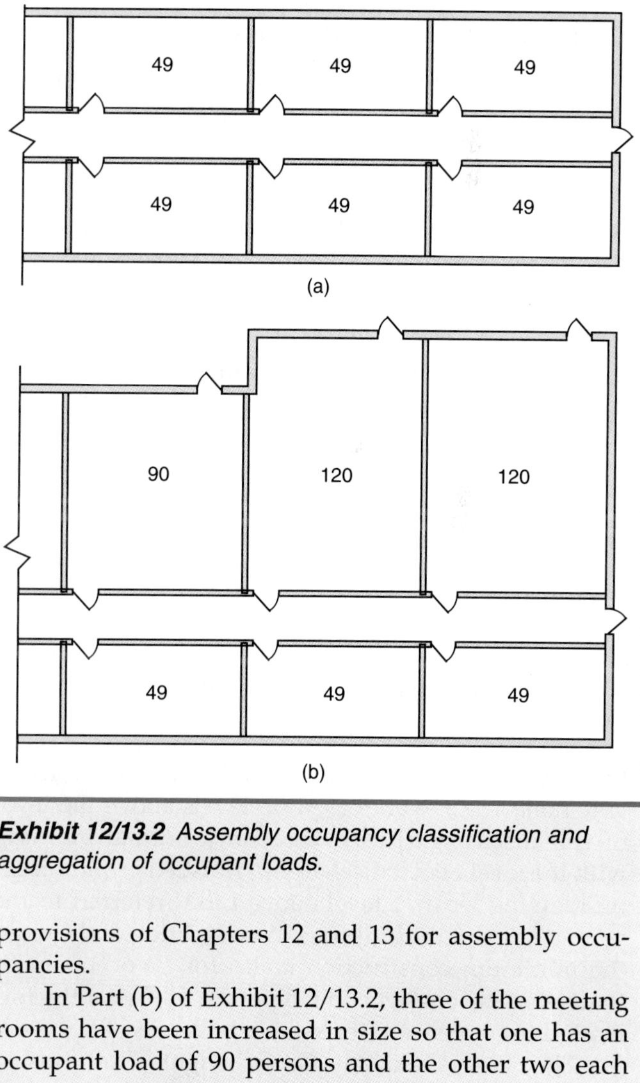


*Exhibit 12/13.2 Assembly occupancy classification and aggregation of occupant loads.*

provisions of Chapters 12 and 13 for assembly occupancies.

In Part (b) of Exhibit 12/13.2, three of the meeting rooms have been increased in size so that one has an occupant load of 90 persons and the other two each have an occupant load of 120 persons. Each of these meeting rooms, considered individually, has an occupant load in excess of the 50-person criterion of 6.1.2.1 so as to create an assembly occupancy. For purposes of applying the provisions of Chapters 12 and 13 to each of the assembly occupancy meeting rooms, the occupant load of each room is considered alone. For example, the requirement of 12/13.2.2.2.3 for panic hardware applies to doors in a required means of egress from an area having an occupant load of 100 or more persons. The panic hardware provisions do not apply to the doors in the meeting room with the 90-person occupant load, but do apply to the doors in the two 120-person rooms and (as explained in the paragraph that follows) to the door from the corridor to the outside.

Additionally, the occupant loads of the three meeting rooms are aggregated to produce an assembly occupancy with a 330-person occupant load for purposes of applying the provisions of Chapters 12 and 13. Per 12/13.3.4.1, an alarm system is required for assembly occupancies with occupant loads of more than 300 persons. The 330-person combined occupant load of the three assembly occupancy meeting rooms mandates the alarm system requirement, although none of the three meeting rooms has a sufficient occupant load by itself to require the installation of an alarm system.

### 12.1.5 Classification of Hazard of Contents.

Contents of assembly occupancies shall be classified in accordance with the provisions of Section 6.2.

### 12.1.6 Minimum Construction Requirements.

Assembly occupancies shall be limited to the building construction types specified in Table 12.1.6, based on the number of stories in height as defined in 4.6.3, unless otherwise permitted by the following *(see 8.2.1)*:

(1) This requirement shall not apply to outdoor grandstands of Type I or Type II construction.
(2) This requirement shall not apply to outdoor grandstands of Type III, Type IV, or Type V construction that meet the requirements of 12.4.8.
(3) This requirement shall not apply to grandstands of noncombustible construction supported by the floor in a building meeting the construction requirements of Table 12.1.6.
(4) This requirement shall not apply to assembly occupancies within mall buildings in accordance with 36.4.4.

### 13.1.5 Classification of Hazard of Contents.

Contents of assembly occupancies shall be classified in accordance with the provisions of Section 6.2.

### 13.1.6 Minimum Construction Requirements.

Assembly occupancies shall be limited to the building construction types specified in Table 13.1.6, based on the number of stories in height as defined in 4.6.3, unless otherwise permitted by the following *(see 8.2.1)*:

(1) This requirement shall not apply to outdoor grandstands of Type I or Type II construction.
(2) This requirement shall not apply to outdoor grandstands of Type III, Type IV, or Type V construction that meet the requirements of 13.4.8.
(3) This requirement shall not apply to grandstands of noncombustible construction supported by the floor in a building meeting the construction requirements of Table 13.1.6.
(4) This requirement shall not apply to assembly occupancies within mall buildings in accordance with 37.4.4.

In the 2006 and earlier editions of the *Code*, Table 12.1.6 and Table 13.1.6 were based on levels above the level of exit discharge (LED). Thus, in a normal building with the level of exit discharge at finished ground level (grade), the term "1 level above LED" referred to the second story of the building. In this edition of the *Code*, the minimum construction tables for all occupancies that regulate construction type are consistently formatted to reference "stories in height." See 4.6.3.

The 1942 Cocoanut Grove Night Club fire in Boston illustrated the effect of a combustible structure, combustible interior finish materials, and a multilevel configuration on the severity of a fire and its death count. The Beverly Hills Supper Club fire in 1977 also illustrated these consequences.[2] See Exhibit 12/13.3.

Based in part on the lessons learned from the Cocoanut Grove fire, the *Code* limits the number of persons in assembly occupancies located in buildings that are not of the highest fire-resistive construction types. Construction Types I(443), I(332), and II(222) represent the most highly fire-resistive forms of construction. Their inherent structural stability under fire makes these construction types acceptable for any assembly occupancy. As the fire resistance of the structure di-

*Table 12.1.6 Construction Type Limitations*

| Construction Type | Sprinklered[b] | Stories Below | Stories in Height[a] | | | | |
|---|---|---|---|---|---|---|---|
| | | | 1 | 2 | 3 | 4 | ≥5 |
| I (442)[c, d, e] | Yes | X | X | X | X | X | X |
| | No | NP | X | X | X | X | X4 |
| I (332)[c, d, e] | Yes | X | X | X | X | X | X |
| | No | NP | X | X | X | X | X4 |
| II (222)[c, d, e] | Yes | X | X | X | X | X | X |
| | No | NP | X | X | X | X | X4 |
| II (111)[c, d, e] | Yes | X1 | X | X | X | X3 | NP |
| | No | NP | X | X | X3 | NP | NP |
| II (000) | Yes | X2 | X | X4 | NP | NP | NP |
| | No | NP | X3 | NP | NP | NP | NP |
| III (211)[d] | Yes | X1 | X | X | X | X3 | NP |
| | No | NP | X | X | X4 | NP | NP |
| III (200) | Yes | X2 | X3 | X4 | NP | NP | NP |
| | No | NP | X3 | NP | NP | NP | NP |
| IV (2HH) | Yes | X1 | X | X | X | X3 | NP |
| | No | NP | X | X | X4 | NP | NP |
| V (111) | Yes | X1 | X | X | X | X3 | NP |
| | No | NP | X | X | X4 | NP | NP |
| V (000) | Yes | X2 | X3 | X4 | NP | NP | NP |
| | No | NP | X3 | NP | NP | NP | NP |

X: Permitted for assembly of any occupant load.

X1: Permitted for assembly of any occupant load, but limited to one story below the level of exit discharge.

X2: Permitted for assembly limited to an occupant load of 1000 or less, and limited to one story below the level of exit discharge.

X3: Permitted for assembly limited to an occupant load of 1000 or less.

X4: Permitted for assembly limited to an occupant load of 300 or less.

NP: Not permitted.

[a] See 4.6.3

[b] Protected by an approved, supervised automatic sprinkler system in accordance with Section 9.7 in the following locations:

(1) Throughout the story of the assembly occupancy

(2) Throughout all stories below the story of the assembly occupancy, including all stories below the level of exit discharge

(3) In the case of an assembly occupancy located below the level of exit discharge, throughout all stories intervening between the story of the assembly occupancy and the level of exit discharge, including the level of exit discharge

[c] Where every part of the structural framework of roofs in Type I or Type II construction is 20 ft (6100 mm) or more above the floor immediately below, omission of all fire protection of the structural members is permitted, including protection of trusses, roof framing, decking, and portions of columns above 20 ft (6100 mm).

[d] In open-air fixed seating facilities, including stadia, omission of fire protection of structural members exposed to the outside atmosphere is permitted where substantiated by an approved engineering analysis.

[e] Where seating treads and risers serve as floors, such seating treads and risers are permitted to be of 1-hour fire resistance–rated construction. Structural members supporting seating treads and risers are required to conform to the requirements of Table 12.1.6. Joints between seating tread and riser units are permitted to be unrated, provided that such joints do not involve separation from areas containing high hazard contents and the facility is constructed and operated in accordance with 12.4.2.

*Table 13.1.6 Construction Type Limitations*

| Construction Type | Sprinklered[b] | Stories Below | Stories in Height[a] 1 | 2 | 3 | 4 | ≥5 |
|---|---|---|---|---|---|---|---|
| I (442)[c, d] | Yes | X | X | X | X | X | X |
| | No | NP | X | X | X | X | X3 |
| I (332)[c, d] | Yes | X | X | X | X | X | X |
| | No | NP | X | X | X | X | X3 |
| II (222)[c, d] | Yes | X | X | X | X | X | X |
| | No | NP | X | X | X | X | X3 |
| II (111)[c, d] | Yes | X1 | X | X | X | X3 | NP |
| | No | NP | X | X | X3 | NP | NP |
| II (000) | Yes | X2 | X | X4 | NP | NP | NP |
| | No | NP | X3 | NP | NP | NP | NP |
| III (211) | Yes | X1 | X | X | X | X3 | NP |
| | No | NP | X | X | X4 | NP | NP |
| III (200) | Yes | X2 | X | X4 | NP | NP | NP |
| | No | NP | X3 | NP | NP | NP | NP |
| IV (2HH) | Yes | X1 | X | X | X | X3 | NP |
| | No | NP | X | X | X4 | NP | NP |
| V (111) | Yes | X1 | X | X | X | X3 | NP |
| | No | NP | X | X | X4 | NP | NP |
| V (000) | Yes | X2 | X | X4 | NP | NP | NP |
| | No | NP | X3 | NP | NP | NP | NP |

X: Permitted for assembly of any occupant load.

X1: Permitted for assembly of any occupant load, but limited to one story below the level of exit discharge.

X2: Permitted for assembly limited to an occupant load of 1000 or less, and limited to one story below the level of exit discharge.

X3: Permitted for assembly limited to an occupant load of 1000 or less.

X4: Permitted for assembly limited to an occupant load of 300 or less.

NP: Not permitted.

[a] See 4.6.3.

[b] Protected by an approved automatic sprinkler system in accordance with Section 9.7 in the following locations:

(1) Throughout the story of the assembly occupancy

(2) Throughout all stories intervening between the story of the assembly occupancy and the level of exit discharge

(3) Throughout the level of exit discharge if there are any openings between the level of exit discharge and the exits serving the assembly occupancy

[c] Where every part of the structural framework of roofs in Type I or Type II construction is 20 ft (6100 mm) or more above the floor immediately below, omission of all fire protection of the structural members is permitted, including protection of trusses, roof framing, decking, and portions of columns above 20 ft (6100 mm).

[d] In open-air fixed seating facilities, including stadia, omission of fire protection of structural members exposed to the outside atmosphere is permitted where substantiated by an approved engineering analysis.

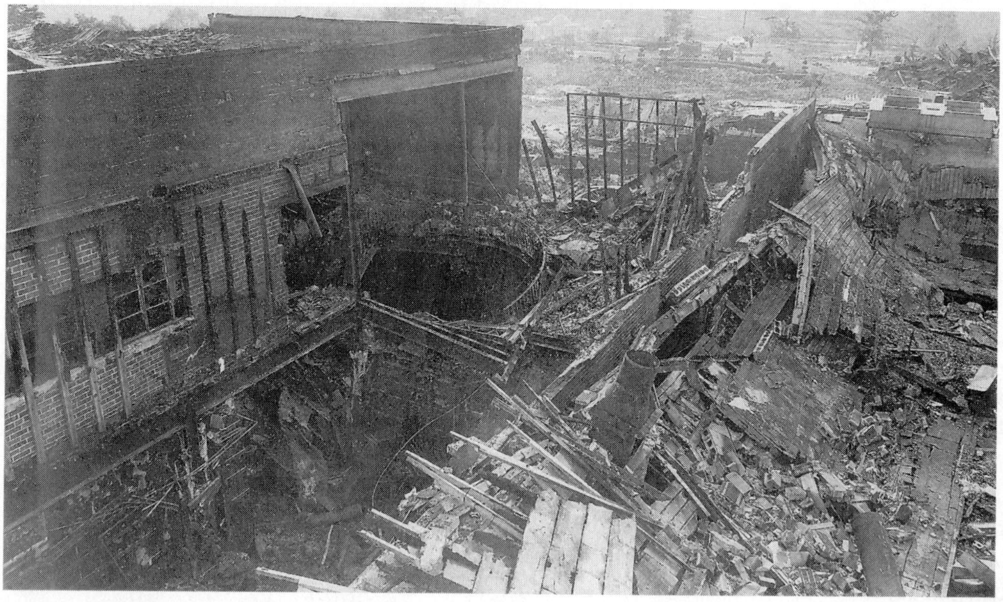

***Exhibit 12/13.3*** *Beverly Hills Supper Club following 1977 fire.*

minishes from Type II(111) to Type V(000) construction, the location of assembly occupancies within the building and the permitted number of occupants are restricted. The construction types referenced in Table 12.1.6 and Table 13.1.6 are based on NFPA 220, *Standard on Types of Building Construction*,[3] which extracts its material from *NFPA 5000®*, *Building Construction and Safety Code®*.[4] See 8.2.1.2 and Table A.8.2.1.2.

Note that Table 12.1.6 and Table 13.1.6 address the location of the assembly occupancy and not the total number of stories in the building. For example, if the building in question were five stories in height, of Type II(111) construction, and sprinklered (to the extent required by footnote b), an assembly occupancy with an occupant load in excess of 1000 persons would be permitted to be located on floors 1 through 3 but not on floors 4 and 5. Assembly occupancies with occupant loads of 1000 or fewer persons could be located on floors 1 through 4 but not on floor 5.

The extent of the required sprinkler protection (see footnote b in Table 12.1.6 and Table 13.1.6) is illustrated in Exhibit 12/13.4 for new construction and in Exhibit 12/13.5 for an existing assembly occupancy building.

In Exhibit 12/13.4, in the building on the left, a new assembly occupancy with an occupant load greater than 300 persons is located on the fifth floor of an eight-story, Type II(222) building. Automatic sprinkler protection is required on the fifth-story assembly occupancy floor and all floors below, including those below grade level. In the building on the right in Exhibit 12/13.4, the assembly occupancy is located in the subbasement, two levels below the level of exit discharge of an eight-story, Type II(222) building. Automatic sprinkler protection is required on the subbasement assembly occupancy floor, the basement level between the subbasement and the level of exit discharge, and the level of exit discharge.

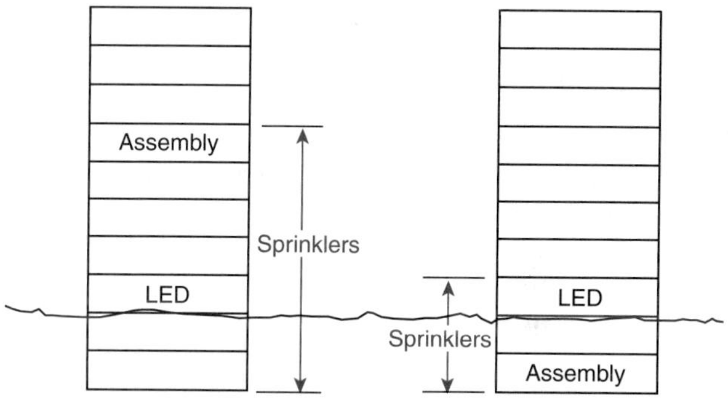


***Exhibit 12/13.4*** *New assembly occupancy building — extent of required sprinkler protection.*

In Exhibit 12/13.5, in the building on the left, an existing assembly occupancy with an occupant load greater than 1000 persons is located on the fifth floor of

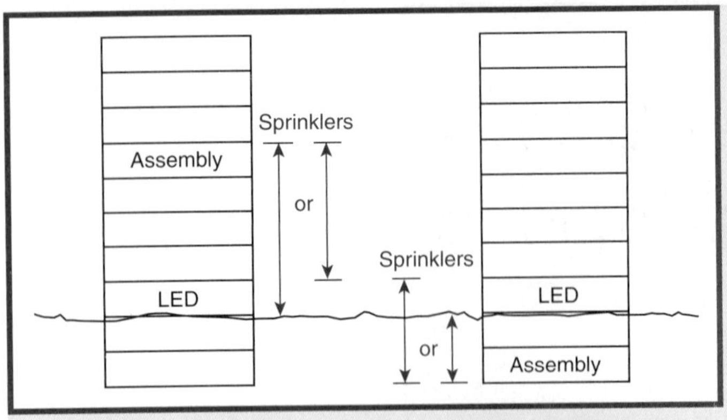


***Exhibit 12/13.5*** *Existing assembly occupancy building — extent of required sprinkler protection.*

an eight-story, Type II(222) building. Automatic sprinkler protection is required on the fifth-story assembly occupancy floor and all floors intervening between the fifth story and the level of exit discharge, including the level of exit discharge if any openings exist between the level of exit discharge and the enclosed exit stairs serving the assembly occupancy. In the building on the right in Exhibit 12/13.5, the assembly occupancy is located in the subbasement, two levels below the level of exit discharge of an eight-story, Type II(222) building. Automatic sprinkler protection is required on the subbasement assembly occupancy floor, the basement level between the subbasement and the level of exit discharge, and the level of exit discharge if any openings exist between the level of exit discharge and the enclosed exit stairs serving the assembly occupancy.

The three primary subsections that address automatic sprinkler protection that might be required in assembly occupancies are 12/13.1.6 (minimum construction requirements), 12/13.3.5 (extinguishment requirements), and 12/13.4.4 (high-rise buildings). Each of these subsections is to be applied independently of the other to determine whether automatic sprinkler protection is required. For example, the provisions of 12/13.3.5 and 12/13.4.4 might not require sprinklers, while the provisions of 12/13.1.6 might require sprinklers for an assembly occupancy with a given occupant load, based on building construction type and location within the building. If one subsection requires sprinklers while the others do not, sprinklers are required to be provided.

### 12.1.7 Occupant Load.

**12.1.7.1* General.** The occupant load, in number of persons for whom means of egress and other provisions are required, shall be determined on the basis of the occupant load factors of Table 7.3.1.2 that are characteristic of the use of the space or shall be determined as the maximum probable population of the space under consideration, whichever is greater.

**A.12.1.7.1** The increase in occupant load above that calculated using occupant load factors from Table 7.3.1.2 is permitted if the provisions of 12.1.7.1 are followed. The owner or operator has the right to submit plans and to be permitted an increase in occupant load if the plans comply with the *Code*. The authority having jurisdiction is permitted to reject the plan for increase in occupant load if the plan is unrealistic, inaccurate, or otherwise does not properly reflect compliance with other *Code* requirements. It is not the intent of the provisions of 12.1.7.1 to prohibit an increase in occupant load solely on the basis of exceeding the limits calculated using occupant load factors from Table 7.3.1.2.

### 13.1.7 Occupant Load.

**13.1.7.1* General.** The occupant load, in number of persons for whom means of egress and other provisions are required, shall be determined on the basis of the occupant load factors of Table 7.3.1.2 that are characteristic of the use of the space or shall be determined as the maximum probable population of the space under consideration, whichever is greater.

**A.13.1.7.1** The increase in occupant load above that calculated using occupant load factors from Table 7.3.1.2 is permitted if the provisions of 13.1.7.1 are followed. The owner or operator has the right to submit plans and to be permitted an increase in occupant load if the plans comply with the *Code*. The authority having jurisdiction is permitted to reject the plan for increase in occupant load if the plan is unrealistic, inaccurate, or otherwise does not properly reflect compliance with other *Code* requirements. It is not the intent of the provisions of 13.1.7.1 to prohibit an increase in occupant load solely on the basis of exceeding the limits calculated using occupant load factors from Table 7.3.1.2.

Existing auditorium and arena structures might not be designed for the added occupant load beyond the fixed seating. The authority having jurisdiction should consider exit access and aisles before permitting additional occupant load in areas using seating such as festival seating or movable seating on the auditorium or arena floor area.

CHAPTER 12 • New

To assist in preventing serious overcrowding incidents in sports arenas, stadia, and similar occupancies, spectator standing room should not be permitted between the seating areas and the playing areas, except in horse race and dog track facilities.

Where a capacity or near-capacity audience is anticipated, all seating should be assigned with tickets showing the section, row, and seat number.

Where standing room is permitted, the capacity of the standing area should meet the following criteria:

(1) The capacity should be determined on the basis of 5 $ft^2$ (0.46 $m^2$) per person.
(2) The capacity should be added to the seating capacity in determining egress requirements.
(3) The capacity should be located to the rear of the seating area.
(4) The capacity should be assigned standing-room-only tickets according to the area designated for the purpose.

The number of tickets sold, or otherwise distributed, should not exceed the aggregate number of seats plus the approved standing room numbers.

**12.1.7.1.1** In areas not in excess of 10,000 $ft^2$ (930 $m^2$), the occupant load shall not exceed one person in 5 $ft^2$ (0.46 $m^2$).

**12.1.7.1.2** In areas in excess of 10,000 $ft^2$ (930 $m^2$), the occupant load shall not exceed one person in 7 $ft^2$ (0.65 $m^2$).

**12.1.7.2 Waiting Spaces.** In theaters and other assembly occupancies where persons are admitted to the building at times when seats are not available, or when the permitted occupant load has been reached based on 12.1.7.1 and persons are allowed to wait in a lobby or similar space until seats or space is available, the following requirements shall apply:

(1) Such use of a lobby or similar space shall not encroach upon the required clear width of exits.
(2) The waiting spaces shall be restricted to areas other than the required means of egress.
(3) Exits shall be provided for the waiting spaces on the basis of one person for each 3 $ft^2$ (0.28 $m^2$) of waiting space area.
(4) Exits for waiting spaces shall be in addition to the exits specified for the main auditorium area and shall conform in construction and arrangement to the general rules for exits given in this chapter.

CHAPTER 13 • Existing

To assist in preventing serious overcrowding incidents in sports arenas, stadia, and similar occupancies, spectator standing room should not be permitted between the seating areas and the playing areas, except in horse race and dog track facilities.

Where a capacity or near-capacity audience is anticipated, all seating should be assigned with tickets showing the section, row, and seat number.

Where standing room is permitted, the capacity of the standing area should meet the following criteria:

(1) The capacity should be determined on the basis of 5 $ft^2$ (0.46 $m^2$) per person.
(2) The capacity should be added to the seating capacity in determining egress requirements.
(3) The capacity should be located to the rear of the seating area.
(4) The capacity should be assigned standing-room-only tickets according to the area designated for the purpose.

The number of tickets sold, or otherwise distributed, should not exceed the aggregate number of seats plus the approved standing room numbers.

**13.1.7.1.1** In areas not in excess of 10,000 $ft^2$ (930 $m^2$), the occupant load shall not exceed one person in 5 $ft^2$ (0.46 $m^2$).

**13.1.7.1.2** In areas in excess of 10,000 $ft^2$ (930 $m^2$), the occupant load shall not exceed one person in 7 $ft^2$ (0.65 $m^2$).

**13.1.7.1.3** The authority having jurisdiction shall be permitted to establish the occupant load as the number of persons for which the existing means of egress is adequate, provided that measures are established to prevent occupancy by a greater number of persons.

**13.1.7.2 Waiting Spaces.** In theaters and other assembly occupancies where persons are admitted to the building at times when seats are not available, or when the permitted occupant load has been reached based on 13.1.7.1 and persons are allowed to wait in a lobby or similar space until seats or space is available, the following requirements shall apply:

(1) Such use of a lobby or similar space shall not encroach upon the required clear width of exits.
(2) The waiting spaces shall be restricted to areas other than the required means of egress.
(3) Exits shall be provided for the waiting spaces on the basis of one person for each 3 $ft^2$ (0.28 $m^2$) of waiting space area.
(4) Exits for waiting spaces shall be in addition to the exits specified for the main auditorium area and shall conform in construction and arrangement to the general rules for exits given in this chapter.

CHAPTER 12 • New

**12.1.7.3 Life Safety Evaluation.** Where the occupant load of an assembly occupancy exceeds 6000, a life safety evaluation shall be performed in accordance with 12.4.1.

**12.1.7.4 Outdoor Facilities.** In outdoor facilities, where approved by the authority having jurisdiction, the number of occupants who are each provided with not less than 15 $ft^2$ (1.4 $m^2$) of lawn surface shall be permitted to be excluded from the maximum occupant load of 6000 of 12.1.7.3 in determining the need for a life safety evaluation.

CHAPTER 13 • Existing

**13.1.7.3 Life Safety Evaluation.** Where the occupant load of an assembly occupancy exceeds 6000, a life safety evaluation shall be performed in accordance with 13.4.1.

**13.1.7.4 Outdoor Facilities.** In outdoor facilities, where approved by the authority having jurisdiction, the number of occupants who are each provided with not less than 15 $ft^2$ (1.4 $m^2$) of lawn surface shall be permitted to be excluded from the maximum occupant load of 6000 of 13.1.7.3 in determining the need for a life safety evaluation.

Occupant load factors appear in Table 7.3.1.2. Note that occupant load factors are provided in Chapter 7, a core chapter, because occupant load is based on the use of the space, not on the occupancy classification. For example, a small conference room for approximately 30 persons located in a business occupancy doesn't have the requisite 50 persons to constitute an assembly occupancy. The occupancy classification is business, but the occupant load of the conference room is calculated using an occupant load factor from Table 7.3.1.2 for an assembly use, not a business use. Thus, the occupant load factors belong in Chapter 7 so that they can be employed based on the use of the space, regardless of the occupancy classification.

Paragraphs 12/13.1.7.1, 12/13.1.7.1.1, and 12/13.1.7.1.2 limit the permitted increase in occupant load to avoid overcrowding, which affects the movement characteristics of the occupants. If people are crowded into a space so that each person occupies less than 7 $ft^2$ (0.65 $m^2$), movement approaches a shuffle; where each person occupies less than 3 $ft^2$ (0.28 $m^2$), "jam point" is approached, and all movement by occupants comes to a virtual stop.

Some *Code* users have questioned why the 5 $ft^2$ (0.46 $m^2$) and 7 $ft^2$ (0.65 $m^2$) maximum packing density factors of 12/13.1.7.1.1 and 12/13.1.7.1.2 are not included as part of Table 7.3.1.2. The occupant load factors in Table 7.3.1.2 are for calculating occupant load based on use of the space, regardless of the occupancy classification. The maximum packing density criteria of 12/13.1.7.1.1 and 12/13.1.7.1.2 are specifically for application to assembly occupancies and, therefore, belong in the assembly occupancy chapters. The requirement of 12/13.1.7.1.2, that the occupant load not exceed one person in 7 $ft^2$ (0.65 $m^2$) of floor area, recognizes that, in assembly venues larger than 10,000 $ft^2$ (930 $m^2$), patrons will crowd the portion of the space that is nearest the attraction (e.g., the space near the performance stage). The uneven distribution of occupants in the space will result in persons near the attraction having less than 7 $ft^2$ (0.65 $m^2$) of area; those occupants furthest from the attraction will have more than 7 $ft^2$ (0.65 $m^2$); and the average for the entire space might be around 5 $ft^2$ (0.46 $m^2$) per person. In venues smaller than 10,000 $ft^2$ (930 $m^2$), patrons are not expected to crowd the stage area, as most of the space provides for reasonable proximity to the attraction. These smaller, more evenly occupied venues are permitted an occupant load calculated at 5 $ft^2$ (0.46 $m^2$) per person.

Note that 13.1.7.1.3, applicable to existing assembly occupancies, has no counterpart in Chapter 12 for new assembly occupancies. Paragraph 13.1.7.1.3 permits the authority having jurisdiction (AHJ) to set aside the calculated occupant load and establish the occupant load of an existing assembly occupancy as the number of persons for which the existing means of egress is adequate. In other words, rather than forcing an existing assembly occupancy to unnecessarily upgrade its egress system, the existing system is permitted to serve, provided that the maximum number of persons present can be effectively regulated. The occupant load is to be posted, and staff is to strictly enforce the posted occupant load. For example, the calculated occupant load — derived by dividing the available floor area by the occupant load factors that represent the uses — might be 1110 persons. Yet, the existing egress system [e.g., three door openings that are each 64 in. (1625 mm) wide] might accommodate only 960 persons. If the AHJ believes that the existing assembly occupancy itself can enforce an occupant load of not more than 960, then an occupant load of 960 can be established. Thus, a fourth exit with capacity for at least 150 persons does not have to be added retroactively. Paragraph 13.1.7.1.3 and 43.4.2 are the only provisions in the *Code* that permit the established occupant load to be less than the calculated occupant load. The exemption was written to recognize that the occupant load factors characteristic of assembly uses are small — such as 7 $ft^2$ or 15 $ft^2$ (0.65 $m^2$ or 1.4 $m^2$) per person — compared to those characteristic of business and residential uses — such as 100 $ft^2$ or 200 $ft^2$ (9.3 $m^2$ or 18.6 $m^2$) per person. These small occupant load factors result in large occupant loads for even modestly sized areas.

Numerous occupant load factors for assembly uses are presented in Table 7.3.1.2. The occupant load factors characteristic of assembly uses reflect the data developed from surveys of typical assembly occupancies. The commentary that follows explains some of these factors.

One of the assembly use occupant load factors is for concentrated use at 7 net $ft^2$ (0.65 net $m^2$) per person. The phrase "one person per 7 net $ft^2$ (0.65 net $m^2$)" means that one person is assumed to be present for each 7 $ft^2$ (0.65 $m^2$) of net floor area that is available to be used by occupants. Another assembly use occupant load factor is for less concentrated use at 15 net $ft^2$ (1.4 net $m^2$) per person. The phrase "one person per 15 net $ft^2$" (1.4 net $m^2$) means that one person is assumed to be present for each 15 $ft^2$ (1.4 $m^2$) of net floor area that is available to be used by occupants. See 3.3.19.2.2 for the definition of *net floor area*.

The term *concentrated use* is intended to describe a condition that has meaning only in comparison to the related term *less concentrated use*. The word *concentrated* relates to the density at which persons can occupy such space. Where furniture precludes persons from occupying the same space taken by the furniture, there will be fewer persons per unit area than if no furniture were present, or if the space occupied by the furniture could simultaneously be occupied by people (e.g., persons seated in chairs).

The 7 $ft^2$ (0.65 $m^2$) concentrated use occupant load factor is based on open floor space with people standing comfortably. This factor also can be used to calculate the occupant load in a multipurpose room where portable chairs are placed for meetings, film viewing, or lectures. The 15 $ft^2$ (1.4 $m^2$) less concentrated use occupant load factor is intended for use where a certain amount of space is occupied by furniture. An example is a space furnished with tables and chairs, as in a restaurant or conference room.

Often a controversy exists regarding where to use an occupant load factor of 7 $ft^2$ (0.65 $m^2$) versus 15 $ft^2$ (1.4 $m^2$). These factors are based on concentrated versus less concentrated use, and the selection of one over the other is based strictly on judgment. Because the occupant load is used in determining the required egress capacity and the construction, alarm, and sprinkler requirements, it is usually safer to provide features for the larger occupant load than to try to enforce, usually with great difficulty, a smaller occupant load limit. Designing the egress system to accommodate the larger occupant load affords the facility with much greater flexibility of use over the life of the building.

The occupant load factor for kitchens has particular application to assembly uses, which are often characterized by food service and an associated kitchen. The kitchen occupant load factor helps to clarify the method of calculating the total occupant load in restaurants and cafeterias where a portion of the floor area is used as a kitchen. Note that the occupant load of the kitchen is calculated by using gross area in accordance with footnote a to Table 7.3.1.2. The 100 gross $ft^2$ (9.3 gross $m^2$) factor takes into consideration the stoves, sinks, counters, and culinary machinery found in a kitchen.

The 100 gross $ft^2$ (9.3 gross $m^2$) associated with the occupant load factor for library stack areas takes into consideration the existence of bookshelves and permanent aisles. Because reading rooms typically have large magazine racks, chairs, tables, couches, and other furnishings that can require considerable space, an occupant load factor of 50 $ft^2$ (4.6 $m^2$) of net area per person is specified for such areas. Exhibit 12/13.6 illustrates a library reading room.

Swimming pools, pool decks, exercise rooms, skating rinks, and casino or gaming rooms are often parts of assembly occupancies. The occupant load factors for such areas are presented in Table 7.3.1.2 to help piece

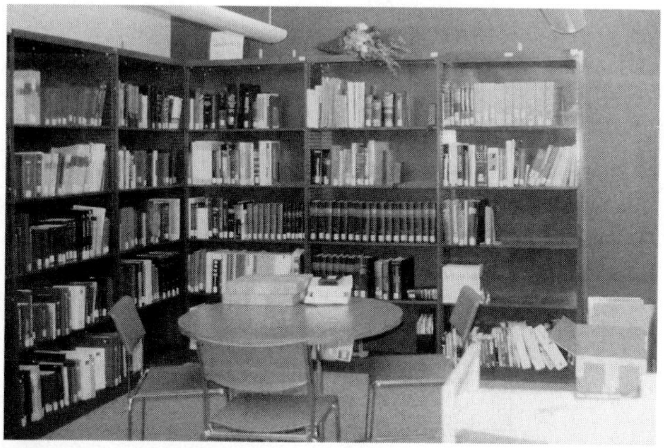

***Exhibit 12/13.6*** *Library reading room for which Code specifies an occupant load factor of 50 $ft^2$ (4.6 $m^2$) net area per person.*

together a realistic occupant load for the entire assembly space.

The occupant load factor for stages is provided because it is necessary to include the occupant load of a stage in the total occupant load. The occupant load factor allows for the occupant load of a stage to be calculated with consistency.

Consideration needs to be given to the actual use of a room or space. A multi-use room might have several occupant loads, with each load applicable to a specific arrangement and use. This situation is especially common in multipurpose rooms in schools and hotels.

Exhibit 12/13.7 illustrates a net 2500 ft$^2$ (net 232 m$^2$) room with two 46 in. (1170 mm) clear width doors. If the room were to be used as a banquet room with tables and chairs, its occupant load would be based on the 15 ft$^2$ (1.4 m$^2$) per person occupant load factor characteristic of a less concentrated use. The occupant load calculation would divide 2500 net ft$^2$ by 15 ft$^2$ (232 net m$^2$ by 1.4 m$^2$) per person for an occupant load of 167 persons. However, if the room were to be used for a stand-up cocktail party with essentially no furniture, the occupant load would be based on the 7 ft$^2$ (0.65 m$^2$) per person factor characteristic of concentrated use. The occupant load calculation would divide 2500 net ft$^2$ by 7 ft$^2$ (232 net m$^2$ by 0.65 m$^2$) per person, for an occupant load of 357 persons. Thus, based on the two planned forms of assembly use, the room has two occupant loads.

The egress capacity from the room is limited by the width available from the two 46 in. (1170 mm) clear width doors. The egress capacity is calculated by dividing the 46 in. (1170 mm) clear width by the 0.2 in. (5 mm) per person capacity factor for level travel, and then multiplying by 2 (because of the two identical doors). The calculation shows the room has an egress capacity of 460 occupants. Because each of the occupant loads calculated is less than the egress capacity, the situation is satisfactory.

As noted in the previous two paragraphs, both egress capacity and occupant load must be considered in establishing the permissible occupant load for a room or area. Exhibit 12/13.8 illustrates a net 3600 ft$^2$ (net 334 m$^2$) room with two 36 in. (915 mm) clear width doors. The egress capacity of the room is calculated by dividing the 36 in. (915 mm) clear width of the doors by the 0.2 in. (5 mm) per person capacity factor for level travel specified by Table 7.3.3.1, and then multiplying by 2. The calculation produces an egress capacity of 360 occupants. However, an occupant load for the same room, calculated based on 7 ft$^2$ (0.65 m$^2$) per person, results in an occupant load of 514 persons. Section 7.3 requires that egress capacity be provided for the occupant load determined by application of the occupant load factor. Therefore, for new assembly occupancies, the egress capacity must be increased to accommodate at least 514 persons, via a minimum of three means of egress as required by 12.2.4.1 and 7.4.1.2. For existing assembly occupancies, either the egress capacity must be increased to accommodate at least 514 persons or the occupant load can be set at 360 occupants — the number of persons for which the existing means of egress is adequate — in accordance with 13.1.7.1.3. The latter occupant load requires specific approval by the authority having jurisdiction

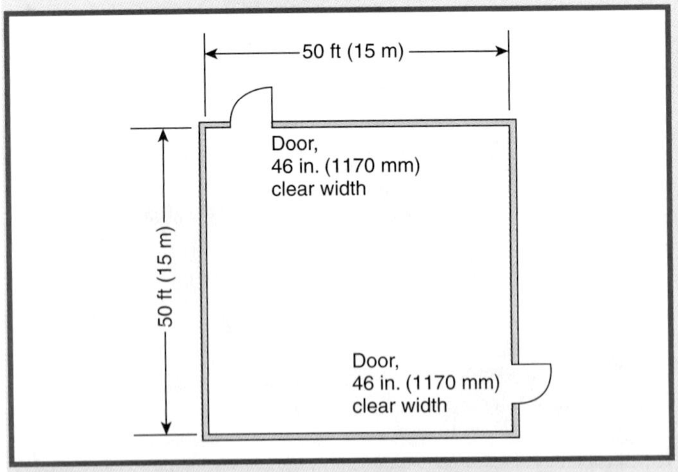


***Exhibit 12/13.7*** *Acceptable scenario where calculated occupant load is less than number of persons that means of egress can safely accommodate.*

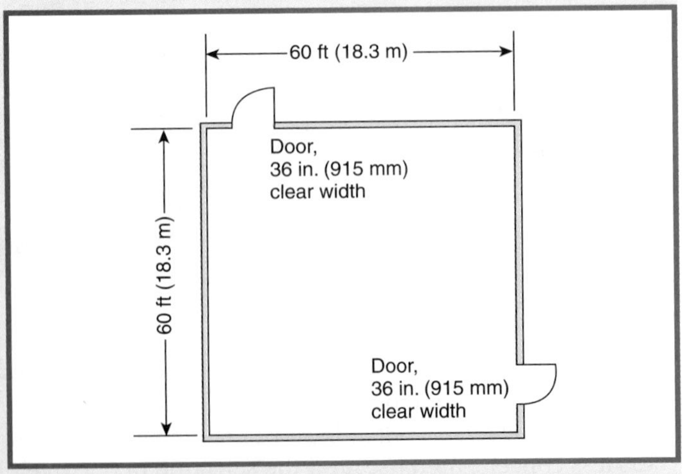


***Exhibit 12/13.8*** *Unacceptable scenario where calculated occupant load is larger than egress capacity.*

(AHJ) after it has been ensured that measures are in place to prevent occupancy by more than 360 persons in the existing assembly occupancy.

The accessibility of a room's exit access doors is as important as the egress capacity of that room. Therefore, where an increase in occupant load is permitted over that established by 12/13.1.7.1, it is required by 7.3.1.3 that adequate aisle accessways and aisles leading to the room exit access doors be provided. Where tables abut an aisle, the spacing must allow for chairs as well as the required aisle width. Consideration should be given to the likelihood that, when occupants leave during an emergency, they might not take time to move chairs out of the aisles. See 12/13.2.5.7.3 and 12/13.2.5.8.3.

Dining and drinking areas make the most frequent use of the provisions of 7.3.1.3 for occupant load increases. There have been large banquet layouts where the occupant load was successfully increased to reflect an occupant load factor of 11 ft$^2$ (1 m$^2$) per person instead of the 15 ft$^2$ (1.4 m$^2$) per person specified by Table 7.3.1.2. In cases where the occupant load is increased above that calculated using the occupant load factor of Table 7.3.1.2, the authority having jurisdiction (AHJ) should require diagrams showing fixture and furniture layouts and should enforce adherence to approved layouts. As noted previously, one room might have several approved occupant loads, depending on the various layouts.

Although 12/13.1.7.1.1 limits occupant density to one person for each available 5 ft$^2$ (0.46 m$^2$), 12/13.1.7.2(3) permits a density of one person per 3 ft$^2$ (0.28 m$^2$) for specially designated waiting spaces. The waiting space cannot be located in, or interfere with, the egress routes from the rest of the assembly occupancy. As shown in Exhibit 12/13.9, such waiting spaces might be associated with a theater where patrons wait for the audience seating chamber to clear of people attending a previous show before entering and taking their seats for the next performance. A similar waiting space might be established to the side of the entrance foyer of a restaurant where diners await a table. Space at a bar where patrons gather to place a drink order does not qualify as a waiting space for purposes of the provisions of 12/13.1.7.2.

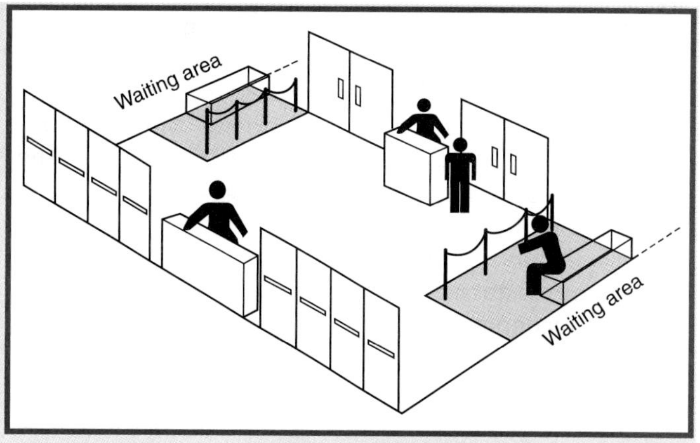


***Exhibit 12/13.9*** *Designated waiting spaces arranged not to encroach on required means of egress.*

The life safety evaluation required for large assembly occupancies by 12/13.1.7.3 recognizes that fixed protection and suppression systems alone do not ensure safe egress where large numbers of people are present. Expected crowd behavior is part of such an evaluation, as is consideration of techniques to manage any behavioral problems. See 12/13.4.1 and, in particular, A.12/13.4.1.3, which outlines the many factors that might need to be considered in a required life safety evaluation.

Paragraph 12/13.1.7.4 recognizes that where outdoor assembly occupancy patrons are each provided with at least 15 ft$^2$ (1.4 m$^2$) of lawn surface, their predicted behavior obviates the need for further scrutiny via a life safety evaluation.

## 12.2 Means of Egress Requirements

### 12.2.1 General.

All means of egress shall be in accordance with Chapter 7 and this chapter.

### 12.2.2 Means of Egress Components.

**12.2.2.1 Components Permitted.** Components of means of egress shall be limited to the types described in 12.2.2.2 through 12.2.2.12.

## 13.2 Means of Egress Requirements

### 13.2.1 General.

All means of egress shall be in accordance with Chapter 7 and this chapter.

### 13.2.2 Means of Egress Components.

**13.2.2.1 Components Permitted.** Components of means of egress shall be limited to the types described in 13.2.2.2 through 13.2.2.12.

CHAPTER 12 • New

CHAPTER 13 • Existing

Paragraph 12/13.2.2.1 limits components within the required means of egress to those detailed in 12/13.2.2.2 through 12/13.2.2.12. Note that it is not required that each component addressed in these paragraphs be used; rather, if a component is used, the provisions of Chapter 7 that apply to the component, as modified by Chapters 12 and 13, must be followed.

Escalators are permitted to be part of a means of egress in existing occupancies (see 13.2.2.8), but they are not recognized as such in new construction. Note that Chapter 7 does not credit escalators that serve within the required means of egress in new construction. These devices can be (and often are) installed in assembly occupancies, but they cannot obstruct or interfere with the required means of egress. However, where a new assembly occupancy is located more than 30 ft (9.1 m) below the level of exit discharge, 12.4.3.3.2 requires a mechanical means of moving people vertically to the level of exit discharge. This requirement can be satisfied via an escalator or an elevator.

**12.2.2.2 Doors.**

**12.2.2.2.1** Doors complying with 7.2.1 shall be permitted.

**12.2.2.2.2** Assembly occupancies with occupant loads of 300 or less in malls *(see 36.4.4.2.2)* shall be permitted to have horizontal or vertical security grilles or doors complying with 7.2.1.4.1(3) on the main entrance/exits.

**12.2.2.2.3** Any door in a required means of egress from an area having an occupant load of 100 or more persons shall be permitted to be provided with a latch or lock only if the latch or lock is panic hardware or fire exit hardware complying with 7.2.1.7, unless otherwise permitted by the following:

(1) This requirement shall not apply to delayed-egress locks as permitted in 12.2.2.2.5.
(2) This requirement shall not apply to access-controlled egress doors as permitted in 12.2.2.2.6.

**12.2.2.2.4** Locking devices complying with 7.2.1.5.4 shall be permitted to be used on a single door or a single pair of doors if both of the following conditions apply:

(1) The door or pair of doors serve as the main exit and the assembly occupancy has an occupant load not greater than 500.
(2) Any latching devices on such a door(s) from an assembly occupancy having an occupant load of 100 or more are released by panic hardware or fire exit hardware.

**12.2.2.2.5** Delayed-egress locks complying with 7.2.1.6.1 shall be permitted on doors other than main entrance/exit doors.

**12.2.2.2.6** Doors in the means of egress shall be permitted to be equipped with an approved access control system complying with 7.2.1.6.2, and such doors shall not be locked from the egress side when the assembly occupancy is occupied. *(See 7.2.1.1.3.)*

**12.2.2.2.7** Elevator lobby exit access door locking in accordance with 7.2.1.6.3 shall be permitted.

**13.2.2.2 Doors.**

**13.2.2.2.1** Doors complying with 7.2.1 shall be permitted.

**13.2.2.2.2** Assembly occupancies with occupant loads of 300 or less in malls *(see 37.4.4.2.2)* shall be permitted to have horizontal or vertical security grilles or doors complying with 7.2.1.4.1(3) on the main entrance/exits.

**13.2.2.2.3** Any door in a required means of egress from an area having an occupant load of 100 or more persons shall be permitted to be provided with a latch or lock only if the latch or lock is panic hardware or fire exit hardware complying with 7.2.1.7, unless otherwise permitted by the following:

(1) This requirement shall not apply to delayed-egress locks as permitted in 13.2.2.2.5.
(2) This requirement shall not apply to access-controlled egress doors as permitted in 13.2.2.2.6.

**13.2.2.2.4** Locking devices complying with 7.2.1.5.4 shall be permitted to be used on a single door or a single pair of doors if both of the following conditions apply:

(1) The door or pair of doors serve as the main exit from assembly occupancies having an occupant load not greater than 600.
(2) Any latching devices on such a door(s) from an assembly occupancy having an occupant load of 100 or more are released by panic hardware or fire exit hardware.

**13.2.2.2.5** Delayed-egress locks complying with 7.2.1.6.1 shall be permitted on doors other than main entrance/exit doors.

**13.2.2.2.6** Doors in the means of egress shall be permitted to be equipped with an approved access control system complying with 7.2.1.6.2, and such doors shall not be locked from the egress side when the assembly occupancy is occupied. *(See 7.2.1.1.3.)*

**13.2.2.2.7** Elevator lobby exit access door locking in accordance with 7.2.1.6.3 shall be permitted.

CHAPTER 12 • New

**12.2.2.2.8** Revolving doors complying with the requirements of 7.2.1.10 shall be permitted.

**12.2.2.2.9** The provisions of 7.2.1.11.1.1 to permit turnstiles where revolving doors are permitted shall not apply.

**12.2.2.2.10** No turnstiles or other devices that restrict the movement of persons shall be installed in any assembly occupancy in such a manner as to interfere with required means of egress facilities.

CHAPTER 13 • Existing

**13.2.2.2.8** Revolving doors complying with the requirements of 7.2.1.10 for new construction shall be permitted.

**13.2.2.2.9** The provisions of 7.2.1.11.1.1 to permit turnstiles where revolving doors are permitted shall not apply.

**13.2.2.2.10** No turnstiles or other devices that restrict the movement of persons shall be installed in any assembly occupancy in such a manner as to interfere with required means of egress facilities.

The provision of 12/13.2.2.2.2 permits, for example, small restaurants in mall buildings to use the security grilles or doors addressed by 7.2.1.4.1(3).

Paragraph 12/13.2.2.2.3 requires doors that latch or lock to be provided with panic hardware or fire exit hardware if the door serves an area having an occupant load of 100 or more persons. The panic hardware (or, for fire-rated doors, the fire exit hardware) releases the latch when occupants depress the actuating bar or push pad, as might occur when a crowd pushes up against a door so as to hinder normal unlatching via turning a doorknob or lever.

In Exhibit 12/13.10, the doors from room A are permitted to be latched or locked and provided with a traditional doorknob or lever to release the latch, as the 60-person occupant load is less than the 100-person threshold. Room B has an occupant load of 110 persons and is provided with two doors to the corridor. The area served by the doors is the entire room (not half the room) with its 110-person occupant load, which exceeds the 100-person threshold. If the doors from room B are provided with a latch or lock, panic hardware (or fire exit hardware if the door has a fire protection rating) is required as the means for releasing the latch or lock. Similarly, the doors from the corridor to the outside serve an area comprised of all the rooms with doors to the corridor. The combined occupant load of those rooms exceeds the 100-person threshold, so panic hardware is required if those doors are provided with a latch or lock. An example of an assembly occupancy that might have no latches or locks on its doors, so as to be exempted from the panic hardware requirement, is a highway tourist information center with a restaurant that is open 24 hours per day, 365 days per year.

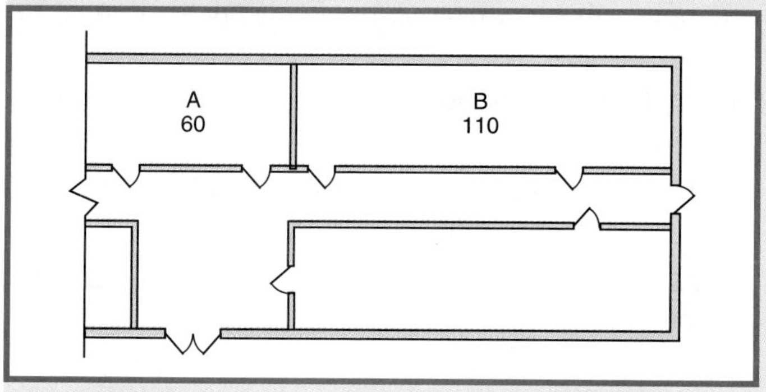


***Exhibit 12/13.10*** *Occupant load determines which doors require panic hardware.*

Paragraph 12/13.2.2.2.4 recognizes the particular key-operated dead bolt lock described in 7.2.1.5.4. Using a key-operated dead bolt lock in an assembly occupancy is permitted where all the conditions of 7.2.1.5.4 and 12/13.2.2.2.4 are met. The assembly occupancy is limited to an occupant load of not more than 500 persons in new assembly occupancies; 600 persons for existing assembly occupancies. Use is limited to the main exit, based on the assumption that the lock will need to be released for the facility to operate. The main exit is limited to a single door or single pair of doors to help ensure that the main exit will be unlocked whenever the building is occupied.

Although delayed-egress locks are addressed by 12/13.2.2.2.3(1) as an exemption to the requirement to provide panic hardware for doors that latch or lock, 12/13.2.2.2.5 further describes the exemption for delayed-egress locks. It permits delayed-egress hardware meeting the requirements of 7.2.1.6.1 to be used on all but the main exit. In addition to other requirements, 7.2.1.6.1 requires that the building be protected throughout by either an approved, supervised automatic sprinkler system or an approved, supervised automatic fire detection system.

Although access-controlled egress doors are permitted by 12/13.2.2.2.3(2) to omit panic hardware for doors that latch or lock, 12/13.2.2.2.6 further describes the permission for access control door-locking systems complying with 7.2.1.6.2.

The provision of 12/13.2.2.2.7 is new for the 2009 edition of the *Code*. It permits use of the elevator lobby exit access door-locking provisions of 7.2.1.6.3. Paragraph 7.2.1.6.3 details 15 criteria that must be met as an alternative to the requirements of 7.4.1.6 that each elevator landing or lobby must have access to at least one exit without the use of a key, a tool, special knowledge, or special effort. See 7.4.1.6 and 7.2.1.6.3.

**12.2.2.3 Stairs.**

**12.2.2.3.1 General.** Stairs complying with 7.2.2 shall be permitted, unless one of the following criteria applies:

(1)* Stairs serving seating that is designed to be repositioned shall not be required to comply with 7.2.2.3.1.

**A.12.2.2.3.1(1)** The seating plan and the means of egress should be reviewed each time the seating is substantially rearranged.

(2) This requirement shall not apply to stages and platforms as permitted by 12.4.5.

**12.2.2.3.2 Catwalk, Gallery, and Gridiron Stairs.**

**12.2.2.3.2.1** Noncombustible grated stair treads and landing floors shall be permitted in means of egress from lighting and access catwalks, galleries, and gridirons.

**12.2.2.3.2.2** Spiral stairs complying with 7.2.2.2.3 shall be permitted in means of egress from lighting and access catwalks, galleries, and gridirons.

**13.2.2.3 Stairs.**

**13.2.2.3.1 General.** Stairs complying with 7.2.2 shall be permitted, unless one of the following criteria applies:

(1)* Stairs serving seating that is designed to be repositioned shall not be required to comply with 7.2.2.3.1.

**A.13.2.2.3.1(1)** The seating plan and the means of egress should be reviewed each time the seating is substantially rearranged.

(2) This requirement shall not apply to stages and platforms as permitted by 13.4.5.

**13.2.2.3.2 Catwalk, Gallery, and Gridiron Stairs.**

**13.2.2.3.2.1** Noncombustible grated stair treads and landing floors shall be permitted in means of egress from lighting and access catwalks, galleries, and gridirons.

**13.2.2.3.2.2** Spiral stairs complying with 7.2.2.2.3 shall be permitted in means of egress from lighting and access catwalks, galleries, and gridirons.

Assembly occupancies with theater-type seating typically use sloped floors to help provide the sight lines needed for viewing the attraction at the front of the room. The floor slope is often sufficient to require stepped aisles, because a ramped aisle would exceed the slope criteria of Table 7.2.5.2(a). The stepped aisles are treated as stairs for purposes of applying the requirements of Chapters 12 and 13. For example, see Table 12/13.2.3.2, and the associated provisions of 12/13.2.3.3, where stairs (i.e., stepped aisles) are sized differently from the criteria in Chapter 7 to account for riser heights in excess of the 7 in. (180 mm) specified for new stairs in Table 7.2.2.2.1.1(a).

Paragraph 7.2.2.3.1.1 requires that stairs within required means of egress be of permanent fixed construction, unless they serve seating that is designed to be repositioned and, thus, are exempted by 12/13.2.2.3.1(1). In some theaters, for example, entire seating sections are moved to accommodate the performance area requirements for a particular presentation. The stairs serving these movable seating sections cannot easily be of fixed permanent construction.

**12.2.2.4 Smokeproof Enclosures.** Smokeproof enclosures complying with 7.2.3 shall be permitted.

**12.2.2.5 Horizontal Exits.** Horizontal exits complying with 7.2.4 shall be permitted.

**12.2.2.6 Ramps.** Ramps complying with 7.2.5 shall be permitted, and the following alternatives shall also apply:

(1) Ramps not part of an accessible means of egress and serving only stages or nonpublic areas shall be permitted to have a slope not steeper than 1 in 8.

**13.2.2.4 Smokeproof Enclosures.** Smokeproof enclosures complying with 7.2.3 shall be permitted.

**13.2.2.5 Horizontal Exits.** Horizontal exits complying with 7.2.4 shall be permitted.

**13.2.2.6 Ramps.** Ramps complying with 7.2.5 shall be permitted.

(2) Ramped aisles not part of an accessible means of egress shall be permitted to have a slope not steeper than 1 in 8.

**12.2.2.7 Exit Passageways.** Exit passageways complying with 7.2.6 shall be permitted.

**12.2.2.8 Reserved.**

**12.2.2.9 Reserved.**

**12.2.2.10 Fire Escape Ladders.**

**12.2.2.10.1** Fire escape ladders complying with 7.2.9 shall be permitted.

**12.2.2.10.2** For ladders serving catwalks, the three-person limitation in 7.2.9.1(3) shall be permitted to be increased to ten persons.

**12.2.2.11 Alternating Tread Devices.** Alternating tread devices complying with 7.2.11 shall be permitted.

**12.2.2.12 Areas of Refuge.** Areas of refuge complying with 7.2.12 shall be permitted.

### 12.2.3 Capacity of Means of Egress.

**12.2.3.1 General.** The capacity of means of egress shall be in accordance with one of the following:

(1) Section 7.3 for other than theater-type seating or smoke-protected assembly seating
(2) 12.2.3.2 for rooms with theater-type seating or similar seating arranged in rows
(3) 12.4.2 for smoke-protected assembly seating

**12.2.3.2* Theater-Type Seating.** Minimum clear widths of aisles and other means of egress serving theater-type seating, or similar seating arranged in rows, shall be in accordance with Table 12.2.3.2.

***Table 12.2.3.2 Capacity Factors***

| | Clear Width per Seat Served | | | |
|---|---|---|---|---|
| | Stairs | | Passageways, Ramps, and Doorways | |
| No. of Seats | in. | mm | in. | mm |
| Unlimited | 0.3 *AB* | 7.6 *AB* | 0.22 *C* | 5.6 *C* |

**A.12.2.3.2** The provisions of 12.2.3.2 should be applied within the audience seating chamber and to the room doors. The capacity of means of egress components encountered after leaving the audience seating chamber, such as concourses, lobbies, exit stair enclosures, and the exit discharge, should be calculated in accordance with Section 7.3.

**13.2.2.7 Exit Passageways.** Exit passageways complying with 7.2.6 shall be permitted.

**13.2.2.8 Escalators and Moving Walks.** Escalators and moving walks complying with 7.2.7 shall be permitted.

**13.2.2.9 Fire Escape Stairs.** Fire escape stairs complying with 7.2.8 shall be permitted.

**13.2.2.10 Fire Escape Ladders.**

**13.2.2.10.1** Fire escape ladders complying with 7.2.9 shall be permitted.

**13.2.2.10.2** For ladders serving catwalks, the three-person limitation in 7.2.9.1(3) shall be permitted to be increased to ten persons.

**13.2.2.11 Alternating Tread Devices.** Alternating tread devices complying with 7.2.11 shall be permitted.

**13.2.2.12 Areas of Refuge.** Areas of refuge complying with 7.2.12 shall be permitted.

### 13.2.3 Capacity of Means of Egress.

**13.2.3.1 General.** The capacity of means of egress shall be in accordance with one of the following:

(1) Section 7.3 for other than theater-type seating or smoke-protected assembly seating
(2) 13.2.3.2 for rooms with theater-type seating or similar seating arranged in rows
(3) 13.4.2 for smoke-protected assembly seating

**13.2.3.2* Theater-Type Seating.** Minimum clear widths of aisles and other means of egress serving theater-type seating, or similar seating arranged in rows, shall be in accordance with Table 13.2.3.2.

***Table 13.2.3.2 Capacity Factors***

| | Clear Width per Seat Served | | | |
|---|---|---|---|---|
| | Stairs | | Passageways, Ramps, and Doorways | |
| No. of Seats | in. | mm | in. | mm |
| Unlimited | 0.3 *AB* | 7.6 *AB* | 0.22 *C* | 5.6 *C* |

**A.13.2.3.2** The provisions of 13.2.3.2 should be applied within the audience seating chamber and to the room doors. The capacity of means of egress components encountered after leaving the audience seating chamber, such as concourses, lobbies, exit stair enclosures, and the exit discharge, should be calculated in accordance with Section 7.3.

CHAPTER 12 • New

**12.2.3.3 Width Modifications.** The minimum clear widths shown in Table 12.2.3.2 shall be modified in accordance with all of the following:

(1) If risers exceed 7 in. in height, the stair width in Table 12.2.3.2 shall be multiplied by factor *A*, where *A* equals the following:

$$A = 1 + \frac{\text{riser height} - 7}{5}$$

(2) If risers exceed 178 mm in height, the stair width in Table 12.2.3.2 shall be multiplied by factor *A*, where *A* equals the following:

$$A = 1 + \frac{\text{riser height} - 178}{125}$$

(3) Stairs not having a handrail within a 30 in. (760 mm) horizontal distance shall be 25 percent wider than otherwise calculated; that is, their width shall be multiplied by factor *B*, where *B* equals the following:

$$B = 1.25$$

(4) Ramps steeper than 1 in 10 slope where used in ascent shall have their width increased by 10 percent; that is, their width shall be multiplied by factor *C*, where *C* equals the following:

$$C = 1.10$$

**12.2.3.4 Lighting and Access Catwalks.** The requirements of 12.2.3.2 and 12.2.3.3 shall not apply to lighting and access catwalks as permitted by 12.4.5.9.

**12.2.3.5 Reserved.**

CHAPTER 13 • Existing

**13.2.3.3 Width Modifications.** The minimum clear widths shown in Table 13.2.3.2 shall be modified in accordance with all of the following:

(1) If risers exceed 7 in. in height, the stair width in Table 13.2.3.2 shall be multiplied by factor *A*, where *A* equals the following:

$$A = 1 + \frac{\text{riser height} - 7}{5}$$

(2) If risers exceed 178 mm in height, the stair width in Table 13.2.3.2 shall be multiplied by factor *A*, where *A* equals the following:

$$A = 1 + \frac{\text{riser height} - 178}{125}$$

(3) Stairs not having a handrail within a 30 in. (760 mm) horizontal distance shall be 25 percent wider than otherwise calculated; that is, their width shall be multiplied by factor *B*, where *B* equals the following:

$$B = 1.25$$

(4) Ramps steeper than 1 in 10 slope where used in ascent shall have their width increased by 10 percent; that is, their width shall be multiplied by factor *C*, where *C* equals the following:

$$C = 1.10$$

**13.2.3.4 Lighting and Access Catwalks.** The requirements of 13.2.3.2 and 13.2.3.3 shall not apply to lighting and access catwalks as permitted by 13.4.5.9.

**13.2.3.5 Bleachers Aisles.** In seating composed entirely of bleachers for which the row-to-row dimension is 28 in. (710 mm) or less, and from which front egress is not limited, aisles shall not be required to exceed 66 in. (1675 mm) in width.

Paragraph 12/13.2.3.2 applies to egress serving theater-type seating or similar seating arranged in rows in assembly occupancies that are not smoke protected. See 12/13.2.3.1(2). If the assembly occupancy provides smoke-protected seating, the provisions of 12/13.4.2 and the capacity factors of Table 12/13.4.2.3 apply.

In using Table 12/13.2.3.2, the capacity factors might need to be adjusted using factors *A*, *B*, and *C*. Stair (i.e., stepped aisle) capacity is calculated at 0.3 in. (7.6 mm) per person only if the riser height and horizontal distance to a handrail meet specific criteria. If the stair riser height exceeds 7 in. (178 mm), the 0.3 in. (7.6 mm) per person factor must be multiplied by factor *A*, which is calculated using the formula in 12/13.2.3.3(1). If the stair does not have a handrail within a 30 in. (760 mm) horizontal distance, the 0.3 in. (7.6 mm) per person factor must be multiplied by factor *B*, which equals 1.25 per 12/13.2.3.3(3). If both the riser geometry and handrail deviations occur, the 0.3 in. (7.6 mm) per person factor must be multiplied by both a factor *A* that is greater than 1.0 and a factor *B* of 1.25.

If the stair riser height does not exceed 7 in. (178 mm), factor *A* is still used but is to equal 1.0. Similarly, if the stair does have a handrail within a 30 in. (760 mm) horizontal distance, factor *B* is still used but is to equal 1.0.

For most occupancies, egress capacity involving

horizontal travel is calculated at 0.2 in. (5 mm) per person. In Table 12/13.2.3.2, egress capacity within the audience seating chamber is penalized by 10 percent to 0.22 in. (5.6 mm) per person. Further, the presence of factor *C* indicates that additional modification of the capacity factor is necessary if the egress travel involves ascending a ramp with a slope steeper than 1 in 10. In such cases, the 0.22 in. (5.6 mm) per person capacity factor must be multiplied by a factor *C* of 1.10 per 12/13.2.3.3(4).

If the travel does not involve ascending a ramp with a slope steeper than 1 in 10, factor *C* is still used but is to equal 1.0.

## Capacity Factor Modification

The comparative examples that follow demonstrate modification of the capacity factors of Table 12/13.2.3.2.

### *Example 1*

**Inch/pound Units.** An auditorium has 5000 seats. It is not smoke protected. One stair is 70 in. wide; riser height is 7 in.; handrails are positioned at each side; an additional handrail runs along the center of the aisle. One ramp is 44 in. wide and rises with a slope of 1 in 12 to the rear exit access door.

The capacity of the stair is determined using the 0.3 *AB* formula from Table 12/13.2.3.2. Because the riser height does not exceed 7 in., factor $A = 1.0$. Because there is a handrail within a 30 in. horizontal distance, factor $B = 1.0$. Substituting gives

$$\text{Stair capacity} = \frac{70\text{ in.}}{(0.300)(1.0)(1.0)\text{ in. per person}}$$
$$= 233\text{ persons}$$

The capacity of the ramp is determined using the 0.22 *C* formula from Table 12/13.2.3.2. Factor *C* must be considered, because the ramp is used in the upward direction for egress. Because the ramp slope does not exceed 1 in 10, factor $C = 1.0$. Substituting gives

$$\text{Ramp capacity} = \frac{44\text{ in.}}{(0.22)(1.0)\text{ in. per person}}$$
$$= 200\text{ persons}$$

**SI Units.** An auditorium has 5000 seats. It is not smoke protected. One stair is 1780 mm wide; riser height is 178 mm; handrails are positioned at each side; an additional handrail runs along the center of the aisle. One ramp is 1120 mm wide and rises with a slope of 1 in 12 to the rear exit access door.

The capacity of the stair is determined using the 7.6 *AB* formula from Table 12/13.2.3.2. Because the riser height does not exceed 178 mm, factor $A = 1.0$. Because there is a handrail within a 760 mm horizontal distance, factor $B = 1.0$. Substituting gives

$$\text{Stair capacity} = \frac{1780\text{ mm}}{(7.6)(1.0)(1.0)\text{ mm per person}}$$
$$= 234\text{ persons}$$

The capacity of the ramp is determined using the 5.6 *C* formula from Table 12/13.2.3.2. Factor *C* must be considered, because the ramp is used in the upward direction for egress. Because the ramp slope does not exceed 1 in 10, factor $C = 1.0$. Substituting gives

$$\text{Ramp capacity} = \frac{1120\text{ mm}}{(5.6)(1.0)\text{ mm per person}}$$
$$= 200\text{ persons}$$

### *Example 2*

**Inch/pound Units.** An auditorium has 5000 seats. It is not smoke protected. One stair is 70 in. wide; riser height is 7.5 in.; handrails are positioned at each side; there is no handrail along the center of the aisle. One ramp is 44 in. wide and rises with a slope of 1 in 9 to the rear exit access door.

The capacity of the stair is determined using the 0.3 *AB* formula from Table 12/13.2.3.2. Because the riser height exceeds 7 in., factor *A* must be calculated using the following formula in 12/13.2.3.3(1):

$$A = 1 + \frac{7.5 - 7.0}{5} = 1.1$$

Because there is no handrail within a 30 in. horizontal distance, factor $B = 1.25$ per 12/13.2.3.3(3). Substituting gives

$$\text{Stair capacity} = \frac{70\text{ in.}}{(0.3)(1.1)(1.25)\text{ in. per person}}$$
$$= 170\text{ persons}$$

The capacity of the ramp is determined using the 0.22 *C* formula from Table 12/13.2.3.2. Because the ramp is used in ascent for egress and the slope exceeds 1 in 10, factor $C = 1.10$ per 12/13.2.3.3(4). Substituting gives

$$\text{Ramp capacity} = \frac{44\text{ in.}}{(0.22)(1.10)\text{ in. per person}}$$
$$= 182\text{ persons}$$

**SI Units.** An auditorium has 5000 seats. It is not smoke protected. One stair is 1780 mm wide; riser

CHAPTER 12 • New

height is 190 mm; handrails are positioned at each side; there is no handrail along the center of the aisle. One ramp is 1120 mm wide and rises with a slope of 1 in 9 to the rear exit access door.

The capacity of the stair is determined using the 7.6 *AB* formula from Table 12/13.2.3.2. Because the riser height exceeds 178 mm, factor *A* must be calculated using the following formula in 12/13.2.3.3(2):

$$A = 1 + \frac{190 - 178}{125} = 1.1$$

Because there is no handrail within a 760 mm horizontal distance, factor $B = 1.25$ per 12/13.2.3.3(3). Substituting gives

$$\text{Stair capacity} = \frac{1780 \text{ mm}}{(7.6)(1.1)(1.25) \text{ mm per person}} = 170 \text{ persons}$$

The capacity of the ramp is determined using the 5.6 *C* formula from Table 12/13.2.3.2. Because the ramp is used in ascent for egress and the slope exceeds 1 in 10, factor $C = 1.10$ per 12/13.2.3.3(4). Substituting gives

$$\text{Ramp capacity} = \frac{1120 \text{ mm}}{(5.6)(1.10) \text{ mm per person}} = 182 \text{ persons}$$

**12.2.3.6 Main Entrance/Exit.**

**12.2.3.6.1** Every assembly occupancy shall be provided with a main entrance/exit.

**12.2.3.6.2** The main entrance/exit width shall be as follows:

(1) The main entrance/exit shall be of a width that accommodates two-thirds of the total occupant load in the following assembly occupancies:
  (a) Bars with live entertainment
  (b) Dance halls
  (c) Discotheques
  (d) Nightclubs
  (e) Assembly occupancies with festival seating
(2) In assembly occupancies, other than those listed in 12.2.3.6.2(1), the main entrance/exit shall be of a width that accommodates one-half of the total occupant load.

**12.2.3.6.3** The main entrance/exit shall be at the level of exit discharge or shall connect to a stairway or ramp leading to a street.

**12.2.3.6.4** Access to the main entrance/exit shall be as follows:

(1) Each level of the assembly occupancy shall have access to the main entrance/exit, and such access shall have the capacity to accommodate two-thirds of the occupant load of such levels in the following assembly occupancies:
  (a) Bars with live entertainment
  (b) Dance halls
  (c) Discotheques
  (d) Nightclubs
  (e) Assembly occupancies with festival seating
(2) In assembly occupancies, other than those listed in 12.2.3.6.4(1), each level of the assembly occupancy

CHAPTER 13 • Existing

**13.2.3.6 Main Entrance/Exit.**

**13.2.3.6.1** Every assembly occupancy shall be provided with a main entrance/exit.

**13.2.3.6.2** The main entrance/exit shall be of a width that accommodates one-half of the total occupant load.

**13.2.3.6.3** The main entrance/exit shall be at the level of exit discharge or shall connect to a stairway or ramp leading to a street.

**13.2.3.6.4 Reserved.**

shall have access to the main entrance/exit, and such access shall have the capacity to accommodate one-half of the occupant load of such levels.

**12.2.3.6.5** Where the main entrance/exit from an assembly occupancy is through a lobby or foyer, the aggregate capacity of all exits from the lobby or foyer shall be permitted to provide the required capacity of the main entrance/exit, regardless of whether all such exits serve as entrances to the building.

**12.2.3.6.6*** In assembly occupancies where there is no well-defined main entrance/exit, exits shall be permitted to be distributed around the perimeter of the building, provided that the total exit width furnishes not less than 100 percent of the width needed to accommodate the permitted occupant load.

**A.12.2.3.6.6** The original *Code* wording exempted sports arenas and railway stations. If an assembly occupancy was not similar to a sports arena or railway station, it was often judged ineligible to use the provision of 12.2.3.6.6. A list of exempted assembly venues also raises the question of why other occupancies are not included and necessitates additions to the list. For example, an exhibit hall of very large size might have several main entrances/exits. A theater extending the width of a block cannot really have a main entrance/exit in one confined location. A restaurant might have a main entrance serving the parking lot and another main entrance for those entering from the street. The authority having jurisdiction needs to determine where such arrangements are acceptable.

**12.2.3.7 Other Exits.** Each level of an assembly occupancy shall have access to the main entrance/exit and shall be provided with additional exits of a width to accommodate not less than one-half of the total occupant load served by that level.

**12.2.3.7.1** Additional exits shall discharge in accordance with 12.2.7.

**12.2.3.7.2** Additional exits shall be located as far apart as practicable and as far from the main entrance/exit as practicable.

**12.2.3.7.3** Additional exits shall be accessible from a cross aisle or a side aisle.

**12.2.3.7.4** In assembly occupancies where there is no well-defined main entrance/exit, exits shall be permitted to be distributed around the perimeter of the building, provided that the total exit width furnishes not less than 100 percent of the width required to accommodate the permitted occupant load.

**13.2.3.6.5** Where the main entrance/exit from an assembly occupancy is through a lobby or foyer, the aggregate capacity of all exits from the lobby or foyer shall be permitted to provide the required capacity of the main entrance/exit, regardless of whether all such exits serve as entrances to the building.

**13.2.3.6.6*** In assembly occupancies where there is no well-defined main entrance/exit, exits shall be permitted to be distributed around the perimeter of the building, provided that the total exit width furnishes not less than 100 percent of the width needed to accommodate the permitted occupant load.

**A.13.2.3.6.6** The original *Code* wording exempted sports arenas and railway stations. If an assembly occupancy was not similar to a sports arena or railway station, it was often judged ineligible to use the provision of 13.2.3.6.6. A list of exempted assembly venues also raises the question of why other occupancies are not included and necessitates additions to the list. For example, an exhibit hall of very large size might have several main entrances/exits. A theater extending the width of a block cannot really have a main entrance/exit in one confined location. A restaurant might have a main entrance serving the parking lot and another main entrance for those entering from the street. The authority having jurisdiction needs to determine where such arrangements are acceptable.

**13.2.3.7 Other Exits.** Each level of an assembly occupancy shall have access to the main entrance/exit and shall be provided with additional exits of a width to accommodate not less than one-half of the total occupant load served by that level.

**13.2.3.7.1** Additional exits shall discharge in accordance with 13.2.7.

**13.2.3.7.2** Additional exits shall be located as far apart as practicable and as far from the main entrance/exit as practicable.

**13.2.3.7.3** Additional exits shall be accessible from a cross aisle or a side aisle.

**13.2.3.7.4** In assembly occupancies where there is no well-defined main entrance/exit, exits shall be permitted to be distributed around the perimeter of the building, provided that the total exit width furnishes not less than 100 percent of the width required to accommodate the permitted occupant load.

CHAPTER 12 • New

CHAPTER 13 • Existing

**12.2.3.8 Minimum Corridor Width.** The width of any exit access corridor serving 50 or more persons shall be not less than 44 in. (1120 mm).

In February of 2003, a fire at The Station nightclub in West Warwick, Rhode Island, claimed 100 patrons' lives. The fire began when pyrotechnics ignited exposed, acoustical foamed plastic panels that lined the walls and ceiling of a platform serving as a stage for the musical group performing to a capacity crowd. Patrons died as the fire spread faster than they could egress the building. More than 30 bodies were found blocking the main entrance/exit. Some reviewers of the disaster might judge the patrons as having panicked, while others might say the patrons behaved rationally in trying to move toward the exit that they had used to enter the nightclub, but their actions created a crowd crush. The facility was far from being *Code* compliant. The pyrotechnic devices (gerbs) used were designed for a venue with a much higher ceiling. The exposed foamed plastic panels lining the walls and ceiling of the performers' platform was a prohibited material and noted as a distinct hazard by existing *Code* requirements applicable to interior wall and ceiling finishes.

The National Institute of Standards and Technology (NIST) issued *Report of the Technical Investigation of The Station Nightclub Fire*.[5] The key findings related to emergency egress included the following:

**1.** The nightclub patrons first recognized danger 24 seconds after the pyrotechnics ignited the foam. The bulk of the crowd began to evacuate around the time that the band stopped playing (30 seconds after ignition).

**2.** About two-thirds of the occupants attempted to leave through the main entrance; many were unsuccessful.

**3.** Prior to 90 seconds into the fire, a crowd crush occurred at the main entrance that almost entirely disrupted the flow of the evacuation through the front exit.

**4.** The event that precipitated the crowd crush likely was related to the arrangement of the single interior door with merging streams of traffic and the pressure to escape the rapidly deteriorating conditions in the main area of the nightclub.

**5.** Measurements in a fire test conducted on a mock-up of a portion of The Station nightclub platform and dance floor produced — within 90 seconds — temperatures, heat fluxes, and combustion gases well in excess of accepted survivability limits.

**6.** A computer simulation of the full nightclub fire suggests that conditions around the dance floor, sunroom, and dart room would have led to severe incapacitation or death within about 90 seconds after ignition of the foam for anyone remaining standing in those areas — and not much longer even for those close to the nightclub floor.

The intent of 12/13.2.3.6 is to require that 50 percent or more of the occupants are able to egress through the same door(s) they used to enter the building. The door through which an occupant enters a building is generally the door most familiar to the occupant. The occupant can be expected to attempt to use that door for emergency egress. The term *main entrance/exit* clarifies that the *Code* intends the main entrance to an assembly occupancy to be designated as the main exit.

The 50 percent main entrance capacity criterion was established prior to 1970. Since the 2006 edition, 12.2.3.6.2 increased to two-thirds the minimum capacity required at the main entrance/exit for new nightclub-type assembly occupancies. The provision was not made retroactively applicable to existing assembly occupancies, as that would have imposed an unreasonable burden.

Note that 12.2.3.7 continues to require that the other exits (i.e., exits other than the main entrance/exit) provide capacity for not less than 50 percent of the occupant load. Thus, new nightclub-type assembly occupancies are required to provide capacity for 117 percent of the occupant load, calculated as $\frac{2}{3} + \frac{1}{2} = 1.17$.

As an example of the requirements of 12/13.2.3.6.2 and 12/13.2.3.7, if a new assembly occupancy (other than a nightclub-type assembly occupancy) or an existing assembly occupancy has an occupant load of 900 persons, the main exit would have to accommodate 450 persons (one-half). The other exits would have to accommodate the remaining 450 persons. For a new nightclub-type assembly occupancy with an occupant load of 900 persons, the main exit would have to accommodate 600 persons (two-thirds), and the other exits would have to accommodate 450 persons (one-half), for a total of 1050 persons (117 percent).

Where the main entrance is through a lobby, a majority of the occupants can be expected to return to the lobby area during emergency egress. If the lobby has additional doors that are not used as entrance doors (e.g., doors A and B in Exhibit 12/13.11), the occupants are likely to use these doors, because they have reached the lobby, with which they are familiar. Thus, 12/13.2.3.6.5 permits all the lobby doors to serve collectively as the required main exit. See Exhibit 12/13.11.

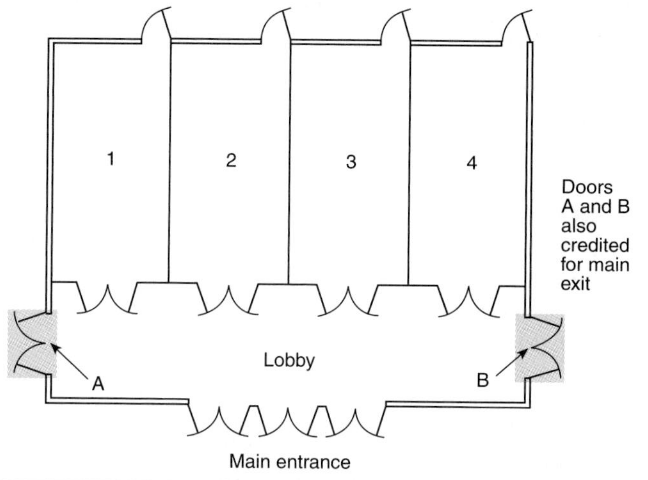


***Exhibit 12/13.11*** *Main entrance/exit.*

Paragraph 12/13.2.3.6.6 acknowledges that some assembly occupancy buildings have no well-defined main entrance/exit. Occupants enter the building by doors in multiple walls. Under emergency egress conditions, all occupants will not attempt to use the same doors, because some occupants are familiar with certain doors, while others are familiar with other doors. In such cases, it is the intent that egress width be distributed among the various exits without any one exit being required to provide 50 percent of the egress capacity. See also 12/13.2.3.7.4.

A major change occurred in the 1991 edition of the *Code* with the deletion of a requirement that exits, other than the main exit, had to accommodate two-thirds of the occupant load, which resulted in a $16\frac{2}{3}$ percent overdesign. For new nightclub-like assembly occupancies, 12.2.3.6.2(1) reinstates the two-thirds concept but applies it to the main entrance/exit, which is expected to experience use by the majority of the occupants, as explained in the previous paragraph.

The minimum 44 in. (1120 mm) width for exit access corridors serving 50 or more persons in new assembly occupancies — required by 12.2.3.8 — allows more than one file of persons to travel along the corridor simultaneously. The minimum width also permits persons capable of traveling at normal speed to pass persons who are slower, rather than queuing behind them.

### 12.2.4* Number of Exits.

**A.12.2.4** It is not the intent to require four means of egress from each level of an assembly occupancy building having a total occupant load of more than 1000 where, individually, the floors have occupant loads of less than 1000.

**12.2.4.1** The number of exits shall be in accordance with Section 7.4, other than exits for fenced outdoor assembly occupancies in accordance with 12.2.4.4.

**12.2.4.2 Reserved.**

**12.2.4.3 Reserved.**

**12.2.4.4** A fenced outdoor assembly occupancy shall have not less than two remote means of egress from the enclosure in accordance with 7.5.1.3, unless otherwise required by one of the following:

(1) If more than 6000 persons are to be served by such means of egress, there shall be not less than three means of egress.

### 13.2.4* Number of Exits.

**A.13.2.4** It is not the intent to require four means of egress from each level of an assembly occupancy building having a total occupant load of more than 1000 where, individually, the floors have occupant loads of less than 1000.

**13.2.4.1** The number of exits shall be in accordance with Section 7.4, other than fenced outdoor assembly occupancies in accordance with 13.2.4.4, unless otherwise permitted by 13.2.4.2 or 13.2.4.3.

**13.2.4.2** Assembly occupancies with occupant loads of 600 or fewer shall have two separate means of egress.

**13.2.4.3** Assembly occupancies with occupant loads greater than 600 but fewer than 1000 shall have three separate means of egress.

**13.2.4.4** A fenced outdoor assembly occupancy shall have not less than two widely separated means of egress from the enclosure, unless otherwise required by one of the following:

(1) If more than 6000 persons are to be served by such means of egress, there shall be not less than three means of egress.

CHAPTER 12 • New

(2) If more than 9000 persons are to be served by such means of egress, there shall be not less than four means of egress.

**12.2.4.5** Balconies or mezzanines having an occupant load not exceeding 50 shall be permitted to be served by a single means of egress, and such means of egress shall be permitted to lead to the floor below.

**12.2.4.6** Balconies or mezzanines having an occupant load exceeding 50, but not exceeding 100, shall have not less than two remote means of egress, but both such means of egress shall be permitted to lead to the floor below.

**12.2.4.7** Balconies or mezzanines having an occupant load exceeding 100 shall have means of egress as described in 7.4.1.

**12.2.4.8** A second means of egress shall not be required from lighting and access catwalks, galleries, and gridirons where a means of escape to a floor or a roof is provided. Ladders, alternating tread devices, or spiral stairs shall be permitted in such means of escape.

CHAPTER 13 • Existing

(2) If more than 9000 persons are to be served by such means of egress, there shall be not less than four means of egress.

**13.2.4.5** Balconies or mezzanines having an occupant load not exceeding 50 shall be permitted to be served by a single means of egress, and such means of egress shall be permitted to lead to the floor below.

**13.2.4.6** Balconies or mezzanines having an occupant load exceeding 50, but not exceeding 100, shall have not less than two remote means of egress, but both such means of egress shall be permitted to lead to the floor below.

**13.2.4.7** Balconies or mezzanines having an occupant load exceeding 100 shall have means of egress as described in 7.4.1.

**13.2.4.8** A second means of egress shall not be required from lighting and access catwalks, galleries, and gridirons where a means of escape to a floor or a roof is provided. Ladders, alternating tread devices, or spiral stairs shall be permitted in such means of escape.

Assembly occupancy spaces, other than on small balconies or mezzanines as detailed in 12/13.2.4.5, are required to be provided with a minimum of two means of egress. Any room occupied for assembly use by at least 50 persons, so as to constitute an assembly occupancy, must be provided with two means of egress from the room (e.g., two exit access doors to a corridor). A room with an occupant load of 49 or fewer persons, used for adult education so as to constitute a business occupancy, has no direct requirement for providing a second exit access from the room. The business occupancy room is permitted a single means of egress (e.g., an exit access door to a corridor), provided that the allowable common path of travel is not exceeded.

As the concentration or number of people in an assembly occupancy increases, the need for simultaneous egressing by a sizable group of occupants increases. Therefore, to reduce jamming at doorways (which might lead to panic and disorder), in accordance with the provisions of Section 7.4, more than two exits are needed for large occupant loads.

By permitting a single means of egress from a small balcony or mezzanine, 12/13.2.4.5 provides a relaxation in requirements for balconies and mezzanines that do not accommodate more than 50 people, such as choir lofts. See also 12/13.2.5.1.2, which increases the permitted common path of travel to 75 ft (23 m) from an area with not more than 50 occupants.

The balconies or mezzanines addressed by 12/13.2.4.6 might typically be found in restaurants or small theaters. The provisions explain that it is important to have two remote means of egress, but, because the total number of occupants does not exceed 100, it is reasonable to permit occupants to egress onto the floor below.

Any balcony or mezzanine that can accommodate more than 100 people, as addressed by 12/13.2.4.7, should be treated as a separate floor with regard to the number of means of egress. Such treatment avoids overloading the means of egress on the floor below and provides mezzanine occupants with independent travel paths in case of fire on the floor below.

Paragraph 12.2.4.4 was revised for the 2006 edition to employ the remoteness criteria of 7.5.1.3. In 13.2.4.4, the existing text was retained so as to require that the two means of egress for fenced outdoor assembly occupancies be "widely separated" — a subjective term that is difficult to enforce consistently.

CHAPTER 12 • New

### 12.2.5 Arrangement of Means of Egress.

**12.2.5.1 General.**

**12.2.5.1.1** Means of egress shall be arranged in accordance with Section 7.5.

**12.2.5.1.2** A common path of travel shall be permitted for the first 20 ft (6100 mm) from any point where the common path serves any number of occupants, and for the first 75 ft (23 m) from any point where the common path serves not more than 50 occupants.

**12.2.5.1.3** Dead-end corridors shall not exceed 20 ft (6100 mm).

**12.2.5.2 Access Through Hazardous Areas.** Means of egress from a room or space for assembly purposes shall not be permitted through kitchens, storerooms, restrooms, closets, platforms, stages, projection rooms, or hazardous areas as described in 12.3.2.

**12.2.5.3 Auditorium and Area Floors.** Where the floor area of auditoriums and arenas is used for assembly occupancy activities/events, not less than 50 percent of the occupant load shall have means of egress provided without passing through adjacent fixed seating areas.

CHAPTER 13 • Existing

### 13.2.5 Arrangement of Means of Egress.

**13.2.5.1 General.**

**13.2.5.1.1** Means of egress shall be arranged in accordance with Section 7.5.

**13.2.5.1.2** A common path of travel shall be permitted for the first 20 ft (6100 mm) from any point where the common path serves any number of occupants, and for the first 75 ft (23 m) from any point where the common path serves not more than 50 occupants.

**13.2.5.1.3** Dead-end corridors shall not exceed 20 ft (6100 mm).

**13.2.5.2 Access Through Hazardous Areas.** Means of egress shall not be permitted through kitchens, storerooms, restrooms, closets, platforms, stages, or hazardous areas as described in 13.3.2.

**13.2.5.3 Reserved.**

The remoteness of exit accesses, exits, and exit discharges is an important concept addressed by Chapter 7. Exit accesses, exits, and exit discharges that are located too close to each other can quickly become unusable during a single fire. The provisions of 4.5.3.1 require remoteness of means of egress paths to the point that a single fire will not simultaneously block two routes. The remoteness requirements of Section 7.5 must be met.

Revolving rooftop assembly occupancies require special consideration; as the structure revolves, exit signs are often lost from view. To provide an unobstructed panoramic view, the exterior ring-shaped floor area revolves around a small stationary interior core where the exits are often located. In many cases, the two exits are too close to each other to meet remoteness criteria. Usually, at least one stairway from the building core involves a horizontal passage on the floor below to transfer occupants from that stairway to the normal, remotely located exit stairways. This transfer, because it is a continuation of the exit stair enclosure within the core, must be made via an exit passageway with a fire resistance rating equal to that required for the exit stair enclosure.

Although exit access and exit placement must meet the remoteness criteria of Section 7.5, it is not practical to require immediate access to egress paths from every point in a building. Rather, occupants are permitted to be forced to travel in only one direction for a limited distance before reaching a point where travel in more than one direction becomes possible. This limited travel in one direction is called *common path of travel* (see definition in 3.3.42). See the commentary associated with A.7.5.1.5.

Paragraph 12/13.2.5.1.2 establishes two allowable common paths of travel limitations as follows:

1. 20 ft (6100 mm), regardless of occupant load
2. 75 ft (23 m) where serving not more than 50 persons

Additionally, 12/13.2.5.5.5 permits a 30 ft (9.1 m) common path of travel between a point within an aisle accessway and the aisle serving a seating row. Paragraph 12/13.4.2.9 permits a 50 ft (15 m) common path of travel in seating areas in smoke-protected assembly seating. Thus, the common path of travel limitations are numerous for assembly occupancies.

The requirement of 12/13.2.5.2 clarifies that exit access travel is not permitted to pass through areas subject to locking or areas presenting a hazard level higher than that normally associated with an assembly occupancy, including platforms and stages.

CHAPTER 12 • New

The provision of 12.2.5.3, which applies only to new assembly occupancies, is intended to reduce the amount of merging and sharing of means of egress by persons in fixed seating areas and those who are forced to travel from the arena floor up into the seating sections to egress the building.

**12.2.5.4 General Requirements for Access and Egress Routes Within Assembly Areas.**

**12.2.5.4.1** Festival seating, as defined in 3.3.221.1, shall be prohibited within a building, unless otherwise permitted by the following:

(1) Festival seating shall be permitted in assembly occupancies having occupant loads of 250 or less.
(2) Festival seating shall be permitted in assembly occupancies where occupant loads exceed 250, provided that an approved life safety evaluation has been performed. *(See 12.4.1.)*

**12.2.5.4.2*** Access and egress routes shall be maintained so that any individual is able to move without undue hindrance, on personal initiative and at any time, from an occupied position to the exits.

**A.12.2.5.4.2** This requirement and the associated requirement of 12.2.5.4.3 have the effect of prohibiting festival seating, unless it truly is a form of seating, such as lawn seating, where generous spaces are commonly maintained between individuals and small groups so that people can circulate freely at any time. Such lawn seating is characterized by densities of about one person per 15 $ft^2$ (1.4 $m^2$). Both requirements prohibit uncontrolled crowd situations, such as in front of stages at rock music concerts where the number and density of people is uncontrolled by architectural or management features.

**12.2.5.4.3*** Access and egress routes shall be maintained so that crowd management, security, and emergency medical personnel are able to reach any individual at any time, without undue hindrance.

**A.12.2.5.4.3** This requirement is intended to facilitate rapid emergency access to individuals who are experiencing a medical emergency, especially in the case of cardiopulmonary difficulties, where there is a need for rapid medical attention from trained personnel. The requirement also addresses the need for security and law enforcement personnel to reach individuals whose behavior is endangering themselves and others.

**12.2.5.4.4*** The width of aisle accessways and aisles shall provide sufficient egress capacity for the number of persons accommodated by the catchment area served by the aisle accessway or aisle in accordance with 12.2.3.2, or for smoke-protected assembly seating in accordance with 12.4.2.

CHAPTER 13 • Existing

**13.2.5.4 General Requirements for Access and Egress Routes Within Assembly Areas.**

**13.2.5.4.1** Festival seating, as defined in 3.3.221.1, shall be prohibited within a building, unless otherwise permitted by the following:

(1) Festival seating shall be permitted in assembly occupancies having occupant loads of 250 or less.
(2) Festival seating shall be permitted in assembly occupancies where occupant loads exceed 250, provided that an approved life safety evaluation has been performed. *(See 13.4.1.)*

**13.2.5.4.2*** Access and egress routes shall be maintained so that any individual is able to move without undue hindrance, on personal initiative and at any time, from an occupied position to the exits.

**A.13.2.5.4.2** This requirement and the associated requirement of 13.2.5.4.3 have the effect of prohibiting festival seating, unless it truly is a form of seating, such as lawn seating, where generous spaces are commonly maintained between individuals and small groups so that people can circulate freely at any time. Such lawn seating is characterized by densities of about one person per 15 $ft^2$ (1.4 $m^2$). Both requirements prohibit uncontrolled crowd situations, such as in front of stages at rock music concerts where the number and density of people is uncontrolled by architectural or management features.

**13.2.5.4.3*** Access and egress routes shall be maintained so that crowd management, security, and emergency medical personnel are able to reach any individual at any time, without undue hindrance.

**A.13.2.5.4.3** This requirement is intended to facilitate rapid emergency access to individuals who are experiencing a medical emergency, especially in the case of cardiopulmonary difficulties, where there is a need for rapid medical attention from trained personnel. The requirement also addresses the need for security and law enforcement personnel to reach individuals whose behavior is endangering themselves and others.

**13.2.5.4.4*** The width of aisle accessways and aisles shall provide sufficient egress capacity for the number of persons accommodated by the catchment area served by the aisle accessway or aisle in accordance with 13.2.3.2, or for smoke-protected assembly seating in accordance with 13.4.2.

CHAPTER 12 • New

**A.12.2.5.4.4** The catchment area served by an aisle accessway or aisle is the portion of the total space that is naturally served by the aisle accessway or aisle. Hence, the requirement for combining the required capacity where paths converge is, in effect, a restatement of the idea of a catchment area. The establishment of catchment areas should be based on a balanced use of all means of egress, with the number of persons in proportion to egress capacity.

**12.2.5.4.5** Where aisle accessways or aisles converge to form a single path of egress travel, the required egress capacity of that path shall be not less than the combined required capacity of the converging aisle accessways and aisles.

**12.2.5.4.6** Those portions of aisle accessways and aisles where egress is possible in either of two directions shall be uniform in required width, unless otherwise permitted by 12.2.5.4.7.

**12.2.5.4.7** The requirement of 12.2.5.4.6 shall not apply to those portions of aisle accessways where the required width, not including the seat space described by 12.2.5.7.3, does not exceed 12 in. (305 mm).

**12.2.5.4.8** In the case of side boundaries for aisle accessways or aisles, other than those for nonfixed seating at tables, the clear width shall be measured to boundary elements such as walls, guardrails, handrails, edges of seating, tables, and side edges of treads, and said measurement shall be made horizontally to the vertical projection of the elements, resulting in the smallest width measured perpendicularly to the line of travel.

CHAPTER 13 • Existing

**A.13.2.5.4.4** The catchment area served by an aisle accessway or aisle is the portion of the total space that is naturally served by the aisle accessway or aisle. Hence, the requirement for combining the required capacity where paths converge is, in effect, a restatement of the idea of a catchment area. The establishment of catchment areas should be based on a balanced use of all means of egress, with the number of persons in proportion to egress capacity.

**13.2.5.4.5** Where aisle accessways or aisles converge to form a single path of egress travel, the required egress capacity of that path shall be not less than the combined required capacity of the converging aisle accessways and aisles.

**13.2.5.4.6** Those portions of aisle accessways and aisles where egress is possible in either of two directions shall be uniform in required width, unless otherwise permitted by 13.2.5.4.7.

**13.2.5.4.7** The requirement of 13.2.5.4.6 shall not apply to those portions of aisle accessways where the required width, not including the seat space described by 13.2.5.7.3, does not exceed 12 in. (305 mm).

**13.2.5.4.8** In the case of side boundaries for aisle accessways or aisles, other than those for nonfixed seating at tables, the clear width shall be measured to boundary elements such as walls, guardrails, handrails, edges of seating, tables, and side edges of treads, and said measurement shall be made horizontally to the vertical projection of the elements, resulting in the smallest width measured perpendicularly to the line of travel.

Festival seating, as addressed in 12/13.2.5.4.1, is illustrated in Exhibit 12/13.12. The low-density arrangement of people depicted, which provides them with the ability to sit directly on the ground or floor and to move relatively easily through and out of the area, likely evolved from outdoor festivals held in open areas. Festival seating has been abused — at both indoor and outdoor events — where the assembled spectators are not controllable in terms of their numbers, location, or behavior. A rock music concert is an example of an event where the festival seating concept might become decidedly unfestive when unmanageable crowds of standing (not seated) people form in front of the stage area and circulation routes through the assembled crowd are completely lost. Injuries caused by bodies crushing against bodies or portions of the structure are likely when this situation occurs.

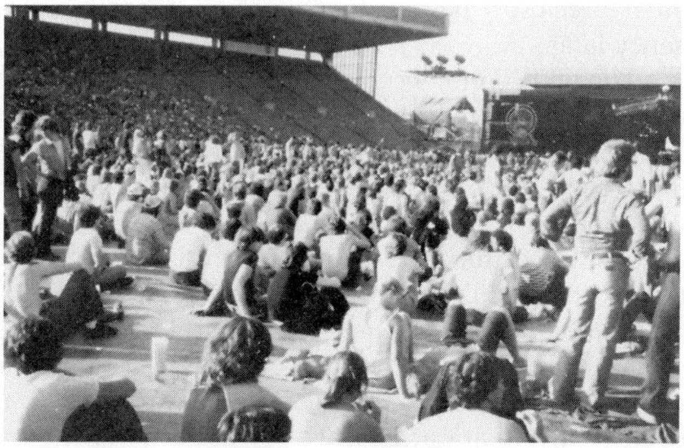

***Exhibit 12/13.12*** *Outdoor festival seating at a rock music concert held in a stadium. (Photograph courtesy of Jake Pauls)*

 

A description of a typical crowd crush is found in a report titled "Observations of Crowd Conditions at Rock Concert in Exhibition Stadium, Toronto, 16 July 1980," by J. L. Pauls.[6] Because the number and arrangement of people in this instance were not controlled throughout the event, there were eventually some 30,000 to 40,000 people distributed unevenly in an area of about 125,000 ft² (10,600 m²). The result was an average density of about 1 person per 3.5 ft² (0.33 m²). However, due to localized crowding at the stage area, several thousand people were at crushing densities of about 1 person per 2 ft² (0.19 m²). Both normal access and emergency access into this congested area were all but impossible, and management efforts to instruct people to move back toward less densely occupied areas proved futile. Incidents such as this led to the requirements of 12/13.2.5.4.1, which prohibit indoor festival seating for more than 250 persons unless an approved life safety evaluation is utilized.

In performance-oriented language, 12/13.2.5.4.2 prohibits overcrowding and the blocking of aisles and other portions of the exit access. See the explanation in A.12/A.13.2.5.4.2.

In addition to providing life safety under fire conditions, the requirements of 12/13.2.5.4.3 address the emergency and nonemergency movement of people. Because of the potential for ingress and egress paths to become blocked by the large crowds characteristic of many assembly occupancies, it is important that crowd management, security, and emergency medical personnel are able to move to any individual without undue hindrance at any time. The ability to deal effectively with an emergency while the problem is small often precludes having to deal with a larger emergency later.

The width referenced in 12/13.2.5.4.4 refers to the egress capacity–driven width requirements of 12/13.2.3. The capacity-related width requirements must be considered along with the other minimum width requirements detailed in 12/13.2.5.6.3. The applicable minimum width requirement is the larger of the widths established by the two sets of requirements.

Exhibit 12/13.13 illustrates how catchment areas would be allotted in the case of a theater with four egress doors having approximately equal egress capacity. Note that catchment area apportionment for normal, nonemergency uses often will make use of only some of the available exit access paths and exits, particularly those provided by the main entrance/exit.

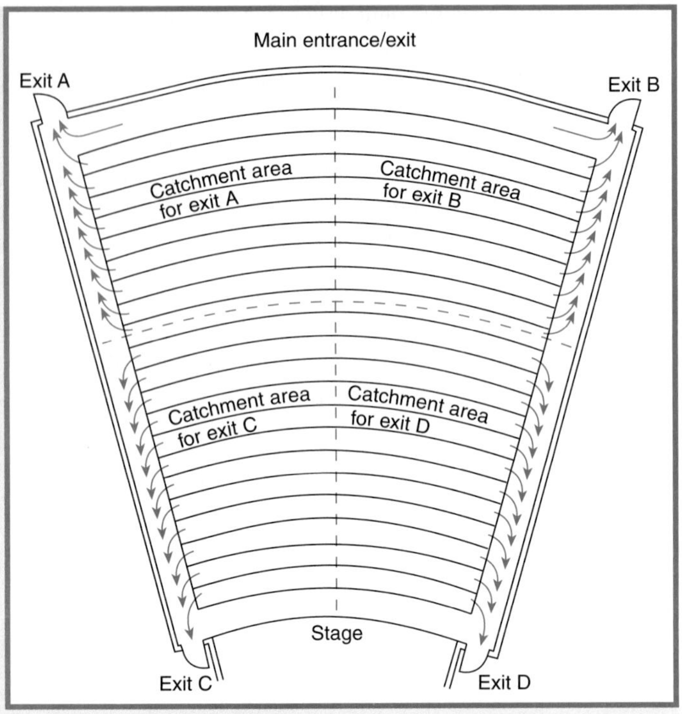


***Exhibit 12/13.13** Catchment areas based on balanced use of all means of egress in proportion to egress capacity.*

This arrangement might be quite different from a catchment area apportionment based on a balanced distribution of people in proportion to the egress capacity of individual exits. Facility management procedures must allow for the difficulties of informing people of, and directing them to, all the available means of egress, especially when normally used, familiar routes become blocked in an emergency.

Note that the phrase "required egress capacity" is used in 12/13.2.5.4.5 to clarify that the combined required width of the egress routes might be smaller than their combined actual widths. Widths that exceed *Code* minimums might be provided voluntarily to facilitate day-to-day operations.

Per 12/13.2.5.4.6, if egress travel is possible in two directions, all portions of the aisle or aisle accessway must meet or exceed the minimum width required for any other portion of the aisle or aisle accessway. Generally, this prohibits aisles and aisle accessways from being hourglass shaped, allowing them to accommodate efficient egress travel that might have to reverse direction because of blockage at one end of the aisle or aisle accessway.

CHAPTER 12 • New

**12.2.5.5* Aisle Accessways Serving Seating Not at Tables.**

**A.12.2.5.5** For purposes of the means of egress requirements of this *Code*, tablet-arm chair seating is not considered seating at tables. Dinner theater–style configurations are required to comply with the aisle accessway provisions applying to seating at tables and the aisle requirements of 12.2.5.6, if the aisles contain steps or are ramped. Generally, if aisles contain steps or are ramped, all of the *Code* requirements for aisles, stairs, and ramps are required to be met. *(Also see 7.1.7 and A.7.1.7.2.)*

**12.2.5.5.1*** The required clear width of aisle accessways between rows of seating shall be determined as follows:

(1) Horizontal measurements shall be made, between vertical planes, from the back of one seat to the front of the most forward projection of the seat immediately behind it.
(2) Where the entire row consists of automatic- or self-rising seats that comply with ASTM F 851, *Standard Test Method for Self-Rising Seat Mechanisms*, the measurement shall be permitted to be made with the seats in the up position.

**A.12.2.5.5.1** Seats having reclining backs are assumed to be in their most upright position when unoccupied.

*Aisle accessway* is defined in 3.3.11 as "the initial portion of an exit access that leads to an aisle." Exhibit 12/13.14 illustrates the aisle accessways formed by rows of chairs. The space between each row of chairs (indicated by the arrows) is an aisle accessway.

The method for measuring the width of an aisle accessway formed by rows of chairs is illustrated in Exhibit 12/13.15. In Part (a) in Exhibit 12/13.15, the seats are not self-rising. In Part (b), the seats are self-rising, as detailed in 12/13.2.5.5.1(2).

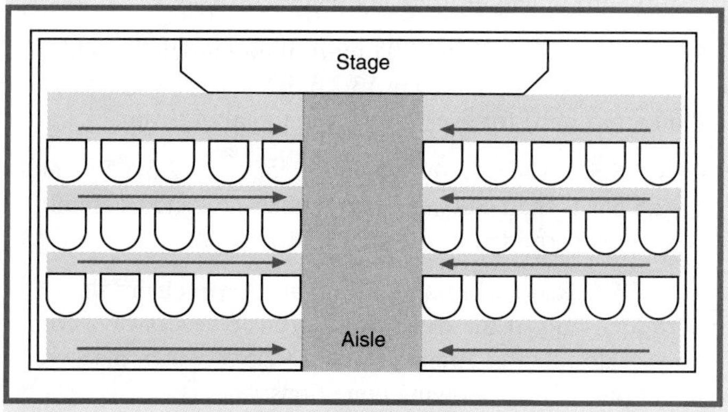


***Exhibit 12/13.14** Aisle accessways.*

CHAPTER 13 • Existing

**13.2.5.5* Aisle Accessways Serving Seating Not at Tables.**

**A.13.2.5.5** For purposes of the means of egress requirements of this *Code*, tablet-arm chair seating is not considered seating at tables. Dinner theater–style configurations are required to comply with the aisle accessway provisions applying to seating at tables and the aisle requirements of 13.2.5.6, if the aisles contain steps or are ramped. Generally, if aisles contain steps or are ramped, all of the *Code* requirements for aisles, stairs, and ramps are required to be met. *(Also see 7.1.7 and A.7.1.7.2.)*

**13.2.5.5.1*** The required clear width of aisle accesses between rows of seating shall be determined as follows:

(1) Horizontal measurements shall be made, between vertical planes, from the back of one seat to the front of the most forward projection of the seat immediately behind it.
(2) Where the entire row consists of automatic- or self--rising seats that comply with ASTM F 851, *Standard Test Method for Self-Rising Seat Mechanisms*, the measurement shall be permitted to be made with the seats in the up position.

**A.13.2.5.5.1** Seats having reclining backs are assumed to be in their most upright position when unoccupied.

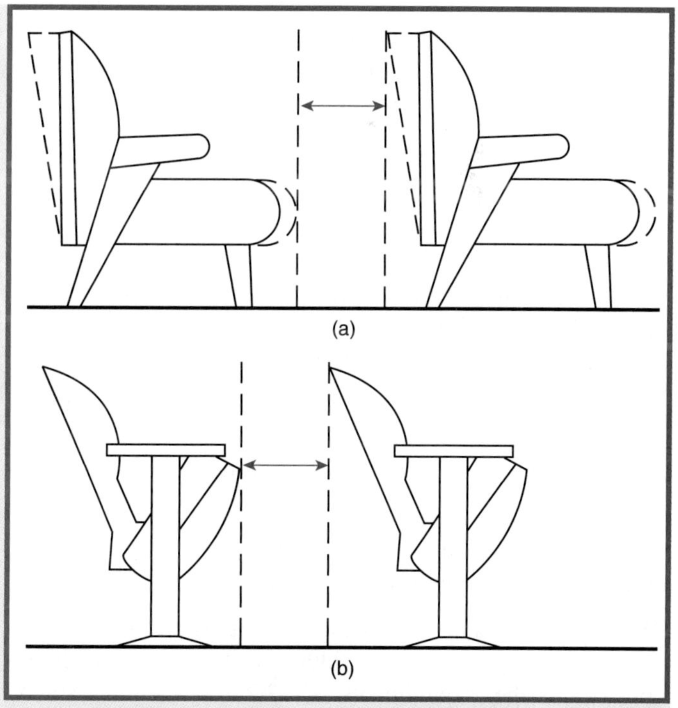


***Exhibit 12/13.15** Measurement of width of aisle accessway formed by rows of chairs.*

CHAPTER 12 • New

**12.2.5.5.2** The aisle accessway between rows of seating shall have a clear width of not less than 12 in. (305 mm), and this minimum shall be increased as a function of row length in accordance with 12.2.5.5.4 and 12.2.5.5.5.

**12.2.5.5.3** If used by not more than four persons, no minimum clear width shall be required for the portion of an aisle accessway having a length not exceeding 6 ft (1830 mm), measured from the center of the seat farthest from the aisle.

**12.2.5.5.4*** Rows of seating served by aisles or doorways at both ends shall not exceed 100 seats per row.

**A.12.2.5.5.4** The system known as *continental seating* has one pair of egress doors provided for every five rows that is located close to the ends of the rows. In previous editions of the *Code*, such egress doors were required to provide a clear width of not less than 66 in. (1675 mm) discharging into a foyer, into a lobby, or to the exterior of the building. This continental seating arrangement can result in egress flow times (i.e., with nominal flow times of approximately 100 seconds, rather than 200 seconds) that are approximately one-half as long as those resulting where side aisles lead to more remote doors. Such superior egress flow time performance is desirable in some situations; however, special attention should be given either to a comparably good egress capacity for other parts of the egress system or to sufficient space to accommodate queuing outside the seating space.

**12.2.5.5.4.1** The 12 in. (305 mm) minimum clear width of aisle accessway specified in 12.2.5.5.2 shall be increased by 0.3 in. (7.6 mm) for every seat over a total of 14 but shall not be required to exceed 22 in. (560 mm).

**12.2.5.5.4.2** The requirement of 12.2.5.5.4.1 shall not apply to smoke-protected assembly seating as permitted by 12.4.2.7.

**12.2.5.5.5** Rows of seating served by an aisle or doorway at one end only shall have a path of travel not exceeding 30 ft (9140 mm) in length from any seat to an aisle.

**12.2.5.5.5.1** The 12 in. (305 mm) minimum clear width of aisle accessway specified in 12.2.5.5.2 shall be increased by 0.6 in. (15 mm) for every seat over a total of seven.

**12.2.5.5.5.2** The requirements of 12.2.5.5.5 and 12.2.5.5.5.1 shall not apply to smoke-protected assembly seating as permitted by 12.4.2.8 and 12.4.2.9.

**12.2.5.5.6** Rows of seating using tablet-arm chairs shall be permitted only if the clear width of aisle accessways complies with the requirements of 12.2.5.5 when measured under one of the following conditions:

(1) The clear width is measured with the tablet arm in the usable position.

CHAPTER 13 • Existing

**13.2.5.5.2** The aisle accessway between rows of seating shall have a clear width of not less than 12 in. (305 mm), and this minimum shall be increased as a function of row length in accordance with 13.2.5.5.4 and 13.2.5.5.5.

**13.2.5.5.3** If used by not more than four persons, no minimum clear width shall be required for the portion of an aisle accessway having a length not exceeding 6 ft (1830 mm), measured from the center of the seat farthest from the aisle.

**13.2.5.5.4*** Rows of seating served by aisles or doorways at both ends shall not exceed 100 seats per row.

**A.13.2.5.5.4** The system known as *continental seating* has one pair of egress doors provided for every five rows that is located close to the ends of the rows. In previous editions of the *Code*, such egress doors were required to provide a clear width of not less than 66 in. (1675 mm) discharging into a foyer, into a lobby, or to the exterior of the building. This continental seating arrangement can result in egress flow times (i.e., with nominal flow times of approximately 100 seconds rather than 200 seconds) that are approximately one-half as long as those resulting where side aisles lead to more remote doors. Such superior egress flow time performance is desirable in some situations; however, special attention should be given either to a comparably good egress capacity for other parts of the egress system or to sufficient space to accommodate queuing outside the seating space.

**13.2.5.5.4.1** The 12 in. (305 mm) minimum clear width of aisle accessway specified in 13.2.5.5.2 shall be increased by 0.3 in. (7.6 mm) for every seat over a total of 14 but shall not be required to exceed 22 in. (560 mm).

**13.2.5.5.4.2** The requirement of 13.2.5.5.4.1 shall not apply to smoke-protected assembly seating as permitted by 13.4.2.7.

**13.2.5.5.5** Rows of seating served by an aisle or doorway at one end only shall have a path of travel not exceeding 30 ft (9140 mm) in length from any seat to an aisle.

**13.2.5.5.5.1** The 12 in. (305 mm) minimum clear width of aisle accessway specified in 13.2.5.5.2 shall be increased by 0.6 in. (15 mm) for every seat over a total of seven.

**13.2.5.5.5.2** The requirements of 13.2.5.5.5 and 13.2.5.5.5.1 shall not apply to smoke-protected assembly seating as permitted by 13.4.2.8 and 13.4.2.9.

**13.2.5.5.6** Rows of seating using tablet-arm chairs shall be permitted only if the clear width of aisle accessways complies with the requirements of 13.2.5.5 when measured under one of the following conditions:

(1) The clear width is measured with the tablet arm in the usable position.

CHAPTER 12 • New

(2) The clear width is measured with the tablet arm in the stored position where the tablet arm automatically returns to the stored position when raised manually to a vertical position in one motion and falls to the stored position by force of gravity.

**12.2.5.5.7** The depth of seat boards shall be not less than 9 in. (230 mm) where the same level is not used for both seat boards and footboards.

**12.2.5.5.8** Footboards, independent of seats, shall be provided so that there is no horizontal opening that allows the passage of a ½ in. (13 mm) diameter sphere.

CHAPTER 13 • Existing

(2) The clear width is measured with the tablet arm in the stored position where the tablet arm automatically returns to the stored position when raised manually to a vertical position in one motion and falls to the stored position by force of gravity.

**13.2.5.5.7** The depth of seat boards shall be not less than 9 in. (230 mm) where the same level is not used for both seat boards and footboards.

**13.2.5.5.8** Footboards, independent of seats, shall be provided so that there is no horizontal opening that allows the passage of a ½ in. (13 mm) diameter sphere.

The text of A.12/A.13.2.5.5.4 relates the expected egress flow time performance of continental seating, as addressed by the *Code* prior to 1988, to the egress flow time performance of the more flexible requirements for egress width related to capacity. See Exhibit 12/13.16 for an example of continental seating. In earlier editions of the *Code*, this arrangement was required where there were more than 14 seats in a row. A maximum of 100 seats was permitted for one row.

Currently, the *Code* permits design flexibility, based on the continental seating principle of variable minimum spacing for rows of seats and row length, using the provisions of 12/13.2.5.5.4.1. As reference

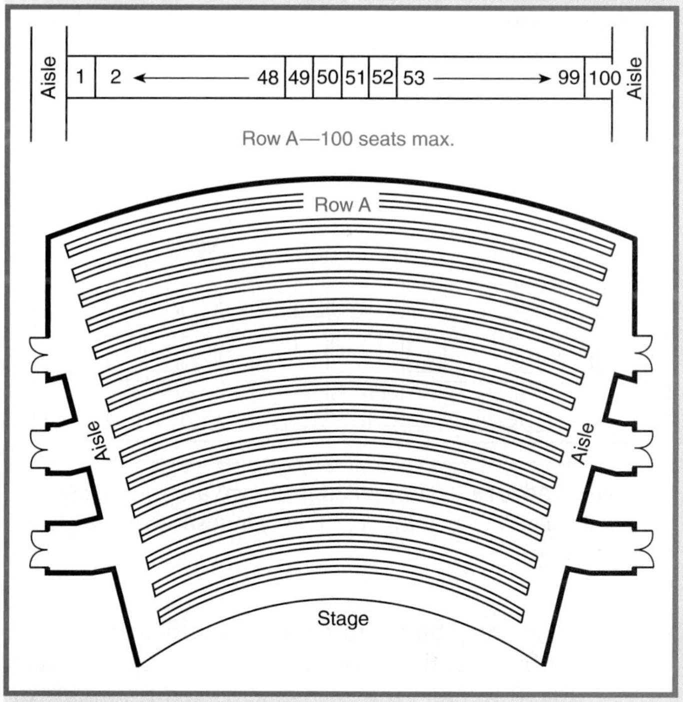


***Exhibit 12/13.16** Arrangement of seats and aisles with continental seating.*

points for each end of the spacing range, the newer requirement uses the previous 12 in. (305 mm) of clearance for rows up to 14 seats in length and 22 in. (560 mm) for rows over 47 seats in length. For example, rows with 47 seats require a clearance of 21.9 in. (555 mm). This clearance is calculated by subtracting 14 from 47 and multiplying the result, 33, by 0.3 in. (7.6 mm) to obtain 9.9 in. (250 mm), which is added to the 12 in. (305 mm) minimum aisle accessway width to obtain the total required clear aisle accessway width of 21.9 in. (555 mm). Because the aisle accessway width is not required to exceed 22 in. (560 mm), rows with 48 to 100 seats require 22 in. (560 mm) of clear aisle accessway width.

The current flexibility, which applies to all seating arranged in rows, is based on the assumption that the egress time required for a seating arrangement will be influenced more by the capacity of routes downstream from the rows of seating than by the rows' clear widths. Subsection 12/13.2.3 provides a standardized method for calculating the widths of those routes serving the space containing the seating. The combination of 12/13.2.3 and 12/13.2.5.5 offers designers of theaters, in particular, a great deal of flexibility in laying out blocks of seating while still requiring a standard of egress flow time performance that is based on traditionally accepted egress performance. Traditional performance, nominally about 200 seconds of flow time, is achieved through the application of specific requirements on aisle and cross-aisle design. For example, rows longer than 14 seats are permitted, and egress door locations can be more flexibly determined than is permitted under the continental seating rules contained in previous *Code* editions.

Exhibit 12/13.17 illustrates the seating layout for a theater with 630 seats in a single unbroken area, with 21 rows ranging uniformly in length from 20 seats at row 1 to 40 seats at row 21. The required minimum

CHAPTER 12 • New | CHAPTER 13 • Existing

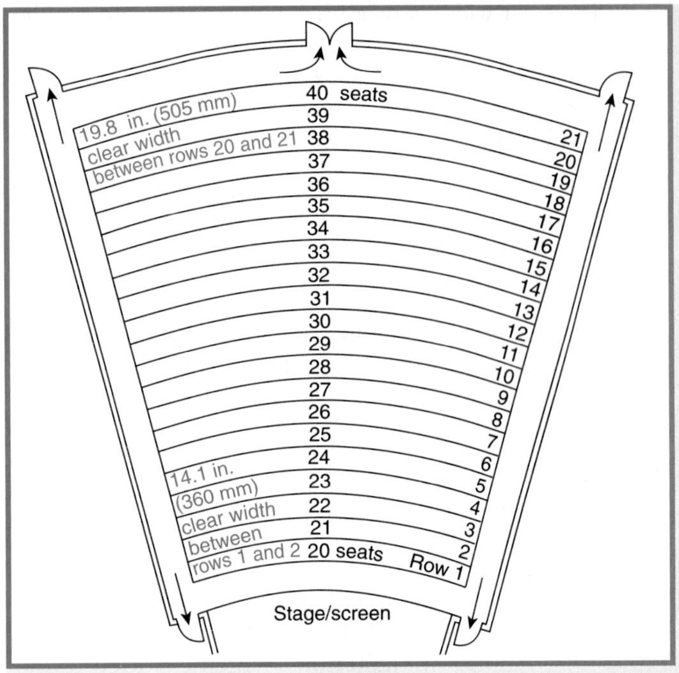


***Exhibit 12/13.17*** *Minimum aisle accessway clear widths.*

aisle accessway clear width between the front row (with 20 seats) and the row behind it (with 21 seats) is 14.1 in. (360 mm), calculated as follows:

$$12 \text{ in.} + [(21 - 14 \text{ seats}) \times 0.3 \text{ in./seat}] = 12 + 2.1 = 14.1 \text{ in.}$$

or

$$305 \text{ mm} + [(21 - 14 \text{ seats}) \times 7.6 \text{ mm/seat}] = 305 + 53 \approx 360 \text{ mm}$$

The required minimum aisle accessway clear width between the back row (with 40 seats) and the row in front of it (with 39 seats) is 19.8 in. (505 mm), calculated as follows:

$$12 \text{ in.} + [(40 - 14 \text{ seats}) \times 0.3 \text{ in./seat}] = 12 + 7.8 = 19.8 \text{ in.}$$

or

$$305 \text{ mm} + [(40 - 14 \text{ seats}) \times 7.6 \text{ mm/seat}] = 305 + 198 \approx 505 \text{ mm}$$

The designer has the option of making the clear widths of all aisle accessways uniform and at least 19.8 in. (505 mm) wide or progressively increasing them from 14.1 in. (360 mm) at the front to 19.8 in. (505 mm) at the back.

For the theater shown in Exhibit 12/13.17, the option of a traditional layout can be used. The traditional arrangement is a maximum of 14 seats per row for rows served by aisles at both ends, and a maximum of 7 seats per row where the row is served by an aisle at only one end and abuts the wall at the other end. This layout would require that more space be devoted to aisles and cross aisles, but this lost space might be partly offset by the minimum 12 in. (305 mm) aisle accessway clear width permitted of such rows of seating.

In a seating row served by an aisle at one end only, the occupant of the seat farthest from the aisle must be able to reach the aisle with not more than 30 ft (9.1 m) of aisle accessway travel in accordance with 12/13.2.5.5.5. Exhibit 12/13.18 illustrates a seating row served by an aisle at one end only where, upon reaching the aisle, it is not immediately possible to move in either of two egress directions because of the obstruction to egress created by the rear wall of the room. The aisle accessway (point *X* to point *Y*) cannot exceed 30 ft (9.1 m). However, upon reaching the aisle, the common path of travel measurement does not end; it continues to point *Z*, which is the first point at which travel in two independent directions becomes possible. Per 12/13.2.5.1.2, the common path of travel (point *X* to point *Z*) is permitted to be 75 ft (23 m), because the area served does not exceed 50 persons (in this case, 28 occupants, based on two rows of seats with 14 seats per row).

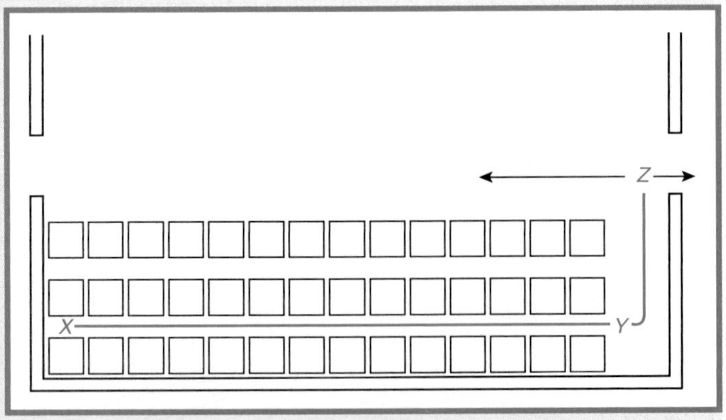


***Exhibit 12/13.18*** *Maximum 30 ft (9.1 m) aisle accessway length (point X to point Y) for seating row served by aisle at one end only.*

In rows of tablet-arm chairs on which the tablet arms are fixed in the in-use position, the chairs must be arranged to meet the row spacing requirements of 12/13.2.5.5. Exhibit 12/13.19 illustrates this provision.

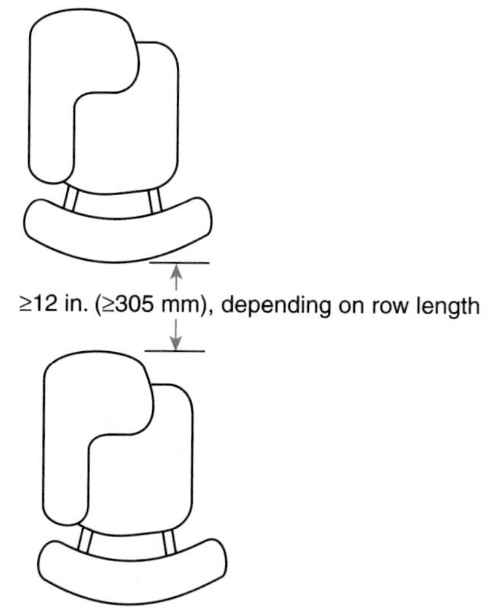


***Exhibit 12/13.19** Minimum spacing between rows of seats with fixed tablet arms.*

Although the clear space between the back of a seat and the leading edge of the tablet arm of a chair located behind that seat varies, depending on row length, in accordance with the requirements of 12/13.2.5.5, the clear space cannot be less than 12 in. (305 mm). Paragraph 12/13.2.5.5.6 addresses tablet-arm chairs with self-storing tablet arms, which present little threat to life safety.

**12.2.5.6 Aisles Serving Seating Not at Tables.**

**12.2.5.6.1 General.**

**12.2.5.6.1.1** Aisles shall be provided so that the number of seats served by the nearest aisle is in accordance with 12.2.5.5.2 through 12.2.5.5.5, unless otherwise permitted by 12.2.5.6.1.2.

**12.2.5.6.1.2** Aisles shall not be required in bleachers, provided that all of the following conditions are met:

(1) Egress from the front row shall not be obstructed by a rail, a guard, or other obstruction.
(2) The row spacing shall be 28 in. (710 mm) or less.
(3) The rise per row, including the first row, shall be 6 in. (150 mm) or less.
(4) The number of rows shall not exceed 16.
(5) The seat spaces shall not be physically defined.
(6) Seat boards that are also used as stepping surfaces for descent shall provide a walking surface with a width not less than 12 in. (305 mm), and, where a depressed footboard exists, the gap between seat boards of adjacent rows shall not exceed 12 in. (305 mm), measured horizontally.
(7) The leading edges of seat boards used as stepping surfaces shall be provided with a contrasting marking stripe so that the location of the leading edge is readily apparent, particularly where viewed in descent, and the following shall also apply:
    (a) The marking stripe shall be not less than 1 in. (25 mm) wide and shall not exceed 2 in. (51 mm) in width.

**13.2.5.6 Aisles Serving Seating Not at Tables.**

**13.2.5.6.1 General.**

**13.2.5.6.1.1** Aisles shall be provided so that the number of seats served by the nearest aisle is in accordance with 13.2.5.5.2 through 13.2.5.5.5, unless otherwise permitted by 13.2.5.6.1.2.

**13.2.5.6.1.2** Aisles shall not be required in bleachers, provided that all of the following conditions are met:

(1) Egress from the front row shall not be obstructed by a rail, a guard, or other obstruction.
(2) The row spacing shall be 28 in. (710 mm) or less.
(3) The rise per row, including the first row, shall be 6 in. (150 mm) or less.
(4) The number of rows shall not exceed 16.
(5) The seat spaces shall not be physically defined.
(6) Seat boards that are also used as stepping surfaces for descent shall provide a walking surface with a width of not less than 12 in. (305 mm), and, where a depressed footboard exists, the gap between seat boards of adjacent rows shall not exceed 12 in. (305 mm), measured horizontally.
(7) The leading edges of seat boards used as stepping surfaces shall be provided with a contrasting marking stripe so that the location of the leading edge is readily apparent, particularly where viewed in descent, and the following shall also apply:
    (a) The marking stripe shall be not less than 1 in. (25 mm) wide and shall not exceed 2 in. (51 mm) in width.

CHAPTER 12 • New

(b) The marking stripe shall not be required where bleacher surfaces and environmental conditions, under all conditions of use, are such that the location of each leading edge is readily apparent, particularly when viewed in descent.

**12.2.5.6.2 Dead-End Aisles.** Dead-end aisles shall not exceed 20 ft (6100 mm) in length, unless otherwise permitted by the following:

(1) A dead-end aisle shall be permitted to exceed 20 ft (6100 mm) in length where seats served by the dead-end aisle are not more than 24 seats from another aisle, measured along a row of seats having a clear width of not less than 12 in. (305 mm) plus 0.6 in. (15 mm) for each additional seat over a total of 7 in the row.
(2) A 16-row, dead-end aisle shall be permitted in folding and telescopic seating and grandstands.
(3) Aisle termination in accordance with 12.4.2.10 for smoke-protected assembly seating shall be permitted.

CHAPTER 13 • Existing

(b) The marking stripe shall not be required where bleacher surfaces and environmental conditions, under all conditions of use, are such that the location of each leading edge is readily apparent, particularly when viewed in descent.

**13.2.5.6.2 Dead-End Aisles.** Dead-end aisles shall not exceed 20 ft (6100 mm) in length, unless otherwise permitted by the following:

(1) A dead-end aisle shall be permitted to exceed 20 ft (6100 mm) in length where seats served by the dead-end aisle are not more than 24 seats from another aisle, measured along a row of seats having a clear width of not less than 12 in. (305 mm) plus 0.6 in. (15 mm) for each additional seat over a total of 7 in the row.
(2) A 16-row, dead-end aisle shall be permitted in folding and telescopic seating and grandstands.
(3) Aisle termination in accordance with 13.4.2.10 for smoke-protected assembly seating shall be permitted.
(4) Bleacher aisles in accordance with 13.2.3.5 shall not be considered as dead-end aisles.

Bleacher seating, as addressed in 12/13.2.5.6.1.2, does not have seat backs. Provided that the row-to-row dimension does not exceed 28 in. (710 mm) and egress is not restricted from the front of the bleacher, occupants can effectively walk on the seating surfaces and not rely on aisles.

Paragraph 12/13.2.5.6.2(1) formally recognizes the inherent redundancy that exists where a block of seating rows is served by more than one aisle, so that the problem created by the blockage of any one aisle can be mitigated by greater movement along rows to reach a more distant aisle. The exemption recognizes that movement along rows (even with the constricted row widths) provides many routes that permit faster movement to alternative aisles than would be possible with a dedicated cross aisle. This exemption is useful in arenas and theaters where it is not easy to provide a cross aisle or a door at the end of an aisle, but where it is relatively easy to reach a remote aisle and its associated exit by moving along the aisle accessways created by the seating rows. Note that 12/13.2.5.6.2(1) requires increased aisle accessway clear width to facilitate travel along the seating rows to reach alternative aisles. At the row length limit of 24 seats, the required aisle accessway clear width for use of this exemption is 22.2 in. (565 mm).

CHAPTER 12 • New

**12.2.5.6.3* Minimum Aisle Width.** The minimum clear width of aisles shall be sufficient to provide egress capacity in accordance with 12.2.3.2 but shall be not less than the following:

(1) 48 in. (1220 mm) for stairs having seating on each side, or 36 in. (915 mm) where the aisle does not serve more than 50 seats

CHAPTER 13 • Existing

**13.2.5.6.3* Minimum Aisle Width.** The minimum clear width of aisles shall be sufficient to provide egress capacity in accordance with 13.2.3.2 but shall be not less than the following:

(1) 42 in. (1065 mm) for stairs having seating on each side, unless otherwise permitted by the following:
    (a) The minimum clear width required by 13.2.5.6.3(1) shall be permitted to be not less than 30 in. (760 mm) for catchment areas having not more than 60 seats.
    (b) The minimum clear width required by 13.2.5.6.3(1) shall be permitted to be not less than 36 in. (915 mm) where an aisle does not serve more than 50 seats.

CHAPTER 12 • New

(2) 36 in. (915 mm) for stairs having seating on only one side

(3) 23 in. (585 mm) between a handrail and seating, or between a guardrail and seating where the aisle is subdivided by a handrail

(4) 42 in. (1065 mm) for level or ramped aisles having seating on both sides, or 36 in. (915 mm) where the aisle does not serve more than 50 seats

(5) 36 in. (915 mm) for level or ramped aisles having seating on only one side

(6) 23 in. (585 mm) between a handrail or a guardrail and seating where the aisle does not serve more than five rows on one side

**A.12.2.5.6.3** It is the intent to permit handrails to project not more than 3½ in. (90 mm) into the clear width of aisles required by 12.2.5.6.3.

CHAPTER 13 • Existing

(2) 36 in. (915 mm) for stairs having seating on only one side, or 30 in. (760 mm) for catchment areas having not more than 60 seats

(3) 20 in. (510 mm) between a handrail and seating or between a guardrail and seating where the aisle is subdivided by a handrail

(4) 42 in. (1065 mm) for level or ramped aisles having seating on both sides, unless otherwise permitted by the following:

(a) The minimum clear width required by 13.2.5.6.3(4) shall be not less than 30 in. (760 mm) for catchment areas having not more than 60 seats.

(b) The minimum clear width required by 13.2.5.6.3(4) shall be not less than 36 in. (915 mm) where an aisle does not serve more than 50 seats.

(5) 36 in. (915 mm) for level or ramped aisles having seating on only one side, or 30 in. (760 mm) for catchment areas having not more than 60 seats

(6) 23 in. (585 mm) between a handrail or a guardrail and seating where the aisle does not serve more than five rows on one side

**A.13.2.5.6.3** It is the intent to permit handrails to project not more than 3½ in. (90 mm) into the clear width of aisles required by 13.2.5.6.3.

Where the minimum aisle width specified by 12/13.2.5.6.3 is wider than that calculated for a required egress capacity, as is often the case, the width specified by 12/13.2.5.6.3 is the minimum required width. The requirements of 12/13.2.5.6.3 take into account the width needed by individuals moving alone or with others, overtaking others, and moving in counterflow past others on aisles. Differing movement behavior and the need for handrails on different walking surfaces, such as stepped aisles versus level aisles, are considered. Exhibit 12/13.20 and Exhibit 12/13.21 illustrate how intensively a 48 in. (1220 mm) aisle stair subdivided by a center handrail can be used. Exhibit 12/13.22 shows an overhead view of a large male walking down a similar aisle stair. Chair seating is shown adjoining the aisle in these photographs.

Paragraph 12/13.2.5.6.3(6) is based on the requirement for handrails in aisle stairs. It specifically addresses the allowance for extending such handrails down the center of aisles for as many as five rows, leaving only about 23 in. (585 mm) of nominal width clear to the side of the handrail. This width is readily used by individuals moving in single or staggered file and can be used with tolerable inconvenience where people must pass each other on the same side of the handrail. This provision of the *Code* might be useful in cases where a short stub aisle is needed to serve rows of seating immediately beside a vomitory.

Generally, the effective width of aisles is often somewhat wider than is necessary for egress stairs or

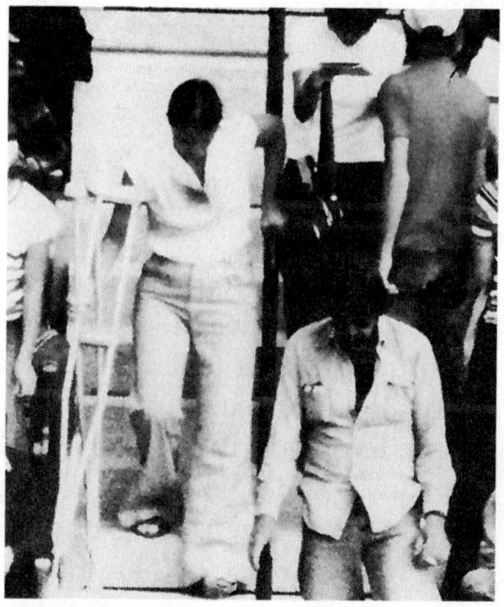

***Exhibit 12/13.20*** *Intensive use of stadium aisle stair, 48 in. (1220 mm) wide with center handrail. (Photograph courtesy of Jake Pauls)*

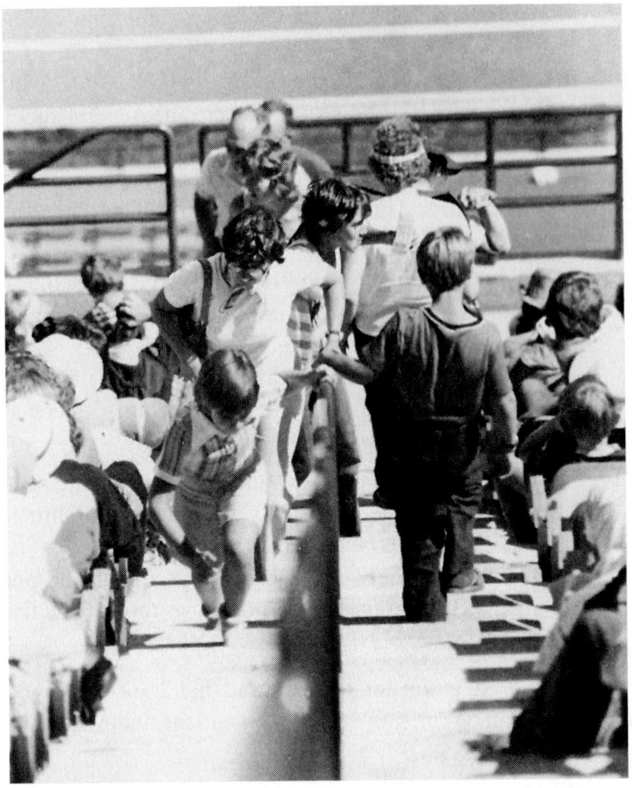

*Exhibit 12/13.21 Intensive use of stadium handrail, approximately 34 in. (865 mm) high, at center of 48 in. (1220 mm) wide aisle stair. (Photograph courtesy of Jake Pauls)*

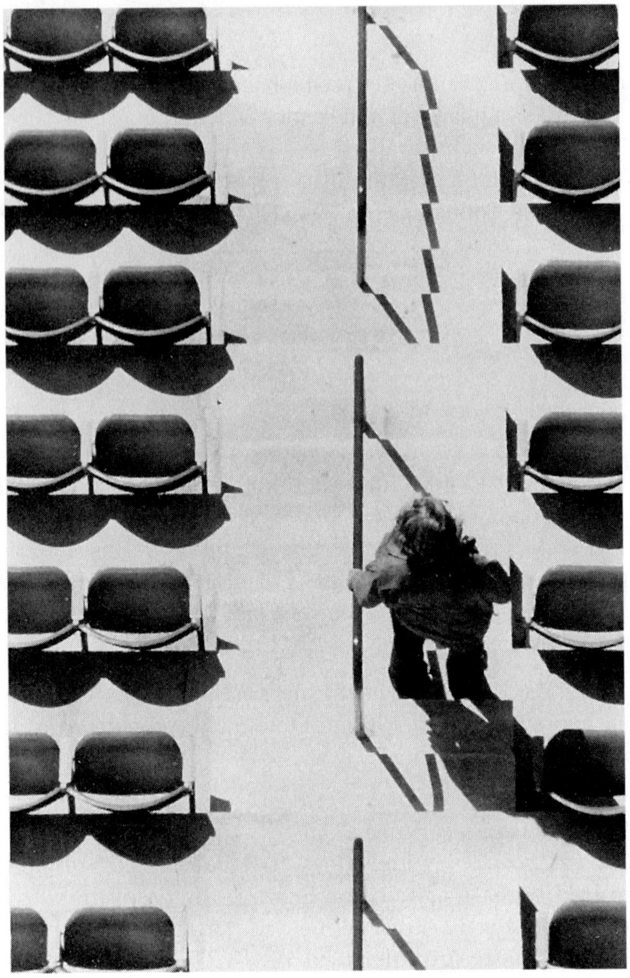

*Exhibit 12/13.22 Overhead view of 48 in. (1220 mm) wide aisle stair with center handrail. (Photograph courtesy of Jake Pauls)*

corridors that are bounded on both sides by wall construction. One important exception to this generalization occurs where many people are attempting to sit on undivided benches or bleachers served by an aisle. The 18 in. (455 mm) spacing usually provided for each person is often too small, and there is a natural tendency for people to extend their legs, hips, and shoulders into a significant part of the aisle width. Therefore, it is prudent when designing for crowded, nonchair seating to increase either the width of the seat per person or the minimum aisle widths to facilitate normal circulation in the aisles under nonemergency conditions. It is expected that the individuals encroaching on the aisle width will stand and move during emergency egress so as to restore the aisle to its full, required egress width.

**12.2.5.6.4* Aisle Stairs and Ramps.** The following shall apply to aisle stairs and ramps:

(1) Aisles having a gradient steeper than 1 in 20, but not steeper than 1 in 8, shall consist of a ramp.
(2) Aisles having a gradient steeper than 1 in 8 shall consist of an aisle stair.

**13.2.5.6.4* Aisle Stairs and Ramps.** The following shall apply to aisle stairs and ramps:

(1) Aisles having a gradient steeper than 1 in 20, but not steeper than 1 in 8, shall consist of a ramp.
(2) Aisles having a gradient steeper than 1 in 8 shall consist of an aisle stair.

CHAPTER 12 • New

(3) The limitation on height between landings in Table 7.2.2.2.1.1(a) and Table 7.2.2.2.1.1(b) shall not apply to aisle stairs.

**A.12.2.5.6.4** Technical information about the convenience and safety of ramps and stairs having gradients in the region of 1 in 8 clearly suggests that the goal should be slopes for ramps that are less steep and combinations of stair risers and treads that are, for example, superior to 4 in. (100 mm) risers and 32 in. (865 mm) treads. This goal should be kept in mind by designers in establishing the gradient of seating areas to be served by aisles.

**12.2.5.6.5 Aisle Stair Treads.** Aisle stair treads shall meet the following criteria:

(1) There shall be no variation in the depth of adjacent treads that exceeds $^3/_{16}$ in. (4.8 mm), unless otherwise permitted by 12.2.5.6.5(2).
(2) Construction-caused nonuniformities in tread depth shall be permitted, provided that the following criteria are met:
  (a) The nonuniformity does not exceed $^3/_8$ in. (10 mm).
  (b) The aisle tread depth is 22 in. (560 mm) or greater.

(3)* Tread depth shall be not less than 11 in. (280 mm).

**A.12.2.5.6.5(3)** Tread depth is more important to stair safety than is riser height. Therefore, in cases where the seating area gradient is less than 5 in 11, it is recommended that the tread dimension be increased beyond 11 in. (280 mm), rather than reducing the riser height. Where the seating area gradient exceeds 8 in 11, it is recommended that the riser height be increased while maintaining a tread depth of not less than 11 in. (280 mm).

(4) All treads shall extend the full width of the aisle.

CHAPTER 13 • Existing

(3) The limitation on height between landings in Table 7.2.2.2.1.1(a) and Table 7.2.2.2.1.1(b) shall not apply to aisle stairs.

**A.13.2.5.6.4** Technical information about the convenience and safety of ramps and stairs having gradients in the region of 1 in 8 clearly suggests that the goal should be slopes for ramps that are less steep and combinations of stair risers and treads that are, for example, superior to 4 in. (100 mm) risers and 32 in. (865 mm) treads. This goal should be kept in mind by designers in establishing the gradient of seating areas to be served by aisles.

**13.2.5.6.5 Aisle Stair Treads.** Aisle stair treads shall meet the following criteria:

(1) There shall be no variation in the depth of adjacent treads that exceeds $^3/_{16}$ in. (4.8 mm), unless otherwise permitted by 13.2.5.6.5(2), (5), or (6).
(2) Construction-caused nonuniformities in tread depth shall be permitted, provided that the following criteria are met:
  (a) The nonuniformity does not exceed $^3/_8$ in. (10 mm).
  (b) The aisle tread depth is 22 in. (560 mm) or greater.

(3)* Tread depth shall be not less than 11 in. (280 mm).

**A.13.2.5.6.5(3)** Tread depth is more important to stair safety than is riser height. Therefore, in cases where the seating area gradient is less than 5 in 11, it is recommended that the tread dimension be increased beyond 11 in. (280 mm), rather than reducing the riser height. Where the seating area gradient exceeds 8 in 11, it is recommended that the riser height be increased while maintaining a tread depth of not less than 11 in. (280 mm).

(4) All treads shall extend the full width of the aisle.
(5)* In aisle stairs where a single intermediate tread is provided halfway between seating platforms, such intermediate treads shall be permitted to be of a relatively smaller but uniform depth but shall be not less than 13 in. (330 mm).

**A.13.2.5.6.5(5)** Completely uniform tread dimensions are preferred over aisle stair designs where tread depths alternate between relatively small intermediate treads between seating platforms and relatively large treads at seating platforms. A larger tread that is level with the seating platform is not needed to facilitate easy access to, and egress from, a row of seating. If this arrangement is used, it is important to provide a tread depth that is better than minimum for the intermediate tread; hence, 13 in. (330 mm) is specified. Where nonuniformities exist due to construction tolerance, they should not exceed $^3/_{16}$ in. (4.8 mm) between adjacent treads.

CHAPTER 12 • New

CHAPTER 13 • Existing

(6) The following shall apply to grandstands, bleachers, and folding and telescopic seating:

(a) Steps shall not be required to be provided in aisles to overcome differences in level unless the gradient exceeds 1 unit of rise in 10 units of run.

(b) Where the rise of the seating platform exceeds 11 in. (280 mm), an intermediate step shall be provided for the full width of the aisle and shall be proportioned to provide two steps of equal rise per platform.

(c) Where the rise of the seating platform exceeds 18 in. (455 mm), two intermediate steps for the full width of the aisle shall be provided and proportioned to provide three steps of equal rise per platform that are uniform and not less than 9 in. (230 mm).

(d) The full length of the nose of each step in the aisle, as required by 13.2.5.6.5(6)(c), shall be conspicuously marked.

The requirements of 12/13.2.5.6.4 address the need to design aisle stairs, for example, with all the attention and care required for stairs in general, plus additional care due to the unique design and use conditions encountered with aisles serving seating arranged in rows. Extra attention is especially necessary where large elevation differences exist between the rows of seating. Paragraph 12/13.2.5.6.4(1) addresses aisles in terms of steepness. Ideally, designing aisles with a gradient of approximately 1 in 8 is to be avoided; however, sight lines might dictate the use of such slopes in some situations. These ramps are relatively steep and problematic for people with walking difficulties. Stairs with a very small rise and long treads also present problems, notably trips and missteps, because the presence of low-height risers might not be evident, especially when a crowd is present. Generally, people using aisles are also distracted because of the unusual aisle length, the presence of other people in the aisles, and the presence of those entering the aisles from adjoining seating rows. Therefore, aisles of any slope must be designed with considerable care and attention to human factors.

Allowing unequal-sized treads within aisle stairs, a practice previously believed to be useful in facilitating access to seat rows, is not permitted by the *Code* for new assembly occupancies. Even with the increased minimum tread size requirement of older editions of the *Code*, the end result (larger treads at the seat row entry level and smaller intermediate treads between seat row levels) was not as beneficial in terms of stair safety as that provided by consistently sized treads. The desirability of uniformly sized treads holds even for treads as large as 20 in. (510 mm) in depth (assuming a relatively low riser height). Handrails (required by 12/13.2.5.6.8) help to compensate for the stretched but consistent stride length that might be needed in such long-tread aisle stairs. It is preferable to keep treads uniform, so that the risk of misstepping, particularly the risk of overstepping on relatively smaller treads, is reduced.

For existing aisle stairs, 13.2.5.6.5(5) continues to recognize an intermediate tread between seating platforms but requires that the intermediate treads be uniform in depth and at least 13 in. (330 mm) deep. This exaggerated depth makes the intermediate tread more obvious and provides a deep surface on which to place one's feet.

Special attention must be given to careful design detailing and construction practice in relation to the placement of treads in aisle stairs. Careful site supervision is recommended to avoid serious problems both in cast-in-place concrete construction and in precast concrete construction of aisle stairs. Field research studies of situations where aisle step dimensions are not consistent indicate that the incidence of missteps rises significantly where tolerances of tread uniformity exceed those specified by 12/13.2.5.6.5.

Paragraph 12/13.2.5.6.5(2) recognizes that construction-caused nonuniformities are unavoidable. It limits such construction-caused nonuniformities to $^{3}/_{8}$ in. (10 mm) and compensates to avoid misstepping by increasing the tread depth to a minimum of 22 in. (560 mm). The increased tread depth will cause most users to change their stepping cadence over that used on stairs with the traditional 11 in. (280 mm) tread depth. The change in cadence should help to heighten the stair user's awareness of nonuniformities in tread depth.

Exhibit 12/13.23 shows a side view of an aisle stair with 11 in. (280 mm) treads used by a person with footwear measuring 12 in. (305 mm) in length. This situation is experienced by 5 percent of adults generally, and it might occur more often in those assembly situations attracting a higher proportion of male adults.

With respect to 12/13.2.5.6.5(1), which requires tread depth to be uniform, apparently no difficulty is experienced in entering or leaving the aisles or in entering or leaving the seat row where three 11 in. (280 mm) treads at each seat row are provided, as shown in Exhibit 12/13.23.

If treads do not extend the full width of the aisle, a pocket (or drop-off) might occur between the side edge of the tread and the side edge of the seat nearest the aisle. The requirement of 12/13.2.5.6.5(4), that treads extend the full width of the aisle, is intended to avoid such drop-offs and prevent missteps and falls.

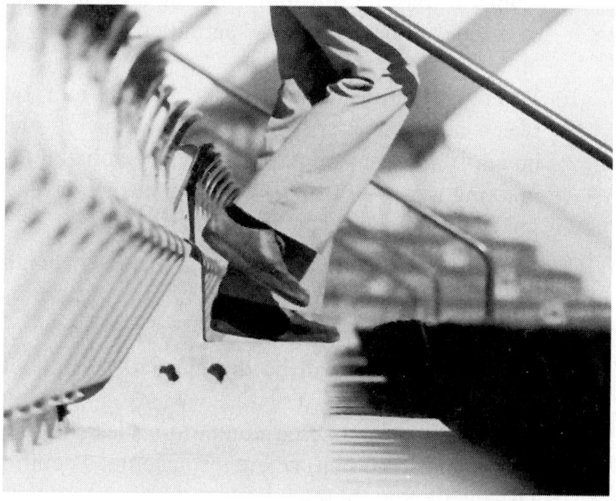

***Exhibit 12/13.23*** *Side view of aisle stair with uniform tread depth of 11 in. (280 mm). (Photograph courtesy of Jake Pauls)*

**12.2.5.6.6 Aisle Stair Risers.** Aisle stair risers shall meet the following criteria:

(1) Riser heights shall be not less than 4 in. (100 mm) in aisle stairs, unless aisle stairs are those in folding and telescopic seating.
(2) The riser height of aisle stairs in folding and telescopic seating shall be permitted to be not less than $3\frac{1}{2}$ in. (90 mm).
(3) Riser heights shall not exceed 8 in. (205 mm), unless otherwise permitted by 12.2.5.6.6(4) or (5).
(4) The riser height of aisle stairs in folding and telescopic seating shall be permitted to be not more than 11 in. (280 mm).
(5) Where the gradient of an aisle is steeper than 8 in. (205 mm) in rise in 11 in. (280 mm) of run for the purpose of maintaining necessary sight lines in the adjoining seating area, the riser height shall be permitted to exceed 8 in. (205 mm) but shall not exceed 9 in. (230 mm).
(6) Riser heights shall be designed to be uniform in each aisle, and the construction-caused nonuniformities shall not exceed $\frac{3}{16}$ in. (4.8 mm) between adjacent risers, unless the conditions of 12.2.5.6.6(7) or (8) are met.
(7) Riser height shall be permitted to be nonuniform as follows:
    (a) The nonuniformity shall be only for the purpose of accommodating changes in gradient necessary to

**13.2.5.6.6 Aisle Stair Risers.** Aisle stair risers shall meet the following criteria:

(1) Riser heights shall be not less than 4 in. (100 mm) in aisle stairs, unless aisle stairs are those in folding and telescopic seating.
(2) The riser height of aisle stairs in folding and telescopic seating shall be permitted to be not less than $3\frac{1}{2}$ in. (90 mm).
(3) Riser heights shall not exceed 8 in. (205 mm), unless otherwise permitted by 13.2.5.6.6(4) or (5).
(4) The riser height of aisle stairs in folding and telescopic seating shall be permitted to be not more than 11 in. (280 mm).
(5) Where the gradient of an aisle is steeper than 8 in. (205 mm) in rise in 11 in. (280 mm) of run for the purpose of maintaining necessary sight lines in the adjoining seating area, the riser height shall be permitted to exceed 8 in. (205 mm) but shall not exceed 11 in. (280 mm).
(6) Riser heights shall be designed to be uniform in each aisle, and the construction-caused nonuniformities shall not exceed $\frac{3}{16}$ in. (4.8 mm) between adjacent risers, unless the conditions of 13.2.5.6.6(7) or (8) are met.
(7) Riser height shall be permitted to be nonuniform as follows:
    (a) The uniformity shall be only for the purpose of accommodating changes in gradient necessary to

**CHAPTER 12 • New**

maintain sight lines within a seating area, in which case the riser height shall be permitted to exceed $^{3}/_{16}$ in. (4.8 mm) in any flight.

(b) Where nonuniformities exceed $^{3}/_{16}$ in. (4.8 mm) between adjacent risers, the exact location of such nonuniformities shall be indicated by a distinctive marking stripe on each tread at the nosing or leading edge adjacent to the nonuniform risers.

(8) Construction-caused nonuniformities in riser height shall be permitted to exceed $^{3}/_{16}$ in. (4.8 mm) where the following criteria are met:

(a) The riser height shall be designed to be nonuniform.
(b) The construction-caused nonuniformities shall not exceed $^{3}/_{8}$ in. (10 mm) where the aisle tread depth is less than 22 in. (560 mm).
(c) The construction-caused nonuniformities shall not exceed $^{3}/_{4}$ in. (19 mm) where the aisle tread depth is 22 in. (560 mm) or greater.
(d) Where nonuniformities exceed $^{3}/_{16}$ in. (4.8 mm) between adjacent risers, the exact location of such nonuniformities shall be indicated by a distinctive marking stripe on each tread at the nosing or leading edge adjacent to the nonuniform risers.

**12.2.5.6.7 Aisle Stair Profile.** Aisle stairs shall comply with the following:

(1) Aisle risers shall be vertical or sloped under the tread projection at an angle not to exceed 30 degrees from vertical.
(2) Tread projection not exceeding $1\frac{1}{2}$ in. (38 mm) shall be permitted.
(3) Tread projection shall be uniform in each aisle, except as otherwise permitted by 12.2.5.6.7(4).
(4) Construction-caused projection nonuniformities not exceeding $^{1}/_{4}$ in. (6.4 mm) shall be permitted.

**CHAPTER 13 • Existing**

maintain sight lines within a seating area, in which case the riser height shall be permitted to exceed $^{3}/_{16}$ in. (4.8 mm) in any flight.

(b) Where nonuniformities exceed $^{3}/_{16}$ in. (4.8 mm) between adjacent risers, the exact location of such nonuniformities shall be indicated by a distinctive marking stripe on each tread at the nosing or leading edge adjacent to the nonuniform risers.

(8) Construction-caused nonuniformities in riser height shall be permitted to exceed $^{3}/_{16}$ in. (4.8 mm) where the following criteria are met:

(a) The riser height shall be designed to be nonuniform.
(b) The construction-caused nonuniformities shall not exceed $^{3}/_{8}$ in. (10 mm) where the aisle tread depth is less than 22 in. (560 mm).
(c) The construction-caused nonuniformities shall not exceed $^{3}/_{4}$ in. (19 mm) where the aisle tread depth is 22 in. (560 mm) or greater.
(d) Where nonuniformities exceed $^{3}/_{16}$ in. (4.8 mm) between adjacent risers, the exact location of such nonuniformities shall be indicated by a distinctive marking stripe on each tread at the nosing or leading edge adjacent to the nonuniform risers.

**13.2.5.6.7 Aisle Stair Profile.** Aisle stairs shall comply with the following:

(1) Aisle risers shall be vertical or sloped under the tread projection at an angle not to exceed 30 degrees from vertical.
(2) Tread projection not exceeding $1\frac{1}{2}$ in. (38 mm) shall be permitted.
(3) Tread projection shall be uniform in each aisle, except as otherwise permitted by 13.2.5.6.7(4).
(4) Construction-caused projection nonuniformities not exceeding $^{1}/_{4}$ in. (6.4 mm) shall be permitted.

At the minimum slope for which the *Code* requires aisle stairs (i.e., slopes steeper than 1 in 8 for which a ramp would be too steep for safe, general use), there is a riser height of 4 in. (100 mm) for which the seat platform is 32 in. (810 mm) deep. At such low riser heights, which present a tripping hazard if people do not detect the risers, the tread nosing marking requirement in 12/13.2.5.6.9 is especially significant.

Editions of the *Code* prior to 1988 permitted new aisle stairs to have a maximum riser height of 11 in. (280 mm). Current editions of the *Code* limit the maximum riser height for new aisle stairs to 9 in. (230 mm). In addition to reducing movement safety, the unusually high risers of some aisle stairs reduce the speed and efficiency of movement, especially in the descending direction. This is taken into account in 12/13.2.3.3 where, for each additional 1 in. (25 mm) of riser height above 7 in. (178 mm), an additional 20 percent must be added to the required capacity-related width of the aisle to satisfy *Code* requirements and achieve an acceptable egress flow time performance.

A special case is made for severely nonuniform riser heights [those beyond the usual $^{3}/_{16}$ in. (4.8 mm) tolerance] in situations where there is a break in the slope of a seating deck to maintain adequate sight lines. The seating deck slope might change incrementally at each row, or, more commonly, a large change might occur at one or more locations. At such locations, there is often a change in the row-to-row elevation that greatly exceeds the $^3/_{16}$ in. (4.8 mm) tolerance. Aisle step riser heights will, as a consequence, change radically at this point. It is the duty of the designer and owner to alert people using the aisle to this unusual change in the riser dimensions. The required marking at each tread is addressed in 12/13.2.5.6.6(7)(b).

Construction-caused nonuniformities in riser height are permitted to exceed $^3/_{16}$ in. (4.8 mm) in accordance with 12/13.2.5.6.6(8). The nonuniformity is permitted to be $^3/_4$ in. (19 mm) where the tread depth is exaggerated to a minimum 22 in. (560 mm). The increased tread depth will cause most users to change their stepping cadence compared to that used on stairs with the traditional 11 in. (280 mm) tread depth. The change in cadence should help to heighten the stair user's awareness of nonuniformities in riser height.

The aisle stair profile provisions of 12/13.2.5.6.7 have been in the *Code* since the 2006 edition. The profile is impacted by the construction tolerance for the seating units, so the criteria are intended to complete the package related to construction-caused nonuniformities addressed in 12/13.2.5.6.5(2) and 12/13.2.5.6.6(8).

**12.2.5.6.8* Aisle Handrails.**

**A.12.2.5.6.8** Failure to provide a handrail within a 30 in. (760 mm) horizontal distance of all required portions of the aisle stair width means that the egress capacity calculation is required to be modified as specified by 12.2.3.3(3). This modification might lead to an increase in the aisle width. Although this increase will compensate for reduced egress efficiency, it does not help individuals walking on such portions of stairs to recover from missteps, other than by possibly marginally reducing the crowding that might exacerbate the problem of falls. *(See also 7.2.2.4.)*

**12.2.5.6.8.1** Ramped aisles having a gradient exceeding 1 in 20 and aisle stairs shall be provided with handrails at one side or along the centerline and shall also be in accordance with 7.2.2.4.4.1, 7.2.2.4.4.5, and 7.2.2.4.4.6.

**12.2.5.6.8.2** Where seating exists on both sides of the aisle, the handrails shall be noncontinuous with gaps or breaks at intervals not exceeding five rows to facilitate access to seating and to allow crossing from one side of the aisle to the other.

**12.2.5.6.8.3** The gaps or breaks permitted by 12.2.5.6.8.2 shall have a clear width of not less than 22 in. (560 mm) and shall not exceed 36 in. (915 mm), measured horizontally, and the handrail shall have rounded terminations or bends.

**12.2.5.6.8.4** Where handrails are provided in the middle of aisle stairs, an additional intermediate rail shall be located approximately 12 in. (305 mm) below the main handrail.

**12.2.5.6.8.5** Handrails shall not be required where otherwise permitted by the following:

(1) Handrails shall not be required for ramped aisles having a gradient not steeper than 1 in 8 and having seating on both sides where the aisle does not serve as an accessible route.



**13.2.5.6.8* Aisle Handrails.**

**A.13.2.5.6.8** Failure to provide a handrail within a 30 in. (760 mm) horizontal distance of all required portions of the aisle stair width means that the egress capacity calculation is required to be modified as specified by 13.2.3.3(3). This modification might lead to an increase in the aisle width. Although this increase will compensate for reduced egress efficiency, it does not help individuals walking on such portions of stairs to recover from missteps, other than by possibly marginally reducing the crowding that might exacerbate the problem of falls. *(See also 7.2.2.4.)*

**13.2.5.6.8.1** Ramped aisles having a gradient exceeding 1 in 12 and aisle stairs shall be provided with handrails at one side or along the centerline and shall also be in accordance with 7.2.2.4.4.1, 7.2.2.4.4.5, and 7.2.2.4.4.6.

**13.2.5.6.8.2** Where seating exists on both sides of the aisle, the handrails shall be noncontinuous with gaps or breaks at intervals not exceeding five rows to facilitate access to seating and to allow crossing from one side of the aisle to the other.

**13.2.5.6.8.3** The gaps or breaks permitted by 13.2.5.6.8.2 shall have a clear width of not less than 22 in. (560 mm) and shall not exceed 36 in. (915 mm), measured horizontally, and the handrail shall have rounded terminations or bends.

**13.2.5.6.8.4** Where handrails are provided in the middle of aisle stairs, an additional intermediate rail shall be located approximately 12 in. (305 mm) below the main handrail.

**13.2.5.6.8.5** Handrails shall not be required where otherwise permitted by the following:

(1) Handrails shall not be required for ramped aisles having a gradient not steeper than 1 in 8 and having seating on both sides.

CHAPTER 12 • New

(2) The requirement for a handrail shall be satisfied by the use of a guard provided with a rail that complies with the graspability requirements for handrails and located at a consistent height between 34 in. and 42 in. (865 mm and 1065 mm), measured as follows:
   (a) Vertically from the top of the rail to the leading edge (nosing) of stair treads
   (b) Vertically from the top of the rail to the adjacent walking surface in the case of a ramp

CHAPTER 13 • Existing

(2) The requirement for a handrail shall be satisfied by the use of a guard provided with a rail that complies with the graspability requirements for handrails and located at a consistent height between 34 in. and 42 in. (865 mm and 1065 mm), measured as follows:
   (a) Vertically from the top of the rail to the leading edge (nosing) of stair treads
   (b) Vertically from the top of the rail to the adjacent walking surface in the case of a ramp

(3) Handrails shall not be required where risers do not exceed 7 in. (180 mm) in height.

The *Code* requires handrails on aisle stairs in new construction, even where riser heights are less than 7 in. (180 mm). This requirement is a result of increased experience with the provision and use of aisle handrails, as well as a general realization that aisles pose unique challenges to users that might go beyond those encountered on other stairs. Exhibit 12/13.20 and Exhibit 12/13.21 illustrate the variety of use conditions in aisles and the extensive use of handrails. Field research studies show that aisle stair handrails have been used about twice as often as handrails provided to meet *Code* requirements for non-aisle stairs. This high level of use is not surprising, given the unusual lengths, varied step geometries, and very complex use conditions of assembly occupancy aisles. Aside from their value in increasing the safety and comfort of people using the aisles, handrails also help to improve egress efficiency. This benefit is taken into account in calculation of egress capacity. See 12/13.2.3.3(3).

The required gaps between sections of center-aisle handrails are illustrated in Exhibit 12/13.22. Spacing such gaps as frequently as every three rows is recommended where there is extensive use of aisles during events. A spacing of up to five rows between gaps might be acceptable where there is little use of the aisles during events and little counterflow at any time. Gap size should be kept at the lower end of the permitted range of 22 in. to 36 in. (560 mm to 915 mm) where the aisles are unusually steep, and handrail use is especially valuable in reducing the risk of falls.

Paragraph 12/13.2.5.6.8.5(2) takes into account the proven utility of handrails that are higher than those normally permitted, even with the increase in handrail height range [from 34 in. to 38 in. (865 mm to 965 mm)] introduced with the 1988 edition of the *Code*. A guardrail that is 42 in. (1065 mm) high (such as at the side of an aisle where there is a vomitory) can be considered a usable handrail if it offers graspability as required for handrails. See 7.2.2.4.4.

**12.2.5.6.9* Aisle Marking.**

**A.12.2.5.6.9** Certain tread cover materials such as plush carpets, which are often used in theaters, produce an inherently well-marked tread nosing under most lighting conditions. On the other hand, concrete treads have nosings with a sharp edge and, especially under outdoor lighting conditions, are difficult to discriminate. Therefore, concrete treads require an applied marking stripe. The slip resistance of such marking stripes should be similar to the rest of the treads, and no tripping hazard should be created; luminescent, self-luminous, and electroluminescent tread markings have the advantage of being apparent in reduced light or in the absence of light.

**12.2.5.6.9.1** A contrasting marking stripe shall be provided on each tread at the nosing or leading edge so that the location of such tread is readily apparent, particularly when viewed in descent.

**13.2.5.6.9* Aisle Marking.**

**A.13.2.5.6.9** Certain tread cover materials such as plush carpets, which are often used in theaters, produce an inherently well-marked tread nosing under most lighting conditions. On the other hand, concrete treads have nosings with a sharp edge and, especially under outdoor lighting conditions, are difficult to discriminate. Therefore, concrete treads require an applied marking stripe. The slip resistance of such marking stripes should be similar to the rest of the treads, and no tripping hazard should be created; luminescent, self-luminous, and electroluminescent tread markings have the advantage of being apparent in reduced light or in the absence of light.

**13.2.5.6.9.1** A contrasting marking stripe shall be provided on each tread at the nosing or leading edge so that the location of such tread is readily apparent, particularly when viewed in descent.

CHAPTER 12 • New

**12.2.5.6.9.2** The marking stripe shall be not less than 1 in. (25 mm) wide and shall not exceed 2 in. (51 mm) in width.

**12.2.5.6.9.3** The marking stripe shall not be required where tread surfaces and environmental conditions, under all conditions of use, are such that the location of each tread is readily apparent, particularly when viewed in descent.

CHAPTER 13 • Existing

**13.2.5.6.9.2** The marking stripe shall be not less than 1 in. (25 mm) wide and shall not exceed 2 in. (51 mm) in width.

**13.2.5.6.9.3** The marking stripe shall not be required where tread surfaces and environmental conditions, under all conditions of use, are such that the location of each tread is readily apparent, particularly when viewed in descent.

Exhibit 12/13.24 illustrates some of the step visibility difficulties that are commonly encountered in outdoor facilities with concrete stair treads. Without the shadows from the handrail posts, there would be little indication of the exact location of each tread nosing. This situation requires the applied nosing markings referred to in 12/13.2.5.6.9. The distractions of the playing field and the unusually long aisle further justify making the steps as obvious as possible. Each situation needs to be carefully evaluated, with mock-ups at the design stage and inspection of actual conditions during use, to determine whether any improvements are warranted in marking and lighting such aisles.

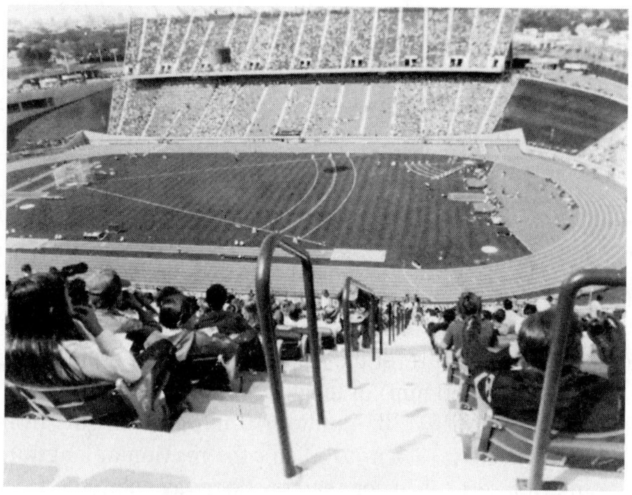

***Exhibit 12/13.24** View down stadium aisle stair with center handrail. (Photograph courtesy of Jake Pauls)*

**12.2.5.7* Aisle Accessways Serving Seating at Tables.**

**A.12.2.5.7** For purposes of the means of egress requirements of this *Code*, seating at counters or at other furnishings is considered to be the same as seating at tables.

**12.2.5.7.1** The required clear width of an aisle accessway shall be not less than 12 in. (305 mm) where measured in accordance with 12.2.5.7.3 and shall be increased as a function of length in accordance with 12.2.5.7.4, unless otherwise permitted by 12.2.5.7.2.

**12.2.5.7.2*** If used by not more than four persons, no minimum clear width shall be required for the portion of an aisle accessway having a length not exceeding 6 ft (1830 mm) and located farthest from an aisle.

**A.12.2.5.7.2** Effectively, where the aisle accessway is bounded by movable seating, the 12 in. (305 mm) minimum width might be increased by about 15 in. to 30 in. (380 mm to 760 mm) as seating is pushed in toward tables. Moreover, it is such movement of chairs during normal and emergency egress situations that makes the zero-clearance allowance workable. The allowance also applies to booth seating where people sitting closest to the aisle normally move out ahead of people farthest from the aisle.

**13.2.5.7* Aisle Accessways Serving Seating at Tables.**

**A.13.2.5.7** For purposes of the means of egress requirements of this *Code*, seating at counters or at other furnishings is considered to be the same as seating at tables.

**13.2.5.7.1** The required clear width of an aisle accessway shall be not less than 12 in. (305 mm) where measured in accordance with 13.2.5.7.3 and shall be increased as a function of length in accordance with 13.2.5.7.4, unless otherwise permitted by 13.2.5.7.2.

**13.2.5.7.2*** If used by not more than four persons, no minimum clear width shall be required for the portion of an aisle accessway having a length not exceeding 6 ft (1830 mm) and located farthest from an aisle.

**A.13.2.5.7.2** Effectively, where the aisle accessway is bounded by movable seating, the 12 in. (305 mm) minimum width might be increased by about 15 in. to 30 in. (380 mm to 760 mm) as seating is pushed in toward tables. Moreover, it is such movement of chairs during normal and emergency egress situations that makes the zero-clearance exception workable. The exception also applies to booth seating where people sitting closest to the aisle normally move out ahead of people farthest from the aisle.

CHAPTER 12 • New

**12.2.5.7.3*** Where nonfixed seating is located between a table and an aisle accessway or aisle, the measurement of required clear width of the aisle accessway or aisle shall be made to a line 19 in. (485 mm), measured perpendicularly to the edge of the table, away from the edge of said table.

**A.12.2.5.7.3** See A.12.2.5.8.3.

**12.2.5.7.4*** The minimum required clear width of an aisle accessway, measured in accordance with 12.2.5.4.8 and 12.2.5.7.3, shall be increased beyond the 12 in. (305 mm) requirement of 12.2.5.7.1 by ½ in. (13 mm) for each additional 12 in. (305 mm) or fraction thereof beyond 12 ft (3660 mm) of aisle accessway length, where measured from the center of the seat farthest from an aisle.

**A.12.2.5.7.4** The minimum width requirement as a function of accessway length is as follows:

(1) 0 in. (0 mm) for the first 6 ft (1830 mm) of length toward the exit
(2) 12 in. (305 mm) for the next 6 ft (1830 mm); that is, up to 12 ft (3660 mm) of length
(3) 12 in. to 24 in. (305 mm to 610 mm) for lengths from 12 ft to 36 ft (3.7 m to 11 m), the maximum length to the closest aisle or egress doorway permitted by 12.2.5.7.5

Any additional width needed for seating is to be added to these widths, as described in 12.2.5.8.3.

**12.2.5.7.5** The path of travel along the aisle accessway shall not exceed 36 ft (11 m) from any seat to the closest aisle or egress doorway.

CHAPTER 13 • Existing

**13.2.5.7.3*** Where nonfixed seating is located between a table and an aisle accessway or aisle, the measurement of required clear width of the aisle accessway or aisle shall be made to a line 19 in. (485 mm), measured perpendicularly to the edge of the table, away from the edge of said table.

**A.13.2.5.7.3** See A.13.2.5.8.3.

**13.2.5.7.4*** The minimum required clear width of an aisle accessway, measured in accordance with 13.2.5.4.8 and 13.2.5.7.3, shall be increased beyond the 12 in. (305 mm) requirement of 13.2.5.7.1 by ½ in. (13 mm) for each additional 12 in. (305 mm) or fraction thereof beyond 12 ft (3660 mm) of aisle accessway length, where measured from the center of the seat farthest from an aisle.

**A.13.2.5.7.4** The minimum width requirement as a function of accessway length is as follows:

(1) 0 in. (0 mm) for the first 6 ft (1830 mm) of length toward the exit
(2) 12 in. (305 mm) for the next 6 ft (1830 mm); that is, up to 12 ft (3660 mm) of length
(3) 12 in. to 24 in. (305 mm to 610 mm) for lengths from 12 ft to 36 ft (3.7 m to 11 m), the maximum length to the closest aisle or egress doorway permitted by 13.2.5.7.5

Any additional width needed for seating is to be added to these widths, as described in 13.2.5.8.3.

**13.2.5.7.5** The path of travel along the aisle accessway shall not exceed 36 ft (11 m) from any seat to the closest aisle or egress doorway.

Paragraph 12/13.2.5.7.2 exempts a portion of the aisle accessway from the minimum width requirement under the specific conditions illustrated in Exhibit 12/13.25. The groupings of four chairs within the first 6 ft (1830 mm) of the aisle accessway are unregulated with respect to spacing. From the 6 ft (1830 mm) point away from the wall to the point where the aisle accessway reaches the aisle, the minimum width requirement of 12/13.2.5.7.1 applies.

Figure A.12/13.2.5.8.3 illustrates the provisions of 12/13.2.5.7.3 and 12/13.2.5.8.3. These requirements provide guidance on how aisle accessways and aisles with movable chairs are to be measured.

Exhibit 12/13.26 illustrates the maximum length of aisle accessway at tables permitted with the minimum 12 in. (305 mm) clear width. The aisle accessway width is greater than or equal to 12 in. (305 mm), with increased spacing of 0.5 in. (13 mm) for each additional 12 in. (305 mm) of aisle accessway beyond the

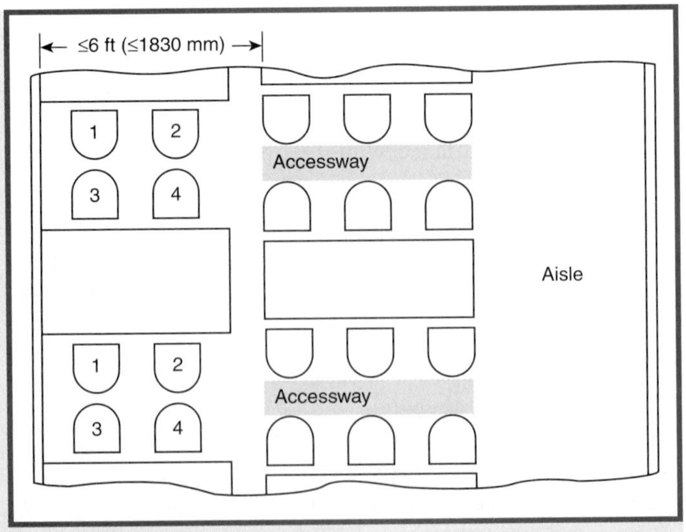


***Exhibit 12/13.25** First 6 ft (1830 mm) of aisle accessway serving four or fewer persons exempted from minimum aisle accessway width.*

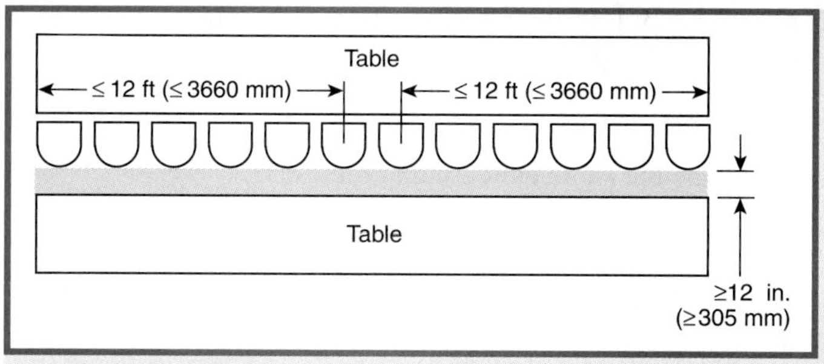


*Exhibit 12/13.26 Minimum aisle accessway at tables.*

initial 12 ft (3660 mm) from the center of the seat farthest from an aisle. In accordance with 12/13.2.5.7.3, the presence of chairs at one side of the aisle accessway increases the table-to-table spacing by 19 in. (485 mm).

Exhibit 12/13.27 illustrates the maximum length permitted for an aisle accessway serving seating at tables. The total length of the table is slightly more than 72 ft (22 m). Seating at longer tables requires a 36 in. (915 mm) aisle in accordance with the minimum width requirements of 12/13.2.5.8.2 instead of an aisle accessway. For the arrangement shown in Exhibit 12/13.27, the aisle accessway clear width, $X$, is 12 in. (305 mm) plus 0.5 in. (13 mm) for each additional 12 in. (305 mm) of aisle accessway beyond the initial 12 ft (3.7 m) from the center seat farthest from an aisle. The aisle accessway clear width is calculated as follows:

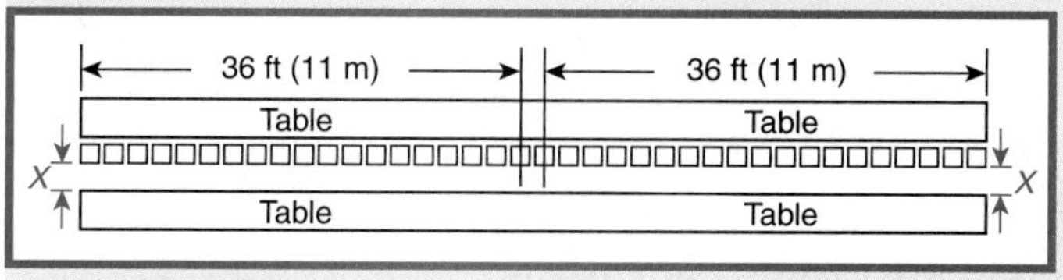


*Exhibit 12/13.27 Maximum 36 ft (11 m) permitted for an aisle accessway serving seating at tables.*

For inch/pound units,

$$\begin{aligned} X &= 12 \text{ in.} + [0.5 \text{ in./ft } (36 \text{ ft} - 12 \text{ ft})] \\ &= 12 \text{ in.} + [0.5 \text{ in./ft } (24 \text{ ft})] \\ &= 12 \text{ in.} + 12 \text{ in.} \\ &= 24 \text{ in.} \end{aligned}$$

For metric units,

$$13 \text{ mm}/305 \text{ mm} = 42.6 \text{ mm/m}$$

$$\begin{aligned} X &= 305 \text{ mm} + [42.6 \text{ mm/m } (11 \text{ m} - 3.7 \text{ m})] \\ &= 305 \text{ mm} + [42.6 \text{ mm/m } (7.3 \text{ m})] \\ &= 615 \text{ mm} \end{aligned}$$

With the 19 in. (485 mm) space required for the chairs, the table-to-table spacing must be ≥ 43 in. (1090 mm).

**12.2.5.8 Aisles Serving Seating at Tables.**

**12.2.5.8.1*** Aisles that contain steps or that are ramped, such as aisles serving dinner theater–style configurations, shall comply with the requirements of 12.2.5.6.

**A.12.2.5.8.1** See 7.1.7 and A.7.1.7.2 for special circulation safety precautions applicable where small elevation differences occur.

**12.2.5.8.2*** The width of aisles serving seating at tables shall be not less than 44 in. (1120 mm) where serving an occupant load exceeding 50, and 36 in. (915 mm) where serving an occupant load of 50 or fewer.

**A.12.2.5.8.2** It is important to make facilities accessible to people using wheelchairs. See ICC/ANSI A117.1, *American National Standard for Accessible and Usable Buildings and Facilities,* which provides guidance on appropriate aisle widths.

**12.2.5.8.3*** Where nonfixed seating is located between a table and an aisle, the measurement of required clear width of the aisle shall be made to a line 19 in. (485 mm), measured perpendicularly to the edge of the table, away from the edge of said table.

**13.2.5.8 Aisles Serving Seating at Tables.**

**13.2.5.8.1*** Aisles that contain steps or that are ramped, such as aisles serving dinner theater–style configurations, shall comply with the requirements of 13.2.5.6.

**A.13.2.5.8.1** See 7.1.7 and A.7.1.7.2 for special circulation safety precautions applicable where small elevation differences occur.

**13.2.5.8.2*** The width of aisles serving seating at tables shall be not less than 44 in. (1120 mm) where serving an occupant load exceeding 50, and 36 in. (915 mm) where serving an occupant load of 50 or fewer.

**A.13.2.5.8.2** It is important to make facilities accessible to people using wheelchairs. See ICC/ANSI A117.1, *American National Standard for Accessible and Usable Buildings and Facilities,* which provides guidance on appropriate aisle widths.

**13.2.5.8.3*** Where nonfixed seating is located between a table and an aisle, the measurement of required clear width of the aisle shall be made to a line 19 in. (485 mm), measured perpendicularly to the edge of the table, away from the edge of said table.

CHAPTER 12 • New

**A.12.2.5.8.3** Figure A.12.2.5.8.3 shows typical measurements involving seating and tables abutting an aisle. For purposes of the means of egress requirements of this *Code*, seating at counters or other furnishings is considered to be the same as seating at tables.

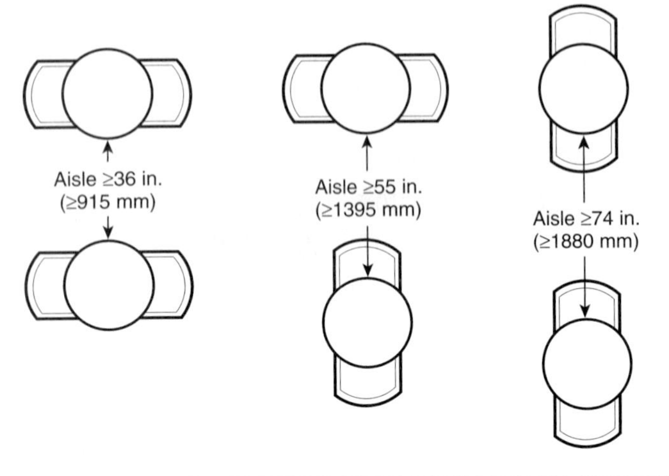


*Figure A.12.2.5.8.3 Seating at Tables Abutting an Aisle.*

**12.2.5.9 Approval of Layouts.**

**12.2.5.9.1** Where required by the authority having jurisdiction, plans drawn to scale showing the arrangement of furnishings or equipment shall be submitted to the authority by the building owner, manager, or authorized agent to substantiate conformance with the provisions of 12.2.5.

**12.2.5.9.2** The layout plans shall constitute the only acceptable arrangement, unless one of the following criteria is met:

(1) The plans are revised.
(2) Additional plans are submitted and approved.
(3) Temporary deviations from the specifications of the approved plans are used, provided that the occupant load is not increased and the intent of 12.2.5.9 is maintained.

**12.2.6 Travel Distance to Exits.**

**12.2.6.1** Travel distance shall be measured in accordance with Section 7.6.

**12.2.6.2** Exits shall be arranged so that the total length of travel from any point to reach an exit shall not exceed 200 ft (61 m) in any assembly occupancy, unless otherwise permitted by the following:

(1) The travel distance shall not exceed 250 ft (76 m) in assembly occupancies protected throughout by an approved, supervised automatic sprinkler system in accordance with Section 9.7.

CHAPTER 13 • Existing

**A.13.2.5.8.3** Figure A.13.2.5.8.3 shows typical measurements involving seating and tables abutting an aisle. Note that, for purposes of the means of egress requirements of this *Code*, seating at counters or other furnishings is considered to be the same as seating at tables.

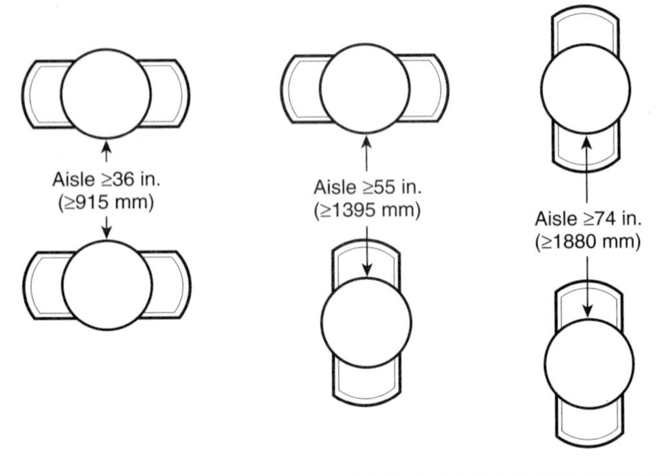


*Figure A.13.2.5.8.3 Seating at Tables Abutting an Aisle.*

**13.2.5.9 Approval of Layouts.**

**13.2.5.9.1** Where required by the authority having jurisdiction, plans drawn to scale showing the arrangement of furnishings or equipment shall be submitted to the authority by the building owner, manager, or authorized agent to substantiate conformance with the provisions of 13.2.5.

**13.2.5.9.2** The layout plans shall constitute the only acceptable arrangement, unless one of the following criteria is met:

(1) The plans are revised.
(2) Additional plans are submitted and approved.
(3) Temporary deviations from the specifications of the approved plans are used, provided that the occupant load is not increased and the intent of 13.2.5.9 is maintained.

**13.2.6 Travel Distance to Exits.**

**13.2.6.1** Travel distance shall be measured in accordance with Section 7.6.

**13.2.6.2** Exits shall be arranged so that the total length of travel from any point to reach an exit shall not exceed 200 ft (61 m) in any assembly occupancy, unless otherwise permitted by the following:

(1) The travel distance shall not exceed 250 ft (76 m) in assembly occupancies protected throughout by an approved automatic sprinkler system in accordance with Section 9.7.

CHAPTER 12 • New

(2) The travel distance requirement shall not apply to smoke-protected assembly seating as permitted by 12.4.2.11, 12.4.2.12, and 12.4.2.13.

Travel distance in assembly occupancies is required to be measured in accordance with Section 7.6. See 7.6.1 through 7.6.6.

Travel distance to exits from balconies or galleries that are served by unenclosed stairways must be measured to include the distance on the slope of the stair in the plane of the nosings and the distance from the bottom of the stair to the exterior exit door at the level of discharge, as illustrated in Exhibit 12/13.28.

### 12.2.7 Discharge from Exits.

**12.2.7.1** Exit discharge shall comply with Section 7.7.

**12.2.7.2** The level of exit discharge shall be measured at the point of principal entrance to the building.

**12.2.7.3** Where the principal entrance to an assembly occupancy is via a terrace, either raised or depressed, such terrace shall be permitted to be considered to be the first story in height for the purposes of Table 12.1.6 where the following criteria are met:

(1) The terrace is at least as long, measured parallel to the building, as the total width of the exit(s) it serves but not less than 60 in. (1525 mm) long.
(2) The terrace is at least as wide, measured perpendicularly to the building, as the exit(s) it serves but not less than 10 ft (3050 mm) wide.
(3) Required stairs leading from the terrace to the finished ground level are protected in accordance with 7.2.2.6.3 or are not less than 10 ft (3050 mm) from the building.

The *Code* specifies that 10 ft (3050 mm) is the minimum terrace depth necessary to allow people to exit the building into a depressed or raised area without causing a jamming effect at the exit. The same result was intended in requiring stairs to be at least 10 ft (3050 mm) from the face of the building, unless they are protected as provided in Chapter 7. The requirements of 12.2.7.3 are illustrated in Exhibit 12/13.29. Assuming that stair D serves exit B plus one-half of entrance A, and that stair E serves exit C plus one-half of entrance A, then X must be equal to or greater than the largest one of the following:

1. 10 ft (3050 mm), per 12.2.7.3(2)
2. 5 ft (1525 mm) + ½ of 14 ft (4270 mm) = 12 ft (3660 mm)
3. 6 ft (1830 mm) + ½ of 14 ft (4270 mm) = 13 ft (3960 mm)

Therefore, $X \geq 13$ ft (3960 mm).

CHAPTER 13 • Existing

(2) The travel distance requirement shall not apply to smoke-protected assembly seating as permitted by 13.4.2.11, 13.4.2.12, and 13.4.2.13.

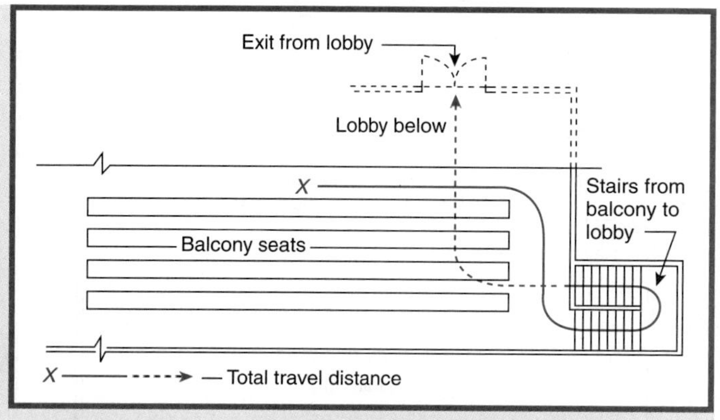


***Exhibit 12/13.28** Measurement of travel distance from balcony with egress by unenclosed stairs.*

### 13.2.7 Discharge from Exits.

**13.2.7.1** Exit discharge shall comply with Section 7.7.

**13.2.7.2** The level of exit discharge shall be measured at the point of principal entrance to the building.

**13.2.7.3** Where the principal entrance to an assembly occupancy is via a terrace, either raised or depressed, such terrace shall be permitted to be considered to be the first story in height for the purposes of Table 13.1.6 where the following criteria are met:

(1) The terrace is at least as long, measured parallel to the building, as the total width of the exit(s) it serves but not less than 60 in. (1525 mm) long.
(2) The terrace is at least as wide, measured perpendicularly to the building, as the exit(s) it serves but not less than 60 in. (1525 mm) wide.
(3) Required stairs leading from the terrace to the finished ground level are protected in accordance with 7.2.2.6.3 or are not less than 10 ft (3050 mm) from the building.

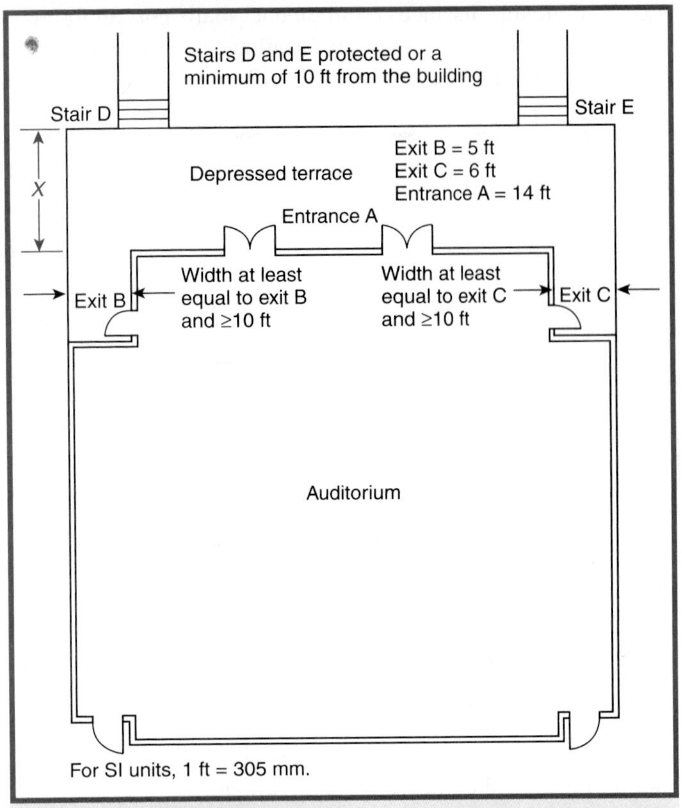


***Exhibit 12/13.29** New assembly occupancy with depressed terrace as principal entrance.*

### 12.2.8 Illumination of Means of Egress.

Means of egress, other than for private party tents not exceeding 1200 $ft^2$ (112 $m^2$), shall be illuminated in accordance with Section 7.8.

### 12.2.9 Emergency Lighting.

**12.2.9.1** Emergency lighting shall be provided in accordance with Section 7.9.

**12.2.9.2** Private party tents not exceeding 1200 $ft^2$ (112 $m^2$) shall not be required to have emergency lighting.

### 12.2.10 Marking of Means of Egress.

**12.2.10.1** Means of egress shall be provided with signs in accordance with Section 7.10.

**12.2.10.2** Exit markings shall not be required on the seating side of vomitories from seating areas where exit marking is

### 13.2.8 Illumination of Means of Egress.

Means of egress, other than for private party tents not exceeding 1200 $ft^2$ (112 $m^2$), shall be illuminated in accordance with Section 7.8.

### 13.2.9 Emergency Lighting.

**13.2.9.1** Emergency lighting, other than that permitted by 13.2.9.3, shall be provided in accordance with Section 7.9.

**13.2.9.2** Private party tents not exceeding 1200 $ft^2$ (112 $m^2$) shall not be required to have emergency lighting.

**13.2.9.3** Assembly occupancies with an occupant load not exceeding 300 and used exclusively for a place of worship shall not be required to have emergency lighting.

### 13.2.10 Marking of Means of Egress.

**13.2.10.1** Means of egress shall be provided with signs in accordance with Section 7.10.

**13.2.10.2** Exit markings shall not be required on the seating side of vomitories from seating areas where exit marking is

CHAPTER 12 • New

provided in the concourse and where such marking is readily apparent from the vomitories.

**12.2.10.3** Evacuation diagrams in accordance with 7.10.8.5 shall be provided.

### 12.2.11 Special Means of Egress Features.

**12.2.11.1 Guards and Railings.**

**12.2.11.1.1* Sight Line–Constrained Rail Heights.** Unless subject to the requirements of 12.2.11.1.2, a fasciae or railing system complying with the guard requirements of 7.2.2.4, and having a height of not less than 26 in. (660 mm), shall be provided where the floor or footboard elevation is more than 30 in. (760 mm) above the floor or the finished ground level below, and where the fasciae or railing system would otherwise interfere with the sight lines of immediately adjacent seating.

CHAPTER 13 • Existing

provided in the concourse and where such marking is readily apparent from the vomitories.

**13.2.10.3** Evacuation diagrams in accordance with 7.10.8.5 shall be provided.

### 13.2.11 Special Means of Egress Features.

**13.2.11.1 Guards and Railings: Boxes, Balconies, and Galleries.** Boxes, balconies, and galleries shall meet the following criteria:

(1) The fasciae of boxes, balconies, and galleries shall rise not less than 26 in. (660 mm) above the adjacent floor or shall have substantial railings not less than 26 in. (660 mm) above the adjacent floor.
(2) The height of the rail above footrests on the adjacent floor immediately in front of a row of seats shall be not less than 26 in. (660 mm), and the following also shall apply:
    (a) Railings at the ends of aisles shall be not less than 36 in. (915 mm) high for the full width of the aisle.
    (b) Railings at the end of aisles shall be not less than 36 in. (915 mm) high at the ends of aisles where steps occur.
(3) Aisle accessways adjacent to orchestra pits and vomitories, and all cross aisles, shall be provided with railings not less than 26 in. (660 mm) above the adjacent floor.
(4) The requirement of 13.2.11.1(3) shall not apply where the backs of seats located at the front of the aisle project 24 in. (610 mm) or more above the adjacent floor of the aisle.
(5) Guardrails shall not be required on the audience side of stages, raised platforms, and other raised floor areas such as runways, ramps, and side stages used for entertainment or presentations.
(6) Permanent guardrails shall not be required at vertical openings in the performance area of stages.
(7) Guardrails shall not be required where the side of an elevated walking surface is required to be open for the normal functioning of special lighting or for access and use of other special equipment.

**A.12.2.11.1.1** This requirement includes provisions of guards and rails at the front of boxes, galleries, and balconies, and at aisle accessways adjacent to vomitories and orchestra pits.

**12.2.11.1.2 At Foot of Aisles.**

**12.2.11.1.2.1** A fasciae or railing system complying with the guard requirements of 7.2.2.4 shall be provided for the full width of the aisle where the foot of the aisle is more than 30 in. (760 mm) above the floor or the finished ground level below.

**12.2.11.1.2.2** The fasciae or railing shall be not less than 36 in. (915 mm) high and shall provide not less than 42 in. (1065 mm), measured diagonally, between the top of the rail and the nosing of the nearest tread.

**12.2.11.1.3 At Cross Aisles.** Guards and railings at cross aisles shall meet the following criteria:

(1) Cross aisles located behind seating rows shall be provided with railings not less than 26 in. (660 mm) above the adjacent floor of the aisle.
(2) The requirement of 12.2.11.1.3(1) shall not apply where the backs of seats located at the front of the aisle project 24 in. (610 mm) or more above the adjacent floor of the aisle.
(3) Where cross aisles exceed 30 in. (760 mm) above the floor or the finished ground level below, guards shall be provided in accordance with 7.2.2.4.

**12.2.11.1.4 At Side and Back of Seating Areas.** Guards complying with the guard requirements of 7.2.2.4 shall be provided with a height not less than 42 in. (1065 mm) above the aisle, aisle accessway, or footboard where the floor elevation exceeds 30 in. (760 mm) above the floor or the finished ground level to the side or back of seating.

**12.2.11.1.5 Below Seating.** Openings between footboards and seat boards shall be provided with intermediate construction so that a 4 in. (100 mm) diameter sphere cannot pass through the opening.

**12.2.11.1.6 Locations Not Requiring Guards.** Guards shall not be required in the following locations:

(1) Guards shall not be required on the audience side of stages, of raised platforms, and of other raised floor areas such as runways, ramps, and side stages used for entertainment or presentations.
(2) Permanent guards shall not be required at vertical openings in the performance area of stages.
(3) Guards shall not be required where the side of an elevated walking surface is required to be open for the normal functioning of special lighting or for access and use of other special equipment.

The requirements for guards and handrails for new assembly seating areas were revised for the 1997 edition of the *Code* and have been carried forward without further change. The requirements for guards and handrails for existing assembly seating areas remained without revision. The provisions for new construction are, thus, different from those applicable to existing facilities. The commentary that follows addresses new installations first and existing arrangements second.

Paragraphs 12.2.11.1.1 and 12.2.11.1.2 clarify that new assembly seating area guards, where the floor is more than 30 in. (760 mm) above the floor or grade below, must comply with the guard requirements of 7.2.2.4. This requirement includes the provision for intermediate rails or balusters to meet the 4 in. (100 mm) diameter sphere requirement of 7.2.2.4.5.3, which is illustrated in Exhibit 12/13.30.

Paragraph 12.2.11.1.1 permits a guard height of 26 in. (660 mm) at the front of seating but not at the foot of aisles. Further, the 26 in. (660 mm) height allowance applies only if a 36 in. (915 mm) height rail [as permitted by 12.2.11.1.2.2 in lieu of the typical 42 in. (1065 mm) height guard detailed in 7.2.2.4.5] would otherwise interfere with sight lines of immediately adjacent seating. Note that the heading for paragraph 12.2.11.1.1 is Sight Line–Constrained Rail Heights. The minimum 26 in. (660 mm) height is illustrated in Exhibit 12/13.30.

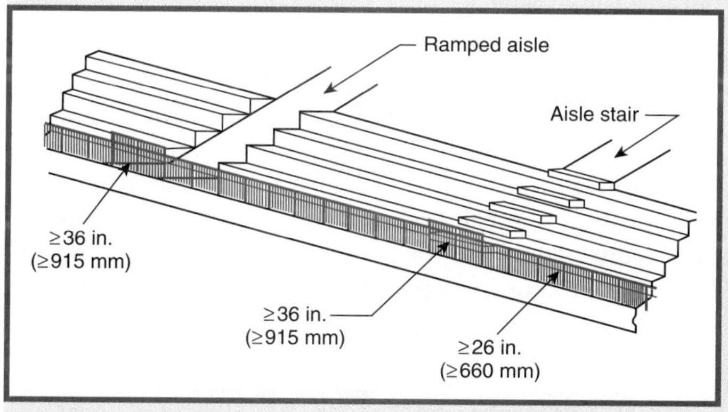


***Exhibit 12/13.30** New assembly occupancy building with railings installed in accordance with 12.2.11.1.1 and 12.2.11.1.2.*

Paragraph 12.2.11.1.2.1 requires that a guard be provided at the foot of an aisle if there is more than a 30 in. (760 mm) vertical distance to fall. Again, such guards must meet the guard requirements of 7.2.2.4.5 and must be at least 36 in. (915 mm) in height. See Exhibit 12/13.30. Where previous editions of the *Code* re-



quired a 42 in. (1065 mm) guard at the foot of a stepped aisle, the current requirement of 12.2.11.1.2.2 is for a minimum 36 in. (915 mm) height and a minimum 42 in. (1065 mm), measured diagonally between the top of the guardrail and the nosing of the nearest step tread. This requirement is illustrated in Exhibit 12/13.31.

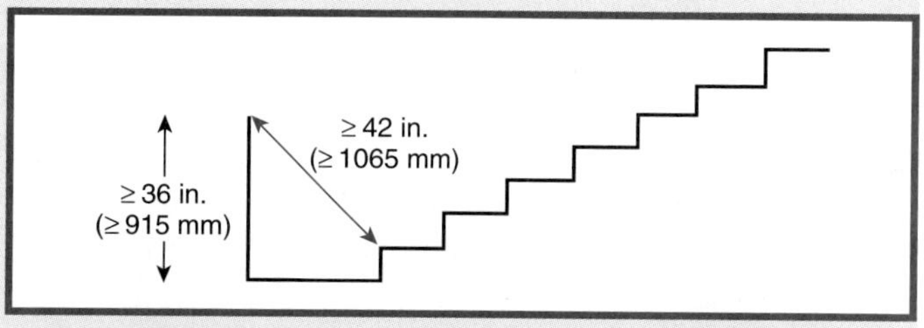


***Exhibit 12/13.31** New assembly occupancy building with railings installed at foot of stepped aisle in accordance with 12.2.11.1.2.2.*

Where there is a stepped aisle, the requirement of 12.2.11.1.2.2 to provide a minimum of 42 in. (1065 mm), measured diagonally between the top of the guardrail and the nosing of the nearest step tread, will force the guardrail height to be greater than 36 in. (915 mm) if the first riser is positioned too close, horizontally, to the guard. For example, if the first riser is positioned 28 in. (710 mm) horizontally from the guard and an 8 in. (205 mm) riser height is used, the minimum 42 in. (1065 mm) diagonal distance requirement will force the guardrail height to be a minimum of 39 in. (990 mm). For the same riser height of 8 in. (205 mm), a 36 in. (915 mm) high guardrail at the foot of the stepped aisle would require that the first step riser be positioned at least 31 in. (785 mm), horizontally, from the guardrail.

Paragraph 13.2.11.1 addresses guards and railings in existing assembly occupancies.

Exhibit 12/13.32 illustrates the requirements of 13.2.11.1(1) and (2). Rail height at the fascia end of a ramped aisle or a stepped aisle must not be less than 36 in. (915 mm).

It is not the intent of the *Code* to reduce the height of guards where sight lines are not a problem, such as with cross aisles at the rear or top of seating areas or where cross aisles are sufficiently below seating that a proper height guard will not interfere with sight lines.

Note that, for existing assembly occupancies, the railings described by 13.2.11.1(1) and (2) are, in fact, railings and not the guards required by 7.2.2.4.5. As depicted in Exhibit 12/13.32, there is no requirement

CHAPTER 12 • New

CHAPTER 13 • Existing

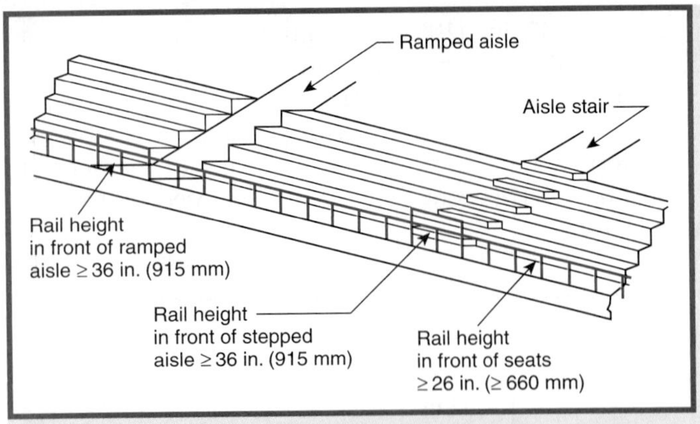


***Exhibit 12/13.32** Existing assembly occupancy building with railings installed in accordance with 13.2.11.1(1) and 13.2.11.1(2).*

for intermediate rails or balusters — the assembly seating rails are not required to meet the 4 in. (100 mm) diameter sphere requirement of 7.2.2.4.5.3. This provision is more lenient than the requirements applicable to new assembly occupancies, where 12.2.11.1 requires a railing system to comply with the guard requirements of 7.2.2.4 (see Exhibit 12/13.30).

The *Code* requires a barrier along the downhill side of a cross aisle for both new construction and existing buildings. The barrier might consist of a rail or the backs of the seats that abut the downhill side of the aisle where the backs project 24 in. (610 mm) or more above the cross aisle. The difference between the 24 in. (610 mm) back height and the required 26 in. (660 mm) railing is not sufficient to require the railing. See Exhibit 12/13.33.

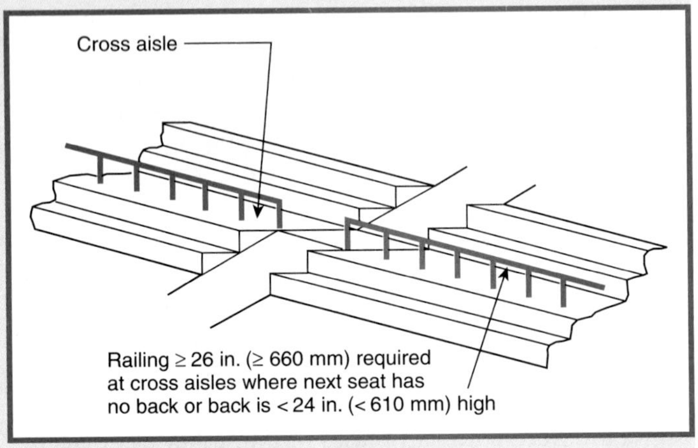


***Exhibit 12/13.33** Barrier for cross aisles.*

**12.2.11.2 Lockups.** Lockups in assembly occupancies shall comply with the requirements of 22.4.5.

**13.2.11.2 Lockups.** Lockups in assembly occupancies, other than approved existing lockups, shall comply with the requirements of 23.4.5.

A *lockup* is defined in 3.3.155 as "an incidental use area in other than a detention and correctional occupancy where occupants are restrained and such occupants are mostly incapable of self-preservation because of security measures not under the occupants' control." Examples of lockups in assembly occupancies include a holding area for customs/immigration violators at an international airport and a holding area for unruly patrons at a sports arena. The provisions of Chapters 12 and 13 alone are not adequate to ensure life safety for those who are detained by security measures not under their control. Lockups in assembly occupancies are required to meet the provisions of 22/23.4.5, which complete the needed package of protection features.

## 12.3 Protection

### 12.3.1 Protection of Vertical Openings.

Any vertical opening shall be enclosed or protected in accordance with Section 8.6, unless otherwise permitted by the following:

(1)* Stairs or ramps shall be permitted to be unenclosed between balconies or mezzanines and main assembly areas located below, provided that the balcony or mezzanine is open to the main assembly area.

## 13.3 Protection

### 13.3.1 Protection of Vertical Openings.

Any vertical opening shall be enclosed or protected in accordance with Section 8.6, unless otherwise permitted by the following:

(1)* Stairs or ramps shall be permitted to be unenclosed between balconies or mezzanines and main assembly areas located below, provided that the balcony or mezzanine is open to the main assembly area.

CHAPTER 12 • New

**A.12.3.1(1)** The allowance for unenclosed stairs or ramps presumes the balcony or mezzanine complies with the other provisions of the *Code,* such as travel distance to exits in accordance with 12.2.6 and numbers of exits in accordance with 12.2.4. For the purposes of this exception, a balcony with glazing that provides a visual awareness of the main assembly area is considered open.

(2) Exit access stairs from lighting and access catwalks, galleries, and gridirons shall not be required to be enclosed.
(3) Assembly occupancies protected by an approved, supervised automatic sprinkler system in accordance with Section 9.7 shall be permitted to have unprotected vertical openings in accordance with 8.6.8.2.

### 12.3.2 Protection from Hazards.

**12.3.2.1 Service Equipment, Hazardous Operations or Processes, and Storage Facilities.**

**12.3.2.1.1** Rooms containing high-pressure boilers, refrigerating machinery of other than the domestic refrigerator type, large transformers, or other service equipment subject to explosion shall meet the following requirements:

(1) Such rooms shall not be located directly under or abutting required exits.
(2) Such rooms shall be separated from other parts of the building by fire barriers in accordance with Section 8.3 having a minimum 1-hour fire resistance rating or shall be protected by automatic extinguishing systems in accordance with Section 8.7.

**12.3.2.1.2** Rooms or spaces for the storage, processing, or use of materials specified in 12.3.2.1.2(1) through (3) shall be protected in accordance with the following:

(1) Separation from the remainder of the building by fire barriers having a minimum 1-hour fire resistance rating or protection of such rooms by automatic extinguishing systems as specified in Section 8.7 in the following areas:

CHAPTER 13 • Existing

**A.13.3.1(1)** The allowance for unenclosed stairs or ramps presumes the balcony or mezzanine complies with the other provisions of the *Code*, such as travel distance to exits in accordance with 13.2.6 and numbers of exits in accordance with 13.2.4. For the purposes of this exception, a balcony with glazing that provides a visual awareness of the main assembly area is considered open.

(2) Exit access stairs from lighting and access catwalks, galleries, and gridirons shall not be required to be enclosed.
(3) Assembly occupancies protected by an approved, supervised automatic sprinkler system in accordance with Section 9.7 shall be permitted to have unprotected vertical openings in accordance with 8.6.8.2.
(4) Use of the following alternative materials shall be permitted where assemblies constructed of such materials are in good repair and free of any condition that would diminish their original fire resistance characteristics:
    (a) Existing wood lath and plaster
    (b) Existing $\frac{1}{2}$ in. (13 mm) gypsum wallboard
    (c) Existing installations of $\frac{1}{4}$ in. (6.3 mm) thick wired glass that are, or are rendered, inoperative and fixed in the closed position
    (d) Other existing materials having similar fire resistance capabilities

### 13.3.2 Protection from Hazards.

**13.3.2.1 Service Equipment, Hazardous Operations or Processes, and Storage Facilities.**

**13.3.2.1.1** Rooms containing high-pressure boilers, refrigerating machinery of other than the domestic refrigerator type, large transformers, or other service equipment subject to explosion shall meet the following requirements:

(1) Such rooms shall not be located directly under or abutting required exits.
(2) Such rooms shall be separated from other parts of the building by fire barriers in accordance with Section 8.3 that have a minimum 1-hour fire resistance rating or shall be protected by automatic extinguishing systems in accordance with Section 8.7.

**13.3.2.1.2** Rooms or spaces for the storage, processing, or use of materials specified in 13.3.2.1.2(1) through (3) shall be protected in accordance with the following:

(1) Separation from the remainder of the building by fire barriers having a minimum 1-hour fire resistance rating or protection of such rooms by automatic extinguishing systems as specified in Section 8.7 in the following areas:

CHAPTER 12 • New

(a) Boiler and furnace rooms, unless otherwise permitted by the following:
  i. The requirement of 12.3.2.1.2(1)(a) shall not apply to rooms enclosing furnaces, heating and air-handling equipment, or compressor equipment with a total aggregate input rating less than 200,000 Btu (211 MJ), provided that such rooms are not used for storage.
  ii. The requirement of 12.3.2.1.2(1)(a) shall not apply to attic locations of the rooms addressed in 12.3.2.1.2(1)(a)(i), provided that such rooms comply with the draftstopping requirements of 8.6.10.

(b) Rooms or spaces used for the storage of combustible supplies in quantities deemed hazardous by the authority having jurisdiction
(c) Rooms or spaces used for the storage of hazardous materials or flammable or combustible liquids in quantities deemed hazardous by recognized standards

(2) Separation from the remainder of the building by fire barriers having a minimum 1-hour fire resistance rating and protection of such rooms by automatic extinguishing systems as specified in Section 8.7 in the following areas:
  (a) Laundries
  (b) Maintenance shops, including woodworking and painting areas
  (c) Rooms or spaces used for processing or use of combustible supplies deemed hazardous by the authority having jurisdiction
  (d) Rooms or spaces used for processing or use of hazardous materials or flammable or combustible liquids in quantities deemed hazardous by recognized standards

(3) Where automatic extinguishing is used to meet the requirements of 12.3.2.1.2(1) or (2), the protection shall be permitted in accordance with 9.7.1.2.

CHAPTER 13 • Existing

(a) Boiler and furnace rooms, unless otherwise protected by the following:
  i. The requirement of 13.3.2.1.2(1)(a) shall not apply to rooms enclosing furnaces, heating and air-handling equipment, or compressor equipment with a total aggregate input rating less than 200,000 Btu (211 MJ), provided that such rooms are not used for storage.
  ii. The requirement of 13.3.2.1.2(1)(a) shall not apply to attic locations of the rooms addressed in 13.3.2.1.2(1)(a)i, provided that such rooms comply with the draftstopping requirements of 8.6.10.

(b) Rooms or spaces used for the storage of combustible supplies in quantities deemed hazardous by the authority having jurisdiction
(c) Rooms or spaces used for the storage of hazardous materials or flammable or combustible liquids in quantities deemed hazardous by recognized standards

(2) Separation from the remainder of the building by fire barriers having a minimum 1-hour fire resistance rating and protection of such rooms by automatic extinguishing systems as specified in Section 8.7 in the following areas:
  (a) Laundries
  (b) Maintenance shops, including woodworking and painting areas
  (c) Rooms or spaces used for processing or use of combustible supplies deemed hazardous by the authority having jurisdiction
  (d) Rooms or spaces used for processing or use of hazardous materials or flammable or combustible liquids in quantities deemed hazardous by recognized standards

(3) Where automatic extinguishing is used to meet the requirements of 13.3.2.1.2(1) or (2), the protection shall be permitted in accordance with 9.7.1.2

The intent of 12/13.3.2.1.2 is to specify the degree of protection necessary for certain hazardous areas. The requirements are separated into three subdivisions: 12/13.3.2.1.2(1) and (2), which are based on the degree of hazard, and 12/13.3.2.1.2(3), which addresses the use of the domestic water supply for sprinklers used to protect the hazardous area. The hazards noted in 12/13.3.2.1.2(1) are required to be enclosed in 1-hour construction *or* be protected by sprinklers. If the sprinkler option is chosen, an enclosure is still required; however, the enclosure need not be fire rated. In new construction, the enclosure must be formed by smoke partitions (see 8.7.1.2 and Section 8.4); existing enclosures must form a membrane against the passage of smoke.

The hazards noted in 12/13.3.2.1.2(2) must be en-

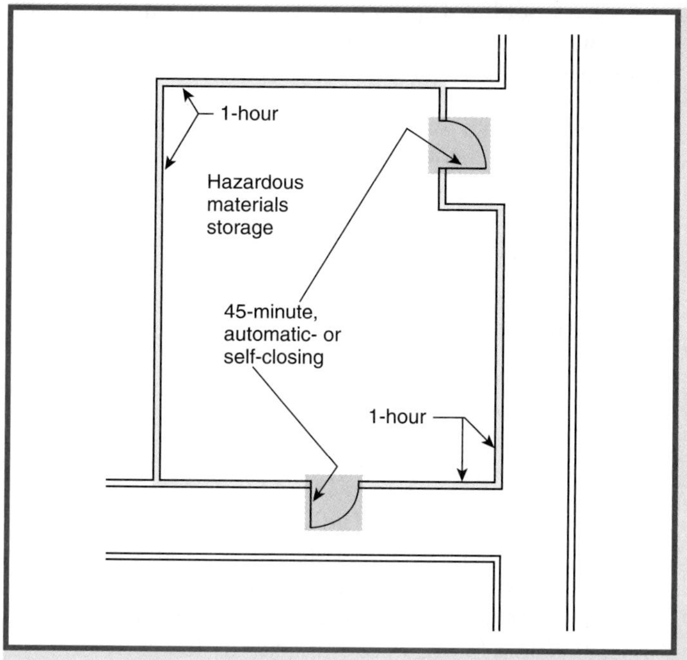


***Exhibit 12/13.34** Protection of hazardous areas using fire-rated enclosure.*

closed in 1-hour construction *and* be protected by automatic sprinklers.

Exhibit 12/13.34 through Exhibit 12/13.36 illustrate the three methods of protection specified by 12/13.3.2.1.2. Exhibit 12/13.34 and Exhibit 12/13.35 illustrate the two options for complying with 12/13.3.2.1.2(1), that is, separation via fire-rated barriers or protection by automatic sprinklers. Exhibit 12/13.36 illustrates the requirement of 12/13.3.2.1.2(2) that both fire resistance–rated separation and automatic sprinkler protection be provided.

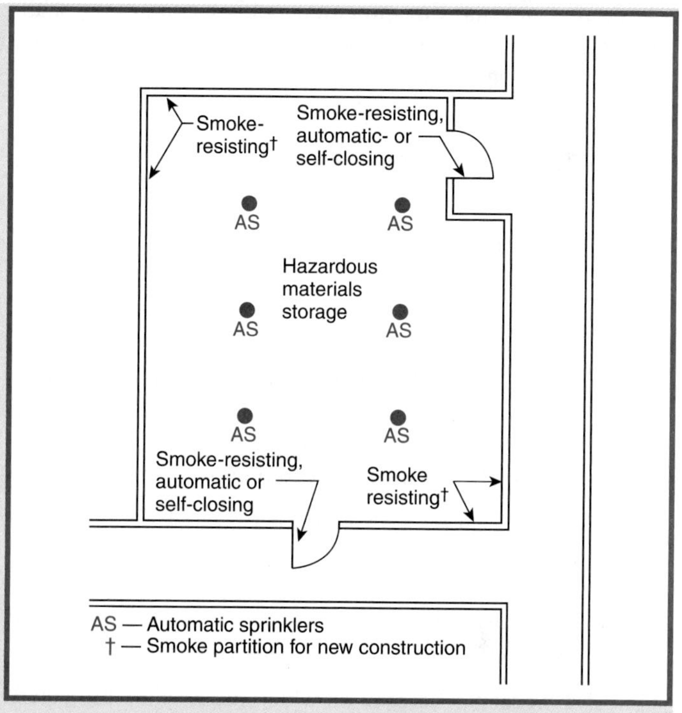


***Exhibit 12/13.35** Protection of hazardous areas using automatic sprinklers.*

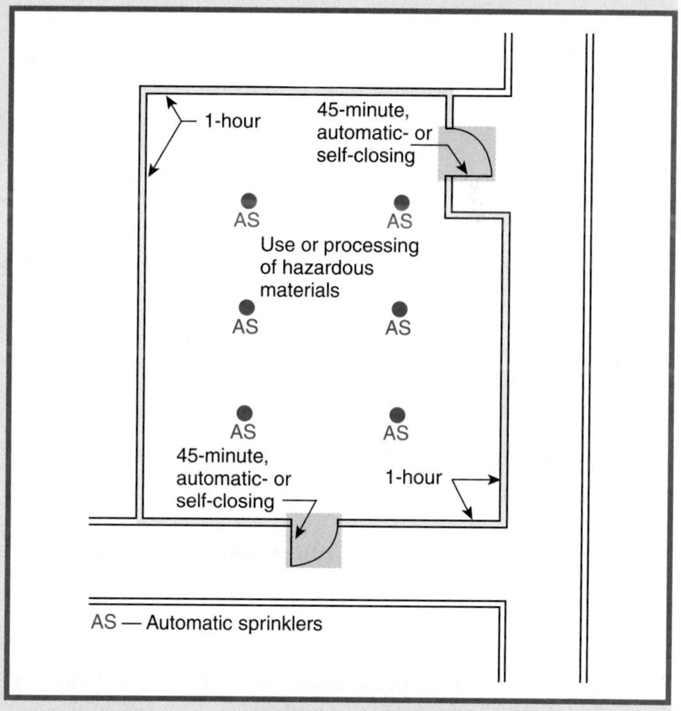


***Exhibit 12/13.36** Protection of hazardous areas using both fire-rated enclosure and automatic sprinklers.*

CHAPTER 12 • New

**12.3.2.2 Cooking Equipment.** Cooking equipment shall be protected in accordance with 9.2.3, unless the cooking equipment is one of the following types:

(1) Outdoor equipment
(2) Portable equipment not flue-connected
(3) Equipment used only for food warming

### 12.3.3 Interior Finish.

**12.3.3.1 General.** Interior finish shall be in accordance with Section 10.2.

**12.3.3.2 Corridors, Lobbies, and Enclosed Stairways.** Interior wall and ceiling finish materials complying with Section 10.2 shall be Class A or Class B in all corridors and lobbies and shall be Class A in enclosed stairways.

**12.3.3.3 Assembly Areas.** Interior wall and ceiling finish materials complying with Section 10.2 shall be Class A or Class B in general assembly areas having occupant loads of more than 300 and shall be Class A, Class B, or Class C in assembly areas having occupant loads of 300 or fewer.

**12.3.3.4 Screens.** Screens on which pictures are projected shall comply with requirements of Class A or Class B interior finish in accordance with Section 10.2.

**12.3.3.5 Interior Floor Finish.**

**12.3.3.5.1** Interior floor finish shall comply with Section 10.2.

**12.3.3.5.2** Interior floor finish in exit enclosures and exit access corridors and in spaces not separated from them by walls complying with 12.3.6 shall be not less than Class II.

**12.3.3.5.3** Interior floor finish shall comply with 10.2.7.1 or 10.2.7.2, as applicable.

### 12.3.4 Detection, Alarm, and Communications Systems.

**12.3.4.1 General.**

**12.3.4.1.1** Assembly occupancies with occupant loads of more than 300 and all theaters with more than one audience-viewing room shall be provided with an approved fire alarm system in accordance with 9.6.1 and 12.3.4, unless otherwise permitted by 12.3.4.1.2.

CHAPTER 13 • Existing

**13.3.2.2 Cooking Equipment.** Cooking equipment shall be protected in accordance with 9.2.3, unless the cooking equipment is one of the following types:

(1) Outdoor equipment
(2) Portable equipment not flue-connected
(3) Equipment used only for food warming

### 13.3.3 Interior Finish.

**13.3.3.1 General.** Interior finish shall be in accordance with Section 10.2.

**13.3.3.2 Corridors, Lobbies, and Enclosed Stairways.** Interior wall and ceiling finish materials complying with Section 10.2 shall be Class A or Class B in all corridors and lobbies and shall be Class A in enclosed stairways.

**13.3.3.3 Assembly Areas.** Interior wall and ceiling finish materials complying with Section 10.2 shall be Class A or Class B in general assembly areas having occupant loads of more than 300 and shall be Class A, Class B, or Class C in assembly areas having occupant loads of 300 or fewer.

**13.3.3.4 Screens.** Screens on which pictures are projected shall comply with requirements of Class A or Class B interior finish in accordance with Section 10.2.

Evaluation of existing interior finish is sometimes difficult. Where flame spread characteristics cannot be readily determined, the questionable material should be removed or treated with approved flame retardants. Where treatment cannot reduce flame spread to the required limits, automatic sprinklers might be provided to help compensate for the deficiency.

**13.3.3.5 Interior Floor Finish.** (No requirements.)

### 13.3.4 Detection, Alarm, and Communications Systems.

**13.3.4.1 General.**

**13.3.4.1.1** Assembly occupancies with occupant loads of more than 300 and all theaters with more than one audience-viewing room shall be provided with an approved fire alarm system in accordance with 9.6.1 and 13.3.4, unless otherwise permitted by 13.3.4.1.2, 13.3.4.1.3, or 13.3.4.1.4.

CHAPTER 12 • New

**12.3.4.1.2** Assembly occupancies that are a part of a multiple occupancy protected as a mixed occupancy *(see 6.1.14)* shall be permitted to be served by a common fire alarm system, provided that the individual requirements of each occupancy are met.

**12.3.4.2 Initiation.**

**12.3.4.2.1** Initiation of the required fire alarm system shall be by both of the following means:

(1) Manual means in accordance with 9.6.2.1(1), unless otherwise permitted by the following:
  (a) The requirement of 12.3.4.2.1(1) shall not apply where initiation is by means of an approved automatic fire detection system in accordance with 9.6.2.1(2) that provides fire detection throughout the building.
  (b) The requirement of 12.3.4.2.1(1) shall not apply where initiation is by means of an approved automatic sprinkler system in accordance with 9.6.2.1(3) that provides fire detection and protection throughout the building.
(2) Where automatic sprinklers are provided, sprinkler system waterflow shall initiate the fire alarm system, even where manual fire alarm boxes are provided in accordance with 12.3.4.2.1(1).

**12.3.4.2.2** The initiating device shall be capable of transmitting an alarm to a receiving station, located within the building, that is constantly attended when the assembly occupancy is occupied.

**12.3.4.2.3*** In assembly occupancies with occupant loads of more than 300, automatic detection shall be provided in all hazardous areas that are not normally occupied, unless such areas are protected throughout by an approved, supervised automatic sprinkler system in accordance with Section 9.7.

**A.12.3.4.2.3** The intent is to require detectors only in nonsprinklered hazardous areas that are unoccupied. When the building is occupied, the detectors in the unoccupied, unsprinklered hazardous areas will initiate occupant notification.

CHAPTER 13 • Existing

**13.3.4.1.2** Assembly occupancies that are a part of a multiple occupancy protected as a mixed occupancy *(see 6.1.14)* shall be permitted to be served by a common fire alarm system, provided that the individual requirements of each occupancy are met.

**13.3.4.1.3** Voice communication or public address systems complying with 13.3.4.3.6 shall not be required to comply with 9.6.1.

**13.3.4.1.4** The requirement of 13.3.4.1.1 shall not apply to assembly occupancies where, in the judgment of the authority having jurisdiction, adequate alternative provisions exist or are provided for the discovery of a fire and for alerting the occupants promptly.

**13.3.4.2 Initiation.**

**13.3.4.2.1** Initiation of the required fire alarm system shall be by both of the following means, and the system shall be provided with an emergency power source:

(1) Manual means in accordance with 9.6.2.1(1), unless otherwise permitted by the following:
  (a) The requirement of 13.3.4.2.1(1) shall not apply where initiation is by means of an approved automatic fire detection system in accordance with 9.6.2.1(2) that provides fire detection throughout the building.
  (b) The requirement of 13.3.4.2.1(1) shall not apply where initiation is by means of an approved automatic sprinkler system in accordance with 9.6.2.1(3) that provides fire detection and protection throughout the building.
(2) Where automatic sprinklers are provided, sprinkler system waterflow shall initiate the fire alarm system, even where manual fire alarm boxes are provided in accordance with 13.3.4.2.1(1).

**13.3.4.2.2** The initiating device shall be capable of transmitting an alarm to a receiving station, located within the building, that is constantly attended when the assembly occupancy is occupied.

**13.3.4.2.3*** In assembly occupancies with occupant loads of more than 300, automatic detection shall be provided in all hazardous areas that are not normally occupied, unless such areas are protected throughout by an approved automatic sprinkler system in accordance with Section 9.7.

**A.13.3.4.2.3** The intent is to require detectors only in nonsprinklered hazardous areas that are unoccupied. Where the building is occupied, the detectors in the unoccupied, unsprinklered hazardous areas will initiate occupant notification.

CHAPTER 12 • New

If the building is unoccupied, the fire in the nonsprinklered hazardous area is not a life safety issue, and the detectors, upon activation, are not required to notify anyone. The signal from a detector is permitted to be sent to a control panel in an area that is occupied when the building is occupied, but that is unoccupied when the building is unoccupied, without the need for central station monitoring or the equivalent.

**12.3.4.3 Notification.** The required fire alarm system shall activate an audible and visible alarm in a constantly attended receiving station within the building when occupied for purposes of initiating emergency action.

**12.3.4.3.1** Positive alarm sequence in accordance with 9.6.3.4 shall be permitted.

**12.3.4.3.2 Reserved.**

**12.3.4.3.3** Occupant notification shall be by means of voice announcements in accordance with 9.6.3.9, initiated by the person in the constantly attended receiving station.

**12.3.4.3.4** Occupant notification shall be by means of visible signals in accordance with 9.6.3.5, initiated by the person in the constantly attended receiving station, unless otherwise permitted by 12.3.4.3.5.

**12.3.4.3.5*** Visible signals shall not be required in the assembly seating area, or the floor area used for the contest, performance, or entertainment, where the occupant load exceeds 1000 and an approved, alternative visible means of occupant notification is provided. *(See 9.6.3.5.7.)*

**A.12.3.4.3.5** Examples of devices that might be used to provide alternative visible means include scoreboards, message boards, and other electronic devices.

**12.3.4.3.6** The announcement shall be permitted to be made via a voice communication or public address system in accordance with 9.6.3.9.2.

**12.3.4.3.7** Where the authority having jurisdiction determines that a constantly attended receiving station is impractical, both of the following shall be provided:

(1) Automatically transmitted evacuation or relocation instructions shall be provided in accordance with *NFPA 72, National Fire Alarm Code.*
(2) The system shall be monitored by a supervising station in accordance with *NFPA 72, National Fire Alarm Code.*

CHAPTER 13 • Existing

If the building is unoccupied, the fire in the nonsprinklered hazardous area is not a life safety issue, and the detectors, upon activation, are not required to notify anyone. The signal from a detector is permitted to be sent to a control panel in an area that is occupied when the building is occupied, but that is unoccupied when the building is unoccupied, without the need for central station monitoring or the equivalent.

**13.3.4.3 Notification.** The required fire alarm system shall activate an audible alarm in a constantly attended receiving station within the building when occupied for purposes of initiating emergency action.

**13.3.4.3.1** Positive alarm sequence in accordance with 9.6.3.4 shall be permitted.

**13.3.4.3.2** A presignal system in accordance with 9.6.3.3 shall be permitted.

**13.3.4.3.3** Occupant notification shall be by means of voice announcements in accordance with 9.6.3.9 initiated by the person in the constantly attended receiving station.

**13.3.4.3.4 Reserved.**

**13.3.4.3.5 Reserved.**

**13.3.4.3.6** The announcement shall be permitted to be made via a voice communication or public address system in accordance with 9.6.3.9.2.

**13.3.4.3.7** Where the authority having jurisdiction determines that a constantly attended receiving station is impractical, automatically transmitted evacuation or relocation instructions shall be provided in accordance with *NFPA 72, National Fire Alarm Code.*

Paragraph 12/13.3.4.1.2 clarifies that a common alarm system can be used within a building that houses occupancies in addition to an assembly occupancy, provided that the system meets the alarm requirements applicable to each of those occupancies. This provision permits an assembly occupancy in a school, hotel, hos-

CHAPTER 12 • New

pital, mall, or other building to be served by the same fire alarm as the predominant occupancy, provided that it also meets the requirements applicable to alarm systems in an assembly occupancy.

Paragraph 13.3.4.1.3 permits an existing voice communication system or public address system installed to comply with 13.3.4.3.6 to be exempt from the installation requirements of *NFPA 72®*, *National Fire Alarm Code®*,[7] including electrical supervision and secondary power. In *Code* editions through 2006, alarm systems in new assembly occupancies were afforded the same exemption under the belief that the daily use of the voice communication system would provide adequate self-supervision and sufficient need to keep the system in good working order. The 2009 edition requires new alarm systems in assembly occupancies to provide occupant notification by means of voice announcements in accordance with 9.6.3.9. The provisions of 9.6.3.9 permit automatically transmitted or live voice evacuation or relocation instructions, used to notify occupants, to comply with either *NFPA 72* or the criteria of 9.6.3.9.2, which require, among other features, secondary power. The text of A.9.6.3.9.2 explains that 9.6.3.9.2 is meant to be used for facilities such as large assembly venues in which the configuration (e.g., large-volume spaces), function, and human behavior (including elevated levels of occupant-generated noise) present challenges with respect to effective occupant notification by standard means in accordance with *NFPA 72*. Because the routine operation of large-venue assembly occupancies demands highly reliant, acoustically capable, and sufficiently audible public address systems, properly trained staff can be relied on to use these public address systems to effect occupant notification.

Paragraph 13.3.4.1.4, which applies only to existing assembly occupancies, specifically allows the authority having jurisdiction (AHJ) to permit the continued use of existing alternative means for discovering fire and alerting occupants — even if such means do not meet the myriad requirements of *NFPA 72*.

The provisions of 12/13.3.4.2.3 recognize that a fire developing in an unoccupied, nonsprinklered, hazardous area while the assembly area is in use could go undiscovered. Although separated by 1-hour fire resistance–rated barriers, these hazardous areas can present a significant hazard to occupants. Because a fire alarm system is already required, the additional requirement for either heat or smoke detection, as appropriate, is not a significant burden. Where sprinkler protection is provided, the fire is expected to be controlled, permitting early detection to be exempted.

The intent of 12/13.3.4.3 is to provide an alarm system that will not elicit a panic reaction from occupants. The panic reaction is avoided by providing a system that will permit activation by pull stations as required by 9.6.2 but that will not sound an audible alarm in the seating or audience areas of the assembly occupancy. In lieu of the audible alarm throughout the assembly occupancy, the system must provide an audible alarm (and, for new installations, a visible alarm) in a constantly attended location. "Constantly attended," in this case, means that the alarm panel must be attended while the assembly occupancy is in use. From that constantly attended location, voice messages that instruct the occupants can be issued via a public address or voice communication system. This method allows for the orderly evacuation of the occupants and the issuance of proper evacuation instructions rather than simply providing an evacuation alarm that might produce panic. The *Code* permits the use of recorded or electronically synthesized evacuation instructions that will automatically be played upon initiation of the system. With the approval of the AHJ, this arrangement is permitted to be used in lieu of the attended station.

**12.3.5 Extinguishment Requirements.**

**12.3.5.1** The following assembly occupancies shall be protected throughout by an approved, supervised automatic sprinkler system in accordance with 9.7.1.1(1):

(1) Bars with live entertainment
(2) Dance halls
(3) Discotheques
(4) Nightclubs
(5) Assembly occupancies with festival seating

CHAPTER 13 • Existing

**13.3.5 Extinguishment Requirements.**

See also 13.1.6, 13.2.6, and 13.3.2.

**13.3.5.1** Where the occupant load exceeds 100, the following assembly occupancies shall be protected throughout by an approved, supervised automatic sprinkler system in accordance with 9.7.1.1(1):

(1) Bars with live entertainment
(2) Dance halls
(3) Discotheques
(4) Nightclubs
(5) Assembly occupancies with festival seating

CHAPTER 12 • New

**12.3.5.2** Any building containing one or more assembly occupancies where the aggregate occupant load of the assembly occupancies exceeds 300 shall be protected by an approved, supervised automatic sprinkler system in accordance with Section 9.7 as follows *(see also 12.1.6, 12.2.6, 12.3.2, and 12.3.6)*:

(1) Throughout the story containing the assembly occupancy
(2) Throughout all stories below the story containing the assembly occupancy
(3) In the case of an assembly occupancy located below the level of exit discharge, throughout all stories intervening between that story and the level of exit discharge, including the level of exit discharge

**12.3.5.3** The requirements of 12.3.5.2 shall not apply to the following:

(1)* Assembly occupancies consisting of a single multipurpose room of less than 12,000 ft$^2$ (1115 m$^2$) that are not used for exhibition or display and are not part of a mixed occupancy

**A.12.3.5.3(1)** It is the intent to permit a single multipurpose room of less than 12,000 ft$^2$ (1115 m$^2$) to have certain small rooms as part of the single room. These rooms could be a kitchen, office, equipment room, and the like. It is also the intent that an addition could be made to an existing building, without requiring that the existing building be sprinklered, where both the new and existing buildings have independent means of egress and a fire-rated separation is provided to isolate one building from the other.

A school gymnasium with egress independent of, and separated from, the school would be included in this exception, as would a function hall attached to a church with a similar egress arrangement.

(2) Gymnasiums, skating rinks, and swimming pools used exclusively for participant sports with no audience facilities for more than 300 persons
(3) Locations in stadia and arenas as follows:
    (a) Over the floor area used for contest, performance, or entertainment
    (b) Over the seating areas
    (c) Over open-air concourses where an approved engineering analysis substantiates the ineffectiveness of the sprinkler protection due to building height and combustible loading
(4) Locations in unenclosed stadia and arenas as follows:
    (a) Press boxes of less than 1000 ft$^2$ (93 m$^2$)
    (b) Storage facilities of less than 1000 ft$^2$ (93 m$^2$) if enclosed with not less than 1-hour fire resistance–rated construction

CHAPTER 13 • Existing

**13.3.5.2** Any assembly occupancy used or capable of being used for exhibition or display purposes shall be protected throughout by an approved automatic sprinkler system in accordance with Section 9.7 where the exhibition or display area exceeds 15,000 ft$^2$ (1400 m$^2$).

**13.3.5.3** The sprinklers specified by 13.3.5.2 shall not be required where otherwise permitted in the following locations:

(1) Locations in stadia and arenas as follows:
    (a) Over the floor area used for contest, performance, or entertainment
    (b) Over the seating areas
    (c) Over open-air concourses where an approved engineering analysis substantiates the ineffectiveness of the sprinkler protection due to building height and combustible loading
(2) Locations in unenclosed stadia and arenas as follows:
    (a) Press boxes of less than 1000 ft$^2$ (93 m$^2$)
    (b) Storage facilities of less than 1000 ft$^2$ (93 m$^2$) if enclosed with not less than 1-hour fire resistance–rated construction

(c) Enclosed areas underneath grandstands that comply with 12.4.8.5

**12.3.5.4** Where another provision of this chapter requires an automatic sprinkler system, the sprinkler system shall be installed in accordance with 9.7.1.1(1).



(c) Enclosed areas underneath grandstands that comply with 13.4.8.5

**13.3.5.4** Where another provision of this chapter requires an automatic sprinkler system, the sprinkler system shall be installed in accordance with 9.7.1.1(1).

Subsection 12/13.3.5 is one of the two primary locations within the chapter where automatic sprinkler protection might be required. The other is 12/13.1.6, which applies to minimum construction requirements. Each of these subsections is to be applied independently to determine whether automatic sprinkler protection is required. For example, if 12/13.1.6 does not require sprinklers for a particular assembly occupancy on the basis of building construction type and location within the building, 12.3.5 might require automatic sprinklers for that assembly occupancy based on use or occupant load, or 13.3.5 might require automatic sprinklers based on use or floor area that is capable of being used for exhibition purposes. If one subsection requires sprinklers and the other does not, sprinklers must be provided.

The requirements of 12.3.5.1 for new nightclub-type assembly occupancies to be sprinklered, and of 13.3.5.1 for existing nightclub-type assembly occupancies with more than a 100-person occupant load to be sprinklered, were added to the *Code* in 2006. The provisions were developed in response to the February 2003 fire at The Station nightclub in West Warwick, Rhode Island, which claimed the lives of 100 patrons. The fire and the key findings related to emergency egress reported by NIST are described in the commentary following 12.2.3.8.

The requirement of 12.3.5.2 for automatic sprinkler protection for new assembly occupancies with an occupant load in excess of 300 persons was prompted by the occurrence of fires involving assembly occupancies, most notably the Beverly Hills Supper Club fire in 1977[8] and the MGM Grand Hotel fire in 1980.[9]

Paragraph 12.3.5.2 was revised for the 2009 edition of the *Code* to clarify that a 300-person occupant load threshold is to be applied to the aggregate occupant load of all the assembly occupancies in the building. For example, if there are two assembly occupancies in the building, and each has an occupant load of 160 persons, the 300-person threshold of 12.3.5.2 is exceeded so as to require sprinklers. The extent of the sprinkler system is addressed by 12.3.5.2 (1), (2), and (3).

The exemptions to the sprinkler requirement of 12.3.5.2, as contained in 12.3.5.3, are important in that they limit the areas or buildings requiring sprinkler protection.

The concepts used in footnote b of Table 12.1.6 and Table 13.1.6 are also used with regard to which areas must be sprinklered — see 12.3.5.2 (1), (2), and (3). If a five-story building has an assembly occupancy on the first floor, the floors above the assembly occupancy are not required to be sprinklered by the assembly occupancy provisions; however, the applicable occupancy chapter might require sprinklering of those floors. If the assembly occupancy were on the fifth floor, then the fifth floor and all floors below it would be required to be sprinklered.

Paragraph 12.3.5.3(1) exempts sprinkler protection for multipurpose assembly occupancies that are contained in one room, have an area of less than 12,000 $ft^2$ (1115 $m^2$), and are not used as an exhibition hall or for a display room. Exhibit and display halls have been shown to be fire and life safety problems because of their high fuel load and potential for rapid fire spread.

The text of A.12.3.5.3(1) clarifies that it is not the intent of 12.3.5.3(1) to prohibit the presence of normal ancillary spaces. However, a number of assembly rooms or a mixed occupancy would not be permitted to use this exemption.

Paragraph 12.3.5.3(2) exempts gymnasiums, skating rinks (including ice and roller rinks), and swimming pools where there is an audience or spectator gallery with an occupant load of 300 or fewer persons. If the skating rink or swimming pool can be floored over and used for other purposes, then the multipurpose room requirements contained in 12.3.5.3(1) might apply. If the spectator gallery has an occupant load greater than 300, then an automatic sprinkler system is required. In effect, 12.3.5.3(2) exempts the participants on the gym floor, on the skating rink, or in the swimming pool from being counted as part of the 300-person threshold at which the provisions of 12.3.5.2 apply.

Two major questions that arise with regard to 12.3.5 deal with multiple occupancies (especially assembly/educational) and multiple assembly occupancies (especially religious halls with multipurpose rooms).

With regard to multiple occupancies, 6.1.14.3 states that, if mixed occupancies provisions are to be used to protect a multiple occupancy, the most stringent requirements applicable to any of the involved occupancies must be provided for all occupancies. Therefore, new schools with assembly occupancies with an occupant load in excess of 300 need to be fully sprinklered, unless the multiple occupancy is treated as separated occupancies in accordance with 6.1.14.4, which would require independent exit access systems and substantial fire-rated separating construction. If separated occupancies can be established, only the assembly occupancy with an occupant load in excess of 300 would need to be sprinklered. Also, multipurpose assembly rooms in a multiple occupancy assembly and educational occupancies building utilizing the separated occupancies provisions of 6.1.14.4 could potentially use 12.3.5.3(1) for exemption from the sprinkler requirement. Paragraph 12.3.5.3(1) emphasizes that the assembly occupancy is essentially a single room and, thus, cannot be part of a multiple occupancy building protected as mixed occupancies in accordance with 6.1.14.3.

Paragraph 12.3.5.3(1) was originally intended for a typical fellowship hall, such as a VFW, American Legion, or Grange hall. Some ancillary rooms, such as kitchens, restrooms, storage rooms, or minor offices, will exist, and it is not the intent that these ancillary spaces disqualify a facility from using this exemption [see A.12.3.5.3(1)]; however, it is the intent that the facility consist essentially of only one major room.

The provisions of 13.3.5.2 — which apply to existing assembly occupancies used or capable of being used for exhibition or display purposes — are not as stringent as those for new assembly occupancies. This requirement would apply to many facilities over 15,000 $ft^2$ (1400 $m^2$), unless fixed seating or similar permanent obstruction to exhibition use is provided.

### 12.3.6 Corridors.

Interior corridors and lobbies shall be constructed in accordance with 7.1.3.1 and Section 8.3, unless otherwise permitted by the following:

(1) Corridor and lobby protection shall not be required where assembly rooms served by the corridor or lobby have at least 50 percent of their exit capacity discharging directly to the outside, independent of corridors and lobbies.
(2) Corridor and lobby protection shall not be required in buildings protected throughout by an approved, supervised automatic sprinkler system in accordance with Section 9.7.
(3) Lobbies serving only one assembly area that meet the requirements for intervening rooms *(see 7.5.1.6)* shall not be required to have a fire resistance rating.
(4) Where the corridor ceiling is an assembly having a 1-hour fire resistance rating where tested as a wall, the corridor walls shall be permitted to terminate at the corridor ceiling.
(5) Corridor and lobby protection shall not be required in buildings protected throughout by an approved, total (complete) coverage smoke detection system providing occupant notification and installed in accordance with Section 9.6.

### 13.3.6 Corridors.

(No requirements.)

The corridor provisions of 12.3.6 apply only to new assembly occupancies.

Paragraph 12.3.6(1) permits corridor protection to be eliminated but requires 50 percent of the egress capacity of each assembly room to be direct to the outside, independent of corridors or lobbies. This

CHAPTER 12 • New

requirement permits theaters, for example, to use nonrated doors between the audience seating chamber and the lobby. Nonrated doors are not required to latch. The absence of the latch helps to avoid the disruptive noise associated with unlatching the door any time an occupant enters or leaves the room.

Paragraph 12.3.6(2) recognizes the excellent record of automatic sprinkler systems to control a fire while the fire is small. However, this exemption requires the entire building, not only the assembly area, to be sprinklered.

Paragraph 12.3.6(3) recognizes the situation where

## 12.4 Special Provisions

### 12.4.1 Life Safety Evaluation.

**12.4.1.1*** Where a life safety evaluation is required by other provisions of the *Code*, it shall comply with the following:

(1) The life safety evaluation shall be performed by persons acceptable to the authority having jurisdiction.
(2) The life safety evaluation shall include a written assessment of safety measures for conditions listed in 12.4.1.2.
(3) The life safety evaluation shall be approved annually by the authority having jurisdiction and shall be updated for special or unusual conditions.

**A.12.4.1.1** Life safety evaluations are examples of performance-based approaches to life safety. In this respect, significant guidance in the form and process of life safety evaluations is provided by Chapter 5, keeping in mind the fire safety emphasis in Chapter 5. Performance criteria, scenarios, evaluation, safety factors, documentation, maintenance, and periodic assessment (including a warrant of fitness) all apply to the broader considerations in a life safety evaluation. A life safety evaluation deals not only with fire but also with storms, collapse, crowd behavior, and other related safety considerations for which a checklist is provided in A.12.4.1.3. Chapter 5 provides guidance, based on fire safety requirements, for establishing a documented case showing that products of combustion in all conceivable fire scenarios will not significantly endanger occupants using means of egress in the facility (for example, due to fire detection, automatic suppression, smoke control, large-volume space, or management procedures). Moreover, means of egress facilities plus facility management capabilities should be adequate to cope with scenarios where certain egress routes are blocked for some reason.

In addition to making realistic assumptions about the capabilities of persons in the facility (e.g., an assembled

CHAPTER 13 • Existing

the lobby serves only one assembly space and where, from a fire safety perspective, it can be considered part of that assembly space.

Paragraph 12.3.6(4) does not exempt the facility from providing fire-rated corridor walls. It permits the rated fire barrier to terminate tight against a ceiling that is constructed to be equivalent to a 1-hour wall.

Paragraph 12.3.6(5) recognizes the excellent record of automatic smoke detection systems in providing early warning. However, this exemption requires the entire building, not only the assembly area, to be equipped with smoke detectors.

## 13.4 Special Provisions

### 13.4.1 Life Safety Evaluation.

**13.4.1.1*** Where a life safety evaluation is required by other provisions of the *Code*, it shall comply with the following:

(1) The life safety evaluation shall be performed by persons acceptable to the authority having jurisdiction.
(2) The life safety evaluation shall include a written assessment of safety measures for conditions listed in 13.4.1.2.
(3) The life safety evaluation shall be approved annually by the authority having jurisdiction and shall be updated for special or unusual conditions.

**A.13.4.1.1** Life safety evaluations are examples of performance-based approaches to life safety. In this respect, significant guidance in the form and process of life safety evaluations is provided by Chapter 5, keeping in mind the fire safety emphasis in Chapter 5. Performance criteria, scenarios, evaluation, safety factors, documentation, maintenance, and periodic assessment (including a warrant of fitness) all apply to the broader considerations in a life safety evaluation. A life safety evaluation deals not only with fire but also with storms, collapse, crowd behavior, and other related safety considerations for which a checklist is provided in A.13.4.1.3. Chapter 5 provides guidance, based on fire safety requirements, for establishing a documented case showing that products of combustion in all conceivable fire scenarios will not significantly endanger occupants using means of egress in the facility (for example, due to fire detection, automatic suppression, smoke control, large-volume space, or management procedures). Moreover, means of egress facilities plus facility management capabilities should be adequate to cope with scenarios where certain egress routes are blocked for some reason.

In addition to making realistic assumptions about the capabilities of persons in the facility (e.g., an assembled

CHAPTER 12 • New

crowd including many disabled persons or persons unfamiliar with the facility), the life safety evaluation should include a factor of safety of not less than 2.0 in all calculations relating to hazard development time and required egress time (the combination of flow time and other time needed to detect and assess an emergency condition, initiate egress, and move along the egress routes). The factor of safety takes into account the possibility that half of the egress routes might not be used (or be usable) in certain situations.

Regarding crowd behavior, the potential hazards created by larger masses of people and greater crowd densities (which can be problematic during ingress, occupancy, and egress) demand that technology be used by designers, managers, and authorities responsible for buildings to compensate for the relaxed egress capacity provisions of Table 12.4.2.3. In very large buildings for assembly use, the hazard of crowd crushes can exceed that of fire or structural failure. Therefore, the building designers, managers, event planners, security personnel, police authorities, and fire authorities, as well as the building construction authorities, should understand the potential problems and solutions, including coordination of their activities. For crowd behavior, this understanding includes factors of space, energy, time, and information, as well as specific crowd management techniques, such as metering. Published guidance on these factors and techniques is found in the *SFPE Handbook of Fire Protection Engineering*, Section 3, Chapter 13, pp. 3-342–3-366 (Proulx, G., "Movement of People"), and the publications referenced therein.

Table 12.2.3.2 and Table 12.4.2.3 are based on a linear relationship between number of seats and nominal flow time, with not less than 200 seconds (3.3 minutes) for 2000 seats plus 1 second for every additional 50 seats up to 25,000. Beyond 25,000 total seats, the nominal flow time is limited to 660 seconds (11 minutes). Nominal flow time refers to the flow time for the most able group of patrons; some groups less familiar with the premises or less able groups might take longer to pass a point in the egress system. Although three or more digits are noted in the tables, the resulting calculations should be assumed to provide only two significant figures of precision.

**12.4.1.2** Life safety evaluations shall include an assessment of the following conditions and related appropriate safety measures:

(1) Nature of the events and the participants and attendees
(2) Access and egress movement, including crowd density problems
(3) Medical emergencies
(4) Fire hazards
(5) Permanent and temporary structural systems
(6) Severe weather conditions

CHAPTER 13 • Existing

crowd including many disabled persons or persons unfamiliar with the facility), the life safety evaluation should include a factor of safety of not less than 2.0 in all calculations relating to hazard development time and required egress time (the combination of flow time and other time needed to detect and assess an emergency condition, initiate egress, and move along the egress routes). This factor of safety takes into account the possibility that half of the egress routes might not be used (or usable) in certain situations.

Regarding crowd behavior, the potential hazards created by larger masses of people and greater crowd densities (which can be problematic during ingress, occupancy, and egress) demand that technology be used by designers, managers, and authorities responsible for buildings to compensate for the relaxed egress capacity provisions of Table 13.4.2.3. In very large buildings for assembly use, the hazard of crowd crushes can exceed that of fire or structural failure. Therefore, the building designers, managers, event planners, security personnel, police authorities, and fire authorities, as well as the building construction authorities, should understand the potential problems and solutions, including coordination of their activities. For crowd behavior, this understanding includes factors of space, energy, time, and information, as well as specific crowd management techniques, such as metering. Published guidance on these factors and techniques is found in the *SFPE Handbook of Fire Protection Engineering*, Section 3, Chapter 13, pp. 3-342–3-366 (Proulx, G., "Movement of People"), and the publications referenced therein.

Table 13.2.3.2 and Table 13.4.2.3 are based on a linear relationship between number of seats and nominal flow time, with not less than 200 seconds (3.3 minutes) for 2000 seats plus 1 second for every additional 50 seats up to 25,000. Beyond 25,000 total seats, the nominal flow time is limited to 660 seconds (11 minutes). Nominal flow time refers to the flow time for the most able group of patrons; some groups less familiar with the premises or less able groups might take longer to pass a point in the egress system. Although three or more digits are noted in the tables, the resulting calculations should be assumed to provide only two significant figures of precision.

**13.4.1.2** Life safety evaluations shall include an assessment of the following conditions and the related appropriate safety measures:

(1) Nature of the events and the participants and attendees
(2) Access and egress movement, including crowd density problems
(3) Medical emergencies
(4) Fire hazards
(5) Permanent and temporary structural systems
(6) Severe weather conditions

CHAPTER 12 • New

(7) Earthquakes
(8) Civil or other disturbances
(9) Hazardous materials incidents within and near the facility
(10) Relationships among facility management, event participants, emergency response agencies, and others having a role in the events accommodated in the facility

**12.4.1.3*** Life safety evaluations shall include assessments of both building systems and management features upon which reliance is placed for the safety of facility occupants, and such assessments shall consider scenarios appropriate to the facility.

**A.12.4.1.3** Factors to be considered in a life safety evaluation include the following:

(1) Nature of the events being accommodated, including the following:
   (a) Ingress, intra-event movement, and egress patterns
   (b) Ticketing and seating policies/practices
   (c) Event purpose (e.g., sports contest, religious meeting)
   (d) Emotional qualities (e.g., competitiveness) of event
   (e) Time of day when event is held
   (f) Time duration of single event
   (g) Time duration of attendees' occupancy of the building
(2) Occupant characteristics and behavior, including the following:
   (a) Homogeneity
   (b) Cohesiveness
   (c) Familiarity with building
   (d) Familiarity with similar events
   (e) Capability (as influenced by factors such as age, physical abilities)
   (f) Socioeconomic factors
   (g) Small minority involved with recreational violence
   (h) Emotional involvement with the event and other occupants
   (i) Use of alcohol or drugs
   (j) Food consumption
   (k) Washroom utilization
(3) Management, including the following:
   (a) Clear, contractual arrangements for facility operation/use as follows:
      i. Between facility owner and operator
      ii. Between facility operator and event promoter
      iii. Between event promoter and performer
      iv. Between event promoter and attendee
      v. With police forces

CHAPTER 13 • Existing

(7) Earthquakes
(8) Civil or other disturbances
(9) Hazardous materials incidents within and near the facility
(10) Relationships among facility management, event participants, emergency response agencies, and others having a role in the events accommodated in the facility

**13.4.1.3*** Life safety evaluations shall include assessments of both building systems and management features upon which reliance is placed for the safety of facility occupants, and such assessments shall consider scenarios appropriate to the facility.

**A.13.4.1.3** Factors to be considered in a life safety evaluation might include the following:

(1) Nature of the events being accommodated, including the following:
   (a) Ingress, intra-event movement, and egress patterns
   (b) Ticketing and seating policies/practices
   (c) Event purpose (e.g., sports contest, religious meeting)
   (d) Emotional qualities (e.g., competitiveness) of event
   (e) Time of day when event is held
   (f) Time duration of single event
   (g) Time duration of attendees' occupancy of the building
(2) Occupant characteristics and behavior, including the following:
   (a) Homogeneity
   (b) Cohesiveness
   (c) Familiarity with building
   (d) Familiarity with similar events
   (e) Capability (as influenced by factors such as age, physical abilities)
   (f) Socioeconomic factors
   (g) Small minority involved with recreational violence
   (h) Emotional involvement with the event and other occupants
   (i) Use of alcohol or drugs
   (j) Food consumption
   (k) Washroom utilization
(3) Management, including the following:
   (a) Clear, contractual arrangements for facility operation/use as follows:
      i. Between facility owner and operator
      ii. Between facility operator and event promoter
      iii. Between event promoter and performer
      iv. Between event promoter and attendee
      v. With police forces

CHAPTER 12 • New

vi. With private security services
vii. With ushering services
(b) Experience with the building
(c) Experience with similar events and attendees
(d) Thorough, up-to-date operations manual
(e) Training of personnel
(f) Supervision of personnel
(g) Communications systems and utilization
(h) Ratios of management and other personnel to attendees
(i) Location/distribution of personnel
(j) Central command location
(k) Rapport between personnel and attendees
(l) Personnel support of attendee goals
(m) Respect of attendees for personnel due to the following:
i. Dress (uniform) standards
ii. Age and perceived experience
iii. Personnel behavior, including interaction
iv. Distinction between crowd management and control
v. Management concern for facility quality (e.g., cleanliness)
vi. Management concern for entire event experience of attendees (i.e., not just during occupancy of the building)

(4) Emergency management preparedness, including the following:
(a) Complete range of emergencies addressed in operations manual
(b) Power loss
(c) Fire
(d) Severe weather
(e) Earthquake
(f) Crowd incident
(g) Terrorism
(h) Hazardous materials
(i) Transportation accident (e.g., road, rail, air)
(j) Communications systems available
(k) Personnel and emergency forces ready to respond
(l) Attendees clearly informed of situation and proper behavior

(5) Building systems, including the following:
(a) Structural soundness
(b) Normal static loads
(c) Abnormal static loads (e.g., crowds, precipitation)
(d) Dynamic loads (e.g., crowd sway, impact, explosion, wind, earthquake)
(e) Stability of nonstructural components (e.g., lighting)

CHAPTER 13 • Existing

vi. With private security services
vii. With ushering services
(b) Experience with the building
(c) Experience with similar events and attendees
(d) Thorough, up-to-date operations manual
(e) Training of personnel
(f) Supervision of personnel
(g) Communications systems and utilization
(h) Ratios of management and other personnel to attendees
(i) Location/distribution of personnel
(j) Central command location
(k) Rapport between personnel and attendees
(l) Personnel support of attendee goals
(m) Respect of attendees for personnel due to the following:
i. Dress (uniform) standards
ii. Age and perceived experience
iii. Personnel behavior, including interaction
iv. Distinction between crowd management and control
v. Management concern for facility quality (e.g., cleanliness)
vi. Management concern for entire event experience of attendees (i.e., not just during occupancy of the building)

(4) Emergency management preparedness, including the following:
(a) Complete range of emergencies addressed in operations manual
(b) Power loss
(c) Fire
(d) Severe weather
(e) Earthquake
(f) Crowd incident
(g) Terrorism
(h) Hazardous materials
(i) Transportation accident (e.g., road, rail, air)
(j) Communications systems available
(k) Personnel and emergency forces ready to respond
(l) Attendees clearly informed of situation and proper behavior

(5) Building systems, including the following:
(a) Structural soundness
(b) Normal static loads
(c) Abnormal static loads (e.g., crowds, precipitation)
(d) Dynamic loads (e.g., crowd sway, impact, explosion, wind, earthquake)
(e) Stability of nonstructural components (e.g., lighting)

(f) Stability of movable (e.g., telescoping) structures
(g) Fire protection
(h) Fire prevention (e.g., maintenance, contents, housekeeping)
(i) Compartmentation
(j) Automatic detection and suppression of fire
(k) Smoke control
(l) Alarm and communications systems
(m) Fire department access routes and response capability
(n) Structural integrity
(o) Weather protection
(p) Wind
(q) Precipitation (attendees rush for shelter or hold up egress of others)
(r) Lightning protection
(s) Circulation systems
(t) Flowline or network analysis
(u) Waywinding and orientation
(v) Merging of paths (e.g., precedence behavior)
(w) Decision/branching points
(x) Route redundancies
(y) Counterflow, crossflow, and queuing situations
(z) Control possibilities, including metering
(aa) Flow capacity adequacy
(bb) System balance
(cc) Movement time performance
(dd) Flow times
(ee) Travel times
(ff) Queuing times
(gg) Route quality
(hh) Walking surfaces (e.g., traction, discontinuities)
(ii) Appropriate widths and boundary conditions
(jj) Handrails, guardrails, and other rails
(kk) Ramp slopes
(ll) Step geometries
(mm) Perceptual aspects (e.g., orientation, signage, marking, lighting, glare, distractions)
(nn) Route choices, especially for vertical travel
(oo) Resting/waiting areas
(pp) Levels of service (overall crowd movement quality)
(qq) Services
(rr) Washroom provision and distribution
(ss) Concessions
(tt) First aid and EMS facilities
(uu) General attendee services

A scenario-based approach to performance-based fire safety is addressed in Chapter 5. In addition to using such scenarios and, more generally, the attention to performance criteria, evaluation, safety factors, documentation, mainte-



(f) Stability of movable (e.g., telescoping) structures
(g) Fire protection
(h) Fire prevention (e.g., maintenance, contents, housekeeping)
(i) Compartmentation
(j) Automatic detection and suppression of fire
(k) Smoke control
(l) Alarm and communications systems
(m) Fire department access routes and response capability
(n) Structural integrity
(o) Weather protection
(p) Wind
(q) Precipitation (attendees rush for shelter or hold up egress of others)
(r) Lightning protection
(s) Circulation systems
(t) Flowline or network analysis
(u) Waywinding and orientation
(v) Merging of paths (e.g., precedence behavior)
(w) Decision/branching points
(x) Route redundancies
(y) Counterflow, crossflow, and queuing situations
(z) Control possibilities, including metering
(aa) Flow capacity adequacy
(bb) System balance
(cc) Movement time performance
(dd) Flow times
(ee) Travel times
(ff) Queuing times
(gg) Route quality
(hh) Walking surfaces (e.g., traction, discontinuities)
(ii) Appropriate widths and boundary conditions
(jj) Handrails, guardrails, and other rails
(kk) Ramp slopes
(ll) Step geometries
(mm) Perceptual aspects (e.g., orientation, signage, marking, lighting, glare, distractions)
(nn) Route choices, especially for vertical travel
(oo) Resting/waiting areas
(pp) Levels of service (overall crowd movement quality)
(qq) Services
(rr) Washroom provision and distribution
(ss) Concessions
(tt) First aid and EMS facilities
(uu) General attendee services

A scenario-based approach to performance-based fire safety is addressed in Chapter 5. In addition to utilizing such scenarios and, more generally, the attention to performance criteria, evaluation, safety factors, documentation, mainte-

**CHAPTER 12 • New**

nance, and periodic assessment required when the Chapter 5 option is used, life safety evaluations should consider scenarios based on characteristics important in assembly occupancies. These characteristics include the following:

(1) Whether there is a local or mass awareness of an incident, event, or condition that might provoke egress
(2) Whether the incident, event, or condition stays localized or spreads
(3) Whether or not egress is desired by facility occupants
(4) Whether there is a localized start to any egress or mass start to egress
(5) Whether exits are available or not available

Examples of scenarios and sets of characteristics that might occur in a facility follow.

*Scenario 1.* Characteristics: mass start, egress desired (by management and attendees), exits not available, local awareness.

Normal egress at the end of an event occurs just as a severe weather condition induces evacuees at the exterior doors to retard or stop their egress. The backup that occurs in the egress system is not known to most evacuees, who continue to press forward, potentially resulting in a crowd crush.

*Scenario 2.* Characteristics: mass start, egress not desired (by management), exits possibly not available, mass awareness.

An earthquake occurs during an event. The attendees are relatively safe in the seating area. The means of egress outside the seating area are relatively unsafe and vulnerable to aftershock damage. Facility management discourages mass egress until the means of egress can be checked and cleared for use.

*Scenario 3.* Characteristics: local start, incident stays local, egress desired (by attendees and management), exits available, mass awareness.

A localized civil disturbance (e.g., firearms violence) provokes localized egress, which is seen by attendees, generally, who then decide to leave also.

*Scenario 4.* Characteristics: mass start, egress desired (by attendees), incident spreads, exits not available, mass awareness.

In an open-air facility unprotected from wind, precipitation, and lightning, sudden severe weather prompts egress to shelter, but not from the facility. The means of egress congest and block quickly as people in front stop once they are under shelter, while people behind them continue to press forward, potentially resulting in a crowd crush.

These scenarios illustrate some of the broader factors to be taken into account when assessing the capability of both building systems and management features on which reliance is placed in a range of situations, not just fire emer-

**CHAPTER 13 • Existing**

nance, and periodic assessment required when the Chapter 5 option is used, life safety evaluations should consider scenarios based on characteristics important in assembly occupancies. These characteristics include the following:

(1) Whether there is a local or mass awareness of an incident, event, or condition that might provoke egress
(2) Whether the incident, event, or condition stays localized or spreads
(3) Whether or not egress is desired by facility occupants
(4) Whether there is a localized start to any egress or mass start to egress
(5) Whether exits are available or not available

Examples of scenarios and sets of characteristics that might occur in a facility follow.

*Scenario 1.* Characteristics: mass start, egress desired (by management and attendees), exits not available, local awareness.

Normal egress at the end of an event occurs just as a severe weather condition induces evacuees at the exterior doors to retard or stop their egress. The backup that occurs in the egress system is not known to most evacuees, who continue to press forward, potentially resulting in a crowd crush.

*Scenario 2.* Characteristics: mass start, egress not desired (by management), exits possibly not available, mass awareness.

An earthquake occurs during an event. The attendees are relatively safe in the seating area. The means of egress outside the seating area are relatively unsafe and vulnerable to aftershock damage. Facility management discourages mass egress until the means of egress can be checked and cleared for use.

*Scenario 3.* Characteristics: local start, incident stays local, egress desired (by attendees and management), exits available, mass awareness.

A localized civil disturbance (e.g., firearms violence) provokes localized egress, which is seen by attendees, generally, who then decide to leave also.

*Scenario 4.* Characteristics: mass start, egress desired (by attendees), incident spreads, exits not available, mass awareness.

In an open-air facility unprotected from wind, precipitation, and lightning, sudden severe weather prompts egress to shelter but not from the facility. The means of egress congest and block quickly as people in front stop once they are under shelter, while people behind them continue to press forward, potentially resulting in a crowd crush.

These scenarios illustrate some of the broader factors to be taken into account when assessing the capability of both building systems and management features on which reliance is placed in a range of situations, not just fire emergencies. Some scenarios also illustrate the conflicting motivations of management and attendees, based on differing perceptions of danger and differing knowledge of hazards, countermeasures, and capabilities. Mass egress might not be the most appropriate life safety strategy in some scenarios, such as Scenario 2.

Table A.12.4.1.3 summarizes the characteristics in the scenarios and provides a framework for developing other characteristics and scenarios that might be important for a particular facility, hazard, occupant type, event, or management.

### 12.4.2* Smoke-Protected Assembly Seating.

The preparation of life safety evaluations will become more common as assembly occupancy designers request approval, from authorities having jurisdiction (AHJ), of designs using the various *Code* provisions that conditionally require a life safety evaluation. For example, to be considered smoke protected and thus be permitted to use the reduced egress capacity criteria of Table 12/13.4.2.3, a building must be sprinklered, be provided with features that prevent it from becoming smoke-logged, and — most important — be assessed using a life safety evaluation conducted in accordance with 12/13.4.1.



gencies. Some scenarios also illustrate the conflicting motivations of management and attendees based on differing perceptions of danger and differing knowledge of hazards, countermeasures, and capabilities. Mass egress might not be the most appropriate life safety strategy in some scenarios, such as Scenario 2.

Table A.13.4.1.3 summarizes the characteristics in the scenarios and provides a framework for developing other characteristics and scenarios that might be important for a particular facility, hazard, occupant type, event, or management.

### 13.4.2* Smoke-Protected Assembly Seating.

The expansive material contained in A.12/A.13.4.1.3 emphasizes that conducting a life safety evaluation is a complex process that should not be attempted by most *Code* practitioners. Such an evaluation must demonstrate that all life safety hazards have been considered and that control measures have been provided to ensure that occupants evacuating the building will not be endangered by conditions developing faster than the time required to clear the means of egress. The AHJ needs to realize that, if an evaluation doesn't cover nearly all of the subjects addressed in A.12/A.13.4.1.3, it should not be approved. A

***Table A.12.4.1.3 Life Safety Evaluation Scenario Characteristics Matrix***

| | | | | | Management | | Occupants | | | | | | |
|---|---|---|---|---|---|---|---|---|---|---|---|---|---|
| Scenario | Local Awareness | Mass Awareness | Incident Localized | Incident Spreads | Egress Desired | Egress Not Desired | Egress Desired | Egress Not Desired | Local Start | Mass Start | Exits Available | Exits Not Available | Other |
| 1 | X | — | — | — | X | — | X | — | — | X | — | X | — |
| 2 | — | X | — | — | — | X | — | — | — | X | — | X | — |
| 3 | — | X | X | — | X | — | X | — | X | — | X | — | — |
| 4 | — | X | — | X | — | — | X | — | — | X | — | X | — |

***Table A.13.4.1.3 Life Safety Evaluation Scenario Characteristics Matrix***

| | | | | | Management | | Occupants | | | | | | |
|---|---|---|---|---|---|---|---|---|---|---|---|---|---|
| Scenario | Local Awareness | Mass Awareness | Incident Localized | Incident Spreads | Egress Desired | Egress Not Desired | Egress Desired | Egress Not Desired | Local Start | Mass Start | Exits Available | Exits Not Available | Other |
| 1 | X | — | — | — | X | — | X | — | — | X | — | X | — |
| 2 | — | X | — | — | — | X | — | — | — | X | — | X | — |
| 3 | — | X | X | — | X | — | X | — | X | — | X | — | — |
| 4 | — | X | — | X | — | — | X | — | — | X | — | X | — |

reduced egress capacity system in accordance with 12/13.4.2.3, but for which the life safety evaluation is inadequate, is itself an inadequate egress system. The reduced capacity factors of Table 12/13.4.2.3 are not to be used as a matter of right; rather, their use needs to be earned by providing a comprehensive life safety evaluation.

**A.12.4.2** Outdoor facilities are not accepted as inherently smoke-protected but must meet the requirements of smoke-protected assembly seating in order to utilize the special requirements for means of egress.

**12.4.2.1** To be considered smoke protected, an assembly seating facility shall comply with the following:

(1) All enclosed areas with walls and ceilings in buildings or structures containing smoke-protected assembly seating shall be protected with an approved, supervised automatic sprinkler system in accordance with Section 9.7, unless otherwise permitted by the following:
   (a) The requirement of 12.4.2.1(1) shall not apply to the floor area used for the contest, performance, or entertainment, provided that the roof construction is more than 50 ft (15 m) above the floor level and use is restricted to low fire hazard uses.
   (b)*Sprinklers shall not be required to be located over the floor area used for contest, performance, or entertainment and over the seating areas where an approved engineering analysis substantiates the ineffectiveness of the sprinkler protection due to building height and combustible loading.

**A.12.4.2.1(1)(b)** The engineering analysis should be part of the life safety evaluation required by 12.4.1.

(2) All means of egress serving a smoke-protected assembly seating area shall be provided with smoke-actuated ventilation facilities or natural ventilation designed as follows:
   (a) The ventilation system shall be designed to maintain the level of smoke at not less than 6 ft (1830 mm) above the floor of the means of egress.
   (b) The ventilation system shall be in accordance with NFPA 92B, *Standard for Smoke Management Systems in Malls, Atria, and Large Spaces*, or, where applicable, NFPA 92A, *Standard for Smoke-Control Systems Utilizing Barriers and Pressure Differences*.

**12.4.2.2** To use the provisions of smoke-protected assembly seating, a facility shall be subject to a life safety evaluation in accordance with 12.4.1.

**12.4.2.3** Minimum clear widths of aisles and other means of egress serving smoke-protected assembly seating shall be in accordance with Table 12.4.2.3.

**A.13.4.2** Outdoor facilities are not accepted as inherently smoke-protected but must meet the requirements of smoke-protected assembly seating in order to use the special requirements for means of egress.

**13.4.2.1** To be considered smoke protected, an assembly seating facility shall comply with the following:

(1) All enclosed areas with walls and ceilings in buildings or structures containing smoke-protected assembly seating shall be protected with an approved automatic sprinkler system in accordance with Section 9.7, unless otherwise permitted by the following:
   (a) The requirement of 13.4.2.1(1) shall not apply to the floor area used for the contest, performance, or entertainment, provided that the roof construction is more than 50 ft (15 m) above the floor level and use is restricted to low fire hazard uses.
   (b)*Sprinklers shall not be required to be located over the floor area used for contest, performance, or entertainment and over the seating areas where an approved engineering analysis substantiates the ineffectiveness of the sprinkler protection due to building height and combustible loading.

**A.13.4.2.1(1)(b)** The engineering analysis should be part of the life safety evaluation required by 13.4.1.

(2) All means of egress serving a smoke-protected assembly seating area shall be provided with smoke-actuated ventilation facilities or natural ventilation designed to maintain the level of smoke at not less than 6 ft (1830 m) above the floor of the means of egress.

**13.4.2.2** To use the provisions of smoke-protected assembly seating, a facility shall be subject to a life safety evaluation in accordance with 13.4.1.

**13.4.2.3** Minimum clear widths of aisles and other means of egress serving smoke-protected assembly seating shall be in accordance with Table 13.4.2.3.

CHAPTER 12 • New

*Table 12.4.2.3 Capacity Factors for Smoke-Protected Assembly Seating*

| No. of Seats | Clear Width per Seat Served | | | |
|---|---|---|---|---|
| | Stairs | | Passageways, Ramps, and Doorways | |
| | in. | mm | in. | mm |
| 2,000 | 0.300 *AB* | 7.6 *AB* | 0.220 *C* | 5.6 *C* |
| 5,000 | 0.200 *AB* | 5.1 *AB* | 0.150 *C* | 3.8 *C* |
| 10,000 | 0.130 *AB* | 3.3 *AB* | 0.100 *C* | 2.5 *C* |
| 15,000 | 0.096 *AB* | 2.4 *AB* | 0.070 *C* | 1.8 *C* |
| 20,000 | 0.076 *AB* | 1.9 *AB* | 0.056 *C* | 1.4 *C* |
| ≥25,000 | 0.060 *AB* | 1.5 *AB* | 0.044 *C* | 1.1 *C* |

**12.4.2.4** Where smoke-protected assembly seating and its means of egress are located wholly outdoors, capacity shall be permitted to be provided in accordance with Table 12.4.2.4.

*Table 12.4.2.4 Capacity Factors for Outdoor Smoke-Protected Assembly Seating*

| Feature | Clear Width per Seat Served | | | |
|---|---|---|---|---|
| | Stairs | | Passageways, Ramps, and Doorways | |
| | in. | mm | in. | mm |
| Outdoor smoke-protected assembly seating | 0.08 *AB* | 2.0 *AB* | 0.06 *C* | 1.5 *C* |

**12.4.2.5** Where using Table 12.4.2.3, the number of seats specified shall be within a single assembly space, and interpolation shall be permitted between the specific values shown. A single seating space shall be permitted to have multiple levels, floors, or mezzanines.

**12.4.2.6** The minimum clear widths shown in Table 12.4.2.3 and Table 12.4.2.4 shall be modified in accordance with all of the following:

(1) If risers exceed 7 in. in height, the stair width in Table 12.4.2.3 and Table 12.4.2.4 shall be multiplied by factor $A$, where $A$ equals the following:

$$A = 1 + \frac{\text{riser height} - 7}{5}$$

CHAPTER 13 • Existing

*Table 13.4.2.3 Capacity Factors for Smoke-Protected Assembly Seating*

| No. of Seats | Clear Width per Seat Served | | | |
|---|---|---|---|---|
| | Stairs | | Passageways, Ramps, and Doorways | |
| | in. | mm | in. | mm |
| 2,000 | 0.300 *AB* | 7.6 *AB* | 0.220 *C* | 5.6 *C* |
| 5,000 | 0.200 *AB* | 5.1 *AB* | 0.150 *C* | 3.8 *C* |
| 10,000 | 0.130 *AB* | 3.3 *AB* | 0.100 *C* | 2.5 *C* |
| 15,000 | 0.096 *AB* | 2.4 *AB* | 0.070 *C* | 1.8 *C* |
| 20,000 | 0.076 *AB* | 1.9 *AB* | 0.056 *C* | 1.4 *C* |
| ≥25,000 | 0.060 AB | 1.5 AB | 0.044 C | 1.1 C |

**13.4.2.4** Where smoke-protected assembly seating and its means of egress are located wholly outdoors, capacity shall be permitted to be provided in accordance with Table 13.4.2.4.

*Table 13.4.2.4 Capacity Factors for Outdoor Smoke-Protected Assembly Seating*

| Feature | Clear Width per Seat Served | | | |
|---|---|---|---|---|
| | Stairs | | Passageways, Ramps, and Doorways | |
| | in. | mm | in. | mm |
| Outdoor smoke-protected assembly seating | 0.08 *AB* | 2.0 *AB* | 0.06 *C* | 1.5 *C* |

**13.4.2.5** Where using Table 13.4.2.3, the number of seats specified shall be within a single assembly space, and interpolation shall be permitted between the specific values shown. A single seating space shall be permitted to have multiple levels, floors, or mezzanines.

**13.4.2.6** The minimum clear widths shown in Table 13.4.2.3 and Table 13.4.2.4 shall be modified in accordance with all of the following:

(1) If risers exceed 7 in. in height, the stair width in Table 13.4.2.3 and Table 13.4.2.4 shall be multiplied by factor $A$, where $A$ equals the following:

$$A = 1 + \frac{\text{riser height} - 7}{5}$$

CHAPTER 12 • New

(2) If risers exceed 178 mm in height, the stair width in Table 12.4.2.3 and Table 12.4.2.4 shall be multiplied by factor $A$, where $A$ equals the following:

$$A = 1 + \frac{\text{riser height} - 178}{125}$$

(3) Stairs not having a handrail within a 30 in. (760 mm) horizontal distance shall be 25 percent wider than otherwise calculated; that is, their width shall be multiplied by factor $B$, where $B$ equals the following:

$$B = 1.25$$

(4) Ramps steeper than 1 in 10 slope where used in ascent shall have their width increased by 10 percent; that is, their width shall be multiplied by factor $C$, where $C$ equals the following:

$$C = 1.10$$

**12.4.2.7** Where smoke-protected assembly seating conforms to the requirements of 12.4.2, for rows of seats served by aisles or doorways at both ends, the number of seats per row shall not exceed 100, and the clear width of not less than 12 in. (305 mm) for aisle accessways shall be increased by 0.3 in. (7.6 mm) for every additional seat beyond the number stipulated in Table 12.4.2.7; however, the minimum clear width shall not be required to exceed 22 in. (560 mm).

***Table 12.4.2.7 Smoke-Protected Assembly Seating Aisle Accessways***

| **Total Number of Seats in the Space** | **Number of Seats per Row Permitted to Have a Clear Width Aisle Accessway of Not Less than 12 in. (305 mm)** | |
|---|---|---|
| | **Aisle or Doorway at Both Ends of Row** | **Aisle or Doorway at One End of Row** |
| <4,000 | 14 | 7 |
| 4,000–6,999 | 15 | 7 |
| 7,000–9,999 | 16 | 8 |
| 10,000–12,999 | 17 | 8 |
| 13,000–15,999 | 18 | 9 |
| 16,000–18,999 | 19 | 9 |
| 19,000–21,999 | 20 | 10 |
| ≥22,000 | 21 | 11 |

**12.4.2.8** Where smoke-protected assembly seating conforms to the requirements of 12.4.2, for rows of seats served by an aisle or doorway at one end only, the aisle accessway clear width of not less than 12 in. (305 mm) shall be increased by 0.6 in. (15 mm) for every additional seat beyond the number stipulated in Table 12.4.2.7; however, the mini-

CHAPTER 13 • Existing

(2) If risers exceed 178 mm in height, the stair width in Table 13.4.2.3 and Table 13.4.2.4 shall be multiplied by factor $A$, where $A$ equals the following:

$$A = 1 + \frac{\text{riser height} - 178}{125}$$

(3) Stairs not having a handrail within a 30 in. (760 mm) horizontal distance shall be 25 percent wider than otherwise calculated; that is, their width shall be multiplied by factor $B$, where $B$ equals the following:

$$B = 1.25$$

(4) Ramps steeper than 1 in 10 slope used in ascent shall have their width increased by 10 percent; that is, their width shall be multiplied by factor $C$, where $C$ equals the following:

$$C = 1.10$$

**13.4.2.7** Where smoke-protected assembly seating conforms to the requirements of 13.4.2, for rows of seats served by aisles or doorways at both ends, the number of seats per row shall not exceed 100, and the clear width of not less than 12 in. (305 mm) for aisle accessways shall be increased by 0.3 in. (7.6 mm) for every additional seat beyond the number stipulated in Table 13.4.2.7; however, the minimum clear width shall not be required to exceed 22 in. (560 mm).

***Table 13.4.2.7 Smoke-Protected Assembly Seating Aisle Accessways***

| **Total Number of Seats in the Space** | **Number of Seats per Row Permitted to Have a Clear Width Aisle Accessway of Not Less than 12 in. (305 mm)** | |
|---|---|---|
| | **Aisle or Doorway at Both Ends of Row** | **Aisle or Doorway at One End of Row** |
| <4,000 | 14 | 7 |
| 4,000–6,999 | 15 | 7 |
| 7,000–9,999 | 16 | 8 |
| 10,000–12,999 | 17 | 8 |
| 13,000–15,999 | 18 | 9 |
| 16,000–18,999 | 19 | 9 |
| 19,000–21,999 | 20 | 10 |
| ≥22,000 | 21 | 11 |

**13.4.2.8** Where smoke-protected assembly seating conforms to the requirements of 13.4.2, for rows of seats served by an aisle or doorway at one end only, the aisle accessway clear width of not less than 12 in. (305 mm) shall be increased by 0.6 in. (15 mm) for every additional seat beyond the number stipulated in Table 13.4.2.7; however, the mini-

CHAPTER 12 • New

mum clear width shall not be required to exceed 22 in. (560 mm).

**12.4.2.9** Smoke-protected assembly seating conforming with the requirements of 12.4.2 shall be permitted to have a common path of travel of 50 ft (15 m) from any seat to a point where a person has a choice of two directions of egress travel.

**12.4.2.10** Where smoke-protected assembly seating conforms to the requirements of 12.4.2, the dead ends in aisle stairs shall not exceed a distance of 21 rows, unless both of the following criteria are met:

(1) The seats served by the dead-end aisle are not more than 40 seats from another aisle.
(2) The 40-seat distance is measured along a row of seats having an aisle accessway with a clear width of not less than 12 in. (305 mm) plus 0.3 in. (7.6 mm) for each additional seat above 7 in the row.

**12.4.2.11** Where smoke-protected assembly seating conforms to the requirements of 12.4.2, the travel distance from each seat to the nearest entrance to an egress vomitory portal or egress concourse shall not exceed 400 ft (122 m).

**12.4.2.12** Where smoke-protected assembly seating conforms to the requirements of 12.4.2, the travel distance from the entrance to the vomitory portal or from the egress concourse to an approved egress stair, ramp, or walk at the building exterior shall not exceed 200 ft (61 m).

**12.4.2.13** The travel distance requirements of 12.4.2.11 and 12.4.2.12 shall not apply to outdoor assembly seating facilities of Type I or Type II construction, where all portions of the means of egress are essentially open to the outside.

CHAPTER 13 • Existing

mum clear width shall not be required to exceed 22 in. (560 mm).

**13.4.2.9** Smoke-protected assembly seating conforming with the requirements of 13.4.2 shall be permitted to have a common path of travel of 50 ft (15 m) from any seat to a point where a person has a choice of two directions of egress travel.

**13.4.2.10** Where smoke-protected assembly seating conforms to the requirements of 13.4.2, the dead ends in aisle stairs shall not exceed a distance of 21 rows, unless both of the following criteria are met:

(1) The seats served by the dead-end aisle are not more than 40 seats from another aisle.
(2) The 40-seat distance is measured along a row of seats having an aisle accessway with a clear width of not less than 12 in. (305 mm) plus 0.3 in. (7.6 mm) for each additional seat above 7 in the row.

**13.4.2.11** Where smoke-protected assembly seating conforms to the requirements of 13.4.2, the travel distance from each seat to the nearest entrance to an egress vomitory portal or egress concourse shall not exceed 400 ft (122 m).

**13.4.2.12** Where smoke-protected assembly seating conforms to the requirements of 13.4.2, the travel distance from the entrance to the vomitory portal or from the egress concourse to an approved egress stair, ramp, or walk at the building exterior shall not exceed 200 ft (61 m).

**13.4.2.13** The travel distance requirements of 13.4.2.11 and 13.4.2.12 shall not apply to outdoor assembly seating facilities of Type I or Type II construction, where all portions of the means of egress are essentially open to the outside.

The *Code* requires that extra caution be taken before a facility is permitted to use the less stringent egress capacity factors contained in Table 12/13.4.2.3 (versus those in Table 12/13.2.3.2). The authority having jurisdiction (AHJ) must approve a life safety evaluation, which should not be undertaken lightly or without special competence in a wide range of life safety issues including, but not limited to, fire safety. See 12/13.4.1.

When conducting the life safety evaluation, the capabilities of the potential occupants must be taken into account (e.g., will the facilities be used by groups of occupants who are unfamiliar with the facility, or who are unable to move quickly and in dense groups?). The need to consider the capabilities of occupants in relation to circulation facility geometry has led to the application of several correction factors detailed in 12/13.4.2.6 for use with the values for clear width in Table 12/13.4.2.3. Maintaining the best possible geometries should be a priority that is heavily emphasized in new facilities. However, the preservation of sight lines often requires stepped aisle riser height to exceed 7 in. (180 mm). Therefore, the correction factor *A* in the table will seldom be 1.0, but correction factors *B* and *C* can often be 1.0. It might not be possible to achieve this level of safety in existing facilities. However, handrails can be retrofitted on aisles and other means of egress to significantly improve occupant safety and comfort. These factors are taken into account here and in other *Code* requirements for means of egress.

The reduction in required egress capacity factors provided by Table 12/13.4.2.3 must be used with caution. The proper balance must be maintained among the relative egress capacities of each part of the means of egress system that occupants encounter as they leave the facility. Otherwise, queuing or waiting at some points other than the point of origin might result.

Attention should be given to the occupants' acceptance of the queue or the wait at their seats before proceeding out of the building; however, if a "downstream" component of the means of egress system is expected to slow the occupant movement, even greater attention should be given to the actual and perceived conditions faced by occupants.

Exhibit 12/13.37 shows egress from a large stadium. The egress performance provided is perceived to be acceptable in terms of time and other factors. Occupants' acceptance of the longer egress flow times, permitted by the *Code* for larger assembly facilities, should be taken into account when performing a life safety evaluation for the building.

Paragraph 12/13.4.2.4 was added to the *Code* in 2006. Table 12/13.4.2.3, which varies the capacity factor based on number of seats, was developed mainly to address indoor arenas. As the number of seats increases in an indoor assembly venue, the area and height of the assembly space increases, so as to increase the overall volume of the space. Large-volume spaces are less susceptible to the effects of a developing fire, including smoke filling. The larger-volume spaces act much the same as outdoor spaces without a roof, especially where smoke control, as required by 12/13.4.2.1(2), is provided. Table 12/13.4.2.4 offers a reduction in the capacity factors for smoke-protected assembly seating venues for which the seating area and its egress system are located wholly outdoors. Such reduction is offered independent of the number

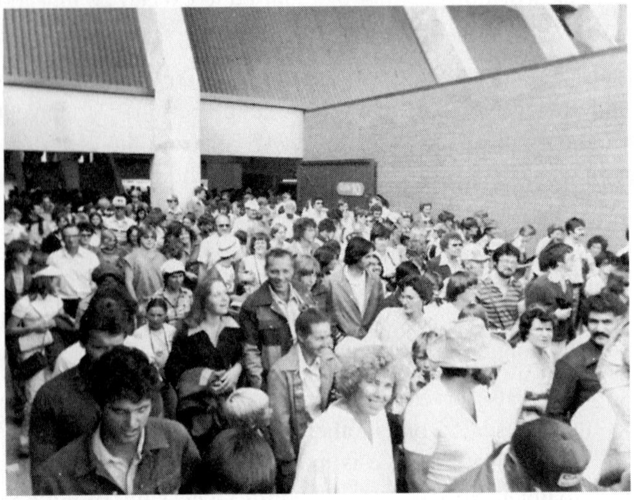

***Exhibit 12/13.37*** *Crowd egress from a large assembly facility that might be eligible for egress capacity factor reductions of Table 12/13.4.2.3. (Photograph courtesy of Jake Pauls)*

of seats. The capacity factors specified in Table 12/13.4.2.4 for the outdoor, smoke-protected assembly seating correlate with those of Table 12/13.4.2.3 for approximately 19,000 seats. Thus, the outdoor, smoke-protected assembly seating capacity factors of Table 12/13.4.2.4 are not as lenient as some specified in Table 12/13.4.2.3, but offer great relief from those capacity factors applicable to traditional, non-smoke-protected seating as required by Table 12/13.2.3.2.

Note that 12/13.4.2.4 applies to outdoor assembly seating only if it is smoke-protected assembly seating. Per 12/13.4.2.2, the outdoor seating qualifies as smoke-protected assembly seating only if a life safety evaluation in accordance with 12/13.4.1 is performed.

### 12.4.3 Limited Access or Underground Buildings.

**12.4.3.1** Limited access or underground buildings shall comply with 12.4.3 and Section 11.7.

**12.4.3.2** Underground buildings or portions of buildings having a floor level more than 30 ft (9140 mm) below the level of exit discharge shall comply with the requirements of 12.4.3.3 through 12.4.3.5, unless otherwise permitted by the following:

(1) This requirement shall not apply to areas within buildings used only for service to the building, such as boiler/heater rooms, cable vaults, and dead storage.

### 13.4.3 Limited Access or Underground Buildings.

Limited access or underground buildings shall comply with Section 11.7.

CHAPTER 12 • New

CHAPTER 13 • Existing

(2) This requirement shall not apply to auditoriums without intervening occupiable levels.

**12.4.3.3** Each level more than 30 ft (9.1 m) below the level of exit discharge shall be divided into not less than two smoke compartments by a smoke barrier complying with Section 8.5 and shall have a minimum 1-hour fire resistance rating.

**12.4.3.3.1** Smoke compartments shall comply with the following:

(1) Each smoke compartment shall have access to not less than one exit without passing through the other required compartment.
(2) Any doors connecting required compartments shall be tight-fitting, minimum 1-hour-rated fire door assemblies designed and installed to minimize smoke leakage and to close and latch automatically upon detection of smoke.

**12.4.3.3.2** Each smoke compartment shall be provided with a mechanical means of moving people vertically, such as an elevator or escalator.

**12.4.3.3.3** Each smoke compartment shall have an independent air supply and exhaust system capable of smoke control or smoke exhaust functions. The system shall be in accordance with NFPA 92A, *Standard for Smoke-Control Systems Utilizing Barriers and Pressure Differences*, or NFPA 92B, *Standard for Smoke Management Systems in Malls, Atria, and Large Spaces*.

**12.4.3.3.4** Throughout each smoke compartment shall be provided an automatic smoke detection system designed such that the activation of any two detectors causes the smoke control system to operate and the building voice alarm to sound.

**12.4.3.4** Any required smoke control or exhaust system shall be provided with a standby power system complying with Article 701 of *NFPA 70, National Electrical Code*.

**12.4.3.5** The building shall be provided with an approved, supervised voice alarm system, in accordance with Section 9.6, that complies with 9.6.3.9 and provides a prerecorded evacuation message.

Recognizing the potential hazard that limited access or underground buildings pose, the *Code* requires new assembly occupancies to comply with Section 11.7. In addition, new assembly occupancies must comply with the provisions of 12.4.3.3 through 12.4.3.5 if the assembly occupancy is more than 30 ft (9.1 m) below the level of exit discharge.

Exemptions are provided for areas used only for service functions (such as boiler rooms or heater rooms) and for assembly occupancies where there is no occupiable intervening level between the assembly occupancy and the level of exit discharge.

The provisions for underground buildings or portions of assembly buildings with an occupiable floor more than 30 ft (9.1 m) below the level of exit discharge (LED) are designed to provide protected areas on the subterranean level. This protection, coupled with a smoke control or smoke exhaust system, will provide sufficient time to egress the building. Elevators or escalators are required in each compartment to help rapidly evacuate the area, as shown in Exhibit 12/13.38. It is believed that elevators or escalators will not, themselves, create a life safety threat because of the other requirements of 12.4.3, including separate smoke compartments and smoke control or exhaust systems. The elevator or escalator is not being considered the required means of egress; normal exits are still required.

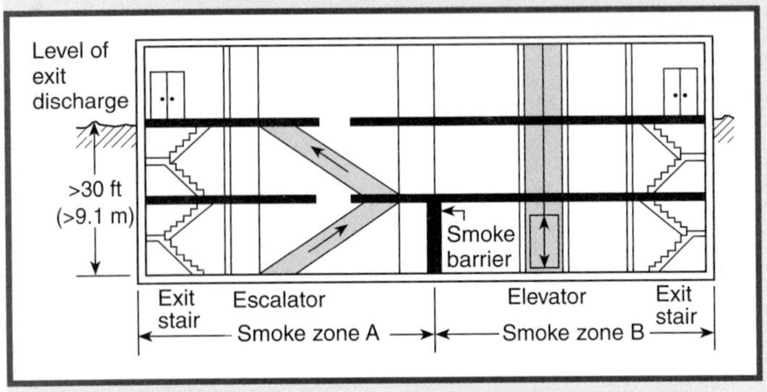


*Exhibit 12/13.38 Escalator and elevator use in assembly occupancy located more than 30 ft (9.1 m) below LED.*

The provision of 12.4.3.3.3 was revised for the 2009 edition of the *Code*. In prior editions, a smoke exhaust rate of not less than six air changes per hour was required. In 2006, NFPA 92A, *Standard for Smoke-Control Systems Utilizing Barriers and Pressure Differences*, was revised and upgraded to the status of a standard.[10] Similarly, in 2005, NFPA 92B, *Standard for Smoke Management Systems in Malls, Atria, and Large Spaces*, was revised and upgraded to the status of a standard.[11] As standards, NFPA 92A and NFPA 92B are permitted to be mandatorily referenced by other NFPA codes and standards. Paragraph 12.4.3.3.3 makes such mandatory reference.

To provide redundancy in the life safety provisions, standby power, as defined in Article 701 of *NFPA 70®, National Electrical Code®*,[12] is required by 12.4.3.4 for the smoke control or exhaust system.

To facilitate orderly evacuation and reduce the possibility of panic, 12.4.3.5 requires the use of a supervised voice alarm system that will sound a prerecorded evacuation message.

### 12.4.4 High-Rise Buildings.

High-rise assembly occupancy buildings and high-rise mixed occupancy buildings that house assembly occupancies in the high-rise portions of the building shall comply with Section 11.8.

High-rise assembly occupancy buildings have the same inherent life safety dangers that are found in other high-rise buildings. Therefore, the protection provided for high-rise buildings in general should be appropriate and applicable to high-rise assembly occupancies and portions of high-rise buildings that are used for assembly occupancy. Note that the sprinkler requirement applies even to existing assembly occupancies located in the high-rise portion of a building. For new assembly occupancies, the complete high-rise building package of Section 11.8 is required. The high-rise building package includes sprinklers, standpipes, voice alarm/communication, standby power, and an emergency command center in addition to the other features required by Chapter 12.

### 12.4.5 Stages and Platforms.

See 3.3.246 and 3.3.195.

**12.4.5.1 Materials and Design.** Materials used in the construction of platforms and stages shall conform to the applicable requirements of the local building code.



### 13.4.4 High-Rise Buildings.

Existing high-rise buildings that house assembly occupancies in high-rise portions of the building shall have the highest level of the assembly occupancy and all levels below protected by an approved, supervised automatic sprinkler system in accordance with Section 9.7. *(See also 13.1.6.)*

### 13.4.5 Stages and Platforms.

See 3.3.246 and 3.3.195.

**13.4.5.1 Materials and Design. (Reserved)**

CHAPTER 12 • New

**12.4.5.2 Platform Construction.**

**12.4.5.2.1** Temporary platforms shall be permitted to be constructed of any materials.

**12.4.5.2.2** The space between the floor and the temporary platform above shall not be used for any purpose other than the electrical wiring to platform equipment.

**12.4.5.2.3** Permanent platforms shall be of the materials required for the building construction type in which the permanent platform is located, except that the finish floor shall be permitted to be of wood in all types of construction.

**12.4.5.2.4** Where the space beneath the permanent platform is used for storage or any purpose other than equipment wiring or plumbing, the floor construction shall not be less than 1-hour fire resistive.

**12.4.5.3 Stage Construction.**

**12.4.5.3.1** Regular stages shall be of the materials required for the building construction type in which they are located. In all cases, the finish floor shall be permitted to be of wood.

**12.4.5.3.2** Legitimate stages shall be constructed of materials required for Type I buildings, except that the area extending from the proscenium opening to the back wall of the stage, and for a distance of 6 ft (1830 mm) beyond the proscenium opening on each side, shall be permitted to be constructed of steel or heavy timber covered with a wood floor not less than $1\frac{1}{2}$ in. (38 mm) in actual thickness.

**12.4.5.3.3** Openings through stage floors shall be equipped with tight-fitting traps with approved safety locks, and such traps shall comply with one of the following:

(1) The traps shall be of wood having an actual thickness of not less than $1\frac{1}{2}$ in. (38 mm).
(2) The traps shall be of a material that provides fire and heat resistance at least equivalent to that provided by wood traps having an actual thickness of not less than $1\frac{1}{2}$ in. (38 mm).

**12.4.5.4 Accessory Rooms.**

**12.4.5.4.1** Workshops, storerooms, permanent dressing rooms, and other accessory spaces contiguous to stages shall be separated from each other and other building areas by 1-hour fire resistance–rated construction and protected openings.

**12.4.5.4.2** The separation requirements of 12.4.5.4.1 shall not be required for stages having a floor area not exceeding 1000 $ft^2$ (93 $m^2$).

**12.4.5.5 Ventilators.** Regular stages in excess of 1000 $ft^2$ (93 $m^2$) and legitimate stages shall be provided with emergency ventilation to provide a means of removing smoke

CHAPTER 13 • Existing

**13.4.5.2 Platform Construction. (Reserved)**

**13.4.5.3 Stage Construction. (Reserved)**

**13.4.5.4 Accessory Rooms. (Reserved)**

**13.4.5.5 Ventilators.** Regular stages in excess of 1000 $ft^2$ (93 $m^2$) and legitimate stages shall be provided with emergency ventilation to provide a means of removing smoke

CHAPTER 12 • New

and combustion gases directly to the outside in the event of a fire, and such ventilation shall be achieved by one or a combination of the methods specified in 12.4.5.5.1 through 12.4.5.5.3.

**12.4.5.5.1 Smoke Control.**

**12.4.5.5.1.1** A means complying with Section 9.3 shall be provided to maintain the smoke level at not less than 6 ft (1830 mm) above the highest level of assembly seating or above the top of the proscenium opening where a proscenium wall and opening protection are provided.

**12.4.5.5.1.2** Smoke control systems used for compliance with 12.4.5.5.1.1 shall be in accordance with NFPA 92B, *Standard for Smoke Management Systems in Malls, Atria, and Large Spaces*, or, where applicable, NFPA 92A, *Standard for Smoke-Control Systems Utilizing Barriers and Pressure Differences*.

**12.4.5.5.1.3** The smoke control system shall be activated independently by each of the following:

(1) Activation of the sprinkler system in the stage area
(2) Activation of smoke detectors over the stage area
(3) Activation by manually operated switch at an approved location

**12.4.5.5.1.4** The emergency ventilation system shall be supplied by both normal and standby power.

**12.4.5.5.1.5** The fan(s) power wiring and ducts shall be located and properly protected to ensure a minimum of 20 minutes of operation in the event of activation.

**12.4.5.5.2 Roof Vents.**

**12.4.5.5.2.1** Two or more vents shall be located near the center of and above the highest part of the stage area.

**12.4.5.5.2.2** The vents shall be raised above the roof and shall provide a net free vent area equal to 5 percent of the stage area.

**12.4.5.5.2.3** Vents shall be constructed to open automatically by approved heat-activated devices, and supplemental means shall be provided for manual operation and periodic testing of the ventilator from the stage floor.

**12.4.5.5.2.4** Vents shall be labeled.

**12.4.5.5.3 Other Means.** Approved, alternate means of re-

CHAPTER 13 • Existing

and combustion gases directly to the outside in the event of a fire, and such ventilation shall be achieved by one or a combination of the methods specified in 13.4.5.5.1 through 13.4.5.5.3.

**13.4.5.5.1 Smoke Control.**

**13.4.5.5.1.1** A means complying with Section 9.3 shall be provided to maintain the smoke level at not less than 6 ft (1830 mm) above the highest level of assembly seating or above the top of the proscenium opening where a proscenium wall and opening protection are provided.

**13.4.5.5.1.2** The smoke control system shall be activated independently by each of the following:

(1) Activation of the sprinkler system in the stage area
(2) Activation of smoke detectors over the stage area
(3) Activation by manually operated switch at an approved location

**13.4.5.5.1.3** The emergency ventilation system shall be supplied by both normal and standby power.

**13.4.5.5.1.4** The fan(s) power wiring and ducts shall be located and properly protected to ensure a minimum of 20 minutes of operation in the event of activation.

**13.4.5.5.2 Roof Vents.**

**13.4.5.5.2.1** Two or more vents shall be located near the center of and above the highest part of the stage area.

**13.4.5.5.2.2** The vents shall be raised above the roof and shall provide a net free vent area equal to 5 percent of the stage area.

**13.4.5.5.2.3** Vents shall be constructed to open automatically by approved heat-activated devices, and supplemental means shall be provided for manual operation and periodic testing of the ventilator from the stage floor.

**13.4.5.5.2.4** Vents shall be labeled.

**13.4.5.5.2.5** Existing roof vents that are not labeled shall be permitted where they open by spring action or force of gravity sufficient to overcome the effects of neglect, rust, dirt, frost, snow, or expansion by heat or warping of the framework, and the following requirements also shall apply:

(1) Glass, if used in vents, shall be protected against falling onto the stage.

moving smoke and combustion gases shall be permitted.

**12.4.5.6 Proscenium Walls.** Legitimate stages shall be completely separated from the seating area by a proscenium wall of not less than 2-hour fire-resistive, noncombustible construction.

**12.4.5.6.1** The proscenium wall shall extend not less than 48 in. (1220 mm) above the roof of the auditorium in combustible construction.

**12.4.5.6.2** All openings in the proscenium wall of a legitimate stage shall be protected by a fire assembly having a minimum $1\frac{1}{2}$-hour fire protection rating.

**12.4.5.6.3** The main proscenium opening used for viewing performances shall be provided with proscenium opening protection as described in 12.4.5.7.

**12.4.5.6.4** Proscenium walls shall not be required in smoke-



(2) A wire screen, if used under the glass, shall be placed so that, if clogged, it does not reduce the required venting area, interfere with the operating mechanism, or obstruct the distribution of water from an automatic sprinkler.
(3) Vents shall be arranged to open automatically by the use of fusible links.
(4) The fusible links and operating cable shall hold each door closed against a minimum 30 lb (133 N) counterforce that shall be exerted on each door through its entire arc of travel and for not less than 115 degrees.
(5) Vents shall be provided with manual control.
(6) Springs, where employed to actuate vent doors, shall be capable of maintaining full required tension.
(7) Springs shall not be stressed more than 50 percent of their rated capacity and shall not be located directly in the airstream nor exposed to the outside.
(8) A fusible link shall be placed in the cable control system on the underside of the vent at or above the roofline, or as approved by the building official.
(9) The fusible link shall be located so as not to be affected by the operation of an automatic sprinkler system.
(10) Remote, manual, or electric controls shall provide for both opening and closing of the vent doors for periodic testing and shall be located at a point on stage designated by the authority having jurisdiction.
(11) Where remote control vents are electrical, power failure shall not affect instant operation of the vent in the event of fire.
(12) Hand winches shall be permitted to be employed to facilitate operation of manually controlled vents.

**13.4.5.5.3 Other Means.** Approved, alternate means of removing smoke and combustion gases shall be permitted.

**13.4.5.6 Proscenium Walls. (Reserved)**

**13.4.5.7 Proscenium Opening Protection.**

CHAPTER 12 • New

protected assembly seating facilities constructed and operated in accordance with 12.4.2.

**12.4.5.7 Proscenium Opening Protection.**

**12.4.5.7.1** Where required by 12.4.5.6, the proscenium opening shall be protected by a listed, minimum 20-minute opening protective assembly, a fire curtain complying with NFPA 80, *Standard for Fire Doors and Other Opening Protectives*, or an approved water curtain complying with NFPA 13, *Standard for the Installation of Sprinkler Systems*.

**12.4.5.7.2** Proscenium opening protection provided by other than a fire curtain shall activate upon automatic detection of a fire and upon manual activation.

**12.4.5.8 Gridiron, Fly Galleries, and Pinrails.**

**12.4.5.8.1** Structural framing designed only for the attachment of portable or fixed theater equipment, gridirons, galleries, and catwalks shall be constructed of materials

CHAPTER 13 • Existing

**13.4.5.7.1** On every legitimate stage, the main proscenium opening used for viewing performances shall be provided with proscenium opening protection as follows:

(1) The proscenium opening protection shall comply with 12.4.5.7.
(2) Asbestos shall be permitted in lieu of a listed fabric.
(3) Manual curtains of any size shall be permitted.

**13.4.5.7.2** In lieu of the protection required by 13.4.5.7.1(1), all the following shall be provided:

(1) A noncombustible opaque fabric curtain shall be arranged so that it closes automatically.
(2) An automatic, fixed waterspray deluge system shall be located on the auditorium side of the proscenium opening and shall be arranged so that the entire face of the curtain will be wetted, and the following requirements also shall apply:
    (a) The system shall be activated by a combination of rate-of-rise and fixed-temperature detectors located on the ceiling of the stage.
    (b) Detectors shall be spaced in accordance with their listing.
    (c) The water supply shall be controlled by a deluge valve and shall be sufficient to keep the curtain completely wet for 30 minutes or until the valve is closed by fire department personnel.
(3) The curtain shall be automatically operated in case of fire by a combination of rate-of-rise and fixed-temperature detectors that also activates the deluge spray system.
(4) Stage sprinklers and vents shall be automatically operated by fusible elements in case of fire.
(5) Operation of the stage sprinkler system or spray deluge valve shall automatically activate the emergency ventilating system and close the curtain.
(6) The curtain, vents, and spray deluge system valve shall also be capable of manual operation.

**13.4.5.7.3** Proscenium opening protection provided by other than a fire curtain in accordance with 12.4.5.7 *[see 13.4.5.7.1(1)]* shall activate upon automatic detection of a fire and upon manual activation.

**13.4.5.8 Gridirons, Fly Galleries, and Pinrails. (Reserved)**

**13.4.5.9 Catwalks.** The clear width of lighting and access catwalks and the means of egress from galleries and consistent with the building construction type, and a fire resistance rating shall not be required.

**12.4.5.8.2** Combustible materials shall be permitted to be used for the floors of galleries and catwalks of all construction types.

**12.4.5.9 Catwalks.** The clear width of lighting and access catwalks and the means of egress from galleries and gridirons shall be not less than 22 in. (560 mm).

**12.4.5.10 Fire Protection.** Every stage shall be protected by an approved, supervised automatic sprinkler system in compliance with Section 9.7.

**12.4.5.10.1** Protection shall be provided throughout the stage and in storerooms, workshops, permanent dressing rooms, and other accessory spaces contiguous to stages.

**12.4.5.10.2** Sprinklers shall not be required for stages 1000 $ft^2$ (93 $m^2$) or less in area and 50 ft (15 m) or less in height where the following criteria are met:

(1) Curtains, scenery, or other combustible hangings are not retractable vertically.
(2) Combustible hangings are limited to borders, legs, a single main curtain, and a single backdrop.

**12.4.5.10.3** Sprinklers shall not be required under stage areas less than 48 in. (1220 mm) in clear height that are used exclusively for chair or table storage and lined on the inside with $^5/_8$ in. (16 mm) Type X gypsum wallboard or the approved equivalent.

**12.4.5.11 Flame-Retardant Requirements.**

**12.4.5.11.1** Combustible scenery of cloth, film, vegetation (dry), and similar materials shall meet the requirements of NFPA 701, *Standard Methods of Fire Tests for Flame Propagation of Textiles and Films.*

**12.4.5.11.2** Foamed plastics *(see definition of cellular or foamed plastic in 3.3.36)* shall be permitted to be used only by specific approval of the authority having jurisdiction.

**12.4.5.11.3** Scenery and stage properties not separated from the audience by proscenium opening protection shall be of noncombustible materials, limited-combustible materials, or fire-retardant-treated wood.

**12.4.5.11.4** In theaters, motion picture theaters, and television stage settings, with or without horizontal projections, and in simulated caves and caverns of foamed plastic, any single fuel package shall have a heat release rate not to exceed 100 kW where tested in accordance with ANSI/UL 1975, *Standard for Fire Tests for Foamed Plastics Used for Decorative Purposes.*

**12.4.5.12* Standpipes.**

gridirons shall be not less than 22 in. (560 mm).

**13.4.5.10 Fire Protection.** Every stage shall be protected by an approved automatic sprinkler system in compliance with Section 9.7.

**13.4.5.10.1** Protection shall be provided throughout the stage and in storerooms, workshops, permanent dressing rooms, and other accessory spaces contiguous to stages.

**13.4.5.10.2** Sprinklers shall not be required for stages 1000 $ft^2$ (93 $m^2$) or less in area where the following criteria are met:

(1) Curtains, scenery, or other combustible hangings are not retractable vertically.
(2) Combustible hangings are limited to borders, legs, a single main curtain, and a single backdrop.

**13.4.5.10.3** Sprinklers shall not be required under stage areas less than 48 in. (1220 mm) in clear height that are used exclusively for chair or table storage and lined on the inside with $^5/_8$ in. (16 mm) Type X gypsum wallboard or the approved equivalent.

**13.4.5.11 Flame-Retardant Requirements.**

**13.4.5.11.1** Combustible scenery of cloth, film, vegetation (dry), and similar materials shall meet the requirements of NFPA 701, *Standard Methods of Fire Tests for Flame Propagation of Textiles and Films.*

**13.4.5.11.2** Foamed plastics *(see definition of cellular or foamed plastic in 3.3.36)* shall be permitted to be used only by specific approval of the authority having jurisdiction.

**13.4.5.11.3** Scenery and stage properties on thrust stages shall be of noncombustible materials, limited-combustible materials, or fire-retardant-treated wood.

**13.4.5.12* Standpipes.**

CHAPTER 12 • New

**A.12.4.5.12** Prior editions of the *Code* required stages to be protected by a Class III standpipe system in accordance with NFPA 14, *Standard for the Installation of Standpipe and Hose Systems*. NFPA 14 requires that Class II and Class III standpipes be automatic — not manual — because they are intended to be used by building occupants. Automatic standpipe systems are required to provide not less than 500 gpm (1890 L/min) at 100 psi (689 kN). This requirement often can be met only if a fire pump is installed. Installation of a fire pump presents an unreasonable burden for the system supplying the two hose outlets at the side of the stage. The revised wording of 12.4.5.12 offers some relief by permitting the hose outlets to be in accordance with NFPA 13, *Standard for the Installation of Sprinkler Systems*.

**12.4.5.12.1** Regular stages over 1000 ft² (93 m²) in area and all legitimate stages shall be equipped with 1½ in. (38 mm) hose lines for first aid fire fighting at each side of the stage.

**12.4.5.12.2** Hose connections shall be in accordance with NFPA 13, *Standard for the Installation of Sprinkler Systems*, unless Class II or Class III standpipes in accordance with NFPA 14, *Standard for the Installation of Standpipe and Hose Systems*, are used.

CHAPTER 13 • Existing

**A.13.4.5.12** Prior editions of the *Code* required stages to be protected by a Class III standpipe system in accordance with NFPA 14, *Standard for the Installation of Standpipe and Hose Systems*. NFPA 14 requires that Class II and Class III standpipes be automatic — not manual — because they are intended to be used by building occupants. Automatic standpipe systems are required to provide not less than 500 gpm (1890 L/min) at 100 psi (689 kN/m²). This requirement often can be met only if a fire pump is installed. Installation of a fire pump presents an unreasonable burden for the system supplying the two hose outlets at the side of the stage. The revised wording of 13.4.5.12 offers some relief by permitting the hose outlets to be in accordance with NFPA 13, *Standard for the Installation of Sprinkler Systems*.

**13.4.5.12.1** Stages over 1000 ft² (93 m²) in area shall be equipped with 1½ in. (38 mm) hose lines for first aid fire fighting at each side of the stage.

**13.4.5.12.2** Hose connections shall be in accordance with NFPA 13, *Standard for the Installation of Sprinkler Systems*, unless Class II or Class III standpipes in accordance with NFPA 14, *Standard for the Installation of Standpipe and Hose Systems*, are used.

Stages pose a host of life safety protection challenges. Scenery might be shifted horizontally, vertically, or both ways. The use of thrust stages and arena stages introduces new challenges.

The classic stage of the past rose high above the proscenium opening to accommodate the rigid asbestos curtain. The high void was a natural place to house combustible scenery for a performance, along with the rigging necessary for handling scene changes. This vertical storage area represented both a high fuel load and a space difficult to reach in case of fire. Many new theaters use a flexible, noncombustible curtain that does not require much height to accommodate it. Scenery on these stages is moved horizontally, thus reducing the distance necessary for storage between the top of the proscenium opening and the stage ceiling. Most combustible scenery is now stored in areas adjacent to the stage. All rigging and lighting is condensed in less vertical space.

Ventilators are addressed in 12/13.4.5.5. The venting requirements of 12/13.4.5.5 apply to regular stages larger than 1000 ft² (93 m²) and to all legitimate stages. Smaller stages, such as those commonly seen in small schools, do not pose the same fire potential as larger stages. See the definitions of *stage* in 3.3.246 and *platform* in 3.3.195.

Paragraph 12/13.4.5.5.1 makes use of performance-oriented language to specify the intended function of smoke control, if smoke control is the method used to provide the required ventilation. The performance criterion is to maintain the smoke level at not less than 6 ft (1830 mm) above the highest level of the assembly seating or above the top of a proscenium opening where a proscenium wall and opening protection are provided. For new installations, the provisions of 12.4.5.5.1.2 require that the smoke control system be in accordance with NFPA 92B, *Standard for Smoke Management Systems in Malls, Atria, and Large Spaces*,[13] or, where applicable, NFPA 92A, *Standard for Smoke-Control Systems Utilizing Barriers and Pressure Differences*.[14]

In lieu of a smoke control system, 12/13.4.5.5 permits roof vents as prescribed by 12/13.4.5.5.2 to provide the required ventilation. For existing vents that are not labeled, 13.4.5.5.2.5 provides prescriptive criteria that help to ensure that the vent will operate as reliably as a vent that is listed.

Paragraph 12/13.4.5.5.3 permits other approved means of removing smoke and combustion gases to fulfill the ventilation requirement of 12/13.4.5.5.

The proscenium opening protection provisions of 12.4.5.7 were revised for the 2009 edition of the *Code* to

CHAPTER 12 • New

reflect that NFPA 80, *Standard for Fire Doors and Other Opening Protectives,*[15] was revised in 2007 to include provisions for fabric fire safety curtains. Paragraph 12.4.5.7.1 permits the proscenium opening protection to be provided by either a fire curtain complying with NFPA 80, an approved water curtain complying with NFPA 13, *Standard for the Installation of Sprinkler Systems,*[16] or a listed, minimum 20-minute opening protective assembly (such as the horizontal-sliding door detailed in 7.2.1.14). Given that the details associated with the fire curtain are detailed in NFPA 80, the prescriptive text on fire curtains that appeared in the *Code* for many editions was deleted. Existing proscenium opening protection, as required by 13.4.5.7, is permitted to meet the criteria applicable to new construction (i.e., 13.4.5.7.1 references 12.4.5.7) or the provisions of 13.4.5.7.2, which have been in the *Code* for many editions.

Regardless of whether a stage has automatic sprinkler protection, standpipes are required on each side of the stage to provide stagehands and the responding fire department with manual fire-fighting capability in the area of a theater where a fire is most likely to occur.

### 12.4.6 Projection Rooms.

**12.4.6.1** Projection rooms shall comply with 12.4.6.2 through 12.4.6.10.

**12.4.6.2** Where cellulose nitrate film is used, the projection room shall comply with NFPA 40, *Standard for the Storage and Handling of Cellulose Nitrate Film.*

**12.4.6.3** Film or video projectors or spotlights utilizing light sources that produce particulate matter, or toxic gases or light sources that produce hazardous radiation, without protective shielding shall be located within a projection room complying with 12.3.2.1.2.

**12.4.6.4** Every projection room shall be of permanent construction consistent with the building construction type in which the projection room is located and shall comply with the following:

(1) Openings shall not be required to be protected.
(2) The room shall have a floor area of not less than 80 $ft^2$ (7.4 $m^2$) for a single machine and not less than 40 $ft^2$ (3.7 $m^2$) for each additional machine.
(3) Each motion picture projector, floodlight, spotlight, or similar piece of equipment shall have a clear working space of not less than 30 in. (760 mm) on each side and at its rear, but only one such space shall be required between adjacent projectors.

**12.4.6.5** The projection room and the rooms appurtenant to it shall have a ceiling height of not less than 7 ft 6 in. (2285 mm).

**12.4.6.6** Each projection room for safety film shall have not less than one out-swinging, self-closing door not less than 30 in. (760 mm) wide and 6 ft 8 in. (2030 mm) high.

**12.4.6.7** The aggregate of ports and openings for projection equipment shall not exceed 25 percent of the area of the wall between the projection room and the auditorium, and all

CHAPTER 13 • Existing

### 13.4.6 Projection Rooms.

**13.4.6.1** Projection rooms shall comply with 13.4.6.2 through 13.4.6.10.

**13.4.6.2** Where cellulose nitrate film is used, the projection room shall comply with NFPA 40, *Standard for the Storage and Handling of Cellulose Nitrate Film.*

**13.4.6.3** Film or video projectors or spotlights utilizing light sources that produce particulate matter, or toxic gases or light sources that produce hazardous radiation, without protective shielding shall be located within a projection room complying with 13.3.2.1.2.

**13.4.6.4** Every projection room shall be of permanent construction consistent with the building construction type in which the projection room is located and shall comply with the following:

(1) Openings shall not be required to be protected.
(2) The room shall have a floor area of not less than 80 $ft^2$ (7.4 $m^2$) for a single machine and not less than 40 $ft^2$ (3.7 $m^2$) for each additional machine.
(3) Each motion picture projector, floodlight, spotlight, or similar piece of equipment shall have a clear working space of not less than 30 in. (760 mm) on each side and at its rear, but only one such space shall be required between adjacent projectors.

**13.4.6.5** The projection room and the rooms appurtenant to it shall have a ceiling height of not less than 7 ft 6 in. (2285 mm).

**13.4.6.6** Each projection room for safety film shall have not less than one out-swinging, self-closing door not less than 30 in. (760 mm) wide and 6 ft 8 in. (2030 mm) high.

**13.4.6.7** The aggregate of ports and openings for projection equipment shall not exceed 25 percent of the area of the wall between the projection room and the auditorium, and all

CHAPTER 12 • New

openings shall be provided with glass or other approved material so as to completely close the opening.

**12.4.6.8** Projection room ventilation shall comply with 12.4.6.8.1 and 12.4.6.8.2.

**12.4.6.8.1 Supply Air.**

**12.4.6.8.1.1** Each projection room shall be provided with adequate air supply inlets arranged to provide well-distributed air throughout the room.

**12.4.6.8.1.2** Air inlet ducts shall provide an amount of air equivalent to the amount of air being exhausted by projection equipment.

**12.4.6.8.1.3** Air shall be permitted to be taken from the outside; from adjacent spaces within the building, provided that the volume and infiltration rate is sufficient; or from the building air-conditioning system, provided that it is arranged to supply sufficient air whether or not other systems are in operation.

**12.4.6.8.2 Exhaust Air.**

**12.4.6.8.2.1 Projection booths shall be permitted to be exhausted through the lamp exhaust system.**

**12.4.6.8.2.2** The lamp exhaust system shall be positively interconnected with the lamp so that the lamp cannot operate unless there is sufficient airflow required for the lamp.

**12.4.6.8.2.3** Exhaust air ducts shall terminate at the exterior of the building in such a location that the exhaust air cannot be readily recirculated into any air supply system.

**12.4.6.8.2.4** The projection room ventilation system shall be permitted also to serve appurtenant rooms, such as the generator room and the rewind room.

**12.4.6.9** Each projection machine shall be provided with an exhaust duct that draws air from each lamp and exhausts it directly to the outside of the building.

**12.4.6.9.1** The lamp exhaust shall be permitted to exhaust air from the projection room to provide room air circulation.

**12.4.6.9.2** Lamp exhaust ducts shall be of rigid materials, except for a flexible connector approved for the purpose.

**12.4.6.9.3** The projection lamp and projection room exhaust systems shall be permitted to be combined but shall not be interconnected with any other exhaust system or return-air system within the buildings.

**12.4.6.9.4** Specifications for electric arc and xenon projection equipment shall comply with 12.4.6.9.4.1 and 12.4.6.9.4.2.

CHAPTER 13 • Existing

openings shall be provided with glass or other approved material so as to completely close the opening.

**13.4.6.8** Projection room ventilation shall comply with 13.4.6.8.1 and 13.4.6.8.2.

**13.4.6.8.1 Supply Air.**

**13.4.6.8.1.1** Each projection room shall be provided with adequate air supply inlets arranged to provide well-distributed air throughout the room.

**13.4.6.8.1.2** Air inlet ducts shall provide an amount of air equivalent to the amount of air being exhausted by projection equipment.

**13.4.6.8.1.3** Air shall be permitted to be taken from the outside; from adjacent spaces within the building, provided that the volume and infiltration rate is sufficient; or from the building air-conditioning system, provided that it is arranged to supply sufficient air whether or not other systems are in operation.

**13.4.6.8.2 Exhaust Air.**

**13.4.6.8.2.1** Projection booths shall be permitted to be exhausted through the lamp exhaust system.

**13.4.6.8.2.2** The lamp exhaust system shall be positively interconnected with the lamp so that the lamp cannot operate unless there is sufficient airflow required for the lamp.

**13.4.6.8.2.3** Exhaust air ducts shall terminate at the exterior of the building in such a location that the exhaust air cannot be readily recirculated into any air supply system.

**13.4.6.8.2.4** The projection room ventilation system shall be permitted also to serve appurtenant rooms, such as the generator room and the rewind room.

**13.4.6.9** Each projection machine shall be provided with an exhaust duct that draws air from each lamp and exhausts it directly to the outside of the building.

**13.4.6.9.1** The lamp exhaust shall be permitted to exhaust air from the projection room to provide room air circulation.

**13.4.6.9.2** Lamp exhaust ducts shall be of rigid materials, except for a flexible connector approved for the purpose.

**13.4.6.9.3** The projection lamp and projection room exhaust systems shall be permitted to be combined but shall not be interconnected with any other exhaust system or return-air system within the buildings.

**13.4.6.9.4** Specifications for electric arc and xenon projection equipment shall comply with 13.4.6.9.4.1 and 13.4.6.9.4.2.

**12.4.6.9.4.1 Electric Arc Projection Equipment.** The exhaust capacity shall be 200 $ft^3$/min (0.09 $m^3$/s) for each lamp connected to the lamp exhaust system, or as recommended by the equipment manufacturer, and auxiliary air shall be permitted to be introduced into the system through a screened opening to stabilize the arc.

**12.4.6.9.4.2 Xenon Projection Equipment.** The lamp exhaust system shall exhaust not less than 300 $ft^3$/min (0.14 $m^3$/s) per lamp, or not less than the exhaust volume required or recommended by the equipment manufacturer, whichever is greater.

**12.4.6.10** Miscellaneous equipment and storage shall be protected as follows:

(1) Each projection room shall be provided with rewind and film storage facilities.
(2) Flammable liquids containers shall be permitted in projection rooms, provided that the following criteria are met:
  (a) There are not more than four containers per projection room.
  (b) No container has a capacity exceeding 16 oz (0.5 L).
  (c) The containers are of a nonbreakable type.
(3) Appurtenant electrical equipment, such as rheostats, transformers, and generators, shall be permitted to be located within the booth or in a separate room of equivalent construction.



**13.4.6.9.4.1 Electric Arc Projection Equipment.** The exhaust capacity shall be 200 $ft^3$/min (0.09 $m^3$/s) for each lamp connected to the lamp exhaust system or as recommended by the equipment manufacturer, and auxiliary air shall be permitted to be introduced into the system through a screened opening to stabilize the arc.

**13.4.6.9.4.2 Xenon Projection Equipment.** The lamp exhaust system shall exhaust not less than 300 $ft^3$/min (0.14 $m^3$/s) per lamp, or not less than the exhaust volume required or recommended by the equipment manufacturer, whichever is greater.

**13.4.6.10** Miscellaneous equipment and storage shall be protected as follows:

(1) Each projection room shall be provided with rewind and film storage facilities.
(2) Flammable liquids containers shall be permitted in projection rooms, provided that the following criteria are met:
  (a) There are not more than four containers per projection room.
  (b) No container has a capacity exceeding 16 oz (0.5 L).
  (c) The containers are of a nonbreakable type.
(3) Appurtenant electrical equipment, such as rheostats, transformers, and generators, shall be permitted to be located within the booth or in a separate room of equivalent construction.

The requirements for projection booths were developed jointly with those of NFPA 40, *Standard for the Storage and Handling of Cellulose Nitrate Film,*[17] and the motion picture industry when cellulose nitrate film was still being used. Although only safety film is now used (except at film festivals or revivals) and the risk level has been reduced, the primary function of the requirements of 12/13.4.6.3 is to enclose the projection booth, eliminating it as an exposure threat to the theater audience.

The intent of 12/13.4.6.3 is to protect the audience from the dangers associated with light sources, such as electric arc or xenon. Where incandescent light is used, projection booths are not required in assembly occupancies. Note that the booth is required based on the light source, not on the use of film.

The provisions of 12/13.4.6.4 apply only to projection booths for the use of cellulose acetate or other safety film. Although openings in the booth do not need to be protected, they must be provided with glass or other approved material that will completely close the opening and prevent gas, dust, or radiation from contaminating the audience seating area.

New projection equipment in new theaters has a console that draws air in at the floor and up through the projection machine, thus eliminating the need to provide ducts near the floor.

The requirements of 12/13.4.6.8 for the ventilation of a projection booth are designed to isolate the booth from the theater, so that any products of combustion created by a fire in a projection booth are not circulated into the theater. This isolation is achieved by providing an independent exhaust system for the booth, making certain that the exhaust outlet on the exterior of the building is located at a point where the air intake for the theater cannot recirculate the exhausted air.

If fresh air for the projection booth's ventilation system is supplied from the general system for the building, it is essential that the combined system be arranged to ensure the required air changes in the booth, even when no air is supplied to the general system of the building.

CHAPTER 12 • New

In 12/13.4.6.9.4, the *Code* specifies the minimum capacity for the exhaust system of a projection machine; however, a greater capacity must be provided where recommended by the manufacturer of the projection equipment. The system must be independent of any other ventilation system in the building housing the theater, but it can be combined with projection room ventilation.

**12.4.7* Special Amusement Buildings.**

**A.12.4.7** Where a special amusement building is installed inside another building, such as within an exhibit hall, the special amusement building requirements apply only to the special amusement building. For example, the smoke detectors required by 12.4.7.4 are not required to be connected to the building's system. Where installed in an exhibit hall, such smoke detectors are also required to comply with the provisions applicable to an exhibit.

**12.4.7.1* General.** Special amusement buildings, regardless of occupant load, shall meet the requirements for assembly occupancies in addition to the requirements of 12.4.7, unless the special amusement building is a multilevel play structure that is not more than 10 ft (3050 mm) in height and has aggregate horizontal projections not exceeding 160 ft$^2$ (15 m$^2$).

**A.12.4.7.1** The aggregate horizontal projections of a multilevel play structure are indicative of the number of children who might be within the structure and at risk from a fire or similar emergency. The word "aggregate" is used in recognition of the fact that the platforms and tubes that make up the multilevel play structure run above each other at various levels. In calculating the area of the projections, it is important to account for all areas that might be expected to be occupied within, on top of, or beneath the components of the structure when the structure is used for its intended function.

**12.4.7.2* Automatic Sprinklers.** Every special amusement building, other than buildings or structures not exceeding 10 ft (3050 mm) in height and not exceeding 160 ft$^2$ (15 m$^2$) in aggregate horizontal projection, shall be protected throughout by an approved, supervised automatic sprinkler system installed and maintained in accordance with Section 9.7.

**A.12.4.7.2** See A.12.4.7.1.

**12.4.7.3 Temporary Water Supply.** Where the special amusement building required to be sprinklered by 12.4.7.2 is movable or portable, the sprinkler water supply shall be permitted to be provided by an approved temporary means.

CHAPTER 13 • Existing

The requirement of 12/13.4.6.10 for the storage and rewinding of film is intended to prevent these operations from taking place outside the projection booth at some less protected location where, if a fire occurred, the exposure to the theater would be significantly greater. All operations that relate to projection activities must be kept within the protected enclosure afforded by the projection booth.

**13.4.7* Special Amusement Buildings.**

**A.13.4.7** Where a special amusement building is installed inside another building, such as within an exhibit hall, the special amusement building requirements apply only to the special amusement building. For example, the smoke detectors required by 13.4.7.4 are not required to be connected to the building's system. Where installed in an exhibit hall, such smoke detectors are also required to comply with the provisions applicable to an exhibit.

**13.4.7.1* General.** Special amusement buildings, regardless of occupant load, shall meet the requirements for assembly occupancies in addition to the requirements of 13.4.7, unless the special amusement building is a multilevel play structure that is not more than 10 ft (3050 mm) in height and has aggregate horizontal projections not exceeding 160 ft$^2$ (15 m$^2$).

**A.13.4.7.1** The aggregate horizontal projections of a multilevel play structure are indicative of the number of children who might be within the structure and at risk from a fire or similar emergency. The word "aggregate" is used in recognition of the fact that the platforms and tubes that make up the multilevel play structure run above each other at various levels. In calculating the area of the projections, it is important to account for all areas that might be expected to be occupied within, on top of, or beneath the components of the structure when the structure is used for its intended function.

**13.4.7.2* Automatic Sprinklers.** Every special amusement building, other than buildings or structures not exceeding 10 ft (3050 mm) in height and not exceeding 160 ft$^2$ (15 m$^2$) in aggregate horizontal projection, shall be protected throughout by an approved, supervised automatic sprinkler system installed and maintained in accordance with Section 9.7.

**A.13.4.7.2** See A.13.4.7.1.

**13.4.7.3 Temporary Water Supply.** Where the special amusement building required to be sprinklered by 13.4.7.2 is movable or portable, the sprinkler water supply shall be permitted to be provided by an approved temporary means.

CHAPTER 12 • New

**12.4.7.4 Smoke Detection.** Where the nature of the special amusement building is such that it operates in reduced lighting levels, the building shall be protected throughout by an approved automatic smoke detection system in accordance with Section 9.6.

**12.4.7.5 Alarm Initiation.** Actuation of any smoke detection system device shall sound an alarm at a constantly attended location on the premises.

**12.4.7.6 Illumination.** Actuation of the automatic sprinkler system, or any other suppression system, or actuation of a smoke detection system having an approved verification or cross-zoning operation capability shall provide for the following:

(1) Increase in illumination in the means of egress to that required by Section 7.8
(2) Termination of any conflicting or confusing sounds and visuals

**12.4.7.7 Exit Marking.**

**12.4.7.7.1** Exit marking shall be in accordance with Section 7.10.

**12.4.7.7.2** Floor proximity exit signs shall be provided in accordance with 7.10.1.6.

**12.4.7.7.3*** In special amusement buildings where mazes, mirrors, or other designs are used to confound the egress path, approved directional exit marking that becomes apparent in an emergency shall be provided.

**A.12.4.7.7.3** Consideration should be given to the provision of directional exit marking on or adjacent to the floor.

**12.4.7.8 Interior Finish.** Interior wall and ceiling finish materials complying with Section 10.2 shall be Class A throughout.

CHAPTER 13 • Existing

**13.4.7.4 Smoke Detection.** Where the nature of the special amusement building is such that it operates in reduced lighting levels, the building shall be protected throughout by an approved automatic smoke detection system in accordance with Section 9.6.

**13.4.7.5 Alarm Initiation.** Actuation of any smoke detection system device shall sound an alarm at a constantly attended location on the premises.

**13.4.7.6 Illumination.** Actuation of the automatic sprinkler system, or any other suppression system, or actuation of a smoke detection system having an approved verification or cross-zoning operation capability shall provide for the following:

(1) Increase in illumination in the means of egress to that required by Section 7.8
(2) Termination of any conflicting or confusing sounds and visuals

**13.4.7.7 Exit Marking.**

**13.4.7.7.1** Exit marking shall be in accordance with Section 7.10.

**13.4.7.7.2** Floor proximity exit signs shall be provided in accordance with 7.10.1.6.

**13.4.7.7.3*** In special amusement buildings where mazes, mirrors, or other designs are used to confound the egress path, approved directional exit marking that becomes apparent in an emergency shall be provided.

**A.13.4.7.7.3** Consideration should be given to the provision of directional exit marking on or adjacent to the floor.

**13.4.7.8 Interior Finish.** Interior wall and ceiling finish materials complying with Section 10.2 shall be Class A throughout.

Any special amusement building is considered an assembly occupancy, even if the occupant load is not more than 50 persons. However, special amusement buildings do not include theaters, movie houses, and other similar types of assembly occupancies.

Paragraph 12/13.4.7.6 addresses the importance of the exits and means of egress being well lighted upon the activation of a smoke detector or suppression system. It is also important that any conflicting or confusing sounds or visuals be stopped and that, where a person's relative position to an exit is changed, additional exit signs be provided.

In special amusement buildings, the provision of directions to an exit is particularly important. Floor proximity exit signs, as required by 12/13.4.7.7.2, should provide patrons an additional tool to assist them in finding their way out under emergency conditions.

## 12.4.8 Grandstands.

## 13.4.8 Grandstands.

The *Life Safety Code* provisions of 12/13.4.8 and 12/13.4.9, concerning bleacher or grandstand seating and folding or telescopic seating, were extracted over several *Code*-revision cycles from NFPA 102, *Standard*

CHAPTER 12 • New

*for Grandstands, Folding and Telescopic Seating, Tents, and Membrane Structures.*[18] In 2006, NFPA 102 was revised to become wholly an extracted-text document with almost all of its content extracted from this *Code* and *NFPA 5000, Building Construction and Safety Code.*[19]

**12.4.8.1 General.** Grandstands shall comply with the provisions of this chapter as modified by 12.4.8.

**12.4.8.2 Seating.**

**12.4.8.2.1** Where grandstand seating without backs is used indoors, rows of seats shall be spaced not less than 22 in. (560 mm) back-to-back.

**12.4.8.2.2** The depth of footboards and seat boards in grandstands shall be not less than 9 in. (230 mm); where the same level is not used for both seat foundations and footrests, footrests independent of seats shall be provided.

**12.4.8.2.3** Seats and footrests of grandstands shall be supported securely and fastened in such a manner that they cannot be displaced inadvertently.

**12.4.8.2.4** Individual seats or chairs shall be permitted only if secured in rows in an approved manner, unless seats do not exceed 16 in number and are located on level floors and within railed-in enclosures, such as boxes.

**12.4.8.2.5** The maximum number of seats permitted between the farthest seat and an aisle in grandstands and bleachers shall not exceed that shown in Table 12.4.8.2.5.

***Table 12.4.8.2.5 Maximum Number of Seats Between Farthest Seat and an Aisle***

| Application | Outdoors | Indoors |
|---|---|---|
| Grandstands | 11 | 6 |
| Bleachers *[See 12.2.5.6.1.2.]* | 20 | 9 |

**12.4.8.3 Special Requirements — Wood Grandstands.**

**12.4.8.3.1** An outdoor wood grandstand shall be erected within not less than two-thirds of its height, and, in no case, within not less than 10 ft (3050 mm), of a building, unless otherwise permitted by the following:

(1) The distance requirement shall not apply to buildings having minimum 1-hour fire resistance–rated construction with openings protected against the fire exposure hazard created by the grandstand.

CHAPTER 13 • Existing

**13.4.8.1 General.**

**13.4.8.1.1** Grandstands shall comply with the provisions of this chapter as modified by 13.4.8.

**13.4.8.1.2** Approved existing grandstands shall be permitted to be continued to be used.

**13.4.8.2 Seating.**

**13.4.8.2.1** Where grandstand seating without backs is used indoors, rows of seats shall be spaced not less than 22 in. (560 mm) back-to-back.

**13.4.8.2.2** The depth of footboards and seat boards in grandstands shall be not less than 9 in. (230 mm); where the same level is not used for both seat foundations and footrests, footrests independent of seats shall be provided.

**13.4.8.2.3** Seats and footrests of grandstands shall be supported securely and fastened in such a manner that they cannot be displaced inadvertently.

**13.4.8.2.4** Individual seats or chairs shall be permitted only if secured firmly in rows in an approved manner, unless seats do not exceed 16 in number and are located on level floors and within railed-in enclosures, such as boxes.

**13.4.8.2.5** The maximum number of seats permitted between the farthest seat and an aisle in grandstands and bleachers shall not exceed that shown in Table 13.4.8.2.5.

***Table 13.4.8.2.5 Maximum Number of Seats Between Farthest Seat and an Aisle***

| Application | Outdoors | Indoors |
|---|---|---|
| Grandstands | 11 | 6 |
| Bleachers *[See 13.2.5.6.1.2.]* | 20 | 9 |

**13.4.8.3 Special Requirements — Wood Grandstands.**

**13.4.8.3.1** An outdoor wood grandstand shall be erected within not less than two-thirds of its height, and, in no case, within not less than 10 ft (3050 mm), of a building, unless otherwise permitted by the following:

(1) The distance requirement shall not apply to buildings having minimum 1-hour fire resistance–rated construction with openings protected against the fire exposure hazard created by the grandstand.

CHAPTER 12 • New

(2) The distance requirement shall not apply where a wall having minimum 1-hour fire resistance–rated construction separates the grandstand from the building.

**12.4.8.3.2** An outdoor wood grandstand unit shall not exceed 10,000 ft$^2$ (929 m$^2$) in finished ground level area or 200 ft (61 m) in length, and the following requirements also shall apply:

(1) Grandstand units of the maximum size shall be placed not less than 20 ft (6100 mm) apart or shall be separated by walls having a minimum 1-hour fire resistance rating.
(2) The number of grandstand units erected in any one group shall not exceed three.
(3) Each group of grandstand units shall be separated from any other group by a wall having minimum 2-hour fire resistance–rated construction extending 24 in. (610 mm) above the seat platforms or by an open space of not less than 50 ft (15 m).

**12.4.8.3.3** The finished ground level area or length required by 12.4.8.3.2 shall be permitted to be doubled where one of the following criteria is met:

(1) Where the grandstand is constructed entirely of labeled fire-retardant-treated wood that has passed the standard rain test, ASTM D 2898, *Standard Test Methods for Accelerated Weathering of Fire-Retardant-Treated Wood for Fire Testing*
(2) Where the grandstand is constructed of members conforming to dimensions for heavy timber construction [Type IV (2HH)]

**12.4.8.3.4** The highest level of seat platforms above the finished ground level or the surface at the front of any wood grandstand shall not exceed 20 ft (6100 mm).

**12.4.8.3.5** The highest level of seat platforms above the finished ground level, or the surface at the front of a portable grandstand within a tent or membrane structure, shall not exceed 12 ft (3660 mm).

**12.4.8.3.6** The height requirements specified in 12.4.8.3.4 and 12.4.8.3.5 shall be permitted to be doubled where constructed entirely of labeled fire-retardant-treated wood that has passed the standard rain test, ASTM D 2898, *Standard Test Methods for Accelerated Weathering of Fire-Retardant-Treated Wood for Fire Testing*, or where constructed of members conforming to dimensions for heavy timber construction [Type IV (2HH)].

**12.4.8.4 Special Requirements — Portable Grandstands.**

**12.4.8.4.1** Portable grandstands shall conform to the requirements of 12.4.8 for grandstands and the requirements of 12.4.8.4.2 through 12.4.8.4.7.

CHAPTER 13 • Existing

(2) The distance requirement shall not apply where a wall having minimum 1-hour fire resistance–rated construction separates the grandstand from the building.

**13.4.8.3.2** An outdoor wood grandstand unit shall not exceed 10,000 ft$^2$ (929 m$^2$) in finished ground level area or 200 ft (61 m) in length, and the following requirements also shall apply:

(1) Grandstand units of the maximum size shall be placed not less than 20 ft (6100 mm) apart or shall be separated by walls having minimum 1-hour fire resistance rating.
(2) The number of grandstand units erected in any one group shall not exceed three.
(3) Each group of grandstand units shall be separated from any other group by a wall having minimum 2-hour fire resistance–rated construction extending 24 in. (610 mm) above the seat platforms or by an open space of not less than 50 ft (15 m).

**13.4.8.3.3** The finished ground level area or length required by 13.4.8.3.2 shall be permitted to be doubled where one of the following criteria is met:

(1) Where the grandstand is constructed entirely of labeled fire-retardant-treated wood that has passed the standard rain test, ASTM D 2898, *Standard Test Methods for Accelerated Weathering of Fire-Retardant-Treated Wood for Fire Testing*
(2) Where the grandstand is constructed of members conforming to dimensions for heavy timber construction [Type IV (2HH)]

**13.4.8.3.4** The highest level of seat platforms above the finished ground level or the surface at the front of any wood grandstand shall not exceed 20 ft (6100 mm).

**13.4.8.3.5** The highest level of seat platforms above the finished ground level, or the surface at the front of a portable grandstand within a tent or membrane structure, shall not exceed 12 ft (3660 mm).

**13.4.8.3.6** The height requirements specified in 13.4.8.3.4 and 13.4.8.3.5 shall be permitted to be doubled where the grandstand is constructed entirely of labeled fire-retardant-treated wood that has passed the standard rain test, ASTM D 2898, *Standard Test Methods for Accelerated Weathering of Fire-Retardant-Treated Wood for Fire Testing*, or where constructed of members conforming to dimensions for heavy timber construction [Type IV (2HH)].

**13.4.8.4 Special Requirements — Portable Grandstands.**

**13.4.8.4.1** Portable grandstands shall conform to the requirements of 13.4.8 for grandstands and the requirements of 13.4.8.4.2 through 13.4.8.4.7.

CHAPTER 12 • New

**12.4.8.4.2** Portable grandstands shall be self-contained and shall have within them all necessary parts to withstand and restrain all forces that might be developed during human occupancy.

**12.4.8.4.3** Portable grandstands shall be designed and manufactured so that, if any structural members essential to the strength and stability of the structure have been omitted during erection, the presence of unused connection fittings shall make the omissions self-evident.

**12.4.8.4.4** Portable grandstand construction shall be skillfully accomplished to produce the strength required by the design.

**12.4.8.4.5** Portable grandstands shall be provided with base plates, sills, floor runners, or sleepers of such area that the permitted bearing capacity of the supporting material is not exceeded.

**12.4.8.4.6** Where a portable grandstand rests directly on a base of such character that it is incapable of supporting the load without appreciable settlement, mud sills of suitable material, having sufficient area to prevent undue or dangerous settlement, shall be installed under base plates, runners, or sleepers.

**12.4.8.4.7** All bearing surfaces of portable grandstands shall be in contact with each other.

**12.4.8.5 Spaces Underneath Grandstands.** Spaces underneath a grandstand shall be kept free of flammable or combustible materials, unless protected by an approved, supervised automatic sprinkler system in accordance with Section 9.7 or unless otherwise permitted by the following:

(1) This requirement shall not apply to accessory uses of 300 $ft^2$ (28 $m^2$) or less, such as ticket booths, toilet facilities, or concession booths, where constructed of noncombustible or fire-resistive construction in otherwise nonsprinklered facilities.
(2) This requirement shall not apply to rooms that are enclosed in not less than 1-hour fire resistance–rated construction and are less than 1000 $ft^2$ (93 $m^2$) in otherwise nonsprinklered facilities.

**12.4.8.6 Guards and Railings.**

**12.4.8.6.1** Railings or guards not less than 42 in. (1065 mm) above the aisle surface or footrest or not less than 36 in. (915 mm) vertically above the center of the seat or seat board surface, whichever is adjacent, shall be provided along those portions of the backs and ends of all grandstands where the seats are more than 48 in. (1220 mm) above the floor or the finished ground level.

CHAPTER 13 • Existing

**13.4.8.4.2** Portable grandstands shall be self-contained and shall have within them all necessary parts to withstand and restrain all forces that might be developed during human occupancy.

**13.4.8.4.3** Portable grandstands shall be designed and manufactured so that, if any structural members essential to the strength and stability of the structure have been omitted during erection, the presence of unused connection fittings shall make the omissions self-evident.

**13.4.8.4.4** Portable grandstand construction shall be skillfully accomplished to produce the strength required by the design.

**13.4.8.4.5** Portable grandstands shall be provided with base plates, sills, floor runners, or sleepers of such area that the permitted bearing capacity of the supporting material is not exceeded.

**13.4.8.4.6** Where a portable grandstand rests directly on a base of such character that it is incapable of supporting the load without appreciable settlement, mud sills of suitable material, having sufficient area to prevent undue or dangerous settlement, shall be installed under base plates, runners, or sleepers.

**13.4.8.4.7** All bearing surfaces shall be in contact with each other.

**13.4.8.5 Spaces Underneath Grandstands.** Spaces underneath a grandstand shall be kept free of flammable or combustible materials, unless protected by an approved, supervised automatic sprinkler system in accordance with Section 9.7 or unless otherwise permitted by the following:

(1) This requirement shall not apply to accessory uses of 300 $ft^2$ (28 $m^2$) or less, such as ticket booths, toilet facilities, or concession booths, where constructed of noncombustible or fire-resistive construction in otherwise nonsprinklered facilities.
(2) This requirement shall not apply to rooms that are enclosed in not less than 1-hour fire resistance–rated construction and are less than 1000 $ft^2$ (93 $m^2$) in otherwise nonsprinklered facilities.

**13.4.8.6 Guards and Railings.**

**13.4.8.6.1** Railings or guards not less than 42 in. (1065 mm) above the aisle surface or footrest or not less than 36 in. (915 mm) vertically above the center of the seat or seat board surface, whichever is adjacent, shall be provided along those portions of the backs and ends of all grandstands where the seats are in excess of 48 in. (1220 mm) above the floor or the finished ground level.

CHAPTER 12 • New

**12.4.8.6.2** The requirement of 12.4.8.6.1 shall not apply where an adjacent wall or fence affords equivalent safeguard.

**12.4.8.6.3** Where the front footrest of any grandstand is more than 24 in. (610 mm) above the floor, railings or guards not less than 33 in. (825 mm) above such footrests shall be provided.

**12.4.8.6.4** The railings required by 12.4.8.6.3 shall be permitted to be not less than 26 in. (660 mm) high in grandstands or where the front row of seats includes backrests.

**12.4.8.6.5** Cross aisles located within the seating area shall be provided with rails not less than 26 in. (660 mm) high along the front edge of the cross aisle.

**12.4.8.6.6** The railings specified by 12.4.8.6.5 shall not be required where the backs of the seats in front of the cross aisle project 24 in. (610 mm) or more above the surface of the cross aisle.

**12.4.8.6.7** Vertical openings between guardrails and footboards or seat boards shall be provided with intermediate construction so that a 4 in. (100 mm) diameter sphere cannot pass through the opening.

**12.4.8.6.8** An opening between the seat board and footboard located more than 30 in. (760 mm) above the finished ground level shall be provided with intermediate construction so that a 4 in. (100 mm) diameter sphere cannot pass through the opening.

### 12.4.9 Folding and Telescopic Seating.

**12.4.9.1 General.** Folding and telescopic seating shall comply with the provisions of this chapter as modified by 12.4.9.

**12.4.9.2 Seating.**

**12.4.9.2.1** The horizontal distance of seats, measured back-to-back, shall be not less than 22 in. (560 mm) for seats without backs, and the following requirements shall also apply:

(1) There shall be a space of not less than 12 in. (305 mm) between the back of each seat and the front of each seat immediately behind it.
(2) If seats are of the chair type, the 12 in. (305 mm) dimension shall be measured to the front edge of the rear seat in its normal unoccupied position.
(3) All measurements shall be taken between plumb lines.

CHAPTER 13 • Existing

**13.4.8.6.2** The requirement of 13.4.8.6.1 shall not apply where an adjacent wall or fence affords equivalent safeguard.

**13.4.8.6.3** Where the front footrest of any grandstand is more than 24 in. (610 mm) above the floor, railings or guards not less than 33 in. (825 mm) above such footrests shall be provided.

**13.4.8.6.4** The railings required by 13.4.8.6.3 shall be permitted to be not less than 26 in. (660 mm) high in grandstands or where the front row of seats includes backrests.

**13.4.8.6.5** Cross aisles located within the seating area shall be provided with rails not less than 26 in. (660 mm) high along the front edge of the cross aisle.

**13.4.8.6.6** The railings specified by 13.4.8.6.5 shall not be required where the backs of the seats in front of the cross aisle project 24 in. (610 mm) or more above the surface of the cross aisle.

**13.4.8.6.7** Vertical openings between guardrails and footboards or seat boards shall be provided with intermediate construction so that a 4 in. (100 mm) diameter sphere cannot pass through the opening.

**13.4.8.6.8** An opening between the seat board and footboard located more than 30 in. (760 mm) above the finished ground level shall be provided with intermediate construction so that a 4 in. (100 mm) diameter sphere cannot pass through the opening.

### 13.4.9 Folding and Telescopic Seating.

**13.4.9.1 General.**

**13.4.9.1.1** Folding and telescopic seating shall comply with the provisions of this chapter as modified by 13.4.9.

**13.4.9.1.2** Approved existing folding and telescopic seating shall be permitted to be continued to be used.

**13.4.9.2 Seating.**

**13.4.9.2.1** The horizontal distance of seats, measured back-to-back, shall be not less than 22 in. (560 mm) for seats without backs, and the following requirements shall also apply:

(1) There shall be a space of not less than 12 in. (305 mm) between the back of each seat and the front of each seat immediately behind it.
(2) If seats are of the chair type, the 12 in. (305 mm) dimension shall be measured to the front edge of the rear seat in its normal unoccupied position.
(3) All measurements shall be taken between plumb lines.

CHAPTER 12 • New

**12.4.9.2.2** The depth of footboards (footrests) and seat boards in folding and telescopic seating shall be not less than 9 in. (230 mm).

**12.4.9.2.3** Where the same level is not used for both seat foundations and footrests, footrests independent of seats shall be provided.

**12.4.9.2.4** Individual chair-type seats shall be permitted in folding and telescopic seating only if firmly secured in groups of not less than three.

**12.4.9.2.5** The maximum number of seats permitted between the farthest seat in an aisle in folding and telescopic seating shall not exceed that shown in Table 12.4.8.2.5.

**12.4.9.3 Guards and Railings.**

**12.4.9.3.1** Railings or guards not less than 42 in. (1065 mm) above the aisle surface or footrest, or not less than 36 in. (915 mm) vertically above the center of the seat or seat board surface, whichever is adjacent, shall be provided along those portions of the backs and ends of all folding and telescopic seating where the seats are more than 48 in. (1220 mm) above the floor or the finished ground level.

**12.4.9.3.2** The requirement of 12.4.9.3.1 shall not apply where an adjacent wall or fence affords equivalent safeguard.

**12.4.9.3.3** Where the front footrest of folding or telescopic seating is more than 24 in. (610 mm) above the floor, railings or guards not less than 33 in. (825 mm) above such footrests shall be provided.

**12.4.9.3.4** The railings required by 12.4.9.3.3 shall be permitted to be not less than 26 in. (660 mm) high where the front row of seats includes backrests.

**12.4.9.3.5** Cross aisles located within the seating area shall be provided with rails not less than 26 in. (660 mm) high along the front edge of the cross aisle.

**12.4.9.3.6** The railings specified by 12.4.9.3.5 shall not be required where the backs of the seats in front of the cross aisle project 24 in. (610 mm) or more above the surface of the cross aisle.

**12.4.9.3.7** Vertical openings between guardrails and footboards or seat boards shall be provided with intermediate construction so that a 4 in. (100 mm) diameter sphere cannot pass through the opening.

**12.4.9.3.8** An opening between the seat board and footboard located more than 30 in. (760 mm) above the finished ground level shall be provided with intermediate construction so that a 4 in. (100 mm) diameter sphere cannot pass through the opening.

CHAPTER 13 • Existing

**13.4.9.2.2** The depth of footboards (footrests) and seat boards in folding and telescopic seating shall be not less than 9 in. (230 mm).

**13.4.9.2.3** Where the same level is not used for both seat foundations and footrests, footrests independent of seats shall be provided.

**13.4.9.2.4** Individual chair-type seats shall be permitted in folding and telescopic seating only if firmly secured in groups of not less than three.

**13.4.9.2.5** The maximum number of seats permitted between the farthest seat in an aisle in folding and telescopic seating shall not exceed that shown in Table 13.4.8.2.5.

**13.4.9.3 Guards and Railings.**

**13.4.9.3.1** Railings or guards not less than 42 in. (1065 mm) above the aisle surface or footrest, or not less than 36 in. (915 mm) vertically above the center of the seat or seat board surface, whichever is adjacent, shall be provided along those portions of the backs and ends of all folding and telescopic seating where the seats are more than 48 in. (1220 mm) above the floor or the finished ground level.

**13.4.9.3.2** The requirement of 13.4.9.3.1 shall not apply where an adjacent wall or fence affords equivalent safeguard.

**13.4.9.3.3** Where the front footrest of folding or telescopic seating is more than 24 in. (610 mm) above the floor, railings or guards not less than 33 in. (825 mm) above such footrests shall be provided.

**13.4.9.3.4** The railings required by 13.4.9.3.3 shall be permitted to be not less than 26 in. (660 mm) high where the front row of seats includes backrests.

**13.4.9.3.5** Cross aisles located within the seating area shall be provided with rails not less than 26 in. (660 mm) high along the front edge of the cross aisle.

**13.4.9.3.6** The railings specified by 13.4.9.3.5 shall not be required where the backs of the seats in front of the cross aisle project 24 in. (610 mm) or more above the surface of the cross aisle.

**13.4.9.3.7** Vertical openings between guardrails and footboards or seat boards shall be provided with intermediate construction so that a 4 in. (100 mm) diameter sphere cannot pass through the opening.

**13.4.9.3.8** An opening between the seat board and footboard located more than 30 in. (760 mm) above the finished ground level shall be provided with intermediate construction so that a 4 in. (100 mm) diameter sphere cannot pass through the opening.

CHAPTER 12 • New

### 12.4.10 Airport Loading Walkways.

**12.4.10.1** Airport loading walkways shall conform to NFPA 415, *Standard on Airport Terminal Buildings, Fueling Ramp Drainage, and Loading Walkways*, and the provisions of 12.4.10.2 and 12.4.10.3.

**12.4.10.2** Doors in the egress path from the aircraft through the airport loading walkway into the airport terminal building shall meet the following criteria:

(1) They shall swing in the direction of egress from the aircraft.
(2)* They shall not be permitted to have delayed-egress locks.

**A.12.4.10.2(2)** Delayed-egress locks on doors from the airport loading walkway into the airport terminal building might compromise life safety due to the limited period of time the airport loading walkway will provide protection for emergency egress. The requirement of 12.4.10.2(2) would not limit the use of access-controlled or delayed-egress hardware from the airport terminal building into the airport loading walkway.

**12.4.10.3** Exit access shall be unimpeded from the airport loading walkway to the nonsecured public areas of the airport terminal building.

CHAPTER 13 • Existing

### 13.4.10 Airport Loading Walkways.

**13.4.10.1** Airport loading walkways shall conform to NFPA 415, *Standard on Airport Terminal Buildings, Fueling Ramp Drainage, and Loading Walkways*, and the provisions of 13.4.10.2 and 13.4.10.3.

**13.4.10.2** Doors in the egress path from the aircraft through the airport loading walkway into the airport terminal building shall meet the following criteria:

(1) They shall swing in the direction of egress from the aircraft.
(2)* They shall not be permitted to have delayed-egress locks.

**A.13.4.10.2(2)** Delayed-egress locks on doors from the airport loading walkway into the airport terminal building might compromise life safety due to the limited period of time the airport loading walkway will provide protection for emergency egress. The requirement of 13.4.10.2(2) would not limit the use of access-controlled or delayed-egress hardware from the airport terminal building into the airport loading walkway.

**13.4.10.3** Exit access shall be unimpeded from the airport loading walkway to the nonsecured public areas of the airport terminal building.

Subsection 12/13.4.10 on airport loading walkways addresses situations unique to airport terminal buildings that present challenges to life safety. Most doors from the airport terminal building to the aircraft loading walkways are not part of the means of egress for occupants of the terminal building, but this does not mean such doors can go unregulated. In most buildings, the egress system functions by getting building occupants to the outside at the public way. At airport terminals, occupants of the loading walkways might be ensured safety only if provided with re-entry into the building, since the fire threat might be outside on the tarmac, as in the case of a spilled fuel fire. The criteria specified in 12/13.4.10 supplement the other provisions of Chapters 12 and 13 to help provide a complete protection package.

## 12.5 Building Services

### 12.5.1 Utilities.

Utilities shall comply with the provisions of Section 9.1.

### 12.5.2 Heating, Ventilating, and Air-Conditioning Equipment.

Heating, ventilating, and air-conditioning equipment shall comply with the provisions of Section 9.2.

### 12.5.3 Elevators, Escalators, and Conveyors.

Elevators, escalators, and conveyors shall comply with the provisions of Section 9.4.

## 13.5 Building Services

### 13.5.1 Utilities.

Utilities shall comply with the provisions of Section 9.1.

### 13.5.2 Heating, Ventilating, and Air-Conditioning Equipment.

Heating, ventilating, and air-conditioning equipment shall comply with the provisions of Section 9.2.

### 13.5.3 Elevators, Escalators, and Conveyors.

Elevators, escalators, and conveyors shall comply with the provisions of Section 9.4.

### 12.5.4 Rubbish Chutes, Incinerators, and Laundry Chutes.

Rubbish chutes, incinerators, and laundry chutes shall comply with the provisions of Section 9.5.

## 12.6 Reserved

## 12.7 Operating Features

### 12.7.1 Means of Egress Inspection.

**12.7.1.1** The building owner or agent shall inspect the means of egress to ensure it is maintained free of obstructions, and correct any deficiencies found, prior to each opening of the building to the public.

**12.7.1.2** The building owner or agent shall prepare and maintain records of the date and time of each inspection on approved forms, listing any deficiencies found and actions taken to correct them.

**12.7.1.3 Inspection of Door Openings.** Door openings shall be inspected in accordance with 7.2.1.15.



### 13.5.4 Rubbish Chutes, Incinerators, and Laundry Chutes.

Rubbish chutes, incinerators, and laundry chutes shall comply with the provisions of Section 9.5.

## 13.6 Reserved

## 13.7 Operating Features

### 13.7.1 Means of Egress Inspection.

**13.7.1.1** The building owner or agent shall inspect the means of egress to ensure it is maintained free of obstructions, and correct any deficiencies found, prior to each opening of the building to the public.

**13.7.1.2** The building owner or agent shall prepare and maintain records of the date and time of each inspection on approved forms, listing any deficiencies found and actions taken to correct them.

**13.7.1.3 Inspection of Door Openings.** Door openings shall be inspected in accordance with 7.2.1.15.

The means of egress features required by Chapters 12 and 13 cannot be ensured to be effective unless maintained. The requirement for inspection and correction of the deficiencies found helps to keep the means of egress features usable. The required record keeping serves as an enforcement tool for the authority having jurisdiction (AHJ) to help ensure such inspection is conducted as specified.

The provision of 12/13.7.1.3 for the inspection of door openings is new to the 2009 edition of the *Code*. The criteria of 7.2.1.15 are formatted to apply only where specifically required by another portion of the *Code*. The inspection requirements apply to doors that are required to swing in the direction of egress travel. Door leaves that are required to swing in the direction of egress travel include those from spaces with an occupant load of 50 or more persons [see 7.2.1.4.2(1)] and those used in an exit enclosure [see 7.2.1.4.2(2)]. This application threshold was chosen to help ensure that the egress doors used most frequently on a normal day-to-day basis and those designed to accommodate larger numbers of occupants under emergency egress or relocation are inspected and tested. Door leaves that get used frequently are more apt to experience wear that adversely affects operability and leads to failure. Door leaves that are infrequently used, like those into exit stair enclosures in high-rise buildings, might be misaligned within their frames so as to be difficult to open within the operating forces requirements of 7.2.1.4.5. The door inspection and testing criteria of 7.2.1.15 are intended to help identify problems with door openings and ensure that such problems are remedied. See 7.2.1.15.

### 12.7.2 Special Provisions for Food Service Operations.

**12.7.2.1** All devices in connection with the preparation of food shall be installed and operated to avoid hazard to the safety of occupants.

### 13.7.2 Special Provisions for Food Service Operations.

**13.7.2.1** All devices in connection with the preparation of food shall be installed and operated to avoid hazard to the safety of occupants.

CHAPTER 12 • New

12.7.2.2 All devices in connection with the preparation of food shall be of an approved type and shall be installed in an approved manner.

12.7.2.3 Food preparation facilities shall be protected in accordance with 9.2.3 and shall not be required to have openings protected between food preparation areas and dining areas.

12.7.2.4 Portable cooking equipment that is not flue-connected shall be permitted only as follows:

(1) Equipment fueled by small heat sources that can be readily extinguished by water, such as candles or alcohol-burning equipment, including solid alcohol, shall be permitted to be used, provided that precautions satisfactory to the authority having jurisdiction are taken to prevent ignition of any combustible materials.
(2) Candles shall be permitted to be used on tables used for food service where securely supported on substantial noncombustible bases located to avoid danger of ignition of combustible materials and only where approved by the authority having jurisdiction.
(3) Candle flames shall be protected.
(4) "Flaming sword" or other equipment involving open flames and flamed dishes, such as cherries jubilee or crêpes suzette, shall be permitted to be used, provided that precautions subject to the approval of the authority having jurisdiction are taken.
(5)* Listed and approved LP-Gas commercial food service appliances shall be permitted to be used where in accordance with NFPA 58, *Liquefied Petroleum Gas Code*.

A.12.7.2.4(5) NFPA 58, *Liquefied Petroleum Gas Code*, permits portable butane-fueled appliances in restaurants and in attended commercial food catering operations where fueled by not more than two 10 oz (0.3 L) LP-Gas capacity, nonrefillable butane containers that have a water capacity not exceeding 1.08 lb (0.5 kg) per container. The containers are required to be directly connected to the appliance, and manifolding of containers is not permitted. Storage of cylinders is also limited to 24 containers, with an additional 24 permitted where protected by a 2-hour fire resistance–rated barrier.

CHAPTER 13 • Existing

13.7.2.2 All devices in connection with the preparation of food shall be of an approved type and shall be installed in an approved manner.

13.7.2.3 Food preparation facilities shall be protected in accordance with 9.2.3 and shall not be required to have openings protected between food preparation areas and dining areas.

13.7.2.4 Portable cooking equipment that is not flue-connected shall be permitted only as follows:

(1) Equipment fueled by small heat sources that can be readily extinguished by water, such as candles or alcohol-burning equipment, including solid alcohol, shall be permitted to be used, provided that precautions satisfactory to the authority having jurisdiction are taken to prevent ignition of any combustible materials.
(2) Candles shall be permitted to be used on tables used for food service where securely supported on substantial noncombustible bases located to avoid danger of ignition of combustible materials and only where approved by the authority having jurisdiction.
(3) Candle flames shall be protected.
(4) "Flaming sword" or other equipment involving open flames and flamed dishes, such as cherries jubilee or crépe suzette, shall be permitted to be used, provided that precautions subject to the approval of the authority having jurisdiction are taken.
(5)* Listed and approved LP-Gas commercial food service appliances shall be permitted to be used where in accordance with NFPA 58, *Liquefied Petroleum Gas Code*.

A.13.7.2.4(5) NFPA 58, *Liquefied Petroleum Gas Code*, permits portable butane-fueled appliances in restaurants and in attended commercial food catering operations where fueled by not in excess of two 10 oz (0.3 L) LP-Gas capacity, nonrefillable butane containers that have a water capacity not exceeding 1.08 lb (0.5 kg) per container. The containers are required to be directly connected to the appliance, and manifolding of containers is not permitted. Storage of cylinders is also limited to 24 containers, with an additional 24 permitted where protected by a 2-hour fire resistance–rated barrier.

An approved type of device, as required by 12/13.7.2.2, is one that, with regard to potential fire hazards, is acceptable to the authority having jurisdiction (AHJ). An "approved manner" of installation means installation acceptable to the AHJ.

The *Code* depends on the automatic extinguishing system mandated by 9.2.3 to control any fire on the cooking surfaces, and, thus, 12/13.7.2.3 does not require enclosure by rated construction.

The list of tragic fires in assembly occupancies caused by "friendly" fire (e.g., alcohol or solid alcohol fires in restaurants, flames used for dramatic effects in theaters) is well documented. The requirements of 12/13.7.2.4 and 12/13.7.3 attempt to prevent a fire by tightly controlling the use of open flame devices.

CHAPTER 12 • New

### 12.7.3 Open Flame Devices and Pyrotechnics.

No open flame devices or pyrotechnic devices shall be used in any assembly occupancy, unless otherwise permitted by the following:

(1) Pyrotechnic special effect devices shall be permitted to be used on stages before proximate audiences for ceremonial or religious purposes, as part of a demonstration in exhibits, or as part of a performance, provided that both of the following criteria are met:
   (a) Precautions satisfactory to the authority having jurisdiction are taken to prevent ignition of any combustible material.
   (b) Use of the pyrotechnic device complies with NFPA 1126, *Standard for the Use of Pyrotechnics Before a Proximate Audience.*
(2) Flame effects before an audience shall be permitted in accordance with NFPA 160, *Standard for the Use of Flame Effects Before an Audience.*
(3) Open flame devices shall be permitted to be used in the following situations, provided that precautions satisfactory to the authority having jurisdiction are taken to prevent ignition of any combustible material or injury to occupants:
   (a)* For ceremonial or religious purposes

**A.12.7.3(3)(a)** Securely supported altar candles in churches that are well separated from any combustible material are permitted. On the other hand, lighted candles carried by children wearing cotton robes present a hazard too great to be permitted. There are many other situations of intermediate hazard where the authority having jurisdiction will have to exercise judgment.

   (b) On stages and platforms where part of a performance
   (c) Where candles on tables are securely supported on substantial noncombustible bases and candle flame is protected
(4) The requirement of 12.7.3 shall not apply to heat-producing equipment complying with 9.2.2.
(5) The requirement of 12.7.3 shall not apply to food service operations in accordance with 12.7.2.
(6) Gas lights shall be permitted to be used, provided that precautions are taken, subject to the approval of the authority having jurisdiction, to prevent ignition of any combustible materials.

### 12.7.4 Furnishings, Decorations, and Scenery.

**12.7.4.1** Fabrics and films used for decorative purposes, all draperies and curtains, and similar furnishings shall be in accordance with the provisions of 10.3.1.

CHAPTER 13 • Existing

### 13.7.3 Open Flame Devices and Pyrotechnics.

No open flame devices or pyrotechnic devices shall be used in any assembly occupancy, unless otherwise permitted by the following:

(1) Pyrotechnic special effect devices shall be permitted to be used on stages before proximate audiences for ceremonial or religious purposes, as part of a demonstration in exhibits, or as part of a performance, provided that both of the following criteria are met:
   (a) Precautions satisfactory to the authority having jurisdiction are taken to prevent ignition of any combustible material.
   (b) Use of the pyrotechnic device complies with NFPA 1126, *Standard for the Use of Pyrotechnics Before a Proximate Audience.*
(2) Flame effects before an audience shall be permitted in accordance with NFPA 160, *Standard for the Use of Flame Effects Before an Audience.*
(3) Open flame devices shall be permitted to be used in the following situations, provided that precautions satisfactory to the authority having jurisdiction are taken to prevent ignition of any combustible material or injury to occupants:
   (a)* For ceremonial or religious purposes

**A.13.7.3(3)(a)** Securely supported altar candles in churches that are well separated from any combustible material, are permitted. On the other hand, lighted candles carried by children wearing cotton robes present a hazard too great to be permitted. There are many other situations of intermediate hazard where the authority having jurisdiction will have to exercise judgment.

   (b) On stages and platforms where part of a performance
   (c) Where candles on tables are securely supported on substantial noncombustible bases and candle flame is protected
(4) The requirement of 13.7.3 shall not apply to heat-producing equipment complying with 9.2.2.
(5) The requirement of 13.7.3 shall not apply to food service operations in accordance with 13.7.2.
(6) Gas lights shall be permitted to be used, provided that precautions are taken, subject to the approval of authority having jurisdiction, to prevent ignition of any combustible materials.

### 13.7.4 Furnishings, Decorations, and Scenery.

**13.7.4.1** Fabrics and films used for decorative purposes, all draperies and curtains, and similar furnishings shall be in accordance with the provisions of 10.3.1.

CHAPTER 12 • New

**12.7.4.2** The authority having jurisdiction shall impose controls on the quantity and arrangement of combustible contents in assembly occupancies to provide an adequate level of safety to life from fire.

**12.7.4.3*** Exposed foamed plastic materials and unprotected materials containing foamed plastic used for decorative purposes or stage scenery shall have a heat release rate not exceeding 100 kW where tested in accordance with ANSI/UL 1975, *Standard for Fire Tests for Foamed Plastics Used for Decorative Purposes.*

**A.12.7.4.3** The phrase "unprotected materials containing foamed plastic" is meant to include foamed plastic items covered by "thermally thin" combustible fabrics or paint. *(See A.10.2.3.4.)*

**12.7.4.4** The requirement of 12.7.4.3 shall not apply to individual foamed plastic items and items containing foamed plastic where the foamed plastic does not exceed 1 lb (0.45 kg) in weight.

### 12.7.5 Special Provisions for Exposition Facilities.

**12.7.5.1 General.** No display or exhibit shall be installed or operated to interfere in any way with access to any required exit or with the visibility of any required exit or required exit sign; nor shall any display block access to fire-fighting equipment.

**12.7.5.2 Materials Not On Display.** A storage room having an enclosure consisting of a smoke barrier having a minimum 1-hour fire resistance rating and protected by an automatic extinguishing system shall be provided for combustible materials not on display, including combustible packing crates used to ship exhibitors' supplies and products.

CHAPTER 13 • Existing

**13.7.4.2** The authority having jurisdiction shall impose controls on the quantity and arrangement of combustible contents in assembly occupancies to provide an adequate level of safety to life from fire.

**13.7.4.3*** Exposed foamed plastic materials and unprotected materials containing foamed plastic used for decorative purposes or stage scenery shall have a heat release rate not exceeding 100 kW where tested in accordance with ANSI/UL 1975, *Standard for Fire Tests for Foamed Plastics Used for Decorative Purposes.*

**A.13.7.4.3** The phrase "unprotected materials containing foamed plastic" is meant to include foamed plastic items covered by "thermally thin" combustible fabrics or paint. *(See A.10.2.3.4.)*

**13.7.4.4** The requirement of 13.7.4.3 shall not apply to individual foamed plastic items and items containing foamed plastic where the foamed plastic does not exceed 1 lb (0.45 kg) in weight.

### 13.7.5 Special Provisions for Exposition Facilities.

**13.7.5.1 General.** No display or exhibit shall be installed or operated to interfere in any way with access to any required exit or with the visibility of any required exit or required exit sign; nor shall any display block access to fire-fighting equipment.

**13.7.5.2 Materials Not on Display.** A storage room having an enclosure consisting of a smoke barrier having a minimum 1-hour fire resistance rating and protected by an automatic extinguishing system shall be provided for combustible materials not on display, including combustible packing crates used to ship exhibitors' supplies and products.

Exposition facilities have problems that differ from those of theaters, restaurants, or other assembly occupancies. They are generally large, multi-use facilities with high ceilings appropriate to their size. Combustible materials are frequently displayed, and the containers in which the exhibits are shipped contribute to the fuel load. Due to the size of exhibition halls, most are required by 12/13.1.6 and 12/13.3.5.2 to be protected by automatic sprinklers.

The authority having jurisdiction (AHJ) at the local level is often working with organizations that exhibit on a national basis and that are unaware of the local fire safety regulations. It is the intent that this *Code* provide the more consistent and universal treatment needed in these occupancies and, at the same time, encourage more uniform enforcement practices.

Prior to the inclusion of 12/13.7.5, the trade show and exposition hall regulations used by many jurisdictions were very similar; however, there was no nationally recognized model code that could be referenced. This lack of a model code presented a hardship, as well as confusion between the local AHJ and persons responsible for the various functions of the trade show or exposition.

To meet the intent of 12/13.7.5.1, it is advisable to have prepared plans or diagrams to show the arrangement of displays or exhibits, including any that are to be suspended from the ceiling or housed within an overhead structure. Displays or exhibits must not interfere with access to any required exit, and they must not conceal exit signs. See Exhibit 12/13.39. A display should not block access to fire-fighting equipment or

CHAPTER 12 • New

CHAPTER 13 • Existing

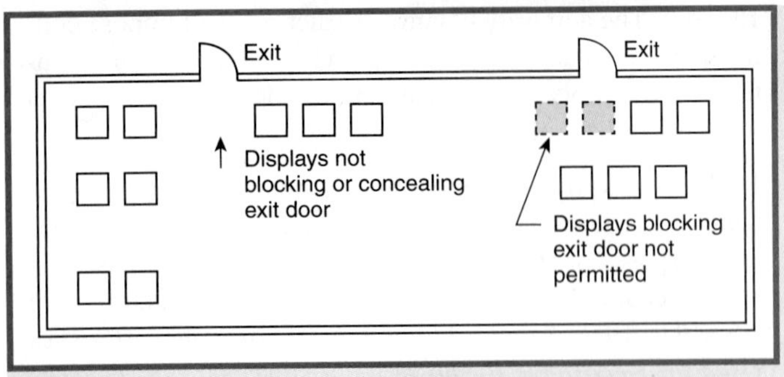


*Exhibit 12/13.39 Arrangement of displays in an exhibition hall.*

interfere with the normal operation of automatic extinguishing equipment or devices for smoke evacuation.

Aisles serving rows of booths are exit accesses; therefore, booths and other temporary construction should be of minimal combustible construction or should be protected to avoid undue hazard of fire that might endanger occupants before they can reach available exits.

Displays or exhibits of combustible material must be limited in quantity to reduce the fuel load to an acceptable level. In accordance with 12/13.7.5.2, excess combustible display material and all other combustible materials that are not in use should be kept in a separate storage room until needed. A separation with a fire resistance rating of 1 hour is required between such a storage room and all other parts of the building, and the room must be protected by an automatic sprinkler system.

**12.7.5.3 Exhibits.**

**12.7.5.3.1** Exhibits shall comply with 12.7.5.3.2 through 12.7.5.3.11.

**12.7.5.3.2** The travel distance within the exhibit booth or exhibit enclosure to an exit access aisle shall not exceed 50 ft (15 m).

**12.7.5.3.3** The upper deck of multilevel exhibits exceeding 300 ft$^2$ (28 m$^2$) shall have not less than two remote means of egress.

**12.7.5.3.4** Exhibit booths shall be constructed of the following:

(1) Noncombustible or limited-combustible materials
(2) Wood exceeding $^1/_4$ in. (6.3 mm) nominal thickness
(3) Wood that is pressure-treated, fire-retardant wood meeting the requirements of NFPA 703, *Standard for Fire Retardant–Treated Wood and Fire-Retardant Coatings for Building Materials*
(4) Flame-retardant materials complying with NFPA 701, *Standard Methods of Fire Tests for Flame Propagation of Textiles and Films*
(5) Textile wall coverings, such as carpeting and similar products used as wall or ceiling finishes, complying with the provisions of 10.2.2 and 10.2.4
(6) Plastics limited to those that comply with 12.3.3 and Section 10.2
(7) Foamed plastics and materials containing foamed plastics having a heat release rate for any single fuel package that does not exceed 100 kW where tested in accordance with ANSI/UL 1975, *Standard for Fire Tests for Foamed Plastics Used for Decorative Purposes*

**13.7.5.3 Exhibits.**

**13.7.5.3.1** Exhibits shall comply with 13.7.5.3.2 through 13.7.5.3.11.

**13.7.5.3.2** The travel distance within the exhibit booth or exhibit enclosure to an exit access aisle shall not exceed 50 ft (15 m).

**13.7.5.3.3** The upper deck of multilevel exhibits exceeding 300 ft$^2$ (28 m$^2$) shall have not less than two remote means of egress.

**13.7.5.3.4** Exhibit booths shall be constructed of the following:

(1) Noncombustible or limited-combustible materials
(2) Wood exceeding $^1/_4$ in. (6.3 mm) nominal thickness
(3) Wood that is pressure-treated, fire-retardant wood meeting the requirements of NFPA 703, *Standard for Fire Retardant–Treated Wood and Fire-Retardant Coatings for Building Materials*
(4) Flame-retardant materials complying with NFPA 701, *Standard Methods of Fire Tests for Flame Propagation of Textiles and Films*
(5) Textile wall coverings, such as carpeting and similar products used as wall or ceiling finishes, complying with the provisions of 10.2.2 and 10.2.4
(6) Plastics limited to those that comply with 13.3.3 and Section 10.2
(7) Foamed plastics and materials containing foamed plastics having a heat release rate for any single fuel package that does not exceed 100 kW where tested in accordance with ANSI/UL 1975, *Standard for Fire Tests for Foamed Plastics Used for Decorative Purposes*

CHAPTER 12 • New

(8) Cardboard, honeycombed paper, and other combustible materials having a heat release rate for any single fuel package that does not exceed 150 kW where tested in accordance with ANSI/UL 1975

**12.7.5.3.5** Curtains, drapes, and decorations shall comply with 10.3.1.

**12.7.5.3.6** Acoustical and decorative material including, but not limited to, cotton, hay, paper, straw, moss, split bamboo, and wood chips shall be flame-retardant treated to the satisfaction of the authority having jurisdiction.

**12.7.5.3.6.1** Materials that cannot be treated for flame retardancy shall not be used.

**12.7.5.3.6.2** Foamed plastics, and materials containing foamed plastics and used as decorative objects such as, but not limited to, mannequins, murals, and signs shall have a heat release rate for any single fuel package that does not exceed 150 kW where tested in accordance with ANSI/UL 1975, *Standard for Fire Tests for Foamed Plastics Used for Decorative Purposes*.

**12.7.5.3.6.3** Where the aggregate area of acoustical and decorative materials is less than 10 percent of the individual floor or wall area, such materials shall be permitted to be used subject to the approval of the authority having jurisdiction.

**12.7.5.3.7** The following shall be protected by automatic extinguishing systems:

(1) Single-level exhibit booths exceeding 300 $ft^2$ (28 $m^2$) and covered with a ceiling
(2) Each level of multilevel exhibit booths, including the uppermost level where the uppermost level is covered with a ceiling

**12.7.5.3.7.1** The requirements of 12.7.5.3.7 shall not apply where otherwise permitted by the following:

(1) Ceilings that are constructed of open grate design or listed dropout ceilings in accordance with NFPA 13, *Standard for the Installation of Sprinkler Systems*, shall not be considered ceilings within the context of 12.7.5.3.7.
(2) Vehicles, boats, and similar exhibited products having over 100 $ft^2$ (9.3 $m^2$) of roofed area shall be provided with smoke detectors acceptable to the authority having jurisdiction.
(3)* The requirement of 12.7.5.3.7(2) shall not apply where fire protection of multilevel exhibit booths is consistent with the criteria developed through a life safety evaluation of the exhibition hall in accordance with 12.4.1, subject to approval of the authority having jurisdiction.

CHAPTER 13 • Existing

(8) Cardboard, honeycombed paper, and other combustible materials having a heat release rate for any single fuel package that does not exceed 150 kW where tested in accordance with ANSI/UL 1975

**13.7.5.3.5** Curtains, drapes, and decorations shall comply with 10.3.1.

**13.7.5.3.6** Acoustical and decorative material including, but not limited to, cotton, hay, paper, straw, moss, split bamboo, and wood chips shall be flame-retardant treated to the satisfaction of the authority having jurisdiction.

**13.7.5.3.6.1** Materials that cannot be treated for flame retardancy shall not be used.

**13.7.5.3.6.2** Foamed plastics, and materials containing foamed plastics and used as decorative objects such as, but not limited to, mannequins, murals, and signs shall have a heat release rate for any single fuel package that does not exceed 150 kW where tested in accordance with ANSI/UL 1975, *Standard for Fire Tests for Foamed Plastics Used for Decorative Purposes*.

**13.7.5.3.6.3** Where the aggregate area of acoustical and decorative materials is less than 10 percent of the individual floor or wall area, such materials shall be permitted to be used subject to the approval of the authority having jurisdiction.

**13.7.5.3.7** The following shall be protected by automatic extinguishing systems:

(1) Single-level exhibit booths exceeding 300 $ft^2$ (28 $m^2$) and covered with a ceiling
(2) Each level of multilevel exhibit booths, including the uppermost level where the uppermost level is covered with a ceiling

**13.7.5.3.7.1** The requirements of 13.7.5.3.7 shall not apply where otherwise permitted by the following:

(1) Ceilings that are constructed of open grate design or listed dropout ceilings in accordance with NFPA 13, *Standard for the Installation of Sprinkler Systems*, shall not be considered ceilings within the context of 13.7.5.3.7.
(2) Vehicles, boats, and similar exhibited products having over 100 $ft^2$ (9.3 $m^2$) of roofed area shall be provided with smoke detectors acceptable to the authority having jurisdiction.
(3)* The requirement of 13.7.5.3.7(2) shall not apply where fire protection of multilevel exhibit booths is consistent with the criteria developed through a life safety evaluation of the exhibition hall in accordance with 13.4.1, subject to approval of the authority having jurisdiction.

CHAPTER 12 • New

**A.12.7.5.3.7.1(3)** See A.12.4.1.1.

**12.7.5.3.7.2** A single exhibit or group of exhibits with ceilings that do not require sprinklers shall be separated by a distance of not less than 10 ft (3050 mm) where the aggregate ceiling exceeds 300 ft² (28 m²).

**12.7.5.3.7.3** The water supply and piping for the sprinkler system shall be permitted to be of an approved temporary means that is provided by a domestic water supply, a standpipe system, or a sprinkler system.

CHAPTER 13 • Existing

**A.13.7.5.3.7.1(3)** See A.13.4.1.1.

**13.7.5.3.7.2** A single exhibit or group of exhibits with ceilings that do not require sprinklers shall be separated by a distance not less than 10 ft (3050 mm) where the aggregate ceiling exceeds 300 ft² (28 m²).

**13.7.5.3.7.3** The water supply and piping for the sprinkler system shall be permitted to be of approved temporary means that is provided by a domestic water supply, a standpipe system, or a sprinkler system.

The requirement of 12/13.7.5.3.2 applies to a standard exhibit booth arrangement, whether constructed of pipe supports and cloth or paper drapes, or whether it is a large exhibit enclosure designed and built from other materials, which could include small booths, open displays, large board displays, or other arrangements. This requirement also includes exhibit enclosures that are created by the arrangement of products such as machinery or vehicles. The intent is that travel distance is not to be more than 50 ft (15 m) for occupants who are inside the enclosure, whether they are employees or patrons. Note that this is not travel distance to an exit, but only to an aisle.

The requirement of 12/13.7.5.3.3 ensures that larger exhibits with a second level will provide at least two means of egress to prevent entrapping occupants on the upper level.

Paragraph 12/13.7.5.3.4 is intended to provide direction to manufacturers of exhibit booths as well as decorators, exhibitors, and authorities having jurisdiction (AHJ). This paragraph focuses on the construction components of the ceilings, walls, and floors of an exhibit booth or display area in addition to the finish treatment. The intent is to regulate the materials used for large signs and display boards; small signs might be considered interior finish materials per the criteria of 10.2.5.3. Paragraph 12/13.7.5.3.4 does not apply to the goods or products that are being displayed.

Plastics are limited to Class A and Class B for wall and ceiling finishes. The intent of 12/13.7.5.3.4(6) is to prohibit the use of foamed plastics because of their inherent burning characteristics, unless they have been tested for heat release rate in accordance with UL 1975, *Standard for Fire Tests for Foamed Plastics Used for Decorative Purposes,*[20] and meet the maximum 100 kW threshold. Foamed plastics are used in sign construction and display boards, and, in some cases, the entire booth is constructed of foamed plastics.

Large booths and multistory booths pose special life safety problems in exhibit halls. A fire in these booths could grow to proportions large enough to have a significant negative impact on the performance of the building's sprinkler system. The intent of 12/13.7.5.3.7 is to provide sprinkler protection in these booths by means of a temporary tap into the existing sprinkler system. Sprinklers should provide the protection necessary to extinguish a fire in its incipient stage, thus reducing the life hazard to occupants.

Paragraph 12/13.7.5.3.7.1(1) is not really an exemption to 12/13.7.5.3.7, because the exemption of sprinklers below dropout ceilings is already permitted by the reference document, NFPA 13, *Standard for the Installation of Sprinkler Systems.*[21] The exemption was added to emphasize that it is not the intent to prohibit this provision of the sprinkler installation standard from being applied.

Paragraph 12/13.7.5.3.7.1(2) exempts large vehicles (i.e., boats, mobile homes, and recreational vehicles) from the sprinkler requirement but requires a smoke detector if the vehicle is larger than 100 ft² (9.3 m²) to provide early warning in the immediate area to allow for orderly evacuation. This provision could most probably be met by single-station, battery-operated smoke alarms.

Paragraph 12/13.7.5.3.7.1(3) permits exposition hall operators to work with the AHJ to devise alternate methods of compliance via the life safety evaluation of 12/13.4.1.

CHAPTER 12 • New

**12.7.5.3.8** Open flame devices within exhibit booths shall comply with 12.7.3.

**12.7.5.3.9** Cooking and food-warming devices in exhibit booths shall comply with 12.7.2 and the following:

CHAPTER 13 • Existing

**13.7.5.3.8** Open flame devices within exhibit booths shall comply with 13.7.3.

**13.7.5.3.9** Cooking and food-warming devices in exhibit booths shall comply with 13.7.2 and the following:

CHAPTER 12 • New

(1) Gas-fired devices shall comply with the following:
   (a) Natural gas-fired devices shall comply with 9.1.1.
   (b) The requirement of 12.7.5.3.9(1)(a) shall not apply to compressed natural gas where permitted by the authority having jurisdiction.
   (c) The use of LP-Gas cylinders shall be prohibited.
   (d) Nonrefillable LP-Gas cylinders shall be approved for use where permitted by the authority having jurisdiction.
(2) The devices shall be isolated from the public by not less than 48 in. (1220 mm) or by a barrier between the devices and the public.
(3) Multi-well cooking equipment using combustible oils or solids shall comply with 9.2.3.
(4) Single-well cooking equipment using combustible oils or solids shall meet the following criteria:
   (a) The equipment shall have lids available for immediate use.
   (b) The equipment shall be limited to 2 $ft^2$ (0.2 $m^2$) of cooking surface.
   (c) The equipment shall be placed on noncombustible surface materials.
   (d) The equipment shall be separated from each other by a horizontal distance of not less than 24 in. (610 mm).
   (e) The requirement of 12.7.5.3.9(4)(d) shall not apply to multiple single-well cooking equipment where the aggregate cooking surface area does not exceed 2 $ft^2$ (0.2 $m^2$).
   (f) The equipment shall be kept at a horizontal distance of not less than 24 in. (610 mm) from any combustible material.
(5) A portable fire extinguisher in accordance with 9.7.4.1 shall be provided within the booth for each device, or an approved automatic extinguishing system shall be provided.

**12.7.5.3.10** Combustible materials within exhibit booths shall be limited to a one-day supply. Storage of combustible materials behind the booth shall be prohibited. *(See 12.7.4.2 and 12.7.5.2.)*

**12.7.5.3.11** Plans for the exposition, in an acceptable form, shall be submitted to the authority having jurisdiction for approval prior to setting up any exhibit.

**12.7.5.3.11.1** The plan shall show all details of the proposed exposition.

**12.7.5.3.11.2** No exposition shall occupy any exposition facility without approved plans.

CHAPTER 13 • Existing

(1) Gas-fired devices shall comply with the following:
   (a) Natural gas-fired devices shall comply with 9.1.1.
   (b) The requirement of 13.7.5.3.9(1)(a) shall not apply to compressed natural gas where permitted by the authority having jurisdiction.
   (c) The use of LP-Gas cylinders shall be prohibited.
   (d) Nonrefillable LP-Gas cylinders shall be approved for use where permitted by the authority having jurisdiction.
(2) The devices shall be isolated from the public by not less than 48 in. (1220 mm) or by a barrier between the devices and the public.
(3) Multi-well cooking equipment using combustible oils or solids shall comply with 9.2.3.
(4) Single-well cooking equipment using combustible oils or solids shall meet the following criteria:
   (a) The equipment shall have lids available for immediate use.
   (b) The equipment shall be limited to 2 $ft^2$ (0.2 $m^2$) of cooking surface.
   (c) The equipment shall be placed on noncombustible surface materials.
   (d) The equipment shall be separated from each other by a horizontal distance of not less than 24 in. (610 mm).
   (e) The requirement of 13.7.5.3.9(4)(d) shall not apply to multiple single-well cooking equipment where the aggregate cooking surface area does not exceed 2 $ft^2$ (0.2 $m^2$).
   (f) The equipment shall be kept at a horizontal distance of not less than 24 in. (610 mm) from any combustible material.
(5) A portable fire extinguisher in accordance with 9.7.4.1 shall be provided within the booth for each device, or an approved automatic extinguishing system shall be provided.

**13.7.5.3.10** Combustible materials within exhibit booths shall be limited to a one-day supply. Storage of combustible materials behind the booth shall be prohibited. *(See 13.7.4.2 and 13.7.5.2.)*

**13.7.5.3.11** Plans for the exposition, in an acceptable form, shall be submitted to the authority having jurisdiction for approval prior to setting up any exhibit.

**13.7.5.3.11.1** The plan shall show all details of the proposed exposition.

**13.7.5.3.11.2** No exposition shall occupy any exposition facility without approved plans.

Open flame devices, as noted in 12/13.7.5.3.8, need to comply with the provisions of 12/13.7.3. Any use of open flames requires the approval of the authority having jurisdiction (AHJ).

The provisions of 12/13.7.5.3.9 recognize the inherent dangers in cooking and food-warming devices that are used in an exhibit hall subject to large, transient crowds.

The provisions of 12/13.7.5.3.9(2) require separation distance or a barrier between the public and the device. The purpose is to guard against the dangers of accidental spills of hot greases or foods and to minimize the potential for ignition of combustibles, especially clothing worn by patrons.

Paragraph 12/13.7.5.3.9(3) requires that multi-vat, or multi-well, cooking equipment comply with NFPA 96, *Standard for Ventilation Control and Fire Protection of Commercial Cooking Operations.*[22]

The intent of requiring the lid in 12/13.7.5.3.9(4)(a) is to provide the operator with a ready method of smothering the fire.

The provisions of 12/13.7.5.3.9(4)(c) are important, because the bottom surface of many devices could be subject to heating to temperatures that could ignite combustible surfaces.

The minimum separation distances in 12/13.7.5.3.9(4)(d) are necessary to minimize the danger of a fire in one device extending into another device; the same principle applies to 12/13.7.5.3.9(4)(f), except that the exposure of concern is to combustible decorations or other products, as opposed to another cooking device.

Paragraph 12/13.7.5.3.9(5) requires a portable extinguisher for each cooking device. The intent is to provide an extinguisher near each cooking device, so the operator is able to access the extinguisher readily if a lid does not extinguish the fire or cannot be applied. It is not the intent to permit all extinguishers to be located in one place. The reference to 9.7.4.1 leads the user to NFPA 10, *Standard for Portable Fire Extinguishers,*[23] which provides the necessary information with regard to the type and size of the appropriate extinguisher.

Paragraph 12/13.7.5.3.10 limits the amount of literature, brochures, boxes, giveaways, and other products that are kept in the exhibit booth. The number of items necessary to constitute a one-day supply obviously varies. However, the AHJ should be able to make a judgment after reviewing the activity anticipated by the exhibitor. Additional supplies and combustible crates (such as those used for shipping) should be kept in a separate storage area having a fire resistance rating of 1 hour and protected by an automatic sprinkler system, as required by 12/13.7.5.2.

The intent of 12/13.7.5.3.11 is to provide the AHJ with a set of plans that shows aisle widths, travel distances, exits, booth locations, display area configurations, types of displays (e.g., cooking, machinery, drapery, arts and crafts), location of fire protection equipment (extinguishers, manual fire alarm boxes, hose cabinets), and lobby and registration area usage. This list is not complete, but it provides some guidance in determining the contents of the plan that should be submitted. The plan should also be drawn to scale. The scale used is not usually critical, provided that it is indicated on the plan.

**12.7.5.4 Vehicles.** Vehicles on display within an exposition facility shall comply with 12.7.5.4.1 through 12.7.5.4.5.

**12.7.5.4.1** All fuel tank openings shall be locked and sealed in an approved manner to prevent the escape of vapors; fuel tanks shall not contain in excess of one-half their capacity or contain in excess of 10 gal (38 L) of fuel, whichever is less.

**12.7.5.4.2** At least one battery cable shall be removed from the batteries used to start the vehicle engine, and the disconnected battery cable shall then be taped.

**12.7.5.4.3** Batteries used to power auxiliary equipment shall be permitted to be kept in service.

**12.7.5.4.4** Fueling or defueling of vehicles shall be prohibited.

**13.7.5.4 Vehicles.** Vehicles on display within an exposition facility shall comply with 13.7.5.4.1 through 13.7.5.4.5.

**13.7.5.4.1** All fuel tank openings shall be locked and sealed in an approved manner to prevent the escape of vapors; fuel tanks shall not contain in excess of one-half their capacity or contain in excess of 10 gal (38 L) of fuel, whichever is less.

**13.7.5.4.2** At least one battery cable shall be removed from the batteries used to start the vehicle engine, and the disconnected battery cable shall then be taped.

**13.7.5.4.3** Batteries used to power auxiliary equipment shall be permitted to be kept in service.

**13.7.5.4.4** Fueling or defueling of vehicles shall be prohibited.

CHAPTER 12 • New

12.7.5.4.5 Vehicles shall not be moved during exhibit hours.

CHAPTER 13 • Existing

13.7.5.4.5 Vehicles shall not be moved during exhibit hours.

Paragraph 12/13.7.5.4 on vehicles is intended to minimize the danger from both fuel and ignition sources.

In accordance with 12/13.7.5.4.1, it is important that fuel tank openings be locked to prevent tampering and accessibility to fuel. It is also important that the tank openings be taped to prevent the escape of flammable vapors. When these *Code* requirements were written, the issue of the quantity of fuel that is permitted in a tank was studied. Some jurisdictions preferred empty tanks to eliminate fuel, while others preferred full tanks to prevent vapors. It was determined that most exhibitors were unaware of the local regulation until they arrived at the exhibit hall. After learning the specific rule (empty or full), exhibitors proceeded to make their adjustment in the adjacent parking area or some other unsuitable area. It is also difficult for the authority having jurisdiction (AHJ) to determine whether a tank is absolutely full or empty. Fueling and defueling by exhibitors outside the hall presented a greater danger than the level of fuel in the tanks, given that the tanks are locked and sealed, and ignition sources are eliminated from the vehicle. However, to avoid excessive quantities of fuel in the exhibition hall, the *Code* does limit the quantity of fuel in tanks.

In accordance with 12/13.7.5.4.2, it is important that at least one of the battery cables be removed from each battery. Many vehicles have more than one battery. The intent is to eliminate the possibility of a spark from the battery that might ignite fuel or surrounding combustibles. Battery cable connectors should be thoroughly taped after they have been removed.

The provision of 12/13.7.5.4.3 permits batteries that cannot be used to start the vehicle to remain in service. These batteries present no more of an ignition hazard than does providing house electrical power to the item on display.

Vehicle movement is addressed in 12/13.7.5.4.5. The movement of vehicles inside the exhibit hall potentially compromises the means of egress by blocking the exit access; vehicles should, therefore, be positioned before the hall is opened to the public. There is also a concern regarding the effects of carbon monoxide inside an exhibit hall that is occupied.

**12.7.5.5 Prohibited Materials.**

**12.7.5.5.1** The following items shall be prohibited within exhibit halls:

(1) Compressed flammable gases
(2) Flammable or combustible liquids
(3) Hazardous chemicals or materials
(4) Class II or greater lasers, blasting agents, and explosives

**12.7.5.5.2** The authority having jurisdiction shall be permitted to allow the limited use of any items specified in 12.7.5.5.1 under special circumstances.

**12.7.5.6 Alternatives.** See Section 1.4.

**13.7.5.5 Prohibited Materials.**

**13.7.5.5.1** The following items shall be prohibited within exhibit halls:

(1) Compressed flammable gases
(2) Flammable or combustible liquids
(3) Hazardous chemicals or materials
(4) Class II or greater lasers, blasting agents, and explosives

**13.7.5.5.2** The authority having jurisdiction shall be permitted to allow the limited use of any items specified in 13.7.5.5.1 under special circumstances.

**13.7.5.6 Alternatives.** See Section 1.4.

Compressed gas containers, as addressed by 12/13.7.5.5.1, are subject to fire damage that could cause an explosion or create a serious threat to life safety. Flammable and combustible liquids compromise life safety by their inherent capability to contribute to rapid fire spread. Hazardous materials present a variety of hazards to life safety, from their flammability to their toxicity. Class II or greater lasers can cause tissue damage to humans, and blasting agents and explosives can cause a large loss of life or injury if handled improperly.

Exhibitors who wish to display explosives, pesticides, or a type of compressed gas container, among other items, can effectively do so without bringing the actual product into the hall by using empty containers instead.

Paragraph 12/13.7.5.5.2 gives the authority having jurisdiction (AHJ) the discretion to permit small amounts of otherwise prohibited materials under special circumstances. For example, an exhibit or trade show for collectors of small arms ammunition or a highly supervised and closed (to the public) vocational trade show using such materials is permitted where special controls and professional supervision are provided.

### 12.7.6* Crowd Managers.

**A.12.7.6** The training program in crowd management should develop a clear appreciation of factors of space, energy, time, and information, as well as specific crowd management techniques, such as metering. Published guidelines on these factors and techniques are found in the *SFPE Handbook of Fire Protection Engineering*, Section 3, Chapter 13.

**12.7.6.1** Assembly occupancies shall be provided with a minimum of one trained crowd manager or crowd manager supervisor. Where the occupant load exceeds 250, additional trained crowd managers or crowd manager supervisors shall be provided at a ratio of one crowd manager or crowd manager supervisor for every 250 occupants, unless otherwise permitted by the following:

(1) This requirement shall not apply to assembly occupancies used exclusively for religious worship with an occupant load not exceeding 2000.
(2) The ratio of trained crowd managers to occupants shall be permitted to be reduced where, in the opinion of the authority having jurisdiction, the existence of an approved, supervised automatic sprinkler system and the nature of the event warrant.

**12.7.6.2** The crowd manager shall receive approved training in crowd management techniques.

### 13.7.6* Crowd Managers.

**A.13.7.6** The training program in crowd management should develop a clear appreciation of factors of space, energy, time, and information, as well as specific crowd management techniques, such as metering. Published guidelines on these factors and techniques are found in the *SFPE Handbook of Fire Protection Engineering*, Section 3, Chapter 13.

**13.7.6.1** Assembly occupancies shall be provided with a minimum of one trained crowd manager or crowd manager supervisor. Where the occupant load exceeds 250, additional trained crowd managers or crowd manager supervisors shall be provided at a ratio of one crowd manager or crowd manager supervisor for every 250 occupants, unless otherwise permitted by the following:

(1) This requirement shall not apply to assembly occupancies used exclusively for religious worship with an occupant load not exceeding 2000.
(2) The ratio of trained crowd managers to occupants shall be permitted to be reduced where, in the opinion of the authority having jurisdiction, the existence of an approved, supervised automatic sprinkler system and the nature of the event warrant.

**13.7.6.2** The crowd manager shall receive approved training in crowd management techniques.

Since the 2006 edition of the *Code*, a minimum of one crowd manager has been required for each assembly occupancy, regardless of occupant load. Where the occupant load exceeds 250, additional crowd managers are required at the specified ratio. In editions prior to 2006, a crowd manager was required only if the occupant load exceeded 1000. The change was made in reaction to The Station nightclub fire addressed in the commentary following 12.2.3.8.

The material in Section 3, Chapter 13, of the third edition of the *SFPE Handbook of Fire Protection Engineering*,[24] which is referenced in A.12/13.7.6, makes a distinction between the required crowd management and the more extreme, but nonmandatory, crowd control. Crowd management meshes the design features of a facility, the established operating features of the facility, and an understanding of the occupants' expected natural behavior in the facility for a specific type of event. Crowd control, on the other hand, is often necessitated when crowd management fails.

Limited options exist with respect to training programs for crowd managers. The International Association of Assembly Managers (http://www.iaam.org) conducts its annual International Crowd Management Conference (ICMC) each October. The conference in 2008 was its twenty-sixth such annual training event. The focus of the conference is on large assembly venues such as arenas and stadia. The Maryland State Fire Marshal's Office provides, at no charge, a crowd management e-course at http://www.firemarshal.state.md.us/crowdmanager/bginfo.html.

CHAPTER 12 • New

### 12.7.7* Drills.

**A.12.7.7** It is important that an adequate number of competent attendants are on duty at all times when the assembly occupancy is occupied.

**12.7.7.1** The employees or attendants of assembly occupancies shall be trained and drilled in the duties they are to perform in case of fire, panic, or other emergency to effect orderly exiting.

**12.7.7.2** Employees or attendants of assembly occupancies shall be instructed in the proper use of portable fire extinguishers and other manual fire suppression equipment where provided.

**12.7.7.3*** In the following assembly occupancies, an audible announcement shall be made, or a projected image shall be shown, prior to the start of each program that notifies occupants of the location of the exits to be used in case of a fire or other emergency:

(1) Theaters
(2) Motion picture theaters
(3) Auditoriums
(4) Other similar assembly occupancies with occupant loads exceeding 300 where there are noncontinuous programs

**A.12.7.7.3** It is not the intent of this provision to require an announcement in bowling alleys, cocktail lounges, restaurants, or places of worship.

**12.7.7.4** The requirement of 12.7.7.3 shall not apply to assembly occupancies in schools where used for nonpublic events.

CHAPTER 13 • Existing

### 13.7.7* Drills.

**A.13.7.7** It is important that an adequate number of competent attendants are on duty at all times when the assembly occupancy is occupied.

**13.7.7.1** The employees or attendants of assembly occupancies shall be trained and drilled in the duties they are to perform in case of fire, panic, or other emergency to effect orderly exiting.

**13.7.7.2** Employees or attendants of assembly occupancies shall be instructed in the proper use of portable fire extinguishers and other manual fire suppression equipment where provided.

**13.7.7.3*** In the following assembly occupancies, an audible announcement shall be made, or a projected image shall be shown, prior to the start of each program that notifies occupants of the location of the exits to be used in case of a fire or other emergency:

(1) Theaters
(2) Motion picture theaters
(3) Auditoriums
(4) Other similar assembly occupancies with occupant loads exceeding 300 where there are noncontinuous programs

**A.13.7.7.3** It is not the intent of this provision to require an announcement in bowling alleys, cocktail lounges, restaurants, or places of worship.

**13.7.7.4** The requirement of 13.7.7.3 shall not apply to assembly occupancies in schools where used for nonpublic events.

The provisions of 12/13.7.7.2 do not require fire extinguishers for life safety in an assembly occupancy. They do specify, however, that if fire extinguishers are provided, the staff must be trained in their use to prevent a false sense of security and possible injury. The authority having jurisdiction (AHJ) determines the extent of this training, whether instruction only or instruction and hands-on use.

The relatively simple requirement of 12/13.7.7.3 for notifying occupants of the location of exits can make a significant difference during an emergency. Note that the requirement does not apply to assembly occupancies where the flow of people is constantly changing, such as in a restaurant. Movie theaters commonly meet the provisions of 12/13.7.7.3 through means of sound and screen projection that are presented prior to the main feature, during the same period that notifications of restroom, trash container, and snack bar locations are made and previews are shown. The same complete message is thereby delivered to each audience without the need for human intervention.

### 12.7.8 Smoking.

**12.7.8.1** Smoking in assembly occupancies shall be regulated by the authority having jurisdiction.

**12.7.8.2** In rooms or areas where smoking is prohibited, plainly visible signs shall be posted that read as follows:

NO SMOKING

### 13.7.8 Smoking.

**13.7.8.1** Smoking in assembly occupancies shall be regulated by the authority having jurisdiction.

**13.7.8.2** In rooms or areas where smoking is prohibited, plainly visible signs shall be posted that read as follows:

NO SMOKING

CHAPTER 12 • New

**12.7.8.3** No person shall smoke in prohibited areas that are so posted, unless permitted by the authority having jurisdiction under both of the following conditions:

(1) Smoking shall be permitted on a stage only where it is a necessary and rehearsed part of a performance.
(2) Smoking shall be permitted only where the smoker is a regular performing member of the cast.

**12.7.8.4** Where smoking is permitted, suitable ashtrays or receptacles shall be provided in convenient locations.

### 12.7.9 Seating.

**12.7.9.1 Secured Seating.**

**12.7.9.1.1** Seats in assembly occupancies accommodating more than 200 persons shall be securely fastened to the floor, except where fastened together in groups of not less than three and as permitted by 12.7.9.2.

**12.7.9.1.2** All seats in balconies and galleries shall be securely fastened to the floor, except in places of religious worship.

CHAPTER 13 • Existing

**13.7.8.3** No person shall smoke in prohibited areas that are so posted, unless permitted by the authority having jurisdiction under both of the following conditions:

(1) Smoking shall be permitted on a stage only where it is a necessary and rehearsed part of a performance.
(2) Smoking shall be permitted only where the smoker is a regular performing member of the cast.

**13.7.8.4** Where smoking is permitted, suitable ashtrays or receptacles shall be provided in convenient locations.

### 13.7.9 Seating.

**13.7.9.1 Secured Seating.**

**13.7.9.1.1** Seats in assembly occupancies accommodating more than 200 persons shall be securely fastened to the floor, except where fastened together in groups of not less than three and as permitted by 13.7.9.2.

**13.7.9.1.2** All seats in balconies and galleries shall be securely fastened to the floor, except in places of religious worship.

The function of 12/13.7.9.1 is to prevent the movement of seats so that aisles, rows, and access to the exits do not become blocked in an assembly occupancy during the jostling that occurs when people flee from a fire.

The provision of 12/13.7.9.1.1 for fastening seats together in groups was revised for the 2009 edition of the *Code*. In prior editions, the seats were required to be fastened together in groups of not less than three and not more than seven. The maximum number of seats in a group was deleted, as it served no practical purpose.

CHAPTER 12 • New

**12.7.9.2 Unsecured Seating.**

**12.7.9.2.1** Seats not secured to the floor shall be permitted in restaurants, night clubs, and other occupancies where fastening seats to the floor might be impracticable.

**12.7.9.2.2** Unsecured seats shall be permitted, provided that, in the area used for seating, excluding such areas as dance floors and stages, there is not more than one seat for each 15 $ft^2$ (1.4 $m^2$) of net floor area, and adequate aisles to reach exits are maintained at all times.

**12.7.9.2.3** Seating diagrams shall be submitted for approval by the authority having jurisdiction to permit an increase in occupant load per 7.3.1.3.

**12.7.9.3 Occupant Load Posting.**

**12.7.9.3.1** Every room constituting an assembly occupancy and not having fixed seats shall have the occupant load of the room posted in a conspicuous place near the main exit from the room.

CHAPTER 13 • Existing

**13.7.9.2 Unsecured Seating.**

**13.7.9.2.1** Seats not secured to the floor shall be permitted in restaurants, night clubs, and other occupancies where fastening seats to the floor might be impracticable.

**13.7.9.2.2** Unsecured seats shall be permitted, provided that, in the area used for seating, excluding such areas as dance floors and stages, there is not more than one seat for each 15 $ft^2$ (1.4 $m^2$) of net floor area, and adequate aisles to reach exits are maintained at all times.

**13.7.9.2.3** Seating diagrams shall be submitted for approval by the authority having jurisdiction to permit an increase in occupant load per 7.3.1.3.

**13.7.9.3 Occupant Load Posting.**

**13.7.9.3.1** Every room constituting an assembly occupancy and not having fixed seats shall have the occupant load of the room posted in a conspicuous place near the main exit from the room.

CHAPTER 12 • New

12.7.9.3.2 Approved signs shall be maintained in a legible manner by the owner or authorized agent.

12.7.9.3.3 Signs shall be durable and shall indicate the number of occupants permitted for each room use.

Paragraph 12/13.7.9.2.3 requires that seating diagrams be provided to the authority having jurisdiction (AHJ) to support a request for an increase in occupant load above that calculated using the occupant load factors of Table 7.3.1.2 characteristic of the uses of the space. Such increase in occupant load must not exceed the limits imposed by 12/13.1.7.

### 12.7.10 Maintenance of Outdoor Grandstands.

12.7.10.1 The owner shall provide for not less than annual inspection and required maintenance of each outdoor grandstand to ensure safe conditions.

12.7.10.2 At least biennially, the inspection shall be performed by a professional engineer, registered architect, or individual certified by the manufacturer.

12.7.10.3 Where required by the authority having jurisdiction, the owner shall provide a copy of the inspection report and certification that the inspection required by 12.7.10.2 has been performed.

### 12.7.11 Maintenance and Operation of Folding and Telescopic Seating.

12.7.11.1 Instructions in both maintenance and operation shall be transmitted to the owner by the manufacturer of the seating or his or her representative.

12.7.11.2 Maintenance and operation of folding and telescopic seating shall be the responsibility of the owner or his or her duly authorized representative and shall include the following:

(1) During operation of the folding and telescopic seats, the opening and closing shall be supervised by responsible personnel who shall ensure that the operation is in accordance with the manufacturer's instructions.
(2) Only attachments specifically approved by the manufacturer for the specific installation shall be attached to the seating.
(3) An annual inspection and required maintenance of each grandstand shall be performed to ensure safe conditions.
(4) At least biennially, the inspection shall be performed by a professional engineer, registered architect, or individual certified by the manufacturer.

CHAPTER 13 • Existing

13.7.9.3.2 Approved signs shall be maintained in a legible manner by the owner or authorized agent.

13.7.9.3.3 Signs shall be durable and shall indicate the number of occupants permitted for each room use.

The provisions of 12/13.7.9.3 for occupant load posting are unique to assembly occupancies. All occupancies use occupant load for capacity calculations to ensure the means of egress system is adequately sized. Assembly occupancies use occupant load for the additional purpose of posting the occupant load as a tool to help avoid overcrowding.

### 13.7.10 Maintenance of Outdoor Grandstands.

13.7.10.1 The owner shall provide for not less than annual inspection and required maintenance of each outdoor grandstand to ensure safe conditions.

13.7.10.2 At least biennially, the inspection shall be performed by a professional engineer, registered architect, or individual certified by the manufacturer.

13.7.10.3 Where required by the authority having jurisdiction, the owner shall provide a copy of the inspection report and certification that the inspection required by 13.7.10.2 has been performed.

### 13.7.11 Maintenance and Operation of Folding and Telescopic Seating.

13.7.11.1 Instructions in both maintenance and operation shall be transmitted to the owner by the manufacturer of the seating or his or her representative.

13.7.11.2 Maintenance and operation of folding and telescopic seating shall be the responsibility of the owner or his or her duly authorized representative and shall include the following:

(1) During operation of the folding and telescopic seats, the opening and closing shall be supervised by responsible personnel who shall ensure that the operation is in accordance with the manufacturer's instructions.
(2) Only attachments specifically approved by the manufacturer for the specific installation shall be attached to the seating.
(3) An annual inspection and required maintenance of each grandstand shall be performed to ensure safe conditions.
(4) At least biennially, the inspection shall be performed by a professional engineer, registered architect, or individual certified by the manufacturer.

CHAPTER 12 • New

### 12.7.12 Clothing.

Clothing and personal effects shall not be stored in corridors, and spaces not separated from corridors, unless otherwise permitted by the following:

(1) This requirement shall not apply to corridors, and spaces not separated from corridors, that are protected by an approved, supervised automatic sprinkler system in accordance with Section 9.7.
(2) This requirement shall not apply to corridors, and spaces not separated from corridors, that are protected by a smoke detection system in accordance with Section 9.6.
(3) This requirement shall not apply to storage in metal lockers, provided that the required egress width is maintained.

CHAPTER 13 • Existing

### 13.7.12 Clothing.

Clothing and personal effects shall not be stored in corridors, and spaces not separated from corridors, unless otherwise permitted by the following:

(1) This requirement shall not apply to corridors, and spaces not separated from corridors, that are protected by an approved automatic sprinkler system in accordance with Section 9.7.
(2) This requirement shall not apply to corridors, and spaces not separated from corridors, that are protected by a smoke detection system in accordance with Section 9.6.
(3) This requirement shall not apply to storage in metal lockers, provided that the required egress width is maintained.

Clothing hung on hooks along corridor walls or on racks in lobbies greatly increases the combustible load and will generally allow flame to spread quickly. Each of the exemptions (control of fire by sprinklers, early warning of incipient stage fire via smoke detection, or isolating fuel packages by locating the clothing in metal lockers) helps to mitigate the chance that a clothing fire would render the exit access unusable. The wording of 12/13.7.12 was revised for the 2009 edition of the *Code* to clarify that the provision applies to clothing in spaces not separated from the corridor as well as in the corridor.

### 12.7.13 Emergency Plans.

**12.7.13.1** Emergency plans shall be provided in accordance with Section 4.8.

**12.7.13.2** Where assembly occupancies are located in the high-rise portion of a building, the emergency plan shall include egress procedures, methods, and preferred evacuation routes for each event considered to be a life safety hazard that could impact the building, including the appropriateness of the use of elevators.

### 13.7.13 Emergency Plans.

**13.7.13.1** Emergency plans shall be provided in accordance with Section 4.8.

**13.7.13.2** Where assembly occupancies are located in the high-rise portion of a building, the emergency plan shall include egress procedures, methods, and preferred evacuation routes for each event considered to be a life safety hazard that could impact the building, including the appropriateness of the use of elevators.

The provisions of 12/13.7.13 for emergency plans are new for the 2009 edition of the *Code*.

### References Cited in Commentary


1. NFPA 130, *Standard for Fixed Guideway Transit and Passenger Rail Systems*, 2007 edition, National Fire Protection Association, Quincy, MA.
2. Best, R., "Tragedy in Kentucky," *Fire Journal®* 72, no. 1 (January 1978) pp. 18–44 and "Reconstruction of a Tragedy," NFPA LS-72, 1978.
3. NFPA 220, *Standard on Types of Building Construction*, 2009 edition, National Fire Protection Association, Quincy, MA.
4. *NFPA 5000®, Building Construction and Safety Code®*, 2009 edition, National Fire Protection Association, Quincy, MA.
5. Grosshandler,W., Bryner, N. and Madrzykowski, D., *Report of the Technical Investigation of The Station Nightclub Fire*, NIST NCST Act Report (NCSTAR) 2, National Institute of Standards and Technology, 100 Bureau Drive, Gaithersburg, MD 20899-1070, June 2005.
6. Pauls, J., "Observations of Crowd Conditions at Rock Concert in Exhibition Stadium, Toronto, 16 July 1980."
7. *NFPA 72®, National Fire Alarm Code®*, 2007 edition, National Fire Protection Association, Quincy, MA.
8. See note 2.
9. Best, R. and Demers, D., "Investigation Report on

the MGM Grand Hotel Fire," NFPA LS-4, 1980 (rev. 1982).
10. NFPA 92A, *Standard for Smoke-Control Systems Utilizing Barriers and Pressure Differences*, 2009 edition, National Fire Protection Association, Quincy, MA.
11. NFPA 92B, *Standard for Smoke Management Systems in Malls, Atria, and Large Spaces*, 2009 edition, National Fire Protection Association, Quincy, MA.
12. *NFPA 70®, National Electrical Code®*, 2008 edition, National Fire Protection Association, Quincy, MA.
13. See note 11.
14. See note 10.
15. NFPA 80, *Standard for Fire Doors and Other Opening Protectives*, 2007 edition, National Fire Protection Association, Quincy, MA.
16. NFPA 13, *Standard for the Installation of Sprinkler Systems*, 2007 edition, National Fire Protection Association, Quincy, MA.
17. NFPA 40, *Standard for the Storage and Handling of Cellulose Nitrate Film*, 2007 edition, National Fire Protection Association, Quincy, MA.
18. NFPA 102, *Standard for Grandstands, Folding and Telescopic Seating, Tents, and Membrane Structures*, editions prior to 2006, National Fire Protection Association, Quincy, MA.
19. See note 4.
20. UL 1975, *Standard for Fire Tests for Foamed Plastics Used for Decorative Purposes*, 2006 edition, Underwriters Laboratories Inc., 333 Pfingsten Road, Northbrook, IL 60062-2096.
21. See note 16.
22. NFPA 96, *Standard for Ventilation Control and Fire Protection of Commercial Cooking Operations*, 2008 edition, National Fire Protection Association, Quincy, MA.
23. NFPA 10, *Standard for Portable Fire Extinguishers*, 2007 edition, National Fire Protection Association, Quincy, MA.
24. DiNenno, P. J., ed., *SFPE Handbook of Fire Protection Engineering*, National Fire Protection Association, Quincy, MA, 3rd edition, 2002.

CHAPTERS 14 AND 15

# New and Existing Educational Occupancies

Chapters 14 and 15 provide the life safety features necessary to protect students in an educational setting such as a school. These chapters apply to educational settings for students in kindergarten through the twelfth grade; they do not apply to college classrooms. The range of student characteristics and self-preservation abilities found in the educational occupancies regulated by Chapters 14 and 15 requires that student fire safety needs be treated differently from those of adults occupying a college classroom.

Many of the life safety requirements applicable to educational occupancies are the result of lessons learned from fires involving schools in which a large loss of life occurred. Fortunately, such fires are now rare. Fatal fires have been extremely rare in educational occupancies for many years. Those fires that do occur tend to involve either employees in accidental fires (e.g., fires caused by cleaning floors with flammable liquids) or, more often, firesetters trapped by their own fires. Children who died in school fires in recent years have been largely limited to juvenile firesetters, acting as individuals or in groups, who are on school grounds after hours without permission.

The protection measures used for educational occupancies recognize the structured environment found in a school. For example, class times, time between classes, and activities during class time are rigidly structured. These factors make it possible to train students to respond to a fire by conducting emergency egress and relocation drills.

Smaller children who might be overwhelmed and pushed aside by older students during a fire emergency evacuation must be housed in classrooms on lower floor levels. Paragraphs 14/15.2.1.2 through 14/15.2.1.4 recognize this problem and establish the criteria to control it. The minimum corridor width requirement (see 14/15.2.3.2) is based on expected student behavior. The wider corridor width accommodates students who are filing out of classrooms and forming parallel lines to proceed down the corridor.

Schools also have one of the more assertive schedules for conducting emergency egress drills (see 14/15.7.2). The drills not only provide a structured fire escape plan, they also help to instill fire-safe behavior for long-term use.

## 14.1 General Requirements

### 14.1.1 Application.

**14.1.1.1** The requirements of this chapter shall apply to new buildings or portions thereof used as educational occupancies. *(See 1.3.1.)*

The provisions for new educational occupancies are addressed in Chapter 14; the provisions for existing educational occupancies (i.e., existing conditions in educational occupancies) are addressed in Chapter 15.

## 15.1 General Requirements

### 15.1.1 Application.

**15.1.1.1** The requirements of this chapter shall apply to existing buildings or portions thereof currently occupied as educational occupancies.

In editions of the *Code* prior to 2006, renovations, additions, and changes of occupancy were required to comply with the requirements for new construction. For educational occupancies, such renovations, additions, and changes of occupancy were required to meet the provisions of Chapter 14, while existing conditions were subject to the provisions of Chapter 15. Chapter 43, Building Rehabilitation, was added in 2006 to promote the adaptive reuse of existing buildings without sacrificing the needed level of life safety. The provisions of Chapter 43 blend the requirements for new construction with those for existing conditions, so as to require additional life safety features as the rehabilitation work category increases in complexity. The rehabilitation work categories are repair, renovation, modification, reconstruction, change of use or occupancy classification, and addition. See 4.6.8, 4.6.12, and Chapter 43.

**14.1.1.2** Educational facilities that do not meet the definition of an educational occupancy shall not be required to comply with this chapter but shall comply with the following requirements:

(1) Instructional building — business occupancy
(2) Classrooms under 50 persons — business occupancy
(3) Classrooms, 50 persons and over — assembly occupancy
(4) Laboratories, instructional — business occupancy
(5) Laboratories, noninstructional — industrial

**15.1.1.2** Educational facilities that do not meet the definition of an educational occupancy shall not be required to comply with this chapter but shall comply with the following requirements:

(1) Instructional building — business occupancy
(2) Classrooms under 50 persons — business occupancy
(3) Classrooms, 50 persons and over — assembly occupancy
(4) Laboratories, instructional — business occupancy
(5) Laboratories, noninstructional — industrial

As defined in Chapter 6 and repeated in 14/15.1.4.1, educational occupancies include those buildings, or portions of buildings, used for educating six or more students for 4 or more hours per day or more than 12 hours per week, but only through the twelfth grade. The provisions of 14/15.1.1.2 recognize that colleges, universities, and similar educational facilities that do not meet the definition of an educational occupancy do not pose the same life safety concerns as elementary and high schools. Because of the maturity of their occupants, college buildings more closely resemble business occupancies.

Paragraph 14/15.1.1.2 also identifies how to classify an occupancy for other educational uses that do not meet the definition of an educational occupancy. Note that the provisions of 14/15.1.1.2(1) through (5) apply only where the educational use does not meet the definition of an educational occupancy. For example, 14/15.1.1.2(3) specifies that a classroom with an occupant load of 50 or more persons be classified as an assembly occupancy only if such classroom is not an educational occupancy. A classroom occupied by 60 eighth-grade students for more than 12 hours per week is an educational occupancy, and not an assembly occupancy, because it meets the definition of an educational occupancy. A classroom occupied by 60 college students is an assembly occupancy in accordance with 14/15.1.1.2(3), as the definition of an educational occupancy applies through only the twelfth grade. A classroom occupied by 49 college students is a business occupancy in accordance with 14/15.1.1.2(2), as the definition of an educational occupancy applies through only the twelfth grade.

### 14.1.2 Multiple Occupancies.

**14.1.2.1 General.** Multiple occupancies shall be in accordance with 6.1.14.

**14.1.2.2 Assembly and Educational.**

**14.1.2.2.1** Spaces subject to assembly occupancy shall comply with Chapter 12, including 12.1.2.2, which provides that, where auditorium and gymnasium egress lead through corridors or stairways also serving as egress for other parts of the building, the egress capacity shall be sufficient to allow simultaneous egress from auditorium and classroom sections.

### 15.1.2 Multiple Occupancies.

**15.1.2.1 General.** Multiple occupancies shall be in accordance with 6.1.14.

**15.1.2.2 Assembly and Educational.**

**15.1.2.2.1** Spaces subject to assembly occupancy shall comply with Chapter 13, including 13.1.2.2, which provides that, where auditorium and gymnasium egress lead through corridors or stairways also serving as egress for other parts of the building, the egress capacity shall be sufficient to allow simultaneous egress from auditorium and classroom sections.

CHAPTER 14 • New

**14.1.2.2.2** In the case of an assembly occupancy of a type suitable for use only by the school occupant load, and therefore not subject to simultaneous occupancy, the same egress capacity shall be permitted to serve both sections.

**14.1.2.3 Dormitory and Classrooms.**

**14.1.2.3.1** Any building used for both classroom and dormitory purposes shall comply with the applicable provisions of Chapter 28 in addition to complying with Chapter 14.

**14.1.2.3.2** Where classroom and dormitory sections are not subject to simultaneous occupancy, the same egress capacity shall be permitted to serve both sections.

CHAPTER 15 • Existing

**15.1.2.2.2** In the case of an assembly occupancy of a type suitable for use only by the school occupant load, and therefore not subject to simultaneous occupancy, the same egress capacity shall be permitted to serve both sections.

**15.1.2.3 Dormitory and Classrooms.**

**15.1.2.3.1** Any building used for both classroom and dormitory purposes shall comply with the applicable provisions of Chapter 29 in addition to complying with Chapter 15.

**15.1.2.3.2** Where classroom and dormitory sections are not subject to simultaneous occupancy, the same egress capacity shall be permitted to serve both sections.

Paragraph 14/15.1.2.1 refers to 6.1.14, which specifies that, where multiple occupancies are to be protected as mixed occupancies, the most stringent requirement applicable to any of the occupancies present is to be applied to all occupancies. For example, one of the occupancies present might have a travel distance limitation stricter than that of the other occupancies present; therefore, the stricter limitation is to be applied throughout the building. An occupancy that differs from the occupancy with the strictest travel distance limit might have the strictest requirements for protection of vertical openings, and these provisions also need to be implemented throughout the building. Similarly, for each subject addressed by the *Code*, a comparison must be made among the requirements applicable to each of the occupancies present, and the strictest requirement must be provided throughout the building.

Paragraph 14/15.1.2.2 addresses multiple occupancies that are part assembly and part educational in recognition of the fact that the occupancy that most typically appears within an educational occupancy building to create a multiple occupancy is an assembly occupancy. Note that 6.1.14.1.2 requires that, where exit access from an occupancy traverses another occupancy, the multiple occupancy must be treated as a mixed occupancy (i.e., the option of protecting the multiple occupancy as separated occupancies is prohibited).

Because of the large numbers of occupants characteristic of both assembly and educational occupancies, it is important that their combined occupant loads be used to size the means of egress system if they share common egress components, such as corridors and exit stair enclosures. The requirement assumes that the classrooms and assembly areas are likely to be occupied simultaneously. For example, classrooms are often used during the evening for adult or remedial education while a school's gymnasium or auditorium is being used by another group. Where simultaneous occupancy does not occur, 14/15.1.2.2.2 permits the shared means of egress to be sized to handle the larger of the uses, either educational or assembly.

Chapters 12 and 13 contain several requirements applicable to assembly occupancies that could have a significant impact on an educational occupancy contained in a multiple-use building if the building is not designed so the occupancies can be treated separately. For example, in new construction, if the mixed use creates a multiple occupancy that is to be protected as a mixed occupancy, the building will most likely have to be sprinklered throughout by applying the provisions of 12.3.5. The other option is to use the separated occupancies provisions of 6.1.14.4 so as to sprinkler only the assembly occupancy [provided that the educational occupancy building is less than 20,000 $ft^2$ (1860 $m^2$) and less than four stories in height so as not to be required to be sprinklered by 14.3.5.1 or 14.3.5.2], but, in such case, the educational occupancy and the assembly occupancy are not permitted to have common exit access. See 6.1.14.1.2.

Subsection 14/15.1.2.3 addresses a situation common to boarding schools where a building is used for both classroom and dormitory purposes. The residential occupancy created by the dormitory is not permitted to be considered incidental to the building being used as an educational occupancy (see 6.1.14.1.3). The occupants of the dormitory have life safety needs that differ from those of the occupants of the classrooms. The provisions of Chapters 28 and 29 need to be applied to the dormitory/classroom building in addition to the educational occupancy provisions of Chapters 14 and 15. For example, smoke alarms are required in the dormitory sleeping rooms to help ensure that the sleeping occupants are awakened upon detection of smoke.

CHAPTER 14 • New

### 14.1.3 Special Definitions.

A list of special terms used in this chapter follows:

(1) **Common Atmosphere.** See 3.3.23.1.
(2) **Flexible Plan and Open Plan Educational or Day-Care Building.** See 3.3.32.6.
(3) **Separate Atmosphere.** See 3.3.23.2.

### 14.1.4 Classification of Occupancy.

See 6.1.3.

**14.1.4.1** Educational occupancies shall include all buildings used for educational purposes through the twelfth grade by six or more persons for 4 or more hours per day or more than 12 hours per week.

**14.1.4.2** Educational occupancies shall include part-day preschools, kindergartens, and other schools whose purpose is primarily educational, even though the children who attend such schools are of preschool age.

**14.1.4.3** In cases where instruction is incidental to some other occupancy, the section of this *Code* governing such other occupancy shall apply.

**14.1.4.4** Other occupancies associated with educational institutions shall be in accordance with the appropriate parts of this *Code*. *(See Chapters 18, 20, 26, 28, 30, 40, and 42 and 6.1.14.)*

CHAPTER 15 • Existing

### 15.1.3 Special Definitions.

A list of special terms used in this chapter follows:

(1) **Common Atmosphere.** See 3.3.23.1.
(2) **Flexible Plan and Open Plan Educational or Day-Care Building.** See 3.3.32.6.
(3) **Separate Atmosphere.** See 3.3.23.2.

### 15.1.4 Classification of Occupancy.

See 6.1.3.

**15.1.4.1** Educational occupancies shall include all buildings used for educational purposes through the twelfth grade by six or more persons for 4 or more hours per day or more than 12 hours per week.

**15.1.4.2** Educational occupancies shall include part-day preschools, kindergartens, and other schools whose purpose is primarily educational, even though the children who attend such schools are of preschool age.

**15.1.4.3** In cases where instruction is incidental to some other occupancy, the section of this *Code* governing such other occupancy shall apply.

**15.1.4.4** Other occupancies associated with educational institutions shall be in accordance with the appropriate parts of this *Code*. *(See Chapters 19, 21, 26, 29, 31, 40, and 42 and 6.1.14.)*

Paragraph 14/15.1.4.1 has the effect of exempting the following three types of schools from the provisions of Chapters 14 and 15:

1. Schools with small numbers of students (fewer than six), such as facilities providing private tutoring or individual lessons
2. Schools with limited operating hours (less than 4 hours per day and not more than 12 hours per week), such as some sports schools or weekend religious instruction schools
3. Schools that educate people above the high school level, as in the case of universities or military training

For purposes of determining occupant load, a classroom area — regardless of whether it is part of an educational occupancy — is still considered an educational use, and the occupant load factors provided for educational uses by Table 7.3.1.2 are to be used to calculate a realistic, maximum, probable occupant load.

Where instruction is incidental in an occupancy other than educational, the requirements for the occupancy in which the instruction takes place are applicable. Church schools used for instruction for a few hours once or twice a week are generally considered part of the assembly occupancy in which instruction takes place.

Paragraph 14/15.1.4.2 classifies part-time day-care facilities as educational occupancies if they primarily provide education in addition to care services. This classification parallels federal guidelines for subsidizing day-care/educational activities at both the federal and state levels. This classification does not describe a typical day-care facility. Chapters 16 and 17 contain special requirements for typical, noneducational day-care facilities.

The requirement of 14/15.1.4.3 does not carry the same significance as it did when places of higher education were encompassed by 14/15.1.4.1 in earlier editions of the *Code*. Paragraph 14/15.1.4.3 could be applied, for example, to an office building or factory in which a few rooms might be used for orientation or instruction in job performance; these rooms are subject to the *Code* requirements for business or industrial occupancies.

The requirement of 14/15.1.4.4 serves as a reminder that other occupancy chapters need to be applied to portions of an educational occupancy campus that do not meet the definition of an educational occupancy. For example, a dormitory where students sleep needs to be classified as a residential occupancy subject to the requirements of Chapter 28 or Chapter 29 for new or existing hotels and dormitories. A heating and air-conditioning plant with its boilers and chillers needs to be classified as an industrial occupancy subject to the requirements of Chapter 40.

### 14.1.5 Classification of Hazard of Contents.

The contents of educational occupancies shall be classified in accordance with the provisions of Section 6.2.

### 15.1.5 Classification of Hazard of Contents.

The contents of educational occupancies shall be classified in accordance with the provisions of Section 6.2.

In general, educational occupancies contain ordinary hazard contents. Some laboratories and storage areas might contain high hazard contents. See Section 7.11 for additional egress requirements for areas with high hazard contents.

### 14.1.6 Minimum Construction Requirements.

(No requirements.)

### 14.1.7 Occupant Load.

**14.1.7.1** The occupant load, in number of persons for whom means of egress and other provisions are required, shall be determined on the basis of the occupant load factors of Table 7.3.1.2 that are characteristic of the use of the space or shall be determined as the maximum probable population of the space under consideration, whichever is greater.

**14.1.7.2** The occupant load of an educational occupancy, or a portion thereof, shall be permitted to be modified from that specified in 14.1.7.1 if the necessary aisles and exits are provided.

**14.1.7.3** An approved aisle or seating diagram shall be required by the authority having jurisdiction to substantiate the modification permitted in 14.1.7.2.

### 15.1.6 Minimum Construction Requirements.

(No requirements.)

### 15.1.7 Occupant Load.

**15.1.7.1** The occupant load, in number of persons for whom means of egress and other provisions are required, shall be determined on the basis of the occupant load factors of Table 7.3.1.2 that are characteristic of the use of the space or shall be determined as the maximum probable population of the space under consideration, whichever is greater.

**15.1.7.2** The occupant load of an educational occupancy, or a portion thereof, shall be permitted to be modified from that specified in 15.1.7.1 if the necessary aisles and exits are provided.

**15.1.7.3** An approved aisle or seating diagram shall be required by the authority having jurisdiction to substantiate the modification permitted in 15.1.7.2.

Because occupant load is calculated on the basis of the use of a space, regardless of occupancy classification, occupant load factors appear in Chapter 7, a general chapter. Occupant load factors for a wide variety of uses are detailed in Table 7.3.1.2.

It is not the intent that occupant load factors be applied to require a minimum area per student for functional purposes. Rather, the occupant load factors are used to determine the occupant load for purposes of sizing the means of egress system. The intent is to require adequate egress capacity for those present. Efficient use of classroom space might result in the presence of a greater number of occupants than that determined by calculation using the occupant load factors of Table 7.3.1.2. Paragraph 14/15.1.7.1 permits the occupant load to be established as the maximum probable population if that number exceeds the number determined by calculation using the occupant load factors. However, the means of egress must adequately accommodate all occupants, and all other requirements dependent on the calculated occupant load must be met.

## 14.2 Means of Egress Requirements

### 14.2.1 General.

**14.2.1.1** Means of egress shall be in accordance with Chapter 7 and Section 14.2.

**14.2.1.2** Rooms normally occupied by preschool, kindergarten, or first-grade students shall be located on a level of exit discharge, unless otherwise permitted by 14.2.1.4.

**14.2.1.3** Rooms normally occupied by second-grade students shall not be located more than one story above a level of exit discharge, unless otherwise permitted by 14.2.1.4.

**14.2.1.4** Rooms or areas located on floor levels other than as specified in 14.2.1.2 and 14.2.1.3 shall be permitted to be used where provided with independent means of egress dedicated for use by the preschool, kindergarten, first-grade, or second-grade students.

The restrictions on the location of rooms used by preschool, kindergarten, or first- or second-grade pupils were developed to avoid the danger of older — and larger — children overrunning the very young on stairs or ramps during a fire or other incident requiring rapid evacuation. The exemption offered by 14/15.2.1.4 recognizes that the younger students — often with the help of teachers and staff — can use the stairs and ramps effectively if they don't have to compete with the older, larger, and faster students. For a definition of the term *level of exit discharge*, see 3.3.77.1.

### 14.2.2 Means of Egress Components.

**14.2.2.1 Components Permitted.** Components of means of egress shall be limited to the types described in 14.2.2.2 through 14.2.2.10.

**14.2.2.2 Doors.**

**14.2.2.2.1** Doors complying with 7.2.1 shall be permitted.

**14.2.2.2.2** Any door in a required means of egress from an area having an occupant load of 100 or more persons shall be permitted to be provided with a latch or lock only if the latch or lock is panic hardware or fire exit hardware complying with 7.2.1.7.

**14.2.2.2.3** Special locking arrangements complying with 7.2.1.6 shall be permitted.

**14.2.2.2.4** Elevator lobby exit access door locking in accordance with 7.2.1.6.3 shall be permitted.

**14.2.2.3* Stairs.** Stairs complying with 7.2.2 shall be permitted.

**A.14.2.2.3** See A.7.2.2.4.4.4 regarding additional handrails on stairs that are used extensively by children 5 years of age or less.



## 15.2 Means of Egress Requirements

### 15.2.1 General.

**15.2.1.1** Means of egress shall be in accordance with Chapter 7 and Section 15.2.

**15.2.1.2** Rooms normally occupied by preschool, kindergarten, or first-grade students shall be located on a level of exit discharge, unless otherwise permitted by 15.2.1.4.

**15.2.1.3** Rooms normally occupied by second-grade students shall not be located more than one story above a level of exit discharge, unless otherwise permitted by 15.2.1.4.

**15.2.1.4** Rooms or areas located on floor levels other than as specified in 15.2.1.2 and 15.2.1.3 shall be permitted to be used where provided with independent means of egress dedicated for use by the preschool, kindergarten, first-grade, or second-grade students.

### 15.2.2 Means of Egress Components.

**15.2.2.1 Components Permitted.** Components of means of egress shall be limited to the types described in 15.2.2.2 through 15.2.2.10.

**15.2.2.2 Doors.**

**15.2.2.2.1** Doors complying with 7.2.1 shall be permitted.

**15.2.2.2.2** Any required exit door subject to use by 100 or more persons shall be permitted to be provided with a latch or lock only if the latch or lock is panic hardware or fire exit hardware complying with 7.2.1.7.

**15.2.2.2.3** Special locking arrangements complying with 7.2.1.6 shall be permitted.

**15.2.2.2.4** Elevator lobby exit access door locking in accordance with 7.2.1.6.3 shall be permitted.

**15.2.2.3* Stairs.** Stairs complying with 7.2.2 shall be permitted.

**A.15.2.2.3** See A.7.2.2.4.4.4 regarding additional handrails on stairs that are used extensively by children 5 years of age or less.

CHAPTER 14 • New

**14.2.2.4 Smokeproof Enclosures.** Smokeproof enclosures complying with 7.2.3 shall be permitted.

**14.2.2.5 Horizontal Exits.** Horizontal exits complying with 7.2.4 shall be permitted.

**14.2.2.6 Ramps.** Ramps complying with 7.2.5 shall be permitted.

**14.2.2.7 Exit Passageways.** Exit passageways complying with 7.2.6 shall be permitted.

**14.2.2.8 Fire Escape Ladders.** Fire escape ladders complying with 7.2.9 shall be permitted.

**14.2.2.9 Alternating Tread Devices.** Alternating tread devices complying with 7.2.11 shall be permitted.

**14.2.2.10 Areas of Refuge.** Areas of refuge complying with 7.2.12 shall be permitted.

CHAPTER 15 • Existing

**15.2.2.4 Smokeproof Enclosures.** Smokeproof enclosures complying with 7.2.3 shall be permitted.

**15.2.2.5 Horizontal Exits.** Horizontal exits complying with 7.2.4 shall be permitted.

**15.2.2.6 Ramps.** Ramps complying with 7.2.5 shall be permitted.

**15.2.2.7 Exit Passageways.** Exit passageways complying with 7.2.6 shall be permitted.

**15.2.2.8 Fire Escape Ladders.** Fire escape ladders complying with 7.2.9 shall be permitted.

**15.2.2.9 Alternating Tread Devices.** Alternating tread devices complying with 7.2.11 shall be permitted.

**15.2.2.10 Areas of Refuge.** Areas of refuge complying with 7.2.12 shall be permitted.

Subsection 14/15.2.2 lists those components acceptable for use in the means of egress serving an educational occupancy. Some of the components described in Chapter 7 were judged to be unacceptable for educational occupancy egress system use. Note that slide escapes, escalators, fire escape stairs, and revolving doors are not permitted to be credited as providing any of the required means of egress in an educational occupancy.

The panic hardware and fire exit hardware provisions of 14/15.2.2.2.2 include application thresholds expressed in terms of occupant load. For new construction, the occupant load addressed by 14.2.2.2.2 is the total occupant load of the area served and not only the required capacity of the door. For example, if an area of a new educational occupancy has an occupant load of 180 persons and is served by three doors, each door is required to have sufficient capacity for 60 persons. However, because the doors serve an overall area with 100 or more persons, any latches on these doors must be arranged to be released by panic hardware or fire exit hardware.

The requirement for panic hardware or fire exit hardware in existing educational occupancies is slightly less restrictive than for new educational occupancies. In accordance with 15.2.2.2.2, panic hardware or fire exit hardware is required only on exit doors rather than all egress doors; therefore, the requirement does not apply to exit access doors — such as corridor doors and smoke barrier doors. In addition, 15.2.2.2.2 establishes its criteria on the basis of the number of people using the door for egress. For example, if a single-story existing educational occupancy building with an occupant load of 180 persons has three exit doors, each door can be considered as providing egress capacity for 60 persons. Because no individual exit door is required to have a capacity for 100 or more occupants, panic hardware is not required for the existing doors.

The provision of 14/15.2.2.2.3 references 7.2.1.6, which, at the time it was written, included only 7.2.1.6.1, which applies to delayed-egress locks, and 7.2.1.6.2, which applies to access-controlled egress doors. The intent of 14/15.2.2.2.3 is to permit the use of both sets of features in educational occupancies. New to the 2009 edition of the *Code* are the provisions of 7.2.1.6.3 for elevator lobby exit access door assemblies locking. The technical committee created 14/15.2.2.2.4 to specifically permit the provisions of 7.2.1.6.3 to be used in educational occupancies. For a future edition of the *Code*, the committee will be asked to create separate paragraphs to permit the use of delayed-egress locking systems, access-controlled egress door assemblies, and elevator lobby exit access door assemblies locking.

To use the provisions for delayed-egress locks, the building must be either fully sprinklered or fully protected by an automatic fire detection system. Although many occupancies recognize use of the Chapter 7 provisions for delayed-egress locks, the original hardware was developed for educational occupancies. Delayed-egress locking provisions were added to Chapter 7 based on hardware development that addresses security concerns in schools.

As explained in the fourth paragraph of this commentary, the provision of 14/15.2.2.2.4 is new to the 2009 edition of the *Code*. It permits use of the elevator lobby exit access door-locking provisions of 7.2.1.6.3. Paragraph 7.2.1.6.3 details 15 criteria that must be met as an alternative to the requirements of 7.4.1.6 that each elevator landing or lobby must have access to at least one exit without the use of a key, a tool, special knowledge, or special effort. See 7.4.1.6 and 7.2.1.6.3.

Since the 2006 edition of the *Code*, 15.2.2.3, applicable to existing stairs, references the provisions of 7.2.2 without further modification. In earlier editions, existing stairs for student use were required to be those stairs that were formerly designated as Class A stairs. Subsection 7.2.2 was revised to eliminate the Class A and Class B designations for existing stairs. The existing stairs provisions in Table 7.2.2.2.1.1(b) permit the formerly designated Class B stairs to suffice for all existing installations.

Although 14/15.2.2.8 and 14/15.2.2.9 permit fire escape ladders and alternating tread devices as components of the means of egress, some Chapter 7 provisions limit the use of such ladders and devices. For example, the provisions of 7.2.9 and 7.2.11 restrict the use of fire escape ladders and alternating tread devices to normally unoccupied areas, such as rooftops, or to mechanical equipment platforms subject to occupancy by not more than three persons who are all capable of using the ladder or alternating tread device.

### 14.2.3 Capacity of Means of Egress.

**14.2.3.1 General.** Capacity of means of egress shall be in accordance with Section 7.3.

**14.2.3.2 Minimum Corridor Width.** Exit access corridors shall have not less than 6 ft (1830 mm) of clear width.

### 15.2.3 Capacity of Means of Egress.

**15.2.3.1 General.** Capacity of means of egress shall be in accordance with Section 7.3.

**15.2.3.2 Minimum Corridor Width.** Exit access corridors shall have not less than 6 ft (1830 mm) of clear width.

Note that the minimum exit access corridor width requirement of 14/15.2.3.2 applies, regardless of the required capacity of the corridor. Based on egress capacity considerations, larger widths might be necessary for corridors handling large numbers of students; see 14/15.2.3.1 and Section 7.3.

The term *clear width* means a 6 ft (1830 mm) wide clear space with no obstructions other than those permitted by 7.3.2.2. Subsection 7.3.2 details the required method for measuring the width of a component of the means of egress. Paragraph 7.3.2.2 permits projections of not more than 4½ in. (114 mm) on each side of the corridor. The projections are permitted to be located at or below a handrail height of 38 in. (965 mm), and the maximum 4 ½ in. (114 mm) encroachment is to be ignored when determining width for use in egress capacity calculations.

The intent of the 6 ft (1830 mm) corridor width requirement is to permit two files of students to move simultaneously, with sufficient room for teachers or monitors to supervise. Extremely short corridor stubs or sections serving only one or two rooms might warrant consideration for some reduction in required width under the equivalency concept of Section 1.4.

### 14.2.4 Number of Exits.

Not less than two separate exits shall be as follows:

(1) Provided on every story
(2) Accessible from every part of every story and mezzanine

### 15.2.4 Number of Exits.

Not less than two separate exits shall be as follows:

(1) Provided on every story
(2) Accessible from every part of every story and mezzanine

Access must be provided to a minimum of two exits, both of which must be located on the floor or story in question. Contrast this requirement with a related provision for industrial occupancies that only one of the required exits be located on the floor or story (see 40.2.4.1.1). Thus, in an educational occupancy, an open exit access stair, if it were permitted without violating the provisions applicable to the protection of vertical openings, would be permitted to serve as exit access only if the requirement for two exits on the floor is first

CHAPTER 14 • New

satisfied. In a multistory educational occupancy building, the requirements of 14/15.2.4 are typically met by providing two properly enclosed exit stairs that can be accessed from all floors above or below the level of exit discharge.

### 14.2.5 Arrangement of Means of Egress.

See also Section 7.5.

**14.2.5.1** Means of egress shall be arranged in accordance with Section 7.5.

**14.2.5.2** No dead-end corridor shall exceed 20 ft (6100 mm), other than in buildings protected throughout by an approved, supervised automatic sprinkler system in accordance with Section 9.7, in which case dead-end corridors shall not exceed 50 ft (15 m).

**14.2.5.3** Limitations on common path of travel shall be in accordance with 14.2.5.3.1 and 14.2.5.3.2.

**14.2.5.3.1** Common path of travel shall not exceed 100 ft (30 m) in a building protected throughout by an approved, supervised automatic sprinkler system in accordance with Section 9.7.

**14.2.5.3.2** Common path of travel shall not exceed 75 ft (23 m) in a building not protected throughout by an approved, supervised automatic sprinkler system in accordance with Section 9.7.

**14.2.5.4** Every room or space larger than 1000 $ft^2$ (93 $m^2$) or with an occupant load of more than 50 persons shall comply with the following:

(1) The room or space shall have a minimum of two exit access doors.
(2) The doors required by 14.2.5.4(1) shall provide access to separate exits.
(3) The doors required by 14.2.5.4(1) shall be permitted to open onto a common corridor, provided that such corridor leads to separate exits located in opposite directions.

CHAPTER 15 • Existing

### 15.2.5 Arrangement of Means of Egress.

**15.2.5.1** Means of egress shall be arranged in accordance with Section 7.5.

**15.2.5.2** No dead-end corridor shall exceed 20 ft (6100 mm), other than in buildings protected throughout by an approved, supervised automatic sprinkler system in accordance with Section 9.7, in which case dead-end corridors shall not exceed 50 ft (15 m).

**15.2.5.3** Limitations on common path of travel shall be in accordance with 15.2.5.3.1 and 15.2.5.3.2.

**15.2.5.3.1** Common path of travel shall not exceed 100 ft (30 m) in a building protected throughout by an approved, supervised automatic sprinkler system in accordance with Section 9.7.

**15.2.5.3.2** Common path of travel shall not exceed 75 ft (23 m) in a building not protected throughout by an approved, supervised automatic sprinkler system in accordance with Section 9.7.

**15.2.5.4** Every room or space larger than 1000 $ft^2$ (93 $m^2$) or with an occupant load of more than 50 persons shall comply with the following:

(1) The room or space shall have a minimum of two exit access doors.
(2) The doors required by 15.2.5.4(1) shall provide access to separate exits.
(3) The doors required by 15.2.5.4(1) shall be permitted to open onto a common corridor, provided that such corridor leads to separate exits located in opposite directions.

Paragraph 7.5.1.1.4 permits individual occupancy chapters to allow, and to set limits for, common paths of travel. Paragraph 14/15.2.5.3 establishes the maximum common path of travel for educational occupancies as 100 ft (30 m), if the building is protected throughout by an approved, supervised automatic sprinkler system, and limits the common path of travel to 75 ft (23 m) where the sprinkler criteria are not met. The 75 ft (23 m) limit is strict enough to help ensure that occupants can safely tolerate traveling in only one direction for a limited distance before reaching a point where travel in independent directions becomes possible. The increase to 100 ft (30 m) recognizes that fire controlled by sprinklers increases the safe travel time along the single available path.

Paragraph 7.5.1.5 permits individual occupancy chapters to establish limits for dead-end corridors. The standard dead-end corridor limitation for educational occupancies in the past has been 20 ft (6100 mm), as permitted by 14/15.2.5.2 — and the limitation still appears reasonable. However, 14/15.2.5.2 permits the dead-end corridor to be increased by 30 ft (9.1 m) to a maximum of 50 ft (15 m) in recognition of the fire-controlling capabilities of a sprinkler system.

A floor arrangement with outside doors or stairways at both ends of a central corridor typically creates no dead-end corridors. Dead-end corridor pockets might be created where stairways are not located at the end of corridors but are located at intermediate points. See Exhibit 14/15.1. Part (a) in Exhibit 14/15.1 indicates no dead-end corridors. This arrangement is preferred but is not always practical in terms of building layout and use. At each end of the corridor in Part (b) of Exhibit 14/15.1, dead-end pockets are shown into which occupants might mistakenly travel, only to have to retrace their path to find an exit. However, the length of the dead-end corridor does not exceed the 20 ft (6100 mm) permitted by 14/15.2.5.2. All classrooms have been arranged so that the common path of travel does not exceed the 75 ft (23 m) limitation of 14/15.2.5.3.2. This arrangement is acceptable. In an educational occupancy building that is protected throughout by an approved, supervised automatic sprinkler system, the 20 ft (6100 mm) dead-end corridor can be increased to 50 ft (15 m); and the 75 ft (23 m) common path of travel can be increased to 100 ft (30 m).

Exhibit 14/15.1 also depicts the provisions of 14/15.2.5.4. In Part (a), two of the rooms are large enough to require a second exit access door. In one case, the room has an occupant load of more than 50 persons; in the other, the room area exceeds 1000 ft² (93 m²). The two doors from each of the two rooms open onto a common corridor but provide access to exits in two different directions.

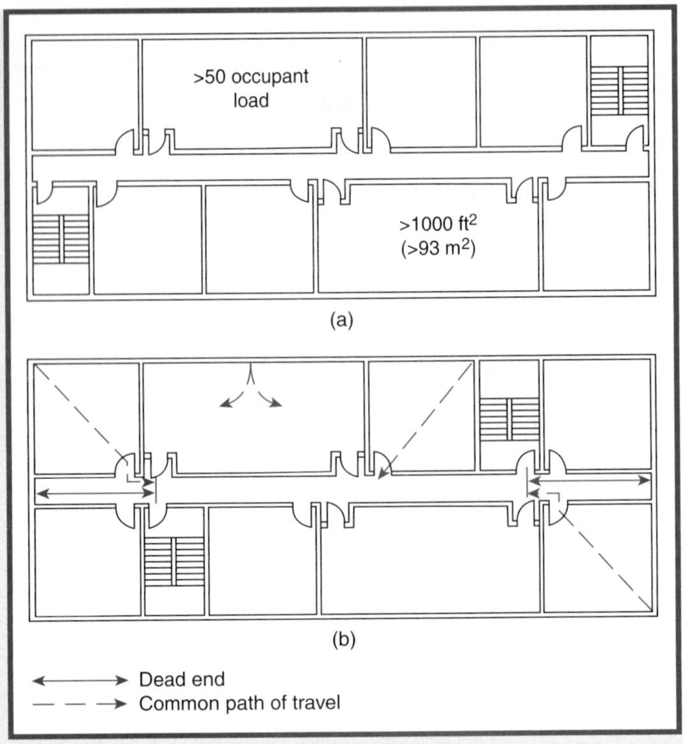


***Exhibit 14/15.1*** *Dead-end corridors, common path of travel, and second exit access from larger rooms.*

**14.2.5.5** Every room that is normally subject to student occupancy shall have an exit access door leading directly to an exit access corridor or exit, unless otherwise permitted by the following:

(1) This requirement shall not apply where an exit door opens directly to the outside or to an exterior balcony or corridor as described in 14.2.5.9.

(2) One room shall be permitted to intervene between a normally occupied student room and an exit access corridor, provided that all of the following criteria are met:

(a) The travel from a room served by an intervening room to the corridor door or exit shall not exceed 75 ft (23 m).

(b) Clothing, personal effects, or other materials deemed hazardous by the authority having jurisdiction shall be stored in metal lockers, provided that they do not obstruct the exit access, or the intervening room shall be sprinklered in accordance with Section 9.7.

**15.2.5.5** Every room that is normally subject to student occupancy shall have an exit access door leading directly to an exit access corridor or exit, unless otherwise permitted by the following:

(1) This requirement shall not apply where an exit door opens directly to the outside or to an exterior balcony or corridor as described in 15.2.5.9.

(2) One room shall be permitted to intervene between a normally occupied student room and an exit access corridor, provided that all of the following criteria are met:

(a) The travel from a room served by an intervening room to the corridor door or exit shall not exceed 75 ft (23 m).

(b) Clothing, personal effects, or other materials deemed hazardous by the authority having jurisdiction shall be stored in metal lockers, provided that they do not obstruct the exit access, or the intervening room shall be sprinklered in accordance with Section 9.7.

**CHAPTER 14 • New**

(c) One of the following means of protection shall be provided:
  i. The intervening room shall have approved fire detection that activates the building alarm.
  ii. The building shall be protected by an approved, supervised automatic sprinkler system in accordance with Section 9.7.

**CHAPTER 15 • Existing**

(c) One of the following means of protection shall be provided:
  i. The intervening room shall have approved fire detection that activates the building alarm.
  ii. The building shall be protected by an approved automatic sprinkler system in accordance with Section 9.7.

(3) Approved existing arrangements shall be permitted to continue in use.

To ensure ready access to the exit access corridor — which is intended to be a safer portion of the exit access than an occupied room with furnishings — 14/15.2.5.5 requires most normally occupied rooms to have a door open directly into an exit access corridor. The use of such a door avoids the need for occupants to pass through intervening rooms that might not be arranged or maintained to allow orderly evacuation.

Normally occupied rooms that have doors opening directly to the outside at grade or to an exterior exit access balcony are exempted from the base requirement. Also exempted are normally occupied rooms having only one intervening room that meets the following criteria:

1. Travel distance through the intervening room to the corridor door is limited to 75 ft (23 m).
2. Personal effects — such as coats and other belongings or other contents deemed hazardous by the authority having jurisdiction (AHJ) — must be kept in metal lockers, or the intervening room must be sprinklered.
3. Either the intervening room is supplied with fire detectors connected to the building alarm system, or the entire building is protected throughout by an approved automatic sprinkler system.

It is the *Code*'s intent that, if metal lockers are chosen as the intervening room fire detection option, smoke detectors, rather than heat detectors, should be selected to provide for rapid occupant notification. However, heat detectors are permitted to be used if nuisance alarms are anticipated (e.g., in automotive or woodworking shops with attached classrooms).

Exhibit 14/15.2 and Exhibit 14/15.3 illustrate several possible intervening room configurations that comply with the *Code*. In Exhibit 14/15.2, Suite A is arranged to comply with 14/15.2.5.5. Each normally occupied room has a door opening either directly to the corridor or to the exterior (opening at grade or to an exterior exit access balcony), as permitted by 14/15.2.5.5(1). The arrangement shown in the lower portion of Exhibit 14/15.2 is permitted, provided that travel distance from the normally occupied rooms to the corridor (from point *X* to point *C*) does not exceed 75 ft (23 m), clothing and other personal effects in the intervening room are stored in metal lockers, and occupant notification is provided in the intervening room by a fire detection system (preferably smoke detection for earliest possible notification).

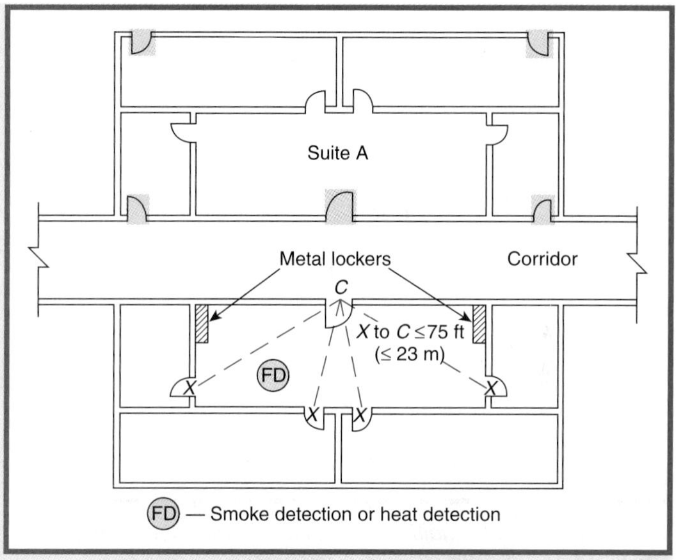


***Exhibit 14/15.2*** *Room arrangements complying with 14/15.2.5.5.*

In Exhibit 14/15.3, Part (a) and Part (b) represent acceptable intervening room arrangements in accordance with 14/15.2.5.5(2). Part (a) depicts the limited travel distance from point *X* to point *C*, along with the intervening room sprinkler system addressed in 14/15.2.5.5(2)(b) and the intervening room fire detection system addressed in 14/15.2.5.5(2)(c)i. Part (b) represents a building protected throughout by an automatic sprinkler system that satisfies both 14/15.2.5.5(2)(b) and 14/15.2.5.5(2)(c)ii. In effect, even the installation within an intervening room of an automatic sprinkler system that is connected to the

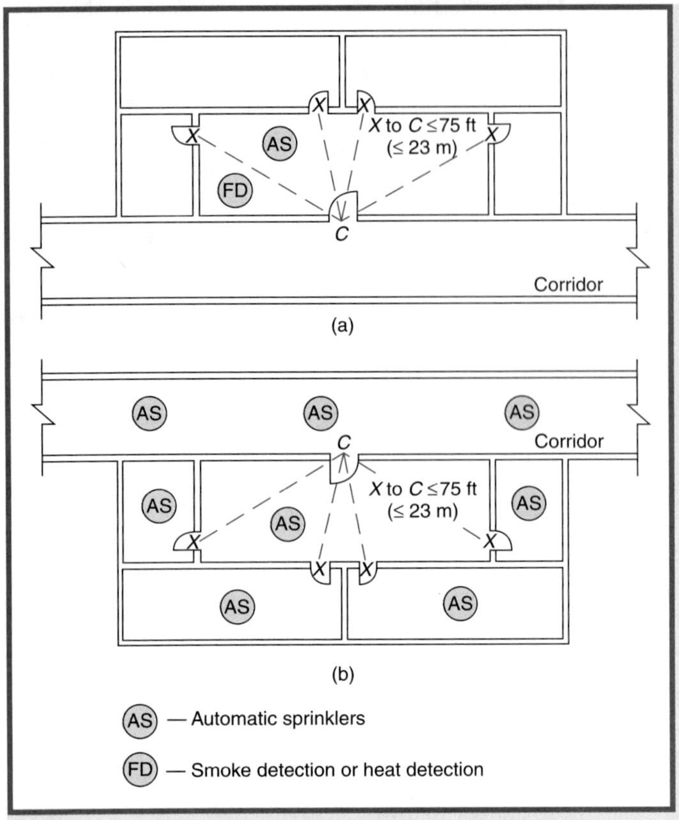


***Exhibit 14/15.3** Additional room arrangements complying with 14/15.2.5.5.*

building fire alarm system would satisfy the criteria of 14/15.2.5.5(2)(c)i, because automatic sprinklers are considered heat detectors. Therefore, this approach would satisfy both 14/15.2.5.5(2)(b) and 14/15.2.5.5(2)(c).

**14.2.5.6** Doors that swing into an exit access corridor shall be arranged to prevent interference with corridor travel. *(See also 7.2.1.4.3.)*

**14.2.5.7** Aisles shall be not less than 30 in. (760 mm) wide.

**14.2.5.8** The space between parallel rows of seats shall not be subject to the minimum aisle width, provided that the number of seats that intervene between any seat and an aisle does not exceed six.

**14.2.5.9*** Exterior exit access shall comply with 7.5.3.

**A.14.2.5.9** A corridor roofed over and enclosed on its long side and open to the atmosphere at the end is permitted to be considered an exterior corridor if either of the following criteria are met:

(1) Clear story openings for the corridor are provided on both sides of the corridor and above adjacent roofs or buildings, and such clear openings are not less than one-half the height of the corridor walls.
(2) The corridor roof has unobstructed openings to the sky not less than 50 percent of the area of the roof.

**15.2.5.6** Doors that swing into an exit access corridor shall be arranged to prevent interference with corridor travel. *(See also 7.2.1.4.3.)*

**15.2.5.7** Aisles shall be not less than 30 in. (760 mm) wide.

**15.2.5.8** The space between parallel rows of seats shall not be subject to the minimum aisle width, provided that the number of seats that intervene between any seat and an aisle does not exceed six.

**15.2.5.9*** Exterior exit access shall comply with 7.5.3.

**A.15.2.5.9** A corridor roofed over and enclosed on its long side and open to the atmosphere at the end is permitted to be considered an exterior corridor if either of the following criteria are met:

(1) Clear story openings for the corridor are provided on both sides of the corridor and above adjacent roofs or buildings, and such clear openings are not less than one-half the height of the corridor walls.
(2) The corridor roof has unobstructed openings to the sky not less than 50 percent of the area of the roof.

CHAPTER 14 • New

The openings detailed in A.14.2.5.9(1) and (2) are to be equally distributed, and, if louvers are installed, they are to be fixed open with a clear area based on the actual openings between louver vanes.

CHAPTER 15 • Existing

The openings detailed in A.15.2.5.9(1) are to be equally distributed, and, if louvers are installed, they are to be fixed open with a clear area based on the actual openings between louver vanes.

Exhibit 14/15.4 illustrates exterior exit access arranged in accordance with 7.5.3. The stairs have been positioned to comply with 7.5.3.3; the arrangement allows an occupant to reach at least one of the stairs without having to travel past an unprotected opening.

Exhibit 14/15.5 and Exhibit 14/15.6 illustrate the use of roofed-over exterior exit access corridors suggested by A.14/A.15.2.5.9. In Exhibit 14/15.5, the openings labeled A, B, C, and D are clear story openings. The building height is 10 ft (3050 mm). For a corridor to be considered an outside corridor, the minimum height for the corridor roof is 5 ft (1525 mm). In this exhibit, the minimum clear story height requirements have been met.

In Exhibit 14/15.6, the alternative to the clear story openings is a roof with unobstructed openings to the sky that are equal to not less than 50 percent of the corridor roof area. The example shown has eight openings. Each opening is 4 ft × 16 ft (1220 mm × 4875 mm), or 64 ft² (5.9 m²). The total corridor roof area is 900 ft² (84 m²). The total unobstructed opening equals 512 ft² (48 m²) — greater than 50 percent of the total roof area. This example is considered an acceptable design.

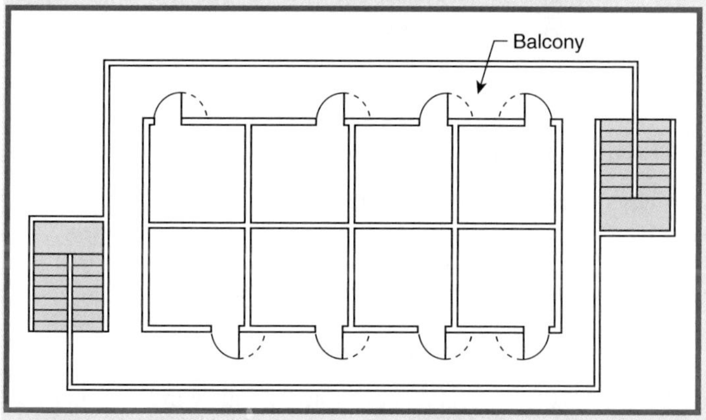


***Exhibit 14/15.4*** *Exterior exit access via balcony and stairs.*

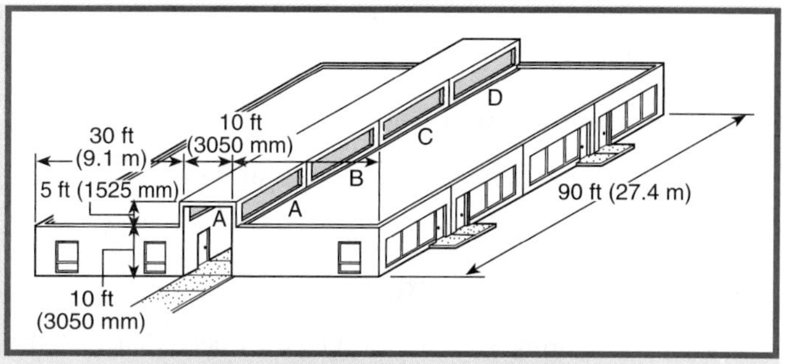


***Exhibit 14/15.5*** *Exterior corridor using clear story openings.*

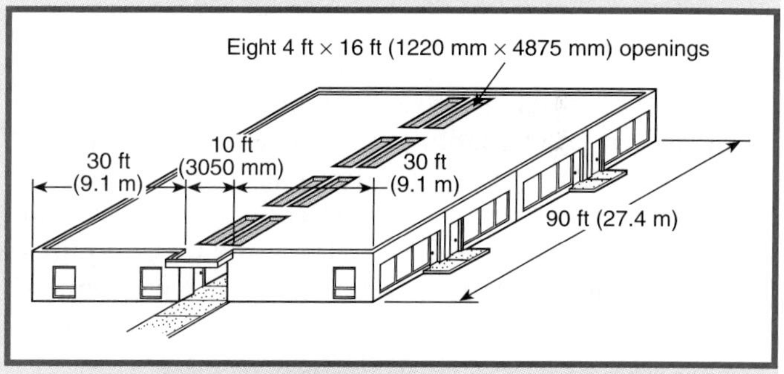


***Exhibit 14/15.6*** *Exterior corridor using roof openings.*

### 14.2.6 Travel Distance to Exits.

Travel distance shall comply with 14.2.6.1 through 14.2.6.3.

**14.2.6.1** Travel distance shall be measured in accordance with Section 7.6.

**14.2.6.2** Travel distance to an exit shall not exceed 150 ft (46 m) from any point in a building, unless otherwise provided in 14.2.6.3. *(See also Section 7.6.)*

**14.2.6.3** Travel distance shall not exceed 200 ft (61 m) in educational occupancies protected throughout by an approved, supervised automatic sprinkler system in accordance with Section 9.7.

### 15.2.6 Travel Distance to Exits.

Travel distance shall comply with 15.2.6.1 through 15.2.6.4.

**15.2.6.1** Travel distance shall be measured in accordance with Section 7.6.

**15.2.6.2** Travel distance to an exit shall not exceed 150 ft (46 m) from any point in a building, unless otherwise permitted by 15.2.6.3 or 15.2.6.4. *(See also Section 7.6.)*

**15.2.6.3** Travel distance shall not exceed 200 ft (61 m) in educational occupancies protected throughout by an approved automatic sprinkler system in accordance with Section 9.7.

CHAPTER 14 • New

### 14.2.7 Discharge from Exits.

Discharge from exits shall be arranged in accordance with Section 7.7.

### 14.2.8 Illumination of Means of Egress.

Means of egress shall be illuminated in accordance with Section 7.8.

### 14.2.9 Emergency Lighting.

Emergency lighting shall be provided in accordance with Section 7.9.

CHAPTER 15 • Existing

**15.2.6.4** Approved existing travel distances shall be permitted to continue in use.

### 15.2.7 Discharge from Exits.

Discharge from exits shall be arranged in accordance with Section 7.7.

### 15.2.8 Illumination of Means of Egress.

Means of egress shall be illuminated in accordance with Section 7.8.

### 15.2.9 Emergency Lighting.

**15.2.9.1** Emergency lighting shall be provided in accordance with Section 7.9, unless otherwise permitted by 15.2.9.2.

**15.2.9.2** Approved existing emergency lighting installations shall be permitted to be continued in use.

In earlier editions of the *Code*, emergency lighting was required in shops, laboratories, assembly use spaces (such as lecture halls, auditoriums, and dining rooms), and interior and windowless portions of educational occupancies. Since the 2003 edition, the *Code* requires that educational occupancies be provided with emergency lighting in accordance with Section 7.9. Paragraph 7.9.1.2 clarifies that the portion of the exit access for which the emergency lighting must be provided includes designated aisles, corridors, and passageways — not all portions of the exit access.

CHAPTER 14 • New

### 14.2.10 Marking of Means of Egress.

Means of egress shall have signs in accordance with Section 7.10.

### 14.2.11 Special Means of Egress Features.

**14.2.11.1* Windows for Rescue.**

**A.14.2.11.1** It is highly desirable that all windows be of a type that can be readily opened from inside and that they are large enough and low enough for use by students, teachers, and fire fighters. Windows are permitted to serve as a supplementary means of emergency escape, particularly where ladders can be raised by fire fighters or others.

**14.2.11.1.1** Every room or space greater than 250 $ft^2$ (23.2 $m^2$) and used for classroom or other educational purposes or normally subject to student occupancy shall have not less than one outside window for emergency rescue that complies with the following, unless otherwise permitted by 14.2.11.1.2:

(1) Such windows shall be openable from the inside without the use of tools and shall provide a clear opening of not less than 20 in. (510 mm) in width, 24 in. (610 mm) in height, and 5.7 $ft^2$ (0.5 $m^2$) in area.

CHAPTER 15 • Existing

### 15.2.10 Marking of Means of Egress.

Means of egress shall have signs in accordance with Section 7.10.

### 15.2.11 Special Means of Egress Features.

**15.2.11.1* Windows for Rescue.**

**A.15.2.11.1** It is highly desirable that all windows be of a type that can be readily opened from inside and that they are large enough and low enough for use by students, teachers, and fire fighters. Windows are permitted to serve as a supplementary means of emergency escape, particularly where ladders can be raised by fire fighters or others.

**15.2.11.1.1** Every room or space greater than 250 $ft^2$ (23.2 $m^2$) and used for classroom or other educational purposes or normally subject to student occupancy shall have not less than one outside window for emergency rescue that complies with the following, unless otherwise permitted by 15.2.11.1.2:

(1) Such windows shall be openable from the inside without the use of tools and shall provide a clear opening of not less than 20 in. (510 mm) in width, 24 in. (610 mm) in height, and 5.7 $ft^2$ (0.5 $m^2$) in area.

CHAPTER 14 • New

(2) The bottom of the opening shall be not more than 44 in. (1120 mm) above the floor, and any latching device shall be capable of being operated from not more than 54 in. (1370 mm) above the finished floor.
(3) The clear opening shall allow a rectangular solid, with a width and height that provides not less than the required 5.7 ft$^2$ (0.5 m$^2$) opening and a depth of not less than 20 in. (510 mm), to pass fully through the opening.
(4) Such windows shall be accessible by the fire department and shall open into an area having access to a public way.

**14.2.11.1.2** The requirements of 14.2.11.1.1 shall not apply to the following:

(1) Buildings protected throughout by an approved, supervised automatic sprinkler system in accordance with Section 9.7
(2) Where the room or space has a door leading directly to the outside of the building
(3) Rooms located four or more stories above the finished ground level

CHAPTER 15 • Existing

(2) The bottom of the opening shall be not more than 44 in. (1120 mm) above the floor, and any latching device shall be capable of being operated from not more than 54 in. (1370 mm) above the finished floor.
(3) The clear opening shall allow a rectangular solid, with a width and height that provides not less than the required 5.7 ft$^2$ (0.5 m$^2$) opening and a depth of not less than 20 in. (510 mm), to pass fully through the opening.

**15.2.11.1.2** The requirements of 15.2.11.1.1 shall not apply to the following:

(1) Buildings protected throughout by an approved automatic sprinkler system in accordance with Section 9.7
(2) Where the room or space has a door leading directly to the outside of the building
(3) Rooms located four or more stories above the finished ground level
(4) Where awning-type or hopper-type windows that are hinged or subdivided to provide a clear opening of not less than 4 ft$^2$ (0.38 m$^2$) or any dimension of not less than 22 in. (560 mm) meet the following criteria:
   (a) Such windows shall be permitted to continue in use.
   (b) Screen walls or devices located in front of required windows shall not interfere with rescue requirements.
(5) Where the room or space complies with the following:
   (a) Doors shall exist that allow travel between adjacent classrooms.
   (b) Doors used to travel from classroom to classroom shall provide one of the following:
      i. Direct access to exits in both directions
      ii. Direct access to an exit in one direction and to a separate smoke compartment that provides access to another exit in the other direction
   (c) The corridor shall be separated from the classrooms by a wall that resists the passage of smoke, and all doors between the classrooms and the corridor shall be self-closing or automatic-closing in accordance with 7.2.1.8.
   (d) The length of travel to exits along such paths shall not exceed 150 ft (46 m).
   (e) Each communicating door shall be marked in accordance with Section 7.10.
   (f) No locking device shall be permitted on the communicating doors.

CHAPTER 14 • New

Small rooms of 250 ft² (23.2 m²) or less, such as those used for music instruction or student counseling, and subject to occupancy by very few students, are exempt from the rescue window requirement.

The dimensions specified for windows used for emergency rescue are based on simulations of emergency rescue conducted by the San Diego Fire Department. Windows providing clear openings of identical dimensions are also required for rescue in dwellings. Exhibit 14/15.7 illustrates two configurations that provide the required area of 5.7 ft² (0.5 m²) and the minimum opening height and width.

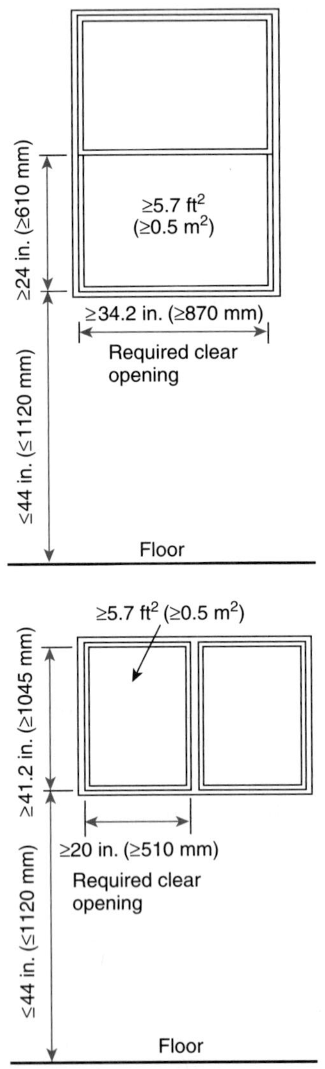


***Exhibit 14/15.7*** *Windows for rescue — minimum required dimension.*

CHAPTER 15 • Existing

Awning-type and hopper-type windows might provide the required opening within the plane of the building exterior wall. However, when the window is open, the sash and glazing are outside that plane and might prevent occupants from passing through the opening. Therefore, the criterion of 14/15.2.11.1.1(3) for providing an opening through which a minimum-size rectangular solid can pass is intended to ensure that occupants can pass through the opening. For existing awning-type windows, 15.2.11.1.2(4) offers some relief from the rectangular solid and minimum-size opening requirements. The exemption in 15.2.11.1.2(4) is provided in acknowledgment of a feature that was formerly recognized by the *Code*. Although the exemption is no longer permitted in new construction, it is still permitted in existing facilities. Exhibit 14/15.8 illustrates the use of 15.2.11.1.2(4).

The *Code* intends that the fire department or others are to assist students, especially over ladders once students have moved through the window opening. Emergency rescue windows used as a supplementary means of escape need to allow small children to utilize the window unaided. Therefore, storm sashes, screens, or devices in front of the windows must be easy to open or remove, and the sills must be low enough for children to reach.

The *Code* also requires that new rescue windows be accessible to the fire department and that occupants, once they escape through the window to the outside, have access to a public way.

Emergency rescue windows are not required if a

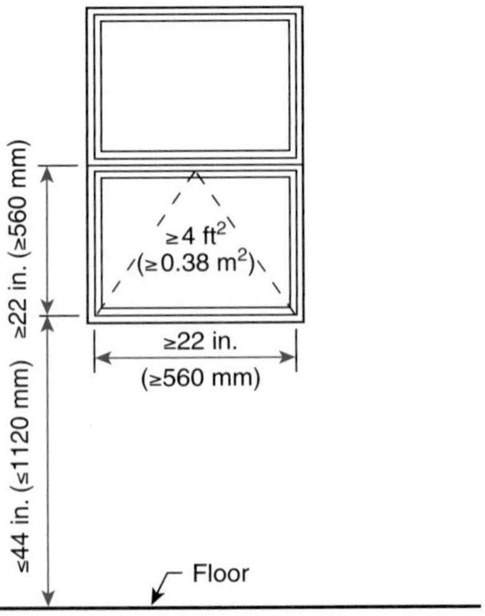


***Exhibit 14/15.8*** *Existing awning window — minimum dimensions permitted by 15.2.11.1.2(4).*

CHAPTER 14 • New | CHAPTER 15 • Existing

classroom has a door leading directly to the outside or if the building is totally sprinklered. Note that 14/115.2.11.1.2(1) requires that the building be protected throughout by an automatic sprinkler system. The purpose of the window is to provide means of escape when the interior corridor is blocked by smoke from a fire in another part of the building. Installing sprinklers in only some rooms does not provide protection from smoke that is emanating from other areas.

Paragraph 15.2.11.1.2(5) applies only in existing buildings. Exhibit 14/15.9 illustrates how the exemption can be used.

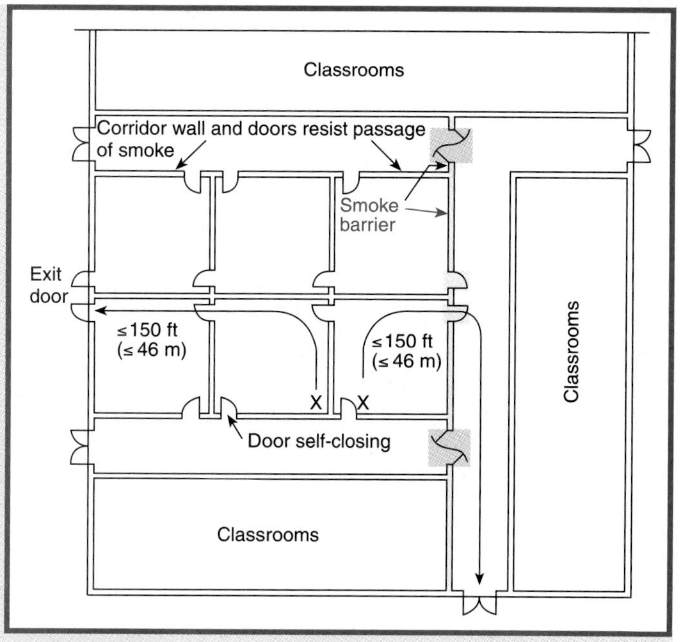


***Exhibit 14/15.9** One method of compensating for windowless classrooms in existing buildings as permitted by 15.2.11.1.2(5).*

**14.2.11.2 Lockups.** Lockups in educational occupancies shall comply with the requirements of 22.4.5.

**15.2.11.2 Lockups.** Lockups in educational occupancies, other than approved existing lockups, shall comply with the requirements of 23.4.5.

A *lockup* is defined in 3.3.155 as "an incidental use area in other than a detention and correctional occupancy where occupants are restrained and such occupants are mostly incapable of self-preservation because of security measures not under the occupants' control." For example, a lockup in an educational occupancy is a room for holding unruly students until police can transport such students to the police station. The provisions of Chapters 14 and 15 alone are not adequate to ensure life safety for those who are detained by security measures not under their control. Lockups in educational occupancies are required to meet the provisions of 22/23.4.5, which complete the needed package of protection features.

## 14.3 Protection

### 14.3.1 Protection of Vertical Openings.

**14.3.1.1** Any vertical opening, other than unprotected vertical openings in accordance with 8.6.8.2, shall be enclosed or protected in accordance with Section 8.6.

**14.3.1.2** Where the provisions of 8.6.6 are used, the requirements of 14.3.5.4 shall be met.

## 15.3 Protection

### 15.3.1 Protection of Vertical Openings.

**15.3.1.1** Any vertical opening, other than unprotected vertical openings in accordance with 8.6.8.2, shall be enclosed or protected in accordance with Section 8.6.

**15.3.1.2** Where the provisions of 8.6.6 are used, the requirements of 15.3.5.4 shall be met.

**15.3.1.3** Stairway enclosures shall not be required under the following conditions:

(1) Where a stairway serves only one adjacent floor, other than a basement

CHAPTER 14 • New

CHAPTER 15 • Existing

(2) Where a stairway is not connected with stairways serving other floors
(3) Where a stairway is not connected with corridors serving other than the two floors involved

Chapters 14 and 15 require all vertical openings, with the exception of an open and unobstructed communicating space connecting three floors or less (see 8.6.6, which often is referred to as the mini-atrium provision), an atrium (see 8.6.7), and a convenience opening (see 8.6.8.2), to be enclosed in accordance with Section 8.6. Although not specified by the communicating space provisions of 8.6.6, 14/15.3.1.2 and 14/15.3.5.4 require a building to be fully sprinklered to permit the maximum three-story unenclosed vertical opening. The convenience opening addressed by 8.6.8.2 might be useful, especially for two-story libraries or offices within schools.

The two-story stair permitted by 15.3.1.3 differs from the convenience opening detailed in 8.6.8.2; paragraph 15.3.1.3 permits an existing two-story school building to have open egress stairs between the first-floor corridor and second-floor corridor. Open egress stairs are not permitted in new construction. Basements are excluded from use of the exemption in 15.3.1.3, because basements usually contain hazardous contents areas with high fuel loads, such as storage rooms, boiler rooms, or workshops.

### 14.3.2 Protection from Hazards.

**14.3.2.1** Rooms or spaces for the storage, processing, or use of materials shall be protected in accordance with the following:

(1) Such rooms or spaces shall be separated from the remainder of the building by fire barriers having a minimum 1-hour fire resistance rating or protected by automatic extinguishing systems as specified in Section 8.7 in the following areas:
   (a) Boiler and furnace rooms, unless such rooms enclose only air-handling equipment
   (b) Rooms or spaces used for the storage of combustible supplies in quantities deemed hazardous by the authority having jurisdiction
   (c) Rooms or spaces used for the storage of hazardous materials or flammable or combustible liquids in quantities deemed hazardous by recognized standards
   (d) Janitor closets *[see also 14.3.2.1(4)]*
(2) Such rooms or spaces shall be separated from the remainder of the building by fire barriers having a minimum 1-hour fire resistance rating and protected by automatic extinguishing systems as specified in Section 8.7 in the following areas:
   (a) Laundries
   (b) Maintenance shops, including woodworking and painting areas
   (c) Rooms or spaces used for processing or use of combustible supplies deemed hazardous by the authority having jurisdiction

### 15.3.2 Protection from Hazards.

**15.3.2.1** Rooms or spaces for the storage, processing, or use of materials shall be protected in accordance with the following:

(1) Such rooms or spaces shall be separated from the remainder of the building by fire barriers having a minimum 1-hour fire resistance rating or protected by automatic extinguishing systems as specified in Section 8.7 in the following areas:
   (a) Boiler and furnace rooms, unless such rooms enclose only air-handling equipment
   (b) Rooms or spaces used for the storage of combustible supplies in quantities deemed hazardous by the authority having jurisdiction
   (c) Rooms or spaces used for the storage of hazardous materials or flammable or combustible liquids in quantities deemed hazardous by recognized standards
   (d) Janitor closets *[see also 15.3.2.1(4)]*
(2) Such rooms or spaces shall be separated from the remainder of the building by fire barriers having a minimum 1-hour fire resistance rating and protected by automatic extinguishing systems as specified in Section 8.7 in the following areas:
   (a) Laundries
   (b) Maintenance shops, including woodworking and painting areas
   (c) Rooms or spaces used for processing or use of combustible supplies deemed hazardous by the authority having jurisdiction

CHAPTER 14 • New

(d) Rooms or spaces used for processing or use of hazardous materials or flammable or combustible liquids in quantities deemed hazardous by recognized standards

(3) Where automatic extinguishing is used to meet the requirements of 14.3.2.1(1) or (2), the protection shall be permitted in accordance with 9.7.1.2.
(4) Where janitor closets addressed in 14.3.2.1(1)(d) are protected in accordance with the sprinkler option of 14.3.2.1(1), the janitor closet doors shall be permitted to have ventilating louvers.

**14.3.2.2** Cooking facilities shall be protected in accordance with 9.2.3. Openings shall not be required to be protected between food preparation areas and dining areas.

**14.3.2.3** Stages and platforms shall be protected in accordance with Chapter 12.

**14.3.2.4 Alcohol-Based Hand-Rub Dispensers.** Alcohol-based hand-rub dispensers shall be protected in accordance with 8.7.3, unless all of the following conditions are met:

(1) Dispensers shall be installed in rooms or spaces separated from corridors and exits.
(2) The maximum individual dispenser fluid capacity shall be as follows:
   (a) 0.32 gal (1.2 L) for dispensers in rooms
   (b) 0.53 gal (2.0 L) for dispensers in suites of rooms
(3) The dispensers shall be separated from each other by horizontal spacing of not less than 48 in. (1220 mm).
(4) Storage of quantities greater than 5 gal (18.9 L) in a single fire compartment shall meet the requirements of NFPA 30, *Flammable and Combustible Liquids Code*.
(5) The dispensers shall not be installed over or directly adjacent to an ignition source.
(6) Dispensers installed directly over carpeted floors shall be permitted only in sprinklered rooms or spaces.

**14.3.2.5** Educational occupancy laboratories using chemicals shall be in accordance with 8.7.4.

CHAPTER 15 • Existing

(d) Rooms or spaces used for processing or use of hazardous materials or flammable or combustible liquids in quantities deemed hazardous by recognized standards

(3) Where automatic extinguishing is used to meet the requirements of 15.3.2.1(1) or (2), the protection shall be permitted in accordance with 9.7.1.2.
(4) Where janitor closets addressed in 15.3.2.1(1)(d) are protected in accordance with the sprinkler option of 15.3.2.1(1), the janitor closet doors shall be permitted to have ventilating louvers.

**15.3.2.2** Cooking facilities shall be protected in accordance with 9.2.3. Openings shall not be required to be protected between food preparation areas and dining areas.

**15.3.2.3** Stages and platforms shall be protected in accordance with Chapter 13.

**15.3.2.4 Alcohol-Based Hand-Rub Dispensers.** Alcohol-based hand-rub dispensers shall be protected in accordance with 8.7.3, unless all of the following conditions are met:

(1) Dispensers shall be installed in rooms or spaces separated from corridors and exits.
(2) The maximum individual dispenser fluid capacity shall be as follows:
   (a) 0.32 gal (1.2 L) for dispensers in rooms
   (b) 0.53 gal (2.0 L) for dispensers in suites of rooms
(3) The dispensers shall be separated from each other by horizontal spacing of not less than 48 in. (1220 mm).
(4) Storage of quantities greater than 5 gal (18.9 L) in a single fire compartment shall meet the requirements of NFPA 30, *Flammable and Combustible Liquids Code*.
(5) The dispensers shall not be installed over or directly adjacent to an ignition source.
(6) Dispensers installed directly over carpeted floors shall be permitted only in sprinklered rooms or spaces.

**15.3.2.5** Educational occupancy laboratories using chemicals shall be in accordance with 8.7.4.

The intent of 14/15.3.2.1 is to specify the degree of protection necessary for certain hazardous contents areas. The hazards noted in 14/15.3.2.1 (1) are required to be enclosed in 1-hour construction or protected by automatic sprinklers. If the sprinkler option is chosen for new construction, an enclosure is still required by 8.7.1.2. However, the enclosure is not required to be rated; it is required to be a smoke partition in accordance with the provisions of Section 8.4.

Where janitor closets abut and are entered from a corridor, a louvered door is usually provided for ventilation. It is necessary to provide these spaces with automatic sprinkler protection, because a fire in the janitor closet might directly affect the usability of the corridor for exit access. Paragraph 9.7.1.2 describes an economical method of providing sprinkler protection for such closets by using the normal building water supply. To achieve this protection at reasonable cost, these sprinklers (not more than six for a given room or space) are permitted to be supplied from the building water supply, if the supply is capable of providing the required flow of water. It is advisable to provide a waterflow switch to initiate an alarm when a sprinkler is opened.

Exhibit 14/15.10 through Exhibit 14/15.12 illustrate the various protection requirements of 14/15.3.2.1.

In accordance with 14/15.3.2.2, openings in the wall between kitchens and dining areas are not restricted and do not need to be protected. The *Code* relies on the specialized automatic extinguishing system required by 9.2.3 to control any fire on the cooking surfaces and, thus, does not require openings between the kitchen and dining areas to be protected.

The provision of 14/15.3.2.3 was revised for the 2009 edition of the *Code* to require that platforms, and not just stages, as addressed in earlier editions, be protected in accordance with the criteria of the assembly occupancies chapters. See 12/13.4.5.

The provisions of 14/15.3.2.4 are new to the 2009 edition of the *Code* and draw from material developed for the health care occupancies chapters to permit alcohol-based hand-rub dispensers. Although health care occupancies have a functional need to position such dispensers in corridors to permit hand sanitizing prior to entering a patient room and again upon leaving, no such need exists for educational occupancies.

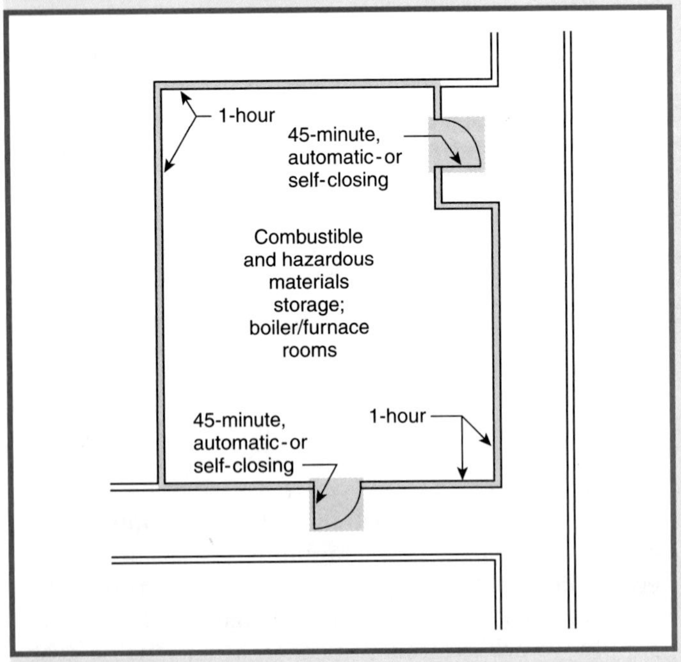


***Exhibit 14/15.10** Protection of hazardous contents areas — rated enclosure complying with 14/15.3.2.1(1).*

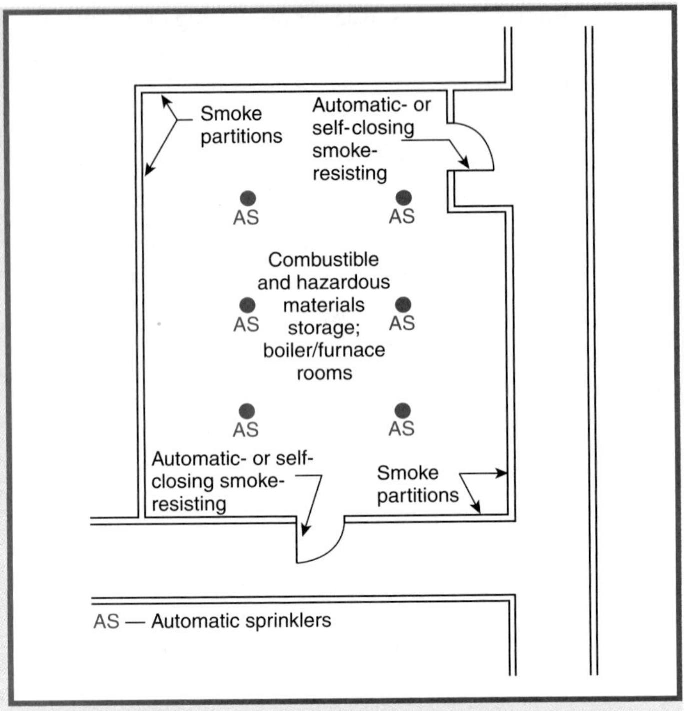


***Exhibit 14/15.11** Protection of new hazardous contents areas — sprinkler protection and smoke partition enclosure complying with 14.3.2.1(1).*

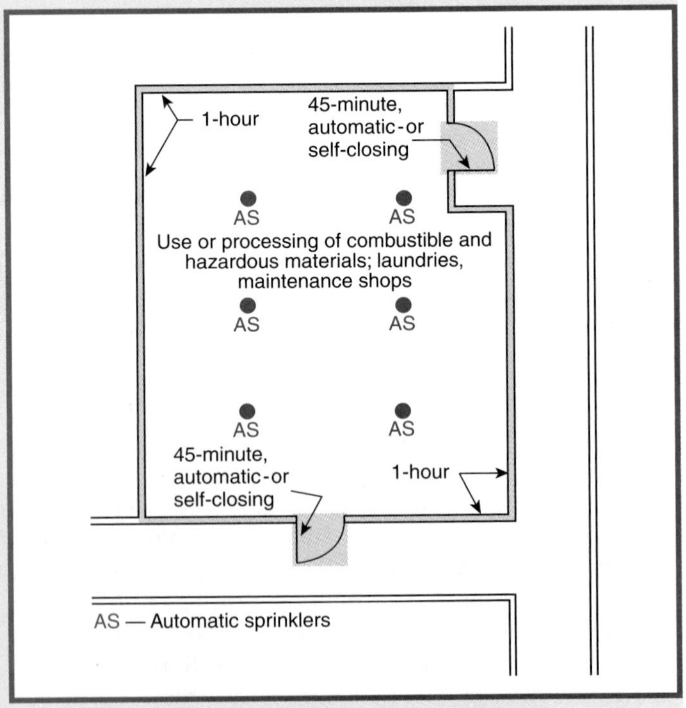


***Exhibit 14/15.12** Protection of hazardous contents areas — separation by 1-hour-rated enclosure and automatic sprinkler protection complying with 14/15.3.2.1(2).*

For educational occupancies, the alcohol-based hand-rub dispensers are permitted only in rooms or spaces separated from the corridor. Prior to the inclusion of the provisions for alcohol-based hand-rub dispensers, the only option available to educational occupancies was to treat the alcohol solutions as flammable liquids subject to the provisions of 8.7.3, which meant the dispensers were prohibited from being placed in student-occupied areas. Dispensers not meeting all the criteria of 14/15.3.2.4(1) through (6) are subject to regulation as flammable liquids in accordance with 8.7.3.

The provision of 14/15.3.2.5 is new to the 2009 edition of the *Code* and recognizes that educational occupancies often have laboratories using chemicals. Laboratories using chemicals need protection in accordance with 8.7.4.

### 14.3.3 Interior Finish.

**14.3.3.1 General.** Interior finish shall be in accordance with Section 10.2.

**14.3.3.2* Interior Wall and Ceiling Finish.** Interior wall and ceiling finish materials complying with Section 10.2 shall be permitted as follows:

(1) Exits — Class A
(2) Other than exits — Class A or Class B
(3) Low-height partitions not exceeding 60 in. (1525 mm) and used in locations other than exits — Class A, Class B, or Class C

**A.14.3.3.2** The definition of interior wall finish is meant to include washroom water closet partitions.

**14.3.3.3 Interior Floor Finish.**

**14.3.3.3.1** Interior floor finish shall comply with Section 10.2.

**14.3.3.3.2** Interior floor finish in exit enclosures and exit access corridors and spaces not separated from them by walls complying with 14.3.6 shall be not less than Class II.

**14.3.3.3.3** Interior floor finish shall comply with 10.2.7.1 or 10.2.7.2, as applicable.

### 15.3.3 Interior Finish.

**15.3.3.1 General.** Interior finish shall be in accordance with Section 10.2.

**15.3.3.2 Interior Wall and Ceiling Finish.** Interior wall and ceiling finish materials complying with Section 10.2 shall be permitted as follows:

(1) Exits — Class A
(2) Corridors and lobbies — Class A or Class B
(3) Low-height partitions not exceeding 60 in. (1525 mm) and used in locations other than exits — Class A, Class B, or Class C

**15.3.3.3 Interior Floor Finish.** (No requirements.)

New interior floor finish is regulated by 14.3.3.3. Floor finish in corridors is susceptible to ignition and flame spread when exposed to a well-developed fire such as might occur if a room fire were to grow to flashover and the room door remained open. Paragraph 14.3.3.3.2 addresses this concern. Paragraph 14.3.3.3.3 references the generalized criteria of 10.2.7.1 and 10.2.7.2, which are intended to identify and prohibit the use of floor finish materials that have little or no resistance to ignition.

### 14.3.4 Detection, Alarm, and Communications Systems.

**14.3.4.1 General.**

**14.3.4.1.1** Educational occupancies shall be provided with a fire alarm system in accordance with Section 9.6.

**14.3.4.1.2** The requirement of 14.3.4.1.1 shall not apply to buildings meeting all of the following criteria:

### 15.3.4 Detection, Alarm, and Communications Systems.

**15.3.4.1 General.**

**15.3.4.1.1** Educational occupancies shall be provided with a fire alarm system in accordance with Section 9.6.

**15.3.4.1.2** The requirement of 15.3.4.1.1 shall not apply to buildings meeting all of the following criteria:

CHAPTER 14 • New

(1) Buildings having an area not exceeding 1000 ft² (93 m²)
(2) Buildings containing a single classroom
(3) Buildings located not less than 30 ft (9.1 m) from another building

CHAPTER 15 • Existing

(1) Buildings having an area not exceeding 1000 ft² (93 m²)
(2) Buildings containing a single classroom
(3) Buildings located not less than 30 ft (9.1 m) from another building

The limited-size, single-classroom building addressed by 14/15.3.4.1.2 does not need an alarm system, because the fire will be immediately obvious to the occupants. Emergency egress can begin upon first notice of fire. A fire within a building located at least 30 ft (9.1 m) from another building should not prove to be detrimental to the occupants of the other building if egress is delayed because no alarm system is provided.

CHAPTER 14 • New

**14.3.4.2 Initiation.**

**14.3.4.2.1 General.** Initiation of the required fire alarm system, other than as permitted by 14.3.4.2.3, shall be by manual means in accordance with 9.6.2.1(1).

**14.3.4.2.2 Automatic Initiation.** In buildings provided with automatic sprinkler protection, the operation of the sprinkler system shall automatically activate the fire alarm system in addition to the initiation means required in 14.3.4.2.1.

**14.3.4.2.3 Alternative Protection System.** Manual fire alarm boxes shall be permitted to be eliminated in accordance with 14.3.4.2.3.1 or 14.3.4.2.3.2.

**14.3.4.2.3.1*** Manual fire alarm boxes shall be permitted to be eliminated where all of the following conditions apply:

(1) Interior corridors are protected by smoke detectors using an alarm verification system as described in *NFPA 72, National Fire Alarm Code*.
(2) Auditoriums, cafeterias, and gymnasiums are protected by heat-detection devices or other approved detection devices.
(3) Shops and laboratories involving dusts or vapors are protected by heat-detection devices or other approved detection devices.
(4) Provision is made at a central point to manually activate the evacuation signal or to evacuate only affected areas.

**A.14.3.4.2.3.1** Occupied portions of the building should have access to a central point for manual activation of the evacuation signal.

CHAPTER 15 • Existing

**15.3.4.2 Initiation.**

**15.3.4.2.1 General.** Initiation of the required fire alarm system shall be by manual means in accordance with 9.6.2.1(1), unless otherwise permitted by the following:

(1) Manual fire alarm boxes shall not be required where permitted by 15.3.4.2.3.
(2) In buildings where all normally occupied spaces are provided with a two-way communication system between such spaces and a constantly attended receiving station from where a general evacuation alarm can be sounded, the manual fire alarm boxes shall not be required, except in locations specifically designated by the authority having jurisdiction.

**15.3.4.2.2 Automatic Initiation.** In buildings provided with automatic sprinkler protection, the operation of the sprinkler system shall automatically activate the fire alarm system in addition to the initiation means required in 15.3.4.2.1.

**15.3.4.2.3 Alternative Protection System.** Manual fire alarm boxes shall be permitted to be eliminated in accordance with 15.3.4.2.3.1 or 15.3.4.2.3.2.

**15.3.4.2.3.1*** Manual fire alarm boxes shall be permitted to be eliminated where all of the following conditions apply:

(1) Interior corridors are protected by smoke detectors using an alarm verification system as described in *NFPA 72, National Fire Alarm Code*.
(2) Auditoriums, cafeterias, and gymnasiums are protected by heat-detection devices or other approved detection devices.
(3) Shops and laboratories involving dusts or vapors are protected by heat-detection devices or other approved detection devices.
(4) Provision is made at a central point to manually activate the evacuation signal or to evacuate only affected areas.

**A.15.3.4.2.3.1** Occupied portions of the building should have access to a central point for manual activation of the evacuation signal.

CHAPTER 14 • New

**14.3.4.2.3.2*** Manual fire alarm boxes shall be permitted to be eliminated where all of the following conditions apply:

(1) The building is protected throughout by an approved, supervised automatic sprinkler system in accordance with Section 9.7.
(2) Provision is made at a central point to manually activate the evacuation signal or to evacuate only affected areas.

**A.14.3.4.2.3.2** Occupied portions of the building should have access to a central point for manual activation of the evacuation signal.

CHAPTER 15 • Existing

**15.3.4.2.3.2*** Manual fire alarm boxes shall be permitted to be eliminated where all of the following conditions apply:

(1) The building is protected throughout by an approved, supervised automatic sprinkler system in accordance with Section 9.7.
(2) Provision is made at a central point to manually activate the evacuation signal or to evacuate only affected areas.

**A.15.3.4.2.3.2** Occupied portions of the building should have access to a central point for manual activation of the evacuation signal.

Paragraph 14/15.3.4.2.3 provides alternatives to the manual fire alarm boxes required by 14/15.3.4.2.1. These alternatives are offered as a means to avoid the nuisance alarms initiated through unauthorized use of the building manual fire alarm boxes. By relying on the automatic initiation that is provided by the detection systems addressed in 14/15.3.4.2.3.1(1) through (3), equivalent protection is provided. By relying on the fire control that is provided by the automatic sprinkler system addressed in 14/15.3.4.2.3.2, equivalent protection is provided.

Paragraph 15.3.4.2.1(2) — which applies only to existing educational occupancies — recognizes an alternative to a dedicated fire alarm system. Where there is a two-way communication system between classrooms and a constantly attended location where a general alarm can be sounded, the requirement for an alarm system — and its requisite manual fire alarm boxes — is exempted. To use this exemption, the authority having jurisdiction (AHJ) must designate those manual fire alarm boxes that are not required. For the purposes of this provision, a "constantly attended" location is a location that is attended while the school building is in use as a school. Compliance might involve providing personnel at this location during night classes, when the regular school office staff is not present. The exemption is not permitted for new construction due to reliability concerns.

CHAPTER 14 • New

**14.3.4.3 Notification.**

**14.3.4.3.1 Occupant Notification.**

**14.3.4.3.1.1*** Occupant notification shall be accomplished automatically in accordance with 9.6.3.

**A.14.3.4.3.1.1** Use of the distinctive three-pulse temporal pattern fire alarm evacuation signal that is required by *NFPA 72, National Fire Alarm Code*, will help educate students to recognize the need to evacuate when they are in other occupancies.

**14.3.4.3.1.2** Positive alarm sequence shall be permitted in accordance with 9.6.3.4.

**14.3.4.3.1.3** Where installed and operated per *NFPA 72, National Fire Alarm Code*, the fire alarm system shall be permitted to be used for other emergency signaling or for class changes.

CHAPTER 15 • Existing

**15.3.4.3 Notification.**

**15.3.4.3.1 Occupant Notification.**

**15.3.4.3.1.1*** Occupant notification shall be accomplished automatically in accordance with 9.6.3.

**A.15.3.4.3.1.1** The audible occupant notification signal for evacuation of an educational occupancy building should be the distinctive three-pulse temporal pattern fire alarm evacuation signal that is required of new systems by *NFPA 72, National Fire Alarm Code*. The temporal pattern will help educate students to recognize the need to evacuate when they are in other occupancies. Existing fire alarm systems should be modified, as feasible, to sound the three-pulse temporal pattern.

**15.3.4.3.1.2** Positive alarm sequence shall be permitted in accordance with 9.6.3.4.

**15.3.4.3.1.3** Where acceptable to the authority having jurisdiction, the fire alarm system shall be permitted to be used for other emergency signaling or for class changes, provided that the fire alarm is distinctive in signal and overrides all other use.

CHAPTER 14 • New

**14.3.4.3.1.4** To prevent students from being returned to a building that is burning, the recall signal shall be separate and distinct from any other signals, and such signal shall be permitted to be given by use of distinctively colored flags or banners.

**14.3.4.3.1.5** If the recall signal required by 14.3.4.3.1.4 is electric, the push buttons or other controls shall be kept under lock, the key for which shall be in the possession of the principal or another designated person in order to prevent a recall at a time when there is an actual fire.

**14.3.4.3.1.6** Regardless of the method of recall signal, the means of giving the recall signal shall be kept under lock.

**14.3.4.3.2 Emergency Forces Notification.** Fire department notification shall be accomplished in accordance with 9.6.4.

### 14.3.5 Extinguishment Requirements.

**14.3.5.1*** Educational occupancy buildings exceeding 20,000 ft$^2$ (1860 m$^2$) shall be protected throughout by an approved, supervised automatic sprinkler system in accordance with Section 9.7.

**A.14.3.5.1** It is the intent to permit use of the criteria of 8.2.1.3(1) to create separate buildings for purposes of limiting educational occupancy building area to not more than 20,000 ft$^2$ (1860 m$^2$).

**14.3.5.2** Educational occupancy buildings four or more stories in height shall be protected throughout by an approved, supervised automatic sprinkler system in accordance with Section 9.7.

**14.3.5.3** Every portion of educational buildings below the level of exit discharge shall be protected throughout by an approved, supervised automatic sprinkler system in accordance with Section 9.7.

CHAPTER 15 • Existing

**15.3.4.3.1.4** To prevent students from being returned to a building that is burning, the recall signal shall be separate and distinct from any other signals, and such signal shall be permitted to be given by use of distinctively colored flags or banners.

**15.3.4.3.1.5** If the recall signal required by 15.3.4.3.1.4 is electric, the push buttons or other controls shall be kept under lock, the key for which shall be in the possession of the principal or another designated person in order to prevent a recall at a time when there is an actual fire.

**15.3.4.3.1.6** Regardless of the method of recall signal, the means of giving the recall signal shall be kept under lock.

**15.3.4.3.2 Emergency Forces Notification.** Wherever any of the school authorities determine that an actual fire exists, they shall immediately call the local fire department using the public fire alarm system or other available facilities.

### 15.3.5 Extinguishment Requirements.

**15.3.5.1** Where student occupancy exists below the level of exit discharge, every portion of such floor shall be protected throughout by an approved automatic sprinkler system in accordance with Section 9.7.

**15.3.5.2** Where student occupancy does not exist on floors below the level of exit discharge, such floors shall be separated from the rest of the building by 1-hour fire resistance–rated construction or shall be protected throughout by an approved automatic sprinkler system in accordance with Section 9.7.

**15.3.5.3** Automatic sprinkler protection shall not be required where student occupancy exists below the level of exit discharge, provided that both of the following criteria are met:

(1) The approval of the authority having jurisdiction shall be required.

CHAPTER 14 • New

14.3.5.4 Buildings with unprotected openings in accordance with 8.6.6 shall be protected throughout by an approved, supervised automatic sprinkler system in accordance with Section 9.7.

14.3.5.5 Where another provision of this chapter requires an automatic sprinkler system, the sprinkler system shall be installed in accordance with 9.7.1.1(1).

CHAPTER 15 • Existing

(2) Windows for rescue and ventilation shall be provided in accordance with 15.2.11.1.

15.3.5.4 Buildings with unprotected openings in accordance with 8.6.6 shall be protected throughout by an approved, supervised automatic sprinkler system in accordance with Section 9.7.

15.3.5.5 Where another provision of this chapter requires an automatic sprinkler system, the sprinkler system shall be installed in accordance with 9.7.1.1(1).

The provisions of 14.3.5.1 and 14.3.5.2 are new to the 2009 edition of the *Code*. Paragraph 14.3.5.1 requires new educational occupancy buildings exceeding 20,000 ft$^2$ (1860 m$^2$) to be sprinklered, as the occupant load characteristic of a building of that size has the potential to place a large number of persons at risk from a single fire. Note that A.14.3.5.1 recognizes the placement of 2-hour or greater vertically aligned fire barriers, in accordance with 8.2.1.3(1), to create separate fire compartments that might be considered the equivalent of separate buildings. Provided that no such fire compartment exceeds the 20,000 ft$^2$ (1860 m$^2$) criterion of 14.3.5.1, sprinklers are not required in the structure that appears from the outside to be a single building with aggregate area in excess of 20,000 ft$^2$ (1860 m$^2$). The text of A.14.3.5.1 is based on the belief that a single fire (see 4.3.2) has the potential to affect only the occupants of the fire compartment in which the fire originates, especially early in the fire.

Paragraph 14.3.5.2 requires new educational occupancy buildings four or more stories in height (see 3.3.250 and 4.6.3) to be sprinklered, as large numbers of occupants are expected to have to travel vertically on stairs to egress the building. Stair travel is slower and more complicated than level travel across a floor. Sprinklers control fires so as to provide additional safe egress time.

The provision of 14.3.5.3 and those of 15.3.5.1 through 15.3.5.3 address the need for sprinklers based on whether there are levels or floors below the level of exit discharge. For new construction, this provision will normally require basements of schools to be sprinklered; for existing educational occupancies, the basement will need to be sprinklered if it is used for student occupancy.

The provisions of 8.6.6, applicable to the communicating space exemption to the requirements for vertical opening protection, are permitted to be used unless prohibited by the applicable occupancy chapter. The provisions of 14/15.3.1, related to vertical opening protection for educational occupancies, do not prohibit the use of 8.6.6 but add one extra requirement for situations where the communicating space exemption of 8.6.6 is used. The requirement is for the educational occupancy building to be protected throughout by an approved, supervised automatic sprinkler system as detailed in 14/15.3.5.4.

### 14.3.6 Corridors.

Corridors shall be separated from other parts of the story by walls having a 1-hour fire resistance rating in accordance with Section 8.3, unless otherwise permitted by the following:

(1) Corridor protection shall not be required where all spaces normally subject to student occupancy have not less than one door opening directly to the outside or to an exterior exit access balcony or corridor in accordance with 7.5.3.
(2) The following shall apply to buildings protected throughout by an approved, supervised automatic sprinkler system in accordance with Section 9.7:

### 15.3.6 Corridors.

Corridors shall be separated from other parts of the story by walls having a minimum ½-hour fire resistance rating in accordance with Section 8.3, unless otherwise permitted by the following:

(1) Corridor protection shall not be required where all spaces normally subject to student occupancy have not less than one door opening directly to the outside or to an exterior exit access balcony or corridor in accordance with 7.5.3.
(2)* The following shall apply to buildings protected throughout by an approved automatic sprinkler system with valve supervision in accordance with Section 9.7:

CHAPTER 14 • New

(a) Corridor walls shall not be required to be rated, provided that such walls form smoke partitions in accordance with Section 8.4.
(b) The provisions of 8.4.3.5 shall not apply to normally occupied classrooms.

(3) Where the corridor ceiling is an assembly having a 1-hour fire resistance rating where tested as a wall, the corridor walls shall be permitted to terminate at the corridor ceiling.
(4) Lavatories shall not be required to be separated from corridors, provided that they are separated from all other spaces by walls having not less than a 1-hour fire resistance rating in accordance with Section 8.3.
(5) Lavatories shall not be required to be separated from corridors, provided that the building is protected throughout by an approved, supervised automatic sprinkler system in accordance with Section 9.7.

CHAPTER 15 • Existing

(a) Corridor walls shall not be required to be rated, provided that such walls form smoke partitions in accordance with Section 8.4.
(b) The provisions of 8.4.3.5 shall not apply to normally occupied classrooms.

**A.15.3.6(2)** This provision permits valve supervision in accordance with Section 9.7, rather than requiring that the entire automatic sprinkler system be electrically supervised. It is intended that the valve supervision be performed electrically, not by chaining and locking the valves in the open position.

(3) Where the corridor ceiling is an assembly having a minimum ½-hour fire resistance rating where tested as a wall, the corridor wall shall be permitted to terminate at the corridor ceiling.
(4) Lavatories shall not be required to be separated from corridors, provided that they are separated from all other spaces by walls having a minimum ½-hour fire resistance rating in accordance with Section 8.3.
(5) Lavatories shall not be required to be separated from corridors, provided that the building is protected throughout by an approved, supervised automatic sprinkler system in accordance with Section 9.7.

Given the protection provided by an automatic sprinkler system installed throughout the building, 14/15.3.6(2)(a) permits the corridor walls to be unrated, provided that they form smoke partitions. See Section 8.4 for applicable criteria. Further, in a provision that is new to the 2009 edition of the *Code*, 14/15.3.6.2(b) permits the door closer to be omitted from corridor doors to normally occupied classrooms. The emergency plan required by 14/15.7.1 and the emergency egress drills required by 14/15.7.2 help to ensure that staff and students, working together as a team, close corridor doors as part of the emergency egress procedure.

Paragraph 14/15.3.6(3) legitimizes the practice of designing a corridor protection system by building a tunnel with walls and ceilings constructed to meet the requirements of a 1-hour-rated wall assembly for new construction and by providing a ½-hour rating for existing assemblies.

The walls and doors that typically separate a school lavatory from the corridor often serve to isolate the lavatory, making incidents of violence or illegal drug use difficult to monitor by staff. In recognition of this problem, and given the typically low fuel loads associated with lavatories, 14/15.3.6(4) exempts the wall separating the lavatory from the corridor from the rated construction requirement, provided that the rated corridor wall continuously separates the lavatory from adjacent rooms. This separation method permits lavatory doors to be omitted from the doorways. Exhibit 14/15.13 illustrates this arrangement.

The intent of 14/15.3.6(5) is to combine parts of the concepts addressed in 14/15.3.6(2) and (4). Where the entire building is protected by automatic sprinklers, the lavatory is permitted to be open to the corridor,

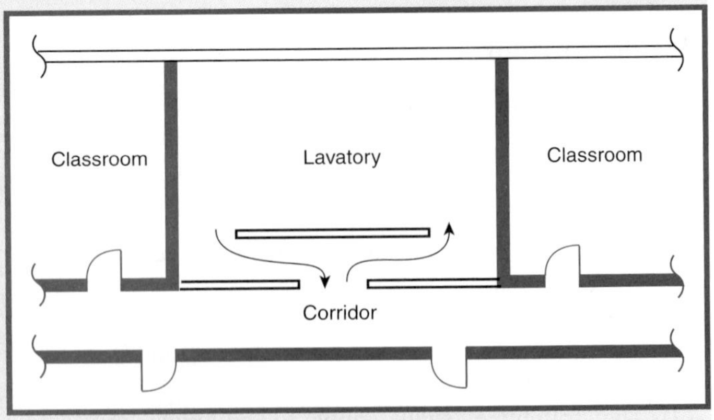


***Exhibit 14/15.13** Lavatory open to corridor but separated from adjacent rooms by continuous, rated corridor wall to building exterior walls.*

and the walls separating the lavatory from other rooms do not need to be fire rated but do need to form smoke partitions. The *Code* language does not fully explain this.

In the 2003 and earlier editions of the *Code*, the provisions of 15.3.6, applicable to existing corridors, permitted existing doors in $\frac{1}{2}$-hour fire resistance–rated corridor walls to be $1\frac{3}{4}$ in. (44 mm) thick solid-bonded wood-core doors or equivalent in lieu of 20-minute fire protection-rated doors. The text was deleted for the 2006 edition, because the subject is adequately addressed as a core chapter provision in 8.3.4.4.

**14.3.7 Subdivision of Building Spaces.**

**14.3.7.1** Educational occupancies shall be subdivided into compartments by smoke partitions having not less than a 1-hour fire resistance rating and complying with Section 8.4 where one or both of the following conditions exist:

(1) The maximum floor area, including the aggregate area of all floors having a common atmosphere, exceeds 30,000 $ft^2$ (2800 $m^2$).
(2) The length or width of the building exceeds 300 ft (91 m).

**14.3.7.2** The requirement of 14.3.7.1 shall not apply to the following:

(1) Where all spaces normally subject to student occupancy have not less than one door opening directly to the outside or to an exterior or exit access balcony or corridor in accordance with 7.5.3
(2) Buildings protected throughout by an approved, supervised automatic sprinkler system in accordance with Section 9.7

**14.3.7.3** The area of any smoke compartment required by 14.3.7.1 shall not exceed 30,000 $ft^2$ (2800 $m^2$), with no dimension exceeding 300 ft (91 m).

**15.3.7 Subdivision of Building Spaces.**

**15.3.7.1** Educational occupancies shall be subdivided into compartments by smoke partitions having not less than a 1-hour fire resistance rating and complying with Section 8.4 where one or both of the following conditions exist:

(1) The maximum area of a compartment, including the aggregate area of all floors having a common atmosphere, exceeds 30,000 $ft^2$ (2800 $m^2$).
(2) The length or width of the building exceeds 300 ft (91 m).

**15.3.7.2** The requirement of 15.3.7.1 shall not apply to the following:

(1) Where all classrooms have exterior exit access in accordance with 7.5.3
(2) Buildings protected throughout by an approved automatic sprinkler system in accordance with Section 9.7

**15.3.7.3** The area of any smoke compartment required by 15.3.7.1 shall not exceed 30,000 $ft^2$ (2800 $m^2$), with no dimension exceeding 300 ft (91 m).

The *Code* requires smoke barriers at maximum intervals of 300 ft (91 m) so that the products of combustion will not affect large numbers of occupants and their exits simultaneously. A primary concern is a situation in which a corridor becomes clogged with smoke, resulting in the loss of the exit access. Rooms with exterior exit access provide the occupants a readily available, alternate means of escape in the event that a corridor fills with smoke.

The excellent record of automatic fire sprinkler systems permits the compartmentation requirements to be exempted in buildings with such systems.

The provision of 14/15.3.7.3 limits the area of a smoke compartment only if such compartmentation is required by 14/15.3.7.1 and not exempted by 14/15.3.7.2.

## 14.4 Special Provisions

### 14.4.1 Limited Access Buildings and Underground Buildings.

Limited access buildings and underground buildings shall comply with Section 11.7.

## 15.4 Special Provisions

### 15.4.1 Limited Access Buildings and Underground Buildings.

Limited access buildings and underground buildings shall comply with Section 11.7.

CHAPTER 14 • New

CHAPTER 15 • Existing

### 14.4.2 High-Rise Buildings.

High-rise buildings shall comply with Section 11.8.

### 15.4.2 High-Rise Buildings.

High-rise buildings shall comply with 11.8.3.1.

An educational occupancy high-rise building poses many of the same problems for occupants and fire-fighting forces that are posed by other occupancies located in high-rise buildings. Thus, the package of protection addressed by Section 11.8 (i.e., automatic sprinkler, standpipe, alarm and communications, standby power, and emergency command center requirements) is mandatorily referenced for new construction; the sprinkler provisions of 11.8.3.1 are mandatorily referenced for existing educational occupancy high-rise buildings.

### 14.4.3 Flexible Plan and Open Plan Buildings.

**14.4.3.1** Flexible plan and open plan buildings shall comply with the requirements of this chapter as modified by 14.4.3.2 through 14.4.3.5.

**14.4.3.2** Each room occupied by more than 300 persons shall have two or more means of egress entering into separate atmospheres.

**14.4.3.3** Where three or more means of egress are required, the number of means of egress permitted to enter into the same atmosphere shall not exceed two.

**14.4.3.4** Flexible plan buildings shall be permitted to have walls and partitions rearranged periodically only if revised plans or diagrams have been approved by the authority having jurisdiction.

**14.4.3.5** Flexible plan buildings shall be evaluated while all folding walls are extended and in use as well as when they are in the retracted position.

### 15.4.3 Flexible Plan and Open Plan Buildings.

**15.4.3.1** Flexible plan and open plan buildings shall comply with the requirements of this chapter as modified by 15.4.3.2 through 15.4.3.5.

**15.4.3.2** Each room occupied by more than 300 persons shall have two or more means of egress entering into separate atmospheres.

**15.4.3.3** Where three or more means of egress are required, the number of means of egress permitted to enter into the same atmosphere shall not exceed two.

**15.4.3.4** Flexible plan buildings shall be permitted to have walls and partitions rearranged periodically only if revised plans or diagrams have been approved by the authority having jurisdiction.

**15.4.3.5** Flexible plan buildings shall be evaluated while all folding walls are extended and in use as well as when they are in the retracted position.

Flexible plan and open plan buildings are addressed in 14/15.4.3. Rooms occupied by more than 300 persons require special treatment in flexible plan and open plan schools. To ensure the safety of this large number of persons occupying one room, means of egress must be arranged so that each of the egress paths traverses atmospheres that are separate from each other. If more than two separate means of egress paths are required, not more than two are permitted to pass through the same atmosphere. See the definition of *separate atmosphere* in 3.3.23.2. Using this arrangement should prevent a single fire from contaminating or blocking all egress routes in an open plan or flexible plan building.

Exhibit 14/15.14 illustrates a room in an open plan building that requires two or more means of egress into separate atmospheres.

In accordance with 14/15.4.3.4, approval of revised plans or diagrams is necessary to avoid the possibility of circuitous egress paths or other arrange-

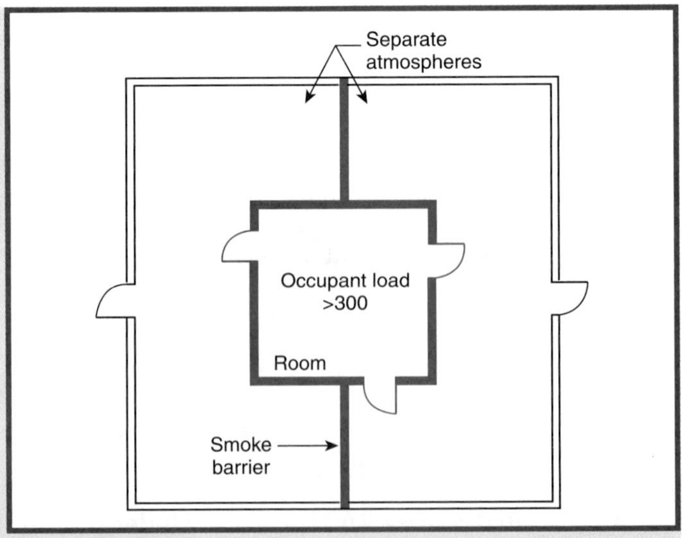


***Exhibit 14/15.14** Room in open plan building requiring two or more means of egress into separate atmospheres.*

CHAPTER 14 • New

ments that do not comply with the intent of the *Code*. Also, flexible plan buildings are required to meet the provisions for corridor protection, as well as those for the subdivision of building spaces, using smoke barriers.

## 14.5 Building Services

### 14.5.1 Utilities.

Utilities shall comply with the provisions of Section 9.1.

### 14.5.2 Heating, Ventilating, and Air-Conditioning Equipment.

**14.5.2.1** Heating, ventilating, and air-conditioning equipment shall comply with the provisions of Section 9.2.

**14.5.2.2** Unvented fuel-fired heating equipment, other than gas space heaters in compliance with NFPA 54/ANSI Z223.1, *National Fuel Gas Code,* shall be prohibited.

It is not in the interest of reasonable life safety to permit unvented fuel-fired equipment in a school building occupied by children; the typical use of such equipment might jeopardize the life safety of the students. Improper venting and potential misuse by students might result in injury to students, especially younger children. Paragraph 14/15.5.2.2 recognizes a special form of gas space heater that — although not vented in the conventional way — can be used safely.

### 14.5.3 Elevators, Escalators, and Conveyors.

Elevators, escalators, and conveyors shall comply with the provisions of Section 9.4.

### 14.5.4 Rubbish Chutes, Incinerators, and Laundry Chutes.

Rubbish chutes, incinerators, and laundry chutes shall comply with the provisions of Section 9.5.

## 14.6 Reserved

## 14.7 Operating Features

### 14.7.1 Emergency Plan.

Emergency plans shall be provided in accordance with Section 4.8.

### 14.7.2 Emergency Egress Drills.

**14.7.2.1*** Emergency egress drills shall be conducted in accordance with Section 4.7 and the applicable provisions of 14.7.2.3 as otherwise provided in 14.7.2.2.

CHAPTER 15 • Existing

## 15.5 Building Services

### 15.5.1 Utilities.

Utilities shall comply with the provisions of Section 9.1.

### 15.5.2 Heating, Ventilating, and Air-Conditioning Equipment.

**15.5.2.1** Heating, ventilating, and air-conditioning equipment shall comply with the provisions of Section 9.2.

**15.5.2.2** Unvented fuel-fired heating equipment, other than gas space heaters in compliance with NFPA 54/ANSI Z223.1, *National Fuel Gas Code*, shall be prohibited.

### 15.5.3 Elevators, Escalators, and Conveyors.

Elevators, escalators, and conveyors shall comply with the provisions of Section 9.4.

### 15.5.4 Rubbish Chutes, Incinerators, and Laundry Chutes.

Rubbish chutes, incinerators, and laundry chutes shall comply with the provisions of Section 9.5.

## 15.6 Reserved

## 15.7 Operating Features

### 15.7.1 Emergency Plan.

Emergency plans shall be provided in accordance with Section 4.8.

### 15.7.2 Emergency Egress Drills.

**15.7.2.1*** Emergency egress drills shall be conducted in accordance with Section 4.7 and the applicable provisions of 15.7.2.3 as otherwise provided by 15.7.2.2.

CHAPTER 14 • New

**A.14.7.2.1** The requirements are, of necessity, general in scope, as it is recognized that they apply to all types of educational occupancies as well as conditions of occupancies, such as truant schools; schools for the mentally handicapped, vision impaired, hearing impaired, and speech impaired; and public schools. It is fully recognized that no one code can meet all the conditions of the various buildings involved, and it will be necessary for site administrators to issue supplements to these requirements, but all supplements should be consistent with these requirements.

**14.7.2.2** Approved training programs designed for education and training and for the practice of emergency egress to familiarize occupants with the drill procedure, and to establish conduct of the emergency egress as a matter of routine, shall be permitted to receive credit on a one-for-one basis for not more than four of the emergency egress drills required by 14.7.2.3, provided that a minimum of four emergency egress drills are completed prior to the conduct of the first such training and practice program.

**14.7.2.3** Emergency egress drills shall be conducted as follows:

(1) Not less than one emergency egress drill shall be conducted every month the facility is in session, unless both of the following criteria are met:
   (a) In climates where the weather is severe, the monthly emergency egress drills shall be permitted to be deferred.
   (b) The required number of emergency egress drills shall be conducted, and not less than four shall be conducted before the drills are deferred.
(2) All occupants of the building shall participate in the drill.
(3) One additional emergency egress drill, other than for educational occupancies that are open on a year-round basis, shall be required within the first 30 days of operation.

**14.7.2.4** All emergency drill alarms shall be sounded on the fire alarm system.

CHAPTER 15 • Existing

**A.15.7.2.1** The requirements are, of necessity, general in scope, as it is recognized that they apply to all types of educational occupancies as well as conditions of occupancies, such as truant schools; schools for the mentally handicapped, vision impaired, hearing impaired, and speech impaired; and public schools. It is fully recognized that no one code can meet all the conditions of the various buildings involved, and it will be necessary for site administrators to issue supplements to these requirements, but all supplements should be consistent with these requirements.

**15.7.2.2** Approved training programs designed for education and training and for the practice of emergency egress to familiarize occupants with the drill procedure, and to establish conduct of the emergency egress as a matter of routine, shall be permitted to receive credit on a one-for-one basis for not more than four of the emergency egress drills required by 15.7.2.3, provided that a minimum of four emergency egress drills are completed prior to the conduct of the first such training and practice program.

**15.7.2.3** Emergency egress drills shall be conducted as follows:

(1) Not less than one emergency egress drill shall be conducted every month the facility is in session, unless both of the following criteria are met:
   (a) In climates where the weather is severe, the monthly emergency egress drills shall be permitted to be deferred.
   (b) The required number of emergency egress drills shall be conducted, and not less than four shall be conducted before the drills are deferred.
(2) All occupants of the building shall participate in the drill.
(3) One additional emergency egress drill, other than for educational occupancies that are open on a year-round basis, shall be required within the first 30 days of operation.

**15.7.2.4** All emergency drill alarms shall be sounded on the fire alarm system.

Emergency egress drills for educational occupancies, particularly those at the grade school level, are essential to ensure an orderly response during a fire. Unfortunately, the predictability of such drills often leads to their ineffectiveness. When an alarm bell sounds and a fire department monitor appears in a corridor, some teachers ignore the bell, assuming that it is a false alarm. If the bell sounds and a fire department monitor is not seen, teachers opt to either evacuate or remain in the building. This decision is made in the hallway. While the bell continues to ring, the students remain in their classrooms. Therefore, when a bell sounds, the primary emphasis should be placed on evacuation, regardless of who is or is not present in the hallways and regardless of whether fire equipment is parked in front of the school. Essentially, the fire department and the school should vary the timing and arrangement of the drills but not the required response, which is orderly evacuation. See also Section 4.7.

CHAPTER 14 • New

CHAPTER 15 • Existing

The provisions of 14/15.7.2.2 are new to the 2009 edition of the *Code* and permit emergency egress training programs to substitute for as many as four of the required monthly emergency egress drills. The mixture of training programs and emergency egress drills might elicit student egress behavior that is superior to that instilled by drills alone. However, at least four egress drills need to be conducted prior to the first training program to ensure that the students have walked the egress route and demonstrated other behavior addressed by the emergency plan. The concept behind the requirement that emergency drills be conducted at the start of the school year is that training without the hands-on instruction accomplished by drilling does not guarantee that students will be familiar with the egress routes and able to interact with others during an emergency evacuation or relocation.

### 14.7.3 Inspection.

**14.7.3.1*** It shall be the duty of principals, teachers, or staff to inspect all exit facilities daily to ensure that all stairways, doors, and other exits are in proper condition.

**A.14.7.3.1** Particular attention should be given to keeping all doors unlocked; keeping doors that serve to protect the safety of paths of egress closed and under no conditions blocked open, such as doors on stairway enclosures; keeping outside stairs and fire escape stairs free from all obstructions and clear of snow and ice; and allowing no accumulation of snow or ice or materials of any kind outside exit doors that might prevent the opening of the door or interfere with rapid escape from the building.

Any condition likely to interfere with safe egress should be corrected immediately, if possible, or otherwise should be reported at once to the appropriate authorities.

**14.7.3.2** Open plan buildings shall require extra surveillance to ensure that exit paths are maintained clear of obstruction and are obvious.

**14.7.3.3 Inspection of Door Openings.** Door openings shall be inspected in accordance with 7.2.1.15.

### 15.7.3 Inspection.

**15.7.3.1*** It shall be the duty of principals, teachers, or staff to inspect all exit facilities daily to ensure that all stairways, doors, and other exits are in proper condition.

**A.15.7.3.1** Particular attention should be given to keeping all doors unlocked; keeping doors that serve to protect the safety of paths of egress closed and under no conditions blocked open, such as doors on stairway enclosures; keeping outside stairs and fire escape stairs free from all obstructions and clear of snow and ice; and allowing no accumulation of snow or ice or materials of any kind outside exit doors that might prevent the opening of the door or interfere with rapid escape from the building.

Any condition likely to interfere with safe egress should be corrected immediately, if possible, or otherwise should be reported at once to the appropriate authorities.

**15.7.3.2** Open plan buildings shall require extra surveillance to ensure that exit paths are maintained clear of obstruction and are obvious.

**15.7.3.3 Inspection of Door Openings.** Door openings shall be inspected in accordance with 7.2.1.15.

Compliance with the requirement of 14/15.7.3.1 for daily inspection of the egress system has benefits that far outweigh the time and resources required to conduct such inspections. The provision was revised for the 2006 edition of the *Code*, and carried forward into this edition, to permit staff other than principals and teachers to make such inspections. The inspection function is often better performed by maintenance personnel who have responsibility for, and intimate working knowledge of, the many building features and systems.

The provision of 14/15.7.3.3 for the inspection of door openings is new to the 2009 edition of the *Code*. The criteria of 7.2.1.15 are formatted to apply only where specifically required by another portion of the *Code*. The inspection requirements apply to doors that are required to swing in the direction of egress travel. Door leaves that are required to swing in the direction of egress travel include those from spaces with an occupant load of 50 or more persons [see 7.2.1.4.2(1)] and those used in an exit enclosure [see 7.2.1.4.2(2)]. This application threshold was chosen to help ensure that the egress doors used most frequently on a normal day-to-day basis and those designed to accommodate larger numbers of occupants under emergency egress or relocation are inspected and tested. Door leaves that get used frequently are more apt to experience wear that adversely affects operability and leads to failure. Door leaves that are infrequently used, like those into exit stair enclosures in high-rise buildings, might be misaligned within their frames so as to be difficult to open within the operating forces requirements of 7.2.1.4.5. The door inspection and testing criteria of 7.2.1.15 are intended to help identify problems with door openings and ensure that such problems are remedied. See 7.2.1.15.

### 14.7.4 Furnishings and Decorations.

**14.7.4.1** Draperies, curtains, and other similar furnishings and decorations in educational occupancies shall be in accordance with the provisions of 10.3.1.

**14.7.4.2** Clothing and personal effects shall not be stored in corridors, unless otherwise permitted by the following:

(1) This requirement shall not apply to corridors protected by an automatic sprinkler system in accordance with Section 9.7.
(2) This requirement shall not apply to corridor areas protected by a smoke detection system in accordance with Section 9.6.
(3) This requirement shall not apply to storage in metal lockers, provided that the required egress width is maintained.

### 15.7.4 Furnishings and Decorations.

**15.7.4.1** Draperies, curtains, and other similar furnishings and decorations in educational occupancies shall be in accordance with the provisions of 10.3.1.

**15.7.4.2** Clothing and personal effects shall not be stored in corridors, unless otherwise permitted by the following:

(1) This requirement shall not apply to corridors protected by an automatic sprinkler system in accordance with Section 9.7.
(2) This requirement shall not apply to corridor areas protected by a smoke detection system in accordance with Section 9.6.
(3) This requirement shall not apply to storage in metal lockers, provided that the required egress width is maintained.

Clothing hung on hooks along corridor walls or on racks in school lobbies greatly increases the combustible load and will generally allow flame to spread quickly. Because Chapters 14 and 15 regulate the interior wall finish for corridors and lobbies, surfaces covered by combustible clothing that would allow flame to spread more quickly than is permitted by wall surfaces should not be created. The three provisions of 14/15.7.4.2 (control of fire by sprinklers, early warning of incipient stage fire via smoke detection, or isolating fuel packages by locating the clothing in metal lockers) help to mitigate the potential for a clothing fire to render the exit access unusable.

**14.7.4.3** Artwork and teaching materials shall be permitted to be attached directly to the walls in accordance with the following:

(1) The artwork and teaching materials shall not exceed 20 percent of the wall area in a building that is not protected throughout by an approved, supervised automatic sprinkler system in accordance with Section 9.7.
(2) The artwork and teaching materials shall not exceed 50 percent of the wall area in a building that is protected throughout by an approved, supervised automatic sprinkler system in accordance with Section 9.7.

**15.7.4.3** Artwork and teaching materials shall be permitted to be attached directly to the walls in accordance with the following:

(1) The artwork and teaching materials shall not exceed 20 percent of the wall area in a building that is not protected throughout by an approved automatic sprinkler system in accordance with Section 9.7.
(2) The artwork and teaching materials shall not exceed 50 percent of the wall area in a building that is protected throughout by an approved automatic sprinkler system in accordance with Section 9.7.

It is advantageous not only to limit the quantity of artwork displayed but also to avoid placing such materials near a room's exit access doors. Because the combustibility of the artwork cannot be effectively controlled, the quantity, in terms of the percentage of wall area covered, is regulated to avoid creating a continuous combustible surface that will spread flame across the room. If the building is protected throughout by automatic sprinklers, the percentage of wall area permitted to be covered with artwork and teaching materials is increased to 50 percent.

The format of 10.3.2 for smoldering ignition testing of upholstered furniture and mattresses was changed beginning with the 2006 edition of the *Code* from a menu-like item requiring adoption by an occupancy chapter to an outright mandate. Paragraph

CHAPTER 14 • New

CHAPTER 15 • Existing

10.3.2 requires smoldering ignition resistance for newly introduced upholstered furniture and mattresses, unless otherwise modified by an occupancy chapter. Given that Chapter 14/15 does not take exception with the requirement of 10.3.2, newly introduced furniture and mattresses in educational occupancies are subject to the smoldering ignition resistance fire testing requirements of 10.3.2. This represents a change for the 2009 edition of the *Code,* as the 2006 edition exempted the testing of upholstered furniture and mattresses in educational occupancies protected throughout by automatic sprinklers. The new requirement has little impact on educational occupancies in the United States, as mattresses have been required to meet comparable federally mandated cigarette ignition testing for many decades, and upholstered furniture is subjected to comparable cigarette ignition testing by American trade associations for the manufacture of institutional and contract upholstered furniture and the manufacturers of residential upholstered furniture.

### 14.7.5 Open Flames.

Approved open flames shall be permitted in laboratories and vocational/technical areas.

### 15.7.5 Open Flames.

Approved open flames shall be permitted in laboratories and vocational/technical areas.

CHAPTERS 16 AND 17

# New and Existing Day-Care Occupancies

Chapters 16 and 17 address not only traditional child day care, but also the growing field of adult day care. In both cases, these chapters recognize that many of the individuals who occupy these facilities are not totally capable of self-preservation. Very young children will require a certain amount of assistance from the day-care staff to help with relocation or evacuation. Likewise, some adults in adult day care will also require staff assistance during a fire emergency. For these reasons, Chapters 16 and 17 mandate select features that anticipate that these occupants will respond to a fire more slowly than is average. The requirements address a range of protection features, including the physical location of the day-care facility as it relates to the highest story used as a day-care occupancy (see Table 16.1.6.1 and Table 17.1.6.1). In reviewing the tables, note that the building construction features become more stringent where the day-care occupancy is located above or below the first story. These tables also establish a threshold at which automatic sprinkler protection is required for a given building construction type and story height used as a day-care occupancy.

The complement of fire alarm systems, sprinkler systems, and other building construction features are addressed in these chapters. Section 16/17.7 addresses the staffing, training, and drilling necessary to carry out an effective and efficient fire emergency response plan.

## 16.1 General Requirements

### 16.1.1* Application.

**A.16.1.1** Day-care occupancies do not provide for the full-time maintenance of a client. Occupancies that provide a primary place of residence are addressed in other occupancy chapters. *(See Chapters 24 through 33.)*

The requirements of Chapter 16 are based on the need to adequately protect the occupants in case of fire. The requirements assume that adequate staffing will be available and are based on staffing similar to that outlined in Table A.16.1.1.

If staff-to-client ratios fall below that suggested by Table A.16.1.1, it is the responsibility of the authority having jurisdiction to determine the additional safeguards beyond the requirements of Chapter 16 that are necessary. Typical additional provisions might include restricting the day-care occupancy to the level of exit discharge, requiring additional smoke detection, requiring automatic sprinkler

## 17.1 General Requirements

### 17.1.1* Application.

**A.17.1.1** Day-care occupancies do not provide for the full-time maintenance of a client. Occupancies that provide a primary place of residence are addressed in other occupancies. *(See Chapters 24 through 33.)*

The requirements of Chapter17 are based on the need to adequately protect the occupants in case of fire. The requirements assume that adequate staffing will be available and are based on staffing similar to that outlined in Table A.17.1.1.

If staff-to-client ratios fall below that suggested by Table A.17.1.1, it is the responsibility of the authority having jurisdiction to determine what additional safeguards beyond the requirements of Chapter 17 are necessary. Typical additional provisions might include restricting the day-care occupancy to the level of exit discharge, requiring additional smoke detection, requiring automatic sprinkler protection,

CHAPTER 16 • New

*Table A.16.1.1 Staffing*

| Staff-to-Client Ratio | Age (mo.) |
|---|---|
| 1:3 | 0–24 |
| 1:4 | 25–36 |
| 1:7 | 37–60 |
| 1:10 | 61–96 |
| 1:12 | ≥97 |
| 1:3 | Clients incapable of self-preservation |

protection, requiring better or additional means of egress, and similar types of provisions, depending on the situation.

**16.1.1.1** The requirements of this chapter shall apply to new buildings or portions thereof used as day-care occupancies. *(See 1.3.1.)*

The provisions for new day-care occupancies are addressed in Chapter 16; the provisions for existing day-care occupancies (i.e., existing conditions in day-care occupancies) are addressed in Chapter 17.

In editions of the *Code* prior to 2006, renovations, additions, and changes of occupancy were required to comply with the requirements for new construction. For day-care occupancies, such renovations, additions, and changes of occupancy were required to meet the provisions of Chapter 16, while existing conditions were subject to the provisions of Chapter 17. Since the 2006 edition of the *Code*, Chapter 43, Building Rehabilitation, has addressed the subject. Chapter 43 was written to promote the adaptive reuse of existing buildings without sacrificing the needed level of life safety. The provisions of Chapter 43 blend the requirements for new construction with those for existing conditions, so as to require additional life safety features as the rehabilitation work category increases in complexity. The rehabilitation work categories are repair, renovation, modification, reconstruction, change of use or occupancy classification, and addition. See 4.6.8, 4.6.12, and Chapter 43.

**16.1.1.2** The requirements of Sections 16.1 through 16.5 and Section 16.7 shall apply to day-care occupancies in which more than 12 clients receive care, maintenance, and supervision by other than their relative(s) or legal guardian(s) for less than 24 hours per day.

**16.1.1.3** The requirements of Section 16.1 (other than 16.1.6) and Sections 16.4 through 16.7 (other than 16.7.4.1) shall apply to day-care homes as defined in 16.1.3.

CHAPTER 17 • Existing

*Table A.17.1.1 Staffing*

| Staff-to-Client Ratio | Age (mo.) |
|---|---|
| 1:3 | 0–24 |
| 1:4 | 25–36 |
| 1:7 | 37–60 |
| 1:10 | 61–96 |
| 1:12 | ≥97 |
| 1:3 | Clients incapable of self-preservation |

requiring better or additional means of egress, and similar types of items, depending on the situation.

**17.1.1.1** The requirements of this chapter shall apply to existing buildings or portions thereof currently occupied as day-care occupancies.

**17.1.1.2** The requirements of Sections 17.1 through 17.5 and Section 17.7 shall apply to existing day-care occupancies in which more than 12 clients receive care, maintenance, and supervision by other than their relative(s) or legal guardian(s) for less than 24 hours per day. An existing day-care occupancy shall be permitted the option of meeting the requirements of Chapter 16 in lieu of Chapter 17. An existing day-care occupancy that meets the requirements of Chapter 16 shall be judged as meeting the requirements of Chapter 17.

**17.1.1.3** The requirements of Section 17.1 (other than 17.1.6) and Sections 17.4 through 17.7 (other than 17.7.4.1) shall apply to existing day-care homes as defined in 17.1.3. An existing day-care home shall be permitted the option of meeting the requirements of Chapter 16 in lieu of Chapter 17. An existing day-care home that meets the requirements of Chapter 16 shall be judged as meeting the requirements of Chapter 17.

CHAPTER 16 • New

**16.1.1.4** Where a facility houses more than one age group or self-preservation capability, the strictest requirements applicable to any group present shall apply throughout the day-care occupancy or building, as appropriate to a given area, unless the area housing such a group is maintained as a separate fire area.

**16.1.1.5** Places of religious worship shall not be required to meet the provisions of this chapter where providing day care while services are being held in the building.

CHAPTER 17 • Existing

**17.1.1.4** Where a facility houses clients of more than one self-preservation capability, the strictest requirements applicable to any group present shall apply throughout the day-care occupancy or building, as appropriate to a given area, unless the area housing such a group is maintained as a separate fire area.

**17.1.1.5** Places of religious worship shall not be required to meet the provisions of this chapter where providing day care while services are being held in the building.

The intent of 16/17.1.1.2 is to differentiate between institutions where clients are in residence 24 hours a day (such as orphanages) and day-care facilities where clients who normally reside at another location are provided care. A facility supplying "total care" for each client would provide laundries, dormitories, cafeterias, and other ancillary services not found in a day-care center. Other occupancy provisions of the *Code* would govern the life safety requirements of such a facility.

Note that, per 17.1.1.2 and 17.1.1.3, an existing day-care center or an existing day-care home meeting the requirements of Chapter 16 is to be judged as meeting the requirements of Chapter 17. Thus, if a new day-care center or day-care home is built in accordance with the requirements of Chapter 16, it later becomes an existing facility. Because the requirements of Chapters 16 and 17 differ, it would be unfair to reexamine the existing facility under the requirements of Chapter 17, because the protection package provided in accordance with Chapter 16 is as good as, if not better than, the package provided by compliance with the requirements of Chapter 17.

The parenthetical expression "(other than 16/17.7.4.1)," as contained in 16/17.1.1.3, clarifies that the provision regulating draperies and curtains for flame propagation does not apply to day-care homes (i.e., day-care facilities with 4 to 12 clients), only to day-care occupancies (i.e., day-care facilities with more than 12 clients).

The provisions of 16/17.1.1.4 tailor the protection package to the client group with the greatest needs. This concept is similar to that applied by 6.1.14.3 to a multiple occupancy protected as a mixed occupancy. Paragraph 6.1.14.3.2 requires that the most stringent *Code* provisions applicable to any of the occupancies present must be applied throughout the facility.

For example, 16.1.6.2 requires smoke partitions in new day-care centers if clients are 2 years old or younger. If any client in a facility is 2 years old or younger, the floors of the building that client occupies must be provided with smoke partitions. A portion of the facility separated from that occupied by a client who is 2 years old or younger is not required to have smoke partitions. A separated fire area is usually constructed with walls that have a fire resistance rating of 2 hours, as required by Table 6.1.14.4.1(a) or Table 6.1.14.4.1(b).

Paragraph 16/17.1.1.5 addresses day care provided within a place of worship while religious services are being held. The parents of the clients of the day-care center would be among those attending a worship service; they and others assembled for the worship service would be expected to assist the day-care staff with any necessary evacuation. The requirements of Chapters 16 and 17, therefore, do not apply under such circumstances. On the other hand, if day-care operations are conducted in the same building while religious services are not being conducted — such as during the work week — the day-care provisions of Chapters 16 and 17 would apply.

### 16.1.2 Multiple Occupancies.

**16.1.2.1** Multiple occupancies shall be in accordance with 6.1.14.

**16.1.2.2** Where the mixed occupancies provisions of 6.1.14.3 are utilized, the provisions of 16.1.2.2.1 and 16.1.2.2.2 shall also apply.

### 17.1.2 Multiple Occupancies.

**17.1.2.1** Multiple occupancies shall be in accordance with 6.1.14.

**17.1.2.2** Where the mixed occupancies provisions of 6.1.14.3 are utilized, the provisions of 17.1.2.2.1 and 17.1.2.2.2 shall also apply.

CHAPTER 16 • New

**16.1.2.2.1 General.** The day-care occupancy shall be separated from the other occupancies by not less than 1-hour fire resistance–rated barriers constructed in accordance with Section 8.3.

**16.1.2.2.2 Day-Care Occupancies in Apartment Buildings.** If the two exit accesses from a day-care occupancy enter the same corridor as an apartment occupancy, the exit accesses shall be separated in the corridor by a smoke partition complying with both of the following:

(1) It shall have not less than a 1-hour fire resistance rating and shall be constructed in accordance with Section 8.4.
(2) It shall be located so that it has an exit on each side.

CHAPTER 17 • Existing

**17.1.2.2.1 General.** The day-care occupancy shall be separated from the other occupancies by not less than 1-hour fire resistance–rated barriers constructed in accordance with Section 8.3.

**17.1.2.2.2 Day-Care Occupancies in Apartment Buildings.** If the two exit accesses from a day-care occupancy enter the same corridor as an apartment occupancy, the exit accesses shall be separated in the corridor by a smoke partition complying with both of the following:

(1) It shall have not less than a 1-hour fire resistance rating and shall be constructed in accordance with Section 8.4.
(2) It shall be located so that it has an exit on each side.

Where a day-care occupancy is located in a building housing another occupancy, the operators of the day-care facility usually have no control over the safety procedures and precautions practiced by that occupancy. Subsection 16/17.1.2 requires additional protection to minimize the clients' exposure to potential hazards outside the day-care occupancy.

A day-care use with more than three clients is not permitted to be considered incidental to a predominant occupancy within the same building, except for a specialized case involving places of religious worship as specified in 16/17.1.1.5. See 6.1.14.1.3(2). Thus, the presence of a day-care use for more than three clients in a building with some other occupancy creates a multiple occupancy. As required by 16/17.1.2.1, the multiple occupancy must be protected in accordance with 6.1.14. Two protection options are offered: the multiple occupancy can be protected as a mixed occupancy, or it can be protected as separated occupancies.

The reason for requiring corridor subdivision by smoke partitions in accordance with Section 8.4 where day-care centers are located in an apartment building, and where the multiple occupancy is protected as a mixed occupancy, is the same as that used in Chapters 18 and 19 for health care facilities. This minimum construction will provide sufficient protection against flame and smoke spread. The 1-hour wall provides a barrier that either will contain a fire within a space for a limited time after the space has been evacuated or will prevent a fire from entering an occupied space for a period of time.

CHAPTER 16 • New

## 16.1.3 Special Definitions.

A list of special terms used in this chapter follows:

(1) **Day-Care Home.** See 3.3.131.1.
(2) **Flexible Plan and Open Plan Educational or Day-Care Building.** See 3.3.32.6.
(3) **Self-Preservation (Day-Care Occupancy).** See 3.3.224.
(4) **Separate Atmosphere.** See 3.3.23.2.

## 16.1.4 Classification of Occupancy.

See 6.1.4.

**16.1.4.1 General.** Occupancies that include part-day preschools, kindergartens, and other schools whose purpose is primarily educational, even though the children who attend such schools are of preschool age, shall comply with the provisions of Chapter 14.

CHAPTER 17 • Existing

## 17.1.3 Special Definitions.

A list of special terms used in this chapter follows:

(1) **Day-Care Home.** See 3.3.131.1.
(2) **Flexible Plan and Open Plan Educational or Day-Care Building.** See 3.3.32.6.
(3) **Self-Preservation (Day-Care Occupancy).** See 3.3.224.
(4) **Separate Atmosphere.** See 3.3.23.2.

## 17.1.4 Classification of Occupancy.

See 6.1.4.

**17.1.4.1 General.** Occupancies that include part-day preschools, kindergartens, and other schools whose purpose is primarily educational, even though the children who attend such schools are of preschool age, shall comply with the provisions of Chapter 15.

CHAPTER 16 • New

16.1.4.2 Adult Day-Care Occupancies.

16.1.4.2.1 Adult day-care occupancies shall include any building or portion thereof used for less than 24 hours per day to house more than three adults requiring care, maintenance, and supervision by other than their relative(s).

16.1.4.2.2 Clients in adult day-care occupancies shall be ambulatory or semiambulatory and shall not be bedridden.

16.1.4.2.3 Clients in adult day-care occupancies shall not exhibit behavior that is harmful to themselves or to others.

**16.1.4.3* Conversions.** A conversion from a day-care home to a day-care occupancy with more than 12 clients shall be permitted only if the day-care occupancy conforms to the requirements of this chapter for new day-care occupancies with more than 12 clients.

**A.16.1.4.3** A conversion from a day-care occupancy with more than 12 clients to a day-care home is not considered a change of occupancy. The resulting day-care home should be permitted to meet the requirements of Chapter 17 for existing day-care homes.

CHAPTER 17 • Existing

17.1.4.2 Adult Day-Care Occupancies.

17.1.4.2.1 Adult day-care occupancies shall include any building or portion thereof used for less than 24 hours per day to house more than three adults requiring care, maintenance, and supervision by other than their relative(s).

17.1.4.2.2 Clients in adult day-care occupancies shall be ambulatory or semiambulatory and shall not be bedridden.

17.1.4.2.3 Clients in adult day-care occupancies shall not exhibit behavior that is harmful to themselves or to others.

**17.1.4.3* Conversions.** A conversion from a day-care home to a day-care occupancy with more than 12 clients shall be permitted only if the day-care occupancy conforms to the requirements of Chapter 16 for new day-care occupancies with more than 12 clients.

**A.17.1.4.3** A conversion from a day-care occupancy with more than 12 clients to a day-care home is not considered a change of occupancy. The resulting day-care home should be permitted to meet the requirements of Chapter 17 for existing day-care homes.

The specific reference to an adult day-care occupancy in 16/17.1.4.2 acknowledges that more and more senior citizens are being cared for in day-care centers similar to child day-care centers. The definition of an adult day-care occupancy includes the characteristics of clients who might be cared for in this type of occupancy. Essentially, the capabilities of adult day-care clients clarify that these occupancies are not nursing homes or old age homes but occupancies used by adults who are capable of self-preservation but who are in need of limited attendance, supervision, or observation.

Earlier editions of the *Code* included several cues for identifying adults who meet the criteria of adult day-care clients as described in the previous paragraph. However, to avoid the implication that medical training is necessary for assessing such adults, these cues were removed from the *Code*. It might be appropriate, however, to use some of the following guidelines from previous editions to determine the acceptability of a client for adult day care:

1. The client does not require medical injections from staff but might require the administration of oral medication by staff when and as prescribed by a licensed medical examiner.
2. The client might require limited supervision, attendance, or observation.
3. The client exhibits acceptable behavior (not harmful to self or others).

Paragraph 16/17.1.4.3 addresses conversions that result in an increase in the number of clients to a number greater than 12. The conversion from a day-care home to a day-care center places a sufficiently greater number of clients at risk so as to justify imposing the requirements for new construction. If the conversion is made in reverse (i.e., from an existing day-care center to a day-care home), fewer clients are placed at risk. The existing protection package for the day-care center would be considered adequate to permit treating the post-conversion day-care home as an existing occupancy.

### 16.1.5 Classification of Hazard of Contents.

The contents of day-care occupancies shall be classified as ordinary hazard in accordance with Section 6.2.

### 17.1.5 Classification of Hazard of Contents.

The contents of day-care occupancies shall be classified as ordinary hazard in accordance with Section 6.2.

CHAPTER 16 • New

## 16.1.6 Minimum Construction Requirements.

**16.1.6.1** Day-care occupancies, other than day-care homes, shall be limited to the building construction types specified in Table 16.1.6.1 based on the number of stories in height as defined in 4.6.3. *(See 8.2.1.)*

**16.1.6.2** Where day-care occupancies, other than day-care homes, with clients who are 24 months or less in age or who are incapable of self-preservation, are located one or more stories above the level of exit discharge, or where day-care occupancies are located two or more stories above the level of exit discharge, smoke partitions shall be provided to divide such stories into not less than two compartments. The smoke partitions shall be constructed in accordance with Section 8.4 but shall not be required to have a fire resistance rating.

CHAPTER 17 • Existing

## 17.1.6 Minimum Construction Requirements.

**17.1.6.1** Day-care occupancies, other than day-care homes, shall be limited to the building construction types specified in Table 17.1.6.1 based on the number of stories in height as defined in 4.6.3. *(See 8.2.1.)*

**17.1.6.2 Reserved.**

***Table 16.1.6.1 Construction Type Limitations***

| | | Stories in Height[a] | | | | | |
|---|---|---|---|---|---|---|---|
| **Construction Type** | **Sprinklered[b]** | **1 Story Below[c]** | **1** | **2** | **3–4** | **>4 but Not High-Rise** | **High-Rise** |
| I (442) | Yes | X | X | X | X | X | X |
| | No | NP | X | X | X | NP | NP |
| I (332) | Yes | X | X | X | X | X | X |
| | No | NP | X | X | X | NP | NP |
| II (222) | Yes | X | X | X | X | X | X |
| | No | NP | X | X | X | NP | NP |
| II (111) | Yes | X | X | X | X | X | NP |
| | No | NP | X | NP | NP | NP | NP |
| II (000) | Yes | X | X | X | X | NP | NP |
| | No | NP | X | NP | NP | NP | NP |
| III (211) | Yes | X | X | X | X | NP | NP |
| | No | NP | X | NP | NP | NP | NP |
| III (200) | Yes | NP | X | X | NP | NP | NP |
| | No | NP | X | NP | NP | NP | NP |
| IV (2HH) | Yes | X | X | X | NP | NP | NP |
| | No | NP | X | NP | NP | NP | NP |
| V (111) | Yes | X | X | X | X | NP | NP |
| | No | NP | X | NP | NP | NP | NP |
| V (000) | Yes | NP | X | X | NP | NP | NP |
| | No | NP | X | NP | NP | NP | NP |

X: Permitted. NP: Not Permitted.

[a] See 4.6.3.

[b] Sprinklered throughout by an approved, supervised automatic sprinkler system in accordance with Section 9.7.

[c] One story below the level of exit discharge.

*Table 17.1.6.1 Construction Type Limitations*

| Construction Type | Sprinklered[b] | Stories in Height[a] | | | | | |
|---|---|---|---|---|---|---|---|
| | | 1 Story Below[c] | 1 | 2 | 3–4 | >4 but Not High-Rise | High-Rise |
| I (442) | Yes | X | X | X | X | X | X |
| | No | X | X | X | X | X | NP |
| I (332) | Yes | X | X | X | X | X | X |
| | No | X | X | X | X | X | NP |
| II (222) | Yes | X | X | X | X | X | X |
| | No | X | X | X | X | X | NP |
| II (111) | Yes | X | X | X | X[d] | X[d] | NP |
| | No | X | X | X[d] | NP | NP | NP |
| II (000) | Yes | X | X | X | NP | NP | NP |
| | No | NP | X | X | NP | NP | NP |
| III (211) | Yes | X | X | X | X[d] | NP | NP |
| | No | X | X | X[d] | NP | NP | NP |
| III (200) | Yes | NP | X | X | NP | NP | NP |
| | No | NP | X | X | NP | NP | NP |
| IV (2HH) | Yes | X | X | X | NP | NP | NP |
| | No | X | X | X | NP | NP | NP |
| V (111) | Yes | X | X | X | X[d] | NP | NP |
| | No | X | X | X[d] | NP | NP | NP |
| V (000) | Yes | NP | X | X | NP | NP | NP |
| | No | NP | X | NP | NP | NP | NP |

X: Permitted. NP: Not Permitted.

[a] See 4.6.3.

[b] Sprinklered throughout by an approved, supervised automatic sprinkler system in accordance with Section 9.7. *(See 17.3.5.).*

[c] One story below the level of exit discharge.

[d] Permitted only if clients capable of self-preservation.

Table 16.1.6.1 and Table 17.1.6.1 coordinate the building construction type, the automatic sprinkler protection, and the highest story occupied as they relate to a day-care center. See 4.6.3, which explains that the number of stories in height is counted starting with the level of exit discharge and ending with the highest occupiable story containing the occupancy considered, which, in this case, is a day-care occupancy. For example, a new or existing day-care center is permitted to be located on the first story (i.e., the level of exit discharge) in any building, regardless of construction type or automatic sprinkler protection. For a new day-care center located on the second story (i.e., one story above the level of exit discharge) in a nonsprinklered building, the building must be of Type I(442), Type I(332), or Type II(222) construction. In the case of an existing day-care center where the clients are capable of self-preservation, Type II(111), Type III(211), and Type V(111) construction are permitted in addition to Type I(442), Type I(332), or Type II(222) construction. If the building is of any other construction type, the day-care center is permitted to be located one story above the level of exit discharge only if the building is protected by automatic sprinklers. For other possible combinations of story height, building construction type, and building sprinklering, see Table 16.1.6.1 and Table 17.1.6.1.

Although Table 16.1.6.1 permits new day-care occupancies on floors above the first story if the building is of the required construction type and is sprinklered, the *Code* recognizes that rapid vertical movement to the level of exit discharge might be difficult. Therefore,

CHAPTER 16 • New

per 16.1.6.2, where clients who are 24 months old or younger, or who are incapable of self-preservation, are located above the level of exit discharge, the floor must be subdivided into two compartments using smoke partitions. The intent is that at least one of the two compartments on the floor is expected to be unaffected by any fire for the time necessary to summon assistance and evacuate, or for the time necessary to control the fire, so that evacuation is unnecessary. This requirement was added to the *Code* in 1994 for new day-care occupancies, but the provision was not applied to existing day-care centers, as there was not sufficient justification to impose the requirement retroactively.

### 16.1.7 Occupant Load.

**16.1.7.1** The occupant load, in number of persons for whom means of egress and other provisions are required, either shall be determined on the basis of the occupant load factors of Table 7.3.1.2 that are characteristic of the use of the space or shall be determined as the maximum probable population of the space under consideration, whichever is greater.

**16.1.7.2** Where the occupant load is determined as the maximum probable population of the space in accordance with 16.1.7.1, an approved aisle, seating, and exiting diagram shall be required by the authority having jurisdiction to substantiate such a modification.

Many jurisdictions that license day-care centers require such facilities to provide a net area of 35 $ft^2$ (3.3 $m^2$) per client for functional reasons other than life safety. In Table 7.3.1.2, the *Code* establishes the 35 $ft^2$ (3.3 $m^2$) net area occupant load factor solely for the purpose of calculating occupant load and associated egress capacity. The occupant load is required to be the maximum number of persons expected to occupy the floor but not less than the number calculated using the occupant load factor.

If a day-care center occupies a portion of a floor on which another occupancy exists, the occupant load for that floor is the sum of the occupant loads of the two occupancies.

## 16.2 Means of Egress Requirements

### 16.2.1 General.

Means of egress shall be in accordance with Chapter 7 and Section 16.2.

### 16.2.2 Means of Egress Components.

**16.2.2.1 Components Permitted.** Components of means of egress shall be limited to the types described in 16.2.2.2 through 16.2.2.10.

**16.2.2.2 Doors.**

**16.2.2.2.1 General.** Doors complying with 7.2.1 shall be permitted.

**16.2.2.2.2 Panic Hardware or Fire Exit Hardware.** Any door in a required means of egress from an area having an

CHAPTER 17 • Existing

### 17.1.7 Occupant Load.

**17.1.7.1** The occupant load, in number of persons for whom means of egress and other provisions are required, either shall be determined on the basis of the occupant load factors of Table 7.3.1.2 that are characteristic of the use of the space or shall be determined as the maximum probable population of the space under consideration, whichever is greater.

**17.1.7.2** Where the occupant load is determined as the maximum probable population of the space in accordance with 17.1.7.1, an approved aisle, seating, and exiting diagram shall be required by the authority having jurisdiction to substantiate such a modification.

## 17.2 Means of Egress Requirements

### 17.2.1 General.

Means of egress shall be in accordance with Chapter 7 and Section 17.2.

### 17.2.2 Means of Egress Components.

**17.2.2.1 Components Permitted.** Components of means of egress shall be limited to the types described in 17.2.2.2 through 17.2.2.10.

**17.2.2.2 Doors.**

**17.2.2.2.1 General.** Doors complying with 7.2.1 shall be permitted.

**17.2.2.2.2 Panic Hardware or Fire Exit Hardware.** Any door in a required means of egress from an area having an

**CHAPTER 16 • New**

occupant load of 100 or more persons shall be permitted to be provided with a latch or lock only if the latch or lock is panic hardware or fire exit hardware complying with 7.2.1.7.

**16.2.2.2.3 Special Locking Arrangements.** Special locking arrangements complying with 7.2.1.6 shall be permitted.

**16.2.2.2.4 Elevator Lobby Exit Access Door Locking.** Elevator lobby exit access door locking in accordance with 7.2.1.6.3 shall be permitted.

**16.2.2.2.5* Closet Doors.** Every closet door latch shall be such that clients can open the door from inside the closet.

**A.16.2.2.2.5** The purpose of this requirement is to prevent arrangements whereby a child can be trapped in a closet. It is intended that this provision be broadly interpreted by the authority having jurisdiction to include equipment such as refrigerators and freezers.

**16.2.2.2.6 Bathroom Doors.** Every bathroom door lock shall be designed to allow opening of the locked door from the outside by an opening device that shall be readily accessible to the staff.

**CHAPTER 17 • Existing**

occupant load of 100 or more persons shall be permitted to be provided with a latch or lock only if the latch or lock is panic hardware or fire exit hardware complying with 7.2.1.7.

**17.2.2.2.3 Special Locking Arrangements.** Special locking arrangements complying with 7.2.1.6 shall be permitted.

**17.2.2.2.4 Elevator Lobby Exit Access Door Locking.** Elevator lobby exit access door locking in accordance with 7.2.1.6.3 shall be permitted.

**17.2.2.2.5* Closet Doors.** Every closet door latch shall be such that clients can open the door from inside the closet.

**A.17.2.2.2.5** The purpose of this requirement is to prevent arrangements where a client can be trapped in a closet. It is intended that this provision be broadly interpreted by the authority having jurisdiction to include equipment such as refrigerators and freezers.

**17.2.2.2.6 Bathroom Doors.** Every bathroom door lock shall be designed to allow opening of the locked door from the outside by an opening device that shall be readily accessible to the staff.

The requirement of 16/17.2.2.2.2 for panic hardware or fire exit hardware is based on the total occupant load of the area served, not on the required capacity of the door. For example, if an area has an occupant load of 120 persons and is served by three doors, each door is required only to have a capacity for 40 persons. However, since each of these doors serves the common area with 100 or more persons, any latches on these doors must be arranged to be released by panic hardware or fire exit hardware. The concept employed recognizes that it is not possible to predict how many occupants will move to any one of the doors serving the area. The number of persons from the assembled group of 100 or more who travel to any one of the doors might be sufficiently large to cause crowding and shoving. Panic hardware and fire exit hardware are designed to release the door latch when building occupants push up against the actuating mechanism (typically a push pad or bar that must extend across at least one-half the width of the door in accordance with 7.2.1.7).

The provision of 16/17.2.2.2.3 references 7.2.1.6, which, at the time it was written, included only 7.2.1.6.1, which applies to delayed-egress locks, and 7.2.1.6.2, which applies to access-controlled egress doors. The intent of 16/17.2.2.2.3 is to permit the use of both sets of features in day-care occupancies. New to the 2009 edition of the *Code* are the provisions of 7.2.1.6.3 for elevator lobby exit access door assemblies locking. The technical committee created 16/17.2.2.2.4 to specifically permit the provisions of 7.2.1.6.3 to be used in educational occupancies. For a future edition of the *Code*, the committee will be asked to create separate paragraphs to permit the use of delayed-egress locking systems, access-controlled egress door assemblies, and elevator lobby exit access door assemblies locking.

To use the provisions for delayed-egress locks, the building must be either fully sprinklered or fully protected by an automatic fire detection system. Although many occupancies recognize use of the Chapter 7 provisions for delayed-egress locks, the original hardware was developed for educational occupancies. Delayed-egress locking provisions were added to Chapter 7 based on hardware development that addresses security concerns in schools. Day-care occupancy clients have many of the same characteristics as educational occupancy students.

**16.2.2.3* Stairs.** Stairs complying with 7.2.2 shall be permitted.

**17.2.2.3* Stairs.** Stairs complying with 7.2.2 shall be permitted.

CHAPTER 16 • New

**A.16.2.2.3** See A.7.2.2.4.4.4 regarding additional handrails on stairs that are used extensively by children 5 years of age or less.

Since the 2006 edition of the *Code*, 17.2.2.3, applicable to existing stairs, references the provisions of 7.2.2 without further modification. In earlier editions, existing stairs for client use were required to be those stairs that were formerly designated as Class A stairs. Subsection 7.2.2 was revised for the 2006 edition to eliminate the Class A and Class B designations for existing stairs. The existing stairs provisions in Table 7.2.2.2.1.1(b) permit the stair features formerly designated for Class B stairs to suffice for all existing installations.

**16.2.2.4 Smokeproof Enclosures.** Smokeproof enclosures complying with 7.2.3 shall be permitted.

**16.2.2.5 Horizontal Exits.** Horizontal exits complying with 7.2.4 shall be permitted.

Paragraph 17.2.2.5.2 requires an existing, nonsprinklered building with a day-care occupancy located above the fifth story to have horizontal exits or smokeproof enclosures to help ensure that clients will survive a fire. The smokeproof enclosures or the areas of refuge created by the horizontal exit provide the occupant protection needed where no sprinklers are provided to control or extinguish the fire. A similar provision does not apply to new day-care centers, because Table 16.1.6.1 requires sprinklers in buildings that house day-care centers above the fourth story.

Table 17.1.6.1 would permit the continued use of an existing day-care center located above the fourth story of a nonsprinklered building if the building were of minimum 2-hour fire resistance–rated construction. However, such continued use would not be permitted within the high-rise portion of that building. If an existing day-care center is located in the high-rise portion of a building [i.e., on a floor more than 75 ft (23 m) above the lowest level of fire department vehicle access — see 3.3.32.7], Table 17.1.6.1 requires sprinkler protection for the entire building and further requires that the building be of minimum 2-hour fire resistance–rated construction. Thus, the provision of 17.2.2.5.2 would apply only where day-care clients occupy floors above the fifth story and not a floor in the high-rise portion of a nonsprinklered building.

**16.2.2.6 Ramps.** Ramps complying with 7.2.5 shall be permitted.

**16.2.2.7 Exit Passageways.** Exit passageways complying with 7.2.6 shall be permitted.

**16.2.2.8 Fire Escape Ladders.** Fire escape ladders complying with 7.2.9 shall be permitted.

CHAPTER 17 • Existing

**A.17.2.2.3** See A.7.2.2.4.4.4 regarding additional handrails on stairs that are used extensively by children 5 years of age and under.

**17.2.2.4 Smokeproof Enclosures.** Smokeproof enclosures complying with 7.2.3 shall be permitted.

**17.2.2.5 Horizontal Exits.**

**17.2.2.5.1** Horizontal exits complying with 7.2.4 shall be permitted.

**17.2.2.5.2** Day-care occupancies located six or more stories above the level of exit discharge shall have horizontal exits to provide areas of refuge, unless the building meets one of the following criteria:

(1) The building is provided with smokeproof enclosures.
(2) The building is protected throughout by an approved, supervised automatic sprinkler system in accordance with Section 9.7.

**17.2.2.6 Ramps.** Ramps complying with 7.2.5 shall be permitted.

**17.2.2.7 Exit Passageways.** Exit passageways complying with 7.2.6 shall be permitted.

**17.2.2.8 Fire Escape Ladders.** Fire escape ladders complying with 7.2.9 shall be permitted.

CHAPTER 16 • New

**16.2.2.9 Alternating Tread Devices.** Alternating tread devices complying with 7.2.11 shall be permitted.

Fire escape ladders and alternating tread devices are permitted egress components for day-care occupancies, but only within the constraints detailed in 7.2.9 and 7.2.11. The provisions of 7.2.9 and 7.2.11 restrict the use of fire escape ladders and alternating tread devices to normally unoccupied areas, such as rooftops, or to mechanical equipment platforms subject to occupancy by not more than three persons who are all capable of using the ladder or alternating tread device. This means that fire escape ladders and alternating tread devices are not egress components permitted within the required means of egress for day-care clients.

**16.2.2.10 Areas of Refuge.** Areas of refuge complying with 7.2.12 shall be permitted.

### 16.2.3 Capacity of Means of Egress.

Capacity of means of egress shall be in accordance with Section 7.3.

### 16.2.4 Number of Exits.

**16.2.4.1** Not less than two separate exits shall be as follows:

(1) Provided on every story
(2) Accessible from every part of every story and mezzanine

**16.2.4.2 Reserved.**

CHAPTER 17 • Existing

**17.2.2.9 Alternating Tread Devices.** Alternating tread devices complying with 7.2.11 shall be permitted.

**17.2.2.10 Areas of Refuge.** Areas of refuge complying with 7.2.12 shall be permitted.

### 17.2.3 Capacity of Means of Egress.

Capacity of means of egress shall be in accordance with Section 7.3.

### 17.2.4 Number of Exits.

**17.2.4.1** Not less than two separate exits shall be as follows:

(1) Provided on every story
(2) Accessible from every part of every story and mezzanine

**17.2.4.2** Where the story below the level of exit discharge is occupied as a day-care occupancy, 17.2.4.2.1 and 17.2.4.2.2 shall apply.

**17.2.4.2.1** One means of egress shall be an outside or interior stair in accordance with 7.2.2. An interior stair, if used, shall serve only the story below the level of exit discharge. The interior stair shall be permitted to communicate with the level of exit discharge; however, the exit route from the level of exit discharge shall not pass through the stair enclosure.

**17.2.4.2.2** The second means of egress shall be permitted to be via an unenclosed stairway separated from the level of exit discharge in accordance with 8.6.5.

**17.2.4.2.3** The path of egress travel on the level of exit discharge shall be protected in accordance with 7.1.3.1, unless one of the following criteria is met:

(1) The path of egress on the level of exit discharge shall be permitted to be unprotected if the level of exit discharge and the level below the level of exit discharge are protected throughout by a smoke detection system.
(2) The path of egress on the level of exit discharge shall be permitted to be unprotected if the level of exit discharge and the level below the level of exit discharge are protected throughout by an approved automatic sprinkler system.

CHAPTER 16 • New

CHAPTER 17 • Existing

Access must be provided to a minimum of two exits, both of which must be located on the floor or story in question. Contrast this requirement with a related provision for industrial occupancies that requires access to two exits but mandates that only one of those required exits be located on the floor or story (see 40.2.4.1.1). Thus, in a day-care occupancy, an open exit access stair, if it were permitted without violating the provisions applicable to the protection of vertical openings, would be permitted to serve as exit access only if the requirement for two exits on the floor is first satisfied. In a multistory day-care occupancy building, the requirements of 16/17.2.4.1 are typically met by providing two properly enclosed exit stairs that can be accessed from all floors.

Paragraph 17.2.4.2 contains requirements for existing day-care centers located below the level of exit discharge. (Similar provisions do not appear in Chapter 16, because Table 16.1.6.1 requires complete sprinklering of the building if a new day-care center is located below the first story.) This requirement helps to ensure that the occupants of the lower level have a protected egress path that doesn't force them to traverse the street floor. The requirement does help but doesn't guarantee safe egress, because a convenience door is permitted from the street floor into the lower level's stair enclosure. If a fire were to occur on the street floor and if someone were to wedge the door open, smoke and other effects of fire could enter the stair designated for use by the occupants of the lower level. Diligent enforcement is needed to ensure that the self-closing door will not be improperly held open. The intent of 17.2.4.2 is illustrated in Exhibit 16/17.1.

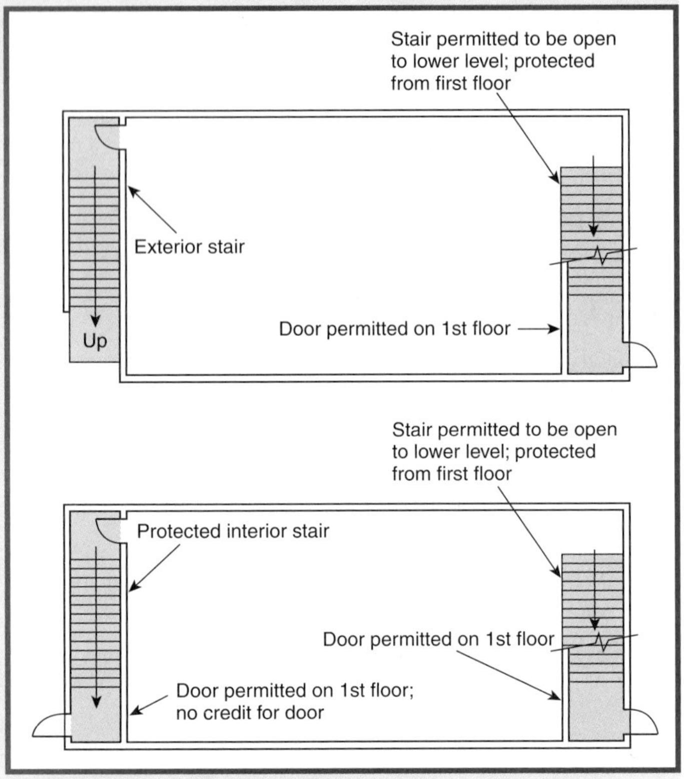


***Exhibit 16/17.1*** *Egress for levels below level of exit discharge — existing day-care occupancies.*

### 16.2.5 Arrangement of Means of Egress.

See also 16.1.6.2.

**16.2.5.1** Means of egress shall be arranged in accordance with Section 7.5.

**16.2.5.2** No dead-end corridor shall exceed 20 ft (6100 mm), other than in buildings protected throughout by an approved, supervised automatic sprinkler system in accordance with Section 9.7, in which case dead-end corridors shall not exceed 50 ft (15 m).

**16.2.5.3** Limitations on common path of travel shall be in accordance with 16.2.5.3.1 and 16.2.5.3.2.

**16.2.5.3.1** Common path of travel shall not exceed 100 ft (30 m) in a building protected throughout by an approved, supervised automatic sprinkler system in accordance with Section 9.7.

### 17.2.5 Arrangement of Means of Egress.

**17.2.5.1** Means of egress shall be arranged in accordance with Section 7.5.

**17.2.5.2** No dead-end corridor shall exceed 20 ft (6100 mm), other than in buildings protected throughout by an approved, supervised automatic sprinkler system in accordance with Section 9.7, in which case dead-end corridors shall not exceed 50 ft (15 m).

**17.2.5.3** Limitations on common path of travel shall be in accordance with 17.2.5.3.1 and 17.2.5.3.2.

**17.2.5.3.1** Common path of travel shall not exceed 100 ft (30 m) in a building protected throughout by an approved, supervised automatic sprinkler system in accordance with Section 9.7.

CHAPTER 16 • New

16.2.5.3.2 Common path of travel shall not exceed 75 ft (23 m) in a building not protected throughout by an approved, supervised automatic sprinkler system in accordance with Section 9.7.

CHAPTER 17 • Existing

17.2.5.3.2 Common path of travel shall not exceed 75 ft (23 m) in a building not protected throughout by an approved, supervised automatic sprinkler system in accordance with Section 9.7.

17.2.5.4 The story used below the level of exit discharge shall be in accordance with 17.2.4.2.

Paragraph 7.5.1.1.4 permits individual occupancy chapters to mandate, and to set limits for, common paths of travel. Paragraph 16/17.2.5.3 establishes the maximum common path of travel for day-care occupancies as 100 ft (30 m), if the building is protected throughout by an approved, supervised automatic sprinkler system, and limits the common path of travel to 75 ft (23 m) where the sprinkler criteria are not met. The 75 ft (23 m) limit is strict enough to help ensure that occupants can safely tolerate traveling in only one direction for a limited distance before reaching a point where travel in independent directions becomes possible. The increase to 100 ft (30 m) recognizes that fire control by sprinklers increases the safe travel time along the single available path.

Paragraph 7.5.1.5 permits individual occupancy chapters to establish limits for dead-end corridors. The dead-end corridor limitation for day-care occupancies is 20 ft (6100 mm), as permitted by 16/17.2.5.2 — and the limitation appears reasonable. However, 16/17.2.5.2 permits the dead-end corridor to be increased by 30 ft (9.1 m) to a maximum of 50 ft (15 m) in recognition of the fire-controlling capabilities of a sprinkler system. A floor arrangement with outside doors or stairways at both ends of a central corridor typically creates no dead-end corridors. Dead-end corridor pockets might be created where stairways are not located at the end of corridors but are located at intermediate points.

### 16.2.6 Travel Distance to Exits.

16.2.6.1 Travel distance shall be measured in accordance with Section 7.6.

16.2.6.2 Travel distance shall meet the following criteria, unless otherwise permitted by 16.2.6.3:

(1) The travel distance between any room door intended as an exit access and an exit shall not exceed 100 ft (30 m).
(2) The travel distance between any point in a room and an exit shall not exceed 150 ft (46 m).
(3) The travel distance between any point in a sleeping room and an exit access door in that room shall not exceed 50 ft (15 m).

16.2.6.3 The travel distance required by 16.2.6.2(1) and (2) shall be permitted to be increased by 50 ft (15 m) in buildings protected throughout by an approved, supervised automatic sprinkler system in accordance with Section 9.7.

### 17.2.6 Travel Distance to Exits.

17.2.6.1 Travel distance shall be measured in accordance with Section 7.6.

17.2.6.2 Travel distance shall meet the following criteria, unless otherwise permitted by 17.2.6.3:

(1) The travel distance between any room door intended as an exit access and an exit shall not exceed 100 ft (30 m).
(2) The travel distance between any point in a room and an exit shall not exceed 150 ft (46 m).
(3) The travel distance between any point in a sleeping room and an exit access door in that room shall not exceed 50 ft (15 m).

17.2.6.3 The travel distance required by 17.2.6.2(1) and (2) shall be permitted to be increased by 50 ft (15 m) in buildings protected throughout by an approved automatic sprinkler system in accordance with Section 9.7.

Exhibit 16/17.2 illustrates the travel distance limitations of 16/17.2.6.

The maximum permitted travel distance from a room door to the nearest exit (e.g., the path from the exit access door to the corridor shown as *C*1 to *E*1 or *C*2 to *E*2) is 100 ft (30 m); if the building is sprinklered, the maximum is extended to 150 ft (46 m) in accordance with 16/17.2.6.3. Note that, for new construction, the *Code* requires that the sprinkler system be supervised to permit the 50 ft (15 m) increase in allowable travel distance.

The maximum travel distance from a point in a sleeping room to an exit access door from that room (path *X*1 to *C*1) is 50 ft (15 m). This travel distance limit within a sleeping room is not permitted to be increased, even if the building is sprinklered.

CHAPTER 16 • New

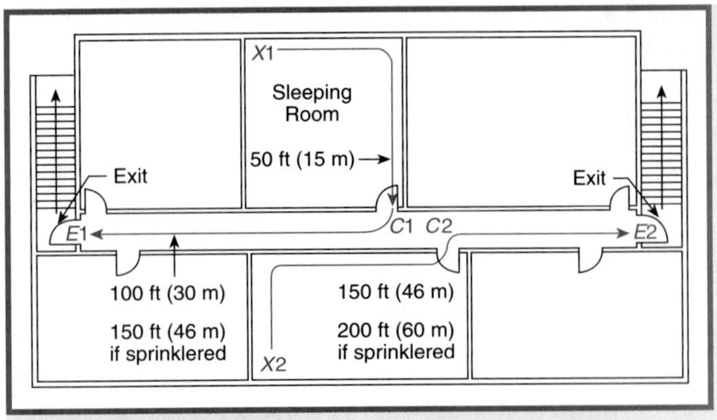


*Exhibit 16/17.2 Maximum travel distance in a day-care occupancy.*

The total travel distance permitted from any point in a sleeping room to an exit (path X1 to E1) is 150 ft (46 m), unless the building is sprinklered, as explained in 16/17.2.6.3. In a sprinklered building, the total permitted travel distance associated with a sleeping room is 200 ft (61 m) only if the full 50 ft (15 m) of within-room exit access and the full 150 ft (46 m) of corridor exit access are used.

For rooms other than sleeping rooms, the total travel distance permitted from any point in a nonsleeping room to an exit (path X2 to E2) is 150 ft (46 m), unless the building is sprinklered, as explained in 16/17.2.6.3. In a sprinklered building, the total permitted travel distance associated with a nonsleeping room is 200 ft (61 m), but not more than 150 ft (46 m) of that total can occur outside the room (path C2 to E2).

### 16.2.7 Discharge from Exits.

Discharge from exits shall be arranged in accordance with Section 7.7.

### 16.2.8 Illumination of Means of Egress.

Means of egress shall be illuminated in accordance with Section 7.8.

### 16.2.9 Emergency Lighting.

Emergency lighting shall be provided in accordance with Section 7.9 in the following areas:

(1) Interior stairs and corridors
(2) Assembly use spaces
(3) Flexible and open plan buildings
(4) Interior or limited access portions of buildings
(5) Shops and laboratories

### 16.2.10 Marking of Means of Egress.

Means of egress shall have signs in accordance with Section 7.10.

### 16.2.11 Special Means of Egress Features.

#### 16.2.11.1 Windows for Rescue.

**16.2.11.1.1** Every room or space normally subject to client occupancy, other than bathrooms, shall have not less than one outside window for emergency rescue that complies with the following, unless otherwise permitted by 16.2.11.1.2:

(1) Such windows shall be openable from the inside without the use of tools and shall provide a clear opening of

CHAPTER 17 • Existing

### 17.2.7 Discharge from Exits.

Discharge from exits shall be arranged in accordance with Section 7.7, unless otherwise provided in 17.2.4.2.

### 17.2.8 Illumination of Means of Egress.

Means of egress shall be illuminated in accordance with Section 7.8.

### 17.2.9 Emergency Lighting.

Emergency lighting shall be provided in accordance with Section 7.9 in the following areas:

(1) Interior stairs and corridors
(2) Assembly use spaces
(3) Flexible and open plan buildings
(4) Interior or limited access portions of buildings
(5) Shops and laboratories

### 17.2.10 Marking of Means of Egress.

Means of egress shall have signs in accordance with Section 7.10.

### 17.2.11 Special Means of Egress Features.

#### 17.2.11.1 Windows for Rescue.

**17.2.11.1.1** Every room or space greater than 250 $ft^2$ (23.2 $m^2$) and normally subject to client occupancy shall have not less than one outside window for emergency rescue that complies with the following, unless otherwise permitted by 17.2.11.1.2:

(1) Such windows shall be openable from the inside without the use of tools and shall provide a clear opening of

not less than 20 in. (510 mm) in width, 24 in. (610 mm) in height, and 5.7 ft$^2$ (0.5 m$^2$) in area.

(2) The bottom of the opening shall be not more than 44 in. (1120 mm) above the floor.

(3) The clear opening shall allow a rectangular solid, with a width and height that provides not less than the required 5.7 ft$^2$ (0.5 m$^2$) opening and a depth of not less than 20 in. (510 mm), to pass fully through the opening.

**16.2.11.1.2** The requirements of 16.2.11.1.1 shall not apply to the following:

(1) Buildings protected throughout by an approved, supervised automatic sprinkler system in accordance with Section 9.7

(2) Where the room or space has a door leading directly to the outside of the building



not less than 20 in. (510 mm) in width, 24 in. (610 mm) in height, and 5.7 ft$^2$ (0.5 m$^2$) in area.

(2) The bottom of the opening shall be not more than 44 in. (1120 mm) above the floor.

(3) The clear opening shall allow a rectangular solid, with a width and height that provides not less than the required 5.7 ft$^2$ (0.5 m$^2$) opening and a depth of not less than 20 in. (510 mm), to pass fully through the opening.

**17.2.11.1.2** The requirements of 17.2.11.1.1 shall not apply to the following:

(1) Buildings protected throughout by an approved, supervised automatic sprinkler system in accordance with Section 9.7

(2) Where the room or space has a door leading directly to the outside of the building

(3) Rooms located four or more stories above the level of exit discharge

(4) Where awning-type or hopper-type windows that are hinged or subdivided to provide a clear opening of not less than 4 ft$^2$ (0.38 m$^2$) or any dimension of not less than 22 in. (560 mm) meet the following criteria:

   (a) Such windows shall be permitted to continue in use.
   (b) Screen walls or devices in front of required windows shall not interfere with normal rescue requirements.

(5) Where the room or space complies with the following:

   (a) Doors shall exist that allow travel between adjacent rooms.
   (b) Doors used to travel from room to room shall provide one of the following:
      i. Direct access to exits in both directions
      ii. Direct access to an exit in one direction and to a separate smoke compartment that provides access to another exit in the other direction
   (c) The corridor shall be separated from the rooms by a wall that resists the passage of smoke, and all doors between the rooms and the corridor shall be self-closing in accordance with 7.2.1.8.
   (d) The length of travel to exits along such paths shall not exceed 150 ft (46 m).
   (e) Each communicating door shall be marked in accordance with Section 7.10.
   (f) No locking device shall be permitted on the communicating doors.

The dimensions specified for windows used for emergency rescue in day-care occupancies, which are identical to those required for secondary escape from dwelling units, are based on simulations of emergency rescue conducted by the San Diego Fire Department. Exhibit 16/17.3 illustrates two configurations that achieve the required area of 5.7 ft$^2$ (0.5 m$^2$).

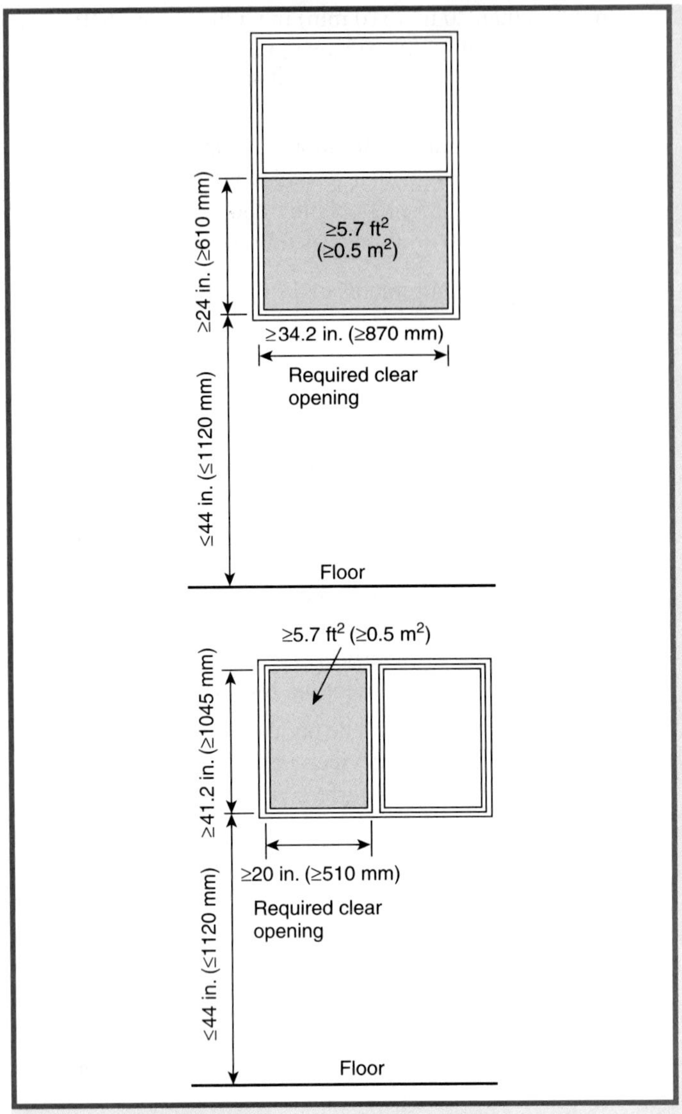


***Exhibit 16/17.3** Windows for rescue or ventilation — minimum dimensions.*

The *Code* assumes that the fire department or others will assist day-care occupancy clients, especially over ladders. If these emergency rescue windows must be used as a supplementary means of escape, the windows should allow younger children to escape unaided. Therefore, storm sashes, screens, or devices in front of the windows must be easy to open or remove, and the sills must be low enough for children to reach.

According to 16/17.2.11.1.2(1) and (2), emergency rescue windows are not required if a room has a door leading directly to the outside or if the building is totally sprinklered.

It might not be practical to use a window above the fourth story as an escape window. Therefore, 17.2.11.1.2(3) exempts windows above the fourth story in existing day-care centers. This exemption will have limited application, because Table 17.1.6.1 requires most day-care centers located above the fourth story to be sprinklered, and, per 17.2.11.1.2(1), sprinklers negate the need for the rescue window. Similarly, the exemption is not needed for new construction, because Table 16.1.6.1 requires day-care centers located above the fourth story to be sprinklered.

Awning-type and hopper-type windows might provide the required opening within the plane of the building's exterior wall. However, when the window is open, the sash and glazing are located outside that plane and might prevent occupants from passing through the opening. Therefore, the criterion of 16/17.2.11.1.1(3) for providing an opening through which a minimum-size rectangular solid can pass is intended to ensure that occupants can pass through the opening. For existing awning-type windows, 17.2.11.1.2(4) offers some relief from the rectangular solid and minimum-size opening requirements. Exhibit 16/17.4 illustrates the use of 17.2.11.1.2(4).

The provisions of 17.2.11.1.2(5) provide an alternative to the rescue windows that is identical to that offered in 15.2.11.1.2(5) for existing educational occupancies and that is illustrated in Exhibit 14/15.9.

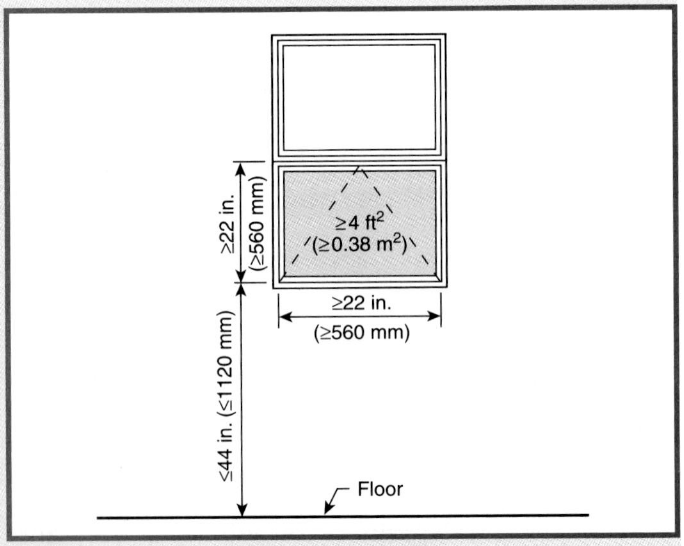


***Exhibit 16/17.4** Existing awning window — minimum dimensions.*

CHAPTER 16 • New

**16.2.11.2 Lockups.** Lockups in day-care occupancies shall comply with the requirements of 22.4.5.

CHAPTER 17 • Existing

**17.2.11.2 Lockups.** Lockups in day-care occupancies, other than approved existing lockups, shall comply with the requirements of 23.4.5.

A *lockup* is defined in 3.3.155 as "an incidental use area in other than a detention and correctional occupancy where occupants are restrained and such occupants are mostly incapable of self-preservation because of security measures not under the occupants' control." It is difficult to provide an example of a lockup in a day-care occupancy, but that does not mean that there will not be a lockup in a day-care occupancy. An example of a lockup in an educational occupancy is a room for holding unruly students until police can transport such students to the police station. The provisions of Chapters 16 and 17 alone are not adequate to ensure life safety for those who are detained by security measures not under their control. Lockups in day-care occupancies are required to meet the provisions of 22/23.4.5, which complete the needed package of protection features.

## 16.3 Protection

### 16.3.1 Protection of Vertical Openings.

Any vertical opening, other than unprotected vertical openings in accordance with 8.6.8.2, shall be enclosed or protected in accordance with Section 8.6.

### 16.3.2 Protection from Hazards.

**16.3.2.1** Rooms or spaces for the storage, processing, or use of materials specified in 16.3.2.1(1) through (3) shall be protected in accordance with the following:

(1) Separation from the remainder of the building by fire barriers having a minimum 1-hour fire resistance rating, or protection of such rooms by automatic extinguishing systems as specified in Section 8.7, in the following areas:
   (a) Boiler and furnace rooms, unless such rooms enclose only air-handling equipment
   (b) Rooms or spaces used for the storage of combustible supplies in quantities deemed hazardous by the authority having jurisdiction
   (c) Rooms or spaces used for the storage of hazardous materials or flammable or combustible liquids in quantities deemed hazardous by recognized standards
   (d) Janitor closets

(2) Separation from the remainder of the building by fire barriers having a minimum 1-hour fire resistance rating and protection of such rooms by automatic extinguishing systems as specified in Section 8.7 in the following areas:
   (a)* Laundries

## 17.3 Protection

### 17.3.1 Protection of Vertical Openings.

Any vertical opening, other than unprotected vertical openings in accordance with 8.6.8.2, shall be enclosed or protected in accordance with Section 8.6.

### 17.3.2 Protection from Hazards.

**17.3.2.1** Rooms or spaces for the storage, processing, or use of materials specified in 17.3.2.1(1) through (3) shall be protected in accordance with the following:

(1) Separation from the remainder of the building by fire barriers having a minimum 1-hour fire resistance rating, or protection of such rooms by automatic extinguishing systems as specified in Section 8.7, in the following areas:
   (a) Boiler and furnace rooms, unless such rooms enclose only air-handling equipment
   (b) Rooms or spaces used for the storage of combustible supplies in quantities deemed hazardous by the authority having jurisdiction
   (c) Rooms or spaces used for the storage of hazardous materials or flammable or combustible liquids in quantities deemed hazardous by recognized standards
   (d) Janitor closets

(2) Separation from the remainder of the building by fire barriers having a minimum 1-hour fire resistance rating and protection of such rooms by automatic extinguishing systems as specified in Section 8.7 in the following areas:
   (a)* Laundries

CHAPTER 16 • New

**A.16.3.2.1(2)(a)** It is not the intent to classify a room with a domestic-type clothes washer and a domestic-type clothes dryer as a laundry.

(b) Maintenance shops, including woodworking and painting areas
(c) Rooms or spaces used for processing or use of combustible supplies deemed hazardous by the authority having jurisdiction
(d) Rooms or spaces used for processing or use of hazardous materials or flammable or combustible liquids in quantities deemed hazardous by recognized standards

(3) Where automatic extinguishing is used to meet the requirements of 16.3.2.1(1) and (2), the protection shall be permitted in accordance with 9.7.1.2.

**16.3.2.2** Janitor closets protected in accordance with 16.3.2.1(1)(d) shall be permitted to have doors fitted with ventilating louvers where the space is protected by automatic sprinklers.

**16.3.2.3** Cooking facilities shall be protected in accordance with 9.2.3, unless otherwise permitted by 16.3.2.4 or 16.3.2.5.

**16.3.2.4** Openings shall not be required to be protected between food preparation areas and dining areas.

**16.3.2.5** Approved domestic cooking equipment used for food warming or limited cooking shall not be required to be protected.

**16.3.2.6 Alcohol-Based Hand-Rub Dispensers.** Alcohol-based hand-rub dispensers shall be protected in accordance with 8.7.3, unless all of the following conditions are met:

(1) Dispensers shall be installed in rooms or spaces separated from corridors and exits.
(2) The maximum individual dispenser fluid capacity shall be as follows:
    (a) 0.32 gal (1.2 L) for dispensers in rooms
    (b) 0.53 gal (2.0 L) for dispensers in suites of rooms
(3) Dispensers shall be separated from each other by horizontal spacing of not less than 48 in. (1220 mm).
(4) Storage of quantities greater than 5 gal (18.9 L) in a single fire compartment shall meet the requirements of NFPA 30, *Flammable and Combustible Liquids Code*.
(5) Dispensers shall not be installed over or directly adjacent to an ignition source.
(6) Dispensers installed directly over carpeted floors shall be permitted only in sprinklered rooms or spaces.

CHAPTER 17 • Existing

**A.17.3.2.1(2)(a)** It is not the intent to classify a room with a domestic-type clothes washer and a domestic-type clothes dryer as a laundry.

(b) Maintenance shops, including woodworking and painting areas
(c) Rooms or spaces used for processing or use of combustible supplies deemed hazardous by the authority having jurisdiction
(d) Rooms or spaces used for processing or use of hazardous materials or flammable or combustible liquids in quantities deemed hazardous by recognized standards

(3) Where automatic extinguishing is used to meet the requirements of 17.3.2.1(1) and (2), the protection shall be permitted in accordance with 9.7.1.2.

**17.3.2.2** Janitor closets protected in accordance with 17.3.2.1(1)(d) shall be permitted to have doors fitted with ventilating louvers where the space is protected by automatic sprinklers.

**17.3.2.3** Cooking facilities shall be protected in accordance with 9.2.3, unless otherwise permitted by 17.3.2.4 or 17.3.2.5.

**17.3.2.4** Openings shall not be required to be protected between food preparation areas and dining areas.

**17.3.2.5** Approved domestic cooking equipment used for food warming or limited cooking shall not be required to be protected.

**17.3.2.6 Alcohol-Based Hand-Rub Dispensers** Alcohol-based hand-rub dispensers shall be protected in accordance with 8.7.3, unless all of the following conditions are met:

(1) Dispensers shall be installed in rooms or spaces separated from corridors and exits.
(2) The maximum individual dispenser fluid capacity shall be as follows:
    (a) 0.32 gal (1.2 L) for dispensers in rooms
    (b) 0.53 gal (2.0 L) for dispensers in suites of rooms
(3) Dispensers shall be separated from each other by horizontal spacing of not less than 48 in. (1220 mm).
(4) Storage of quantities greater than 5 gal (18.9 L) in a single fire compartment shall meet the requirements of NFPA 30, *Flammable and Combustible Liquids Code*.
(5) Dispensers shall not be installed over or directly adjacent to an ignition source.
(6) Dispensers installed directly over carpeted floors shall be permitted only in sprinklered rooms or spaces.

The intent of 16/17.3.2.1 is to specify the degree of protection necessary for certain hazardous contents areas. The hazards noted in 16/17.3.2.1(1) are required to be enclosed in 1-hour construction or protected by automatic sprinklers. In new construction, if the sprinkler option were chosen, 8.7.1.2 would still require an enclosure comprised of smoke partitions.

Exhibit 16/17.5 through Exhibit 16/17.7 illustrate the various protection requirements of 16/17.3.2.1.

The provisions of 16/17.3.2.6 are new to the 2009 edition of the *Code* and draw from material developed for the health care occupancies chapters to permit alcohol-based hand-rub dispensers. Although health care occupancies have a functional need to position such dispensers in corridors to permit hand sanitizing prior to entering a patient room and again upon leaving, no such need exists for day-care occupancies. For day-care occupancies, the alcohol-based hand-rub dispensers are permitted only in rooms or spaces separated from the corridor. Prior to the inclusion of the provisions for alcohol-based hand-rub dispensers, the only option available to day-care occupancies was to treat the alcohol solutions as flammable liquids subject to the provisions of 8.7.3, which meant the dispensers were prohibited from being placed in client-occupied areas. Dispensers not meeting all the criteria of 16/17.3.2.6(1) through (6) are subject to regulation as flammable liquids in accordance with 8.7.3.

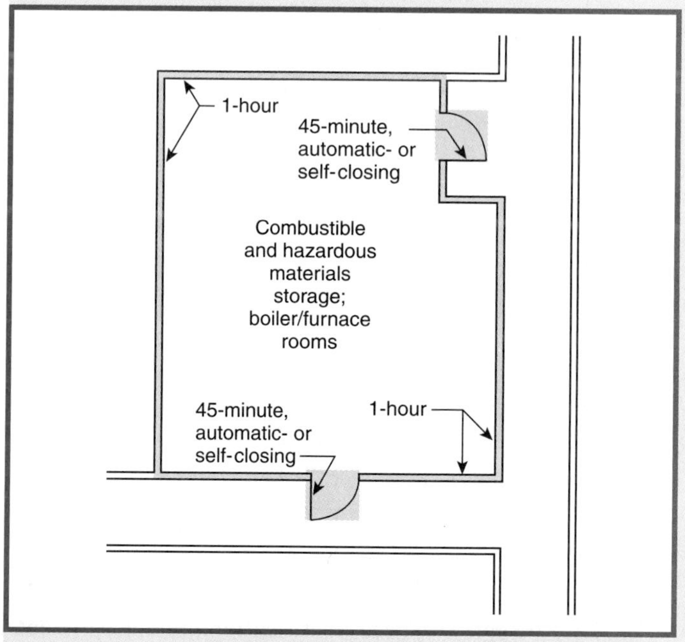


***Exhibit 16/17.5** Protection of hazardous contents areas — rated enclosure complying with 16/17.3.2.1(1).*

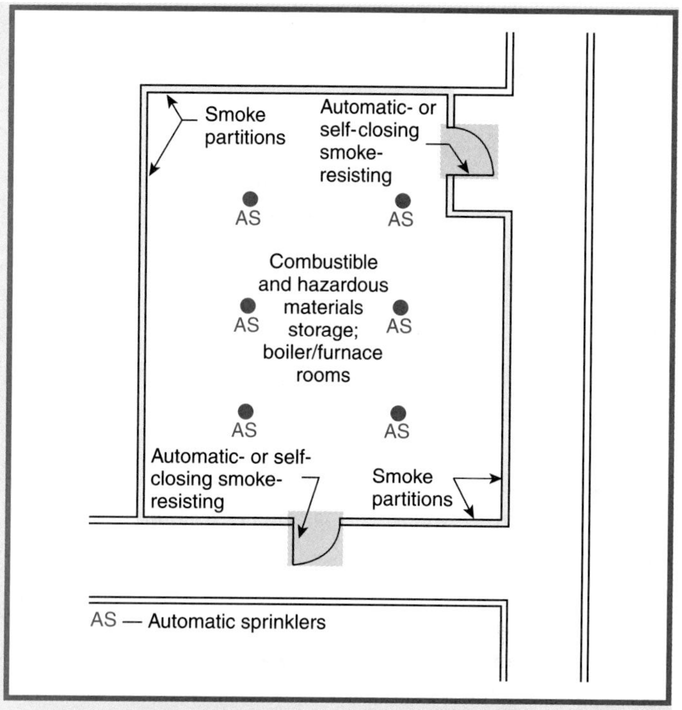


***Exhibit 16/17.6** Protection of new hazardous contents areas — sprinkler protection and smoke partition enclosure complying with 16.3.2.1(1).*

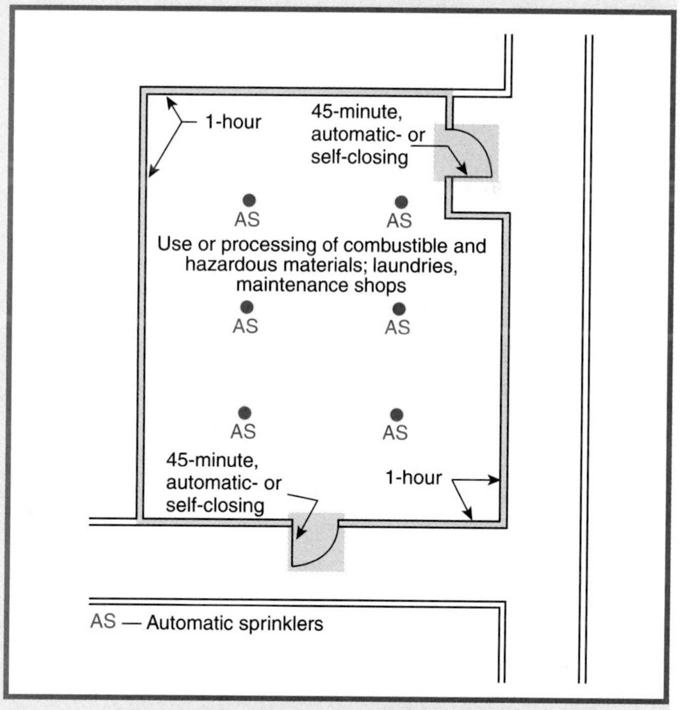


***Exhibit 16/17.7** Protection of hazardous areas — rated enclosure and sprinkler protection complying with 16/17.3.2.1(2).*

CHAPTER 16 • New

### 16.3.3 Interior Finish.

**16.3.3.1 General.** Interior finish shall be in accordance with Section 10.2.

**16.3.3.2 Interior Wall and Ceiling Finish.** Interior wall and ceiling finish materials complying with Section 10.2 shall be Class A in stairways, corridors, and lobbies; in all other occupied areas, interior wall and ceiling finish shall be Class A or Class B.

**16.3.3.3 Interior Floor Finish.**

**16.3.3.3.1** Interior floor finish shall comply with Section 10.2.

**16.3.3.3.2** Interior floor finish in exit enclosures and exit access corridors and spaces not separated from them by walls complying with 14.3.6 shall be not less than Class II.

**16.3.3.3.3** Interior floor finish shall comply with 10.2.7.1 or 10.2.7.2, as applicable.

### 16.3.4 Detection, Alarm, and Communications Systems.

**16.3.4.1 General.** Day-care occupancies, other than day-care occupancies housed in one room having at least one door opening directly to the outside at grade plane or to an exterior exit access balcony in accordance with 7.5.3, shall be provided with a fire alarm system in accordance with Section 9.6.

**16.3.4.2 Initiation.** Initiation of the required fire alarm system shall be by manual means and by operation of any required smoke detectors and required sprinkler systems. *(See 16.3.4.5.)*

**16.3.4.3 Occupant Notification.**

**16.3.4.3.1** Occupant notification shall be in accordance with 9.6.3.

**16.3.4.3.2** Positive alarm sequence shall be permitted in accordance with 9.6.3.4.

**16.3.4.3.3** Where occupant notification appliances are provided in all occupied rooms and corridors, the private operating mode as described in *NFPA 72, National Fire Alarm Code*, shall be permitted to be used in either or both of the following locations:

(1) Occupied rooms
(2) Corridors

**16.3.4.4 Emergency Forces Notification.** Fire department notification shall be accomplished in accordance with 9.6.4.

CHAPTER 17 • Existing

### 17.3.3 Interior Finish.

**17.3.3.1 General.** Interior finish shall be in accordance with Section 10.2.

**17.3.3.2 Interior Wall and Ceiling Finish.** Interior wall and ceiling finish materials complying with Section 10.2 shall be Class A or Class B throughout.

**17.3.3.3 Interior Floor Finish.** (No requirements.)

### 17.3.4 Detection, Alarm, and Communications Systems.

**17.3.4.1 General.** Day-care occupancies, other than day-care occupancies housed in one room, shall be provided with a fire alarm system in accordance with Section 9.6.

**17.3.4.2 Initiation.** Initiation of the required fire alarm system shall be by manual means and by operation of any required smoke detectors and required sprinkler systems. *(See 17.3.4.5.)*

**17.3.4.3 Occupant Notification.**

**17.3.4.3.1** Occupant notification shall be in accordance with 9.6.3.

**17.3.4.3.2** Positive alarm sequence shall be permitted in accordance with 9.6.3.4.

**17.3.4.3.3** Where occupant notification appliances are provided in all occupied rooms and corridors, the private operating mode as described in *NFPA 72, National Fire Alarm Code*, shall be permitted to be used in either or both of the following locations:

(1) Occupied rooms
(2) Corridors

**17.3.4.4 Emergency Forces Notification.** Fire department notification, other than for day-care occupancies with not more than 100 clients, shall be accomplished in accordance with 9.6.4.

CHAPTER 16 • New

**16.3.4.5 Detection.** A smoke detection system in accordance with Section 9.6 shall be installed in day-care occupancies, other than those housed in one room having at least one door opening directly to the outside at grade plane or to an exterior exit access balcony in accordance with 7.5.3, and such system shall comply with both of the following:

(1) Detectors shall be installed on each story in front of the doors to the stairways and in the corridors of all floors occupied by the day-care occupancy.
(2) Detectors shall be installed in lounges, recreation areas, and sleeping rooms in the day-care occupancy.

CHAPTER 17 • Existing

**17.3.4.5 Detection.** A smoke detection system in accordance with Section 9.6 shall be installed in day-care occupancies, other than those housed in one room or those housing clients capable of self-preservation where no sleeping facilities are provided, and such system shall comply with both of the following:

(1) Detectors shall be installed on each story in front of the doors to the stairways and in the corridors of all floors occupied by the day-care occupancy.
(2) Detectors shall be installed in lounges, recreation areas, and sleeping rooms in the day-care occupancy.

New day-care centers, other than those housed in a single room having a door opening directly to the outside at grade plane or to an exterior exit access balcony, are required to have a fire alarm system. Existing day-care centers, other than those housed in a single room, are required to have a fire alarm system. The alarm system is for purposes of occupant notification and fire department notification. Existing day-care centers are exempt from the fire department notification requirement if there are 100 or fewer clients.

Neither new nor existing day-care centers are permitted to use a presignal system (see 9.6.3.3). A delay in occupant notification is permitted only if positive alarm sequence in accordance with 9.6.3.4 is provided. Positive alarm sequence includes some fail-safe features not found in presignal systems. For example, if the person staffing the control panel does not acknowledge the signal, general occupant notification occurs automatically. Also, if a second initiation device reports a fire condition to the control panel, the delay ends and general occupant notification occurs immediately.

Some day-care centers make provisions for clients to nap. Also, parents who work at night might place their children in day-care centers for the purpose of sleeping through the night. Regardless of whether occupants sleep in the center, the smoke detectors required by 16/17.3.4.5 will provide critical extra time to evacuate clients. The requirement for smoke detection does not apply to new day-care centers housed in a single room having a door opening directly to the outside at grade plane or to an exterior exit access balcony, where a fire will be obvious simultaneously to all occupants. Similarly, the requirement for smoke detection does not apply to existing day-care centers housed in a single room or where the clients are capable of self-preservation and there are no sleeping facilities.

CHAPTER 16 • New

### 16.3.5 Extinguishment Requirements.

**16.3.5.1** Any required sprinkler systems shall be in accordance with Section 9.7.

**16.3.5.2** Required sprinkler systems shall be installed in accordance with 9.7.1.1(1).

**16.3.5.3** Buildings with unprotected openings in accordance with 8.6.6 shall be protected throughout by an approved, supervised automatic sprinkler system in accordance with Section 9.7.

### 16.3.6 Corridors.

Every interior corridor shall be constructed of walls having not less than a 1-hour fire resistance rating in accordance with Section 8.3, unless otherwise permitted by the following:

(1) Corridor protection shall not be required where all spaces normally subject to client occupancy have not

CHAPTER 17 • Existing

### 17.3.5 Extinguishment Requirements.

**17.3.5.1** Any required sprinkler system shall be in accordance with Section 9.7.

**17.3.5.2** Required sprinkler systems, other than approved existing systems, shall be installed in accordance with 9.7.1.1(1).

**17.3.5.3** Buildings with unprotected openings in accordance with 8.6.6 shall be protected throughout by an approved, supervised automatic sprinkler system in accordance with Section 9.7.

### 17.3.6 Corridors.

Every interior corridor shall be constructed of walls having a minimum ½-hour fire resistance rating in accordance with Section 8.3, unless otherwise permitted by the following:

(1) Corridor protection shall not be required where all spaces normally subject to student occupancy have not

CHAPTER 16 • New

less than one door opening directly to the outside or to an exterior exit access balcony or corridor in accordance with 7.5.3.

(2) In buildings protected throughout by an approved, supervised automatic sprinkler system in accordance with Section 9.7, corridor walls shall not be required to be rated, provided that such walls form smoke partitions in accordance with Section 8.4.

(3) Where the corridor ceiling is an assembly having a 1-hour fire resistance rating where tested as a wall, the corridor walls shall be permitted to terminate at the corridor ceiling.

(4) Lavatories shall not be required to be separated from corridors, provided that they are separated from all other spaces by walls having not less than a 1-hour fire resistance rating in accordance with Section 8.3.

(5) Lavatories shall not be required to be separated from corridors, provided that the building is protected throughout by an approved, supervised automatic sprinkler system in accordance with Section 9.7.

CHAPTER 17 • Existing

less than one door opening directly to the outside or to an exterior exit access balcony or corridor in accordance with 7.5.3.

(2) In buildings protected throughout by an approved automatic sprinkler system with valve supervision in accordance with Section 9.7, corridor walls shall not be required to be rated, provided that such walls form smoke partitions in accordance with Section 8.4.

(3) Where the corridor ceiling is an assembly having a minimum ½-hour fire resistance rating where tested as a wall, the corridor walls shall be permitted to terminate at the corridor ceiling.

(4) Lavatories shall not be required to be separated from corridors, provided that they are separated from all other spaces by walls having a minimum ½-hour fire resistance rating in accordance with Section 8.3.

(5) Lavatories shall not be required to be separated from corridors, provided that the building is protected throughout by an approved, supervised automatic sprinkler system in accordance with Section 9.7.

Given the protection provided by an automatic sprinkler system installed throughout the building, 16/17.3.6(2) permits the corridor walls to be unrated, provided that they form smoke partitions. See Section 8.4 for applicable criteria.

Paragraph 16/17.3.6(3) legitimizes the practice of designing a corridor protection system by building a tunnel with walls and ceilings constructed to meet the requirements of a 1-hour-rated wall assembly for new construction and by providing a ½-hour rating for existing assemblies.

The walls and doors that typically separate a lavatory from the corridor often serve to isolate the lavatory, making it difficult for staff to monitor the lavatory. In recognition of this problem, and given the typically low fuel loads associated with lavatories, 16/17.3.6(4) exempts the wall separating the lavatory from the corridor from the rated construction requirement, provided that the rated corridor wall continuously separates the lavatory from adjacent rooms.

The intent of 16/17.3.6(5) is to combine parts of the concepts addressed in 16/17.3.6(2) and (4). Where the entire building is protected by automatic sprinklers, the lavatory is permitted to be open to the corridor, and the walls separating the lavatory from other rooms do not need to be fire rated but do need to form smoke partitions. The *Code* language does not fully explain this.

In the 2003 and earlier editions of the *Code*, the provisions of 17.3.6, applicable to existing corridors, permitted existing doors in ½-hour fire resistance–rated corridor walls to be 1¾ in. (44 mm) thick solid-bonded wood-core doors or equivalent in lieu of 20-minute fire protection–rated doors. The text was deleted for the 2006 edition because the subject is adequately addressed as a core chapter provision in 8.3.4.4.

## 16.4 Special Provisions

### 16.4.1 Limited Access Buildings and Underground Buildings.

Limited access buildings and underground buildings shall comply with Section 11.7.

## 17.4 Special Provisions

### 17.4.1 Limited Access Buildings and Underground Buildings.

Limited access buildings and underground buildings shall comply with Section 11.7.

CHAPTER 16 • New

### 16.4.2 High-Rise Buildings.

High-rise buildings that house day-care occupancies on floors more than 75 ft (23 m) above the lowest level of fire department vehicle access shall comply with Section 11.8.

Subsection 16/17.4.2 requires compliance with Section 11.8 (i.e., automatic sprinkler, standpipe, alarm and communications, standby power, and emergency command center requirements) where a day-care center is located on a floor above 75 ft (23 m), regardless of whether the center is new or existing.

### 16.4.3 Flexible Plan and Open Plan Buildings.

**16.4.3.1** Flexible plan and open plan buildings shall comply with the requirements of this chapter as modified by 16.4.3.2 through 16.4.3.5.

**16.4.3.2** Flexible plan buildings shall be permitted to have walls and partitions rearranged periodically only if revised plans or diagrams have been approved by the authority having jurisdiction.

**16.4.3.3** Flexible plan buildings shall be evaluated while all folding walls are extended and in use as well as when they are in the retracted position.

**16.4.3.4** Each room occupied by more than 300 persons shall have two or more means of egress entering into separate atmospheres.

**16.4.3.5** Where three or more means of egress are required from a single room, the number of means of egress permitted to enter into a common atmosphere shall not exceed two.

## 16.5 Building Services

### 16.5.1 Utilities.

**16.5.1.1** Utilities shall comply with the provisions of Section 9.1.

**16.5.1.2** Special protective covers for all electrical receptacles shall be installed in all areas occupied by clients.

### 16.5.2 Heating, Ventilating, and Air-Conditioning Equipment.

**16.5.2.1** Heating, ventilating, and air-conditioning equipment shall be in accordance with Section 9.2.

**16.5.2.2** Unvented fuel-fired heating equipment, other than gas space heaters in compliance with NFPA 54/ANSI Z223.1, *National Fuel Gas Code*, shall be prohibited.

CHAPTER 17 • Existing

### 17.4.2 High-Rise Buildings.

High-rise buildings that house day-care occupancies on floors more than 75 ft (23 m) above the lowest level of fire department vehicle access shall comply with Section 11.8.

The requirement of 16/17.4.2 will force careful review when considering the placement of a new day-care center above 75 ft (23 m) in an existing high-rise building. If the building does not already comply with the requirements of Section 11.8, it will need to be brought into compliance.

### 17.4.3 Flexible Plan and Open Plan Buildings.

**17.4.3.1** Flexible plan and open plan buildings shall comply with the requirements of this chapter as modified by 17.4.3.2 and 17.4.3.3.

**17.4.3.2** Flexible plan buildings shall be permitted to have walls and partitions rearranged periodically only if revised plans or diagrams have been approved by the authority having jurisdiction.

**17.4.3.3** Flexible plan buildings shall be evaluated while all folding walls are extended and in use as well as when they are in the retracted position.

## 17.5 Building Services

### 17.5.1 Utilities.

**17.5.1.1** Utilities shall comply with the provisions of Section 9.1.

**17.5.1.2** Special protective covers for all electrical receptacles shall be installed in all areas occupied by clients.

### 17.5.2 Heating, Ventilating, and Air-Conditioning Equipment.

**17.5.2.1** Heating, ventilating, and air-conditioning equipment shall be in accordance with Section 9.2.

**17.5.2.2** Unvented fuel-fired heating equipment, other than gas space heaters in compliance with NFPA 54/ANSI Z223.1, *National Fuel Gas Code,* shall be prohibited.

CHAPTER 16 • New

16.5.2.3 Any heating equipment in spaces occupied by clients shall be provided with partitions, screens, or other means to protect clients from hot surfaces and open flames; if solid partitions are used to provide such protection, provisions shall be made to ensure adequate air for combustion and ventilation for the heating equipment.

### 16.5.3 Elevators, Escalators, and Conveyors.

Elevators, escalators, and conveyors, other than those in day-care homes, shall comply with the provisions of Section 9.4.

### 16.5.4 Rubbish Chutes, Incinerators, and Laundry Chutes.

Rubbish chutes, incinerators, and laundry chutes, other than those in day-care homes, shall comply with the provisions of Section 9.5.

CHAPTER 17 • Existing

17.5.2.3 Any heating equipment in spaces occupied by clients shall be provided with partitions, screens, or other means to protect clients from hot surfaces and open flames; if solid partitions are used to provide such protection, provisions shall be made to ensure adequate air for combustion and ventilation for the heating equipment.

### 17.5.3 Elevators, Escalators, and Conveyors.

Elevators, escalators, and conveyors, other than those in day-care homes, shall comply with the provisions of Section 9.4.

### 17.5.4 Rubbish Chutes, Incinerators, and Laundry Chutes.

Rubbish chutes, incinerators, and laundry chutes, other than those in day-care homes, shall comply with the provisions of Section 9.5.

Paragraph 16/17.5.1.2 requires that protective covers be provided and maintained on all electrical receptacles to avoid serious injuries resulting from clients inserting objects into such receptacles.

The interest of reasonable life safety is not served by permitting the use of unvented fuel-fired equipment in buildings occupied by day-care center clients. Thus, 16/17.5.2.2 prohibits such equipment, with the exception of a special form of gas space heater that can be used safely.

Day-care center clients do not always understand the dangers of hot surfaces; paragraph 16/17.5.2.3 recognizes the importance of providing safeguards to protect clients from the hot surfaces of heating equipment. It is important that such safeguards allow adequate air for combustion, as incomplete or inadequate combustion could cause serious injury or death.

CHAPTER 16 • New

## 16.6 Day-Care Homes

### 16.6.1 General Requirements.

**16.6.1.1 Application.**

**16.6.1.1.1** The requirements of Section 16.6 shall apply to new buildings or portions thereof used as day-care homes. *(See 1.3.1.)*

**16.6.1.1.2** The requirements of Section 16.6 shall apply to day-care homes in which more than 3, but not more than 12, clients receive care, maintenance, and supervision by other than their relative(s) or legal guardian(s) for less than 24 hours per day, generally within a dwelling unit. *(See also 16.6.1.4.)*

CHAPTER 17 • Existing

## 17.6 Day-Care Homes

### 17.6.1 General Requirements.

**17.6.1.1 Application.**

**17.6.1.1.1 Reserved.**

**17.6.1.1.2*** The requirements of Section 17.6 shall apply to existing day-care homes in which more than 3, but not more than 12, clients receive care, maintenance, and supervision by other than their relative(s) or legal guardian(s) for less than 24 hours per day, generally within a dwelling unit. An existing day-care home shall be permitted the option of meeting the requirements of Section 16.6 in lieu of Section 17.6. Any existing day-care home that meets the requirements of Chapter 16 shall be judged as meeting the requirements of this chapter. *(See also 17.6.1.4.)*

CHAPTER 16 • New

16.6.1.1.3 Where a facility houses more than one age group or one self-preservation capability, the strictest requirements applicable to any group present shall apply throughout the day-care home or building, as appropriate to a given area, unless the area housing such a group is maintained as a separate fire area.

16.6.1.1.4 Facilities that supervise clients on a temporary basis with a parent or guardian in close proximity shall not be required to meet the provisions of Section 16.6.

16.6.1.1.5 Places of religious worship shall not be required to meet the provisions of Section 16.6 where operating a day-care home while services are being held in the building.

**16.6.1.2 Multiple Occupancies.** See 16.1.2.

**16.6.1.3 Definitions.** See 16.1.3.

**16.6.1.4 Classification of Occupancy.**

**16.6.1.4.1 Subclassification of Day-Care Homes.** Subclassification of day-care homes shall comply with 16.6.1.4.1.1 and 16.6.1.4.1.2.

**16.6.1.4.1.1 Family Day-Care Home.** A family day-care home shall be a day-care home in which more than three, but fewer than seven, clients receive care, maintenance, and supervision by other than their relative(s) or legal guardian(s) for less than 24 hours per day, generally within a dwelling unit.

**16.6.1.4.1.2 Group Day-Care Home.** A group day-care home shall be a day-care home in which not less than 7, but not more than 12, clients receive care, maintenance, and supervision by other than their relative(s) or legal guardian(s) for less than 24 hours per day, generally within a dwelling unit.

**16.6.1.4.2* Conversions.** A conversion from a day-care home to a day-care occupancy with more than 12 clients shall be permitted only if the day-care occupancy conforms to the requirements of Chapter 16 for new day-care occupancies with more than 12 clients.

A.16.6.1.4.2 A conversion from a day-care occupancy with more than 12 clients to a day-care home is not considered a change of occupancy. The resulting day-care home should be permitted to meet the requirements of Chapter 17 for existing day-care homes.

CHAPTER 17 • Existing

A.17.6.1.1.2 Day-care homes do not provide for the full-time maintenance of a client. Day-care occupancies that provide a primary place of residence are addressed in other day-care occupancy chapters. *(See Chapters 24 through 33.)*

17.6.1.1.3 Where a facility houses clients of more than one self-preservation capability, the strictest requirements applicable to any group present shall apply throughout the day-care home or building, as appropriate to a given area, unless the area housing such a group is maintained as a separate fire area.

17.6.1.1.4 Facilities that supervise clients on a temporary basis with a parent or guardian in close proximity shall not be required to meet the provisions of Section 17.6.

17.6.1.1.5 Places of religious worship shall not be required to meet the provisions of Section 17.6 where operating a day-care home while services are being held in the building.

**17.6.1.2 Multiple Occupancies.** See 17.1.2.

**17.6.1.3 Definitions.** See 17.1.3.

**17.6.1.4 Classification of Occupancy.**

**17.6.1.4.1 Subclassification of Day-Care Homes.** Subclassification of day-care homes shall comply with 17.6.1.4.1.1 and 17.6.1.4.1.2.

**17.6.1.4.1.1 Family Day-Care Home.** A family day-care home shall be a day-care home in which more than three, but fewer than seven, clients receive care, maintenance, and supervision by other than their relative(s) or legal guardian(s) for less than 24 hours per day, generally within a dwelling unit.

**17.6.1.4.1.2 Group Day-Care Home.** A group day-care home shall be a day-care home in which not less than 7, but not more than 12, clients receive care, maintenance, and supervision by other than their relative(s) or legal guardian(s) for less than 24 hours per day, generally within a dwelling unit.

**17.6.1.4.2* Conversions.** A conversion from a day-care home to a day-care occupancy with more than 12 clients shall be permitted only if the day-care occupancy conforms to the requirements of Chapter 16 for new day-care occupancies with more than 12 clients.

A.17.6.1.4.2 A conversion from a day-care occupancy with more than 12 clients to a day-care home is not considered a change of occupancy. The resulting day-care home should be permitted to meet the requirements of Chapter 17 for existing day-care homes.

CHAPTER 16 • New

CHAPTER 17 • Existing

Section 16/17.6 addresses both family day-care homes (4 to 6 clients) and group day-care homes (7 to 12 clients). Where the requirements vary between the two sizes of day-care homes, Section 16/17.6 references the applicable size.

The provisions of Section 16/17.6 recognize that day-care homes are typically located in residential settings. However, a day-care home, whether a family day-care home or a group day-care home, is to be treated via the day-care home requirements of Section 16/17.6 even if it is located in a nonresidential setting, such as an office building.

Day-care homes and group day-care homes are often found in buildings primarily composed of apartment, mercantile, business, or assembly occupancies. Where a day-care home is located in a building housing another occupancy, the operators of the day-care home usually have no control over the safety procedures and precautions practiced outside the day-care home. Thus, 6.1.14.1.3 does not permit a day-care home with four or more clients to be considered incidental to another occupancy. This means that the day-care home provisions of the *Code* must be followed, because the provisions applicable to the predominant occupancy might not be adequate to protect the day-care home clients.

**16.6.1.5 Classification of Hazard of Contents.** See 16.1.5.

**16.6.1.6 Location and Construction.** No day-care home shall be located more than one story below the level of exit discharge.

**16.6.1.7 Occupant Load.**

**16.6.1.7.1** In family day-care homes, the following shall apply:

(1) The minimum staff-to-client ratio shall be not less than one staff for up to six clients, including the caretaker's own children under age six.
(2) There shall be not more than two clients incapable of self-preservation.

**16.6.1.7.2** In group day-care homes, the following shall apply:

(1) The minimum staff-to-client ratio shall be not less than two staff for up to 12 clients.
(2) There shall be not more than 3 clients incapable of self-preservation.
(3) The staff-to-client ratio shall be permitted to be modified by the authority having jurisdiction where safeguards in addition to those specified by Section 16.6 are provided.

### 16.6.2 Means of Escape Requirements.

**16.6.2.1 General.** Means of escape shall comply with Section 24.2.

**16.6.2.2 Reserved.**

**16.6.2.3 Reserved.**

**16.6.2.4 Number of Means of Escape.** The number of means of escape shall comply with Section 24.2 and 16.6.2.4.1 through 16.6.2.4.4.

**17.6.1.5 Classification of Hazard of Contents.** See 17.1.5.

**17.6.1.6 Location and Construction.** No day-care home shall be located more than one story below the level of exit discharge.

**17.6.1.7 Occupant Load.**

**17.6.1.7.1** In family day-care homes, the following shall apply:

(1) The minimum staff-to-client ratio shall be not less than one staff for up to six clients, including the caretaker's own children under age six.
(2) There shall be not more than two clients incapable of self-preservation.

**17.6.1.7.2** In group day-care homes, the following shall apply:

(1) The minimum staff-to-client ratio shall be not less than two staff for up to 12 clients.
(2) There shall be not more than 3 clients incapable of self-preservation.
(3) The staff-to-client ratio shall be permitted to be modified by the authority having jurisdiction where safeguards in addition to those specified by Section 17.6 are provided.

### 17.6.2 Means of Escape Requirements.

**17.6.2.1 General.** Means of escape shall comply with Section 24.2.

**17.6.2.2 Reserved.**

**17.6.2.3 Reserved.**

**17.6.2.4 Number of Means of Escape.** The number of means of escape shall comply with Section 24.2 and 17.6.2.4.1 through 17.6.2.4.4.

CHAPTER 16 • New

**16.6.2.4.1** In group day-care homes, every story occupied by clients shall have not less than two remotely located means of escape.

**16.6.2.4.2** Every room used for sleeping, living, or dining purposes shall comply with the following:

(1) There shall be not less than two means of escape, not less than one of which shall be a door or stairway providing a means of unobstructed travel to the outside of the building at street or the finished ground level.
(2) The second means of escape shall be permitted to be a window in accordance with 16.2.11.1.
(3) No room or space that is accessible only by a ladder or folding stairs or through a trap door shall be occupied for living or sleeping purposes.

**16.6.2.4.3** In group day-care homes where spaces on the story above the level of exit discharge are used by clients, not less than one means of escape shall be an exit discharging directly to the outside, and the second means of escape shall be permitted to be a window in accordance with 16.2.11.1.

**16.6.2.4.4** Where clients occupy a story below the level of exit discharge, not less than one means of escape shall be an exit discharging directly to the outside, the vertical travel to the finished ground level shall not exceed 8 ft (2440 mm), and the second means of escape shall be permitted to be a window in accordance with 16.2.11.1.

CHAPTER 17 • Existing

**17.6.2.4.1** In group day-care homes, every story occupied by clients shall have not less than two remotely located means of escape.

**17.6.2.4.2** Every room used for sleeping, living, or dining purposes shall comply with the following:

(1) There shall be not less than two means of escape, not less than one of which shall be a door or stairway providing a means of unobstructed travel to the outside of the building at street or the finished ground level.
(2) The second means of escape shall be permitted to be a window in accordance with 17.2.11.1.
(3) No room or space that is accessible only by a ladder or folding stairs or through a trap door shall be occupied for living or sleeping purposes.

**17.6.2.4.3** In group day-care homes where spaces on the story above the level of exit discharge are used by clients, not less than one means of escape shall be an exit discharging directly to the outside, and the second means of escape shall be permitted to be a window in accordance with 17.2.11.1.

**17.6.2.4.4** Where clients occupy a story below the level of exit discharge, not less than one means of escape shall be an exit discharging directly to the outside, the vertical travel to the finished ground level shall not exceed 8 ft (2440 mm), and the second means of escape shall be permitted to be a window in accordance with 17.2.11.1.

The concept of means of escape is well developed in Chapter 24 for one- and two-family dwellings. However, 16/17.6.2.4.3 and 16/17.6.2.4.4 require the primary means of escape to discharge directly to the outside if day-care home clients occupy the second story or basement.

If an open stair serves the second story of a typical single-family dwelling, the requirement of 16/17.6.2.4.3 mandates that the second story is to be served by an enclosed exit stair or an exterior stair (not a fire escape) if clients are occupying the second story. See also 16/17.6.3.1.

The requirement of 16/17.6.2.4.4 is similar to that of 16/17.6.2.4.3 for a second story and mandates that, where clients are below the level of exit discharge, at least one true exit is to be provided. In addition, per the requirements of 16/17.6.3.1, any stairway to the first floor requires a minimum 20-minute fire protection–rated door as a separation between the stair and the first floor.

As illustrated in Exhibit 16/17.8, where a group day-care home is located in a basement, an exit is required that opens directly to the outside, with vertical travel to the ground level not exceeding 8 ft (2440 mm). If a stairway to the story above were provided, it would have to be cut off from the basement by a fire barrier containing a door with a fire protection rating of at least 20 minutes. This separation is required at the top or bottom of the stair, but not at both. See also 16/17.6.3.1.

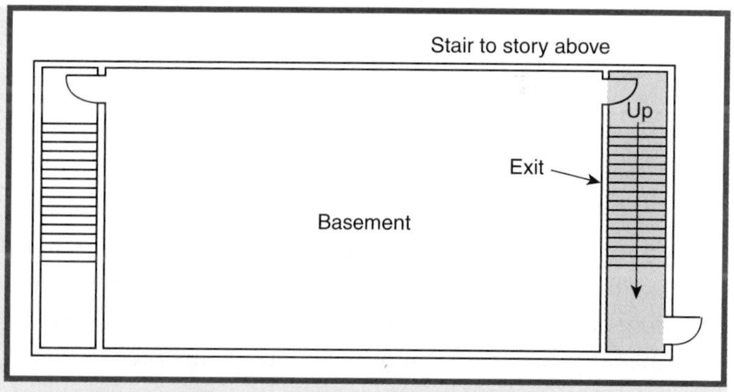


***Exhibit 16/17.8*** *Egress requirements for group day-care home occupying basement.*

**CHAPTER 16 • New**

**16.6.2.5 Arrangement of Means of Escape.**

**16.6.2.5.1** A story used above or below the level of exit discharge shall be in accordance with 16.6.2.4.3 and 16.6.2.4.4.

**16.6.2.5.2** For group day-care homes, means of escape shall be arranged in accordance with Section 7.5.

**16.6.2.5.3** No dead-end corridors shall exceed 20 ft (6100 mm).

**16.6.2.5.4** Doors in means of escape shall be protected from obstructions, including snow and ice.

**CHAPTER 17 • Existing**

**17.6.2.5 Arrangement of Means of Escape.**

**17.6.2.5.1** A story used above or below the level of exit discharge shall be in accordance with 17.6.2.4.3 or 17.6.2.4.4.

**17.6.2.5.2** For group day-care homes, means of escape shall be arranged in accordance with Section 7.5.

**17.6.2.5.3** No dead-end corridor shall exceed 20 ft (6100 mm), other than in buildings protected throughout by an approved, supervised automatic sprinkler system in accordance with Section 9.7, in which case dead-end corridors shall not exceed 50 ft (15 m).

**17.6.2.5.4** Doors in means of escape shall be protected from obstructions, including snow and ice.

Since the 2006 edition of the *Code*, the title of 16/17.6.2.5 and its provisions have reflected that day-care homes are required to be provided with means of escape, not means of egress. The provision of 16/17.6.2.5.4 is presented for completeness, because the means of egress provisions of Chapter 7 related to maintaining the egress path free of obstructions, including snow and ice, do not automatically apply to means of escape.

**CHAPTER 16 • New**

**16.6.2.6 Travel Distance.** Travel distance shall comply with 16.6.2.6.1 through 16.6.2.6.3.

**16.6.2.6.1** Travel distance shall be measured in accordance with Section 7.6.

**16.6.2.6.2** Travel distance shall meet the following criteria, unless otherwise permitted by 16.6.2.6.3:

(1) The travel distance between any room door intended as an exit access and an exit shall not exceed 100 ft (30 m).
(2) The travel distance between any point in a room and an exit shall not exceed 150 ft (46 m).
(3) The travel distance between any point in a sleeping room and an exit access to that room shall not exceed 50 ft (15 m).

**16.6.2.6.3** The travel distance required by 16.6.2.6.2(1) and (2) shall be permitted to be increased by 50 ft (15 m) in buildings protected throughout by an approved, supervised automatic sprinkler system in accordance with Section 9.7.

**16.6.2.7 Discharge from Exits.** See 16.6.2.4.

**16.6.2.8 Illumination of Means of Egress.** Means of egress shall be illuminated in accordance with Section 7.8.

**16.6.2.9 Emergency Lighting.** (No requirements.)

**16.6.2.10 Marking of Means of Egress.** (No requirements.)

### 16.6.3 Protection.

**16.6.3.1 Protection of Vertical Openings.**

**16.6.3.1.1** For group day-care homes, the doorway between the level of exit discharge and any story below shall be

**CHAPTER 17 • Existing**

**17.6.2.6 Travel Distance.** Travel distance shall comply with 17.6.2.6.1 through 17.6.2.6.3.

**17.6.2.6.1** Travel distance shall be measured in accordance with Section 7.6.

**17.6.2.6.2** Travel distance shall meet the following criteria, unless otherwise permitted by 17.6.2.6.3:

(1) The travel distance between any room door intended as an exit access and an exit shall not exceed 100 ft (30 m).
(2) The travel distance between any point in a room and an exit shall not exceed 150 ft (46 m).
(3) The travel distance between any point in a sleeping room and an exit access to that room shall not exceed 50 ft (15 m).

**17.6.2.6.3** The travel distance required by 17.6.2.6.2(1) and (2) shall be permitted to be increased by 50 ft (15 m) in buildings protected throughout by an approved, supervised automatic sprinkler system in accordance with Section 9.7.

**17.6.2.7 Discharge from Exits.** See 17.6.2.4.

**17.6.2.8 Illumination of Means of Egress.** Means of egress shall be illuminated in accordance with Section 7.8.

**17.6.2.9 Emergency Lighting.** (No requirements.)

**17.6.2.10 Marking of Means of Egress.** (No requirements.)

### 17.6.3 Protection.

**17.6.3.1 Protection of Vertical Openings.**

**17.6.3.1.1** For group day-care homes, the doorway between the level of exit discharge and any story below shall be

CHAPTER 16 • New

equipped with a fire door assembly having a 20-minute fire protection rating.

**16.6.3.1.2** Where the story above the level of exit discharge is used for sleeping purposes, there shall be a fire door assembly having a 20-minute fire protection rating at the top or bottom of each stairway.

**16.6.3.2 Protection from Hazards.**

**16.6.3.2.1 Alcohol-Based Hand-Rub Dispensers.** Alcohol-based hand-rub dispensers shall be protected in accordance with 8.7.3, unless all of the following conditions are met:

(1) Dispensers shall be installed in rooms or spaces separated from corridors and exits.
(2) The maximum individual dispenser fluid capacity shall be as follows:
   (a) 0.32 gal (1.2 L) for dispensers in rooms
   (b) 0.53 gal (2.0 L) for dispensers in suites of rooms
(3) Dispensers shall be separated from each other by horizontal spacing of not less than 48 in. (1220 mm).
(4) Storage of quantities greater than 5 gal (18.9 L) in a single fire compartment shall meet the requirements of NFPA 30, *Flammable and Combustible Liquids Code*.
(5) Dispensers shall not be installed over or directly adjacent to an ignition source.
(6) Dispensers installed directly over carpeted floors shall be permitted only in sprinklered rooms or spaces.

CHAPTER 17 • Existing

equipped with a fire door assembly having a 20-minute fire protection rating.

**17.6.3.1.2** Where the story above the level of exit discharge is used for sleeping purposes, there shall be a fire door assembly having a 20-minute fire protection rating at the top or bottom of each stairway, unless otherwise permitted by 17.6.3.1.3.

**17.6.3.1.3** Approved existing self-closing $1^3/_4$ in. (44 mm) thick, solid-bonded wood doors without rated frames shall be permitted to continue in use.

**17.6.3.2 Protection from Hazards.**

**17.6.3.2.1 Alcohol-Based Hand-Rub Dispensers.** Alcohol-based hand-rub dispensers shall be protected in accordance with 8.7.3, unless all of the following conditions are met:

(1) Dispensers shall be installed in rooms or spaces separated from corridors and exits.
(2) The maximum individual dispenser fluid capacity shall be as follows:
   (a) 0.32 gal (1.2 L) for dispensers in rooms
   (b) 0.53 gal (2.0 L) for dispensers in suites of rooms
(3) Dispensers shall be separated from each other by horizontal spacing of not less than 48 in. (1220 mm).
(4) Storage of quantities greater than 5 gal (18.9 L) in a single fire compartment shall meet the requirements of NFPA 30, *Flammable and Combustible Liquids Code*.
(5) Dispensers shall not be installed over or directly adjacent to an ignition source.
(6) Dispensers installed directly over carpeted floors shall be permitted only in sprinklered rooms or spaces.

See the last paragraph of the commentary following 16/17.3.2.6(6).

CHAPTER 16 • New

**16.6.3.2.2 Reserved.**

**16.6.3.3 Interior Finish.**

**16.6.3.3.1 General.** Interior finish shall be in accordance with Section 10.2.

**16.6.3.3.2 Interior Wall and Ceiling Finish.**

**16.6.3.3.2.1** Interior wall and ceiling finish materials complying with Section 10.2 shall be Class A or Class B in corridors, stairways, lobbies, and exits. In the exits of family day-care homes, interior wall and ceiling finish materials in accordance with Section 10.2 shall be Class A or Class B.

CHAPTER 17 • Existing

**17.6.3.2.2 Reserved.**

**17.6.3.3 Interior Finish.**

**17.6.3.3.1 General.** Interior finish shall be in accordance with Section 10.2.

**17.6.3.3.2 Interior Wall and Ceiling Finish.**

**17.6.3.3.2.1** Interior wall and ceiling finish materials complying with Section 10.2 shall be Class A or Class B in exits.

CHAPTER 16 • New

**16.6.3.3.2.2** Interior wall and ceiling finish materials complying with Section 10.2 shall be Class A, Class B, or Class C in occupied spaces.

**16.6.3.3.3 Interior Floor Finish.**

**16.6.3.3.3.1** Interior floor finish shall comply with Section 10.2.

**16.6.3.3.3.2** Interior floor finish in exit enclosures shall be not less than Class II.

**16.6.3.3.3.3** Interior floor finish shall comply with 10.2.7.1 or 10.2.7.2, as applicable.

**16.6.3.4 Detection, Alarm, and Communications Systems.**

**16.6.3.4.1** Smoke alarms shall be installed within day-care homes in accordance with 9.6.2.10.

**16.6.3.4.2** Where a day-care home is located within a building of another occupancy, such as in an apartment building or office building, any corridors serving the day-care home shall be provided with a smoke detection system in accordance with Section 9.6.

**16.6.3.4.3** Single-station or multiple-station smoke alarms or smoke detectors shall be provided in all rooms used for sleeping in accordance with 9.6.2.10.

CHAPTER 17 • Existing

**17.6.3.3.2.2** Interior wall and ceiling finish materials complying with Section 10.2 shall be Class A, Class B, or Class C in occupied spaces.

**17.6.3.3.3 Interior Floor Finish.** (No requirements.)

**17.6.3.4 Detection, Alarm, and Communications Systems.**

**17.6.3.4.1** Smoke alarms shall be installed within day-care homes in accordance with 9.6.2.10.

**17.6.3.4.2** Where a day-care home is located within a building of another occupancy, such as in an apartment building or office building, any corridors serving the day-care home shall be provided with a smoke detection system in accordance with Section 9.6.

**17.6.3.4.3** Single-station or multiple-station smoke alarms or smoke detectors shall be provided in all rooms used for sleeping in accordance with 9.6.2.10, other than as permitted by 17.6.3.4.4.

**17.6.3.4.4** Approved existing battery-powered smoke alarms, rather than house electrical service–powered smoke alarms required by 17.6.3.4.3, shall be permitted where the facility has testing, maintenance, and battery replacement programs that ensure reliability of power to the smoke alarms.

The provisions of 16/17.6.3.4 are as follows:

1. To provide smoke alarms within the day-care home
2. To provide a smoke detection system in the corridor serving the day-care home in a building of mixed occupancy
3. To require that smoke alarms or smoke detectors be installed in each sleeping room

**16.6.3.5 Extinguishment Requirements.** Any required sprinkler systems shall be in accordance with Section 9.7 and shall be installed in accordance with 9.7.1.1(1), (2), or (3), as appropriate with respect to the scope of the installation standard.

## 16.7 Operating Features

Section 16/17.7 is positioned to follow the provisions of Section 16/17.6, applicable to day-care homes, but has applicability both to day-care occupancies and day-care homes, unless otherwise specified. For example, the provisions of 16/17.7.4.1, applicable to limiting the flame propagation of draperies and curtains, is a requirement for day-care occupancies only, not day-care homes. See 16/17.1.1.3 and 16/17.7.4.1.

dance with Section 9.6.

**17.6.3.4.3** Single-station or multiple-station smoke alarms or smoke detectors shall be provided in all rooms used for sleeping in accordance with 9.6.2.10, other than as permitted by 17.6.3.4.4.

**17.6.3.4.4** Approved existing battery-powered smoke alarms, rather than house electrical service–powered smoke alarms required by 17.6.3.4.3, shall be permitted where the facility has testing, maintenance, and battery replacement programs

CHAPTER 16 • New

16.7.1* Emergency Plans.

Emergency plans shall be provided in accordance with Section 4.8.

**A.16.7.1** The requirements are, of necessity, general in scope, because it is recognized that they apply to all types of day-care occupancies as well as conditions of occupancies, such as truant day-care occupancies; occupancies for the mentally handicapped, vision impaired, hearing impaired, and speech impaired; adult day-care; care of infants; and day-care occupancies. It is fully recognized that no one code can meet all the conditions of the various buildings involved, and it will be necessary for site administrators, through the written fire emergency response plan, to issue supplements to these requirements; however, all supplements should be consistent with these requirements. Additionally, it is recommended that fire safety be a part of the educational programs of the occupancy for clients.

Fire emergency response plans need to be written and made available to all employees, including temporary or substitute staff, so that all employees know what is expected of them during a fire emergency. The elements needed in the written plan should be identified in coordination with the authority having jurisdiction.

The facility fire emergency response plan might be a module of a facility disaster plan that covers other emergencies.

The proper safeguarding of clients during a fire emergency requires prompt and effective response by the facility employees in accordance with the fire emergency response plan. Duties covered under the plan should be assigned by position rather than by employee name. Such assignment ensures that, in the absence of an employee, the duties of the position will be performed by a substitute or temporary employee assigned to the position. Temporary or substitute employees should be instructed in advance regarding their duties under the plan for the position to which they are assigned.

Written fire emergency response plans should include, but should not be limited to, information for employees regarding methods and devices available for alerting occupants of a fire emergency. Employees should know how the fire department is to be alerted. Even where automatic systems are expected to alert the fire department, the written plan should provide for backup alerting procedures by staff. Other responses of employees to a fire emergency should include the following:

(1) Removal of clients in immediate danger to areas of safety, as set forth in the plan
(2) Methods of using building features to confine the fire and its byproducts to the room or area of origin

CHAPTER 17 • Existing

17.7.1* Emergency Plans.

Emergency plans shall be provided in accordance with Section 4.8.

**A.17.7.1** The requirements are, of necessity, general in scope, because it is recognized that they apply to all types of day-care occupancies as well as conditions of occupancies, such as truant day-care occupancies; occupancies for the mentally handicapped, vision impaired, hearing impaired, and speech impaired; adult day-care; care of infants; and day-care occupancies. It is fully recognized that no one code can meet all the conditions of the various buildings involved, and it will be necessary for site administrators, through the written fire emergency response plan, to issue supplements to these requirements; however, all supplements should be consistent with these requirements. Additionally, it is recommended that fire safety be a part of the educational programs of the occupancy for clients.

Fire emergency response plans need to be written and made available to all employees, including temporary or substitute staff, so that all employees know what is expected of them during a fire emergency. The elements needed in the written plan should be identified in coordination with the authority having jurisdiction.

The facility fire emergency response plan might be a module of a facility disaster plan that covers other emergencies.

The proper safeguarding of clients during a fire emergency requires prompt and effective response by the facility employees in accordance with the fire emergency response plan. Duties covered under the plan should be assigned by position rather than by employee name. Such assignment ensures that, in the absence of an employee, the duties of the position will be performed by a substitute or temporary employee assigned to the position. Temporary or substitute employees should be instructed in advance regarding their duties under the plan for the position to which they are assigned.

Written fire emergency response plans should include, but should not be limited to, information for employees about methods and devices available for alerting occupants of a fire emergency. Employees should know how the fire department is to be alerted. Even where automatic systems are expected to alert the fire department, the written plan should provide for backup alerting procedures by staff. Other responses of employees to a fire emergency should include the following:

(1) Removal of clients in immediate danger to areas of safety, as set forth in the plan
(2) Methods of using building features to confine the fire and its byproducts to the room or area of origin

(3) Control of actions and behaviors of clients during removal or evacuation activities and at predetermined safe assembly areas

The written plan should state clearly the facility policy regarding the actions staff are to take or not take to extinguish a fire. It should also incorporate the emergency egress and relocation drill procedures set forth in 16.7.2.

For additional guidance on emergency plans, see NFPA 1600, *Standard on Disaster/Emergency Management and Business Continuity Programs*. This standard establishes a common set of criteria for disaster management, emergency management, and business continuity programs.

### 16.7.2 Emergency Egress and Relocation Drills.

**16.7.2.1*** Emergency egress and relocation drills shall be conducted in accordance with Section 4.7 and the applicable provisions of 16.7.2.2.

**A.16.7.2.1** The requirements are, of necessity, general in scope, because it is recognized that they apply to all types of day-care occupancies as well as conditions of occupancies, such as truant day-care occupancies; day-care occupancies for the mentally handicapped, vision impaired, hearing impaired, and speech impaired. It is fully recognized that no one code can meet all the conditions of the various buildings involved, and it will be necessary for site administrators to issue supplements to these requirements, but all supplements should be consistent with these requirements.

**16.7.2.2** Emergency egress and relocation drills shall be conducted as follows:

(1) Not less than one emergency egress and relocation drill shall be conducted every month the facility is in session, unless both of the following criteria are met:
   (a) In climates where the weather is severe, the monthly emergency egress and relocation drills shall be permitted to be deferred.
   (b) The required number of emergency egress and relocation drills shall be conducted, and not less than four shall be conducted before the drills are deferred.
(2) All occupants of the building shall participate in the drill.
(3) One additional emergency egress and relocation drill, other than for day-care occupancies that are open on a year-round basis, shall be required within the first 30 days of operation.



(3) Control of actions and behaviors of clients during removal or evacuation activities and at predetermined safe assembly areas

The written plan should state clearly the facility policy regarding the actions staff are to take or not take to extinguish a fire. It should also incorporate the emergency egress and relocation drill procedures set forth in 17.7.2.

For additional guidance on emergency plans, see NFPA 1600, *Standard on Disaster/Emergency Management and Business Continuity Programs*. This standard establishes a common set of criteria for disaster management, emergency management, and business continuity programs.

### 17.7.2 Emergency Egress and Relocation Drills.

**17.7.2.1*** Emergency egress and relocation drills shall be conducted in accordance with Section 4.7 and the applicable provisions of 17.7.2.2.

**A.17.7.2.1** The requirements are, of necessity, general in scope, because it is recognized that they apply to all types of day-care occupancies as well as conditions of occupancies, such as truant day-care occupancies; day-care occupancies for the mentally handicapped, vision impaired, hearing impaired, and speech impaired. It is fully recognized that no one code can meet all the conditions of the various buildings involved, and it will be necessary for site administrators to issue supplements to these requirements, but all supplements should be consistent with these requirements.

**17.7.2.2** Emergency egress and relocation drills shall be conducted as follows:

(1) Not less than one emergency egress and relocation drill shall be conducted every month the facility is in session, unless both of the following criteria are met:
   (a) In climates where the weather is severe, the monthly emergency egress and relocation drills shall be permitted to be deferred.
   (b) The required number of emergency egress and relocation drills shall be conducted, and not less than four shall be conducted before the drills are deferred.
(2) All occupants of the building shall participate in the drill.
(3) One additional emergency egress and relocation drill, other than for day-care occupancies that are open on a year-round basis, shall be required within the first 30 days of operation.

Emergency egress drills for day-care occupancies are essential to ensure an orderly response of staff and clients during a fire. The fire department and the day-care facility should vary the timing and arrangement of the drills but not the required response, which is orderly evacuation. See also Section 4.7.

CHAPTER 16 • New

### 16.7.3 Inspections.

**16.7.3.1** Fire prevention inspections shall be conducted monthly by a trained senior member of the staff, after which a copy of the latest inspection report shall be posted in a conspicuous place in the day-care facility.

**16.7.3.2*** It shall be the duty of site administrators and staff members to inspect all exit facilities daily to ensure that all stairways, doors, and other exits are in proper condition.

**A.16.7.3.2** Particular attention should be given to keeping all doors unlocked; keeping doors that serve to protect the safety of paths of egress closed and under no conditions blocked open, such as doors on stairway enclosures; keeping outside stairs and fire escape stairs free from all obstructions and clear of snow and ice; and allowing no accumulation of snow or ice or materials of any kind outside exit doors that might prevent the opening of the door or interfere with rapid escape from the building.

**16.7.3.3** Open plan buildings shall require extra surveillance to ensure that exit paths are maintained clear of obstruction and are obvious.

**16.7.3.4 Inspection of Door Openings.** Door openings shall be inspected in accordance with 7.2.1.15.

CHAPTER 17 • Existing

### 17.7.3 Inspections.

**17.7.3.1** Fire prevention inspections shall be conducted monthly by a trained senior member of the staff, after which a copy of the latest inspection report shall be posted in a conspicuous place in the day-care facility.

**17.7.3.2*** It shall be the duty of site administrators and staff members to inspect all exit facilities daily to ensure that all stairways, doors, and other exits are in proper condition.

**A.17.7.3.2** Particular attention should be given to keeping all doors unlocked; keeping doors that serve to protect the safety of paths of egress closed and under no conditions blocked open, such as doors on stairway enclosures; keeping outside stairs and fire escape stairs free from all obstructions and clear of snow and ice; and allowing no accumulation of snow or ice or materials of any kind outside exit doors that might prevent the opening of the door or interfere with rapid escape from the building.

**17.7.3.3** Open plan buildings shall require extra surveillance to ensure that exit paths are maintained clear of obstruction and are obvious.

**17.7.3.4 Inspection of Door Openings.** Door openings shall be inspected in accordance with 7.2.1.15.

Compliance with the requirement of 16/17.7.3.2 for daily inspection of the egress system has benefits that far outweigh the time and resources required to conduct such inspections. Staff members are permitted to conduct such inspections. Staff members typically are well acquainted with the building features and operations of the facility.

The provision of 16/17.7.3.4 for the inspection of door openings is new to the 2009 edition of the *Code*. The criteria of 7.2.1.15 are formatted to apply only where specifically required by another portion of the *Code*. The inspection requirements apply to doors that are required to swing in the direction of egress travel. Door leaves that are required to swing in the direction of egress travel include those from spaces with an occupant load of 50 or more persons [see 7.2.1.4.2(1)] and those used in an exit enclosure [see 7.2.1.4.2(2)]. This application threshold was chosen to help ensure that the egress doors used most frequently on a normal day-to-day basis and those designed to accommodate larger numbers of occupants under emergency egress or relocation are inspected and tested. Door leaves that get used frequently are more apt to experience wear that adversely affects operability and leads to failure. Doors leaves that are infrequently used, such as those into exit stair enclosures in high-rise buildings, might be misaligned within their frames so as to be difficult to open within the operating forces requirements of 7.2.1.4.5. The door inspection and testing criteria of 7.2.1.15 are intended to help identify problems with door openings and ensure that such problems are remedied. See 7.2.1.15.

### 16.7.4 Furnishings and Decorations.

**16.7.4.1** Draperies, curtains, and other similar furnishings and decorations in day-care occupancies shall be in accordance with the provisions of 10.3.1.

**16.7.4.2** Clothing and personal effects shall not be stored in corridors, unless otherwise permitted by the following:

(1) This requirement shall not apply to corridors protected by an automatic sprinkler system in accordance with Section 9.7.

a copy of the latest inspection report shall be posted in a conspicuous place in the day-care facility.

**17.7.3.2*** It shall be the duty of site administrators and staff members to inspect all exit facilities daily to ensure that all stairways, doors, and other exits are in proper condition.

**A.17.7.3.2** Particular attention should be given to keeping all doors unlocked; keeping doors that serve to protect the safety of paths of egress closed and under no conditions blocked open, such as doors on stairway enclosures; keeping outside stairs and fire escape stairs free from all obstructions

CHAPTER 16 • New

(2) This requirement shall not apply to corridor areas protected by a smoke detection system in accordance with Section 9.6.
(3) This requirement shall not apply to storage in metal lockers, provided that the required egress width is maintained.

CHAPTER 17 • Existing

(2) This requirement shall not apply to corridor areas protected by a smoke detection system in accordance with Section 9.6.
(3) This requirement shall not apply to storage in metal lockers, provided that the required egress width is maintained.

Clothing hung on hooks along corridor walls greatly increases the combustible load and will generally allow flame to spread quickly. Because Chapters 16 and 17 regulate the interior wall finish for corridors and lobbies, surfaces covered by combustible clothing that would allow flame to spread more quickly than is permitted by wall surfaces should not be created. The three provisions of 16/17.7.4.2 (control of fire by sprinklers, early warning of incipient stage fire via smoke detection, or isolating fuel packages by locating the clothing in metal lockers) help to mitigate the potential for a clothing fire to render the exit access unusable.

**16.7.4.3** Artwork and teaching materials shall be permitted to be attached directly to the walls in accordance with the following:

(1) The artwork and teaching materials shall not exceed 20 percent of the wall area in a building that is not protected throughout by an approved, supervised automatic sprinkler system in accordance with Section 9.7.
(2) The artwork and teaching materials shall not exceed 50 percent of the wall area in a building that is protected throughout by an approved, supervised automatic sprinkler system in accordance with Section 9.7.

lance to ensure that exit paths are maintained clear of obstruction and are obvious.

**17.7.3.4 Inspection of Door Openings.** Door openings shall be inspected in accordance with 7.2.1.15.

### 17.7.4 Furnishings and Decorations.

**17.7.4.1** Draperies, curtains, and other similar furnishings and decorations in day-care occupancies shall be in accordance with the provisions of 10.3.1.

**17.7.4.2** Clothing and personal effects shall not be stored in

It is advantageous not only to limit the quantity of artwork displayed but also to avoid placing such materials near a room's exit access doors. Because the combustibility of the artwork cannot be effectively controlled, the quantity, in terms of the percentage of wall area covered, is regulated to avoid creating a continuous combustible surface that will spread flame across the room. If the building is protected throughout by automatic sprinklers, the percentage of wall area permitted to be covered with artwork and teaching materials is increased to 50 percent.

**16.7.4.4** The provision of 10.3.2 for cigarette ignition resistance of newly introduced upholstered furniture and mattresses shall not apply to day-care homes.

corridors, unless otherwise permitted by the following:

(1) This requirement shall not apply to corridors protected by an automatic sprinkler system in accordance with

The format of 10.3.2 was changed for the 2006 edition of the *Code* from a menu-like item requiring adoption by an occupancy chapter to an outright mandate. Paragraph 10.3.2 requires smoldering ignition resistance for newly introduced upholstered furniture and mattresses, unless otherwise modified by an occupancy chapter. Paragraph 16/17.7.4.4 clarifies that furniture and mattresses in day-care homes (i.e., 4 to 12 clients), but not day-care occupancies (i.e., more than 12 clients), are exempted from fire testing for smoldering ignition resistance.

### 16.7.5* Day-Care Staff.

Adequate adult staff shall be on duty in the facility and alert at all times where clients are present.

**A.16.7.5** It is the intent that the requirement for adequate adult staff to be awake at all times when clients are present

Section 9.7.
(2) This requirement shall not apply to corridor areas protected by a smoke detection system in accordance with Section 9.6.
(3) This requirement shall not apply to storage in metal lockers, provided that the required egress width is main-

CHAPTER 16 • New

be applied to family day-care and group day-care homes that are operated at night, as well as day-care occupancies.

It is beyond the scope of the *Code* to specify a minimum staff-to-client ratio, but 16/17.7.5 clearly requires that adequate adult staff be on duty and alert in the facility at all times when clients are present. The mandatory language of 16/17.7.5 mandates that staff be on duty and alert; the text of A.16/A.17.7.5 clarifies that, in order to be alert, staff must be awake. The overall protection package of Chapters 16 and 17 relies heavily on staff action. The staff-to-client ratios on which the other provisions of the chapter were developed are summarized in A.16/A.17.1.1.

CHAPTER 17 • Existing

tained.

**17.7.4.3** Artwork and teaching materials shall be permitted to be attached directly to the walls in accordance with the following:

(1) The artwork and teaching materials shall not exceed 20 percent of the wall area in a building that is not protected throughout by an approved automatic sprinkler system in accordance with Section 9.7.
(2) The artwork and teaching materials shall not exceed 50 percent of the wall area in a building that is protected throughout by an approved automatic sprinkler system in accordance with Section 9.7.

**17.7.4.4** The provision of 10.3.2 for cigarette ignition resistance of newly introduced upholstered furniture and mattresses shall not apply to day-care homes.

### 17.7.5* Day-Care Staff.

Adequate adult staff shall be on duty in the facility and alert at all times where clients are present.

**A.17.7.5** It is the intent that the requirement for adequate adult staff to be awake at all times when clients are present be applied to family day-care and group day-care homes that are operated at night, as well as day-care occupancies.

CHAPTERS 18 AND 19

# New and Existing Health Care Occupancies

Life safety in health care occupancies is so encompassing that it includes nearly the entire gamut of systems, options, and features addressed in the core chapters. Unlike most other buildings and use groups addressed by the *Code*, the least desirable emergency action in a health care occupancy is the wholesale relocation or evacuation of patients. For this reason, a "defend-in-place" strategy is used.

The defend-in-place strategy is implemented using a "total concept" approach. As detailed in 18/19.1.1.3, the total concept approach provides an assortment of features that are deemed necessary to avoid the movement of patients to the outside during a fire. Of course, those patients who might be perilously close to the effects of the fire are given a range of protection features, such as being moved to an adjacent smoke compartment on the same floor.

Requirements for allowable building construction types, sprinklers, alarm and detection systems, and staff training work in harmony to help ensure that a patient can be safely and adequately protected, regardless of where a fire starts.

Chapters 18 and 19 also address provisions under which doors are permitted to be locked. Examples of conditions that might justify door locking for the protection of patients or the public are provided in A.18/A.19.1.1.1.5. The criteria of the exemptions are detailed within the door provisions of 18/19.2.2.2.

Staff action is an integral part of the life safety features required in a health care facility. The proper response from staff in terms of availability, actions, and management of a fire can readily influence the outcome of a fire. Health care facility staff are charged with the responsibility of preserving the safety of their charges, whether that involves informing patients who are not in jeopardy from the fire or helping to relocate those who are.

Staff training, coupled with the traditional built-in systems and features (e.g., construction; compartmentation; interior finish; alarm, detection, and sprinkler systems; and control of contents and furnishings), provides one of the safest environments for one of the most vulnerable population groups addressed by the *Code*.

## 18.1 General Requirements

Chapters 18 and 19 cover the requirements for health care occupancies. Prior to the 1976 edition of the *Code*, these occupancies were grouped with penal facilities (currently addressed by Chapters 22 and 23) and were known as "institutional occupancies."

Health care occupancies are those facilities used on an inpatient basis for the medical care or treatment of four or more persons suffering from physical or mental illness, disease, or infirmity, and for the care of infants, convalescents, or infirm aged persons.

## 19.1 General Requirements

The health care occupancies addressed in Chapters 18 and 19 include the following:

1. Hospitals
2. Nursing homes
3. Limited care facilities

Hospitals, nursing homes, and limited care facilities provide sleeping facilities for occupants incapable of self-preservation due to age, physical or mental disabilities, or security measures not under their control.

Ambulatory health care facilities differ from health care occupancies in that they provide health care services on an outpatient basis; they are addressed separately in Chapters 20 and 21.

**18.1.1 Application.**

**18.1.1.1 General.**

**18.1.1.1.1*** The requirements of this chapter shall apply to new buildings or portions thereof used as health care occupancies. *(See 1.3.1.)*

**19.1.1 Application.**

**19.1.1.1 General.**

**19.1.1.1.1*** The requirements of this chapter shall apply to existing buildings or portions thereof currently occupied as health care occupancies, unless the authority having jurisdiction has determined equivalent safety has been provided in accordance with Section 1.4.

**A.18.1.1.1.1** In determining equivalency for conversions, modernizations, renovations, or unusual design concepts of hospitals or nursing homes, the authority having jurisdiction is permitted to accept evaluations based on the health care occupancies for safety evaluation system (FSES) of NFPA 101A, *Guide on Alternative Approaches to Life Safety*, utilizing the parameters for new construction.

**A.19.1.1.1.1** In determining equivalency for existing hospitals or nursing homes, the authority having jurisdiction is permitted to accept evaluations based on the health care occupancies fire safety evaluation system (FSES) of NFPA 101A, *Guide on Alternative Approaches to Life Safety*, utilizing the parameters for existing buildings.

The provisions for new health care occupancies are addressed in Chapter 18; the provisions for existing health care occupancies (i.e., existing conditions in health care occupancies) are addressed in Chapter 19.

In editions of the *Code* prior to 2006, renovations, additions, and change of occupancy were required to comply with the requirements for new construction. For health care occupancies, such renovations, additions, and changes of occupancy were required to meet the provisions of Chapter 18, while existing conditions were subject to the provisions of Chapter 19. With the 2006 edition of the *Code*, Chapter 43, Building Rehabilitation, was added. The chapter was written to promote the adaptive reuse of existing buildings without sacrificing the needed level of life safety. The provisions of Chapter 43 blend the requirements for new construction with those for existing conditions, so as to require additional life safety features as the rehabilitation work category increases in complexity. The rehabilitation work categories are repair, renovation, modification, reconstruction, change of use or occupancy classification, and addition. See 4.6.8, 4.6.12, and Chapter 43.

Chapters 18 and 19 are not intended to limit the methods that an authority having jurisdiction (AHJ) might use to determine equivalency. However, as noted in A.18/A.19.1.1.1.1, NFPA 101A, *Guide on Alternative Approaches to Life Safety*,[1] provides an "equivalency system" that uses numerical values to analyze the fire safety effectiveness of a building design and arrangement. This system, known as the fire safety evaluation system (FSES), provides a method for evaluating alternative designs as options to literal *Code* compliance. It is not the intent of the *Code* to limit equivalency evaluations solely to this system. The AHJ does retain the power to evaluate and approve alternative designs on the basis of appropriate supporting data, whether or not the FSES is used to aid in that evaluation. Paragraph A.18/A.19.1.1.1.1 in no way mandates the use of the FSES, nor does it require the AHJ to accept the results of an evaluation using the system.

The FSES is a tool to help determine equivalency — it should not be used to circumvent *Code* requirements. *Code* requirements must be met, or equivalent safety must be provided by alternative means approved by the AHJ. Although the FSES was developed primarily to evaluate alternative designs in existing buildings, it is particularly useful in determining equivalency for unusual design concepts and has applicability to new construction as well.

The 2007 edition of NFPA 101A was calibrated so that its measurement tools would compare alternative designs against the requirements of the 2006 edition of the *Life Safety Code*. It does not measure equivalency against the requirements of the 2009 edition of the *Code* and, therefore, must not be used to measure such equivalency. At the time this handbook went to press, the 2010 edition of NFPA 101A was being processed via the NFPA consensus-based standards-making process. The 2010 edition, to be published late in 2009, will include the proper calibration of the health care occupancies FSES for measuring equivalency against the requirements of Chapter 18/19 of the 2009 edition of the *Code*.

**18.1.1.1.2** The requirements established by this chapter shall apply to the design of all new hospitals, nursing homes, and limited care facilities. The term *hospital*, wherever used in this *Code*, shall include general hospitals, psychiatric hospitals, and specialty hospitals. The term *nursing home*, wherever used in this *Code*, shall include nursing and convalescent homes, skilled nursing facilities, intermediate care facilities, and infirmaries in homes for the aged. Where requirements vary, the specific subclass of health care occupancy that shall apply is named in the paragraph pertaining thereto. The requirements established by Chapter 20 shall apply to all new ambulatory health care facilities. The operating feature requirements established by Section 18.7 shall apply to all health care occupancies.

**18.1.1.1.3** The health care facilities regulated by this chapter shall be those that provide sleeping accommodations for their occupants and are occupied by persons who are mostly incapable of self-preservation because of age, because of physical or mental disability, or because of security measures not under the occupants' control.

**18.1.1.1.4** Buildings, or sections of buildings, that primarily house patients who, in the opinion of the governing body of the facility and the governmental agency having jurisdiction, are capable of exercising judgment and appropriate physical action for self-preservation under emergency conditions shall be permitted to comply with chapters of this *Code* other than Chapter 18.

**18.1.1.1.5*** It shall be recognized that, in buildings housing certain patients, it might be necessary to lock doors and bar windows to confine and protect building inhabitants.

**A.18.1.1.1.5** There are many reasons why doors in the means of egress in health care occupancies might need to be locked for the protection of the patients or the public. Examples of conditions that might justify door locking include dementia, mental health, infant care, pediatric care, or patients under court detention order requiring medical treatment in a health care facility. See 18.2.2.2.5 for details on door locking.

**18.1.1.1.6** Buildings, or sections of buildings, that house older persons and that provide activities that foster continued independence but that do not include services distinctive to health care occupancies *(see 18.1.3)*, as defined in 3.3.178.7, shall be permitted to comply with the requirements of other chapters of this *Code*, such as Chapters 30 or 32.



**19.1.1.1.2** The requirements established by this chapter shall apply to all existing hospitals, nursing homes, and limited care facilities. The term *hospital*, wherever used in this *Code*, shall include general hospitals, psychiatric hospitals, and specialty hospitals. The term *nursing home*, wherever used in this *Code*, shall include nursing and convalescent homes, skilled nursing facilities, intermediate care facilities, and infirmaries in homes for the aged. Where requirements vary, the specific subclass of health care occupancy that shall apply is named in the paragraph pertaining thereto. The requirements established by Chapter 21 shall apply to all existing ambulatory health care facilities. The operating features requirements established by Section 19.7 shall apply to all health care occupancies.

**19.1.1.1.3** The health care facilities regulated by this chapter shall be those that provide sleeping accommodations for their occupants and are occupied by persons who are mostly incapable of self-preservation because of age, because of physical or mental disability, or because of security measures not under the occupants' control.

**19.1.1.1.4** Buildings, or sections of buildings, that primarily house patients who, in the opinion of the governing body of the facility and the governmental agency having jurisdiction, are capable of exercising judgment and appropriate physical action for self-preservation under emergency conditions shall be permitted to comply with chapters of the *Code* other than Chapter 19.

**19.1.1.1.5*** It shall be recognized that, in buildings housing certain patients, it might be necessary to lock doors and bar windows to confine and protect building inhabitants.

**A.19.1.1.1.5** There are many reasons why doors in the means of egress in health care occupancies might need to be locked for the protection of the patients or the public. Examples of conditions that might justify door locking include dementia, mental health, infant care, pediatric care, or patients under court detention order requiring medical treatment in a health care facility. See 19.2.2.2.5 for details on door locking.

**19.1.1.1.6** Buildings, or sections of buildings, that house older persons and that provide activities that foster continued independence but do not include services distinctive to health care occupancies *(see 19.1.3)*, as defined in 3.3.178.7, shall be permitted to comply with the requirements of other chapters of this *Code*, such as Chapters 31 or 33.

CHAPTER 18 • New

**18.1.1.1.7** Facilities that do not provide housing on a 24-hour basis for their occupants shall be classified as other occupancies and shall be covered by other chapters of this *Code*.

**18.1.1.1.8*** The requirements of this chapter shall apply based on the assumption that staff is available in all patient-occupied areas to perform certain fire safety functions as required in other paragraphs of this chapter.

**A.18.1.1.1.8** The *Code* recognizes that certain functions necessary for the life safety of building occupants — such as the detection of fire and associated products of combustion, the closing of corridor doors, the operation of manual fire alarm devices, and the removal of patients from the room of fire origin — require the intervention of facility staff. It is not the intent of 18.1.1.1.8 to specify the levels or locations of staff necessary to meet this requirement.

CHAPTER 19 • Existing

**19.1.1.1.7** Facilities that do not provide housing on a 24-hour basis for their occupants shall be classified as other occupancies and shall be covered by other chapters of this *Code*.

**19.1.1.1.8*** The requirements of this chapter shall apply based on the assumption that staff is available in all patient-occupied areas to perform certain fire safety functions as required in other paragraphs of this chapter.

**A.19.1.1.1.8** The *Code* recognizes that certain functions necessary for the life safety of building occupants — such as the detection of fire and associated products of combustion, the closing of corridor doors, the operation of manual fire alarm devices, and the removal of patients from the room of fire origin — require the intervention of facility staff. It is not the intent of 19.1.1.1.8 to specify the levels or locations of staff necessary to meet this requirement.

Paragraphs 18/19.1.1.1.2 through 18/19.1.1.1.8 contain general material applicable to health care occupancies. Occupants in a health care facility are housed primarily for treatment of mental or physical infirmities, though they might be restrained. If occupants are restrained for penal or correctional purposes, the building would be classified as a detention and correctional occupancy, and the provisions of Chapters 22 and 23 would apply. However, see A.18/A.19.1.1.1.5, which recognizes that patients under court detention order might receive medical treatment in a health care occupancy where doors are locked.

If a building is used for the treatment or housing of patients, including those with mental disabilities or older persons (see 18/19.1.1.1.4 and 18/19.1.1.1.6), the building can be classified as an occupancy other than health care under the following conditions:

1. Occupants are not restrained by locked doors or other devices.
2. Patients are ambulatory.
3. Occupants are capable of perceiving threats and taking appropriate action for self-preservation.

Occupants of health care facilities are considered to be incapable of self-preservation (see 18/19.1.1.1.3) due to age, physical or mental disabilities, or security measures not under their control. A significant number of occupants in health care facilities are assumed to be nonambulatory or bedridden. Other occupants, while capable of self-movement, might have impaired judgment.

Although locked exit doors and barred windows are undesirable in terms of life safety, the *Code* recognizes that, in some cases, such measures are necessary for the protection of the patients or the public. In these instances, provisions need to be made for the continuous supervision and prompt release of those restrained (see 18/19.1.1.1.5). Release of occupants should be achieved by a system capable of automatically unlocking doors in the means of egress or by continuously available attendants equipped with keys. In either case, continuous supervision is considered essential. Also see 18/19.2.2.2.4 through 18/19.2.2.2.6, which were revised for the 2009 edition to permit locked doors for the following conditions:

1. Door locking for the clinical needs of patients who require specialized security measures
2. Door locking where patients pose a security threat
3. Door locking where patient needs require specialized protective measures for their safety

The *Code* assumes that staff will be in continuous attendance in all health care facilities. In fact, staff are assigned certain critical functions during a fire emergency, such as rescuing patients from the room of origin, closing the door to the room, and activating the fire alarm system. The *Code* does not specify minimum staff/patient ratios, because such provisions are included in licensing criteria, and compliance with licensing criteria will normally satisfy the *Code*. Paragraph 18/19.1.1.1.8, in effect, mandates that staff be present. A staff person should be situated to supervise each smoke compartment housing patients. A nursing station located to allow visual supervision of two or more smoke compartments is considered adequate. If, because of some unusual arrangement, staff is not available 24 hours a day to provide supervision, alternative means should be provided to ensure an adequate level of fire safety that is in compliance with the *Code*.

**18.1.1.2* Goals and Objectives.** The goals and objectives of Sections 4.1 and 4.2 shall be met with due consideration for functional requirements, which are accomplished by limiting the development and spread of a fire emergency to the room of fire origin and reducing the need for occupant evacuation, except from the room of fire origin.

**A.18.1.1.2** This objective is accomplished in the context of the physical facilities, the type of activities undertaken, the provisions for the capabilities of staff, and the needs of all occupants through requirements directed at the following:

(1) Prevention of ignition
(2) Detection of fire
(3) Control of fire development
(4) Confinement of the effects of fire
(5) Extinguishment of fire
(6) Provision of refuge or evacuation facilities, or both
(7) Staff reaction

**18.1.1.3 Total Concept.**

**18.1.1.3.1** All health care facilities shall be designed, constructed, maintained, and operated to minimize the possibility of a fire emergency requiring the evacuation of occupants.

**18.1.1.3.2** Because the safety of health care occupants cannot be ensured adequately by dependence on evacuation of the building, their protection from fire shall be provided by appropriate arrangement of facilities; adequate, trained staff; and development of operating and maintenance procedures composed of the following:

(1) Design, construction, and compartmentation
(2) Provision for detection, alarm, and extinguishment
(3) Fire prevention procedures and planning, training, and drilling programs for the isolation of fire, transfer of occupants to areas of refuge, or evacuation of the building



**19.1.1.2* Goals and Objectives.** The goals and objectives of Sections 4.1 and 4.2 shall be met with due consideration for functional requirements, which are accomplished by limiting the development and spread of a fire emergency to the room of fire origin and reducing the need for occupant evacuation, except from the room of fire origin.

**A.19.1.1.2** This objective is accomplished in the context of the physical facilities, the type of activities undertaken, the provisions for the capabilities of staff, and the needs of all occupants through requirements directed at the following:

(1) Prevention of ignition
(2) Detection of fire
(3) Control of fire development
(4) Confinement of the effects of fire
(5) Extinguishment of fire
(6) Provision of refuge or evacuation facilities, or both
(7) Staff reaction

**19.1.1.3 Total Concept.**

**19.1.1.3.1** All health care facilities shall be designed, constructed, maintained, and operated to minimize the possibility of a fire emergency requiring the evacuation of occupants.

**19.1.1.3.2** Because the safety of health care occupants cannot be ensured adequately by dependence on evacuation of the building, their protection from fire shall be provided by appropriate arrangement of facilities; adequate, trained staff; and development of operating and maintenance procedures composed of the following:

(1) Design, construction, and compartmentation
(2) Provision for detection, alarm, and extinguishment
(3) Fire prevention procedures and planning, training, and drilling programs for the isolation of fire, transfer of occupants to areas of refuge, or evacuation of the building

The well-being of an individual located in the room of fire origin can be reasonably ensured only through complete control of that environment, including construction materials, wall and ceiling finishes, furnishings, decorations, clothing, linens, bedding, and the like. However, no code can prevent injury resulting from a person's careless actions.

Although an effort should be made to protect the individual through fire prevention, the primary goal of the requirements of Chapters 18 and 19, as stated in 4.1.1(1), is to limit fire size so as to protect individuals not intimate with the initial fire development. In accordance with the goal of 4.1.1(2), the same protection scheme should have the benefit of additionally improving the survivability of those occupants who are intimate with the initial fire development.

Vertical movement of patients within a health care facility is an inefficient, time-consuming process. In

CHAPTER 18 • New

CHAPTER 19 • Existing

particular, patients in critical care areas might be connected to life-support equipment, making movement difficult and, in some cases, impossible. The provisions of Chapters 18 and 19, therefore, are based on a defend-in-place strategy, which minimizes the probability of a fire dictating vertical movement of occupants. Barriers are required to provide for the horizontal movement of patients to safe areas on a single floor level and to maintain a manageable limit on the number of occupants exposed to any single fire. Vertical means of egress (stairs, in particular) should be considered as egress routes for visitors and staff who are not directly involved with patient relocation and as a "last line of defense" for the movement of patients.

**18.1.1.4 Additions, Conversions, Modernization, Renovation, and Construction Operations.**

**19.1.1.4 Additions, Conversions, Modernization, Renovation, and Construction Operations.**

The provisions of 4.6.8.3 through 4.6.8.5 explain the effect rehabilitation is permitted to have on existing features. The rehabilitation must not reduce existing life safety features that do not meet the requirements for new construction but that exceed the requirements for existing buildings. The rehabilitation is permitted to decrease existing life safety features only if such features are in excess of that required for new construction. For example, a portion of an existing hospital with a 6 ft (1830 mm) wide corridor is to be renovated. Although the hospital is an existing building and existing health care occupancies require minimum 4 ft (1220 mm) wide corridors in accordance with 19.2.3.4, the 6 ft (1830 mm) wide corridor must be maintained, since 18.2.3.4, applicable to new construction, requires a minimum 8 ft (2440 mm) corridor width. Conversely, if a portion of an existing hospital with a 10 ft (3050 mm) wide corridor is to be altered, the corridor is permitted to be reduced to 8 ft (2440 mm) wide, which is the minimum requirement for new construction in accordance with 18.2.3.4.

**18.1.1.4.1 Additions.** Additions shall be separated from any existing structure not conforming to the provisions within Chapter 19 by a fire barrier having not less than a 2-hour fire resistance rating and constructed of materials as required for the addition. *(See 4.6.12 and 4.6.8.)*

**18.1.1.4.1.1** Communicating openings in dividing fire barriers required by 18.1.1.4.1 shall be permitted only in corridors and shall be protected by approved self-closing fire door assemblies. *(See also Section 8.3.)*

**18.1.1.4.1.2** Doors in barriers required by 18.1.1.4.1 shall normally be kept closed, unless otherwise permitted by 18.1.1.4.1.3.

**18.1.1.4.1.3** Doors shall be permitted to be held open if they meet the requirements of 18.2.2.2.7.

**19.1.1.4.1 Additions.** Additions shall be separated from any existing structure not conforming to the provisions within Chapter 19 by a fire barrier having not less than a 2-hour fire resistance rating and constructed of materials as required for the addition. *(See 4.6.12 and 4.6.8.)*

**19.1.1.4.1.1** Communicating openings in dividing fire barriers required by 19.1.1.4.1 shall be permitted only in corridors and shall be protected by approved self-closing fire door assemblies. *(See also Section 8.3.)*

**19.1.1.4.1.2** Doors in barriers required by 19.1.1.4.1 shall normally be kept closed, unless otherwise permitted by 19.1.1.4.1.3.

**19.1.1.4.1.3** Doors shall be permitted to be held open if they meet the requirements of 19.2.2.2.7.

Paragraph 18/19.1.1.4.1 establishes separation criteria for additions to existing structures where those structures do not conform to the provisions of Chapter 19. However, if the existing building does meet the provisions of Chapter 19, a new addition complying with Chapter 18 would not be required to be separated from the existing structure.

If additions are required to be separated from existing portions of buildings, barriers must be constructed of assemblies that provide not less than a 2-hour fire resistance rating. If the structural framing of the addition or the existing buildings consists of assemblies that provide less than 2-hour fire resistance, special provision must be made to ensure that the necessary separation will be maintained for a 2-hour period.

Exhibit 18/19.1 illustrates the provisions of 18/19.1.1.4.1. In Part (a), the new addition that complies with Chapter 18 must be separated from the existing portion of the building that does not comply with the requirements of Chapter 19 for existing health care occupancies. In Part (b), the new addition that complies with Chapter 18 is permitted to be open to the existing portion of the building that complies with the requirements of Chapter 19.

Materials used in the construction of the separation barrier required by 18/19.1.1.4.1 should meet the standards applicable to the addition under construction. That is, if the addition is required to be constructed of noncombustible or limited-combustible materials (construction Type I or Type II), the materials used in the barrier should be noncombustible or limited-combustible as defined in NFPA 220, *Standard on Types of Building Construction.*[2] Conversely, if the addition is permitted to be constructed of combustible materials, combustible materials are permitted to be used in the fire-rated barrier.

Openings in fire barriers separating additions that comply with Chapter 18 from portions of the building not in compliance with the requirements of Chapter 19 are limited to those that are absolutely necessary — that is, cross-corridor doors (see 18/19.1.1.4.1.1). Openings are required to be protected by $1\frac{1}{2}$-hour fire protection–rated door assemblies. The fire doors are required to be self-closing and to remain closed; they are permitted, however, to be held open by an automatic release device in accordance with 18/19.2.2.2.7. In Part (a) of Exhibit 18/19.1, no openings, other than the cross-corridor doors, would be permitted in the separating barrier. This means there can be no penetrations by ductwork. A convenience door between two rooms on opposite sides of the barrier also would be prohibited. However, as shown in Part (b) of Exhibit 18/19.1, if the existing section of the building is in compliance with the requirements of Chapter 19, no fire-rated separating barrier is required. Therefore, unlimited openings are permitted, as depicted in Part (b) of Exhibit 18/19.1 by the four doors in the room walls between the new and existing portions of the building.

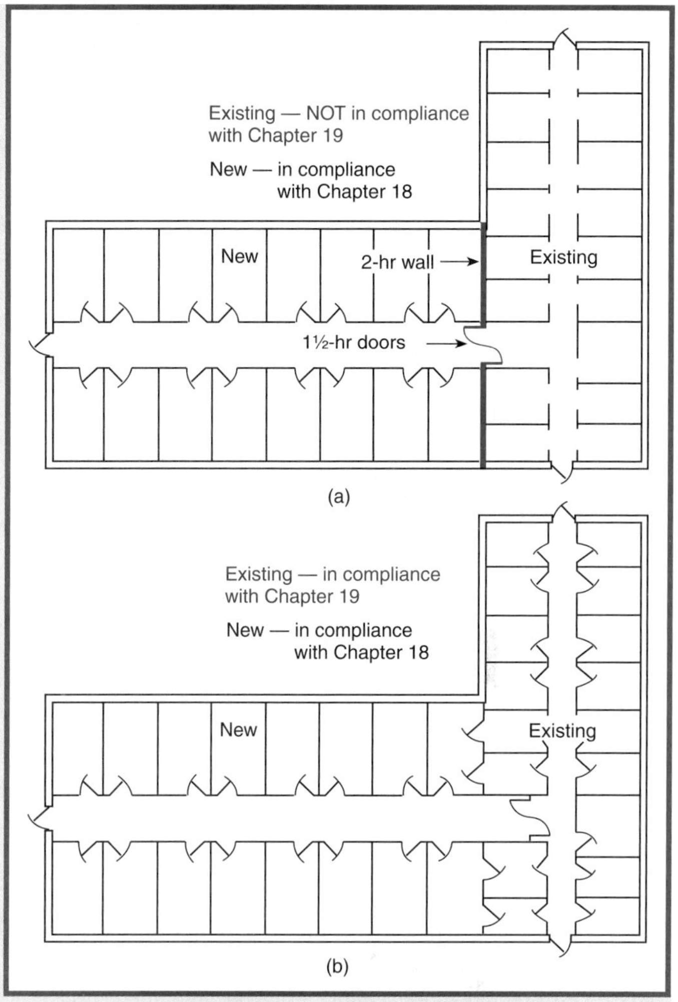


***Exhibit 18/19.1*** *Separation of new construction from existing building.*

**18.1.1.4.2 Changes of Use or Occupancy Classification.** Changes of use or occupancy classification shall comply with 4.6.12, unless otherwise permitted by the following:

(1) A change from a hospital to a nursing home or from a nursing home to a hospital shall not be considered a change in occupancy classification or a change in use.
(2) A change from a hospital or nursing home to a limited care facility shall not be considered a change in occupancy classification or a change in use.

**19.1.1.4.2 Changes of Use or Occupancy Classification.** Changes of use or occupancy classification shall comply with 4.6.12, unless otherwise permitted by the following:

(1) A change from a hospital to a nursing home or from a nursing home to a hospital shall not be considered a change in occupancy classification or a change in use.
(2) A change from a hospital or nursing home to a limited care facility shall not be considered a change in occupancy classification or a change in use.

CHAPTER 18 • New

(3) A change from a hospital or nursing home to an ambulatory health care facility shall not be considered a change in occupancy classification or a change in use.

Paragraph 18/19.1.1.4.2 provides exemptions to the provisions of 4.6.12 related to change of occupancy classification or change of use. Exemptions offered by 18/19.1.1.4.2(1) through (3) address changes from one health care occupancy subclassification to another health care occupancy subclassification. The exemptions state that the specific changes addressed are not meant to invoke the provisions for change of occupancy or change of use. Provided that the change in subclassification is from a subclassification that is heavily regulated by the *Code* to a subclassification that is either less regulated or at least as regulated (e.g., hospital to ambulatory health care, or hospital to nursing home, respectively), the resulting facility is not subject to the change of occupancy or change of use provisions of 4.6.12. However, if the change is in the opposite direction — for example, from an ambulatory health care facility, which the *Code* regulates with a modest package of requirements, to a hospital or nursing home, which the *Code* regulates via an extensive package of requirements — then the resulting facility is subject to the change of occupancy or change of use provisions of 4.6.12.

**18.1.1.4.3 Rehabilitation.**

**18.1.1.4.3.1** For purposes of the provisions of this chapter, the following shall apply:

(1) A major rehabilitation shall involve the modification of more than 50 percent, or more than 4500 $ft^2$ (420 $m^2$), of the area of the smoke compartment.
(2) A minor rehabilitation shall involve the modification of not more than 50 percent, and not more than 4500 $ft^2$ (420 $m^2$), of the area of the smoke compartment.

**18.1.1.4.3.2** Work that is exclusively plumbing, mechanical, fire protection system, electrical, medical gas, or medical equipment work shall not be included in the computation of the modification area within the smoke compartment.

**18.1.1.4.3.3*** Where major rehabilitation is done in a nonsprinklered smoke compartment, the automatic sprinkler requirements of 18.3.5 shall apply to the smoke compartment undergoing the rehabilitation, and, in cases where the building is not protected throughout by an approved automatic sprinkler system, the requirements of 18.4.3.2, 18.4.3.3, and 18.4.3.8 shall also apply.

**A.18.1.1.4.3.3** For the purpose of this requirement, a floor that is not divided by a smoke barrier is considered one smoke compartment. Where automatic sprinklers are retrofitted into existing nonsprinklered buildings, the construction alternatives for sprinklers provided in this *Code* are intended to apply to the renovated area.

**18.1.1.4.3.4*** Where minor rehabilitation is done in a nonsprinklered smoke compartment, the requirements of 18.3.5.1 shall not apply, but, in such cases, the rehabilitation shall not reduce life safety below the level required for new

CHAPTER 19 • Existing

(3) A change from a hospital or nursing home to an ambulatory health care facility shall not be considered a change in occupancy classification or a change in use.

**19.1.1.4.3 Rehabilitation.**

**19.1.1.4.3.1** For purposes of the provisions of this chapter, the following shall apply:

(1) A major rehabilitation shall involve the modification of more than 50 percent, or more than 4500 $ft^2$ (420 $m^2$), of the area of the smoke compartment.
(2) A minor rehabilitation shall involve the modification of not more than 50 percent, and not more than 4500 $ft^2$ (420 $m^2$), of the area of the smoke compartment.

**19.1.1.4.3.2** Work that is exclusively plumbing, mechanical, fire protection system, electrical, medical gas, or medical equipment work shall not be included in the computation of the modification area within the smoke compartment.

**19.1.1.4.3.3*** Where major rehabilitation is done in a nonsprinklered smoke compartment, the automatic sprinkler requirements of 18.3.5 shall apply to the smoke compartment undergoing the rehabilitation, and, in cases where the building is not protected throughout by an approved automatic sprinkler system, the requirements of 18.4.3.2, 18.4.3.3, and 18.4.3.8 shall also apply.

**A.19.1.1.4.3.3** For the purpose of this requirement, a floor that is not divided by a smoke barrier is considered one smoke compartment. Where automatic sprinklers are retrofitted into existing nonsprinklered buildings, the construction alternatives for sprinklers provided in this *Code* are intended to apply to the renovated area.

**19.1.1.4.3.4*** Where minor rehabilitation is done in a nonsprinklered smoke compartment, the requirements of 18.3.5.1 shall not apply, but, in such cases, the rehabilitation shall not reduce life safety below the level required for new

CHAPTER 18 • New

buildings or below the level of the requirements of 18.4.3 for nonsprinklered smoke compartment rehabilitation. *(See 4.6.8.)*

**A.18.1.1.4.3.4** In minor rehabilitation, only the rehabilitation itself — not the entire smoke compartment or building — is required to be brought up to the requirements for new nonsprinklered facilities.

CHAPTER 19 • Existing

buildings or below the level of the requirements of 18.4.3 for nonsprinklered smoke compartment rehabilitation. *(See 4.6.8.)*

**A.19.1.1.4.3.4** In minor rehabilitation, only the rehabilitation itself is required to be brought up to the requirements for new nonsprinklered facilities, not the entire smoke compartment or building.

Automatic sprinkler protection is required for all new health care facilities (see 18.3.5.1) and existing nursing homes (see 19.3.5.1). Existing hospitals might be nonsprinklered. Where major rehabilitation is made in a nonsprinklered existing facility, in addition to performing those planned renovations in accordance with the requirements for new construction, 18/19.1.1.4.3.3 requires that the smoke compartment in which the major rehabilitation occurs be sprinklered. Therefore, although the rehabilitation was not originally planned to include the installation of sprinklers, such installation is required within the smoke compartment being rehabilitated.

Paragraph 18/19.1.1.4.3.1 defines major and minor rehabilitation with reference to the term *modification*. The definition of the term *modification* in 3.3.168 originated in Chapter 15, Building Rehabilitation, of *NFPA 5000®, Building Construction and Safety Code®*,[3] which served as the basis for Chapter 43, Building Rehabilitation, that was added to the *Code* in 2006. The Chapter 43 hierarchy of rehabilitation methods includes repair, renovation, modification, reconstruction, change of use or occupancy classification, and addition. Repair and renovation do not require classification as a major rehabilitation. Change of use or occupancy classification is addressed in the commentary following 18/19.1.1.4.2(3) with respect to 18/19.1.1.4.2.

Modification and reconstruction can require major rehabilitation classification, depending on the floor area involved, as detailed in 18/19.1.1.4.3.1(1). Note that, per 18/19.1.1.4.3.2, work that is exclusively plumbing, mechanical, fire protection system, electrical, medical gas, or medical equipment work is not included in the computation of the modification area within the smoke compartment undergoing the rehabilitation.

Minor rehabilitation — as defined by 18/19.1.1.4.3.1(2) — does not mandate the requirement for installing sprinklers. Only that smoke compartment undergoing major rehabilitation is required to be sprinklered at the time of rehabilitation. Therefore, if a floor of a hospital is subdivided into three smoke compartments and only one smoke compartment is undergoing major rehabilitation, only that particular smoke compartment would require sprinkler installation. Over the course of a few years of undergoing multiple major rehabilitation projects, the entire building would eventually be fully sprinklered. Because the building undergoing major rehabilitation in only one smoke compartment would then be only partially protected with sprinklers, the construction requirements of 18.4.3.2 for nonsprinklered buildings must be met, egress capacity must be based on the nonsprinklered criteria of 18.4.3.3 in the nonsprinklered portions of the building, and smoke dampers are required where ducts penetrate required smoke barriers per 18.4.3.8. [For example, stair capacity is calculated at 0.6 in. (15 mm) per person, rather than the typical 0.3 in. (7.6 mm) per person.] Smoke dampers are permitted to be omitted for ducted penetrations of smoke barriers only where the smoke compartments on both sides of the smoke barrier are fully sprinklered as specified in 18.4.3.8.

**18.1.1.4.4 Construction, Repair, and Improvement Operations.** See 4.6.11.

**19.1.1.4.4 Construction, Repair, and Improvement Operations.** See 4.6.11.

The introduction of workers, other than regular employees, and activities associated with rehabilitation creates unusual risks for fire in health care occupancies. Special precautions should be taken to guard against the potential exposure created by the introduction of flammable substances or by other hazardous practices that could pose a threat to occupants. See 4.6.11.3.

Temporary fire-resistant barriers should be erected to separate rehabilitation areas and associated activity

CHAPTER 18 • New

from the functioning areas of the existing buildings. Care should be taken to ensure that these temporary barriers do not block means of egress for the existing building and that all existing equipment for fire protection and all portions of the required means of egress are maintained in full working order. See 4.6.11.1.

### 18.1.2 Multiple Occupancies.

**18.1.2.1** Multiple occupancies shall be in accordance with 6.1.14.

**18.1.2.2*** Sections of health care facilities shall be permitted to be classified as other occupancies, provided that they meet all of the following conditions:

(1) They are not intended to serve health care occupants for purposes of housing, treatment, or customary access by patients incapable of self-preservation.
(2) They are separated from areas of health care occupancies by construction having a minimum 2-hour fire resistance rating in accordance with 8.2.1.3.
(3) The construction type and supporting construction of the health care occupancy is based on the story on which it is located in the building in accordance with the provisions of 18.1.6 and Table 18.1.6.1.
(4) The construction type of the areas of the building enclosing the other occupancies is based on the applicable occupancy chapters of this *Code*.

**A.18.1.2.2** Doctors' offices and treatment and diagnostic facilities that are intended solely for outpatient care and are physically separated from facilities for the treatment or care of inpatients, but that are otherwise associated with the management of an institution, might be classified as business occupancies rather than health care occupancies.

**18.1.2.3*** Ambulatory care facilities, medical clinics, and similar facilities that are contiguous to health care occupancies, but are primarily intended to provide outpatient services, shall be permitted to be classified as business occupancies or ambulatory health care facilities, provided that the facilities are separated from the health care occupancy by construction having a minimum 2-hour fire resistance rating, and the facility is not intended to provide services simultaneously for four or more inpatients who are litterborne.

**A.18.1.2.3** It is the intent that these requirements apply to mobile, transportable, and relocatable structures (in accor-

CHAPTER 19 • Existing

Adequate escape facilities should be provided and continuously maintained for the use of construction workers. See 4.6.11.2, A.4.6.11.2, and NFPA 241, *Standard for Safeguarding Construction, Alteration, and Demolition Operations.*[4]

### 19.1.2 Multiple Occupancies.

**19.1.2.1** Multiple occupancies shall be in accordance with 6.1.14.

**19.1.2.2*** Sections of health care facilities shall be permitted to be classified as other occupancies, provided that they meet all of the following conditions:

(1) They are not intended to serve health care occupants for purposes of housing, treatment, or customary access by patients incapable of self-preservation.
(2) They are separated from areas of health care occupancies by construction having a minimum 2-hour fire resistance rating in accordance with 8.2.1.3.
(3) The construction type and supporting construction of the health care occupancy is based on the story on which it is located in the building in accordance with the provisions of 19.1.6 and Table 19.1.6.1.
(4) The construction type of the areas of the building enclosing the other occupancies is based on the applicable occupancy chapters of this *Code*.
(5) For other than previously approved occupancy separation arrangements, the entire building is protected throughout by an approved, supervised automatic sprinkler system in accordance with Section 9.7.

**A.19.1.2.2** Doctors' offices and treatment and diagnostic facilities that are intended solely for outpatient care and are physically separated from facilities for the treatment or care of inpatients, but that are otherwise associated with the management of an institution, might be classified as business occupancies rather than health care occupancies.

**19.1.2.3*** Ambulatory care facilities, medical clinics, and similar facilities that are contiguous to health care occupancies, but are primarily intended to provide outpatient services, shall be permitted to be classified as business occupancies or ambulatory health care facilities, provided that the facilities are separated from the health care occupancy by not less than 2-hour fire resistance–rated construction, and the facility is not intended to provide services simultaneously for four or more inpatients who are litterborne.

**A.19.1.2.3** It is the intent of the *Code* that these requirements apply to mobile, transportable, and relocatable strucdance with 1.3.2) where such structures are used to provide shared medical services on an extended or a temporary basis. Where properly separated from the health care occupancy and intended to provide services simultaneously for three or fewer health care patients who are litterborne, the level of protection for such structures should be based on the appropriate occupancy classification of other chapters of this *Code*. Mobile, transportable, or relocatable structures that are not separated from a contiguous health care occupancy, or that are intended to provide services simultaneously for four or more health care patients who are litterborne, should be classified and designed as health care occupancies.

**18.1.2.4** All means of egress from health care occupancies that traverse non-health-care spaces shall conform to the requirements of this *Code* for health care occupancies, unless otherwise permitted by 18.1.2.5.

**18.1.2.5** Exit through a horizontal exit into other contiguous occupancies that do not conform to health care egress provisions, but that do comply with requirements set forth in the appropriate occupancy chapter of this *Code*, shall be permitted, provided that both of the following criteria apply:

(1) The occupancy does not contain high hazard contents.
(2) The horizontal exit complies with the requirements of 18.2.2.5.

**18.1.2.6** Egress provisions for areas of health care facilities that correspond to other occupancies shall meet the corresponding requirements of this *Code* for such occupancies, and, where the clinical needs of the occupant necessitate the locking of means of egress, staff shall be present for the supervised release of occupants during all times of use.

**18.1.2.7** Auditoriums, chapels, staff residential areas, or other occupancies provided in connection with health care facilities shall have means of egress provided in accordance with other applicable sections of this *Code*.

**18.1.2.8** Any area with a hazard of contents classified higher than that of the health care occupancy and located in the same building shall be protected as required by 18.3.2.

**18.1.2.9** Non-health care–related occupancies classified as containing high hazard contents shall not be permitted in buildings housing health care occupancies.



tures (in accordance with 1.3.2) when such structures are used to provide shared medical services on an extended or a temporary basis. Where properly separated from the health care occupancy and intended to provide services simultaneously for three or fewer health care patients who are litterborne, the level of protection for such structures should be based on the appropriate occupancy classification of other chapters of this *Code*. Mobile, transportable, or relocatable structures that are not separated from a contiguous health care occupancy, or that are intended to provide services simultaneously for four or more health care patients who are litterborne, should be classified and designed as health care occupancies.

**19.1.2.4** All means of egress from health care occupancies that traverse non-health-care spaces shall conform to the requirements of this *Code* for health care occupancies, unless otherwise permitted by 19.1.2.5.

**19.1.2.5** Exit through a horizontal exit into other contiguous occupancies that do not conform to health care egress provisions, but that do comply with requirements set forth in the appropriate occupancy chapter of this *Code*, shall be permitted, provided that both of the following criteria apply:

(1) The occupancy does not contain high hazard contents.
(2) The horizontal exit complies with the requirements of 19.2.2.5.

**19.1.2.6** Egress provisions for areas of health care facilities that correspond to other occupancies shall meet the corresponding requirements of this *Code* for such occupancies, and, where the clinical needs of the occupant necessitate the locking of means of egress, staff shall be present for the supervised release of occupants during all times of use.

**19.1.2.7** Auditoriums, chapels, staff residential areas, or other occupancies provided in connection with health care facilities shall have means of egress provided in accordance with other applicable sections of this *Code*.

**19.1.2.8** Any area with a hazard of contents classified higher than that of the health care occupancy and located in the same building shall be protected as required by 19.3.2.

**19.1.2.9** Non-health care–related occupancies classified as containing high hazard contents shall not be permitted in buildings housing health care occupancies.

Paragraph 18/19.1.2.1 directs the user to the multiple occupancies provisions of 6.1.14, which permit protecting multiple occupancies either as mixed occupancies or as separated occupancies. The provisions of 18/19.1.2.2 through 18/19.1.2.9 have the effect of modifying those of 6.1.14 for the very specific situations described.

Paragraphs 18/19.1.2.2 and 18/19.1.2.3 contain criteria for classifying spaces as other occupancies, although those spaces are located in buildings used primarily for health care purposes. For example, 18/19.1.2.2 permits offices to be classified as business occupancies, cafeterias to be classified as assembly occupancies, or dormitories for other than inpatients to be classified as residential occupancies, provided that the requirements of 18/19.1.2.2(1) through (4), and 19.1.2.2(5) where applicable, are met.

The provisions of 18/19.1.2.2 were revised for the 2009 edition of the *Code*. Paragraph 18/19.1.2.2(1) notes that customary access by patients incapable of self-preservation is not permitted within the other occupancy. This paragraph is intended to permit an occasional ambulatory inpatient to visit a doctor's office in an adjacent business occupancy, for example, without requiring classification of the business occupancy as a health care facility. Further, emergency egress from the health care occupancy into the other occupancy is permitted, because emergency egress is not considered customary access (see 18/19.1.2.4 and 18/19.1.2.5).

Paragraph 18/19.1.2.2(2) requires that the other occupancy be separated from the health care occupancy by construction having a minimum 2-hour fire resistance rating. The fire barrier is permitted to be vertically aligned (i.e., a wall assembly where the occupancies are located in adjacent spaces on the same floor) or horizontally aligned (i.e., a floor assembly where the occupancies are located on different, but adjacent, floors). The reference to the provisions of 8.2.1.3 was added to the 2009 edition to clarify that the separating barrier is permitted to be the demarcation point between different building construction types only if it is vertically aligned (i.e., a wall assembly and not a floor assembly). For example, where floors constructed of unprotected wood frame, Type V(000) construction are positioned above floors of Type II(222) construction, the provisions of 8.2.1.3 require the overall building to be classified as Type V(000) construction (i.e., the lesser fire-resistive type), even where the two types of construction are separated by a minimum 2-hour fire resistance–rated floor/ceiling assembly.

Paragraphs 18/19.1.2.2(3) and (4) are new to the 2009 edition of the *Code*. They clarify that, for purposes of applying the building construction requirements of 18/19.1.6 and Table 18/19.1.6.1, the story height of a non-health care occupancy located above a health care occupancy can be ignored. For example, where Table 18.1.6.1 limits a new health care occupancy building of Type II(000) construction to being not more than one story in height, a three-story Type II(000) building would be permitted if the following conditions were met:

1. The health care occupancy occupies only the first story.
2. A business occupancy occupies the second and third stories [note that 38.1.6, applicable to new business occupancies, has no minimum construction requirements, so the Type II(000) construction is permitted in accordance with 18.1.2.2(4)].
3. The floor/ceiling assembly (and the structural frame that supports the floor assembly) between the first and second stories has a minimum 2-hour fire resistance rating.

If the requirements of 18/19.1.2.2 are not met, the area would be considered a multiple occupancy requiring protection as mixed occupancies. The most restrictive life safety requirements applicable to any one occupancy present would be required for all the occupancies. In most cases, the requirements of the health care occupancy would be stricter than those of the other occupancies, requiring that health care occupancy requirements be met throughout the building. Such generalization should not lead to compliance only with Chapters 18 and 19, as each provision of the applicable occupancy chapters needs to be compared and the most stringent identified and implemented. See 6.1.14.3.2.

Paragraph 18/19.1.2.3 addresses a subject similar to that of 18/19.1.2.2 but specifically covers ambulatory care facilities, medical clinics, and similar areas that primarily provide outpatient services and are associated with, or attached to, a health care facility. If these facilities are separated by 2-hour fire resistance–rated construction, they are permitted to be classified as ambulatory health care facilities or as business occupancies, whichever applies. The provisions applicable to business occupancies and ambulatory health care facilities are based on the assumption that most people are treated on an outpatient basis. If four or more litterborne inpatients are treated simultaneously, the facility must meet the requirements for health care occupancies. Conversely, if three or fewer litterborne inpatients are present in the outpatient facility on a regular basis, the facility would be classified as an occupancy other than health care.

Paragraph 18/19.1.2.4 specifies that the means of egress from health care occupancies that traverse non-health-care spaces must conform to the requirements for health care occupancies. However, an exemption is permitted by 18/19.1.2.5 where a 2-hour separating barrier is provided to meet the requirements for a horizontal exit. Where a 2-hour barrier serves as a horizontal exit, it is acceptable to exit from a health care occupancy into a different occupancy if the other occupancy complies with the *Code* provisions applicable to that occupancy and does not contain high hazard contents. For example, if a horizontal exit is provided between a hospital and a business occupancy, inpatients are permitted to exit into the business occupancy through a horizontal exit. In this instance, corridor width, corridor partitions, stairway details, and similar features must conform to the provisions of either Chapter 38 or Chapter 39, which address business occupancies. However, the horizontal exit must comply with all the requirements of 18/19.2.2.5, which include provisions in addition to those required by the core provisions of 7.2.4 applicable to horizontal exits.

Health care occupancy patients are sometimes moved to nonmedical areas — such as a chapel for religious services or an auditorium for recreation — that typically do not meet the provisions applicable to health care occupancies. Paragraph 18/19.1.2.6 permits such areas to be regulated by the provisions applicable to the corresponding occupancy (which would be an assembly occupancy, in the case of chapels or auditoriums). Paragraph 18/19.1.2.6 addresses a subject similar to that addressed in 18/19.1.2.7 but adds the requirement that, where the clinical needs of the occupants necessitate the locking of doors, staff must be present for the supervised unlocking of doors and release of occupants. This additional requirement ensures that procedures are in place for the ready release of occupants.

Auditoriums, chapels, and other areas separated from the health care occupancy by construction meeting the criteria of 6.1.14.4 for separated occupancies are permitted to be designed in accordance with the appropriate occupancy chapter governing their use, rather than in accordance with those applicable to the health care occupancy.

Paragraph 18/19.1.2.8 regulates spaces in other occupancies in the same building as a health care facility that, although comprising only a portion of the facility, contain more hazardous materials (in quantity or type) than are usually found in health care occupancies. Spaces such as rooms used for the storage of combustible materials, trash collection rooms, gift shops, and paint shops must be protected in accordance with 18/19.3.2.

Paragraph 18/19.1.2.9 prohibits another occupancy, such as storage, that contains highly hazardous contents, such as flammable liquids, from being located in a building housing a health care occupancy. This paragraph limits use, based on occupancy classification, with regard to hazard of contents. For example, the paragraph does not intend to exclude laboratory operations from being part of a health care facility. The intent is to prevent a portion of a hospital from being designed and used as an educational or research facility — which would be classified as an educational occupancy, business occupancy, or possibly an industrial occupancy — where laboratories use and store sizable quantities of flammable liquids.

### 18.1.3 Special Definitions.

A list of special terms used in this chapter follows:

(1) **Ambulatory Health Care Occupancy.** See 3.3.178.1.
(2) **Hospital.** See 3.3.133.
(3) **Limited Care Facility.** See 3.3.82.2.
(4) **Nursing Home.** See 3.3.131.2.

### 19.1.3 Special Definitions.

A list of special terms used in this chapter follows:

(1) **Ambulatory Health Care Occupancy.** See 3.3.178.1.
(2) **Hospital.** See 3.3.133.
(3) **Limited Care Facility.** See 3.3.82.2.
(4) **Nursing Home.** See 3.3.131.2.

Section 3.3 defines the terms *hospital, nursing home,* and *limited care facility*. Each must house four or more people incapable of self-preservation on a 24-hour basis to be classified as a health care occupancy.

Occupants of hospitals or nursing homes are assumed to be nonambulatory and incapable of self-preservation. In making this judgment, due consideration should be given to the use of physical restraints and tranquilizing drugs, which can render occupants immobile. Variable staffing criteria and levels of care differentiate hospitals from nursing homes. The difference between nursing homes and limited care facilities is less clear.

Although limited care facilities house four or more occupants incapable of self-preservation due to age or physical or mental limitations, occupants are generally considered to be ambulatory and to require only limited assistance during emergency evacuation. Buildings that house ambulatory occupants who are mentally handicapped or undergoing treatment for alcohol or drug dependency and who can be expected to evacuate a structure with limited assistance meet the criteria for limited care facilities. Day-care facilities that provide day care for the aged, children, mentally handicapped, or others would be classified as other than health care. See Chapters 16 and 17.

Although age itself is not sufficient justification for developing a separate subclassification for a health care occupancy, the elderly pose a unique problem in the achievement of fire safety. Experiences in buildings where the elderly are housed demonstrate that the response of the elderly to a fire might not be in the interest of self-preservation. Upon discovering a fire, elderly occupants might ignore it, become transfixed by it, or seek refuge from it in their rooms and fail to notify anyone of the fire. In some cases, the elderly have resisted efforts to remove them from the building and familiar surroundings.

Terms such as *residential*, *lodging* and *boarding*, and *custodial care* were used in the health care occupancy chapters of earlier editions of the *Code* but have been deleted to avoid confusion with the residential board and care occupancy classification addressed by Chapters 32 and 33. Board and care facilities, personal care homes, halfway houses, assisted living, or similar facilities house occupants who might require medication and personal care but do not require the close supervision and services typical of the occupants in a health care facility. Therefore, these facilities would be classified as residential board and care occupancies. Occupant capability must be carefully evaluated to determine whether application of health care criteria (contained in Chapters 18 and 19) or application of lesser safeguards associated with residential board and care occupancies (prescribed by Chapters 32 and 33) are more appropriate.

Prior to the 1981 edition of the *Code*, occupancies that offered medical services on an outpatient basis would have been regulated within the chapter covering business occupancies. The threat to life in an outpatient facility where four or more patients might be subject to medical procedures requiring general anesthesia, treatments such as hemodialysis, or freestanding emergency service is significantly greater than that typical of a business occupancy. Conversely, application of the requirements for health care facilities that contemplate 24-hour care would be unnecessarily restrictive. In establishing the occupancy classification of an ambulatory health care occupancy, the intent was to develop requirements that fall between the restrictions applicable to business occupancies and health care occupancies (i.e., inpatient health care) in terms of the level of life safety provided. See Chapters 20 and 21.

### 18.1.4 Classification of Occupancy.

See 6.1.5 and 18.1.3.

### 18.1.5 Classification of Hazard of Contents.

The classification of hazard of contents shall be as defined in Section 6.2.

### 18.1.6 Minimum Construction Requirements.

**18.1.6.1** Health care occupancies shall be limited to the building construction types specified in Table 18.1.6.1, unless otherwise permitted by 18.1.6.2 through 18.1.6.7. *(See 8.2.1.)*

**18.1.6.2** Any building of Type I(442), Type I(332), Type II(222), or Type II(111) construction shall be permitted to include roofing systems involving combustible supports, decking, or roofing, provided that the following criteria are met:

(1) The roof covering shall meet Class A requirements in accordance with NFPA 256, *Standard Methods of Fire Tests of Roof Coverings*.

### 19.1.4 Classification of Occupancy.

See 6.1.5 and 19.1.3.

### 19.1.5 Classification of Hazard of Contents.

The classification of hazard of contents shall be as defined in Section 6.2.

### 19.1.6 Minimum Construction Requirements.

**19.1.6.1** Health care occupancies shall be limited to the building construction types specified in Table 19.1.6.1, unless otherwise permitted by 19.1.6.2 through 19.1.6.7. *(See 8.2.1.)*

**19.1.6.2*** Any building of Type I(442), Type I(332), Type II(222), or Type II(111) construction shall be permitted to include roofing systems involving combustible supports, decking, or roofing, provided that the following criteria are met:

(1) The roof covering shall meet Class C requirements in accordance with NFPA 256, *Standard Methods of Fire Tests of Roof Coverings*.

*Table 18.1.6.1 Construction Type Limitations*

| Construction Type | Sprinklered‡ | Total Number of Stories of Building† | | | |
|---|---|---|---|---|---|
| | | 1 | 2 | 3 | ≥4 |
| I (442) | Yes | X | X | X | X |
| | No | NP | NP | NP | NP |
| I (332) | Yes | X | X | X | X |
| | No | NP | NP | NP | NP |
| II (222) | Yes | X | X | X | X |
| | No | NP | NP | NP | NP |
| II (111) | Yes | X | X | X | NP |
| | No | NP | NP | NP | NP |
| II (000) | Yes | X | NP | NP | NP |
| | No | NP | NP | NP | NP |
| III (211) | Yes | X | NP | NP | NP |
| | No | NP | NP | NP | NP |
| III (200) | Yes | NP | NP | NP | NP |
| | No | NP | NP | NP | NP |
| IV (2HH) | Yes | X | NP | NP | NP |
| | No | NP | NP | NP | NP |
| V (111) | Yes | X | NP | NP | NP |
| | No | NP | NP | NP | NP |
| V (000) | Yes | NP | NP | NP | NP |
| | No | NP | NP | NP | NP |

X: Permitted NP: Not permitted.

† Basements are not counted as stories.

‡ Sprinklered throughout by an approved, supervised automatic sprinkler system in accordance with Section 9.7. *(See 18.3.5.)*

(2) The roof shall be separated from all occupied portions of the building by a noncombustible floor assembly having not less than a 2-hour fire resistance rating that includes not less than 2½ in. (63 mm) of concrete or gypsum fill.
(3) The structural elements supporting the 2-hour fire resistance–rated floor assembly specified in 18.1.6.2(2) shall be required to have only the fire resistance rating required of the building.

**18.1.6.3** Any building of Type I(442), Type I(332), Type II(222), or Type II(111) construction shall be permitted to include roofing systems involving combustible supports, decking, or roofing, provided that the following criteria are met:

(1) The roof covering shall meet Class A requirements in accordance with NFPA 256, *Standard Methods of Fire Tests of Roof Coverings.*

(2) The roof shall be separated from all occupied portions of the building by a noncombustible floor assembly that includes not less than 2½ in. (63 mm) of concrete or gypsum fill.
(3) The attic or other space shall be either unoccupied or protected throughout by an approved automatic sprinkler system.

**A.19.1.6.2** Unoccupied space, for the purposes of 19.1.6.2(3), is space not normally occupied by persons, fuel-fired equipment, or hazardous contents.

**19.1.6.3** Any building of Type I(442), Type I(332), Type II(222), or Type II(111) construction shall be permitted to include roofing systems involving combustible supports, decking, or roofing, provided that the following criteria are met:

(1) The roof covering shall meet Class A requirements in accordance with NFPA 256, *Standard Methods of Fire Tests of Roof Coverings.*

*Table 19.1.6.1 Construction Type Limitations*

| | | Total Number of Stories of Building† | | | |
|---|---|---|---|---|---|
| **Construction Type** | **Sprinklered‡** | **1** | **2** | **3** | **≥4** |
| I (442) | Yes | X | X | X | X |
| | No | X | X | X | X |
| I (332) | Yes | X | X | X | X |
| | No | X | X | X | X |
| II (222) | Yes | X | X | X | X |
| | No | X | X | X | X |
| II (111) | Yes | X | X | X | NP |
| | No | X | NP | NP | NP |
| II (000) | Yes | X | X | NP | NP |
| | No | NP | NP | NP | NP |
| III (211) | Yes | X | X | NP | NP |
| | No | NP | NP | NP | NP |
| III (200) | Yes | X | NP | NP | NP |
| | No | NP | NP | NP | NP |
| IV (2HH) | Yes | X | X | NP | NP |
| | No | NP | NP | NP | NP |
| V (111) | Yes | X | X | NP | NP |
| | No | NP | NP | NP | NP |
| V (000) | Yes | X | NP | NP | NP |
| | No | NP | NP | NP | NP |

X: Permitted. NP: Not permitted.

†Basements are not counted as stories.

‡Sprinklered throughout by an approved, supervised automatic sprinkler system in accordance with Section 9.7. *(See 19.3.5.)*

(2) The roof/ceiling assembly shall be constructed with fire-retardant-treated wood meeting the requirements of NFPA 220, *Standard on Types of Building Construction.*
(3) The roof/ceiling assembly shall have the required fire resistance rating for the type of construction.

**18.1.6.4** Interior nonbearing walls in buildings of Type I or Type II construction shall be constructed of noncombustible or limited-combustible materials, unless otherwise permitted by 18.1.6.5.

**18.1.6.5** Interior nonbearing walls required to have a minimum 2-hour fire resistance rating shall be permitted to be of fire-retardant-treated wood enclosed within noncombustible or limited-combustible materials, provided that such walls are not used as shaft enclosures.

**18.1.6.6** Fire-retardant-treated wood that serves as supports for the installation of fixtures and equipment shall be permitted to be installed behind noncombustible or limited-combustible sheathing.

(2) The roof/ceiling assembly shall be constructed with fire-retardant-treated wood meeting the requirements of NFPA 220, *Standard on Types of Building Construction.*
(3) The roof/ceiling assembly shall have the required fire resistance rating for the type of construction.

**19.1.6.4** Interior nonbearing walls in buildings of Type I or Type II construction shall be constructed of noncombustible or limited-combustible materials, unless otherwise permitted by 19.1.6.5.

**19.1.6.5** Interior nonbearing walls required to have a minimum 2-hour fire resistance rating shall be permitted to be fire-retardant-treated wood enclosed within noncombustible or limited-combustible materials, provided that such walls are not used as shaft enclosures.

**19.1.6.6** Fire-retardant-treated wood that serves as supports for the installation of fixtures and equipment shall be permitted to be installed behind noncombustible or limited-combustible sheathing.

CHAPTER 18 • New

**18.1.6.7** All buildings with more than one level below the level of exit discharge shall have all such lower levels separated from the level of exit discharge by not less than Type II(111) construction.

CHAPTER 19 • Existing

**19.1.6.7** Each exterior wall of frame construction and all interior stud partitions shall be firestopped to cut off all concealed draft openings, both horizontal and vertical, between any cellar or basement and the first floor, and such firestopping shall consist of wood not less than 2 in. (51 mm) (nominal) thick or shall be of noncombustible material.

Table 18/19.1.6.1 is applied relative to building construction types. See NFPA 220, *Standard on Types of Building Construction*, and *NFPA 5000, Building Construction and Safety Code*, for definitions of construction types. Table A.8.2.1.2 summarizes the details associated with Type I through Type V construction.

Table 18/19.1.6.1 is formatted differently than the minimum construction requirements table of the ___.1.6 subsection of other occupancy chapters. Table 18/19.1.6.1 establishes building construction type limitations based on the total number of stories in a building; the other minimum construction tables establish criteria in terms of "stories in height," as established by 4.6.3. Table 18/19.1.6.1 is applied to health care occupancies by starting the story count with the level of exit discharge and ending with the highest occupiable story, even if that story is not used as a health care occupancy. [Note that a building can have only one level of exit discharge, as defined in 3.3.77.1.] A five-story building where the first story is used as a health care occupancy and the second through fifth stories are used as business occupancies is treated as a five-story building for purposes of applying Table 18/19.1.6.1 for health care occupancies. For occupancies, other than health care, that regulate building construction type (e.g., assembly occupancies), the applicable table is applied to the number of stories in height, with the story count starting with the level of exit discharge and ending with the highest occupiable story containing the occupancy considered. A five-story building where the first story is used as an assembly occupancy and the second through fifth stories are used as business occupancies is treated as a one-story building for purposes of applying Table 12/13.1.6 for assembly occupancies.

The provisions of 18/19.1.2.2 have the effect of modifying the application of Table 18/19.1.6.1 so as to permit its application based on number of "stories in height," rather than "total number of stories of building," where an occupancy other than health care is positioned above the stories used as health care occupancies and the floor/ceiling assembly (and all supporting construction) that separates the two occupancies is a minimum 2-hour fire resistance–rated barrier. See 18/19.1.2.2 and the associated commentary that follows 18/19.1.2.9.

Exhibit 18/19.2 illustrates the application of the provisions of Table 18.1.6.1 to two buildings whose plans are being reviewed prior to construction. Each building is to house a health care occupancy on the first story and business occupancies on the second through fifth stories. Each building is to be of Type II(111) construction and protected throughout by automatic sprinklers in accordance with 18.3.5.1. In applying the construction requirements of Table 18.1.6.1 to Building A, the appropriate cell is located where the row for Type II (111) under "Construction Type" and "Yes" under "Sprinklered" intersects with the column for ≥ 4 under "Total Number of Stories of Building." The intersection cell, "NP," means that the new health care occupancy is not permitted to be located in the five-story Type II(111) building. Next, the construction requirements of Table 18.1.6.1 are applied in conjunction with those of 18.1.2.2 to Building B. Building B, in addition to having the features of Building A, has a 2-hour fire resistance–rated floor/ceiling assembly separating the first and second stories in accordance with 18.1.2.2(2). In accordance with 18.1.2.2(3), Table 18.1.6.1 is applied with respect to the number of stories in height, and not to the total number of stories in the

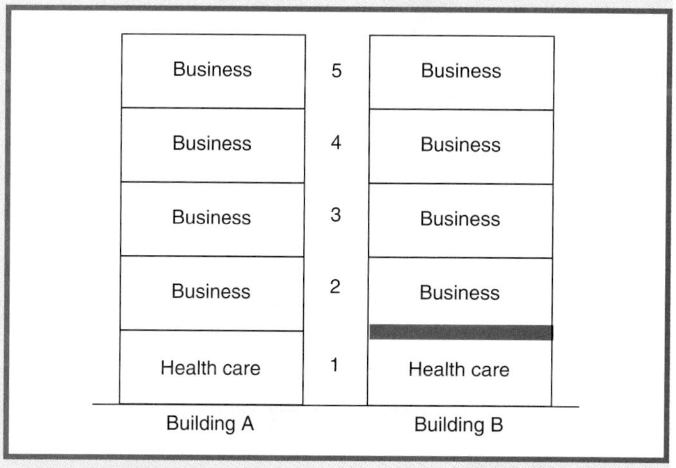


***Exhibit 18/19.2*** *Applying provisions of Table 18.1.6.1 to total number of stories and to number of stories in height.*

building, which is 1, given that the health care occupancy occupies only the first story. In Table 18.1.6.1, the appropriate cell is located where the row for Type II (111) under "Construction Type" and "Yes" under "Sprinklered" intersects with the column for 1 under "Total Number of Stories of Building." The intersection cell, "X", means that the new health care occupancy is permitted to be located on the first story of the five-story Type II(111) building because of the presence of the 2-hour floor/ceiling assembly that separates the health care occupancy from the business occupancies.

In certain areas, it has been common practice to erect a building with a flat, concrete roof deck. A wood deck on a wood frame peaked roof is then added for weather protection. Paragraph 18/19.1.6.2 contains an exemption that permits, under certain conditions, construction of such a combustible roof system on a multistory building without affecting the classification of the building construction. In other words, a Type I or Type II building, which by definition has a roof constructed wholly of noncombustible materials, is permitted to retain its Type I or Type II classification and have a combustible wood "roof" in accordance with the provisions of 18/19.1.6.2.

The exemption detailed in 19.1.6.2(3) specifies that the existing attic space must be unoccupied or protected with automatic sprinklers. The word "unoccupied" is meant to disallow routine, regular use of the attic, which might increase the likelihood of fire or add a "fuel load" to the nonsprinklered space. Office or combustible storage spaces, for example, would be prohibited. The word "unoccupied" is not intended to prohibit the presence of mechanical equipment requiring periodic maintenance, such as air-handling units. Although 8.2.3.3 requires fire-rated assemblies to be supported by fire-rated structural members, 18.1.6.2 specifically exempts the 2-hour fire resistance–rated floor assembly (that separates the roof from the occupied floors below) from having to be supported on the floors below by 2-hour-rated structural members, if the required fire resistance rating of the building is less than 2 hours.

Paragraph 18/19.1.6.3 is similar to 18/19.1.6.2 in permitting the roofing system to include combustible supports, decking, or roofing, but is specific to the use of fire-retardant-treated wood.

Although NFPA 220, *Standard on Types of Building Construction*, does not set combustibility requirements for nonbearing interior walls and partitions, 18/19.1.6.4 adds requirements that exceed those of NFPA 220. Paragraph 18/19.1.6.4 adds that, in Type I and Type II construction, all nonbearing interior walls and partitions must be constructed of noncombustible or limited-combustible materials. The terms *noncombustible (material)* and *limited-combustible (material)* are defined within NFPA 220, and the definitions are repeated in Chapter 3 of the *Code* for easy reference. See 3.3.160.3 and 3.3.160.2.

Paragraph 18/19.1.6.5 supplements 18/19.1.6.4 in permitting fire-retardant-treated wood to be used within the core of minimum 2-hour fire resistance–rated interior nonbearing walls where the sheathing of such walls is of noncombustible or limited-combustible materials. Similarly, 18/19.1.6.6 permits fire-retardant-treated wood used for supporting fixtures to be used within the core of walls and partitions similarly sheathed.

### 18.1.7 Occupant Load.

The occupant load, in number of persons for whom means of egress and other provisions are required, either shall be determined on the basis of the occupant load factors of Table 7.3.1.2 that are characteristic of the use of the space or shall be determined as the maximum probable population of the space under consideration, whichever is greater.

## 18.2 Means of Egress Requirements

### 18.2.1 General.

Every aisle, passageway, corridor, exit discharge, exit location, and access shall be in accordance with Chapter 7, unless otherwise modified by 18.2.2 through 18.2.11.



### 19.1.7 Occupant Load.

The occupant load, in number of persons for whom means of egress and other provisions are required, either shall be determined on the basis of the occupant load factors of Table 7.3.1.2 that are characteristic of the use of the space or shall be determined as the maximum probable population of the space under consideration, whichever is greater.

## 19.2 Means of Egress Requirements

### 19.2.1 General.

Every aisle, passageway, corridor, exit discharge, exit location, and access shall be in accordance with Chapter 7, unless otherwise modified by 19.2.2 through 19.2.11.

CHAPTER 18 • New

### 18.2.2* Means of Egress Components.

**A.18.2.2** In planning egress, arrangements should be made to transfer patients from one section of a floor to another section of the same floor that is separated by a fire barrier or smoke barrier in such a manner that patients confined to their beds can be transferred in their beds. Where the building design will allow, the section of the corridor containing an entrance or elevator lobby should be separated from corridors leading from it by fire or smoke barriers. Such arrangement, where the lobby is centrally located, will, in effect, produce a smoke lock, placing a double barrier between the area to which patients might be taken and the area from which they need to be evacuated because of threatening smoke and fire.

**18.2.2.1 Components Permitted.** Components of means of egress shall be limited to the types described in 18.2.2.2 through 18.2.2.10.

**18.2.2.2 Doors.**

**18.2.2.2.1** Doors complying with 7.2.1 shall be permitted.

**18.2.2.2.2** Locks shall not be permitted on patient sleeping room doors, unless otherwise permitted by the following:

(1) Key-locking devices that restrict access to the room from the corridor and that are operable only by staff from the corridor side shall be permitted, provided that such devices do not restrict egress from the room.
(2) Locks complying with 18.2.2.2.5 shall be permitted.

CHAPTER 19 • Existing

### 19.2.2 Means of Egress Components.

**19.2.2.1 Components Permitted.** Components of means of egress shall be limited to the types described in 19.2.2.2 through 19.2.2.10.

**19.2.2.2 Doors.**

**19.2.2.2.1** Doors complying with 7.2.1 shall be permitted.

**19.2.2.2.2** Locks shall not be permitted on patient sleeping room doors, unless otherwise permitted by the following:

(1) Key-locking devices that restrict access to the room from the corridor and that are operable only by staff from the corridor side shall be permitted, provided that such devices do not restrict egress from the room.
(2) Locks complying with 19.2.2.2.5 shall be permitted.

Paragraphs 18/19.2.2.2.1 through 18/19.2.2.2.10 address the door provisions of 7.2.1 and provide any modifications particular to health care occupancies.

In the 1991 and earlier editions of the *Code*, numerous provisions of Chapters 18 and 19 specified minimum door width requirements as a leaf width rather than as a clear width. For example, doors from patient rooms to the corridor in new construction were required to be 44 in. (1120 mm) wide. The intent was that, after allowing for the stops built into the door frame and the thickness of the protruding hinge stile edge, a 44 in. (1120 mm) wide door leaf would provide approximately 41½ in. (1055 mm) of clear, unobstructed width. However, there was no requirement for the door to swing a minimum of 90 degrees from the plane of the door opening, so the intended 41½ in. (1055 mm) of clear, unobstructed width was not ensured. Since the 1994 edition of the *Code*, all minimum door width requirements for new health care occupancies have been specified as clear, unobstructed width. For existing doors in health care occupancies, all minimum door width requirements have been specified as clear, unobstructed width, but exceptions continue to recognize existing doors with the minimum door leaf widths previously specified.

The provisions of 18/19.2.2.2.2 address the locking of patient sleeping room doors. The provisions of 18/19.2.2.2.4 address the locking of doors other than patient sleeping room doors. Where a door-locking option detailed elsewhere in 18/19.2.2.2 is appropriate for use on any egress door, permission to use the option appears in both 18/19.2.2.2.2 and 18/19.2.2.2.4. For example, both 18/19.2.2.2.2(2) and 18/19.2.2.2.4(1) recognize the use of the door-locking provisions of 18/19.2.2.2.5.

Paragraph 18/19.2.2.2.2(1) permits access from the corridor to a patient sleeping room to be limited via a locked door that staff can unlock with keys they keep readily available. Limited access would permit, for example, patient isolation rooms to have doors locked from the corridor side only, so that other patients could not wander into the room and thus endanger themselves. However, the patient within the isolation room with the door locked from the corridor side needs to be able to open the door from the room side without the use of a key or tool.

Paragraphs 18/19.2.2.2.2(2) and 18/19.2.2.2.4(1) recognize use of the provisions of 18/19.2.2.2.5, which were expanded for the 2009 edition of the *Code* to address door locking where patients pose a security threat and where patient needs require specialized protective measures for their safety, as well as door locking for the clinical needs of patients as allowed by earlier editions.

**18.2.2.2.3** Doors not located in a required means of egress shall be permitted to be subject to locking.

**18.2.2.2.4** Doors within a required means of egress shall not be equipped with a latch or lock that requires the use of a tool or key from the egress side, unless otherwise permitted by the following:

(1) Locks complying with 18.2.2.2.5 shall be permitted.
(2)* Delayed-egress locks complying with 7.2.1.6.1 shall be permitted.

**A.18.2.2.2.4(2)** Where delayed-egress locks complying with 7.2.1.6.1 are used, the provisions of 18.2.2.2.5 are not required.

(3)* Access-controlled egress doors complying with 7.2.1.6.2 shall be permitted.

**A.18.2.2.2.4(3)** Where access-controlled egress doors complying with 7.2.1.6.2 are used, the provisions of 18.2.2.2.5 are not required.

(4) Elevator lobby exit access door locking in accordance with 7.2.1.6.3 shall be permitted.



**19.2.2.2.3** Doors not located in a required means of egress shall be permitted to be subject to locking.

**19.2.2.2.4** Doors within a required means of egress shall not be equipped with a latch or lock that requires the use of a tool or key from the egress side, unless otherwise permitted by the following:

(1) Locks complying with 19.2.2.2.5 shall be permitted.
(2)* Delayed-egress locks complying with 7.2.1.6.1 shall be permitted.

**A.19.2.2.2.4(2)** Where delayed-egress locks complying with 7.2.1.6.1 are used, the provisions of 19.2.2.2.5 are not required.

(3)* Access-controlled egress doors complying with 7.2.1.6.2 shall be permitted.

**A.19.2.2.2.4(3)** Where access-controlled egress doors complying with 7.2.1.6.2 are used, the provisions of 19.2.2.2.5 are not required.

(4) Elevator lobby exit access door locking in accordance with 7.2.1.6.3 shall be permitted.
(5) Approved existing door-locking installations shall be permitted.

Paragraph 18/19.2.2.2.4(2) addresses the delayed-egress lock described in 7.2.1.6.1. Paragraph 7.2.1.6.1 specifies detailed requirements for delayed-egress locking hardware, including the requirement that the building be protected throughout by automatic sprinklers or automatic fire detection. The exemption permits the use of the delayed-egress lock on any door in a health care facility. Editions of the *Code* prior to 2009 permitted only one delayed-egress lock along any egress path. The restriction was deleted, as there was not adequate substantiation to retain it.

Paragraph 18/19.2.2.2.4(3) addresses access-controlled egress door assemblies described in 7.2.1.6.2. Paragraph 7.2.1.6.2 specifies detailed requirements for doors where ingress is restricted so as to require an electronic key but for which egress is not restricted, as a motion detector is provided to sense a building occupant's approach toward the egress door and unlock the door automatically.

Paragraph 18/19.2.2.2.4(4) is new to the 2009 edition of the *Code*. It permits use of the elevator lobby exit access door-locking provisions of 7.2.1.6.3. Paragraph 7.2.1.6.3 details 15 criteria that must be met as an alternative to the requirements of 7.4.1.6 that each elevator landing or lobby must have access to at least one exit without the use of a key, a tool, special knowledge, or special effort. See 7.4.1.6 and 7.2.1.6.3.

Paragraph 19.2.2.2.4(5) recognizes existing door-locking arrangements that do not meet the provisions of 19.2.2.2.4(1), (2), (3), or (4) where approved by the authority having jurisdiction (AHJ). For example, the AHJ might permit an existing door-locking system that was installed to reduce the potential for infant abduction but does not meet all the criteria of 19.2.2.2.5.2

CHAPTER 18 • New

to be continued in use. Note that the provision does not relate to previously approved systems (see 3.3.198). Rather, approval of the current AHJ must be

**18.2.2.2.5** Door-locking arrangements shall be permitted in accordance with either 18.2.2.2.5.1 or 18.2.2.2.5.2.

**18.2.2.2.5.1*** Door-locking arrangements shall be permitted where the clinical needs of patients require specialized security measures or where patients pose a security threat, provided that one of the following criteria is met:

(1) Staff can readily unlock doors at all times in accordance with 18.2.2.2.6.
(2) The provisions of 18.2.2.2.5.2 are met.

**A.18.2.2.2.5.1** Psychiatric units, Alzheimer units, and dementia units are examples of areas with patients who might have clinical needs that justify door locking. Forensic units and detention units are examples of areas with patients who might pose a security threat. Where Alzheimer or dementia patients in nursing homes are not housed in specialized units, the provisions of 18.2.2.2.5.1 should not apply. *(See 18.2.2.2.5.2.)*

**18.2.2.2.5.2** Door-locking arrangements shall be permitted where patient special needs require specialized protective measures for their safety, provided that all of the following criteria are met:

(1) Staff can readily unlock doors at all times in accordance with 18.2.2.2.6.
(2) A total (complete) smoke detection system is provided throughout the locked space in accordance with 9.6.2.9, or locked doors can be remotely unlocked at an approved, constantly attended location within the locked space.
(3)* The building is protected throughout by an approved, supervised automatic sprinkler system in accordance with 18.3.5.1.

**A.18.2.2.2.5.2(3)** Where locked doors in accordance with 18.2.2.2.5.2 are proposed for an existing building that is not sprinklered throughout, the authority having jurisdiction might consider permitting the installation based on an analysis of the extent of sprinkler protection provided. Sprinklered areas should include, at a minimum, the secured compartment and compartments that the occupants of the secured compartment must travel through to egress the building.

(4) The locks are electrical locks that fail safely so as to release upon loss of power to the device.

CHAPTER 19 • Existing

secured in order to permit the existing door-locking system to remain in use.

**19.2.2.2.5** Door-locking arrangements shall be permitted in accordance with either 19.2.2.2.5.1 or 19.2.2.2.5.2.

**19.2.2.2.5.1*** Door-locking arrangements shall be permitted where the clinical needs of patients require specialized security measures or where patients pose a security threat, provided that one of the following criteria is met:

(1) Staff can readily unlock doors at all times in accordance with 19.2.2.2.6.
(2) The provisions of 19.2.2.2.5.2 are met.

**A.19.2.2.2.5.1** Psychiatric units, Alzheimer units, and dementia units are examples of areas with patients who might have clinical needs that justify door locking. Forensic units and detention units are examples of areas with patients who might pose a security threat. Where Alzheimer or dementia patients in nursing homes are not housed in specialized units, the provisions of 19.2.2.2.5.1 should not apply. *(See 19.2.2.2.5.2.)*

**19.2.2.2.5.2*** Door-locking arrangements shall be permitted where patient special needs require specialized protective measures for their safety, provided that all of the following are met:

(1) Staff can readily unlock doors at all times in accordance with 19.2.2.2.6.
(2) A total (complete) smoke detection system is provided throughout the locked space in accordance with 9.6.2.9, or locked doors can be remotely unlocked at an approved, constantly attended location within the locked space.
(3)* The building is protected throughout by an approved, supervised automatic sprinkler system in accordance with 19.3.5.1.

**A.19.2.2.2.5.2(3)** Where locked doors in accordance with 19.2.2.2.5.2 are proposed for an existing building that is not sprinklered throughout, the authority having jurisdiction might consider permitting the installation based on an analysis of the extent of sprinkler protection provided. Sprinklered areas should include, at a minimum, the secured compartment and compartments that the occupants of the secured compartment must travel through to egress the building.

(4) The locks are electrical locks that fail safely so as to release upon loss of power to the device.

CHAPTER 18 • New

(5) The locks release by independent activation of each of the following:
   (a) Activation of the smoke detection system required by 18.2.2.2.5.2(2)
   (b) Waterflow in the automatic sprinkler system required by 18.2.2.2.5.2(3)

The provisions of 18/19.2.2.2.5 address features that must be met in order to lock doors for the following conditions:

1. Door locking for the clinical needs of patients who require specialized security measures
2. Door locking where patients pose a security threat
3. Door locking where patient needs require specialized protective measures for their safety

Paragraph 18/19.2.2.2.5.1 addresses the locking of patient sleeping room doors where patient clinical needs require specialized security measures or where patients pose a security threat. Health care facilities might need to lock patient room doors against egress for functional purposes involving the clinical needs of patients or to prevent patients from harming other building occupants. For example, if certain patients require confinement because they would otherwise leave their rooms and endanger themselves or others, locking patient room doors would provide specialized security. If patient room doors are locked against egress for patient clinical needs or where patients pose a security threat, the provisions of 18/19.2.2.2.5.1 offer two options, with the detailed provisions for carrying out the options specified in subsequent paragraphs.

One option is to provide for staff to readily unlock doors at all times as addressed by 18/19.2.2.2.6, such as might be done by having staff carry keys at all times so as to be able to unlock doors immediately. The other option is to employ the criteria of 18/19.2.2.2.5.2, which are new to the 2009 edition of the *Code,* and address door locking where patient special needs require specialized protective measures. The level of protection provided by compliance with 18/19.2.2.2.5.2 is more than adequate to address door locking where patient clinical needs require specialized security measures or where patients pose a security threat.

The provisions of 18/19.2.2.2.5.2 are new to the 2009 edition of the *Code* and permit doors to be locked where patient special needs require specialized protective measures for their safety. For example, the provisions of 18/19.2.2.2.5.2 might be used on the doors of a newborn infant nursery or nursery wing of a building to reduce the potential for infant abduction. The protective systems required are extensive, as detailed in 18/19.2.2.2.5.2(1) through (5), and blend together staff action, smoke detection, sprinkler protection, fail-safe locks, and lock release via multiple independent actions.

**A.18.2.2.2.5.2** Pediatric units, maternity units, Alzheimer units, dementia units, and emergency departments are examples of areas where patients might have special needs that justify door locking.

**18.2.2.2.6** Doors that are located in the means of egress and are permitted to be locked under other provisions of 18.2.2.2.5 shall comply with the following:

(1) Provisions shall be made for the rapid removal of occupants by means of one of the following:
   (a) Remote control of locks
   (b) Keying of all locks to keys carried by staff at all times
   (c) Other such reliable means available to the staff at all times
(2) Only one locking device shall be permitted on each door.

CHAPTER 19 • Existing

(5) The locks release by independent activation of each of the following:
   (a) Activation of the smoke detection system required by 19.2.2.2.5.2(2)
   (b) Waterflow in the automatic sprinkler system required by 19.2.2.2.5.2(3)

**A.19.2.2.2.5.2** Pediatric units, maternity units, Alzheimer units, dementia units, and emergency departments are examples of areas where patients might have special needs that justify door locking.

**19.2.2.2.6** Doors that are located in the means of egress and are permitted to be locked under other provisions of 19.2.2.2.5 shall comply with the following:

(1) Provisions shall be made for the rapid removal of occupants by means of one of the following:
   (a) Remote control of locks
   (b) Keying of all locks to keys carried by staff at all times
   (c) Other such reliable means available to the staff at all times
(2) Only one locking device shall be permitted on each door.

CHAPTER 18 • New

CHAPTER 19 • Existing

(3) More than one lock shall be permitted on each door, subject to approval of the authority having jurisdiction.

In buildings where the locking of doors is necessary, continuous staff supervision must be provided in order to comply with the performance-based requirements of 18/19.2.2.2.6. Provisions must be made for the prompt release of persons who are restrained either by equipping staff with keys, by providing remote unlocking capabilities for doors, or by other reliable means available to staff at all times. If staff relies on the use of keys, a master key system for facilitating the quick release of occupants should be considered. In existing buildings, given the approval of the authority having jurisdiction, 19.2.2.2.6(3) permits more than one lock on a door.

**18.2.2.2.7*** Any door in an exit passageway, stairway enclosure, horizontal exit, smoke barrier, or hazardous area enclosure (except boiler rooms, heater rooms, and mechanical equipment rooms) shall be permitted to be held open only by an automatic release device that complies with 7.2.1.8.2. The automatic sprinkler system and the fire alarm system, and the systems required by 7.2.1.8.2, shall be arranged to initiate the closing action of all such doors throughout the smoke compartment or throughout the entire facility.

**A.18.2.2.2.7** It is desirable to keep doors in exit passageways, stair enclosures, horizontal exits, smoke barriers, and required enclosures around hazardous areas closed at all times to impede the travel of smoke and fire gases. Functionally, however, this involves decreased efficiency and limits patient observation by the staff of a facility. To accommodate such needs, it is practical to presume that such doors will be kept open, even to the extent of employing wood chocks and other makeshift devices. Doors in exit passageways, horizontal exits, and smoke barriers should, therefore, be equipped with automatic hold-open devices activated by the methods described, regardless of whether the original installation of the doors was predicated on a policy of keeping them closed.

**18.2.2.2.8** Where doors in a stair enclosure are held open by an automatic release device as permitted in 18.2.2.2.7, initiation of a door-closing action on any level shall cause all doors at all levels in the stair enclosure to close.

**19.2.2.2.7*** Any door in an exit passageway, stairway enclosure, horizontal exit, smoke barrier, or hazardous area enclosure shall be permitted to be held open only by an automatic release device that complies with 7.2.1.8.2. The automatic sprinkler system, if provided, and the fire alarm system, and the systems required by 7.2.1.8.2, shall be arranged to initiate the closing action of all such doors throughout the smoke compartment or throughout the entire facility.

**A.19.2.2.2.7** It is desirable to keep doors in exit passageways, stair enclosures, horizontal exits, smoke barriers, and required enclosures around hazardous areas closed at all times to impede the travel of smoke and fire gases. Functionally, however, this involves decreased efficiency and limits patient supervision by the staff of a facility. To accommodate such needs, it is practical to presume that such doors will be kept open, even to the extent of employing wood chocks and other makeshift devices. Doors in exit passageways, horizontal exits, and smoke barriers should, therefore, be equipped with automatic hold-open devices actuated by the methods described, regardless of whether the original installation of the doors was predicated on a policy of keeping them closed.

**19.2.2.2.8** Where doors in a stair enclosure are held open by an automatic release device as permitted in 19.2.2.2.7, initiation of a door-closing action on any level shall cause all doors at all levels in the stair enclosure to close.

Paragraph 18/19.2.2.2.7 modifies the requirements of 7.2.1.8.2 addressing automatic-closing doors. According to 7.2.1.8.2 and *NFPA 72®, National Fire Alarm Code®*,[5] the doors must be designed to close automatically by actuation of smoke detectors installed to detect smoke on either side of the door. In addition, where health care occupancy doors that are required to be self-closing are held open, an automatic device must close doors (either throughout the affected smoke compartment or throughout the building) upon operation of the building fire alarm system and upon operation of the building sprinkler system. As a further safeguard for stair enclosures, any automatic action that closes a stair enclosure door on one level must close the doors on the other levels of that stair enclosure in accordance with 18/19.2.2.2.8.

CHAPTER 18 • New

**18.2.2.2.9** High-rise health care occupancies shall comply with the re-entry provisions of 7.2.1.5.7.

Paragraph 18.2.2.2.9 regulates stairway re-entry in new health care occupancies having occupied floor levels more than 75 ft (23 m) above the lowest level of fire department access. In doing so, the *Code* exempts new low-rise health care occupancies from the requirements of 7.2.1.5.7. Stair doors in new high-rise health care facilities must allow for re-entry in accordance with Chapter 7. All stair doors must be unlocked, or they must be interlocked with the building fire alarm to unlock automatically in the event of alarm actuation. As for all occupancies, use of 7.2.1.5.7.1 is permitted. Paragraph 7.2.1.5.7.1 permits stair doors to be locked, provided that the following requirements are met:

1. A minimum of two doors are maintained unlocked.
2. There are no more than four intervening floors between unlocked doors.
3. Re-entry is possible at either of the two top floor levels that provides access to a different exit.
4. Unlocked doors are appropriately marked on the stairwell side.
5. Locked doors have signage regarding the location of unlocked doors.

Existing health care occupancies — even those that are in high-rise buildings — are exempt from the stairwell re-entry provisions (see 19.2.2.2.9).

**18.2.2.2.10** Horizontal-sliding doors shall be permitted in accordance with 18.2.2.2.10.1 or 18.2.2.2.10.2.

**18.2.2.2.10.1** Horizontal-sliding doors, as permitted by 7.2.1.14, that are not automatic-closing shall be limited to a single leaf and shall have a latch or other mechanism that ensures that the doors will not rebound into a partially open position if forcefully closed.

**18.2.2.2.10.2** Horizontal-sliding doors serving an occupant load of fewer than 10 shall be permitted, provided that all of the following criteria are met:

(1) The area served by the door has no high hazard contents.
(2) The door is readily operable from either side without special knowledge or effort.
(3) The force required to operate the door in the direction of door travel is not more than 30 lbf (133 N) to set the door in motion and is not more than 15 lbf (67 N) to close the door or open it to the minimum required width.
(4) The door assembly complies with any required fire protection rating, and, where rated, is self-closing or automatic-closing by means of smoke detection in accordance with 7.2.1.8 and is installed in accordance with NFPA 80, *Standard for Fire Doors and Other Opening Protectives*.

CHAPTER 19 • Existing

**19.2.2.2.9*** Existing health care occupancies shall be exempt from the re-entry provisions of 7.2.1.5.7.

**A.19.2.2.2.9** Doors to the enclosures of interior stair exits should be arranged to open from the stair side at not less than every third floor so that it will be possible to leave the stairway at such floor if fire renders the lower part of the stair unusable during egress or if occupants seek refuge on another floor.

**19.2.2.2.10** Horizontal-sliding doors shall be permitted in accordance with 19.2.2.2.10.1 or 19.2.2.2.10.2.

**19.2.2.2.10.1** Horizontal-sliding doors, as permitted by 7.2.1.14, that are not automatic-closing shall be limited to a single leaf and shall have a latch or other mechanism that ensures that the doors will not rebound into a partially open position if forcefully closed.

**19.2.2.2.10.2** Horizontal-sliding doors serving an occupant load of fewer than 10 shall be permitted, provided that all of the following criteria are met:

(1) The area served by the door has no high hazard contents.
(2) The door is readily operable from either side without special knowledge or effort.
(3) The force required to operate the door in the direction of door travel is not more than 30 lbf (133 N) to set the door in motion and is not more than 15 lbf (67 N) to close the door or open it to the minimum required width.
(4) The door assembly complies with any required fire protection rating, and, where rated, is self-closing or automatic-closing by means of smoke detection in accordance with 7.2.1.8 and is installed in accordance with NFPA 80, *Standard for Fire Doors and Other Opening Protectives*.

CHAPTER 18 • New

(5) Where corridor doors are required to latch, the doors are equipped with a latch or other mechanism that ensures that the doors will not rebound into a partially open position if forcefully closed.

CHAPTER 19 • Existing

(5) Where corridor doors are required to latch, the doors are equipped with a latch or other mechanism that ensures that the doors will not rebound into a partially open position if forcefully closed.

Paragraph 18/19.2.2.2.10.1 establishes requirements exceeding those of 7.2.1.14 for horizontal-sliding doors. If the special form of sliding door addressed in 7.2.1.14 is to be closed manually, the door must consist of a single leaf to avoid openings at the meeting edges of the two leafs, and provisions must be made, by use of a latch or other means, to prevent the door from contacting the frame and rebounding to a partially open position when closed forcefully. The requirements of 7.2.1.14 should be closely reviewed. The sliding door described is highly specialized, and all requirements of 7.2.1.14 must be met. One unique requirement that differentiates this special door from a typical horizontal-sliding door is that it must slide to the side to allow passage through the door opening when force is applied in the direction of egress travel to the door actuator.

Paragraph 18/19.2.2.2.10.2 permits traditional horizontal-sliding doors (as contrasted with the special form of sliding door addressed in 7.2.1.14) to serve within the required means of egress. A nearly identical set of provisions for horizontal-sliding doors appears in 7.2.1.4.1(4)(c), which is new to the 2009 edition of the *Code* and was modeled after 18/19.2.2.2.10.2. The horizontal-sliding door is permitted as an exemption to the requirement of 7.2.1.4.1 that any door in a means of egress be of the swinging type. By limiting the use of the horizontal-sliding door to serving an occupant load of fewer than 10, the provision relies on staff assistance to help ensure that the door will be operated correctly, so as to open to the full required width. Horizontal-sliding doors are frequently used within suites, including critical care units. Such doors do not need to be installed with a breakaway feature, as they are not required to be of the swinging type. The requirement of 18/19.2.2.2.10.2(5) was revised for the 2009 edition to clarify that the latching criterion applies only where the doors are corridor doors that are required to latch, so as not to have applicability to horizontal-sliding doors, for example, within suites.

**18.2.2.3 Stairs.** Stairs complying with 7.2.2 shall be permitted.

**18.2.2.4 Smokeproof Enclosures.** Smokeproof enclosures complying with 7.2.3 shall be permitted.

**18.2.2.5 Horizontal Exits.** Horizontal exits complying with 7.2.4 and the modifications of 18.2.2.5.1 through 18.2.2.5.7 shall be permitted.

**18.2.2.5.1** Accumulation space shall be provided in accordance with 18.2.2.5.1.1 and 18.2.2.5.1.2.

**18.2.2.5.1.1** Not less than 30 net ft$^2$ (2.8 net m$^2$) per patient in a hospital or nursing home, or not less than 15 net ft$^2$ (1.4 net m$^2$) per resident in a limited care facility, shall be provided within the aggregated area of corridors, patient rooms, treatment rooms, lounge or dining areas, and other similar areas on each side of the horizontal exit.

**18.2.2.5.1.2** On stories not housing bedridden or litterborne patients, not less than 6 net ft$^2$ (0.56 net m$^2$) per occupant shall be provided on each side of the horizontal exit for the total number of occupants in adjoining compartments.

**18.2.2.5.2** The total egress capacity of the other exits (stairs, ramps, doors leading outside the building) shall not

**19.2.2.3 Stairs.** Stairs complying with 7.2.2 shall be permitted.

**19.2.2.4 Smokeproof Enclosures.** Smokeproof enclosures complying with 7.2.3 shall be permitted.

**19.2.2.5 Horizontal Exits.** Horizontal exits complying with 7.2.4 and the modifications of 19.2.2.5.1 through 19.2.2.5.4 shall be permitted.

**19.2.2.5.1** Accumulation space shall be provided in accordance with 19.2.2.5.1.1 and 19.2.2.5.1.2.

**19.2.2.5.1.1** Not less than 30 net ft$^2$ (2.8 net m$^2$) per patient in a hospital or nursing home, or not less than 15 net ft$^2$ (1.4 net m$^2$) per resident in a limited care facility, shall be provided within the aggregated area of corridors, patient rooms, treatment rooms, lounge or dining areas, and other similar areas on each side of the horizontal exit.

**19.2.2.5.1.2** On stories not housing bedridden or litterborne patients, not less than 6 net ft$^2$ (0.56 net m$^2$) per occupant shall be provided on each side of the horizontal exit for the total number of occupants in adjoining compartments.

**19.2.2.5.2** The total egress capacity of the other exits (stairs, ramps, doors leading outside the building) shall not

CHAPTER 18 • New

be reduced below one-third of that required for the entire area of the building.

**18.2.2.5.3** A single door shall be permitted in a horizontal exit if the following conditions apply:

(1) The exit serves one direction only.
(2) Such door is a swinging door or a horizontal-sliding door complying with 7.2.1.14.
(3) The door is not less than $41\frac{1}{2}$ in. (1055 mm) in clear width.

**18.2.2.5.4** A horizontal exit involving a corridor 8 ft (2440 mm) or more in width and serving as a means of egress from both sides of the doorway shall have the opening protected by a pair of swinging doors arranged to swing in opposite directions from each other, with each door having a clear width of not less than $41\frac{1}{2}$ in. (1055 mm), or by a horizontal-sliding door that complies with 7.2.1.14 and provides a clear width of not less than 6 ft 11 in. (2110 mm).

**18.2.2.5.5** A horizontal exit involving a corridor 6 ft (1830 mm) or more in width and serving as a means of egress from both sides of the doorway shall have the opening protected by a pair of swinging doors, arranged to swing in opposite directions from each other, with each door having a clear width of not less than 32 in. (810 mm), or by a horizontal-sliding door that complies with 7.2.1.14 and provides a clear width of not less than 64 in. (1625 mm).

**18.2.2.5.6** An approved vision panel shall be required in each horizontal exit door.

**18.2.2.5.7** Center mullions shall be prohibited in horizontal exit door openings.

CHAPTER 19 • Existing

be reduced below one-third of that required for the entire area of the building.

**19.2.2.5.3*** A door in a horizontal exit shall not be required to swing with egress travel as specified in 7.2.4.3.8(1).

**A.19.2.2.5.3** The waiver of the requirement for doors to swing in the direction of egress travel is based on the assumption that, in this occupancy, there is no possibility of a panic rush that might prevent the opening of doors that swing against egress travel.

A desirable arrangement, which is possible with corridors 8 ft (2440 mm) or more in width, is to have two 42 in. (1070 mm) doors, normally closed, each swinging with the egress travel (in opposite directions).

**19.2.2.5.4** Door openings in horizontal exits shall be protected by one of the following methods:

(1) Such door openings shall be protected by a swinging door providing a clear width of not less than 32 in. (810 mm).
(2) Such door openings shall be protected by a horizontal-sliding door that complies with 7.2.1.14 and provides a clear width of not less than 32 in. (810 mm).
(3) Such door openings shall be protected by an existing 34 in. (865 mm) swinging door.

Special recognition is given to horizontal travel and the use of horizontal exits in health care facilities because of practical difficulties involving vertical egress travel, such as on stairways. Horizontal exits are permitted to provide up to two-thirds of the total required egress capacity for a given fire area — an extension of the one-half of total egress capacity limitation of 7.2.4.1.2. Every floor and every fire section must have at least one exit consisting of a door leading directly outside the building, an interior stair, an outside stair, a smokeproof enclosure, a ramp, or an exit passageway (see 18/19.2.4.3). No fire area can be served by horizontal exits only (see 18/19.2.2.5.2). In the event a horizontal exit also serves as a smoke barrier, see the commentary following A.18/19.2.4.3, and also see 18/19.3.7.

The requirements for horizontal exits in 18/19.2.2.5 are illustrated in Exhibit 18/19.3 through Exhibit 18/19.5.

Doors in new horizontal exits are required to swing in the direction of egress travel. In the case of a fire barrier that serves as a new horizontal exit for two adjoining fire areas, a pair of doors arranged with each leaf to swing in a direction opposite from the other, or some equivalent arrangement, must be used. If a fire barrier serves as a horizontal exit from only one fire

CHAPTER 18 • New

CHAPTER 19 • Existing

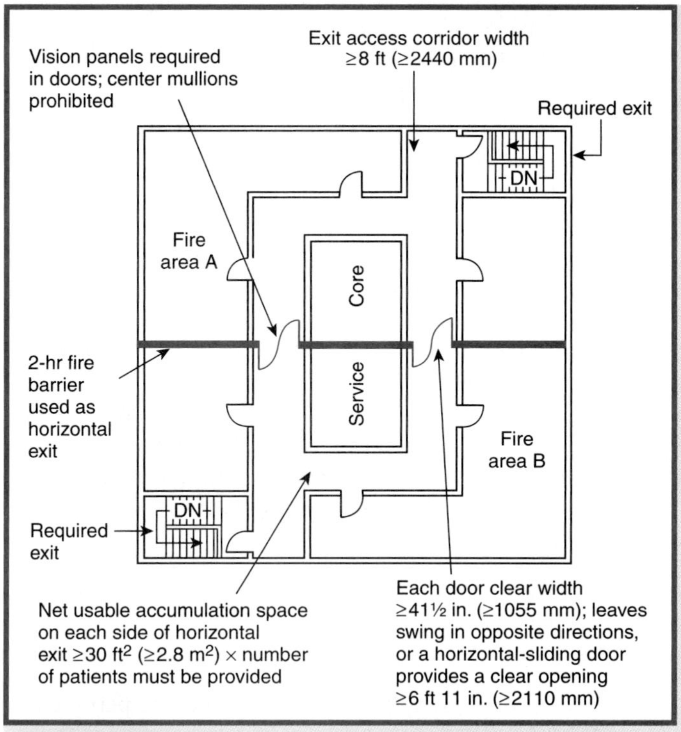


***Exhibit 18/19.3*** *Horizontal exit in a new general hospital or nursing home.*

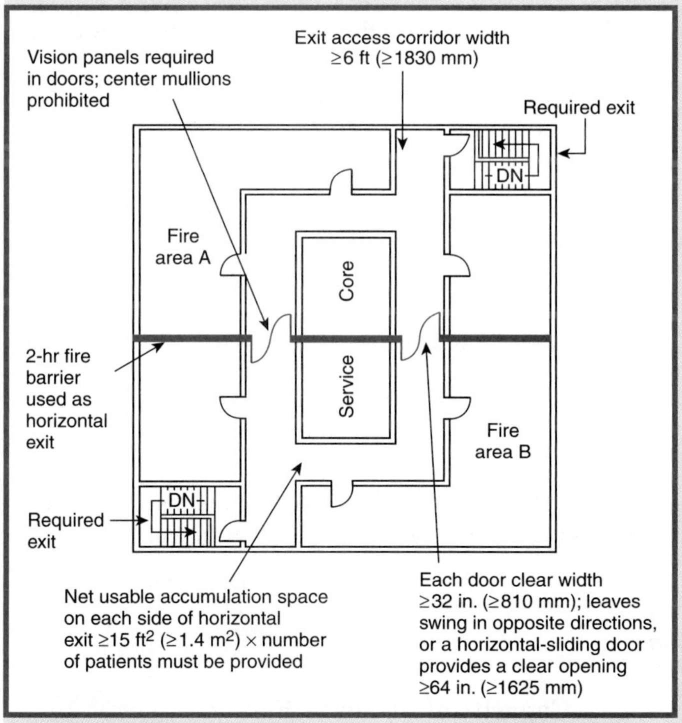


***Exhibit 18/19.4*** *Horizontal exit in a new limited care facility or psychiatric hospital.*

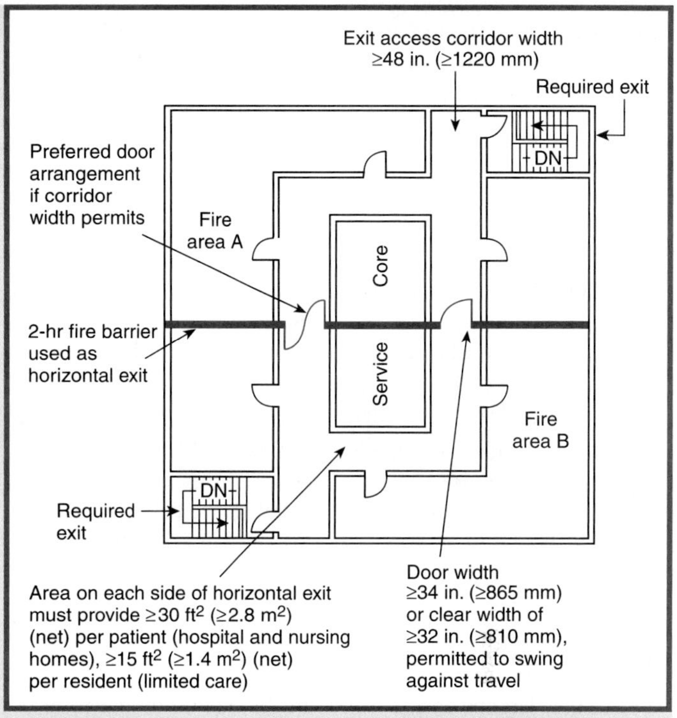


***Exhibit 18/19.5*** *Horizontal exit in an existing health care occupancy.*

area, the door opening is permitted to be protected by a single door providing 41½ in. (1055 mm) clear width in new hospitals and nursing homes or 32 in. (810 mm) clear width in new limited care facilities. See Exhibit 18/19.3.

The *Code* recognizes the use of sliding doors complying with 7.2.1.14 for the protection of openings in horizontal exits. The use of power-operated sliding doors results in an obstruction-free opening for normal traffic while providing adequate fire protection for openings under fire emergency conditions.

Corridors in new limited care facilities and new psychiatric hospitals are required to be 6 ft (1830 mm) wide; therefore, it would not be practical to install a pair of 41½ in. (1055 mm) clear width doors to protect corridor openings in a horizontal exit. Recognizing this practical consideration and that no obstructions, such as mullions mounted at the center of a two-door opening, are permitted, doors protecting openings in horizontal exits of such facilities are required to provide a minimum 32 in. (810 mm) clear width. See Exhibit 18/19.4.

Prohibiting center mullions in new construction provides one, large, usable door opening where two

CHAPTER 18 • New

doors are positioned within a door frame and eliminates any obstructions that would restrict the movement of patients in beds, in wheelchairs, or on gurneys.

The *Code* permits corridors in existing health care occupancies to be 48 in. (1220 mm) wide, and it is, therefore, impractical in many instances to install a pair of cross-corridor doors in a horizontal exit. However, the 48 in. (1220 mm) corridor width will allow the opening of a single door against the flow of travel with minimal difficulty. A power-operated sliding door might be used to reduce problems associated with door swing. The *Code* permits sliding doors complying with 7.2.1.14 for the protection of openings in horizontal exits. The use of power-operated sliding doors results in an obstruction-free opening for normal traffic while still providing adequate fire protection for openings.

In the case of an existing fire barrier serving as a horizontal exit for two adjoining fire areas, and where corridor widths will allow, a pair of doors arranged with each leaf to swing in a direction opposite from the other should be used. Each leaf in the pair of doors must either be a minimum of 34 in. (865 mm) wide or provide a clear opening of 32 in. (810 mm). See Exhibit 18/19.5.

New horizontal exits installed in an existing facility are subject to the rehabilitation provisions of Chapter 43. The category of rehabilitation work associated with the addition of a door is classified as modification in accordance with 43.2.2.1.3. Per 43.5.1.3, the newly constructed element must comply with the requirements applicable to new construction. Thus, the new horizontal exit door must be installed in accordance with Chapter 18.

**18.2.2.6 Ramps.**

**18.2.2.6.1** Ramps complying with 7.2.5 shall be permitted.

**18.2.2.6.2** Ramps enclosed as exits shall be of sufficient width to provide egress capacity in accordance with 18.2.3.

CHAPTER 19 • Existing

**19.2.2.6 Ramps.**

**19.2.2.6.1** Ramps complying with 7.2.5 shall be permitted.

**19.2.2.6.2** Ramps enclosed as exits shall be of sufficient width to provide egress capacity in accordance with 19.2.3.

Ramps with a slope minimally graduated so as not to be dangerous for use in both normal and emergency traffic require so much space that they would be impracticable in most situations. They are, however, the only practicable method of moving bedridden patients from one story to another, except by elevators, which may not be available during fire conditions. The best plan is to provide for horizontal egress to another smoke compartment on the same floor, minimizing the need for complete evacuation.

Ramps might be the best means for providing egress from doors two or three steps above or below grade level (see 7.1.7) and might compensate for minor differences in floor levels between adjoining sections of buildings. Such ramps must be constructed in accordance with 18/19.2.2.6 and 7.2.5.

CHAPTER 18 • New

**18.2.2.7 Exit Passageways.** Exit passageways complying with 7.2.6 shall be permitted.

**18.2.2.8 Fire Escape Ladders.** Fire escape ladders complying with 7.2.9 shall be permitted.

**18.2.2.9 Alternating Tread Devices.** Alternating tread devices complying with 7.2.11 shall be permitted.

**18.2.2.10 Areas of Refuge.** Areas of refuge used as part of a required accessible means of egress shall comply with 7.2.12.

## 18.2.3 Capacity of Means of Egress.

**18.2.3.1** The capacity of means of egress shall be in accordance with Section 7.3.

CHAPTER 19 • Existing

**19.2.2.7 Exit Passageways.** Exit passageways complying with 7.2.6 shall be permitted.

**19.2.2.8 Fire Escape Ladders.** Fire escape ladders complying with 7.2.9 shall be permitted.

**19.2.2.9 Alternating Tread Devices.** Alternating tread devices complying with 7.2.11 shall be permitted.

**19.2.2.10 Areas of Refuge.** Areas of refuge used as part of a required accessible means of egress shall comply with 7.2.12.

## 19.2.3 Capacity of Means of Egress.

**19.2.3.1** The capacity of means of egress shall be in accordance with Section 7.3.

CHAPTER 18 • New

**18.2.3.2 Reserved.**

**18.2.3.3 Reserved.**

**18.2.3.4*** Aisles, corridors, and ramps required for exit access in a hospital or nursing home shall be not less than 8 ft (2440 mm) in clear and unobstructed width, unless otherwise permitted by the following:

(1)* Aisles, corridors, and ramps in adjunct areas not intended for the housing, treatment, or use of inpatients shall be not less than 44 in. (1120 mm) in clear and unobstructed width.

**A.18.2.3.4(1)** Occupant characteristics are an important factor to be evaluated in setting egress criteria. Egress components in nonpatient use areas, such as administrative office spaces, should be evaluated based on actual use. A clear corridor width of not less than 44 in. (1120 mm) is specified, assuming occupants in nonpatient areas will be mobile and capable of evacuation without assistance.

(2) Where the corridor width is at least 6 ft (1830 mm), projections not more than 6 in. (150 mm) from the corridor wall, above the handrail height, shall be permitted for the installation of hand-rub dispensing units in accordance with 18.3.2.6.
(3) Where the corridor width is at least 6 ft (1830 mm), projections shall be permitted in corridors, at both sides of the corridor, as follows:
   (a) Each projection shall not exceed a depth of 6 in. (150 mm).
   (b) Each projection shall not exceed a length of 36 in. (915 mm).
   (c) Each projection shall be positioned not less than 40 in. (1015 mm) above the floor.
   (d) Each projection shall have not less than 48 in. (1220 mm) horizontal separation from adjacent projections.
(4)* Exit access within a room or suite of rooms complying with the requirements of 18.2.5 shall be permitted.

**A.18.2.3.4(4)** Exit access should be arranged to avoid any obstructions to the convenient removal of nonambulatory

CHAPTER 19 • Existing

**19.2.3.2** The capacity of means of egress providing travel by means of stairs shall be 0.6 in. (15 mm) per person, and the capacity of means of egress providing horizontal travel (without stairs) by means such as doors, ramps, or horizontal exits shall be $^1/_2$ in. (13 mm) per person, unless otherwise permitted by 19.2.3.3.

**19.2.3.3** The capacity of means of egress in health care occupancies protected throughout by an approved, supervised automatic sprinkler system in accordance with 19.3.5.7 shall be 0.3 in. (7.6 mm) per person for travel by means of stairs and 0.2 in. (5 mm) per person for horizontal travel without stairs.

**19.2.3.4*** Any required aisle, corridor, or ramp shall be not less than 48 in. (1220 mm) in clear width where serving as means of egress from patient sleeping rooms, unless otherwise permitted by the following:

(1) Aisles, corridors, and ramps in adjunct areas not intended for the housing, treatment, or use of inpatients shall be not less than 44 in. (1120 mm) in clear and unobstructed width.
(2) Where corridor width is at least 6 ft (1830 mm), projections not more than 6 in. (150 mm) from the corridor wall, above the handrail height, shall be permitted for the installation of hand-rub dispensing units in accordance with 19.3.2.6.
(3) Where the corridor width is at least 6 ft (1830 mm), projections shall be permitted in corridors, at both sides of the corridor, as follows:
   (a) Each projection shall not exceed a depth of 6 in. (150 mm).
   (b) Each projection shall not exceed a length of 36 in. (915 mm).
   (c) Each projection shall be positioned not less than 40 in. (1015 mm) above the floor.
   (d) Each projection shall have not less than 48 in. (1220 mm) horizontal separation from adjacent projections.
(4) Exit access within a room or suite of rooms complying with the requirements of 19.2.5 shall be permitted.

CHAPTER 18 • New

persons carried on stretchers or on mattresses serving as stretchers.

**A.18.2.3.4** It is not the intent that the required corridor width be maintained clear and unobstructed at all times. Projections into the required width are permitted by 7.3.2.2. It is not the intent that 18.2.3.4 supersede 7.3.2.2. Also, it is recognized that wheeled items in use (such as food service carts, housekeeping carts, gurneys, beds, and similar items) and wheeled crash carts not in use (because they need to be immediately accessible during a clinical emergency) are encountered in health care occupancy corridors. The health care occupancy's fire plan and training program should address the relocation of these items during a fire. Note that "not in use" is not the same as "in storage." Storage is not permitted to be open to the corridor, unless it meets one of the provisions permitted by 18.3.6.1 and is not a hazardous area.

**18.2.3.5** Aisles, corridors, and ramps required for exit access in a limited care facility or hospital for psychiatric care shall be not less than 6 ft (1830 mm) in clear and unobstructed width, unless otherwise permitted by the following:

(1)* Aisles, corridors, and ramps in adjunct areas not intended for the housing, treatment, or use of inpatients shall be not less than 44 in. (1120 mm) in clear and unobstructed width.

**A.18.2.3.5(1)** See A.18.2.3.4(1).

(2) Where the corridor width is at least 6 ft (1830 mm), projections not more than 6 in. (150 mm) from the corridor wall, above the handrail height, shall be permitted for the installation of hand-rub dispensing units in accordance with 18.3.2.6.
(3) Where the corridor width is at least 6 ft (1830 mm), projections shall be permitted in corridors, at both sides of the corridor, as follows:
   (a) Each projection shall not exceed a depth of 6 in. (150 mm).
   (b) Each projection shall not exceed a length of 36 in. (915 mm).
   (c) Each projection shall be positioned not less than 40 in. (1015 mm) above the floor.
   (d) Each projection shall have not less than 48 in. (1220 mm) horizontal separation from adjacent projections.
(4)* Exit access within a room or suite of rooms complying with the requirements of 18.2.5 shall be permitted.

**A.18.2.3.5(4)** See A.18.2.3.4(4).

**18.2.3.6** The minimum clear width for doors in the means of egress from sleeping rooms; diagnostic and treatment

CHAPTER 19 • Existing

**A.19.2.3.4** It is not the intent that the required corridor width be maintained clear and unobstructed at all times. Projections into the required width are permitted by 7.3.2.2. It is not the intent that 19.2.3.4 supersede 7.3.2.2. Also, it is recognized that wheeled items in use (such as food service carts, housekeeping carts, gurneys, beds, and similar items) and wheeled crash carts not in use (because they need to be immediately accessible during a clinical emergency) are encountered in health care occupancy corridors. The health care occupancy's fire plan and training program should address the relocation of these items during a fire. Note that "not in use" is not the same as "in storage." Storage is not permitted to be open to the corridor, unless it meets one of the provisions permitted by 19.3.6.1 and is not a hazardous area.

**19.2.3.5** The aisle, corridor, or ramp shall be arranged to avoid any obstructions to the convenient removal of nonambulatory persons carried on stretchers or on mattresses serving as stretchers.

**19.2.3.6** The minimum clear width for doors in the means of egress from hospitals, nursing homes, limited care faciliareas, such as x-ray, surgery, or physical therapy; and nursery rooms shall be as follows:

(1) Hospitals and nursing homes — $41\frac{1}{2}$ in. (1055 mm)
(2) Psychiatric hospitals and limited care facilities — 32 in. (810 mm)

**18.2.3.7** The requirements of 18.2.3.6 shall not apply where otherwise permitted by the following:

(1) Doors that are located so as not to be subject to use by any health care occupant shall be not less than 32 in. (810 mm) in clear width.
(2) Doors in exit stair enclosures shall be not less than 32 in. (810 mm) in clear width.
(3) Doors serving newborn nurseries shall be not less than 32 in. (810 mm) in clear width.
(4) Where a pair of doors is provided, the following criteria shall be met:
    (a) Not less than one of the doors shall provide not less than a 32 in. (810 mm) clear width opening.
    (b) A rabbet, bevel, or astragal shall be provided at the meeting edge.
    (c) The inactive door leaf shall have an automatic flush bolt to provide positive latching.



ties, psychiatric hospital sleeping rooms, and diagnostic and treatment areas, such as x-ray, surgery, or physical therapy, shall be not less than 32 in. (810 mm) wide.

**19.2.3.7** The requirement of 19.2.3.6 shall not apply where otherwise permitted by the following:

(1) Existing 34 in. (865 mm) doors shall be permitted.
(2) Existing 28 in. (710 mm) corridor doors in facilities where the fire plans do not require evacuation by bed, gurney, or wheelchair shall be permitted.

The method used in calculating egress capacity acknowledges that increasing the width of egress systems results in increasing the occupant flow through that system. The provisions of 19.2.3.2 and 19.2.3.3 (as well as the reference 18.2.3.1 makes to Section 7.3) compute stair egress capacity in sprinklered health care occupancies on the basis of 0.3 in. (7.6 mm) per person. Therefore, a 44 in. (1120 mm) stair provides egress capacity for 146 persons [44 in./0.3 in. per person (1120 mm/7.6 mm per person) = 146 persons]. Similarly, a 50 in. (1270 mm) stair provides capacity for 167 persons. In nonsprinklered existing health care occupancies, stair egress capacity is computed on the basis of 0.6 in. (15 mm) per person. The capacity of level surfaces and doors in fully sprinklered health care occupancy smoke compartments is computed on the basis of 0.2 in. (5 mm) per person, and on 0.5 in. (13 mm) per person in nonsprinklered existing health care occupancy smoke compartments. Egress capacity calculations must use clear width as specified in 7.2.1.2.

In earlier editions of the *Code*, egress capacity for health care occupancies was calculated using more conservative egress capacity factors. For example, stair capacity for nonsprinklered health care occupancies was calculated on the basis of 1 in. (25 mm) per person, rather than the current factor of 0.3 in. (7.6 mm) per person, based on the belief that extra width was needed to create space that could serve as a refuge area. The capacity of health care egress system components was set conservatively in recognition of the slow rate of travel for patients and the fact that space was needed for patients on litters and in wheelchairs.

Recent editions of the *Code* use a different concept for egress system design in health care occupancies. Life safety from fire in health care facilities relies on a defend-in-place principle. Horizontal exits or smoke barriers are used to subdivide each story to provide an area of refuge on each story without requiring travel by means of stairs. Flow rates for exits (capacity) are established on the assumption that able-bodied staff, visitors, and ambulatory patients will principally use exit stairs for emergency evacuation. Nonambulatory patients will remain in the building, and those on the floor of fire origin will be moved horizontally to an area of refuge. The defend-in-place principle is complemented by the requirement that all new health care facilities be fully protected by automatic sprinklers.

Corridor width is addressed in 18/19.2.3.4 and 18.2.3.5. Exit access corridors in new hospitals and nursing homes are required to be at least 8 ft (2440 mm) in clear width, based on the assumption that, during a fire emergency, some patients might require movement on litters or in wheelchairs. Also, multiple files of persons should be able to use the corridor at one time, with those who move more quickly passing those who move more slowly. Exit access corridors in existing health care occupancies are required to be at least 48 in. (1220 mm) in clear width. This specified minimum leaves little safety margin. Care is necessary to prevent carts, furnishings, and other materials from obstructing or interfering with potential occupant movement. In both new and existing facilities, a minimum corridor width of 44 in. (1120 mm) is considered acceptable within areas not subject to use by inpatients, such as administrative office spaces, where occupants are assumed to be mobile and capable of evacuation without assistance.

Exhibit 18/19.6 and Exhibit 18/19.7 illustrate the minimum clear width requirements of 18/19.2.3.4 and 18.2.3.5. For new limited care facilities and psychiatric hospitals, which, by definition, involve patients who are more ambulatory than those in general hospitals

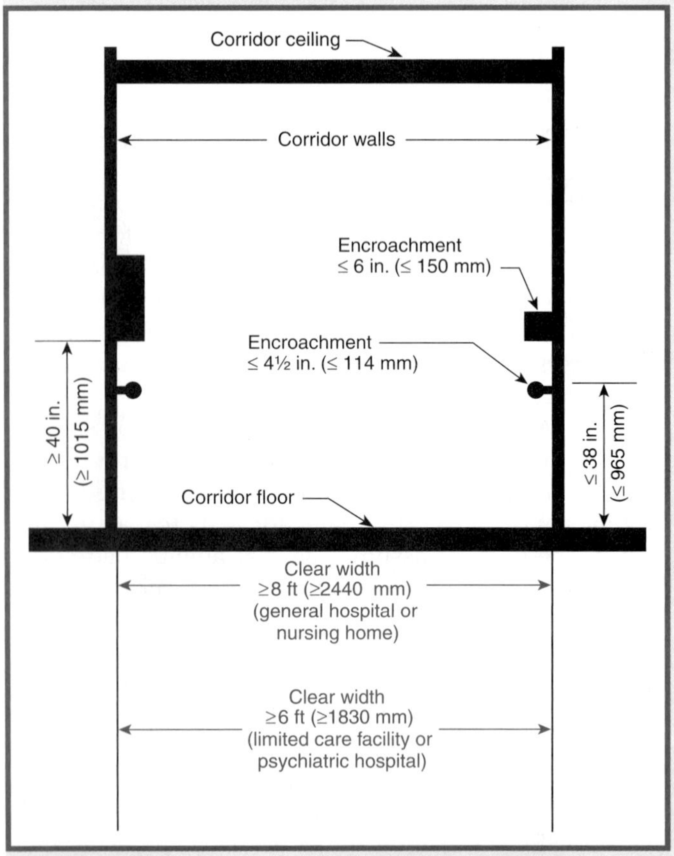


***Exhibit 18/19.6*** *Exit access corridor in new health care facility.*

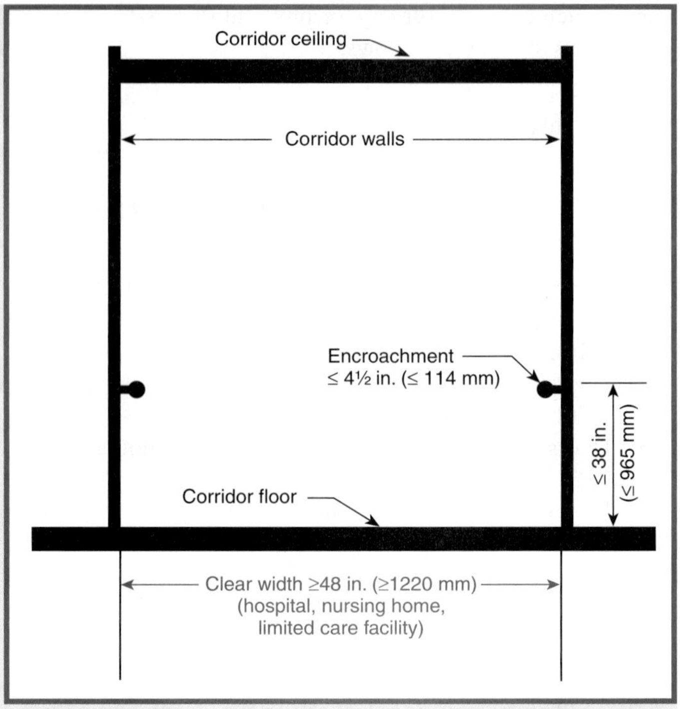


***Exhibit 18/19.7*** *Exit access corridor in existing health care facility.*

and nursing homes, the required corridor width is 6 ft (1830 mm), as opposed to the minimum 8 ft (2440 mm) in new general hospitals and nursing homes.

The actual corridor width is permitted to be considered as the clear width if handrail encroachment does not exceed $4\frac{1}{2}$ in. (114 mm) on each side of the corridor (see 7.3.2.2).

The provisions of 18/19.2.3.4(2) and (3) and 18.2.3.5(2) and (3) were new to the 2006 edition of the *Code*. Provided that the corridor is at least 6 ft (1830 mm) wide, additional encroachments are permitted without having to consider the clear width to be anything less than the actual width. The projections permitted by 18/19.2.3.4(2) and 18.2.3.5(2) are for the installation of hand-rub solution dispensing units as further addressed in 18/19.3.2.6. The projections permitted by 18/19.2.3.4(3) and 18.2.3.5(3) are for unspecified items meeting the criteria of 18/19.2.3.4(3) (a) through 18/19.2.3.4(3) (d) and 18.2.3.5(3) (a) through 18.2.3.5(3) (d). Such projections might be for the installation of charting stations, flat-panel information screens, disposal units for sharps, surface-mounted lighting fixtures, or artwork. Exhibit 18/19.8 illustrates the mounting height, spacing, and projection limita-

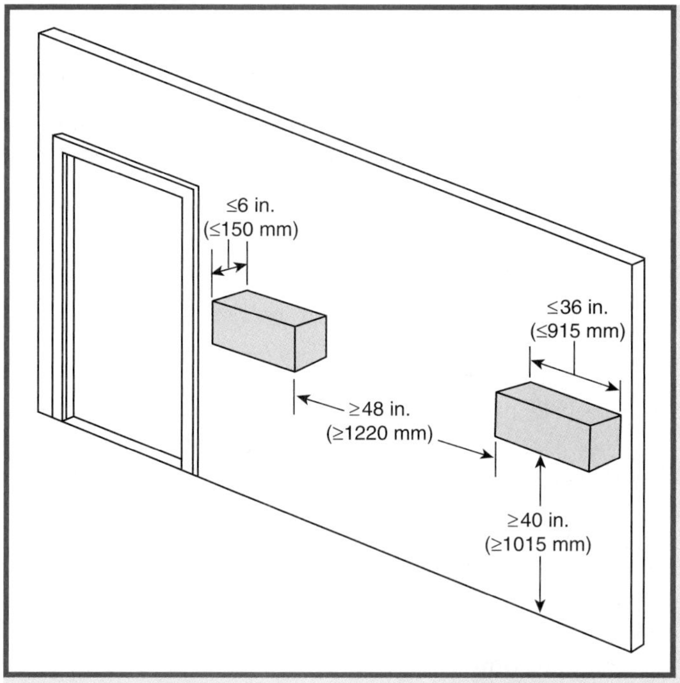


***Exhibit 18/19.8*** *Permitted corridor projections.*

tions for the projections permitted by 18/19.2.3.4(3) and 18.2.3.5(3).

In editions of the *Code* prior to 1994, numerous health care occupancy provisions specified minimum requirements for door widths as a leaf width rather than as a clear width. For example, new doors from patient rooms to the corridor were required to be 44 in. (1120 mm) wide; existing doors were required to be 34 in. (865 mm) wide. The intent was that, after allowing for the stops built into the door frame and for the thickness of the protruding hinge stile edge, a 44 in. (1120 mm) wide door leaf would provide approximately $41\frac{1}{2}$ in. (1055 mm) of clear, unobstructed width; a 34 in. (865 mm) wide door leaf would provide approximately 32 in. (810 mm) of clear, unobstructed width. However, there was no requirement for the door to swing a minimum of 90 degrees from the plane of the door opening, so the intended clear, unobstructed width was not ensured. Since the 1994 edition, minimum door width requirements for health care occupancies have been specified as clear, unobstructed width; exemptions continue to recognize existing doors with the minimum door leaf widths previously specified. Exhibit 18/19.9 illustrates door leaf measurement, rather than clear opening measurement, as permitted by 19.2.3.7(1). Paragraph 19.2.2.5.4(3), applicable to horizontal exit doors, and 19.3.7.10, applicable to smoke barrier doors, also permit existing doors to provide the minimum required width via a door leaf measurement.

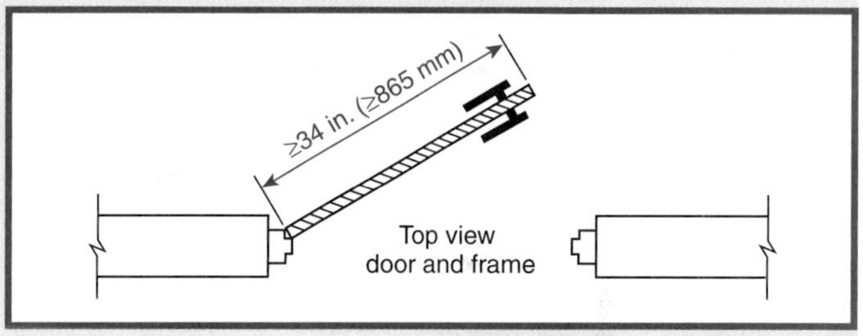


***Exhibit 18/19.9*** *Minimum door (leaf) width measurement for existing doors.*

### 18.2.4 Number of Exits.

**18.2.4.1** Not less than two exits shall be provided on every story.

**18.2.4.2** Not less than two separate exits shall be accessible from every part of every story.

**18.2.4.3*** Not less than two exits shall be accessible from each smoke compartment, and egress shall be permitted through an adjacent compartment(s) but shall not require return through the compartment of fire origin.

**A.18.2.4.3** An exit is not necessary for each individual smoke compartment if there is access to an exit through other smoke compartments without passing through the smoke compartment of fire origin.

### 19.2.4 Number of Exits.

**19.2.4.1** Not less than two exits shall be provided on every story.

**19.2.4.2** Not less than two separate exits shall be accessible from every part of every story.

**19.2.4.3*** Not less than two exits shall be accessible from each smoke compartment, and egress shall be permitted through an adjacent compartment(s) but shall not require return through the compartment of fire origin.

**A.19.2.4.3** An exit is not necessary for each individual smoke compartment if there is access to an exit through other smoke compartments without passing through the smoke compartment of fire origin.

Exhibit 18/19.10 can be used to illustrate the application of 18/19.2.4.1 and 18/19.2.4.2. The four exits depicted (i.e., exit stair 1, exit stair 2, horizontal exit 1, and horizontal exit 2) meet the requirement of 18/19.2.4.1 that not less than two exits be provided on the story. Occupants of all areas on the story have access to not less than two separate exits as required by 18/19.2.4.2. For example, occupants of area A have access to exit stair 1 and horizontal exit 1. If horizontal exit 1 were replaced by a wall with no door openings, occupants of area A would have access to only one exit in violation of the requirement of 18/19.2.4.2.

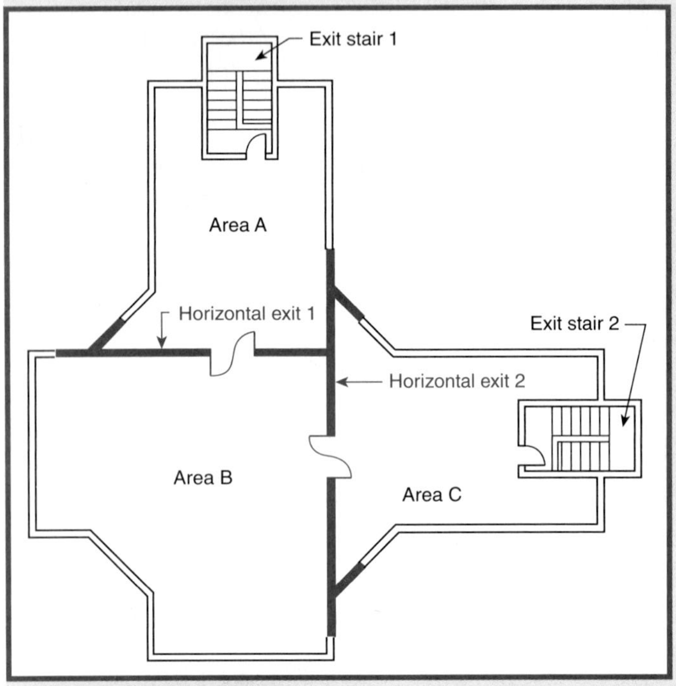


***Exhibit 18/19.10** Minimum of two exits accessible from all parts of floor.*

Horizontal exits 1 and 2 divide the floor into three fire compartments, areas A, B, and C. An enclosed exit stair (i.e., an exit other than a horizontal exit) is provided from areas A and C; area B is provided with two horizontal exits. Paragraph 18/19.2.4.2 requires that area B must be provided with at least one exit other than a horizontal exit. Area B is deficient in that it has no exit other than horizontal exits. Without this additional exit, area B is required by 18/19.2.4.3 to be considered part of one of the adjoining areas — either part of an enlarged area A, in which case horizontal exit 1 would receive no credit for providing egress capacity, or part of an enlarged area C, in which case horizontal exit 2 would receive no credit for providing egress capacity.

Exhibit 18/19.11 can be used to illustrate the application of 18/19.2.4.3. Smoke barrier 1 and smoke barrier 2 divide the floor into three smoke compartments — area A, area B, and area C. Access to two exits is provided from each smoke compartment. For area A, exit stair 1 provides access to one exit, and traveling through smoke barrier 1 into area B provides access to the second exit, exit stair 2. For area B, exit stair 2 provides access to one exit, and traveling through smoke barrier 1 into area A provides access to the second exit, exit stair 1. For area C, the two remotely located pairs of doors in smoke barrier 2 provide access to exit stair 1 in area A and exit stair 2 in area B, but passage into area B is required. Area C is deficient in that both of its exit accesses require passage into area B, which might be the smoke compartment of fire origin. To satisfy the provision of 18/19.2.4.3 — that egress not require return through the smoke compartment of fire origin — either an exit stair can be added to area C, or the door at Z can be relocated to position XX.

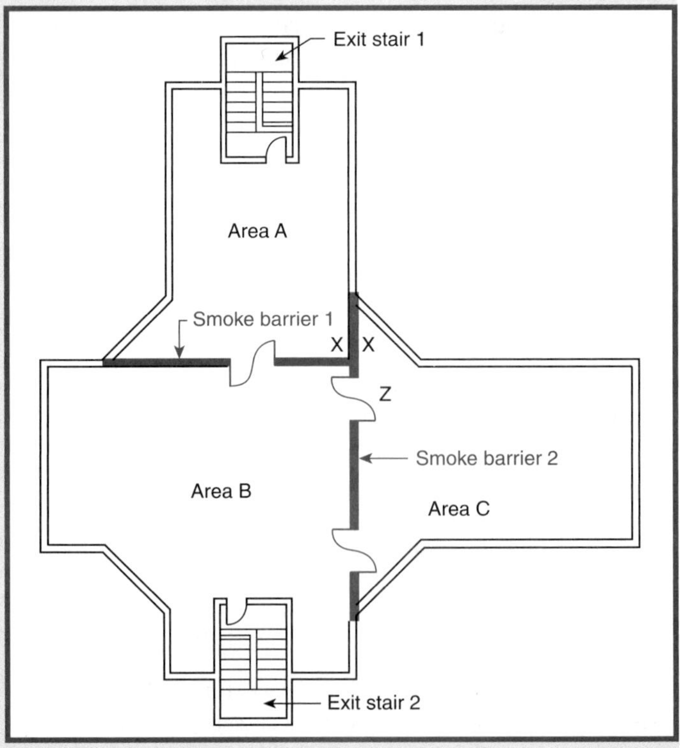


***Exhibit 18/19.11** Arrangement of exits for smoke compartments formed by smoke barriers.*

**CHAPTER 18 • New**

### 18.2.5 Arrangement of Means of Egress.

**18.2.5.1 General.** Arrangement of means of egress shall comply with Section 7.5.

**18.2.5.2 Dead-End Corridors.** Dead-end corridors shall not exceed 30 ft (9.1 m).

**18.2.5.3 Common Path of Travel.** Common path of travel shall not exceed 100 ft (30 m).

**CHAPTER 19 • Existing**

### 19.2.5 Arrangement of Means of Egress.

**19.2.5.1 General.** Arrangement of means of egress shall comply with Section 7.5.

**19.2.5.2* Dead-End Corridors.** Existing dead-end corridors not exceeding 30 ft (9.1 m) shall be permitted. Existing dead-end corridors exceeding 30 ft (9.1 m) shall be permitted to continue in use if it is impractical and unfeasible to alter them.

**A.19.2.5.2** Every exit or exit access should be arranged, if practical and feasible, so that no corridor has a dead end exceeding 30 ft (9.1 m).

**19.2.5.3 Reserved.**

An existing dead-end corridor, in excess of 30 ft (9.1 m), is permitted to remain in use if it is impractical and unfeasible to alter it. Exhibit 18/19.12 illustrates the maximum 30 ft (9.1 m) dead-end corridor limitation imposed by 18.2.5.2 and the maximum 100 ft (30 m) common path of travel limitation imposed by 18.2.5.3 on new construction in health care occupancies. The common path of travel limitation is new to the 2009 edition of the *Code* and was not made retroactive to existing common path of travel arrangements. However, existing common path of travel arrangements continue to be addressed indirectly by the requirements of 19.2.5.5, which require a room to be provided with a second exit access door where the room exceeds 1000 ft² (230 m²) and is used for sleeping or the room exceeds 2500 ft² (230 m²) and is not used for sleeping.

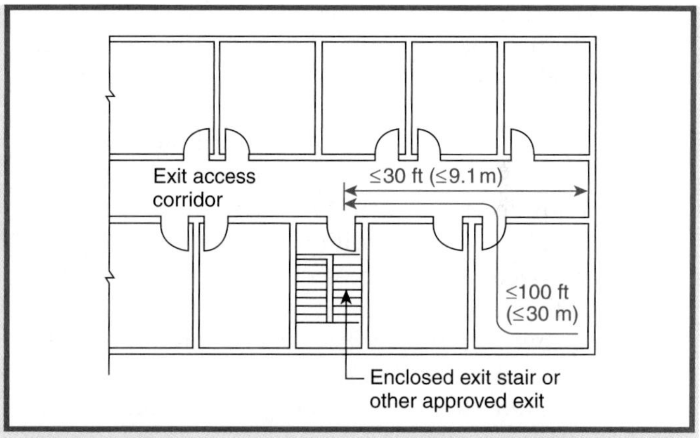


***Exhibit 18/19.12*** *Dead-end corridor and common path of travel limitations in a new health care occupancy.*

**18.2.5.4* Intervening Rooms or Spaces.** Every corridor shall provide access to not less than two approved exits in accordance with Sections 7.4 and 7.5 without passing through any intervening rooms or spaces other than corridors or lobbies.

**A.18.2.5.4** The term *intervening rooms or spaces* means rooms or spaces serving as a part of the required means of egress from another room.

**19.2.5.4* Intervening Rooms or Spaces.** Every corridor shall provide access to not less than two approved exits in accordance with Sections 7.4 and 7.5 without passing through any intervening rooms or spaces other than corridors or lobbies.

**A.19.2.5.4** The term *intervening rooms or spaces* means rooms or spaces serving as a part of the required means of egress from another room.

Paragraph 18/19.2.5.4 specifically prohibits an exit access arrangement that takes an occupant into a corridor and then requires passage through an occupiable space, such as another patient sleeping or treatment room, to gain access to a required exit. Once an occupant reaches the exit access corridor, that corridor is thought to be a safer portion of the exit access than an occupiable room because of the features required by 18/19.3.6. The occupant must be able to reach an exit without having to leave the safety provided by the corridor.

The requirement of 18/19.2.5.4 is commonly violated in existing buildings that lose general access to an exit following a building rehabilitation project in which the end of a wing is turned into a suite. Prior to the creation of the suite, the existing exit stair enclosure located at the end of the wing was accessible to all occupants of the floor via the corridor running the length of the floor. After the rehabilitation, the exit stair is located within the suite and only the occupants of the suite are credited with having access to the exit. The occupants outside the suite would have to enter the suite to access the exit stair in violation of the provision of 18/19.2.5.4.

CHAPTER 18 • New

### 18.2.5.5 Two Means of Egress.

**18.2.5.5.1** Sleeping rooms of more than 1000 $ft^2$ (93 $m^2$) shall have not less than two exit access doors remotely located from each other.

**18.2.5.5.2** Non-sleeping rooms of more than 2500 $ft^2$ (230 $m^2$) shall have not less than two exit access doors remotely located from each other.

CHAPTER 19 • Existing

### 19.2.5.5 Two Means of Egress.

**19.2.5.5.1** Sleeping rooms of more than 1000 $ft^2$ (93 $m^2$) shall have not less than two exit access doors remotely located from each other.

**19.2.5.5.2** Non-sleeping rooms of more than 2500 $ft^2$ (230 $m^2$) shall have not less than two exit access doors remotely located from each other.

The provision of 18/19.2.5.5.1 requires a second exit access door from any sleeping room that exceeds 1000 $ft^2$ (93 $m^2$). The provision of 18/19.2.5.5.2 requires a second exit access door from any non-sleeping room that exceeds 2500 $ft^2$ (230 $m^2$). The provision of 18/19.2.5.5.2 appears to be new to the 2009 edition of the *Code* but was a requirement for many editions prior to 2006. The provisions of 18/19.2.5 were extensively rewritten for the 2006 edition to address suites as one aggregated set of provisions, and the earlier requirement was inadvertently positioned only with the suites requirements of 18/19.2.5.7. The addition of 18/19.2.5.5.2 to the 2009 edition reinstates the requirement for a second exit access door for any non-sleeping room that exceeds 2500 $ft^2$ (230 $m^2$).

The two exit access doors required by 18/19.2.5.5.1 and 18/19.2.5.5.2 are required to be remotely located from each other in accordance with 7.5.1.3. Paragraphs 7.5.1.3.2 and 7.5.1.3.3 address the one-half and one-third diagonal measurement criteria for other than existing situations (see 7.5.1.3.5). Exhibit 18/19.13 depicts a patient sleeping room in a new health care occupancy that exceeds the 1000 $ft^2$ (93 $m^2$) threshold and a non-sleeping room in a new health care occupancy that exceeds the 2500 $ft^2$ (230 $m^2$) threshold, so that each room requires a second exit access door. The two exit access doors must be separated by a distance, *d*, that is at least one-third the room diagonal measurement, *D*, because the new health care occupancy must be sprinklered. See 7.5.1.3.3.

The requirement for a second exit access door from the large area room is another way of addressing the concern on which common path of travel limitations are based. That concern is that a large area with only one exit access door might allow a fire near the door to grow to such a size that, by the time the room occupant approaches the door, it will no longer provide a tenable egress path. Any new common path of travel is regulated by 18.2.5.3 and 18.2.5.5. Any existing common path of travel is regulated by 19.2.5.5. See the commentary following 18/19.2.5.3.

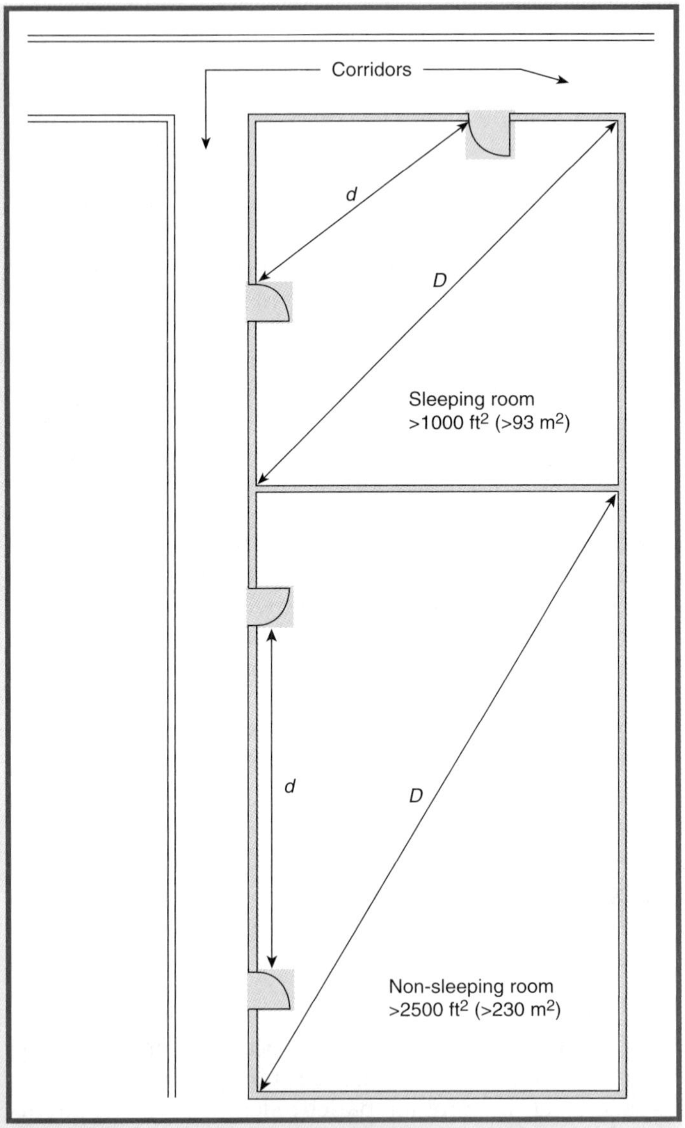


***Exhibit 18/19.13** Two exit access doors required for a sleeping room exceeding 1000 $ft^2$ (93 $m^2$) and a non-sleeping room exceeding 2500 $ft^2$ (230 $m^2$).*

CHAPTER 18 • New

18.2.5.6 Corridor Access.

**18.2.5.6.1*** Every habitable room shall have an exit access door leading directly to an exit access corridor, unless otherwise provided in 18.2.5.6.2, 18.2.5.6.3, and 18.2.5.6.4.

**A.18.2.5.6.1** For the purposes of this paragraph, it is the intent that "habitable rooms" not include individual bathrooms, closets, and similar spaces, as well as briefly occupied work spaces, such as control rooms in radiology and small storage rooms in a pharmacy.

**18.2.5.6.2** Exit access from a patient sleeping room with not more than eight patient beds shall be permitted to pass through one intervening room to reach an exit access corridor, provided that the intervening room is equipped with an approved automatic smoke detection system in accordance with Section 9.6.

**18.2.5.6.3** Rooms having an exit door opening directly to the outside from the room at the finished ground level shall not be required to have an exit access door leading directly to an exit access corridor.

**18.2.5.6.4** Rooms within suites complying with 18.2.5.7 shall not be required to have an exit access door leading directly to an exit access corridor.

CHAPTER 19 • Existing

19.2.5.6 Corridor Access.

**19.2.5.6.1*** Every habitable room shall have an exit access door leading directly to an exit access corridor, unless otherwise provided in 19.2.5.6.2, 19.2.5.6.3, and 19.2.5.6.4.

**A.19.2.5.6.1** For the purposes of this paragraph, it is the intent that "habitable rooms" not include individual bathrooms, closets, and similar spaces, as well as briefly occupied work spaces, such as control rooms in radiology and small storage rooms in a pharmacy.

**19.2.5.6.2** Exit access from a patient sleeping room with not more than eight patient beds shall be permitted to pass through one intervening room to reach an exit access corridor, provided that the intervening room is equipped with an approved automatic smoke detection system in accordance with Section 9.6, or the furnishings and furniture, in combination with all other combustibles within the area, are of such minimum quantity and arrangements that a fully developed fire is unlikely to occur.

**19.2.5.6.3** Rooms having an exit door opening directly to the outside from the room at the finished ground level shall not be required to have an exit access door leading directly to an exit access corridor.

**19.2.5.6.4** Rooms within suites complying with 19.2.5.7 shall not be required to have an exit access door leading directly to an exit access corridor.

The term *habitable room* is used in 18/19.2.5.6.1 in lieu of the term *patient sleeping room* to clarify that all occupied rooms in a health care facility must have direct access to a corridor leading to an exit (or must be arranged to comply with one of the exemptions).

Exhibit 18/19.14 illustrates the intent of 18/19.2.5.6. The intervening room is permitted between room A and the corridor, because room A has an exit door directly to the outside at ground level, as addressed in 18/19.2.5.6.3. The intervening room is permitted between sleeping room B and the corridor if it meets the maximum eight-bed exemption of 18/19.2.5.6.2, or if it complies with the sleeping suite provisions of 18/19.2.5.7.2. The intervening room is permitted between the examination room C and the corridor if it complies with the non-sleeping suite provisions of 18/19.2.5.7.3.

Exit access from a patient sleeping room to the corridor is permitted to pass through an intervening room in accordance with 18/19.2.5.6.2. See Exhibit 18/19.15. Locking hardware on the two doors in the path to the corridor is permitted only under the special conditions addressed by 18/19.2.2.2.2. If the maximum eight-bed patient room (including the intervening room) exceeds 1000 ft² (93 m²), a second exit access door, remote from the first, is required in accordance with 18/19.2.5.5.1.

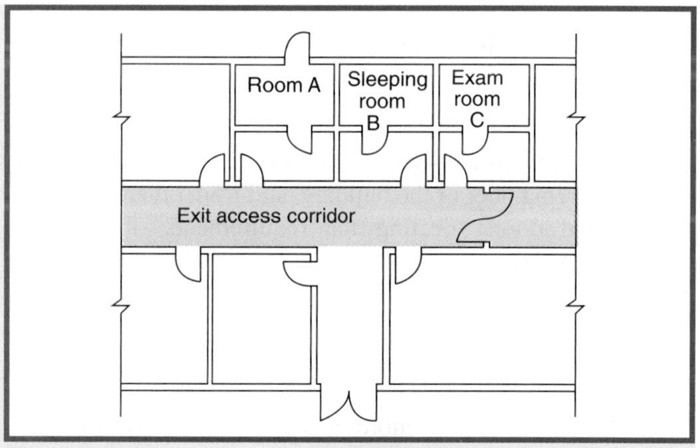


***Exhibit 18/19.14** Direct access to corridor from habitable rooms.*

CHAPTER 18 • New | CHAPTER 19 • Existing

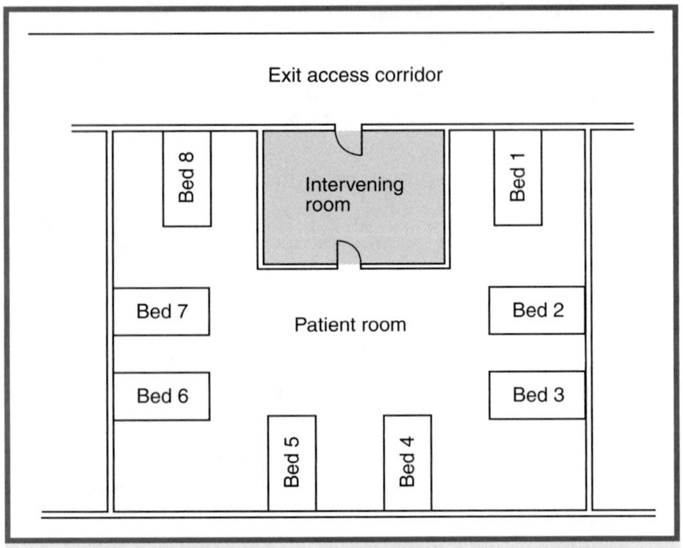


***Exhibit 18/19.15*** *Intervening room between maximum eight-bed patient sleeping room and corridor.*

**18.2.5.7 Suites.**

**19.2.5.7 Suites.**

In editions of the *Code* prior to 2006, the provisions for suites of rooms were dispersed as parts of subsections of Chapters 18 and 19. The suite provisions were extensively revised for the 2006 edition. The applicable criteria were revised, grouped, and formatted so as to appear as a complete package in 18/19.2.5.7. Paragraph 18/19.2.5.7.1 is general and applies to all suites; 18/19.2.5.7.2 addresses sleeping suites; and 18/19.2.5.7.3 covers non-sleeping suites.

**18.2.5.7.1 General.**

**18.2.5.7.1.1 Suite Permission.** Suites complying with 18.2.5.7 shall be permitted to be used to meet the corridor access requirements of 18.2.5.6.

**18.2.5.7.1.2* Suite Separation.** Suites shall be separated from the remainder of the building, and from other suites, by walls and doors meeting the requirements of 18.3.6.2 through 18.3.6.5.

**A.18.2.5.7.1.2** Two or more contiguous suites with an aggregate area not exceeding the suite size limitations of 18.2.5.7.2.3 and 18.2.5.7.3.3 are permitted to be considered a single suite, so as not to require separation from each other.

**19.2.5.7.1 General.**

**19.2.5.7.1.1 Suite Permission.** Suites complying with 19.2.5.7 shall be permitted to be used to meet the corridor access requirements of 19.2.5.6.

**19.2.5.7.1.2* Suite Separation.** Suites shall be separated from the remainder of the building, and from other suites, by one of the following:

(1) Walls and doors meeting the requirements of 19.3.6.2 through 19.3.6.5
(2) Existing approved barriers and doors that limit the transfer of smoke

**A.19.2.5.7.1.2** Two or more contiguous suites with an aggregate area not exceeding the suite size limitation of 19.2.5.7.2.3 and 19.2.5.7.3.3 are permitted to be considered a single suite, so as not to require separation from each other. The intent of 19.2.5.7.1.2(2) is to continue to permit suites that have smoke-resisting walls separating them from the rest of the building, even though the walls might not have a fire resistance rating. This requirement includes walls that comply with 19.3.6.2.4, even though sprinkler protection is not provided.

CHAPTER 18 • New

**18.2.5.7.1.3 Suite Hazardous Contents Areas.**

**(A)*** Intervening rooms shall not be hazardous areas as defined by 18.3.2.

**A.18.2.5.7.1.3(A)** The term *intervening room* means a room serving as a part of the required means of egress from another room.

**(B)** Hazardous areas within a suite shall be separated from the remainder of the suite in accordance with 18.3.2.1, unless otherwise provided in 18.2.5.7.1.3(C).

**(C)*** Hazardous areas within a suite shall not be required to be separated from the remainder of the suite where complying with all of the following:

(1) The suite is primarily a hazardous area.
(2) The suite is protected by an approved automatic smoke detection system in accordance with Section 9.6.
(3) The suite is separated from the rest of the health care facility as required for a hazardous area by 18.3.2.1.

**A.18.2.5.7.1.3(C)** Examples of suites that might be hazardous areas are medical records and pharmaceutical suites.

**18.2.5.7.1.4 Suite Subdivision.** The subdivision of suites shall be by means of noncombustible or limited-combustible partitions or partitions constructed with fire-retardant-treated wood enclosed with noncombustible or limited-combustible materials, and such partitions shall not be required to be fire rated.

CHAPTER 19 • Existing

**19.2.5.7.1.3 Suite Hazardous Contents Areas.**

**(A)*** Intervening rooms shall not be hazardous areas as defined by 19.3.2.

**A.19.2.5.7.1.3(A)** The term *intervening room* means a room serving as a part of the required means of egress from another room.

**(B)** Hazardous areas within a suite shall be separated from the remainder of the suite in accordance with 19.3.2.1, unless otherwise provided in 19.2.5.7.1.3(C) or 19.2.5.7.1.3(D).

**(C)*** Hazardous areas within a suite shall not be required to be separated from the remainder of the suite where complying with both of the following:

(1) The suite is primarily a hazardous area.
(2) The suite is separated from the rest of the health care facility as required for a hazardous area by 19.3.2.1.

**A.19.2.5.7.1.3(C)** Examples of suites that might be hazardous areas are medical records and pharmaceutical suites.

**(D)*** Spaces containing sterile surgical materials limited to a one-day supply in operating suites or similar spaces that are sprinklered in accordance with 19.3.5.7 shall be permitted to be open to the remainder of the suite without separation.

**A.19.2.5.7.1.3(D)** It is the intent that the provision of 19.2.5.7.1.3(D) apply only where the quantities of combustibles occupy an area exceeding 50 ft$^2$ (4.6 m$^2$) so as to be a hazardous contents area. Where quantities of combustibles occupy less than 50 ft$^2$ (4.6 m$^2$), there is no restriction on quantity.

**19.2.5.7.1.4 Suite Subdivision.** The subdivision of suites shall be by means of noncombustible or limited-combustible partitions or partitions constructed with fire-retardant-treated wood enclosed with noncombustible or limited-combustible materials, and such partitions shall not be required to be fire rated.

Suite A, as illustrated in Exhibit 18/19.16, is separated, in accordance with 18/19.2.5.7.1.2, from both the corridor and the abutting rooms (e.g., suite B and room C) by walls and doors meeting the corridor separation criteria of 18/19.3.6. Walls and partitions within the suite subdivide the space in accordance with 18/19.2.5.7.1.4. The storage room is classified as a hazardous area and is further isolated from the suite, the corridor, and the abutting suite in accordance with 18/19.3.2.1.

The suite provisions are widely used to create a grouping of rooms and spaces that functions effectively, because such suites are exempted from other *Code* provisions that might adversely affect the functional needs. For example, in Exhibit 18/19.16, the space used to access the open-front cubicles is

CHAPTER 18 • New

CHAPTER 19 • Existing

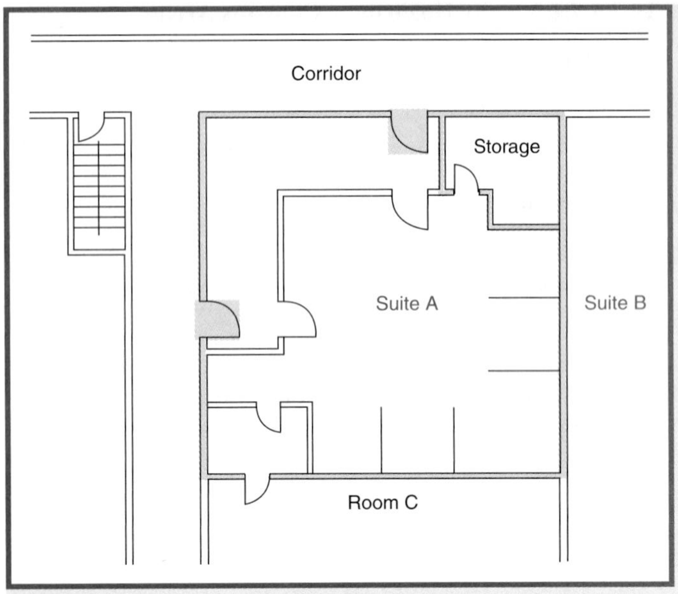


***Exhibit 18/19.16** Suite subdivision and separation in accordance with 18/19.2.5.7.1.*

considered to be circulation space and not a corridor. Therefore, the corridor provisions of 18/19.3.6 do not apply within the suite. Therefore, the cubicles can remain open to the suite circulation space without the need for walls and doors. The openness permitted by the suite provisions is needed for the functional purposes of patient monitoring and care.

**18.2.5.7.2 Sleeping Suites.** Sleeping suites shall be in accordance with the following:

(1) Sleeping suites for patient care shall comply with the provisions of 18.2.5.7.2.1 through 18.2.5.7.2.4.
(2) Sleeping suites not for patient care shall comply with the provisions of 18.2.5.7.4.

**18.2.5.7.2.1 Sleeping Suite Arrangement.**

**(A)*** Occupants of habitable rooms within sleeping suites shall have exit access to a corridor complying with 18.3.6 without having to pass through more than one intervening room.

**A.18.2.5.7.2.1(A)** For the purposes of this paragraph, it is the intent that "habitable rooms" not include individual bathrooms, closets, and similar spaces, as well as briefly occupied work spaces, such as control rooms in radiology and small storage rooms in a pharmacy. The term *intervening room* means a room serving as a part of the required means of egress from another room.

**(B)** Sleeping suites shall be provided with constant staff supervision within the suite.

**(C)** Sleeping suites shall be arranged in accordance with one of the following:

(1)* Patient sleeping rooms within sleeping suites shall provide one of the following:

(a) The patient sleeping rooms shall be arranged to allow for direct supervision from a normally at-

**19.2.5.7.2 Sleeping Suites.** Sleeping suites shall be in accordance with the following:

(1) Sleeping suites for patient care shall comply with the provisions of 19.2.5.7.2.1 through 19.2.5.7.2.4.
(2) Sleeping suites not for patient care shall comply with the provisions of 19.2.5.7.4.

**19.2.5.7.2.1 Sleeping Suite Arrangement.**

**(A)*** Occupants of habitable rooms within sleeping suites shall have exit access to a corridor complying with 19.3.6 without having to pass through more than one intervening room.

**A.19.2.5.7.2.1(A)** For the purposes of this paragraph, it is the intent that *habitable rooms* not include individual bathrooms, closets, and similar spaces, as well as briefly occupied work spaces, such as control rooms in radiology and small storage rooms in a pharmacy. The term *intervening room* means a room serving as a part of the required means of egress from another room.

**(B)** Sleeping suites shall be provided with constant staff supervision within the suite.

**(C)** Sleeping suites shall be arranged in accordance with one of the following:

(1)* Patient sleeping rooms within sleeping suites shall provide one of the following:

(a) The patient sleeping rooms shall be arranged to allow for direct supervision from a normally attended location within the suite, such as is provided by glass walls, and cubicle curtains shall be permitted.

(b) Any patient sleeping rooms without the direct supervision required by 18.2.5.7.2.1(C)(1)(a) shall be provided with smoke detection in accordance with Section 9.6 and 18.3.4.

**A.18.2.5.7.2.1(C)(1)** The interior partitions or walls might extend full height to the ceiling, provided that they do not obscure visual supervision of the suite. Where they do obscure visual supervision, see 18.2.5.7.2.1(C)(2).

(2) Sleeping suites shall be provided with a total coverage (complete) automatic smoke detection system in accordance with 9.6.2.9 and 18.3.4.

**18.2.5.7.2.2 Sleeping Suite Number of Means of Egress.**

**(A)** Sleeping suites of more than 1000 ft$^2$ (93 m$^2$) shall have not less than two exit access doors remotely located from each other.

**(B)*** One means of egress from the suite shall be directly to a corridor complying with 18.3.6.

**A.18.2.5.7.2.2(B)** Where only one means of egress is required from the suite, it needs to be provided by a door opening directly to a corridor complying with 18.3.6.

**(C)*** For suites requiring two means of egress, one means of egress from the suite shall be permitted to be into another suite, provided that the separation between the suites complies with the corridor requirements of 18.3.6.2 through 18.3.6.5.

**A.18.2.5.7.2.2(C)** Where the second exit access for a sleeping suite is through an adjacent suite, it is the intent that the 100 ft (30 m) travel distance limitation in the suite be applied only to the suite under consideration.

**18.2.5.7.2.3 Sleeping Suite Maximum Size.**

**(A)** Sleeping suites shall not exceed 5000 ft$^2$ (460 m$^2$), unless otherwise provided in 18.2.5.7.2.3(B).

**(B)** Sleeping suites greater than 5000 ft$^2$ (460 m$^2$) and not exceeding 7500 ft$^2$ (700 m$^2$) shall be permitted where both of the following are provided in the suite:

(1)* Direct visual supervision in accordance with 18.2.5.7.2.1(C)(1)(a)

**A.18.2.5.7.2.3(B)(1)** The alternative of 18.2.5.7.2.1(C)(1)(b) is not to be applied, since 18.2.5.7.2.3(B)(2) requires total coverage automatic smoke detection for the suite that exceeds 5000 ft$^2$ (460 m$^2$) but does not exceed 7500 ft$^2$ (700 m$^2$).



tended location within the suite, such as is provided by glass walls, and cubicle curtains shall be permitted.

(b) Any patient sleeping rooms without the direct supervision required by 19.2.5.7.2.1(C)(1)(a) shall be provided with smoke detection in accordance with Section 9.6 and 19.3.4.

**A.19.2.5.7.2.1(C)(1)** The interior partitions or walls might extend full height to the ceiling, provided that they do not obscure visual supervision of the suite. Where they do obscure visual supervision, see 19.2.5.7.2.1(C)(2).

(2) Sleeping suites shall be provided with a total coverage (complete) automatic smoke detection system in accordance with 9.6.2.9 and 19.3.4.

**19.2.5.7.2.2 Sleeping Suite Number of Means of Egress.**

**(A)** Sleeping suites of more than 1000 ft$^2$ (93 m$^2$) shall have not less than two exit access doors remotely located from each other.

**(B)*** One means of egress from the suite shall be directly to a corridor complying with 19.3.6.

**A.19.2.5.7.2.2(B)** Where only one means of egress is required from the suite, it needs to be provided by a door opening directly to a corridor complying with 19.3.6.

**(C)*** For suites requiring two means of egress, one means of egress from the suite shall be permitted to be into another suite, provided that the separation between the suites complies with the corridor requirements of 19.3.6.2 through 19.3.6.5.

**A.19.2.5.7.2.2(C)** Where the second exit access for a sleeping suite is through an adjacent suite, it is the intent that the 100 ft (30 m) travel distance limitation in the suite be applied only to the suite under consideration.

**19.2.5.7.2.3 Sleeping Suite Maximum Size.**

**(A)** Sleeping suites shall not exceed 5000 ft$^2$ (460 m$^2$), unless otherwise provided in 19.2.5.7.2.3(B).

**(B)** Sleeping suites greater than 5000 ft$^2$ (460 m$^2$) and not exceeding 7500 ft$^2$ (700 m$^2$) shall be permitted where all of the following are provided in the suite:

(1)* Direct visual supervision in accordance with 19.2.5.7.2.1(C)(1)(a)

**A.19.2.5.7.2.3(B)(1)** The alternative of 19.2.5.7.2.1(C)(1)(b) is not to be applied, since 19.2.5.7.2.3(B)(2) requires total coverage automatic smoke detection for the suite that exceeds 5000 ft$^2$ (460 m$^2$) but does not exceed 7500 ft$^2$ (700 m$^2$).

**CHAPTER 18 • New**

(2) Total coverage (complete) automatic smoke detection in accordance with 9.6.2.9 and 18.3.4

**18.2.5.7.2.4 Sleeping Suite Travel Distance.**

**(A)** Travel distance between any point in a sleeping suite and an exit access door from that suite shall not exceed 100 ft (30 m).

**(B)** Travel distance between any point in a sleeping suite and an exit shall not exceed 200 ft (61 m).

**CHAPTER 19 • Existing**

(2) Total coverage (complete) automatic smoke detection in accordance with 9.6.2.9 and 19.3.4
(3) Approved, electrically supervised sprinkler system protection complying with 19.3.5.7

**19.2.5.7.2.4 Sleeping Suite Travel Distance.**

**(A)** Travel distance between any point in a sleeping suite and an exit access door from that suite shall not exceed 100 ft (30 m).

**(B)** Travel distance between any point in a sleeping suite and an exit shall not exceed the following:

(1) 150 ft (46 m) if the building is not protected throughout by an approved electrically supervised sprinkler system complying with 19.3.5.7
(2) 200 ft (61 m) if the building is protected throughout by an approved electrically supervised sprinkler system complying with 19.3.5.7

Sleeping suites for patient care are addressed by 18/19.2.5.7.2 through 18/19.2.5.7.2.4. Sleeping suites not for patient care (e.g., staff sleeping suites) are addressed by 18/19.2.5.7.4.

Exhibit 18/19.17 illustrates the provision of 18/19.2.5.7.2 through 18/19.2.5.7.2.4, applicable to sleeping suites for patient care. For purposes of Exhibit 18/19.17, the building is protected throughout by an electrically supervised automatic sprinkler system in accordance with 18/19.3.5. For sleeping suites not used for patient care, see 18/19.2.5.7.2(2) and 18/19.2.5.7.4.

The features of sleeping suite A in Exhibit 18/19.17 are outlined in paragraphs 1 through 6.

**1.** The suite is more than 1000 ft² (93 m²), so as to require a second exit access door in accordance with 18/19.2.5.7.2.2(A). One of the two required exit access doors is provided at point A2; the other is provided at point A4. The doors are permitted to open onto a common corridor but are required to be remotely located from each other (see 7.5.1.3).

**2.** The door to the corridor at point A4 satisfies the requirement of 18/19.2.5.7.2.1(A); that is, that occupants of habitable rooms within the sleeping suite be provided with exit access to the corridor without having to pass through more than one intervening room. For example, the travel from the room at point 2 through the circulation space at the center of suite A is considered traveling through one intervening room. The circulation space connects directly to the corridor via the door at point A4 without requiring travel through any additional intervening rooms. Travel from any of the patient beds at points 4, 5, and 6 (which are provided with cubicle curtains that can be drawn across the open cubicle front for privacy) through the circulation space to the corridor door at point A4 is not considered to involve passing through any intervening room. Although travel from the room at point 2, through the circulation space, and continuing through the additional intervening room at point 1 would involve passing through more than one intervening room, the issue is moot, as the corridor exit access door at point A4, by itself, fulfills the requirement of 18/19.2.5.7.2.1(A).

**3.** The door to the corridor at point A4 also satisfies the requirement of 18/19.2.5.7.2.2(B). The intent of 18/19.2.5.7.2.2(B) is to prohibit the situation where all exit access routes from the suite would require travel through other suites. At least one of the exit access doors must provide direct access from the suite to the corridor.

**4.** The provision of 18/19.2.5.7.2.1(C)(1) is met in consideration of the following:

**a.** Direct supervision of the room at point 1 is not required, because the room is not used for sleeping.
**b.** Direct supervision of the room at point 2 is provided via the glass vision panels in the wall separating it from the circulation space.
**c.** Direct supervision of the beds at points 4, 5, and 6 is provided, because the patient bed areas are open to the circulation space for other than the

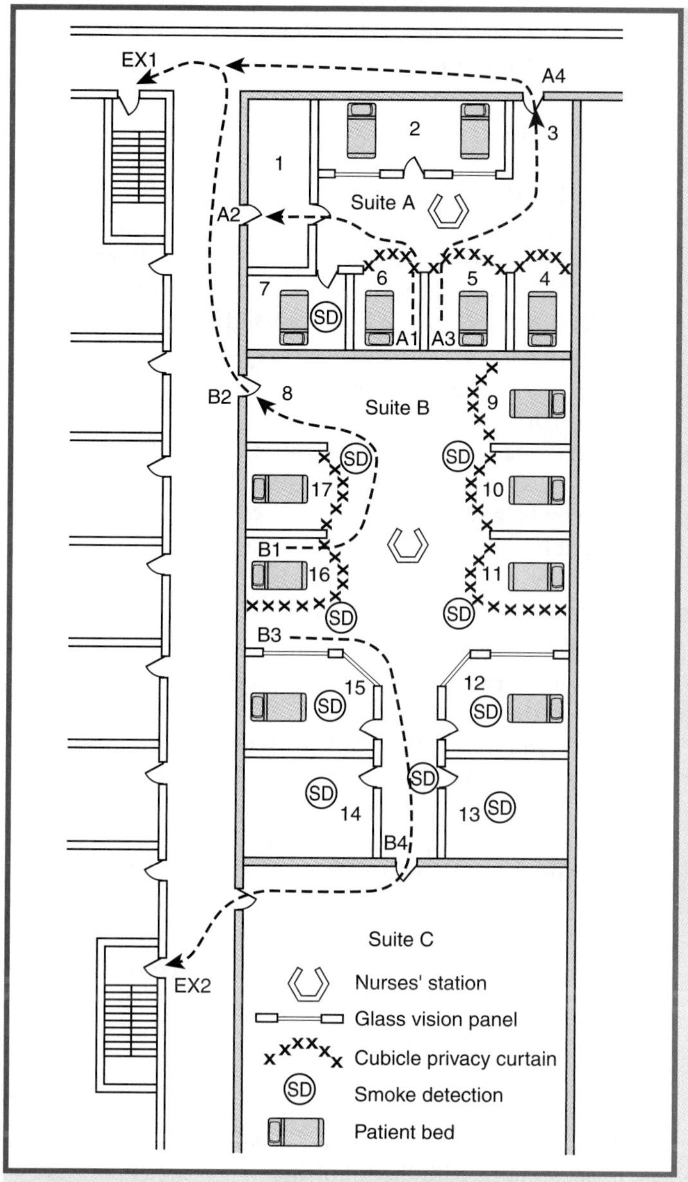


*Exhibit 18/19.17 Sleeping suites for patient care.*

condition where the cubicle curtains are drawn across the open cubicle front for privacy, as permitted by 18/19.2.5.7.2.1(C)(1)(a).

**d.** Direct supervision of the room at point 7 is not feasible, so smoke detection is provided within the room in accordance with the alternative permitted by 18/19.2.5.7.2.1(C)(1)(b).

**5.** The suite is not more than 5000 ft² (460 m²), so as to comply with 18/19.2.5.7.2.3(A) and be exempted from the additional provisions of 18/19.2.5.7.2.3(B).

**6.** The portion of the travel distance from any point within the suite to an exit access door from the suite (e.g., from point A1 to A2 or from point A3 to A4) is not more than 100 ft (30 m) in accordance with 18/19.2.5.7.2.4(A). The overall travel distance from any point within the suite to the nearest exit (e.g., from point A1 to EX1 or from point A3 to EX1) in the sprinklered building is not more than 200 ft (61 m) in accordance with 18.2.5.7.2.4(B) or 19.2.5.7.2.4(B)(2). If the suite were an existing sleeping suite in a nonsprinklered building, the overall travel distance from point A1 to EX1 or from point A3 to EX1 would be limited to 150 ft (46 m) in accordance with 19.2.5.7.2.4(B)(1).

The features of sleeping suite B in Exhibit 18/19.17 are outlined in paragraphs 1 through 6.

**1.** The suite is more than 1000 ft² (93 m²), so as to require a second exit access door in accordance with 18/19.2.5.7.2.2(A). One of the two required exit access doors is provided at point B2; the other is provided by the door at point B4 that opens into suite C, as permitted by 18/19.2.5.7.2.2(C). Note that the separation between suite B and suite C must comply with the corridor requirements of 18/19.3.6.2 through 18/19.3.6.5. In other words, the separation between the suites is treated the same as the walls separating the suites from the corridor. Additionally, the suite is more than 5000 ft² (460 m²), but not more than 7500 ft² (700 m²), as addressed in paragraph 5.

**2.** The door to the corridor at point B2 satisfies the requirement of 18/19.2.5.7.2.1(A); that is, that occupants of habitable rooms within the sleeping suite be provided with exit access to the corridor without having to pass through more than one intervening room. For example, the travel from any of the rooms at points 12 through 15 through the circulation space at the center of suite B is considered traveling through one intervening room. The circulation space connects directly to the corridor via the door at point B2 without requiring travel through any additional intervening rooms. Travel from any of the patient beds at points 9 through 11 and 16 and 17 (which are provided with cubicle curtains that can be drawn across the open cubicle front for privacy), through the circulation space to the corridor door at point B2, is not considered to involve passing through any intervening room.

**3.** The door to the corridor at point B2 also satisfies the requirement of 18/19.2.5.7.2.2(B). The intent of 18/19.2.5.7.2.2(B) is to prohibit the situation where all exit access routes from the suite would require travel

CHAPTER 18 • New

through other suites. At least one of the exit access doors must provide direct access from the suite to the corridor. As noted in paragraph 1, the other exit access door is provided by the door at point B4 that opens into suite C, as permitted by 18/19.2.5.7.2.2(C).

**4.** The provision of 18/19.2.5.7.2.1(C)(1) is met in consideration of the following:

**a.** Direct supervision of the rooms at points 13 and 14 is not required, because the rooms are not used for sleeping.

**b.** Direct supervision of the rooms at points 12 and 15 is provided via the glass vision panels in the wall separating it from the circulation space. As explained in paragraph 5, the suite is required to be provided throughout with smoke detection and with direct visual supervision of all sleeping rooms, because the suite exceeds 5000 ft² (460 m²). The presence of the smoke detection system does not exempt the requirement for direct supervision.

**c.** Direct supervision of the beds at points 9 through 11 and 16 and 17 is provided, because the patient bed areas are open to the circulation space for other than the condition where the cubicle curtains are drawn across the open cubicle front for privacy, as permitted by 18/19.2.5.7.2.1(C)(1)(a). Again, as explained in paragraph 5, the suite is required to be provided throughout with smoke detection, and with direct visual supervision of all sleeping rooms, because the suite exceeds 5000 ft² (460 m²). The presence of the smoke detection system does not exempt the requirement for direct supervision.

CHAPTER 19 • Existing

**5.** The suite is more than 5000 ft² (460 m²), but not more than 7500 ft² (700 m²), which would require compliance with the provisions of 18/19.2.5.7.2.3(B), because the suite would exceed the area limitation of 18/19.2.5.7.2.3(A). As noted in the introduction to Exhibit 18/19.17, the building is protected throughout by an electrically supervised automatic sprinkler system in accordance with 18/19.3.5. Paragraph 18/19.2.5.7.2.3(B)(2) requires sleeping suites larger than 5000 ft² (460 m²) to be protected by a total coverage automatic smoke detection system (see 9.6.2.9). Further, 18/19.2.5.7.2.3(B)(1) requires direct visual supervision in accordance with 18/19.2.5.7.2.1(C)(1)(a), which has the effect of precluding the use of the smoke detection alternative of 18/19.2.5.7.2.1(C)(1)(b). In other words, a sleeping suite in excess of 5000 ft² (460 m²) must be provided with direct visual supervision of all sleeping rooms, regardless of the fact that the suite also has a smoke detection system.

**6.** The portion of the travel distance from any point within the suite to an exit access door from the suite (e.g., from point B1 to B2 or from point B3 to B4) is not more than 100 ft (30 m) in accordance with 18/19.2.5.7.2.4(A). The overall travel distance from any point within the suite to the nearest exit (e.g., from point B1 to EX1 or from point B3 to EX2) in the sprinklered building is not more than 200 ft (61 m) in accordance with 18.2.5.7.2.4(B) or 19.2.5.7.2.4(B)(2). If the suite were an existing sleeping suite in a nonsprinklered building, the overall travel distance from point B1 to EX1 or from point B3 to EX2 would be limited to 150 ft (46 m) in accordance with 19.2.5.7.2.4(B)(1).

**18.2.5.7.3 Non-Sleeping Suites.** Non-sleeping suites shall be in accordance with the following:

(1) Non-sleeping suites for patient care shall comply with the provisions of 18.2.5.7.3.1 through 18.2.5.7.3.4.
(2) Non-sleeping suites not for patient care shall comply with the provisions of 18.2.5.7.4.

**18.2.5.7.3.1* Non-Sleeping Suite Arrangement.** Occupants of habitable rooms within non-sleeping suites shall have exit access to a corridor complying with 18.3.6 without having to pass through more than two intervening rooms.

**A.18.2.5.7.3.1** The term *intervening room* means a room serving as a part of the required means of egress from another room.

**18.2.5.7.3.2 Non-Sleeping Suite Number of Means of Egress.**

**19.2.5.7.3 Non-Sleeping Suites.** Non-sleeping suites shall be in accordance with the following:

(1) Non-sleeping suites for patient care shall comply with the provisions of 19.2.5.7.3.1 through 19.2.5.7.3.4.
(2) Non-sleeping suites not for patient care shall comply with the provisions of 19.2.5.7.4

**19.2.5.7.3.1* Non-Sleeping Suite Arrangement.** Occupants of habitable rooms within non-sleeping suites shall have exit access to a corridor complying with 19.3.6 without having to pass through more than two intervening rooms.

**A.19.2.5.7.3.1** The term *intervening room* means a room serving as a part of the required means of egress from another room.

**19.2.5.7.3.2 Non-Sleeping Suite Number of Means of Egress.**

CHAPTER 18 • New

**(A)** Non-sleeping suites of more than 2500 ft² (230 m²) shall have not less than two exit access doors remotely located from each other.

**(B)*** One means of egress from the suite shall be directly to a corridor complying with 18.3.6.

**A.18.2.5.7.3.2(B)** Where only one means of egress is required from the suite, it needs to be provided by a door opening directly to a corridor complying with 18.3.6.

**(C)*** For suites requiring two means of egress, one means of egress from the suite shall be permitted to be into another suite, provided that the separation between the suites complies with the corridor requirements of 18.3.6.2 through 18.3.6.5.

**A.18.2.5.7.3.2(C)** Where the second exit access for a non-sleeping suite is through an adjacent suite, it is the intent that the adjacent suite not be considered an intervening room.

**18.2.5.7.3.3 Non-Sleeping Suite Maximum Size.** Non-sleeping suites shall not exceed 10,000 ft² (930 m²).

**18.2.5.7.3.4 Non-Sleeping Suite Travel Distance.**

**(A)** Travel distance within a non-sleeping suite to an exit access door from the suite shall not exceed the following:

(1) 100 ft (30 m) where the suite is arranged with one intervening room
(2) 50 ft (15 m) where the suite is arranged with two intervening rooms

**(B)** Travel distance between any point in a non-sleeping suite and an exit shall not exceed 200 ft (61 m).

CHAPTER 19 • Existing

**(A)** Non-sleeping suites of more than 2500 ft² (230 m²) shall have not less than two exit access doors remotely located from each other.

**(B)*** One means of egress from the suite shall be directly to a corridor complying with 19.3.6.

**A.19.2.5.7.3.2(B)** Where only one means of egress is required from the suite, it needs to be provided by a door opening directly to a corridor complying with 19.3.6.

**(C)*** For suites requiring two means of egress, one means of egress from the suite shall be permitted to be into another suite, provided that the separation between the suites complies with the corridor requirements of 19.3.6.2 through 19.3.6.5.

**A.19.2.5.7.3.2(C)** Where the second exit access for a non-sleeping suite is through an adjacent suite, it is the intent that the adjacent suite not be considered an intervening room.

**19.2.5.7.3.3 Non-Sleeping Suite Maximum Size.** Non-sleeping suites shall not exceed 10,000 ft² (930 m²).

**19.2.5.7.3.4 Non-Sleeping Suite Travel Distance.**

**(A)** Travel distance within a non-sleeping suite to an exit access door from the suite shall not exceed the following:

(1) 100 ft (30 m) where the suite is arranged with one intervening room
(2) 50 ft (15 m) where the suite is arranged with two intervening rooms

**(B)** Travel distance between any point in a non-sleeping suite and an exit shall not exceed the following:

(1) 150 ft (46 m) if the building is not protected throughout by an approved electrically supervised sprinkler system complying with 19.3.5.7
(2) 200 ft (61 m) if the building is protected throughout by an approved electrically supervised sprinkler system complying with 19.3.5.7

Exhibit 18/19.18 illustrates the provision of 18/19.2.5.7.3, applicable to non-sleeping suites for patient care. For purposes of the illustration, the building is protected throughout by an electrically supervised automatic sprinkler system in accordance with 18/19.3.5. For non-sleeping suites not used for patient care, see 18/19.2.5.7.3(2) and 18/19.2.5.7.4.

The features of non-sleeping suite D in Exhibit 18/19.18 are outlined in paragraphs 1 through 5.

**1.** The suite is more than 2500 ft² (230 m²), so as to require a second exit access door in accordance with 18/19.2.5.7.3.2(A). One of the two required exit access doors is provided at point D2; the other is provided at point D4. The doors are permitted to open onto a common corridor but are required to be remotely located from each other (see 7.5.1.3).

**2.** The corridor exit access door at either point D2 or point D4 can be used to satisfy the requirement of 18/19.2.5.7.3.1; that is, that occupants of habitable rooms within the non-sleeping suite be provided with exit access to the corridor without having to pass through more than two intervening rooms. For example, the travel from the room at point D1 through the circulation space at the center of suite D is considered

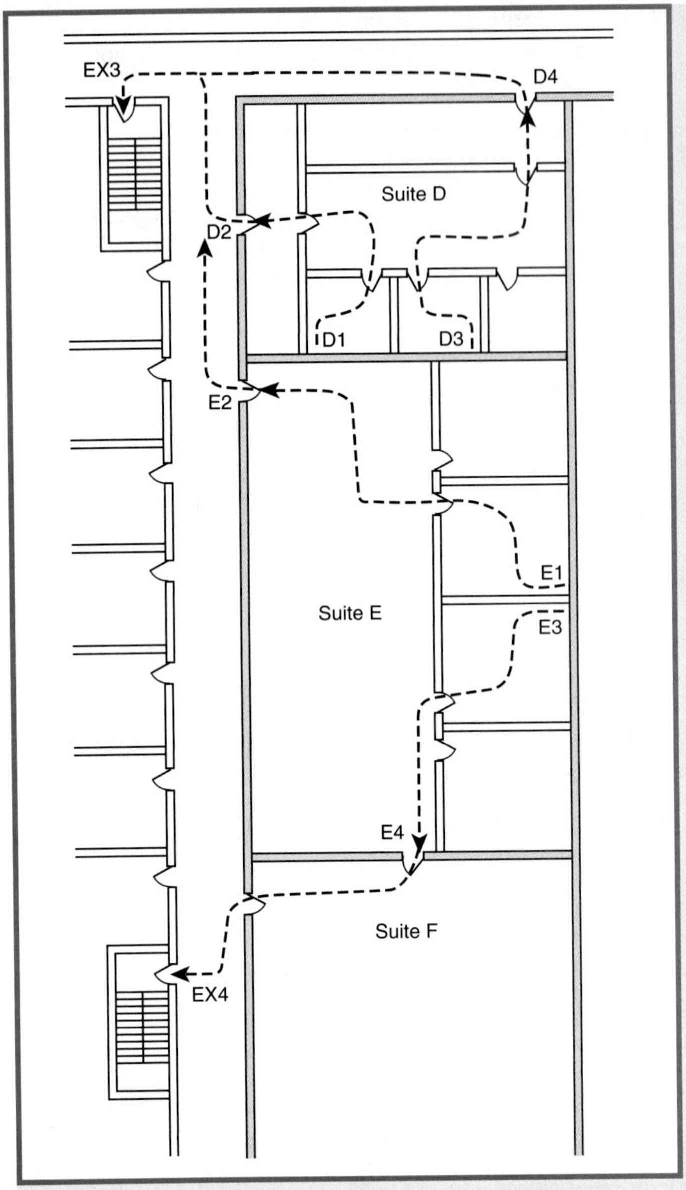


***Exhibit 18/19.18*** *Non-sleeping suites for patient care.*

traveling through one intervening room. The travel from the circulation space through the room adjacent to the corridor door at point D2 is considered traveling through a second intervening room. Similarly, the travel from the room at point D3 through the circulation space and its adjacent room to a corridor door at point D4 is considered traveling through two intervening rooms.

**3.** The corridor exit access door at either point D2 or point D4 can be used to satisfy the requirement of 18/19.2.5.7.3.2(B). The intent of 18/19.2.5.7.3.2(B) is to prohibit the situation where all exit access routes from the suite would require travel through other suites. At least one of the exit access doors must provide direct access from the suite to the corridor.

**4.** Non-sleeping suite D does not exceed 10,000 ft$^2$ (930 m$^2$), as required by 18/19.2.5.7.3.3.

**5.** The portion of the travel distance from any point within the suite to an exit access door from the suite (e.g., from point D1 to D2 or from point D3 to D4) is not more than 50 ft (15 m) in accordance with 18/19.2.5.7.3.4(A)(2), based on the presence of a second intervening room. The overall travel distance from any point within the suite to the nearest exit (e.g., from point D1 to EX3 or from point D3 to EX3) in the sprinklered building is not more than 200 ft (61 m) in accordance with 18.2.5.7.3.4(B) or 19.2.5.7.3.4(B)(2). If the suite were an existing non-sleeping suite used for patient care in a nonsprinklered building, the overall travel distance from point D1 to EX3, or from point D3 to EX3, would be limited to 150 ft (46 m) in accordance with 19.2.5.7.3.4(B)(1).

The features of non-sleeping suite E, used for patient care, in Exhibit 18/19.18 are outlined in paragraphs 1 through 5.

**1.** The suite is more than 2500 ft$^2$ (230 m$^2$), so as to require a second exit access door in accordance with 18/19.2.5.7.3.2(A). One of the two required exit access doors is provided at point E2; the other is provided by the door at point E4 that opens into suite F, as permitted by 18/19.2.5.7.3.2(C). Note that the separation between suite E and suite F must comply with the corridor requirements of 18/19.3.6.2 through 18/19.3.6.5. In other words, the separation between the suites is treated the same as the walls separating the suites from the corridor.

**2.** The corridor exit access door at point E2 satisfies the requirement of 18/19.2.5.7.3.1; that is, that occupants of habitable rooms within the non-sleeping suite be provided with exit access to the corridor without having to pass through more than two intervening rooms. For example, the travel from the room at point E1 through the circulation space, shown at the left of suite E, to the corridor door at point E2 is considered traveling through one intervening room. The arrangement shown with only one intervening room satisfies 18/19.2.5.7.3.1, which permits travel through two intervening rooms.

**3.** The corridor exit access door at point E2 satisfies the requirement of 18/19.2.5.7.3.2(B). The intent of

18/19.2.5.7.3.2(B) is to prohibit the situation where all exit access routes from the suite would require travel through other suites. At least one of the exit access doors must provide direct access from the suite to the corridor.

**4.** Non-sleeping suite E does not exceed 10,000 $ft^2$ (930 $m^2$), as required by 18/19.2.5.7.3.3.

**5.** The portion of the travel distance from any point within the suite to an exit access door from the suite (e.g., from point E1 to E2 or from point E3 to E4) is not more than 100 ft (30 m), in accordance with 18/19.2.5.7.3.4(A)(1), based on the presence of only one intervening room. The overall travel distance from any point within the suite to the nearest exit (e.g., from point E1 to EX3 or from point E3 to EX4) in the sprinklered building is not more than 200 ft (61 m) in accordance with 18.2.5.7.3.4(B) or 19.2.5.7.3.4(B)(2). If the suite were an existing non-sleeping suite in a nonsprinklered building, the overall travel distance from point E1 to EX3, or from point E3 to EX4, would be limited to 150 ft (46 m) in accordance with 19.2.5.7.3.4(B)(1).

**18.2.5.7.4 Non-Patient-Care Suites.** The egress provisions for non-patient-care suites shall be in accordance with the primary use and occupancy of the space, except that in no case shall the maximum travel distance to an exit from within the suite exceed 200 ft (61 m).

**19.2.5.7.4 Non-Patient-Care Suites.** The egress provisions for non-patient-care suites shall be in accordance with the primary use and occupancy of the space, except that in no case shall the maximum travel distance to an exit from within the suite exceed 200 ft (61 m).

The provisions of 18/19.2.5.7.4 are new to the 2009 edition of the *Code*. The provisions, in conjunction with 18/19.2.5.7.2(2) and 18/19.2.5.7.3(2), clarify that suites not used for patient care are to be addressed by the requirements applicable to the primary use of the space. The requirements applicable to the primary use of the space are to be used regardless of whether the suite is considered incidental to the primary occupancy (i.e., a health care occupancy), so as to be subject to the provisions of Chapter 18/19 in accordance with 6.1.14.1.3. For example, if an existing suite in a hospital is used for medical records storage so as to constitute an existing ordinary hazard storage use, and the building is sprinklered, the maximum 100 ft (30 m) common path of travel limitation of Table 42.2.5 for ordinary hazard storage would apply, even though Chapter 19 for existing health care occupancies establishes no maximum common path of travel. The provisions of 19.2.5.7.4 limit the travel distance from the existing medical records storage suite, as used in this example, to its nearest exit to not more than 200 ft (61 m), which is a stricter requirement than the 400 ft (122 m) travel distance limitation imposed by Table 42.2.6 for ordinary hazard storage in a sprinklered building.

### 18.2.6 Travel Distance to Exits.

**18.2.6.1** Travel distance shall be measured in accordance with Section 7.6.

**18.2.6.2** Travel distance shall comply with 18.2.6.2.1 through 18.2.6.2.4.

**18.2.6.2.1** The travel distance between any point in a room and an exit shall not exceed 200 ft (61 m).

**18.2.6.2.2 Reserved.**

**18.2.6.2.3** The travel distance between any point in a health care sleeping room and an exit access door in that room shall not exceed 50 ft (15 m).

### 19.2.6 Travel Distance to Exits.

**19.2.6.1** Travel distance shall be measured in accordance with Section 7.6.

**19.2.6.2** Travel distance shall comply with 19.2.6.2.1 through 19.2.6.2.4.

**19.2.6.2.1** The travel distance between any point in a room and an exit shall not exceed 150 ft (46 m), unless otherwise permitted by 19.2.6.2.2.

**19.2.6.2.2** The maximum travel distance specified in 19.2.6.2.1 shall be permitted to be increased by 50 ft (15 m) in buildings protected throughout by an approved, supervised automatic sprinkler system in accordance with 19.3.5.7.

**19.2.6.2.3** The travel distance between any point in a health care sleeping room and an exit access door in that room shall not exceed 50 ft (15 m).

CHAPTER 18 • New

**18.2.6.2.4** The travel distance within suites shall be in accordance with 18.2.5.7.

Travel distance limitations for suites, as addressed in 18/19.2.6.2.4, are included within the suites provisions of 18/19.2.5.7. See the commentary and exhibits that follow 18.2.5.7.2.4(B) and 19.2.5.7.2.4(B)(2) for sleeping suites and 18.2.5.7.3.4(B) and 19.2.5.7.3.4(B)(2) for non-sleeping suites.

Exhibit 18/19.19 illustrates the travel distance limitations set by 18/19.2.6.2.1 through 18/19.2.6.2.3, applicable to other than suites. Travel distance is measured only to the nearest exit (point EX in Exhibit 18/19.19), not to the second exit required by 18/19.2.4.1, which is not shown in the exhibit. The smoke barrier depicted is not an exit, although travel through the cross-corridor door opening in the smoke barrier, into the adjoining smoke compartment, and along the corridor, will eventually lead to the second required exit.

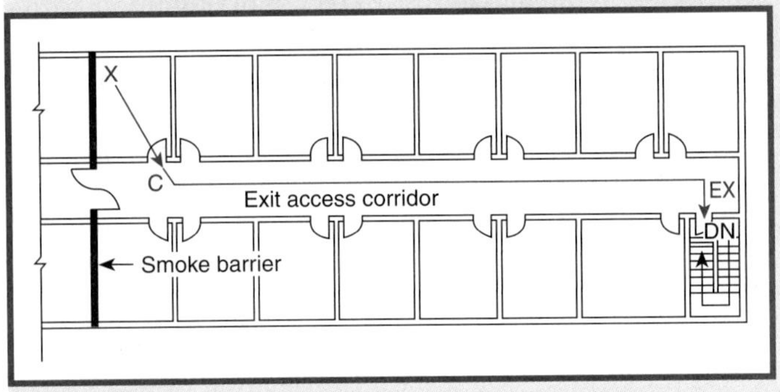


***Exhibit 18/19.19*** *Travel distance measurement.*

CHAPTER 19 • Existing

**19.2.6.2.4** The travel distance within suites shall be in accordance with 19.2.5.7.

In evaluating travel distance for sleeping rooms, the two tests outlined in paragraphs 1 and 2 are required.

**1.** *Is the travel distance within the sleeping room excessive?* Regardless of the presence of sprinklers, 18/19.2.6.2.3 limits this travel distance (X to C in Exhibit 18/19.19) to 50 ft (15 m). If a fire were to start in a patient sleeping room, the ability to leave the room quickly would be important. Provided that the travel within the room does not exceed 50 ft (15 m), it should be possible to learn quickly of the fire within such a room and move, or be moved, to the corridor before the fire grows to such size that it would block patient and staff access to the door to the corridor. The 50 ft (15 m) travel distance restriction within a room applies only to sleeping rooms.

**2.** *Is the overall travel distance excessive?* For new construction and sprinklered existing buildings, 18/19.2.6.2.1 and 19.2.6.2.2 limit the total travel distance (X to EX in Exhibit 18/19.19) to 200 ft (61 m). For nonsprinklered existing buildings, the total travel distance is limited to 150 ft (46 m) per 19.2.6.2.1.

For non-sleeping rooms, travel distance is evaluated by a single test of whether the overall travel distance is excessive. For new construction and sprinklered existing buildings, 18/19.2.6.2.1 and 19.2.6.2.2 limit the total travel distance (X to EX in Exhibit 18/19.19) to 200 ft (61 m). For nonsprinklered existing buildings, the distance is limited to 150 ft (46 m) per 19.2.6.2.1.

### 18.2.7 Discharge from Exits.

Discharge from exits shall be arranged in accordance with Section 7.7.

### 18.2.8 Illumination of Means of Egress.

Means of egress shall be illuminated in accordance with Section 7.8.

### 18.2.9 Emergency Lighting.

**18.2.9.1** Emergency lighting shall be provided in accordance with Section 7.9.

**18.2.9.2** Buildings equipped with, or in which patients require the use of, life-support systems *(see 18.5.1.3)* shall have emergency lighting equipment supplied by the life safety branch of the electrical system as described in NFPA 99, *Standard for Health Care Facilities.*

### 19.2.7 Discharge from Exits.

Discharge from exits shall be arranged in accordance with Section 7.7.

### 19.2.8 Illumination of Means of Egress.

Means of egress shall be illuminated in accordance with Section 7.8.

### 19.2.9 Emergency Lighting.

**19.2.9.1** Emergency lighting shall be provided in accordance with Section 7.9.

**19.2.9.2 Reserved.**

CHAPTER 18 • New

### 18.2.10 Marking of Means of Egress.

**18.2.10.1** Means of egress shall have signs in accordance with Section 7.10.

**18.2.10.2 Reserved.**

**18.2.10.3** Illumination of required exit and directional signs in buildings equipped with, or in which patients use, life-support systems *(see 18.5.1.3)* shall be provided as follows:

(1) Illumination shall be supplied by the life safety branch of the electrical system as described in NFPA 99, *Standard for Health Care Facilities*.
(2) Self-luminous exit signs complying with 7.10.4 shall be permitted.

CHAPTER 19 • Existing

### 19.2.10 Marking of Means of Egress.

**19.2.10.1** Means of egress shall have signs in accordance with Section 7.10, unless otherwise permitted by 19.2.10.2.

**19.2.10.2** Where the path of egress travel is obvious, signs shall not be required in one-story buildings with an occupant load of fewer than 30 persons.

Each new health care facility equipped with, or requiring the use of, life-support systems is required by 18.2.10.3 to have the marking of the means of egress and emergency lighting supplied by the life safety branch of the electrical systems described in NFPA 99, *Standard for Health Care Facilities*.[6]

A facility would not be required to have an emergency generator if the building were a freestanding unit in which, as a normal practice, all the following apply:

1. Management maintains admitting and discharge policies that preclude the provision of care for any patient or resident who might need to be sustained by electrical life-support equipment, such as respirators or suction apparatus.
2. No surgical treatment requiring general anesthesia is offered.
3. Battery-operated systems or equipment is provided to maintain power to exit lights and illumination of egress corridors, stairways, medical preparation areas, and the like for a minimum of $1\frac{1}{2}$ hours.

Additionally, battery power would be required to be supplied to all alarm systems. For additional information, refer to NFPA 99, *Standard for Health Care Facilities*.

NFPA 99 requires that emergency power supplies be arranged and protected to minimize the possibility of a single incident affecting both normal and emergency power supplies simultaneously. Circuits are to be run separately. Emergency and normal circuits are "joined" at the transfer switch, so damage to the transfer switch would interrupt normal and emergency power supplies simultaneously. The transfer switch is, therefore, a critical item and should be separated from any potential source of fire, including the emergency generator and attendant fuel supply.

### 18.2.11 Special Means of Egress Features.

**(Reserved)**

### 19.2.11 Special Means of Egress Features.

**(Reserved)**

## 18.3 Protection

### 18.3.1 Protection of Vertical Openings.

Any vertical opening shall be enclosed or protected in accordance with Section 8.6, unless otherwise modified by 18.3.1.1 through 18.3.1.8.

**18.3.1.1 Reserved.**

## 19.3 Protection

### 19.3.1 Protection of Vertical Openings.

Any vertical opening shall be enclosed or protected in accordance with Section 8.6, unless otherwise modified by 19.3.1.1 through 19.3.1.8.

**19.3.1.1** Where enclosure is provided, the construction shall have not less than a 1-hour fire resistance rating.

CHAPTER 18 • New

**18.3.1.2** Unprotected vertical openings in accordance with 8.6.8.2 shall be permitted.

**18.3.1.3** Subparagraph 8.6.7(1)(b) shall not apply to patient sleeping and treatment rooms.

**18.3.1.4** Multilevel patient sleeping areas in psychiatric facilities shall be permitted without enclosure protection between levels, provided that all of the following conditions are met:

(1) The entire normally occupied area, including all communicating floor levels, is sufficiently open and unobstructed so that a fire or other dangerous condition in any part is obvious to the occupants or supervisory personnel in the area.
(2) The egress capacity provides simultaneously for all the occupants of all communicating levels and areas, with all communicating levels in the same fire area being considered as a single floor area for purposes of determination of required egress capacity.
(3) The height between the highest and lowest finished floor levels does not exceed 13 ft (3960 mm), and the number of levels is permitted to be unrestricted.

**18.3.1.5** Unprotected openings in accordance with 8.6.6 shall not be permitted.

**18.3.1.6 Reserved.**

**18.3.1.7** A door in a stair enclosure shall be self-closing and shall normally be kept in the closed position, unless otherwise permitted by 18.3.1.8.

**18.3.1.8** Doors in stair enclosures shall be permitted to be held open under the conditions specified by 18.2.2.2.7 and 18.2.2.2.8.

CHAPTER 19 • Existing

**19.3.1.2** Unprotected vertical openings in accordance with 8.6.8.2 shall be permitted.

**19.3.1.3** Subparagraph 8.6.7(1)(b) shall not apply to patient sleeping and treatment rooms.

**19.3.1.4** Multilevel patient sleeping areas in psychiatric facilities shall be permitted without enclosure protection between levels, provided that all of the following conditions are met:

(1) The entire normally occupied area, including all communicating floor levels, is sufficiently open and unobstructed so that a fire or other dangerous condition in any part is obvious to the occupants or supervisory personnel in the area.
(2) The egress capacity provides simultaneously for all the occupants of all communicating levels and areas, with all communicating levels in the same fire area being considered as a single floor area for purposes of determination of required egress capacity.
(3) The height between the highest and lowest finished floor levels does not exceed 13 ft (3960 mm), and the number of levels is permitted to be unrestricted.

**19.3.1.5** Unprotected openings in accordance with 8.6.6 shall not be permitted.

**19.3.1.6** Where a full enclosure of a stairway that is not a required exit is impracticable, the required enclosure shall be permitted to be limited to that necessary to prevent a fire originating in any story from spreading to any other story.

**19.3.1.7** A door in a stair enclosure shall be self-closing and shall normally be kept in the closed position, unless otherwise permitted by 19.3.1.8.

**19.3.1.8** Doors in stair enclosures shall be permitted to be held open under the conditions specified by 19.2.2.2.7 and 19.2.2.2.8.

Subsection 18/19.3.1 specifies protection levels required to maintain floor-to-floor separation in health care facilities. For new construction, 18.3.1 references Section 8.6, which requires 2-hour enclosures around vertical openings connecting more than three stories in buildings. One-hour enclosure of vertical openings is required in all other new health care occupancies. For existing health care occupancies, 19.3.1.1 requires 1-hour enclosure of vertical openings. Note that this requirement is more than the ½ hour required by 8.6.5(3) for existing enclosures of vertical openings. Health care occupancies employ a defend-in-place strategy that recognizes the difficulty in evacuating patients to the outside. Thus, the ½ hour typically permitted for existing enclosures in existing buildings is not applicable to existing health care occupancies.

Per 19.3.1.6, if an existing stairway is not used as an exit and full enclosure is not possible, the enclosure is permitted to be limited to that necessary to prevent fire or smoke originating in any one story from spreading to another story. For example, in a two-story building, the stair might be enclosed at the first-floor level and left open at the second-floor level.

Paragraph 18/19.3.1.2 references the permitted convenience opening described in 8.6.8.2 and illustrated in Exhibit 18/19.20. This exemption applies to

CHAPTER 18 • New

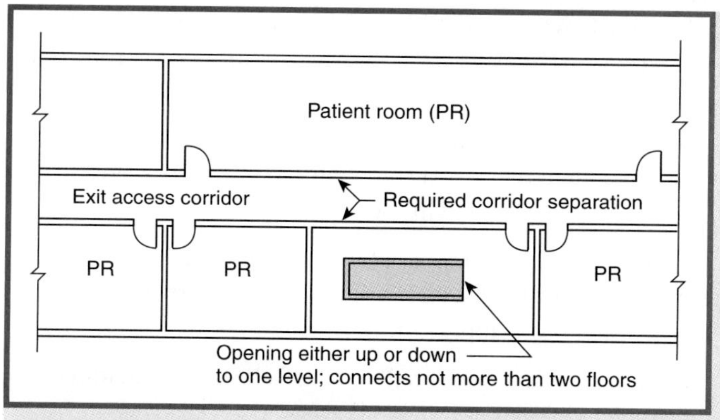


*Exhibit 18/19.20 Permitted convenience opening.*

any nonconcealed vertical opening, not only to a convenience stair. This exemption would permit a light well to connect two stories or permit a stair to connect two levels of a medical library, a file storage area, or an administrative office, for example. The exemption would not permit omission of firestopping around pipe penetrations of a floor slab or omission of protection for duct penetrations.

CHAPTER 19 • Existing

Paragraph 18/19.3.1.3 modifies the atrium provisions of 8.6.7(1)(b) for applicability to health care occupancies. Patient sleeping and treatment rooms must be separated from the atrium by partitions complying with 8.6.7(1) or 8.6.7(1)(c) — either 1-hour-rated walls or glass protected by closely spaced sprinklers.

Paragraph 18/19.3.1.4 recognizes the vertical openings inherent in multilevel patient sleeping areas similar to those described for detention and correctional occupancies in 22.4.4.6 and 23.3.1.2.

Paragraph 18/19.3.1.7 requires fire doors protecting openings in stairway enclosures to be self-closing and normally maintained in a closed position. However, 18/19.3.1.8 permits stairway doors meeting specified conditions to be held open by an automatic-closing device. If stair enclosure doors are not automatic-closing in accordance with 7.2.1.8.2 (see 18/19.2.2.2.7), they should be provided with a sign that states "Fire Exit — Keep Door Closed," as they are susceptible to being chocked open because there is no electromagnet to hold the door in the open position.

### 18.3.2 Protection from Hazards.

**18.3.2.1* Hazardous Areas.** Any hazardous areas shall be protected in accordance with Section 8.7, and the areas described in Table 18.3.2.1 shall be protected as indicated.

**A.18.3.2.1** Provisions for the enclosure of rooms used for charging linen chutes and waste chutes or for rooms into which these chutes empty are provided in Section 9.5.

*Table 18.3.2.1 Hazardous Area Protection*

| Hazardous Area Description | Protection/ Separation† |
|---|---|
| Boiler and fuel-fired heater rooms | 1 hour |
| Central/bulk laundries larger than 100 ft$^2$ (9.3 m$^2$) | 1 hour |
| Laboratories employing flammable or combustible materials in quantities less than those that would be considered a severe hazard | See 18.3.6.3.11. |
| Laboratories that use hazardous materials that would be classified as a severe hazard in accordance with NFPA 99, *Standard for Health Care Facilities* | 1 hour |
| Paint shops employing hazardous substances and materials in quantities less than those that would be classified as a severe hazard | 1 hour |
| Physical plant maintenance shops | 1 hour |
| Rooms with soiled linen in volume exceeding 64 gal (242 L) | 1 hour |
| Storage rooms larger than 50 ft$^2$ (4.6 m$^2$) but not exceeding 100 ft$^2$ (9.3 m$^2$) and storing combustible material | See 18.3.6.3.11. |
| Storage rooms larger than 100 ft$^2$ (9.3 m$^2$) and storing combustible material | 1 hour |
| Rooms with collected trash in volume exceeding 64 gal (242 L) | 1 hour |

†Minimum fire resistance rating.

### 19.3.2 Protection from Hazards.

**19.3.2.1 Hazardous Areas.** Any hazardous areas shall be safeguarded by a fire barrier having a 1-hour fire resistance rating or shall be provided with an automatic extinguishing system in accordance with 8.7.1.

CHAPTER 18 • New

CHAPTER 19 • Existing

**19.3.2.1.1** An automatic extinguishing system, where used in hazardous areas, shall be permitted to be in accordance with 19.3.5.9.

**19.3.2.1.2*** Where the sprinkler option of 19.3.2.1 is used, the areas shall be separated from other spaces by smoke partitions in accordance with Section 8.4.

**A.19.3.2.1.2** Penetrations of hazardous area walls located above ceilings that comply with Section 8.4 are not required to be sealed to comply with 19.3.2.1.2.

**19.3.2.1.3** The doors shall be self-closing or automatic-closing.

**19.3.2.1.4** Doors in rated enclosures shall be permitted to have nonrated, factory- or field-applied protective plates extending not more than 48 in. (1220 mm) above the bottom of the door.

**19.3.2.1.5** Hazardous areas shall include, but shall not be restricted to, the following:

(1) Boiler and fuel-fired heater rooms
(2) Central/bulk laundries larger than 100 $ft^2$ (9.3 $m^2$)
(3) Paint shops
(4) Repair shops
(5) Rooms with soiled linen in volume exceeding 64 gal (242 L)
(6) Rooms with collected trash in volume exceeding 64 gal (242 L)
(7) Rooms or spaces larger than 50 $ft^2$ (4.6 $m^2$), including repair shops, used for storage of combustible supplies and equipment in quantities deemed hazardous by the authority having jurisdiction
(8) Laboratories employing flammable or combustible materials in quantities less than those that would be considered a severe hazard

**18.3.2.2* Laboratories.** Laboratories employing quantities of flammable, combustible, or hazardous materials that are considered as a severe hazard shall be protected in accordance with NFPA 99, *Standard for Health Care Facilities.*

**A.18.3.2.2** The hazard level of a laboratory is considered severe if quantities of flammable, combustible, or hazardous materials are present that are capable of sustaining a fire of sufficient magnitude to breach a 1-hour fire separation. See the NFPA *Fire Protection Handbook* for guidance.

**18.3.2.3 Anesthetizing Locations.** Anesthetizing locations shall be protected in accordance with NFPA 99, *Standard for Health Care Facilities.*

**18.3.2.4 Medical Gas.** Medical gas storage and administration areas shall be protected in accordance with NFPA 99, *Standard for Health Care Facilities.*

**19.3.2.2* Laboratories.** Laboratories employing quantities of flammable, combustible, or hazardous materials that are considered as a severe hazard shall be protected in accordance with NFPA 99, *Standard for Health Care Facilities.*

**A.19.3.2.2** The hazard level of a laboratory is considered severe if quantities of flammable, combustible, or hazardous materials are present that are capable of sustaining a fire of sufficient magnitude to breach a 1-hour fire separation. See NFPA *Fire Protection Handbook* for guidance.

**19.3.2.3 Anesthetizing Locations.** Anesthetizing locations shall be protected in accordance with NFPA 99, *Standard for Health Care Facilities.*

**19.3.2.4 Medical Gas.** Medical gas storage and administration areas shall be protected in accordance with NFPA 99, *Standard for Health Care Facilities.*

CHAPTER 18 • New

**18.3.2.5 Cooking Facilities.**

**18.3.2.5.1** Cooking facilities shall be protected in accordance with 9.2.3, unless otherwise permitted by 18.3.2.5.2.

**18.3.2.5.2*** Where domestic cooking equipment is used for food warming or limited cooking, protection or separation of food preparation facilities shall not be required.

**A.18.3.2.5.2** This provision is intended to permit small appliances used for reheating, such as microwave ovens, hot plates, toasters, and nourishment centers to be exempt from the requirements for commercial cooking equipment.

CHAPTER 19 • Existing

**19.3.2.5 Cooking Facilities.**

**19.3.2.5.1** Cooking facilities shall be protected in accordance with 9.2.3, unless otherwise permitted by 19.3.2.5.2.

**19.3.2.5.2*** Where domestic cooking equipment is used for food warming or limited cooking, protection or separation of food preparation facilities shall not be required.

**A.19.3.2.5.2** This provision is intended to permit small appliances used for reheating, such as microwave ovens, hot plates, toasters, and nourishment centers, to be exempt from the requirements for commercial cooking equipment.

Hazardous areas are spaces containing materials that, due to their basic nature (as in the case of flammable liquids), or because of the quantity of combustible materials involved, represent a significantly higher hazard than would otherwise be typical in the general areas of health care facilities.

A list of typically hazardous areas is included in Table 18.3.2.1 and in 19.3.2.1.5. The lists are meant to be representative, not inclusive. The general reference in 18/19.3.2.1 to Section 8.7 provides the authority having jurisdiction (AHJ) with the opportunity to regulate any space judged to represent a significantly higher hazard than most spaces.

Chapter 18 requires automatic sprinkler protection throughout all new health care facilities. Therefore, all hazardous spaces in new construction must be sprinklered. Where a hazardous area is judged to represent a severe exposure, such as in the case of boiler rooms, laundries, paint shops, and soiled linen rooms, 1-hour fire resistance–rated separation is also necessary. Hazardous areas that are not judged to be severe also require a separation, but the separation is permitted to use a non-fire-rated smoke partition in accordance with Section 8.4 (see 8.7.1.2). Doors protecting openings in such partitions must be tight-fitting and equipped with a closing device (see 18.3.6.3.11 and 8.4.3.5). Door openings in 1-hour fire resistance–rated barriers must be protected with $^3/_4$-hour fire protection–rated door assemblies.

In existing health care occupancies, hazardous areas must be separated from other areas by barriers having a 1-hour fire resistance rating, complete with approved fire doors protecting door openings; otherwise, automatic sprinkler protection must be installed. If automatic sprinkler protection is provided, the hazardous area must still be separated from the rest of the building by non-fire-rated smoke partitions in accordance with Section 8.4. See 19.3.2.1.2.

Note that, in Table 18.3.2.1 and in 19.3.2.1.5, the entries related to soiled linen and collected trash were revised for the 2009 edition of the *Code*. In editions prior to 2009, the list included the terms *soiled linen rooms* and *trash collection rooms*. The authority having jurisdiction was at a disadvantage in getting the provisions of 18/19.3.2 applied to rooms that were not identified as soiled linen rooms or trash collection rooms but that had significant soiled linen or trash present, albeit in a minority of the overall room area, as some of the rooms were large. The new criteria for soiled linen and collected trash apply to rooms where the soiled linen or collected trash volume exceeds 64 gal (242 L). Facilities operators have the option, for example, of protecting multiple rooms on a floor as hazardous areas, so as to permit the introduction of soiled linen (or collected trash) into any of those rooms, or of protecting one room as a hazardous area and limiting the placement of soiled linen (or collected trash) to that room only. Designers of new facilities will most likely opt to protect multiple rooms to ensure flexibility in use once the facility is operating.

Provisions for the enclosure of rooms used for charging linen and waste chutes, or for the rooms into which these chutes empty, are provided in Section 9.5. The enclosure requirements of 9.5.1 supplement the provisions of 9.5.2 for installing and maintaining the rubbish chutes and laundry chutes in accordance with NFPA 82, *Standard on Incinerators and Waste and Linen Handling Systems and Equipment*.[7]

If flammable liquids are handled or stored, NFPA 30, *Flammable and Combustible Liquids Code*,[8] must be consulted to establish the minimum criteria necessary to mitigate this hazard. Provisions for the use and storage of flammable gases and oxygen are covered in NFPA 99, *Standard for Health Care Facilities*.

Paragraph 19.3.2.1.4 recognizes the benefit of protective plates for the protection of doors that are frequently assaulted with carts and other wheeled vehicles. Without the exemption, the minimum 45-minute fire protection–rated doors to hazardous area rooms would be subject to the requirements of 8.3.3, which, via a mandatory reference to NFPA 80, *Standard for Fire Doors and Other Opening Protectives*,[9] would not permit the field application of protective plates to fire-rated doors. The field application of protective plates must be accomplished without reducing the fire performance of the door — such as might result if the door is drilled through its entire thickness for the installation of through-bolts.

Laboratories are addressed in 18/19.3.2.2. Laboratories that contain ordinary combustibles and flammable liquids in sufficient quantity to threaten a 1-hour fire separation [e.g., wood-equivalent fuel loads in the range of 5 lb/ft$^2$ to 10 lb/ft$^2$ (25 kg/m$^2$ to 50 kg/m$^2$)] are considered a severe hazard. Laboratories posing a severe hazard must be protected in accordance with NFPA 99, *Standard for Health Care Facilities*. Protection would include 1-hour fire resistance–rated separation and automatic sprinkler protection.

If fuel loads of lesser amounts are involved and quantities of flammable liquids are limited, laboratories would simply be considered hazardous areas and would be adequately protected by the automatic sprinklers required in all new health care occupancies. In existing health care occupancies, either 1-hour separation or automatic sprinkler protection would be required.

Commercial cooking equipment is addressed in 18/19.3.2.5. It must be installed and protected in accordance with NFPA 96, *Standard for Ventilation Control and Fire Protection of Commercial Cooking Operations*.[10] A regularly serviced, fixed, automatic fire-extinguishing system would be required for the protection of cooking surfaces and exhaust and duct systems where cooking operations involve the potential for grease-laden vapors. Paragraph 18/19.3.2.5.2 exempts domestic cooking equipment used for food warming or limited cooking from the specialized extinguishment requirements of NFPA 96 and the separation requirements of 18/19.3.2.1.

**18.3.2.6* Alcohol-Based Hand-Rub Dispensers.** Alcohol-based hand-rub dispensers shall be protected in accordance with 8.7.3, unless all of the following conditions are met:

(1) Where dispensers are installed in a corridor, the corridor shall have a minimum width of 6 ft (1830 mm).
(2) The maximum individual dispenser fluid capacity shall be as follows:
    (a) 0.32 gal (1.2 L) for dispensers in rooms, corridors, and areas open to corridors
    (b) 0.53 gal (2.0 L) for dispensers in suites of rooms
(3) Where aerosol containers are used, the maximum capacity of the aerosol dispenser shall be 18 oz. (0.51 kg) and shall be limited to Level 1 aerosols as defined in NFPA 30B, *Code for the Manufacture and Storage of Aerosol Products*.
(4) Dispensers shall be separated from each other by horizontal spacing of not less than 48 in. (1220 mm).
(5) Not more than an aggregate 10 gal (37.8 L) of alcohol-based hand-rub solution or 1135 oz (32.2 kg) of Level 1 aerosols, or a combination of liquids and Level 1 aerosols not to exceed, in total, the equivalent of 10 gal (37.8 L) or 1135 oz (32.2 kg,) shall be in use outside of a storage cabinet in a single smoke compartment.
(6) Storage of quantities greater than 5 gal (18.9 L) in a single smoke compartment shall meet the requirements of NFPA 30, *Flammable and Combustible Liquids Code*.

**19.3.2.6* Alcohol-Based Hand-Rub Dispensers.** Alcohol-based hand-rub dispensers shall be protected in accordance with 8.7.3, unless all of the following conditions are met:

(1) Where dispensers are installed in a corridor, the corridor shall have a minimum width of 6 ft (1830 mm).
(2) The maximum individual dispenser fluid capacity shall be as follows:
    (a) 0.32 gal (1.2 L) for dispensers in rooms, corridors, and areas open to corridors
    (b) 0.53 gal (2.0 L) for dispensers in suites of rooms
(3) Where aerosol containers are used, the maximum capacity of the aerosol dispenser shall be 18 oz. (0.51 kg) and shall be limited to Level 1 aerosols as defined in NFPA 30B, *Code for the Manufacture and Storage of Aerosol Products*.
(4) Dispensers shall be separated from each other by horizontal spacing of not less than 48 in. (1220 mm).
(5) Not more than an aggregate 10 gal (37.8 L) of alcohol-based hand-rub solution or 1135 oz (32.2 kg) of Level 1 aerosols, or a combination of liquids and Level 1 aerosols not to exceed, in total, the equivalent of 10 gal (37.8 L) or 1135 oz (32.2 kg,) shall be in use outside of a storage cabinet in a single smoke compartment.
(6) Storage of quantities greater than 5 gal (18.9 L) in a single smoke compartment shall meet the requirements of NFPA 30, *Flammable and Combustible Liquids Code*.

CHAPTER 18 • New

(7) Dispensers shall not be installed in the following locations:
   (a) Above an ignition source for a horizontal distance of 1 in. (25 mm) to each side of the ignition source
   (b) To the side of an ignition source within a 1 in. (25 mm) horizontal distance from the ignition source
   (c) Beneath an ignition source within a 1 in. (25 mm) vertical distance from the ignition source
(8) Dispensers installed directly over carpeted floors shall be permitted only in sprinklered smoke compartments.

**A.18.3.2.6** Extensive research, including fire modeling, has indicated that alcohol-based hand-rub solutions can be safely installed in corridors of health care facilities, provided that certain other precautions are taken. The total quantities of flammable liquids in any area should comply with the provisions of other recognized codes, including NFPA 1, *Fire Code*, and NFPA 30, *Flammable and Combustible Liquids Code*. In addition, special consideration should be given to the following:

(1) Obstructions created by the installation of hand-rub solution dispensers
(2) Location of dispensers with regard to adjacent combustible materials and potential sources of ignition, especially where dispensers are mounted on walls of combustible construction
(3) Requirements for other fire protection features, including complete automatic sprinkler protection, to be installed throughout the compartment
(4) Amount and location of the flammable solutions, both in use and in storage, particularly with respect to potential for leakage or failure of the dispenser

CHAPTER 19 • Existing

(7) Dispensers shall not be installed in the following locations:
   (a) Above an ignition source for a horizontal distance of 1 in. (25 mm) to each side of the ignition source
   (b) To the side of an ignition source within a 1 in. (25 mm) horizontal distance from the ignition source
   (c) Beneath an ignition source within a 1 in. (25 mm) vertical distance from the ignition source
(8) Dispensers installed directly over carpeted floors shall be permitted only in sprinklered smoke compartments.

**A.19.3.2.6** Extensive research, including fire modeling, has indicated that alcohol-based hand-rub solutions can be safely installed in corridors of health care facilities, provided that certain other precautions are taken. The total quantities of flammable liquids in any area should comply with the provisions of other recognized codes, including NFPA 1, *Fire Code*, and NFPA 30, *Flammable and Combustible Liquids Code*. In addition, special consideration should be given to the following:

(1) Obstructions created by the installation of hand-rub solution dispensers
(2) Location of dispensers with regard to adjacent combustible materials and potential sources of ignition, especially where dispensers are mounted on walls of combustible construction
(3) Requirements for other fire protection features, including complete automatic sprinkler protection, to be installed throughout the compartment
(4) Amount and location of the flammable solutions, both in use and in storage, particularly with respect to potential for leakage or failure of the dispenser

The provisions for alcohol-based hand-rub dispensers were added to the *Code* for the 2006 edition and revised for the 2009 edition. Prior to the inclusion of the provisions for alcohol-based hand-rub dispensers, the only option available was to treat the alcohol solutions as flammable liquids subject to the provisions of 8.7.3, which meant the dispensers were prohibited from being placed in patient areas, especially in corridors. The provisions of 18/19.3.2.6 permit limited use of such dispensers in corridors, rooms, and suites. Dispensers not meeting all the criteria of 18/19.3.2.6(1) through (8) are subject to regulation as flammable liquids in accordance with 8.7.3.

The NFPA *101* public proposal[11] submitted by the American Society for Healthcare Engineering of the American Hospital Association, recommending the provisions for alcohol-based hand-rub dispensers, provided the history behind the quantity limits established. The related text from the proposal reads as follows:

> The Centers for Disease Control and Prevention (CDC) on October 25, 2002, issued the *Guidelines for Hand Hygiene in Health-Care Settings*,[12] which highly recommends the placement of alcohol-based hand-rub solutions in convenient locations of patient care areas of health care organizations. Clinical studies indicate that the frequency of handwashing or antiseptic handwashing by personnel is affected by the accessibility of hand-hygiene facilities. By permitting the installation of hand-rub dispensers immediately outside the patient/residence bedroom or within suites of

rooms, the overall efficacy of staff use has been proven to increase by over 20 percent.

According to the CDC more that 88,000 patient deaths per year are attributed to hospital-acquired infections and one of the principal methodologies for reducing this statistic is by the expanded use of alcohol-based hand-rub solutions. These products have been found to be more effective for standard hand-washing or hand antisepsis by health care workers than soap or antimicrobial soaps.

To address the fire hazard of introducing additional alcohol-based materials, a fire-modeling project was initiated to study the overall effects of placing dispensers in corridors and suites of rooms. This modeling was accomplished using the Fire Dynamics Simulator (FDS) Version 3.1 published by the National Institute of Standards and Technology (NIST). Using the results of the FDS model, the potential hazards were evaluated by reviewing the data for tenability of the space, ignition of adjacent fuel loads/combustibles, and sprinkler activation.

The tenability value used in the report was chosen to be conservative. The fire modeling showed that up to 0.3-gallon (1.2-Liter) container size in a corridor and up to a 0.5-gallon (2-liter) container size in a suite location to be acceptable for either Ethyl or Isopropyl Alcohol based products. Except for a scenario that modeled the 0.3-gallon (1.2-Liter) Isopropyl Alcohol container in a 6-ft (1830-mm) wide corridor with all doors closed, all of the results with realistic conditions showed no issues. For that one scenario, the visibility did drop below the stated threshold, but since visibility is not an immediate health concern and it did not occur until the very end of the fire's burn time (final 15 seconds), only to improve dramatically to twice the allowable value, we feel that this is still an acceptable result. The scenario with the 6-ft (1830-mm) corridors and all doors closed, which is a very extreme case compared to actual conditions, does show some concerns compared to our tenability criteria. The results showed that the corridor remained below the visibility and CO thresholds established. The temperature in scenario with 6-ft (1830-mm) corridors and all doors closed did drop below the tenability threshold (which has a factor of safety of 10) but not significantly. This scenario helps to prove that the hazard is acceptable.

The results clearly indicate the 0.5-gallon (2-liter) container size to be unacceptable in a corridor location. In addition, the results also indicate the scenario with a carpeted floor is a concern due to visibility problems. The scenario showed that the visibility in the corridor dropped slightly below our assigned threshold. The carpet scenario is based on assumptions (soot and CO yields) that are not validated via any test data or other available data sources. The yields used are based on engineering judgment and need further study to make a firm recommendation. Visibility, unlike other tenability areas (for example, temperature or toxicity), is based on a number of factors, has limited real life test data, and is very subjective. The resources available have a wide range of values that could be considered acceptable based on various factors, such as type of smoke (irritating vs. non-irritating), travel distances, familiarity with escape routes, etc.

The results showed that none of the fuel targets put into the models would ignite based on the design fires chosen. This indicates the proposed spacing to be reasonable to prevent additional dispensers from becoming involved in the fire. Sprinkler activation was not predicted for most of the scenarios modeled. When the sprinklers actuated it was most often after the conditions had exceeded the tenability thresholds and typically with the larger 0.5-gallon (2-liter) spills. Due to the lack of sprinkler activation, it is important to address the hazard from products of combustion such as smoke or CO more than the hazards from heat or the actual fire.

Note that, in addition to the criteria of 18/19.3.2.6(1) through (8), the alcohol-based hand-rub dispensers are limited to encroaching not more than 6 in. (150 mm) into the minimum 6 ft (1830 mm) width corridor in accordance with 18/19.2.3.4(2). Exhibit 18/19.21 illustrates an alcohol-based hand-rub dispenser installed on a corridor wall in accordance with the provisions of 18/19.3.2.6(1) through (8) and 18/19.2.3.4(2).

The provisions of 18/19.3.2.6 were expanded for

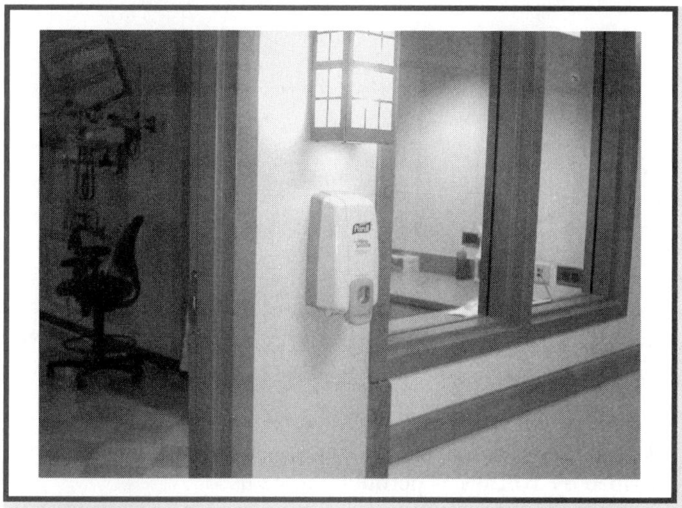

*Exhibit 18/19.21 Alcohol-based hand-rub dispenser located in corridor.*

the 2009 edition of the *Code* to permit aerosol-based dispensers, as the original provisions added to the 2006 edition addressed only liquid/gel dispensers. The criteria of 18/19.3.2.6(3) and (5), related to aerosol containers, were substantiated by a 2007 Consumer Specialty Products Association (CSPA) report by David Fredrickson titled "Alcohol Based Hand Sanitizers — Level 1 Aerosol Products."[13] The report concluded that aerosol hand sanitizer containers, limited to the capacities and quantities addressed in 18/19.3.2.6(3) and (5), can be safely used in corridors for the following reasons:

1. Level 1 aerosol is treated as a Class III commodity.
2. The calculated chemical heats of combustion of the aerosol products are well under the boundary between Level 1 and Level 2 aerosols.
3. The chemical heat of combustion is equal to or lower than that for the liquid/gel products currently permitted.
4. The proposed aerosol container capacity is less than half the quantity currently permitted for liquids/gels.
5. The structural integrity of the aerosol container is substantially better than that in which liquids/gels are packaged, and the container is not combustible.
6. The thermal integrity of the aerosol container prevents the aerosol product from being exposed to fire until air temperatures reach well above 200°F (93°C) — temperatures that would make the corridor unusable.

The provision of 18/19.3.2.6(7) is new to the 2009 edition of the *Code* and replaces a requirement that prohibited the dispenser from being positioned over or directly adjacent to an ignition source, as such language was too subjective to be enforced consistently. Exhibit 18/19.22 illustrates the area, above and to the side of an ignition source, from which alcohol-based hand-rub dispensers are prohibited from being located.

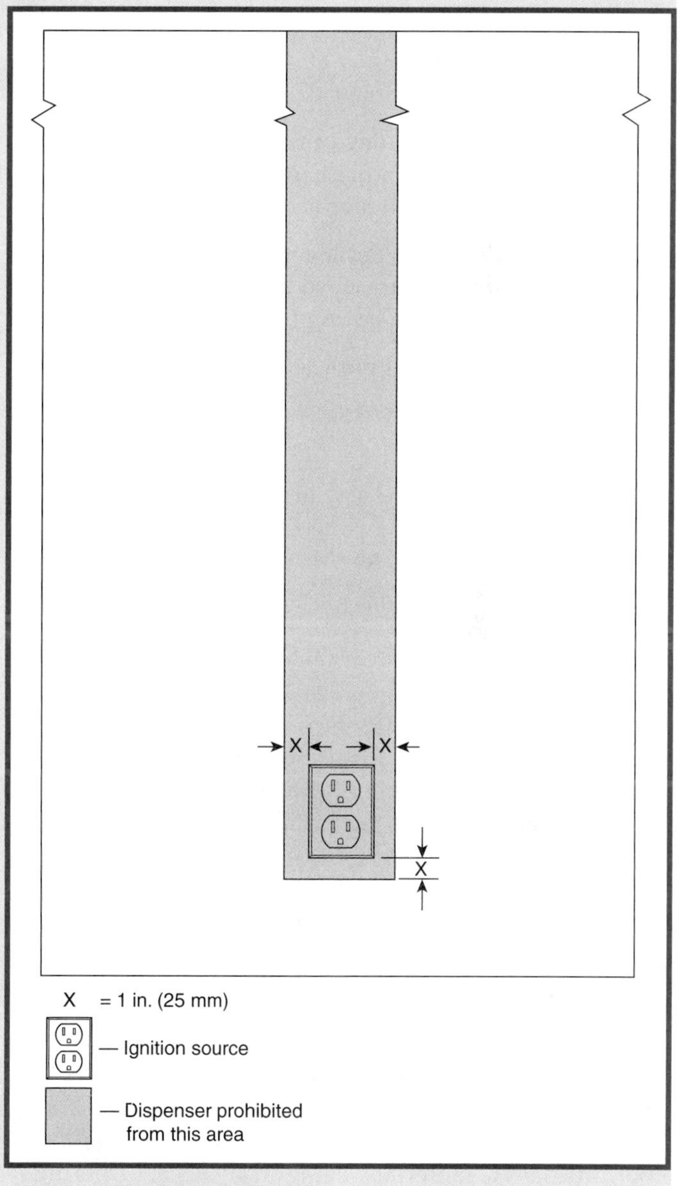


*Exhibit 18/19.22 Prohibited location for alcohol-based hand-rub dispenser with respect to an ignition source.*

CHAPTER 18 • New

**18.3.2.7 Heliports.** Buildings that house health care occupancies, as indicated in 18.1.1.1.2, and have rooftop heliports shall be protected in accordance with NFPA 418, *Standard for Heliports*.

### 18.3.3 Interior Finish.

**18.3.3.1 General.** Interior finish shall be in accordance with Section 10.2.

**18.3.3.2* Interior Wall and Ceiling Finish.** Interior wall and ceiling finish materials complying with Section 10.2 shall be permitted throughout if Class A, except as indicated in 18.3.3.2.1 or 18.3.3.2.2.

**A.18.3.3.2** The reductions in class of interior finish prescribed by 10.2.8.1 are permitted to be used.

**18.3.3.2.1** Walls and ceilings shall be permitted to have Class A or Class B interior finish in individual rooms having a capacity not exceeding four persons.

**18.3.3.2.2** Corridor wall finish not exceeding 48 in. (1220 mm) in height that is restricted to the lower half of the wall shall be permitted to be Class A or Class B.

**18.3.3.3 Interior Floor Finish.**

**18.3.3.3.1** Interior floor finish shall comply with Section 10.2.

**18.3.3.3.2** Interior floor finish in exit enclosures and exit access corridors and spaces not separated from them by walls complying with 18.3.6 shall be Class I or Class II.

**18.3.3.3.3** Interior floor finish shall comply with 10.2.7.1 or 10.2.7.2, as applicable.

CHAPTER 19 • Existing

### 19.3.3 Interior Finish.

**19.3.3.1 General.** Interior finish shall be in accordance with Section 10.2.

**19.3.3.2* Interior Wall and Ceiling Finish.** Existing interior wall and ceiling finish materials complying with Section 10.2 shall be permitted to be Class A or Class B.

**A.19.3.3.2** The reduction in class of interior finish prescribed by 10.2.8.1 is permitted to be used.

**19.3.3.3 Interior Floor Finish.** No restrictions shall apply to existing interior floor finish.

New interior finishes on walls and ceilings are limited to Class A materials, with the exception of small rooms (see 18.3.3.2.1) and the lower portion of corridor walls (see 18.3.3.2.2). However, if the new interior wall and ceiling finish material is installed in a sprinklered smoke compartment (all new health care occupancies are required to be sprinklered by 18.3.5.1), the Class A requirement can be relaxed to Class B per the provisions of 10.2.8.1. Existing interior finish materials are permitted to be Class A or Class B without requiring sprinkler protection.

Paragraph 18.3.3.2.1 permits Class B interior wall and ceiling finish materials in rooms with a capacity of four or fewer persons, but, again, the presence of automatic sprinklers would relax this requirement to permit Class C materials. Paragraph 18.3.3.2.2 permits wall finish in corridors to be of Class B materials where located 48 in. (1220 mm) or less above the floor, but, once again, the presence of automatic sprinklers would relax this requirement to permit Class C materials. This provision recognizes fire research that has shown the finish on the lower half of the wall to be far less significant in its influence on early fire growth than the finish on the upper half.[14] In the case of textile materials on walls or ceilings, 10.2.4.1 would take precedence and require automatic sprinkler protection in conjunction with Class A materials, or such wall and ceiling materials must be proven safe by specialized fire testing.

Existing interior finishes on walls and ceilings are limited solely on the basis of flame spread. Paragraph 10.2.3.4(4) exempts existing interior finishes from the limitations based on smoke development.

Paragraph 10.2.6.1 makes provision for application of approved fire-retardant coatings to existing interior finish materials for the purpose of reducing the flame spread characteristics to an acceptable level. The commentary following 10.2.6.2 offers additional guidance.

It has been shown that floor coverings will not spread a fire until the fire approaches flashover (see A.10.2.7.3 and associated commentary). Automatic sprinklers will activate well in advance of any significant involvement of a floor covering. Paragraph 18.3.3.2 has the effect of regulating new interior floor finish in exit enclosures and exit access corridors only in nonsprinklered areas, as 10.2.8.2 permits the Class II criterion to be reduced to no rating where sprinkler protection is provided. Existing floor finish materials are permitted to continue to be used.

### 18.3.4 Detection, Alarm, and Communications Systems.

**18.3.4.1 General.** Health care occupancies shall be provided with a fire alarm system in accordance with Section 9.6.

**18.3.4.2* Initiation.**

**A.18.3.4.2** It is not the intent of this *Code* to require single-station smoke detectors that might be required by local codes to be connected to or to initiate the building fire alarm system.

**18.3.4.2.1** Initiation of the required fire alarm systems shall be by manual means in accordance with 9.6.2 and by means of any required sprinkler system waterflow alarms, detection devices, or detection systems, unless otherwise permitted by 18.3.4.2.2.

**18.3.4.2.2** Manual fire alarm boxes in patient sleeping areas shall not be required at exits if located at all nurses' control stations or other continuously attended staff location, provided that both of the following criteria are met:

(1) Such manual fire alarm boxes are visible and continuously accessible.
(2) Travel distances required by 9.6.2.5 are not exceeded.

**18.3.4.3 Notification.** Positive alarm sequence in accordance with 9.6.3.4 shall be permitted.

**18.3.4.3.1 Occupant Notification.** Occupant notification shall be accomplished automatically in accordance with 9.6.3, unless otherwise modified by the following:

(1) Paragraph 9.6.3.2.3 shall not be permitted to be used.
(2)* In lieu of audible alarm signals, visible alarm-indicating appliances shall be permitted to be used in critical care areas.



### 19.3.4 Detection, Alarm, and Communications Systems.

**19.3.4.1 General.** Health care occupancies shall be provided with a fire alarm system in accordance with Section 9.6.

**19.3.4.2* Initiation.**

**A.19.3.4.2** It is not the intent of this *Code* to require single-station smoke detectors, which might be required by local codes, to be connected to or to initiate the building fire alarm system.

**19.3.4.2.1** Initiation of the required fire alarm systems shall be by manual means in accordance with 9.6.2 and by means of any required sprinkler system waterflow alarms, detection devices, or detection systems, unless otherwise permitted by 19.3.4.2.2 through 19.3.4.2.4.

**19.3.4.2.2** Manual fire alarm boxes in patient sleeping areas shall not be required at exits if located at all nurses' control stations or other continuously attended staff location, provided that both of the following criteria are met:

(1) Such manual fire alarm boxes are visible and continuously accessible.
(2) Travel distances required by 9.6.2.5 are not exceeded.

**19.3.4.2.3** Fixed extinguishing systems protecting commercial cooking equipment in kitchens that are protected by a complete automatic sprinkler system shall not be required to initiate the fire alarm system.

**19.3.4.2.4** Detectors required by 19.7.5.3 and 19.7.5.5 shall not be required to initiate the fire alarm system.

**19.3.4.3 Notification.** Positive alarm sequence in accordance with 9.6.3.4 shall be permitted in health care occupancies protected throughout by an approved, supervised automatic sprinkler system in accordance with 9.7.1.1(1).

**19.3.4.3.1 Occupant Notification.** Occupant notification shall be accomplished automatically in accordance with 9.6.3, unless otherwise modified by the following:

(1)* In lieu of audible alarm signals, visible alarm-indicating appliances shall be permitted to be used in critical care areas.

CHAPTER 18 • New

**A.18.3.4.3.1(2)** It is the intent of this provision to permit a visible fire alarm signal instead of an audible signal to reduce interference between the fire alarm and medical equipment monitoring alarms.

**18.3.4.3.2 Emergency Forces Notification.**

**18.3.4.3.2.1** Fire department notification shall be accomplished in accordance with 9.6.4.

**18.3.4.3.2.2 Reserved.**

**18.3.4.3.3 Annunciation and Annunciation Zoning.**

**18.3.4.3.3.1** Annunciation and annunciation zoning shall be provided in accordance with 9.6.7, unless otherwise permitted by 18.3.4.3.3.2 or 18.3.4.3.3.3.

**18.3.4.3.3.2** The alarm zone shall be permitted to coincide with the permitted area for smoke compartments.

**18.3.4.3.3.3** The provision of 9.6.7.4.3, which permits sprinkler system waterflow to be annunciated as a single building zone, shall be prohibited.

**18.3.4.4 Fire Safety Functions.** Operation of any activating device in the required fire alarm system shall be arranged to accomplish automatically any control functions to be performed by that device. *(See 9.6.5.)*

**18.3.4.5 Detection.**

**18.3.4.5.1 General.** Detection systems, where required, shall be in accordance with Section 9.6.

**18.3.4.5.2 Detection in Spaces Open to Corridors.** See 18.3.6.1.

CHAPTER 19 • Existing

**A.19.3.4.3.1(1)** It is the intent of this provision to permit a visible fire alarm signal instead of an audible signal to reduce interference between the fire alarm and medical equipment monitoring alarms.

(2) Where visual devices have been installed in patient sleeping areas in place of an audible alarm, they shall be permitted where approved by the authority having jurisdiction.

**19.3.4.3.2 Emergency Forces Notification.**

**19.3.4.3.2.1** Fire department notification shall be accomplished in accordance with 9.6.4.

**19.3.4.3.2.2** Smoke detection devices or smoke detection systems equipped with reconfirmation features shall not be required to automatically notify the fire department, unless the alarm condition is reconfirmed after a period not exceeding 120 seconds.

**19.3.4.4 Fire Safety Functions.** Operation of any activating device in the required fire alarm system shall be arranged to accomplish automatically any control functions to be performed by that device. *(See 9.6.5.)*

**19.3.4.5 Detection.**

**19.3.4.5.1 Corridors.** An approved automatic smoke detection system in accordance with Section 9.6 shall be installed in all corridors of limited care facilities, unless otherwise permitted by the following:

(1) Where each patient sleeping room is protected by an approved smoke detection system, and a smoke detector is provided at smoke barriers and horizontal exits in accordance with Section 9.6, the corridor smoke detection system shall not be required on the patient sleeping room floors.
(2) Smoke compartments protected throughout by an approved, supervised automatic sprinkler system in accordance with 19.3.5.7 shall be permitted.

**19.3.4.5.2 Detection in Spaces Open to Corridors.** See 19.3.6.1.

**18.3.4.5.3* Nursing Homes.** An approved automatic smoke detection system shall be installed in corridors throughout smoke compartments containing patient sleeping rooms and in spaces open to corridors as permitted in nursing homes by 18.3.6.1, unless otherwise permitted by the following:

(1) Corridor systems shall not be required where each patient sleeping room is protected by an approved smoke detection system.
(2) Corridor systems shall not be required where patient room doors are equipped with automatic door-closing devices with integral smoke detectors on the room side installed in accordance with their listing, provided that the integral detectors provide occupant notification.

**A.18.3.4.5.3** The requirement for smoke detectors in spaces open to the corridors eliminates the requirements of 18.3.6.1(1)(c), (2)(b), and (5)(b) for direct supervision by the facility staff of nursing homes.

A manual fire alarm system is required by 18/19.3.4.1 and 18/19.3.4.2. Manual fire alarm boxes are normally located along the natural routes of egress and are also located to cover all portions of the building. Paragraph 18/19.3.4.2.2 permits manual fire alarm boxes, under certain conditions, to be located only at continuously attended staff positions in sleeping areas. This arrangement provides the opportunity for prompt notification of fire without requiring staff to leave their normal workstations. In new installations, it would normally be desirable to have manual fire alarm boxes at all attended staff locations and at entrances to exits, because the additional cost of the extra fire alarm boxes would be minimal. However, the exemptions recognize that the fire alarm boxes located near the exits might lead to nuisance alarms if patients misuse them.

Manual fire alarm boxes should be located so that those qualified to send an alarm can summon aid without having to leave their zone of ordinary activity or pass out of the sight and hearing of people immediately exposed to, or in direct view of, a fire. The operation of a manual fire alarm box should automatically summon attendants who can assist in removing physically helpless occupants and controlling mentally disabled occupants.

The alarm system initiation required by 18/19.3.4.2 is permitted to be incorporated into an automatic system equipped to detect a fire and initiate an alarm.

Paragraph 19.3.4.2.4 addresses smoke detectors installed for a special purpose — to provide an exemption to paragraphs 19.7.5.3 and 19.7.5.5, which require that newly introduced upholstered furniture and mattresses be resistant to cigarette ignition and have limited rates of heat release. Paragraph 19.3.4.2.4 exempts such smoke detectors from having to initiate the building alarm system.

Paragraph 18/19.3.4.3 permits positive alarm sequence in accordance with 9.6.3.4 in sprinklered health care occupancies (see 18.3.5.1 and 19.3.4.3). The criteria for positive alarm sequence are detailed in *NFPA 72, National Fire Alarm Code,* and include the criteria specified in paragraphs 1 through 4.

**1.** The signal from an automatic fire detection device selected for positive alarm sequence operation must be acknowledged at the control unit by trained personnel within 15 seconds of annunciation in order to initiate the alarm investigation phase. If the signal is not acknowledged within 15 seconds, notification signals in accordance with the building evacuation or relocation plan and remote signals must be automatically and immediately activated (i.e., immediate occupant notification and emergency force notification must occur).

**2.** Trained personnel have up to 180 seconds during the alarm investigation phase to evaluate the fire condition and reset the system. If the system is not reset during the investigation phase, notification signals in accordance with the building evacuation or relocation plan and remote signals must be automatically and immediately activated (i.e., immediate occupant notification and emergency force notification must occur).

**3.** If a second automatic fire detector selected for positive alarm sequence is actuated during the alarm investigation phase, notification signals in accordance with the building evacuation or relocation plan and remote signals must be automatically and immediately activated (i.e., immediate occupant notification and emergency force notification must occur).

**4.** If any other initiating device is actuated (e.g., a manual fire alarm box), notification signals in accordance with the building evacuation or relocation plan and remote signals must be automatically and immediately activated (that is, immediate occupant notification and emergency force notification must occur).

Occupant notification (see 18/19.3.4.3.1) and emergency forces notification (see 18/19.3.4.3.2) can be delayed during the 180-second alarm investigation phase associated with the positive alarm sequence permitted by 18/19.3.4.3.

Actuation of the fire alarm must initiate the operation of alerting devices throughout the affected zone or building, as appropriate. See 9.6.3.6.2 and 9.6.3.6.3, which address occupant notification by zone. Visible alerting devices are permitted to substitute for audible devices in critical care areas. See A.18.3.4.3.1(2) and A.19.3.4.3.1(1).

Although 18/19.3.4.3.1 requires occupant notification, coded messages are permitted to be used to notify staff and trained responders. As part of their emergency duties, staff will then keep patients and visitors informed of expected actions.

Paragraph 18.3.4.3.1(1) specifically prohibits new health care occupancies from using 9.6.3.2.3, which exempts detectors at doors used for the exclusive operation of automatic door release from the requirements for occupant notification. Note that the use of 9.6.3.2.1 and 9.6.3.2.2, which exempt detectors used for recalling elevators or closing dampers from initiating occupant notification, respectively, is not prohibited. Although such detectors must be arranged to initiate the health care occupancy alarm system in accordance with 18.3.4.2.1, subsequent, automatic occupant notification is not required.

Emergency forces notification is addressed in 18/19.3.4.3.2. An independent study by the National Bureau of Standards (currently the National Institute of Standards and Technology) indicates a high rate of nuisance alarms for smoke detectors installed in health care facilities.[15] The study determined that 4.4 nuisance alarms occurred per 100 smoke detectors per year. Further, approximately 14 nuisance alarms occurred for every actual alarm. Because of the high incidence of nuisance alarms, 18/19.3.4.3 permits positive alarm sequence in accordance with 9.6.3.4. With positive alarm sequence, provided that a person at the alarm system control unit acknowledges the signal within 15 seconds of annunciation and no additional automatic fire detector is actuated, emergency forces notification can be delayed for 180 seconds while trained personnel investigate the alarm to evaluate the fire condition and reset the system. Further, 19.3.4.3.2.2 permits the continued use of an existing alarm system feature that delays fire department notification for up to 120 seconds where smoke detectors or smoke detection systems are equipped with a reconfirmation feature. However, staff notification, as required by 19.3.4.3.1, cannot be delayed by the existing smoke detection system with reconfirmation feature.

The alarm must automatically transmit to a point outside the facility. If the fire department legally committed to serve the facility does not permit automatic alarm transmission, arrangements are to be made for the prompt notification of the fire department or such other assistance as may be available in the case of fire or other emergency. Paragraph 9.6.4.2 lists various acceptable methods for automatically notifying the fire department. The fire department should also be called manually to verify and confirm the automatic transmission of the alarm. In larger facilities, this might be the responsibility of the facility telephone operator; in smaller facilities, it might be the responsibility of the nursing staff.

The provision of 18.3.4.3.3.3 is new to the 2009 edition of the *Code*. It prohibits sprinkler system water flow from being annunciated as a single building zone. The prohibition was written in reaction to the addition of 9.6.7.4.3, which permits such single-zone annunciation so as not to prohibit a so-called sprinkler system "birdcage" piping configuration, in which the sprinkler branch lines are run vertically through the building, rather than horizontally, providing an economical installation alternative. The resulting piping network resembles a birdcage, thus the name. With such a piping configuration, it is not practical to provide waterflow devices for every floor, since each branch line typically serves multiple floors. Therefore, a single waterflow device is provided on the supply piping ahead of the branch lines, resulting in the sprinkler system being annunciated as a single zone. Such an arrangement has the potential to increase the time required for emergency responders to locate the fire and is inconsistent with the protection level mandated for health care occupancies.

Paragraph 19.3.4.5.1 requires smoke detectors in the corridors of existing limited care facilities. Staffing levels in hospitals and nursing homes reasonably ensure discovery of a fire at an early stage. In existing hospitals and nursing homes, it is considered reasonable to rely on staff to sound the alarm.

Paragraph 18.3.4.5.3 requires corridor smoke detection systems in new nursing homes. The justification for the creation of this requirement stated that corridor smoke detectors are needed for redundancy, since, in some fire scenarios, the corridor detector might be the first device to provide notification of fire, and the cost of installing a corridor smoke detection system as part of new construction is minor.

Subsection 18/19.3.4 addresses required fire alarm equipment. Reliability is of primary importance; therefore, electrical supervision of the system and system components is specified by reference to Section 9.6. In the event of circuit fault, component failure, or other trouble, continuous trouble indication is required and should be provided at a constantly attended location.

### 18.3.5 Extinguishment Requirements.

**18.3.5.1*** Buildings containing health care occupancies shall be protected throughout by an approved, supervised automatic sprinkler system in accordance with Section 9.7, unless otherwise permitted by 18.3.5.5.

**A.18.3.5.1** In areas where the replenishment of water supplies is not immediately available from on-site sources, alternate provisions for the water-fill rate requirements of NFPA 13, *Standard for the Installation of Sprinkler Systems*, and NFPA 22, *Standard for Water Tanks for Private Fire Protection*, that are acceptable to the authority having jurisdiction should be provided. Appropriate means for the replenishment of these supplies from other sources, such as fire department tankers, public safety organizations, or other independent contractors should be incorporated into the overall fire safety plan of the facility.

With automatic sprinkler protection required throughout new health care facilities and quick-response sprinklers required in smoke compartments containing patient sleeping rooms, a fire and its life-threatening byproducts can be reduced, thereby allowing the defend-in-place concept to continue. The difficulty in maintaining the proper integrity of life safety elements has been considered, and it has been judged that the probability of a sprinkler system operating as designed is equal to or greater than other life safety features.

**18.3.5.2 Reserved.**

**18.3.5.3 Reserved.**

### 19.3.5 Extinguishment Requirements.

**19.3.5.1** Buildings containing nursing homes shall be protected throughout by an approved, supervised automatic sprinkler system in accordance with Section 9.7, unless otherwise permitted by 19.3.5.5.

**19.3.5.2** High-rise buildings shall comply with 19.4.2.

**19.3.5.3** Where required by 19.1.6, buildings containing hospitals or limited care facilities shall be protected throughout by an approved, supervised automatic sprinkler system in accordance with Section 9.7, unless otherwise permitted by 19.3.5.5.

CHAPTER 18 • New

**18.3.5.4** The sprinkler system required by 18.3.5.1 shall be installed in accordance with 9.7.1.1(1).

**18.3.5.5** In Type I and Type II construction, alternative protection measures shall be permitted to be substituted for sprinkler protection without causing a building to be classified as nonsprinklered in specified areas where the authority having jurisdiction has prohibited sprinklers.

**18.3.5.6*** Listed quick-response or listed residential sprinklers shall be used throughout smoke compartments containing patient sleeping rooms.

**A.18.3.5.6** The requirements for use of quick-response sprinklers intend that quick-response sprinklers be the predominant type of sprinkler installed in the smoke compartment. It is recognized, however, that quick-response sprinklers might not be approved for installation in all areas, such as those where NFPA 13, *Standard for the Installation of Sprinkler Systems*, requires sprinklers of the intermediate- or high-temperature classification. It is not the intent of the 18.3.5.6 requirements to prohibit the use of standard sprinklers in limited areas of a smoke compartment where intermediate- or high-temperature sprinklers are required.

Where the installation of quick-response sprinklers is impracticable in patient sleeping room areas, appropriate equivalent protection features acceptable to the authority having jurisdiction should be provided. It is recognized that the use of quick-response sprinklers might be limited in facilities housing certain types of patients or by the installation limitations of quick-response sprinklers.

**18.3.5.7 Reserved.**

CHAPTER 19 • Existing

**19.3.5.4*** The sprinkler system required by 19.3.5.1 or 19.3.5.3 shall be installed in accordance with 9.7.1.1(1).

**A.19.3.5.4** It is not the intent to require existing standard sprinklers in existing sprinkler systems to be replaced with listed quick-response or listed residential sprinklers. It is the intent that new sprinkler systems installed in existing buildings comply with the requirements of Chapter 18, including 18.3.5.6.

**19.3.5.5** In Type I and Type II construction, alternative protection measures shall be permitted to be substituted for sprinkler protection in specified areas where the authority having jurisdiction has prohibited sprinklers, without causing a building to be classified as nonsprinklered.

**19.3.5.6 Reserved.**

**19.3.5.7*** Where this *Code* permits exceptions for fully sprinklered buildings or smoke compartments, the sprinkler system shall meet the following criteria:

(1) It shall be in accordance with Section 9.7.
(2) It shall be installed in accordance with 9.7.1.1(1), unless it is an approved existing system.
(3) It shall be electrically connected to the fire alarm system.
(4) It shall be fully supervised.
(5) In Type I and Type II construction, where the authority having jurisdiction has prohibited sprinklers, approved alternative protection measures shall be permitted to be substituted for sprinkler protection in specified areas without causing a building to be classified as nonsprinklered.

**A.19.3.5.7** It is intended that any valve that controls automatic sprinklers in the building or portions of the building, including sectional and floor control valves, be electrically supervised. Valves that control isolated sprinkler heads, such as in laundry and trash chutes, are not required to be electrically supervised. Appropriate means should be provided to ensure that valves that are not electrically supervised remain open.

**18.3.5.8 Reserved.**

**19.3.5.8*** Where this *Code* permits exceptions for fully sprinklered buildings or smoke compartments and specifically references this paragraph, the sprinkler system shall meet the following criteria:

(1) It shall be installed throughout the building or smoke compartment in accordance with Section 9.7.
(2) It shall be installed in accordance with 9.7.1.1(1), unless it is an approved existing system.
(3) It shall be electrically connected to the fire alarm system.
(4) It shall be fully supervised.
(5) It shall be equipped with listed quick-response or listed residential sprinklers throughout all smoke compartments containing patient sleeping rooms.
(6) Standard-response sprinklers shall be permitted to be continued to be used in approved existing sprinkler systems where quick-response and residential sprinklers were not listed for use in such locations at the time of installation.
(7) Standard-response sprinklers shall be permitted for use in hazardous areas protected in accordance with 19.3.2.1.

**A.19.3.5.8** The provisions of 19.3.5.8(6) and (7) are not intended to supplant NFPA 13, *Standard for the Installation of Sprinkler Systems*, which requires that residential sprinklers with more than a 10°F (5.6°C) difference in temperature rating not be mixed within a room. Currently there are no additional prohibitions in NFPA 13 on the mixing of sprinklers having different thermal response characteristics. Conversely, there are no design parameters to make practical the mixing of residential and other types of sprinklers.

**18.3.5.9 Reserved.**

**19.3.5.9** Isolated hazardous areas shall be permitted to be protected in accordance with 9.7.1.2. For new installations in existing health care occupancies, where more than two sprinklers are installed in a single area, waterflow detection shall be provided to sound the building fire alarm or to notify, by a signal, any constantly attended location, such as PBX, security, or emergency room, at which the necessary corrective action shall be taken.

**18.3.5.10*** Sprinklers in areas where cubicle curtains are installed shall be in accordance with NFPA 13, *Standard for the Installation of Sprinkler Systems*.

**19.3.5.10*** Newly introduced cubicle curtains in sprinklered areas shall be installed in accordance with NFPA 13, *Standard for the Installation of Sprinkler Systems*.

**CHAPTER 18 • New**

**A.18.3.5.10** For the proper operation of sprinkler systems, cubicle curtains and sprinkler locations need to be coordinated. Improperly designed systems might obstruct the sprinkler spray from reaching the fire or might shield the heat from the sprinkler. Many options are available to the designer including, but not limited to, hanging the cubicle curtains 18 in. (455 mm) below the sprinkler deflector; using a ½ in. (13 mm) diagonal mesh or a 70 percent open weave top panel that extends 18 in. (455 mm) below the sprinkler deflector; or designing the system to have a horizontal and minimum vertical distance that meets the requirements of NFPA 13, *Standard for the Installation of Sprinkler Systems*. The test data that form the basis of the NFPA 13 requirements are from fire tests with sprinkler discharge that penetrated a single privacy curtain.

**18.3.5.11** Portable fire extinguishers shall be provided in all health care occupancies in accordance with 9.7.4.1.

**CHAPTER 19 • Existing**

**A.19.3.5.10** For the proper operation of sprinkler systems, cubicle curtains and sprinkler locations need to be coordinated. Improperly designed systems might obstruct the sprinkler spray from reaching the fire or might shield the heat from the sprinkler. Many options are available to the designer including, but not limited to, hanging the cubicle curtains 18 in. (455 mm) below the sprinkler deflector; using ½ in. (13 mm) diagonal mesh or a 70 percent open weave top panel that extends 18 in. (455 mm) below the sprinkler deflector; or designing the system to have a horizontal and minimum vertical distance that meets the requirements of NFPA 13, *Standard for the Installation of Sprinkler Systems*. The test data that forms the basis of the NFPA 13 requirements is from fire tests with sprinkler discharge that penetrated a single privacy curtain.

**19.3.5.11** Portable fire extinguishers shall be provided in all health care occupancies in accordance with 9.7.4.1.

Paragraph 18.3.5.1 requires automatic sprinkler protection throughout all new health care facilities; 18.3.5.6 requires the use of quick-response or residential sprinklers throughout all smoke compartments containing patient sleeping rooms.

Paragraph 19.3.5.1 was added to the *Code* for the 2006 edition and requires automatic sprinkler protection throughout all existing nursing homes. The NFPA *101* public proposal[16] recommending the sprinklering of all existing nursing homes was received from the American Health Care Association (AHCA). The substantiation provided by AHCA to support its proposal reads as follows:

> Until 2003, the fire safety record for nursing homes has been excellent. For the past 20 years the average number of fire deaths in nursing homes from multiple death fires has averaged one death per year. For the past 10 years, the average has been 0.3 deaths per year, less than one death per year. Unfortunately, in 2003 there have been two multiple death nursing home fires. There is nothing more important to the American Health Care Association than to insure the protection of patients entrusted in the care of our member facilities. Although compliance with the *Life Safety Code*, including in nonsprinklered buildings, has proven over the last 20 years to provide a very high level of fire safety, the two recent nursing home multiple death fires require us to reevaluate nursing home fire safety requirements. Following review of all the multiple death nursing home fires since Medicare/Medicaid Regulations adopted the *Life Safety Code* in 1970, it is our opinion that having sprinklers installed in all nursing homes will significantly reduce, if not eliminate, multiple death nursing home fires.
>
> Approximately 25 percent of the nursing homes in the United States are not fully sprinklered and our data shows that it will cost approximately 1 billion dollars to retrofit sprinklers in all nonsprinklered nursing homes. This is a significant cost and local, state, and federal governments must work with the nursing home profession to find a way to pay for this. These funds must be available to providers well in advance of the required date for compliance.
>
> Like cost, compliance must be considered when requiring that all nursing homes be fully sprinklered. There must be a reasonable period of time allowed for that, taking into consideration the enormous undertaking of the task, which may necessitate the safe temporary relocation of patients and will also impact the fire sprinkler industry.
>
> It is important that the proposed Annex note be included to recognize the excellent fire/life safety record of existing sprinkler systems using standard sprinkler heads and the lack of a need to replace these existing sprinkler heads with quick response or residential heads.

Paragraph 19.3.5.2 references the existing health care occupancies high-rise building sprinkler requirement of 19.4.2 that is new to the 2009 edition of the *Code*. Without the cross-reference, the user who consults 19.3.5 to identify the sprinkler requirements applicable to existing health care occupancies might miss the requirement that is located in the chapter subsection on high-rise buildings.

Where sprinkler protection is specified, complete building coverage in accordance with the provisions of NFPA 13, *Standard for the Installation of Sprinkler Systems*,[17] is required (see 18/19.3.5.4). The *Code* does not exempt any area of the building from sprinkler protection (see Section 9.7). However, where automatic sprinkler protection is omitted from certain spaces in Type I and Type II construction at the mandate of the authority having jurisdiction (AHJ), and the AHJ approves alternative protective measures, the building is still considered fully protected throughout in accordance with the 18/19.3.5.5. Sprinklers are permitted to be omitted only from areas in buildings of fire-rated, noncombustible construction, locations believed to have sufficient structural fire resistance to outlast most fires. Use of alternative protective measures should be carefully evaluated to ensure protection equivalent to that provided by automatic sprinklers. Where other automatic fire-extinguishing systems are used as an alternative to sprinklers for specific spaces, it is suggested that the spaces also be separated by fire resistance–rated construction from the remainder of the building that is protected by automatic sprinklers.

The word "supervised," as used in 18/19.3.5.1, means that a distinct supervisory signal must be provided to a constantly attended location in the event of any malfunction or action that would impair sprinkler performance. Supervision must be provided, for example, for water supply and sprinkler control valves, fire pump power and running conditions, water tank levels and temperatures, pressure in pressure tanks, air pressure in dry-pipe systems, building temperature, and city water pressure. Supervision should include all sprinkler sectional control valves, in addition to main control valves. See also 9.7.2.

The intent of 19.3.5.7 is to permit the deletion of redundant features of fire protection within an individual smoke compartment that is sprinklered. Paragraph 19.3.5.7, for example, could be used to permit higher flame spread for interior wall/ceiling finish or nonrated corridor partitions within the sprinklered smoke compartment. In a limited care facility, the corridor smoke detection could be eliminated within the sprinklered smoke compartment as detailed in 19.3.4.5.1(2). However, certain general building protection features must be maintained, unless the building is fully sprinklered. For example, no relaxation in exit features (see Section 19.2) or building construction requirements (see 19.1.6) should be granted, unless the building is fully protected by automatic sprinklers.

Paragraph 19.3.5.8 provides sprinkler system criteria, which other sections of the chapter can require by reference, for permitting exemptions to requirements where automatic sprinkler protection is provided that utilizes quick-response sprinklers throughout smoke compartments having sleeping rooms. For example, 19.3.7.3(2) permits elimination of dampers in ducts penetrating smoke barriers where compartments on both sides of the barriers are sprinkler protected under certain conditions. This paragraph permits elimination of dampers where compartments not used for patient sleeping are sprinklered, using either standard-response or quick-response sprinklers, or where compartments having patient sleeping rooms use quick-response or residential sprinklers.

The exemption provided by 19.3.5.8(6), for use of standard-response sprinklers in lieu of quick-response or residential sprinklers, has been used for purposes not intended by the *Code*. When the exemption was written for the 1991 edition of the *Code*, it addressed the case where quick-response or residential sprinklers were installed throughout the smoke compartment, except in locations where the listing of the sprinkler prohibited its use. For example, the earliest quick-response sprinklers were not listed for use under sloped ceilings, in skylights, or in high ambient temperature areas. The exemption has been editorially revised over multiple editions of the *Code* so as to become unclear and subject to misapplication. The exemption has been misapplied to situations where the smoke compartment is sprinklered with standard-response sprinklers that were installed prior to the advent of quick-response or residential sprinklers. The exemption is not intended to "grandfather" such existing systems. Where another provision of Chapter 19 references 19.3.5.8, such reference is made because the presence of quick-response or residential sprinklers is needed to afford the intended level of life safety. The technical committee agenda for the next revision cycle will include the subject of revising the exemption to express the original intent.

CHAPTER 18 • New

## 18.3.6 Corridors.

Subsection 18/19.3.6 essentially stipulates that all areas that contain combustibles in sufficient quantities to produce a life-threatening fire must be separated from exit access corridors by partitions. Corridor partitions in new health care occupancies and sprinklered existing health care occupancies must be able to limit the transfer of smoke but need not be fire rated. In nonsprinklered existing health care occupancies, the corridor partitions must have a minimum ½-hour fire resistance rating.

A summary of the provisions of 18/19.3.6 follows.

1. Paragraph 18/19.3.6.1 establishes requirements for corridor partitions (walls) to be provided, complete with numerous exemptions.
2. Paragraph 18/19.3.6.2 establishes construction requirements for corridor partitions.
3. Paragraph 18/19.3.6.3 establishes requirements for doors in corridor partitions.
4. Paragraph 18/19.3.6.4 addresses transfer grilles.
5. Paragraph 18/19.3.6.5 permits miscellaneous openings, such as mail slots.

**18.3.6.1 Corridor Separation.** Corridors shall be separated from all other areas by partitions complying with 18.3.6.2 through 18.3.6.5 *(see also 18.2.5.4)*, unless otherwise permitted by the following:

(1) Spaces shall be permitted to be unlimited in area and open to the corridor, provided that the following criteria are met:

(a) The spaces are not used for patient sleeping rooms, treatment rooms, or hazardous areas.
(b) The corridors onto which the spaces open in the same smoke compartment are protected by an electrically supervised automatic smoke detection system in accordance with 18.3.4, or the smoke compartment in which the space is located is protected throughout by quick-response sprinklers.
(c) The open space is protected by an electrically supervised automatic smoke detection system in accordance with 18.3.4, or the entire space is arranged and located to allow direct supervision by the facility staff from a nurses' station or similar space.
(d) The space does not obstruct access to required exits.

(2) Waiting areas shall be permitted to be open to the corridor, provided that the following criteria are met:

(a) The aggregate waiting area in each smoke compartment does not exceed 600 ft² (55.7 m²).
(b) Each area is protected by an electrically supervised automatic smoke detection system in accordance with 18.3.4, or each area is arranged and located to allow direct supervision by the facility staff from a nursing station or similar space.
(c) The area does not obstruct access to required exits.

CHAPTER 19 • Existing

## 19.3.6 Corridors.

**19.3.6.1 Corridor Separation.** Corridors shall be separated from all other areas by partitions complying with 19.3.6.2 through 19.3.6.5 *(see also 19.2.5.4)*, unless otherwise permitted by the following:

(1) Smoke compartments protected throughout by an approved, supervised automatic sprinkler system in accordance with 19.3.5.8 shall be permitted to have spaces that are unlimited in size and open to the corridor, provided that the following criteria are met:

(a) The spaces are not used for patient sleeping rooms, treatment rooms, or hazardous areas.
(b) The corridors onto which the spaces open in the same smoke compartment are protected by an electrically supervised automatic smoke detection system in accordance with 19.3.4, or the smoke compartment in which the space is located is protected throughout by quick-response sprinklers.
(c) The open space is protected by an electrically supervised automatic smoke detection system in accordance with 19.3.4, or the entire space is arranged and located to allow direct supervision by the facility staff from a nurses' station or similar space.
(d) The space does not obstruct access to required exits.

(2) In smoke compartments protected throughout by an approved, supervised automatic sprinkler system in accordance with 19.3.5.8, waiting areas shall be permitted to be open to the corridor, provided that the following criteria are met:

(a) The aggregate waiting area in each smoke compartment does not exceed 600 ft² (55.7 m²).
(b) Each area is protected by an electrically supervised automatic smoke detection system in accordance with 19.3.4, or each area is arranged and located to allow direct supervision by the facility staff from a nursing station or similar space.
(c) The area does not obstruct access to required exits.

**CHAPTER 18 • New**

(3)* This requirement shall not apply to spaces for nurses' stations.

**A.18.3.6.1(3)** A typical nurses' station would normally contain one or more of the following with associated furniture and furnishings:

(1) Charting area
(2) Clerical area
(3) Nourishment station
(4) Storage of small amounts of medications, medical equipment and supplies, clerical supplies, and linens
(5) Patient monitoring and communication equipment

(4) Gift shops not exceeding 500 ft$^2$ (46.4 m$^2$) shall be permitted to be open to the corridor or lobby.

(5) In a limited care facility, group meeting or multipurpose therapeutic spaces shall be permitted to open to the corridor, provided that the following criteria are met:

(a) The space is not a hazardous area.
(b) The space is protected by an electrically supervised automatic smoke detection system in accordance with 18.3.4, or the space is arranged and located to allow direct supervision by the facility staff from the nurses' station or similar location.
(c) The space does not obstruct access to required exits.

**CHAPTER 19 • Existing**

(3)* This requirement shall not apply to spaces for nurses' stations.

**A.19.3.6.1(3)** A typical nurses' station would normally contain one or more of the following with associated furniture and furnishings:

(1) Charting area
(2) Clerical area
(3) Nourishment station
(4) Storage of small amounts of medications, medical equipment and supplies, clerical supplies, and linens
(5) Patient monitoring and communication equipment

(4) Gift shops not exceeding 500 ft$^2$ (46.4 m$^2$) shall be permitted to be open to the corridor or lobby, provided that one of the following criteria is met:

(a) The building is protected throughout by an approved automatic sprinkler system in accordance with Section 9.7.
(b) The gift shop is protected throughout by an approved automatic sprinkler system in accordance with Section 9.7, and storage is separately protected.

(5) Limited care facilities in smoke compartments protected throughout by an approved, supervised automatic sprinkler system in accordance with 19.3.5.8 shall be permitted to have group meeting or multipurpose therapeutic spaces open to the corridor, provided that the following criteria are met:

(a) The space is not a hazardous area.
(b) The space is protected by an electrically supervised automatic smoke detection system in accordance with 19.3.4, or the space is arranged and located to allow direct supervision by the facility staff from the nurses' station or similar location.
(c) The space does not obstruct access to required exits.

(6) Spaces, other than patient sleeping rooms, treatment rooms, and hazardous areas, shall be permitted to be open to the corridor and unlimited in area, provided that the following criteria are met:

(a) The space and the corridors onto which it opens, where located in the same smoke compartment, are protected by an electrically supervised automatic smoke detection system in accordance with 19.3.4.
(b)*Each space is protected by automatic sprinklers, or the furnishings and furniture, in combination with all other combustibles within the area, are of such minimum quantity and arrangement that a fully developed fire is unlikely to occur.

CHAPTER 18 • New

CHAPTER 19 • Existing

**A.19.3.6.1(6)(b)** A fully developed fire (flashover) occurs if the rate of heat release of the burning materials exceeds the capability of the space to absorb or vent that heat. The ability of common lining (wall, ceiling, and floor) materials to absorb heat is approximately 0.75 Btu/ft$^2$ (0.07 kJ/m$^2$) of lining. The venting capability of open doors or windows is in excess of 20 Btu/ft$^2$ (1.95 kJ/m$^2$) of opening. In a fire that has not reached flashover conditions, fire will spread from one furniture item to another only if the burning item is close to another furniture item. For example, if individual furniture items have heat release rates of 500 Btu/s (525 kW) and are separated by 12 in. (305 mm) or more, the fire is not expected to spread from item to item, and flashover is unlikely to occur. *(See also the NFPA Fire Protection Handbook.)*

(c) The space does not obstruct access to required exits.

(7)* Waiting areas shall be permitted to be open to the corridor, provided that the following criteria are met:

(a) Each area does not exceed 600 ft$^2$ (55.7 m$^2$).
(b) The area is equipped with an electrically supervised automatic smoke detection system in accordance with 19.3.4.
(c) The area does not obstruct any access to required exits.

**A.19.3.6.1(7)** This provision permits waiting areas to be located across the corridor from each other, provided that neither area exceeds the 600 ft$^2$ (55.7 m$^2$) limitation.

(8) Group meeting or multipurpose therapeutic spaces, other than hazardous areas, that are under continuous supervision by facility staff shall be permitted to be open to the corridor, provided that the following criteria are met:

(a) Each area does not exceed 1500 ft$^2$ (139 m$^2$).
(b) Not more than one such space is permitted per smoke compartment.
(c) The area is equipped with an electrically supervised automatic smoke detection system in accordance with 19.3.4.
(d) The area does not obstruct access to required exits.

Paragraph 18/19.3.6.1 requires that all spaces be separated from corridors by partitions. The intent is to limit the risk of exposing the corridor to fire. Exemptions are provided to permit specific areas to be open to the corridor. Paragraphs 18.3.6.1(1) through (5) and 19.3.6.1(1) through (8) specify those areas that are permitted to be open to corridors.

Paragraph 18/19.3.6.1(1) contains provisions that permit unlimited size spaces, such as recreation/lounge/waiting areas [or wheelchair and gurney storage alcoves not larger than 50 ft$^2$ (4.6 m$^2$), so as not to constitute a hazardous area], to be open to the corridor. New health care occupancies are offered this exemption because they are sprinklered; existing health care occupancies must be sprinklered in order to use the exemption. The staff must visually supervise the open space from a permanent staff location, or equivalent early warning of fire must be provided by an electrically supervised smoke detection system within the open space. Interconnected corridors that are not separated from the open space must be equipped with an electrically supervised smoke detection system, or the sprinklers throughout the smoke compartment must be quick-response sprinklers. Exhibit 18/19.23 illustrates the provisions of 18/19.3.6.1(1). The black-filled circles at the left of the figure depict quick-response sprinklers; the unfilled circles at the right of the figure depict standard-response sprinklers. In the smoke compartment at the left, which includes patient sleeping rooms, the open space has direct supervision from the nurses' station located across the corridor. In the smoke compartment at the right, which contains no patient sleeping rooms, none of the three open spaces has direct supervision, so each space is equipped with smoke detection (denoted by X); because the sprinklers in this compartment are standard-response sprinklers, the required smoke detection must be extended into the corridor of that smoke compartment.

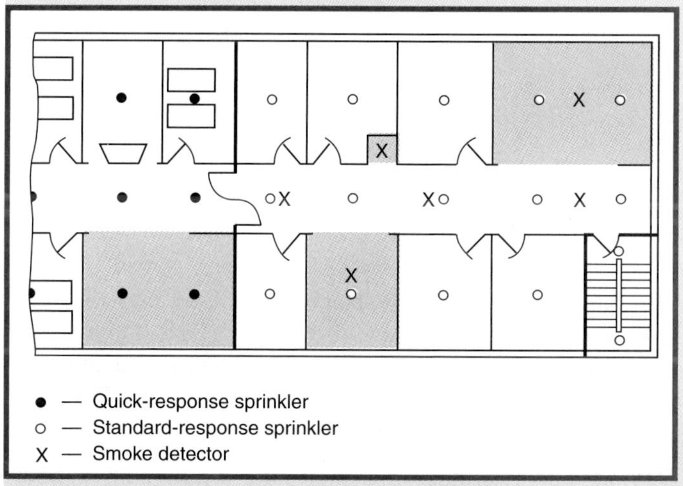


***Exhibit 18/19.23** Spaces permitted to be open to the corridor.*

In Exhibit 18/19.23, the smallest of the three open spaces at the right of the figure is meant to depict a wheelchair and gurney storage alcove not larger than 50 ft² (4.6 m²). By limiting the alcove size to not more than 50 ft² (4.6 m²) and restricting its use to the storage of wheelchairs and gurneys, such space is not a hazardous area [see Table 18.3.2.1 and 19.3.2.1.5(7)]. The open space created by the alcove meets the use limitation of 18/19.3.6.1(1)(a) by not being used for patient sleeping, for patient treatment, or as a hazardous area. Smoke detection of the space is required in accordance with 18/19.3.6.1(1)(c) because of the lack of direct supervision by staff, but the smoke detector shown in the exhibit could be omitted if the corridor detectors were positioned to cover the storage alcove in accordance with the spacing provisions of *NFPA 72, National Fire Alarm Code*, and the listing of the smoke detectors.

Waiting areas that are open to the corridor and whose aggregate area exceeds 600 ft² (55.7 m²) in any smoke compartment are permitted only if the provisions of 18/19.3.6.1(1) are met. Provided that the waiting areas that are open to the corridor do not exceed 600 ft² (55.7 m²) in aggregate area in any smoke compartment, they are permitted to meet the less-demanding criteria of 18/19.3.6.1(2). The smoke compartment utilizing the open space exemption must be sprinklered, and, where the smoke compartment is used for patient sleeping, the sprinklers must be quick-response sprinklers (see 18.3.5.6 and 19.3.5.8). Each waiting area must be located to allow direct visual supervision by the staff or be equipped with an electrically supervised automatic smoke detection system. In all cases, waiting spaces must be arranged so as not to obstruct access to exits. Exhibit 18/19.24 illustrates the provisions of 18/19.3.6.1(2). The waiting space at the left of the compartment receives direct supervision from the nurses' station located across the corridor. The waiting space at the right of the compartment has no direct supervision and, therefore, must be provided with smoke detection (denoted by X).

Although 18/19.3.6.1(1) does not permit treatment spaces to be open to corridors, and 18/19.3.6.1(2) lim-

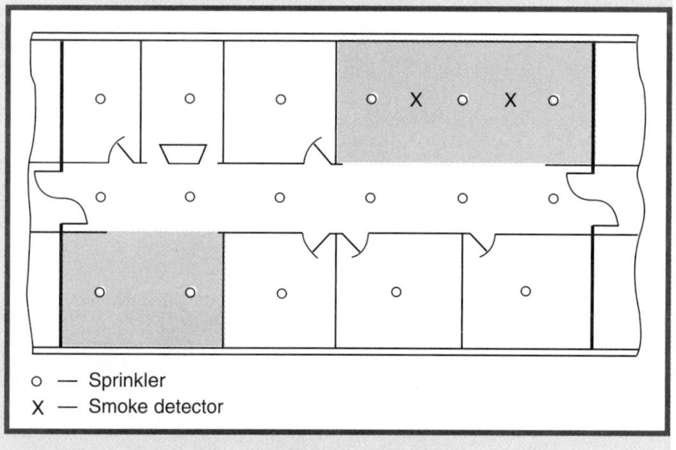


***Exhibit 18/19.24** Waiting spaces of limited aggregate area that are open to the corridor.*

CHAPTER 18 • New

its the open spaces for use as waiting areas, 18/19.3.6.1(5) permits group meeting or multipurpose therapeutic spaces to be open to corridors in limited care facilities. Where the sprinklered smoke compartment utilizing the open space exemption is used for patient sleeping, the sprinklers must be quick-response sprinklers (see 18.3.5.6 and 19.3.5.8). These spaces are not permitted to be hazardous areas or to obstruct access to required exits.

Paragraphs 18/19.3.6.1(1), (2), and (5) require that the open space be supervised by the staff or be protected by a smoke detection system. Staff supervision is important; it allows the staff to see, hear, or smell a developing fire or to prevent the ignition of a fire by virtue of their presence. The use of closed-circuit television or mirrors does not offer all the protection provided by staff and should not be relied on as a substitute for direct supervision. Adequate supervision is not provided if the staff cannot readily supervise the space without special effort (e.g., by looking around a corner).

CHAPTER 19 • Existing

Areas used for charting and communication by staff are permitted to be open to the corridor, as are nurses' stations. See 18/19.3.6.1(3).

Gift shops are addressed in 18/19.3.6.1(4). Many gift shops, particularly those containing combustible storage and having sizable retail areas, pose a hazard well beyond that which is considered normal to patient-occupied spaces and, thus, merit special protection. However, it is recognized that many small retail areas [e.g., less than 500 ft$^2$ (46.4 m$^2$)] constitute a relatively minor hazard that is mitigated adequately by automatic sprinkler protection. Paragraph 18/19.3.6.1(4) provides the facility some flexibility in the design and operation of gift shops. The gift shop must be sprinklered, and, for existing health care occupancy buildings that are not sprinklered throughout, any storage associated with the gift shop must be protected in a separate room. Where the stored materials are combustible and the storage room exceeds 50 ft$^2$ (4.6 m$^2$), such room must be protected as a hazardous area in accordance with 19.3.2.1.5(7).

**18.3.6.2* Construction of Corridor Walls.**

**A.18.3.6.2** It is the intent of the *Code* that there be no required fire resistance or area limitations for vision panels in corridor walls and doors.

An architectural, exposed, suspended-grid acoustical tile ceiling with penetrating items, such as sprinkler piping and sprinklers; ducted HVAC supply and return-air diffusers; speakers; and recessed lighting fixtures, is capable of limiting the transfer of smoke.

**18.3.6.2.1** Corridor walls shall be permitted to terminate at the ceiling where the ceiling is constructed to limit the transfer of smoke.

**18.3.6.2.2** No fire resistance rating shall be required for corridor walls.

**18.3.6.2.3** Corridor walls shall form a barrier to limit the transfer of smoke.

**19.3.6.2 Construction of Corridor Walls.**

**19.3.6.2.1** Corridor walls shall be continuous from the floor to the underside of the floor or roof deck above; through any concealed spaces, such as those above suspended ceilings; and through interstitial structural and mechanical spaces, unless otherwise permitted by 19.3.6.2.4 through 19.3.6.2.8.

**19.3.6.2.2*** Corridor walls shall have a minimum $^1/_2$-hour fire resistance rating.

**A.19.3.6.2.2** The intent of the minimum $^1/_2$-hour fire resistance rating for corridor partitions is to require a nominal fire rating, particularly where the fire rating of existing partitions cannot be documented. Examples of acceptable partition assemblies would include, but are not limited to, $^1/_2$ in. (13 mm) gypsum board, wood lath and plaster, gypsum lath, or metal lath and plaster.

**19.3.6.2.3*** Corridor walls shall form a barrier to limit the transfer of smoke.

**A.19.3.6.2.3** The purpose of extending a corridor wall above a lay-in ceiling or through a concealed space is to provide a barrier to limit the passage of smoke. The intent of 19.3.6.2.3 is not to require light-tight barriers above lay-in ceilings or to require an absolute seal of the room from the corridor. Small holes, penetrations, or gaps around items such as ductwork, conduit, or telecommunication lines should not affect the ability of this barrier to limit the passage of smoke.

**19.3.6.2.4*** In smoke compartments protected throughout by an approved, supervised automatic sprinkler system in accordance with 19.3.5.7, a corridor shall be permitted to be separated from all other areas by non-fire-rated partitions and shall be permitted to terminate at the ceiling where the ceiling is constructed to limit the transfer of smoke.

**A.19.3.6.2.4** An architectural, exposed, suspended-grid acoustical tile ceiling with penetrating items, such as sprinkler piping and sprinklers; ducted HVAC supply and return-air diffusers; speakers; and recessed lighting fixtures, is capable of limiting the transfer of smoke.

**19.3.6.2.5** Existing corridor partitions shall be permitted to terminate at ceilings that are not an integral part of a floor construction if 60 in. (1525 mm) or more of space exists between the top of the ceiling subsystem and the bottom of the floor or roof above, provided that all the following criteria are met:

(1) The ceiling is part of a fire-rated assembly tested to have a minimum 1-hour fire resistance rating in compliance with the provisions of Section 8.3.
(2) The corridor partitions form smoke-tight joints with the ceilings, and joint filler, if used, is noncombustible.
(3) Each compartment of interstitial space that constitutes a separate smoke area is vented, in a smoke emergency, to the outside by mechanical means having the capacity to provide not less than two air changes per hour but, in no case, a capacity less than 5000 $ft^3/min$ (2.35 $m^3/s$).
(4) The interstitial space is not used for storage.
(5) The space is not used as a plenum for supply, exhaust, or return air, except as noted in 19.3.6.2.5(3).

**19.3.6.2.6*** Existing corridor partitions shall be permitted to terminate at monolithic ceilings that resist the passage of smoke where there is a smoke-tight joint between the top of the partition and the bottom of the ceiling.

**A.19.3.6.2.6** Monolithic ceilings are continuous horizontal membranes composed of noncombustible or limited-combustible materials, such as plaster or gypsum board, with seams or cracks permanently sealed.

**19.3.6.2.7** Fixed fire window assemblies in accordance with Section 8.3 shall be permitted in corridor walls, unless otherwise permitted in 19.3.6.2.8.

**19.3.6.2.8** There shall be no restrictions in area and fire resistance of glass and frames in smoke compartments protected throughout by an approved, supervised automatic sprinkler system in accordance with 19.3.5.7.

The building construction types addressed by 18/19.1.6.1 might affect the choice of materials used to construct corridor walls/partitions. For example, corridor construction materials in buildings of Type I or Type II construction must be either noncombustible or limited-combustible, as required by 18/19.1.6.4.

In new health care occupancies and sprinklered existing health care occupancies, corridor walls need not be fire rated but must be constructed to resist the passage of smoke. Corridor walls in such buildings are permitted to terminate at ceilings, provided that the wall and ceiling resist the passage of smoke. Where suspended ceilings are provided, partitions are permitted to terminate at the suspended ceiling without any additional special protection if the suspended ceiling will resist the passage of smoke. The ability of the ceiling to resist the passage of smoke must be carefully evaluated, and guidance is provided in A.18.3.6.2 and A.19.3.6.2.4. There are no restrictions in terms of area or fire resistance for glazing used in these non-fire-rated corridor partitions. These requirements are illustrated in Exhibit 18/19.25.

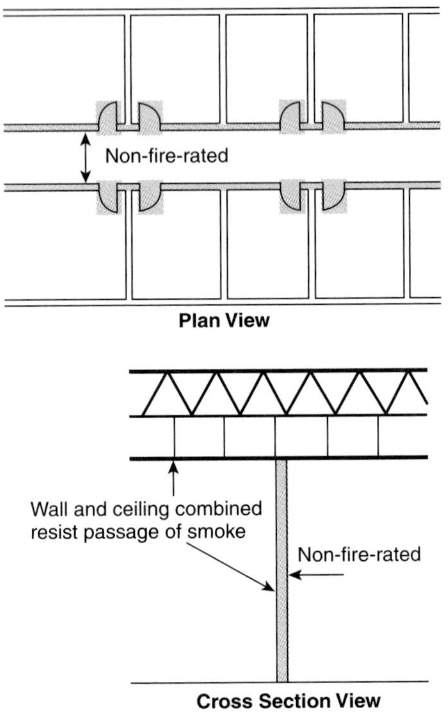


*Exhibit 18/19.25 Corridor walls in new health care occupancies and existing, sprinklered health care occupancies.*

Editions of the *Code* prior to 1997 required that corridor walls in nonsprinklered health care occupancies have a minimum 20-minute fire resistance rating. The change to a minimum ½-hour fire resistance rating was not meant to implement a more stringent requirement. Rather, the intent was to correlate with a change made in Chapter 8, where the range of fire resistance ratings that had previously been 20-minute, ½-hour, and ¾-hour ratings was simplified to the single category of a ½-hour fire resistance rating. See the explanation in A.8.3.1(4) for determining that existing walls in good condition, which previously received credit for providing a 20-minute rating, provide a ½-hour rating. It is not the intent to throw into noncompliance existing walls that were previously judged to meet the former 20-minute rating criterion.

In nonsprinklered existing health care occupancies, corridor walls must be constructed of assemblies having a minimum fire resistance rating of ½ hour. In setting the requirements for ½-hour corridor wall partitions, it was intended to accept the separation provided by existing partitions of any substantial construction that are capable of serving as a barrier for a short period of time — without requiring documentation of a specific fire rating. The ½-hour rating is intended to permit partitions of wood lath and plaster, ½ in. (13 mm) gypsum board, and similar materials. Ordinary glass would not be permitted in corridor walls of nonsprinklered health care occupancies.

Fire-rated existing corridor partitions must be constructed to extend continuously through all concealed spaces — for example, through to the floor or roof deck above a suspended ceiling. This requirement is illustrated in Exhibit 18/19.26.

Openings in corridor partitions in nonsprinklered smoke compartments must be suitably protected to

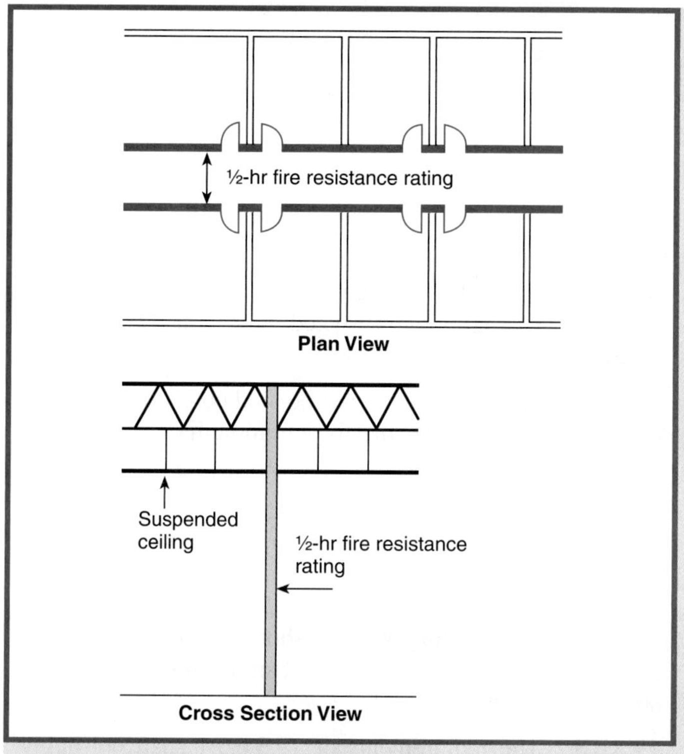


***Exhibit 18/19.26*** *Corridor walls in existing, nonsprinklered health care smoke compartment.*

maintain corridor separation. Fixed fire windows are permitted by 19.3.6.2.7, which references Section 8.3. Section 8.3 requires compliance with NFPA 80, *Standard for Fire Doors and Other Opening Protectives.* Fire-rated, $^1/_4$ in. (6 mm) thick wired glass is limited to a maximum of 1296 in.$^2$ (0.84 m$^2$) set in approved metal frames. Each wired glass panel is limited to a maximum dimension of 54 in. (1370 mm). The glass should be labeled and should be well embedded in putty, with all exposed joints between the metal and the glass struck and pointed. A number of wired glass panels can be used in a single partition, provided that each 1296 in.$^2$ (0.84 m$^2$) section is separated from adjacent panels by a steel or other approved metal mullion. Fire-rated glazing, other than $^1/_4$ in. (6 mm) wired glass, should be installed in accordance with the manufacturer's instructions and listing. The use of fire-rated glazing in a partition reduces the fire resistance capability of the partition because of radiant energy transfer through the glass panel. The excessive use of glazing in corridor walls of nonsprinklered smoke compartments, therefore, should be avoided. In sprinklered smoke compartments, there are no restrictions on the use of glass and glazing in corridor walls (see 19.3.6.2.8).

Paragraph 19.3.6.2.5 specifies criteria for terminating existing corridor partitions at ceilings where the interstitial space above the ceiling meets certain criteria. However, the minimum $^1/_2$-hour fire resistance rating of the corridor walls still applies. The walls are permitted to terminate at a ceiling that has been tested as a portion of a floor/ceiling or roof/ceiling assembly having a fire resistance rating of 1 hour or more. Each compartment located above such a ceiling must be equipped with an automatic mechanical smoke exhaust system that is capable of providing a minimum of two air changes per hour but exhausting not less than 5000 ft$^3$/min (2.35 m$^3$/s). See the additional criteria in 19.3.6.2.5(1) through (5).

Where a monolithic ceiling composed of noncombustible materials, such as plaster or gypsum board with permanently sealed seams forming a continuous horizontal membrane, is provided, existing partitions are permitted to terminate at the underside of the ceiling in accordance with 19.3.6.2.6.

**18.3.6.3* Corridor Doors.**

**A.18.3.6.3** While it is recognized that closed doors serve to maintain tenable conditions in a corridor and adjacent patient rooms, such doors, which, under normal or fire conditions, are self-closing, might create a special hazard for the personal safety of a room occupant. Such closed doors might present a problem of delay in discovery, confining fire products beyond tenable conditions.

Because it is critical for responding staff members to be able to immediately identify the specific room involved, it is suggested that approved automatic smoke detection that is interconnected with the building fire alarm be considered for rooms having doors equipped with closing devices. Such

**19.3.6.3 Corridor Doors.**

CHAPTER 18 • New

detection is permitted to be located at any approved point within the room. When activated, the detector is required to provide a warning that indicates the specific room of involvement by activation of a fire alarm annunciator, nurse call system, or any other device acceptable to the authority having jurisdiction.

**18.3.6.3.1*** Doors protecting corridor openings shall be constructed to resist the passage of smoke, and the following also shall apply:

(1) Compliance with NFPA 80, *Standard for Fire Doors and Other Opening Protectives*, shall not be required.
(2) A clearance between the bottom of the door and the floor covering not exceeding 1 in. (25 mm) shall be permitted for corridor doors.
(3) Doors to toilet rooms, bathrooms, shower rooms, sink closets, and similar auxiliary spaces that do not contain flammable or combustible material shall not be required to be constructed to resist the passage of smoke.

**A.18.3.6.3.1** Gasketing of doors should not be necessary to achieve resistance to the passage of smoke if the door is relatively tight-fitting.

**18.3.6.3.2 Reserved.**

**18.3.6.3.3 Reserved.**

**18.3.6.3.4 Reserved.**

**18.3.6.3.5** Doors shall be self-latching and provided with positive latching hardware.

CHAPTER 19 • Existing

**19.3.6.3.1*** Doors protecting corridor openings in other than required enclosures of vertical openings, exits, or hazardous areas shall be doors constructed to resist the passage of smoke and shall be constructed of materials such as the following:

(1) $1\frac{3}{4}$ in. (44 mm) thick, solid-bonded core wood
(2) Material that resists fire for a minimum of 20 minutes

**A.19.3.6.3.1** Gasketing of doors should not be necessary to achieve resistance to the passage of smoke if the door is relatively tight-fitting.

**19.3.6.3.2** The requirements of 19.3.6.3.1 shall not apply where otherwise permitted by the following:

(1) Doors to toilet rooms, bathrooms, shower rooms, sink closets, and similar auxiliary spaces that do not contain flammable or combustible materials shall not be required to comply with 19.3.6.3.1.
(2) In smoke compartments protected throughout by an approved, supervised automatic sprinkler system in accordance with 19.3.5.7, the door construction materials requirements of 19.3.6.3.1 shall not be mandatory, but the doors shall be constructed to resist the passage of smoke.

**19.3.6.3.3** Compliance with NFPA 80, *Standard for Fire Doors and Other Opening Protectives*, shall not be required.

**19.3.6.3.4** A clearance between the bottom of the door and the floor covering not exceeding 1 in. (25 mm) shall be permitted for corridor doors.

**19.3.6.3.5*** Doors shall be provided with a means for keeping the door closed that is acceptable to the authority having jurisdiction, and the following requirements also shall apply:

(1) The device used shall be capable of keeping the door fully closed if a force of 5 lbf (22 N) is applied at the latch edge of the door.
(2) Roller latches shall be prohibited on corridor doors in buildings not fully protected by an approved automatic sprinkler system in accordance with 19.3.5.7.

**A.19.3.6.3.5** While it is recognized that closed doors serve to maintain tenable conditions in a corridor and adjacent patient rooms, such doors, which, under normal or fire conditions, are self-closing, might create a special hazard for the personal safety of a room occupant. Such closed doors might present a problem of delay in discovery, confining fire products beyond tenable conditions.

Because it is critical for responding staff members to be able to immediately identify the specific room involved, it is suggested that approved automatic smoke detection that is interconnected with the building fire alarm be considered for rooms having doors equipped with closing devices. Such detection is permitted to be located at any approved point within the room. When activated, the detector is required to provide a warning that indicates the specific room of involvement by activation of a fire alarm annunciator, nurse call system, or any other device acceptable to the authority having jurisdiction.

In existing buildings, use of the following options reasonably ensures that patient room doors will be closed and remain closed during a fire:

(1) Doors should have positive latches, and a suitable program that trains staff to close the doors in an emergency should be established.
(2) It is the intent of the *Code* that no new installations of roller latches be permitted; however, repair or replacement of roller latches is not considered a new installation.
(3) Doors protecting openings to patient sleeping or treatment rooms, or spaces having a similar combustible loading, might be held closed using a closer exerting a closing force of not less than 5 lbf (22 N) on the door latch stile.

**18.3.6.3.6** Doors to toilet rooms, bathrooms, shower rooms, sink closets, and similar auxiliary spaces that do not contain flammable or combustible materials shall not be required to meet the latching requirements of 18.3.6.3.5.

**19.3.6.3.6** The requirements of 19.3.6.3.5 shall not apply where otherwise permitted by the following:

(1) Doors to toilet rooms, bathrooms, shower rooms, sink closets, and similar auxiliary spaces that do not contain flammable or combustible materials shall not be required to comply with 19.3.6.3.5.
(2) Existing roller latches demonstrated to keep the door closed against a force of 5 lbf (22 N) shall be permitted to be kept in service.

**18.3.6.3.7** Powered doors that comply with the requirements of 7.2.1.9 shall not be required to meet the latching requirements of 18.3.6.3.5, provided that:

(1) The door is equipped with a means for keeping the door closed that is acceptable to the authority having jurisdiction
(2) The device used is capable of keeping the door fully closed if a force of 5 lbf (22 N) is applied at the latch edge of a swinging door and applied in any direction to a sliding or folding door.

**19.3.6.3.7** Powered doors that comply with the requirements of 7.2.1.9 shall be considered as complying with the requirements of 19.3.6.3.5 provided the door is equipped with a means for keeping the door closed that is acceptable to the authority having jurisdiction and the device used is capable of keeping the door fully closed if a force of 5 lbf (22 N) is applied at the latch edge of a swinging door and applied in any direction to a sliding or folding door.

CHAPTER 18 • New

**18.3.6.3.8** Corridor doors utilizing an inactive leaf shall have automatic flush bolts on the inactive leaf to provide positive latching.

**18.3.6.3.9** Roller latches shall be prohibited.

**18.3.6.3.10*** Doors shall not be held open by devices other than those that release when the door is pushed or pulled.

**A.18.3.6.3.10** Doors should not be blocked open by furniture, door stops, chocks, tie-backs, drop-down or plunger-type devices, or other devices that necessitate manual unlatching or releasing action to close. Examples of hold-open devices that release when the door is pushed or pulled are friction catches or magnetic catches.

**18.3.6.3.11** Door-closing devices shall not be required on doors in corridor wall openings other than those serving required exits, smoke barriers, or enclosures of vertical openings and hazardous areas.

**18.3.6.3.12*** Nonrated, factory- or field-applied protective plates, unlimited in height, shall be permitted.

**A.18.3.6.3.12** It is not the intent of 18.3.6.3.12 to prohibit the application of push plates, hardware, or other attachments on corridor doors in health care occupancies.

**18.3.6.3.13** Dutch doors shall be permitted where they conform to 18.3.6.3 and meet the following criteria:

(1) Both the upper leaf and lower leaf are equipped with a latching device.
(2) The meeting edges of the upper and lower leaves are quipped with an astragal, a rabbet, or a bevel.
(3) Where protecting openings in enclosures around hazardous areas, the doors comply with NFPA 80, *Standard for Fire Doors and Other Opening Protectives.*

CHAPTER 19 • Existing

**19.3.6.3.8 Reserved.**

**19.3.6.3.9 Reserved.**

**19.3.6.3.10*** Doors shall not be held open by devices other than those that release when the door is pushed or pulled.

**A.19.3.6.3.10** Doors should not be blocked open by furniture, door stops, chocks, tie-backs, drop-down or plunger-type devices, or other devices that necessitate manual unlatching or releasing action to close. Examples of hold-open devices that release when the door is pushed or pulled are friction catches or magnetic catches.

**19.3.6.3.11** Door-closing devices shall not be required on doors in corridor wall openings other than those serving required exits, smoke barriers, or enclosures of vertical openings and hazardous areas.

**19.3.6.3.12*** Nonrated, factory- or field-applied protective plates, unlimited in height, shall be permitted.

**A.19.3.6.3.12** It is not the intent of 19.3.6.3.12 to prohibit the application of push plates, hardware, or other attachments on corridor doors in health care occupancies.

**19.3.6.3.13** Dutch doors shall be permitted where they conform to 19.3.6.3 and meet the following criteria:

(1) Both the upper leaf and lower leaf are equipped with a latching device.
(2) The meeting edges of the upper and lower leaves are equipped with an astragal, a rabbet, or a bevel.
(3) Where protecting openings in enclosures around hazardous areas, the doors comply with NFPA 80, *Standard for Fire Doors and Other Opening Protectives.*

**19.3.6.3.14** Door frames shall be labeled, shall be of steel construction, or shall be of other materials in compliance with the provisions of Section 8.3, unless otherwise permitted by 19.3.6.3.15.

**19.3.6.3.15** Door frames in smoke compartments protected throughout by an approved, supervised automatic sprinkler system in accordance with 19.3.5.7 shall not be required to comply with 19.3.6.3.14.

**19.3.6.3.16** Fixed fire window assemblies in accordance with Section 8.3 shall be permitted in corridor doors.

**19.3.6.3.17** Restrictions in area and fire resistance of glass and frames required by Section 8.3 shall not apply in smoke compartments protected throughout by an approved, supervised automatic sprinkler system in accordance with 19.3.5.7.

CHAPTER 18 • New

**18.3.6.4 Transfer Grilles.**

**18.3.6.4.1** Transfer grilles, regardless of whether they are protected by fusible link–operated dampers, shall not be used in corridor walls or doors, unless otherwise permitted by 18.3.6.4.2.

**18.3.6.4.2** Doors to toilet rooms, bathrooms, shower rooms, sink closets, and similar auxiliary spaces that do not contain flammable or combustible materials shall be permitted to have ventilating louvers or to be undercut.

**18.3.6.5 Openings.**

**18.3.6.5.1** In other than smoke compartments containing patient bedrooms, miscellaneous openings, such as mail slots, pharmacy pass-through windows, laboratory pass-through windows, and cashier pass-through windows, shall be permitted to be installed in vision panels or doors without special protection, provided that both of the following criteria are met:

(1) The aggregate area of openings per room does not exceed 80 in.$^2$ (0.05 m$^2$).
(2) The openings are installed at or below half the distance from the floor to the room ceiling.

**18.3.6.5.2 Reserved.**

CHAPTER 19 • Existing

**19.3.6.4 Transfer Grilles.**

**19.3.6.4.1** Transfer grilles, regardless of whether they are protected by fusible link–operated dampers, shall not be used in corridor walls or doors.

**19.3.6.4.2** Doors to toilet rooms, bathrooms, shower rooms, sink closets, and similar auxiliary spaces that do not contain flammable or combustible materials shall be permitted to have ventilating louvers or to be undercut.

**19.3.6.5 Openings.**

**19.3.6.5.1** Miscellaneous openings, such as mail slots, pharmacy pass-through windows, laboratory pass-through windows, and cashier pass-through windows, shall be permitted to be installed in vision panels or doors without special protection, provided that both of the following criteria are met:

(1) The aggregate area of openings per room does not exceed 20 in.$^2$ (0.015 m$^2$).
(2) The openings are installed at or below half the distance from the floor to the room ceiling.

**19.3.6.5.2** The alternative requirements of 19.3.6.5.1 shall not apply where otherwise modified by the following:

(1) Openings in smoke compartments containing patient bedrooms shall not be permitted to be installed in vision panels or doors without special protection.
(2) For rooms protected throughout by an approved, supervised automatic sprinkler system in accordance with 19.3.5.7, the aggregate area of openings per room shall not exceed 80 in.$^2$ (0.05 m$^2$).

Paragraphs 18.3.6.3.1(2) and 19.3.6.3.4 permit a maximum 1 in. (25 mm) clearance between the bottom of corridor doors (other than doors required in enclosures of vertical openings, exits, and hazardous areas) and the upper surface of the floor-covering material. The paragraph avoids using the word "undercut," because of the negative connotation that word conjures. It is not the intent to permit the door to be deliberately undercut for purposes of making the building heating, ventilating, and air-conditioning system function. That practice is prohibited by NFPA 90A, *Standard for the Installation of Air-Conditioning and Ventilating Systems.*[18] Also see 18/19.3.6.4, which addresses the concept by prohibiting transfer grilles in corridor walls.

Paragraph 18.3.6.3.5 requires that doors in corridor walls in new health care occupancies be self-latching and that the latch provide positive latching. The purpose is to ensure that doors, once closed by staff, will latch against the frame automatically, without staff having to set such latch and, once latched, remain closed until a deliberate unlatching action is initiated, such as turning a lever handle. Roller latches are not permitted in new health care occupancies (see 18.3.6.3.9).

Paragraph 18.3.6.3.7 exempts powered doors in compliance with 7.2.1.9 from having to be self-latching and positive-latching where complying with performance-based criteria that ensure that the closed door functions equivalently to one that is self-latching and positive-latching.

Paragraph 18.3.6.3.8 requires that new corridor doors utilizing an inactive leaf be provided with

CHAPTER 18 • New

CHAPTER 19 • Existing

automatic flush bolts on the inactive leaf so that positive latching is provided without staff having to throw a manual flush bolt, ensuring that the door stays closed.

Doors protecting openings in non-fire-rated corridor partitions — as permitted in new and existing sprinklered health care occupancies — must be able to resist the passage of smoke but are not required to have a fire protection rating. Door-closing devices are not required, except on doors protecting openings in exit enclosures, horizontal exits, vertical openings, or required enclosures of hazardous areas. There are no restrictions — in terms of area or fire rating for glazing used in corridor doors — in new and sprinklered existing health care occupancies.

Patient room corridor doors are not required to have a fire protection rating in new and sprinklered existing health care occupancies. In existing nonsprinklered health care occupancies, the door need not be a true 20-minute fire protection–rated assembly; rather, it is permitted to be a substantial door, such as those constructed of $1^3/_4$ in. (44 mm) thick, solid-bonded core wood. Some consider these doors to be equivalent to 20-minute fire protection–rated doors for which the self-closer has been omitted. If the doors were truly 20-minute fire protection–rated assemblies, field-applied protective plates would be prohibited. Paragraph 18/19.3.6.3.12 reminds the user that factory- or field-applied protective plates are permitted without any height restriction.

Existing corridor doors are not specifically required to be provided with a positive latch. However, they must be capable of being closed and maintained closed against a force of 5 lbf (22 N), applied at the latch edge of the door. In nonsprinklered buildings, roller latches are not permitted. Where positive latches are used, doors must be equipped with a latch that cannot be held in the retracted position. See 19.3.6.3.5.

Corridor doors in nonsprinklered smoke compartments in existing health care occupancies are required to be installed in steel frames, or frames in compliance with Section 8.3, which would include frames typical of a 20-minute fire protection–rated door assembly, such as might be provided by a heavy wood frame. In accordance with 19.3.6.3.16 and Section 8.3, fixed wired glass vision panels are permitted but must not exceed an area of 1296 in.$^2$ (0.84 m$^2$) [maximum dimension of 54 in. (1370 mm)] and must be set in approved metal frames. Other fire-rated glazing must be used in accordance with its listing. Labeled door frames and closing devices are not required, except on doors protecting openings in exit enclosures, horizontal exits, vertical openings, or required enclosures of hazardous areas.

Paragraph 18/19.3.6.4 addresses transfer grilles in corridor walls. The use of an exit access corridor as an exhaust-air, a supply-air, or a return-air plenum for the building air-handling system is not permitted. Corridor doors are not permitted to be deliberately undercut to facilitate transfer of air, but a maximum 1 in. (25 mm) clearance is permitted at the bottom of the door in accordance with 18.3.6.3.1(2) and 19.3.6.3.4. Transfer grilles are not permitted in corridor walls (see 18/19.3.6.4.1) or corridor doors. Also see NFPA 90A, *Standard for the Installation of Air-Conditioning and Ventilating Systems*. However, sink closets, bathrooms, and toilets can have doors equipped with a fixed grille or louver to allow exhaust air to be "made up" from the corridor [see 18.3.6.3.1(3) and 19.3.6.3.2(1)], provided that the space is not used for the storage of flammable or combustible supplies. When using this exemption for sink closets, caution must be exercised to ensure that the closet is not used for the storage of combustibles.

Paragraph 18/19.3.6.5 establishes restrictions for miscellaneous openings in corridor walls. For practical reasons, many small openings are required in corridor walls for use as mail slots, as cashier windows, and as pass-throughs to laboratory or pharmacy spaces. Paragraph 18/19.3.6.5 permits such openings. Openings are not permitted in smoke compartments having sleeping rooms. In other sprinklered smoke compartments, the opening must be limited to a maximum of 80 in.$^2$ (0.05 m$^2$) and must be located in the lower half of the partition. In existing, nonsprinklered, nonsleeping smoke compartments, the opening size is limited to 20 in.$^2$ (0.015 m$^2$).

**18.3.7* Subdivision of Building Spaces.**

**A.18.3.7** See A.18.2.2.

**18.3.7.1** Buildings containing health care facilities shall be subdivided by smoke barriers *(see 18.2.4.3)*, unless otherwise permitted by 18.3.7.2, as follows:

**19.3.7 Subdivision of Building Spaces.**

**19.3.7.1** Smoke barriers shall be provided to divide every story used for sleeping rooms for more than 30 patients into not less than two smoke compartments *(see 19.2.4.3)*, and the following also shall apply:

CHAPTER 18 • New

(1) To divide every story used by inpatients for sleeping or treatment into not less than two smoke compartments
(2) To divide every story having an occupant load of 50 or more persons, regardless of use, into not less than two smoke compartments
(3) To limit the size of each smoke compartment required by 18.3.7.1(1) and (2) to an area not exceeding 22,500 ft$^2$ (2100 m$^2$), unless the area is an atrium separated in accordance with 8.6.7, in which case no limitation in size is required
(4) To limit the travel distance from any point to reach a door in the required smoke barrier to a distance not exceeding 200 ft (61 m)

**18.3.7.2** The smoke barrier subdivision requirement of 18.3.7.1 shall not apply to the following:

(1) Stories that do not contain a health care occupancy located directly above the health care occupancy
(2) Areas that do not contain a health care occupancy and that are separated from the health care occupancy by a fire barrier complying with 7.2.4.3
(3) Stories that do not contain a health care occupancy and that are more than one story below the health care occupancy
(4) Open-air parking structures protected throughout by an approved, supervised automatic sprinkler system in accordance with Section 9.7

**18.3.7.3** Any required smoke barrier shall be constructed in accordance with Section 8.5 and shall have a minimum 1-hour fire resistance rating, unless otherwise permitted by the following:

(1) This requirement shall not apply where an atrium is used, and both of the following criteria also shall apply:
   (a) Smoke barriers shall be permitted to terminate at an atrium wall constructed in accordance with 8.6.7(1)(c).
   (b) Not less than two separate smoke compartments shall be provided on each floor.
(2)* Smoke dampers shall not be required in duct penetrations of smoke barriers in fully ducted heating, ventilating, and air-conditioning systems.

**A.18.3.7.3(2)** Where the smoke control system design requires dampers so that the system will function effectively, it is not the intent of the provision to permit the damper to be omitted.

This provision is not intended to prevent the use of plenum returns where ducting is used to return air from a

CHAPTER 19 • Existing

(1) The size of any such smoke compartment shall not exceed 22,500 ft$^2$ (2100 m$^2$), and the travel distance from any point to reach a door in the required smoke barrier shall not exceed 200 ft (61 m).
(2) Where neither the length nor width of the smoke compartment exceeds 150 ft (46 m), the travel distance to reach the smoke barrier door shall not be limited.
(3) The area of an atrium separated in accordance with 8.6.7 shall not be limited in size.

**19.3.7.2** For purposes of the requirements of 19.3.7, the number of health care occupants shall be determined by actual count of patient bed capacity.

**19.3.7.3** Any required smoke barrier shall be constructed in accordance with Section 8.5 and shall have a minimum ½-hour fire resistance rating, unless otherwise permitted by the following:

(1) This requirement shall not apply where an atrium is used, and both of the following criteria also shall apply:
   (a) Smoke barriers shall be permitted to terminate at an atrium wall constructed in accordance with 8.6.7(1)(c).
   (b) Not less than two separate smoke compartments shall be provided on each floor.
(2)* Smoke dampers shall not be required in duct penetrations of smoke barriers in fully ducted heating, ventilating, and air-conditioning systems where an approved, supervised automatic sprinkler system in accordance with 19.3.5.8 has been provided for smoke compartments adjacent to the smoke barrier.

**A.19.3.7.3(2)** Where the smoke control system design requires dampers in order that the system functions effectively, it is not the intent of the exception to permit the damper to be omitted.

This provision is not intended to prevent the use of plenum returns where ducting is used to return air from a

CHAPTER 18 • New

ceiling plenum through smoke barrier walls. Short stubs or jumper ducts are not acceptable. Ducting is required to connect at both sides of the opening and to extend into adjacent spaces away from the wall. The intent is to prohibit open-air transfers at or near the smoke barrier walls.

**18.3.7.4** Materials and methods of construction used for required smoke barriers shall not reduce the required fire resistance rating.

**18.3.7.5** Accumulation space shall be provided in accordance with 18.3.7.5.1 and 18.3.7.5.2.

**18.3.7.5.1** Not less than 30 net ft$^2$ (2.8 net m$^2$) per patient in a hospital or nursing home, or not less than 15 net ft$^2$ (1.4 net m$^2$) per resident in a limited care facility, shall be provided within the aggregate area of corridors, patient rooms, treatment rooms, lounge or dining areas, and other low hazard areas on each side of the smoke barrier.

**18.3.7.5.2** On stories not housing bedridden or litterborne patients, not less than 6 net ft$^2$ (0.56 net m$^2$) per occupant shall be provided on each side of the smoke barrier for the total number of occupants in adjoining compartments.

**18.3.7.6*** Doors in smoke barriers shall be substantial doors, such as 1¾ in. (44 mm) thick, solid-bonded wood-core doors, or shall be of construction that resists fire for a minimum of 20 minutes, and shall meet the following requirements:

(1) Nonrated factory- or field-applied protective plates, unlimited in height, shall be permitted.
(2) Cross-corridor openings in smoke barriers shall be protected by a pair of swinging doors or a horizontal-sliding door complying with 7.2.1.14, unless otherwise permitted by 18.3.7.7.
(3) The swinging doors addressed by 18.3.7.6(2) shall be arranged so that each door swings in a direction opposite from the other.
(4) The minimum clear width for swinging doors shall be as follows:
    (a) Hospitals and nursing homes — 41½ in. (1055 mm)
    (b) Psychiatric hospitals and limited care facilities — 32 in. (810 mm)
(5) The minimum clear width opening for horizontal-sliding doors shall be as follows:
    (a) Hospitals and nursing homes — 6 ft 11 in. (2110 mm)
    (b) Psychiatric hospitals and limited care facilities — 64 in. (1625 mm)
(6) The clearance under the bottom of smoke barrier doors shall not exceed ¾ in. (19 mm).

CHAPTER 19 • Existing

ceiling plenum through smoke barrier walls. Short stubs or jumper ducts are not acceptable. Ducting is required to connect at both sides of the opening and to extend into adjacent spaces away from the wall. The intent is to prohibit open-air transfers at or near the smoke barrier walls.

**19.3.7.4 Reserved.**

**19.3.7.5** Accumulation space shall be provided in accordance with 19.3.7.5.1 and 19.3.7.5.2.

**19.3.7.5.1** Not less than 30 net ft$^2$ (2.8 net m$^2$) per patient in a hospital or nursing home, or not less than 15 net ft$^2$ (1.4 net m$^2$) per resident in a limited care facility, shall be provided within the aggregate area of corridors, patient rooms, treatment rooms, lounge or dining areas, and other low hazard areas on each side of the smoke barrier.

**19.3.7.5.2** On stories not housing bedridden or litterborne patients, not less than 6 net ft$^2$ (0.56 net m$^2$) per occupant shall be provided on each side of the smoke barrier for the total number of occupants in adjoining compartments.

**19.3.7.6** Openings in smoke barriers shall be protected using one of the following methods:

(1) Fire-rated glazing
(2) Wired glass panels in steel frames
(3) Doors, such as 1¾ in. (44 mm) thick, solid-bonded wood core doors
(4) Construction that resists fire for a minimum of 20 minutes.

**19.3.7.6.1*** Nonrated factory- or field-applied protective plates, unlimited in height, shall be permitted.

**A.19.3.7.6.1** It is not the intent of 19.3.7.6.1 to prohibit the application of push plates, hardware, or other attachments on smoke barrier doors in health care occupancies.

**19.3.7.6.2** Doors shall be permitted to have fixed fire window assemblies in accordance with Section 8.5.

**A.18.3.7.6** Smoke barrier doors are intended to provide access to adjacent zones. The pair of cross-corridor doors are required to be opposite swinging. Access to both zones is required.

It is not the intent of 18.3.7.6 to prohibit the application of push plates, hardware, or other attachments on some barrier doors in health care occupancies.

**18.3.7.7** Cross-corridor openings in smoke barriers that are not in required means of egress from a health care space shall be permitted to be protected by a single-leaf door.

**19.3.7.7 Reserved.**

**18.3.7.8*** Doors in smoke barriers shall comply with 8.5.4 and shall be self-closing or automatic-closing in accordance with 18.2.2.2.7.

**19.3.7.8*** Doors in smoke barriers shall comply with Section 8.5 and shall be self-closing or automatic-closing in accordance with 19.2.2.2.7. Such doors in smoke barriers shall not be required to swing with egress travel. Positive latching hardware shall not be required.

**A.18.3.7.8** Smoke barriers might include walls having door openings other than cross-corridor doors. There is no restriction in the *Code* regarding which doors or how many doors form part of a smoke barrier. For example, doors from the corridor to individual rooms are permitted to form part of a smoke barrier.

**A.19.3.7.8** Smoke barriers might include walls having door openings other than cross-corridor doors. There is no restriction in the *Code* regarding which doors or how many doors form part of a smoke barrier. For example, doors from the corridor to individual rooms are permitted to form part of a smoke barrier.

**18.3.7.9*** Vision panels consisting of fire-rated glazing or wired glass panels in approved frames shall be provided in each cross-corridor swinging door and at each cross-corridor horizontal-sliding door in a smoke barrier.

**A.18.3.7.9** It is not the intent to require the frame to be a listed assembly.

**19.3.7.9** Door openings in smoke barriers shall be protected using one of the following methods:

(1) Swinging door providing a clear width of not less than 32 in. (810 mm)
(2) Horizontal-sliding door complying with 7.2.1.14 and providing a clear width of not less than 32 in. (810 mm)

**18.3.7.10** Vision panels in doors in smoke barriers, if provided, shall be of fire-rated glazing or wired glass in approved frames.

**19.3.7.10** The requirement of 19.3.7.9 shall not apply to existing 34 in. (865 mm) doors.

**18.3.7.11*** Rabbets, bevels, or astragals shall be required at the meeting edges, and stops shall be required at the head and sides of door frames in smoke barriers. Positive latching hardware shall not be required. Center mullions shall be prohibited.

**A.18.3.7.11** Split astragals (i.e., astragals installed on both door leaves) are also considered astragals.

Paragraph 18.3.7.1 requires that all floors of a building housing a new health care occupancy — other than those meeting one of the four exemptions offered by 18.3.7.2 — be subdivided into smoke compartments.

Per 18.3.7.1(1), any floor used by inpatients for sleeping or treatment must be subdivided into at least two smoke compartments, regardless of floor size or number of patients. Also, 18.3.7.1(2) requires any floor with an occupant load of 50 or more persons, regardless of size or use, to be subdivided into at least two smoke compartments, using smoke barriers. However, 18.3.7.2(1) through (4) provide exemptions for some non-health care occupancy floors.

Exhibit 18/19.27 illustrates the use of 18.3.7.1(1) and (2) and the four exemptions of 18.3.7.2.

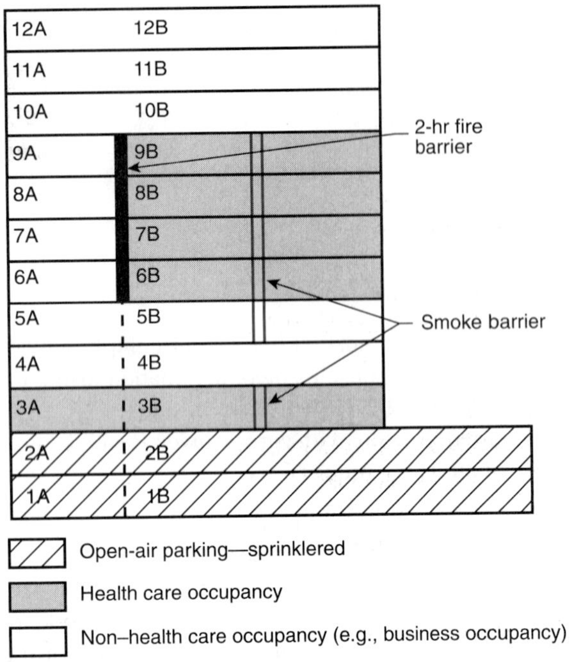


***Exhibit 18/19.27*** *Smoke barriers for new health care occupancy buildings.*

The following requirements are illustrated in Exhibit 18/19.27:

1. Floors 10 through 12 do not contain a health care occupancy and are located above the health care occupancy — per 18.3.7.2(1), they do not require smoke barriers.
2. Floors 6B through 9B are health care occupancy floors used for inpatient sleeping or treatment — per 18.3.7.1(1), they must be subdivided by smoke barriers.
3. Floors 6A through 9A do not contain a health care occupancy and are separated from the health care occupancy by 2-hour fire resistance–rated barriers complying with the provisions of 7.2.4.3, applicable to horizontal exit fire barriers — per 18.3.7.2(2), they do not require smoke barriers.
4. Floor 5 does not contain a health care occupancy and does not meet 18.3.7.2(3), because it is not more than one story below the health care occupancy — per 18.3.7.1(2), it must be subdivided by smoke barriers if it has an occupant load of 50 or more persons.
5. Floor 4 does not contain a health care occupancy and is more than one story below the health care occupancy — per 18.3.7.2(3), it does not require smoke barriers.
6. Floor 3 is a health care occupancy floor used for inpatient sleeping or treatment — per 18.3.7.1(1), it must be subdivided by smoke barriers.
7. Floors 1 and 2 are used as an open-air parking structure and are protected by a supervised automatic sprinkler system — even though floor 2 is located immediately below a health care occupancy floor, 18.3.7.2(4) exempts these floors from the smoke barrier requirement.

For existing health care occupancies, the introductory portion of 19.3.7.1 requires smoke barriers only for the purpose of subdividing stories having sleeping rooms for more than 30 patients. Subdivision is not required on treatment floors (provided that there are no sleeping rooms), regardless of floor area or number of patients. Patient bed capacity is to be used to determine the number of patients per story (see 19.3.7.2).

Paragraphs 18.3.7.1(3) and (4) and 19.3.7.1(1) do not present criteria related to whether smoke barriers are required in a building. Rather, they specify dimensional criteria for smoke compartments where the presence of smoke barriers is required by 18.3.7.1(1) and (2) or the introductory portion of 19.3.7.1. The maximum area of any smoke compartment created by subdividing the floor cannot exceed 22,500 $ft^2$ (2100 $m^2$). If the compartment were perfectly square, this would involve a 150 ft × 150 ft (46 m × 46 m) area. However, to provide the facility and designer with flexibility in the arrangement of smoke compartments, the arbitrary 150 ft (46 m) length and width limits of earlier editions were replaced in 1991 by a 200 ft (61 m) travel limitation from any point in the smoke compartment to a door in the smoke barrier [see 18.3.7.1(4) and 19.3.7.1(1)]. Smoke compartments must be designed so that a person is able to reach a smoke barrier door within a distance of travel of 200 ft (61 m) from any point in a compartment, measured along the natural path of travel in accordance with 7.6.1. However, the travel limitation is exempted by 19.3.7.1(2) for existing smoke compartments where neither the length nor width of the smoke compartment exceeds 150 ft (46 m).

In Exhibit 18/19.28, the construction of one smoke barrier divides the floor into two smoke compartments. If either smoke compartment — one consisting of the combination of areas A and B and the other consisting of area C — exceeds 22,500 $ft^2$ (2100 $m^2$) or re-

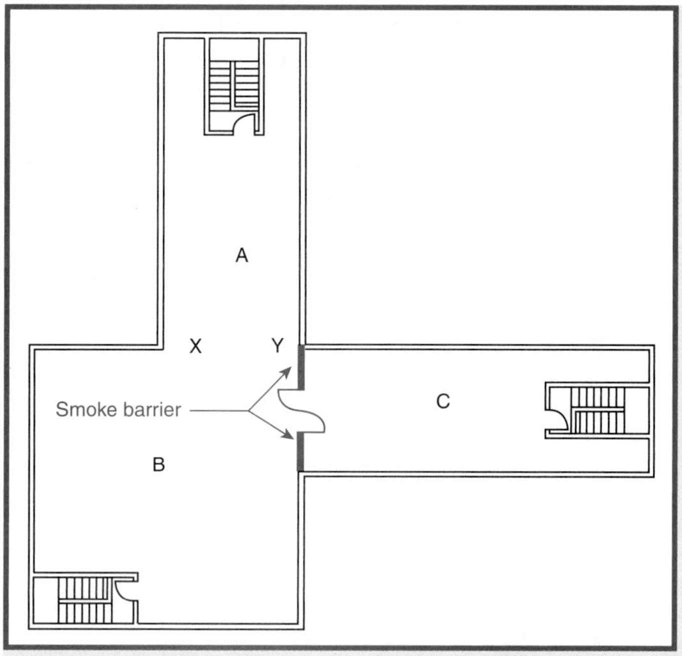


**Exhibit 18/19.28** *Smoke barrier dividing floor into two smoke compartments.*

quires occupant travel in excess of 200 ft (61 m) to reach the doors in the smoke barrier, further subdivision using additional smoke barriers is required [unless both are existing smoke compartments and neither the compartment length nor width exceeds 150 ft (46 m)]. Assuming that the smoke compartment consisting of the combination of areas A and B is too large to meet the specified conditions, a second smoke barrier extending from point X to point Y might provide a logical solution.

Exhibit 18/19.29 illustrates the travel distance limitation to a door in a smoke barrier. Although the room positioned at the top of the exhibit between the smoke barrier and the enclosed exit stair has a short travel distance to an exit (*X* to *E*), the enclosed exit stair is not usable by those incapable of self-preservation. Therefore, the distance of travel to the doors in the smoke barrier (*X* to *E* to *B*) must not exceed 200 ft (61 m). For the existing smoke compartment, the 200 ft (61 m) criterion would be exempted if neither the smoke compartment length nor the width exceeds 150 ft (46 m). For this floor plan, an additional pair of doors in the smoke barrier where it crosses the corridor in the top half of the exhibit might provide a logical solution to a smoke compartment travel distance problem.

Horizontal exits are permitted to be substituted

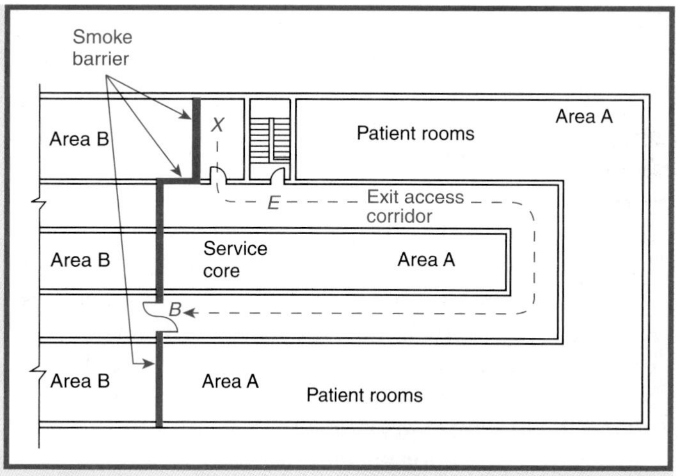


**Exhibit 18/19.29** *Limited travel distance to door in smoke barrier.*

for smoke barriers. In such cases, the horizontal exit would also have to be constructed to comply with the smoke barrier requirements. See 7.2.4 and Section 8.5.

Areas open to atriums are not permitted to be used for patient sleeping or treatment areas (see 18/19.3.1.3). Atrium smoke compartments arranged in accordance with 8.6.7 are not limited in size.

Paragraphs 18.3.7.6 through 18.3.7.11 and 19.3.7.6 through 19.3.7.10 address smoke barrier doors. Although the cross-corridor smoke barrier doors in new health care occupancies are required to resist the penetration of fire for at least 20 minutes, they are not required to have a true fire protection rating. Similarly, the smoke barrier doors in existing health care occupancies are not required to have a true fire protection rating. Yet, some incorrectly consider these $1^3/_4$ in. (44 mm) thick, solid-bonded wood doors to be 20-minute fire protection–rated doors from which the latch has been omitted. If the door were truly a 20-minute fire protection–rated assembly, field-applied protective plates would be prohibited. Paragraphs 18.3.7.6(1) and 19.3.7.6.1 remind the user that factory- or field-applied protective plates are permitted without any height restriction.

During a fire, the emergency evacuation of patients in a health care facility is an inefficient, time-consuming process. Realistically, if patients must be moved, sizable numbers of occupants can be relocated only through horizontal travel. Smoke barriers and horizontal exits used to subdivide a building serve the following three purposes fundamental to the protection of inpatients:

1. They limit the spread of fire and smoke.
2. They limit the number of occupants exposed to a single fire.
3. They provide for the horizontal relocation of patients by creating a safe area on the same floor level.

The smoke barrier requirements result in a floor's area being divided by a barrier into a minimum of two compartments. Although not stated in the *Code*, it would be desirable to subdivide health care facilities in such a way as to have separate banks of elevators in different smoke zones. If evacuation of the building becomes necessary, patients can first be moved horizontally to a temporary area of refuge and then be removed from the floor via elevators.

In new health care occupancies, the openings between the meeting edges of pairs of smoke barrier doors and between the doors and frames must be minimized to retard the transfer of smoke. Because 18.3.7.6(3) requires swinging doors to swing in opposite directions from each other, the protection at the meeting edge does not create a door-closing coordination problem and, therefore, is simple to provide. An overlapping astragal plate on the leading edge of one of the doors will usually suffice for compliance with 18.3.7.11.

Dampers are not required in ducted penetrations of smoke barriers in new health care occupancies, as addressed in 18.3.7.3(2). This exemption anticipates that automatic sprinklers will limit fire size and that duct systems will also inhibit the transfer of smoke. This exemption does not prohibit the installation of smoke dampers, nor does it permit the omission of the smoke damper if the damper is required for other reasons. For example, if the building has a smoke control system that needs a smoke damper at the smoke barrier, then such a damper must be installed. An automatic-closing damper, activated by a smoke detector, would be required to protect a transfer grille.

Note that, for existing smoke barriers, the combination fire/smoke dampers required in 8.5.5.2 are permitted to be omitted in engineered smoke control systems if the system design is such that a damper is not required at that point. Paragraph 19.3.7.3(2) also permits deletion of dampers in ducted penetrations of smoke barriers where compartments adjacent to the barrier are protected by automatic sprinklers (quick-response sprinklers in any smoke compartments used for patient sleeping). This exemption would not be permitted if an engineered smoke control system required a damper at this point. Openings for transfer grilles require automatic-closing dampers.

Exhibit 18/19.30 and Exhibit 18/19.31 illustrate some of the detailed requirements of 18/19.3.7 for subdividing building spaces through the use of smoke barriers.

In Exhibit 18/19.32, the smoke barrier require-

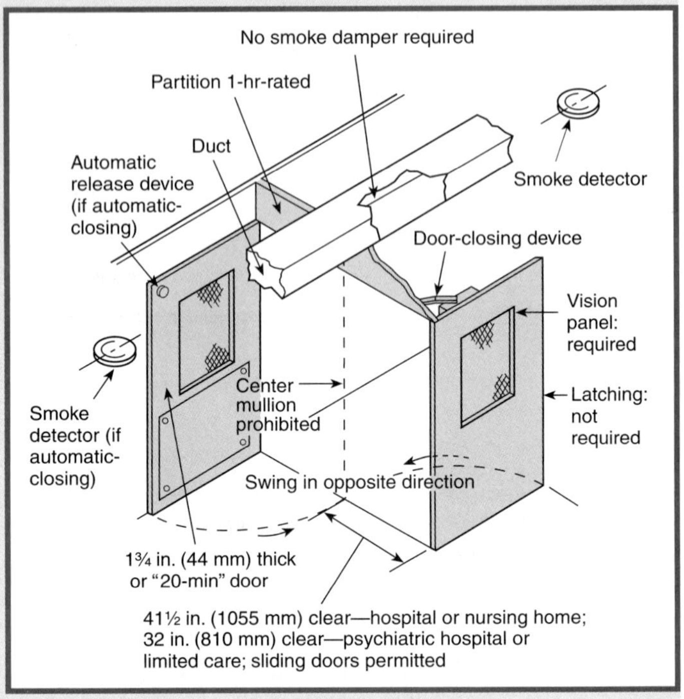


***Exhibit 18/19.30*** *Details of new smoke barrier.*

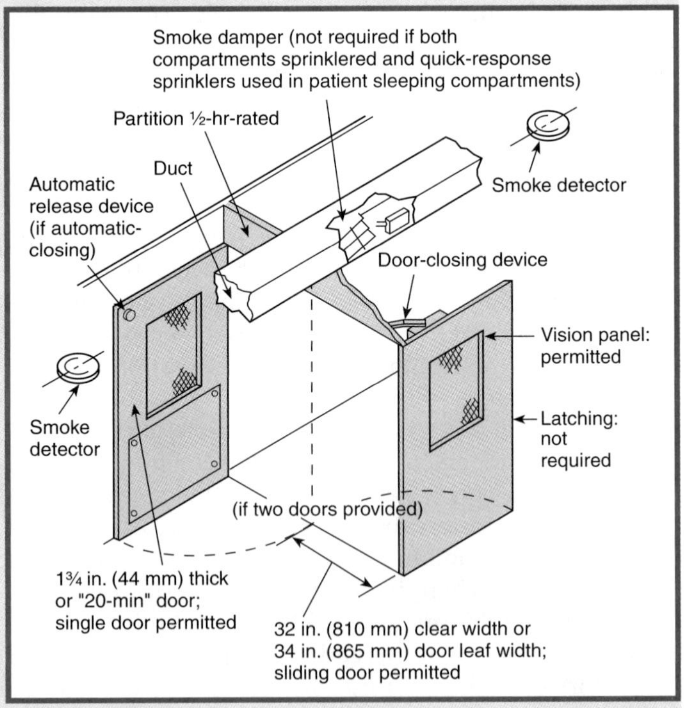


***Exhibit 18/19.31*** *Details of existing smoke barrier.*

CHAPTER 18 • New | CHAPTER 19 • Existing

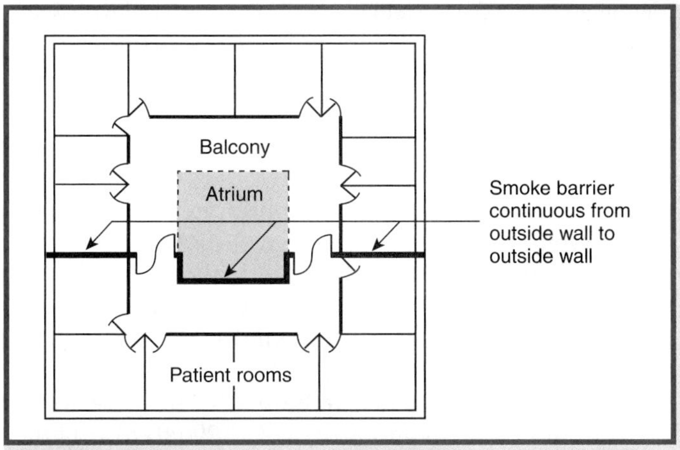


***Exhibit 18/19.32*** *Smoke compartments in atrium building.*

ment for a building with an atrium is satisfied by running the smoke barrier partition directly through the building from one outside wall to the opposite outside wall and hugging one edge of the open atrium space. In Exhibit 18/19.33, 18/19.3.7.1(3) is used to permit the smoke compartment containing the atrium to be unlimited in size. The patient floor is divided into three smoke compartments by locating two smoke barriers away from the atrium opening and thus preserving the visual impact of the atrium. The center smoke compartment, which includes the atrium, is not limited in size, but the distance of travel from any point to a smoke barrier door is limited to 200 ft (61 m).

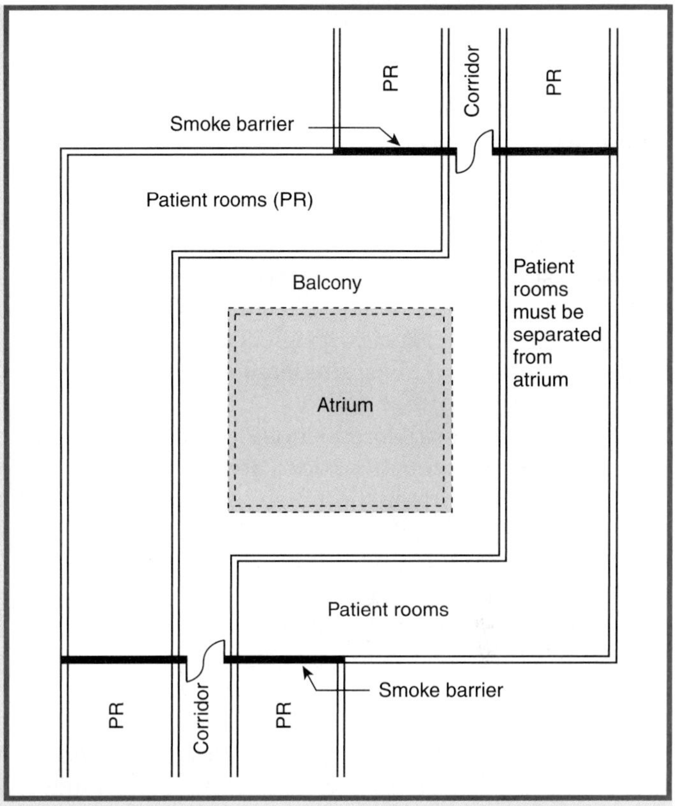


***Exhibit 18/19.33*** *Atrium smoke compartment with unlimited area.*

### 18.3.8 Special Protection Features. (Reserved)

Editions of the *Code* prior to 1994 required an outside door or outside window in each room where patients sleep, and the outside window was required to be operable so as to provide venting. In 1994, the operability requirement was deleted, but the outside door or outside window requirement remained. The requirement for an outside window or outside door was deleted for the 2009 edition, as the total concept approach of 18/19.1.1.3 can be achieved without reliance on such opening.

### 19.3.8 Special Protection Features. (Reserved)

## 18.4 Special Provisions

### 18.4.1 Limited Access Buildings.

Limited access buildings or limited access portions of buildings shall not be used for patient sleeping rooms and shall comply with Section 11.7.

### 18.4.2 High-Rise Buildings.

High-rise buildings shall comply with Section 11.8.

## 19.4 Special Provisions

### 19.4.1 Limited Access Buildings.

See Section 11.7 for requirements for limited access buildings.

### 19.4.2 High-Rise Buildings.

All high-rise buildings containing health care occupancies shall be protected throughout by an approved, supervised

CHAPTER 18 • New

CHAPTER 19 • Existing

automatic sprinkler system installed in accordance with Section 9.7 within 12 years of the adoption of this *Code*.

**18.4.3 Nonsprinklered Existing Smoke Compartment Rehabilitation.**

Chapter 18 requires that new health care occupancies be protected throughout by approved, supervised automatic sprinkler systems. However, in establishing the sprinkler requirement, the Technical Committee on Health Care Occupancies realized that rehabilitation often takes place in nonsprinklered existing buildings. The commentary that follows A.18/19.1.1.4.3.4 explains that nonsprinklered smoke compartments undergoing major rehabilitation are required to be sprinklered as part of the rehabilitation project, but nonsprinklered smoke compartments undergoing minor rehabilitation are not required to be sprinklered just because the rehabilitation occurs. Paragraph 18.1.1.4.3.4 confirms that, where minor rehabilitation is done in a nonsprinklered smoke compartment, the sprinkler requirements of 18.3.5.1 do not apply. Additionally, 18.1.1.4.3.4 requires that the rehabilitation must not reduce life safety below the level required for new buildings or below the level of the requirements of 18.4.3 for nonsprinklered smoke compartment rehabilitation. Similarly, 18.4.3.1 completes the reference trail by requiring that, where a modification in a nonsprinklered smoke compartment is exempted by the provisions of 18.1.1.4.3.4 from the sprinkler requirement of 18.3.5.1, the requirements of 18.4.3.2 through 18.4.3.8 must be met.

The requirements of 18.4.3.2 through 18.4.3.8 provide additional criteria needed for the proper protection of nonsprinklered existing building rehabilitation. For example, 18.4.3.4.2 limits travel distance to 150 ft (46 m) where the travel is not wholly within sprinklered smoke compartments. If the renovation in the nonsprinklered building is predicated on the provisions of 18.2.6.2.1, the travel distance limitation could mistakenly be interpreted to be 200 ft (61 m) between any point in a room and an exit. The 200 ft (61 m) limitation is intended to apply only to sprinklered buildings.

Subsection 18.4.3 serves as a repository for provisions that were contained in the chapter for new health care occupancies before 1991, when sprinklers were mandated for all new health care occupancies. Its provisions remind the user that the requirements interspersed throughout Chapter 18 are predicated on the presence of sprinkler protection. If sprinklers are not installed, additional requirements must be met in an attempt to achieve a level of life safety approaching that provided in a sprinklered building. However, even if all the former specifications for nonsprinklered buildings are met, the overall level of life safety will not necessarily be the same as that provided in a sprinklered facility. When the 1991 edition of the *Code* presented the first requirement for sprinklering of all new health care occupancies, the overall level of life safety was elevated from that provided by compliance with the nonsprinklered building option.

**18.4.3.1* General.** Where a modification in a nonsprinklered smoke compartment is exempted by the provisions of 18.1.1.4.3.4 from the sprinkler requirement of 18.3.5.1, the requirements of 18.4.3.2 through 18.4.3.8 shall apply.

**A.18.4.3.1** For example, the provisions of 18.1.1.4.3.1(2) and 18.1.1.4.3.4 do not require the installation of sprinklers if the modification involves less than 50 percent of the area of the smoke compartment and less than 4500 $ft^2$ (420 $m^2$) of the area of the smoke compartment.

**18.4.3.2 Minimum Construction Requirements (Nonsprinklered Smoke Compartment Rehabilitation).** Health care occupancies in buildings not protected throughout by an approved, supervised automatic sprinkler system in accordance with 19.3.5.7 shall be limited to the building construction types specified in Table 18.4.3.2.

*Table 18.4.3.2 Construction Type Limitations (Nonsprinklered Buildings)*

| | | Total Number of Stories of Building[†] | | | |
|---|---|---|---|---|---|
| **Construction Type** | **Sprinklered** | **1** | **2** | **3** | **≥4** |
| I (442) | Yes | NA | NA | NA | NA |
| | No | X | X | X | X |
| I (332) | Yes | NA | NA | NA | NA |
| | No | X | X | X | X |
| II (222) | Yes | NA | NA | NA | NA |
| | No | X | X | X | X |
| II (111) | Yes | NA | NA | NA | NA |
| | No | X | NP | NP | NP |
| II (000) | Yes | NA | NA | NA | NA |
| | No | NP | NP | NP | NP |
| III (211) | Yes | NA | NA | NA | NA |
| | No | NP | NP | NP | NP |
| III (200) | Yes | NA | NA | NA | NA |
| | No | NP | NP | NP | NP |
| IV (2HH) | Yes | NA | NA | NA | NA |
| | No | NP | NP | NP | NP |
| V (111) | Yes | NA | NA | NA | NA |
| | No | NP | NP | NP | NP |
| V (000) | Yes | NA | NA | NA | NA |
| | No | NP | NP | NP | NP |

NA: Not applicable. X: Permitted. NP: Not permitted.

[†]Basements are not counted as stories.

**18.4.3.3 Capacity of Means of Egress (Nonsprinklered Smoke Compartment Rehabilitation).** The capacity of the means of egress serving the modification area shall be as follows:

(1) $^1/_2$ in. (13 mm) per person for horizontal travel, without stairs, by means such as doors, ramps, or level floor surfaces
(2) 0.6 in. (15 mm) per person for travel by means of stairs

**18.4.3.4 Travel Distance (Nonsprinklered Smoke Compartment Rehabilitation).**

**18.4.3.4.1** The travel distance between any room door required as an exit access and an exit shall not exceed the following:

(1) 150 ft (46 m) where the travel is wholly within smoke compartments protected throughout by an approved, supervised automatic sprinkler system in accordance with 19.3.5.7
(2) 100 ft (30 m) where the travel is not wholly within smoke compartments protected throughout by an approved, supervised automatic sprinkler system in accordance with 19.3.5.7

**18.4.3.4.2** The travel distance between any point in a room and an exit shall not exceed the following:

(1) 200 ft (61 m) where the travel is wholly within smoke compartments protected throughout by an approved supervised sprinkler system in accordance with 19.3.5.7
(2) 150 ft (46 m) where the travel is not wholly within smoke compartments protected throughout by an approved supervised sprinkler system in accordance with 19.3.5.7

**18.4.3.5 Hazardous Area Protection (Nonsprinklered Smoke Compartment Rehabilitation).** Where a new hazardous area is formed in an existing nonsprinklered smoke compartment, the hazardous area itself shall be protected as indicated in Table 18.4.3.5.

***Table 18.4.3.5 Hazardous Area Protection (Nonsprinklered Buildings)***

| Hazardous Area Description | Protection†/ Separation |
|---|---|
| Boiler and fuel-fired heater rooms | 1 hour and sprinklers |
| Central/bulk laundries larger than 100 ft² (9.3 m²) | 1 hour and sprinklers |
| Laboratories employing flammable or combustible materials in quantities less than those that would be considered a severe hazard | 1 hour and sprinklers *(Also see 18.4.3.7.2.2.)* |
| Laboratories that use hazardous materials that would be classified as a severe hazard in accordance with NFPA 99, *Standard for Health Care Facilities* | 1 hour and sprinklers |
| Paint shops employing hazardous substances and materials in quantities less than those that would be classified as a severe hazard | 1 hour and sprinklers |
| Physical plant maintenance shops | 1 hour and sprinklers |
| Soiled linen rooms | 1 hour and sprinklers |
| Storage rooms larger than 50 ft² (4.6 m²) but not exceeding 100 ft² (9.3 m²) and storing combustible material | 1 hour or sprinklers *(Also see 18.4.3.7.2.2.)* |
| Storage rooms larger than 100 ft² (9.3 m²) and storing combustible material | 1 hour and sprinklers |
| Trash collection rooms | 1 hour and sprinklers |

†Minimum fire resistance rating.

**18.4.3.6 Interior Finish (Nonsprinklered Smoke Compartment Rehabilitation).**

**18.4.3.6.1 General.** Interior finish within the modification area shall be in accordance with Section 10.2.

**18.4.3.6.2 Interior Wall and Ceiling Finish.** Newly installed interior wall and ceiling finish materials complying with Section 10.2 shall be permitted throughout nonsprinklered smoke compartments if the materials are Class A, except as otherwise permitted in 18.4.3.6.2.1 or 18.4.3.6.2.2.

**18.4.3.6.2.1** Walls and ceilings shall be permitted to have Class A or Class B interior finish in individual rooms having a capacity not exceeding four persons.

**18.4.3.6.2.2** Corridor wall finish not exceeding 48 in. (1220 mm) in height and restricted to the lower half of the wall shall be permitted to be Class A or Class B.

**18.4.3.6.3 Interior Floor Finish.**

**18.4.3.6.3.1** Newly installed interior floor finish shall comply with Section 10.2.

**18.4.3.6.3.2** The requirements for newly installed interior floor finish in exit enclosures and corridors not separated from them by walls complying with 19.3.5.7 shall be as follows:

(1) Unrestricted in smoke compartments protected throughout by an approved, supervised automatic sprinkler system in accordance with 19.3.5.7
(2) Not less than Class I in smoke compartments not protected throughout by an approved, supervised automatic sprinkler system in accordance with 19.3.5.7

**18.4.3.7 Corridors (Nonsprinklered Smoke Compartment Rehabilitation).**

**18.4.3.7.1 Construction of Corridor Walls.**

**18.4.3.7.1.1** Where the smoke compartment being modified is not protected throughout by an approved, supervised automatic sprinkler system in accordance with 19.3.5.7, corridor walls shall comply with the following, as modified by 18.4.3.7.1.2:

(1) They shall have a minimum $^1/_2$-hour fire resistance rating.
(2) They shall be continuous from the floor to the underside of the floor or roof deck above.
(3) They shall resist the passage of smoke.

**18.4.3.7.1.2** The requirements of 18.4.3.7.1.1 shall be permitted to be modified for conditions permitted by 19.3.6.1(3) and (4) and 19.3.6.1(6) through (8).

CHAPTER 18 • New

**18.4.3.7.2 Corridor Doors.**

**18.4.3.7.2.1** Where the smoke compartment being modified is not protected throughout by an approved, supervised automatic sprinkler system in accordance with 19.3.5.7, the following shall apply:

(1) Doors protecting corridor openings shall be constructed of $1\frac{3}{4}$ in. (44 mm) thick, solid-bonded core wood or of construction that resists the passage of fire for a minimum of 20 minutes.
(2) Door frames shall be labeled or of steel construction.
(3) Existing roller latches demonstrated to keep the door closed against a force of 5 lbf (22 N) shall be permitted.

**18.4.3.7.2.2** Door-closing devices shall be required on doors in corridor wall openings serving smoke barriers or enclosures of exits, hazardous contents areas, or vertical openings.

**18.4.3.8 Subdivision of Building Space (Nonsprinklered Smoke Compartment Rehabilitation).** Subparagraph 18.3.7.3(2) shall be permitted only where adjacent smoke compartments are protected throughout by an approved, supervised automatic sprinkler system in accordance with 18.3.5.4 and 18.3.5.6.

## 18.5 Building Services

### 18.5.1 Utilities.

**18.5.1.1** Utilities shall comply with the provisions of Section 9.1.

**18.5.1.2** Power for alarms, emergency communications systems, and illumination of generator set locations shall be in accordance with the essential electrical system requirements of NFPA 99, *Standard for Health Care Facilities*.

**18.5.1.3** Any health care occupancy, as indicated in 18.1.1.1.2, that normally uses life-support devices shall have electrical systems designed and installed in accordance with NFPA 99, *Standard for Health Care Facilities*, unless the facility uses life-support equipment for emergency purposes only.

### 18.5.2 Heating, Ventilating, and Air-Conditioning.

**18.5.2.1** Heating, ventilating, and air-conditioning shall comply with the provisions of Section 9.2 and shall be installed in accordance with the manufacturer's specifications, unless otherwise modified by 18.5.2.2.

**18.5.2.2*** Any heating device, other than a central heating plant, shall be designed and installed so that combustible

CHAPTER 19 • Existing

## 19.5 Building Services

### 19.5.1 Utilities.

**19.5.1.1** Utilities shall comply with the provisions of Section 9.1.

**19.5.1.2** Existing installations shall be permitted to be continued in service, provided that the systems do not present a serious hazard to life.

### 19.5.2 Heating, Ventilating, and Air-Conditioning.

**19.5.2.1** Heating, ventilating, and air-conditioning shall comply with the provisions of Section 9.2 and shall be installed in accordance with the manufacturer's specifications, unless otherwise modified by 19.5.2.2.

**19.5.2.2*** Any heating device, other than a central heating plant, shall be designed and installed so that combustible

CHAPTER 18 • New

material cannot be ignited by the device or its appurtenances, and the following requirements shall also apply:

(1) If fuel-fired, such heating devices shall comply with the following:
   (a) They shall be chimney connected or vent connected.
   (b) They shall take air for combustion directly from outside.
   (c) They shall be designed and installed to provide for complete separation of the combustion system from the atmosphere of the occupied area.
(2) Any heating device shall have safety features to immediately stop the flow of fuel and shut down the equipment in case of either excessive temperatures or ignition failure.

**A.18.5.2.2** For both new and existing buildings, it is the intent to permit the installation and use of fireplace stoves and room heaters utilizing solid fuel as defined in NFPA 211, *Standard for Chimneys, Fireplaces, Vents, and Solid Fuel–Burning Appliances*, provided that all such devices are installed, maintained, and used in accordance with the appropriate provisions of that standard and all manufacturers' specifications. These requirements are not intended to permit freestanding solid fuel–burning appliances such as freestanding wood-burning stoves.

**18.5.2.3** The requirements of 18.5.2.2 shall not apply where otherwise permitted by the following:

(1) Approved, suspended unit heaters shall be permitted in locations other than means of egress and patient sleeping areas, provided that both of the following criteria are met:
   (a) Such heaters are located high enough to be out of the reach of persons using the area.
   (b) Such heaters are equipped with the safety features required by 18.5.2.2.
(2) Fireplaces shall be permitted and used only in areas other than patient sleeping areas, provided that all of the following criteria are met:
   (a) Such areas are separated from patient sleeping spaces by construction having not less than a 1-hour fire resistance rating.
   (b) The fireplace complies with the provisions of 9.2.2.
   (c) The fireplace is equipped with the following:
      i. Hearth raised not less than 4 in. (100 mm)
      ii. Fireplace enclosure guaranteed against breakage up to a temperature of 650°F (343°C) and constructed of heat-tempered glass or other approved material

CHAPTER 19 • Existing

material cannot be ignited by the device or its appurtenances, and the following requirements also shall apply:

(1) If fuel-fired, such heating devices shall comply with the following:
   (a) They shall be chimney connected or vent connected.
   (b) They shall take air for combustion directly from the outside.
   (c) They shall be designed and installed to provide for complete separation of the combustion system from the atmosphere of the occupied area.
(2) Any heating device shall have safety features to immediately stop the flow of fuel and shut down the equipment in case of either excessive temperature or ignition failure.

**A.19.5.2.2** For both new and existing buildings, it is the intent to permit the installation and use of fireplace stoves and room heaters using solid fuel as defined in NFPA 211, *Standard for Chimneys, Fireplaces, Vents, and Solid Fuel–-Burning Appliances*, provided that all such devices are installed, maintained, and used in accordance with the appropriate provisions of that standard and all manufacturers' specifications. These requirements are not intended to permit freestanding solid fuel–burning appliances such as freestanding wood-burning stoves.

**19.5.2.3** The requirements of 19.5.2.2 shall not apply where otherwise permitted by the following:

(1) Approved, suspended unit heaters shall be permitted in locations other than means of egress and patient sleeping areas, provided that both of the following criteria are met:
   (a) Such heaters are located high enough to be out of the reach of persons using the area.
   (b) Such heaters are equipped with the safety features required by 19.5.2.2(2).
(2) Fireplaces shall be permitted and used only in areas other than patient sleeping areas, provided that all of the following criteria are met:
   (a) Such areas are separated from patient sleeping spaces by construction having not less than a 1-hour fire resistance rating.
   (b) The fireplace complies with the provisions of 9.2.2.
   (c) The fireplace is equipped with a fireplace enclosure guaranteed against breakage up to a temperature of 650°F (343°C) and constructed of heat-tempered glass or other approved material.

CHAPTER 18 • New

(3) If, in the opinion of the authority having jurisdiction, special hazards are present, a lock on the enclosure specified in 18.5.2.3(2)(c)(ii) and other safety precautions shall be permitted to be required.

### 18.5.3 Elevators, Escalators, and Conveyors.

Elevators, escalators, and conveyors shall comply with the provisions of Section 9.4.

CHAPTER 19 • Existing

(3) If, in the opinion of the authority having jurisdiction, special hazards are present, a lock on the enclosure specified in 19.5.2.3(2)(c) and other safety precautions shall be permitted to be required.

### 19.5.3 Elevators, Escalators, and Conveyors.

Elevators, escalators, and conveyors shall comply with the provisions of Section 9.4.

Paragraphs 18/19.5.2.1 through 18/19.5.2.3 specify safeguards for air-conditioning, ventilating, heating, and other service equipment to minimize the possibility of such devices serving as a source of ignition. Fuel-fired heating devices, except central heating systems, must be designed to provide complete separation of the combustion system from the occupied spaces. Air for combustion must be taken directly from the outside.

A major concern is preventing the ignition of clothing, bedclothes, furniture, and other furnishings by a heating device. Therefore, 18/19.7.8 prohibits portable heating devices in areas used by patients.

Paragraph 18/19.5.3 requires elevators to comply with Section 9.4, which mandates the Fire Fighters' Emergency Operations features required in ASME A17.1/CSA B44, *Safety Code for Elevators and Escalators*,[19] for new elevator installations, and ASME A17.3, *Safety Code for Existing Elevators and Escalators*,[20] for existing elevator installations. Phase 1 of the fire fighter's emergency operations requires elevators to be recalled to a designated floor (e.g., the main entrance level lobby or, alternately, to some other floor if smoke is detected in the main entrance level lobby) upon detection of smoke in the elevator machine room, the elevator hoistway, or the elevator lobbies on each floor the elevators serve. Phase 1 recall helps to ensure that the elevators are called out of service, so as not to be misused by building occupants once smoke has reached an elevator lobby and its associated elevator shaft doors, or when smoke is present in the elevator machine room or hoistway. Phase 1 also provides for the elevators to be waiting at the designated floor for emergency service personnel use upon their arrival.

The ASME A17.1/CSA B44 and ASME A17.3 codes prohibit elevators from being recalled by other than smoke detection in the elevator machine room, the hoistway, or the elevator lobbies. Therefore, the elevator should not be recalled upon initiation of the building fire alarm system. This is consistent with the provision of 9.6.3.2.1 of this *Code*, which does not require the elevator recall smoke detectors to activate the building evacuation alarm, provided that the smoke detectors initiate a supervisory signal at a constantly attended location. Therefore, elevators will remain in service in parts of the building not affected by the fire and might constitute a valuable, supplemental means for evacuating patients from health care occupancies. In some cases, using an elevator might be the only feasible way to move critically ill patients or patients in restraining devices.

Elevators, however, have many inherent weaknesses that tend to limit reliability. Elevator access doors are designed with operating tolerances that allow smoke transfer into the shaft. During a fire, a power failure might cause an elevator to stop between floors, trapping its passengers.

Many of these elevator weaknesses can be minimized by providing emergency power, separating the elevator lobby from other building spaces, using rated construction, providing an emergency smoke control system, and pressurizing the elevator shaft and adjacent lobbies. These countermeasures represent good fire protection judgment but are not requirements of this *Code*.

Through emergency planning and staff training, the potential problem of crowded elevators might be avoided. Emergency plans can make effective use of elevators by transferring patients through a horizontal exit, for example, to a separate fire area. Within the separate fire area, a staged evacuation program could be instituted, with the elevators taking patients to the ground level, allowing horizontal movement to the outside.

CHAPTER 18 • New

### 18.5.4 Rubbish Chutes, Incinerators, and Laundry Chutes.

**18.5.4.1** Rubbish chutes, incinerators, and laundry chutes shall comply with the provisions of Section 9.5, unless otherwise specified in 18.5.4.2.

**18.5.4.2*** The fire resistance rating of chute charging rooms and chute discharging rooms shall not be required to exceed 1 hour.

**A.18.5.4.2** The minimum 1-hour fire resistance–rated room permitted by 18.5.4.2 is a deviation from the provisions of NFPA 82, *Standard on Incinerators and Waste and Linen Handling Systems and Equipment.* NFPA 82 requires the charging room and the discharge room to have the same fire rating as required for the shaft enclosing the chute. In fully sprinklered health care occupancies, the 1-hour-rated rooms required by 18.5.4.2 provide the needed protection.

**18.5.4.3** Any rubbish chute or linen chute, including pneumatic rubbish and linen systems, shall be provided with automatic extinguishing protection in accordance with Section 9.7. *(See Section 9.5.)*

**18.5.4.4** Any rubbish chute shall discharge into a trash collection room used for no other purpose and shall be protected in accordance with Section 8.7.

**18.5.4.5** Incinerators shall not be directly flue-fed, nor shall any floor-charging chute directly connect with the combustion chamber.

## 18.6 Reserved

## 18.7* Operating Features

**A.18.7** Health care occupants have, in large part, varied degrees of physical disability, and their removal to the outside, or even their disturbance caused by moving, is inexpedient or impractical in many cases, except as a last resort. Similarly, recognizing that there might be an operating necessity for the restraint of the mentally ill, often by use of barred windows and locked doors, fire exit drills are usually extremely disturbing, detrimental, and frequently impracticable.

In most cases, fire exit drills, as ordinarily practiced in other occupancies, cannot be conducted in health care occupancies. Fundamentally, superior construction, early discovery and extinguishment of incipient fires, and prompt

CHAPTER 19 • Existing

### 19.5.4 Rubbish Chutes, Incinerators, and Laundry Chutes.

**19.5.4.1** Existing rubbish chutes or linen chutes, including pneumatic rubbish and linen systems, that open directly onto any corridor shall be sealed by fire-resistive construction to prevent further use or shall be provided with a fire door assembly having a minimum 1-hour fire protection rating. All new chutes shall comply with Section 9.5.

**19.5.4.2 Reserved.**

**19.5.4.3** Any rubbish chute or linen chute, including pneumatic rubbish and linen systems, shall be provided with automatic extinguishing protection in accordance with Section 9.7. *(See Section 9.5.)*

**19.5.4.4** Any rubbish chute shall discharge into a trash collection room used for no other purpose and shall be protected in accordance with Section 8.7.

**19.5.4.5** Existing flue-fed incinerators shall be sealed by fire-resistive construction to prevent further use.

## 19.6 Reserved

## 19.7* Operating Features

**A.19.7** Health care occupants have, in large part, varied degrees of physical disability, and their removal to the outside, or even their disturbance caused by moving, is inexpedient or impractical in many cases, except as a last resort. Similarly, recognizing that there might be an operating necessity for the restraint of the mentally ill, often by use of barred windows and locked doors, fire exit drills are usually extremely disturbing, detrimental, and frequently impracticable.

In most cases, fire exit drills, as ordinarily practiced in other occupancies, cannot be conducted in health care occupancies. Fundamentally, superior construction, early discovery and extinguishment of incipient fires, and prompt

CHAPTER 18 • New

notification need to be relied on to reduce the occasion for evacuation of buildings of this class to a minimum.

### 18.7.1 Evacuation and Relocation Plan and Fire Drills.

**18.7.1.1** The administration of every health care occupancy shall have, in effect and available to all supervisory personnel, written copies of a plan for the protection of all persons in the event of fire, for their evacuation to areas of refuge, and for their evacuation from the building when necessary.

**18.7.1.2** All employees shall be periodically instructed and kept informed with respect to their duties under the plan required by 18.7.1.1.

**18.7.1.3** A copy of the plan required by 18.7.1.1 shall be readily available at all times in the telephone operator's location or at the security center.

**18.7.1.4*** Fire drills in health care occupancies shall include the transmission of a fire alarm signal and simulation of emergency fire conditions.

**A.18.7.1.4** Many health care occupancies conduct fire drills without disturbing patients by choosing the location of the simulated emergency in advance and by closing the doors to patients' rooms or wards in the vicinity prior to initiation of the drill. The purpose of a fire drill is to test and evaluate the efficiency, knowledge, and response of institutional personnel in implementing the facility fire emergency plan. Its purpose is not to disturb or excite patients. Fire drills should be scheduled on a random basis to ensure that personnel in health care facilities are drilled not less than once in each 3-month period.

Drills should consider the ability to move patients to an adjacent smoke compartment. Relocation can be practiced using simulated patients or empty wheelchairs.

**18.7.1.5** Infirm or bedridden patients shall not be required to be moved during drills to safe areas or to the exterior of the building.

**18.7.1.6** Drills shall be conducted quarterly on each shift to familiarize facility personnel (nurses, interns, maintenance engineers, and administrative staff) with the signals and emergency action required under varied conditions.

**18.7.1.7** When drills are conducted between 9:00 p.m. (2100 hours) and 6:00 a.m. (0600 hours), a coded announcement shall be permitted to be used instead of audible alarms.

**18.7.1.8** Employees of health care occupancies shall be instructed in life safety procedures and devices.

CHAPTER 19 • Existing

notification need to be relied on to reduce the occasion for evacuation of buildings of this class to a minimum.

### 19.7.1 Evacuation and Relocation Plan and Fire Drills.

**19.7.1.1** The administration of every health care occupancy shall have, in effect and available to all supervisory personnel, written copies of a plan for the protection of all persons in the event of fire, for their evacuation to areas of refuge, and for their evacuation from the building when necessary.

**19.7.1.2** All employees shall be periodically instructed and kept informed with respect to their duties under the plan required by 19.7.1.1.

**19.7.1.3** A copy of the plan required by 19.7.1.1 shall be readily available at all times in the telephone operator's location or at the security center.

**19.7.1.4*** Fire drills in health care occupancies shall include the transmission of a fire alarm signal and simulation of emergency fire conditions.

**A.19.7.1.4** Many health care occupancies conduct fire drills without disturbing patients by choosing the location of the simulated emergency in advance and by closing the doors to patients' rooms or wards in the vicinity prior to initiation of the drill. The purpose of a fire drill is to test and evaluate the efficiency, knowledge, and response of institutional personnel in implementing the facility fire emergency plan. Its purpose is not to disturb or excite patients. Fire drills should be scheduled on a random basis to ensure that personnel in health care facilities are drilled not less than once in each 3-month period.

Drills should consider the ability to move patients to an adjacent smoke compartment. Relocation can be practiced using simulated patients or empty wheelchairs.

**19.7.1.5** Infirm or bedridden patients shall not be required to be moved during drills to safe areas or to the exterior of the building.

**19.7.1.6** Drills shall be conducted quarterly on each shift to familiarize facility personnel (nurses, interns, maintenance engineers, and administrative staff) with the signals and emergency action required under varied conditions.

**19.7.1.7** When drills are conducted between 9:00 p.m. (2100 hours) and 6:00 a.m. (0600 hours), a coded announcement shall be permitted to be used instead of audible alarms.

**19.7.1.8** Employees of health care occupancies shall be instructed in life safety procedures and devices.

The life safety provisions applicable to health care occupancies involve more than fixed building features and systems. Life safety in this defend-in-place occupancy relies heavily on staff readiness and action. The evacuation and relocation plan and fire drill provisions of 18/19.7.1 provide the foundation for carrying out the needed staff duties, as detailed in 18/19.7.2.

The former requirement for patient beds to be on wheels or casters was deleted from the *Code* in 1991. Ordinary practice in health care occupancies is to move patients through the hospital on narrow beds, on gurneys, on carts, or in wheelchairs. The furniture in patient rooms — chairs, nightstands, food trays/tables, and medical equipment — must be moved out of the way to allow patient beds to be turned and moved out of the room. Moving patients in this way requires extra staff time that is usually unavailable during a fire. Emphasis should be placed on the quick movement of patients who are in the room of fire origin, as well as others who are directly exposed to the fire. Patient movement in fire emergencies is often achieved by dragging occupants on bedding, as opposed to moving beds.

### 18.7.2 Procedure in Case of Fire.

**18.7.2.1* Protection of Patients.**

**A.18.7.2.1** Each facility has specific characteristics that vary sufficiently from other facilities to prevent the specification of a universal emergency procedure. The recommendations that follow, however, contain many of the elements that should be considered and adapted, as appropriate, to the individual facility.

Upon discovery of fire, personnel should immediately take the following action:

(1) If any person is involved in the fire, the discoverer should go to the aid of that person, calling aloud an established code phrase, which provides for both the immediate aid of any endangered person and the transmission of an alarm.
(2) Any person in the area, upon hearing the code called aloud, should activate the building fire alarm using the nearest manual fire alarm box.
(3) If a person is not involved in the fire, the discoverer should activate the building fire alarm using the nearest manual fire alarm box.
(4) Personnel, upon hearing the alarm signal, should immediately execute their duties as outlined in the facility fire safety plan.
(5) The telephone operator should determine the location of the fire as indicated by the audible signal.
(6) In a building equipped with an uncoded alarm system, a person on the floor of fire origin should be responsible for promptly notifying the facility telephone operator of the fire location.
(7) If the telephone operator receives a telephone alarm reporting a fire from a floor, the operator should regard that alarm in the same fashion as an alarm received over the fire alarm system and should immediately notify the fire department and alert all facility personnel of the place of fire and its origin.

### 19.7.2 Procedure in Case of Fire.

**19.7.2.1* Protection of Patients.**

**A.19.7.2.1** Each facility has specific characteristics that vary sufficiently from other facilities to prevent the specification of a universal emergency procedure. The recommendations that follow, however, contain many of the elements that should be considered and adapted, as appropriate, to the individual facility.

Upon discovery of fire, personnel should immediately take the following action:

(1) If any person is involved in the fire, the discoverer should go to the aid of that person, calling aloud an established code phrase, which provides for both the immediate aid of any endangered person and the transmission of an alarm.
(2) Any person in the area, upon hearing the code called aloud, should activate the building fire alarm using the nearest manual fire alarm box.
(3) If a person is not involved in the fire, the discoverer should activate the building fire alarm using the nearest manual fire alarm box.
(4) Personnel, upon hearing the alarm signal, should immediately execute their duties as outlined in the facility fire safety plan.
(5) The telephone operator should determine the location of the fire as indicated by the audible signal.
(6) In a building equipped with an uncoded alarm system, a person on the floor of fire origin should be responsible for promptly notifying the facility telephone operator of the fire location.
(7) If the telephone operator receives a telephone alarm reporting a fire from a floor, the operator should regard that alarm in the same fashion as an alarm received over the fire alarm system and should immediately notify the fire department and alert all facility personnel of the place of fire and its origin.

CHAPTER 18 • New

(8) If the building fire alarm system is out of order, any person discovering a fire should immediately notify the telephone operator by telephone, and the operator should then transmit this information to the fire department and alert the building occupants.

**18.7.2.1.1** For health care occupancies, the proper protection of patients shall require the prompt and effective response of health care personnel.

**18.7.2.1.2** The basic response required of staff shall include the following:

(1) Removal of all occupants directly involved with the fire emergency
(2) Transmission of an appropriate fire alarm signal to warn other building occupants and summon staff
(3) Confinement of the effects of the fire by closing doors to isolate the fire area
(4) Relocation of patients as detailed in the health care occupancy's fire safety plan

**18.7.2.2 Fire Safety Plan.** A written health care occupancy fire safety plan shall provide for the following:

(1) Use of alarms
(2) Transmission of alarms to fire department
(3) Emergency phone call to fire department
(4) Response to alarms
(5) Isolation of fire
(6) Evacuation of immediate area
(7) Evacuation of smoke compartment
(8) Preparation of floors and building for evacuation
(9) Extinguishment of fire

**18.7.2.3 Staff Response.**

**18.7.2.3.1** All health care occupancy personnel shall be instructed in the use of and response to fire alarms.

**18.7.2.3.2** All health care occupancy personnel shall be instructed in the use of the code phrase to ensure transmission of an alarm under the following conditions:

(1) When the individual who discovers a fire must immediately go to the aid of an endangered person
(2) During a malfunction of the building fire alarm system

**18.7.2.3.3** Personnel hearing the code announced shall first activate the building fire alarm using the nearest manual fire alarm box and then shall execute immediately their duties as outlined in the fire safety plan.

CHAPTER 19 • Existing

(8) If the building fire alarm system is out of order, any person discovering a fire should immediately notify the telephone operator by telephone, and the operator should then transmit this information to the fire department and alert the building occupants.

**19.7.2.1.1** For health care occupancies, the proper protection of patients shall require the prompt and effective response of health care personnel.

**19.7.2.1.2** The basic response required of staff shall include the following:

(1) Removal of all occupants directly involved with the fire emergency
(2) Transmission of an appropriate fire alarm signal to warn other building occupants and summon staff
(3) Confinement of the effects of the fire by closing doors to isolate the fire area
(4) Relocation of patients as detailed in the health care occupancy's fire safety plan

**19.7.2.2 Fire Safety Plan.** A written health care occupancy fire safety plan shall provide for the following:

(1) Use of alarms
(2) Transmission of alarms to fire department
(3) Emergency phone call to fire department
(4) Response to alarms
(5) Isolation of fire
(6) Evacuation of immediate area
(7) Evacuation of smoke compartment
(8) Preparation of floors and building for evacuation
(9) Extinguishment of fire

**19.7.2.3 Staff Response.**

**19.7.2.3.1** All health care occupancy personnel shall be instructed in the use of and response to fire alarms.

**19.7.2.3.2** All health care occupancy personnel shall be instructed in the use of the code phrase to ensure transmission of an alarm under the following conditions:

(1) When the individual who discovers a fire must immediately go to the aid of an endangered person
(2) During a malfunction of the building fire alarm system

**19.7.2.3.3** Personnel hearing the code announced shall first activate the building fire alarm using the nearest manual fire alarm box and then shall execute immediately their duties as outlined in the fire safety plan.

In addition to the requirements of 18/19.7.2, evacuation plans should stress that the doors of as many patient rooms as possible be closed to block smoke spreading from a fire and, if possible, to confine the fire in a room. This single action taken by the staff (i.e., manually closing the doors) achieves the level of

CHAPTER 18 • New

safety to life mandated by the *Code* in Chapters 18 and 19.

In many fatal fires in health care facilities, staff either did not close doors or someone reopened them; the fire spread was sizable, and the loss of life was

CHAPTER 19 • Existing

high. Emphasis must be placed on training staff to sound an alarm, to rescue patients (as needed), and then to close all doors. The closing of doors historically has had the most significant effect on limiting the spread of fire and smoke.

### 18.7.3 Maintenance of Exits.

**18.7.3.1** Proper maintenance shall be provided to ensure the dependability of the method of evacuation selected.

**18.7.3.2** Health care occupancies that find it necessary to lock exits shall, at all times, maintain an adequate staff qualified to release locks and direct occupants from the immediate danger area to a place of safety in case of fire or other emergency.

### 18.7.4* Smoking.

Smoking regulations shall be adopted and shall include not less than the following provisions:

(1) Smoking shall be prohibited in any room, ward, or individual enclosed space where flammable liquids, combustible gases, or oxygen is used or stored and in any other hazardous location, and such areas shall be posted with signs that read NO SMOKING or shall be posted with the international symbol for no smoking.
(2) In health care occupancies where smoking is prohibited and signs are prominently placed at all major entrances, secondary signs with language that prohibits smoking shall not be required.
(3) Smoking by patients classified as not responsible shall be prohibited.
(4) The requirement of 18.7.4(3) shall not apply where the patient is under direct supervision.
(5) Ashtrays of noncombustible material and safe design shall be provided in all areas where smoking is permitted.
(6) Metal containers with self-closing cover devices into which ashtrays can be emptied shall be readily available to all areas where smoking is permitted.

**A.18.7.4** The most rigid discipline with regard to prohibition of smoking might not be nearly as effective in reducing incipient fires from surreptitious smoking as the open recognition of smoking, with provision of suitable facilities for smoking. Proper education and training of the staff and attendants in the ordinary fire hazards and their abatement is unquestionably essential. The problem is a broad one, varying with different types and arrangements of buildings; the effectiveness of rules of procedure, which need to be flexible, depends in large part on the management.

### 19.7.3 Maintenance of Exits.

**19.7.3.1** Proper maintenance shall be provided to ensure the dependability of the method of evacuation selected.

**19.7.3.2** Health care occupancies that find it necessary to lock exits shall, at all times, maintain an adequate staff qualified to release locks and direct occupants from the immediate danger area to a place of safety in case of fire or other emergency.

### 19.7.4* Smoking.

Smoking regulations shall be adopted and shall include not less than the following provisions:

(1) Smoking shall be prohibited in any room, ward, or individual enclosed space where flammable liquids, combustible gases, or oxygen is used or stored and in any other hazardous location, and such areas shall be posted with signs that read NO SMOKING or shall be posted with the international symbol for no smoking.
(2) In health care occupancies where smoking is prohibited and signs are prominently placed at all major entrances, secondary signs with language that prohibits smoking shall not be required.
(3) Smoking by patients classified as not responsible shall be prohibited.
(4) The requirement of 19.7.4(3) shall not apply where the patient is under direct supervision.
(5) Ashtrays of noncombustible material and safe design shall be provided in all areas where smoking is permitted.
(6) Metal containers with self-closing cover devices into which ashtrays can be emptied shall be readily available to all areas where smoking is permitted.

**A.19.7.4** The most rigid discipline with regard to prohibition of smoking might not be nearly as effective in reducing incipient fires from surreptitious smoking as the open recognition of smoking, with provision of suitable facilities for smoking. Proper education and training of the staff and attendants in the ordinary fire hazards and their abatement is unquestionably essential. The problem is a broad one, varying with different types and arrangements of buildings; the effectiveness of rules of procedure, which need to be flexible, depends in large part on the management.

CHAPTER 18 • New

The provision of 18/19.7.4(1), related to areas where smoking is prohibited, was revised for the 2009 edition of the *Code* to add the words "or individual enclosed space." The revision clarifies that smoking is to be regulated on a space by space basis. For example, smoking is to be prohibited from a room where flammable liquids are stored, but not from the other rooms within the same smoke compartment where those rooms do not meet the criteria of 18/19.7.4(1) for the prohibition of smoking.

### 18.7.5 Furnishings, Mattresses, and Decorations.

**18.7.5.1*** Draperies, curtains, and other loosely hanging fabrics and films serving as furnishings or decorations in health care occupancies shall be in accordance with the provisions of 10.3.1 *(see 18.3.5.10)*, and the following also shall apply:

(1) Such curtains shall include cubicle curtains.
(2) Such curtains shall not include curtains at showers.
(3) Such draperies and curtains shall not include draperies and curtains at windows in patient sleeping rooms.

**A.18.7.5.1** In addition to the provisions of 10.3.1, which deal with ignition resistance, additional requirements with respect to the location of cubicle curtains relative to sprinkler placement are included in NFPA 13, *Standard for the Installation of Sprinkler Systems.*

**18.7.5.2** Newly introduced upholstered furniture within health care occupancies shall comply with one of the following provisions:

(1) The furniture shall meet the criteria specified in 10.3.2.1 and 10.3.3.
(2) The furniture shall be in a building protected throughout by an approved, supervised automatic sprinkler system in accordance with 9.7.1.1(1).

**18.7.5.3 Reserved.**

**18.7.5.4** Newly introduced mattresses within health care occupancies shall comply with one of the following provisions:

(1) The mattresses shall meet the criteria specified in 10.3.2.2 and 10.3.4.
(2) The mattresses shall be in a building protected throughout by an approved, supervised automatic sprinkler system in accordance with 9.7.1.1(1).

CHAPTER 19 • Existing

### 19.7.5 Furnishings, Mattresses, and Decorations.

**19.7.5.1*** Draperies, curtains, and other loosely hanging fabrics and films serving as furnishings or decorations in health care occupancies shall be in accordance with the provisions of 10.3.1 *(see 19.3.5.10)*, and the following also shall apply:

(1) Such curtains shall include cubicle curtains.
(2) Such curtains shall not include curtains at showers.
(3) Such draperies and curtains shall not include draperies and curtains at windows in patient sleeping rooms in sprinklered smoke compartments.

**A.19.7.5.1** In addition to the provisions of 10.3.1, which deal with ignition resistance, additional requirements with respect to the location of cubicle curtains relative to sprinkler placement are included in NFPA 13, *Standard for the Installation of Sprinkler Systems.*

**19.7.5.2** Newly introduced upholstered furniture within health care occupancies shall comply with one of the following provisions, unless otherwise provided in 19.7.5.3:

(1) The furniture shall meet the criteria specified in 10.3.2.1 and 10.3.3.
(2) The furniture shall be in a building protected throughout by an approved, supervised automatic sprinkler system in accordance with 9.7.1.1(1).

**19.7.5.3** The requirements of 19.7.5.2, 10.3.2.1, and 10.3.3 shall not apply to upholstered furniture belonging to the patient in sleeping rooms of nursing homes where the following criteria are met:

(1) A smoke detector shall be installed where the patient sleeping room is not protected by automatic sprinklers.
(2) Battery-powered single-station smoke detectors shall be permitted.

**19.7.5.4** Newly introduced mattresses within health care occupancies shall comply with one of the following provisions, unless otherwise provided in 19.7.5.5:

(1) The mattresses shall meet the criteria specified in 10.3.2.2 and 10.3.4.
(2) The mattresses shall be in a building protected throughout by an approved, supervised automatic sprinkler system in accordance with 9.7.1.1(1).

**18.7.5.5 Reserved.**

**18.7.5.6** Combustible decorations shall be prohibited in any health care occupancy, unless one of the following criteria is met:

(1) They are flame-retardant.
(2)* They are decorations, such as photographs and paintings, in such limited quantities that a hazard of fire development or spread is not present.

**A.18.7.5.6(2)** When determining if the hazard for fire development or spread is present, consideration should be given to whether the building or area being evaluated is sprinklered.

**18.7.5.7** Soiled linen or trash collection receptacles shall not exceed 32 gal (121 L) in capacity and shall meet the following requirements:

(1) The average density of container capacity in a room or space shall not exceed 0.5 gal/ft$^2$ (20.4 L/m$^2$ ).
(2) A capacity of 32 gal (121 L) shall not be exceeded within any 64 ft$^2$ (16 m$^2$) area.
(3)* Mobile soiled linen or trash collection receptacles with capacities greater than 32 gal (121 L) shall be located in a room protected as a hazardous area when not attended.

**A.18.7.5.7(3)** It is not the intent to permit collection receptacles with a capacity greater than 32 gal (121 L) to be positioned at or near a nurses' station based on the argument that such nurses' station is constantly attended. The large collection receptacle itself needs to be actively attended by staff. Staff might leave the large receptacle in the corridor outside a patient room while entering the room to collect soiled linen or trash, but staff is expected to return to the receptacle, move on to the next room, and repeat the collection function. Where staff is not actively collecting material for placement in the receptacle, the receptacle is to be moved to a room protected as a hazardous area.

(4) Container size and density shall not be limited in hazardous areas.



**19.7.5.5** The requirements of 19.7.5.4, 10.3.2.2, and 10.3.4 shall not apply to mattresses belonging to the patient in sleeping rooms of nursing homes where the following criteria are met:

(1) A smoke detector shall be installed where the patient sleeping room is not protected by automatic sprinklers.
(2) Battery-powered single-station smoke detectors shall be permitted.

**19.7.5.6** Combustible decorations shall be prohibited in any health care occupancy, unless one of the following criteria is met:

(1) They are flame-retardant.
(2)* They are decorations, such as photographs and paintings, in such limited quantities that a hazard of fire development or spread is not present.

**A.19.7.5.6(2)** When determining if the hazard for fire development or spread is present, consideration should be given to whether the building or area being evaluated is sprinklered.

**19.7.5.7** Soiled linen or trash collection receptacles shall not exceed 32 gal (121 L) in capacity, and the following also shall apply:

(1) The average density of container capacity in a room or space shall not exceed 0.5 gal/ft$^2$ (20.4 L/m$^2$).
(2) A capacity of 32 gal (121 L) shall not be exceeded within any 64 ft$^2$ (6 m$^2$) area.
(3)* Mobile soiled linen or trash collection receptacles with capacities greater than 32 gal (121 L) shall be located in a room protected as a hazardous area when not attended.

**A.19.7.5.7(3)** It is not the intent to permit collection receptacles with a capacity greater than 32 gal (121 L) to be positioned at or near a nurses' station based on the argument that such nurses' station is constantly attended. The large collection receptacle itself needs to be actively attended by staff. Staff might leave the large receptacle in the corridor outside a patient room while entering the room to collect soiled linen or trash, but staff is expected to return to the receptacle, move on to the next room, and repeat the collection function. Where staff is not actively collecting material for placement in the receptacle, the receptacle is to be moved to a room protected as a hazardous area.

(4) Container size and density shall not be limited in hazardous areas.

CHAPTER 18 • New

CHAPTER 19 • Existing

Cigarette ignition–resistance testing — as detailed in 10.3.2 — and rate of heat release testing — as detailed in 10.3.3 and 10.3.4 — are required by 18/19.7.5.2 and 18/19.7.5.4 for newly introduced upholstered furniture and newly introduced mattresses in health care occupancies, unless the building is fully sprinklered. However, these requirements would seldom apply in new health care occupancies, because 18.3.5.1 requires new health care occupancies to be sprinklered. Unlike new health care occupancies, which are required to be sprinklered, many existing facilities are not sprinklered. Yet, government regulations require that patients be permitted to take their own furniture with them to a nursing home, and such movement of existing furniture into the facility mandates the requirement that applies to newly introduced upholstered furniture and newly introduced mattresses. Paragraphs 19.7.5.3 and 19.7.5.5 offer nonsprinklered existing health care facilities another option — providing smoke detection within the patient room. If early warning is provided to staff, then an incipient stage fire might be extinguished manually almost as quickly as would occur automatically in a room that is sprinklered.

Paragraph 18/19.7.5.7 establishes maximum trash container sizes and placement densities permitted within a room. Containers larger than that specified, or grouped containers exceeding the density-per-room criterion, present a hazard greater than that associated with the normal furnishings of a health care occupancy room.

Large, mobile soiled linen or trash receptacles can be moved along the corridor as collections occur but must be attended by staff. If housekeeping staff, for example, must leave the area, the container must be stored in a room designed and maintained as a hazardous area in accordance with 18/19.3.2.1. The text of A.18/A.19.7.5.7(3) clarifies that receptacles positioned at nurses' stations are not to be considered as being attended.

Exhibit 18/19.34 illustrates the requirements of 18/19.7.5.7.

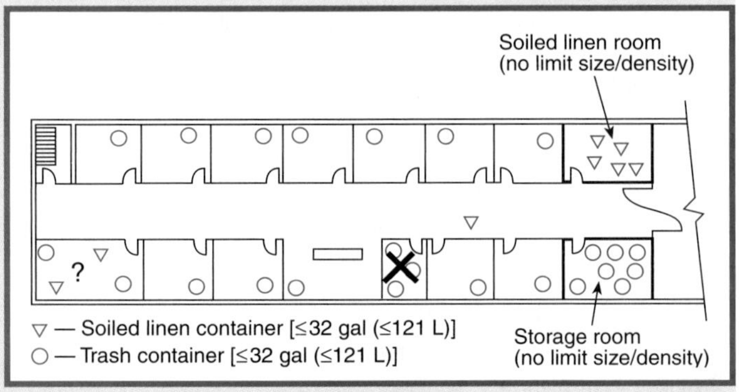


***Exhibit 18/19.34*** *Allowable soiled linen or trash collection receptacles.*

## 18.7.6 Maintenance and Testing.

See 4.6.13.

## 18.7.7 Engineered Smoke Control Systems.

**18.7.7.1** New engineered smoke control systems shall be designed, installed, tested, and maintained in accordance with NFPA 92A, *Standard for Smoke-Control Systems Utilizing Barriers and Pressure Differences*, and NFPA 92B, *Standard for Smoke Management Systems in Malls, Atria, and Large Spaces*, as applicable.

**18.7.7.2** Test documentation shall be maintained on the premises at all times.

## 19.7.6 Maintenance and Testing.

See 4.6.13.

## 19.7.7* Engineered Smoke Control Systems.

**A.19.7.7** Two documents that provide recognized engineering principles for the testing of smoke control systems are NFPA 92A, *Standard for Smoke-Control Systems Utilizing Barriers and Pressure Differences*, and NFPA 92B, *Standard for Smoke Management Systems in Malls, Atria, and Large Spaces*.

**19.7.7.1** Existing engineered smoke control systems, unless specifically exempted by the authority having jurisdiction, shall be tested in accordance with established engineering principles.

**19.7.7.2** Systems not meeting the performance requirements of such testing shall be continued in operation only with the specific approval of the authority having jurisdiction.

CHAPTER 18 • New

### 18.7.8 Portable Space-Heating Devices.

Portable space-heating devices shall be prohibited in all health care occupancies, unless both of the following criteria are met:

(1) Such devices are permitted to be used only in nonsleeping staff and employee areas.
(2) The heating elements of such devices do not exceed 212°F (100°C).

### 18.7.9 Construction, Repair, and Improvement Operations.

**18.7.9.1** Construction, repair, and improvement operations shall comply with 4.6.11.

**18.7.9.2** The means of egress in any area undergoing construction, repair, or improvements shall be inspected daily for compliance with 7.1.10.1 and shall also comply with NFPA 241, *Standard for Safeguarding Construction, Alteration, and Demolition Operations.*

CHAPTER 19 • Existing

### 19.7.8 Portable Space-Heating Devices.

Portable space-heating devices shall be prohibited in all health care occupancies, unless both of the following criteria are met:

(1) Such devices are used only in nonsleeping staff and employee areas.
(2) The heating elements of such devices do not exceed 212°F (100°C).

### 19.7.9 Construction, Repair, and Improvement Operations.

**19.7.9.1** Construction, repair, and improvement operations shall comply with 4.6.11.

**19.7.9.2** The means of egress in any area undergoing construction, repair, or improvements shall be inspected daily for compliance with 7.1.10.1 and shall also comply with NFPA 241, *Standard for Safeguarding Construction, Alteration, and Demolition Operations.*

## References Cited in Commentary


1. NFPA 101A, *Guide on Alternative Approaches to Life Safety*, 2007 edition, National Fire Protection Association, Quincy, MA. The 2010 edition of NFPA 101A corresponds with the 2009 edition of the *Life Safety Code.*
2. NFPA 220, *Standard on Types of Building Construction*, 2009 edition, National Fire Protection Association, Quincy, MA.
3. *NFPA 5000®, Building Construction and Safety Code®*, 2009 edition, National Fire Protection Association, Quincy, MA.
4. NFPA 241, *Standard for Safeguarding Construction, Alteration, and Demolition Operations*, 2004 edition, National Fire Protection Association, Quincy, MA.
5. *NFPA 72®, National Fire Alarm Code®*, 2007 edition, National Fire Protection Association, Quincy, MA.
6. NFPA 99, *Standard for Health Care Facilities*, 2005 edition, National Fire Protection Association, Quincy, MA.
7. NFPA 82, *Standard on Incinerators and Waste and Linen Handling Systems and Equipment*, 2004 edition, National Fire Protection Association, Quincy, MA.
8. NFPA 30, *Flammable and Combustible Liquids Code*, 2008 edition, National Fire Protection Association, Quincy, MA.
9. NFPA 80, *Standard for Fire Doors and Other Opening Protectives*, 2007 edition, National Fire Protection Association, Quincy, MA.
10. NFPA 96, *Standard for Ventilation Control and Fire Protection of Commercial Cooking Operations*, 2008 edition, National Fire Protection Association, Quincy, MA.
11. 2005 June Association Meeting, Building Code Committee and Safety to Life Committee Reports on Proposals, Proposal 101-393, p. 101–141, 2004, National Fire Protection Association, Quincy, MA.
12. Centers for Disease Control and Prevention, *Guidelines for Hand Hygiene in Health-Care Settings*, Morbidity and Mortality Weekly Report (MMWR), October 25, 2002, vol. 51, no. RR-16, U.S. Department of Health and Human Services, Atlanta, GA.
13. Fredrickson, D. L., "Alcohol Based Hand Sanitizers — Level 1 Aerosol Products," Consumer Specialty Products Association (CSPA), 900 17th St NW, Washington, DC 20006, January 2007.
14. Christian, W. J. and Waterman, T. E., "Flame Spread in Corridors: Effects of Location and Area of Wall Finish," *Fire Journal®* 65, no. 4 (July 1971): 25–32.
15. Bukowski, R. W. and Istvan, S. M., "A Survey of Field Experience with Smoke Detectors in Health Care Facilities," NBSIR 80-2130, Center for Fire Research, National Bureau of Standards, October 1980.

16. 2005 June Association Meeting, Building Code Committee and Safety to Life Committee Reports on Proposals, Proposal 101-449, pp. 101-160–101-161, 2004, National Fire Protection Association, Quincy, MA.
17. NFPA 13, *Standard for the Installation of Sprinkler Systems*, 2007 edition, National Fire Protection Association, Quincy, MA.
18. NFPA 90A, *Standard for the Installation of Air-Conditioning and Ventilating Systems*, 2009 edition, National Fire Protection Association, Quincy, MA.
19. ASME A17.1/CSA B44, *Safety Code for Elevators and Escalators*, 2007 edition, American Society of Mechanical Engineers, Three Park Avenue, New York, NY 10016-5990.
20. ASME A17.3, *Safety Code for Existing Elevators and Escalators*, 2005 edition, American Society of Mechanical Engineers, Three Park Avenue, New York, NY 10016-5990.

CHAPTERS 20 AND 21

# New and Existing Ambulatory Health Care Occupancies

Chapters 20 and 21 address the needs of occupants of facilities that provide medical treatment on an outpatient basis. The patient treatment is not merely a routine medical visit, such as to a doctor's office, but rather a procedure that renders the patient incapable of self-preservation or a procedure that requires anesthesia that renders the patient incapable of self-preservation. Ambulatory health care occupancies also provide treatment to patients who arrive at the facility incapable of self-preservation, as might be rendered at an emergency care center that is not part of a hospital. Although these descriptions might seem to resemble a situation that one would associate with a hospital, the major difference is that an ambulatory health care facility does not provide care for any individual for an elapsed time of 24 hours or more. Rather, a patient receives treatment and then leaves the facility. Patients suffering complications that would prevent them from leaving the ambulatory health care facility would typically be transported and admitted to a hospital that provides care on a 24-hour basis.

There is also an important distinction concerning the number of occupants required to constitute classification as an ambulatory health care occupancy — that number being four or more (see the definition of the term *ambulatory health care occupancy* in 3.3.178.1). The Centers for Medicare and Medicaid Services (CMS) play an important role in the government financing of health care services in the United States. CMS applies a stricter definition of ambulatory health care occupancy than NFPA by requiring a surgical center for one or more patients to be classified as an ambulatory health care occupancy. NFPA's four-person criterion applies to all forms of ambulatory health care occupancies.

The provisions for ambulatory health care occupancies are based on a combination of requirements — some from those that are applicable to hospitals and some from direct references to the provisions of Chapters 38 and 39 for business occupancies. If an outpatient medical facility does not meet the definition of the term *ambulatory health care occupancy,* it generally needs to comply only with the requirements for a business occupancy.

Commentary Table 20/21.1 differentiates among health care, ambulatory health care, and business occupancies on the basis of the patient load and care provided. Incapability of self-preservation might be the result of the use of general anesthesia, a treatment such as dialysis, or an injury or illness that brings the

***Commentary Table 20/21.1 Occupancy Classification Comparison***

| Factor | Chapters 18/19 Health Care Occupancies | Chapters 20/21 Ambulatory Health Care Occupancies | Chapters 38/39 Business Occupancies |
|---|---|---|---|
| Number of patients rendered incapable of self-preservation | 4 or more[1] | 4 or more[2] | 3 or fewer |
| Care provided on a 24-hour basis? | Yes | No | No |

[1]Incapability of self-preservation might exist prior to admission and be unrelated to the treatment provided (see 18/19.1.1.1.3).

[2]Incapability of self-preservation might exist prior to admission but be related to the treatment provided [see 3.3.178.1, item (2)].

patient to the ambulatory health care facility for treatment. Based on the information in Commentary Table 20/21.1, if a dentist administers general anesthesia to not more than three patients simultaneously, the dentist's office would be classified as a business occupancy. If the dentist expands the simultaneous administration of general anesthesia to a fourth patient, then the more stringent requirements for ambulatory health care occupancies would apply.

## 20.1 General Requirements

### 20.1.1 Application.

#### 20.1.1.1 General.

**20.1.1.1.1** The requirements of this chapter shall apply to new buildings or portions thereof used as ambulatory health care occupancies. *(See 1.3.1.)*

The provisions for new ambulatory health care occupancies are addressed in Chapter 20; the provisions for existing ambulatory health care occupancies (i.e., existing conditions in ambulatory health care occupancies) are addressed in Chapter 21.

In editions of the *Code* prior to 2006, renovations, additions, and changes of occupancy were required to comply with the requirements for new construction. For ambulatory health care occupancies, such renovations, additions, and changes of occupancy were required to meet the provisions of Chapter 20, while existing conditions were subject to the provisions of Chapter 21. Since the 2006 edition of the *Code,* Chapter 43, Building Rehabilitation, has addressed the subject differently than before. The chapter was written to promote the adaptive reuse of existing buildings without sacrificing the needed level of life safety. The provisions of Chapter 43 blend the requirements for new construction with those for existing conditions, so as to require additional life safety features as the rehabilitation work category increases in complexity. The rehabilitation work categories are repair, renovation, modification, reconstruction, change of use or occupancy classification, and addition. See 4.6.8, 4.6.12, and Chapter 43.

**20.1.1.1.2** Ambulatory health care facilities shall comply with the provisions of Chapter 38 and this chapter, whichever are more stringent.

Ambulatory health care facilities exhibit some of the occupancy characteristics of business occupancies and some of the characteristics of health care occupancies. Chapters 20 and 21 prescribe a level of life safety from fire that is greater than that typically specified for business occupancies but less than that typically found in hospitals, nursing homes, and limited care facilities. See the commentary following 18/19.1.3(4).

Ambulatory health care facilities are required to comply with the provisions of Chapters 38 and 39 pertaining to business occupancies and those contained within Chapters 20 and 21. Where Chapter 38 or Chapter 39 and Chapter 20 or Chapter 21 address a feature in different ways, the stricter application (typically that addressed by Chapter 20 or Chapter 21) governs. Chapters 20 and 21 also address features that are not covered by Chapters 38 and 39 (e.g., subdivision of building space via smoke barriers, as addressed in 20/21.3.7) but that are similar to those required for health care occupancies by Chapters 18 and 19.

As an example, Exhibit 20/21.1 is a plan of a single-story, nonsprinklered, existing office building. Tenants C and D occupy a small portion of the floor. Most of the first-floor area (spaces A and B, located on opposite sides of the corridor) is available for leasing to one or more tenants. A kidney dialysis center (an ambulatory health care occupancy) plans to take space A; a multilawyer law practice (a business occupancy)



## 21.1 General Requirements

### 21.1.1 Application.

#### 21.1.1.1 General.

**21.1.1.1.1** The requirements of this chapter shall apply to existing buildings or portions thereof currently occupied as an ambulatory health care occupancy.

**21.1.1.1.2** Ambulatory health care facilities shall comply with the provisions of Chapter 39 and this chapter, whichever are more stringent.

CHAPTER 20 • New

CHAPTER 21 • Existing

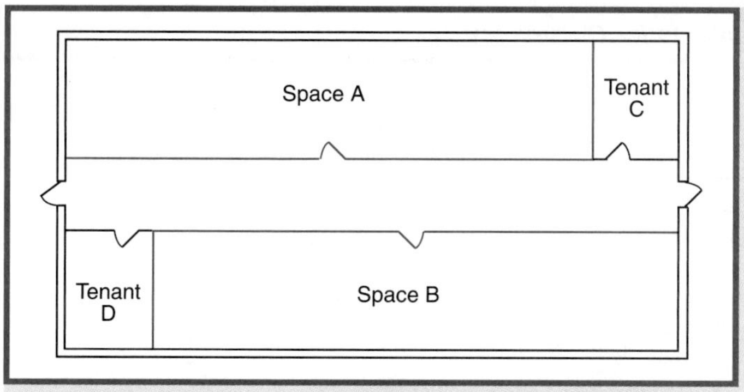


***Exhibit 20/21.1*** *Occupancy classification dependent on tenant use.*

plans to take space B. The previous tenants of both space A and space B used their leased space as offices (business occupancies).

The lawyers' office is classified as a business occupancy; and because its occupancy classification represents no change from that of the previous tenant, it is further classified as an existing business occupancy. The lawyers' office must, therefore, meet the requirements of Chapter 39, which apply to existing business occupancies. The kidney dialysis center will render four or more patients simultaneously incapable of self-preservation [see 3.3.178.1, item (1)]; it is classified as an ambulatory health care occupancy. Because that occupancy classification represents a change of occupancy from that of the previous tenant, 43.7.2.1 requires that the hazard category of the new occupancy be compared against that of the previous occupancy. Per Table 43.7.3, both ambulatory health care and business occupancies are hazard category 3. So, per 43.7.2.1(1), the kidney dialysis center must meet the requirements of Chapter 21, which apply to existing ambulatory health care occupancies, and those of Chapter 39, which apply to existing business occupancies. The additional provision of 43.7.2.1(2), related to compliance with the sprinkler and alarm system provisions applicable to new construction, has no real effect in this case, as the sprinkler and alarm provisions of Chapter 20 are not stricter than those of Chapter 21.

Commentary Table 20/21.2 contrasts some of the *Code* provisions that apply to the kidney dialysis center and the lawyers' office addressed in the preceding paragraph.

**20.1.1.1.3** This chapter establishes life safety requirements, in addition to those required in Chapter 38, that shall apply to the design of all ambulatory health care occupancies as defined in 3.3.178.1.

**20.1.1.1.4** Buildings, or sections of buildings, that primarily house patients who, in the opinion of the governing body of the facility and the governmental agency having jurisdiction, are capable of exercising judgment and appropriate physical action for self-preservation under emergency conditions shall be permitted to comply with chapters of this *Code* other than Chapter 20.

**20.1.1.1.5** It shall be recognized that, in buildings providing treatment for certain types of patients or having detention rooms or a security section, it might be necessary to lock doors and bar windows to confine and protect building inhabitants. In such instances, the authority having jurisdiction shall make appropriate modifications to those sections of this *Code* that would otherwise require means of egress to be kept unlocked.

**20.1.1.1.6*** The requirements of this chapter shall apply based on the assumption that staff is available in all patient-occupied areas to perform certain fire safety functions as required in other paragraphs of this chapter.

**A.20.1.1.1.6** The *Code* recognizes that certain functions necessary for the life safety of building occupants, such as

**21.1.1.1.3** This chapter establishes life safety requirements, in addition to those required in Chapter 39, that shall apply to the design of all ambulatory health care occupancies as defined in 3.3.178.1.

**21.1.1.1.4** Buildings, or sections of buildings, that primarily house patients who, in the opinion of the governing body of the facility and the governmental agency having jurisdiction, are capable of exercising judgment and appropriate physical action for self-preservation under emergency conditions shall be permitted to comply with chapters of this *Code* other than Chapter 21.

**21.1.1.1.5** It shall be recognized that, in buildings providing treatment for certain types of patients or having detention rooms or a security section, it might be necessary to lock doors and bar windows to confine and protect building inhabitants. In such instances, the authority having jurisdiction shall make appropriate modifications to those sections of this *Code* that would otherwise require means of egress to be kept unlocked.

**21.1.1.1.6*** The requirements of this chapter shall apply based on the assumption that staff is available in all patient-occupied areas to perform certain fire safety functions as required in other paragraphs of this chapter.

**A.21.1.1.1.6** The *Code* recognizes that certain functions necessary for the life safety of building occupants, such as

**Commentary Table 20/21.2 Comparison of Applicable Requirements for Occupancy**

| Building Feature | New Kidney Dialysis Center ["existing" ambulatory health care occupancy per 43.7.2.1(1)] | New Lawyers' Office [existing business occupancy] |
|---|---|---|
| Egress door locking | Addressed by 21.1.1.1.5; doors permitted to be locked to confine and protect patients, but AHJ must make modifications to permit locked doors | Doors not permitted to be locked while space is occupied in accordance with 7.2.1.5.1 |
| Minimum construction | Regulated by 21.1.6, but because building is single story, any NFPA 220 construction type is acceptable (see 21.1.6.1) | No regulation |
| Automatic door closing | In addition to release via methods of 7.2.1.8 (smoke detection, power failure, manual action), initiation of required fire alarm must release hold-open devices in accordance with 21.2.2.4 | Hold-open devices released via methods of 7.2.1.8 (smoke detection, power failure, manual action) |
| Door width | Minimum 32 in. (810 mm) clear width or 34 in. (865 mm) in leaf width in accordance with 21.2.3.4 | Minimum 28 in. (710 mm) door leaf width in accordance with 7.2.1.2.3.2(4) |
| Number of exits | Minimum of two in accordance with 21.2.4 | Single exit permitted per 39.2.4 |
| Number of exit accesses | Minimum of two exit access doors from suite of more than 2500 $ft^2$ (232 $m^2$) in accordance with 21.2.4.2, or if common path of travel with single door would be excessive (see 39.2.5.3) | Second exit access door required from suite if common path of travel with single door would be excessive (see 39.2.5.3) |
| Travel distance | Considered in two segments in accordance with 21.2.6.2; room door to exit travel (typically corridor travel) limited to 100 ft (30 m); total travel limited to 150 ft (46 m) | Considered in one segment in accordance with 39.2.6; total travel limited to 200 ft (61 m) |
| Emergency lighting | Required within center and its egress paths by 21.2.9.1 | Required by 39.2.9.1 only if single floor has occupant load of 1000 or more persons |
| Alarm system | Provisions of 20.3.4 and 38.3.4 apply [per 43.7.2.1(2)]; alarm system required within center by 20.3.4 (manual fire alarm boxes, automatic occupant notification, fire department notification) | Required by 39.3.4 only if single floor has occupant load of 1000 or more persons; automatic initiation permitted to substitute for all but one manual fire alarm box; occupant notification permitted to come from attended location; fire department notification not required |
| Automatic sprinklers | Provisions of 20.3.5 and 38.3.5 apply [per 43.7.2.1(2)], but neither requires sprinklers | Provision of 39.3.5 applies, but sprinklers not required |
| Smoke compartmentation | Required by 21.3.7; separation required from other tenants; subdivision by smoke barriers within center, unless <5000 $ft^2$ (<465 $m^2$) and smoke detection or <10,000 $ft^2$ (<929 $m^2$) and sprinklers | No regulation |
| Evacuation and relocation plan | Required by 21.7.1 | No regulation |
| Staff procedures in case of fire | Required by 21.7.2 | No regulation |
| Control of furnishings | Required by 21.7.5 for curtains, upholstered furniture, mattresses, trash receptacles | No regulation |

the closing of corridor doors, the operation of manual fire alarm devices, and the removal of patients from the room of fire origin, require the intervention of facility staff. It is not the intent of 20.1.1.1.6 to specify the levels or locations of staff necessary to meet this requirement.

**20.1.1.2* Goals and Objectives.** The goals and objectives of Sections 4.1 and 4.2 shall be met with due consideration for functional requirements, which are accomplished by limiting the development and spread of a fire emergency to the room of fire origin and reducing the need for occupant evacuation, except from the room of fire origin.

**A.20.1.1.2** This objective is accomplished in the context of the physical facilities, the type of activities undertaken, the provisions for the capabilities of staff, and the needs of all occupants through requirements directed at the following:

(1) Prevention of ignition
(2) Detection of fire
(3) Control of fire development
(4) Confinement of the effects of fire
(5) Extinguishment of fire
(6) Provision of refuge or evacuation facilities, or both
(7) Staff reaction

**20.1.1.3 Total Concept.**

**20.1.1.3.1** All ambulatory health care facilities shall be designed, constructed, maintained, and operated to minimize the possibility of a fire emergency requiring the evacuation of occupants.

**20.1.1.3.2** Because the safety of ambulatory health care occupants cannot be ensured adequately by dependence on evacuation of the building, their protection from fire shall be provided by appropriate arrangement of facilities; adequate, trained staff; and development of operating and maintenance procedures composed of the following:

(1) Design, construction, and compartmentation
(2) Provision for detection, alarm, and extinguishment
(3) Fire prevention and planning, training, and drilling programs for the isolation of fire, transfer of occupants to areas of refuge, or evacuation of the building

**20.1.1.4 Additions, Conversions, Modernization, Renovation, and Construction Operations.**

**20.1.1.4.1 Additions.**

**20.1.1.4.1.1** Additions shall be separated from any existing structure not conforming to the provisions within Chapter 21 by a fire barrier having not less than a 2-hour fire resistance rating and constructed of materials as required for the addition. *(See 4.6.5 and 4.6.8.)*



the closing of corridor doors, the operation of manual fire alarm devices, and the removal of patients from the room of fire origin, require the intervention of facility staff. It is not the intent of 21.1.1.1.6 to specify the levels or locations of staff necessary to meet this requirement.

**21.1.1.2* Goals and Objectives.** The goals and objectives of Sections 4.1 and 4.2 shall be met with due consideration for functional requirements, which are accomplished by limiting the development and spread of a fire emergency to the room of fire origin and reducing the need for occupant evacuation, except from the room of fire origin.

**A.21.1.1.2** This objective is accomplished in the context of the physical facilities, the type of activities undertaken, the provisions for the capabilities of staff, and the needs of all occupants through requirements directed at the following:

(1) Prevention of ignition
(2) Detection of fire
(3) Control of fire development
(4) Confinement of the effects of fire
(5) Extinguishment of fire
(6) Provision of refuge or evacuation facilities, or both
(7) Staff reaction

**21.1.1.3 Total Concept.**

**21.1.1.3.1** All ambulatory health care facilities shall be designed, constructed, maintained, and operated to minimize the possibility of a fire emergency requiring the evacuation of occupants.

**21.1.1.3.2** Because the safety of ambulatory health care occupants cannot be ensured adequately by dependence on evacuation of the building, their protection from fire shall be provided by appropriate arrangement of facilities; adequate, trained staff; and development of operating and maintenance procedures composed of the following:

(1) Design, construction, and compartmentation
(2) Provision for detection, alarm, and extinguishment
(3) Fire prevention and planning, training, and drilling programs for the isolation of fire, transfer of occupants to areas of refuge, or evacuation of the building

**21.1.1.4 Additions, Conversions, Modernization, Renovation, and Construction Operations.**

**21.1.1.4.1 Additions.**

**21.1.1.4.1.1** Additions shall be separated from any existing structure not conforming to the provisions within Chapter 21 by a fire barrier having not less than a 2-hour fire resistance rating and constructed of materials as required for the addition. *(See 4.6.5 and 4.6.8.)*

CHAPTER 20 • New

**20.1.1.4.1.2** Doors in barriers required by 20.1.1.4.1.1 shall normally be kept closed, unless otherwise permitted by 20.1.1.4.1.3.

**20.1.1.4.1.3** Doors shall be permitted to be held open if they meet the requirements of 20.2.2.4.

**20.1.1.4.2 Changes of Occupancy.** A change from a hospital or nursing home to an ambulatory health care occupancy shall not be considered a change in occupancy or occupancy subclassification.

**20.1.1.4.3 Renovations, Alterations, and Modernizations.** See 4.6.8.

**20.1.1.4.4 Construction, Repair, and Improvement Operations.** See 4.6.11.

CHAPTER 21 • Existing

**21.1.1.4.1.2** Doors in barriers required by 21.1.1.4.1.1 shall normally be kept closed, unless otherwise permitted by 21.1.1.4.1.3.

**21.1.1.4.1.3** Doors shall be permitted to be held open if they meet the requirements of 21.2.2.4.

**21.1.1.4.2 Changes of Occupancy.** A change from a hospital or nursing home to an ambulatory health care occupancy shall not be considered a change in occupancy or occupancy subclassification.

**21.1.1.4.3 Renovations, Alterations, and Modernizations.** See 4.6.8.

**21.1.1.4.4 Construction, Repair, and Improvement Operations.** See 4.6.11.

Paragraph 20/21.1.1.4.1 establishes separation criteria for additions to existing structures that do not conform to the provisions of Chapter 21. However, if an existing building meets the provisions of Chapter 21, the new addition that complies with Chapter 20 would not be required to be separated from the existing portion of the newly enlarged building.

Where additions are required to be separated from existing portions of buildings, barriers must be constructed of assemblies providing a minimum 2-hour fire resistance rating.

### 20.1.2 Multiple Occupancies.

**20.1.2.1** Multiple occupancies shall be in accordance with 6.1.14.

### 21.1.2 Multiple Occupancies.

**21.1.2.1** Multiple occupancies shall be in accordance with 6.1.14.

Paragraph 20/21.1.2.1 directs the user to the multiple occupancies provisions of 6.1.14, which permit protecting multiple occupancies either as mixed occupancies or as separated occupancies. Where the multiple occupancy is protected via the provisions of 6.1.14.4 for separated occupancies, the required number of hours of fire-rated separation is specified by Table 6.1.14.4.1(a) or Table 6.1.14.4.1(b). The most common occupancies to abut an ambulatory health care occupancy are health care occupancies and business occupancies. The required separation between an ambulatory health care occupancy and a health care occupancy is 2 hours; between an ambulatory health care occupancy and a business occupancy, the required separation is 1 hour.

The provisions of 20/21.1.2.2 through 20/21.1.2.7 have the effect of modifying those of 6.1.14 for the very specific situations described.

**20.1.2.2*** Sections of ambulatory health care facilities shall be permitted to be classified as other occupancies, provided that they meet all of the following conditions:

(1) They are not intended to serve ambulatory health care occupants for purposes of treatment or customary access by patients incapable of self-preservation.
(2) They are separated from areas of ambulatory health care occupancies by construction having a minimum 1-hour fire resistance rating.

**A.20.1.2.2** Doctors' offices and treatment and diagnostic facilities that are intended solely for outpatient care and are

**21.1.2.2*** Sections of ambulatory health care facilities shall be permitted to be classified as other occupancies, provided that they meet all of the following conditions:

(1) They are not intended to serve ambulatory health care occupants for purposes of treatment or customary access by patients incapable of self-preservation.
(2) They are separated from areas of ambulatory health care occupancies by construction having a minimum 1-hour fire resistance rating.

**A.21.1.2.2** Doctors' offices and treatment and diagnostic facilities that are intended solely for outpatient care and are

CHAPTER 20 • New

physically separated from facilities for the treatment or care of inpatients, but are otherwise associated with the management of an institution, might be classified as business occupancies rather than health care occupancies.

**20.1.2.3** All means of egress from ambulatory health care occupancies that traverse nonambulatory health care spaces shall conform to requirements of this *Code* for ambulatory health care occupancies, unless otherwise permitted by 20.1.2.4.

**20.1.2.4** Exit through a horizontal exit into other contiguous occupancies that do not conform to ambulatory health care egress provisions but that do comply with requirements set forth in the appropriate occupancy chapter of this *Code* shall be permitted, provided that the occupancy does not contain high hazard contents.

**20.1.2.5** Egress provisions for areas of ambulatory health care facilities that correspond to other occupancies shall meet the corresponding requirements of this *Code* for such occupancies, and, where the clinical needs of the occupant necessitate the locking of means of egress, staff shall be present for the supervised release of occupants during all times of use.

**20.1.2.6** Any area with a hazard of contents classified higher than that of the ambulatory health care occupancy and located in the same building shall be protected as required in 20.3.2.

**20.1.2.7** Non-health care–related occupancies classified as containing high hazard contents shall not be permitted in buildings housing ambulatory health care occupancies.

### 20.1.3 Definition — Ambulatory Health Care Occupancy.

See 3.3.178.1.

CHAPTER 21 • Existing

physically separated from facilities for the treatment or care of inpatients, but that are otherwise associated with the management of an institution, might be classified as business occupancies rather than health care occupancies.

**21.1.2.3** All means of egress from ambulatory health care occupancies that traverse nonambulatory health care spaces shall conform to the requirements of this *Code* for ambulatory health care occupancies, unless otherwise permitted by 21.1.2.4.

**21.1.2.4** Exit through a horizontal exit into other contiguous occupancies that do not conform with ambulatory health care egress provisions but that do comply with requirements set forth in the appropriate occupancy chapter of this *Code* shall be permitted, provided that the occupancy does not contain high hazard contents.

**21.1.2.5** Egress provisions for areas of ambulatory health care facilities that correspond to other occupancies shall meet the corresponding requirements of this *Code* for such occupancies, and, where the clinical needs of the occupant necessitate the locking of means of egress, staff shall be present for the supervised release of occupants during all times of use.

**21.1.2.6** Any area with a hazard of contents classified higher than that of the ambulatory health care occupancy and located in the same building shall be protected as required in 21.3.2.

**21.1.2.7** Non-health care–related occupancies classified as containing high hazard contents shall not be permitted in buildings housing ambulatory health care occupancies.

### 21.1.3 Definition — Ambulatory Health Care Occupancy.

See 3.3.178.1.

Prior to the 1981 edition of the *Code,* occupancies that offered medical services on an outpatient basis were regulated by the chapter covering business occupancies. The threat to life in an outpatient facility where four or more patients might be subject to medical procedures requiring general anesthesia, treatments such as hemodialysis, or freestanding emergency or urgent care is significantly greater than that typical of a business occupancy. Conversely, application of the requirements for health care facilities that contemplate 24-hour care would be unnecessarily restrictive. In establishing the occupancy classification of an ambulatory health care facility, the intent was to develop requirements that fall between the provisions applicable to business occupancies and those applicable to inpatient health care facilities in terms of the level of life safety provided.

### 20.1.4 Classification of Occupancy.

See 6.1.6 and 20.1.3.

### 21.1.4 Classification of Occupancy.

See 6.1.6 and 21.1.3.

CHAPTER 20 • New

### 20.1.5 Classification of Hazard of Contents.

The classification of hazard of contents shall be as defined in Section 6.2.

### 20.1.6 Minimum Construction Requirements.

**20.1.6.1** Ambulatory health care occupancies shall be limited to the building construction types specified in Table 20.1.6.1, unless otherwise permitted by 20.1.6.6. *(See 8.2.1.)*

*Table 20.1.6.1 Construction Type Limitations*

| Construction Type | Sprinklered‡ | Stories in Height† 1 | Stories in Height† ≥2 |
|---|---|---|---|
| I (442) | Yes | X | X |
| | No | X | X |
| I (332) | Yes | X | X |
| | No | X | X |
| II (222) | Yes | X | X |
| | No | X | X |
| II (111) | Yes | X | X |
| | No | X | X |
| II (000) | Yes | X | X |
| | No | X | NP |
| III (211) | Yes | X | X |
| | No | X | X |
| III (200) | Yes | X | X |
| | No | X | NP |
| IV (2HH) | Yes | X | X |
| | No | X | X |
| V (111) | Yes | X | X |
| | No | X | X |
| V (000) | Yes | X | X |
| | No | X | NP |

X: Permitted. NP: Not permitted.

† See 4.6.3.

‡ Sprinklered throughout by an approved, supervised automatic sprinkler system in accordance with Section 9.7. *(See 20.3.5.)*

**20.1.6.2** Any level below the level of exit discharge shall be separated from the level of exit discharge by not less than Type II(111), Type III(211), or Type V(111) construction *(see 8.2.1)*, unless both of the following criteria are met:

(1) Such levels are under the control of the ambulatory health care facility.
(2) Any hazardous spaces are protected in accordance with Section 8.7.

CHAPTER 21 • Existing

### 21.1.5 Classification of Hazard of Contents.

The classification of hazard of contents shall be as defined in Section 6.2.

### 21.1.6 Minimum Construction Requirements.

**21.1.6.1** Ambulatory health care occupancies shall be limited to the building construction types specified in Table 21.1.6.1, unless otherwise permitted by 21.1.6.6. *(See 8.2.1.)*

*Table 21.1.6.1 Construction Type Limitations*

| Construction Type | Sprinklered‡ | Stories in Height† 1 | Stories in Height† ≥2 |
|---|---|---|---|
| I (442) | Yes | X | X |
| | No | X | X |
| I (332) | Yes | X | X |
| | No | X | X |
| II (222) | Yes | X | X |
| | No | X | X |
| II (111) | Yes | X | X |
| | No | X | X |
| II (000) | Yes | X | X |
| | No | X | NP |
| III (211) | Yes | X | X |
| | No | X | X |
| III (200) | Yes | X | X |
| | No | X | NP |
| IV (2HH) | Yes | X | X |
| | No | X | X |
| V (111) | Yes | X | X |
| | No | X | X |
| V (000) | Yes | X | X |
| | No | X | NP |

X: Permitted. NP: Not permitted.

† See 4.6.3.

‡ Sprinklered throughout by an approved, supervised automatic sprinkler system in accordance with Section 9.7. *(See 21.3.5.)*

**21.1.6.2** Any level below the level of exit discharge shall be separated from the level of exit discharge by not less than Type II(111), Type III(211), or Type V(111) construction *(see 8.2.1)*, unless both of the following criteria are met:

(1) Such levels are under the control of the ambulatory health care facility.
(2) Any hazardous spaces are protected in accordance with Section 8.7.

CHAPTER 20 • New

20.1.6.3 Interior nonbearing walls in buildings of Type I or Type II construction shall be constructed of noncombustible or limited-combustible materials, unless otherwise permitted by 20.1.6.4.

20.1.6.4 Interior nonbearing walls required to have a minimum 2-hour fire resistance rating shall be permitted to be fire-retardant-treated wood enclosed within noncombustible or limited-combustible materials, provided that such walls are not used as shaft enclosures.

20.1.6.5 All buildings with more than one level below the level of exit discharge shall have all such lower levels separated from the level of exit discharge by not less than Type II(111) construction.

20.1.6.6 Where new ambulatory health care occupancies are located in existing buildings, the authority having jurisdiction shall be permitted to accept construction systems of lesser fire resistance than that required by 20.1.6.1 through 20.1.6.5, provided that it can be demonstrated to the authority's satisfaction that prompt evacuation of the facility can be achieved in case of fire or that the exposing occupancies and materials of construction present no threat of fire penetration from such occupancy to the ambulatory health care facility or to the collapse of the structure.

CHAPTER 21 • Existing

21.1.6.3 Interior nonbearing walls in buildings of Type I or Type II construction shall be constructed of noncombustible or limited-combustible materials, unless otherwise permitted by 21.1.6.4.

21.1.6.4 Interior nonbearing walls required to have a minimum 2-hour fire resistance rating shall be permitted to be fire-retardant-treated wood enclosed within noncombustible or limited-combustible materials, provided that such walls are not used as shaft enclosures.

21.1.6.5 All buildings with more than one level below the level of exit discharge shall have all such lower levels separated from the level of exit discharge by not less than Type II(111) construction.

21.1.6.6 In existing buildings, the authority having jurisdiction shall be permitted to accept construction systems of lesser fire resistance than that required by 21.1.6.1 through 21.1.6.5, provided that it can be demonstrated to the authority's satisfaction that prompt evacuation of the facility can be achieved in case of fire or that the exposing occupancies and materials of construction present no threat of fire penetration from such occupancy to the ambulatory health care facility or to the collapse of the structure.

Table 20/21.1.6.1 is applied relative to building construction types. See NFPA 220, *Standard on Types of Building Construction*,[1] and *NFPA 5000®*, *Building Construction and Safety Code®*,[2] for definitions of construction types. Table A.8.2.1.2 summarizes the details associated with Type I through Type V construction.

Table 20/21.1.6.1 establishes building construction type limitations based on the number of "stories in height" as established by 4.6.3. Table 20/21.1.6.1 is applied to ambulatory health care occupancies by starting the story count with the level of exit discharge and ending with the highest story used as an ambulatory health care occupancy. (Note that a building can have only one level of exit discharge, as defined in 3.3.77.1.)

Although NFPA 220, *Standard on Types of Building Construction*, does not set combustibility requirements for nonbearing interior walls and partitions, 20/21.1.6.3 adds requirements that exceed those of NFPA 220. Paragraph 20/21.1.6.3 adds that, in Type I and Type II construction, all nonbearing interior walls and partitions must be constructed of noncombustible or limited-combustible materials. The terms *noncombustible (material)* and *limited-combustible (material)* are defined within NFPA 220, and the definitions are repeated in Chapter 3 of the *Code* for easy reference. See 3.3.160.3 and 3.3.160.2.

Paragraph 20/21.1.6.4 supplements 20/21.1.6.3 in permitting fire-retardant-treated wood to be used within the core of maximum 2-hour fire resistance–rated interior nonbearing walls where the sheathing of such walls is of noncombustible or limited-combustible materials.

Paragraph 20.1.6.6 permits flexibility in the construction requirements that apply to a new ambulatory health care facility that is placed in an existing building. Paragraph 21.1.6.6 provides similar flexibility for existing facilities. Adequate supporting data must be supplied to the authority having jurisdiction (AHJ) to justify a reduction in fire-rated construction.

### 20.1.7 Occupant Load.

See 38.1.7.

### 21.1.7 Occupant Load.

See 39.1.7.

CHAPTER 20 • New

## 20.2 Means of Egress Requirements

### 20.2.1 General.

Every aisle, passageway, corridor, exit discharge, exit location, and access shall be in accordance with Chapter 7, unless otherwise modified by 20.2.2 through 20.2.11.

### 20.2.2 Means of Egress Components.

**20.2.2.1** Components of means of egress shall be limited to the types described in 38.2.2.

**20.2.2.2** Special locking arrangements complying with 7.2.1.6 shall be permitted.

**20.2.2.3** Elevator lobby exit access door locking in accordance with 7.2.1.6.3 shall be permitted.

**20.2.2.4** Any door required to be self-closing shall be permitted to be held open only by an automatic release device that complies with 7.2.1.8.2. The required manual fire alarm system and the systems required by 7.2.1.8.2 shall be arranged to initiate the closing action of all such doors throughout the smoke compartment or throughout the entire facility.

**20.2.2.5** Where doors in a stair enclosure are held open by an automatic release device as permitted in 20.2.2.4, initiation of a door-closing action on any level shall cause all doors at all levels in the stair enclosure to close.

CHAPTER 21 • Existing

## 21.2 Means of Egress Requirements

### 21.2.1 General.

Every aisle, passageway, corridor, exit discharge, exit location, and access shall be in accordance with Chapter 7, unless otherwise modified by 21.2.2 through 21.2.11.

### 21.2.2 Means of Egress Components.

**21.2.2.1** Components of means of egress shall be limited to the types described in 39.2.2.

**21.2.2.2** Special locking arrangements complying with 7.2.1.6 shall be permitted.

**21.2.2.3** Elevator lobby exit access door locking in accordance with 7.2.1.6.3 shall be permitted.

**21.2.2.4** Any door required to be self-closing shall be permitted to be held open only by an automatic release device that complies with 7.2.1.8.2. The required manual fire alarm system and the systems required by 7.2.1.8.2 shall be arranged to initiate the closing action of all such doors throughout the smoke compartment or throughout the entire facility.

**21.2.2.5** Where doors in a stair enclosure are held open by an automatic release device as permitted in 21.2.2.4, initiation of a door-closing action on any level shall cause all doors at all levels in the stair enclosure to close.

The provision of 20/21.2.2.3 is new to the 2009 edition of the *Code*. It permits use of the elevator lobby exit access door-locking provisions of 7.2.1.6.3. Paragraph 7.2.1.6.3 details 15 criteria that must be met as an alternative to the requirements of 7.4.1.6 that each elevator landing or lobby must have access to at least one exit without the use of a key, a tool, special knowledge, or special effort. See 7.4.1.6 and 7.2.1.6.3.

It is desirable to keep doors in exit enclosures, stair enclosures, horizontal exits, smoke barriers, and hazardous areas closed at all times to impede the spread of smoke and gases caused by a fire. However, some doors will be kept open for reasons of operating efficiency or comfort. Where doors in required fire or smoke barriers are to be held open, they must be equipped with automatic devices designed to close the doors by the methods described in 20/21.2.2.4 and 7.2.1.8.2.

The automatic device must cause the doors to close (either throughout the smoke compartment or throughout the facility) by operation of the manual fire alarm system. The doors must also be designed to close by actuation of smoke detectors in the vicinity of the door opening. See 7.2.1.8.2.

It is especially important in facilities providing ambulatory health care to maintain floor-to-floor separation. Doors protecting openings in a stair enclosure can be held open by an automatic device only if arranged to close as specified in the first paragraph of this commentary. Initiation of any action that causes a door to close at one level must cause all doors protecting openings within that stair enclosure to close in accordance with 20/21.2.2.5. Because the doors in the exit stair enclosure are rated fire door assemblies, they will latch when the closing device brings each door to its closed position.

### 20.2.3 Capacity of Means of Egress.

**20.2.3.1** The capacity of any required means of egress shall be determined in accordance with the provisions of 38.2.3.

### 21.2.3 Capacity of Means of Egress.

**21.2.3.1** The capacity of any required means of egress shall be determined in accordance with the provisions of 39.2.3.

CHAPTER 20 • New

**20.2.3.2** The clear width of any corridor or passageway required for exit access shall be not less than 44 in. (1120 mm).

**20.2.3.3** Where minimum corridor width is 6 ft (1830 mm), projections not more than 6 in. (150 mm) from the corridor wall, above the handrail height, shall be permitted for the installation of hand-rub dispensing units in accordance with 20.3.2.6.

**20.2.3.4** Doors in the means of egress from diagnostic or treatment areas, such as x-ray, surgical, or physical therapy, shall provide a clear width of not less than 32 in. (810 mm).

CHAPTER 21 • Existing

**21.2.3.2** The clear width of any corridor or passageway required for exit access shall be not less than 44 in. (1120 mm).

**21.2.3.3** Where minimum corridor width is 6 ft (1830 mm), projections not more than 6 in. (150 mm) from the corridor wall, above the handrail height, shall be permitted for the installation of hand-rub dispensing units in accordance with 21.3.2.6.

**21.2.3.4** Doors in the means of egress from diagnostic or treatment areas, such as x-ray, surgical, or physical therapy, shall provide a clear width of not less than 32 in. (810 mm), unless such doors are existing 34 in. (865 mm) doors.

The capacity of the means of egress in ambulatory health care facilities is determined on the basis of provisions in Chapters 38 and 39 that address business occupancies. Paragraph 38/39.2.3.1 refers to Section 7.3, which requires the capacity of level exit components to be computed on the basis of 0.2 in. (5 mm) per person; stair capacity is computed using 0.3 in. (7.6 mm) per person. These capacities are the same as permitted within sprinklered hospitals, nursing homes, and limited care facilities. Even if the ambulatory health care facility is not sprinklered, these capacity factors are considered adequate, based on the assumption that the majority of occupants will be ambulatory.

Although greater corridor widths might be required for functional purposes, the minimum width for corridors used as common exit access in ambulatory health care facilities is 44 in. (1120 mm), in accordance with 20/21.2.3.2. This width, which is significantly less than that required in new hospitals, nursing homes, and limited care facilities (see 18.2.3.4 and 18.2.3.5), and somewhat less than required in existing hospitals, nursing homes, and limited care facilities (see 19.2.3.4), is specified on the assumption that most occupants will be ambulatory. The minimum 44 in. (1120 mm) corridor width specified by 20/21.2.3.2 is stricter than that of 38/39.2.3.2 for business occupancies in that business occupancies are required to have a minimum 44 in. (1120 mm) corridor width only where such corridor serves an occupant load of 50 or more.

Paragraph 20/21.2.3.3 has been in the *Code* since the 2006 edition. It provides for hand-rub dispensing units, in accordance with 20/21.3.2.6, to project a maximum of 6 in. (150 mm) into corridors, above handrail height [i.e., above 38 in. (965 mm)], provided that such corridors are at least 6 ft (1830 mm) wide. See 20/21.3.2.6. The encroachment is permitted, provided that it does not exceed 6 in. (150 mm), without having to consider the clear width of the corridor as measuring less than its actual width.

In many instances, doors wider than 32 in. (810 mm) clear width will be required for functional purposes. Paragraph 20/21.2.3.4 addresses doors that provide access to common hallways and corridors. The 32 in. (810 mm) minimum clear width, which is significantly less than that required in new hospitals and nursing homes, is specified on the assumption that most occupants will be ambulatory or moving in wheelchairs. A 32 in. (810 mm) clear width door opening is sufficiently wide to accommodate a wheelchair user. Per 21.2.3.4, an existing 34 in. (865 mm) door [i.e., the door leaf width is 34 in. (865 mm)] is considered as providing the required 32 in. (810 mm) opening width, although there is no assurance that the existing door can be opened a full 90 degrees.

CHAPTER 20 • New

### 20.2.4 Number of Exits.

**20.2.4.1** Not less than two exits of the types described in 38.2.2 that are remotely located from each other shall be provided for each floor or fire section of the building.

**20.2.4.2** Any room and any suite of rooms of more than 2500 ft$^2$ (232 m$^2$) shall have not less than two exit access doors remotely located from each other.

CHAPTER 21 • Existing

### 21.2.4 Number of Exits.

**21.2.4.1** Not less than two exits of the types described in 39.2.2 that are remotely located from each other shall be provided for each floor or fire section of the building.

**21.2.4.2** Any room and any suite of rooms of more than 2500 ft$^2$ (232 m$^2$) shall have not less than two exit access doors remotely located from each other.

CHAPTER 20 • New

**20.2.4.3** Not less than two exits of the types described in 38.2.2 shall be accessible from each smoke compartment.

**20.2.4.4** Egress from smoke compartments addressed in 20.2.4.3 shall be permitted through adjacent compartments but shall not require return through the compartment of fire origin.

### 20.2.5 Arrangement of Means of Egress.

See 38.2.5.

### 20.2.6 Travel Distance to Exits.

**20.2.6.1** Travel distance shall be measured in accordance with Section 7.6.

**20.2.6.2** Travel distance shall be as follows:

(1) The travel distance between any room door required as an exit access and an exit shall not exceed 100 ft (30 m).
(2) The travel distance between any point in a room and an exit shall not exceed 150 ft (46 m).
(3) The maximum travel distance in 20.2.6.2(1) or (2) shall be permitted to be increased by 50 ft (15 m) in buildings protected throughout by an approved automatic sprinkler system in accordance with Section 9.7.

CHAPTER 21 • Existing

**21.2.4.3** Not less than two exits of the types described in 39.2.2 shall be accessible from each smoke compartment.

**21.2.4.4** Egress from smoke compartments addressed in 21.2.4.3 shall be permitted through adjacent compartments but shall not require return through the compartment of fire origin.

### 21.2.5 Arrangement of Means of Egress.

See 39.2.5.

### 21.2.6 Travel Distance to Exits.

**21.2.6.1** Travel distance shall be measured in accordance with Section 7.6.

**21.2.6.2** Travel distance shall be as follows:

(1) The travel distance between any room door required as an exit access and an exit shall not exceed 100 ft (30 m).
(2) The travel distance between any point in a room and an exit shall not exceed 150 ft (46 m).
(3) The maximum travel distance in 21.2.6.2(1) or (2) shall be permitted to be increased by 50 ft (15 m) in buildings protected throughout by an approved automatic sprinkler system in accordance with Section 9.7.

Travel distance is measured only to the nearest exit, not to both exits. The requirements of 20/21.2.6.2 are illustrated in Exhibit 20/21.2.

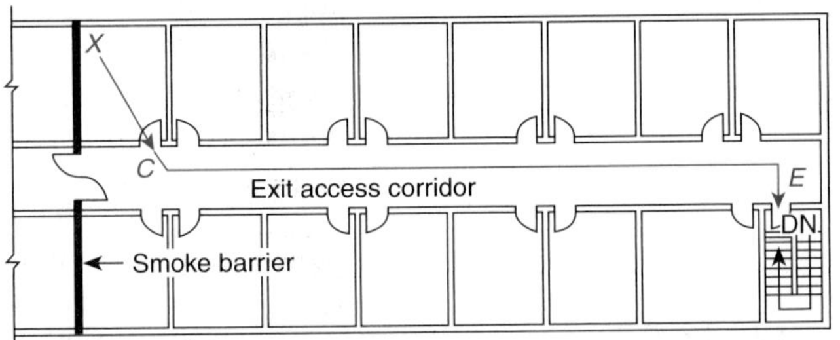


Maximum distance:

C→E — ≤100 ft (≤30 m) [≤150 ft (≤46 m) if building is sprinklered]

X→E — ≤150 ft (≤46 m) [≤200 ft (≤61 m) if building is sprinklered]

***Exhibit 20/21.2*** *Travel distance limitations for an ambulatory health care occupancy.*

### 20.2.7 Discharge from Exits.

See 38.2.7.

### 20.2.8 Illumination of Means of Egress.

Means of egress shall be illuminated in accordance with Section 7.8.

### 21.2.7 Discharge from Exits.

See 39.2.7.

### 21.2.8 Illumination of Means of Egress.

Means of egress shall be illuminated in accordance with Section 7.8.

CHAPTER 20 • New

### 20.2.9 Emergency Lighting and Essential Electrical Systems.

**20.2.9.1** Emergency lighting shall be provided in accordance with Section 7.9.

**20.2.9.2** Where general anesthesia or life-support equipment is used, each ambulatory health care facility shall be provided with an essential electrical system in accordance with NFPA 99, *Standard for Health Care Facilities*, unless otherwise permitted by the following:

(1) Where battery-operated equipment is provided and acceptable to the authority having jurisdiction
(2) Where a facility uses life-support equipment for emergency purposes only

CHAPTER 21 • Existing

### 21.2.9 Emergency Lighting and Essential Electrical Systems.

**21.2.9.1** Emergency lighting shall be provided in accordance with Section 7.9.

**21.2.9.2** Where general anesthesia or life-support equipment is used, each ambulatory health care facility shall be provided with an essential electrical system in accordance with NFPA 99, *Standard for Health Care Facilities*, unless otherwise permitted by the following:

(1) Where battery-operated equipment is provided and acceptable to the authority having jurisdiction
(2) Where a facility uses life-support equipment for emergency purposes only

All ambulatory health care facilities are required to be equipped with emergency lighting. If medical procedures requiring general anesthesia are practiced, or if life-support equipment is used for other than emergency purposes only, ambulatory health care facilities are required to be served by electrical systems meeting the criteria for essential electrical systems, as detailed in NFPA 99, *Standard for Health Care Facilities*.[3]

A facility would not be required to have an emergency generator if the building is a freestanding unit and if, as a normal practice, the following conditions apply:

1. Management maintains policies that preclude the provision of care for any patient who might need to be sustained by electrical life-support equipment, such as respirators or suction apparatus.
2. No surgical treatment requiring general anesthesia is offered.
3. Battery-operated systems or equipment are provided that maintain power to exit lights and illumination for egress corridors, stairways, medical preparation areas, and the like for a minimum of $1\frac{1}{2}$ hours, with battery power required to be supplied to all alarm systems.

### 20.2.10 Marking of Means of Egress.

Means of egress shall have signs in accordance with Section 7.10.

### 20.2.11 Special Means of Egress Features.

**20.2.11.1 Reserved.**

**20.2.11.2 Lockups.** Lockups in ambulatory health care occupancies shall comply with the requirements of 22.4.5.

### 21.2.10 Marking of Means of Egress.

Means of egress shall have signs in accordance with Section 7.10.

### 21.2.11 Special Means of Egress Features.

**21.2.11.1 Reserved.**

**21.2.11.2 Lockups.** Lockups in ambulatory health care occupancies, other than approved existing lockups, shall comply with the requirements of 23.4.5.

## 20.3 Protection

### 20.3.1 Protection of Vertical Openings.

See 38.3.1.

### 20.3.2 Protection from Hazards.

See 38.3.2.

## 21.3 Protection

### 21.3.1 Protection of Vertical Openings.

See 39.3.1.

### 21.3.2 Protection from Hazards.

See 39.3.2.

CHAPTER 20 • New

**20.3.2.1 Doors.** Doors to hazardous areas shall be self-closing or automatic-closing in accordance with 20.2.2.4.

**20.3.2.2 Laboratories.** Laboratories employing quantities of flammable, combustible, or hazardous materials that are considered as a severe hazard shall be protected in accordance with NFPA 99, *Standard for Health Care Facilities*.

**20.3.2.3 Anesthetizing Locations.** Anesthetizing locations shall be protected in accordance with NFPA 99, *Standard for Health Care Facilities*.

**20.3.2.4 Cooking Facilities.** Cooking facilities shall be protected in accordance with 9.2.3, unless otherwise permitted by 20.3.2.5.

**20.3.2.5 Domestic Cooking Equipment.** Where domestic cooking equipment is used for food warming or limited cooking, protection or separation of food preparation facilities shall not be required.

**20.3.2.6* Alcohol-Based Hand-Rub Dispensers.** Alcohol-based hand-rub dispensers shall be protected in accordance with 8.7.3, unless all of the following conditions are met:

(1) Where dispensers are installed in a corridor, the corridor shall have a minimum width of 6 ft (1830 mm).
(2) The maximum individual dispenser fluid capacity shall be as follows:
    (a) 0.32 gal (1.2 L) for dispensers in rooms, corridors, and areas open to corridors
    (b) 0.53 gal (2.0 L) for dispensers in suites of rooms
(3) Dispensers shall be separated from one another by horizontal spacing of not less than 48 in. (1220 mm).
(4) Not more than an aggregate 10 gal (37.8 L) of alcohol-based hand-rub solution shall be in use outside of a storage cabinet in a single smoke compartment.
(5) Storage of quantities greater than 5 gal (18.9 L) in a single smoke compartment shall meet the requirements of NFPA 30, *Flammable and Combustible Liquids Code*.
(6) Dispensers shall not be installed in the following locations:
    (a) Above an ignition source for a horizontal distance of 1 in. (25 mm) to each side of the ignition source
    (b) To the side of an ignition source within a 1 in. (25 mm) horizontal distance from the ignition source
    (c) Beneath an ignition source within a 1 in. (25 mm) vertical distance from the ignition source
(7) Dispensers installed directly over carpeted floors shall be permitted only in sprinklered smoke compartments.

CHAPTER 21 • Existing

**21.3.2.1 Doors.** Doors to hazardous areas shall be self-closing or automatic-closing in accordance with 21.2.2.4.

**21.3.2.2 Laboratories.** Laboratories employing quantities of flammable, combustible, or hazardous materials that are considered as a severe hazard shall be protected in accordance with NFPA 99, *Standard for Health Care Facilities*.

**21.3.2.3 Anesthetizing Locations.** Anesthetizing locations shall be protected in accordance with NFPA 99, *Standard for Health Care Facilities*.

**21.3.2.4 Cooking Facilities.** Cooking facilities shall be protected in accordance with 9.2.3, unless otherwise permitted by 21.3.2.5.

**21.3.2.5 Domestic Cooking Equipment.** Where domestic cooking equipment is used for food warming or limited cooking, protection or separation of food preparation facilities shall not be required.

**21.3.2.6* Alcohol-Based Hand-Rub Dispensers.** Alcohol-based hand-rub dispensers shall be protected in accordance with 8.7.3, unless all of the following conditions are met:

(1) Where dispensers are installed in a corridor, the corridor shall have a minimum width of 6 ft (1830 mm).
(2) The maximum individual dispenser fluid capacity shall be as follows:
    (a) 0.32 gal (1.2 L) for dispensers in rooms, corridors, and areas open to corridors
    (b) 0.53 gal (2.0 L) for dispensers in suites of rooms
(3) Dispensers shall be separated from one another by horizontal spacing of not less than 48 in. (1220 mm).
(4) Not more than an aggregate 10 gal (37.8 L) of alcohol-based hand-rub solution shall be in use outside of a storage cabinet in a single smoke compartment.
(5) Storage of quantities greater then 5 gal (18.9 L) in a single smoke compartment shall meet the requirements of NFPA 30, *Flammable and Combustible Liquids Code*.
(6) Dispensers shall not be installed in the following locations:
    (a) Above an ignition source for a horizontal distance of 1 in. (25 mm) to each side of the ignition source
    (b) To the side of an ignition source within a 1 in. (25 mm) horizontal distance from the ignition source
    (c) Beneath an ignition source within a 1 in. (25 mm) vertical distance from the ignition source
(7) Dispensers installed directly over carpeted floors shall be permitted only in sprinklered smoke compartments.

Laboratories that contain ordinary combustibles and flammable liquids in sufficient quantity to threaten a 1-hour fire separation [e.g., wood-equivalent fuel loads in the range of 5 lb/ft$^2$ to 10 lb/ft$^2$ (25 kg/m$^2$ to 50 kg/m$^2$)] are considered to be a severe hazard. Laboratories representing a severe hazard must be protected in accordance with NFPA 99, *Standard for Health Care Facilities.* Protection would include 1-hour fire resistance separation and automatic sprinkler protection.

Where fuel loads of lesser amounts are involved and quantities of flammable liquids are limited, laboratories would simply be considered hazardous contents areas and would require either 1-hour separation or automatic sprinkler protection. See 38/39.3.2.

The provisions of 20/21.3.2.6 have been in the *Code* since the 2006 edition. Prior to the inclusion of the provisions for alcohol-based hand-rub dispensers, the only option available was to treat the alcohol solutions as flammable liquids subject to the provisions of 8.7.3, which meant the dispensers were prohibited from being placed in patient areas, especially in corridors. The provisions of 20/21.3.2.6 permit limited use of such dispensers in corridors, rooms, and suites. Dispensers not meeting all the criteria of 20/21.3.2.6(1) through (7) are subject to regulation as flammable liquids in accordance with 8.7.3. Note that, in addition to the criteria of 20/21.3.2.6(1) through (7), the alcohol-based hand-rub dispensers are limited to encroaching not more than 6 in. (150 mm) into the minimum 6 ft (1830 mm) width corridor, and such encroachment must be above handrail height [i.e., above 38 in. (965 mm)] in accordance with 20/21.2.3.3.

The provision of 20/21.3.2.6(6) is new to the 2009 edition of the *Code* and replaces a requirement that prohibited the dispenser from being positioned over or directly adjacent to an ignition source, as such language was too subjective to be enforced consistently. Exhibit 20/21.3 illustrates the area, above and to the side of an ignition source, from which alcohol-based hand-rub dispensers are prohibited from being located.

The provisions for alcohol-based hand-rub dispensers for health care occupancies were expanded for the 2009 edition of the *Code* to permit aerosol-based dispensers, as the original provisions added to the 2006 edition addressed only liquid/gel dispensers [see 18/19.3.2.6(3) and (5)]. The change for Chapter 18/19 was proposed during the first phase [i.e., the Report on Proposals (ROP) phase] of the revision process that produced the 2009 edition but was rejected due to lack

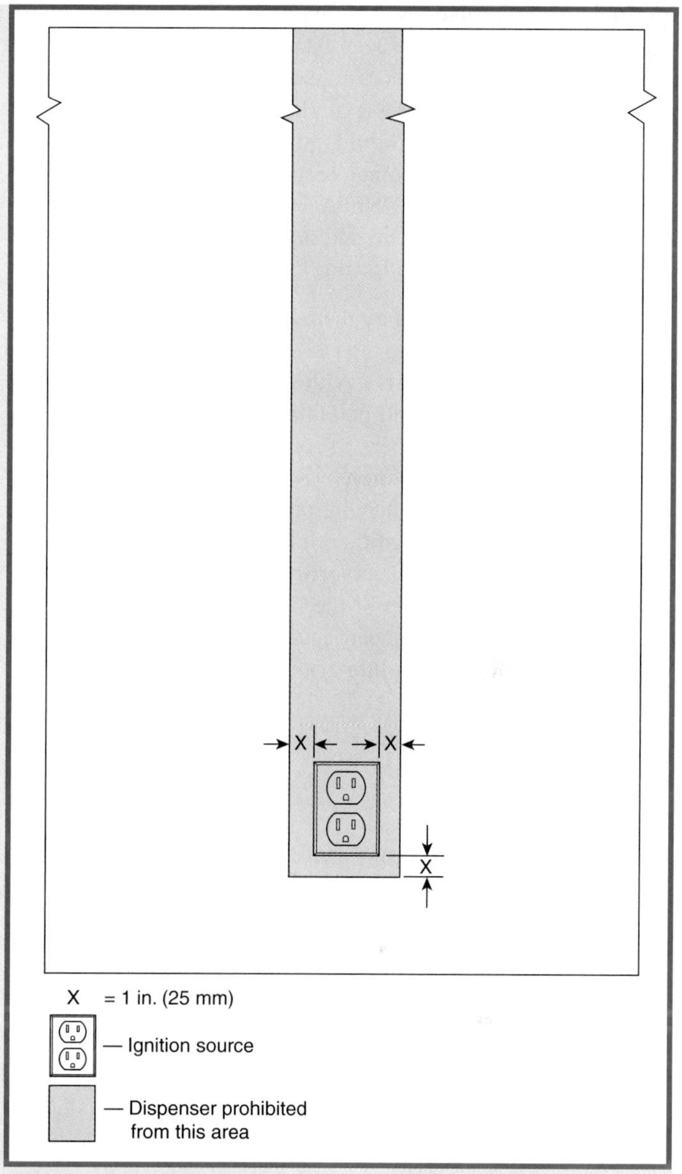


***Exhibit 20/21.3*** *Prohibited location for alcohol-based hand-rub dispenser with respect to an ignition source.*

of technical substantiation. In response to a public comment that included the report addressed in the commentary following A.18/A.19.3.2.6(4), the technical committee accepted the change during the second phase [i.e., the Report on Comments (ROC) phase] of the revision process. The technical committee was not permitted to process a similar change to permit aerosol-based dispensers in Chapter 20/21 for ambulatory health care occupancies, despite its desire to do so during the ROC phase, because the subject had not been raised during the ROP phase.

CHAPTER 20 • New

**A.20.3.2.6** Extensive research, including fire modeling, has indicated that alcohol-based hand-rub solutions can be safely installed in corridors of health care facilities, provided that certain other precautions are taken. The total quantities of flammable liquids in any area should comply with the provisions of other recognized codes, including NFPA 1, *Fire Code*, and NFPA 30, *Flammable and Combustible Liquids Code*. In addition, special consideration should be given to the following:

(1) Obstructions created by the installation of hand-rub solution dispensers
(2) Location of dispensers with regard to adjacent combustible materials and potential sources of ignition, especially where dispensers are mounted on walls of combustible construction
(3) Requirements for other fire protection features, including complete automatic sprinkler protection, to be installed throughout the compartment
(4) Amount and location of the flammable solutions, both in use and in storage, particularly with respect to potential for leakage or failure of the dispenser

### 20.3.3 Interior Finish.

See 38.3.3.

### 20.3.4 Detection, Alarm, and Communications Systems.

**20.3.4.1 General.** Ambulatory health care facilities shall be provided with fire alarm systems in accordance with Section 9.6, except as modified by 20.3.4.2 through 20.3.4.4.

**20.3.4.2 Initiation.** Initiation of the required fire alarm systems shall be by manual means in accordance with 9.6.2 and by means of any detection devices or detection systems required.

**20.3.4.3 Notification.** Positive alarm sequence in accordance with 9.6.3.4 shall be permitted.

**20.3.4.3.1 Occupant Notification.** Occupant notification shall be accomplished automatically, without delay, in accordance with 9.6.3 upon operation of any fire alarm activating device.

**20.3.4.3.2 Emergency Forces Notification.**

**20.3.4.3.2.1** Fire department notification shall be accomplished in accordance with 9.6.4.

**20.3.4.3.2.2 Reserved.**

CHAPTER 21 • Existing

**A.21.3.2.6** Extensive research, including fire modeling, has indicated that alcohol-based hand-rub solutions can be safely installed in corridors of health care facilities, provided that certain other precautions are taken. The total quantities of flammable liquids in any area should comply with the provisions of other recognized codes, including NFPA 1, *Fire Code*, and NFPA 30, *Flammable and Combustible Liquids Code*. In addition, special consideration should be given to the following:

(1) Obstructions created by the installation of hand-rub solution dispensers
(2) Location of dispensers with regard to adjacent combustible materials and potential sources of ignition, especially where dispensers are mounted on walls of combustible construction
(3) Requirements for other fire protection features, including complete automatic sprinkler protection, to be installed throughout the compartment
(4) Amount and location of the flammable solutions, both in use and in storage, particularly with respect to potential for leakage or failure of the dispenser

### 21.3.3 Interior Finish.

See 39.3.3.

### 21.3.4 Detection, Alarm, and Communications Systems.

**21.3.4.1 General.** Ambulatory health care facilities shall be provided with fire alarm systems in accordance with Section 9.6, except as modified by 21.3.4.2 through 21.3.4.4.

**21.3.4.2 Initiation.** Initiation of the required fire alarm systems shall be by manual means in accordance with 9.6.2 and by means of any detection devices or detection systems required.

**21.3.4.3 Notification.** Positive alarm sequence in accordance with 9.6.3.4 shall be permitted.

**21.3.4.3.1 Occupant Notification.** Occupant notification shall be accomplished automatically, without delay, in accordance with 9.6.3 upon operation of any fire alarm activating device.

**21.3.4.3.2 Emergency Forces Notification.**

**21.3.4.3.2.1** Fire department notification shall be accomplished in accordance with 9.6.4.

**21.3.4.3.2.2** Smoke detection devices or smoke detection systems equipped with reconfirmation features shall not be required to automatically notify the fire department, unless the alarm condition is reconfirmed after a period not exceeding 120 seconds.

**20.3.4.4 Fire Safety Functions.** Operation of any activating device in the required fire alarm system shall be arranged to accomplish automatically, without delay, any control functions required to be performed by that device. *(See 9.6.5.)*

**21.3.4.4 Fire Safety Functions.** Operation of any activating device in the required fire alarm system shall be arranged to accomplish automatically, without delay, any control functions required to be performed by that device. *(See 9.6.5.)*

Paragraphs 20/21.3.4.1 through 20/21.3.4.4 address required fire alarm equipment. Reliability is of prime importance; therefore, electrical supervision of the system and system components is specified via the reference to Section 9.6. In the event of circuit fault, component failure, or other trouble, a continuous trouble indication signal is required and should be provided at a constantly attended location.

Paragraphs 20/21.3.4.1 and 20/21.3.4.2 require a manual fire alarm system. Manual fire alarm boxes should be located along the natural routes of egress and cover all portions of the building. They should be located so that those qualified to send an alarm can summon aid without having to leave their zone of ordinary activities or pass beyond the view and hearing of people immediately exposed to, or in direct view of, a fire. The operation of a manual fire alarm box should automatically summon attendants to assist in moving occupants.

Actuation of any required fire or smoke detector, activation of a required sprinkler system, or operation of a manual fire alarm box must automatically, without delay, initiate the alarm system and sound audible alarm devices within the building. Presignal systems are not permitted (see 9.6.3.3); positive alarm sequence is permitted (see 9.6.3.4).

The criteria for positive alarm sequence are detailed in *NFPA 72*®, *National Fire Alarm Code*®,[4] and include the following:

1. The signal from an automatic fire detection device selected for positive alarm sequence operation must be acknowledged at the control unit by trained personnel within 15 seconds of annunciation in order to initiate the alarm investigation phase.
2. If the signal is not acknowledged within 15 seconds, notification signals in accordance with the building evacuation or relocation plan and remote signals must be automatically and immediately activated (i.e., immediate occupant notification and emergency forces notification must occur).
3. Trained personnel have up to 180 seconds during the alarm investigation phase to evaluate the fire condition and reset the system.
4. If the system is not reset during the investigation phase, notification signals in accordance with the building evacuation or relocation plan and remote signals must be automatically and immediately activated (i.e., immediate occupant notification and emergency forces notification must occur).
5. If a second automatic fire detector selected for positive alarm sequence is actuated during the alarm investigation phase, notification signals in accordance with the building evacuation or relocation plan and remote signals must be automatically and immediately activated (i.e., immediate occupant notification and emergency forces notification must occur).
6. If any other initiating device is actuated (e.g., a manual fire alarm box), notification signals in accordance with the building evacuation or relocation plan and remote signals must be automatically and immediately activated (i.e., immediate occupant notification and emergency forces notification must occur).

The alarm must automatically transmit to a point outside the facility. If automatic transmission of the alarm to the fire department legally committed to serve the facility is not permitted, arrangements need to be made for the prompt notification of the fire department or such other assistance as is available in the case of fire or other emergency. Paragraph 9.6.4.2 lists various methods acceptable for automatically notifying the fire department. The fire department should also be called manually to verify and confirm the automatic transmission of the alarm. In larger facilities, this might be the responsibility of the facility telephone operator. In smaller facilities, it might be the responsibility of the medical staff. Actuation of the fire alarm must initiate the operation of audible alerting devices that sound throughout the affected zone or building.

CHAPTER 20 • New

### 20.3.5 Extinguishment Requirements.

See 38.3.5.

**20.3.5.1** Isolated hazardous areas shall be permitted to be protected in accordance with 9.7.1.2.

**20.3.5.2** Where more than two sprinklers are installed in a single area for protection in accordance with 9.7.1.2, waterflow detection shall be provided to sound the building fire alarm or to notify, by a signal, any constantly attended location, such as PBX, security, or emergency room, at which the necessary corrective action shall be taken.

**20.3.5.3** Portable fire extinguishers shall be provided in ambulatory health care facilities in accordance with 9.7.4.1.

### 20.3.6 Corridors.

**20.3.6.1 General.** See 38.3.6.

**20.3.6.2 Openings.**

**20.3.6.2.1** Miscellaneous openings, such as mail slots, pharmacy pass-through windows, laboratory pass-through windows, and cashier pass-through windows, shall be permitted to be installed in vision panels or doors without special protection, provided that both of the following criteria are met:

(1) The aggregate area of openings per room does not exceed 20 in.$^2$ (0.015 m$^2$).
(2) The openings are installed at or below half the distance from the floor to the room ceiling.

**20.3.6.2.2** For rooms protected throughout by an approved, supervised automatic sprinkler system in accordance with Section 9.7, the aggregate area of openings per room shall not exceed 80 in.$^2$ (0.05 m$^2$).

### 20.3.7 Subdivision of Building Space.

**20.3.7.1** Ambulatory health care facilities shall be separated from other tenants and occupancies and shall meet the following requirements:

(1) Walls shall have not less than a 1-hour fire resistance rating and shall extend from the floor slab below to the floor or roof slab above.
(2) Doors shall be constructed of not less than 1$^3/_4$ in. (44 mm) thick, solid-bonded wood core or the equivalent and shall be equipped with positive latches.
(3) Doors shall be self-closing and shall be kept in the closed position, except when in use.
(4) Any windows in the barriers shall be of fixed fire window assemblies in accordance with Section 8.3.

CHAPTER 21 • Existing

### 21.3.5 Extinguishment Requirements.

See 39.3.5.

**21.3.5.1** Isolated hazardous areas shall be permitted to be protected in accordance with 9.7.1.2.

**21.3.5.2** For new installations in existing ambulatory health care facilities, where more than two sprinklers are installed in a single area for protection in accordance with 9.7.1.2, waterflow detection shall be provided to sound the building fire alarm or to notify, by a signal, any constantly attended location, such as PBX, security, or emergency room, at which the necessary corrective action shall be taken.

**21.3.5.3** Portable fire extinguishers shall be provided in ambulatory health care facilities in accordance with 9.7.4.1.

### 21.3.6 Corridors.

(No requirements.)

### 21.3.7 Subdivision of Building Space.

**21.3.7.1** Ambulatory health care facilities shall be separated from other tenants and occupancies and shall meet the following requirements:

(1) Walls shall have not less than a 1-hour fire resistance rating and shall extend from the floor slab below to the floor or roof slab above.
(2) Doors shall be constructed of not less than 1$^3/_4$ in. (44 mm) thick, solid-bonded wood core or the equivalent and shall be equipped with positive latches.
(3) Doors shall be self-closing and shall be kept in the closed position, except when in use.
(4) Any windows in the barriers shall be of fixed fire window assemblies in accordance with Section 8.3.

CHAPTER 20 • New

**20.3.7.2** Every story of an ambulatory health care facility shall be divided into not less than two smoke compartments, unless otherwise permitted by the following:

(1) This requirement shall not apply to facilities of less than 5000 $ft^2$ (465 $m^2$) that are protected by an approved automatic smoke detection system.
(2) This requirement shall not apply to facilities of less than 10,000 $ft^2$ (929 $m^2$) that are protected throughout by an approved, supervised automatic sprinkler system installed in accordance with Section 9.7.
(3) An area in an adjoining occupancy shall be permitted to serve as a smoke compartment for an ambulatory health care facility if the following criteria are met:

   (a) The separating wall and both compartments meet the requirements of 20.3.7.
   (b) The ambulatory health care facility is less than 22,500 $ft^2$ (2100 $m^2$).
   (c) Access from the ambulatory health care facility to the other occupancy is unrestricted.

**20.3.7.3** Smoke compartments shall not exceed an area of 22,500 $ft^2$ (2100 $m^2$), and the travel distance from any point to reach a door in a smoke barrier shall not exceed 200 ft (61 m).

**20.3.7.4** The area of an atrium separated in accordance with 8.6.7 shall not be limited in size.

**20.3.7.5** Required smoke barriers shall be constructed in accordance with Section 8.5 and shall have a minimum 1-hour fire resistance rating, unless otherwise permitted by 20.3.7.6.

**20.3.7.6** Smoke dampers shall not be required in duct penetrations of smoke barriers in fully ducted heating, ventilating, and air-conditioning systems for buildings protected throughout by an approved, supervised automatic sprinkler system in accordance with Section 9.7.

**20.3.7.7** Windows in the smoke barrier shall be of fixed fire window assemblies in accordance with Section 8.3.

**20.3.7.8** Not less than 15 net $ft^2$ (1.4 net $m^2$) per ambulatory health care facility occupant shall be provided within the aggregate area of corridors, patient rooms, treatment rooms, lounges, and other low hazard areas on each side of the smoke compartment for the total number of occupants in adjoining compartments.

**20.3.7.9*** Doors in smoke barriers shall be not less than $1^3/_4$ in. (44 mm) thick, solid-bonded wood core or the equivalent and shall be self-closing or automatic-closing in accordance with 20.2.2.4.

CHAPTER 21 • Existing

**21.3.7.2** Every story of an ambulatory health care facility shall be divided into not less than two smoke compartments, unless otherwise permitted by the following:

(1) This requirement shall not apply to facilities of less than 5000 $ft^2$ (465 $m^2$) that are protected by an approved automatic smoke detection system.
(2) This requirement shall not apply to facilities of less than 10,000 $ft^2$ (929 $m^2$) that are protected throughout by an approved, supervised automatic sprinkler system installed in accordance with Section 9.7.
(3) An area in an adjoining occupancy shall be permitted to serve as a smoke compartment for an ambulatory health care facility if the following criteria are met:

   (a) The separating wall and both compartments meet the requirements of 21.3.7.
   (b) The ambulatory health care facility is less than 22,500 $ft^2$ (2100 $m^2$).
   (c) Access from the ambulatory health care facility to the other occupancy is unrestricted.

**21.3.7.3 Reserved.**

**21.3.7.4 Reserved.**

**21.3.7.5** Required smoke barriers shall be constructed in accordance with Section 8.5 and shall have a minimum 1-hour fire resistance rating, unless otherwise permitted by 21.3.7.6.

**21.3.7.6** Smoke dampers shall not be required in duct penetrations of smoke barriers in fully ducted heating, ventilating, and air-conditioning systems for buildings protected throughout by an approved, supervised automatic sprinkler system in accordance with Section 9.7.

**21.3.7.7** Windows in the smoke barrier shall be of fixed fire window assemblies in accordance with Section 8.3.

**21.3.7.8 Reserved.**

**21.3.7.9*** Doors in smoke barriers shall be not less than $1^3/_4$ in. (44 mm) thick, solid-bonded wood core or the equivalent and shall be self-closing or automatic-closing in accordance with 21.2.2.4.

CHAPTER 20 • New

**A.20.3.7.9** Smoke barriers might include walls having door openings other than cross-corridor doors. There is no restriction in the *Code* regarding which doors or how many doors form part of a smoke barrier. For example, doors from the corridor to individual rooms are permitted to form part of a smoke barrier.

**20.3.7.10** Positive latching hardware shall not be required on smoke barrier cross-corridor doors.

**20.3.7.11** A vision panel consisting of fire-rated glazing or wired glass panels in approved frames shall be provided in each cross-corridor swinging door and at each cross-corridor horizontal-sliding door in a smoke barrier.

**20.3.7.12** Vision panels in doors in smoke barriers, if provided, shall be of fire-rated glazing or wired glass in approved frames.

**20.3.7.13*** Rabbets, bevels, or astragals shall be required at the meeting edges, and stops shall be required at the head and sides of door frames in smoke barriers.

**A.20.3.7.13** Split astragals (i.e., astragals installed on both door leaves) are also considered astragals.

**20.3.7.14** Center mullions shall be prohibited in smoke barrier door openings.

CHAPTER 21 • Existing

**A.21.3.7.9** Smoke barriers might include walls having door openings other than cross-corridor doors. There is no restriction in the *Code* regarding which doors or how many doors form part of a smoke barrier. For example, doors from the corridor to individual rooms are permitted to form part of a smoke barrier.

**21.3.7.10** Positive latching hardware shall not be required on smoke barrier cross-corridor doors.

Ambulatory health care facilities are frequently located within buildings used for a variety of purposes. Placing these facilities within buildings containing hazardous occupancies should be avoided. If located within a multiple-use building, the ambulatory health care facility must be separated from adjacent tenants and occupancies by minimum 1-hour fire resistance–rated partitions in accordance with 20/21.3.7.1. Doors protecting openings in such partitions must be of at least $1^3/_4$ in. (44 mm) thick, solid-bonded wood core or of equivalent construction; that is, a door that will resist fire for a minimum of 20 minutes. The doors must be equipped with positive latching hardware of a type that cannot be held in the retracted position. Roller latches are not a form of positive latching and, therefore, are not permitted. The doors must be self-closing and normally maintained in the closed position, or, if the doors are to be held open, an automatic device must be used as specified in 20/21.2.2.4.

Glazing within doors and partitions will generally involve a maximum area of 1296 in.$^2$ (0.84 m$^2$) of wired glass, set in approved metal frames. Each wired glass panel should be limited to a maximum dimension of 54 in. (1370 mm). The glass should be labeled, be $^1/_4$ in. (6 mm) thick, and be well embedded in putty, with all exposed joints between the metal and the glass struck and pointed (see NFPA 80, *Standard for Fire Doors and Other Opening Protectives*[5]). A number of wired glass panels are permitted to be used in a single partition, provided that each 1296 in.$^2$ (0.84 m$^2$) section is separated from adjacent panels by a metal mullion. The excessive use of wired glass panels should be avoided. The use of wired glass panels in a partition reduces the effectiveness of the partition, because radiant energy transfer readily occurs through the glass panel. Other fire-rated glazing is available and, where used, should be installed in accordance with the manufacturer's instructions and listing.

Partitions separating ambulatory health care facilities from other occupancies must extend from the floor to the floor or roof deck above, extending completely through concealed spaces above suspended ceilings, for example. The partition must form a continuous barrier. Openings around penetrations involving building services should be adequately protected to maintain the 1-hour separation. Special attention should be paid to penetrations involving air-handling ducts. In general, steel ducts will not require a fire damper. Penetrations involving nonmetallic ducts or aluminum ducts should be carefully evaluated. Fire dampers should be provided to protect duct penetrations where the projected fire exposure is judged sufficient to jeopardize the required separation because of the duct penetration. The possible movement of air from space to space under conditions of system operation and conditions of system shutdown should be evaluated for both conditions. If there is a significant potential for the transfer of smoke from an adjacent space to the ambulatory health care facility, or from the ambulatory health care facility to a corridor, fire dampers should be provided for duct penetrations, even though the *Code* does not specifically require such protection. See Exhibit 20/21.4.

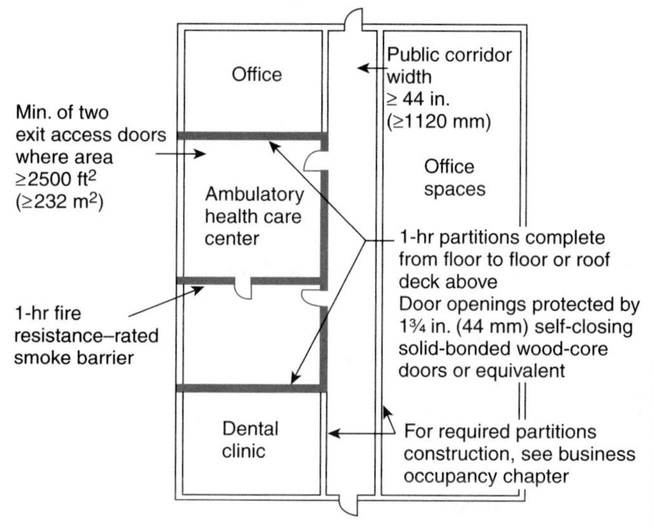


***Exhibit 20/21.4*** *Separation and subdivision requirements for an ambulatory health care facility.*

The requirements of 20.3.7.2 through 20.3.7.14 and 21.3.7.2 through 21.3.7.10 for subdividing building spaces through the use of smoke barriers are illustrated in Exhibit 20/21.4 and Exhibit 20/21.5. Smoke barriers are not required if the ambulatory health care center meets either of the following conditions:

1. Its area is less than 5000 ft² (465 m²), and it is protected by an automatic smoke detection system.
2. Its area is less than 10,000 ft² (929 m²), and it is protected by an automatic sprinkler system.

Further, 20/21.3.7.2(3) permits the smoke barrier to be located — under specific criteria — at the wall that separates the ambulatory health care center from a neighboring tenant space of some other occupancy

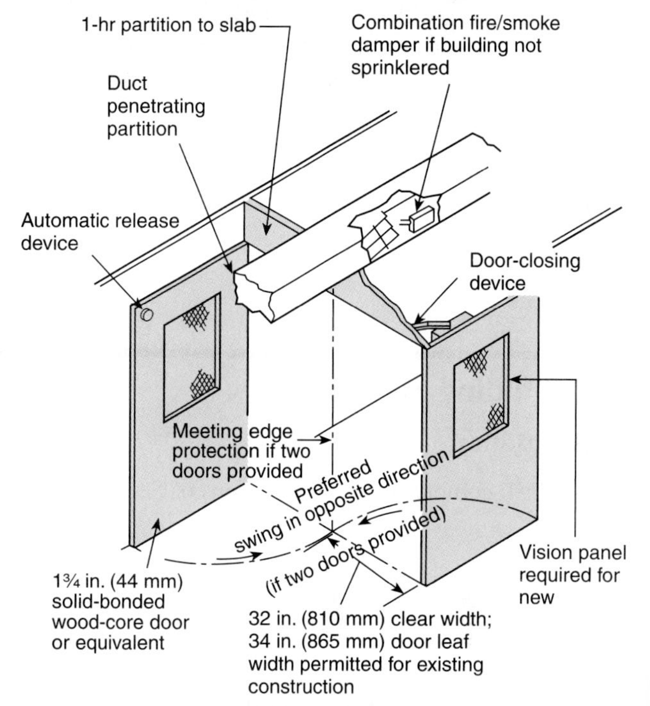


***Exhibit 20/21.5*** *Smoke barrier and associated openings protection for an ambulatory health care facility.*

classification. In other words, if the smoky condition is located within the ambulatory health care occupancy, patients can be moved to a safe smoke compartment in the neighboring space for which access is unrestricted.

During a fire, the emergency evacuation of patients in an ambulatory health care facility can be an inefficient, time-consuming process. Realistically, if nonambulatory patients must be moved, any number of occupants can be relocated, but only readily relocated through horizontal travel. Smoke barriers used to subdivide a building serve the following three purposes fundamental to the protection of patients:

1. They limit the spread of fire and fire-produced contaminants.
2. They limit the number of occupants exposed to a single fire.
3. They provide for horizontal relocation of patients by creating an area of refuge on the same floor level.

The provisions of 21.3.7 for existing smoke barrier cross-corridor doors were revised for the 2009 edition of the *Code* to delete the requirement for a vision panel. The requirement had been added to the 2003 edition without technical substantiation for such a retroactive change, which had the unintended effect of rendering formerly compliant door arrangements noncompliant. The deletion of the requirement for a vision panel re-

## 20.4 Special Provisions

See Section 38.4.

## 20.5 Building Services

### 20.5.1 Utilities.

Utilities shall comply with the provisions of Section 9.1.

### 20.5.2 Heating, Ventilating, and Air-Conditioning.

**20.5.2.1** Heating, ventilating, and air-conditioning shall comply with the provisions of Section 9.2 and shall be installed in accordance with the manufacturer's specifications, unless otherwise modified by 20.5.2.2.

**20.5.2.2** If fuel-fired, heating devices shall comply with the following:

(1) They shall be chimney connected or vent connected.
(2) They shall take air for combustion directly from the outside.
(3) They shall be designed and installed to provide for complete separation of the combustion system from the atmosphere of the occupied area.

**20.5.2.2.1** Any heating device shall have safety features to immediately stop the flow of fuel and shut down the equipment in case of either excessive temperature or ignition failure.

**20.5.2.2.2** Approved, suspended unit heaters shall be permitted in locations other than means of egress and patient treatment areas, provided that both of the following criteria are met:

(1) Such heaters are located high enough to be out of the reach of persons using the area.
(2) Such heaters are equipped with the safety features required by 20.5.2.2.1.



turns the *Code* text to that of the 1981 edition — the first to address ambulatory health care occupancies.

## 21.4 Special Provisions

See Section 39.4.

## 21.5 Building Services

### 21.5.1 Utilities.

**21.5.1.1** Utilities shall comply with the provisions of Section 9.1.

**21.5.1.2** Existing installations shall be permitted to be continued in service, provided that the systems do not present a serious hazard to life.

### 21.5.2 Heating, Ventilating, and Air-Conditioning.

**21.5.2.1** Heating, ventilating, and air-conditioning shall comply with the provisions of Section 9.2 and shall be in accordance with the manufacturer's specifications, unless otherwise modified by 21.5.2.2.

**21.5.2.2** If fuel-fired, heating devices shall comply with the following:

(1) They shall be chimney connected or vent connected.
(2) They shall take air for combustion directly from the outside.
(3) They shall be designed and installed to provide for complete separation of the combustion system from the atmosphere of the occupied area.

**21.5.2.2.1** Any heating device shall have safety features to immediately stop the flow of fuel and shut down the equipment in case of either excessive temperature or ignition failure.

**21.5.2.2.2** Approved, suspended unit heaters shall be permitted in locations other than means of egress and patient treatment areas, provided that both of the following criteria are met:

(1) Such heaters are located high enough to be out of the reach of persons using the area.
(2) Such heaters are equipped with the safety features required by 21.5.2.2.1.

CHAPTER 20 • New

### 20.5.3 Elevators, Escalators, and Conveyors.

Elevators, escalators, and conveyors shall comply with the provisions of Section 9.4.

### 20.5.4 Rubbish Chutes, Incinerators, and Laundry Chutes.

Rubbish chutes, incinerators, and laundry chutes shall comply with the provisions of Section 9.5.

CHAPTER 21 • Existing

### 21.5.3 Elevators, Escalators, and Conveyors.

Elevators, escalators, and conveyors shall comply with the provisions of Section 9.4.

### 21.5.4 Rubbish Chutes, Incinerators, and Laundry Chutes.

Rubbish chutes, incinerators, and laundry chutes shall comply with the provisions of Section 9.5.

Paragraphs 20/21.5.2.1 and 20/21.5.2.2 specify safeguards for air-conditioning, ventilating, heating, and other service equipment in order to minimize the possibility of such devices serving as a source of ignition. Fuel-fired heating devices, except central heating systems, must be designed to provide complete separation of the combustion system from the occupied spaces. Air for combustion must be taken directly from the outside.

A major concern is preventing the ignition of clothing, bedclothes, furniture, and other furnishings by a heating device. Therefore, 20/21.7.8 prohibits portable heating devices in areas used by patients.

Paragraph 20/21.5.3 requires elevators to comply with Section 9.4, which mandates the Fire Fighters' Emergency Operations features required in ASME A17.1/CSA B44, *Safety Code for Elevators and Escalators*,[6] for new elevator installations, and ASME A17.3, *Safety Code for Existing Elevators and Escalators*,[7] for existing elevator installations. Phase 1 of the fire fighter's emergency operations requires elevators to be recalled to a designated floor (e.g., the main entrance level lobby or, alternately, to some other floor if smoke is detected in the main entrance level lobby) upon detection of smoke in the elevator machine room, the elevator hoistway, or the elevator lobbies on each floor the elevators serve. Phase 1 recall helps to ensure that the elevators are called out of service, so as not to be misused by building occupants once smoke has reached an elevator lobby and its associated elevator shaft doors, or when smoke is present in the elevator machine room or hoistway. Phase 1 also provides for the elevators to be waiting at the designated floor for emergency service personnel use upon their arrival.

The ASME A17.1 and A17.3 codes prohibit elevators from being recalled by other than smoke detection in the elevator machine room, the hoistway, or the elevator lobbies. Therefore, the elevator should not be recalled upon initiation of the building fire alarm system. This is consistent with the provision of 9.6.3.2.1 of this *Code,* which does not require the elevator recall smoke detectors to activate the building evacuation alarm, provided that the smoke detectors initiate a supervisory signal at a constantly attended location. Therefore, elevators will remain in service in parts of the building not affected by the fire and might constitute a valuable, supplemental means for evacuating patients from health care occupancies. In some cases, using an elevator might be the only feasible way to move patients who are unable to use the exit stairs.

Elevators, however, have many inherent weaknesses that tend to limit reliability. Elevator access doors are designed with operating tolerances that allow smoke transfer into the shaft. During a fire, a power failure might cause an elevator to stop between floors, trapping its passengers.

Many of these elevator weaknesses can be minimized by providing emergency power, separating the elevator lobby from other building spaces using rated construction, providing an emergency smoke control system, and pressurizing the elevator shaft and adjacent lobbies. These countermeasures represent good fire protection judgment but are not requirements of this *Code.*

Through emergency planning and staff training, the potential problem of crowded elevators might be avoided. Emergency plans can make effective use of elevators by transferring patients through a horizontal exit, for example, to a separate fire area. Within the separate fire area, a staged evacuation program could be instituted, with the elevators taking patients to the ground level, allowing horizontal movement to the outside.

## 20.6 Reserved

## 21.6 Reserved

CHAPTER 20 • New

## 20.7* Operating Features

**A.20.7** Health care occupants have, in large part, varied degrees of physical disability, and their removal to the outside, or even their disturbance caused by moving, is inexpedient or impractical in many cases, except as a last resort. Similarly, recognizing that there might be an operating necessity for the restraint of the mentally ill, often by use of barred windows and locked doors, fire exit drills are usually extremely disturbing, detrimental, and frequently impracticable.

In most cases, fire exit drills, as ordinarily practiced in other occupancies, cannot be conducted in health care occupancies. Fundamentally, superior construction, early discovery and extinguishment of incipient fires, and prompt notification need to be relied on to reduce the occasion for evacuation of buildings of this class to a minimum.

### 20.7.1 Evacuation and Relocation Plan and Fire Drills.

**20.7.1.1** The administration of every ambulatory health care facility shall have, in effect and available to all supervisory personnel, written copies of a plan for the protection of all persons in the event of fire, for their evacuation to areas of refuge, and for their evacuation from the building when necessary.

**20.7.1.2** All employees shall be periodically instructed and kept informed with respect to their duties under the plan required by 20.7.1.1.

**20.7.1.3** A copy of the plan required by 20.7.1.1 shall be readily available at all times in the telephone operator's location or at the security center.

**20.7.1.4*** Fire drills in ambulatory health care facilities shall include the transmission of a fire alarm signal and simulation of emergency fire conditions.

**A.20.7.1.4** Many health care occupancies conduct fire drills without disturbing patients by choosing the location of the simulated emergency in advance and by closing the doors to patients' rooms or wards in the vicinity prior to the initiation of the drill. The purpose of a fire drill is to test and evaluate the efficiency, knowledge, and response of institutional personnel in implementing the facility fire emergency plan. Its purpose is not to disturb or excite patients. Fire drills should be scheduled on a random basis to ensure that personnel in health care facilities are drilled not less than once in each 3-month period.

Drills should consider the ability to move patients to an adjacent smoke compartment. Relocation can be practiced using simulated patients or empty wheelchairs.

CHAPTER 21 • Existing

## 21.7* Operating Features

**A.21.7** Health care occupants have, in large part, varied degrees of physical disability, and their removal to the outside, or even their disturbance caused by moving, is inexpedient or impractical in many cases, except as a last resort. Similarly, recognizing that there might be an operating necessity for the restraint of the mentally ill, often by use of barred windows and locked doors, fire exit drills are usually extremely disturbing, detrimental, and frequently impracticable.

In most cases, fire exit drills, as ordinarily practiced in other occupancies, cannot be conducted in health care occupancies. Fundamentally, superior construction, early discovery and extinguishment of incipient fires, and prompt notification needs to be relied on to reduce the occasion for evacuation of buildings of this class to a minimum.

### 21.7.1 Evacuation and Relocation Plan and Fire Drills.

**21.7.1.1** The administration of every ambulatory health care facility shall have, in effect and available to all supervisory personnel, written copies of a plan for the protection of all persons in the event of fire, for their evacuation to areas of refuge, and for their evacuation from the building when necessary.

**21.7.1.2** All employees shall be periodically instructed and kept informed with respect to their duties under the plan required by 21.7.1.1.

**21.7.1.3** A copy of the plan required by 21.7.1.1 shall be readily available at all times in the telephone operator's location or at the security center.

**21.7.1.4*** Fire drills in ambulatory health care facilities shall include the transmission of a fire alarm signal and simulation of emergency fire conditions.

**A.21.7.1.4** Many health care occupancies conduct fire drills without disturbing patients by choosing the location of the simulated emergency in advance and by closing the doors to patients' rooms or wards in the vicinity prior to initiation of the drill. The purpose of a fire drill is to test and evaluate the efficiency, knowledge, and response of institutional personnel in implementing the facility fire emergency plan. Its purpose is not to disturb or excite patients. Fire drills should be scheduled on a random basis to ensure that personnel in health care facilities are drilled not less than once in each 3-month period.

Drills should consider the ability to move patients to an adjacent smoke compartment. Relocation can be practiced using simulated patients or empty wheelchairs.

CHAPTER 20 • New

**20.7.1.5** Patients shall not be required to be moved during drills to safe areas or to the exterior of the building.

**20.7.1.6** Drills shall be conducted quarterly on each shift to familiarize facility personnel (nurses, interns, maintenance engineers, and administrative staff) with the signals and emergency action required under varied conditions.

**20.7.1.7** When drills are conducted between 9:00 p.m. (2100 hours) and 6:00 a.m. (0600 hours), a coded announcement shall be permitted to be used instead of audible alarms.

**20.7.1.8** Employees of ambulatory health care facilities shall be instructed in life safety procedures and devices.

### 20.7.2 Procedure in Case of Fire.

#### 20.7.2.1* Protection of Patients.

**A.20.7.2.1** Each facility has specific characteristics that vary sufficiently from other facilities to prevent the specification of a universal emergency procedure. The recommendations that follow, however, contain many of the elements that should be considered and adapted, as appropriate, to the individual facility.

Upon discovery of fire, personnel should immediately take the following action:

(1) If any person is involved in the fire, the discoverer should go to the aid of that person, calling aloud an established code phrase, which provides for both the immediate aid of any endangered person and the transmission of an alarm.
(2) Any person in the area, upon hearing the code called aloud, should activate the building fire alarm using the nearest manual fire alarm box.
(3) If a person is not involved in the fire, the discoverer should activate the building fire alarm using the nearest manual fire alarm box.
(4) Personnel, upon hearing the alarm signal, should immediately execute their duties as outlined in the facility fire safety plan.
(5) The telephone operator should determine the location of the fire as indicated by the audible signal.
(6) In a building equipped with an uncoded alarm system, a person on the floor of fire origin should be responsible for promptly notifying the facility telephone operator of the fire location.
(7) If the telephone operator receives a telephone alarm reporting a fire from a floor, the operator should regard that alarm in the same fashion as an alarm received over the fire alarm system and should immediately notify the fire department and alert all facility personnel of the place of fire and its origin.

CHAPTER 21 • Existing

**21.7.1.5** Patients shall not be required to be moved during drills to safe areas or to the exterior of the building.

**21.7.1.6** Drills shall be conducted quarterly on each shift to familiarize facility personnel (nurses, interns, maintenance engineers, and administrative staff) with the signals and emergency action required under varied conditions.

**21.7.1.7** When drills are conducted between 9:00 p.m. (2100 hours) and 6:00 a.m. (0600 hours), a coded announcement shall be permitted to be used instead of audible alarms.

**21.7.1.8** Employees of ambulatory health care facilities shall be instructed in life safety procedures and devices.

### 21.7.2 Procedure in Case of Fire.

#### 21.7.2.1* Protection of Patients.

**A.21.7.2.1** Each facility has specific characteristics that vary sufficiently from other facilities to prevent the specification of a universal emergency procedure. The recommendations that follow, however, contain many of the elements that should be considered and adapted, as appropriate, to the individual facility.

Upon discovery of fire, personnel should immediately take the following action:

(1) If any person is involved in the fire, the discoverer should go to the aid of that person, calling aloud an established code phrase, which provides for both the immediate aid of any endangered person and the transmission of an alarm.
(2) Any person in the area, upon hearing the code called aloud, should activate the building fire alarm using the nearest manual fire alarm box.
(3) If a person is not involved in the fire, the discoverer should activate the building fire alarm using the nearest manual fire alarm box.
(4) Personnel, upon hearing the alarm signal, should immediately execute their duties as outlined in the facility fire safety plan.
(5) The telephone operator should determine the location of the fire as indicated by the audible signal.
(6) In a building equipped with an uncoded alarm system, a person on the floor of fire origin should be responsible for promptly notifying the facility telephone operator of the fire location.
(7) If the telephone operator receives a telephone alarm reporting a fire from a floor, the operator should regard that alarm in the same fashion as an alarm received over the fire alarm system and should immediately notify the fire department and alert all facility personnel of the place of fire and its origin.

(8) If the building fire alarm system is out of order, any person discovering a fire should immediately notify the telephone operator by telephone, and the operator should then transmit this information to the fire department and alert the building occupants.

**20.7.2.1.1** For ambulatory health care facilities, the proper protection of patients shall require the prompt and effective response of ambulatory health care personnel.

**20.7.2.1.2** The basic response required of staff shall include the following:

(1) Removal of all occupants directly involved with the fire emergency
(2) Transmission of an appropriate fire alarm signal to warn other building occupants and summon staff
(3) Confinement of the effects of the fire by closing doors to isolate the fire area
(4) Relocation of patients as detailed in the facility's fire safety plan

**20.7.2.2 Fire Safety Plan.** A written fire safety plan shall provide for the following:

(1) Use of alarms
(2) Transmission of alarms to fire department
(3) Response to alarms
(4) Isolation of fire
(5) Evacuation of immediate area
(6) Evacuation of smoke compartment
(7) Preparation of floors and building for evacuation
(8) Extinguishment of fire

**20.7.2.3 Staff Response.**

**20.7.2.3.1** All personnel shall be instructed in the use of and response to fire alarms.

**20.7.2.3.2** All health care personnel shall be instructed in the use of the code phrase to ensure transmission of an alarm under the following conditions:

(1) When the individual who discovers a fire must immediately go to the aid of an endangered person
(2) During a malfunction of the building fire alarm system

**20.7.2.3.3** Personnel hearing the code announced shall first activate the building fire alarm using the nearest fire alarm box and then shall execute immediately their duties as outlined in the fire safety plan.

### 20.7.3 Maintenance of Exits.

**20.7.3.1** Proper maintenance shall be provided to ensure the dependability of the method of evacuation selected.



(8) If the building fire alarm system is out of order, any person discovering a fire should immediately notify the telephone operator by telephone, and the operator should then transmit this information to the fire department and alert the building occupants.

**21.7.2.1.1** For ambulatory health care facilities, the proper protection of patients shall require the prompt and effective response of ambulatory health care personnel.

**21.7.2.1.2** The basic response required of staff shall include the following:

(1) Removal of all occupants directly involved with the fire emergency
(2) Transmission of an appropriate fire alarm signal to warn other building occupants and summon staff
(3) Confinement of the effects of the fire by closing doors to isolate the fire area
(4) Relocation of patients as detailed in the facility's fire safety plan

**21.7.2.2 Fire Safety Plan.** A written fire safety plan shall provide for the following:

(1) Use of alarms
(2) Transmission of alarms to fire department
(3) Response to alarms
(4) Isolation of fire
(5) Evacuation of immediate area
(6) Evacuation of smoke compartment
(7) Preparation of floors and building for evacuation
(8) Extinguishment of fire

**21.7.2.3 Staff Response.**

**21.7.2.3.1** All personnel shall be instructed in the use of and response to fire alarms.

**21.7.2.3.2** All health care personnel shall be instructed in the use of the code phrase to ensure transmission of an alarm under the following conditions:

(1) When the individual who discovers a fire must immediately go to the aid of an endangered person
(2) During a malfunction of the building fire alarm system

**21.7.2.3.3** Personnel hearing the code announced shall first activate the building fire alarm using the nearest fire alarm box and then shall execute immediately their duties as outlined in the fire safety plan.

### 21.7.3 Maintenance of Exits.

**21.7.3.1** Proper maintenance shall be provided to ensure the dependability of the method of evacuation selected.

CHAPTER 20 • New

20.7.3.2 Ambulatory health care occupancies that find it necessary to lock exits shall, at all times, maintain an adequate staff qualified to release locks and direct occupants from the immediate danger area to a place of safety in case of fire or other emergency.

### 20.7.4* Smoking.

Smoking regulations shall be adopted and shall include not less than the following provisions:

(1) Smoking shall be prohibited in any room, ward, or compartment where flammable liquids, combustible gases, or oxygen is used or stored and in any other hazardous location, and such areas shall be posted with signs that read NO SMOKING or shall be posted with the international symbol for no smoking.
(2) In ambulatory health care facilities where smoking is prohibited and signs are placed at all major entrances, secondary signs with language that prohibits smoking shall not be required.
(3) Smoking by patients classified as not responsible shall be prohibited.
(4) The requirement of 20.7.4(3) shall not apply where the patient is under direct supervision.
(5) Ashtrays of noncombustible material and safe design shall be provided in all areas where smoking is permitted.
(6) Metal containers with self-closing cover devices into which ashtrays can be emptied shall be readily available to all areas where smoking is permitted.

A.20.7.4 The most rigid discipline with regard to prohibition of smoking might not be nearly as effective in reducing incipient fires from surreptitious smoking as the open recognition of smoking, with provision of suitable facilities for smoking. Proper education and training of the staff and attendants in the ordinary fire hazards and their abatement is unquestionably essential. The problem is a broad one, varying with different types and arrangements of buildings; the effectiveness of rules of procedure, which need to be flexible, depends in large part on the management.

### 20.7.5 Furnishings, Mattresses, and Decorations.

20.7.5.1* Draperies, curtains, and other loosely hanging fabrics and films serving as furnishings or decorations in ambulatory health care occupancies shall be in accordance with the provisions of 10.3.1, and the following also shall apply:

(1) Such curtains shall include cubicle curtains.
(2) Such curtains shall not include curtains at showers.

CHAPTER 21 • Existing

21.7.3.2 Ambulatory health care occupancies that find it necessary to lock exits shall, at all times, maintain an adequate staff qualified to release locks and direct occupants from the immediate danger area to a place of safety in case of fire or other emergency.

### 21.7.4* Smoking.

Smoking regulations shall be adopted and shall include not less than the following provisions:

(1) Smoking shall be prohibited in any room, ward, or compartment where flammable liquids, combustible gases, or oxygen is used or stored and in any other hazardous location, and such areas shall be posted with signs that read NO SMOKING or shall be posted with the international symbol for no smoking.
(2) In ambulatory health care facilities where smoking is prohibited and signs are placed at all major entrances, secondary signs with language that prohibits smoking shall not be required.
(3) Smoking by patients classified as not responsible shall be prohibited.
(4) The requirement of 21.7.4(3) shall not apply where the patient is under direct supervision.
(5) Ashtrays of noncombustible material and safe design shall be provided in all areas where smoking is permitted.
(6) Metal containers with self-closing cover devices into which ashtrays can be emptied shall be readily available to all areas where smoking is permitted.

A.21.7.4 The most rigid discipline with regard to prohibition of smoking might not be nearly as effective in reducing incipient fires from surreptitious smoking as the open recognition of smoking, with provision of suitable facilities for smoking. Proper education and training of the staff and attendants in the ordinary fire hazards and their abatement is unquestionably essential. The problem is a broad one, varying with different types and arrangements of buildings; the effectiveness of rules of procedure, which need to be flexible, depends in large part on the management.

### 21.7.5 Furnishings, Mattresses, and Decorations.

21.7.5.1* Draperies, curtains and other loosely hanging fabrics and films serving as furnishings or decorations in ambulatory health care occupancies shall be in accordance with the provisions of 10.3.1, and the following also shall apply:

(1) Such curtains shall include cubicle curtains.
(2) Such curtains shall not include curtains at showers.

CHAPTER 20 • New

**A.20.7.5.1** In addition to the provisions of 10.3.1, which deal with ignition resistance, additional requirements with respect to the location of cubicle curtains relative to sprinkler placement are included in NFPA 13, *Standard for the Installation of Sprinkler Systems.*

**20.7.5.2** Newly introduced upholstered furniture shall comply with 10.3.2.1 and one of the following provisions:

(1) The furniture shall meet the criteria specified in 10.3.3.
(2) The furniture shall be in a building protected throughout by an approved, supervised automatic sprinkler system in accordance with 9.7.1.1(1).

**20.7.5.3** Newly introduced mattresses shall comply with 10.3.2.2 and one of the following provisions:

(1) The mattresses shall meet the criteria specified in 10.3.4.
(2) The mattresses shall be in a building protected throughout by an approved, supervised automatic sprinkler system in accordance with 9.7.1.1(1).

**20.7.5.4** Combustible decorations shall be prohibited, unless one of the following criteria is met:

(1) They are flame-retardant.
(2) They are decorations, such as photographs and paintings, in such limited quantities that a hazard of fire development or spread is not present.

**20.7.5.5** Soiled linen or trash collection receptacles shall not exceed 32 gal (121 L) in capacity, and the following also shall apply:

(1) The average density of container capacity in a room or space shall not exceed 0.5 gal/ft$^2$ (20.4 L/m$^2$).
(2) A capacity of 32 gal (121 L) shall not be exceeded within any 64 ft$^2$ (6 m$^2$) area.
(3) Mobile soiled linen or trash collection receptacles with capacities greater than 32 gal (121 L) shall be located in a room protected as a hazardous area when not attended.
(4) Container size and density shall not be limited in hazardous areas.

CHAPTER 21 • Existing

**A.21.7.5.1** In addition to the provisions of 10.3.1, which deal with ignition resistance, additional requirements with respect to the location of cubicle curtains relative to sprinkler placement are included in NFPA 13, *Standard for the Installation of Sprinkler Systems.*

**21.7.5.2** Newly introduced upholstered furniture shall comply with 10.3.2.1 and one of the following provisions:

(1) The furniture shall meet the criteria specified in 10.3.3.
(2) The furniture shall be in a building protected throughout by an approved, supervised automatic sprinkler system in accordance with 9.7.1.1(1).

**21.7.5.3** Newly introduced mattresses shall comply with 10.3.2.2 and one of the following provisions:

(1) The mattresses shall meet the criteria specified in 10.3.4.
(2) The mattresses shall be in a building protected throughout by an approved, supervised automatic sprinkler system in accordance with 9.7.1.1(1).

**21.7.5.4** Combustible decorations shall be prohibited, unless one of the following criteria is met:

(1) They are flame-retardant.
(2) They are decorations, such as photographs and paintings, in such limited quantities that a hazard of fire development or spread is not present.

**21.7.5.5** Soiled linen or trash collection receptacles shall not exceed 32 gal (121 L) in capacity, and the following also shall apply:

(1) The average density of container capacity in a room or space shall not exceed 0.5 gal/ft$^2$ (20.4 L/m$^2$).
(2) A capacity of 32 gal (121 L) shall not be exceeded within any 64 ft$^2$ (6 m$^2$) area.
(3) Mobile soiled linen or trash collection receptacles with capacities greater than 32 gal (121 L) shall be located in a room protected as a hazardous area when not attended.
(4) Container size and density shall not be limited in hazardous areas.

Cigarette ignition–resistance testing, as detailed in 10.3.2, is required by 20/21.7.5.2 and 20/21.7.5.3 for newly introduced upholstered furniture and newly introduced mattresses in ambulatory health care occupancies, regardless of the presence of sprinkler protection. Rate of heat release testing, as detailed in 10.3.3 and 10.3.4, is required by 20/21.7.5.2 and 20/21.7.5.3 for newly introduced upholstered furniture and newly introduced mattresses in ambulatory health care occupancies, unless the building is sprinklered throughout.

Paragraph 20/21.7.5.5 establishes maximum trash container sizes and placement densities permitted within a room. Containers larger than those specified, or grouped containers exceeding the density per room criterion, present a hazard greater than that associated with the normal furnishing of an ambulatory health care center room.

CHAPTER 20 • New | CHAPTER 21 • Existing

Large, mobile soiled linen or trash receptacles can be moved along the corridor as collections occur but must be attended by staff. If housekeeping staff, for example, must leave the area, the container must be stored in a room designed and maintained as a hazardous area in accordance with 20/21.3.2. Exhibit 20/21.6 illustrates the requirements of 20/21.7.5.5.

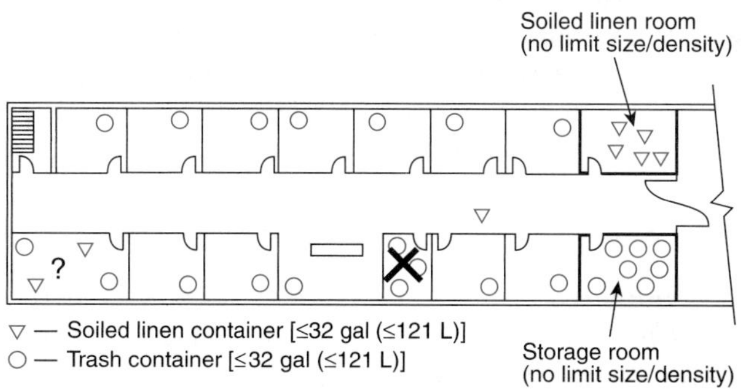


***Exhibit 20/21.6*** *Allowable soiled linen or trash collection receptacles.*

## CHAPTER 20 • New

### 20.7.6 Maintenance and Testing.

See 4.6.13.

### 20.7.7* Engineered Smoke Control Systems.

**A.20.7.7** Two documents that provide recognized engineering principles for the testing of smoke control systems are NFPA 92A, *Standard for Smoke-Control Systems Utilizing Barriers and Pressure Differences*, and NFPA 92B, *Standard for Smoke Management Systems in Malls, Atria, and Large Spaces*.

**20.7.7.1** New engineered smoke control systems shall be tested in accordance with established engineering principles and shall meet the performance requirements of such testing prior to acceptance.

**20.7.7.2** Following acceptance, all engineered smoke control systems shall be tested periodically in accordance with recognized engineering principles.

**20.7.7.3** Test documentation shall be maintained on the premises at all times.

### 20.7.8 Portable Space-Heating Devices.

Portable space-heating devices shall be prohibited in all ambulatory health care occupancies, unless both of the following criteria are met:

(1) Such devices are used only in nonsleeping staff and employee areas.
(2) The heating elements of such devices do not exceed 212°F (100°C).

### 20.7.9 Construction, Repair, and Improvement Operations.

**20.7.9.1** Construction, repair, and improvement operations shall comply with 4.6.11.

## CHAPTER 21 • Existing

### 21.7.6 Maintenance and Testing.

See 4.6.13.

### 21.7.7* Engineered Smoke Control Systems.

**A.21.7.7** Two documents that provide recognized engineering principles for the testing of smoke control systems are NFPA 92A, *Standard for Smoke-Control Systems Utilizing Barriers and Pressure Differences*, and NFPA 92B, *Standard for Smoke Management Systems in Malls, Atria, and Large Spaces*.

**21.7.7.1** New engineered smoke control systems shall be tested in accordance with established engineering principles and shall meet the performance requirements of such testing prior to acceptance.

**21.7.7.2** Following acceptance, all engineered smoke control systems shall be tested periodically in accordance with recognized engineering principles.

**21.7.7.3** Test documentation shall be maintained on the premises at all times.

### 21.7.8 Portable Space-Heating Devices.

Portable space-heating devices shall be prohibited in all ambulatory health care occupancies, unless both of the following criteria are met:

(1) Such devices are used only in nonsleeping staff and employee areas.
(2) The heating elements of such devices do not exceed 212°F (100°C).

### 21.7.9 Construction, Repair, and Improvement Operations.

**21.7.9.1** Construction, repair, and improvement operations shall comply with 4.6.11.

CHAPTER 20 • New

**20.7.9.2** The means of egress in any area undergoing construction, repair, or improvements shall be inspected daily for compliance with 7.1.10.1 and shall also comply with NFPA 241, *Standard for Safeguarding Construction, Alteration, and Demolition Operations.*

CHAPTER 21 • Existing

**21.7.9.2** The means of egress in any area undergoing construction, repair, or improvements shall be inspected daily for compliance with 7.1.10.1 and shall also comply with NFPA 241, *Standard for Safeguarding Construction, Alteration, and Demolition Operations.*

## References Cited in Commentary


1. NFPA 220, *Standard on Types of Building Construction*, 2009 edition, National Fire Protection Association, Quincy, MA.
2. *NFPA 5000®, Building Construction and Safety Code®*, 2009 edition, National Fire Protection Association, Quincy, MA.
3. NFPA 99, *Standard for Health Care Facilities*, 2005 edition, National Fire Protection Association, Quincy, MA.
4. *NFPA 72®, National Fire Alarm Code®*, 2007 edition, National Fire Protection Association, Quincy, MA.
5. NFPA 80, *Standard for Fire Doors and Other Opening Protectives*, 2007 edition, National Fire Protection Association, Quincy, MA.
6. ASME A17.1/CSA B44, *Safety Code for Elevators and Escalators*, 2007 edition, American Society of Mechanical Engineers, Three Park Avenue, New York, NY 10016-5990.
7. ASME A17.3, *Safety Code for Existing Elevators and Escalators*, 2005 edition, American Society of Mechanical Engineers, Three Park Avenue, New York, NY 10016-5990.

CHAPTERS 22 AND 23

# New and Existing Detention and Correctional Occupancies

Detention and correctional occupancies apply the total concept approach to life safety — complete with a defend-in-place strategy — much as is done for health care occupancies. Unlike people in health care occupancies, whose incapability of self-preservation is due to medical conditions, those in detention and correctional occupancies are incapable of self-preservation because of security restrictions. Security restrictions prevent, to a large extent, free and customary movement and access to other areas of a building. In general, many of the normal features needed in a detention facility are nearly the exact opposite of what the *Code* attempts to provide for other occupancies. The use of locked doors, often with key-operated locks (see 22/23.2.11.2 and 22/23.2.11.3); egress components for which use is restricted or traffic flow is constricted, such as a sally port (see 22/23.2.5.4); and discharge of exits onto other than public ways (see 22/23.2.7.1) are features not usually permitted in other occupancies.

Chapters 22 and 23 impose limitations on the degree of locking that can be used. These limits form a classification scheme based on the appropriate use condition. In general, the amount of restriction (e.g., Use Condition I is free egress and Use Condition V is contained; see 22/23.1.4.1) in the detention and correctional facility dictates the use of acceptable locking methods and means of egress features not permitted in other occupancies. As in a health care facility, those unique features necessary to protect the occupants *in place* include construction, compartmentation, alarm and detection, and staff facilitation to help lead or direct occupants to safe areas within the premises of the detention facility campus.

Section 22/23.7 provides routine operating requirements, such as 24-hour staffing; means for resident notification of staff in an emergency; preparation and maintenance of evacuation plans; staff training in the use of portable fire extinguishers; storage of combustible personal property; presence of heat-producing appliances; control of flammability of draperies, curtains, mattresses, and upholstered furniture; and visual and tactile identification of keys necessary for unlocking doors within the means of egress. Because locking doors — which is necessary for the intended function of the facility — is contrary to the basic *Code* tenet that the means of egress system is under the control of building occupants, the presence of properly trained staff is paramount to providing a level of life safety equivalent to that provided in other occupancies. Section 22/23.7 requires the necessary staffing and training that — where combined with the *Code* requirements of the core chapters and the remainder of Chapter 22 or Chapter 23 — achieve the necessary level of life safety.

## 22.1 General Requirements

### 22.1.1 Application.

#### 22.1.1.1 General.

**22.1.1.1.1** The requirements of this chapter shall apply to new buildings or portions thereof used as detention or correctional occupancies. *(See 1.3.1.)*

## 23.1 General Requirements

### 23.1.1 Application.

#### 23.1.1.1 General.

**23.1.1.1.1** The requirements of this chapter shall apply to existing buildings or portions thereof currently occupied as detention or correctional occupancies.

CHAPTER 22 • New

CHAPTER 23 • Existing

The provisions for new detention and correctional occupancies are addressed in Chapter 22; the provisions for existing detention and correctional occupancies (i.e., existing conditions in detention and correctional occupancies) are addressed in Chapter 23.

In editions of the *Code* prior to 2006, renovations, additions, and changes of occupancy were required to comply with the requirements for new construction. For detention and correctional occupancies, such renovations, additions, and changes of occupancy were required to meet the provisions of Chapter 22, while existing conditions were subject to the provisions of Chapter 23. Since the 2006 edition of the *Code,* Chapter 43, Building Rehabilitation, has addressed the subject in a different way. The chapter was written to promote the adaptive reuse of existing buildings without sacrificing the needed level of life safety. The provisions of Chapter 43 blend the requirements for new construction with those for existing conditions, so as to require additional life safety features as the rehabilitation work category increases in complexity. The rehabilitation work categories are repair, renovation, modification, reconstruction, change of use or occupancy classification, and addition. See 4.6.8, 4.6.12, and Chapter 43.

**22.1.1.1.2** This chapter establishes life safety requirements that shall apply to the design of all new detention and correctional facilities, other than the following:

(1) Use Condition I facilities protected as residential occupancies in accordance with 22.1.4.3
(2)* Facilities determined to have equivalent safety provided in accordance with Section 1.4

**A.22.1.1.1.2(2)** In determining equivalency for conversions, modernizations, renovations, or unusual design concepts of detention and correctional facilities, the authority having jurisdiction is permitted to accept evaluations based on the detention and correctional occupancies fire safety evaluation system (FSES) of NFPA 101A, *Guide on Alternative Approaches to Life Safety*, utilizing the parameters for new construction.

**22.1.1.1.3** Detention and correctional occupancies shall include those used for purposes such as correctional institutions, detention facilities, community residential centers, training schools, work camps, and substance abuse centers where occupants are confined or housed under some degree of restraint or security.

**22.1.1.1.4*** Detention and correctional occupancies shall include those that provide sleeping facilities for one or more residents and are occupied by persons who are generally prevented from taking self-preservation action because of security measures not under the occupants' control.

**A.22.1.1.1.4** It is not the intent to classify as detention and correctional occupancies the areas of health care occupancies in which doors are locked against patient egress where needed for the clinical needs of the patients. For example, a dementia treatment center can be adequately protected by the health care occupancies requirements of Chapter 18. *[See 18.1.1.1.5, 18.2.2.2.2, 18.2.2.2.4(1), and 18.2.2.2.6.]*

**23.1.1.1.2** This chapter establishes life safety requirements that shall apply to all existing detention and correctional facilities, other than the following:

(1) Use Condition I facilities protected as residential occupancies in accordance with 23.1.4.3
(2)* Facilities determined to have equivalent safety provided in accordance with Section 1.4

**A.23.1.1.1.2(2)** In determining equivalency for existing detention and correctional facilities, the authority having jurisdiction is permitted to accept evaluations based on the detention and correctional occupancies fire safety evaluation system (FSES) of NFPA 101A, *Guide on Alternative Approaches to Life Safety*, utilizing the parameters for existing buildings.

**23.1.1.1.3** Detention and correctional occupancies shall include those used for purposes such as correctional institutions, detention facilities, community residential centers, training schools, work camps, and substance abuse centers where occupants are confined or housed under some degree of restraint or security.

**23.1.1.1.4*** Detention and correctional occupancies shall include those that provide sleeping facilities for one or more residents and are occupied by persons who are generally prevented from taking self-preservation action because of security measures not under the occupants' control.

**A.23.1.1.1.4** It is not the intent to classify as detention and correctional occupancies the areas of health care occupancies in which doors are locked against patient egress where needed for the clinical needs of the patients. For example, a dementia treatment center can be adequately protected by the health care occupancies requirements of Chapter 19. *[See 19.1.1.1.5, 19.2.2.2.2, 19.2.2.2.4(1), and 19.2.2.2.6.]*

CHAPTER 22 • New

The one-resident threshold requirement of 22.1.1.1.4 is not meant to force a residential occupancy, where security is imposed on one or more occupants, to be reclassified as a detention and correctional occupancy.

**22.1.1.1.5*** Lockups in other than detention and correctional occupancies and health care occupancies shall comply with the requirements of 22.4.5.

**A.22.1.1.1.5** Lockups in which persons are detained with some degree of security imposed on them are common in many occupancies. Examples include the following:

(1) Immigration and naturalization facilities at border crossings
(2) Customs facilities at international airports
(3) Prisoner holding facilities at courthouses
(4) Local police department holding areas
(5) Security offices at sports stadia
(6) Security offices at shopping mall complexes

CHAPTER 23 • Existing

The one-resident threshold requirement of 23.1.1.1.4 is not meant to force a residential occupancy, where security is imposed on one or more occupants, to be reclassified as a detention and correctional occupancy.

**23.1.1.1.5*** Lockups, other than approved existing lockups, in other than detention and correctional occupancies and health care occupancies shall comply with the requirements of 23.4.5.

**A.23.1.1.1.5** Lockups in which persons are detained with some degree of security imposed on them are common in many occupancies. Examples include the following:

(1) Immigration and naturalization facilities at border crossings
(2) Customs facilities at international airports
(3) Prisoner holding facilities at courthouses
(4) Local police department holding areas
(5) Security offices at sports stadia
(6) Security offices at shopping mall complexes

Since the 2006 edition of the *Code*, the definition of the term *detention and correctional occupancy* has applied at the threshold of one or more persons (see 3.3.178.5, 6.1.7.1, and 22/23.1.1.1.4). Formerly, the threshold was four or more persons. This change was made for correlation with the provisions for lockups in other than detention and correctional occupancies, as addressed in 22/23.1.1.1.5 and 22/23.4.5, that have appeared in the *Code* since the 2006 edition. The provisions for lockups are needed for application, even when only one person is detained, as the locked doors characteristic of such detention deny the occupant free egress as required by 7.2.1.5. A lockup in an occupancy other than detention and correctional that detains any individual for more than 24 hours is required to be classified as a detention and correctional occupancy (see 22/23.4.5.1.2) and is subject to the provisions of Chapter 22 or Chapter 23. Thus, the provisions of Chapters 22 and 23 needed to apply to one or more residents.

CHAPTER 22 • New

**22.1.1.2 Total Concept.**

**22.1.1.2.1** All detention and correctional facilities shall be designed, constructed, maintained, and operated to minimize the possibility of a fire emergency.

**22.1.1.2.2** Because the safety of all occupants in detention and correctional facilities cannot be adequately ensured solely by dependence on evacuation of the building, their protection from fire shall be provided by appropriate arrangement of facilities; adequate, trained staff; and development of operating, security, and maintenance procedures composed of the following:

(1) Design, construction, and compartmentation
(2) Provision for detection, alarm, and extinguishment
(3) Fire prevention and planning, training, and drilling programs for the isolation of fire and the transfer of occupants to areas of refuge, for evacuation of the building, or for protection of the occupants in place

CHAPTER 23 • Existing

**23.1.1.2 Total Concept.**

**23.1.1.2.1** All detention and correctional facilities shall be designed, constructed, maintained, and operated to minimize the possibility of a fire emergency.

**23.1.1.2.2** Because the safety of all occupants in detention and correctional facilities cannot be adequately ensured solely by dependence on evacuation of the building, their protection from fire shall be provided by appropriate arrangement of facilities; adequate, trained staff; and development of operating, security, and maintenance procedures composed of the following:

(1) Design, construction, and compartmentation
(2) Provision for detection, alarm, and extinguishment
(3) Fire prevention and planning, training, and drilling programs for the isolation of fire and the transfer of occupants to areas of refuge, for evacuation of the building, or for protection of the occupants in place

CHAPTER 22 • New

(4) Provision of security to the degree necessary for the safety of the public and the occupants of the facility

**22.1.1.3 Additions.** Additions shall be separated from any existing structure not conforming with the provisions of Chapter 23 by a fire barrier having not less than a 2-hour fire resistance rating constructed to the requirements of the addition, and the following also shall apply:

(1) Doors in such partitions shall normally be kept closed.
(2) Doors in such partitions shall be permitted to be held open if they meet the requirements of 7.2.1.8.2.

**22.1.1.4 Modernizations or Renovations.**

**22.1.1.4.1** Modernizations and renovations shall be in accordance with 4.6.8, unless otherwise permitted by 22.1.1.4.2.

**22.1.1.4.2** In nonsprinklered existing buildings, modernizations or renovations shall be permitted to comply with the nonsprinklered options contained in 22.4.4 in lieu of the sprinkler requirement of 22.3.5.2.

CHAPTER 23 • Existing

(4) Provision of security to the degree necessary for the safety of the public and the occupants of the facility

**23.1.1.3 Additions.** Additions shall be separated from any existing structure not conforming with the provisions of this chapter by a fire barrier having not less than a 2-hour fire resistance rating constructed to the requirements of the addition, and the following also shall apply:

(1) Doors in such partitions shall normally be kept closed.
(2) Doors shall be permitted to be held open if they meet the requirements of 7.2.1.8.2.

**23.1.1.4 Modernizations or Renovations.**

**23.1.1.4.1** Modernizations and renovations shall be in accordance with 4.6.8, unless otherwise permitted by 23.1.1.4.2.

**23.1.1.4.2** In nonsprinklered existing buildings, modernizations or renovations shall be permitted to comply with the nonsprinklered options contained in 22.4.4 in lieu of the sprinkler requirement of 22.3.5.2.

Although 22/23.1.1.1.2 states that Chapters 22 and 23 establish life safety requirements for detention and correctional facilities, the chapters focus primarily on life safety requirements for the residential portions of these occupancies.

Paragraph 22/23.1.1.1.2(1) exempts Use Condition I facilities from the requirements of Chapters 22 and 23 if such facilities are protected as residential occupancies. In accordance with 22/23.1.4.1, which defines the five resident user category groups, Use Condition I provides residents with free movement from sleeping areas and other spaces where access or occupancy is permitted to the exterior by a means of an egress system that meets the same requirements as would be provided for occupants of hotel, dormitory, apartment, or lodging or rooming house occupancies. Because locked doors have not been imposed on the residents of a Use Condition I detention or correctional occupancy, such a facility does not require the protect-in-place strategy and associated requirements of Chapters 22 and 23. For information on the protection of Use Condition I facilities, 22/23.1.1.1.2(1) and 22/23.1.4.3(1) refer the user to the residential occupancy chapters of the *Code* in lieu of the provisions of Chapters 22 and 23.

Paragraph 22/23.1.1.1.2(2) permits use of the equivalency provisions of Section 1.4 for compliance with the intended level of life safety, rather than having to meet the requirements of Chapters 22 and 23. The 2010 edition of NFPA 101A, *Guide on Alternative Approaches to Life Safety*,[1] will provide information on one possible equivalency system for use in detention and correctional occupancies. The measurement system of the 2010 edition of NFPA 101A, which is to be published late in 2009, will be calibrated against the requirements of the 2009 edition of the *Life Safety Code*; the fire safety evaluation systems contained in the 2007 edition of NFPA 101A were calibrated against the requirements of the 2006 edition of the *Code*.

The fire safety evaluation system (FSES) for detention and correctional occupancies contained in NFPA 101A provides a method in which the user assigns numerical values to various building parameters. The individual values are totaled and compared with established values. Using this system, alternative designs can be evaluated as options to literal *Code* compliance. The *Code* does not intend to limit acceptable equivalency evaluations solely to those based on the FSES in NFPA 101A. The authority having jurisdiction (AHJ) retains the discretion — in accordance with Section 1.4 — to evaluate and approve alternative designs on the basis of appropriate supporting data. Also, Section 4.4 of the *Code* permits the use of the performance-based option for the design of a complete life safety system in accordance with Chapter 5.

Both A.6.1.7.1 and 22/23.1.1.1.3 reflect the current terminology for various forms of detention and correctional occupancies. The terms *adult correctional institutions, adult local detention facilities, adult community residential centers, juvenile detention facilities, juvenile training schools, adult and juvenile work camps*, and *adult and juvenile substance abuse centers* are used in place of terms such as *reformatories* and *houses of correction.*

Residents of detention and correctional occupancies and patients in health care occupancies are judged to be incapable of self-preservation during a fire emergency. In the case of a health care occupancy patient, incapability is due to physical or mental illness or infirmity. The detention and correctional occupancy resident, although most likely ambulatory or able-bodied, is incapable of self-preservation due to imposed security measures that are beyond the resident's control. In both cases, the occupants might have to await staff action before moving to an exit, another fire compartment, or another smoke compartment. Impediments to adequate egress are further compounded in detention and correctional occupancies by the reluctance of staff to unlock doors leading to the outside. Thus, horizontal movement within the facility to another fire compartment or smoke compartment might be the only means of egress system that the resident is allowed to use in a fire emergency, regardless of how many exit doors to the outside are installed. Therefore, use of the "total concept" described in 22/23.1.1.2 is critical.

The total concept, as used in 22/23.1.1.2, establishes a protect-in-place or defend-in-place strategy. This strategy mandates requirements that minimize the need for building evacuation by restricting the development and spread of a fire emergency to the room of fire origin. The total concept is desirable because safety cannot be ensured by relying on a means of egress system that is predicated on the use of evacuation but for which locks either cannot or will not be unlocked in a timely manner. The requirements (e.g., see Section 22/23.7) first try to prevent ignition and, when fires do occur, set out to detect them (e.g., see 22/23.3.4.4). Other requirements aim to control the speed with which a fire will develop (e.g., see 22/23.3.3), and still others serve to confine the effects of fire. Sprinkler, standpipe, and portable fire extinguisher requirements facilitate the extinguishment of fire. Provisions are made for refuge areas by encouraging the use of horizontal exits and by requiring smoke barriers. Heavy reliance is placed on staff reaction. All these requirements fit together to minimize the need for evacuation. This is the "total concept."

Additions to existing facilities are addressed in 22/23.1.1.3. Buildings that comply with the requirements for existing detention and correctional occupancies in accordance with Chapter 23 do not require separation from new additions used as detention and correctional occupancies.

Note that, unlike similar requirements that apply to health care occupancies (see 18/19.1.1.4.1.1), the positioning of doors in the separating fire barriers is not restricted to cross-corridor locations. Doors must be kept closed, unless they meet the requirements for automatic closing found in 7.2.1.8.2.

Exhibit 22/23.1 illustrates the requirements of 22/23.1.1.3. If the existing portion of the building meets the requirements of Chapter 23, the new addition could be open to the existing building.

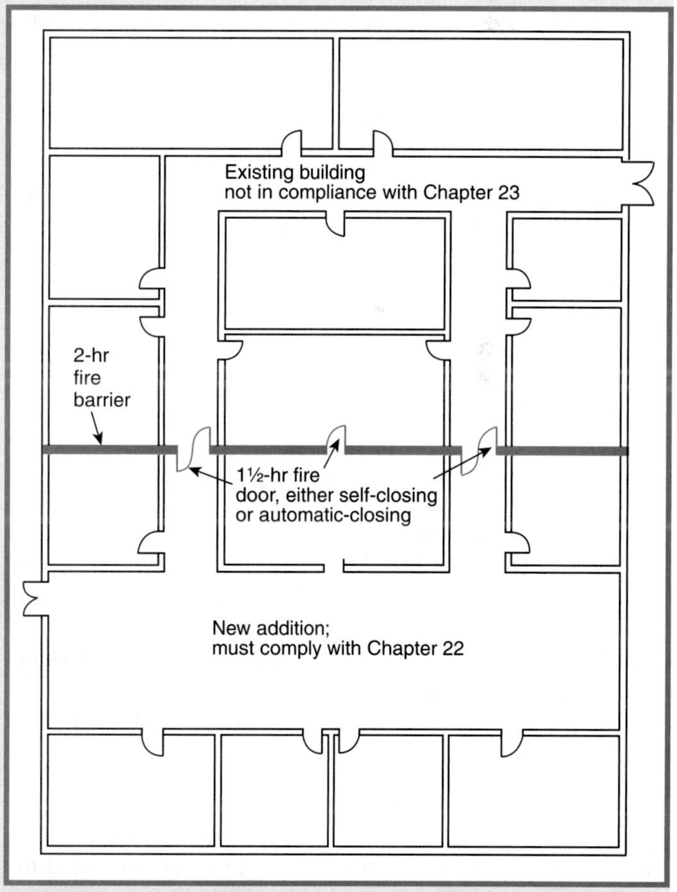


***Exhibit 22/23.1** Separation required between new addition complying with Chapter 22 and existing building not complying with requirements of Chapter 23.*

CHAPTER 22 • New

### 22.1.2* Multiple Occupancies.

**A.22.1.2** Detention and correctional facilities are a complex of structures, each serving a definite and usually different purpose. In many institutions, all, or almost all, the occupancy-type classifications found in this *Code* are represented. Means of egress and other features are governed by the type of occupancy classification and the hazard of occupancy, unless specific exemptions are made.

All buildings and structures are to be classified using Chapter 22 and Section 6.1 as a guide, subject to the ruling of the authority having jurisdiction where a question arises concerning the proper classification of any individual building or structure.

Use condition classification of the institution, as well as of individual areas within the complex, is always to be considered by the authority having jurisdiction.

**22.1.2.1** Multiple occupancies shall be in accordance with 6.1.14.

**22.1.2.2** Egress provisions for areas of detention and correctional facilities that correspond to other occupancies shall meet the corresponding requirements of this *Code* for such occupancies as modified by 22.1.2.2.1 and 22.1.2.2.2.

**22.1.2.2.1** Where security operations necessitate the locking of required means of egress, staff in the building shall be provided with a means for the supervised release of occupants during all times of use.

**22.1.2.2.2*** Where security operations necessitate the locking of required means of egress, the following shall apply:

(1) Detention-grade hardware meeting the requirements of ASTM F 1577, *Standard Test Methods for Detention Locks for Swinging Doors*, shall be provided on swinging doors within the required means of egress.
(2) Sliding doors within the required means of egress shall be designed and engineered for detention and correctional use, and lock cylinders shall meet the cylinder test requirements of ASTM F 1577.

**A.22.1.2.2.2** Key-operated locking hardware of a lesser grade than institutional grade hardware might not be suitable for the heavy use to which such locks are expected to be subjected.

**22.1.2.3** Sections of detention and correctional facilities shall be permitted to be classified as other occupancies, provided that they meet all of the following conditions:

CHAPTER 23 • Existing

### 23.1.2* Multiple Occupancies.

**A.23.1.2** Detention and correctional facilities are a complex of structures, each serving a definite and usually different purpose. In many institutions all, or almost all, of the occupancy-type classifications found in this *Code* are represented. Means of egress and other features are governed by the type of occupancy classification and the hazard of occupancy, unless specific exemptions are made.

All buildings and structures are to be classified using Chapter 23 and Section 6.1 as a guide, subject to the ruling of the authority having jurisdiction where there is a question as to the proper classification of any individual building or structure.

Use condition classification of the institution, as well as of individual areas within the complex, is always to be considered by the authority having jurisdiction.

**23.1.2.1** Multiple occupancies shall be in accordance with 6.1.14.

**23.1.2.2** Egress provisions for areas of detention and correctional facilities that correspond to other occupancies shall meet the corresponding requirements of this *Code* for such occupancies as modified by 23.1.2.2.1.

**23.1.2.2.1*** Where security operations necessitate the locking of required means of egress, staff in the building shall be provided with the means for the supervised release of occupants during all times of use.

**A.23.1.2.2.1** Key-operated locking hardware should be of institutional grade. Lesser grade hardware might not be suitable for the heavy use to which such locks are expected to be subjected.

**23.1.2.2.2 Reserved.**

**23.1.2.3** Sections of detention and correctional facilities shall be permitted to be classified as other occupancies, provided that they meet all of the following conditions:

CHAPTER 22 • New

(1) They are not intended to serve residents for sleeping purposes.
(2) They are separated from areas of detention or correctional occupancies by construction having not less than a 2-hour fire resistance rating.

**22.1.2.4** All means of egress from detention and correctional occupancies that traverse other use areas shall, as a minimum, conform to the requirements of this *Code* for detention and correctional occupancies, unless otherwise permitted by 22.1.2.5.

**22.1.2.5** Egress through a horizontal exit into other contiguous occupancies that do not conform with detention and correctional occupancy egress provisions but that do comply with requirements set forth in the appropriate occupancy chapter of this *Code* shall be permitted, provided that both of the following criteria apply:

(1) The occupancy shall not contain high hazard contents.
(2) The horizontal exit shall comply with the requirements of 22.2.2.5.

**22.1.2.6** Any area with a hazard of contents classified higher than that of the detention or correctional occupancy and located in the same building shall be protected as required in 22.3.2.

**22.1.2.7** Nondetention- or noncorrectional-related occupancies classified as containing high hazard contents shall not be permitted in buildings housing detention or correctional occupancies.

CHAPTER 23 • Existing

(1) They are not intended to serve residents for sleeping purposes.
(2) They are separated from areas of detention or correctional occupancies by construction having not less than a 2-hour fire resistance rating.

**23.1.2.4** All means of egress from detention and correctional occupancies that traverse other use areas shall, as a minimum, conform to the requirements of this *Code* for detention and correctional occupancies, unless otherwise permitted by 23.1.2.5.

**23.1.2.5** Egress through a horizontal exit into other contiguous occupancies that do not conform to detention and correctional occupancy egress provisions but that do comply with requirements set forth in the appropriate occupancy chapter of this *Code* shall be permitted, provided that both of the following criteria apply:

(1) The occupancy shall not contain high hazard contents.
(2) The horizontal exit shall comply with the requirements of 23.2.2.5.

**23.1.2.6** Any area with a hazard of contents classified higher than that of the detention or correctional occupancy and located in the same building shall be protected as required in 23.3.2.

**23.1.2.7** Nondetention- or noncorrectional-related occupancies classified as containing high hazard contents shall not be permitted in buildings housing detention or correctional occupancies.

Paragraph 22/23.1.2.1 directs the user to the multiple occupancies provisions of 6.1.14, which permit protecting multiple occupancies either as mixed occupancies or as separated occupancies. Where the multiple occupancy is protected via the provisions of 6.1.14.4 for separated occupancies, the required number of hours of fire-rated separation is specified by Table 6.1.14.4.1(a) or Table 6.1.14.4.1(b). Note that, per Table 6.1.14.4.1(a) and Table 6.1.14.4.1(b), the 2-hour separation required between detention/correctional occupancies and other occupancies is not permitted to be reduced to a 1-hour separation due to the presence of sprinklers. The protect-in-place strategy being used needs to help ensure tenable conditions for more than 1 hour under fire conditions.

The provisions of 22/23.1.2.2 through 22/23.1.2.7 have the effect of modifying those of 6.1.14 for the very specific situations described.

Paragraph 22/23.1.2.2 addresses areas of detention and correctional facilities that correspond to other occupancies. Yet, the detailed provisions of Chapters 22 and 23 apply mainly to the sleeping and living areas of the detention and correctional facility. Although the work areas resemble a typical industrial occupancy, the requirements of Chapter 40, Industrial Occupancies, cannot be applied by themselves, because doors within the required means of egress of a detention and correctional occupancy are locked for security. Therefore, the concepts of Chapters 22 and 23 should be implemented in locked industrial work areas to ensure that the necessary trained staff who control locks are present to facilitate immediate, supervised release of occupants in the event of fire or a similar emergency.

In addition, some areas of a large facility might correspond to another occupancy classification. For example, a gymnasium would be considered an assembly occupancy (Chapters 12 and 13). If locked doors are required, prompt unlocking and release are critical. Additionally, the requirement of 22.1.2.2.2 for detention-grade hardware increases the reliability of

CHAPTER 22 • New

CHAPTER 23 • Existing

the hardware over that which would normally be installed in nondetention occupancies.

Release of locked doors is permitted to be achieved by a remotely activated system capable of unlocking all doors in the means of egress or by a sufficient number of attendants who are continuously on duty, provided with keys, and stationed in the immediate area of all locked means of egress doors. Continuous staff supervision is essential.

Paragraph 22/23.1.2.3 permits portions of a detention and correctional occupancy to be classified as some other occupancy, provided that certain safeguards are implemented. For example, administrative offices or maintenance areas that are not customarily used by residents as sleeping areas and are separated by 2-hour fire resistance–rated construction could be classified as business or industrial occupancies. In many cases, "trustees" might be employed in these areas. Their presence in these areas would be permitted, provided that they have the freedom of egress found in an unlocked environment.

Paragraph 22/23.1.2.3(2) requires that, if a detention or correctional occupancy is located in a building of another classification, the detention or correctional occupancy must be separated from the other occupancy by construction having a fire resistance rating of 2 hours. This requirement would apply to a small detention facility in which detainees sleep that is located in a combination county courthouse/office/police building. In accordance with 22/23.7.1.1, the detention area must be staffed 24 hours per day. The remainder of the building, especially office areas, might not be occupied at night. A fire that originates and develops in an unoccupied area will not threaten the occupants of the detention facility as readily, due to the protection provided by the required 2-hour fire resistance–rated barrier.

Paragraph 22/23.1.2.4 addresses detention and correctional occupancy egress paths that traverse other use areas. The means of egress from detention and correctional occupancies that traverse other types of spaces must conform to the requirements for detention and correctional occupancies. However, if a 2-hour fire barrier and the associated opening protectives located between a detention or correctional occupancy and another occupancy (e.g., business) qualify as a horizontal exit (see 22/23.2.2.5 and 7.2.4), the means of egress system in the business occupancy needs to comply only with the appropriate requirements contained in Chapters 38 and 39. See 22/23.1.2.5.

Paragraph 22/23.1.2.6 regulates those spaces that have more hazardous contents — in quantity or type — than are usually found in a detention and correctional occupancy. Spaces, such as rooms used for the storage of highly combustible materials, trash collection rooms, and paint shops, must be protected in accordance with 22/23.3.2.

Paragraph 22/23.1.2.7 prohibits another occupancy with highly hazardous contents — such as flammable liquids storage — from being located in a building housing detention and correctional occupancies. The intent of this paragraph is not to exclude normal storage, but to prevent the conversion of a portion of a detention and correctional facility to a warehouse that contains a larger quantity or a more hazardous type of combustible material than normally would be expected in a detention and correctional occupancy. This requirement applies principally to residential areas. For example, industrial areas that are part of the overall detention and correctional facility but are located in a nonresidential-use building can have flammable liquids as part of the industrial process.

### 22.1.3 Special Definitions.

A list of special terms used in this chapter follows:

(1) **Detention and Correctional Residential Housing Area.** See 3.3.19.1.
(2) **Sally Port (Security Vestibule).** See 3.3.220.

### 22.1.4 Classification of Occupancy.

See 6.1.7.

**22.1.4.1*** For application of the life safety requirements of this chapter, the resident user category shall be divided into the groups specified in 22.1.4.1.1 through 22.1.4.1.5.

### 23.1.3 Special Definitions.

A list of special terms used in this chapter follows:

(1) **Detention and Correctional Residential Housing Area.** See 3.3.19.1.
(2) **Sally Port (Security Vestibule).** See 3.3.220.

### 23.1.4 Classification of Occupancy.

See 6.1.7.

**23.1.4.1*** For application of the life safety requirements that follow, the resident user category shall be divided into the groups specified in 23.1.4.1.1 through 23.1.4.1.5.

## CHAPTER 22 • New

**A.22.1.4.1** Users and occupants of detention and correctional facilities at various times can be expected to include staff, visitors, and residents. The extent and nature of facility utilization vary according to the type of facility, its function, and its programs.

Figure A.22.1.4.1 illustrates the five use conditions.

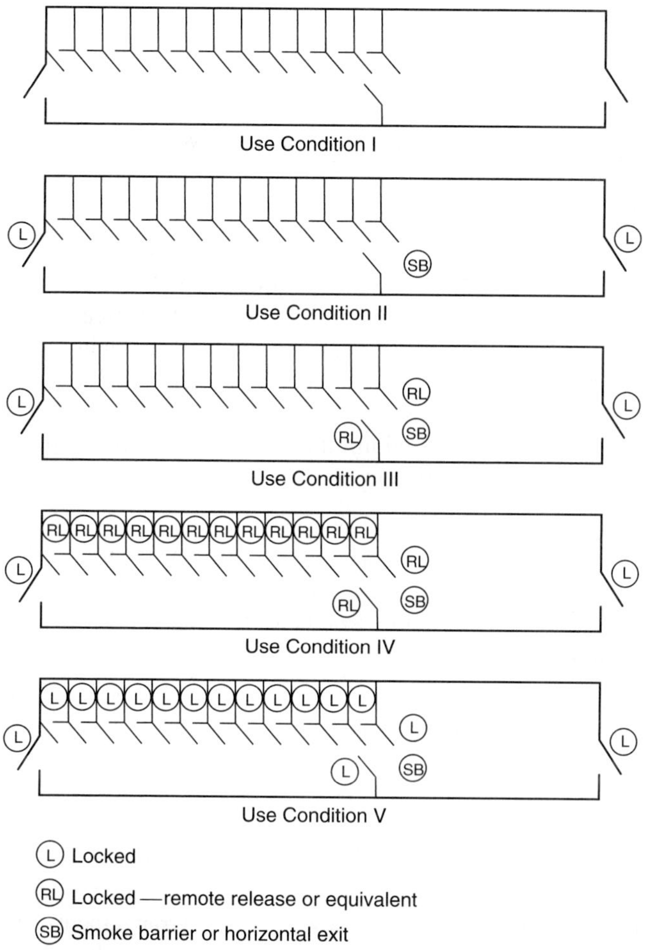


***Figure A.22.1.4.1*** *Detention and Correctional Use Conditions.*

**22.1.4.1.1 Use Condition I — Free Egress.** Use Condition I shall be defined as a condition under which free movement is allowed from sleeping areas and other spaces where access or occupancy is permitted to the exterior via means of egress that meet the requirements of the *Code*.

**22.1.4.1.2 Use Condition II — Zoned Egress.** Use Condition II shall be defined as a condition under which free movement is allowed from sleeping areas and any other occupied smoke compartment to one or more other smoke compartments.

## CHAPTER 23 • Existing

**A.23.1.4.1** Users and occupants of detention and correctional facilities at various times can be expected to include staff, visitors, and residents. The extent and nature of facility utilization will vary according to the type of facility, its function, and its programs.

Figure A.23.1.4.1 illustrates the five use conditions.

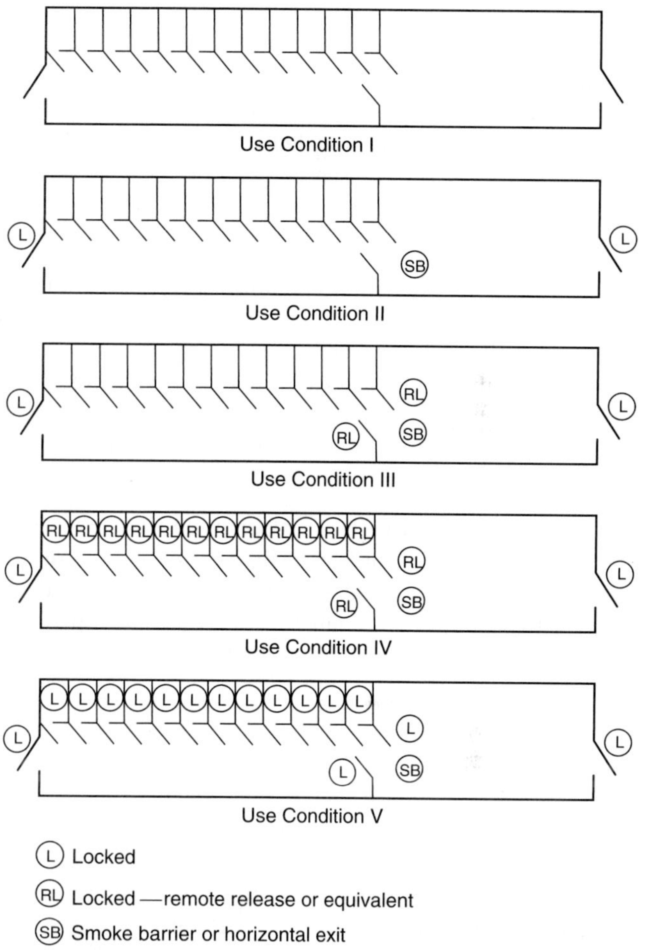


***Figure A.23.1.4.1*** *Detention and Correctional Use Conditions.*

**23.1.4.1.1 Use Condition I — Free Egress.** Use Condition I shall be defined as a condition under which free movement is allowed from sleeping areas and other spaces where access or occupancy is permitted to the exterior via means of egress meeting the requirements of this *Code*.

**23.1.4.1.2 Use Condition II — Zoned Egress.** Use Condition II shall be defined as a condition under which free movement is allowed from sleeping areas and any other occupied smoke compartment to one or more other smoke compartments.

CHAPTER 22 • New

**22.1.4.1.3 Use Condition III — Zoned Impeded Egress.** Use Condition III shall be defined as a condition under which free movement is allowed within individual smoke compartments, such as within a residential unit comprised of individual sleeping rooms and a group activity space, with egress impeded by remote-controlled release of means of egress from such a smoke compartment to another smoke compartment.

**22.1.4.1.4 Use Condition IV — Impeded Egress.** Use Condition IV shall be defined as a condition under which free movement is restricted from an occupied space, and remote-controlled release is provided to allow movement from all sleeping rooms, activity spaces, and other occupied areas within the smoke compartment to another smoke compartment.

**22.1.4.1.5 Use Condition V — Contained.** Use Condition V shall be defined as a condition under which free movement is restricted from an occupied space, and staff-controlled manual release at each door is provided to allow movement from all sleeping rooms, activity spaces, and other occupied areas within the smoke compartment to another smoke compartment.

**22.1.4.2*** To be classified as Use Condition III or Use Condition IV, the arrangement, accessibility, and security of the release mechanism(s) used for emergency egress shall be such that the minimum available staff, at any time, can promptly release the locks.

**A.22.1.4.2** Prompt operation is intended to be accomplished in the period of time between detection of fire either by the smoke detector(s) required by 22.3.4.4 or by other means, whichever occurs first, and the advent of intolerable conditions forcing emergency evacuation. Fire tests have indicated that the time available is a function of the volume and height of the space involved and the rate of fire development. In traditional one-story corridor arrangements, the time between detection by smoke detectors and the advent of lethal conditions down to head height can be as short as approximately 3 minutes. In addition, it should be expected that approximately 1 minute will be required to evacuate all the occupants of a threatened smoke compartment once the locks are released. In such a case, a prompt release time would be 2 minutes.

**22.1.4.3** Areas housing occupancies corresponding to Use Condition I shall conform to one of the following:

(1) Requirements of residential occupancies under this *Code*
(2)* Requirements of this chapter for Use Condition II facilities, provided that the staffing requirements of Section 22.7 are met

CHAPTER 23 • Existing

**23.1.4.1.3 Use Condition III — Zoned Impeded Egress.** Use Condition III shall be defined as a condition under which free movement is allowed within individual smoke compartments, such as within a residential unit comprised of individual sleeping rooms and a group activity space, with egress impeded by remote-controlled release of means of egress from such a smoke compartment to another smoke compartment.

**23.1.4.1.4 Use Condition IV — Impeded Egress.** Use Condition IV shall be defined as a condition under which free movement is restricted from an occupied space, and remote-controlled release is provided to allow movement from all sleeping rooms, activity spaces, and other occupied areas within the smoke compartment to another smoke compartment.

**23.1.4.1.5 Use Condition V — Contained.** Use Condition V shall be defined as a condition under which free movement is restricted from an occupied space, and staff-controlled manual release at each door is provided to allow movement from all sleeping rooms, activity spaces, and other occupied areas within the smoke compartment to another smoke compartment.

**23.1.4.2*** To be classified as Use Condition III or Use Condition IV, the arrangement, accessibility, and security of the release mechanism(s) used for emergency egress shall be such that the minimum available staff, at any time, can promptly release the locks.

**A.23.1.4.2** Prompt operation is intended to be accomplished in the period of time between detection of fire either by the smoke detector(s) required by 23.3.4.4 or by other means, whichever occurs first, and the advent of intolerable conditions forcing emergency evacuation. Fire tests have indicated that the time available is a function of the volume and height of the space involved and the rate of fire development. In traditional one-story corridor arrangements, the time between detection by smoke detectors and the advent of lethal conditions down to head height can be as short as approximately 3 minutes. In addition, it should be expected that approximately 1 minute will be required to evacuate all the occupants of a threatened smoke compartment once the locks are released. In such a case, a prompt release time would be 2 minutes.

**23.1.4.3** Areas housing occupancies corresponding to Use Condition I shall conform to one of the following:

(1) Requirements of residential occupancies under this *Code*
(2)* Requirements of this chapter for Use Condition II facilities, provided that the staffing requirements of Section 23.7 are met

CHAPTER 22 • New

**A.22.1.4.3(2)** If the Use Condition I facility conforms to the requirements of residential occupancies under this *Code*, there are no staffing requirements. If the Use Condition I facility conforms to the requirements of Use Condition II facilities as permitted by this provision, staffing is required in accordance with 22.7.1.

CHAPTER 23 • Existing

**A.23.1.4.3(2)** If the Use Condition I facility conforms to the requirements of residential occupancies under this *Code*, there are no staffing requirements. If the Use Condition I facility conforms to the requirements of Use Condition II facilities as permitted by this exception, staffing is required in accordance with 23.7.1.

Use Condition I facilities have no physical restrictions, such as locks, on the means of egress. The occupants are capable of self-preservation. An example is a work release center in which the doors are not locked. See Figure A.22/A.23.1.4.1. Because the means of egress system is kept unlocked, occupants are as free to escape a fire emergency as occupants of any other residential type of occupancy. Therefore, Use Condition I detention and correctional occupancies are exempted from the requirements of Chapters 22 and 23 if they meet the requirements of some other occupancy chapter, such as Chapter 28 or Chapter 29 for hotels and dormitories. See 22/23.1.4.3 and 22/23.1.1.1.2(1).

The residents of a Use Condition II facility have the freedom to move within the building, including the freedom to move from their rooms, across the smoke barrier, and into a separate smoke compartment. Locked doors that are permitted to be unlocked manually at the door impede movement through the exit door in the exterior wall to the outside. See Figure A.22/A.23.1.4.1.

The residents of a Use Condition III facility are free to move outside their rooms but are confined to the smoke compartment that contains their rooms. Locked doors within the smoke barrier that are equipped with remote-control release impede movement to an adjoining smoke compartment. Locked doors that are permitted to be unlocked manually at the door impede movement through the exit door in the exterior wall to the outside. See Figure A.22/A.23.1.4.1.

The residents of Use Condition IV facilities are locked in their sleeping rooms. Locks on sleeping room doors must be equipped with remote-control release. Locked doors within the smoke barrier that are equipped with remote-control release impede movement to an adjoining smoke compartment. Locked doors that are permitted to be unlocked manually at the door impede movement through the exit door in the exterior wall to the outside. See Figure A.22/A.23.1.4.1.

In Use Condition V facilities, all locks are manually operated at the individual door. See Figure A.22/A.23.1.4.1. The unlocking process places a heavy demand on staff to open doors in an emergency and severely restricts the movement of residents of Use Condition V facilities. Therefore, the most stringent requirements of Chapters 22 and 23 are applied to such facilities.

As part of the definitions of Use Condition II through Use Condition V, reference is made to smoke compartments and the type of locking (none, remote release, or manual operation) used for smoke barrier doors. A facility without a smoke barrier can still qualify as meeting the requirements for one of these use conditions by providing for movement to a location judged to be equivalent to a smoke compartment, such as (1) a public way, (2) a building separated from the space in question by either adequate fire resistance–rated construction or distance, or (3) an adequately sized outside holding area located at a safe distance. The locking operation of the door to this alternative location cannot be more stringent than that permitted for the smoke barrier door of the corresponding use condition — no locking for Use Condition II, remote release for Use Condition III and Use Condition IV, and manual operation for Use Condition V. See also 22/23.3.7.

Note that, in Figure A.22/A.23.1.4.1, "Locked" designates that such doors are arranged to require a manual unlocking operation at the door.

The major requirements of 22/23.1.4.2, applicable to Use Condition III and Use Condition IV facilities, are that the area must be under continuous supervision and a sufficient number of staff must be present and have the necessary keys readily available to release the locks.

The intent of 22/23.1.4.3 is that detention and correctional occupancies in which the occupants are not locked in at any time are permitted to be classified as residential occupancies if they meet the requirements of Chapter 26, Chapter 28, Chapter 29, Chapter 30, or Chapter 31, as appropriate. Those buildings that permit free egress, although used as correctional occupancies, are not classified as detention and correctional occupancies under this *Code*. A facility equipped with locking devices on its doors cannot be classified as Use Condition I, because the locks could be used in the future. Instead, depending on the locks' mode of operation — remote or manual — the corresponding use condition should be assigned and the requirements of Chapter 22 or Chapter 23 followed. A facility should be classified as Use Condition I only if the locking devices are physically removed.

In lieu of following the requirements for a normal residential occupancy, as detailed in Chapter 26, Chapter 28, Chapter 29, Chapter 30, or Chapter 31, a Use Condition I facility is permitted to comply with the Chapter 22 or Chapter 23 provisions applicable to a Use Condition II facility. This exemption permits the entire facility, which might have a variety of use conditions, to be measured against the requirements of Chapter 22 or Chapter 23 without having to make special use of the residential occupancy chapters. However, as A.22/A.23.1.4.3(2) advises, if the requirements applicable to Use Condition II are used, staffing is required. Proper protection would not be ensured by mixing the provisions of a residential occupancy chapter — Chapter 28 or Chapter 29, for example, for which the hotel provisions do not rely on staff action — with those of Chapters 22 and 23 applicable to Use Condition II facilities, for which heavy reliance is placed on staff action. In other words, the *Code* requires full compliance with either the requirements applicable to a residential occupancy or those applicable to a detention and correctional occupancy — not a self-prescribed mixing of options.

### 22.1.5 Classification of Hazard of Contents.

The classification of hazard of contents shall be as defined in Section 6.2.

### 23.1.5 Classification of Hazard of Contents.

The classification of hazard of contents shall be as defined in Section 6.2.

### 22.1.6 Minimum Construction Requirements.

**22.1.6.1** Detention and correctional occupancies shall be limited to the building construction types specified in Table 22.1.6.1. *(See 8.2.1.)*

### 23.1.6 Minimum Construction Requirements.

**23.1.6.1** Detention and correctional occupancies shall be limited to the building construction types specified in Table 23.1.6.1 *(see*8.2.1)*.

***Table 22.1.6.1 Construction Type Limitations***

| | | Stories in Height[†] | | | | | |
|---|---|---|---|---|---|---|---|
| **Construction Type** | **Sprinklered[‡]** | **1 With Basement** | **1 Without Basement** | **2** | **3** | **> 3 But Not High-Rise** | **High-Rise** |
| I (442) | Yes | X | X | X | X | X | X |
| | No | NP | NP | NP | NP | NP | NP |
| I (332) | Yes | X | X | X | X | X | X |
| | No | NP | NP | NP | NP | NP | NP |
| II (222) | Yes | X | X | X | X | X | X |
| | No | NP | NP | NP | NP | NP | NP |
| II (111) | Yes | X | X | X | NP | NP | NP |
| | No | NP | NP | NP | NP | NP | NP |
| II (000) | Yes | X | X | X | NP | NP | NP |
| | No | NP | NP | NP | NP | NP | NP |
| III (211) | Yes | X | X | X | NP | NP | NP |
| | No | NP | NP | NP | NP | NP | NP |
| III (200) | Yes | X | X | X | NP | NP | NP |
| | No | NP | NP | NP | NP | NP | NP |
| IV (2HH) | Yes | X | X | X | NP | NP | NP |
| | No | NP | NP | NP | NP | NP | NP |
| V (111) | Yes | X | X | X | NP | NP | NP |
| | No | NP | NP | NP | NP | NP | NP |
| V (000) | Yes | X | X | X | NP | NP | NP |
| | No | NP | NP | NP | NP | NP | NP |

X: Permitted for Use Conditions II, III, IV, and V. *(See 22.1.4.3 for Use Condition I.)*
NP: Not permitted.
[†]See 4.6.3.
[‡] Sprinklered throughout by an approved, supervised automatic sprinkler system in accordance with 9.7.1.1(1). *(See 22.3.5.)*

*Table 23.1.6.1 Construction Type Limitations*

| Construction Type | Sprinklered[b] | Stories in Height [a] | | | | | |
|---|---|---|---|---|---|---|---|
| | | 1 With Basement | 1 Without Basement | 2 | 3 | >3 But Not High-Rise | High-Rise |
| I (442)[c, d] | Yes | X | X | X | X | X | X |
| | No | X | X | X | X | X | NP |
| I (332)[c, d] | Yes | X | X | X | X | X | X |
| | No | X | X | X | X | X | NP |
| II (222)[c, d] | Yes | X | X | X | X | X | X |
| | No | X | X | X | X | X | NP |
| II (111)[c, d] | Yes | X | X | X | X | X | X |
| | No | X1 | X | X1 | NP | NP | NP |
| II (000)[d] | Yes | X | X | X | X | X | X |
| | No | X1 | X1 | NP | NP | NP | NP |
| III (211)[d] | Yes | X | X | X | X | X | X |
| | No | X1 | X | X1 | NP | NP | NP |
| III (200)[d] | Yes | X | X | X | X | X | X |
| | No | X1 | X1 | NP | NP | NP | NP |
| IV (2HH)[d] | Yes | X | X | X | X | X | X |
| | No | X1 | X | X1 | NP | NP | NP |
| V (111)[d] | Yes | X | X | X | X | X | X |
| | No | X1 | X | X1 | NP | NP | NP |
| V (000)[d] | Yes | X | X | X | X | X | X |
| | No | X1 | X1 | NP | NP | NP | NP |

NP: Not permitted.

X: Permitted for Use Conditions II, III, IV, and V. *(See 23.1.4.3 for Use Condition I.)*

X1: Permitted for Use Conditions II, III, and IV. Use Condition V not permitted. *(See 23.1.4.3 for Use Condition I.)*

[a] See 4.6.3.

[b] Entire building is protected throughout by an approved, supervised automatic sprinkler system in accordance with 9.7.1.1(1). *(See 23.3.5.)*

[c] Any building of Type I, Type II(222), or Type II(111) construction is permitted to include roofing systems involving combustible or steel supports, decking, or roofing, provided that all of the following are met:

(1) The roof covering meets not less than Class C requirements in accordance with NFPA 256, *Standard Methods of Fire Tests of Roof Coverings.*

(2) The roof is separated from all occupied portions of the building by a noncombustible floor assembly that includes not less than $2^1/_2$ in. (64 mm) of concrete or gypsum fill, and the attic or other space so developed meets one of the following requirements:

(a) It is unoccupied.

(b) It is protected throughout by an approved automatic sprinkler system.

[d] In determining building construction type, exposed steel roof members located 16 ft (4875 mm) or more above the floor of the highest cell is permitted to be disregarded.

**22.1.6.2** All interior walls and partitions in Type I or Type II construction shall be of noncombustible or limited-combustible materials.

**23.1.6.2** A residential housing area complying with 23.3.1.2 shall be considered as one story in height for purposes of applying 23.1.6.1.

Table 22/23.1.6.1 is applied relative to building construction types. See NFPA 220, *Standard on Types of Building Construction,*[2] and *NFPA 5000®, Building Construction and Safety Code®,*[3] for definitions of construction types. Table A.8.2.1.2 summarizes the details associated with Type I through Type V construction.

Table 22/23.1.6.1 establishes building construction type limitations based on the number of "stories in height," as established by 4.6.3. Table 22/23.1.6.1 is applied to detention and correctional occupancies by starting the story count with the level of exit discharge and ending with the highest story used as a detention and correctional occupancy. (Note that a building can have only one level of exit discharge, as defined in 3.3.77.1.)

Table 22/23.1.6.1 prohibits certain building construction types from being constructed and occupied for detention and correctional occupancy use, even if protected by automatic sprinklers. The automatic sprinkler requirements contained in Table 22/23.1.6.1 are based on construction type. Automatic sprinkler protection also is required for new construction by 22.3.5.2. High-rise detention and correctional occupancy buildings are required to be sprinklered by 22/23.4.3.

Maintaining the integrity of building construction under fire conditions is mandated, because detention and correctional facility residents are incapable of self-preservation due to security requirements imposed by the facility. Thus, although NFPA 220 does not regulate the combustibility of interior nonbearing walls and partitions, 22.1.6.2 permits credit to be taken for Type I or Type II construction in new detention and correctional occupancies only if such interior walls and partitions are of noncombustible or limited-combustible construction. The terms *noncombustible (material)* and *limited-combustible (material)* are defined in 3.3.160.3 and 3.3.160.2.

The provisions of 22.4.4.6 and 23.3.1.2 address multilevel housing areas for which the vertical separation between the lowest floor level and the uppermost floor level does not exceed 13 ft (3960 mm), without limiting the number of levels. See Figure A.22.4.4.6.4 and Figure A.23.3.1.2.3. A multilevel housing area meeting all the requirements of 22.4.4.6 and 23.3.1.2 is treated as being one story in height for purposes of determining required building construction type in accordance with 22/23.1.6.1, as permitted by 22.4.4.2.2 and 23.1.6.2.

The *Code* recognizes that locked doors to the outside will be reluctantly unlocked, slowly unlocked, or never unlocked. Therefore, the *Code* relies on the defend-in-place or protect-in-place strategy addressed in the commentary on 22/23.1.1.2 following 22/23.1.1.4.2. Paragraph 22/23.1.6.1 establishes minimum construction requirements to help ensure the structural integrity of the building for the time required to release residents to the outside or hold them in a safe fire compartment or smoke compartment.

### 22.1.7 Occupant Load.

The occupant load, in number of persons for whom means of egress and other provisions are required, either shall be determined on the basis of the occupant load factors of Table 7.3.1.2 that are characteristic of the use of the space or shall be determined as the maximum probable population of the space under consideration, whichever is greater.

### 23.1.7 Occupant Load.

The occupant load, in number of persons for whom means of egress and other provisions are required, either shall be determined on the basis of the occupant load factors of Table 7.3.1.2 that are characteristic of the use of the space or shall be determined as the maximum probable population of the space under consideration, whichever is greater.

Paragraph 22/23.1.7 references the use of the occupant load factors of Table 7.3.1.2, from which an occupant load can be determined. The means of egress system must be sized to handle whichever is larger: the number of persons intended to occupy the space or the number of persons calculated by using the occupant load factors.

The *Code* intends that the occupant load factors be used only for sizing the means of egress, not for limiting the number of persons within a space. If a means of egress can accommodate an occupant load larger than that calculated using the occupant load factor characteristic of the use of the space, the *Code* does not prohibit such a load. In a facility with excess means of egress capacity, other considerations, such as plumbing codes or sanitary codes, sociological factors, and common sense, will help determine the maximum occupant load.

## 22.2 Means of Egress Requirements

### 22.2.1 General.

Means of egress shall comply with Chapter 7, unless otherwise provided or modified by Section 22.2.

## 23.2 Means of Egress Requirements

### 23.2.1 General.

Means of egress shall comply with Chapter 7, unless otherwise provided or modified by Section 23.2.

CHAPTER 22 • New

## 22.2.2 Means of Egress Components.

**22.2.2.1 Components Permitted.** Components of means of egress shall be limited to the types described in 22.2.2.2 through 22.2.2.11.

**22.2.2.2 Doors.** Doors complying with 7.2.1 shall be permitted, unless otherwise provided by 22.2.11.

**22.2.2.3 Stairs.**

**22.2.2.3.1** Stairs shall be permitted as follows:

(1) Stairs complying with 7.2.2 shall be permitted.
(2) Noncombustible grated stair treads and landing floors shall be permitted.

**22.2.2.3.2** Spiral stairs complying with 7.2.2.2.3 shall be permitted for access to and between staff locations.

**22.2.2.4 Smokeproof Enclosures.** Smokeproof enclosures complying with 7.2.3 shall be permitted.

**22.2.2.5 Horizontal Exits.** Horizontal exits complying with 7.2.4 and the modifications of 22.2.2.5.1 and 22.2.2.5.2 shall be permitted.

**22.2.2.5.1** Not less than 6 $ft^2$ (0.55 $m^2$) of accessible space per occupant shall be provided on each side of the horizontal exit for the total number of people in adjoining compartments.

**22.2.2.5.2*** Horizontal exits shall be permitted to comprise 100 percent of the exits required, provided that an exit, other than a horizontal exit, located in another (not necessarily adjacent) fire compartment is accessible without returning through the compartment of fire origin.

**A.22.2.2.5.2** An exit is not necessary from each individual fire compartment or smoke compartment if there is access to an exit through other fire compartments or smoke compartments without passing through the fire compartment or smoke compartment of fire origin.

CHAPTER 23 • Existing

## 23.2.2 Means of Egress Components.

**23.2.2.1 Components Permitted.** Components of means of egress shall be limited to the types described in 23.2.2.2 through 23.2.2.11.

**23.2.2.2 Doors.** Doors complying with 7.2.1 shall be permitted, unless otherwise provided in 23.2.11.

**23.2.2.3 Stairs.**

**23.2.2.3.1** Stairs shall be permitted as follows:

(1) Stairs complying with 7.2.2 shall be permitted.
(2) Noncombustible grated stair treads and landing floors shall be permitted.

**23.2.2.3.2** Spiral stairs complying with 7.2.2.2.3 shall be permitted for access to and between staff locations.

**23.2.2.4 Smokeproof Enclosures.** Smokeproof enclosures complying with 7.2.3 shall be permitted.

**23.2.2.5 Horizontal Exits.** Horizontal exits complying with 7.2.4 and the modifications of 23.2.2.5.1 through 23.2.2.5.4 shall be permitted.

**23.2.2.5.1** Not less than 6 $ft^2$ (0.55 $m^2$) of accessible space per occupant shall be provided on each side of the horizontal exit for the total number of people in adjoining compartments.

**23.2.2.5.2*** Horizontal exits shall be permitted to comprise 100 percent of the exits required, provided that an exit, other than a horizontal exit, located in another (not necessarily adjacent) fire compartment is accessible without returning through the compartment of fire origin.

**A.23.2.2.5.2** An exit is not necessary from each individual fire compartment if there is access to an exit through other fire compartments without passing through the fire compartment of fire origin.

**23.2.2.5.3*** Ducts shall be permitted to penetrate horizontal exits in accordance with 7.2.4.3.5(3) if protected by combination fire dampers/smoke leakage–rated dampers that meet the smoke damper actuation requirements of 8.5.5.

**A.23.2.2.5.3** This provision is intended to promote the use of horizontal exits in detention and correctional occupancies. Horizontal exits provide an especially effective egress system for an occupancy in which the occupants, due to security concerns, are not commonly released to the outside. This provision offers a *Code*-specified equivalent alternative to the requirement of 7.2.4.3.5 that horizontal exits are not to be penetrated by ducts. The intended continuity of the fire resistance–rated and smoke-resisting barrier is maintained by requiring that duct penetrations of horizontal exits be protected by combination fire damper/smoke leakage–rated

**CHAPTER 22 • New** | **CHAPTER 23 • Existing**

dampers that close upon activation of a smoke detector and a heat-actuated mechanism before the barrier's ability to resist the passage of smoke and fire is compromised.

**23.2.2.5.4** A door in a horizontal exit shall not be required to swing with egress travel as specified in 7.2.4.3.8(1).

**22.2.2.6 Ramps.** Ramps complying with 7.2.5 shall be permitted.

**23.2.2.6 Ramps.** Ramps complying with 7.2.5 shall be permitted.

**22.2.2.7 Exit Passageways.** Exit passageways complying with 7.2.6 shall be permitted.

**23.2.2.7 Exit Passageways.** Exit passageways complying with 7.2.6 shall be permitted.

**22.2.2.8 Reserved.**

**23.2.2.8 Fire Escape Stairs.** Fire escape stairs complying with 7.2.8 shall be permitted.

**22.2.2.9 Fire Escape Ladders.** Fire escape ladders complying with 7.2.9 shall be permitted.

**23.2.2.9 Fire Escape Ladders.** Fire escape ladders complying with 7.2.9 shall be permitted.

**22.2.2.10 Alternating Tread Devices.** Alternating tread devices complying with 7.2.11 shall be permitted.

**23.2.2.10 Alternating Tread Devices.** Alternating tread devices complying with 7.2.11 shall be permitted.

**22.2.2.11 Areas of Refuge.** Areas of refuge complying with 7.2.12 shall be permitted.

**23.2.2.11 Areas of Refuge.** Areas of refuge complying with 7.2.12 shall be permitted.

Chapters 22 and 23 recognize the following means of egress components, as described in Chapter 7:

1. Doors (7.2.1)
2. Stairs (7.2.2)
3. Smokeproof enclosures (7.2.3)
4. Horizontal exits (7.2.4)
5. Ramps (7.2.5)
6. Exit passageways (7.2.6)
7. Fire escape ladders (7.2.9)
8. Alternating tread devices (7.2.11)
9. Areas of refuge (7.2.12)

Chapter 23 also recognizes existing fire escape stairs (7.2.8). However, Chapters 22 and 23 often modify the provisions of Chapter 7 applicable to those means of egress components. For example, although the Chapter 7 provisions that apply to horizontal exits would limit a horizontal exit to providing a maximum of 50 percent of the number of exits or 50 percent of the total egress capacity, Chapters 22 and 23 encourage the voluntary use of horizontal exits by permitting up to 100 percent of the exits to be reached by way of horizontal exits if additional criteria can be met.

Chapter 7 considers escalators and moving walks as acceptable means of egress only if they are part of an existing occupancy and are specifically recognized by an occupancy chapter. They are not permitted in the means of egress system of a detention and correctional occupancy. Chapters 22 and 23 do not recognize slide escapes as part of an egress system. Areas of refuge (see 7.2.12) might be used to provide accessible means of egress as required for new facilities in accordance with the provisions of 7.5.4.

Older editions of the *Code* contained a provision in Chapters 22 and 23 that exempted handrails and guards from the requirement for intermediate rails designed to keep children from falling through the spaces between rails. The exemption still applies to detention and correctional occupancies [see 7.2.2.4.5.3(2)]. The rationale for this exemption is that only adults or older juveniles use these facilities, and intermediate railings might impact functional requirements by interfering with visual observation by staff.

Grated stair treads and grated landing floors are recognized as usable in detention and correctional occupancies, because occupant reluctance to walk on such surfaces is not expected. Similarly, the potential for small shoe heels getting caught in the grated surfaces is greatly reduced in detection and correctional occupancies.

Paragraph 22/23.2.2.3.2 permits spiral stairs conforming to 7.2.2.2.3 for staff use only. These provisions prohibit a spiral stair from being part of the required means of egress system within areas occupied by residents.

Paragraph 22/23.2.2.4 permits a smokeproof enclosure to serve as part of the means of egress system in detention and correctional occupancies if that enclo-

CHAPTER 22 • New

CHAPTER 23 • Existing

sure meets the requirements of 7.2.3. However, the smokeproof enclosure is not required. An example of an occupancy requiring a smokeproof enclosure can be found in 31.2.11.1, in which nonsprinklered, existing high-rise apartment buildings are required to be provided with smokeproof enclosures in accordance with 7.2.3.

Horizontal exits are addressed in 22/23.2.2.5. Although 7.2.4 requires only 3 $ft^2$ (0.28 $m^2$) of accessible space per occupant on each side of the horizontal exit, 22/23.2.2.5.1 requires 6 $ft^2$ (0.55 $m^2$) per occupant. The reasons for this requirement include the possible conflicts among the residents, the anticipated extended time spent in the refuge area, and the fact that horizontal exits are permitted to comprise 100 percent of required exits in detention and correctional occupancies in accordance with 22/23.2.2.5.2.

Paragraph 22/23.2.2.5.2 permits horizontal exits to comprise 100 percent of the exits from any fire compartment, provided that it is not necessary to travel through the compartment of fire origin to reach a door to the outside — that is, the compartment is not "dead ended."

In Exhibit 22/23.2, horizontal exits correctly comprise 100 percent of the total exits from fire compartments B, C, and D. Compartment F would require the addition of an exit door that opens directly to the outside in order to reach the outside of the building without traveling through fire compartment E. Compartments A and E comply with the *Code*, using one horizontal exit and one exit door directly to the exterior of the building.

Due to the practical difficulties of using vertical exit travel to the outside in detention and correctional occupancies, including the reluctance of staff to unlock doors, special recognition is given to horizontal travel and the use of horizontal exits. As previously explained, 100 percent of the total required egress capacity for a given fire area is permitted to be provided by horizontal exits. In the event a horizontal exit also serves as a smoke barrier, refer to 22/23.2.4.2 and 22/23.3.7.

Paragraph 7.2.4.3.5 states that fire barriers used in creating a horizontal exit are prohibited from penetration by ducts. To promote the use of horizontal exits in

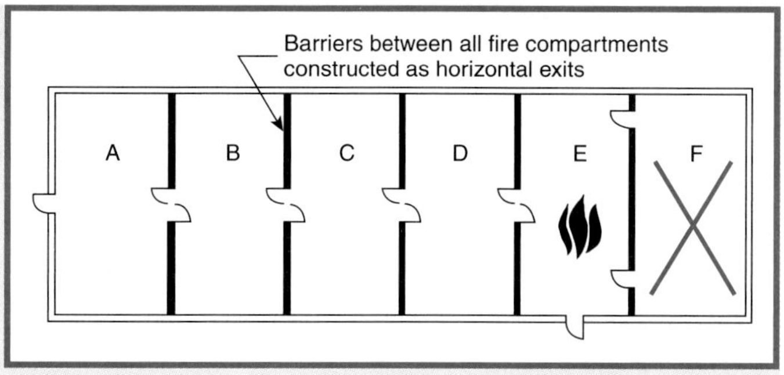


***Exhibit 22/23.2** Horizontal exit fire compartment arrangement.*

detention and correctional occupancies, without burdening a facility with regard to duct penetrations, 22.4.4.3 and 23.2.2.5.3 and the corresponding exemption in 7.2.4.3.5(3) were developed. If smoke detection is used to shut a combination fire damper/smoke leakage–rated damper early in a fire, the fire- and smoke-resisting features of the horizontal exit can be reestablished at points where ducts penetrate the barrier.

Paragraphs 22/23.2.2.6, 22/23.2.2.7, 22/23.2.2.9, and 22/23.2.2.10 do not mandate the use of ramps, exit passageways, fire escape ladders, or alternating tread devices. Rather, these paragraphs recognize ramps, exit passageways, fire escape ladders, or alternating tread devices as part of the means of egress system only if they meet the applicable requirements of 7.2.5 through 7.2.11. Further, 23.2.2.8 recognizes the use of existing fire escape stairs in accordance with 7.2.8. Note that 7.2.9 and 7.2.11 restrict the use of fire escape ladders and alternative tread devices, respectively, to spaces such as normally unoccupied roofs and equipment platforms. In addition, use is restricted to a maximum of three persons who are all capable of using the ladder or device.

Paragraph 22/23.2.2.11 does not mandate the use of areas of refuge but does recognize an area of refuge as part of the means of egress system only if it meets the requirements of 7.2.12. Areas of refuge will often be used to meet the requirements for accessible means of egress mandated for new facilities by 7.5.4 in areas accessible to persons with severe mobility impairments.

### 22.2.3 Capacity of Means of Egress.

**22.2.3.1** The capacity of any required means of egress shall be in accordance with Section 7.3.

### 23.2.3 Capacity of Means of Egress.

**23.2.3.1** The capacity of any required means of egress shall be in accordance with Section 7.3.

CHAPTER 22 • New

**22.2.3.2** Aisles, corridors, and ramps required for egress shall be not less than 48 in. (1220 mm) in width.

**22.2.3.3** Residents' sleeping room door widths shall be permitted to comply with 22.2.11.4.

### 22.2.4 Number of Exits.

See also Section 7.4.

**22.2.4.1** Not less than two separate exits shall meet the following criteria:

(1) They shall be provided on every story.
(2) They shall be accessible from every part of every story, fire compartment, or smoke compartment; however, exit access travel shall be permitted to be common for the distances permitted as common path of travel by 22.2.5.3.

**22.2.4.2** Not less than one approved exit shall be accessible from each fire compartment and each required smoke compartment into which residents are potentially moved in a fire emergency, with the exits arranged so that egress is possible without returning through the zone of fire origin.

### 22.2.5 Arrangement of Means of Egress.

See also Section 7.5.

**22.2.5.1** Every sleeping room shall have a door leading directly to an exit access corridor, unless otherwise permitted by the following:

(1) The requirement of 22.2.5.1 shall not apply if there is an exit door opening directly to the outside from a room at the finished ground level.
(2) One adjacent room, such as a day room, a group activity space, or other common space, shall be permitted to intervene, and the following also shall apply:
    (a) Where sleeping rooms directly adjoin a day room or group activity space that is used for access to an exit, such sleeping rooms shall be permitted to open directly to the day room or space.
    (b) Sleeping rooms permitted to open directly to the day room or space shall be permitted to be separated in elevation by a one-half story or full story height.

CHAPTER 23 • Existing

**23.2.3.2** Aisles, corridors, and ramps required for egress shall be not less than 36 in. (915 mm) in width.

**23.2.3.3** Residents' sleeping room door widths shall be permitted to comply with 23.2.11.4.

### 23.2.4 Number of Exits.

See also Section 7.4.

**23.2.4.1*** Not less than two separate exits shall meet the following criteria:

(1) They shall be provided on every story.
(2) They shall be accessible from every part of every story, fire compartment, or smoke compartment; however, exit access travel shall be permitted to be common for the distances permitted as common path of travel by 23.2.5.3.

**A.23.2.4.1** Multilevel and multitiered residential housing areas meeting the requirements of 23.3.1.2 and 23.3.1.3 are considered one story. Therefore, two exits are not required from each level; only access to two exits is required.

**23.2.4.2*** Not less than one approved exit shall be accessible from each fire compartment and each required smoke compartment into which residents are potentially moved in a fire emergency, with the exits arranged so that egress is possible without returning through the zone of fire origin.

**A.23.2.4.2** An exit is not necessary from each individual fire compartment and smoke compartment if there is access to an exit through other fire compartments or smoke compartments without passing through the fire compartment or smoke compartment of fire origin.

### 23.2.5 Arrangement of Means of Egress.

See also Section 7.5.

**23.2.5.1** Every sleeping room shall have a door leading directly to an exit access corridor, unless otherwise permitted by the following:

(1) The requirement of 23.2.5.1 shall not apply if there is an exit door opening directly to the outside from a room at the finished ground level.
(2) One adjacent room, such as a day room, a group activity space, or other common space, shall be permitted to intervene, and the following also shall apply:
    (a) Where sleeping rooms directly adjoin a day room or group activity space that is used for access to an exit, such sleeping rooms shall be permitted to open directly to the day room or space.
    (b) Sleeping rooms permitted to open directly to the day room or space shall be permitted to be separated in elevation by a one-half story or full story height.

CHAPTER 22 • New

**22.2.5.2** No exit or exit access shall contain a corridor, a hallway, or an aisle having a pocket or dead end exceeding 50 ft (15 m) for Use Condition II, Use Condition III, or Use Condition IV and 20 ft (6100 mm) for Use Condition V.

**22.2.5.3** A common path of travel shall not exceed 100 ft (30 m).

**22.2.5.4** A sally port shall be permitted in a means of egress where there are provisions for continuous and unobstructed travel through the sally port during an emergency egress condition.

CHAPTER 23 • Existing

**23.2.5.2*** Existing dead-end corridors are undesirable and shall be altered wherever possible so that exits are accessible in not less than two different directions from all points in aisles, passageways, and corridors.

**A.23.2.5.2** Every exit or exit access should be arranged, if feasible, so that no corridor or aisle has a pocket or dead end exceeding 50 ft (15 m) for Use Conditions II, III, and IV and 20 ft (6100 mm) for Use Condition V.

**23.2.5.3** A common path of travel shall not exceed 50 ft (15 m), unless otherwise permitted by the following:

(1) A common path of travel shall be permitted for the first 100 ft (30 m) in smoke compartments protected throughout by an approved automatic sprinkler system in accordance with 23.3.5.3.
(2) A common path of travel shall be permitted to exceed 50 ft (15 m) in multilevel residential housing units in which each floor level, considered separately, has not less than one-half of its individual required egress capacity accessible by exit access leading directly out of that level without traversing another communicating floor level.
(3)* Approved existing common paths of travel that exceed 50 ft (15 m) shall be permitted to continue to be used.

**A.23.2.5.3(3)** In determining whether to approve the existing common path of travel that exceeds 50 ft (15 m), the authority having jurisdiction should ensure that the common path is not in excess of the travel distance permitted by 23.2.6.

**23.2.5.4** A sally port shall be permitted in a means of egress where there are provisions for continuous and unobstructed travel through the sally port during an emergency egress condition.

Exhibit 22/23.3 illustrates the use of 22/23.2.5.1(2), which permits one adjacent room to intervene between a sleeping room and the exit access corridor. Sleeping rooms are permitted to be separated in elevation from the day room by one-half to one story. See 22/23.2.5.1(2)(b).

Exhibit 22/23.4 illustrates the dead-end corridor requirements of 22.2.5.2 applicable to new detention and correctional facilities. In Use Condition V, resident room doors are individually key-locked, and the allowable dead-end corridor length is reduced from 50 ft (15 m) to 20 ft (6100 mm). For existing facilities, 23.2.5.2 advises that dead-end corridors are undesirable but sets no maximum depth for existing dead ends.

Exhibit 22/23.5 illustrates a common path of travel. If distance X to C exceeds 50 ft (15 m) [100 ft (30 m), if the smoke compartment is sprinklered as is required for new construction], a second exit access is required for the upper level per 22/23.2.5.3. If the multilevel housing area is large, the common path of travel limitation might require a second, remote exit access door to the corridor.

Paragraphs 23.2.5.3(2) and (3) introduce criteria that recognize existing common paths of travel that exceed the 50 ft (15 m) limitation contained in the base paragraph and the 100 ft (30 m) limitation permitted in sprinklered smoke compartments by 23.2.5.3(1). Paragraph 23.2.5.3(2) offers some relief to existing facilities with lengthy common paths of travel on individual levels of multilevel residential housing units, provided that at least half the occupant load of any level can be

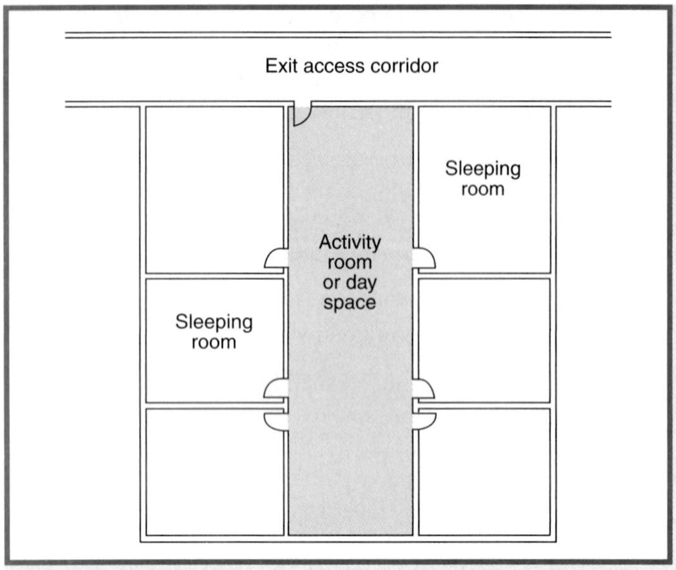


***Exhibit 22/23.3*** *One intervening room between sleeping room and exit access corridor.*

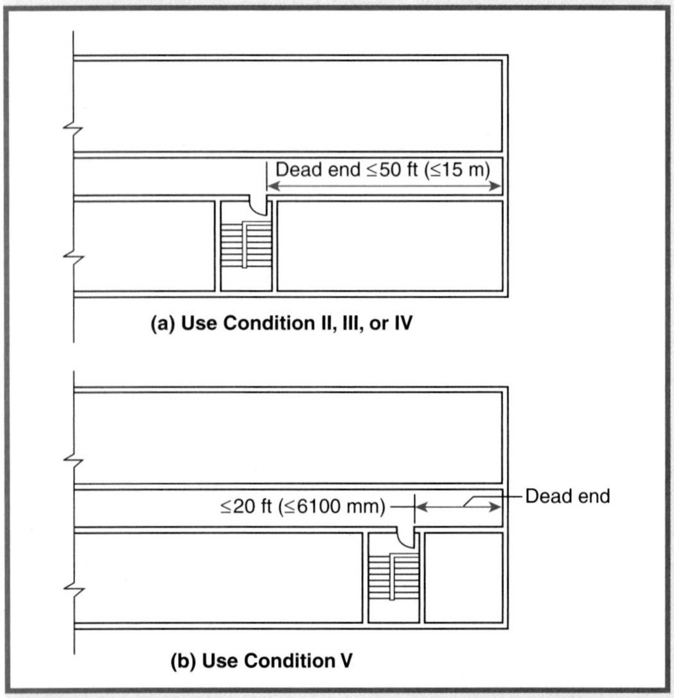


***Exhibit 22/23.4*** *Maximum dead-end corridor for new construction.*

accommodated by exit access leading directly from that level without traveling on any other level that is open to that housing unit. This exemption affords the residents of any level with an exit access that leads to an exit without being exposed to the fire on another

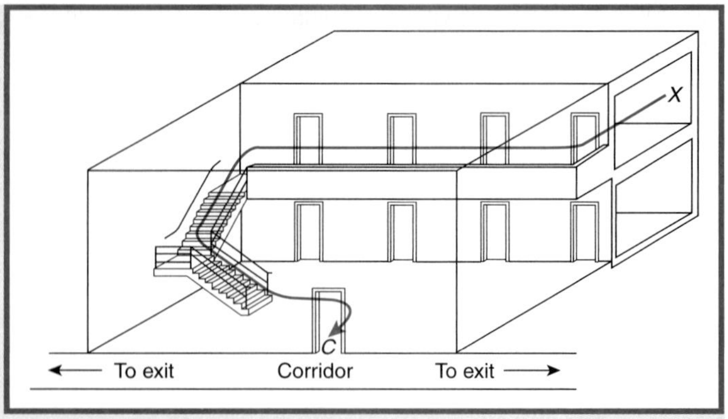


***Exhibit 22/23.5*** *Common path of travel.*

level of the housing unit. Paragraph 23.2.5.3(3) permits existing, excessively long common paths of travel to continue to be used only if specifically approved by the authority having jurisdiction (AHJ).

A security vestibule, called a *sally port*, is addressed in 22/23.2.5.4. A sally port is designed so that, during routine and non-fire-emergency conditions, the door at one end of the vestibule is securely locked whenever the door at the opposite end is open. When one door is opened, the door through which entrance is made is closed and locked; the door at the opposite end is then unlocked and opened to provide egress from the vestibule. The sally port acts as a security device that prevents a continuous flow of people from "storming" the exits. Under fire conditions, a sally port would severely restrict the egress flow of occupants and prevent hose lines from being run through the openings. Therefore, if a sally port is to be permitted as part of a required means of egress, the door controls must be capable of being overridden to allow continuous and unobstructed passage in accordance with 22/23.2.5.4. Exhibit 22/23.6 depicts a sally port.

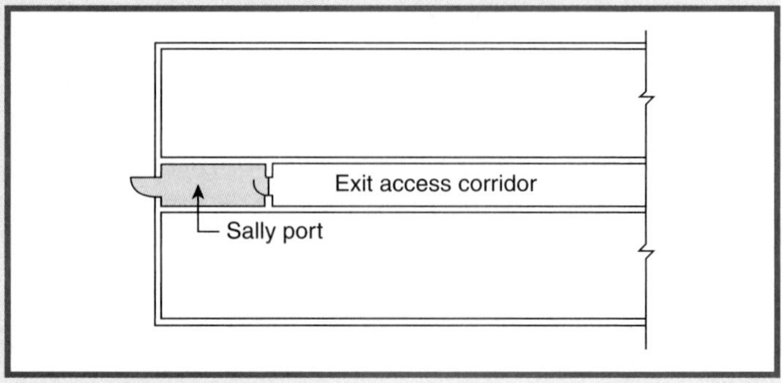


***Exhibit 22/23.6*** *A sally port or security vestibule.*

CHAPTER 22 • New

### 22.2.6 Travel Distance to Exits.

Travel distance shall comply with 22.2.6.1 through 22.2.6.7.

**22.2.6.1** Travel distance shall be measured in accordance with Section 7.6.

**22.2.6.2** The travel distance between any room door required as an exit access and an exit shall not exceed 150 ft (46 m).

**22.2.6.3 Reserved.**

**22.2.6.4** The travel distance between any point in a room and an exit shall not exceed 200 ft (61 m).

**22.2.6.5 Reserved.**

**22.2.6.6** The travel distance between any point in a sleeping room to the door in that room shall not exceed 50 ft (15 m), unless otherwise permitted by 22.2.6.7.

**22.2.6.7** The maximum travel distance limitation of 22.2.6.6 shall be permitted to be increased to 100 ft (30 m) in open dormitories, provided that the following criteria are met:

(1) The enclosing walls of the dormitory space shall be of smoke-tight construction.
(2) Not less than two exit access doors remotely located from each other shall be provided where travel distance to the exit access door from any point within the dormitory exceeds 50 ft (15 m).

CHAPTER 23 • Existing

### 23.2.6 Travel Distance to Exits.

Travel distance shall comply with 23.2.6.1 through 23.2.6.7.

**23.2.6.1** Travel distance shall be measured in accordance with Section 7.6.

**23.2.6.2** The travel distance between any room door required as an exit access and an exit or smoke barrier shall not exceed 100 ft (30 m), unless otherwise permitted by 23.2.6.3.

**23.2.6.3** The maximum travel distance limitations of 23.2.6.2 shall be permitted to be increased by 50 ft (15 m) in buildings protected throughout by an approved automatic sprinkler system in accordance with 23.3.5.3 or a smoke control system.

**23.2.6.4** The travel distance between any point in a room and an exit or smoke barrier shall not exceed 150 ft (46 m), unless otherwise permitted by 23.2.6.5.

**23.2.6.5** The maximum travel distance limitations of 23.2.6.4 shall be permitted to be increased by 50 ft (15 m) in buildings protected throughout by an approved automatic sprinkler system in accordance with 23.3.5.3 or a smoke control system.

**23.2.6.6** The travel distance between any point in a sleeping room to the door of that room shall not exceed 50 ft (15 m), unless otherwise permitted by 23.2.6.7.

**23.2.6.7** The maximum travel distance limitations of 23.2.6.6 shall be permitted to be increased to 100 ft (30 m) in open dormitories, provided that the following criteria are met:

(1) The enclosing walls of the dormitory space shall be of smoke-tight construction.
(2) Not less than two exit access doors remotely located from each other shall be provided where travel distance to the exit access door from any point within the dormitory exceeds 50 ft (15 m).

Exhibit 22/23.7 illustrates the travel distance requirements of 22/23.2.6. Travel distance is measured to the closest exit only, not to both of the exits required by 22/23.2.4. Travel distance is measured along the natural path of travel [see 7.6.1(1)]. The term *sprinklered*, as used in the exhibit, means that the entire building is protected by a complete, approved automatic extinguishing system. New detention and correctional occupancies are required to be sprinklered; thus, they are permitted the longer travel distances. The term *smoke control*, as used in the exhibit, means that the entire building is equipped with a system to control the movement of smoke in accordance with Section 9.3.

CHAPTER 22 • New

### 22.2.7 Discharge from Exits.

**22.2.7.1** Exits shall be permitted to discharge into a fenced or walled courtyard, provided that not more than two walls

CHAPTER 23 • Existing

### 23.2.7 Discharge from Exits.

**23.2.7.1** Exits shall be permitted to discharge into a fenced or walled courtyard, provided that not more than two walls

**CHAPTER 22 • New**

of the courtyard are the building walls from which egress is being made.

**22.2.7.2** Enclosed yards or courts used for exit discharge in accordance with 22.2.7.1 shall be of sufficient size to accommodate all occupants at a distance of not less than 50 ft (15 m) from the building while providing a net area of 15 $ft^2$ (1.4 $m^2$) per person.

**22.2.7.3** All exits shall be permitted to discharge through the level of exit discharge.

**22.2.7.4** The requirements of 7.7.2 shall be waived, provided that not more than 50 percent of the exits discharge into a single fire compartment separated from other compartments by construction having not less than a 1-hour fire resistance rating.

**CHAPTER 23 • Existing**

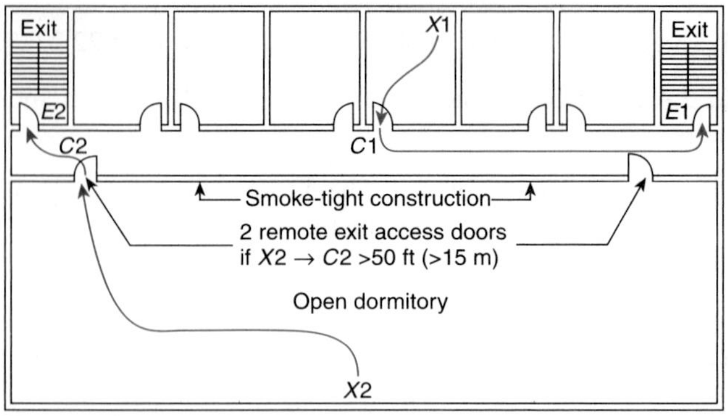


Maximum distance:

*X1*→*C1* ≤50 ft (≤15 m)
*X2*→*C2* ≤100 ft (≤30 m)
*C1*→*E1*, *C2*→*E2* ≤100 ft (≤30 m) [≤150 ft (≤46 m) if sprinklered or equipped with smoke control]
*X1*→*E1* ≤150 ft (≤46 m) [≤200 ft (≤61 m) if sprinklered or equipped with smoke control]
*X2*→*E2* ≤200 ft (≤61 m) [≤250 ft (≤76 m) if sprinklered or equipped with smoke control]

***Exhibit 22/23.7*** *Travel distance to exits in detention and correctional occupancies.*

of the courtyard are the building walls from which egress is being made.

**23.2.7.2** Enclosed yards or courts used for exit discharge in accordance with 23.2.7.1 shall be of sufficient size to accommodate all occupants at a distance of not less than 50 ft (15 m) from the building while providing a net area of 15 $ft^2$ (1.4 $m^2$) per person.

**23.2.7.3** All exits shall be permitted to discharge through the level of exit discharge.

**23.2.7.4** The requirements of 7.7.2 shall be waived, provided that not more than 50 percent of the exits discharge into a single fire compartment separated from other compartments by construction having not less than a 1-hour fire resistance rating.

**23.2.7.5** Where all exits are permitted to discharge through areas on the level of discharge, the following criteria shall be met:

(1) A smoke barrier shall be provided to divide that level into not less than two compartments, with not less than one exit discharging into each compartment.
(2) Each smoke compartment shall have an exit discharge to the building exterior.
(3) The level of discharge shall be provided with automatic sprinkler protection.

(4) Any other portion of the level of discharge with access to the discharge area shall be provided with automatic sprinkler protection or shall be separated from the discharge area in accordance with the requirements for the enclosure of exits. *(See 7.1.3.2.1.)*

Exhibit 22/23.8 and Exhibit 22/23.9 illustrate the requirements of 22/23.2.7.1 and 22/23.2.7.2.

The provisions of 7.7.2 establish criteria under which up to 50 percent of the required exits, in either number or capacity, are permitted to discharge through the level of exit discharge, with the other 50 percent required to discharge directly to the outside. Because of security concerns and the belief that doors to the exterior will not be readily unlocked in detention and correctional occupancies, 22/23.2.7.3 and 22/23.2.7.4 permit 100 percent of the exits to discharge through the level of exit discharge. This exemption is permitted if a minimum 1-hour fire resistance–rated separation that creates at least two fire compartments is provided on the level of exit discharge. Not more than one-half of the exits is permitted to discharge into any one fire compartment.

Paragraph 23.2.7.5 permits a smoke barrier to be substituted for a fire barrier in an existing facility if certain conditions can be met. The travel route along the level of exit discharge must be sprinklered, and the route must be separated from nonsprinklered portions of the level of exit discharge by fire barriers meeting the fire resistance rating requirements applicable to exit enclosures.

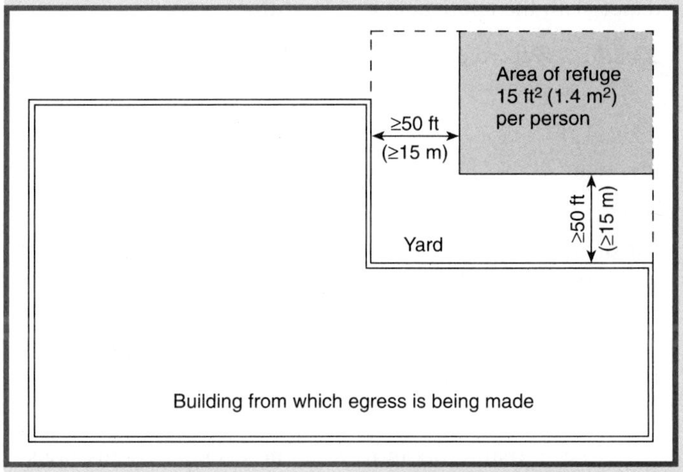


***Exhibit 22/23.8*** *Exit discharge into fenced yard with minimum separation distance from building.*

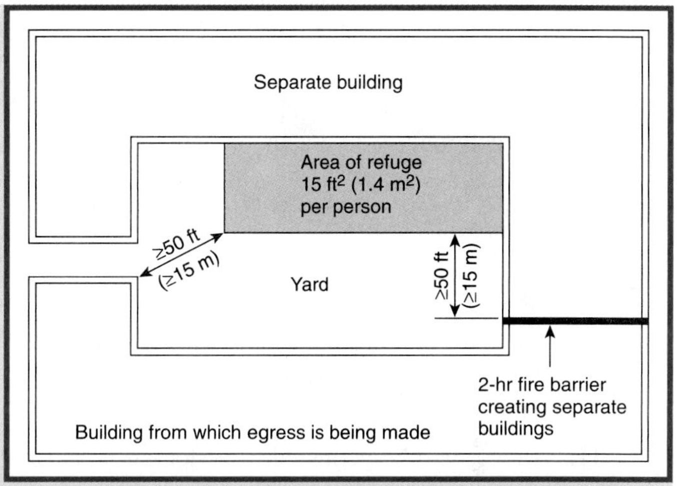


***Exhibit 22/23.9*** *Exit discharge into an enclosed yard with minimum separation distance from "building" from which egress is being made.*

### 22.2.8 Illumination of Means of Egress.

Means of egress shall be illuminated in accordance with Section 7.8.

### 22.2.9 Emergency Lighting.

Emergency lighting shall be provided in accordance with Section 7.9.

### 23.2.8 Illumination of Means of Egress.

Means of egress shall be illuminated in accordance with Section 7.8.

### 23.2.9 Emergency Lighting.

**23.2.9.1** Emergency lighting shall be provided in accordance with Section 7.9, unless otherwise permitted by 23.2.9.2.

**23.2.9.2** Emergency lighting of not less than a 1-hour duration shall be permitted to be provided.

CHAPTER 22 • New

### 22.2.10 Marking of Means of Egress.

Exit marking shall be provided as follows:

(1) Exit signs shall be provided in areas accessible to the public in accordance with Section 7.10.
(2) Exit signs shall not be required in detention and correctional residential housing areas. *(See 3.3.19.1.)*

The exemption of exit signs in sleeping areas of detention and correctional occupancies recognizes that persons occupying such areas are familiar with those portions of the facility and know the location of exits.

### 22.2.11 Special Features.

**22.2.11.1** Doors within means of egress shall be in accordance with Chapter 7, unless otherwise provided in 22.2.11.2 through 22.2.11.12.

**22.2.11.2** Doors shall be permitted to be locked in accordance with the applicable use condition.

**22.2.11.3** Where egress doors are locked with key-operated locks, the provisions of 22.7.7 shall apply.

**22.2.11.4*** Doors to resident sleeping rooms shall be not less than 28 in. (710 mm) in clear width.

**A.22.2.11.4** It might be necessary to provide a certain number of resident sleeping rooms with doors providing a clear width of not less than 32 in. (810 mm) *(see 7.2.1.2)* in order to comply with the requirements for the physically handicapped. Such sleeping rooms should be located where there is a direct accessible route to the exterior or to an area of safe refuge. *(See 22.3.7.)*

**22.2.11.5 Reserved.**

**22.2.11.6** Doors in a means of egress shall be permitted to be of the horizontal-sliding type, provided that the force necessary to slide the door to its fully open position does not exceed 50 lbf (222 N) where a force of 50 lbf (222 N) is simultaneously applied perpendicular to the door.

**22.2.11.7** Doors from areas of refuge to the exterior shall be permitted to be locked with key locks in lieu of locking methods described in 22.2.11.8, the keys to unlock such doors shall be maintained and available at the facility at all times, and the locks shall be operable from the outside.

**22.2.11.8*** Any remote-control release used in a means of egress shall be provided with a reliable means of operation to release locks on all doors and shall be remotely located

CHAPTER 23 • Existing

### 23.2.10 Marking of Means of Egress.

Exit marking shall be provided as follows:

(1) Exit signs shall be provided in areas accessible to the public in accordance with Section 7.10.
(2) Exit signs shall not be required in detention and correctional residential housing areas. *(See 3.3.19.1.)*

Other portions of the facility might not be as familiar to residents and visitors and, thus, must have proper exit marking in accordance with 22/23.2.10.

### 23.2.11 Special Features.

**23.2.11.1** Doors within means of egress shall be in accordance with Chapter 7, unless otherwise provided in 23.2.11.2 through 23.2.11.10.

**23.2.11.2** Doors shall be permitted to be locked in accordance with the applicable use condition.

**23.2.11.3** Where egress doors are locked with key-operated locks, the provisions of 23.7.7 shall apply.

**23.2.11.4*** Doors to resident sleeping rooms shall be not less than 28 in. (710 mm) in clear width.

**A.23.2.11.4** It might be necessary to provide a certain number of resident sleeping rooms with doors providing a clear width of not less than 32 in (810 mm) *(see 7.2.1.2)* in order to comply with the requirements for the physically handicapped. Such sleeping rooms should be located where there is a direct accessible route to the exterior or to an area of safe refuge. *(See 23.3.7.)*

**23.2.11.5** Existing doors to resident sleeping rooms housing four or fewer residents shall be permitted to be not less than 19 in. (485 mm) in clear width.

**23.2.11.6** Doors in a means of egress shall be permitted to be of the horizontal-sliding type, provided that the force necessary to slide the door to its fully open position does not exceed 50 lbf (222 N) where a force of 50 lbf (222 N) is simultaneously applied perpendicular to the door.

**23.2.11.7** Doors from areas of refuge to the exterior shall be permitted to be locked with key locks in lieu of locking methods described in 23.2.11.8, the keys to unlock such doors shall be maintained and available at the facility at all times, and the locks shall be operable from the outside.

**23.2.11.8*** Any remote-control release used in a means of egress shall be provided with a reliable means of operation to release locks on all doors and shall be remotely located

CHAPTER 22 • New

from the resident living areas, unless otherwise permitted by 22.2.11.8.2.

**A.22.2.11.8** A remote position is generally a control point where a number of doors can be unlocked simultaneously, either mechanically or electrically. In areas where there are a number of sleeping rooms, it is impractical for attendants to unlock doors individually. Doors in an exit should be unlocked prior to unlocking sleeping room doors. Sight and sound supervision of resident living areas can be by means of camera and communications systems.

This section of the *Code* does not intend to prohibit Use Condition V facilities, nor does it intend to limit Use Condition V facilities to 10 manually released locks.

**22.2.11.8.1** The remote location of a remote-control release used in a means of egress shall provide sight and sound supervision of the resident living areas.

**22.2.11.8.2** Remote-control locking and unlocking of occupied rooms in Use Condition IV shall not be required, provided that both of the following criteria are met:

(1) Not more than 10 locks need to be unlocked to relocate all occupants from one smoke compartment to an area of refuge as promptly as is required where remote-control unlocking is used. *(See 22.3.7.9 for requirements for smoke barrier doors.)*
(2) Unlocking of all necessary locks is accomplished with not more than two separate keys.

**22.2.11.9** All remote-control release–operated doors shall be provided with a redundant means of operation as follows:

(1) Power-operated sliding doors or power-operated locks shall be constructed so that, in the event of power failure, a manual mechanical means to release and open the doors is provided at each door, and either emergency power arranged in accordance with 7.9.2.3 is provided for the power operation or a remote-control manual mechanical release is provided.
(2) Mechanically operated sliding doors or mechanically operated locks shall be provided with a manual mechanical means at each door to release and open the door.

**22.2.11.10** The provisions of 7.2.1.5.7 for stairway re-entry shall not apply.

**22.2.11.11** Doors unlocked by means of remote control under emergency conditions shall not automatically relock

CHAPTER 23 • Existing

from the resident living area, unless otherwise permitted by 23.2.11.8.2.

**A.23.2.11.8** A remote position is generally a control point where a number of doors can be unlocked simultaneously, either mechanically or electrically. In areas where there are a number of sleeping rooms, it is impractical for attendants to unlock doors individually. Doors in an exit should be unlocked prior to unlocking sleeping room doors. Sight and sound supervision of resident living areas can be by means of camera and communications systems.

This section of the *Code* does not intend to prohibit Use Condition V facilities, nor does it intend to limit Use Condition V facilities to 10 manually released locks.

**23.2.11.8.1** The remote location of a remote-control release used in a means of egress shall provide sight and sound supervision of the resident living areas.

**23.2.11.8.2** Remote-control locking and unlocking of occupied rooms in Use Condition IV shall not be required, provided that both of the following criteria are met:

(1) Not more than 10 locks need to be unlocked to relocate all occupants from one smoke compartment to an area of refuge as promptly as is required where remote-control unlocking is used. *(See 23.3.7.9 for requirements for smoke barrier doors.)*
(2) Unlocking of all necessary locks is accomplished with not more than two separate keys.

**23.2.11.9** All remote-control release–operated doors shall be provided with a redundant means of operation as follows:

(1) Power-operated sliding doors or power-operated locks shall be constructed so that, in the event of power failure, a manual mechanical means to release and open the doors is provided at each door, and either emergency power arranged in accordance with 7.9.2.3 is provided for the power operation or a remote-control manual mechanical release is provided.
(2) A combination of the emergency power–operated release of selected individual doors and remote-control manual mechanical ganged release specified in 23.2.11.9(1) shall be permitted without mechanical release means at each door.
(3) Mechanically operated sliding doors or mechanically operated locks shall be provided with a manual mechanical means at each door to release and open the door.

**23.2.11.10** The provisions of 7.2.1.5.7 for stairway re-entry shall not apply.

when closed, unless specific action is taken at the remote-control location to enable doors to relock.

**22.2.11.12** Emergency power shall be provided for all electric power–operated sliding doors and electric power–-operated locks, unless otherwise permitted by 22.2.11.12.2.

**22.2.11.12.1** The emergency power shall be arranged to automatically operate within 10 seconds upon failure of normal power and to maintain the necessary power source for a minimum of $1^1/_2$ hours.

**22.2.11.12.2** The emergency power specified in 22.2.11.12 shall not be required in facilities with 10 or fewer locks complying with 22.2.11.8.2.

The provision of 22/23.2.11.2 overrides the Chapter 7 requirement that all doors within the required means of egress be unlocked from the side from which egress is to be made and that they be under full control of the building occupants. It recognizes that, to function as intended, a detention and correctional occupancy uses various means of locking. Paragraph 22/23.2.11.2 permits only that degree of locking that is appropriate to a specific use condition. Therefore, a Use Condition II facility, which has more lenient life safety requirements than a Use Condition V facility, cannot contain sleeping rooms that must be individually locked by key. A Use Condition V facility must comply with a more stringent set of requirements than a Use Condition II facility and is permitted to have individual doors manually locked by key.

Paragraph 22/23.2.11.3 references the use of the door inspection provisions of 22/23.7.7. The requirement recognizes that inspection is needed for doors with key-operated locks, especially if the operation of such locks does not occur on a regular basis.

Paragraphs 22/23.2.11.4 and 23.2.11.5 permit door-opening widths smaller than the 32 in. (810 mm) clear width required by 7.2.1.2.3.2 as an operational-based need. Wider door openings make it difficult for staff to prevent residents from "storming" the opening.

Paragraph 7.2.1.4.1 requires that all doors in a means of egress be side-hinged or pivoted-swinging. Paragraph 7.2.1.4.1(4)(c) permits horizontal-sliding door assemblies serving a room or area with an occupant load of fewer than 10, unless prohibited by the applicable occupancy chapter. Although Chapter 22/23 does not prohibit the use of 7.2.1.4.1(4)(c), the provision of 22/23.2.11.6 has the effect of modifying the criteria of 7.2.1.4.1(4)(c). Paragraph 22/23.2.11.6 permits the use of sliding doors, without the 10-person threshold of 7.2.1.4.1(4)(c), but limits the force required to slide the door to its fully open position to not more than a 50 lbf (222 N) where a force of 50 lbf (222 N) is simultaneously applied perpendicular to the door. The requirement is based on helping to ensure that the door can be opened when someone is trying to bind the door in its track by applying a force perpendicular to the door so as to make the door inoperative. The force criteria of 22/23.2.11.6 are meant to be applied to the sliding door addressed by 7.2.1.4.1(4)(c). In addition, 7.2.1.4.1(4)(b) recognizes the limited use of other horizontal-sliding doors in accordance with the provisions of 7.2.1.14. Sliding doors are more desirable, from an operations standpoint, than swinging doors, because residents can use swinging doors as weapons.

Paragraph 22/23.2.11.7 requires that keys be maintained and available. The word "available" means that keys are readily accessible to staff for use at any time for evacuation of occupants. It is important that the following requirements are met:

1. The keys needed to evacuate occupants are accessible at all times.
2. The staff is trained in the location and use of keys.
3. The staff has authorization and standing orders to immediately unlock doors that lead from smoke compartments to the exterior during fire emergency conditions.

Authorizing staff to unlock doors avoids time lost awaiting authorization from administrative authorities before doors are unlocked.

In 22/23.2.11.8, use of the term *remotely located* means outside the area where occupants are restrained. It is not necessary to locate the remote unlocking mechanism in a separate fire area, although doing so might be beneficial. Doors within the exit should be unlocked prior to unlocking sleeping room doors. This precaution prevents jamming of the exit door caused by several people exerting pressure on it.

Paragraph 22/23.2.11.8.2 serves as an exemption to 22/23.2.11.8. It applies to facilities that are seeking classification as Use Condition IV but that have need for up to 10 locks that must be manually released at the door. Where Use Condition IV requires remote locking, it must be provided, except as addressed by the exemption. The exemption permits up to 10 manual locks to allow occupants to move to another fire compartment or smoke compartment while permitting the facility to qualify as having provided remote release. The use of a limited number of manual locks (a maximum of 10), in addition to the possibility of hundreds of remotely released locks within the same facility, does not impose a Use Condition V classification. This exemption might apply in situations involving fewer than 10 doors if a door is secured with more than 1 lock.

Exhibit 22/23.10 and Exhibit 22/23.11 depict two typical arrangements that illustrate the exemption of 22/23.2.11.8.2. In Exhibit 22/23.10, each door is equipped with a single key-operated lock. In Exhibit 22/23.11, a door with a single key-operated lock secures multiple door areas. One manual lock, in addition to the 9 shown in the exhibit, would be permitted, but the lock cannot be located on the smoke barrier door if the smoke compartment contains more than 20 persons, in accordance with 22/23.3.7.9.

The provisions of 22/23.2.11.8.2 have been misinterpreted as meaning that a Use Condition V detention/correctional facility (which, by definition, requires manual unlocking of each door) is limited to a maximum of 10 such manual locks. A Use Condition V facility is permitted to have an unlimited number of manual locks. In fact, 22/23.2.11.8.2 applies only to Use Condition IV facilities and permits a facility to retain its classification as Use Condition IV (i.e., remote release), provided that there are 10 or fewer manually released locks and that unlocking can be achieved with a maximum of two keys.

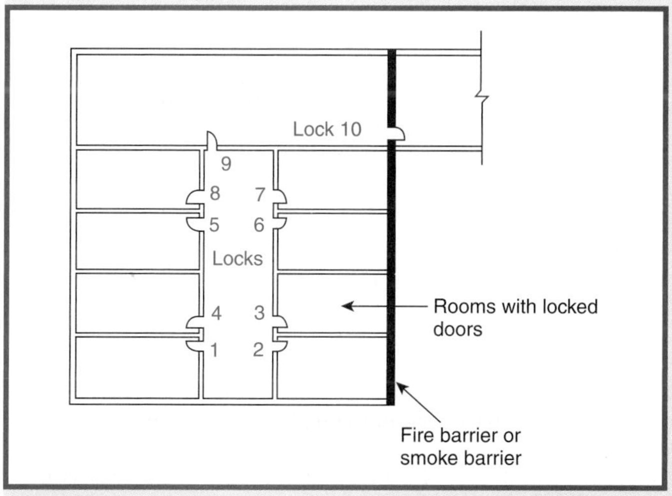


***Exhibit 22/23.10*** *Example of manually unlocked locks permitted within smoke compartment of Use Condition IV facility.*

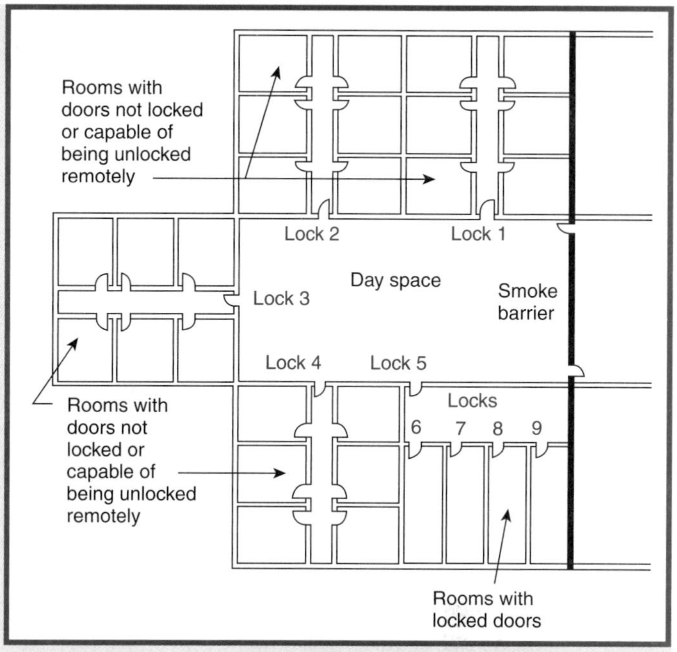


***Exhibit 22/23.11*** *Another example of manually unlocked locks permitted within smoke compartment of Use Condition IV facility.*

The speed with which the doors can be unlocked and the occupants moved to a safe location is critical. If the 10 locks cannot be rapidly released by manual unlocking due to staffing restrictions or for any other reason, remote unlocking must be used. If doors are equipped with locking devices, it is assumed that the locks will be used, and they must be counted as part of the total number of locks.

Paragraph 22.2.11.11, applicable to new facilities, requires that, once doors are remotely unlocked under emergency conditions, they cannot automatically relock if they reclose, unless deliberate action is taken to lock them. This deliberate action can be taken at the individual door or at the remote location. This safety measure prevents occupants from being mistakenly locked into a room during emergency egress.

CHAPTER 22 • New

## 22.3 Protection

### 22.3.1 Protection of Vertical Openings.

Any vertical opening shall be enclosed or protected in accordance with Section 8.6, unless otherwise permitted by the following:

(1) Unprotected vertical openings in accordance with 8.6.8.2 shall be permitted.
(2)* In residential housing area smoke compartments, unprotected vertical openings shall be permitted in accordance with the conditions of 8.6.6, provided that the height between the lowest and highest finished floor levels does not exceed 23 ft (7010 mm), and the following also shall be permitted:
   (a) The number of levels shall not be restricted.
   (b) Residential housing areas subdivided in accordance with 22.3.8 shall be permitted to be considered as part of the communicating space.
   (c) The separation shall not be required to have a fire resistance rating. *[See 8.6.6(4)(b).]*

**A.22.3.1(2)** For purposes of providing control valves and waterflow devices, multilevel residential housing areas complying with this provision are considered to be one story.

CHAPTER 23 • Existing

## 23.3 Protection

### 23.3.1 Protection of Vertical Openings.

**23.3.1.1** Any vertical opening shall be enclosed or protected in accordance with Section 8.6, unless otherwise permitted by the following:

(1) Unprotected vertical openings in accordance with 8.6.8.2 shall be permitted.
(2) In residential housing area smoke compartments protected throughout by an approved automatic sprinkler system in accordance with 23.3.5.3, unprotected vertical openings shall be permitted in accordance with the conditions of 8.6.6, provided that the height between the lowest and highest finished floor levels does not exceed 23 ft (7010 mm), and the following also shall be permitted:
   (a) The number of levels shall not be restricted.
   (b) Residential housing areas subdivided in accordance with 23.3.8 shall be permitted to be considered as part of the communicating space.
   (c) The separation shall not be required to have a fire resistance rating. *[See 8.6.6(4)(b).]*
(3) The requirement of 23.3.1.1 shall not apply to multilevel residential housing areas in accordance with 23.3.1.2.
(4) Where full enclosure is impractical, the required enclosure shall be permitted to be limited to that necessary to prevent a fire originating in any story from spreading to any other story.
(5) Enclosures in detention and correctional occupancies shall have a minimum 1-hour fire resistance rating and shall be protected throughout by an approved automatic sprinkler system in accordance with 23.3.5.3.

**23.3.1.2** Multilevel residential housing areas without enclosure protection between levels shall be permitted, provided that the conditions of 23.3.1.2.1 through 23.3.1.2.3 are met.

**23.3.1.2.1*** The entire normally occupied area, including all communicating floor levels, shall be sufficiently open and unobstructed so that a fire or other dangerous condition in any part is obvious to the occupants or supervisory personnel in the area.

**A.23.3.1.2.1** It is not the intent of this requirement to restrict room face separations, which restrict visibility from the common space into individual sleeping rooms.

**23.3.1.2.2** Egress capacity shall simultaneously accommodate all occupants of all communicating levels and areas, with all communicating levels in the same fire area considered as a single floor area for purposes of determining required egress capacity.

**23.3.1.2.3*** The height between the highest and lowest finished floor levels shall not exceed 13 ft (3960 mm). The number of levels shall not be restricted.

**A.23.3.1.2.3** The vertical separation between the lowest floor level and the uppermost floor level is not to exceed 13 ft (3960 mm). Figure A.23.3.1.2.3 illustrates how the height is to be determined.

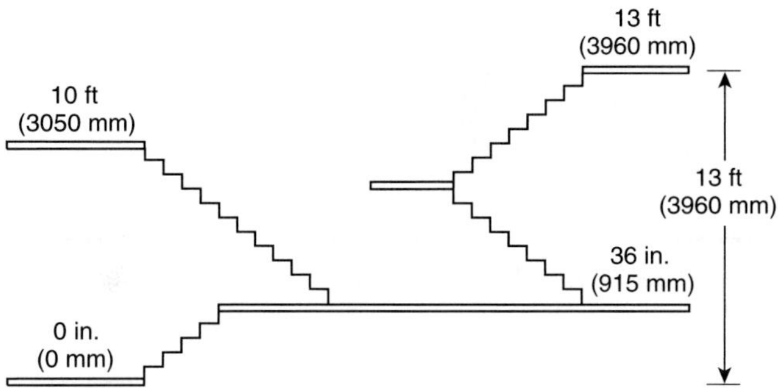


***Figure A.23.3.1.2.3*** *Vertical Height Measurement.*

**23.3.1.3*** A multitiered, open cell block shall be considered as a one-story building where one of the following criteria is met:

(1) A smoke control system is provided to maintain the level of smoke from potential cell fires at not less than 60 in. (1525 mm) above the floor level of any occupied tier involving space that is classified as follows:
    (a) Use Condition IV or Use Condition V
    (b) Use Condition III, unless all persons housed in such space can pass through a free access smoke barrier or freely pass below the calculated smoke level with not more than 50 ft (15 m) of travel from their cells
(2) The entire building, including cells, is provided with complete automatic sprinkler protection in accordance with 23.3.5.3.

Subsection 22/23.3.1 specifies the protection required to maintain floor-to-floor separation, which helps to prevent the products of combustion from moving vertically through the building.

The convenience stair addressed by 8.6.8.2, and recognized by 22.3.1(1) and 23.3.1.1(1), is illustrated in Exhibit 22/23.12 and Exhibit 22/23.13.

Paragraph 8.6.6(1) addresses a vertical opening that is permitted to connect not more than three floor levels. Paragraphs 22.3.1(2) and 23.3.1.1(2) address typical multilevel housing areas that use staggered, partial levels, as depicted in Exhibit 22/23.14. The exemption modifies the three-floor restriction of 8.6.6(1) by permitting a 23 ft (7010 mm) height limitation between the lowest and highest finished floor levels to allow greater flexibility in the design and use of detention and correctional occupancies. The exemption applies only to facilities with residential housing areas that are protected throughout by automatic sprinklers.

Paragraphs 22.3.1(2)(b) and 23.3.1.1(2)(b) clarify that a residential housing unit that complies with the

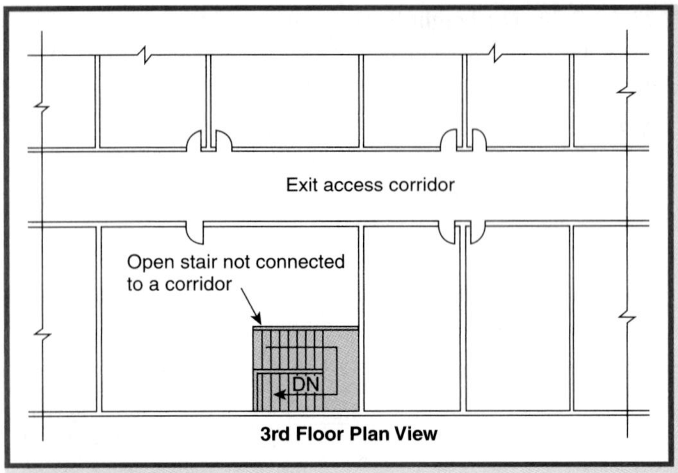


***Exhibit 22/23.12*** *Plan view of unenclosed convenience stair.*

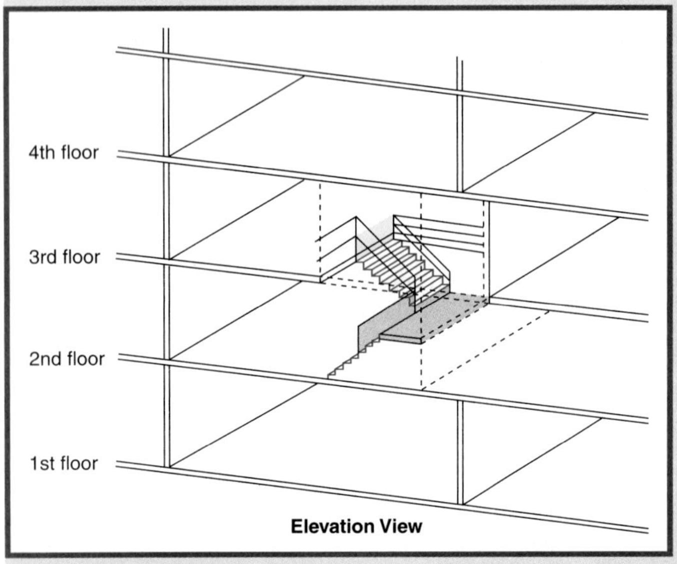


***Exhibit 22/23.13*** *Elevation view of convenience stair.*

requirements of Table 22/23.3.8 is considered to be part of the communicating space addressed by 8.6.6. This clarification prevents the *Code* user from needlessly complying with 8.6.6(4), which would require a fully sprinklered residential area to be separated from all rooms abutting a communicating space (e.g., a day room with a high ceiling) by means of a smoke barrier. If this clarification were not made, all openings, including doors, from resident sleeping rooms to the day space would be required to have smoke-resistant

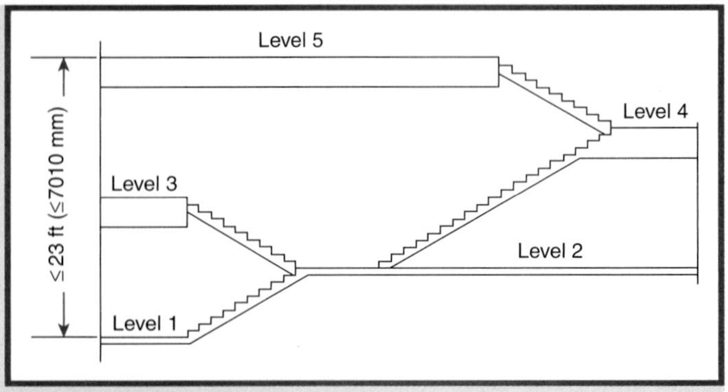


***Exhibit 22/23.14*** *Unprotected vertical openings in sprinklered housing area.*

opening protectives. Such a requirement would place an undue burden on such residential housing units. Instead of requiring smoke barriers between each resident sleeping room and the day space, the *Code* judges that adequate life safety is provided if the residential housing unit is subdivided in accordance with the provisions of 22/23.3.8. Also, compliance with 8.6.6(8) would then be impractical. Paragraph 8.6.6(4)(b) prevents 22.3.1(2)(b) and 23.3.1.1(2)(b) from conflicting with the provisions of 8.6.6(4).

Whereas 22.3.1(2) and 23.3.1.1(2) permit multilevel housing areas with a maximum 23 ft (7010 mm) height between the lowest and the highest finished floor levels if the housing areas are fully sprinklered, 23.3.1.2 permits similar vertical openings in nonsprinklered, existing multilevel housing areas but limits the height of the area served by the openings to 13 ft (3960 mm).

Paragraph 23.3.1.3 addresses an existing multitiered open cell block. A multitiered open cell block in excess of 23 ft (7010 mm) in height, measured between the lowest and highest finished floor levels [see 23.3.1.1(2)], could not be built in compliance with the *Life Safety Code*. However, the provisions of 23.3.1.3 continue to recognize existing, multitiered open cell blocks if (1) smoke control is provided to deal with the limited amount of smoke that a sprinkler-controlled fire generates or (2) automatic sprinkler protection is provided. In addition to the information on smoke control provided in A.23.3.1.3, see the detailed commentary following A.8.6.7(6) on the subject of atrium smoke control. The physics associated with smoke development, spread, and control in a multitiered open cell block is similar to that of an atrium.

**A.23.3.1.3** A recommended method of calculating the expected level of smoke in a smoke removal–equipped cell block follows.

This method for calculating the expected level of smoke has been developed from data experimentally produced in full-scale burnouts of test cells. The test cells were sized, loaded with fuel, and constructed to represent severe conditions of heavily fuel-loaded [approximately 6 $lb/ft^2$ (29 $kg/m^2$)] cells as found in prison locations. The filling rate and temperature of the effluent gas and smoke have been calculated using the data from these tests and established formulae from plume dynamics.

The application of the method described in A.23.3.1.3 should be limited to situations where there is not less than 10 ft (3050 mm) from the floor level to the lowest acceptable level of smoke accumulation *(Z)*; the reservoir above the lowest acceptable level for *Z* is at least 20 percent of the *Z* dimension; the length of the cell block is not less than *Z*; and the fan is not less than 10 ft (3050 mm) higher than the floor of the highest cell.

The determination of smoke removal requirements is based on the dimensions of the cell opening. Where more than one cell opening is involved, the larger size on the level being calculated should be used.

The fan size, temperature rating, and operations means can be determined by the procedure that follows:

*Acceptable Smoke Level.* Determine the lowest acceptable level of smoke accumulation in accordance with 23.3.1.3. The vertical distance between that level and the floor level of the lowest open cell is the value of *Z* to be used in connection with Figure A.23.3.1.3(a).

*Characteristic Cell Opening.* Determine the opening of the cell face. Where there is more than one size of cell opening, use the largest. Match the actual opening to those shown in Figure A.23.3.1.3(b), and use the corresponding curve from Figure A.23.3.1.3(a). If there is no match between the size and shape of the opening and Figure A.23.3.1.3(a), interpolate between the curves. If the opening exceeds 6 ft × 6 ft (1830 mm × 1830 mm), use the curve for a 6 ft × 6 ft (1830 mm × 1830 mm) opening. This curve represents the maximum burning situation, and increasing the size of the opening will not increase the actual burning rate.

*Exhaust Fan Rate.* Determine the exhaust fan capacity needed to extract smoke at a rate that will maintain the smoke level at a point higher than *Z*. This is the rate shown on the baseline of Figure A.23.3.1.3(a) corresponding to the level of *Z* on the vertical axis for the solid line (ventilation rate) curve appropriate to the cell door size. This exhaust capability needs to be provided at a point higher than *Z*.

*Intake Air.* Provide intake air openings that either exist or are automatically provided at times of emergency smoke removal. These openings are to be located at or near the baseline of the cell block to allow for intake air at the rate to be vented by the fan. The openings provided shall be sufficient to avoid a friction load that can reduce the exhaust

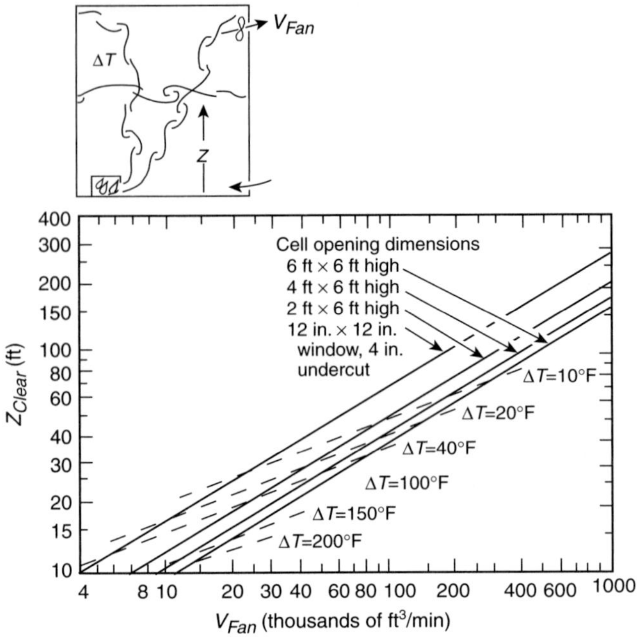


For SI units, 1 ft = 0.3048 m; 1 in. = 25.4 mm;
(°F −32) ÷ 1.8 = °C; 1 ft³/min = 0.00047 m³/s

$\Delta T$ = Temperature of upper layer gases above ambient
$Z_{Clear}$ = Distance from cell floor to smoke layer
$V_{Fan}$ = Fan discharge capacity (as installed)

Solid lines: Ventilation rate curves
Dashed lines: Constant temperature rise curves

***Figure A.23.3.1.3(a)*** *Cell Block Smoke Control Ventilation Curves.*

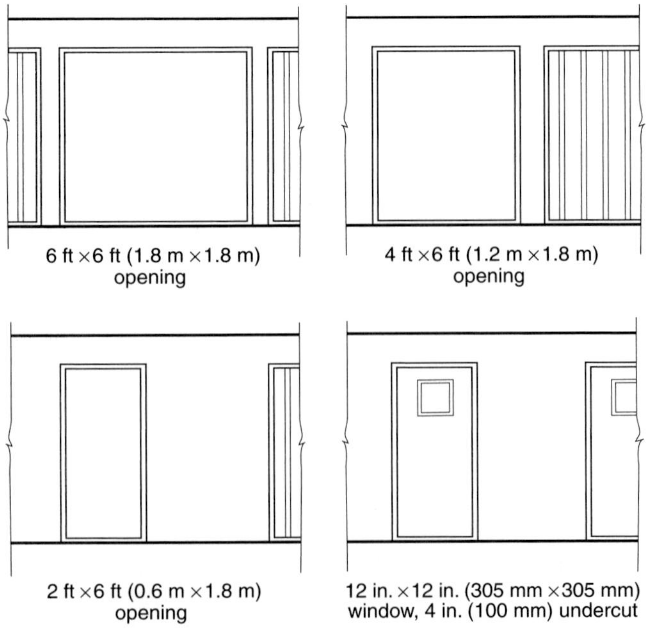


***Figure A.23.3.1.3(b)*** *Typical Cell Openings.*

efficiency. Standard air-handling design criteria are used in making this calculation.

*Fan Temperature Rating.* Determine the potential temperature of gases that the fan might be required to handle by measuring the distance from the floor of the highest cell to the centerline of the fan, or fan ports if the fan is in a duct or similar arrangement. Determine the intersection of the new $Z$ value with the appropriate ventilation rate curve (solid line) from Figure A.23.3.1.3(a). Estimate the temperature rise by interpolating along the appropriate ventilation rate curve and between the constant temperature rise curves (dashed lines) from Figure A.23.3.1.3(a). Provide all elements of the exhaust system that are to be above the acceptable smoke level with the capability to effectively operate with the indicated increase in temperature.

*Operation of Exhaust System.* Arrange the emergency exhaust system to initiate automatically on detection of smoke, on operation of a manual fire alarm system, or by direct manual operation. The capability to manually start the automatic exhaust system should be provided in a guard post in the cell block, at another control location, or both. Where appropriate, the emergency exhaust fans are permitted to be used for comfort ventilation as well as for serving their emergency purposes.

### 22.3.2 Protection from Hazards.

**22.3.2.1*** Any hazardous area shall be protected in accordance with Section 8.7. The areas described in Table 22.3.2.1 shall be protected as indicated.

***Table 22.3.2.1 Hazardous Area Protection***

| Hazardous Area Description | Separation/Protection† |
|---|---|
| Areas not incidental to resident housing | 2 hours |
| Boiler and fuel-fired heater rooms | 1 hour |
| Central or bulk laundries >100 ft² (>9.3 m²) | 1 hour |
| Commercial cooking equipment | In accordance with 9.2.3 |
| Commissaries | Smoke resistant |
| Employee locker rooms | Smoke resistant |
| Hobby/handicraft shops | Smoke resistant |
| Maintenance shops | Smoke resistant |
| Padded cells | 1 hour |
| Soiled linen rooms | 1 hour |
| Storage rooms >50 ft² (>4.6 m²) in area but ≤100 ft² (≤9.3 m²) in area storing combustible material | Smoke resistant |
| Storage rooms >100 ft² (>9.3 m²) storing combustible materials | 1 hour |
| Trash collection rooms | 1 hour |

† Minimum fire resistance rating.

### 23.3.2 Protection from Hazards.

**23.3.2.1*** Any hazardous area shall be protected in accordance with Section 8.7. The areas described in Table 23.3.2.1 shall be protected as indicated.

***Table 23.3.2.1 Hazardous Area Protection***

| Hazardous Area Description | Separation/Protection† |
|---|---|
| Areas not incidental to resident housing | 2 hours |
| Boiler and fuel-fired heater rooms | 1 hour or sprinklers |
| Central or bulk laundries >100 ft² (>9.3 m²) | 1 hour or sprinklers |
| Commercial cooking equipment | In accordance with 9.2.3 |
| Commissaries | 1 hour or sprinklers |
| Employee locker rooms | 1 hour or sprinklers |
| Hobby/handicraft shops | 1 hour or sprinklers |
| Maintenance shops | 1 hour or sprinklers |
| Padded cells | 1 hour and sprinklers |
| Soiled linen rooms | 1 hour or sprinklers |
| Storage rooms >50 ft² (>4.6 m²) in area storing combustible material | 1 hour or sprinklers |
| Trash collection rooms | 1 hour or sprinklers |

†Minimum fire resistance rating.

**A.22.3.2.1** Furnishings are usually the first items ignited in a detention and correctional environment. The type, quantity, and arrangement of furniture and other combustibles are important factors in determining how fast the fire will develop. Furnishings, including upholstered items and wood items, such as wardrobes, desks, and bookshelves, might provide sufficient fuel to result in room flashover, which is the full fire involvement of all combustibles within a room once sufficient heat has been built up within the room.

Combustible loading in any room opening onto a residential housing area should be limited to reduce the potential for room flashover. Rooms in which fuel loads are not controlled, thereby creating a potential for flashover, should be considered hazardous areas. Where fire-rated separation is provided, doors to such rooms, including sleeping rooms, should be self-closing.

It is strongly recommended that padded cells not be used due to their fire record. However, recognizing that they will be used in some cases, provisions for the protection of padded cells are provided. It is recognized that the minimum $^3/_4$-hour fire protection–rated fire door will be violated with the "plant on" of the padding, but a minimum $^3/_4$-hour fire protection–rated fire door should be the base of the assembly.

**22.3.2.2** Where Table 22.3.2.1 requires separations to be smoke resistant, the provision of 8.7.1.2 shall not apply.

**22.3.2.3** Hazardous areas determined by the authority having jurisdiction as not incidental to residents' housing shall be separated by 2-hour fire resistance–rated barriers in conjunction with automatic sprinkler protection.

**22.3.2.4** Where cooking facilities are protected in accordance with 9.2.3, kitchens shall not be required to be provided with roomwide protection.



**A.23.3.2.1** It is strongly recommended that padded cells not be used due to their fire record. However, recognizing that they will be used in some cases, provisions for the protection of padded cells are provided. It is recognized that the minimum $^3/_4$-hour fire protection–rated fire door will be violated with the "plant on" of the padding, but a minimum $^3/_4$-hour fire protection–rated fire door should be the base of the assembly.

**23.3.2.2 Reserved.**

**23.3.2.3** Hazardous areas determined by the authority having jurisdiction as not incidental to residents' housing shall be separated by 2-hour fire resistance–rated barriers in conjunction with automatic sprinkler protection.

**23.3.2.4** Where cooking facilities are protected in accordance with 9.2.3, kitchens shall not be required to be provided with roomwide protection.

Hazardous areas in detention and correctional occupancies are spaces with contents that, due to their nature — as in the case of flammable liquids — or because of the quantity of combustible materials involved, represent a significantly higher hazard than would otherwise be typical of detention and correctional occupancies. Paragraph 22/23.3.2.1 requires hazardous areas to be protected. The protection required by Table 22.3.2.1 for hazardous areas in new facilities was specified knowing that new facilities must be sprinklered. Thus, where Table 22.3.2.1 requires smoke-resistant separation — for example, for employee locker rooms — the actual protection is that provided by both the sprinkler system and the smoke-resistant walls. Similarly, where Table 22.3.2.1 requires 1-hour fire resistance–rated separation, the actual protection is that provided by both the sprinkler system and the fire-rated walls. For existing facilities, the areas listed in Table 23.3.2.1 must be protected by the specified fire resistance–rated separation, sprinklering, or combination of separation and sprinklering.

Paragraph 22.3.2.2 specifies that, where Table 22.3.2.1 requires hazardous area separations to be smoke resistant, it is not the intent to provide a smoke partition in accordance with 8.7.1.2. Rather, a qualitative, lesser level of performance is expected of the required smoke-resistant separation. Such performance is to be judged by the authority having jurisdiction (AHJ).

Padded cells are considered to be severe hazard areas due to high heat release, high rate of combustion, and the quantity of smoke produced by padding materials. Therefore, padded cells must be protected by automatic sprinklers and be separated by 1-hour construction.

Where flammable liquids are handled or stored, NFPA 30, *Flammable and Combustible Liquids Code*,[4] should be consulted to establish the minimum criteria necessary to mitigate this hazard. See also 8.7.3.

Even typical housing area furnishings can provide the combustible loading that will allow room flashover to occur. The potential for flashover should be considered, particularly for nonsprinklered multilevel housing areas permitted by 23.3.1.2. Flashover on a lower level could rapidly deteriorate the tenability of conditions on upper levels, as the products of combustion bank down from the ceiling of the housing area, affecting residents of the upper levels before they can use the means of egress system.

### 22.3.3 Interior Finish.

**22.3.3.1 General.** Interior finish shall be in accordance with Section 10.2.

**22.3.3.2 Interior Wall and Ceiling Finish.** Interior wall and ceiling finish materials complying with Section 10.2 shall be Class A or Class B in corridors, in exits, and in any space not separated from corridors and exits by partitions capable of retarding the passage of smoke; and Class A, Class B, or Class C in all other areas. The provisions of 10.2.8.1 shall not apply.

**22.3.3.3 Interior Floor Finish.**

**22.3.3.3.1** Interior floor finish shall comply with Section 10.2.

**22.3.3.3.2** Interior floor finish in exit enclosures and exit access corridors shall be not less than Class II. The provisions of 10.2.8.2 shall not apply.

**22.3.3.3.3** Interior floor finish shall comply with 10.2.7.1 or 10.2.7.2, as applicable.

### 23.3.3 Interior Finish.

**23.3.3.1 General.** Interior finish shall be in accordance with Section 10.2.

**23.3.3.2 Interior Wall and Ceiling Finish.** Interior wall and ceiling finish materials complying with Section 10.2 shall be Class A or Class B in corridors, in exits, and in any space not separated from corridors and exits by partitions capable of retarding the passage of smoke; and Class A, Class B, or Class C in all other areas.

**23.3.3.3 Interior Floor Finish.**

**23.3.3.3.1** Interior floor finish complying with Section 10.2 shall be Class I or Class II in corridors and exits.

**23.3.3.3.2** Existing floor finish material of Class A or Class B in nonsprinklered smoke compartments and Class A, Class B, or Class C in sprinklered smoke compartments shall be permitted to be continued to be used, provided that it has been evaluated based on tests performed in accordance with 10.2.3.

Paragraph 22/23.3.3.2 imposes stricter interior wall and ceiling finish requirements in exits, corridors, and spaces not separated from the corridor than it does in other use areas. To apply the less stringent requirements within the use areas, the required separation need be only a partition capable of retarding the passage of smoke. The partition must be of substantial construction but is not required to have a fire resistance rating.

Paragraph 23.3.3.3.2 recognizes existing interior floor finish materials that have been tested in accordance with the test procedures specified in 10.2.3.4 for wall and ceiling finish materials (i.e., ASTM E 84, *Standard Test Method for Surface Burning Characteristics of Building Materials*,[5] or ANSI/UL 723, *Standard for Test for Surface Burning Characteristics of Building Materials*[6]) as an exemption to the requirement of 10.2.7 that testing of floor finish materials be performed per NFPA 253, *Standard Method of Test for Critical Radiant Flux of Floor Covering Systems Using a Radiant Heat Energy Source*.[7] ASTM E 84 and ANSI/UL 723 contain the flame spread and smoke development measurement method currently used to evaluate interior wall and ceiling finish materials in accordance with the requirements of Section 10.2. Prior to the 1981 edition of the *Code*, floor finish was tested in accordance with ASTM E 84. Paragraph 23.3.3.3.2 permits material that was tested and approved by this method to remain in use.

CHAPTER 22 • New

## 22.3.4 Detection, Alarm, and Communications Systems.

**22.3.4.1 General.** Detention and correctional occupancies shall be provided with a fire alarm system in accordance with Section 9.6, except as modified by 22.3.4.2 through 22.3.4.4.3.

**22.3.4.2 Initiation.**

**22.3.4.2.1** Initiation of the required fire alarm system shall be by manual means in accordance with 9.6.2, by means of any required detection devices or detection systems, and by means of waterflow alarm in the sprinkler system required by 22.3.5.2, unless otherwise permitted by the following:

(1) Manual fire alarm boxes shall be permitted to be locked, provided that staff is present within the area when it is occupied and staff has keys readily available to unlock the boxes.
(2) Manual fire alarm boxes shall be permitted to be located in a staff location, provided that both of the following criteria are met:
   (a) The staff location is attended when the building is occupied.
   (b) The staff attendant has direct supervision of the sleeping area.

**22.3.4.2.2*** Use of the provision of 9.6.1.8.1.3 shall be permitted only as an exemption to 9.6.1.8.1(2) and (3).

**A.22.3.4.2.2** Where the fire alarm control unit is in an area that is not continuously occupied, automatic smoke detection is needed at the control unit. The provision of 22.3.4.2.2 exempts the smoke detection only at the notification appliance circuit power extenders and the supervising station transmitting equipment.

**22.3.4.3 Notification.**

**22.3.4.3.1 Occupant Notification.** Occupant notification shall be accomplished automatically in accordance with 9.6.3, and the following also shall apply:

(1) A positive alarm sequence shall be permitted in accordance with 9.6.3.4.
(2)* Any smoke detectors required by this chapter shall be permitted to be arranged to alarm at a constantly attended location only and shall not be required to accomplish general occupant notification.

**A.22.3.4.3.1(2)** The staff at the constantly attended location should have the capability to promptly initiate the general alarm function and contact the fire department or have direct communication with a control room or other location that can initiate the general alarm function and contact the fire department.

CHAPTER 23 • Existing

## 23.3.4 Detection, Alarm, and Communications Systems.

**23.3.4.1 General.** Detention and correctional occupancies shall be provided with a fire alarm system in accordance with Section 9.6, except as modified by 23.3.4.2 through 23.3.4.4.4.

**23.3.4.2 Initiation.**

**23.3.4.2.1** Initiation of the required fire alarm system shall be by manual means in accordance with 9.6.2 and by means of any required detection devices or detection systems, unless otherwise permitted by the following:

(1) Manual fire alarm boxes shall be permitted to be locked, provided that staff is present within the area when it is occupied and staff has keys readily available to unlock the boxes.
(2) Manual fire alarm boxes shall be permitted to be located in a staff location, provided that both of the following criteria are met:
   (a) The staff location is attended when the building is occupied.
   (b) The staff attendant has direct supervision of the sleeping area.

**23.3.4.2.2*** Use of the provision of 9.6.1.8.1.3 shall be permitted only as an exemption to 9.6.1.8.1(2) and (3).

**A.23.3.4.2.2** Where the fire alarm control unit is in an area that is not continuously occupied, automatic smoke detection is needed at the control unit. The provision of 23.3.4.2.2 exempts the smoke detection only at the notification appliance circuit power extenders and the supervising station transmitting equipment.

**23.3.4.3 Notification.**

**23.3.4.3.1 Occupant Notification.** Occupant notification shall be accomplished automatically in accordance with 9.6.3, and the following also shall apply:

(1) A positive alarm sequence shall be permitted in accordance with 9.6.3.4.
(2)* Any smoke detectors required by this chapter shall be permitted to be arranged to alarm at a constantly attended location only and shall not be required to accomplish general occupant notification.

**A.23.3.4.3.1(2)** The staff at the constantly attended location should have the capability to promptly initiate the general alarm function and contact the fire department or have direct communication with a control room or other location that can initiate the general alarm function and contact the fire department.

CHAPTER 22 • New

22.3.4.3.2 **Emergency Forces Notification.**

**22.3.4.3.2.1** Fire department notification shall be accomplished in accordance with 9.6.4, unless otherwise permitted by the following:

(1) A positive alarm sequence shall be permitted in accordance with 9.6.3.4.
(2) Any smoke detectors required by this chapter shall not be required to transmit an alarm to the fire department.
(3) This requirement shall not apply where staff is provided at a constantly attended location that meets one of the following criteria:
   (a) It has the capability to promptly notify the fire department.
   (b) It has direct communication with a control room having direct access to the fire department.

**22.3.4.3.2.2** Where the provision of 22.3.4.3.2.1(3) is utilized, the fire plan, as required by 22.7.1.3, shall include procedures for logging of alarms and immediate notification of the fire department.

**22.3.4.4* Detection.** An approved automatic smoke detection system shall be in accordance with Section 9.6, as modified by 22.3.4.4.1 through 22.3.4.4.3, throughout all resident sleeping areas and adjacent day rooms, activity rooms, or contiguous common spaces.

**A.22.3.4.4** Examples of contiguous common spaces are galleries and corridors.

**22.3.4.4.1** Smoke detectors shall not be required in sleeping rooms with four or fewer occupants.

**22.3.4.4.2** Other arrangements and positioning of smoke detectors shall be permitted to prevent damage or tampering, or for other purposes.

**22.3.4.4.2.1** Other arrangements, as specified in 22.3.4.4.2, shall be capable of detecting any fire, and the placement of detectors shall be such that the speed of detection is equivalent to that provided by the spacing and arrangements required by the installation standards referenced in Section 9.6.

**22.3.4.4.2.2** Detectors shall be permitted to be located in exhaust ducts from cells, behind grilles, or in other locations.

**22.3.4.4.2.3** The equivalent performance of the design permitted by 22.3.4.4.2.2 shall be acceptable to the authority having jurisdiction in accordance with the equivalency concepts specified in Section 1.4.

CHAPTER 23 • Existing

**23.3.4.3.2 Emergency Forces Notification.**

**23.3.4.3.2.1** Fire department notification shall be accomplished in accordance with 9.6.4, unless otherwise permitted by the following:

(1) A positive alarm sequence shall be permitted in accordance with 9.6.3.4.
(2) Any smoke detectors required by this chapter shall not be required to transmit an alarm to the fire department.
(3) This requirement shall not apply where staff is provided at a constantly attended location that meets one of the following criteria:
   (a) It has the capability to promptly notify the fire department.
   (b) It has direct communication with a control room having direct access to the fire department.

**23.3.4.3.2.2** Where the provision of 23.3.4.3.2.1(3) is utilized, the fire plan, as required by 23.7.1.3, shall include procedures for logging of alarms and immediate notification of the fire department.

**23.3.4.4 Detection.** An approved automatic smoke detection system shall be in accordance with Section 9.6, as modified by 23.3.4.4.1 through 23.3.4.4.4, throughout all resident housing areas.

**23.3.4.4.1** Smoke detectors shall not be required in sleeping rooms with four or fewer occupants in Use Condition II or Use Condition III.

**23.3.4.4.2** Other arrangements and positioning of smoke detectors shall be permitted to prevent damage or tampering, or for other purposes.

**23.3.4.4.2.1** Other arrangements, as specified in 23.3.4.4.2, shall be capable of detecting any fire, and the placement of detectors shall be such that the speed of detection is equivalent to that provided by the spacing and arrangements required by the installation standards referenced in Section 9.6.

**23.3.4.4.2.2** Detectors shall be permitted to be located in exhaust ducts from cells, behind grilles, or in other locations.

**23.3.4.4.2.3** The equivalent performance of the design permitted by 23.3.4.4.2.2 shall be acceptable to the authority having jurisdiction in accordance with the equivalency concepts specified in Section 1.4.

CHAPTER 22 • New

**22.3.4.4.3*** Smoke detectors shall not be required in Use Condition II open dormitories where staff is present within the dormitory whenever the dormitory is occupied.

**A.22.3.4.4.3** An open dormitory is a dormitory that is arranged to allow staff to observe the entire dormitory area at one time.

CHAPTER 23 • Existing

**23.3.4.4.3*** Smoke detectors shall not be required in Use Condition II open dormitories where staff is present within the dormitory whenever the dormitory is occupied and the building is protected throughout by an approved, supervised automatic sprinkler system in accordance with 23.3.5.3.

**A.23.3.4.4.3** An open dormitory is a dormitory that is arranged to allow staff to observe the entire dormitory area at one time.

**23.3.4.4.4** In smoke compartments protected throughout by an approved automatic sprinkler system in accordance with 23.3.5.3, smoke detectors shall not be required, except in corridors, common spaces, and sleeping rooms with more than four occupants.

In the 2003 and some other earlier editions of the *Code*, alarm systems for detention and correctional occupancies were required to be provided with a secondary power supply in accordance with *NFPA 72®, National Fire Alarm Code®*.[8] The deletion of the requirement for the 2006 edition was not a technical change, as the provision was redundant and already required by *NFPA 72*. Paragraph 22/23.3.4.1 references the use of Section 9.6, which mandates the use of *NFPA 72*. However, the deletion made for the 2006 edition was incomplete and left a remnant of the requirement (i.e., 23.3.4.1.2 of the 2006 edition), which has been deleted for the 2009 edition.

Given that new detention and correctional facilities must be sprinklered, 22.3.4.2.1 requires a waterflow alarm as one of the means for initiating the fire alarm system.

The provision of 22/23.3.4.2.2 is new to the 2009 edition of the *Code*. It was written in response to the new provision of 9.6.1.8.1.2 that permits smoke detection to be omitted from the vicinity of fire alarm system controls where the building is sprinklered. The effect of 22/23.3.4.2.2 is to require smoke detection at the fire alarm control unit, regardless of whether the building is sprinklered.

By being silent on the subject, 22/23.3.4.3.1 does not permit presignal systems. Rather, notification must be provided without delay in accordance with 9.6.3, or the more reliable form of presignal — called positive alarm sequence — can be used if complying with 9.6.3.4. However, to avoid numerous nuisance alarms, smoke detectors are exempted from sounding a general alarm.

Where the fire department is not equipped to receive alarms or where direct transmission to the fire department is not permitted, the provisions of 22/23.3.4.3.2 require that arrangements be made for the prompt notification of the fire department. One means of notification is by an approved central station alarm system. Subsection 9.6.4 provides several options for notifying the fire department automatically. Where smoke detectors are provided, they are not required to sound the fire alarm or to transmit a signal to the fire department, but are required to sound an alarm at a constantly attended location, unless otherwise specified.

Paragraph 22/23.3.4.4.3 is an exemption to the smoke detection system requirement. It applies to Use Condition II open dormitories where staff are present within the dormitory whenever the dormitory is occupied. Note that Use Condition II facilities must allow free movement from sleeping areas to another smoke compartment. The concept employed is one of relying on awake and alert staff within the dormitory to act as human fire detectors, provide early warning, and allow residents to move into a safe smoke compartment.

### 22.3.5 Extinguishment Requirements.

**22.3.5.1** High-rise buildings shall comply with 22.4.3.

**22.3.5.2** All buildings classified as Use Condition II, Use Condition III, Use Condition IV, or Use Condition V shall be protected throughout by an approved, supervised automatic sprinkler system in accordance with 22.3.5.3.

### 23.3.5 Extinguishment Requirements.

**23.3.5.1** High-rise buildings shall comply with 23.4.3.

**23.3.5.2*** Where required by Table 23.1.6.1, facilities shall be protected throughout by an approved, supervised automatic sprinkler system in accordance with 23.3.5.3.

**A.23.3.5.2** Where the openings in ceilings or partitions are $^1/_4$ in. (6.3 mm) or larger in the smallest dimension, where the thickness or depth of the material does not exceed the smallest dimension of the openings, and where such openings constitute not less than 70 percent of the area of the ceiling or partition material, the disruption of sprinkler spray patterns is permitted to be disregarded.

**22.3.5.3** The automatic sprinkler system required by 22.3.5.2 shall be as follows:

(1) In accordance with Section 9.7
(2) Installed in accordance with 9.7.1.1(1)
(3) Electrically connected to the fire alarm system
(4) Fully supervised

**22.3.5.4** Portable fire extinguishers shall be provided in accordance with 9.7.4.1, unless otherwise permitted by the following:

(1)* Access to portable fire extinguishers shall be permitted to be locked.

**A.22.3.5.4(1)** Where access to portable fire extinguishers is locked, staff should be present on a 24-hour basis and should have keys readily available to unlock access to the extinguishers. Where supervision of sleeping areas is from a 24-hour attended staff location, portable fire extinguishers are permitted to be provided at the staff location in lieu of the sleeping area.

(2) Portable fire extinguishers shall be permitted to be located at staff locations only.

**22.3.5.5** Standpipe and hose systems shall be provided in accordance with 9.7.4.2 as follows, unless otherwise permitted by 22.3.5.6:

(1) Class I standpipe systems shall be provided for any building three or more stories in height.
(2) Class III standpipe and hose systems shall be provided for all nonsprinklered buildings three or more stories in height.

**22.3.5.6** The requirements of 22.3.5.5 shall not apply where otherwise permitted by the following:

(1) Formed hose, 1 in. (25 mm) in diameter, on hose reels shall be permitted to provide Class II service.
(2) Separate Class I and Class II systems shall be permitted in lieu of a Class III system.

**23.3.5.3** Where this *Code* permits exceptions for fully sprinklered detention and correctional occupancies or sprinklered smoke compartments, the sprinkler system shall be as follows:

(1) In accordance with Section 9.7
(2) Installed in accordance with 9.7.1.1(1)
(3) Electrically connected to the fire alarm system
(4) Fully supervised

**23.3.5.4** Portable fire extinguishers shall be provided in accordance with 9.7.4.1, unless otherwise permitted by the following:

(1)* Access to portable fire extinguishers shall be permitted to be locked.

**A.23.3.5.4(1)** Where access to portable fire extinguishers is locked, staff should be present on a 24-hour basis and should have keys readily available to unlock access to the extinguishers. Where supervision of sleeping areas is from a 24-hour attended staff location, portable fire extinguishers are permitted to be provided at the staff location in lieu of the sleeping area.

(2) Portable fire extinguishers shall be permitted to be located at staff locations only.

**23.3.5.5** Standpipe and hose systems shall be provided in accordance with 9.7.4.2 as follows, unless otherwise permitted by 23.3.5.6:

(1) Class I standpipe systems shall be provided for any building three or more stories in height.
(2) Class III standpipe and hose systems shall be provided for all nonsprinklered buildings three or more stories in height.

**23.3.5.6** The requirements of 23.3.5.5 shall not apply where otherwise permitted by the following:

(1) Formed hose, 1 in. (25 mm) in diameter, on hose reels shall be permitted to provide Class II service.
(2) Separate Class I and Class II systems shall be permitted in lieu of a Class III system.

Paragraph 22.3.5.1, applicable to new facilities in high-rise buildings, refers to 22.4.3, which, in turn, mandatorily references 11.8.3 — which addresses those high-rise building provisions applicable to automatic sprinkler systems and standpipes. Paragraph 23.3.5.1, applicable to existing facilities in high-rise buildings, refers to 23.4.3, which, in turn, mandates an automatic sprinkler system, but not standpipes. For both new and existing facilities, a sprinkler control valve and waterflow device must be provided for each floor. The control valve facilitates maintaining other zones of the sprinkler system operative when one zone is being serviced. The waterflow device provides staff with an indication of where sprinkler water is flowing in the building.

Paragraph 22.3.5.2 requires that new detention and correctional occupancies be protected throughout by approved, supervised automatic sprinkler systems. However, in establishing the sprinkler requirement, the Technical Committee on Detention and Correctional Occupancies realized that rehabilitation, modernizations, and renovations might take place in nonsprinklered existing buildings. Thus, 22.4.4 provides additional criteria needed for the proper protection of nonsprinklered existing building renovations.

Where automatic sprinklers are installed to comply with the *Code*, the system must be a complete, approved automatic sprinkler system installed in accordance with NFPA 13, *Standard for the Installation of Sprinkler Systems*.[9] The use of manually operated sprinklers is not recognized by the *Code*. Informal surveys of detention and correctional occupancy staff indicate no significant problems with the installation, maintenance, and use of automatic sprinkler systems in detention and correctional facilities. The system must also be supervised in accordance with the requirements of 9.7.2 to comply with the *Code*.

Exhibit 22/23.15 illustrates a typical institutional sprinkler. The sprinkler body and frame are designed to prevent residents from hanging items or themselves from the sprinkler.

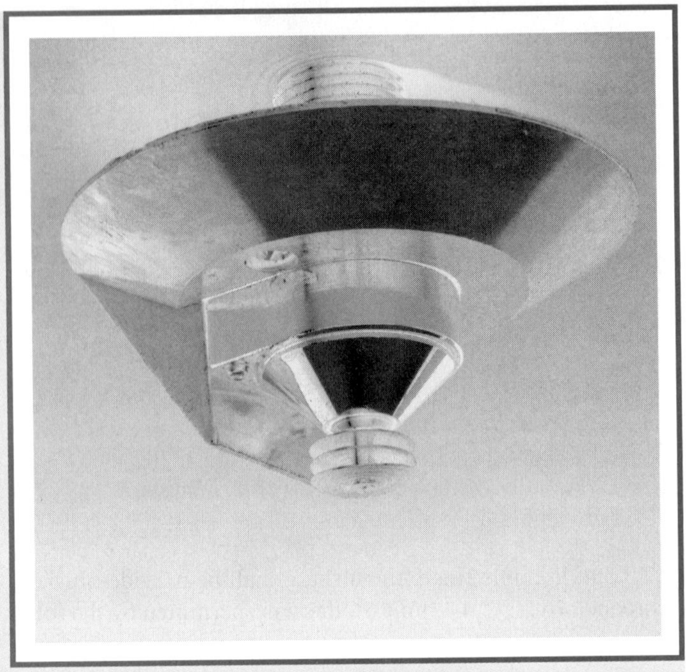

***Exhibit 22/23.15*** *Typical institutional sprinkler.*

Paragraph 22/23.3.5.4(1) permits portable fire extinguishers to be locked away. Time is critical when using extinguishers; therefore, keys must be carried by the staff or be readily accessible.

The requirements of 22/23.3.5.5 for standpipes intend that $2^1/_2$ in. (63 mm) hose connections be available for fire department use in any detention and correctional occupancy more than two stories in height. In addition, if such buildings are nonsprinklered, $1^1/_2$ in. (38 mm) connections and hose for staff and resident use are also required.

Paragraph 22/23.3.5.6(1) permits the use of 1 in. (25 mm) formed rubber hose in place of the fabric-jacketed, rubber-lined hose normally required in standpipe systems. The rubber hose is normally stored on reels and is easier to use.

### 22.3.6 Corridors.

See 22.3.8.

### 22.3.7 Subdivision of Building Spaces.

**22.3.7.1** Smoke barriers shall be provided to divide every story used for sleeping by residents, or any other story having an occupant load of 50 or more persons, into not less

### 23.3.6 Corridors.

See 23.3.8.

### 23.3.7 Subdivision of Building Spaces.

**23.3.7.1*** Smoke barriers shall be provided to divide every story used for sleeping by 10 or more residents, or any other story having an occupant load of 50 or more persons, into

CHAPTER 22 • New

than two compartments, unless otherwise permitted by the following:

(1) Protection shall be permitted to be accomplished using horizontal exits. *(See 7.2.4.)*
(2)* The requirement for subdivision of building space shall be permitted to be fulfilled by one of the following:
   (a) Smoke compartments having exit to a public way, where such exit serves only one area and has no openings to other areas
   (b) Building separated from the resident housing area by a 2-hour fire resistance rating or 50 ft (15 m) of open space
   (c) Secured, open area having a holding space located 50 ft (15 m) from the housing area that provides 15 $ft^2$ (1.4 $m^2$) or more of refuge area for each person (resident, staff, visitors) potentially present at the time of a fire

**A.22.3.7.1(2)** A door to the outside, by itself, does not meet the intent of this provision if emergency operating procedures do not provide for the door to be unlocked when needed. In cases where use of the door is not ensured, a true smoke barrier per the base requirement of 22.3.7.1 would be needed.

**22.3.7.2** Doors used to access the areas specified in 22.3.7.1(2)(a), (b), and (c) shall meet the requirements for doors at smoke barriers for the applicable use condition.

**22.3.7.3** Where smoke barriers are required by 22.3.7.1, they shall be provided as follows:

(1) They shall limit the occupant load to not more than 200 residents in any smoke compartment.
(2) They shall limit the travel distance to a door in a smoke barrier as follows:
   (a) The distance from any room door required as exit access shall not exceed 150 ft (46 m).
   (b) The distance from any point in a room shall not exceed 200 ft (61 mm).

**22.3.7.4 Reserved.**

CHAPTER 23 • Existing

not less than two compartments, unless otherwise permitted by the following:

(1) Protection shall be permitted to be accomplished using horizontal exits. *(See 7.2.4.)*
(2)* The requirement for subdivision of building space shall be permitted to be fulfilled by one of the following:
   (a) Smoke compartments having exit to a public way, where such exit serves only one area and has no openings to other areas
   (b) Building separated from the resident housing area by a 2-hour fire resistance rating or 50 ft (15 m) of open space
   (c) Secured, open area having a holding space located 50 ft (15 m) from the housing area that provides 15 $ft^2$ (1.4 $m^2$) or more of refuge area for each person (resident, staff, visitors) potentially present at the time of a fire

**A.23.3.7.1** Consideration can be given for large open areas that might be permitted to function as smoke sinks as an alternative to the installation of more than one smoke barrier as required by 23.3.7.1. Vertical movement downward to an area of refuge might be permitted by the authority having jurisdiction in lieu of horizontal movement.

**A.23.3.7.1(2)** A door to the outside, by itself, does not meet the intent of this provision if emergency operating procedures do not provide for the door to be unlocked when needed. In cases where use of the door is not ensured, a true smoke barrier per the base requirement of 23.3.7.1 would be needed.

**23.3.7.2** Doors used to access the areas specified in 23.3.7.1(2)(a), (b), and (c) shall meet the requirements for doors at smoke barriers for the applicable use condition.

**23.3.7.3** Where smoke barriers are required by 23.3.7.1, they shall be provided as follows:

(1) They shall limit the occupant load to not more than 200 residents in any smoke compartment.
(2)* They shall limit the travel distance to a door in a smoke barrier, unless otherwise permitted by 23.3.7.4, as follows:
   (a) The distance from any room door required as exit access shall not exceed 100 ft (30 m).
   (b) The distance from any point in a room shall not exceed 150 ft (46 m).

**A.23.3.7.3(2)** Consideration should be given to increasing the travel distance to a smoke barrier to coincide with existing range lengths and exits.

**23.3.7.4** The maximum travel distance to a door in a smoke barrier shall be permitted to be increased by 50 ft (15 m) in

CHAPTER 22 • New

**22.3.7.5*** Any required smoke barrier shall be constructed in accordance with Section 8.5, shall be of substantial construction, and shall have structural fire resistance.

**A.22.3.7.5** Structural fire resistance is defined as the ability of the assembly to stay in place and maintain structural integrity without consideration of heat transmission. Twelve-gauge steel plate suitably framed and stiffened meets this requirement.

**22.3.7.6** Openings in smoke barriers shall be protected in accordance with Section 8.5, unless otherwise permitted by the following:

(1)* The total number of vision panels in any barrier shall not be restricted.

**A.22.3.7.6(1)** As an example, a smoke barrier is permitted to consist of fire-rated glazing panels mounted in a security grille arrangement.

(2) Sliding doors in smoke barriers that are designed to normally be kept closed and are remotely operated from a continuously attended location shall not be required to be self-closing.

**22.3.7.7** Not less than 6 net ft$^2$ (0.55 net m$^2$) per occupant shall be provided on each side of the smoke barrier for the total number of occupants in adjoining compartments, and this space shall be readily available wherever occupants are moved across the smoke barrier in a fire emergency.

**22.3.7.8** Doors shall provide resistance to the passage of smoke. Swinging doors shall be self-latching, or the opening resistance of the door shall be not less than 5 lbf (22 N).

**22.3.7.9** Doors in smoke barriers shall conform with the requirements for doors in means of egress as specified in Section 22.2 and shall have locking and release arrangements according to the applicable use condition. The provisions of 22.2.11.8.2 shall not be used for smoke barrier doors serving a smoke compartment containing more than 20 persons.

**22.3.7.10** Vision panels shall be provided in smoke barriers at points where the barrier crosses an exit access corridor.

**22.3.7.11** Smoke dampers shall be provided in accordance with 8.5.5, unless otherwise permitted by 22.3.7.12.

**22.3.7.12** Arrangements and positioning of smoke detectors required by 22.3.7.11 shall be permitted to prevent damage

CHAPTER 23 • Existing

smoke compartments protected throughout by an approved automatic sprinkler system in accordance with 23.3.5.3 or an automatic smoke control system.

**23.3.7.5*** Any required smoke barrier shall be constructed in accordance with Section 8.5, shall be of substantial construction, and shall have a structural fire resistance.

**A.23.3.7.5** Structural fire resistance is defined as the ability of the assembly to stay in place and maintain structural integrity without consideration of heat transmission. Twelve-gauge steel plate suitably framed and stiffened meets this requirement.

**23.3.7.6** Openings in smoke barriers shall be protected in accordance with Section 8.5, unless otherwise permitted by the following:

(1)* The total number of vision panels in any barrier shall not be restricted.

**A.23.3.7.6(1)** As an example, a smoke barrier is permitted to consist of fire-rated glazing panels mounted in a security grille arrangement.

(2) Sliding doors in smoke barriers that are designed to normally be kept closed and are remotely operated from a continuously attended location shall not be required to be self-closing.

**23.3.7.7** Not less than 6 net ft$^2$ (0.55 net m$^2$) per occupant shall be provided on each side of the smoke barrier for the total number of occupants in adjoining compartments, and this space shall be readily available wherever occupants are moved across the smoke barrier in a fire emergency.

**23.3.7.8** Doors shall provide resistance to the passage of smoke. Swinging doors shall be self-latching, or the opening resistance of the door shall be not less than 5 lbf (22 N). Such doors shall not be required to swing in the direction of egress travel.

**23.3.7.9** Doors in smoke barriers shall conform with the requirements for doors in means of egress as specified in Section 23.2 and shall have locking and release arrangements according to the applicable use condition. The provisions of 23.2.11.8.2 shall not be used for smoke barrier doors serving a smoke compartment containing more than 20 persons.

**23.3.7.10** Vision panels shall be provided in smoke barriers at points where the barrier crosses an exit access corridor.

**23.3.7.11** Smoke dampers shall be provided in accordance with 8.5.5, unless otherwise permitted by 23.3.7.12.

**23.3.7.12** Arrangements and positioning of smoke detectors required by 23.3.7.11 shall be permitted to prevent damage

CHAPTER 22 • New

or tampering, or for other purposes, provided that the following criteria are met:

(1) Such arrangements shall be capable of detecting any fire.
(2) The placement of detectors shall be such that the speed of detection is equivalent to that provided by the spacing and arrangement required by *NFPA 72, National Fire Alarm Code*, as referenced in 8.5.5.7.1.

CHAPTER 23 • Existing

or tampering, or for other purposes, provided that the following criteria are met:

(1) Such arrangements shall be capable of detecting any fire.
(2) The placement of detectors shall be such that the speed of detection is equivalent to that provided by the spacing and arrangement required by *NFPA 72, National Fire Alarm Code*, as referenced in 8.5.5.7.1.

Smoke barriers and horizontal exits used to subdivide a building serve the following three purposes that are fundamental to the protection of occupants:

1. They limit the spread of fire and fire-produced contaminants.
2. They limit the number of occupants exposed to a single fire.
3. They provide for horizontal relocation of occupants by creating a safe area on the same floor.

The requirements of 22/23.3.7.1 and 22/23.3.7.3 for subdividing building spaces are illustrated in Exhibit 22/23.16. Exhibit 22/23.17 illustrates the requirements of 22/23.3.7.1(2). In Exhibit 22/23.17, the door from the resident housing building to the yard can be locked only to the degree that a smoke barrier door can be locked for the applicable use condition.

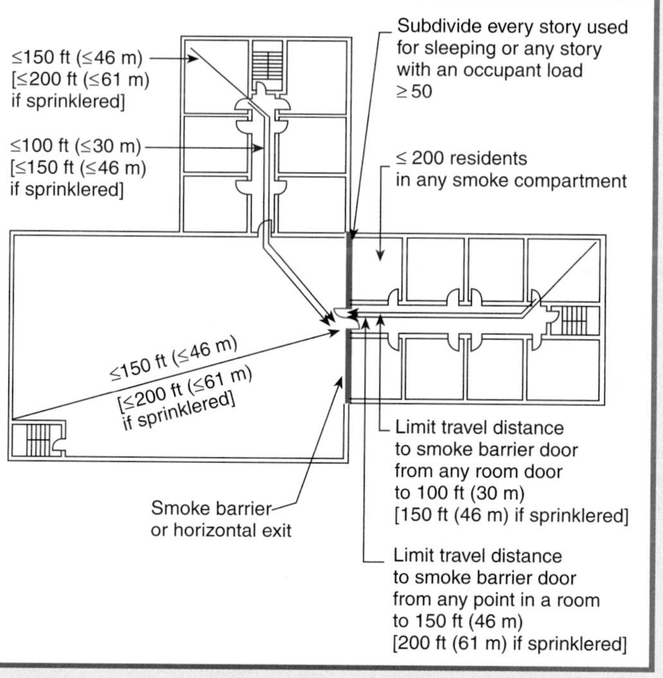


***Exhibit 22/23.16** Subdivision of building spaces into smoke compartments using smoke barriers.*

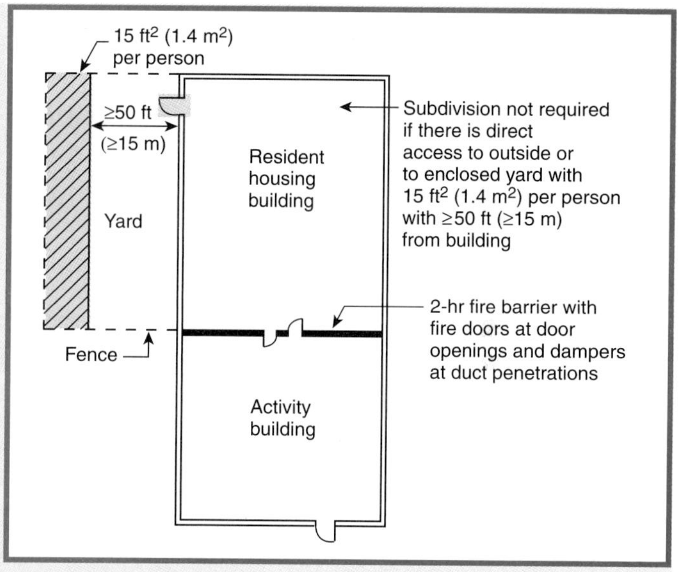


***Exhibit 22/23.17** Alternatives to subdivision by smoke barriers.*

Although it does not specify a required fire resistance rating, 22/23.3.7.5 requires smoke barriers to have structural fire resistance. The intent is to eliminate the use of highly combustible or flimsy materials, such as plastic sheeting, that might possibly limit smoke movement but that have little structural integrity.

The doors in the required smoke barriers must resist the passage of smoke for the same reason that smoke barriers must resist the passage of smoke. The door constructed of materials that resist the passage of smoke will stop smoke from traveling across the door opening only if the door remains tightly closed. Therefore, 22/23.3.7.8 requires that the door, which 8.5.4.4 requires to be either self-closing or automatic-closing, also must be self-latching or must provide a 5 lbf (22 N) resistance to opening, as a minimum. This combination of requirements should help to ensure that the door will be closed under smoke conditions and remain closed, even under the pressures generated by a fire, to resist the passage of smoke.

CHAPTER 22 • New | CHAPTER 23 • Existing

The provisions of 22/23.2.11.8.2 permit up to 10 locks that require manual unlocking in a timely fashion and still be considered as providing the degree of remote unlocking necessary to satisfy the requirements of a Use Condition IV facility — as opposed to a Use Condition V facility. However, 22/23.3.7.9 does not permit locks on smoke barrier doors to be part of the maximum 10 manually unlocked locks where a smoke compartment houses more than 20 persons. This limitation emphasizes the importance of maintaining a means of egress system within a Use Condition IV facility (i.e., where remote release is required) housing more than 20 persons per smoke compartment that allows resident movement to another smoke compartment without having to manually release the lock on the smoke barrier door. A manually released lock on the smoke barrier door would force a reclassification of the facility to Use Condition V and compliance with the more stringent requirements applicable to that classification.

### 22.3.8* Special Protection Features — Subdivision of Resident Housing Spaces.

Subdivision of facility spaces shall comply with Table 22.3.8.

### 23.3.8* Special Protection Features — Subdivision of Resident Housing Spaces.

Subdivision of facility spaces shall comply with Table 23.3.8.

*Table 22.3.8 Subdivision of Resident Housing Spaces*

| Feature | Use Condition II | Use Condition III | | Use Condition IV | | Use Condition V |
|---|---|---|---|---|---|---|
| Room to room separation | NR | NR | | NR | | SR |
| Room face to corridor separation | NR | NR | | NR | | SR |
| Room face to common space separation | NR | NR ≤50 ft (≤15 m)† | SR >50 ft (>15 m)† | NR ≤50 ft (≤15 m)† | SR >50 ft (>15 m)† | SR |
| Common space to corridor separation | NR | NR | | NR | | SR |
| Total openings in solid room face where room face is required to be smoke resistant or fire rated‡ | 0.85 ft² (0.08 m²) | 0.85 ft² (0.08 m²) | | 0.85 ft² (0.08 m²) | | 0.85 ft² (0.08 m²) where meeting one of the following:<br>(1) Kept in closed position, except when in use by staff<br>(2) Closable from the inside<br>(3) Provided with smoke control |

NR: No requirement. SR: Smoke resistant.

Notes:

(1) Doors in openings in partitions required to be smoke resistant (SR) in accordance with Table 22.3.8 are required to be substantial doors of construction that resists the passage of smoke. Latches and door closers are not required on cell doors.

(2) Under Use Condition II, Use Condition III, or Use Condition IV, a space subdivided by open construction (any combination of grating doors and grating walls or solid walls) is permitted to be considered one room if housing not more than 16 persons. The perimeter walls of such space are required to be of smoke-resistant construction. Smoke detection is required to be provided in such space. Under Use Condition IV, common walls between sleeping areas within the space are required to be smoke resistant, and grating doors and fronts are permitted to be used. Under Use Condition II and Use Condition III, open dormitories are permitted to house more than 16 persons, as permitted by other sections of this chapter.

(3) Where barriers are required to be smoke resistant (SR), the provisions of Sections 8.4 and 8.5 do not apply.

†Travel distance through the common space to the exit access corridor.

‡"Total openings in solid room face" include all openings (for example, undercuts, food passes, grilles), the total of which is not to exceed 0.85 ft² (0.08 m²). All openings are required to be 36 in. (915 mm) or less above the floor.

*Table 23.3.8 Subdivision of Resident Housing Spaces*

| | Use Condition | | | | | | | |
|---|---|---|---|---|---|---|---|---|
| | II | | III | | IV | | V | |
| Feature | NS | AS | NS | AS | NS | AS | NS | AS |
| Room to room separation | NR | NR | NR | NR | SR | NR | SR | SR[a] |
| Room face to corridor separation | NR | NR | SR[b] | NR | SR[b] | NR | FR[b] | SR[a] |
| Room face to common space separation | NR | NR | NR ≤50 ft (≤15 m)[c]<br>SR[b] >50 ft (>15 m)[c] | NR ≤50 ft (≤15 m)[c]<br>SR[b] >50 ft (>15 m)[c] | SR[b] | NR ≤50 ft (≤15 m)[c]<br>SR[a] >50 ft (>15 m)[c] | SR[b] | SR[a] |
| Common space to corridor separation | SR | NR | SR | NR | SR | NR | FR | SR[a] |
| Total openings in solid room face where room face is required to be smoke resistant or fire rated[d] | 0.85 ft$^2$ (0.08 m$^2$) | | 0.85 ft$^2$ (0.08 m$^2$) | | 0.85 ft$^2$ (0.08 m$^2$) | | 0.85 ft$^2$ (0.08 m$^2$) where meeting one of the following:<br>(1) Kept in closed position, except when in use by staff<br>(2) Closable from the inside<br>(3) Provided with smoke control | |

NS: Not protected by automatic sprinklers. AS: Protected by automatic sprinklers. NR: No requirement. SR: Smoke resistant. FR: Minimum 1-hour fire resistance rating.

Notes:

(1) Doors in openings in partitions required to be fire rated (FR) in accordance with Table 23.3.8, in other than required enclosures of exits or hazardous areas, are required to be substantial doors of construction that resists fire for a minimum of 20 minutes. Vision panels with wired glass or glass with not less than 45-minute fire-rated glazing are permitted. Latches and door closers are not required on cell doors.

(2) Doors in openings in partitions required to be smoke resistant (SR) in accordance with Table 23.3.8 are required to be substantial doors of construction that resists the passage of smoke. Latches and door closers are not required on cell doors.

(3) Under Use Condition II, Use Condition III, or Use Condition IV, a space subdivided by open construction (any combination of grating doors and grating walls or solid walls) is permitted to be considered one room if housing not more than 16 persons. The perimeter walls of such space are required to be of smoke-resistant construction. Smoke detection is required to be provided in such space. Under Use Condition IV, common walls between sleeping areas within the space are required to be smoke resistant, and grating doors and fronts are permitted to be used. Under Use Condition II and Use Condition III, open dormitories are permitted to house more than 16 persons, as permitted by other sections of this chapter.

(4) Where barriers are required to be smoke resistant (SR), the provisions of Sections 8.4 and 8.5 do not apply.

[a]Might be no requirement (NR) where one of the following is provided:

(1) Approved automatic smoke detection system installed in all corridors and common spaces

(2) Multitiered cell blocks meeting the requirements of 23.3.1.3

[b]Might be no requirement (NR) in multitiered, open cell blocks meeting the requirements of 23.3.1.3.

[c]Travel distance through the common space to the exit access corridor.

[d]"Total openings in solid room face" include all openings (for example, undercuts, food passes, grilles), the total of which are not to exceed 0.85 ft$^2$ (0.08 m$^2$). All openings are required to be 36 in. (915 mm) or less above the floor.

CHAPTER 22 • New

**A.22.3.8** The requirements in Table 22.3.8 for smoke-resistant separations include taking the necessary precautions to restrict the spread of smoke through the air-handling system. However, the intent is not that smoke dampers are required to be provided for each opening. Smoke dampers would be one acceptable method; however, other techniques, such as allowing the fans to continue to run with 100 percent supply and 100 percent exhaust, would be acceptable.

CHAPTER 23 • Existing

**A.23.3.8** The requirements in Table 23.3.8 for smoke-resistant and fire-rated separations include taking the necessary precautions to restrict the spread of smoke through the air-handling system. However, the intent is not that smoke dampers are required to be provided for each opening. Smoke dampers would be one acceptable method; however, other techniques, such as allowing the fans to continue to run with 100 percent supply and 100 percent exhaust, would be acceptable.

Paragraph 22/23.3.8 provides for the separation of areas where residents are housed. This separation serves two basic needs: (1) it keeps a fire and its products confined to the area of origin, and (2) it protects those occupants located outside the area of origin. Table 22/23.3.8 establishes individual requirements based on the use condition involved. If a common wall is used for different purposes, such as "room face to corridor" and "common space to corridor," the most restrictive requirement needs to be applied to the entire wall. Table 22/23.3.8 and its notes specify a wide variety of options in addition to the locking options previously detailed in Chapters 22 and 23. Note 2 to Table 22.3.8 and note 3 to Table 23.3.8 also permit space that has been subdivided to be treated as a single room. In combination with the various locking options, this exemption can facilitate day-to-day operations.

## 22.4 Special Provisions

### 22.4.1 Limited Access Structures.

The provisions of Section 11.7 for limited access structures shall not apply.

## 23.4 Special Provisions

### 23.4.1 Limited Access Structures.

**23.4.1.1** Limited access structures used as detention and correctional occupancies shall comply with 23.4.1.2, unless otherwise permitted by the following:

(1) The provisions of Section 11.7 for limited access structures shall not apply.
(2) The requirement of 23.4.1.1 shall not apply to buildings protected throughout by an approved automatic sprinkler system in accordance with 23.3.5.3.

**23.4.1.2** Any one of the following means shall be provided to evacuate smoke from the smoke compartment of fire origin:

(1) Operable windows on not less than two sides of the building, spaced not more than 30 ft (9.1 m) apart, that provide openings with dimensions of not less than 22 in. (560 mm) in width and 24 in. (610 mm) in height
(2)* Manual or automatic smoke vents

**A.23.4.1.2(2)** The automatic smoke venting should be in accordance with NFPA 204, *Standard for Smoke and Heat Venting*, for light hazard occupancies.

(3) Engineered smoke control system
(4) Mechanical exhaust system providing not less than six air changes per hour
(5) Other method acceptable to the authority having jurisdiction

CHAPTER 22 • New

## 22.4.2 Underground Buildings.

See Section 11.7 for requirements for underground buildings.

## 22.4.3 High-Rise Buildings.

High-rise buildings shall comply with 11.8.3.

CHAPTER 23 • Existing

## 23.4.2 Underground Buildings.

See Section 11.7 for requirements for underground buildings.

## 23.4.3 High-Rise Buildings.

Existing high-rise buildings shall be protected throughout by an approved, supervised automatic sprinkler system in accordance with 23.3.5.3. A sprinkler control valve and a waterflow device shall be provided for each floor.

Paragraph 23.4.1.2 provides a variety of options for evacuating smoke from the smoke compartment of fire origin in limited access buildings.

Paragraph 23.4.3 retroactively requires existing, high-rise detention and correctional occupancy buildings to be protected throughout by approved, supervised automatic sprinkler systems. Additionally, a sprinkler control valve and waterflow device must be provided for each floor. The control valve facilitates keeping other zones of the sprinkler system operative when one zone is being serviced. The waterflow device provides staff with an indication of where sprinkler water is flowing in the building. Levels of a high-rise multilevel housing area complying with 23.3.1.2 and 23.3.1.3 do not constitute multiple floors and, thus, are not required to be provided with individual control valves and waterflow devices on each level.

## 22.4.4 Nonsprinklered Existing Building Renovations.

**22.4.4.1 General.** Modernizations or renovations of nonsprinklered existing buildings shall be permitted to meet the requirements of this chapter, as modified by 22.4.4.2 through 22.4.4.13, in lieu of the sprinkler requirement of 22.3.5.2.

## 23.4.4 Reserved.

Chapter 22 requires that new detention and correctional occupancies be protected throughout by approved, supervised automatic sprinkler systems. However, in establishing the sprinkler requirement, the Technical Committee on Detention and Correctional Occupancies realized that rehabilitation often might take place in nonsprinklered existing buildings. Thus, 22.4.4 provides additional criteria needed for the proper protection of nonsprinklered existing building renovations. For example, 22.4.4.5.2 establishes for nonsprinklered buildings a maximum travel distance of 150 ft (46 m) between any point in a room and an exit. If a renovation in a nonsprinklered building were to be predicated on the provisions of 22.2.6.4, the travel distance limitation would mistakenly be interpreted to be 200 ft (61 m) between any point in a room and an exit. The 200 ft (61 m) allowance is intended to apply only to sprinklered buildings.

Subsection 22.4.4 serves as a repository for provisions that were contained in Chapter 22 before sprinklers were mandated for new construction. Its provisions remind the user that the requirements interspersed throughout Chapter 22 are predicated on the presence of sprinkler protection. If sprinklers are not installed, additional requirements must be met in an attempt to achieve a level of life safety approaching that provided in a sprinklered building. However, even if all the former specifications for nonsprinklered buildings are met, the overall level of life safety will not necessarily be the same as that provided in a sprinklered facility. When the 1997 edition of the *Code* presented the first requirement for sprinklering of all new detention and correctional occupancies, the overall level of life safety was elevated from that provided by compliance with the nonsprinklered building option.

**22.4.4.2 Minimum Construction Requirements (Nonsprinklered Buildings).**

**22.4.4.2.1** Detention and correctional occupancies in nonsprinklered buildings shall be limited to the building construction types specified in Table 22.4.4.2.1. *(See 8.2.1.)*

**22.4.4.2.2** A residential housing area complying with 22.4.4.6 shall be considered as one story in height for purposes of applying Table 22.4.4.2.1.

**22.4.4.3* Horizontal Exit Duct Penetrations (Nonsprinklered Buildings).** Ducts shall be permitted to penetrate horizontal exits in accordance with 7.2.4.3.5(3) if protected by combination fire dampers/smoke leakage–rated dampers that meet the smoke damper actuation requirements of 8.5.5.

**A.22.4.4.3** This provision is intended to promote the use of horizontal exits in detention and correctional occupancies. Horizontal exits provide an especially effective egress system for an occupancy in which the occupants, due to security concerns, are not commonly released to the outside.

***Table 22.4.4.2.1 Construction Type Limitations — Nonsprinklered Buildings***

| | | Stories in Height† | | | | | |
|---|---|---|---|---|---|---|---|
| Construction Type | Sprinklered | 1 With Basement | 1 Without Basement | 2 | 3 | >3 But Not High-Rise | High-Rise |
| I (442) | Yes | NA | NA | NA | NA | NA | NA |
| | No | X | X | X | X | X | NP |
| I (332) | Yes | NA | NA | NA | NA | NA | NA |
| | No | X | X | X | X | X | NP |
| II (222) | Yes | NA | NA | NA | NA | NA | NA |
| | No | X | X | X | X | X | NP |
| II (111) | Yes | NA | NA | NA | NA | NA | NA |
| | No | X1 | X | X1 | NP | NP | NP |
| II (000) | Yes | NA | NA | NA | NA | NA | NA |
| | No | NP | NP | NP | NP | NP | NP |
| III (211) | Yes | NA | NA | NA | NA | NA | NA |
| | No | X1 | X1 | X1 | NP | NP | NP |
| III (200) | Yes | NA | NA | NA | NA | NA | NA |
| | No | NP | NP | NP | NP | NP | NP |
| IV (2HH) | Yes | NA | NA | NA | NA | NA | NA |
| | No | X1 | X1 | X1 | NP | NP | NP |
| V (111) | Yes | NA | NA | NA | NA | NA | NA |
| | No | X1 | X1 | X1 | NP | NP | NP |
| V (000) | Yes | NA | NA | NA | NA | NA | NA |
| | No | NP | NP | NP | NP | NP | NP |

NA: Not applicable. NP: Not permitted.

X: Permitted for Use Conditions II, III, IV, and V. *(See 22.1.4.3 for Use Condition I.)*

X1: Permitted for Use Conditions II, III, and IV. Use Condition V not permitted.

† See 4.6.3.

This provision offers a *Code*-specified equivalent alternative to the requirement of 7.2.4.3.5 that horizontal exits are not to be penetrated by ducts in nonsprinklered buildings. The intended continuity of the fire resistance–rated and smoke-resisting barrier is maintained by requiring that duct penetrations of horizontal exits be protected by combination fire damper/smoke leakage–rated dampers that will close upon activation of a smoke detector and a heat-actuated mechanism before the barrier's ability to resist the passage of smoke and fire is compromised.

**22.4.4.4 Common Path of Travel (Nonsprinklered Buildings).** A common path of travel shall not exceed 50 ft (15 m).

**22.4.4.5 Travel Distance to Exits (Nonsprinklered Buildings).**

**22.4.4.5.1** The travel distance between any room door required as an exit access and an exit shall not exceed 100 ft (30 m).

**22.4.4.5.2** The travel distance between any point in a room and an exit shall not exceed 150 ft (46 m).

**22.4.4.6 Protection of Vertical Openings (Nonsprinklered Buildings).**

**22.4.4.6.1** Multilevel residential housing areas without enclosure protection between levels shall be permitted, provided that the conditions of 22.4.4.6.2 through 22.4.4.6.4 are met.

**22.4.4.6.2*** The entire normally occupied area, including all communicating floor levels, shall be sufficiently open and unobstructed so that a fire or other dangerous condition in any part is obvious to the occupants or supervisory personnel in the area.

**A.22.4.4.6.2** It is not the intent of this requirement to restrict room face separations, which restrict visibility from the common space into individual sleeping rooms.

**22.4.4.6.3** Egress capacity shall simultaneously accommodate all occupants of all communicating levels and areas, with all communicating levels in the same fire area considered as a single floor area for purposes of determining required egress capacity.

**22.4.4.6.4*** The height between the highest and lowest finished floor levels shall not exceed 13 ft (3960 mm). The number of levels shall not be restricted.

**A.22.4.4.6.4** The vertical separation between the lowest floor level and the uppermost floor level is not to exceed 13 ft (3960 mm). Figure A.22.4.4.6.4 illustrates how the height is to be determined.

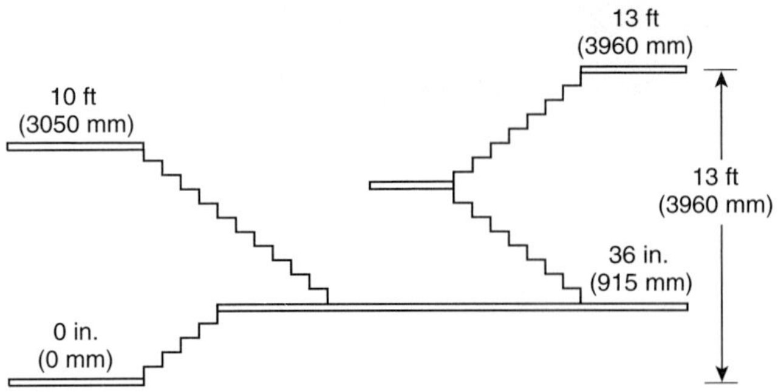


*Figure A.22.4.4.6.4 Vertical Height Measurement.*

**22.4.4.7 Hazardous Areas (Nonsprinklered Buildings).** Any hazardous area shall be protected in accordance with Section 8.7. The areas described in the Table 22.4.4.7 shall be protected as indicated.

*Table 22.4.4.7 Hazardous Area Protection — Nonsprinklered Buildings*

| Hazardous Area Description | Separation/Protection† |
|---|---|
| Areas not incidental to resident housing | 2 hours |
| Boiler and fuel-fired heater rooms | 2 hours or 1 hour and sprinklers |
| Central or bulk laundries >100 $ft^2$ (>9.3 $m^2$) | 2 hours or 1 hour and sprinklers |
| Commercial cooking equipment | In accordance with 9.2.3 |
| Commissaries | 1 hour or sprinklers |
| Employee locker rooms | 1 hour or sprinklers |
| Hobby/handicraft shops | 1 hour or sprinklers |
| Maintenance shops | 1 hour or sprinklers |
| Padded cells | 2 hours or 1 hour and sprinklers |
| Soiled linen rooms | 2 hours or 1 hour and sprinklers |
| Storage rooms >50 $ft^2$ (>4.6 $m^2$) in area but ≤100 $ft^2$ (≤9.3 $m^2$) in area storing combustible material | 1 hour or sprinklers |
| Storage rooms >100 $ft^2$ (>9.3 $m^2$) storing combustible materials | 2 hours or 1 hour and sprinklers |
| Trash collection rooms | 2 hours or 1 hour and sprinklers |

† Minimum fire resistance rating

**22.4.4.8 Interior Finish (Nonsprinklered Buildings).**

**22.4.4.8.1 Interior Wall and Ceiling Finish.** Interior wall and ceiling finish materials complying with Section 10.2

shall be Class A in corridors, in exits, and in any space not separated from corridors and exits by partitions capable of retarding the passage of smoke; and Class A, Class B, or Class C in all other areas.

**22.4.4.8.2 Interior Floor Finish.**

**22.4.4.8.2.1** Interior floor finish shall comply with Section 10.2.

**22.4.4.8.2.2** Interior floor finish in exit enclosures and exit access corridors shall be not less than Class I.

**22.4.4.8.2.3** Interior floor finish shall comply with 10.2.7.1 or 10.2.7.2, as applicable.

**22.4.4.9 Detection, Alarm, and Communications Systems (Nonsprinklered Buildings).**

**22.4.4.9.1 Initiation.** Initiation of the fire alarm system required by 22.3.4.1 shall be by manual means in accordance with 9.6.2 and by means of any required detection devices or detection systems, unless otherwise permitted by the following:

(1) Manual fire alarm boxes shall be permitted to be locked, provided that staff is present within the area when it is occupied and staff has keys readily available to unlock the boxes.
(2) Manual fire alarm boxes shall be permitted to be located in a staff location, provided that both of the following criteria are met:
    (a) The staff location is attended when the building is occupied.
    (b) The staff attendant has direct supervision of the sleeping area.

**22.4.4.9.2 Detection.** An approved automatic smoke detection system shall be in accordance with Section 9.6, as modified by 22.4.4.9.2.1 and 22.4.4.9.2.2, throughout all resident sleeping areas and adjacent day rooms, activity rooms, or contiguous common spaces.

**22.4.4.9.2.1** Smoke detectors shall not be required in sleeping rooms with four or fewer occupants in Use Condition II or Use Condition III.

**22.4.4.9.2.2** Other arrangements and positioning of smoke detectors shall be permitted to prevent damage or tampering, or for other purposes. Such arrangements shall be capable of detecting any fire, and the placement of detectors shall be such that the speed of detection is equivalent to that provided by the spacing and arrangements required by the installation standards referenced in Section 9.6. Detectors shall be permitted to be located in exhaust ducts from cells, behind grilles, or in other locations. The equivalent performance of the design, however, shall be acceptable to the authority having jurisdiction in accordance with the equivalency concepts specified in Section 1.4.

**22.4.4.10 Subdivision of Building Spaces (Nonsprinklered Buildings).** Where smoke barriers are required by 22.3.7.1, they shall be provided as follows:

(1) They shall limit the occupant load to not more than 200 residents in any smoke compartment.
(2) They shall limit the travel distance to a door in a smoke barrier as follows:
    (a) The distance from any room door required as exit access shall not exceed 100 ft (30 m).
    (b) The distance from any point in a room shall not exceed 150 ft (46 m).

**22.4.4.11* Subdivision of Resident Housing Spaces (Nonsprinklered Buildings).** Subdivision of facility spaces shall comply with Table 22.4.4.11.

**A.22.4.4.11** The requirements in Table 22.4.4.11 for smoke-resistant and fire-rated separations include taking the necessary precautions to restrict the spread of smoke through the air-handling system. However, the intent is that smoke dampers are required to be provided for each opening. Smoke dampers would be one acceptable method; however, other techniques, such as allowing the fans to continue to run with 100 percent supply and 100 percent exhaust, would be acceptable.

**22.4.4.12 Limited Access Structures (Nonsprinklered Buildings).**

**22.4.4.12.1** Limited access structures used as detention and correctional occupancies shall comply with 22.4.4.12.2. The provisions of Section 11.7 for limited access structures shall not apply.

**22.4.4.12.2** Any one of the following means shall be provided to evacuate smoke from the smoke compartment of fire origin:

(1) Operable windows on not less than two sides of the building, spaced not more than 30 ft (9.1 m) apart, that provide openings with dimensions of not less than 22 in. (560 mm) in width and 24 in. (610 mm) in height
(2)* Manual or automatic smoke vents

**A.22.4.4.12.2(2)** The automatic smoke venting should be in accordance with NFPA 204, *Standard for Smoke and Heat Venting*, for light hazard occupancies.

(3) Engineered smoke control system
(4) Mechanical exhaust system providing not less than six air changes per hour
(5) Other method acceptable to the authority having jurisdiction

*Table 22.4.4.11 Subdivision of Resident Housing Spaces — Nonsprinklered Buildings*

| | Use Condition | | | |
|---|---|---|---|---|
| **Feature** | **II** | **III** | **IV** | **V** |
| Room to room separation | NR | NR | SR | FR(½) |
| Room face to corridor separation | SR | SR | SR | FR |
| Room face to common space separation | NR | NR ≤50 ft (≤15 m)† / SR >50 ft (>15 m)† | SR | FR |
| Common space to corridor separation | FR | FR | FR | FR |
| Total openings in solid room face where room face is required to be smoke resistant or fire rated‡ | 0.85 $ft^2$ (0.08 $m^2$) | 0.85 $ft^2$ (0.08 $m^2$) | 0.85 $ft^2$ (0.08 $m^2$) | 0.85 $ft^2$ (0.08 $m^2$) where meeting one of the following:<br>(1) Kept in closed position, except when in use by staff<br>(2) Closable from the inside<br>(3) Provided with smoke control |

NR: No requirement. SR: Smoke resistant. FR(½): Minimum ½-hour fire resistance rating. FR: Minimum 1-hour fire resistance rating.

Notes:

(1) Doors in openings in partitions required to be fire rated [FR(½), FR] in accordance with Table 22.4.4.11, in other than required enclosures of exits or hazardous areas, are required to be substantial doors of construction that resists fire for a minimum of 20 minutes. Vision panels with wired glass or glass with not less than 45-minute fire-rated glazing are permitted. Latches and door closers are not required on cell doors.

(2) Doors in openings in partitions required to be smoke resistant (SR) in accordance with Table 22.4.4.11 are required to be substantial doors of construction that resists the passage of smoke. Latches and door closers are not required on cell doors.

(3) Under Use Condition II, Use Condition III, or Use Condition IV, a space subdivided by open construction (any combination of grating doors and grating walls or solid walls) is permitted to be considered one room if housing not more than 16 persons. The perimeter walls of such space are required to be of smoke-resistant construction. Smoke detection is required to be provided in such space. Under Use Condition IV, common walls between sleeping areas within the space are required to be smoke resistant, and grating doors and fronts are permitted to be used. In Use Condition II and Use Condition III, open dormitories are permitted to house more than 16 persons, as permitted by other sections of this chapter.

(4) Where barriers are required to be smoke resistant (SR), the provisions of Sections 8.4 and 8.5 do not apply.

†Travel distance through the common space to the exit access corridor.

‡"Total openings in solid room face" include all openings (for example, undercuts, food passes, grilles), the total of which is not to exceed 0.85 $ft^2$ (0.08 $m^2$). All openings are required to be 36 in. (915 mm) or less above the floor.

**22.4.4.13* Furnishings, Mattresses, and Decorations (Nonsprinklered Buildings).**

**A.22.4.4.13** Personal property provides combustible contents for fire development. Therefore, adequate controls are needed to limit the quantity and combustibility of fuels available to burn to reduce the probability of room flashover. The provisions of 22.4.4.13 will not, by themselves, prevent room flashover if personal property controls are not provided.

**22.4.4.13.1** Newly introduced upholstered furniture within detention and correctional occupancies shall be tested in accordance with the provisions of 10.3.2.1(2) and 10.3.3.

**22.4.4.13.2*** Newly introduced mattresses within detention and correctional occupancies shall be tested in accordance with the provisions of 10.3.2.2 and 10.3.4.

**A.22.4.4.13.2** Mattresses used in detention and correctional facilities should be evaluated with regard to the fire hazards of the environment. The potential for vandalism and excessive wear and tear also should be taken into account when evaluating the fire performance of the mattress. ASTM F 1870, *Standard Guide for Selection of Fire Test Methods for the Assessment of Upholstered Furnishings in Detention and Correctional Facilities*, provides guidance for this purpose.

### 22.4.5 Lockups.

**22.4.5.1 General.**

**22.4.5.1.1** Lockups in occupancies, other than detention and correctional occupancies and health care occupancies, where the holding area has capacity for more than 50 detainees shall be classified as detention and correctional occupancies and shall comply with the requirements of Chapter 22.

**22.4.5.1.2** Lockups in occupancies, other than detention and correctional occupancies and health care occupancies, where any individual is detained for 24 or more hours shall be classified as detention and correctional occupancies and shall comply with the requirements of Chapter 22.

**22.4.5.1.3** Lockups in occupancies, other than detention and correctional occupancies and health care occupancies, where the holding area has capacity for not more than 50 detainees, and where no individual is detained for 24 hours or more, shall comply with 22.4.5.1.4 or 22.4.5.1.5.

**22.4.5.1.4** The lockup shall be permitted to comply with the requirements for the predominant occupancy in which the lockup is placed, provided that all of the following criteria are met:

(1) Doors and other physical restraints to free egress by detainees can be readily released by staff within 2 minutes of the onset of a fire or similar emergency.
(2) Staff is in sufficient proximity to the lockup so as to be able to effect the 2-minute release required by 22.4.5.1.4(1) whenever detainees occupy the lockup.
(3) Staff is authorized to effect the release required by 22.4.5.1.4(1).
(4) Staff is trained and practiced in effecting the release required by 22.4.5.1.4(1).

### 23.4.5 Lockups.

**23.4.5.1 General.**

**23.4.5.1.1** Lockups in occupancies, other than detention and correctional occupancies and health care occupancies, where the holding area has capacity for more than 50 detainees shall be classified as detention and correctional occupancies and shall comply with the requirements of Chapter 23.

**23.4.5.1.2** Lockups in occupancies, other than detention and correctional occupancies and health care occupancies, where any individual is detained for 24 or more hours shall be classified as detention and correctional occupancies and shall comply with the requirements of Chapter 23.

**23.4.5.1.3** Lockups in occupancies, other than detention and correctional occupancies and health care occupancies, where the holding area has capacity for not more than 50 detainees, and where no individual is detained for 24 hours or more, shall comply with 23.4.5.1.4 or 23.4.5.1.5.

**23.4.5.1.4** The lockup shall be permitted to comply with the requirements for the predominant occupancy in which the lockup is placed, provided that all of the following criteria are met:

(1) Doors and other physical restraints to free egress by detainees can be readily released by staff within 2 minutes of the onset of a fire or similar emergency.
(2) Staff is in sufficient proximity to the lockup so as to be able to effect the 2-minute release required by 23.4.5.1.4(1) whenever detainees occupy the lockup.
(3) Staff is authorized to effect the release required by 23.4.5.1.4(1).
(4) Staff is trained and practiced in effecting the release required by 23.4.5.1.4(1).

CHAPTER 22 • New

(5) Where the release required by 22.4.5.1.4(1) is effected by means of remote release, detainees are not to be restrained from evacuating without the assistance of others.

**22.4.5.1.5** Where the lockup does not comply with all the criteria of 22.4.5.1.4, the requirements of 22.4.5.2 shall be met.

**22.4.5.2 Alternate Provisions.**

**22.4.5.2.1** The requirements applicable to the predominant occupancy in which the lockup is placed shall be met.

**22.4.5.2.2** Where security operations necessitate the locking of required means of egress, the following shall apply:

(1) Detention-grade hardware meeting the requirements of ASTM F 1577, *Standard Test Methods for Detention Locks for Swinging Doors*, shall be provided on swinging doors within the required means of egress.
(2) Sliding doors within the required means of egress shall be designed and engineered for detention and correctional use, and lock cylinders shall meet the cylinder test requirements of ASTM F 1577.

**22.4.5.2.3** The lockup shall be provided with a complete smoke detection system in accordance with 9.6.2.9.

**22.4.5.2.4** Where the requirements applicable to the predominant occupancy do not mandate a fire alarm system, the lockup shall be provided with a fire alarm system meeting the following criteria:

(1) The alarm system shall be in accordance with Section 9.6.
(2) Initiation of the alarm system shall be accomplished by all of the following:
    (a) Manual fire alarm boxes in accordance with 9.6.2
    (b) Smoke detection system required by 22.4.5.2.3
    (c) Automatic sprinkler system required by the provisions applicable to the predominant occupancy
(3) Staff and occupant notification shall be provided automatically in accordance with 9.6.3.
(4) Emergency force notification shall be provided in accordance with 9.6.4.

CHAPTER 23 • Existing

(5) Where the release required by 23.4.5.1.4(1) is effected by means of remote release, detainees are not to be restrained from evacuating without the assistance of others.

**23.4.5.1.5** Where the lockup does not comply with all the criteria of 23.4.5.1.4, the requirements of 23.4.5.2 shall be met.

**23.4.5.2 Alternate Provisions.**

**23.4.5.2.1** The requirements applicable to the predominant occupancy in which the lockup is placed shall be met.

**23.4.5.2.2** Where security operations necessitate the locking of required means of egress, the following shall apply:

(1) Detention-grade hardware meeting the requirements of ASTM F 1577, *Standard Test Methods for Detention Locks for Swinging Doors*, shall be provided on swinging doors within the required means of egress.
(2) Sliding doors within the required means of egress shall be designed and engineered for detention and correctional use, and lock cylinders shall meet the cylinder test requirements of ASTM F 1577.

**23.4.5.2.3** The lockup shall be provided with a complete smoke detection system in accordance with 9.6.2.9.

**23.4.5.2.4** Where the requirements applicable to the predominant occupancy do not require a fire alarm system, the lockup shall be provided with a fire alarm system meeting the following criteria:

(1) The alarm system shall be in accordance with Section 9.6.
(2) Initiation of the alarm system shall be accomplished by all of the following:
    (a) Manual fire alarm boxes in accordance with 9.6.2
    (b) Smoke detection system required by 23.4.5.2.3
    (c) Automatic sprinkler system required by the provisions applicable to the predominant occupancy
(3) Staff and occupant notification shall be provided automatically in accordance with 9.6.3.
(4) Emergency force notification shall be provided in accordance with 9.6.4.

As stated in A.22/A.23.2.1.1.1.5, lockups in which persons are detained with some degree of security imposed on them are common in many types of occupancies. Examples include the following:

1. Immigration and naturalization facilities at border crossings
2. Customs facilities at international airports
3. Prisoner holding facilities at courthouses
4. Local police department holding areas
5. Security offices at sports stadia
6. Security offices at shopping mall complexes

Most of the occupancy chapters were written to provide life safety for the ambulatory and unrestrained occupant population characteristic of the occupancy, and not for those who are detained. The health care occupancy chapters utilize a defend-in-place strategy that addresses door locking and staff interaction, so as to obviate the need for any additional criteria for areas where occupants might be detained. Other occupancy chapters (such as those applicable to dwellings, lodging or rooming houses, and small residential board and care facilities) address buildings that are sufficiently limited in size, so that the presence of a lockup is rare. The occupancies that mandate use of the provisions of 22/23.4.5 are as follows:

1. Assembly occupancies (12.2.11.2, 13.2.11.2)
2. Educational occupancies (14.2.11.2, 15.2.11.2)
3. Day-care occupancies (16.2.11.2, 17.2.11.2)
4. Ambulatory health care occupancies (20.2.11.2, 21.2.11.2)
5. Hotels and dormitories (28.2.11.2, 29.2.11.2)
6. Apartment buildings (30.2.11.2, 31.2.11.2)
7. Residential board and care occupancies (large) (32.3.2.11.2, 33.3.2.11.2)
8. Mercantile occupancies (36.2.11.2, 37.2.11.2)
9. Business occupancies (38.2.11.2, 39.2.11.2)
10. Industrial occupancies (40.2.11.2)
11. Storage occupancies (42.2.11.2)

Where the occupancy chapters applicable to existing conditions reference the requirements of 23.4.5, an exemption is provided for approved existing lockups. If the authority having jurisdiction (AHJ) approves the existing arrangement as meeting the *Code*'s intent, further upgrading is not required.

The provisions of 22/23.4.5 for lockups were written to serve as a bridge between the rigorous, defend-in-place provisions applicable to detention and correctional occupancy residential housing areas, as detailed in Chapters 22 and 23, and the provisions applicable to the predominant occupancy in which the lockup is present. The provisions for lockups are meant to apply to holding areas of limited capacity in which no individual is detained for 24 or more hours. Paragraph 22/23.4.5.1.1 establishes that, if the holding area has capacity for more than 50 detainees, it must be classified as a detention and correctional occupancy. Similarly, 22/23.4.5.1.2 mandates that, if any individual is detained for 24 or more hours, the holding area must be classified as a detention and correctional occupancy. Once classified as a detention and correctional occupancy, the holding area is subject to the provisions of Section 22/23.1 through 22/23.4.4 and Section 22/23.5 through Section 22/23.7. Therefore, the holding area is classified as a lockup, and subject to the provisions of 22/23.4.5.1.4 through 22/23.4.5.2.4, only if it has capacity for not more than 50 detainees and no individual is detained for 24 hours or more.

Exhibit 22/23.18 outlines the test for determining occupancy classification and the applicable set of requirements for lockups (other than approved existing lockups) in any of the 11 occupancies listed previously in this commentary.

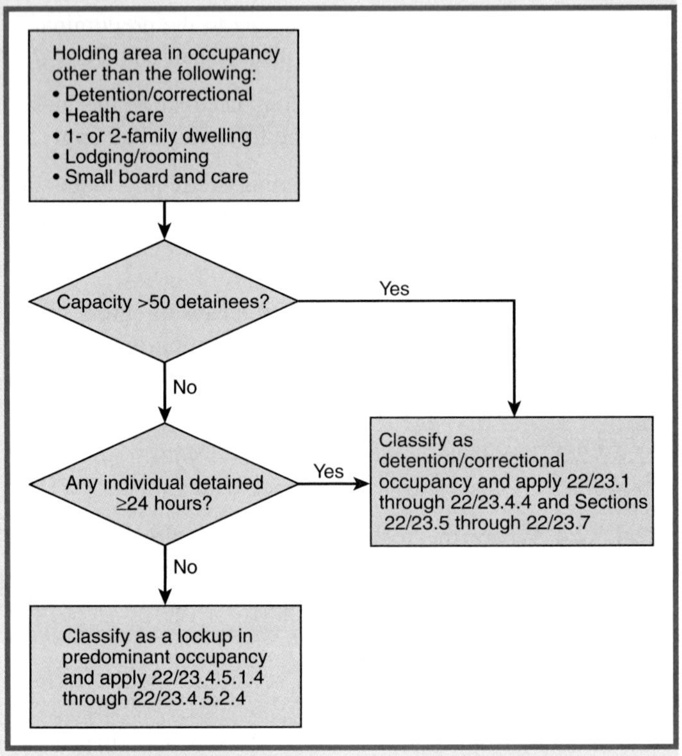


***Exhibit 22/23.18*** *Flowchart for lockup occupancy classification and applicable provisions.*

Lockups subject to the provisions of 22/23.4.5.1.4 through 22/23.4.5.2.4 are offered two methods for compliance as specified in paragraphs 1 and 2, which follow.

**1.** Paragraph 22/23.4.5.1.4, where used, requires a system of safeguards, so that doors and physical restraints to free egress by detainees can be readily released, by trained staff with the authority to effect such release, within 2 minutes of the onset of a fire or similar emergency. This method of compliance will apply to holding areas that either (1) are staffed at all times when detainees are present or (2) have staff in close proximity and the detection and notification technology needed to summon such staff immediately upon the onset of an emergency. Note that 22/23.4.5.1.4(5) does not prohibit the remote release of doors, but, in such cases, detainees are not permitted to be restrained, as might be the case where a detainee is handcuffed to a post.

**2.** Paragraph 22/23.4.5.1.5 and the alternate provisions of 22/23.4.5.2 offer a second method of compliance for which all the criteria of the 2-minute release option of 22/23.4.5.1.4 are not satisfied. This alternate set of provisions relies heavily on the presence of a complete smoke detection system within the lockup and its use to summon staff and emergency forces personnel via the alarm system, which is required even if otherwise exempted for the predominant occupancy. If the *Code* provisions applicable to the predominant occupancy require sprinkler protection, waterflow in the sprinkler system must initiate the required alarm system, but this provision, by itself, does not mandate sprinkler protection. The option also imposes requirements for detention-grade door hardware for reliability concerns.

## 22.5 Building Services

### 22.5.1 Utilities.

**22.5.1.1** Utilities shall comply with the provisions of Section 9.1.

**22.5.1.2** Alarms, emergency communications systems, and the illumination of generator set locations shall be provided with emergency power in accordance with *NFPA 70, National Electrical Code*.

### 22.5.2 Heating, Ventilating, and Air-Conditioning.

**22.5.2.1** Heating, ventilating, and air-conditioning equipment shall comply with the provisions of Section 9.2 and shall be installed in accordance with the manufacturer's specifications, unless otherwise modified by 22.5.2.2.

**22.5.2.2** Portable space-heating devices shall be prohibited, unless otherwise permitted by 22.5.2.4.

**22.5.2.3** Any heating device, other than a central heating plant, shall be designed and installed so that combustible material cannot be ignited by the device or its appurtenances, and the following requirements also shall apply:

(1) If fuel-fired, such heating devices shall comply with the following:

  (a) They shall be chimney connected or vent connected.



## 23.5 Building Services

### 23.5.1 Utilities.

**23.5.1.1** Utilities shall comply with the provisions of Section 9.1.

**23.5.1.2** Alarms, emergency communications systems, and the illumination of generator set installations shall be provided with emergency power in accordance with *NFPA 70, National Electrical Code*, unless otherwise permitted by 23.5.1.3.

**23.5.1.3** Systems complying with earlier editions of *NFPA 70, National Electrical Code*, and not presenting a life safety hazard shall be permitted to continue to be used.

### 23.5.2 Heating, Ventilating, and Air-Conditioning.

**23.5.2.1** Heating, ventilating, and air-conditioning equipment shall comply with the provisions of Section 9.2 and shall be installed in accordance with the manufacturer's specifications, unless otherwise permitted by the following:

(1) The requirement of 23.5.2.1 shall not apply where otherwise modified by 23.5.2.2.
(2) Systems complying with earlier editions of the applicable codes and not presenting a life safety hazard shall be permitted to continue to be used.

**23.5.2.2** Portable space-heating devices shall be prohibited, unless otherwise permitted by 23.5.2.4.

**23.5.2.3** Any heating device, other than a central heating plant, shall be designed and installed so that combustible material cannot be ignited by the device or its appurtenances, and the following requirements also shall apply:

(1) If fuel-fired, such heating devices shall comply with the following:

  (a) They shall be chimney connected or vent connected.

CHAPTER 22 • New

(b) They shall take air for combustion directly from outside.
(c) They shall be designed and installed to provide for complete separation of the combustion system from the atmosphere of the occupied area.

(2) The heating system shall have safety devices to immediately stop the flow of fuel and shut down the equipment in case of either excessive temperatures or ignition failure.

**22.5.2.4** Approved, suspended unit heaters shall be permitted in locations other than means of egress and sleeping areas, provided that both of the following criteria are met:

(1) Such heaters are located high enough to be out of the reach of persons using the area.
(2) Such heaters are vent connected and equipped with the safety devices required by 22.5.2.3(2).

**22.5.2.5** Combustion and ventilation air for boiler, incinerator, or heater rooms shall be taken directly from, and discharged directly to, the outside.

### 22.5.3 Elevators, Escalators, and Conveyors.

Elevators, escalators, and conveyors shall comply with the provisions of Section 9.4.

### 22.5.4 Rubbish Chutes, Incinerators, and Laundry Chutes.

**22.5.4.1** Rubbish chutes, incinerators, and laundry chutes shall comply with the provisions of Section 9.5.

**22.5.4.2** Rubbish chutes and linen chutes, including pneumatic rubbish and linen systems, shall be provided with automatic extinguishing protection in accordance with Section 9.7.

**22.5.4.3** Trash chutes shall discharge into a trash collection room used for no other purpose and protected in accordance with Section 8.7.

**22.5.4.4** Incinerators shall not be directly flue-fed, and floor chutes shall not directly connect with the combustion chamber.

## 22.6 Reserved

CHAPTER 23 • Existing

(b) They shall take air for combustion directly from outside.
(c) They shall be designed and installed to provide for complete separation of the combustion system from the atmosphere of the occupied area.

(2) The heating system shall have safety devices to immediately stop the flow of fuel and shut down the equipment in case of either excessive temperatures or ignition failure.

**23.5.2.4** Approved, suspended unit heaters shall be permitted in locations other than means of egress and sleeping areas, provided that both of the following criteria are met:

(1) Such heaters are located high enough to be out of the reach of persons using the area.
(2) Such heaters are vent connected and equipped with the safety devices required by 23.5.2.3(2).

**23.5.2.5** Combustion and ventilation air for boiler, incinerator, or heater rooms shall be taken directly from, and discharged directly to, the outside.

### 23.5.3 Elevators, Escalators, and Conveyors.

Elevators, escalators, and conveyors shall comply with the provisions of Section 9.4.

### 23.5.4 Rubbish Chutes, Incinerators, and Laundry Chutes.

**23.5.4.1** Rubbish chutes, incinerators, and laundry chutes shall comply with the provisions of Section 9.5.

**23.5.4.2** Rubbish chutes and linen chutes, including pneumatic rubbish and linen systems, shall be provided with automatic extinguishing protection in accordance with Section 9.7.

**23.5.4.3** Trash chutes shall discharge into a trash collection room used for no other purpose and protected in accordance with Section 8.7.

**23.5.4.4** Incinerators shall not be directly flue-fed, and floor chutes shall not directly connect with the combustion chamber.

## 23.6 Reserved

## 22.7 Operating Features

### 22.7.1 Attendants, Evacuation Plan, and Fire Drills.

**22.7.1.1** Detention and correctional facilities, or those portions of facilities having such occupancy, shall be provided with 24-hour staffing, and the following requirements also shall apply:

(1) Staff shall be within three floors or a 300 ft (91 m) horizontal distance of the access door of each resident housing area.
(2) For Use Condition III, Use Condition IV, and Use Condition V, the arrangement shall be such that the staff involved starts the release of locks necessary for emergency evacuation or rescue and initiates other necessary emergency actions within 2 minutes of alarm.
(3) The following shall apply to areas in which all locks are unlocked remotely in compliance with 22.2.11.8:
    (a) Staff shall not be required to be within three floors or 300 ft (91 m) of the access door.
    (b) The 10-lock, manual key exemption of 22.2.11.8.2 shall not be permitted to be used in conjunction with the alternative requirement of 22.7.1.1(3)(a).

**22.7.1.2*** Provisions shall be made so that residents in Use Condition III, Use Condition IV, and Use Condition V shall be able to notify staff of an emergency.

**A.22.7.1.2** This requirement is permitted to be met by electronic or oral monitoring systems, visual monitoring, call signals, or other means.

**22.7.1.3*** The administration of every detention or correctional facility shall have, in effect and available to all supervisory personnel, written copies of a plan for the protection of all persons in the event of fire, for their evacuation to areas of refuge, and for evacuation from the building when necessary.

**A.22.7.1.3** Periodic, coordinated training should be conducted and should involve detention and correctional facility personnel and personnel of the fire department legally committed to serving the facility.

**22.7.1.3.1** All employees shall be instructed and drilled with respect to their duties under the plan.

**22.7.1.3.2** The plan shall be coordinated with, and reviewed by, the fire department legally committed to serve the facility.

**22.7.1.4** Employees of detention and correctional occupancies shall be instructed in the proper use of portable fire extinguishers and other manual fire suppression equipment.

## 23.7 Operating Features

### 23.7.1 Attendants, Evacuation Plan, and Fire Drills.

**23.7.1.1** Detention and correctional facilities, or those portions of facilities having such occupancy, shall be provided with 24-hour staffing, and the following requirements also shall apply:

(1) Staff shall be within three floors or a 300 ft (91 m) horizontal distance of the access door of each resident housing area.
(2) For Use Condition III, Use Condition IV, and Use Condition V, the arrangement shall be such that the staff involved starts the release of locks necessary for emergency evacuation or rescue and initiates other necessary emergency actions within 2 minutes of alarm.
(3) The following shall apply to areas in which all locks are unlocked remotely in compliance with 23.2.11.8:
    (a) Staff shall not be required to be within three floors or 300 ft (91 m) of the access door.
    (b) The 10-lock, manual key exemption of 23.2.11.8.2 shall not be permitted to be used in conjunction with the alternative requirement of 23.7.1.1(3)(a).

**23.7.1.2*** Provisions shall be made so that residents in Use Condition III, Use Condition IV, and Use Condition V shall be able to notify staff of an emergency.

**A.23.7.1.2** This requirement is permitted to be met by electronic or oral monitoring systems, visual monitoring, call signals, or other means.

**23.7.1.3*** The administration of every detention or correctional facility shall have, in effect and available to all supervisory personnel, written copies of a plan for the protection of all persons in the event of fire, for their evacuation to areas of refuge, and for evacuation from the building when necessary.

**A.23.7.1.3** Periodic, coordinated training should be conducted and should involve detention and correctional facility personnel and personnel of the fire department legally committed to serving the facility.

**23.7.1.3.1** All employees shall be instructed and drilled with respect to their duties under the plan.

**23.7.1.3.2** The plan shall be coordinated with, and reviewed by, the fire department legally committed to serve the facility.

**23.7.1.4** Employees of detention and correctional occupancies shall be instructed in the proper use of portable fire extinguishers and other manual fire suppression equipment.

CHAPTER 22 • New

22.7.1.4.1 The training specified in 22.7.1.4 shall be provided to new staff promptly upon commencement of duty.

22.7.1.4.2 Refresher training shall be provided to existing staff at not less than annual intervals.

### 22.7.2 Combustible Personal Property.

Books, clothing, and other combustible personal property allowed in sleeping rooms shall be stored in closable metal lockers or an approved fire-resistant container.

### 22.7.3 Heat-Producing Appliances.

The number of heat-producing appliances, such as toasters and hot plates, and the overall use of electrical power within a sleeping room shall be controlled by facility administration.

### 22.7.4* Furnishings, Mattresses, and Decorations.

**A.22.7.4** Personal property provides combustible contents for fire development. Therefore, adequate controls are needed to limit the quantity and combustibility of the fuels available to burn to reduce the probability of room flashover. The provisions of 22.7.4 will not, by themselves, prevent room flashover if personal property controls are not provided.

**22.7.4.1** Draperies and curtains, including privacy curtains, in detention and correctional occupancies shall be in accordance with the provisions of 10.3.1.

**22.7.4.2** Newly introduced upholstered furniture within detention and correctional occupancies shall be tested in accordance with the provisions of 10.3.2.1(2).

**22.7.4.3** Newly introduced mattresses within detention and correctional occupancies shall be tested in accordance with the provisions of 10.3.2.2.

**22.7.4.4** Combustible decorations shall be prohibited in any detention or correctional occupancy unless flame-retardant.

**22.7.4.5** Wastebaskets and other waste containers shall be of noncombustible or other approved materials. Waste containers with a capacity exceeding 20 gal (76 L) shall be pro-

CHAPTER 23 • Existing

**23.7.1.4.1** The training specified in 23.7.1.4 shall be provided to new staff promptly upon commencement of duty.

**23.7.1.4.2** Refresher training shall be provided to existing staff at not less than annual intervals.

### 23.7.2 Combustible Personal Property.

Books, clothing, and other combustible personal property allowed in sleeping rooms shall be stored in closable metal lockers or an approved fire-resistant container.

### 23.7.3 Heat-Producing Appliances.

The number of heat-producing appliances, such as toasters and hot plates, and the overall use of electrical power within a sleeping room shall be controlled by facility administration.

### 23.7.4* Furnishings, Mattresses, and Decorations.

**A.23.7.4** Personal property provides combustible contents for fire development. Therefore, adequate controls are needed to limit the quantity and combustibility of the fuels available to burn to reduce the probability of room flashover. The provisions of 23.7.4 will not, by themselves, prevent room flashover if personal property controls are not provided.

**23.7.4.1** Draperies and curtains, including privacy curtains, in detention and correctional occupancies shall be in accordance with the provisions of 10.3.1.

**23.7.4.2** Newly introduced upholstered furniture within detention and correctional occupancies shall be tested in accordance with the provisions of 10.3.2.1(2) and 10.3.3.

**23.7.4.3*** Newly introduced mattresses within detention and correctional occupancies shall be tested in accordance with the provisions of 10.3.2.2 and 10.3.4.

**A.23.7.4.3** Mattresses used in detention and correctional facilities should be evaluated with regard to the fire hazards of the environment. The potential for vandalism and excessive wear and tear also should be taken into account when evaluating the fire performance of the mattress. ASTM F 1870, *Standard Guide for Selection of Fire Test Methods for the Assessment of Upholstered Furnishings in Detention and Correctional Facilities*, provides guidance for this purpose.

**23.7.4.4** Combustible decorations shall be prohibited in any detention or correctional occupancy unless flame-retardant.

**23.7.4.5** Wastebaskets and other waste containers shall be of noncombustible or other approved materials. Waste containers with a capacity exceeding 20 gal (76 L) shall be pro-

CHAPTER 22 • New

vided with a noncombustible lid or lid of other approved material.

### 22.7.5 Keys.

All keys necessary for unlocking doors installed in a means of egress shall be individually identified by both touch and sight.

### 22.7.6 Portable Space-Heating Devices.

Portable space-heating devices shall be prohibited in all detention and correctional occupancies.

### 22.7.7 Door Inspection.

Doors and door hardware in means of egress shall be inspected monthly by an appropriately trained person. The inspection shall be documented.

CHAPTER 23 • Existing

vided with a noncombustible lid or lid of other approved material.

### 23.7.5 Keys.

All keys necessary for unlocking doors installed in a means of egress shall be individually identified by both touch and sight.

### 23.7.6 Portable Space-Heating Devices.

Portable space-heating devices shall be prohibited in all detention and correctional occupancies.

### 23.7.7 Door Inspection.

Doors and door hardware in means of egress shall be inspected monthly by an appropriately trained person. The inspection shall be documented.

Paragraph 22/23.7.1.2 requires that residents in Use Condition III, Use Condition IV, and Use Condition V facilities be able to notify staff of an emergency. Use Condition IV and Use Condition V facilities rely on staff action to release locks to allow residents to leave their rooms; Use Condition III, Use Condition IV, and Use Condition V facilities rely on staff action to release locks to allow residents to move to an adjacent smoke compartment. The staff needs to be made aware of fire conditions early in a fire. Thus, in case residents discover a fire before automatic detection devices are initiated, they need a means of notifying staff.

A properly designed and well-tested fire emergency plan, as required by 22/23.7.1.3, is important in detention and correctional occupancies where residents depend heavily on staff performance for safety under fire conditions.

The provisions of 22/23.7.4 make use of the menu of provisions in Section 10.3 that apply to furnishings and contents, particularly those that address upholstered furniture and mattresses. Nevertheless, the control of combustible personal property is needed to limit fire development in sprinklered facilities and prevent the occurrence of room flashover in nonsprinklered facilities. Paragraph 22/23.7.2 provides staff with the authority to regulate the quantities of personal property in sleeping rooms.

The provisions of 22/23.7.4.1 through 22/23.7.4.5 are the most rigorous regulations of contents and furnishings provided by this *Code*. It is appropriate that these provisions be applied to detention and correctional occupancies in consideration of the protect-in-place strategy required of these occupancies by the *Code* and the reluctance of staff to unlock doors to allow residents to move to the outside.

Draperies and curtains must be flame resistant in accordance with 10.3.1, which requires flame propagation performance criteria per NFPA 701, *Standard Methods of Fire Tests for Flame Propagation of Textiles and Films*.[10]

Paragraphs 22/23.7.4.2 and 22/23.7.4.3 require newly introduced upholstered furniture and mattresses to be resistant to cigarette ignition, regardless of whether the facility is sprinklered. Paragraphs 23.7.4.2 and 22.7.4.3 also have the effect of limiting the rate of heat release for newly introduced upholstered furniture and mattresses in nonsprinklered detention and correctional facilities.

For the 2006 edition of the *Code*, 10.3.2.1 and 10.3.2.2 were revised to remove a provision that exempted the cigarette ignition–resistance testing of upholstered furniture and mattresses in sprinklered buildings. The Technical Committee on Detention and Correctional Occupancies learned of the change, agreed that such testing was needed to address smoldering ignition (even in a sprinklered building), and permitted it to take effect on the provisions of 23.7.4.2 and 23.7.4.3. However, the committee overlooked the need for a correlative change to 22.7.4.2 and 22.7.4.3 to require cigarette ignition–resistance testing for upholstered furniture and mattresses in new detention and correctional occupancies. The revision made to

22.7.4.2 and 22.7.4.3 for the 2009 edition corrects the oversight.

The provision of 22/23.7.7 was added to the *Code* for the 2006 edition. Detention and correctional occupancies make extensive use of doors — especially locked doors — for security reasons. It is particularly important in these occupancies that doors and door hardware be inspected regularly.

## References Cited in Commentary


1. NFPA 101A, *Guide on Alternative Approaches to Life Safety*, 2007 edition, National Fire Protection Association, Quincy, MA. (The edition of NFPA 101A that corresponds with the 2009 *Life Safety Code* will be the 2010 edition.)
2. NFPA 220, *Standard on Types of Building Construction*, 2009 edition, National Fire Protection Association, Quincy, MA.
3. *NFPA 5000®, Building Construction and Safety Code®*, 2009 edition, National Fire Protection Association, Quincy, MA.
4. NFPA 30, *Flammable and Combustible Liquids Code*, 2008 edition, National Fire Protection Association, Quincy, MA.
5. ASTM E 84, *Standard Test Method for Surface Burning Characteristics of Building Materials*, 2004 edition, ASTM International, 100 Barr Harbor Drive, P.O. Box C700, West Conshohocken, PA 19428-2959.
6. ANSI/UL 723, *Standard for Test for Surface Burning Characteristics of Building Materials*, 2003 edition, Revised 2005, Underwriters Laboratories Inc., 333 Pfingsten Road, Northbrook, IL 60062-2096.
7. NFPA 253, *Standard Method of Test for Critical Radiant Flux of Floor Covering Systems Using a Radiant Heat Energy Source*, 2006 edition, National Fire Protection Association, Quincy, MA.
8. *NFPA 72®, National Fire Alarm Code®*, 2007 edition, National Fire Protection Association, Quincy, MA.
9. NFPA 13, *Standard for the Installation of Sprinkler Systems*, 2007 edition, National Fire Protection Association, Quincy, MA.
10. NFPA 701, *Standard Methods of Fire Tests for Flame Propagation of Textiles and Films*, 2004 edition, National Fire Protection Association, Quincy, MA.

CHAPTER 24

# One- and Two-Family Dwellings

Although most people feel safest in their homes, fire deaths in the home account for some 80 percent of all fatalities attributable to fire in the United States. Chapter 24 highlights a number of factors that significantly mitigate the fire problem. A key and unique component that is addressed in this chapter, and that is selectively applied to the other residential chapters, is means of escape (see Section 24.2). The concept of means of escape focuses on providing a second way out of an occupied room or space within a living unit, regardless of whether it is a single-family home or a dwelling unit within an apartment building. Means of escape features do not need to meet the high standards and criteria that apply to the means of egress. In short, means of escape is an important yet broadly applied concept that is intended to reduce the chance of occupants becoming trapped in a room or space if the primary egress route is unavailable.

Recognizing that the greatest number of fire fatalities occurs in what has historically been the least regulated occupancy, the *Code*, in a major shift from earlier editions, now requires, since the 2006 edition, all new one- and two-family dwellings to be protected by automatic sprinkler systems. Residential sprinkler systems have a phenomenal record of success in preventing fire deaths and injuries. Although residential sprinkler systems are designed exclusively to protect life, and not necessarily property, many homes and personal possessions have, in fact, been saved from the devastating effects of fire thanks to their installation.

While the 2006 edition of the *Code*, along with the 2006 edition of *NFPA 5000®, Building Construction and Safety Code®*,[1] were the first model codes in the United States to require sprinklers in new one- and two-family dwellings, numerous communities paved the way by enacting local sprinkler legislation. For example, Scottsdale, Arizona, was among the first cities in the United States to mandate sprinklers in new homes effective January 1, 1986. Ten years later, a report titled "Automatic Sprinklers: A 10 Year Study — A Detailed History of the Effects of the Automatic Sprinkler Code in Scottsdale, Arizona"[2] (commonly known as the *Scottsdale Report*), was published. The report provides compelling data to support the economic feasibility of mandating automatic sprinklers in dwellings. See the commentary following 24.3.5.1 for further discussion of the *Scottsdale Report*.

Prince Georges County, Maryland, is another community that is largely recognized as a leader for its residential sprinkler mandate, which became effective on January 1, 1992.

In addition to sprinklers in new one- and two-family dwellings, Chapter 24 regulates interior wall and ceiling finish and mandates the installation of smoke alarms. As is the case in other residential occupancies, these features work together to greatly improve the safety of occupants.

## 24.1 General Requirements

### 24.1.1 Application.

**24.1.1.1*** The requirements of this chapter shall apply to one- and two-family dwellings, which shall include those buildings containing not more than two dwelling units in which each dwelling unit is occupied by members of a single family with not more than three outsiders, if any, accommodated in rented rooms.

**A.24.1.1.1** The *Code* specifies that wherever there are three or more living units in a building, the building is considered an apartment building and is required to comply with either Chapter 30 or Chapter 31, as appropriate. A townhouse unit is considered to be an apartment building if there are three or more units in the building. The type of wall required between units in order to consider them as separate buildings is normally established by the authority having jurisdiction. If the units are separated by a wall of sufficient fire resistance and structural integrity to be considered as separate buildings, the provisions of Chapter 24 apply to each townhouse. Condominium status is a form of ownership, not occupancy; for example, there are condominium warehouses, condominium apartments, and condominium offices.

The provisions of 24.1.1.1 state that, in one- and two-family dwellings, each dwelling unit can be "occupied by members of a single family with not more than three outsiders." The *Code* does not define the term *family*. The definition of *family* is subject to federal, state, and local regulations and might not be restricted to a person or a couple (two people) and their children. The following examples aid in differentiating between a single-family dwelling and a lodging or rooming house:

(1) An individual or a couple (two people) who rent a house from a landlord and then sublease space for up to three individuals should be considered a family renting to a maximum of three outsiders, and the house should be regulated as a single-family dwelling in accordance with Chapter 24.
(2) A house rented from a landlord by an individual or a couple (two people) in which space is subleased to 4 or more individuals, but not more than 16, should be considered and regulated as a lodging or rooming house in accordance with Chapter 26.
(3) A residential building that is occupied by 4 or more individuals, but not more than 16, each renting from a landlord, without separate cooking facilities, should be considered and regulated as a lodging or rooming house in accordance with Chapter 26.

Considerable debate has centered on the term *family*. It is not the intent of 24.1.1.1 to define the term; however, A.24.1.1.1 provides assistance in determining where the term is inappropriate and another chapter of the *Code* is to be used. If more than three outsiders are accommodated in rented rooms within a dwelling unit, the occupancy should be classified as a lodging or rooming house and should meet the requirements of Chapter 26. The reasoning behind this classification guideline is that outsiders do not tend to keep each other as informed as family members do with regard to conditions within the building. In addition, when occupying their rooms, they more often keep their room doors closed than do family members. The lack of communication and reduced openness and awareness justify the additional alarm system, vertical opening, and corridor wall and door requirements that apply to lodging or rooming houses.

**24.1.1.2** The requirements of this chapter shall apply to new buildings and to existing or modified buildings according to the provisions of 1.3.1 of this *Code*.

### 24.1.2 Multiple Occupancies.

**24.1.2.1** Multiple occupancies shall be in accordance with 6.1.14.

**24.1.2.2** No dwelling unit of a residential occupancy shall have its sole means of egress pass through any nonresidential occupancy in the same building, unless otherwise permitted by 24.1.2.2.1 or 24.1.2.2.2.

**24.1.2.2.1** In buildings that are protected by an automatic sprinkler system in accordance with Section 9.7, dwelling units of a residential occupancy shall be permitted to have their sole means of egress pass through a nonresidential occupancy in the same building, provided that the following criteria are met:

(1) The dwelling unit of the residential occupancy shall comply with Chapter 24.
(2) The sole means of egress from the dwelling unit of the residential occupancy shall not pass through a high hazard contents area as defined in 6.2.2.4.

**24.1.2.2.2** In buildings that are not protected by an automatic sprinkler system in accordance with Section 9.7, dwelling units of a residential occupancy shall be permitted to have their sole means of egress pass through a nonresidential occupancy in the same building, provided that the following criteria are met:

(1) The sole means of egress from the dwelling unit of the residential occupancy to the exterior shall be separated from the remainder of the building by fire barriers having a minimum 1-hour fire resistance rating.
(2) The dwelling unit of the residential occupancy shall comply with Chapter 24.
(3) The sole means of egress from the dwelling unit of the residential occupancy shall not pass through a high hazard contents area as defined in 6.2.2.4.

**24.1.2.3** Multiple dwelling units of a residential occupancy shall be permitted to be located above a nonresidential occupancy only where one of the following conditions exists:

(1) Where the dwelling unit of the residential occupancy and exits therefrom are separated from the nonresidential occupancy by construction having a minimum 1-hour fire resistance rating
(2) Where the nonresidential occupancy is protected throughout by an approved, supervised automatic sprinkler system in accordance with Section 9.7
(3) Where the nonresidential occupancy is protected by an automatic fire detection system in accordance with Section 9.6

One- and two-family dwellings are commonly found above stores, offices, and restaurants. Locating these occupancies in proximity to each other presents a life safety challenge for the occupants of the residential dwellings. The typical configuration of these buildings creates the potential for a significant time lapse before occupants of the residential dwellings become aware of an emergency in another part of the building and take the necessary action. The provisions of 24.1.2.2 and 24.1.2.3 are intended to provide added protection for the residential occupancy during that time lapse. Therefore, these requirements are intended to apply wherever such a mixture of occupancies exists, whether in new construction or existing buildings.

### 24.1.3 Special Definitions.

Special terms applicable to this chapter are defined in Chapter 3 of this *Code*. Where necessary, other terms are defined in the text.

### 24.1.4 Classification of Occupancy.

See 6.1.8 and 24.1.1.1.

### 24.1.5 Classification of Hazard of Contents.

The contents of residential occupancies shall be classified as ordinary hazard in accordance with 6.2.2.

NFPA 13, *Standard for the Installation of Sprinkler Systems*,[3] classifies the contents of a dwelling as *light hazard* for the purpose of designing automatic sprinkler systems. NFPA 13 classifies hazard on the basis of the challenge to the extinguishing capability of the automatic sprinkler system (light); hazard classification in this *Code* is based on the threat to life or life safety (ordinary).

### 24.1.6 Minimum Construction Requirements.

(No special requirements.)

### 24.1.7 Occupant Load.

(No requirements.)

## 24.2* Means of Escape Requirements

**A.24.2** The phrase "means of escape" indicates a way out of a residential unit that does not conform to the strict definition of means of egress but does meet the intent of the definition by providing an alternative way out of a building. *(See the definition of means of escape in 3.3.162.)*

### 24.2.1 General.

The provisions of Chapter 7 shall not apply to means of escape, unless specifically referenced in this chapter.

In 24.2.1, the term *means of escape* is used in contrast to the usual term *means of egress*, because the escape paths required for a dwelling need not be the true exit access, exit, and exit discharge required for buildings intended to be occupied by the general public. The concept of means of escape is fully developed in Section 24.2. The intent is that at least one means of escape (primary) be of a high degree of quality that is similar to the means of egress components described in Chapter 7. Homes rarely have an exit arrangement complying with Chapter 7. The door through which occupants normally enter and leave the dwelling can typically serve as the primary means of escape. Another way out of the dwelling, such as through a large, operable window, is needed as the secondary means of escape. A secondary means of escape needs to be available for use if the route involving the primary means of escape becomes unusable during a fire or similar emergency.

Only the means of escape requirements of Chapter 24 are required to be met, unless Chapter 24 specifically references a means of egress provision of Chapter 7. For example, 24.2.5.1 mandatorily references the use of the provisions of 7.2.2 and 7.2.5 for stairs, ramps, and their associated guards and handrails.

### 24.2.2 Number and Types of Means of Escape.

**24.2.2.1 Number of Means of Escape.**

**24.2.2.1.1** In dwellings or dwelling units of two rooms or more, every sleeping room and every living area shall have not less than one primary means of escape and one secondary means of escape.

See the definition of *living area* in 3.3.19.5.

The benefit of providing a primary and a secondary means of escape is based on the same concept as the requirements for two means of egress in other occupancies. The presence of two independent means of escape reduces the probability of a person becoming trapped by fire.

**24.2.2.1.2** A secondary means of escape shall not be required where one of the following conditions are met:

(1) The bedroom or living area has a door leading directly to the outside of the building at or to the finished ground level.

(2) The dwelling unit is protected throughout by an approved automatic sprinkler system in accordance with 24.3.5.

The sprinkler system referred to in 24.2.2.1.2(2) must be installed in accordance with one of the following standards:

1. NFPA 13, *Standard for the Installation of Sprinkler Systems*
2. NFPA 13D, *Standard for the Installation of Sprinkler Systems in One- and Two-Family Dwellings and Manufactured Homes*[4]
3. NFPA 13R, *Standard for the Installation of Sprinkler Systems in Residential Occupancies up to and Including Four Stories in Height*[5]

The sprinkler provision in 24.2.2.1.2(2) is probably the most practical and common way to avoid providing secondary means of escape. The sprinkler provision might be used, for example, in an underground dwelling without windows or in a dwelling where the windows do not comply with 24.2.2.3.3. Since new one- and two-family dwellings are required to be sprinklered per 24.3.5.1, they are exempt from the requirement for secondary means of escape.

**24.2.2.2 Primary Means of Escape.** The primary means of escape shall be a door, stairway, or ramp providing a means of unobstructed travel to the outside of the dwelling unit at street or the finished ground level.

A door, stairway, or ramp providing a means of unobstructed travel to the outside is usually provided for the functional purposes of entering and leaving the dwelling. Therefore, the requirement for a primary means of escape is almost automatically met in a typical dwelling.

Where an attic bedroom is accessible only by means of a trap door or folding ladder, the room does not meet the *Code* requirements for primary means of escape. Such bedrooms must be provided with direct stair access. See 24.2.5.6.

The primary means of escape from a dwelling unit in an apartment building, or from a guest room in a hotel, is permitted to lead to a means of egress, such as a corridor leading to exit stairs complying with Chapter 7.

**24.2.2.3 Secondary Means of Escape.** The secondary means of escape, other than an existing approved means of escape, shall be one of the means specified in 24.2.2.3.1 through 24.2.2.3.3.

**24.2.2.3.1** It shall be a door, stairway, passage, or hall providing a way of unobstructed travel to the outside of the dwelling at street or the finished ground level that is independent of and remote from the primary means of escape.

**24.2.2.3.2** It shall be a passage through an adjacent nonlockable space, independent of and remote from the primary means of escape, to any approved means of escape.

**24.2.2.3.3*** It shall be an outside window or door operable from the inside without the use of tools, keys, or special effort and shall provide a clear opening of not less than 5.7 $ft^2$ (0.53 $m^2$). The width shall be not less than 20 in. (510 mm), and the height shall be not less than 24 in. (610 mm). The bottom of the opening shall be not more than 44 in. (1120 mm) above the floor. Such means of escape shall be acceptable where one of the following criteria is met:

(1) The window shall be within 20 ft (6100 mm) of the finished ground level.
(2) The window shall be directly accessible to fire department rescue apparatus as approved by the authority having jurisdiction.
(3) The window or door shall open onto an exterior balcony.
(4) Windows having a sill height below the adjacent finished ground level shall be provided with a window well meeting the following criteria:
   (a) The window well shall have horizontal dimensions that allow the window to be fully opened.
   (b) The window well shall have an accessible net clear opening of not less than 9 $ft^2$ (0.82 $m^2$) with a length and width of not less than 36 in. (915 mm).
   (c) A window well with a vertical depth of more than 44 in. (1120 mm) shall be equipped with an approved permanently affixed ladder or with steps meeting the following criteria:
      i. The ladder or steps shall not encroach more than 6 in. (150 mm) into the required dimensions of the window well.
      ii. The ladder or steps shall not be obstructed by the window.

**A.24.2.2.3.3** A window with dimensions of 20 in. × 24 in. (510 mm × 610 mm) has an opening of 3.3 $ft^2$ (0.31 $m^2$), which is less than the required 5.7 $ft^2$ (0.53 $m^2$). Therefore, either the height or width needs to exceed the minimum requirement to provide the required clear area. *[See Figure A.24.2.2.3.3.]*

The purpose of the secondary means of escape is to provide an occupant with an alternate escape route when fire or smoke blocks the primary means of escape from the dwelling unit. The three types of sec-

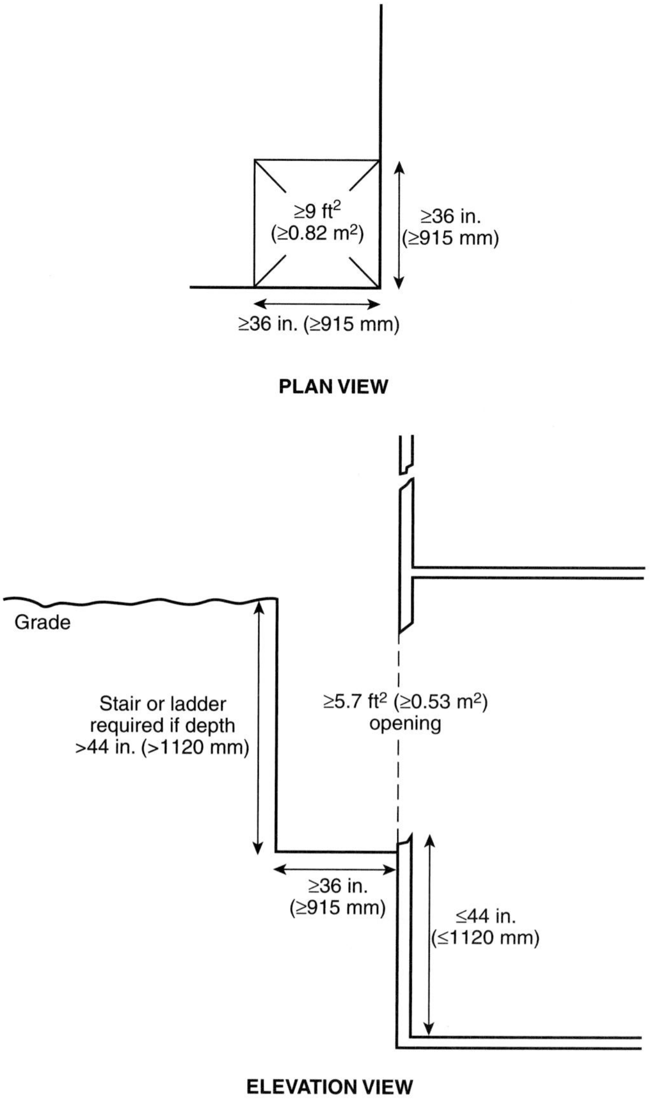


*Figure A.24.2.2.3.3 Escape Window Utilizing a Window Well.*

ondary means of escape permitted by 24.2.2.3 are outlined in paragraphs 1 through 3:

**1.** As stated in 24.2.2.3.1, the door, stairway, passage, or hall serving as the secondary means of escape must be independent of, and remote from, the primary means of escape required by 24.2.2.2. Exhibit 24.1 illustrates a dwelling unit where none of the windows complies with the requirements of 24.2.2.3.3 and a nonlockable door is located between bedrooms 2 and 3. As a result, both the primary and secondary means of escape from bedrooms 2 and 3 lead into the same hallway. A fire in or near this hallway would affect both means of escape from these rooms. Note that if

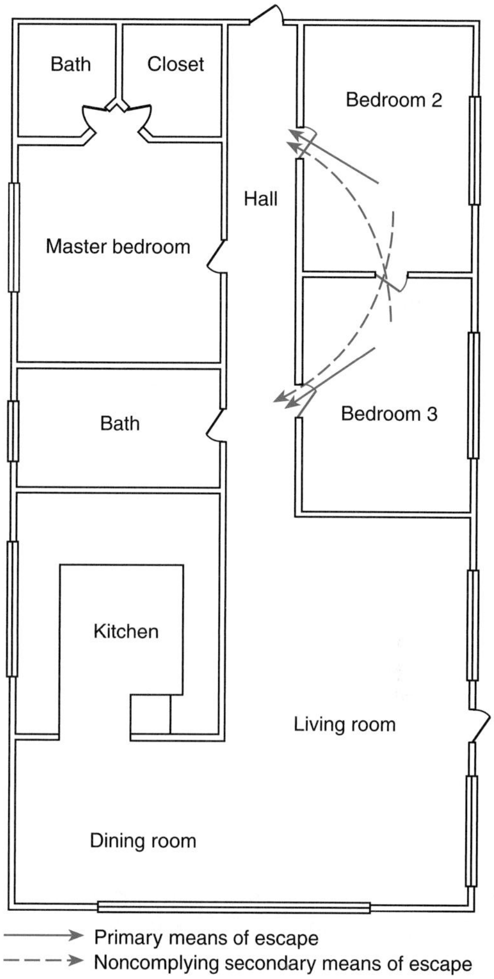


***Exhibit 24.1*** *Noncomplying secondary means of escape arrangement.*

the hallway within the dwelling unit is separated from all living spaces and leads to two separate ways out of the dwelling unit, it might be judged that the hallway does, in fact, lead to two separate, independent, and remote means of escape.

Two doors leading out of a sleeping room might not be practical or effective in most single-family dwellings. In the apartment illustrated in Exhibit 24.2, bedrooms 1 and 2 each have a window that does not comply (WNC) as a secondary means of escape. In bedroom 1, a door that meets the criteria of being independent and remote from the main door provides the secondary means of escape. Bedrooms 2 and 3 are provided with compliant windows (W) as their secondary means of escape, and the living space has a compliant sliding glass door to the balcony.

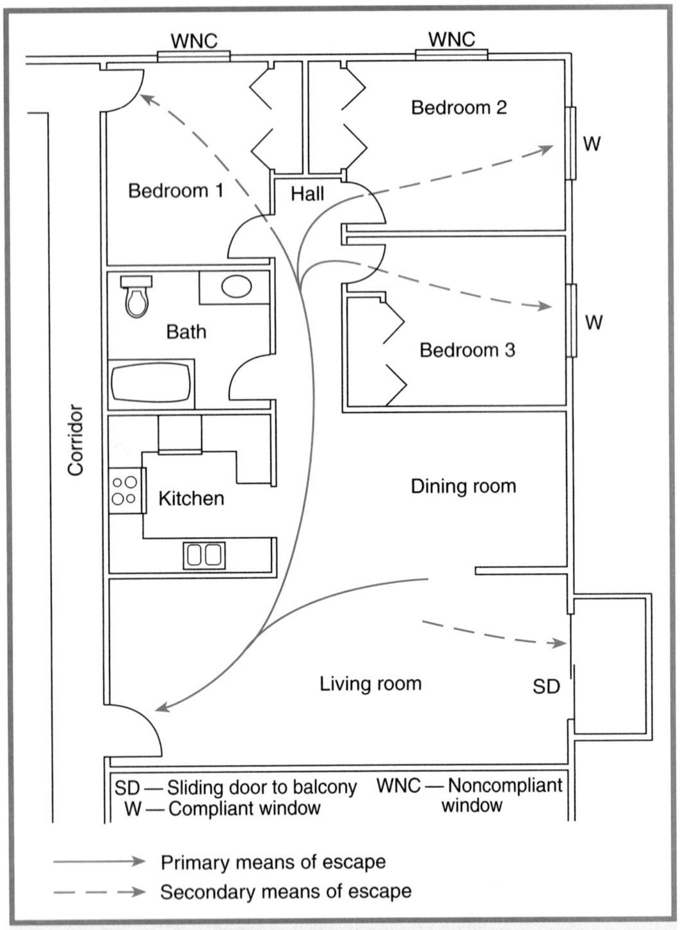


***Exhibit 24.2*** *Secondary means of escape arrangement complying with 24.2.2.*

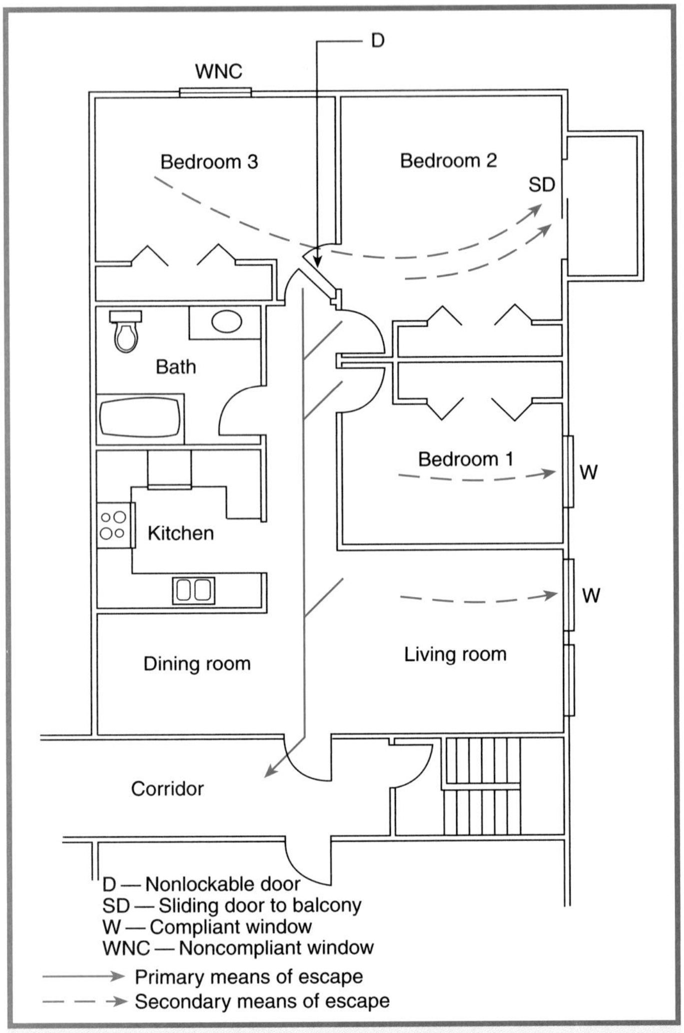


***Exhibit 24.3*** *Alternative secondary means of escape arrangement complying with 24.2.2.*

**2.** Passage through an adjacent nonlockable space, as addressed by 24.2.2.3.2, is illustrated in Exhibit 24.3. In this exhibit, bedroom 3 has a window that does not comply with the provisions of 24.2.2.3.3; however, there is a compliant door between bedrooms 3 and 2 that provides a secondary means of escape to the balcony using the compliant sliding door in bedroom 2.

**3.** The use of an operable window providing an opening of the minimum dimensions specified in 24.2.2.3.3 is the secondary means of escape most often provided. Exhibit 24.4 illustrates the minimum dimensions required for escape windows. Note that a window providing only the minimum width and minimum height dimensions specified by 24.2.2.3.3 does not provide the required minimum area; if either the minimum width or minimum height dimension is used, the other dimension must be increased to achieve the minimum area requirement. This requirement also is illustrated in Exhibit 24.4.

The outside window addressed in 24.2.2.3.3 must comply with one of the four accessibility arrangements outlined in paragraphs 1 through 4.

**1.** The first arrangement makes it possible for an occupant to drop from the window, because the window must be within 20 ft (6100 mm) of the finished ground level.

**2.** The second arrangement relies on the fire department to rescue an occupant from a window that is within reach of rescue apparatus. Such rescue can be achieved either by means of truck-mounted aerial ladders, by ground ladders, or by other means acceptable to the authority having jurisdiction (AHJ).

**3.** The third arrangement allows an occupant to reach an exterior balcony to breathe fresh air while

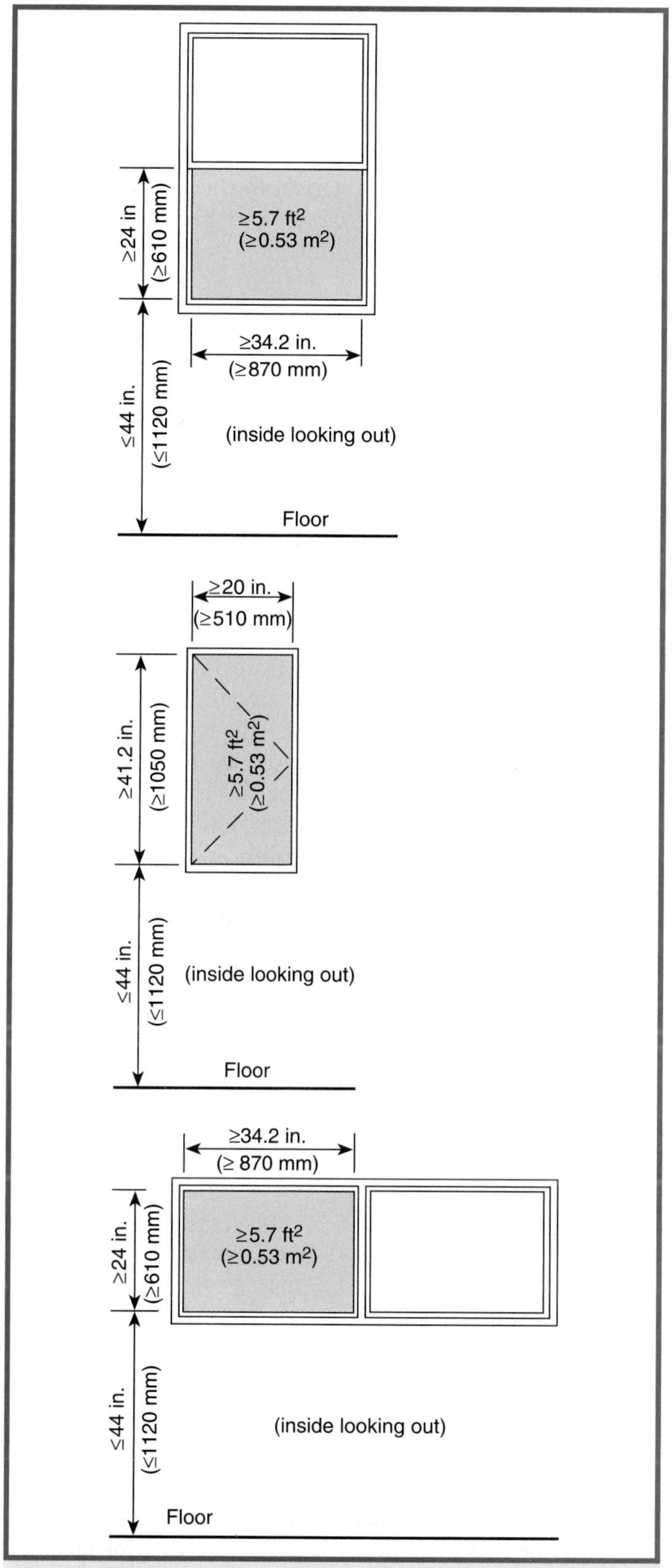


***Exhibit 24.4*** *Escape window minimum opening dimensions.*

awaiting either rescue or fire extinguishment. This method could be used where the balcony is not within reach of rescue apparatus. See Exhibit 24.2 and Exhibit 24.3 for examples of secondary means of escape utilizing balconies.

**4.** The fourth arrangement recognizes the increasing trend of developing or converting basements into living space, such as home offices, playrooms, or sleeping areas. Fire in these areas or the areas above them could easily block the primary means of escape, which is usually a single stair to the upper level. This option provides requirements for the size of the window well, in addition to the window size, to provide sufficient space to operate the window and move up to grade level.

Existing secondary means of escape — such as existing windows that do not meet the strict dimensional requirements of 24.2.2.3.3 — are permitted by 24.2.2.3 to continue to be used subject to the approval of the AHJ. This provision limits the impact on existing buildings, unless the means of escape is of extremely poor quality.

**24.2.2.3.4** Ladders or steps that comply with the requirements of 24.2.2.3.3(4)(c) shall be exempt from the requirements of 7.2.2.

**24.2.2.4 Two Primary Means of Escape.** In buildings, other than existing buildings and other than those protected throughout by an approved, supervised automatic sprinkler system in accordance with 24.3.5, every story more than 2000 ft$^2$ (185 m$^2$) in area within the dwelling unit shall be provided with two primary means of escape remotely located from each other.

### 24.2.3 Arrangement of Means of Escape.

Any required path of travel in a means of escape from any room to the outside shall not pass through another room or apartment not under the immediate control of the occupant of the first room or through a bathroom or other space subject to locking.

A means of escape that relies on travel through an adjacent space might not be usable if the door separating the spaces is locked against escape. One- and two-family dwellings can have rooms occupied by up to three outsiders or could be arranged so that a second family must escape through the living space of the first family. This arrangement is often found in older homes that were not originally built as duplexes but that were later converted to such an arrangement. Any spaces through which escape will occur must be under the control of the person escaping.

### 24.2.4 Doors.

**24.2.4.1** Doors in the path of travel of a means of escape, other than bathroom doors in accordance with 24.2.4.2 and doors serving a room not exceeding 70 $ft^2$ (6.5 $m^2$), shall be not less than 28 in. (710 mm) wide.

**24.2.4.2** Bathroom doors and doors serving a room not exceeding 70 $ft^2$ (6.5 $m^2$) shall be not less than 24 in. (610 mm) wide.

Although Chapter 7 requires 32 in. (810 mm) clear width doors in new construction and 28 in. (710 mm) wide doors in existing buildings, 24.2.4.1 permits the use of 28 in. (710 mm) wide doors [24 in. (610 mm) for bathrooms per 24.2.4.2] in both new and existing one- and two-family dwellings. This measurement, as illustrated in Exhibit 24.5, is a leaf width measurement of the door, not a clear width measurement of the door opening. In addition to one- and two-family dwellings, this requirement applies to doors within the guest rooms and guest suites of lodging or rooming houses, hotels and dormitories, and dwelling units of apartment buildings.

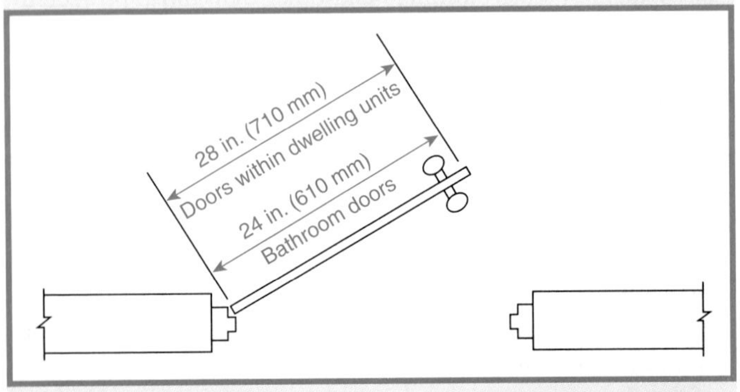


***Exhibit 24.5*** *Minimum width of doors within a dwelling unit.*

The 28 in. (710 mm) wide doors specified in 24.2.4.1 are used in some dwelling designs, but ease of access and the need to move furniture and appliances usually dictate a larger size.

**24.2.4.3** Doors shall be not less than 6 ft 6 in. (1980 mm) in nominal height.

**24.2.4.4** Every closet door latch shall be such that children can open the door from inside the closet.

**24.2.4.5** Every bathroom door shall be designed to allow opening from the outside during an emergency when locked.

During a fire, children will often seek refuge in bathrooms and closets. The provisions of 24.2.4.4 and 24.2.4.5 for releasing the latch from the inside and the lock from the outside of closet and bathroom doors allow for escape and facilitate rescue by parents or emergency responders.

**24.2.4.6** Doors shall be swinging or sliding.

**24.2.4.7*** No door in any means of escape shall be locked against egress when the building is occupied. All locking devices that impede or prohibit egress or that cannot be easily disengaged shall be prohibited.

**A.24.2.4.7** It is the intent of this requirement that security measures, where installed, do not prevent egress.

Dwelling units are prohibited from having any door locked against egress while the dwelling unit is occupied in accordance with 24.2.4.7. This requirement permits a door to have a locking device that allows the door to be opened from within the building for the purpose of escape but that does not allow the door to be opened from outside the building. Ordinary double-cylinder locks and key-operated chain locks do not meet this requirement. Several multiple-death fires have occurred when a door lock could not be released because the key could not be found.

The prohibition on locking applies only to doors or windows that are part of the required means of escape system. Often, the rear door of a dwelling is not part of the required escape system, and, therefore, such a door is permitted to be equipped with a double-cylinder key-operated lock.

**24.2.4.8** Floor levels at doors in the primary means of escape shall comply with 7.2.1.3, unless otherwise permitted by the following:

(1) In existing buildings, where the door discharges to the outside or to an exterior balcony or exterior exit access, the floor level outside the door shall be permitted to be one step lower than the inside, but shall not be in excess of 8 in. (205 mm).
(2) In new buildings, where the door discharges to the outside or to an exterior exit access, an exterior landing with not more than a 7 in. (180 mm) drop below the door threshold and a minimum dimension of 36 in. (915 mm) or the width of the door leaf, whichever is smaller, shall be permitted.

(3) A door at the top of an interior stair shall be permitted to open directly at a stair, provided that the door does not swing over the stair and the door serves an area with an occupant load of fewer than 50 persons.

**24.2.4.9** Forces to open doors shall comply with 7.2.1.4.5.

**24.2.4.10** Latching devices for doors shall comply with 7.2.1.5.9.

## 24.2.5 Stairs, Ramps, and Guards.

**24.2.5.1** Stairs, ramps, guards, and handrails shall be in accordance with 7.2.2 for stairs, 7.2.2.4 for guards, and 7.2.5 for ramps, as modified by 24.2.5.1.1 through 24.2.5.1.3.

**24.2.5.1.1** The provisions of 7.2.2.5, 7.2.5.5, and 7.7.3 shall not apply.

**24.2.5.1.2** If serving as a secondary means of escape, stairs complying with the fire escape requirements of Table 7.2.8.4.1(a) or Table 7.2.8.4.1(b) shall be permitted.

**24.2.5.1.3** If serving as a secondary means of escape, ramps complying with the existing ramp requirements of Table 7.2.5.2(b) shall be permitted.

Prior to the 2003 edition of the *Code*, stairs in dwelling units were permitted to have a geometry modified from that required in Chapter 7; new stairs were previously permitted to have maximum riser heights of 7¾ in. (195 mm) and minimum tread depths of 10 in. (255 mm). The provision to allow for modified tread and riser geometry for new stairs in dwelling units has been removed from the *Code* on the basis of data that suggests stairs not meeting the dimensional criteria in Chapter 7 are less safe to navigate than those that do, under both normal and emergency egress conditions. As such, all new stairs in dwelling units must meet the Chapter 7 dimensional criteria: maximum 7 in. (180 mm) risers and minimum 11 in. (280 mm) treads. Existing stairs are permitted to meet the criteria in Table 7.2.2.2.1.1(b).

It is important to keep in mind that carpeting might be installed on the stairs following construction of the stair itself, and after the home is occupied. Carpeting might have an adverse impact on the effective tread depth. Exhibit 24.6 illustrates the effect of carpeting on the stepping surface of the stair. Designing the stairs to the minimum geometry is insufficient; consideration must be given to floor coverings. If carpeting is to be installed on stairs, the determination of compliance with the dimensional requirements of the *Code* should be made after it is installed.

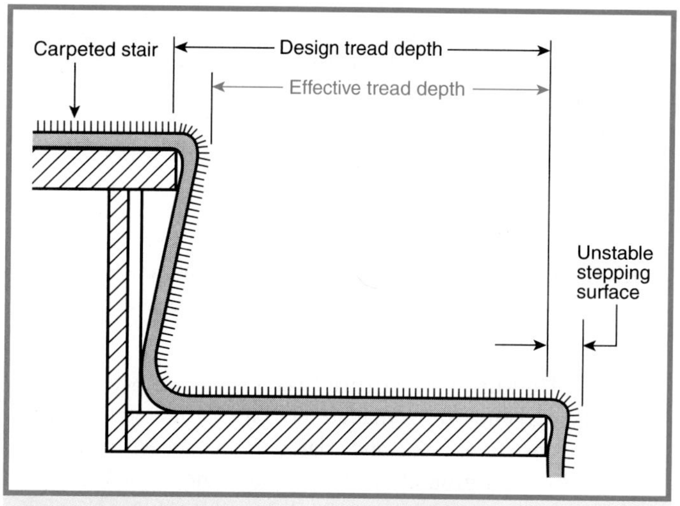


***Exhibit 24.6** Effect of carpeting on tread depth.*

**24.2.5.2** Interior stairways shall be provided with means capable of providing artificial light at the minimum level specified by 7.8.1.3 for exit stairs, measured at the center of treads and on landing surfaces within 24 in. (610 mm) of step nosings.

**24.2.5.3** For interior stairways, manual lighting controls shall be reachable and operable without traversing any step of the stair.

**24.2.5.4** The clear width of stairs, landings, ramps, balconies, and porches shall be not less than 36 in. (915 mm), measured in accordance with 7.3.2.

**24.2.5.5** Spiral stairs and winders in accordance with 7.2.2.2.3 and 7.2.2.2.4 shall be permitted within a single dwelling unit.

**24.2.5.6** No sleeping rooms or living areas shall be accessible only by a ladder, a stair ladder, an alternating tread device, or folding stairs or through a trap door.

## 24.2.6 Hallways.

**24.2.6.1** The width of hallways, other than existing approved hallways, which shall be permitted to continue to be used, shall be not less than 36 in. (915 mm).

**24.2.6.2** The height of hallways, other than existing approved hallways, which shall be permitted to continue to be used, shall be not less than 7 ft (2135 mm) nominal, with clearance below projections from the ceiling of not less than 6 ft 8 in. (2030 mm) nominal.

Within the dwelling unit, headroom clearance is regulated only in the hallways. Such regulation helps to ensure that the space above head height can accumulate smoke early in the fire to allow safe escape through the hallway, which will help to prevent the need for occupants to crawl near floor level to avoid the descending smoke layer.

### 24.2.7 Bulkheads.

**24.2.7.1 Bulkhead Enclosures.** Where provided, bulkhead enclosures shall provide direct access to the basement from the exterior.

**24.2.7.2 Bulkhead Enclosure Stairways.** Stairways serving bulkhead enclosures that are not part of the required primary means of escape, and that provide access from the outside finished ground level to the basement, shall be exempt from the provisions of 24.2.5.1 when the maximum height from the basement finished floor level to the finished ground level adjacent to the stairway does not exceed 8 ft (2440 mm), and the finished ground level opening to the stairway is covered by a bulkhead enclosure with hinged doors or other approved means.

## 24.3 Protection

### 24.3.1 Protection of Vertical Openings.

(No requirements.)

### 24.3.2 Reserved.

### 24.3.3 Interior Finish.

**24.3.3.1 General.** Interior finish shall be in accordance with Section 10.2.

**24.3.3.2 Interior Wall and Ceiling Finish.** Interior wall and ceiling finish materials complying with Section 10.2 shall be Class A, Class B, or Class C.

**24.3.3.3 Interior Floor Finish.** (No requirements.)

**24.3.3.4 Contents and Furnishings.** Contents and furnishings shall not be required to comply with Section 10.3.

### 24.3.4 Detection, Alarm, and Communications Systems.

Smoke alarms or a smoke detection system shall be provided in accordance with either 24.3.4.1 or 24.3.4.2, as modified by 24.3.4.3.

**24.3.4.1*** Smoke alarms shall be installed in accordance with 9.6.2.10 in the following locations:

(1) All sleeping rooms
(2)* Outside of each separate sleeping area, in the immediate vicinity of the sleeping rooms
(3) On each level of the dwelling unit, including basements

**A.24.3.4.1** Paragraph 11.5.1.3 of *NFPA 72, National Fire Alarm Code*, contains related requirements. They specify that, where the interior floor area for a given level of a dwelling unit, excluding garage areas, is greater than 1000 $ft^2$ (93 $m^2$), smoke alarms are to be installed as follows:

(1) All points on the ceiling are to have a smoke alarm within a distance of 30 ft (9.1 m), measured along a path of travel, or have one smoke alarm per 500 $ft^2$ (46.5 $m^2$) of floor area. One smoke alarm per 500 $ft^2$ (46.5 $m^2$) is calculated by dividing the total interior floor area per level by 500 $ft^2$ (46.5 $m^2$).
(2) Where dwelling units include great rooms or vaulted/cathedral ceilings extending over multiple floors, smoke alarms located on the upper floor that are intended to protect the aforementioned area are permitted to be considered as part of the lower floor(s) protection scheme used to meet the requirements of A.24.3.4.1(1).

**A.24.3.4.1(2)** Paragraphs 11.5.1.1(2) and 11.5.1.2 of *NFPA 72, National Fire Alarm Code*, contain related requirements. The requirement of 11.5.1.1(2) specifies that an alarm is to be installed outside of each separate dwelling unit sleeping area, within 21 ft (6.4 m) of any door to a sleeping room, with the distance measured along a path of travel. The requirement in 11.5.1.2 specifies that, where the area addressed in 11.5.1.1(2) is separated from the adjacent living areas by a door, a smoke alarm is to be installed in the area between the door and the sleeping rooms, and additional alarms are to be installed on the living area side of the door.

**24.3.4.2** Dwelling units shall be protected by an approved smoke detection system in accordance with Section 9.6 and equipped with an approved means of occupant notification.

**24.3.4.3** In existing one- and two-family dwellings, approved smoke alarms powered by batteries shall be permitted.

The reference to 9.6.2.10 in 24.3.4.1 requires smoke alarms to be hard-wired into the electrical system of the home or to be plug-in alarms. The provision of 24.3.4.3, which permits battery-powered smoke alarms in existing dwellings, gives dwelling occupants relief from retrofit requirements while providing needed protection. However, occupants of dwellings that use battery-operated smoke alarms must ensure that those alarms are tested and maintained properly. NFPA analysis has shown that 30 percent of smoke alarms were inoperative in homes that had smoke alarms and that had experienced fire. The primary reason for smoke alarm failure is that the battery was removed to avoid nuisance alarms. NFPA public education programs, such as the *Learn Not to Burn*® program, are effective tools for promoting proper smoke alarm maintenance.

Regardless of the power source, it is important that smoke alarms be properly located. Exhibit 24.7 and Exhibit 24.8 illustrate the required locations of the smoke alarms per 24.3.4. Further information on the mounting, location, spacing, and performance of smoke alarms is found in A.24.3.4.1(2) of this *Code* and Chapter 11 of *NFPA 72*®, *National Fire Alarm Code*®.[6]

Note that effective with the 2009 edition, the *Code* now requires smoke alarms to be located in sleeping rooms of both new and existing one- and two-family dwellings. In existing buildings, the smoke alarms are permitted to be battery-powered as indicated by 24.3.4.3.

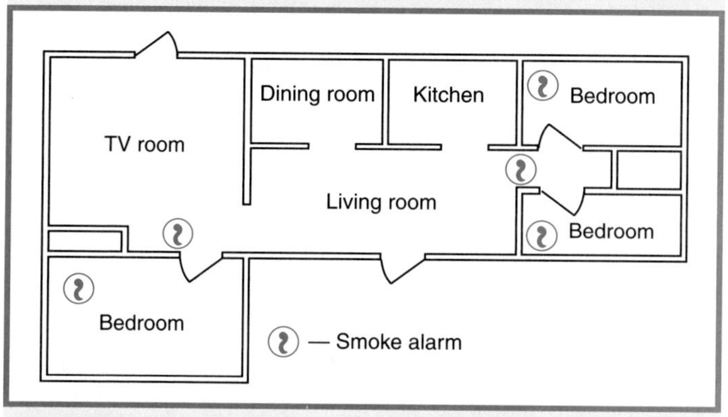


***Exhibit 24.7*** *Required smoke alarm locations.*

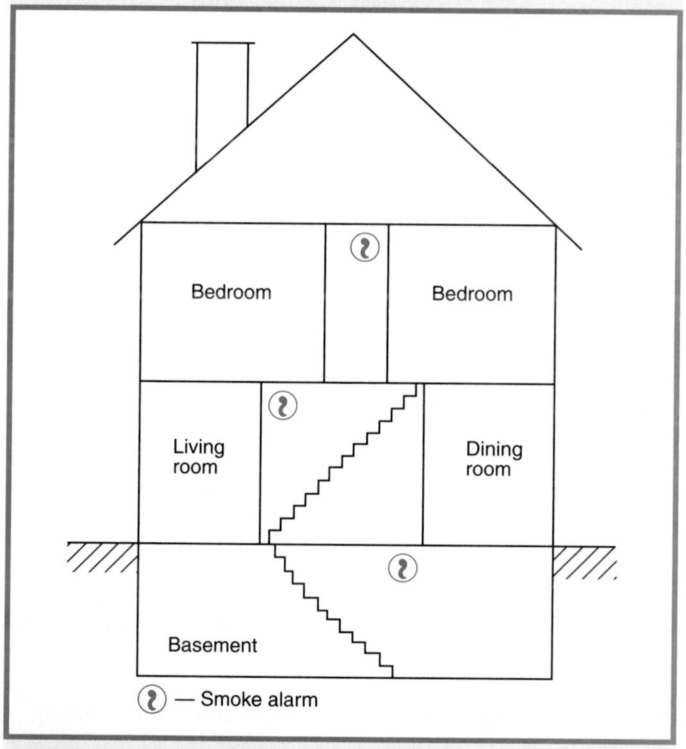


***Exhibit 24.8*** *Required smoke alarm placement per level.*

### 24.3.5* Extinguishment Requirements.

**A.24.3.5** Automatic sprinklers are recognized as an excellent addition to homes to enhance life safety and property protection. Automatic sprinklers can be part of a comprehensive package of fire protection and can assist in the overall master planning of a community. Where all of the buildings within an area are sprinklered, including the single-family dwellings, the response times and personnel of local fire departments can be established at different levels than if the buildings were not sprinklered, saving considerable amounts of tax dollars. When whole developments are sprinklered, water mains, hydrant spacing, road widths, and building density can be altered to help alleviate the economic impact of the sprinklers.

**24.3.5.1** All new one- and two-family dwellings shall be protected throughout by an approved automatic sprinkler system in accordance with 24.3.5.2.

In response to the unacceptable number of fire deaths occurring in one- and two-family dwellings on an annual basis (an average of 2,580 civilian fire deaths per year for the period 2000–2004 in the United States[7]), the *Code,* starting with the 2006 edition, now requires all new one- and two-family dwellings to be protected by automatic sprinkler systems. While the requirement for sprinkler systems in one- and two-family dwellings was new to the 2006 edition of the *Code*, the concept of residential sprinkler protection is not. As part of its decision to mandate sprinklers in new one- and two-family dwellings, the NFPA Technical Committee on Residential Occupancies evaluated economic and sprinkler success data from communities such as Scottsdale, Arizona, and Prince Georges County, Maryland, which have required sprinklers in new homes since 1986 and 1992, respectively. Data from the *Scottsdale Report* has been updated to January 1, 2001, expanding its scope from 10 to 15 years. Some of the highlights of the updated report follow.

1. 41,408 homes (more than 50 percent of the homes in Scottsdale) were protected by automatic sprinklers.
2. Since the sprinkler ordinance was implemented, 598 home fires occurred — 49 of those were in sprinklered homes.

a. No fatalities occurred in the sprinklered homes.
b. 13 people died in homes with no sprinklers.

3. Water damage was less in homes protected by sprinklers.
   a. Ninety-two percent of the fires in sprinklered homes were controlled by one or two sprinklers.
   b. Sprinkler systems discharged an average of 341 gal (1291 L) of water per fire.
   c. In nonsprinklered homes, fire fighter hose streams discharged an average of 2935 gal (11,110 L) of water per fire.
4. Fire damage was less in sprinklered homes.
   a. The average loss per fire in sprinklered homes was $2,166 (1986–2001, 49 fires).
   b. The average loss per fire in nonsprinklered homes was $45,019 (1998–2001, 86 fires).
5. Technological advances have made residential sprinklers less costly and easier to install.
   a. On national average, sprinkler systems add between 1 percent and 1.5 percent to the total cost of the construction of a home.
   b. In Scottsdale, the average installation cost was $0.80 per square foot ($8.61 per square meter) of floor area.

**24.3.5.2** Where an automatic sprinkler system is installed, either for total or partial building coverage, the system shall be in accordance with Section 9.7; in buildings of four or fewer stories in height above grade plane, systems in accordance with NFPA 13R, *Standard for the Installation of Sprinkler Systems in Residential Occupancies up to and Including Four Stories in Height*, and with NFPA 13D, *Standard for the Installation of Sprinkler Systems in One- and Two-Family Dwellings and Manufactured Homes*, shall also be permitted.

NFPA 13D, *Standard for the Installation of Sprinkler Systems in One- and Two-Family Dwellings and Manufactured Homes*, was developed after extensive research that included full-scale fire tests. It introduced the concept of a quick-response residential sprinkler. Unlike its industrial standard spray sprinkler counterpart, which is inherently slow to fuse its relatively massive eutectic solder element, a quick-response residential sprinkler operates very quickly once its rated temperature is reached. Quick-response sprinklers begin to control a fire early in its growth. In addition to being quick to respond, residential sprinklers (as mandated by NFPA 13D) have a specifically designed spray pattern that delivers water to nearly the full height of the walls of small rooms that are typical of residential occupancies. An example of a residential sprinkler is depicted in Exhibit 24.9.

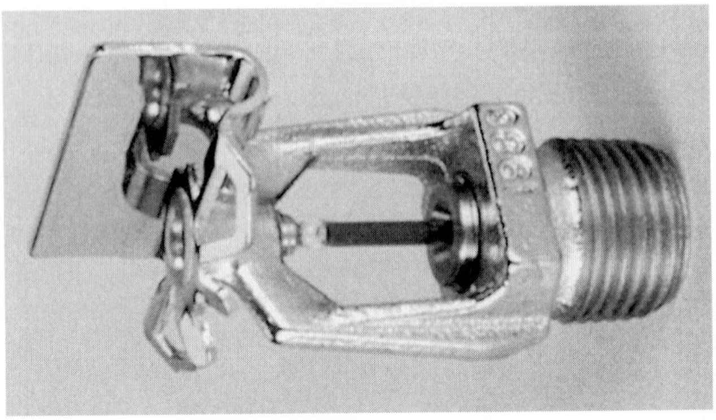

***Exhibit 24.9*** *Viking Model M-1 Horizontal Sidewall Residential Sprinkler. (Photo courtesy of Viking)*

NFPA 13R, *Standard for the Installation of Sprinkler Systems in Residential Occupancies up to and Including Four Stories in Height*, addresses residential sprinklers that incorporate the quick-response sprinkler technology described in the preceding paragraph. NFPA 13R thus extends the technological and economic benefits of an NFPA 13D-type system to larger residential buildings, while requiring additional provisions that are commensurate with increased building size that will help to ensure improved protection against injury and life loss to building residents — including those occupying the room of fire origin. Note that where one- and two-family dwellings are protected with automatic sprinkler systems, they are permitted to meet the requirements of NFPA 13, NFPA 13D, or NFPA 13R.

## 24.4 Reserved

## 24.5 Building Services

### 24.5.1 Heating, Ventilating, and Air-Conditioning.

**24.5.1.1** Heating, ventilating, and air-conditioning equipment shall comply with the provisions of Section 9.2.

**24.5.1.2** Unvented fuel-fired heaters shall not be used unless they are listed and approved.

**24.5.2 Reserved.**

## References Cited in Commentary


1. *NFPA 5000®, Building Construction and Safety Code®*, 2009 edition, National Fire Protection Association, Quincy, MA.
2. Assistant Chief Jim Ford, "Automatic Sprinklers: A 10 Year Study — A Detailed History of the Effects of the Automatic Sprinkler Code in Scottsdale, Arizona," City of Scottsdale/Rural-Metro Fire Department/Home Fire Sprinkler Fire Coalition, 1997.
3. NFPA 13, *Standard for the Installation of Sprinkler Systems*, 2007 edition, National Fire Protection Association, Quincy, MA.
4. NFPA 13D, *Standard for the Installation of Sprinkler Systems in One- and Two-Family Dwellings and Manufactured Homes*, 2007 edition, National Fire Protection Association, Quincy, MA.
5. NFPA 13R, *Standard for the Installation of Sprinkler Systems in Residential Occupancies up to and Including Four Stories in Height*, 2007 edition, National Fire Protection Association, Quincy, MA.
6. *NFPA 72®, National Fire Alarm Code®*, 2007 edition, National Fire Protection Association, Quincy, MA.
7. Ahrens, M. *Home Structure Fires*, February 2007, Fire Analysis and Research Division, National Fire Protection Association, Quincy, MA.

# CHAPTER 25

# Reserved

Typically, the occupancy chapters are paired so that the even-numbered chapter in the pair addresses new facilities of the occupancy type and the odd-numbered chapter addresses existing facilities of the occupancy type. Chapter 24, which precedes this chapter, addresses both new and existing one- and two-family dwellings in a single chapter. Chapter 25 has been reserved to permit the chapter on lodging or rooming houses to be assigned an even number (i.e., Chapter 26). The reserved chapter number might be used at a future date if the requirements for one- and two-family dwellings are split into a pair of chapters — one for new construction and one for existing buildings.

CHAPTER 26

# Lodging or Rooming Houses

Chapter 26 addresses the requirements for both new and existing lodging or rooming houses. These facilities provide sleeping accommodations for 16 or fewer occupants on a transient basis. While some users of the *Code* might confuse lodging or rooming facilities with a hotel occupancy — or a board and care facility — the primary differences among the occupancies center on the total number of occupants served and the nature of any personal care that is provided. While some of these facilities might provide what appear to be longer-term, daily living accommodations, other facilities, such as a bed-and-breakfast facility, might provide accommodations on a short-term basis. If a bed-and-breakfast facility serves more than 16 occupants, it would be appropriate to use Chapters 28 and 29 for hotels and dormitories to evaluate the requisite life safety features.

Commentary Table 26.1 is a guide to the appropriate occupancy chapter for multitenant residential occupancies.

## 26.1 General Requirements

### 26.1.1 Application.

**26.1.1.1*** The requirements of this chapter shall apply to buildings that provide sleeping accommodations for 16 or fewer persons on either a transient or permanent basis, with or without meals, but without separate cooking facilities for individual occupants, except as provided in Chapter 24.

**A.26.1.1.1** Bed and breakfast occupancies with more than 3, but fewer than 17, occupants are considered lodging and rooming houses.

If sleeping accommodations for more than 16 people are provided, the occupancy is classified as a hotel or dormitory. The reference to Chapter 24 in 26.1.1.1 concerns the provision that permits rooms to be occupied by a maximum of three outsiders in addition to family members in one- and two-family dwellings without changing the occupancy classification. Many of the facilities that house more than three outsiders but fewer than 16 people ordinarily would not be considered lodging or rooming houses but, nevertheless, do meet the definition — for example, a fire station that has a bunk room. A fire station with bunking facilities would normally be considered a multiple occupancy, depending on the arrangement of the facility. For example, the fire station in Exhibit 26.1 would be classified as a multiple occupancy with mixed uses, because it contains assembly, business, lodging or rooming, industrial, and storage occupancies. By applying the

***Commentary Table 26.1 Comparative Factors for Classification of Residential Occupancies***

| Factor | Chapter 26 Lodging or Rooming Houses | Chapters 28 and 29 Hotels and Dormitories | Chapters 30 and 31 Apartment Buildings | Chapters 32 and 33 Residential Board and Care |
|---|---|---|---|---|
| Occupants of a transient nature? | Yes | Yes | No | No |
| Number of occupants in facility? | 16 or fewer | More than 16 | As few as 3; application based on presence of 3 or more independent dwelling units | 4 or more |
| Personal care services provided? | No | No | No | Yes |

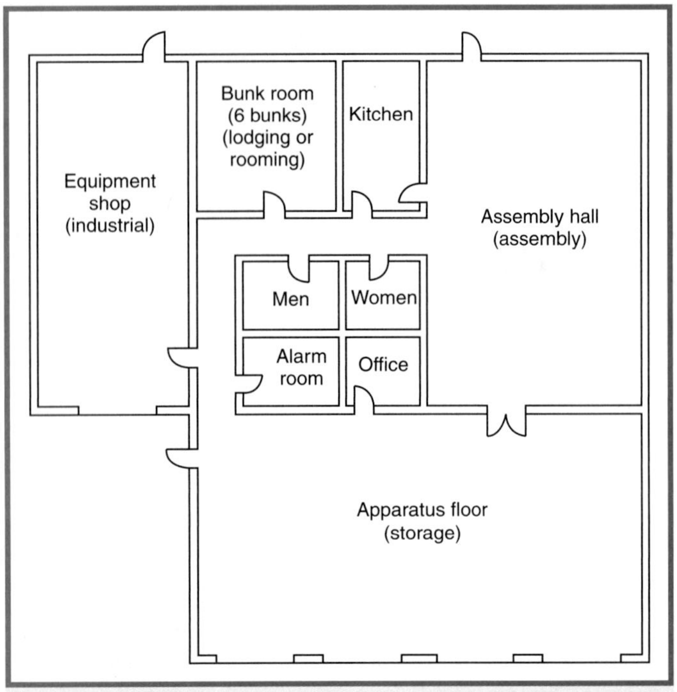


*Exhibit 26.1 Fire station that is a mixed occupancy.*

most restrictive requirements, this building would require automatic sprinklers via the provisions of 26.3.6.1. If additional exits are added to provide separate means of egress for the bunk room, equipment shop, assembly hall, and apparatus bay and the various uses are separated in accordance with 6.1.14.4, as shown in Exhibit 26.2, the building is considered a multiple occupancy with separated uses, and the provisions for the occupancy within each space would be applied separately.

**26.1.1.2** The requirements of this chapter shall apply to new buildings and to existing or modified buildings according to the provisions of 1.3.1 of this *Code*.

### 26.1.2 Multiple Occupancies.

**26.1.2.1** Multiple occupancies shall be in accordance with 6.1.14.

**26.1.2.2** No lodging or rooming house shall have its sole means of egress pass through any nonresidential occupancy in the same building, unless otherwise permitted by 26.1.2.2.1 or 26.1.2.2.2.

**26.1.2.2.1** In buildings that are protected by an automatic sprinkler system in accordance with Section 9.7, lodging or rooming houses shall be permitted to have their sole means of egress pass through a nonresidential occupancy in the same building, provided that the following criteria are met:

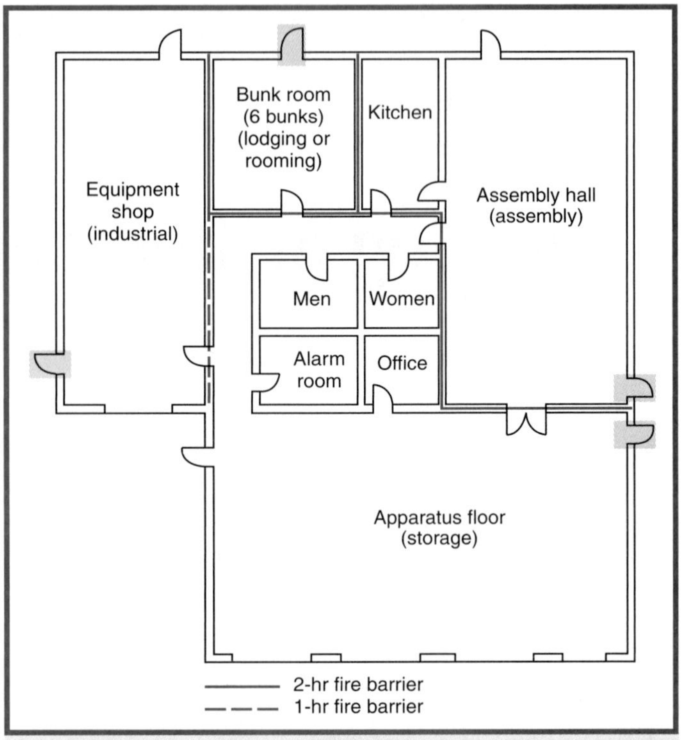


*Exhibit 26.2 Fire station that is a multiple occupancy with separated uses.*

(1) The lodging or rooming house shall comply with Chapter 26.
(2) The sole means of egress from the lodging or rooming house shall not pass through a high hazard contents area, as defined in 6.2.2.4.

**26.1.2.2.2** In buildings that are not protected by an automatic sprinkler system in accordance with Section 9.7, lodging or rooming houses shall be permitted to have their sole means of egress pass through a nonresidential occupancy in the same building, provided that all of the following criteria are met:

(1) The sole means of egress from the lodging or rooming house to the exterior shall be separated from the remainder of the building by fire barriers having a minimum 1-hour fire resistance rating.
(2) The lodging or rooming house shall comply with Chapter 26.
(3) The sole means of egress from the lodging or rooming house shall not pass through a high hazard contents area, as defined in 6.2.2.4.

**26.1.2.3** Lodging or rooming houses shall be permitted to be located above a nonresidential occupancy only where one of the following conditions exists:

(1) Where the lodging or rooming house and exits therefrom are separated from the nonresidential occupancy

by construction having a minimum 1-hour fire resistance rating

(2) Where the nonresidential occupancy is protected throughout by an approved, supervised automatic sprinkler system in accordance with Section 9.7

(3) Where the lodging or rooming house is located above a nonresidential occupancy, and the nonresidential occupancy is protected by an automatic fire detection system in accordance with Section 9.6

A nonresidential occupancy located below a lodging or rooming house presents a life safety challenge for the occupants of the residential space. The typical configuration of these buildings creates the potential for a significant time lapse before occupants of the residential occupancy become aware of an emergency in another part of the building and take the necessary action. The provisions of 26.1.2.2 and 26.1.2.3 are intended to provide added protection for the residential occupancy during that time lapse. Therefore, these requirements are intended to apply wherever this mixture of occupancies exists, whether in new construction or in existing buildings.

### 26.1.3 Special Definitions.

Special terms applicable to this chapter are defined in Chapter 3. Where necessary, other terms are defined in the text.

### 26.1.4 Classification of Occupancy.

See 6.1.8 and 26.1.1.1.

### 26.1.5 Classification of Hazard of Contents.

The contents of residential occupancies shall be classified as ordinary hazard in accordance with 6.2.2.

NFPA 13, *Standard for the Installation of Sprinkler Systems*,[1] classifies the contents of a lodging or rooming house as light hazard for the purpose of designing automatic sprinkler systems. The difference in classification in the *Code* is based on the threat to life or life safety (ordinary), as opposed to the challenge to the extinguishing capability of the automatic sprinkler system (light).

### 26.1.6 Minimum Construction Requirements.

(No special requirements.)

### 26.1.7 Occupant Load.

See 26.1.1.1.

## 26.2 Means of Escape Requirements

### 26.2.1 Number and Types of Means of Escape.

**26.2.1.1 Primary Means of Escape.**

**26.2.1.1.1** Every sleeping room and living area shall have access to a primary means of escape complying with Chapter 24 and located to provide a safe path of travel to the outside.

**26.2.1.1.2** Where the sleeping room is above or below the level of exit discharge, the primary means of escape shall be an interior stair in accordance with 26.2.2, an exterior stair, a horizontal exit in accordance with 7.2.4, or an existing fire escape stair in accordance with 7.2.8.

The concept of means of escape has been fully developed in Chapter 24. Provisions for means of escape — rather than means of egress — are specified in 26.2.1.1.1 and 26.2.1.1.2, because the escape paths required for a lodging or rooming house are more similar to those provided for a residential dwelling than those for publically occupied or commercial buildings.

The *Code* requires at least one means of escape from levels above or below the level of exit discharge to be an enclosed interior stair, an exterior stair, a horizontal exit, or an existing fire escape. The intent is that at least one means of escape (primary) be of a high degree of quality that is similar to the means of egress components described in Chapter 7. Most lodging or rooming houses are converted homes that rarely have a means of egress arrangement complying with Chapter 7. However, the *Code* recognizes the issue of public liability associated with lodging guests and includes requirements in Chapter 26 that provide a level of escape quality higher than that normally found in a single-family home.

The protection of the primary means of escape as required by 26.2.1.1 — often accomplished by the protection of vertical openings in accordance with 26.2.2 and 26.3.1 — is the major distinction between the requirements applicable to one- and two-family dwellings and those applicable to lodging or rooming houses. Another distinction is the requirement in 26.3.6.1 for the provision of automatic sprinklers in new lodging or rooming houses. By protecting the escape path from exposure to unprotected vertical openings — such as the unenclosed stairs normally found in single-family dwellings — the *Code* helps to ensure that the occupants of a lodging or rooming house can reach a point of safety. This protection is important, because the occupants of a lodging or rooming house characteristically occupy their rooms with the doors closed. Therefore, they lack the awareness of emergency conditions that is experienced by members of a family who live together within a dwelling where doors are usually open.

Exhibit 26.3 through Exhibit 26.7 illustrate possible methods of complying with the means of escape provisions of 26.2.1.1, as affected by the provisions of 26.2.2 and 26.3.1.

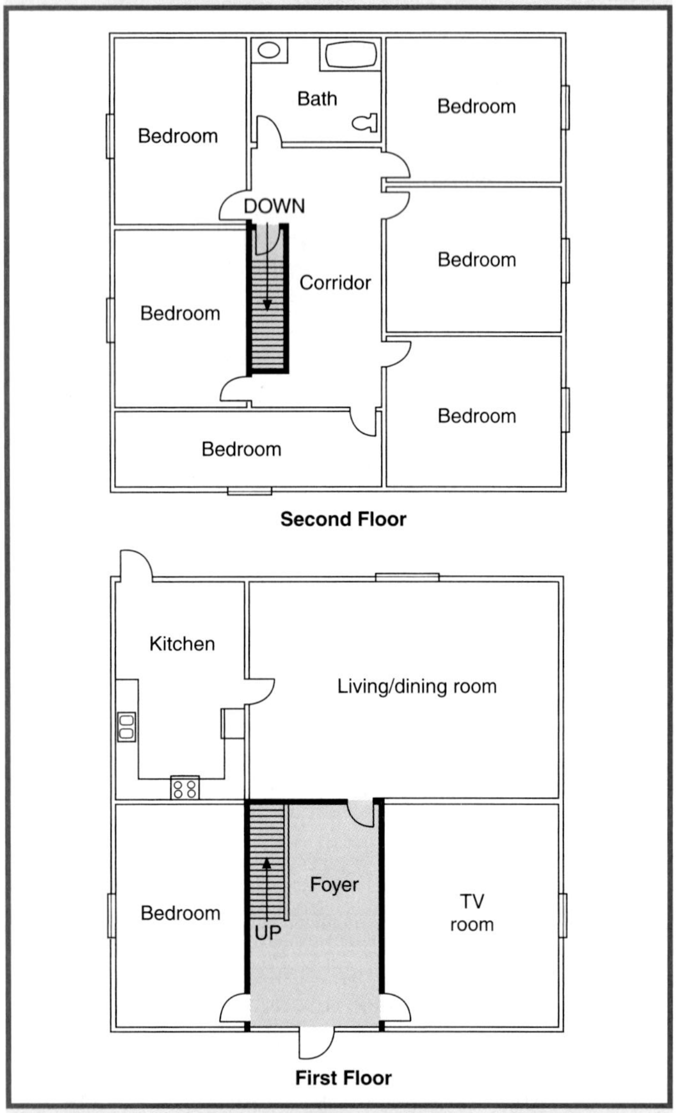


***Exhibit 26.3** Means of escape — existing nonsprinklered lodging or rooming house.*

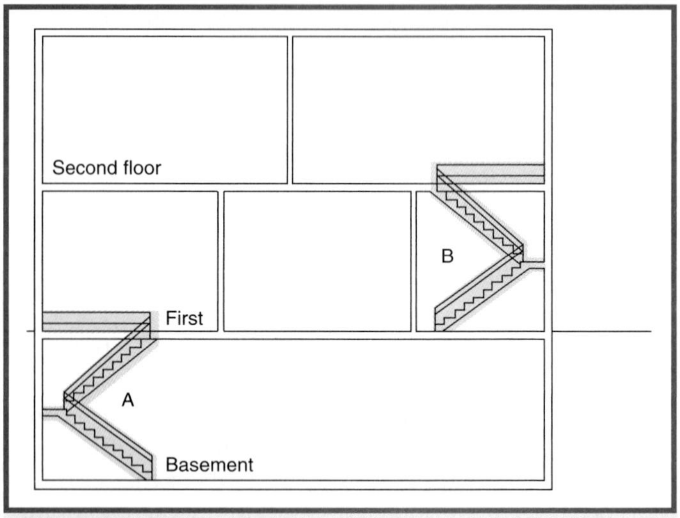


***Exhibit 26.4** Means of escape — two-story stairway.*

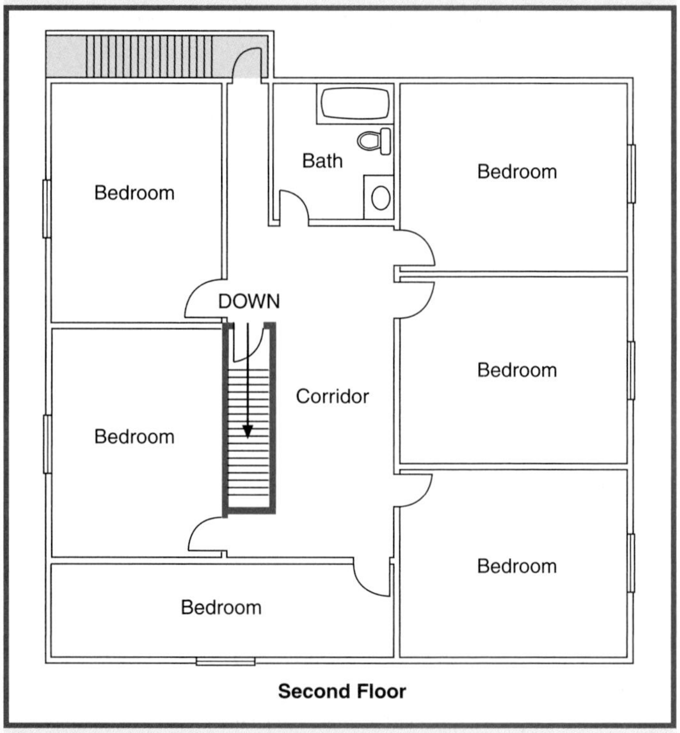


***Exhibit 26.5** Means of escape — outside stair use.*

**26.2.1.2 Secondary Means of Escape.** In addition to the primary route, each sleeping room and living area shall have a second means of escape in accordance with 24.2.2, unless the sleeping room or living area has a door leading directly outside the building with access to the finished ground level or to a stairway that meets the requirements for exterior stairs in 26.2.1.1.2.

The *Code* specifies that the secondary means of escape must comply with 24.2.2. Secondary means of escape is exempted by 24.2.2.1.2 if the building is sprinklered in accordance with NFPA 13, *Standard for the Installation of Sprinkler Systems;* NFPA 13R, *Standard for the In-*

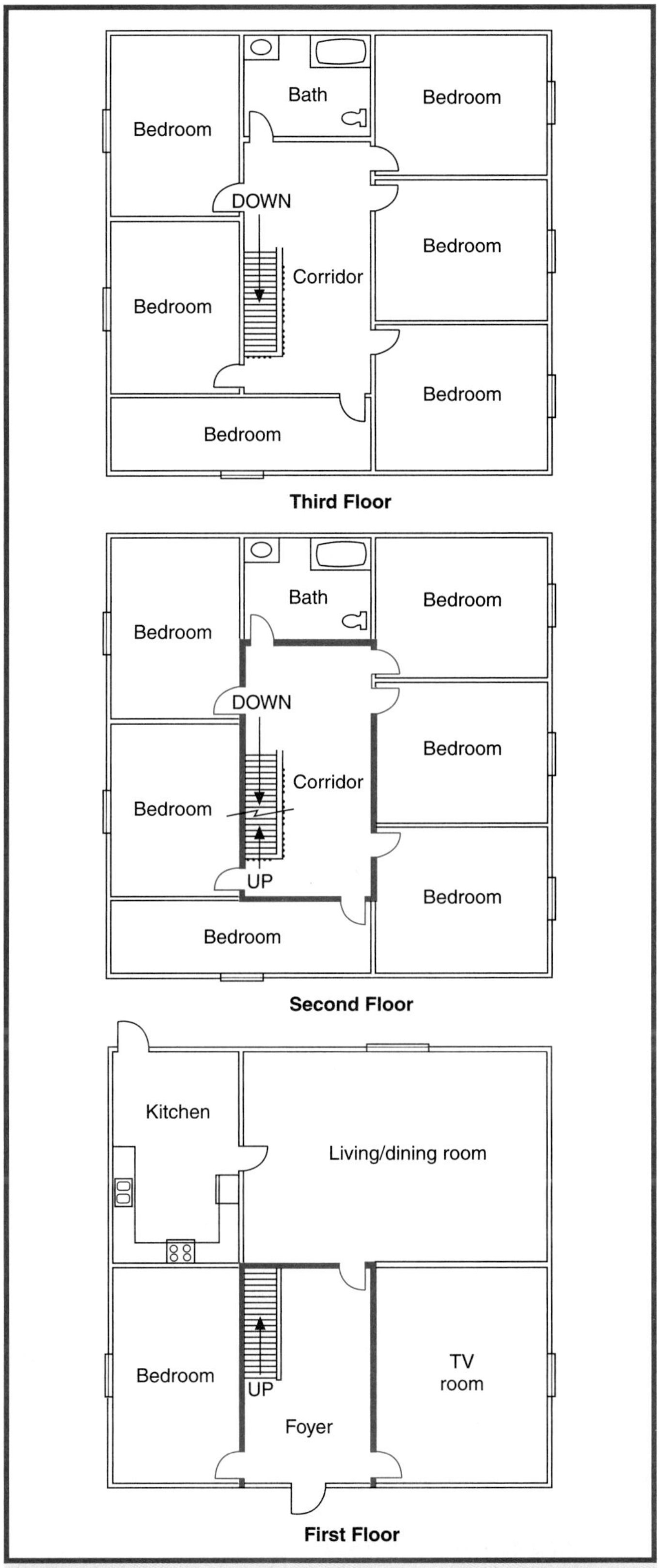


**Exhibit 26.6** *Means of escape — three-story sprinklered lodging or rooming house.*

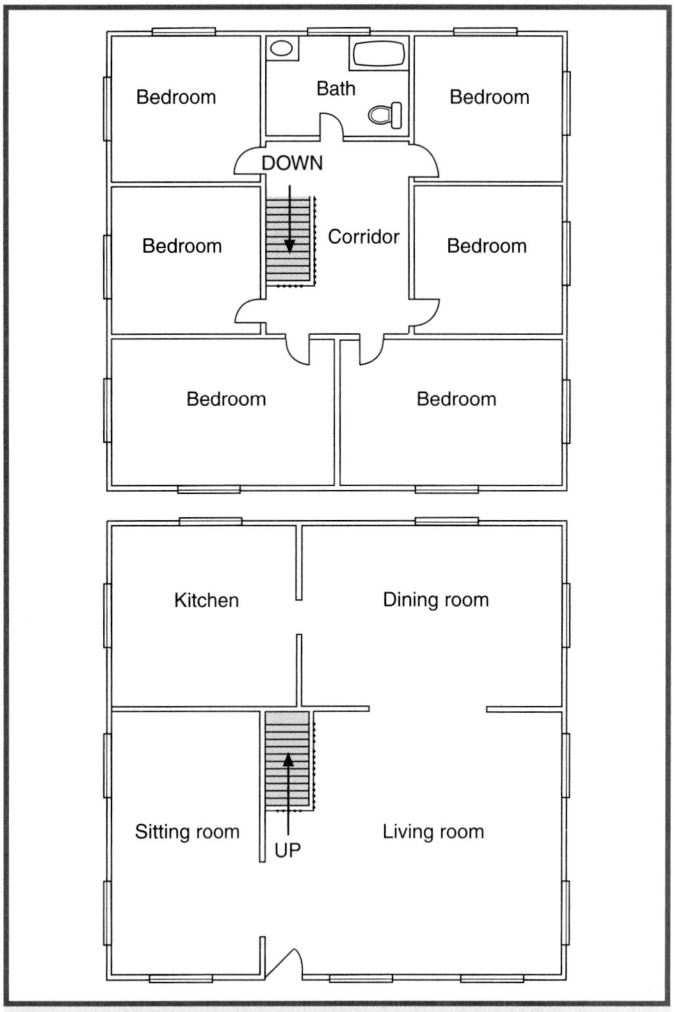


**Exhibit 26.7** *Means of escape — two-story sprinklered bed-and-breakfast facility.*

*stallation of Sprinkler Systems in Residential Occupancies up to and Including Four Stories in Height*[2]; or NFPA 13D, *Standard for the Installation of Sprinkler Systems in One- and Two-Family Dwellings and Manufactured Homes.*[3] Because most new lodging or rooming houses are required to be protected with sprinklers in accordance with 26.3.6.1, secondary means of escape will seldom be required. An exception is that where a stair is left unenclosed per the sprinkler allowance of 26.3.1.1.3, secondary means of escape must be provided. Where existing, nonsprinklered lodging or rooming houses are deficient with respect to secondary means of escape, protection of vertical openings, or required door closers on sleeping room doors, the installation of automatic sprinklers provides a viable alternative to correcting such deficiencies individually.

**26.2.1.3 Two Primary Means of Escape.** In other than existing buildings and those protected throughout by an approved, supervised automatic sprinkler system in accordance with 26.3.6, every story more than 2000 $ft^2$ (185 $m^2$) in area, or with travel distance to the primary means of escape more than 75 ft (23 m), shall be provided with two primary means of escape remotely located from each other.

### 26.2.2 Stairways.

**26.2.2.1** Interior stairways, other than those in accordance with 26.2.2.2 or 26.2.2.3, shall comply with 7.2.2.5.3 and shall be enclosed by fire barriers having a minimum ½-hour fire resistance rating, with all openings protected with smoke-actuated automatic-closing or self-closing doors having a fire resistance comparable to that required for the enclosure.

**26.2.2.2** Where an interior stair connects the street floor with the story next above or below only, but not with both, the interior stair shall be required to be enclosed only on the street floor.

**26.2.2.3** Stairways shall be permitted to be unenclosed in accordance with 26.3.1.1.2 and 26.3.1.1.3.

In Exhibit 26.3, an enclosed interior stair in accordance with 26.2.2.1 is shown on the first floor. The stair discharges directly to the outside and serves as the primary means of escape for this nonsprinklered rooming house. The entry foyer is separated from the rest of the first floor by walls with a ½-hour fire resistance rating, and the doors are self-closing with a 20-minute fire protection rating. The entry foyer cannot be used for any other purpose, such as a lounge for the occupants. Walls with a ½-hour fire resistance rating and a self-closing door with a 20-minute fire protection rating also enclose the stairs on the second floor. The walls and door provide the necessary separation between the second-floor corridor and the vertical opening. Compliant windows in all sleeping and living spaces provide the secondary means of escape. Note that if the stair illustrated in Exhibit 26.3 connects only the street floor and the floor above (or floor below), it is permitted to be open to other than the street floor per 26.2.2.2.

Exhibit 26.4 illustrates the use of 26.2.2.2. To meet the criteria for this provision, stairs A and B connect only two floors and are separated from the rest of the first floor. Stair A cannot extend to the second floor, and stair B cannot extend to the basement. The arrangement of stair A protects the residents on the first and second floors from fire and smoke in the basement. The arrangement of stair B protects the residents on the second floor from fire and smoke on the street-level floor.

**26.2.2.4** Winders in accordance with 7.2.2.2.4 shall be permitted.

### 26.2.3 Doors.

**26.2.3.1** Doors in a means of escape, other than bathroom doors in accordance with 26.2.3.2, and paths of travel in a means of escape shall be not less than 28 in. (710 mm) wide.

**26.2.3.2** Bathroom doors shall be not less than 24 in. (610 mm) wide.

**26.2.3.3** Every closet door latch shall be such that it can be readily opened from the inside in case of emergency.

**26.2.3.4** Every bathroom door shall be designed to allow opening from the outside during an emergency when locked.

**26.2.3.5** Door-locking arrangements shall comply with either 26.2.3.5.1 or 26.2.3.5.2.

**26.2.3.5.1*** No door in any means of escape shall be locked against egress when the building is occupied.

**A.26.2.3.5.1** It is the intent of this requirement that security measures, where installed, do not prevent egress.

**26.2.3.5.2** Delayed-egress locks complying with 7.2.1.6.1 shall be permitted, provided that not more than one such device is located in any one escape path.

A lodging or rooming house is prohibited by 26.2.3.5.1 from having any door locked against egress (escape) while the building is occupied. This requirement permits a door to have a locking device that allows the door to be opened from within the building for the purpose of escape but does not permit the door to be opened from outside the building. Ordinary double-cylinder locks and chain locks do not meet these provisions.

The language of 7.2.1.5.2 is clear: locks, if provided, must not require the use of a key, a tool, or special knowledge or effort for operation from the egress side. This requirement prohibits double-cylinder locks and chain locks that require a key to operate the door from the inside. The use of a simple operation to open a door is required by 7.2.1.5.9; locks that require two-handed knobs and similar operations are prohibited.

Chapter 7 recognizes the need for security chains or rods on guest room doors and permits one releasing device in addition to the doorknob or lever. The typical guest room door has three devices: a latch, a lock, and a security chain or rod. However, the *Code* permits only two releasing actions for new installations. This requirement is met by using a latch and lock set equipped with a lock bolt that automatically retracts when the latch handle is turned from the inside; therefore, only one releasing action is needed for the two devices. The second action is the release of the security chain or rod. However, neither device requires the use of a key, a tool, or special knowledge or effort. In existing installations, three releasing devices are permitted: the security device, the lock, and the latch.

The use of the delayed-egress lock detailed in 7.2.1.6.1 is recognized by 26.2.3.5.2, provided that not more than one such device is encountered in any single escape path. Use of a delayed-egress lock requires that the building be protected throughout by either an automatic sprinkler system or a fire detection system. The 15-second or 30-second delay permitted by 7.2.1.6.1 does not affect the immediate release of the lock upon activation of the sprinklers or detectors, or upon loss of power to the lock. This device helps provide the security needed for doors that are used infrequently in lodging or rooming houses. At the same time, doors remain available for emergency use. Chains and padlocks do not provide this protection.

**26.2.3.6** Doors serving a single dwelling unit shall be permitted to be provided with a lock in accordance with 7.2.1.5.6.

## 26.3 Protection

### 26.3.1 Protection of Vertical Openings.

**26.3.1.1** Vertical openings shall comply with 26.3.1.1.1, 26.3.1.1.2, or 26.3.1.1.3.

**26.3.1.1.1** Vertical openings shall be protected so that no primary escape route is exposed to an unprotected vertical opening.

**26.3.1.1.1.1** The vertical opening shall be considered protected if the opening is cut off and enclosed in a manner that provides a smoke- and fire-resisting capability of not less than ½ hour.

**26.3.1.1.1.2** Any doors or openings shall have a smoke- and fire-resisting capability equivalent to that of the enclosure and shall be automatic-closing on detection of smoke or shall be self-closing.

**26.3.1.1.2** In buildings three or fewer stories in height that are protected throughout by an approved automatic sprinkler system in accordance with 26.3.6, unprotected vertical openings shall be permitted, provided that a primary means of escape from each sleeping area is provided that does not pass through a portion of a lower floor, unless such portion is separated from all spaces on that floor by construction having a minimum ½-hour fire resistance rating.

**26.3.1.1.3** Stair enclosures shall not be required in buildings two or fewer stories in height where both of the following conditions exist:

(1) The building is protected throughout by an approved, supervised automatic sprinkler system in accordance with 26.3.6.1.
(2) The allowance of 24.2.2.1.2 to omit a secondary means of escape is not used.

In Exhibit 26.5, an outside stair is used as the primary means of escape. Compliant windows in each of the bedrooms provide the secondary means of escape. The interior stair in this arrangement is just a convenience stair, independent of the required means of escape. If no sprinkler system is provided, the stairs must be enclosed in accordance with 26.3.1.1.1, as depicted in Exhibit 26.5. If a sprinkler system is provided, either 26.3.1.1.2 or 26.3.1.1.3 is permitted to be applied.

A vertical opening of up to three stories is permitted by 26.3.1.1.2 to be unprotected in a fully sprinklered, maximum three-story lodging or rooming house, provided that the primary means of escape is separated on the lower floor(s). Exhibit 26.6 illustrates a three-story, sprinklered lodging or rooming house. The stairs are open from the first floor to the third floor. However, ½-hour fire resistance–rated walls separate the living spaces from the stairs on the first and second floors.

In bed-and-breakfast facilities, it is often important to retain the historical integrity or homelike ambience of the building. Separation or enclosure of a decorative main stair would effectively eliminate the characteristics that draw people to these facilities. On the other hand, it is necessary to provide appropriate protection to guests. Exhibit 26.7 illustrates a two-story bed-and-breakfast facility that is protected with automatic sprinklers. Once again, the stair serves as the primary means of escape. In this case, 26.3.1.1.3 is used to permit the stair to remain unenclosed on both levels. It is important to note that the use of this provision has an impact on the secondary means of escape. Even though 24.2.2.1.2 permits the elimination of the secondary means of escape in fully sprinklered buildings, 26.3.1.1.3(2) specifically prohibits the use of 24.2.2.1.2 if the automatic sprinklers are used for the purpose of protecting the vertical opening. The result is that all windows from the sleeping rooms or living areas must comply as a secondary means of escape if this arrangement is to be permitted.

**26.3.1.2*** Exterior stairs shall be protected against blockage caused by fire within the building.

**A.26.3.1.2** Such protection can be accomplished by separation by physical distance, arrangement of the stairs, protection of the openings exposing the stairs, or a combination thereof.

### 26.3.2 Reserved.

### 26.3.3 Interior Finish.

**26.3.3.1 General.** Interior finish shall be in accordance with Section 10.2.

**26.3.3.2 Interior Wall and Ceiling Finish.** Interior wall and ceiling finish materials complying with Section 10.2 shall be Class A, Class B, or Class C.

**26.3.3.3 Interior Floor Finish.**

**26.3.3.3.1** Newly installed interior floor finish shall comply with Section 10.2.

**26.3.3.3.2** Newly installed interior floor finish shall comply with 10.2.7.1 or 10.2.7.2, as applicable.

### 26.3.4 Detection, Alarm, and Communications Systems.

**26.3.4.1 General.**

**26.3.4.1.1** Lodging and rooming houses, other than those meeting 26.3.4.1.2, shall be provided with a fire alarm system in accordance with Section 9.6.

**26.3.4.1.2** A fire alarm system in accordance with Section 9.6 shall not be required in existing lodging and rooming houses that have an existing smoke detection system meeting or exceeding the requirements of 26.3.4.5.1 where that detection system includes not less than one manual fire alarm box per floor arranged to initiate the smoke detection alarm.

In existing lodging or rooming houses, 26.3.4.1.2 permits existing multiple-station smoke detectors and a manual fire alarm box arranged as a system to substitute for a standard fire alarm system in accordance with *NFPA 72®*, *National Fire Alarm Code®*.[4]

**26.3.4.2 Initiation.** Initiation of the required fire alarm system shall be by manual means in accordance with 9.6.2, or by alarm initiation in accordance with 9.6.2.1(3) in buildings protected throughout by an approved automatic sprinkler system in accordance with 26.3.6.

**26.3.4.3 Notification.** Occupant notification shall be provided automatically in accordance with 9.6.3, as modified by 26.3.4.3.1 and 26.3.4.3.2.

**26.3.4.3.1*** Visible signals for the hearing impaired shall not be required where the proprietor resides in the building and there are five or fewer rooms for rent.

**A.26.3.4.3.1** The proprietor is the owner or owner's agent with responsible charge.

**26.3.4.3.2** Positive alarm sequence in accordance with 9.6.3.4 shall be permitted.

**26.3.4.4 Detection. (Reserved)**

**26.3.4.5 Smoke Alarms.**

**26.3.4.5.1** Approved single-station smoke alarms, other than existing smoke alarms meeting the requirements of 26.3.4.5.3, shall be installed in accordance with 9.6.2.10 in every sleeping room.

**26.3.4.5.2** In other than existing buildings, the smoke alarms required by 26.3.4.5.1 shall be interconnected in accordance with 9.6.2.10.3.

**26.3.4.5.3** Existing battery-powered smoke alarms, rather than house electric-powered smoke alarms, shall be permitted where the facility has demonstrated to the authority having jurisdiction that the testing, maintenance, and battery replacement programs will ensure reliability of power to the smoke alarms.

Paragraph 26.3.4.5.1 requires the installation of a smoke alarm in each sleeping room. This requirement applies retroactively to existing lodging or rooming houses, as well as to new construction.

While 26.3.4.5.3 permits existing battery-powered smoke alarms to remain in place if approved by the authority having jurisdiction (AHJ), newly installed smoke alarms must be powered by the building electrical service. This requirement applies to both new and existing lodging or rooming houses in accordance with 9.6.2.9.

**26.3.4.6* Protection of Fire Alarm System.** The provision of 9.6.1.8.1.3 shall not apply to the smoke detection required at each fire alarm control unit by 9.6.1.8.1(1).

**A.26.3.4.6** It is the intent that smoke detection be provided at each fire alarm control unit, regardless of the presence of sprinkler protection.

### 26.3.5 Separation of Sleeping Rooms.

**26.3.5.1** All sleeping rooms shall be separated from escape route corridors by smoke partitions in accordance with Section 8.4.

**26.3.5.2** There shall be no louvers or operable transoms in corridor walls.

**26.3.5.3** Air passages shall not penetrate corridor walls, unless they are properly installed heating and utility installations other than transfer grilles.

**26.3.5.4** Transfer grilles shall be prohibited in corridor walls.

**26.3.5.5** Doors shall be provided with latches or other mechanisms suitable for keeping the doors closed.

**26.3.5.6** Doors shall not be arranged to prevent the occupant from closing the door.

**26.3.5.7** In buildings other than those protected throughout by an approved automatic sprinkler system in accordance with 26.3.6, doors shall be self-closing or automatic-closing upon detection of smoke.

The requirements of 26.3.5 are similar to those for corridor walls and doors in hotels and apartment buildings; however, no fire resistance rating is required. Unlike hotels and apartment buildings, door closers are exempted in sprinklered lodging or rooming houses. See Exhibit 26.8.

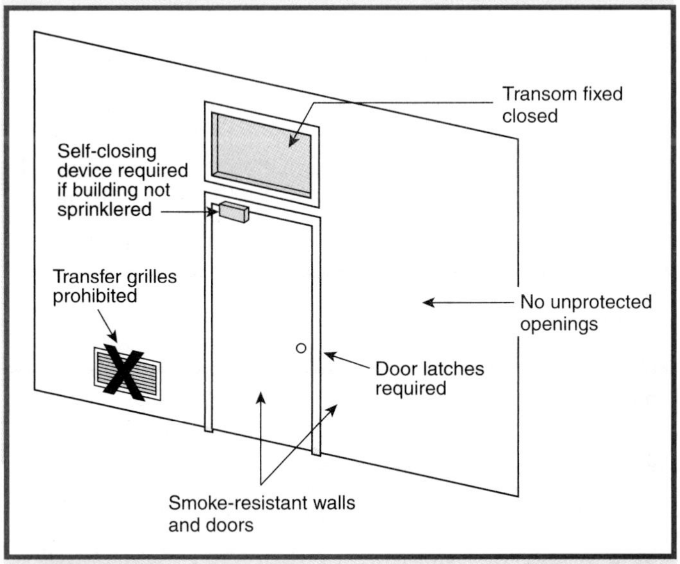


***Exhibit 26.8** Sleeping room/escape route separation.*

### 26.3.6 Extinguishment Requirements.

**26.3.6.1** All new lodging or rooming houses, other than those meeting the requirements of 26.3.6.2, shall be protected throughout by an approved automatic sprinkler system in accordance with 26.3.6.3.

**26.3.6.2** An automatic sprinkler system shall not be required where every sleeping room has a door opening directly to the outside of the building at street or the finished ground level, or has a door opening directly to the outside leading to an exterior stairway that meets the requirements of 26.2.1.1.2.

Exhibit 26.9 illustrates an arrangement where each room has a door leading directly to an exterior balcony and exterior stairs to grade. Per 26.2.1.2, this design eliminates the requirement for a secondary means of escape. Therefore, no protection of the interior stairs is required. If no sleeping rooms are located on the first floor, or if the first-floor sleeping rooms are arranged to discharge directly outside, an automatic sprinkler system is not required in the building.

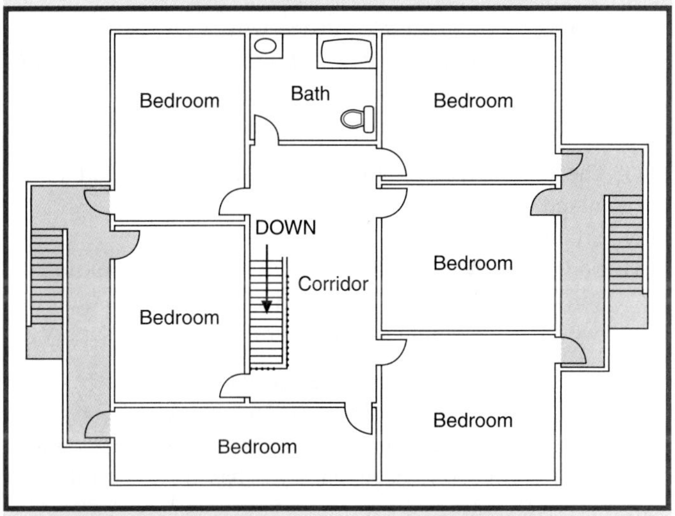


***Exhibit 26.9** Means of escape — nonsprinklered lodging or rooming house.*

With the exception of those lodging or rooming houses in which each sleeping room has a door providing direct access to the exterior at grade or to an exterior stairway, new lodging or rooming houses must be protected throughout with an approved automatic sprinkler system.

If a new lodging or rooming house is part of a multiple occupancy and the occupancies are mixed, the entire mixed occupancy is required to be sprinklered. To waive this requirement, the occupancies would have to be arranged so that the lodging or rooming house is treated as a separate occupancy in accordance with 6.1.14.4. This arrangement would require the exit access for each occupancy to be separate. Doors that open directly to the outside from each of the occupancies usually achieve such independent exit access.

**26.3.6.3** Where an automatic sprinkler system is required or is used as an alternative method of protection, either for total or partial building coverage, the system shall be in accordance with Section 9.7 and 26.3.6.3.1 through 26.3.6.3.6.

**26.3.6.3.1** Activation of the automatic sprinkler system shall actuate the fire alarm system in accordance with Section 9.6.

**26.3.6.3.2** In buildings four or fewer stories above grade plane, systems in accordance with NFPA 13R, *Standard for the Installation of Sprinkler Systems in Residential Occupancies up to and Including Four Stories in Height*, shall be permitted.

**26.3.6.3.3*** Systems in accordance with NFPA 13D, *Standard for the Installation of Sprinkler Systems in One- and Two-Family Dwellings and Manufactured Homes*, shall be permitted where the following requirements are met:

(1) The lodging or rooming house shall not be part of a mixed occupancy.
(2) Entrance foyers shall be sprinklered.
(3) Lodging or rooming houses with sleeping accommodations for more than eight occupants shall be treated as two-family dwellings with regard to the water supply.

**A.26.3.6.3.3** The decision to permit the use of the criteria from NFPA 13D, *Standard for the Installation of Sprinkler Systems in One- and Two-Family Dwellings and Manufactured Homes*, in these occupancies is based on the following:

(1) The desire to obtain a level of fire suppression and control that is approximately equivalent to that delivered by residential facilities protected by such systems *(see A.1.1 in NFPA 13D)*
(2) The fact that potential fire exposure and challenge to the suppression system in a small lodging and rooming occupancy is of the same nature and no more severe than that found in residences

Because there is such a wide variety of buildings that might fall into the classification of lodging or rooming houses, it is necessary to provide references to all three of the standards for the installation of automatic sprinkler systems.

The use of NFPA 13R, *Standard for the Installation of Sprinkler Systems in Residential Occupancies up to and Including Four Stories in Height,* is appropriate for many lodging or rooming houses.

In certain lodging or rooming house occupancies, the use of NFPA 13D, *Standard for the Installation of Sprinkler Systems in One- and Two-Family Dwellings and Manufactured Homes,* is also appropriate. Some lodging or rooming houses might be similar in physical configuration to a one- or two-family dwelling, whereas others are not. For example, an NFPA 13D system would be appropriate for a single-family dwelling that is used as a bed-and-breakfast (lodging or rooming house classification for purposes of applying this *Code*) but not for a fire station with a bunk room. The provision of 26.3.6.3.3(3) refers to the requirement in NFPA 13D specifying that, in multipurpose piping systems, where common water supply connections serve more than one dwelling unit, 5 gpm (19 L/min) must be added to the sprinkler system demand to determine the size of common piping and the size of the total water supply requirements where no provision is made to prevent flow into the domestic water system upon operation of a sprinkler (see Section 6.3 of NFPA 13D).

**26.3.6.3.4** In buildings sprinklered in accordance with NFPA 13, *Standard for the Installation of Sprinkler Systems*, closets less than 12 $ft^2$ (1.1 $m^2$) in area in individual dwelling units shall not be required to be sprinklered.

**26.3.6.3.5** In buildings sprinklered in accordance with NFPA 13, *Standard for the Installation of Sprinkler Systems*, closets that contain equipment such as washers, dryers, furnaces, or water heaters shall be sprinklered, regardless of size.

**26.3.6.3.6** In existing lodging or rooming houses, sprinkler installations shall not be required in closets not exceeding 24 $ft^2$ (2.2 $m^2$) and in bathrooms not exceeding 55 $ft^2$ (5.1 $m^2$).

## 26.4 Reserved

## 26.5 Building Services

### 26.5.1 Utilities.

Utilities shall comply with the provisions of Section 9.1.

### 26.5.2 Heating, Ventilating, and Air-Conditioning.

**26.5.2.1** Heating, ventilating, and air-conditioning equipment shall comply with the provisions of Section 9.2.

**26.5.2.2** Unvented fuel-fired heaters, other than gas space heaters in compliance with NFPA 54, *National Fuel Gas Code*, shall not be used.

### 26.5.3 Elevators, Escalators, and Conveyors.

Elevators, escalators, and conveyors shall comply with the provisions of Section 9.4.

## 26.6 Reserved

## 26.7 Operating Features

### 26.7.1 Contents and Furnishings.

**26.7.1.1** Contents and furnishings shall not be required to comply with Section 10.3.

**26.7.1.2** Furnishings or decorations of an explosive or highly flammable character shall not be used.

**26.7.1.3** Fire-retardant coatings shall be maintained to retain the effectiveness of the treatment under service conditions encountered in actual use.

### References Cited in Commentary

1. NFPA 13, *Standard for the Installation of Sprinkler Systems*, 2007 edition, National Fire Protection Association, Quincy, MA.
2. NFPA 13R, *Standard for the Installation of Sprinkler Systems in Residential Occupancies up to and Including Four Stories in Height*, 2007 edition, National Fire Protection Association, Quincy, MA.
3. NFPA 13D, *Standard for the Installation of Sprinkler Systems in One- and Two-Family Dwellings and Manufactured Homes*, 2007 edition, National Fire Protection Association, Quincy, MA.
4. *NFPA 72®, National Fire Alarm Code®*, 2007 edition, National Fire Protection Association, Quincy, MA.

CHAPTER 27

# Reserved

Typically, the occupancy chapters are paired so that the even-numbered chapter in the pair addresses new facilities of the occupancy type and the odd-numbered chapter addresses existing facilities of the occupancy type. Chapter 26, which precedes this chapter, addresses both new and existing lodging or rooming houses in a single chapter. Chapter 27 has been reserved to permit the chapter on new hotels and dormitories to be assigned an even number (i.e., Chapter 28). The reserved chapter number might be used at a future date if the requirements for lodging or rooming houses are split into a pair of chapters — one for new construction and one for existing buildings.

CHAPTERS 28 AND 29

# New and Existing Hotels and Dormitories

Chapters 28 and 29 address residential occupancies that are primarily transient in nature. Hotel and motel accommodations that are mainly used for stays of relatively short duration fit into this category. Dormitory occupancies, although typically used for up to nine months of near-continuous occupancy in the case of a college dormitory, are also regulated by these chapters.

The hotel and dormitory classification is one of five residential occupancy types addressed by the *Life Safety Code*. Other residential occupancies include one- and two-family dwellings (Chapter 24), lodging or rooming houses (Chapter 26), apartment buildings (Chapters 30 and 31), and residential board and care occupancies (Chapters 32 and 33).

The common principle of life safety that is applied to all residential occupancies addressed by Chapters 24 through 33 is highlighted by 6.1.8.1, which states that residential occupancies are those occupancies in which sleeping accommodations are provided for purposes other than health care or detention and correction. The presence of sleeping occupants is central to the provisions of Chapters 24 through 33, because occupants who are asleep will be unaware of a developing fire and, when awakened to be alerted to the emergency, might be somewhat confused. The definition of the term *residential occupancy* in 6.1.8.1 also differentiates between sleeping occupants in residential occupancies and those in health care or detention and correctional occupancies, which are also characterized by the occupants' incapability of self-preservation. The provisions of Chapters 24 through 33 are also based on the presence of hazards (such as cooking and heating equipment) in residential occupancies and the degree to which occupants are familiar with their living space. Occupants might have little or no familiarity, as in the case of the transient residents of hotels, or they might have the total familiarity that is common to residents of single-family dwellings.

Unfamiliar surroundings and the possibility of being asleep when a fire occurs are factors that jeopardize the safety of hotel guests in particular. Hotels pose an additional problem, because typical hotel building configurations often require escaping guests to traverse an interior corridor, which subsequently might expose them to the heat and smoke of corridor and room fires. In recognition of these potential hazards, the *Code* requires most new hotels and dormitories to be protected throughout by approved, supervised automatic sprinkler systems.

In recent years, hotels and motels have experienced a steady reduction in the number of fires, civilian casualties, and civilian injuries. Part of the explanation for these reductions is the increasing percentage of hotels that use smoke detection and automatic sprinkler systems. From 2002 to 2005, hotels and motels averaged 3900 structure fires per year, as reported to fire departments across the United States. These fires resulted in a yearly average of 11 civilian deaths and 144 civilian injuries. These numbers are down from the previous 4-year averages (1999 to 2002) of 4600 structure fires per year, 16 civilian deaths per year, and 190 civilian injuries. These figures do not include lodging or rooming houses or residential board and care facilities, which are defined for fire-reporting purposes as facilities that are limited to fewer than 16 occupants.

CHAPTER 28 • New

## 28.1 General Requirements

### 28.1.1 Application.

**28.1.1.1** The requirements of this chapter shall apply to new buildings or portions thereof used as hotel or dormitory occupancies. *(See 1.3.1.)*

**28.1.1.2** Any dormitory divided into suites of rooms, with one or more bedrooms opening into a living room or study that has a door opening into a common corridor serving a number of suites, shall be classified as an apartment building.

**28.1.1.3** The term *hotel*, wherever used in this *Code*, shall include a hotel, an inn, a club, a motel, a bed and breakfast, or any other structure meeting the definition of hotel.

CHAPTER 29 • Existing

## 29.1 General Requirements

### 29.1.1 Application.

**29.1.1.1** The requirements of this chapter shall apply to existing buildings or portions thereof currently occupied as hotel or dormitory occupancies, unless meeting the requirement of 29.1.1.2.

**29.1.1.2** Any dormitory divided into suites of rooms, with one or more bedrooms opening into a living room or study that has a door opening into a common corridor serving a number of suites, shall be classified as an apartment building.

**29.1.1.3** The term *hotel*, wherever used in this *Code*, shall include a hotel, an inn, a club, a motel, a bed and breakfast, or any other structure meeting the definition of hotel.

Chapters 28 and 29 apply to various operations that do not specifically use the term *hotel* but are considered such by definition. The terms *dormitory* and *hotel* are defined in 3.3.59 and 3.3.134, respectively. In some cases, Chapters 28 and 29 apply even if the identification of the occupancy suggests the application of a different chapter. For example, a "rooming house" that accommodates more than 16 people is classified as a hotel.

Conversely, some operations that one might expect to be covered by Chapters 28 and 29 are not. For example, 28/29.1.1.2 recognizes that the common dormitory design in which a group of bedrooms opens into a study or living room duplicates a typical apartment design in which several bedrooms open into a living room or kitchen. Because the design and the risk of fire are similar, the *Code* treats this arrangement as an apartment building, despite the lack of individual kitchens. Exhibit 28/29.1 illustrates the arrangement of a dormitory suite that would be treated as an apartment.

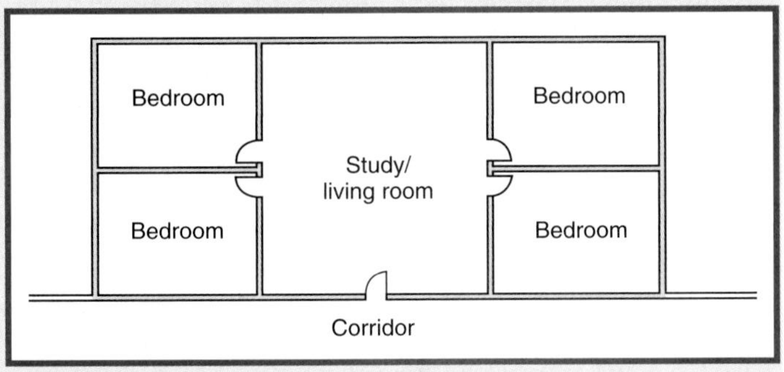


***Exhibit 28/29.1*** *Dormitory suite apartment.*

### 28.1.2 Multiple Occupancies.

**28.1.2.1** Multiple occupancies shall be in accordance with 6.1.14.

**28.1.2.2** No hotel or dormitory shall have its sole means of egress pass through any nonresidential occupancy in the same building, unless otherwise permitted by 28.1.2.2.1 or 28.1.2.2.2.

**28.1.2.2.1** In buildings that are protected by an automatic sprinkler system in accordance with Section 9.7, hotels and dormitories shall be permitted to have their sole means of egress pass through a nonresidential occupancy in the same building, provided that the following criteria are met:

### 29.1.2 Multiple Occupancies.

**29.1.2.1** Multiple occupancies shall be in accordance with 6.1.14.

**29.1.2.2** No hotel or dormitory shall have its sole means of egress pass through any nonresidential occupancy in the same building, unless otherwise permitted by 29.1.2.2.1 or 29.1.2.2.2.

**29.1.2.2.1** In buildings that are protected by an automatic sprinkler system in accordance with Section 9.7, hotels and dormitories shall be permitted to have their sole means of egress pass through a nonresidential occupancy in the same building, provided that the following criteria are met:

CHAPTER 28 • New

(1) The hotel or dormitory shall comply with Chapter 28.
(2) The sole means of egress from the hotel or dormitory shall not pass through a high hazard contents area, as defined in 6.2.2.4.

**28.1.2.2.2** In buildings that are not protected by an automatic sprinkler system in accordance with Section 9.7, hotels and dormitories shall be permitted to have their sole means of egress pass through a nonresidential occupancy in the same building, provided that the following criteria are met:

(1) The sole means of egress from the hotel or dormitory to the exterior shall be separated from the remainder of the building by fire barriers having a minimum 1-hour fire resistance rating.
(2) The hotel or dormitory shall comply with Chapter 28.
(3) The sole means of egress from the hotel or dormitory shall not pass through a high hazard contents area, as defined in 6.2.2.4.

CHAPTER 29 • Existing

(1) The hotel or dormitory shall comply with Chapter 29.
(2) The sole means of egress from the hotel or dormitory shall not pass through a high hazard contents area, as defined in 6.2.2.4.

**29.1.2.2.2** In buildings that are not protected by an automatic sprinkler system in accordance with Section 9.7, hotels and dormitories shall be permitted to have their sole means of egress pass through a nonresidential occupancy in the same building, provided that the following criteria are met:

(1) The sole means of egress from the hotel or dormitory to the exterior shall be separated from the remainder of the building by fire barriers having a minimum 1-hour fire resistance rating.
(2) The hotel or dormitory shall comply with Chapter 29.
(3) The sole means of egress from the hotel or dormitory shall not pass through a high hazard contents area, as defined in 6.2.2.4.

Residential occupancies often exist in buildings that also house assembly, mercantile, or business occupancies. These nonresidential occupancies might pose an additional threat, because they are not typically occupied after regular business hours. An undetected fire in an unoccupied area has the potential to affect the tenability of the residential portion of the building before occupants can be awakened and take the appropriate actions for safe egress. Therefore, the requirements of 28/29.1.2 help to ensure that it is safe to have hotels or dormitories within such multiple occupancy buildings by providing the necessary protection where treated as mixed occupancies and separation where treated as separated occupancies.

**28.1.3 Special Definitions.**

A list of special terms used in this chapter follows:

(1) **Dormitory.** See 3.3.59.
(2) **Guest Room.** See 3.3.121.
(3) **Guest Suite.** See 3.3.255.1.
(4) **Hotel.** See 3.3.134.

**29.1.3 Special Definitions.**

A list of special terms used in this chapter follows:

(1) **Dormitory.** See 3.3.59.
(2) **Guest Room.** See 3.3.121.
(3) **Guest Suite.** See 3.3.255.1.
(4) **Hotel.** See 3.3.134.

In the definition of *dormitory* in 3.3.59, the wording "without individual cooking facilities" refers to the absence of cooking equipment, excluding small appliances, such as coffee makers and microwave ovens, in any room or unit of a dormitory. If such equipment is present throughout a facility, the occupancy should be classified as an apartment building. The wording "with or without meals" recognizes the presence of a central cafeteria used to serve meals for the occupants of a dormitory.

The requirements of Chapters 28 and 29 often are worded to apply specifically within a guest room or guest suite. The first sentence of A.3.3.59 clarifies that, where the chapters use the terms *guest room* and *guest suite*, the intent is that the requirement also be applied to dormitory rooms used for sleeping and living purposes.

A residential occupancy with sleeping accommodations for more than 16 persons, even if referred to as a lodging or rooming house by its operators, is classified as a hotel and is regulated under the provisions of Chapter 28 or Chapter 29. In A.3.3.134, which addresses the definition of the term *hotel*, the reference to a 30-day time period helps to define *transient*. Where guest rooms or guest suites have individual cooking facilities, the appropriate occupancy classification is as an apartment building. However, certain facilities (e.g., extended-stay hotels) might contain the potential for hazards associated with both a hotel (unfamiliarity with surroundings) and an apartment building (higher fuel load, greater number of ignition sources, and travel through multiple rooms). In such cases, the authority having jurisdiction (AHJ) might classify the building as a mixed occupancy (hotel and apartment building) and apply the more restrictive requirements.

**28.1.4 Classification of Occupancy.**

See 6.1.8 and 28.1.3.

**29.1.4 Classification of Occupancy.**

See 6.1.8 and 29.1.3.

**28.1.5 Classification of Hazard of Contents.**

**28.1.5.1** The contents of residential occupancies shall be classified as ordinary hazard in accordance with 6.2.2.

**28.1.5.2** For the design of automatic sprinkler systems, the classification of contents in NFPA 13, *Standard for the Installation of Sprinkler Systems*, shall apply.

**29.1.5 Classification of Hazard of Contents.**

**29.1.5.1** The contents of residential occupancies shall be classified as ordinary hazard in accordance with 6.2.2.

**29.1.5.2** For the design of automatic sprinkler systems, the classification of contents in NFPA 13, *Standard for the Installation of Sprinkler Systems*, shall apply.

NFPA 13, *Standard for the Installation of Sprinkler Systems*,[1] classifies the contents of a hotel or dormitory occupancy building as light hazard for the purpose of designing automatic sprinkler systems. Classification in the *Code*, noted in 28/29.1.5.1, is based on the threat to life or life safety (ordinary) rather than the challenge to the extinguishing capability of the automatic sprinkler system (light).

**28.1.6 Minimum Construction Requirements.**

(No special requirements.)

**29.1.6 Minimum Construction Requirements.**

(No special requirements.)

Although Chapters 28 and 29 do not establish minimum construction requirements, if the hotel contains an assembly occupancy, which is fairly common, Chapters 12 and 13 do establish minimum construction requirements, based on the location of the assembly occupancy within the building. See 12/13.1.6 for construction requirements for assembly occupancies.

**28.1.7 Occupant Load.**

The occupant load, in number of persons for whom means of egress and other provisions are required, shall be determined on the basis of the occupant load factors of Table 7.3.1.2 that are characteristic of the use of the space or shall be determined as the maximum probable population of the space under consideration, whichever is greater.

**29.1.7 Occupant Load.**

The occupant load, in number of persons for whom means of egress and other provisions are required, shall be determined on the basis of the occupant load factors of Table 7.3.1.2 that are characteristic of the use of the space or shall be determined as the maximum probable population of the space under consideration, whichever is greater.

Subsection 28/29.1.7 requires the occupant load to be determined in accordance with the occupant load factors in Table 7.3.1.2. Note that the occupant load factors for residential use do not preclude the need for providing egress capacity from concentrated sleeping areas (e.g., bunk rooms) based on the maximum probable population, rather than on the calculated occupant load using the floor area. If the actual population of a bunk room exceeds one person per 200 $ft^2$ (18.6 $m^2$), the egress capacity features (e.g., door widths) must be designed based on the actual number of occupants. See Section 7.3 for further details on the use of occupant load for determining the capacity of the means of egress.

The occupant load calculations for areas of hotels used for nonresidential purposes are based on the occupant load factors applicable to the use of the area.

CHAPTER 28 • New

## 28.2 Means of Egress Requirements

### 28.2.1 General.

**28.2.1.1** Means of egress from guest rooms or guest suites to the outside of the building shall be in accordance with Chapter 7 and this chapter.

**28.2.1.2** Means of escape within the guest room or guest suite shall comply with the provisions of Section 24.2 for one- and two-family dwellings.

**28.2.1.3** For the purpose of application of the requirements of Chapter 24, the terms *guest room* and *guest suite* shall be synonymous with the terms *dwelling unit* or *living unit*.

CHAPTER 29 • Existing

## 29.2 Means of Egress Requirements

### 29.2.1 General.

**29.2.1.1** Means of egress from guest rooms or guest suites to the outside of the building shall be in accordance with Chapter 7 and this chapter.

**29.2.1.2** Means of escape within the guest room or guest suite shall comply with the provisions of Section 24.2 for one- and two-family dwellings.

**29.2.1.3** For the purpose of application of the requirements of Chapter 24, the terms *guest room* and *guest suite* shall be synonymous with the terms *dwelling unit* or *living unit*.

Every guest room or guest suite must comply with Section 24.2, which addresses means of escape in one- and two-family dwellings, in accordance with 28/29.2.1. This mandatory reference to Section 24.2 is important for several reasons. First, it establishes a requirement for two means of escape from every sleeping room and living area of a guest suite having two rooms or more. Several acceptable types of secondary means of escape are established in 24.2.2.3, the most common of which is an operable window with specified minimum opening dimensions. No secondary means of escape is required if a guest suite is protected by an automatic sprinkler system. Note that 24.2.2.1.2 does not require that the entire building be sprinklered, only that the guest suite deficient with respect to the secondary means of escape be sprinklered. However, a mandate for complete building sprinkler protection might be specified elsewhere, as in 28/29.3.5.1.

A second important provision of Section 24.2 is that the means of egress provisions of Chapter 7 do not apply within the guest room or guest suite unless they are specifically referenced. For example, the minimum width of means of escape doors within a guest room or guest suite is 28 in. (710 mm), rather than the 32 in. (810 mm) minimum width specified for means of egress by Chapter 7. The requirement of Chapter 7 applies to the door from the room or suite to the common corridor, because this door is the transition point at which means of escape ends and the standard means of egress begins. Chapter 24 also permits the use of winders and spiral stairs within a guest room or guest suite, and the provisions of Chapter 24 for headroom apply within the guest room or guest suite, superseding those of Chapter 7. See the commentary on Chapter 24 for additional information on means of escape from dwelling units.

### 28.2.2 Means of Egress Components.

#### 28.2.2.1 General.

**28.2.2.1.1** Components of means of egress shall be limited to the types described in 28.2.2.2 through 28.2.2.12.

**28.2.2.1.2** In buildings, other than high-rise buildings, that are protected throughout by an approved, supervised automatic sprinkler system in accordance with 28.3.5, exit enclosures shall have a minimum 1-hour fire resistance rating, and doors shall have a minimum 1-hour fire protection rating.

### 29.2.2 Means of Egress Components.

#### 29.2.2.1 General.

**29.2.2.1.1** Components of means of egress shall be limited to the types described in 29.2.2.2 through 29.2.2.12.

**29.2.2.1.2** In buildings, other than high-rise buildings, that are protected throughout by an approved automatic sprinkler system in accordance with 29.3.5, exit enclosures shall have a minimum 1-hour fire resistance rating, and doors shall have a minimum 1-hour fire protection rating.

CHAPTER 28 • New

CHAPTER 29 • Existing

The general provisions of 28/29.2.2 for the means of egress components in hotels and dormitories modify the provisions of Chapter 7 in the following two areas:

1. Limits on the components of the means of egress
2. Protection of the means of egress

First, a general reference to the components of the means of egress in Chapter 7 is made in 28/29.2.1.1 in place of repeating its myriad provisions. Most of these components are permitted in both new and existing hotels and dormitories. Some of the components are permitted to be used in accordance with the provisions of Chapter 7 and the additional provisions of Chapters 28 and 29. For example, 28/29.2.2.2.2.2 permits the use of delayed-egress locks in accordance with 7.2.1.6.1 if not more than one such device is located in any single egress path. In addition, 28/29.2.2.2.2.4 permits the use of elevator lobby exit access door locking in accordance with 7.2.1.6.3, which is new to the 2009 edition of the *Code*.

If not permitted, no reference to an egress component is made in the specific occupancy chapter. For example, escalators and fire escape stairs are only permitted in existing hotels. Therefore, 29.2.2.8 and 29.2.2.9 contain specific references to such components, while 28.2.2.8 and 28.2.2.9 are reserved and contain no such reference. Neither chapter permits the use of slide escapes; consequently, no reference to slide escapes is made within the means of egress sections of either chapter.

Second, Chapter 28 recognizes the relatively low fuel loads of hotels and modifies the exit enclosure requirements of Chapter 7. In other than high-rise buildings, 28.2.2.1.2 permits a fire resistance rating of 1 hour for exit enclosures and other vertical openings (see 28.3.1.1.3), regardless of the number of stories connected, provided that the building is protected throughout by an approved, supervised automatic sprinkler system. See 29.3.1 for the unique vertical opening protection criteria for existing hotels and dormitories.

Because the *Code* currently requires most new hotels and dormitories to be protected throughout by an approved automatic sprinkler system, a 1-hour fire resistance–rated exit enclosure will typically be permitted in other than high-rise buildings. However, if 28.3.5.2 — which exempts certain building arrangements from the sprinkler requirement — is utilized, the 1-hour-rated enclosure option of 28.2.2.1.2 is not permitted. This situation dictates a default to the Chapter 7 exit enclosure requirements, which, because they are based on the number of stories connected by the exit enclosure, might require 2-hour fire resistance–rated enclosures. See 7.1.3.2 for requirements for exits.

The reduction to a 1-hour fire resistance–rated enclosure for exits is not permitted for assembly, mercantile, or business occupancies and, therefore, cannot be used where mixed hotel/assembly, hotel/mercantile, or hotel/business occupancies are involved. In facilities of four or more stories, where hotel occupancies and other occupancies are adequately separated in accordance with 6.1.14.4 and treated independently, a 1-hour exit enclosure in the hotel portion and a 2-hour enclosure elsewhere might be permitted.

Exhibit 28/29.2 illustrates the modification to the requirements for protection of exit enclosures and other vertical openings in a fully sprinklered non-high-rise building. The provision for the 1-hour exit enclosure does not apply to other occupancies in a hotel complex or in mixed occupancies.

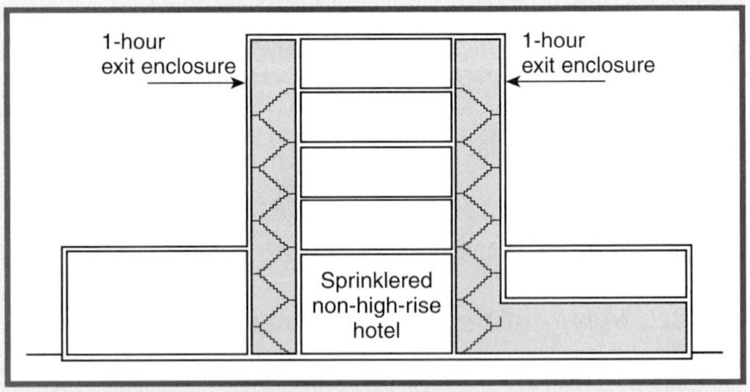


***Exhibit 28/29.2*** *Exit enclosure separation — sprinklered non-high-rise building.*

**28.2.2.2 Doors.**

**28.2.2.2.1** Doors complying with 7.2.1 shall be permitted.

**28.2.2.2.2** Door-locking arrangements shall comply with 28.2.2.2.2.1, 28.2.2.2.2.2, 28.2.2.2.2.3, or 28.2.2.2.2.4.

**28.2.2.2.2.1** No door in any means of egress shall be locked against egress when the building is occupied.

**29.2.2.2 Doors.**

**29.2.2.2.1** Doors complying with 7.2.1 shall be permitted.

**29.2.2.2.2** Door-locking arrangements shall comply with 29.2.2.2.2.1, 29.2.2.2.2.2, 29.2.2.2.2.3, or 29.2.2.2.2.4.

**29.2.2.2.2.1** No door in any means of egress shall be locked against egress when the building is occupied.

CHAPTER 28 • New

**28.2.2.2.2.2** Delayed-egress locks complying with 7.2.1.6.1 shall be permitted, provided that not more than one such device is located in any one egress path.

**28.2.2.2.2.3** Access-controlled egress doors complying with 7.2.1.6.2 shall be permitted.

**28.2.2.2.2.4** Elevator lobby exit access door locking in accordance with 7.2.1.6.3 shall be permitted.

CHAPTER 29 • Existing

**29.2.2.2.2.2** Delayed-egress locks complying with 7.2.1.6.1 shall be permitted, provided that not more than one such device is located in any one egress path.

**29.2.2.2.2.3** Access-controlled egress doors complying with 7.2.1.6.2 shall be permitted.

**29.2.2.2.2.4** Elevator lobby exit access door locking in accordance with 7.2.1.6.3 shall be permitted.

Hotels and dormitories are prohibited from having any door locked against egress while the building is occupied. This requirement permits a door to be equipped with a locking device that allows the door to be opened from within the building for the purpose of egress but does not allow the door to be opened from outside the building.

The language of 7.2.1.5.2 is clear: Locks, if provided, must not require the use of a key, a tool, or special knowledge or effort for operation from the egress side of the building. This requirement prohibits double-cylinder locks and chain locks that require a key to operate the door from the inside. The use of a simple operation to open a door is required by 7.2.1.5.9; locks that require two-handed knobs and similar operations are prohibited.

Hotel room doors provide security for the occupants in the room. Recognizing this additional function, Chapter 7 permits the use of security chains or rods, as well as locks, on hotel room doors and also permits releasing devices in addition to the doorknob or lever. The permitted number of additional releasing actions differs for new and existing buildings. One additional releasing action is permitted for new construction, and two additional actions are permitted in existing buildings (see 7.2.1.5.9.3 and 7.2.1.5.9.4).

The typical hotel room door has three devices: a latch, a lock, and a security chain or rod. This arrangement is permitted in existing buildings, provided that only two additional releasing operations are needed for unlocking and unlatching the door. This arrangement would also be permitted in new construction, provided that the latch and lock set are interconnected so that the lock bolt and the latch will retract simultaneously when the latch handle is turned from the inside; thus, only one releasing action is needed for the two devices. The second action is the release of the security chain or rod. The overriding requirement for any of these devices is that they not require the use of a key, a tool, or special knowledge or effort to operate.

The use of the delayed-egress lock detailed in 7.2.1.6.1 is recognized in 28/29.2.2.2.2.2 if not more than one such lock is located in any single egress path. The use of a delayed-egress lock requires that an automatic sprinkler or automatic fire detection system protect the building throughout. The 15-second or 30-second delay permitted by 7.2.1.6.1 does not affect the immediate release of the lock upon activation of sprinklers or detectors or upon loss of power to the lock. The delay device provides the security needed for doors that are used infrequently. At the same time, the door remains available for emergency use. Chains and padlocks do not provide these safety features.

The use of elevator lobby exit access door locking detailed in 7.2.1.6.3, which is new to the 2009 edition of the *Code*, is recognized by 28/29.2.2.2.2.4. This provision allows an elevator to open to an elevator lobby from which access to an exit stair is required to pass through normally locked doors. Although the floors of most hotels are arranged so that elevators open to lobbies that are directly connected to corridors serving the guest rooms, and in turn provide direct access to exit stairs, there may be arrangements where it is desirable to have a "secure" floor in which occupants step off the elevator into a reception area. The provisions of 7.2.1.6.3 permit access to the required exits to be through normally locked doors subject to the additional protection criteria specified therein. See the commentary following 7.2.1.6.3 for additional details on elevator lobby exit access door locking.

Selected exit stair enclosure doors are permitted to be locked to prevent re-entry from the stairwell side by 7.2.1.5.7, while other stair enclosure doors must remain unlocked. If the selected re-entry provisions are not used, one of the other two options specified by 7.2.1.5.7 must be used for stair enclosures serving five or more stories. Doors are permitted to be locked to prevent re-entry from the stairwell if initiation of the building fire alarm system automatically unlocks the door; otherwise, all stair enclosure doors must remain unlocked at all times.

CHAPTER 28 • New

**28.2.2.2.3** Revolving doors complying with 7.2.1.10 shall be permitted.

**28.2.2.2.4** Horizontal-sliding doors, as permitted by 7.2.1.14, shall not be used across corridors.

Note that the special form of horizontal-sliding door detailed in 7.2.1.14 is prohibited for cross-corridor installations in both new and existing hotels and dormitories in accordance with 28/29.2.2.2.4.

**28.2.2.3 Stairs.** Stairs complying with 7.2.2 shall be permitted.

**28.2.2.4 Smokeproof Enclosures.** Smokeproof enclosures complying with 7.2.3 shall be permitted.

**28.2.2.5 Horizontal Exits.** Horizontal exits complying with 7.2.4 shall be permitted.

**28.2.2.6 Ramps.** Ramps complying with 7.2.5 shall be permitted.

**28.2.2.7 Exit Passageways.** Exit passageways complying with 7.2.6 shall be permitted.

**28.2.2.8 Reserved.**

**28.2.2.9 Reserved.**

**28.2.2.10 Fire Escape Ladders.** Fire escape ladders complying with 7.2.9 shall be permitted.

**28.2.2.11 Alternating Tread Devices.** Alternating tread devices complying with 7.2.11 shall be permitted.

**28.2.2.12 Areas of Refuge.**

**28.2.2.12.1** Areas of refuge complying with 7.2.12 shall be permitted, as modified by 28.2.2.12.2.

**28.2.2.12.2*** In buildings protected throughout by an approved, supervised automatic sprinkler system in accordance with 28.3.5, the two accessible rooms or spaces separated from each other by smoke-resistive partitions in accordance with the definition of area of refuge in 3.3.20 shall not be required.

**A.28.2.2.12.2** The provision of 28.2.2.12.2 permits the entire floor to serve as an area of refuge where it is protected

CHAPTER 29 • Existing

**29.2.2.2.3** Revolving doors complying with 7.2.1.10 shall be permitted.

**29.2.2.2.4** Horizontal-sliding doors, as permitted by 7.2.1.14, shall not be used across corridors.

**29.2.2.3 Stairs.** Stairs complying with 7.2.2 shall be permitted.

**29.2.2.4 Smokeproof Enclosures.** Smokeproof enclosures complying with 7.2.3 shall be permitted.

**29.2.2.5 Horizontal Exits.** Horizontal exits complying with 7.2.4 shall be permitted.

**29.2.2.6 Ramps.** Ramps complying with 7.2.5 shall be permitted.

**29.2.2.7 Exit Passageways.** Exit passageways complying with 7.2.6 shall be permitted.

**29.2.2.8* Escalators.** Escalators previously approved as a component in a means of egress shall be permitted to continue to be considered in compliance.

**A.29.2.2.8** Due to the nature of escalators, they are no longer acceptable as a component in a means of egress. However, because many escalators have been used for exit access and exit discharge in the past, they are permitted to continue to be considered in compliance. Very few escalators have ever been installed in a manner to qualify as an exit. For information on escalator protection and requirements, see previous editions of the *Code*.

**29.2.2.9 Fire Escape Stairs.** Fire escape stairs complying with 7.2.8 shall be permitted.

**29.2.2.10 Fire Escape Ladders.** Fire escape ladders complying with 7.2.9 shall be permitted.

**29.2.2.11 Alternating Tread Devices.** Alternating tread devices complying with 7.2.11 shall be permitted.

**29.2.2.12 Areas of Refuge.**

**29.2.2.12.1** Areas of refuge complying with 7.2.12 shall be permitted, as modified by 28.2.2.12.2.

**29.2.2.12.2*** In buildings protected throughout by an approved, supervised automatic sprinkler system in accordance with 29.3.5, the two accessible rooms or spaces separated from each other by smoke-resistive partitions in accordance with the definition of area of refuge in 3.3.20 shall not be required.

**A.29.2.2.12.2** The provision of 29.2.2.12.2 permits the entire floor to serve as an area of refuge where it is protected

CHAPTER 28 • New

in accordance with 28.3.5. The provision is acceptable because supervised automatic sprinkler systems have built-in signals for monitoring features of the system, such as the opening and closing of water control valves. Such systems also monitor pump power supplies, water tank levels, and conditions that will impair the satisfactory operation of the sprinkler system. Because of these monitoring features, supervised automatic sprinkler systems have a high level of satisfactory performance and response to fire conditions.

In new hotels and dormitories, areas accessible to persons with severe mobility impairment must be provided with accessible means of egress per 7.5.4.1. For stories above the level of exit discharge, where providing ramps is usually not feasible, areas of refuge (see 7.2.12) will typically be used to meet the requirements for accessible means of egress. A story of a fully sprinklered hotel or dormitory is permitted to be considered an area of refuge by 28.2.2.12.2, even if an occupant does not have access to any of the guest rooms and is confined to the exit access corridor. Due to the effectiveness of the sprinkler system, an occupant with mobility impairment should be able to remain on the floor without experiencing untenable conditions. However, because locked guest room doors create inaccessibility to spaces other than the corridor, the corridor effectively serves as the area of refuge.

### 28.2.3 Capacity of Means of Egress.

**28.2.3.1** The capacity of means of egress shall be in accordance with Section 7.3.

**28.2.3.2** Street floor exits shall be sufficient for the occupant load of the street floor plus the required capacity of stairs and ramps discharging onto the street floor.

When occupants from upper floors are discharged from exit stair enclosures onto the street floor (in accordance with 7.7.2) and mix with occupants of the street floor in attempting egress to the exterior, the result is an increased demand on street-floor egress components, such as exit doors. Street-floor exits must be sized to handle the combined capacity in accordance with 28/29.2.3.2.

Exhibit 28/29.3 illustrates the traditional grand lobby design found in many hotels in which multiple exit stairs and street-floor exits converge at one or two exterior door locations. The required aggregate capacity of doors A and B is based on the number of people expected to use them. Assuming that the street floor has an occupant load of 400 persons and each of the two enclosed exit stairs (i.e., stair 1 and stair 2) discharging into the street floor has a required capacity of 200 persons (i.e., a maximum of 50 percent of the

CHAPTER 29 • Existing

in accordance with 29.3.5. The provision is acceptable because supervised automatic sprinkler systems have built-in signals for monitoring features of the system, such as the opening and closing of water control valves. Such systems also monitor pump power supplies, water tank levels, and conditions that will impair the satisfactory operation of the sprinkler system. Because of these monitoring features, supervised automatic sprinkler systems have a high level of satisfactory performance and response to fire conditions.

Existing hotels and dormitories are exempt from the provisions of 7.5.4.1; therefore, areas of refuge are not required but are permitted to serve as means of egress components. If an area of refuge is used within an existing hotel, 29.2.2.12.2 permits a story of a fully sprinklered hotel or dormitory to be considered an area of refuge, even if an occupant does not have access to any of the guest rooms and is confined to the exit access corridor.

### 29.2.3 Capacity of Means of Egress.

**29.2.3.1** The capacity of means of egress shall be in accordance with Section 7.3.

**29.2.3.2** Street floor exits shall be sufficient for the occupant load of the street floor plus the required capacity of stairs and ramps discharging onto the street floor.

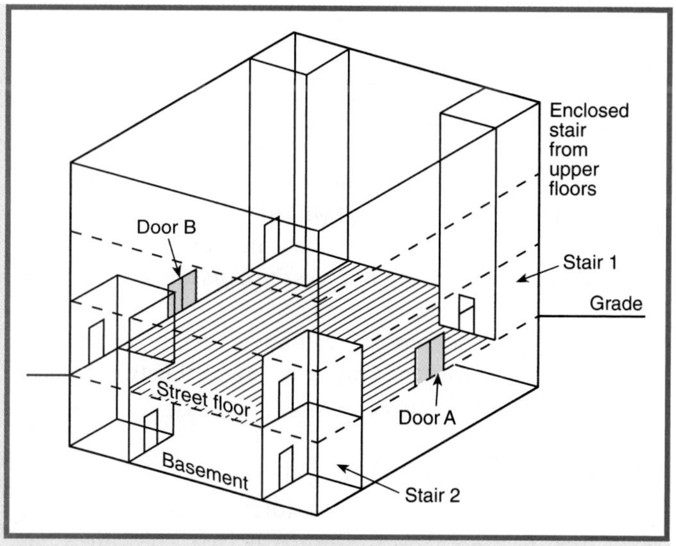


***Exhibit 28/29.3** Egress capacity for street floor.*

CHAPTER 28 • New

CHAPTER 29 • Existing

400-person occupant load of the second or third floor via stair 1 and a maximum of 50 percent of the 400-person occupant load of the basement via stair 2), the required egress capacity for the street floor would be 800 persons. The unobstructed door or level travel width required to accommodate 800 persons is 13 ft 4 in. (4065 mm). The opening provided by each pair of doors, A and B, needs to be 6 ft 8 in. (2030 mm) in clear, unobstructed width.

**28.2.3.3*** Corridors, other than those within individual guest rooms or individual guest suites, shall be of sufficient width to accommodate the required occupant load and shall be not less than 44 in. (1120 mm).

**A.28.2.3.3** The exemption contained in 28.2.3.3 applies to corridors within an individual room or suite and does not apply where a suite can be subdivided and rented separately.

### 28.2.4 Number of Exits.

**28.2.4.1** In buildings other than those complying with 28.2.4.2, not less than two separate exits shall be provided on each story. *(See also Section 7.4.)*

**28.2.4.2** A single exit shall be permitted in buildings where the total number of stories does not exceed four, provided that all of the following conditions are met:

(1) There are four or fewer guest rooms or guest suites per story.
(2) The building is protected throughout by an approved, supervised automatic sprinkler system in accordance with 28.3.5.
(3) The exit stairway does not serve more than one-half of a story below the level of exit discharge.
(4) The travel distance from the entrance door of any guest room or guest suite to an exit does not exceed 35 ft (10.7 m).
(5) The exit stairway is completely enclosed or separated from the rest of the building by barriers having a minimum 1-hour fire resistance rating.
(6) All openings between the exit stairway enclosure and the building are protected with self-closing door assemblies having a minimum 1-hour fire protection rating.
(7) All corridors serving as access to exits have a minimum 1-hour fire resistance rating.
(8) Horizontal and vertical separation having a minimum ½-hour fire resistance rating is provided between guest rooms or guest suites.

### 29.2.4 Number of Exits.

**29.2.4.1** In buildings other than those complying with 29.2.4.2, not less than two exits shall be accessible from every floor, including floors below the level of exit discharge and floors occupied for public purposes.

**29.2.4.2** A single exit shall be permitted in buildings where the total number of stories does not exceed four, provided that all of the following conditions are met:

(1) There are four or fewer guest rooms or guest suites per story.
(2) The building is protected throughout by an approved, supervised automatic sprinkler system in accordance with 29.3.5.
(3) The exit stairway does not serve more than one-half of a story below the level of exit discharge.
(4) The travel distance from the entrance door of any guest room or guest suite to an exit does not exceed 35 ft (10.7 m).
(5) The exit stairway is completely enclosed or separated from the rest of the building by barriers having a minimum 1-hour fire resistance rating.
(6) All openings between the exit stairway enclosure and the building are protected with self-closing door assemblies having a minimum 1-hour fire protection rating.
(7) All corridors serving as access to exits have a minimum 1-hour fire resistance rating.
(8) Horizontal and vertical separation having a minimum ½-hour fire resistance rating is provided between guest rooms or guest suites.

Although 28.2.4.1 requires a minimum of two exits on every story in new hotels and dormitories, and 29.2.4.1 requires access to a minimum of two separate exits from each floor in existing hotels and dormitories, 7.4.1.2 requires a third exit when the occupant load of a floor exceeds 500 and a fourth exit when it exceeds 1000. The requirement of 7.4.1.2 will probably have little effect on modern hotel design practices, because floors large enough to accommodate more than 500 persons would probably be provided with more than two exits, based on travel distance limit considerations (see 28/29.2.6).

**28.2.5 Arrangement of Means of Egress.**

**28.2.5.1** Access to all required exits shall be in accordance with Section 7.5, as modified by 28.2.5.2.

**28.2.5.2** The distance between exits addressed by 7.5.1.3 shall not apply to common nonlooped exit access corridors in buildings that have corridor doors from the guest room or guest suite that are arranged such that the exits are located in opposite directions from such doors.

**28.2.5.3** In buildings not protected throughout by an approved, supervised automatic sprinkler system in accordance with 28.3.5, common paths of travel shall not exceed 35 ft (10.7 m); travel within a guest room or guest suite shall not be included when calculating common path of travel.

**28.2.5.4** In buildings protected throughout by an approved, supervised automatic sprinkler system in accordance with 28.3.5, common path of travel shall not exceed 50 ft (15 m); travel within a guest room or guest suite shall not be included when determining common path of travel.

**28.2.5.5** In buildings not protected throughout by an approved, automatic sprinkler system in accordance with 28.3.5, dead-end corridors shall not exceed 35 ft (10.7 m).

**28.2.5.6** In buildings protected throughout by an approved, supervised automatic sprinkler system in accordance with 28.3.5, dead-end corridors shall not exceed 50 ft (15 m).

**28.2.5.7** Any guest room or any guest suite of rooms in excess of 2000 $ft^2$ (185 $m^2$) shall be provided with not less than two exit access doors remotely located from each other.

**29.2.5 Arrangement of Means of Egress.**

**29.2.5.1** Access to all required exits shall be in accordance with Section 7.5.

**29.2.5.2 Reserved.**

**29.2.5.3** In buildings not protected throughout by an approved, supervised automatic sprinkler system in accordance with 29.3.5, common paths of travel shall not exceed 35 ft (10.7 m); travel within a guest room or guest suite shall not be included when calculating common path of travel.

**29.2.5.4** In buildings protected throughout by an approved, supervised automatic sprinkler system in accordance with 29.3.5, common path of travel shall not exceed 50 ft (15 m); travel within a guest room or guest suite shall not be included when determining common path of travel.

**29.2.5.5** Dead-end corridors shall not exceed 50 ft (15 m).

The provisions for the arrangement of the means of egress for hotels differ significantly from the provisions in Chapter 7. The first difference appears in 28.2.5.2, which addresses the remoteness of exits. Applying the remoteness of exits provisions of 7.5.1.3 could result in a corridor that is longer than is necessary for the efficient use of the space. Some relief is offered by 28.2.5.2. Exhibit 28/29.4 helps to clarify the intent of 28.2.5.2. In Part (a) of Exhibit 28/29.4, all four guest rooms/guest suites have access to two exits immediately upon leaving the guest room/guest suite and entering the exit access corridor — that is, there is no common path of travel within the corridor from any of the apartments. This arrangement meets the provisions of 28.2.5.2. Contrast this arrangement with that depicted in Part (b) of Exhibit 28/29.4, where only guest rooms/guest suites A and B have access to two exits immediately upon leaving the guest room/guest suite and entering the exit access corridor. The other guest rooms/guest suites do not have immediate access to two exits. This arrangement does not meet the provisions of 28.2.5.2.

The concepts underlying the limitations imposed on common paths of travel and dead-end corridors are similar but not identical to those explained in the commentary on 7.5.1.5. Because of modifications made by Chapters 28 and 29 in defining where common path of travel begins, the difference between common paths of travel and dead-end corridors is less pronounced for hotels and dormitories. For most other occupancies,

CHAPTER 28 • New

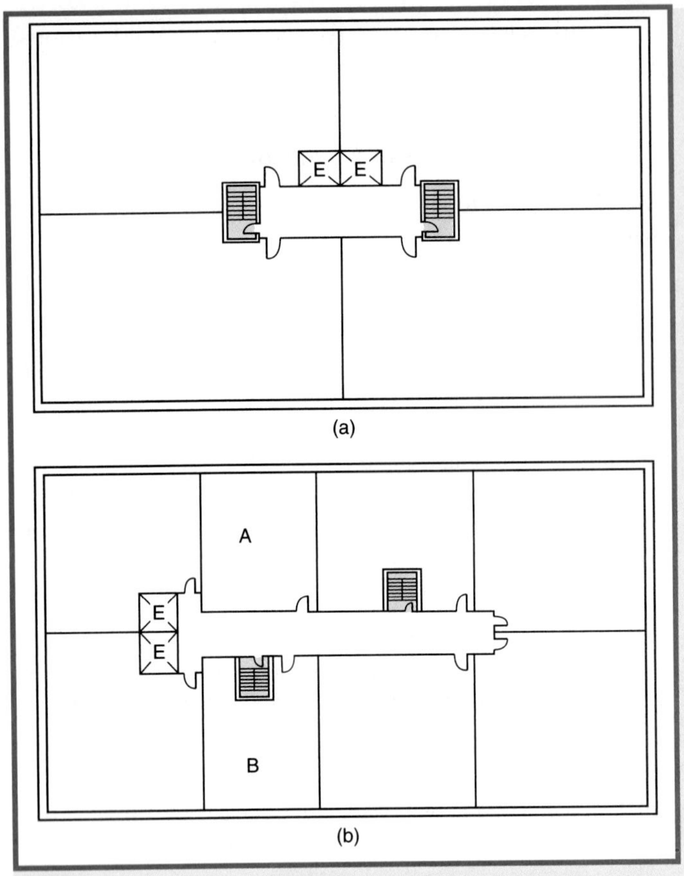


**Exhibit 28/29.4** *New hotels/dormitories — exit remoteness.*

common path of travel is measured from the most remote point subject to occupancy to the point where occupants have a choice of traveling in independent directions (see 7.5.1.1.4 and the definition of *common path of travel* in 3.3.42). In hotels, the travel within the guest room, though regulated by 28/29.2.6.1 and 28/29.2.6.2 for distance, is not included as part of the common path of travel, because the path of travel within the guest room is considered means of escape, rather than means of egress. Therefore, common path of travel, as illustrated by the solid arrows in Exhibit 28/29.5, is measured from the room door to the point where occupants have a choice of traveling in independent directions. This depiction can be thought of as a modified common path of travel, because measurement does not extend into the guest room or guest suite.

CHAPTER 29 • Existing

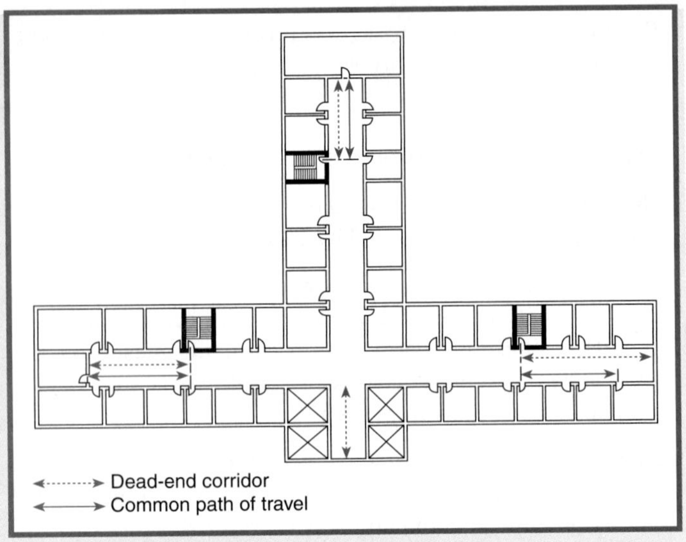


**Exhibit 28/29.5** *Modified common path of travel and dead-end corridors in a hotel.*

The distances permitted for common path of travel in new and existing hotels also differ. Because most new hotels are required to be sprinklered (see 28.3.5.1), the 35 ft (10.7 m) modified common path of travel and dead-end corridor limitations permitted by 28.2.5.3 and 28.2.5.5 will usually be supplanted by the 50 ft (15 m) limitation permitted by 28.2.5.4 and 28.2.5.6. However, if a building can comply with 28.3.5.2, which exempts sprinklers, the 35 ft (10.7 m) common path of travel and dead-end corridor limitations would apply.

In existing hotels, automatic sprinklers are not generally required. However, if the building is protected throughout by an approved, supervised automatic sprinkler system, the common path of travel is permitted to be 50 ft (15 m), which is the same distance permitted for the length of existing dead-end corridors, regardless of the presence of automatic sprinklers.

Although not considered part of the common path of travel, travel within a guest room or a guest suite in a new hotel is regulated indirectly by 28.2.5.7, which limits the area of rooms or suites with a single exit access to not larger than 2000 ft$^2$ (185 m$^2$). See also 28/29.2.6.1 and 28/29.2.6.2 for travel distance limitations within guest rooms and guest suites.

### 28.2.6 Travel Distance to Exits.

**28.2.6.1** Travel distance within a guest room or guest suite to a corridor door shall not exceed 75 ft (23 m) in buildings

### 29.2.6 Travel Distance to Exits.

**29.2.6.1** Travel distance within a guest room or guest suite to a corridor door shall not exceed 75 ft (23 m) in buildings

CHAPTER 28 • New

not protected by an approved, supervised automatic sprinkler system in accordance with 28.3.5.

**28.2.6.2** Travel distance within a guest room or guest suite to a corridor door shall not exceed 125 ft (38 m) in buildings protected by an approved, supervised automatic sprinkler system in accordance with 28.3.5.

**28.2.6.3** Travel distance from the corridor door of any guest room or guest suite to the nearest exit shall comply with 28.2.6.3.1, 28.2.6.3.2, or 28.2.6.3.3.

**28.2.6.3.1** Travel distance from the corridor door of any guest room or guest suite to the nearest exit, measured in accordance with Section 7.6, shall not exceed 100 ft (30 m).

**28.2.6.3.2** Travel distance from the corridor door of any guest room or guest suite to the nearest exit, measured in accordance with Section 7.6, shall not exceed 200 ft (61 m) for exterior ways of exit access arranged in accordance with 7.5.3.

**28.2.6.3.3** Travel distance from the corridor door of any guest room or guest suite to the nearest exit shall comply with 28.2.6.3.3.1 and 28.2.6.3.3.2.

**28.2.6.3.3.1** Travel distance from the corridor door of any guest room or guest suite to the nearest exit shall be measured in accordance with Section 7.6 and shall not exceed 200 ft (61 m) where the exit access and any portion of the building that is tributary to the exit access are protected throughout by an approved, supervised automatic sprinkler system in accordance with 28.3.5.

**28.2.6.3.3.2** Where the building is not protected throughout by an approved, supervised automatic sprinkler system, the 200 ft (61 m) travel distance shall be permitted within any portion of the building that is protected by an approved, supervised automatic sprinkler system, provided that the sprinklered portion of the building is separated from any nonsprinklered portion by fire barriers having a fire resistance rating as follows:

(1) Minimum 1-hour fire resistance rating for buildings three or fewer stories in height
(2) Minimum 2-hour fire resistance rating for buildings four or more stories in height

CHAPTER 29 • Existing

not protected by an approved, supervised automatic sprinkler system in accordance with 29.3.5.

**29.2.6.2** Travel distance within a guest room or guest suite to a corridor door shall not exceed 125 ft (38 m) in buildings protected by an approved, supervised automatic sprinkler system in accordance with 29.3.5.

**29.2.6.3** Travel distance from the corridor door of any guest room or guest suite to the nearest exit shall comply with 29.2.6.3.1, 29.2.6.3.2, or 29.2.6.3.3.

**29.2.6.3.1** Travel distance from the corridor door of any guest room or guest suite to the nearest exit, measured in accordance with Section 7.6, shall not exceed 100 ft (30 m).

**29.2.6.3.2** Travel distance from the corridor door of any guest room or guest suite to the nearest exit, measured in accordance with Section 7.6, shall not exceed 200 ft (61 m) for exterior ways of exit access arranged in accordance with 7.5.3.

**29.2.6.3.3** Travel distance from the corridor door of any guest room or guest suite to the nearest exit shall comply with 29.2.6.3.3.1 and 29.2.6.3.3.2.

**29.2.6.3.3.1** Travel distance from the corridor door of any guest room or guest suite to the nearest exit shall be measured in accordance with Section 7.6 and shall not exceed 200 ft (61 m) where the exit access and any portion of the building that is tributary to the exit access are protected throughout by an approved, supervised automatic sprinkler system in accordance with 29.3.5.

**29.2.6.3.3.2** Where the building is not protected throughout by an approved, supervised automatic sprinkler system, the 200 ft (61 m) travel distance shall be permitted within any portion of the building that is protected by an approved, supervised automatic sprinkler system, provided that the sprinklered portion of the building is separated from any nonsprinklered portion by fire barriers having a fire resistance rating as follows:

(1) Minimum 1-hour fire resistance rating for buildings three or fewer stories in height
(2) Minimum 2-hour fire resistance rating for buildings four or more stories in height

The travel distance limitations specified in 28/29.2.6 are divided into the following two portions of the overall travel distance:

1. Travel within a room or suite of rooms to the room door
2. Travel from the corridor door to the nearest exit

This concept and the distance limitations specified in 28/29.2.6 are illustrated in Exhibit 28/29.6. If the travel distance within a room or suite of rooms is excessive, an additional remote door to the corridor can usually be added to correct the deficiency. Excessive travel distance within the corridor can usually be corrected by adding another exit.

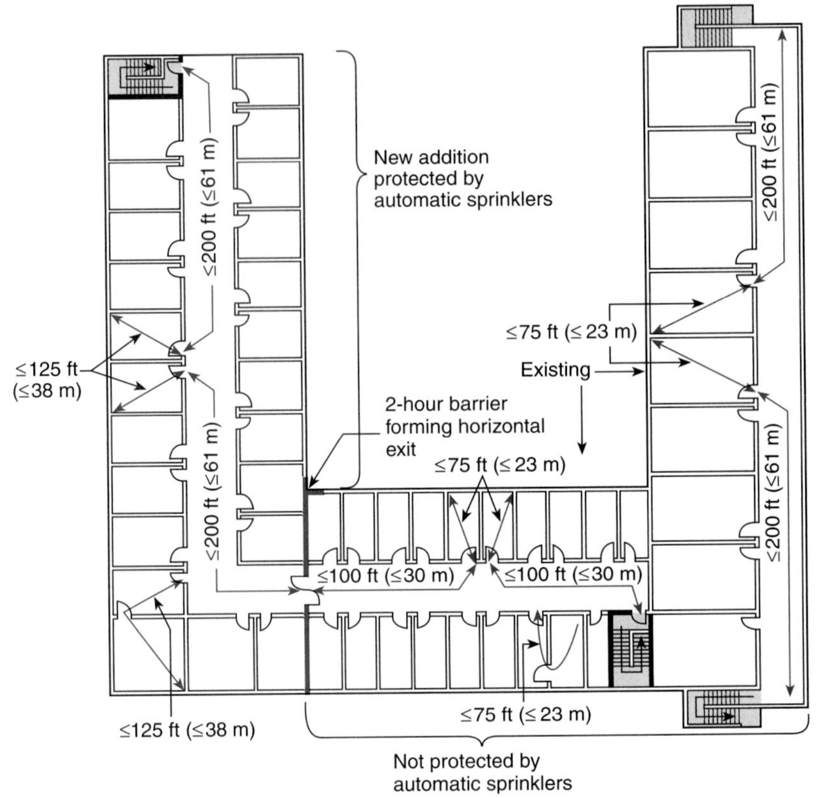


***Exhibit 28/29.6*** *Travel distance measurement and limitations in hotels.*

## 28.2.7 Discharge from Exits.

**28.2.7.1** Exit discharge shall comply with Section 7.7.

**28.2.7.2*** Any required exit stair that is located so that it is necessary to pass through the lobby or other open space to reach the outside of the building shall be continuously enclosed down to a level of exit discharge or to a mezzanine within a lobby at a level of exit discharge.

**A.28.2.7.2** Where open stairways are permitted, they are considered as exit access to exits rather than as exits, and the requirements for travel distance to exits include the travel on such stairs. *(See 7.6.2.)*

**28.2.7.3** The distance of travel from the termination of the exit enclosure to an exterior door leading to a public way shall not exceed 100 ft (30 m).

## 29.2.7 Discharge from Exits.

**29.2.7.1** Exit discharge shall comply with Section 7.7.

**29.2.7.2*** Any required exit stair that is located so that it is necessary to pass through the lobby or other open space to reach the outside of the building shall be continuously enclosed down to a level of exit discharge or to a mezzanine within a lobby at a level of exit discharge.

**A.29.2.7.2** Where open stairways or escalators are permitted, they are considered as exit access to exits rather than as exits, and the requirements for travel distance to exits include the travel on such stairs and escalators. *(See 7.6.2.)*

**29.2.7.3** The distance of travel from the termination of the exit enclosure to an exterior door leading to a public way shall not exceed 150 ft (46 m) in buildings protected throughout by an approved automatic sprinkler system in accordance with 29.3.5 and shall not exceed 100 ft (30 m) in all other buildings.

Section 7.7 permits a maximum of 50 percent of the number and capacity of exits to discharge through the street floor under limited conditions (see 7.7.2). Paragraph 28/29.2.7.2 modifies the restrictions of Section 7.7 by treating an exit that discharges onto a mezzanine within the lobby of a hotel (with subsequent open stair travel to the lobby floor on the level of exit discharge) as equivalent to an exit that discharges directly into the lobby at the level of exit discharge. Therefore, 50 percent of the exits can discharge onto a mezzanine; the other 50 percent must discharge directly outside. However, the distance from the termination of the exit enclosure to the exterior door is limited to a maximum of 100 ft (30 m) in new buildings (see 28.2.7.3). In existing buildings, the same 100 ft (30 m) limitation applies, unless the building is protected with automatic sprinklers, in which case the distance can be extended to 150 ft (46 m) (see 29.2.7.3). The part of the exit discharge that occurs within the building is depicted in Exhibit 28/29.7 by the arrow that connects the door at stair 1 with the lobby door to the outside. See also the commentary following 7.7.2.7.

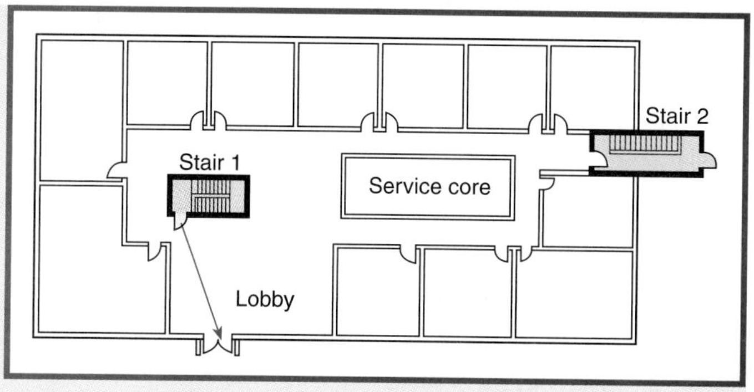


*Exhibit 28/29.7 Exit discharge through street level.*

### 28.2.8 Illumination of Means of Egress.

Means of egress shall be illuminated in accordance with Section 7.8.

### 28.2.9 Emergency Lighting.

**28.2.9.1** Emergency lighting in accordance with Section 7.9 shall be provided.

**28.2.9.2** The requirement of 28.2.9.1 shall not apply where each guest room or guest suite has an exit direct to the outside of the building at street or the finished ground level.

### 28.2.10 Marking of Means of Egress.

Means of egress shall have signs in accordance with Section 7.10.

### 28.2.11 Special Means of Egress Features.

**28.2.11.1 Reserved.**

**28.2.11.2 Lockups.** Lockups in hotel and dormitory occupancies shall comply with the requirements of 22.4.5.

### 29.2.8 Illumination of Means of Egress.

Means of egress shall be illuminated in accordance with Section 7.8.

### 29.2.9 Emergency Lighting.

**29.2.9.1** Emergency lighting in accordance with Section 7.9 shall be provided in all buildings with more than 25 rooms.

**29.2.9.2** The requirement of 29.2.9.1 shall not apply where each guest room or guest suite has an exit direct to the outside of the building at street or the finished ground level.

### 29.2.10 Marking of Means of Egress.

Means of egress shall have signs in accordance with Section 7.10.

### 29.2.11 Special Means of Egress Features.

**29.2.11.1 Reserved.**

**29.2.11.2 Lockups.** Lockups in hotel and dormitory occupancies, other than approved existing lockups, shall comply with the requirements of 23.4.5.

## 28.3 Protection

### 28.3.1 Protection of Vertical Openings.

**28.3.1.1** Vertical openings shall comply with 28.3.1.1.1 through 28.3.1.2.

**28.3.1.1.1** Vertical openings shall be enclosed or protected in accordance with Section 8.6.

## 29.3 Protection

### 29.3.1 Vertical Openings.

**29.3.1.1** Vertical openings shall comply with 29.3.1.1.1 through 29.3.1.2.

**29.3.1.1.1** Vertical openings shall be enclosed or protected in accordance with Section 8.6.

CHAPTER 28 • New

**28.3.1.1.2** Vertical openings in accordance with 8.6.8.2 shall be permitted.

**28.3.1.1.3** In buildings, other than high-rise buildings, that are protected throughout by an approved, supervised automatic sprinkler system in accordance with 28.3.5, the walls enclosing vertical openings shall have a minimum 1-hour fire resistance rating, and doors shall have a minimum 1-hour fire protection rating.

CHAPTER 29 • Existing

**29.3.1.1.2** Vertical openings in accordance with 8.6.8.2 shall be permitted.

**29.3.1.1.3** In buildings, other than high-rise buildings, that are protected throughout by an approved automatic sprinkler system in accordance with 29.3.5, and in which exits and required ways of travel thereto are adequately safeguarded against fire and smoke within the building, or where every individual room has direct access to an exterior exit without passing through any public corridor, the protection of vertical openings that are not part of required exits shall not be required where approved by the authority having jurisdiction and where such openings do not endanger required means of egress.

**29.3.1.1.4** In buildings two or fewer stories in height, unprotected openings shall be permitted by the authority having jurisdiction to continue to be used where the building is protected throughout by an approved automatic sprinkler system in accordance with 29.3.5.

New hotels and dormitories, except those in buildings not more than three stories in height where all guest sleeping rooms have a door to the exterior at grade or to an exterior exit access balcony, must be protected throughout by an approved, supervised automatic sprinkler system (see 28.3.5.1 and 28.3.5.2). Therefore, most new non-high-rise hotels and dormitories, by virtue of their compliance with the sprinkler requirements of 28.3.5.1, are permitted to use the 1-hour vertical enclosure protection option in accordance with 28.3.1.1.3, regardless of the number of stories the vertical opening connects. See also the commentary following 28/29.2.2.1.2 for discussion on the requirements for exits.

The protection of vertical openings in existing hotels is achieved by means of a performance approach. Openings must be either enclosed in accordance with Section 8.6, or they must satisfy the objectives of 4.5.6. Note, however, that no such performance approach is provided for new hotels.

The provisions of 28/29.3.1.1.2 are the same and permit an open stair connecting a maximum of two levels within a guest suite. This stair is permitted to serve as a means of escape (see 8.6.8.2 for the provisions for convenience openings).

Existing unprotected openings in non-high-rise buildings are permitted by 29.3.1.1.3 under the following conditions:

1. Openings are approved by the authority having jurisdiction (AHJ).
2. The building is fully sprinklered.
3. Exits and exit accesses are adequately safeguarded against fire and smoke in the remainder of the building.
4. In lieu of the condition in item 3, every room has direct access to an exterior exit that does not require travel through a public corridor.
5. Shafts that enclose required exit stairs are protected.

Existing unprotected vertical openings are permitted by 29.3.1.1.4 under the following conditions:

1. Openings are approved by the AHJ.
2. The building is not more than two stories.
3. The building is fully sprinklered.

**28.3.1.2** No floor below the level of exit discharge used only for storage, heating equipment, or purposes other than residential occupancy shall have unprotected openings to floors used for residential purposes.

**29.3.1.2** No floor below the level of exit discharge used only for storage, heating equipment, or purposes other than residential occupancy shall have unprotected openings to floors used for residential purposes.

CHAPTER 28 • New

### 28.3.2 Protection from Hazards.

**28.3.2.1 General.** All rooms containing high-pressure boilers, refrigerating machinery, transformers, or other service equipment subject to possible explosion shall not be located directly under or directly adjacent to exits and shall be effectively cut off from other parts of the building as specified in Section 8.7.

**28.3.2.2 Hazardous Areas.**

**28.3.2.2.1** Any hazardous area shall be protected in accordance with Section 8.7.

**28.3.2.2.2** The areas described in Table 28.3.2.2.2 shall be protected as indicated.

*Table 28.3.2.2.2 Hazardous Area Protection*

| Hazardous Area Description | Separation/Protection[a] |
|---|---|
| Boiler and fuel-fired heater rooms serving more than a single guest room or guest suite | 1 hour and sprinklers |
| Employee locker rooms | 1 hour or sprinklers |
| Gift or retail shops | 1 hour or sprinklers |
| Bulk laundries | 1 hour and sprinklers |
| Guest laundries ≤100 $ft^2$ (≤9.3 $m^2$) outside of guest rooms or guest suites | 1 hour or sprinklers[b] |
| Guest laundries >100 $ft^2$ (>9.3 $m^2$) outside of guest rooms or guest suites | 1 hour and sprinklers |
| Maintenance shops | 1 hour and sprinklers |
| Storage rooms[c] | 1 hour or sprinklers |
| Trash collection rooms | 1 hour and sprinklers |

[a] Minimum fire resistance rating.

[b]Where sprinklers are provided, the separation specified in 8.7.1.2 and 28.3.2.2.3 is not required.

[c]Where storage areas not exceeding 24 $ft^2$ (2.2 $m^2$) are directly accessible from the guest room or guest suite, no separation or protection is required.

**28.3.2.2.3** Where sprinkler protection without fire-rated separation is used, areas shall be separated from other spaces by smoke partitions complying with Section 8.4.

CHAPTER 29 • Existing

### 29.3.2 Protection from Hazards.

**29.3.2.1 General.** All rooms containing high-pressure boilers, refrigerating machinery, transformers, or other service equipment subject to possible explosion shall not be located directly under or directly adjacent to exits and shall be effectively cut off from other parts of the building as specified in Section 8.7.

**29.3.2.2 Hazardous Areas.**

**29.3.2.2.1** Any hazardous area shall be protected in accordance with Section 8.7.

**29.3.2.2.2** The areas described in Table 29.3.2.2.2 shall be protected as indicated.

*Table 29.3.2.2.2 Hazardous Area Protection*

| Hazardous Area Description | Separation/Protection[a] |
|---|---|
| Boiler and fuel-fired heater rooms serving more than a single guest room or guest suite | 1 hour or sprinklers |
| Employee locker rooms | 1 hour or sprinklers |
| Gift or retail shops >100 $ft^2$ (>9.3 $m^2$) | 1 hour or sprinklers[b] |
| Bulk laundries | 1 hour or sprinklers |
| Guest laundries >100 $ft^2$ (>9.3 $m^2$) outside of guest rooms or guest suites | 1 hour or sprinklers[b] |
| Maintenance shops | 1 hour and sprinklers |
| Rooms or spaces used for storage of combustible supplies and equipment in quantities deemed hazardous by the authority having jurisdiction[c] | 1 hour or sprinklers |
| Trash collection rooms | 1 hour and sprinklers |

[a] Minimum fire resistance rating.

[b]Where sprinklers are provided, the separation specified in 8.7.1.2 and 29.3.2.2.3 shall not be required.

[c]Where storage areas not exceeding 24 $ft^2$ (2.2 $m^2$) are directly accessible from the guest room or guest suite, no separation or protection is required.

**29.3.2.2.3** Where sprinkler protection without fire-rated separation is used, areas shall be separated from other spaces by smoke partitions complying with Section 8.4.

Note the differences in the hazardous area protection requirements for new and existing hotels. In new construction, many areas are required to be separated by construction with a 1-hour fire resistance rating and to be protected by automatic sprinklers. In existing buildings, automatic sprinklers are often used as an

CHAPTER 28 • New

alternative to rated construction, with the exception of trash collection rooms and maintenance shops, where both protection methods are required.

While the lists that appear in Table 28.3.2.2.2 and Table 29.3.2.2.2 provide specific direction for certain hazardous contents areas, they are not all-inclusive. Other areas that are deemed hazardous need to be provided with the appropriate level of protection in accordance with Section 8.7.

**28.3.3 Interior Finish.**

**28.3.3.1 General.** Interior finish shall be in accordance with Section 10.2.

**28.3.3.2 Interior Wall and Ceiling Finish.** Interior wall and ceiling finish materials complying with Section 10.2 shall be permitted as follows:

(1) Exit enclosures — Class A
(2) Lobbies and corridors — Class A or Class B
(3) Other spaces — Class A, Class B, or Class C

**28.3.3.3 Interior Floor Finish.**

**28.3.3.3.1** Interior floor finish shall comply with Section 10.2.

**28.3.3.3.2** Interior floor finish in exit enclosures and exit access corridors and spaces not separated from them by walls complying with 28.3.6.1 shall be not less than Class II.

**28.3.3.3.3** Interior floor finish shall comply with 10.2.7.1 or 10.2.7.2, as applicable.

**28.3.4 Detection, Alarm, and Communications Systems.**

**28.3.4.1 General.** A fire alarm system in accordance with Section 9.6, except as modified by 28.3.4.2 through 28.3.4.6, shall be provided.

**28.3.4.2 Initiation.** The required fire alarm system shall be initiated by each of the following:

(1) Manual means in accordance with 9.6.2
(2) Manual fire alarm box located at the hotel desk or other convenient central control point under continuous supervision by responsible employees
(3) Required automatic sprinkler system
(4) Required automatic detection system other than sleeping room smoke detectors

CHAPTER 29 • Existing

**29.3.3 Interior Finish.**

**29.3.3.1 General.** Interior finish shall be in accordance with Section 10.2.

**29.3.3.2 Interior Wall and Ceiling Finish.** Interior wall and ceiling finish materials complying with Section 10.2 shall be permitted as follows:

(1) Exit enclosures — Class A or Class B
(2) Lobbies and corridors — Class A or Class B
(3) Other spaces — Class A, Class B, or Class C

**29.3.3.3 Interior Floor Finish.** In nonsprinklered buildings, newly installed interior floor finish in exits and exit access corridors shall be not less than Class II in accordance with 10.2.7.

**29.3.4 Detection, Alarm, and Communications Systems.**

**29.3.4.1 General.** A fire alarm system in accordance with Section 9.6, except as modified by 29.3.4.2 through 29.3.4.6, shall be provided in buildings, other than those where each guest room has exterior exit access in accordance with 7.5.3 and the building is three or fewer stories in height.

**29.3.4.2 Initiation.** The required fire alarm system shall be initiated by each of the following:

(1) Manual means in accordance with 9.6.2, unless there are other effective means to activate the fire alarm system, such as complete automatic sprinkler or automatic detection systems, with manual fire alarm box in accordance with 29.3.4.2(2) required
(2) Manual fire alarm box located at the hotel desk or other convenient central control point under continuous supervision by responsible employees
(3) Required automatic sprinkler system
(4) Required automatic detection system other than sleeping room smoke detectors

CHAPTER 28 • New

28.3.4.3 **Notification.**

**28.3.4.3.1*** Occupant notification shall be provided automatically in accordance with 9.6.3.

**A.28.3.4.3.1** Visible signaling appliances might be governed by provisions of federal regulations in 28 CFR 36, Appendix A, "Americans with Disabilities Act Accessibility Guidelines for Buildings and Facilities," Section 4.28, Alarms.

**28.3.4.3.2** Positive alarm sequence in accordance with 9.6.3.4 shall be permitted.

**28.3.4.3.3*** Guest rooms and guest suites specifically required and equipped to accommodate hearing-impaired individuals shall be provided with a visible notification appliance.

**A.28.3.4.3.3** A quantity of such rooms and suites might be required to be equipped to accommodate hearing-impaired individuals based on the total number of rooms in a transient lodging facility. *(See 28 CFR 36, Appendix A, "Americans with Disabilities Act Accessibility Guidelines for Buildings and Facilities.")*

**28.3.4.3.4** In occupiable areas, other than guest rooms and guest suites, visible notification appliances shall be provided.

**28.3.4.3.5** Annunciation and annunciation zoning in accordance with 9.6.7 shall be provided in buildings three or more stories in height or having more than 50 guest rooms or guest suites. Annunciation shall be provided at a location readily accessible from the primary point of entry for emergency response personnel.

**28.3.4.3.6** Emergency forces notification shall be provided in accordance with 9.6.4.

CHAPTER 29 • Existing

**29.3.4.3 Notification.**

**29.3.4.3.1** Occupant notification shall be provided automatically in accordance with 9.6.3.

**29.3.4.3.2** Positive alarm sequence in accordance with 9.6.3.4, and a presignal system in accordance with 9.6.3.3, shall be permitted.

**29.3.4.3.3 Reserved.**

**29.3.4.3.4 Reserved.**

**29.3.4.3.5 Reserved.**

**29.3.4.3.6*** Provisions shall be made for the immediate notification of the public fire department by telephone or other means in case of fire, and, where there is no public fire department, notification shall be made to the private fire brigade.

**A.29.3.4.3.6** The provision for immediate notification of the public fire department is intended to include, but is not limited to, all of the arrangements in 9.6.4.2. Other arrangements that depend on a clerk or other member of the staff to notify the fire department might also be permitted. In such cases, however, it is essential that a trained staff member and an immediately available means of calling the fire department are continuously available. If a telephone is to be used, it should not be of any type or arrangement that requires a coin or the unlocking of a device to contact the fire department.

The *Code* requires that, in addition to the normal distribution of manual fire alarm boxes (pull stations, see 9.6.2), the front desk, telephone operator's location, or similar location must also be equipped with a manual fire alarm box. The intent is that a manual fire alarm box is to be available at the location where staff would receive notification of an emergency phoned in by a guest.

The smoke alarms installed in sleeping rooms are usually single-station alarms that are provided for the sole purpose of notifying the occupants of the presence of smoke within that room. Thus, the alarms are not a part of a required automatic detection system and are not required to initiate the building alarm system. The *Code*, in fact, prohibits guest room smoke alarms from activating the system to prevent numerous activations that could pose a nuisance alarm problem in hotels (see 9.6.2.10.4). Smoke alarms are available that annunciate at a central point, alert the occupants of the room, and notify management of a problem in that room without sounding an alarm throughout the building.

The provision of 29.3.4.2(1) eliminates the requirements for manual fire alarm boxes to be located so that all portions of a building are within 200 ft (61 m) of a manual fire alarm box (see 9.6.2) in existing hotels where an automatic sprinkler system or an automatic fire detection system is provided throughout the building. The alarm system is still required; only the requirement for additional manual fire alarm boxes is eliminated.

The location of audible alarm devices in hotels affects their audibility. In most new construction, corridor walls are of such character (soundproof) that a sounding device would be needed in each guest room or guest suite to meet the performance criterion for audibility throughout the building. The use of sounding devices only in the corridor might necessitate their operation at dangerous sound levels to awaken guests in their rooms. The permitted use of positive alarm sequence by 28/29.3.4.3.2 recognizes a technology similar to a presignal system but with additional fail-safe features. See the commentary on 9.6.3.4 for a discussion on positive alarm sequence.

Presignal systems have repeatedly been involved in delaying alarms in multiple-death fires and are not permitted in new construction. However, the occurrence of nuisance alarms in hotels is real, and presignal systems continue to be permitted in existing buildings. Therefore, if the presignal is to be transmitted to a building staff location (e.g., the front desk), 9.6.3.3 specifies that it must be received by trained staff. As a result, hotel employees assigned to signal-receiving locations must be well trained with respect to fire alarm signals and proper staff response to an alarm.

Direct fire alarm connection to the fire department by one of the methods recognized by 9.6.4 is required in new hotels and dormitories, as specified by 28.3.4.3.6; this provision is new to the 2009 edition of the *Code*. In existing hotels and dormitories, provisions must be made to notify the fire department by telephone or other approved means. This requirement can usually be met by providing a telephone at the hotel's front desk or other normally staffed location. The telephone addressed in A.29.3.4.3.6 needs to be equipped for direct outside dial without going through a switchboard and should not be a pay phone.

Single-station smoke alarms powered by the building's electrical system are required in each sleeping room and living area located in a guest room or guest suite. The intent is to alert the occupant of the room to the presence of a fire originating in that room or suite. Normally, the alarms are not tied into the building fire alarm [see 28/29.3.4.2(4)]. The expected course of action is as follows:

1. The smoke alarm alerts the occupant of the room; the occupant leaves the room.
2. The self-closing device on the corridor door returns the door to its closed and latched position.
3. The occupant pulls a manual fire alarm box, thereby initiating the building alarm system; the occupant proceeds to an exit and leaves the building.
4. If the occupant fails to sound the alarm manually, compensation is provided in new construction by corridor smoke detectors or by automatic sprinklers (see 28.3.4.4 for corridor smoke detection requirements in new, nonsprinklered hotels and dormitories).

In addition to requiring a smoke alarm in each sleeping room, a smoke alarm is required in each living area within the guest room or guest suite. These alarms are required for the following two reasons:

1. The living area is often used for sleeping, even if such use was not the original intent.
2. Most sleeping rooms are arranged so that a fire in the living area will rapidly block escape from the sleeping area.

If a corridor smoke detection system is provided, it must be maintained, since the system is required for new construction, unless the building is sprinklered.

**28.3.4.4 Detection.** A corridor smoke detection system in accordance with Section 9.6 shall be provided in buildings other than those protected throughout by an approved, supervised automatic sprinkler system in accordance with 28.3.5.3.

**28.3.4.5* Smoke Alarms.** An approved single-station smoke alarm shall be installed in accordance with 9.6.2.10 in every guest room and every living area and sleeping room within a guest suite.

**A.28.3.4.5** Caution needs to be exercised in locating smoke alarms with regard to their proximity to bathrooms, cooking facilities, and HVAC outlets in order to prevent nuisance alarms.

**28.3.4.6* Protection of Fire Alarm System.** The provision of 9.6.1.8.1.3 shall not apply to the smoke detection required at each fire alarm control unit by 9.6.1.8.1(1).

**A.28.3.4.6** It is the intent that smoke detection be provided at each fire alarm control unit, regardless of the presence of sprinkler protection.

### 28.3.5 Extinguishment Requirements.

**28.3.5.1** All buildings, other than those complying with 28.3.5.2, shall be protected throughout by an approved, supervised automatic sprinkler system in accordance with 28.3.5.3.

**28.3.5.2** Automatic sprinkler protection shall not be required in buildings where all guest sleeping rooms or guest suites have a door opening directly to either of the following:

(1) Outside at the street or the finished ground level
(2) Exterior exit access arranged in accordance with 7.5.3 in buildings three or fewer stories in height

**28.3.5.3** Where an automatic sprinkler system is installed, either for total or partial building coverage, the system shall be in accordance with Section 9.7, as modified by 28.3.5.4. In buildings four or fewer stories above grade plane, systems in accordance with NFPA 13R, *Standard for the Installation of Sprinkler Systems in Residential Occupancies up to and Including Four Stories in Height*, shall be permitted.



**29.3.4.4 Detection. (Reserved)**

**29.3.4.5* Smoke Alarms.** An approved single-station smoke alarm shall be installed in accordance with 9.6.2.10 in every guest room and every living area and sleeping room within a guest suite.

**A.29.3.4.5** Caution needs to be exercised in locating smoke alarms with regard to their proximity to bathrooms, cooking facilities, and HVAC outlets in order to prevent nuisance alarms.

**29.3.4.5.1** The smoke alarms shall not be required to be interconnected.

**29.3.4.5.2** Single-station smoke alarms without a secondary (standby) power source shall be permitted.

**29.3.4.6* Protection of Fire Alarm System.** The provision of 9.6.1.8.1.3 shall not apply to the smoke detection required at each fire alarm control unit by 9.6.1.8.1(1).

**A.29.3.4.6** It is the intent that smoke detection be provided at each fire alarm control unit, regardless of the presence of sprinkler protection.

### 29.3.5 Extinguishment Requirements.

**29.3.5.1** All high-rise buildings, other than those where each guest room or guest suite has exterior exit access in accordance with 7.5.3, shall be protected throughout by an approved, supervised automatic sprinkler system in accordance with 29.3.5.3.

**29.3.5.2 Reserved.**

**29.3.5.3*** Where an automatic sprinkler system is installed, either for total or partial building coverage, the system shall be in accordance with Section 9.7, as modified by 29.3.5.4 and 29.3.5.5. In buildings four or fewer stories above grade plane, systems in accordance with NFPA 13R, *Standard for the Installation of Sprinkler Systems in Residential Occupancies up to and Including Four Stories in Height*, shall be permitted.

**A.29.3.5.3** Although not required by the *Code*, the use of residential sprinklers or quick-response sprinklers is encouraged

CHAPTER 28 • New

CHAPTER 29 • Existing

for new installations of sprinkler systems within dwelling units, apartments, and guest rooms. Caution should be exercised, as the system needs to be designed for the sprinkler being used.

**28.3.5.4** The provisions for draft stops and closely spaced sprinklers in NFPA 13, *Standard for the Installation of Sprinkler Systems*, shall not be required for openings complying with 8.6.8.2 where the opening is within the guest room or guest suite.

**28.3.5.5 Reserved.**

**28.3.5.6** Listed quick-response or listed residential sprinklers shall be used throughout guest rooms and guest room suites.

**28.3.5.7** Open parking structures that comply with NFPA 88A, *Standard for Parking Structures*, and are contiguous with hotels or dormitories shall be exempt from the sprinkler requirements of 28.3.5.1.

**28.3.5.8** In buildings other than those protected throughout with an approved, supervised automatic sprinkler system in accordance with 28.3.5.3, portable fire extinguishers shall be provided as specified in 9.7.4.1 in hazardous areas addressed by 28.3.2.2.

**29.3.5.4** The provisions for draft stops and closely spaced sprinklers in NFPA 13, *Standard for the Installation of Sprinkler Systems*, shall not be required for openings complying with 8.6.8.2 where the opening is within the guest room or guest suite.

**29.3.5.5** In guest rooms and in guest room suites, sprinkler installations shall not be required in closets not exceeding 24 $ft^2$ (2.2 $m^2$) and in bathrooms not exceeding 55 $ft^2$ (5.1 $m^2$).

**29.3.5.6 Reserved.**

**29.3.5.7 Reserved.**

**29.3.5.8** In buildings other than those protected throughout with an approved, supervised automatic sprinkler system in accordance with 29.3.5.3, portable fire extinguishers shall be provided as specified in 9.7.4.1 in hazardous areas addressed by 29.3.2.2.

New hotels and dormitories must be protected throughout by an approved, supervised automatic sprinkler system, unless they are three or fewer stories in height and all guest rooms have doors to the exterior at grade or to exterior exit access balconies. The disproportionate percentage of deaths associated with residential occupancies and the conditions precipitating these fatalities in hotel settings (the need to wake sleeping occupants and escape in unfamiliar surroundings) prompted the *Code* mandate that most new hotels have automatic sprinkler systems installed.

One objective of the *Code* is to protect occupants who are not intimate with the initial fire development from loss of life and improve the survivability of those who are intimate with the fire development, as stated in 4.1.1. Based on this objective, new hotels are required to use quick-response or residential sprinklers throughout guest rooms and guest suites per 28.3.5.6. The technology associated with quick-response and residential sprinklers helps to maintain tenability within the room of fire origin.

Automatic sprinklers are not required in all existing hotels and dormitories. Requirements for such systems, if they are installed, are specified by 29.3.5.3. Other portions of Chapter 29 offer significant incentives for installing sprinklers. Examples include a reduction in the fire resistance rating of exit enclosures (29.2.2.1.2) and an increase in common path of travel (29.2.5.4) and travel distance (29.2.6.2 and 29.2.6.3.3.1). In addition, the presence of sprinklers influences requirements addressing exit discharge (29.2.7), vertical openings (29.3.1), hazardous areas (29.3.2), interior finish (29.3.3), corridors (29.3.6), and smoke barriers (29.3.7).

Per 29.3.5.1, an automatic sprinkler system is required in existing high-rise hotels and dormitories, unless every guest room or guest suite has exterior exit access. The presence of exterior exit access eliminates the need to traverse a corridor where conditions might not remain tenable.

CHAPTER 28 • New

### 28.3.6 Corridors.

**28.3.6.1 Walls.**

**28.3.6.1.1** Exit access corridor walls shall comply with 28.3.6.1.2 or 28.3.6.1.3.

**28.3.6.1.2** In buildings not complying with 28.3.6.1.3, exit access corridor walls shall consist of fire barriers in accordance with Section 8.3 that have not less than a 1-hour fire resistance rating.

**28.3.6.1.3** In buildings protected throughout by an approved, supervised automatic sprinkler system in accordance with 28.3.5, corridor walls shall have a minimum $\frac{1}{2}$-hour fire resistance rating.

**28.3.6.2 Doors.**

**28.3.6.2.1** Doors that open onto exit access corridors shall have not less than a 20-minute fire protection rating in accordance with Section 8.3.

**28.3.6.2.2 Reserved.**

**28.3.6.2.3** Doors that open onto exit access corridors shall be self-closing and self-latching.

**28.3.6.3 Unprotected Openings.**

**28.3.6.3.1** Unprotected openings, other than those from spaces complying with 28.3.6.3.2, shall be prohibited in exit access corridor walls and doors.

**28.3.6.3.2** Spaces shall be permitted to be unlimited in area and open to the corridor, provided that the following criteria are met:

(1) The space is not used for guest rooms or guest suites or hazardous areas.
(2) The building is protected throughout by an approved, supervised automatic sprinkler system in accordance with 28.3.5.
(3) The space does not obstruct access to required exits.

**28.3.6.4 Transoms, Louvers, or Transfer Grilles.** Transoms, louvers, or transfer grilles shall be prohibited in walls or doors of exit access corridors.

CHAPTER 29 • Existing

### 29.3.6 Corridors.

**29.3.6.1 Walls.**

**29.3.6.1.1** Exit access corridor walls shall comply with either 29.3.6.1.2 or 29.3.6.1.3.

**29.3.6.1.2** In buildings not complying with 29.3.6.1.3, exit access corridor walls shall consist of fire barriers in accordance with 8.2.3 having a minimum $\frac{1}{2}$-hour fire resistance rating.

**29.3.6.1.3** In buildings protected throughout by an approved automatic sprinkler system in accordance with 29.3.5, no fire resistance rating shall be required, but the walls and all openings therein shall resist the passage of smoke.

**29.3.6.2 Doors.**

**29.3.6.2.1** Doors that open onto exit access corridors, other than those complying with 8.3.4 or in buildings meeting the requirements of 29.3.6.2.2, shall have a minimum 20-minute fire protection rating in accordance with Section 8.3.

**29.3.6.2.2** Where automatic sprinkler protection is provided in the corridor in accordance with 31.3.5.9 through 31.3.5.10, doors shall not be required to have a fire protection rating but shall resist the passage of smoke and be equipped with latches to keep doors tightly closed.

**29.3.6.2.3** Doors that open onto exit access corridors shall be self-closing and self-latching.

**29.3.6.3 Unprotected Openings.**

**29.3.6.3.1** Unprotected openings, other than those from spaces complying with 29.3.6.3.2, shall be prohibited in exit access corridor walls and doors.

**29.3.6.3.2** Spaces shall be permitted to be unlimited in area and open to the corridor, provided that the following criteria are met:

(1) The space is not used for guest rooms or guest suites or hazardous areas.
(2) The space is protected throughout by an approved automatic sprinkler system in accordance with 29.3.5.
(3) The space does not obstruct access to required exits.

**29.3.6.4 Transoms, Louvers, or Transfer Grilles.**

**29.3.6.4.1** Transoms, louvers, or transfer grilles shall be prohibited in walls or doors of exit access corridors, unless meeting the requirements of 29.3.6.4.2, 29.3.6.4.3, or 29.3.6.4.4.

**29.3.6.4.2** Existing transoms shall be permitted but shall be fixed in the closed position and shall be covered or otherwise protected to provide a fire resistance rating not less than that of the wall in which they are installed.

**29.3.6.4.3** The requirement of 29.3.6.4.1 shall not apply where a corridor smoke detection system is provided that, when sensing smoke, sounds the building alarm and shuts down return or exhaust fans that draw air into the corridor from the guest rooms. The transfer grille or louver shall be located in the lower one-third of the wall or door height.

**29.3.6.4.4** The requirement of 29.3.6.4.1 shall not apply to buildings protected throughout by an approved automatic sprinkler system complying with 29.3.5 or buildings with corridor sprinkler protection in accordance with 31.3.5.9 through 31.3.5.10. The transfer grille or louver shall be located in the lower one-third of the wall or door height.

The provisions of 28/29.3.6 reflect concern for providing safety to persons occupying guest rooms during a fire. The minimum fire resistance rating (1 hour for new hotels and dormitories; ½ hour for existing hotels and dormitories) required for corridor wall construction is intended to prevent fire from moving from the corridor to a room or spreading from a room to the corridor.

Although the reduction to a ½-hour fire resistance rating — as permitted by 28.3.6.1.3 — would result in little savings in new construction, it could be useful in the rehabilitation of existing structures that are required to meet the provisions for new construction (see 4.6.8 and Chapter 43). Most existing lath and plaster walls provide 20-minute to 30-minute fire resistance ratings. If automatic sprinkler protection is provided throughout the building, the existing walls should not have to be replaced.

In existing buildings with automatic sprinklers, corridor walls are required only to resist the passage of smoke (see 29.3.6.1.3).

The fire-rated corridor door required by 28/29.3.6.2 provides a level of protection commensurate with the expected fuel load in the room and the fire resistance of the corridor wall construction. The purpose is to box a fire out of a room or to box it within the room by means of corridor wall and door construction. Fuel load studies conducted by the former National Bureau of Standards (now the National Institute of Standards and Technology) demonstrated that residential occupancies typically have fuel loads capable of sustaining a fire for approximately 20 minutes to 30 minutes.

Paragraph 29.3.6.2.2 permits a nonrated door that resists the passage of smoke in buildings that have corridor sprinkler protection installed in accordance with Option 3 for apartment buildings. See 31.3.5.9 and the commentary following 30.3.5.12 and 31.3.5.13 for information on apartment building Option 3 corridor sprinkler requirements. In Exhibit 28/29.8 and Exhibit 28/29.9, the self-closing door is needed to complete the separation established by the fire resistance–rated corridor wall. No provisions permit omission of the self-closing device on the door. Although an existing wall is not required to be fire rated if sprinkler protec-

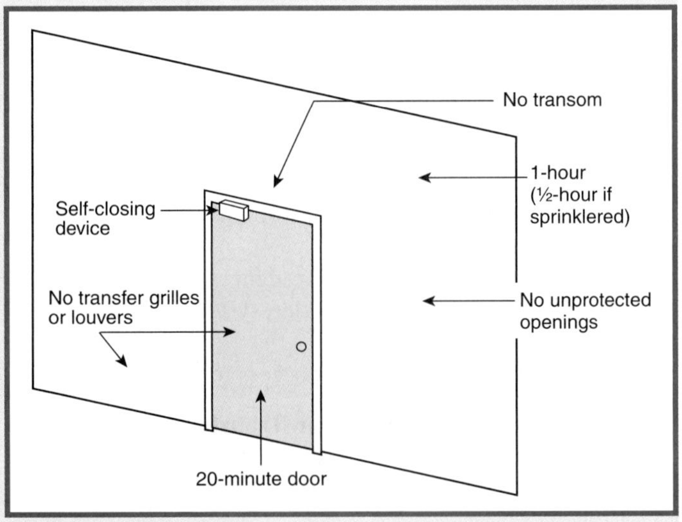


***Exhibit 28/29.8** Protection of guest room corridors and openings in new hotels and dormitories.*

CHAPTER 28 • New | CHAPTER 29 • Existing

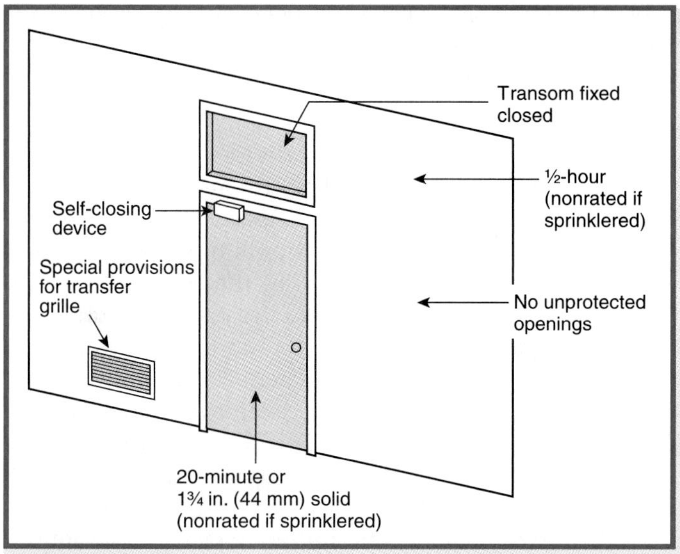


***Exhibit 28/29.9** Protection of guest room corridors and openings in existing hotels and dormitories.*

tion is provided, the wall needs to be solid and resist the passage of smoke.

A 20-minute fire protection rating is required for guest room corridor doors in new hotels and dormitories and those that are existing and nonsprinklered. NFPA 80, *Standard for Fire Doors and Other Opening Protectives,*[2] requires a fire-rated door to be self-closing; however, the requirement for self-closing doors is important enough to be repeated in 28/29.3.6.2.3, rather than relying only on the referenced document.

Self-closers on corridor doors should be properly maintained to ensure that the doors fully close and positively latch on their own. Carpeting and pressure differences created by air-handling systems can interfere with the operation of door closers. If a room door does not completely close under fire conditions, smoke, heat, and other toxic products of combustion can quickly render the corridor untenable.

NFPA 90A, *Standard for the Installation of Air-Conditioning and Ventilating Systems,*[3] prohibits corridors in hotels from being used as a portion of the system for supply, return, or exhaust air.

Operable transoms are prohibited in hotels based on multiple-death fires in which transoms allowed fire and smoke to move through corridors and into occupied rooms. However, existing hotels built prior to 1950 often use corridors for supply or return air. The *Code* continues to recognize this practice for existing hotels if the specific conditions of 29.3.6.4 are met.

### 28.3.7 Subdivision of Building Spaces.

Buildings shall be subdivided in accordance with 28.3.7.1 or 28.3.7.2.

**28.3.7.1** In buildings not protected throughout by an approved, supervised automatic sprinkler system, each hotel guest room, including guest suites, and dormitory room shall be separated from other guest rooms or dormitory rooms by walls and floors constructed as fire barriers having a minimum 1-hour fire resistance rating.

**28.3.7.2** In buildings protected throughout by an approved, supervised automatic sprinkler system, each hotel guest room, including guest suites, and dormitory room shall be separated from other guest rooms or dormitory rooms by walls and floors constructed as fire barriers having a minimum ½-hour fire resistance rating.

**28.3.7.3** Doors in the barriers required by 28.3.7.1 and 28.3.7.2 shall have a fire protection rating of not less than 20 minutes and shall not be required to be self-closing.

### 29.3.7 Subdivision of Building Spaces.

In buildings other than those meeting the requirements of 29.3.7.1, 29.3.7.2, or 29.3.7.3, every guest room floor shall be divided into not less than two smoke compartments of approximately the same size by smoke partitions in accordance with Section 8.4.

**29.3.7.1** Smoke partitions shall not be required in buildings protected throughout by an approved automatic sprinkler system in accordance with 29.3.5 or a corridor sprinkler system conforming to 31.3.5.9 through 31.3.5.10.

**29.3.7.2** Smoke partitions shall not be required where each guest room is provided with exterior ways of exit access arranged in accordance with 7.5.3.

**29.3.7.3** Smoke partitions shall not be required where the aggregate corridor length on each floor is not more than 150 ft (46 m).

CHAPTER 28 • New

CHAPTER 29 • Existing

**29.3.7.4** Additional smoke partitions shall be provided so that the travel distance from a guest room corridor door to a smoke partition shall not exceed 150 ft (46 m).

In new hotels and dormitories, a ½-hour fire resistance–rated separation (1-hour-rated separation if not sprinklered) between guest rooms, guest suites, and dormitory rooms is necessary to confine a fire to the room of fire origin. Hotel guest rooms are frequently provided with connecting doors to allow multiple rooms to be used by a single family or group and to allow for access between the rooms. The requirement for a fire barrier separation between the rooms, therefore, necessitates the use of a fire protection–rated door assembly for at least one of the doors in any guest room-to-guest room opening. The required fire protection rating for such a door is ⅓ hour in both sprinklered and nonsprinklered buildings, and no self-closer is required in accordance with 28.3.7.3.

All but relatively small floors of nonsprinklered existing buildings must be subdivided into two smoke compartments per 29.3.7. This requirement provides for horizontal movement of occupants, limits the number of rooms, and, therefore, limits the number of occupants exposed to a single fire that might render a corridor untenable. Because no fire resistance rating is required for the smoke partition and smoke dampers are not required, the requirement is not overly burdensome in typical hotel or dormitory construction. The exemption for automatic sprinklers reflects the excellent life-loss record of buildings equipped with sprinkler protection.

A horizontal exit is permitted to be used to comply with 29.3.7 and, thereby, to serve more than one function.

**28.3.8 Special Protection Features. (Reserved)**

**29.3.8 Special Protection Features. (Reserved)**

## 28.4 Special Provisions

### 28.4.1 High-Rise Buildings.

**28.4.1.1** High-rise buildings shall comply with Section 11.8.

**28.4.1.2*** Emergency plans in accordance with Section 4.8 shall be provided and shall include the following:

(1) Egress procedures
(2) Methods
(3) Preferred evacuation routes for each event, including appropriate use of elevators

**A.28.4.1.2** See 4.8.2.1(4).

## 29.4 Special Provisions

### 29.4.1 High-Rise Buildings.

**29.4.1.1** High-rise buildings shall comply with 29.3.5.1.

**29.4.1.2*** Emergency plans in accordance with Section 4.8 shall be provided and shall include the following:

(1) Egress procedures
(2) Methods
(3) Preferred evacuation routes for each event, including appropriate use of elevators

**A.29.4.1.2** See 4.8.2.1(4).

In response to recommendations from the NFPA High-Rise Building Safety Advisory Committee following the September 11, 2001, terrorist attacks on the World Trade Center in New York City and the Pentagon in Arlington, Virginia, the provisions of 28/29.4.1.2, which are new to the 2009 edition of the *Code*, require both new and existing high-rise hotels and dormitories to be provided with emergency plans. See the extensive provisions of A.4.8.2.1 and A.4.8.2.1(3) and the associated commentary, which are also new to the 2009 edition, for details on the items that should be included in the emergency plan and a primer on the development of evacuation strategies for specific buildings.

**28.4.2 Reserved.**

**29.4.2 Reserved.**

## 28.5 Building Services

### 28.5.1 Utilities.

Utilities shall comply with the provisions of Section 9.1.

### 28.5.2 Heating, Ventilating, and Air-Conditioning.

**28.5.2.1** Heating, ventilating, and air-conditioning equipment shall comply with the provisions of Section 9.2, except as otherwise required in this chapter.

**28.5.2.2** Unvented fuel-fired heaters, other than gas space heaters in compliance with NFPA 54, *National Fuel Gas Code*, shall not be used.

### 28.5.3 Elevators, Escalators, and Conveyors.

**28.5.3.1** Elevators, escalators, and conveyors shall comply with the provisions of Section 9.4.

**28.5.3.2*** In high-rise buildings, one elevator shall be provided with a protected power supply and shall be available for use by the fire department in case of emergency.

**A.28.5.3.2** "Protected power supply" means a source of electrical energy of sufficient capacity to allow proper operation of the elevator and its associated control and communications systems. The power supply's point of origin, system of distribution, type and size of overcurrent protection, degree of isolation from other portions of the building electrical system, and degree of mechanical protection should be such that it is unlikely that the supply would be disrupted at any but the advanced stages of building fire involvement or by structural collapse.

A protected power supply might consist of, and should provide, not less than the level of reliability associated with an electrical distribution system with service equipment located and installed in accordance with 230.72(B) and 230.82(5) of *NFPA 70, National Electrical Code*. The distribution system is not to have any other connection to the building electrical distribution system. A protected power supply is not required to incorporate two sources of energy or automatic transfer capability from a normal to an emergency source; for example, an alternate set of service conductors.

The number and type of elevators to be connected to a protected power supply should be limited, or the characteristics of the protected power supply should be selected to ensure conformance to 230.95 of NFPA 70, without the provision of ground fault protection for the supply.

An elevator installation supplied by a protected power supply should comply with Article 620 of NFPA 70 and ASME A17.1/CSA B44, *Safety Code for Elevators and*



## 29.5 Building Services

### 29.5.1 Utilities.

Utilities shall comply with the provisions of Section 9.1.

### 29.5.2 Heating, Ventilating, and Air-Conditioning.

**29.5.2.1** Heating, ventilating, and air-conditioning equipment shall comply with the provisions of Section 9.2, except as otherwise required in this chapter.

**29.5.2.2** Unvented fuel-fired heaters, other than gas space heaters in compliance with NFPA 54, *National Fuel Gas Code*, shall not be used.

### 29.5.3 Elevators, Escalators, and Conveyors.

Elevators, escalators, and conveyors shall comply with the provisions of Section 9.4.

*Escalators*. The energy absorption means should always be connected on the load side of the disconnecting means. The energy absorption means should not consist of loads likely to become inoperative or disconnected under the conditions assumed to exist when the elevator is under the control of fire department personnel. Examples of such loads include light and power loads external to the elevator equipment room.

### 28.5.4 Rubbish Chutes, Incinerators, and Laundry Chutes.

Rubbish chutes, incinerators, and laundry chutes shall comply with the provisions of Section 9.5.

## 28.6 Reserved

## 28.7 Operating Features

### 28.7.1 Hotel Emergency Organization.

**28.7.1.1*** Employees of hotels shall be instructed and drilled in the duties they are to perform in the event of fire, panic, or other emergency.

**A.28.7.1.1** Employers are obligated to determine the degree to which employees are to participate in emergency activities. Regulations of the U.S. Department of Labor (OSHA) govern these activities and provide options for employers, from total evacuation to aggressive structural fire fighting by employee brigades. *(For additional information, see 29 CFR 1910, Subparts E and L, "OSHA Regulations for Emergency Procedures and Fire Brigades.")*

**28.7.1.2*** Drills of the emergency organization shall be held at quarterly intervals and shall cover such points as the operation and maintenance of the available first aid fire appliances, the testing of devices to alert guests, and a study of instructions for emergency duties.

**A.28.7.1.2** Emergencies should be assumed to have arisen at various locations in the occupancy in order to train employees in logical procedures.

### 28.7.2 Emergency Duties.

Upon discovery of a fire, employees shall carry out the following duties:

(1) Activation of the facility fire protection signaling system, if provided



### 29.5.4 Rubbish Chutes, Incinerators, and Laundry Chutes.

Rubbish chutes, incinerators, and laundry chutes shall comply with the provisions of Section 9.5.

## 29.6 Reserved

## 29.7 Operating Features

### 29.7.1 Hotel Emergency Organization.

**29.7.1.1*** Employees of hotels shall be instructed and drilled in the duties they are to perform in the event of fire, panic, or other emergency.

**A.29.7.1.1** Employers are obligated to determine the degree to which employees are to participate in emergency activities. Regulations of the U.S. Department of Labor (OSHA) govern these activities and provide options for employers, from total evacuation to aggressive structural fire fighting by employee brigades. *(For additional information, see 29 CFR 1910, Subparts E and L, "OSHA Regulations for Emergency Procedures and Fire Brigades.")*

**29.7.1.2*** Drills of the emergency organization shall be held at quarterly intervals and shall cover such points as the operation and maintenance of the available first aid fire appliances, the testing of devices to alert guests, and a study of instructions for emergency duties.

**A.29.7.1.2** Emergencies should be assumed to have arisen at various locations in the occupancy in order to train employees in logical procedures.

### 29.7.2 Emergency Duties.

Upon discovery of a fire, employees shall carry out the following duties:

(1) Activation of the facility fire protection signaling system, if provided

CHAPTER 28 • New

(2) Notification of the public fire department
(3) Other action as previously instructed

### 28.7.3 Drills in Dormitories.

Emergency egress and relocation drills shall be regularly conducted in accordance with Section 4.7.

### 28.7.4 Emergency Instructions for Residents or Guests.

**28.7.4.1*** A floor diagram reflecting the actual floor arrangement, exit locations, and room identification shall be posted in a location and manner acceptable to the authority having jurisdiction on, or immediately adjacent to, every guest room door in hotels and in every resident room in dormitories.

**A.28.7.4.1** Floor diagrams should reflect the actual floor arrangement and should be oriented with the actual direction to the exits.

CHAPTER 29 • Existing

(2) Notification of the public fire department
(3) Other action as previously instructed

### 29.7.3 Drills in Dormitories.

Emergency egress and relocation drills shall be regularly conducted in accordance with Section 4.7.

### 29.7.4 Emergency Instructions for Residents or Guests.

**29.7.4.1*** A floor diagram reflecting the actual floor arrangement, exit locations, and room identification shall be posted in a location and manner acceptable to the authority having jurisdiction on, or immediately adjacent to, every guest room door in hotels and in every resident room in dormitories.

**A.29.7.4.1** Floor diagrams should reflect the actual floor arrangement and should be oriented with the actual direction to the exits.

The manner in which the information specified in 28/29.7.4.1 is to be posted and the nature of its contents are at the discretion of the authority having jurisdiction (AHJ) and depend on the building, its layout, and the protection provided.

**28.7.4.2*** Fire safety information shall be provided to allow guests to make the decision to evacuate to the outside, to evacuate to an area of refuge, to remain in place, or to employ any combination of the three options.

**A.28.7.4.2** Factors for developing the fire safety information include such items as construction type, suppression systems, alarm and detection systems, building layout, and building HVAC systems.

### 28.7.5 Emergency Plans.

Emergency plans in accordance with Section 4.8 shall be provided.

### 28.7.6 Contents and Furnishings.

**28.7.6.1** New draperies, curtains, and other similar loosely hanging furnishings and decorations shall be flame resistant as demonstrated by testing in accordance with NFPA 701, *Standard Methods of Fire Tests for Flame Propagation of Textiles and Films.*

**28.7.6.2 Upholstered Furniture and Mattresses.**

**28.7.6.2.1** Newly introduced upholstered furniture shall meet the criteria specified in 10.3.2.1 and 10.3.3.

**29.7.4.2*** Fire safety information shall be provided to allow guests to make the decision to evacuate to the outside, to evacuate to an area of refuge, to remain in place, or to employ any combination of the three options.

**A.29.7.4.2** Factors for developing the fire safety information include such items as construction type, suppression systems, alarm and detection systems, building layout, and building HVAC systems.

### 29.7.5 Emergency Plans.

Emergency plans in accordance with Section 4.8 shall be provided.

### 29.7.6 Contents and Furnishings.

**29.7.6.1** New draperies, curtains, and other similar loosely hanging furnishings and decorations shall be flame resistant as demonstrated by testing in accordance with NFPA 701, *Standard Methods of Fire Tests for Flame Propagation of Textiles and Films.*

**29.7.6.2 Upholstered Furniture and Mattresses.**

**29.7.6.2.1** Newly introduced upholstered furniture shall meet the criteria specified in 10.3.2.1 and 10.3.3.

CHAPTER 28 • New

**28.7.6.2.2** Newly introduced mattresses shall meet the criteria specified in 10.3.2.2 and 10.3.4.

**28.7.6.3** Furnishings or decorations of an explosive or highly flammable character shall not be used.

**28.7.6.4** Fire-retardant coatings shall be maintained to retain the effectiveness of the treatment under service conditions encountered in actual use.

CHAPTER 29 • Existing

**29.7.6.2.2** Newly introduced mattresses shall meet the criteria specified in 10.3.2.2 and 10.3.4.

**29.7.6.3** Furnishings or decorations of an explosive or highly flammable character shall not be used.

**29.7.6.4** Fire-retardant coatings shall be maintained to retain the effectiveness of the treatment under service conditions encountered in actual use.

## References Cited in Commentary

1. NFPA 13, *Standard for the Installation of Sprinkler Systems*, 2007 edition, National Fire Protection Association, Quincy, MA.
2. NFPA 80, *Standard for Fire Doors and Other Opening Protectives*, 2007 edition, National Fire Protection Association, Quincy, MA.
3. NFPA 90A, *Standard for the Installation of Air-Conditioning and Ventilating Systems*, 2009 edition, National Fire Protection Association, Quincy, MA.

CHAPTERS 30 AND 31

# New and Existing Apartment Buildings

The apartment building classification is one of five residential occupancy types addressed by the *Life Safety Code*. Other residential occupancies include one- and two-family dwellings, lodging or rooming houses, hotels and dormitories, and residential board and care occupancies.

The common principle of life safety that is applied to all residential occupancies addressed by Chapters 24 through 33 is highlighted by 6.1.8.1, which states that residential occupancies are those occupancies in which sleeping accommodations are provided for purposes other than health care or detention and correction. The presence of sleeping occupants is central to the provisions of Chapters 24 through 33, because occupants who are asleep will be unaware of a developing fire and, when awakened to be alerted to the emergency, might be somewhat confused. The definition of the term *residential occupancy* in 6.1.8.1 also differentiates between sleeping occupants in residential occupancies and those in health care or detention and correctional occupancies, which are also characterized by the occupants' incapability of self-preservation. The provisions of Chapters 24 through 33 are also based on the presence of hazards (such as cooking and heating equipment) in residential occupancies and the degree to which occupants are familiar with their living space. Occupants might have little or no familiarity, as in the case of the transient residents of hotels, or they might have the total familiarity that is common to residents of single-family dwellings.

Apartment buildings pose a problem from a life safety perspective, because the typical building configuration often requires an escaping resident to traverse an interior corridor, which subsequently might expose the resident to the heat and smoke of a corridor or dwelling unit fire. In recognition of these potential hazards, the *Code* requires most new apartment buildings to be protected throughout by an approved, supervised automatic sprinkler system.

From 2000 to 2004, apartment buildings accounted for an average of 94,700 structure fires per year, as reported to U.S. fire departments. This number represents approximately 25 percent of the 375,200 total home fires per year on average for the period. Apartment building fires resulted in an average of 390 civilian deaths per year (13 percent of all home fire deaths) and 3890 civilian injuries per year (27 percent of all home fire injuries). The number of apartment building fires and resulting deaths and injuries are in general trending downward, likely due to the increasing use of electrically powered smoke alarms and automatic sprinkler systems.

The causes of apartment building fires differ significantly from one- and two-family dwelling fires in building equipment areas. Data from 2000 through 2004 indicate heating and electrical equipment accounted for 22 percent of the fires in one- and two-family dwellings, while accounting for only 10 percent of the fires in apartment buildings. This difference is most likely due to the centralized arrangement of the heating and electrical systems typical of most apartment buildings. Equipment fires are usually the result of poor maintenance or human error. Heating and electrical systems tend to be more closely regulated, maintained, and supervised in apartment buildings, which results in a reduced chance of equipment malfunction.

The number of fires caused by occupants (e.g., those due to cooking and smoking) is high in both categories of home structures.

These data demonstrate the importance of applying the *Code* to apartment buildings to help ensure fire safety, but they also demonstrate the continuing need for public education regarding the causes and prevention of home fires.

CHAPTER 30 • New

## 30.1 General Requirements

### 30.1.1 Application.

**30.1.1.1** The requirements of this chapter shall apply to new buildings or portions thereof used as apartment occupancies. *(See 1.3.1.)*

CHAPTER 31 • Existing

## 31.1* General Requirements

**A.31.1** See Table A.31.1.

### 31.1.1 Application.

**31.1.1.1** The requirements of this chapter shall apply to existing buildings or portions thereof currently occupied as apartment occupancies. In addition, the building shall meet the requirements of one of the following options:

(1) Option 1, buildings without fire suppression or detection systems
(2) Option 2, buildings provided with a complete approved automatic fire detection and notification system in accordance with 31.3.4.4
(3) Option 3, buildings provided with approved automatic sprinkler protection in selected areas, as described in 31.3.5.9
(4) Option 4, buildings protected throughout by an approved automatic sprinkler system

Due to the disproportionate percentage of deaths associated with residential occupancies, the *Code*, with some exceptions, mandates sprinkler protection in new apartment buildings. For existing apartment buildings, the *Code* provides four alternative protection packages referred to as *options*.

The options specify the varying degrees to which an apartment building is protected by fire detection or fire suppression systems as follows:

1. Option 1 — no suppression or detection systems
2. Option 2 — total automatic fire detection and notification (although 31.3.4.5.1 requires single-station smoke alarms within each apartment unit, such smoke alarms are not part of a system and are not located in all areas of the building; therefore, their presence does not signify an Option 2 apartment building)
3. Option 3 — partial sprinkler protection (mainly corridor sprinklers — see 31.3.5.9)
4. Option 4 — protection throughout by means of an automatic sprinkler system (see 31.3.5.10)

In recognition of the life safety benefits associated with a properly installed and maintained sprinkler system, an Option 4 apartment building is exempted from the various *Code* provisions required of Option 1 through Option 3 apartment buildings. The benefits of such exemptions include the following:

1. Increased travel distance allowances
2. Reduction in required corridor fire resistance ratings
3. Decreased interior finish requirements
4. Exemption from the smoke compartmentation requirement

The protection requirements for new apartment buildings are equivalent to Option 4.

Table A.31.1 summarizes the different protection packages required, depending on whether an existing apartment building follows Option 1, Option 2, Option 3, or Option 4.

This comprehensive approach is an attempt to codify system design. Although a total system would consist of many alternatives, the systems detailed in Options 1 through 4 are more limited, because only four options are available. However, the user can identify the most appropriate option, based on the existing building's size, height, and arrangement. The options provide an opportunity to coordinate the safety approach that best fits a building, rather than adapting a building to a single codified set of criteria.

**30.1.1.2** The term *apartment building*, wherever used in this *Code*, shall include an apartment house, a tenement, a garden apartment, or any other structure meeting the definition of apartment building.

**31.1.1.2** The term *apartment building*, wherever used in this *Code*, shall include an apartment house, a tenement, a garden apartment, or any other structure meeting the definition of apartment building.

***Table A.31.1 Alternate Requirements for Existing Apartment Buildings According to Protection Provided***

| Feature | No Suppression or Detection System Option 1 | Complete Automatic Fire Detection Option 2 | Automatic Sprinkler Protection in Selected Areas Option 3 | Automatic Sprinkler Protection Throughout per NFPA 13 (with exceptions) Option 4 |
|---|---|---|---|---|
| **Exit Access** | | | | |
| Travel distance from apartment door to exit | 100 ft (30 m) | 150 ft (45 m) | 150 ft (45 m) | 200 ft (61 m) |
| Travel distance within apartment | 75 ft (23 m) | 125 ft (38 m) | 75 ft (23 m) | 125 ft (38 m) |
| Smoke barrier required *(See 31.3.7.)* | R | R | R | NR |
| Maximum single path corridor distance | 35 ft (10.7 m) | 35 ft (10.7 m) | 35 ft (10.7 m) | 35 ft (10.7 m) |
| Maximum dead end | 50 ft (15 m) | 50 ft (15 m) | 50 ft (15 m) | 50 ft (15 m) |
| *Corridor fire resistance* | | | | |
| Walls | ½ hr | ½ hr | ½ hr | ½ hr |
| Doors (fire protection rating) | 20 min. or 1¾ in. (44 mm) thick | 20 min. or 1¾ in. (44 mm) thick | Smoke resisting | Smoke resisting |
| **Interior Finish** | | | | |
| Lobbies and corridors | A or B | A or B | A or B | A, B, or C |
| Other spaces | A, B, or C | A, B, or C | A, B, or C | A, B, or C |
| Floors in corridors | I or II | I or II | NR | NR |
| **Exits** | | | | |
| *Wall fire resistance* | | | | |
| 1–3 stories† | 1 hr | 1 hr | 1 hr | 1 hr |
| >3 stories† | 2 hr | 2 hr | 2 hr | 1 hr |
| *Smokeproof enclosures* | | | | |
| Not high-rise | NR | NR | NR | NR |
| High-rise | R | R | R | NR |
| *Door fire resistance* | | | | |
| 1–3 stories† | 1 hr | 1 hr | 1 hr | 1 hr |
| >3 stories† | 1½ hr | 1½ hr | 1½ hr | 1 hr |
| *Interior finish* | | | | |
| Walls and ceilings | A or B | A or B | A or B | A, B, or C |
| Floors | I or II | I or II | I or II | NR |
| **Within Living Unit (Apartment)** | | | | |
| Escape windows, per Section 24.2 *(See 31.2.1.)* | R | R | R | NR |
| **Alarm System** | | | | |
| >3 stories or >11 units† | Manual initiation | Manual and auto initiation | Manual and auto initiation | Manual and auto initiation |
| >2 stories or >50 units† | Annunciator panel | Annunciator panel | Annunciator panel | Annunciator panel |

R: Required *(see Code for details and exemptions)*. NR: No requirements.

† Number of stories in height.

CHAPTER 30 • New

## 30.1.2 Multiple Occupancies.

**30.1.2.1** Multiple occupancies shall be in accordance with 6.1.14.

**30.1.2.2** No dwelling unit of an apartment building shall have its sole means of egress pass through any nonresidential occupancy in the same building, unless otherwise permitted by 30.1.2.2.1 or 30.1.2.2.2.

**30.1.2.2.1** In buildings that are protected by an automatic sprinkler system in accordance with Section 9.7, dwelling units of an apartment building shall be permitted to have their sole means of egress pass through a nonresidential occupancy in the same building, provided that the following criteria are met:

(1) The dwelling unit of the apartment building shall comply with Chapter 30.
(2) The sole means of egress from the dwelling unit of the apartment building shall not pass through a high hazard contents area, as defined in 6.2.2.4.

**30.1.2.2.2** In buildings that are not protected by an automatic sprinkler system in accordance with Section 9.7, dwelling units of an apartment building shall be permitted to have their sole means of egress pass through a nonresidential occupancy in the same building, provided that the following criteria are met:

(1) The sole means of egress from the dwelling unit of the apartment building to the exterior shall be separated from the remainder of the building by fire barriers having a minimum 1-hour fire resistance rating.
(2) The dwelling unit of the apartment building shall comply with Chapter 30.
(3) The sole means of egress from the dwelling unit of the apartment building shall not pass through a high hazard contents area, as defined in 6.2.2.4.

**30.1.2.3** Multiple dwelling units shall be permitted to be located above a nonresidential occupancy only where one of the following conditions exists:

(1) Where the dwelling units of the residential occupancy and exits therefrom are separated from the nonresidential occupancy by construction having a minimun 1-hour fire resistance rating
(2) Where the nonresidential occupancy is protected throughout by an approved, supervised automatic sprinkler system in accordance with Section 9.7

CHAPTER 31 • Existing

## 31.1.2 Multiple Occupancies.

**31.1.2.1** Multiple occupancies shall be in accordance with 6.1.14.

**31.1.2.2** No dwelling unit of an apartment building shall have its sole means of egress pass through any nonresidential occupancy in the same building, unless otherwise permitted by 31.1.2.2.1 or 31.1.2.2.2.

**31.1.2.2.1** In buildings that are protected by an automatic sprinkler system in accordance with Section 9.7, dwelling units of an apartment building shall be permitted to have their sole means of egress pass through a nonresidential occupancy in the same building, provided that the following criteria are met:

(1) The dwelling unit of the apartment building shall comply with Chapter 31.
(2) The sole means of egress from the dwelling unit of the apartment building shall not pass through a high hazard contents area, as defined in 6.2.2.4.

**31.1.2.2.2** In buildings that are not protected by an automatic sprinkler system in accordance with Section 9.7, dwelling units of an apartment building shall be permitted to have their sole means of egress pass through a nonresidential occupancy in the same building, provided that the following criteria are met:

(1) The sole means of egress from the dwelling unit of the apartment building to the exterior shall be separated from the remainder of the building by fire barriers having a minimum 1-hour fire resistance rating.
(2) The dwelling unit of the apartment building shall comply with Chapter 31.
(3) The sole means of egress from the dwelling unit of the apartment building shall not pass through a high hazard contents area, as defined in 6.2.2.4.

**31.1.2.3** Multiple dwelling units shall be permitted to be located above a nonresidential occupancy only where one of the following conditions exists:

(1) Where the dwelling units of the residential occupancy and exits therefrom are separated from the nonresidential occupancy by construction having a minimum 1-hour fire resistance rating
(2) Where the nonresidential occupancy is protected throughout by an approved, supervised automatic sprinkler system in accordance with Section 9.7
(3) Where not more than two dwelling units are located above a nonresidential occupancy that is protected by an automatic fire detection system in accordance with Section 9.6

CHAPTER 30 • New

CHAPTER 31 • Existing

Residential occupancies often exist in buildings that also house assembly, mercantile, or business occupancies. These nonresidential occupancies might pose an additional threat, because they are not typically occupied after regular business hours. An undetected fire in an unoccupied area has the potential to affect the tenability of the residential portion of the building before occupants can be awakened and take the appropriate actions for safe egress. Therefore, the requirements of 30/31.1.2 help to ensure that it is safe to have apartments within these multiple occupancy buildings by providing the necessary protection and separation.

### 30.1.3 Special Definitions.

**30.1.3.1 General.** Special terms applicable to this chapter are defined in Chapter 3. Where necessary, other terms are defined in the text.

**30.1.3.2 Apartment Building.** See 3.3.32.3.

### 31.1.3 Special Definitions.

**31.1.3.1 General.** Special terms applicable to this chapter are defined in Chapter 3. Where necessary, other terms are defined in the text.

**31.1.3.2 Apartment Building.** See 3.3.32.3.

The text of A.3.3.32.3, which is associated with the definition of *apartment building*, clarifies how town house–type apartments — particularly those under condominium ownership — should be classified for application of the *Code*. It is often mistakenly believed that condominiums are a form of occupancy rather than a form of ownership.

### 30.1.4 Classification of Occupancy.

See 6.1.8 and 30.1.3.

### 30.1.5 Classification of Hazard of Contents.

The contents of residential occupancies shall be classified as ordinary hazard in accordance with 6.2.2.

### 31.1.4 Classification of Occupancy.

See 6.1.8 and 31.1.3.

### 31.1.5 Classification of Hazard of Contents.

The contents of residential occupancies shall be classified as ordinary hazard in accordance with 6.2.2.

NFPA 13, *Standard for the Installation of Sprinkler Systems*,[1] classifies the contents of an apartment building as light hazard for the purpose of designing automatic sprinkler systems. The *Code* classifies the contents of an apartment building as ordinary hazard (see 30/31.1.5) on the basis of the threat to life or life safety, rather than the challenge to the extinguishing capability of the automatic sprinkler system (light hazard).

### 30.1.6 Minimum Construction Requirements.

(No special requirements.)

### 30.1.7 Occupant Load.

The occupant load, in number of persons for whom means of egress and other provisions are required, shall be determined on the basis of the occupant load factors of Table 7.3.1.2 that are characteristic of the use of the space or shall be determined as the maximum probable population of the space under consideration, whichever is greater.

### 31.1.6 Minimum Construction Requirements.

(No special requirements.)

### 31.1.7 Occupant Load.

The occupant load, in number of persons for whom means of egress and other provisions are required, shall be determined on the basis of the occupant load factors of Table 7.3.1.2 that are characteristic of the use of the space or shall be determined as the maximum probable population of the space under consideration, whichever is greater.

The occupant load calculations for areas of apartment buildings used for nonresidential purposes is based on the occupant load factors applicable to the use of the area. For example, the occupant load of an area consisting of apartment dwelling units is calculated using 200 $ft^2$ (18.6 $m^2$) per person; an area used for a building management office is calculated using 100 $ft^2$ (9.3 $m^2$) per person, the appropriate factor for business use (see Table 7.3.1.2).

## 30.2 Means of Egress Requirements

### 30.2.1 General.

**30.2.1.1** Means of egress from dwelling units to the outside of the building shall be in accordance with Chapter 7 and this chapter.

**30.2.1.2** Means of escape within the dwelling unit shall comply with the provisions of Section 24.2 for one- and two-family dwellings.

## 31.2 Means of Egress Requirements

### 31.2.1 General.

**31.2.1.1** Means of egress from dwelling units to the outside of the building shall be in accordance with Chapter 7 and this chapter.

**31.2.1.2** Means of escape within the dwelling unit shall comply with the provisions of Section 24.2 for one- and two-family dwellings.

Per 30/31.2.1.2, every dwelling unit is required to comply with Section 24.2, which addresses means of escape in one- and two-family dwellings. This mandatory reference to Section 24.2 is important for several reasons. First, it establishes a requirement for two means of escape from every sleeping room and living area of a dwelling unit having two rooms or more. Several acceptable types of secondary means of escape are established in 24.2.2.3, the most common of which is an operable window with specified minimum opening dimensions. No secondary means of escape is required if a dwelling unit is protected by an automatic sprinkler system. Note that 24.2.2.1.2 does not require the entire building to be sprinklered, only the dwelling unit that is deficient with respect to the secondary means of escape. However, a mandate for complete building sprinkler protection, such as that in 30.3.5.1, might be specified elsewhere.

A second important provision of Section 24.2 is that the means of egress provisions of Chapter 7 do not apply within the dwelling units unless they are specifically referenced. For example, the minimum width of means of escape doors within a dwelling unit is 28 in. (710 mm), rather than the 32 in. (810 mm) minimum width specified by Chapter 7 for means of egress. The requirements of Chapter 7 apply to the door from the dwelling unit to the common corridor, because this door is the transition point at which means of escape ends and the standard means of egress begins. Chapter 24 also permits the use of winders and spiral stairs within a dwelling unit, and the provisions of Chapter 24 for headroom apply within the dwelling unit, superseding those of Chapter 7. See the commentary on Chapter 24 for additional information on means of escape from dwelling units.

The means of egress provisions of Chapter 7 are applied from the dwelling unit to the outside of the building. Many of the items contained in Section 30/31.2 are provisions that Chapter 7 provides as options that might be specifically recognized by an occupancy chapter; for example, 30/31.2.2.2.2.2 permits the use of delayed-egress locks in accordance with 7.2.1.6.1, with the additional proviso that not more than one such device is encountered in any single egress path. In other cases, a feature addressed by Chapter 7 is not permitted to be used in the means of egress of apartment buildings, because it is not specifically permitted by Section 30/31.2. The absence of slide escapes in the list of acceptable means of egress components in 30/31.2.2 is an example of a component that is not permitted. Also, Section 30/31.2 limits the degree to which Chapter 7 features can be used, such as the provision of maximum lengths for dead-end corridors and common paths of travel addressed in 30/31.2.5.

### 30.2.2 Means of Egress Components.

#### 30.2.2.1 General.

**30.2.2.1.1** Components of means of egress shall be limited to the types described in 30.2.2.2 through 30.2.2.12.

### 31.2.2 Means of Egress Components.

#### 31.2.2.1 General.

**31.2.2.1.1** Components of means of egress shall be limited to the types described in 31.2.2.2 through 31.2.2.12.

CHAPTER 30 • New

**30.2.2.1.2** In buildings protected throughout by an approved, supervised automatic sprinkler system in accordance with 30.3.5, exit enclosures shall have a minimum 1-hour fire resistance rating, and doors shall have a minimum 1-hour fire protection rating.

CHAPTER 31 • Existing

**31.2.2.1.2** In buildings using Option 4, exit enclosures shall have a minimum 1-hour fire resistance rating, and doors shall have a minimum 1-hour fire protection rating.

**31.2.2.1.3** In non-high-rise buildings using Option 2, Option 3, or Option 4, exit stair doors shall be permitted to be $1^3/_4$ in. (44 mm) thick, solid-bonded wood-core doors that are self-closing and self-latching and in wood frames not less than $^3/_4$ in. (19 mm) thick.

The general provisions for the means of egress components in apartment buildings modify the provisions of Chapter 7 in the following two areas:

1. Limits on the components of the means of egress
2. Protection of the means of egress

First, a general reference to the components of the means of egress in Chapter 7 is made in 30/31.2.2.1.1 in place of repeating its myriad provisions. Most of these components are permitted in both new and existing apartment buildings. Some of the components are permitted to be used in accordance with the provisions of Chapter 7 and the additional provisions of Chapters 30 and 31. For example, delayed-egress locks are permitted by 30/31.2.2.2.2.2, which permits their use in accordance with 7.2.1.6.1 if not more than one device is located in any single egress path. In addition, 30/31.2.2.2.2.4 permits the use of elevator lobby exit access door locking in accordance with 7.2.1.6.3, which is new to the 2009 edition of the *Code*.

If not permitted, no reference to an egress component is made in the specific occupancy chapter. For example, escalators and fire escape stairs are only permitted as means of egress components in existing apartment buildings. Therefore, 31.2.2.8 and 31.2.2.9 contain specific references to such components, while 30.2.2.8 and 30.2.2.9 are reserved and contain no such reference. Neither chapter permits the use of slide escapes; consequently, no reference to slide escapes is made within the means of egress sections of either chapter.

Second, Chapter 30 recognizes the relatively low fuel loads of apartment buildings and permits a fire resistance rating of 1 hour for exit enclosures and other vertical openings (see 30.2.2.1.2 and 30.3.1.1.4) in new apartment buildings protected throughout by an approved, supervised automatic sprinkler system, regardless of the number of stories connected by the exit stair or other vertical opening. See 31.3.1.1 for exemptions from the requirements for vertical opening protection in existing apartment buildings.

The reduction to a 1-hour fire resistance–rated enclosure for exits is not permitted for assembly, mercantile, or business occupancies and, therefore, is not permitted to be used where the exit serves mixed apartment/assembly, apartment/mercantile, or apartment/business occupancies. In facilities of four or more stories, where apartment occupancies and other occupancies are adequately separated and treated independently in accordance with 6.1.14.4, 1-hour exit enclosures in the apartment portion and 2-hour enclosures elsewhere might be permitted.

Exhibit 30/31.1 illustrates the modification to the requirements for protection of exit enclosures and other vertical openings in a fully sprinklered apartment building.

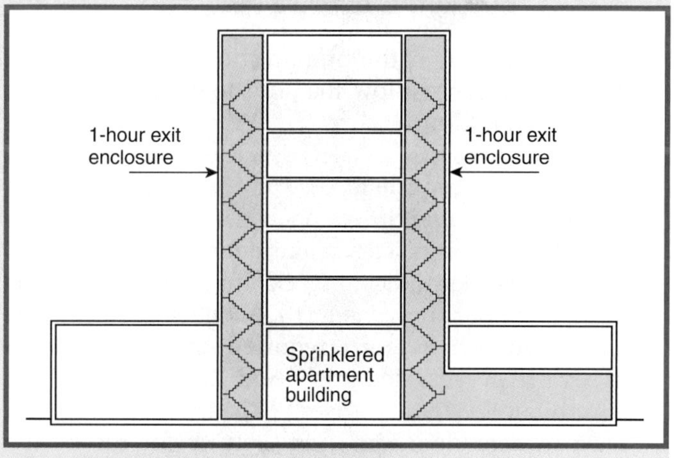


*Exhibit 30/31.1 Exit enclosure separation — sprinklered apartment building.*

**30.2.2.2 Doors.**

**30.2.2.2.1** Doors complying with 7.2.1 shall be permitted.

**31.2.2.2 Doors.**

**31.2.2.2.1** Doors complying with 7.2.1 shall be permitted.

**CHAPTER 30 • New**

**30.2.2.2.2** Door-locking arrangements shall comply with 30.2.2.2.2.1, 30.2.2.2.2.2, 30.2.2.2.2.3, or 30.2.2.2.2.4.

**30.2.2.2.2.1*** No door in any means of egress shall be locked against egress when the building is occupied.

**A.30.2.2.2.2.1** It is the intent of this requirement that security measures, where installed, should not prevent egress.

**30.2.2.2.2.2** Delayed-egress locks complying with 7.2.1.6.1 shall be permitted, provided that not more than one such device is located in any one egress path.

**30.2.2.2.2.3** Access-controlled egress doors complying with 7.2.1.6.2 shall be permitted.

**30.2.2.2.2.4** Elevator lobby exit access door locking in accordance with 7.2.1.6.3 shall be permitted.

**30.2.2.2.3** Revolving doors complying with 7.2.1.10 shall be permitted.

**30.2.2.2.4** Horizontal-sliding doors, as permitted by 7.2.1.14, shall not be used across corridors.

**30.2.2.2.5** Apartment occupancies shall be exempt from the re-entry provisions of 7.2.1.5.7 where the exit enclosure serves directly only one dwelling unit per floor, and such exit is a smokeproof enclosure in accordance with 7.2.3.

**CHAPTER 31 • Existing**

**31.2.2.2.2** Door-locking arrangements shall comply with 30.2.2.2.2.1, 30.2.2.2.2.2, 30.2.2.2.2.3, or 31.2.2.2.2.4.

**31.2.2.2.2.1** No door in any means of egress shall be locked against egress when the building is occupied.

**31.2.2.2.2.2** Delayed-egress locks complying with 7.2.1.6.1 shall be permitted, provided that not more than one such device is located in any one egress path.

**31.2.2.2.2.3** Access-controlled egress doors complying with 7.2.1.6.2 shall be permitted.

**31.2.2.2.2.4** Elevator lobby exit access door locking in accordance with 7.2.1.6.3 shall be permitted.

**31.2.2.2.3** Revolving doors complying with 7.2.1.10 shall be permitted.

**31.2.2.2.4** Horizontal-sliding doors, as permitted by 7.2.1.14, shall not be used across corridors.

**31.2.2.2.5** Apartment occupancies protected throughout by an approved, supervised automatic sprinkler system shall be exempt from the re-entry provisions of 7.2.1.5.7 where the exit enclosure serves directly only one dwelling unit per floor, and such exit is a smokeproof enclosure in accordance with 7.2.3.

Apartment buildings are prohibited from having any door locked against egress while the building is occupied. This requirement permits a door to be equipped with a locking device that allows the door to be opened from within the building for the purpose of egress but does not allow the door to be opened from outside the building.

The language of 7.2.1.5.2 is clear: Locks, if provided, must not require the use of a key, a tool, or special knowledge or effort for operation from the egress side of the building. This requirement prohibits double-cylinder locks and chain locks that require a key to operate the door from the inside. The use of a simple operation to open a door is required by 7.2.1.5.9; locks that require two-handed knobs and similar operations are prohibited.

Apartment doors provide security for the occupants in the dwelling unit. Recognizing this additional function, Chapter 7 permits the use of security chains or rods, as well as locks, on apartment doors and also permits releasing devices in addition to the doorknob or lever. The permitted number of additional releasing actions differs for new and existing buildings. One additional releasing action is permitted for new apartment buildings, and two additional actions are permitted in existing apartment buildings (see 7.2.1.5.9.3 and 7.2.1.5.9.4).

The typical apartment door has three devices: a latch, a lock, and a security chain or rod. This arrangement is permitted in existing buildings, provided that only two additional releasing operations are necessary. This arrangement would also be permitted in new construction, provided that the latch and lock set are interconnected so that the lock bolt and the latch will retract simultaneously when the latch handle is turned from the inside; thus, only one releasing action is needed for the two devices. The second action is the release of the security chain or rod. The overriding requirement for any of these devices is that they not require the use of a key, a tool, or special knowledge or effort to operate.

The use of the delayed-egress lock detailed in 7.2.1.6.1 is recognized in 30/31.2.2.2.2.2 if not more than one such lock is located in any single egress path. The use of a delayed-egress lock requires that the building be protected throughout by either an auto-

CHAPTER 30 • New

CHAPTER 31 • Existing

matic sprinkler system or an automatic fire detection system. The 15-second or 30-second delay permitted by 7.2.1.6.1 does not affect the immediate release of the lock upon activation of sprinklers or detectors or upon loss of power to the lock. The delay device provides the security needed for doors that are used infrequently. At the same time, the door remains available for emergency use. Chains and padlocks do not provide these safety features.

The use of elevator lobby exit access door locking detailed in 7.2.1.6.3, which is new to the 2009 edition of the *Code*, is recognized by 30/31.2.2.2.2.4. This provision allows an elevator to open to an elevator lobby from which access to an exit stair is required to pass through normally locked doors. Although the floors of most apartment buildings are arranged so that elevators open to lobbies that are directly connected to corridors serving the apartments, and in turn provide direct access to exit stairs, there may be arrangements where it is desirable to have a "secure" floor in which occupants step off the elevator into a reception area. The provisions of 7.2.1.6.3 permit access to the required exits to be through normally locked doors subject to the additional protection criteria specified therein. See the commentary following 7.2.1.6.3 for additional details on elevator lobby exit access door locking.

Selected exit stair enclosure doors are permitted to be locked against re-entry from the stairwell side by 7.2.1.5.7, while other stair enclosure doors must remain unlocked. If the selected re-entry provisions are not used, one of the other two options specified by 7.2.1.5.7 must be used for stair enclosures serving five or more stories. Doors are permitted to be locked to prevent re-entry if initiation of the building fire alarm system automatically unlocks the door; otherwise, all stair enclosure doors must remain unlocked at all times.

Note that 30/31.2.2.2.4 restricts the use of the special form of horizontal-sliding door to a greater extent than 7.2.1.14 by prohibiting cross-corridor installations.

A provision that first appeared in the 2003 edition of the *Code* permits the locking of stairway doors against re-entry in sprinklered apartment buildings if the stair serves only one dwelling unit per floor and the stair enclosure is constructed as a smokeproof enclosure in accordance with 7.2.3 (see 30/31.2.2.2.5). This provision is intended to accommodate stairs that open directly to the dwelling units on all floors where re-entry would be impractical from a security standpoint; the only means to provide re-entry would be into another resident's apartment or condominium. The presence of automatic sprinklers, the construction of the stair as a smokeproof enclosure, and the limitation of permitting the stair to serve only one dwelling unit per floor combine to minimize the probability that conditions in the stair will become untenable.

**30.2.2.3 Stairs.**

**30.2.2.3.1** Stairs complying with 7.2.2 shall be permitted.

**30.2.2.3.2 Reserved.**

**30.2.2.3.3** Spiral stairs complying with 7.2.2.2.3 shall be permitted within a single dwelling unit.

**30.2.2.3.4** Winders complying with 7.2.2.2.4 shall be permitted within a single dwelling unit.

**31.2.2.3 Stairs.**

**31.2.2.3.1** Stairs complying with 7.2.2 shall be permitted.

**31.2.2.3.2** Within any individual dwelling unit, unless protected by an approved automatic sprinkler system in accordance with 31.3.5, stairs more than one story above or below the entrance floor level of the dwelling unit shall not be permitted.

**31.2.2.3.3** Spiral stairs complying with 7.2.2.2.3 shall be permitted within a single dwelling unit.

**31.2.2.3.4** Winders complying with 7.2.2.2.4 shall be permitted.

No level of an apartment unit in a nonsprinklered existing building is permitted to be located more than one story away from a dwelling unit entrance per 31.2.2.3.2. This requirement would usually prohibit an apartment unit from encompassing more than three stories: main, upper, and lower. However, if an apartment has entrances at more than one level, or if the building is sprinklered, more than three stories are permitted. A similar provision appears in 30.3.1.3, which applies to all vertical openings in new apartment buildings. Because 30/31.3.1.1.3 permits only two levels within an apartment unit to be open to each other in accordance with 8.6.8.2, the third level must be separated in accordance with Section 8.6.

CHAPTER 30 • New

**30.2.2.4 Smokeproof Enclosures.** Smokeproof enclosures complying with 7.2.3 shall be permitted.

**30.2.2.5 Horizontal Exits.** Horizontal exits complying with 7.2.4 shall be permitted.

**30.2.2.6 Ramps.** Ramps complying with 7.2.5 shall be permitted.

**30.2.2.7 Exit Passageways.** Exit passageways complying with 7.2.6 shall be permitted.

**30.2.2.8 Reserved.**

**30.2.2.9 Reserved.**

**30.2.2.10 Fire Escape Ladders.** Fire escape ladders complying with 7.2.9 shall be permitted.

**30.2.2.11 Alternating Tread Devices.** Alternating tread devices complying with 7.2.11 shall be permitted.

**30.2.2.12 Areas of Refuge.**

**30.2.2.12.1** Areas of refuge complying with 7.2.12 shall be permitted, as modified by 30.2.2.12.2.

**30.2.2.12.2*** In buildings protected throughout by an approved, supervised automatic sprinkler system in accordance with 30.3.5, the two accessible rooms or spaces separated from each other by smoke-resistive partitions in accordance with the definition of area of refuge in 3.3.20 shall not be required.

**A.30.2.2.12.2** The provision of 30.2.2.12.2 permits the entire floor to serve as an area of refuge where it is protected in accordance with 31.3.5. The provision is acceptable because supervised automatic sprinkler systems have built-in signals for monitoring features of the system, such as the opening and closing of water control valves. Such systems also monitor pump power supplies, water tank levels, and conditions that will impair the satisfactory operation of the sprinkler system. Because of these monitoring features, supervised automatic sprinkler systems have a high level of satisfactory performance and response to fire conditions.

CHAPTER 31 • Existing

**31.2.2.4 Smokeproof Enclosures.** Smokeproof enclosures complying with 7.2.3 shall be permitted. *(See also 31.2.11.1.)*

**31.2.2.5 Horizontal Exits.** Horizontal exits complying with 7.2.4 shall be permitted.

**31.2.2.6 Ramps.** Ramps complying with 7.2.5 shall be permitted.

**31.2.2.7 Exit Passageways.** Exit passageways complying with 7.2.6 shall be permitted.

**31.2.2.8* Escalators.** Escalators previously approved as a component in the means of egress shall be permitted to continue to be considered as in compliance.

**A.31.2.2.8** Due to the nature of escalators, they are no longer acceptable as a component in a means of egress. However, because many escalators have been used for exit access and exit discharge in the past, they are permitted to continue to be considered in compliance. Very few escalators have ever been installed in a manner to qualify as an exit. For information on escalator protection and requirements, see previous editions of the *Code*.

**31.2.2.9 Fire Escape Stairs.** Fire escape stairs complying with 7.2.8 shall be permitted.

**31.2.2.10 Fire Escape Ladders.** Fire escape ladders complying with 7.2.9 shall be permitted.

**31.2.2.11 Alternating Tread Devices.** Alternating tread devices complying with 7.2.11 shall be permitted.

**31.2.2.12 Areas of Refuge.**

**31.2.2.12.1** Areas of refuge complying with 7.2.12 shall be permitted, as modified by 31.2.2.12.2.

**31.2.2.12.2*** In buildings protected throughout by an approved, supervised automatic sprinkler system in accordance with 31.3.5, the two accessible rooms or spaces separated from each other by smoke-resistive partitions in accordance with the definition of area of refuge in 3.3.20 shall not be required.

**A.31.2.2.12.2** The provision of 31.2.2.12.2 permits the entire floor to serve as an area of refuge where it is protected in accordance with 31.3.5. The provision is acceptable because supervised automatic sprinkler systems have built-in signals for monitoring features of the system, such as the opening and closing of water control valves. Such systems also monitor pump power supplies, water tank levels, and conditions that will impair the satisfactory operation of the sprinkler system. Because of these monitoring features, supervised automatic sprinkler systems have a high level of satisfactory performance and response to fire conditions.

Areas within new apartment buildings that are accessible to persons with severe mobility impairment must be provided with accessible means of egress per 7.5.4.1. Existing apartment buildings are exempt from the provisions of 7.5.4.1. Therefore, areas of refuge are not required in existing apartment buildings but are permitted to serve within the means of egress.

For stories above the level of exit discharge, where providing ramps is usually not feasible, areas of refuge (see 7.2.12) will typically be used to meet the requirements for accessible means of egress in new apartment buildings. A story of a fully sprinklered apartment building is permitted by 30/31.2.2.12.2 to be considered an area of refuge, even if an occupant does not have access to any of the apartment units. Due to the effectiveness of the sprinkler system, an occupant with mobility impairment should be able to remain on the floor without experiencing untenable conditions. However, because locked apartment unit doors create inaccessibility to spaces other than the corridor, the corridor effectively serves as the area of refuge.

### 30.2.3 Capacity of Means of Egress.

**30.2.3.1** The capacity of means of egress shall be in accordance with Section 7.3.

**30.2.3.2** Street floor exits shall be sufficient for the occupant load of the street floor plus the required capacity of stairs and ramps discharging onto the street floor.

**30.2.3.3** Corridors with a required capacity of more than 50 persons, as defined in Section 7.3, shall be of sufficient width to accommodate the required occupant load but have a width of not less than 44 in. (1120 mm).

**30.2.3.4** Corridors with a required capacity of not more than 50 persons, as defined in Section 7.3, shall be not less than 36 in. (915 mm) in width.

### 31.2.3 Capacity of Means of Egress.

**31.2.3.1** The capacity of means of egress shall be in accordance with Section 7.3.

**31.2.3.2** Street floor exits shall be sufficient for the occupant load of the street floor plus the required capacity of stairs and ramps discharging onto the street floor.

When occupants from upper floors are discharged from exit stair enclosures onto the street floor (in accordance with 7.7.2) and mix with occupants of the street floor in attempting egress to the exterior, the result is an increased demand on street-floor egress components, such as exit doors. Therefore, street-floor exits must be sized to handle the combined capacity in accordance with 30/31.2.3.2.

Exhibit 30/31.2 illustrates a lobby design that might be found in apartment buildings in which multiple exit stairs and street-floor exits converge at one or two exterior door locations. The required aggregate capacity of doors A and B is based on the number of people expected to use them. Assuming that the street floor has an occupant load of 400 persons and each of the two enclosed exit stairs (i.e., stair 1 and stair 2) discharging into the street floor has a required capacity of 200 persons (i.e., a maximum of 50 percent of the 400-person occupant load of the second or third floor via stair 1 and a maximum of 50 percent of the 400-person

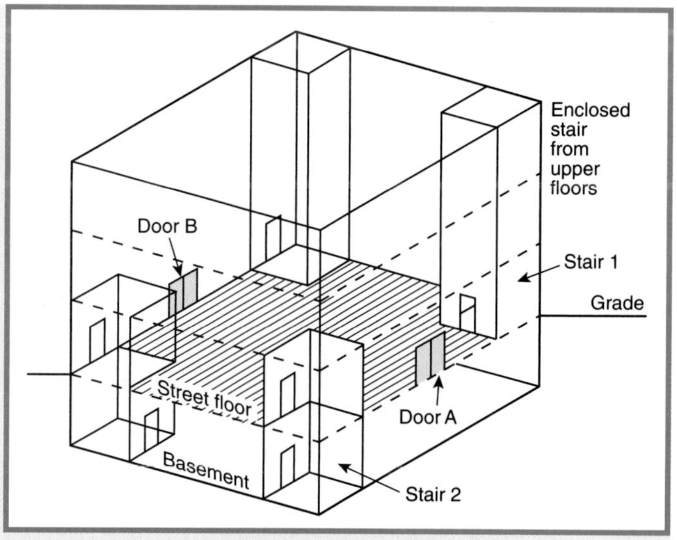


***Exhibit 30/31.2** Egress capacity for street level.*

occupant load of the basement via stair 2), the required egress capacity for the street floor would be 800 persons. The unobstructed door or level travel width required to accommodate 800 persons is 13 ft 4 in. (4065

**30.2.4 Number of Exits.**

The minimum number of exits shall comply with 30.2.4.1, 30.2.4.2, or 30.2.4.4. *(See also Section 7.4.)*

**30.2.4.1** Every dwelling unit shall have access to at least two separate exits remotely located from each other as required by 7.5.1.

**30.2.4.2** A single exit shall be permitted from a dwelling unit, provided that one of the following conditions is met:

(1) The dwelling unit has an exit door opening directly to the street or yard at the finished ground level.
(2) The dwelling unit has direct access to an outside stair that complies with 7.2.2 and serves a maximum of two units, both of which are located on the same story.
(3) The dwelling unit has direct access to an interior stair that serves only that unit and is separated from all other portions of the building by fire barriers having a minimum 1-hour fire resistance rating, with no opening therein.

**30.2.4.3 Reserved.**

**30.2.4.4** A single exit shall be permitted in buildings where the total number of stories does not exceed four, provided that all of the following conditions are met:



mm). The opening provided by each pair of doors, A and B, needs to be 6 ft 8 in. (2030 mm) in clear, unobstructed width.

**31.2.4 Number of Exits.**

The minimum number of exits shall comply with 31.2.4.1, 31.2.4.2, 31.2.4.3, 31.2.4.4, or 31.2.4.5.

**31.2.4.1** Every dwelling unit shall have access to not less than two separate exits remotely located from each other as required by 7.5.1. *(See also Section 7.4.)*

**31.2.4.2** A single exit shall be permitted from a dwelling unit, provided that one of the following conditions is met:

(1) The dwelling unit has an exit door opening directly to the street or yard at the finished ground level.
(2) The dwelling unit has direct access to an outside stair that complies with 7.2.2 and serves not more than two units, both located on the same story.
(3) The dwelling unit has direct access to an interior stair that serves only that unit and is separated from all other portions of the building by fire barriers having a minimum 1-hour fire resistance rating, with no opening therein.

**31.2.4.3** A single exit shall be permitted in buildings where the total number of stories does not exceed four, provided that all of the following conditions are met:

(1) The building is protected throughout by an approved, supervised automatic sprinkler system in accordance with 31.3.5.
(2) The exit stairway does not serve more than one-half of a story below the level of exit discharge.
(3) The travel distance from the entrance door of any dwelling unit to an exit does not exceed 35 ft (10.7 m).
(4) The exit stairway is completely enclosed or separated from the rest of the building by barriers having a minimum 1-hour fire resistance rating.
(5) All openings between the exit stairway enclosure and the building are protected with self-closing doors having a minimum 1-hour fire protection rating.
(6) All corridors serving as access to exits have a minimum ½-hour fire resistance rating.
(7) Horizontal and vertical separation having a minimum ½-hour fire resistance rating is provided between dwelling units.

**31.2.4.4** A single exit shall be permitted in buildings where the total number of stories does not exceed three, provided that all of the following conditions are met:

CHAPTER 30 • New

(1) There are four or fewer dwelling units per story.
(2) The building is protected throughout by an approved, supervised automatic sprinkler system in accordance with 30.3.5.
(3) The exit stairway does not serve more than one-half story below the level of exit discharge.
(4) The travel distance from the entrance door of any dwelling unit to an exit does not exceed 35 ft (10.7 m).
(5) The exit stairway is completely enclosed or separated from the rest of the building by barriers having a minimum 1-hour fire resistance rating.
(6) All openings between the exit stairway enclosure and the building are protected with self-closing door assemblies having a minimum 1-hour fire protection rating.
(7) All corridors serving as access to exits have a minimum 1-hour fire resistance rating.
(8) Horizontal and vertical separation having a minimum ½-hour fire resistance rating is provided between dwelling units

CHAPTER 31 • Existing

(1) The exit stairway does not serve more than one-half of a story below the level of exit discharge.
(2) The travel distance from the entrance door of any dwelling unit to an exit does not exceed 35 ft (10.7 m).
(3) The exit stairway is completely enclosed or separated from the rest of the building by barriers having a minimum 1-hour fire resistance rating.
(4) All openings between the exit stairway enclosure and the building are protected with self-closing doors having a minimum 1-hour fire protection rating.
(5) All corridors serving as access to exits have a minimum 20-minute fire resistance rating.
(6) Horizontal and vertical separation having a minimum ½-hour fire resistance rating is provided between dwelling units.

**31.2.4.5** A building of any height with not more than four dwelling units per floor, with a smokeproof enclosure in accordance with the requirements of 7.2.3 or outside stair as the exit, where such exit is immediately accessible to all dwelling units served thereby, shall be permitted to have a single exit. *Immediately accessible* means that the travel distance from the entrance door of any dwelling unit to an exit shall not exceed 20 ft (6100 mm).

A single means of egress is permitted by 30/31.2.4.2 under the conditions of paragraphs 1 through 3, which follow.

**1.** The living unit has an exit leading directly to the street or yard at ground level. This arrangement is common in the case of town houses or row houses. Under this arrangement, the front door is the only required exit, so no provisions for a rear door are required. If a rear door is provided, it does not have to meet the locking or other requirements of the *Code.*

**2.** The apartment has direct access to an outside stair serving a maximum of two apartments, both of which are on the same floor. The outside stair must be separated from the interior of the building, as detailed in 7.2.2.6.3. This arrangement is detailed in Exhibit 30/31.3.

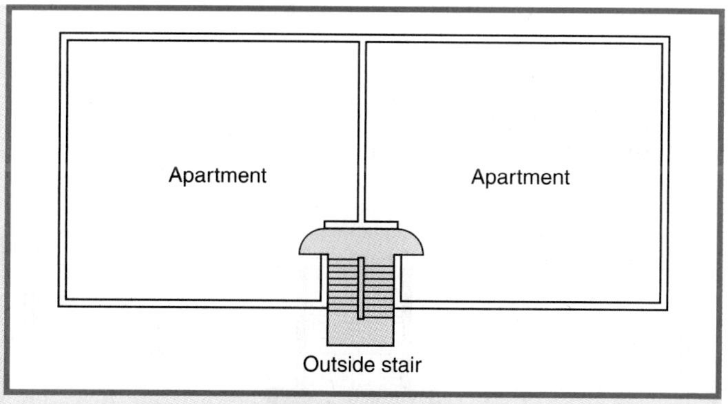


***Exhibit 30/31.3** Outside stair serving two apartment units.*

**3.** The single exit is a private stairway serving one apartment only and is separated from all abutting apartment units, including those on lower floors, by 1-hour–rated construction. Note that this stairway is required to be separated only from other spaces by the required 1-hour construction; it is not required to be separated from the apartment unit that it serves. This arrangement is detailed in Exhibit 30/31.4.

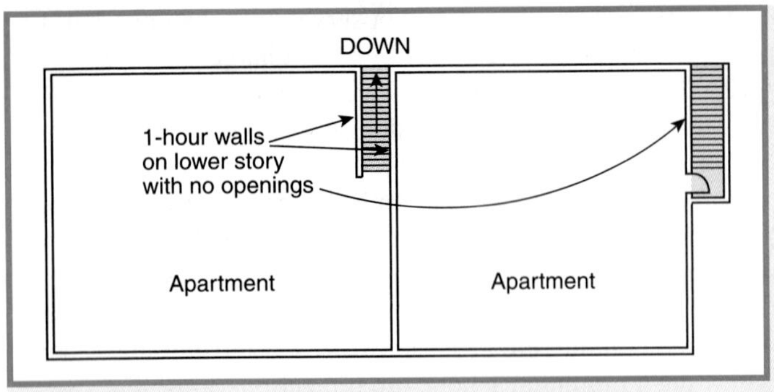


***Exhibit 30/31.4*** *Stair serving one apartment unit.*

Garden-type apartment buildings, where the apartment unit entrance doors open either directly into a single exit stair enclosure or into a vestibule or short corridor leading to a single, enclosed exit stair, are addressed by 30.2.4.4. In other situations, the stair is open to the exterior or is enclosed by glass at the front of the building. A single exit under this arrangement is permitted if additional conditions can be met.

Exhibit 30/31.5 illustrates the provisions of 30.2.4.4 where the following requirements are met:

1. The building must be sprinklered in accordance with 30.3.5.
2. The building must be not more than four stories high.
3. The building must have not more than four apartment units per floor.
4. The single exit stair must be separated from the building by construction with a minimum 1-hour fire resistance rating.
5. The exit enclosure doors (E) must be 1-hour fire protection–rated and self-closing, as are apartment unit doors (A), if they open directly into the exit enclosure.

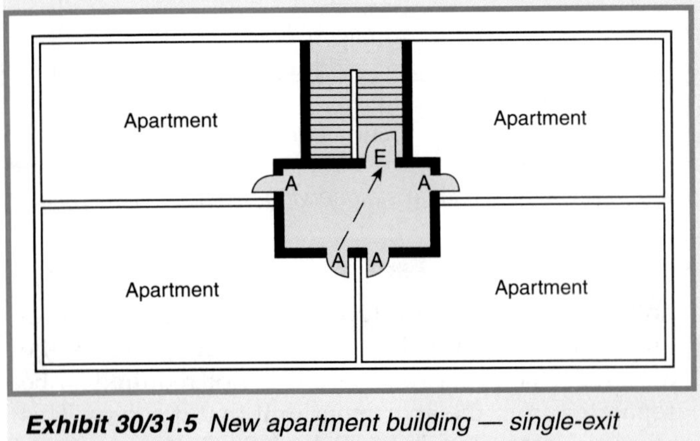


***Exhibit 30/31.5*** *New apartment building — single-exit arrangement.*

6. If the apartment unit doors (A) open into a corridor, they must be 20-minute fire protection rated.

A frequent violation of the provision for a single exit is the use of nonrated doors and the lack of door closers. The travel distance from the apartment unit door to the exit enclosure door (A to E) is not permitted to exceed 35 ft (10.7 m). Both horizontal and vertical 30-minute fire resistance–rated separation are required between apartment units.

For existing apartment buildings, similar criteria are provided in 31.2.4.3; however, 31.2.4.3 differs by not limiting the number of apartment units per floor, as depicted in Exhibit 30/31.6, and by permitting the corridor fire resistance rating to be $\frac{1}{2}$ hour instead of 1 hour.

The provision of 31.2.4.4 is similar to that of 31.2.4.3 in that it permits a single exit from a typical garden-type apartment building. However, the apartment building is not required to be sprinklered and is limited to a height of not more than three stories.

The provision of 31.2.4.5 for existing apartment buildings describes an uncommon arrangement. Note that there are no height limitations, but only four apartment units per floor are permitted. Furthermore, apartments must have immediate access to a smokeproof enclosure or to an outside stair that meets the requirements of a smokeproof enclosure. The exemptions to the requirements for outside stairs in Chapter 7 for unprotected openings that expose a stair would not apply in this case, because the *Code* specifically references 7.2.3 on smokeproof enclosures. Unprotected openings that expose the stair are prohibited by 7.2.3.

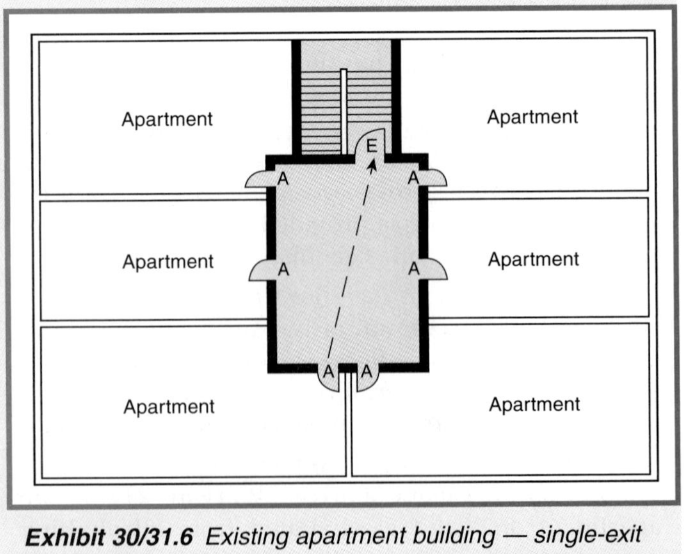


***Exhibit 30/31.6*** *Existing apartment building — single-exit arrangement.*

CHAPTER 30 • New

### 30.2.5 Arrangement of Means of Egress.

**30.2.5.1** Access to all required exits shall be in accordance with Section 7.5, as modified by 30.2.5.2.

**30.2.5.2** The distance between exits addressed by 7.5.1.3 shall not apply to nonlooped exit access corridors in buildings that have corridor doors from the dwelling units that are arranged such that the exits are located in opposite directions from such doors.

**30.2.5.3** Common path of travel shall comply with 30.2.5.3.1 or 30.2.5.3.2.

**30.2.5.3.1** No common path of travel shall exceed 35 ft (10.7 m) in buildings not protected throughout by an approved, supervised automatic sprinkler system installed in accordance with 30.3.5. Travel within a dwelling unit shall not be included when calculating common path of travel.

**30.2.5.3.2** No common path of travel shall exceed 50 ft (15 m) in buildings protected throughout by an approved, supervised automatic sprinkler system installed in accordance with 30.3.5. Travel within a dwelling unit shall not be included when determining common path of travel.

**30.2.5.4** Dead-end corridors shall be limited in accordance with either 30.2.5.4.1 or 30.2.5.4.2.

**30.2.5.4.1** Dead-end corridors shall not exceed 35 ft (10.7 m) in buildings not protected throughout by an approved automatic sprinkler system in accordance with 30.3.5.

**30.2.5.4.2** Dead-end corridors shall not exceed 50 ft (15 m) in buildings protected throughout by an approved, supervised automatic sprinkler system in accordance with 30.3.5.

CHAPTER 31 • Existing

### 31.2.5 Arrangement of Means of Egress.

**31.2.5.1** Access to all required exits shall be in accordance with Section 7.5.

**31.2.5.2 Reserved.**

**31.2.5.3** Common path of travel shall comply with 31.2.5.3.1 or 31.2.5.3.2.

**31.2.5.3.1** No common path of travel shall exceed 35 ft (10.7 m) in buildings not protected throughout by an approved, supervised automatic sprinkler system installed in accordance with 31.3.5. Travel within a dwelling unit shall not be included when calculating common path of travel.

**31.2.5.3.2** No common path of travel shall exceed 50 ft (15 m) in buildings protected throughout by an approved, supervised automatic sprinkler system installed in accordance with 31.3.5. Travel within a dwelling unit shall not be included when calculating common path of travel.

**31.2.5.4** Dead-end corridors shall not exceed 50 ft (15 m).

The provisions for the arrangement of the means of egress in apartment buildings differ significantly from the provisions in Chapter 7. The first difference appears in 30.2.5.2, which addresses the remoteness of exits. Applying the exit remoteness provisions of 7.5.1.3 could result in a corridor that is longer than is necessary for the efficient use of the space. Some relief is offered by 30.2.5.2. Exhibit 30/31.7 helps to clarify the intent of 30.2.5.2. In Part (a) of Exhibit 30/31.7, all four dwelling units have access to two exits immediately upon leaving the dwelling unit and entering the exit access corridor — that is, there is no common path of travel within the corridor from any of the apartments. This arrangement meets the provisions of 30.2.5.2. Contrast this arrangement with that depicted in Part (b) of Exhibit 30/31.7, where only dwelling units A and B have access to two exits immediately upon leaving the dwelling unit and entering the exit access corridor. This arrangement does not meet the provisions of 30.2.5.2.

The concepts underlying the limitations imposed on common paths of travel and dead-end corridors are similar but not identical to those explained in the commentary on 7.5.1.5. Because of modifications made by Chapters 30 and 31 in defining where common path of travel begins, the difference between common paths of travel and dead-end corridors is less pronounced for apartment buildings. For most other occupancies, common path of travel is measured from the most remote point subject to occupancy to the point where occupants have a choice of traveling in independent directions (see 7.5.1.1.4 and the definition of *common path of travel* in 3.3.42). For apartment buildings, the travel distance within the dwelling unit, though regulated by 30/31.2.6, is not included as part of the common path of travel. Therefore, common path of travel,

CHAPTER 30 • New

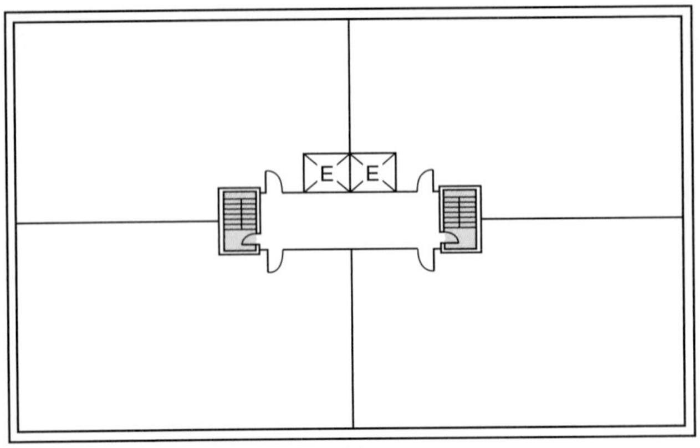


(a)

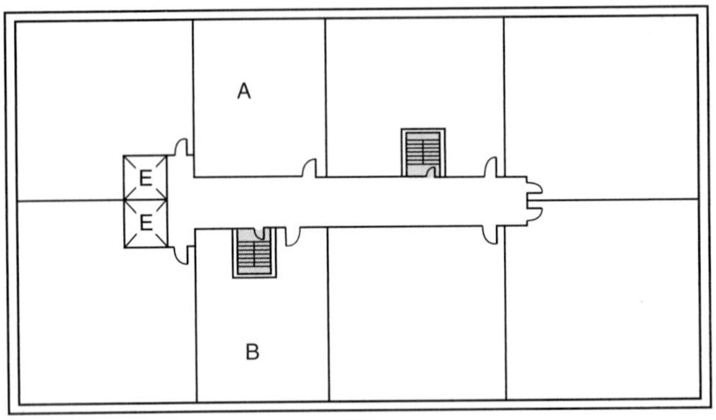


(b)

*Exhibit 30/31.7 New apartment buildings — exit remoteness.*

as illustrated by the solid arrows in Exhibit 30/31.8, is measured from the room door to the point where occupants have a choice of traveling in independent directions. This depiction can be thought of as a modified common path of travel, because measurement does not extend into the dwelling unit.

The distances permitted for common path of travel in new and existing apartment buildings also

CHAPTER 31 • Existing

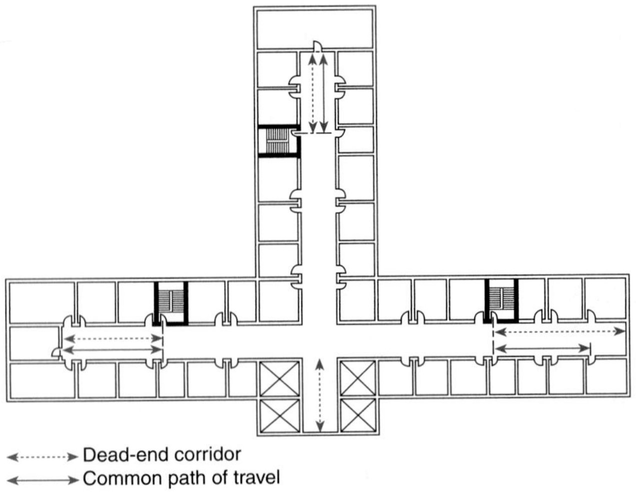


*Exhibit 30/31.8 Modified common path of travel and dead-end corridors in an apartment building.*

differ. Because new apartment buildings are required to be sprinklered without exception (see 30.3.5.1), the 35 ft (10.7 m) modified common path of travel and dead-end corridor limitations permitted by 30.2.5.3.1 and 30.2.5.4.1 will usually be supplanted by the 50 ft (15 m) limitation permitted by 30.2.5.3.2 and 30.2.5.4.2. The 35 ft (10.7 m) criterion for nonsprinklered buildings is maintained for the purpose of applying Chapter 30 to the rehabilitation of existing, nonsprinklered apartment buildings as specified by Chapter 43.

In most existing apartment buildings, automatic sprinklers are not required. However, if the building is protected throughout by an approved, supervised automatic sprinkler system, the common path of travel is permitted to be 50 ft (15 m), which is the same distance permitted for the length of existing dead-end corridors, regardless of the presence of automatic sprinklers.

### 30.2.6 Travel Distance to Exits.

Travel distance shall be measured in accordance with Section 7.6.

**30.2.6.1** Travel distance within a dwelling unit (apartment) to a corridor door shall not exceed 75 ft (23 m) in buildings not protected throughout by an approved, supervised automatic sprinkler system installed in accordance with 30.3.5.

### 31.2.6 Travel Distance to Exits.

Travel distance shall be measured in accordance with Section 7.6.

**31.2.6.1** Travel distance within a dwelling unit (apartment) to a corridor door shall not exceed the following limits:

(1) For buildings using Option 1 or Option 3, 75 ft (23 m)
(2) For buildings using Option 2 or Option 4, 125 ft (38 m)

CHAPTER 30 • New

**30.2.6.2** Travel distance within a dwelling unit (apartment) to a corridor door shall not exceed 125 ft (38 m) in buildings protected throughout by an approved, supervised automatic sprinkler system installed in accordance with 30.3.5.

**30.2.6.3** The travel distance from a dwelling unit (apartment) entrance door to the nearest exit shall be limited in accordance with 30.2.6.3.1, 30.2.6.3.2, or 30.2.6.3.3.

**30.2.6.3.1** The travel distance from a dwelling unit (apartment) entrance door to the nearest exit shall not exceed 100 ft (30 m).

**30.2.6.3.2** In buildings protected throughout by an approved, supervised automatic sprinkler system installed in accordance with 30.3.5, the travel distance from a dwelling unit (apartment) entrance door to the nearest exit shall not exceed 200 ft (61 m).

**30.2.6.3.3** The travel distance from a dwelling unit (apartment) entrance door to the nearest exit shall not exceed 200 ft (61 m) for exterior ways of exit access arranged in accordance with 7.5.3.

**30.2.6.4** The travel distance, from areas other than those within living units, to the exit, shall not exceed 200 ft (61 m), or 250 ft (76 m) in buildings protected throughout by an approved, supervised automatic sprinkler system installed in accordance with 30.3.5.5.

CHAPTER 31 • Existing

**31.2.6.2** The travel distance from a dwelling unit (apartment) entrance door to the nearest exit shall not exceed the following limits, as modified by 31.2.6.3:

(1) For buildings using Option 1, 100 ft (30 m)
(2) For buildings using Option 2 or Option 3, 150 ft (46 m)
(3) For buildings using Option 4, 200 ft (61 m)

**31.2.6.3** Travel distance to exits shall not exceed 200 ft (61 m) for exterior ways of exit access arranged in accordance with 7.5.3.

**31.2.6.4** The travel distance, from areas other than those within living units, to the exit shall not exceed 200 ft (61 m), or 250 ft (76 m) in buildings protected throughout by an approved, supervised automatic sprinkler system installed in accordance with 31.3.5.

The travel distance limitations specified in 30/31.2.6 divide the measurement into the following two portions of the overall travel distance:

1. Travel within an apartment unit to the door to the common space of the building
2. Travel from the corridor door to the nearest exit

If the travel distance within an apartment unit is excessive, an additional remote door to the corridor can usually be added to correct the deficiency. The presence of automatic sprinklers or the use of exterior ways of exit access modifies travel distance requirements. In existing buildings, the presence of a fire detection and notification system or a partial sprinkler system (Option 2 or Option 3) also modifies travel distance requirements, though not to the extent of a complete automatic sprinkler system (Option 4).

Many apartment buildings have common activity rooms, lounges, lobbies, and similar spaces that are neither dwelling units, as addressed by 30.2.6.1 and 30.2.6.2, nor exit access corridor–like spaces, as addressed by 30.2.6.3. Travel distance limitations from areas other than those within dwelling units of new apartment buildings are established by 30.2.6.4. The maximum 200 ft (61 m) travel distance allowance, which can be increased to 250 ft (76 m) in sprinklered buildings, treats the travel distance in one continuous measurement. For example, the travel distance limitation would apply to the full distance of travel through an activity room and the associated exit access corridors to the exit.

### 30.2.7 Discharge from Exits.

Exit discharge shall comply with Section 7.7.

### 31.2.7 Discharge from Exits.

Exit discharge shall comply with Section 7.7.

CHAPTER 30 • New

### 30.2.8 Illumination of Means of Egress.

Means of egress shall be illuminated in accordance with Section 7.8.

### 30.2.9 Emergency Lighting.

Emergency lighting in accordance with Section 7.9 shall be provided in all buildings four or more stories in height, or with more than 12 dwelling units, unless every dwelling unit has a direct exit to the outside of the building at the finished ground level.

### 30.2.10 Marking of Means of Egress.

Means of egress shall have signs in accordance with Section 7.10 in all buildings requiring more than one exit.

### 30.2.11 Special Means of Egress Features.

**30.2.11.1 Reserved.**

**30.2.11.2 Lockups.** Lockups in apartment buildings shall comply with the requirements of 22.4.5.

CHAPTER 31 • Existing

### 31.2.8 Illumination of Means of Egress.

Means of egress shall be illuminated in accordance with Section 7.8.

### 31.2.9 Emergency Lighting.

Emergency lighting in accordance with Section 7.9 shall be provided in all buildings four or more stories in height or with more than 12 dwelling units, unless every dwelling unit has a direct exit to the outside of the building at grade level.

### 31.2.10 Marking of Means of Egress.

Means of egress shall have signs in accordance with Section 7.10 in all buildings requiring more than one exit.

### 31.2.11 Special Means of Egress Features.

**31.2.11.1* High-Rise Buildings.** In high-rise buildings using Option 1, Option 2, or Option 3, smokeproof enclosures shall be provided in accordance with 7.2.3.

**A.31.2.11.1** The provision of 31.2.11 recognizes the need to provide smoke control in existing buildings. Smokeproof enclosures can be accomplished without the use of a vestibule in accordance with 7.2.3.

**31.2.11.2 Lockups.** Lockups in apartment buildings, other than approved existing lockups, shall comply with the requirements of 23.4.5.

Emergency lighting is required in both new and existing apartment buildings if the building either has more than 12 dwelling units or is more than three stories in height. The provision of 30/31.2.9 exempting emergency lighting does not apply to all apartment buildings with exterior exit access but only to those where each apartment unit has direct exit at grade (no vertical travel). In accordance with Section 7.9, where it is required, emergency lighting must be provided in designated portions of the means of egress, but not within individual dwelling units (apartments). Designated components include corridors, exit stairs, and the exit discharge. Omission of emergency lighting in the exit discharge outside the building is a frequent *Code* violation.

Existing, nonsprinklered high-rise apartment buildings are affected by 31.2.11.1. If smokeproof enclosures meeting 7.2.3 are not already provided, it might be more practical to add sprinkler protection to the entire building, so as to meet Option 4, than to modify stairs to meet the requirements for smokeproof enclosures.

## 30.3 Protection

### 30.3.1 Protection of Vertical Openings.

**30.3.1.1** Vertical openings shall comply with 30.3.1.1.1 through 30.3.1.3.

**30.3.1.1.1** Vertical openings shall be enclosed or protected in accordance with Section 8.6.

## 31.3 Protection

### 31.3.1 Protection of Vertical Openings.

**31.3.1.1** Vertical openings shall comply with 31.3.1.1.1 through 31.3.1.2.

**31.3.1.1.1** Vertical openings shall be enclosed or protected in accordance with Section 8.6.

CHAPTER 30 • New

30.3.1.1.2 Where the provisions of 8.6.6 are used, the requirements of 30.3.5.7 shall be met.

30.3.1.1.3 Vertical openings in accordance with 8.6.8.2 shall be permitted.

30.3.1.1.4 In buildings protected throughout by an approved, supervised automatic sprinkler system in accordance with 30.3.5, walls enclosing vertical openings shall have a minimum 1-hour fire resistance rating, and the doors shall have a minimum 1-hour fire protection rating.

30.3.1.2 No floor below the level of exit discharge used only for storage, heating equipment, or purposes other than residential occupancy and open to the public shall have unprotected openings to floors used for residential purposes.

30.3.1.3 Within any individual dwelling unit, unless protected by an approved automatic sprinkler system in accordance with 30.3.5, vertical openings more than one story above or below the entrance floor level of the dwelling unit shall not be permitted.

CHAPTER 31 • Existing

**31.3.1.1.2 Reserved.**

31.3.1.1.3 Vertical openings in accordance with 8.6.8.2 shall be permitted.

31.3.1.1.4 In buildings protected throughout by an approved automatic sprinkler system in accordance with 31.3.5, and in which exits and required ways of travel thereto are adequately safeguarded against fire and smoke within the building, or where every individual room has direct access to an exterior exit without passing through any public corridor, the protection of vertical openings that are not part of required exits shall not be required.

31.3.1.2 No floor below the level of exit discharge used only for storage, heating equipment, or purposes other than residential occupancy and open to the public shall have unprotected openings to floors used for residential purposes.

The protection of vertical openings is provided by a reference to Section 8.6 for both new and existing apartment buildings. However, automatic sprinkler protection is required throughout new apartment buildings where the building has a communicating space in accordance with 8.6.6.

The provision of 30/31.3.1.1.3 has traditionally permitted an unenclosed stair to be located within an apartment unit (living unit) for the purpose of connecting two adjacent stories. The open stair typically serves as means of escape for occupants of a living unit. The provisions of 8.6.8.2 do not permit the opening to serve as required means of egress. It is not the *Code*'s intent to prohibit an open stair from serving as means of escape for occupants of a dwelling unit.

In the case of a three-story apartment unit, only two of the three stories can be connected by an open stair. The stair connecting the third level must be enclosed in accordance with Section 8.6.

Atria are permitted in both new and existing apartment buildings (see 8.6.7). However, 8.6.7 requires total automatic sprinkler protection in buildings with atria. Therefore, an existing apartment building would be permitted to have an atrium only where Option 4 (complete sprinkler protection) is used.

All new apartment buildings must be protected throughout by an approved, supervised automatic sprinkler system. Prior to the 2009 edition of the *Code*, some apartment buildings with means of egress directly to the outside from every apartment, much like a detached single-family home, were exempt from the requirement for automatic sprinklers. However, since the 2006 edition of the *Code*, new one- and two-family dwellings are required to be sprinklered (see 24.3.5.1). As such, there is no justification to permit the omission of sprinklers from new apartment buildings with egress arrangements that resemble those of one- and two-family dwellings.

CHAPTER 30 • New

### 30.3.2 Protection from Hazards.

**30.3.2.1 Hazardous Areas.** Any hazardous area shall be protected in accordance with Section 8.7.

30.3.2.1.1 The areas described in Table 30.3.2.1.1 shall be protected as indicated.

CHAPTER 31 • Existing

### 31.3.2 Protection from Hazards.

**31.3.2.1 Hazardous Areas.** Any hazardous area shall be protected in accordance with Section 8.7.

31.3.2.1.1 The areas described in Table 31.3.2.1.1 shall be protected as indicated.

CHAPTER 30 • New

*Table 30.3.2.1.1 Hazardous Area Protection*

| Hazardous Area Description | Separation/Protection† |
|---|---|
| Boiler and fuel-fired heater rooms serving more than a single dwelling unit | 1 hour and sprinklers |
| Employee locker rooms | 1 hour or sprinklers |
| Gift or retail shops | 1 hour or sprinklers |
| Bulk laundries | 1 hour and sprinklers |
| Laundries ≤100 $ft^2$ (≤9.3 $m^2$) outside of dwelling units | 1 hour or sprinklers‡ |
| Laundries >100 $ft^2$ (>9.3 $m^2$) outside of dwelling units | 1 hour and sprinklers |
| Maintenance shops | 1 hour and sprinklers |
| Storage rooms outside of dwelling units | 1 hour or sprinklers |
| Trash collection rooms | 1 hour and sprinklers |

†Minimum fire resistance rating.

‡Where sprinklers are provided, the separation specified in 8.7.1.2 and 30.3.2.1.2 is not required.

**30.3.2.1.2** Where sprinkler protection without fire-rated separation is used, areas shall be separated from other spaces by smoke partitions complying with Section 8.4.

Note the differences in the hazardous area protection requirements for new and existing apartment buildings as specified in Table 30.3.2.1.1 and Table 31.3.2.1.1. In new apartment buildings, many of the areas are required to be separated by construction with a 1-hour fire resistance rating and protected by automatic sprinklers. In existing apartment buildings, automatic sprinklers are sometimes used as an alternative to the separation requirement.

**30.3.2.2 Reserved.**

### 30.3.3 Interior Finish.

**30.3.3.1 General.** Interior finish shall be in accordance with Section 10.2.

**30.3.3.2 Interior Wall and Ceiling Finish.** Interior wall and ceiling finish materials complying with Section 10.2 shall be permitted as follows:

(1) Exit enclosures — Class A
(2) Lobbies and corridors — Class A or Class B
(3) Other spaces — Class A, Class B, or Class C

CHAPTER 31 • Existing

*Table 31.3.2.1.1 Hazardous Area Protection*

| Hazardous Area Description | Separation/Protection† |
|---|---|
| Boiler and fuel-fired heater rooms serving more than a single dwelling unit | 1 hour or sprinklers |
| Employee locker rooms | 1 hour or sprinklers |
| Gift or retail shops >100 $ft^2$ (>9.3 $m^2$) | 1 hour or sprinklers‡ |
| Bulk laundries | 1 hour or sprinklers |
| Laundries >100 $ft^2$ (>9.3 $m^2$) outside of dwelling units | 1 hour or sprinklers‡ |
| Maintenance shops | 1 hour or sprinklers |
| Rooms or spaces used for storage of combustible supplies and equipment in quantities deemed hazardous by the authority having jurisdiction | 1 hour or sprinklers |
| Trash collection rooms | 1 hour or sprinklers |

†Minimum fire resistance rating.

‡Where sprinklers are provided, the separation specified in 8.7.1.2 and 31.3.2.1.2 is not required.

**31.3.2.1.2** Where sprinkler protection without fire-rated separation is used, areas shall be separated from other spaces by smoke partitions complying with Section 8.4.

Although the lists that appear in Table 30.3.2.1.1 and Table 31.3.2.1.1 provide specific direction for certain hazardous contents areas, they are not all-inclusive. Other areas that are deemed hazardous need to be provided with the appropriate level of protection in accordance with Section 8.7.

**31.3.2.2 Reserved.**

### 31.3.3 Interior Finish.

**31.3.3.1 General.** Interior finish shall be in accordance with Section 10.2.

**31.3.3.2 Interior Wall and Ceiling Finish.** Interior wall and ceiling finish materials complying with 10.2 shall be permitted as follows:

(1) Exit enclosures — Class A or Class B
(2) Lobbies and corridors — Class A or Class B
(3) Other spaces — Class A, Class B, or Class C

CHAPTER 30 • New

**30.3.3.3 Interior Floor Finish.**

**30.3.3.3.1** Interior floor finish shall comply with Section 10.2.

**30.3.3.3.2** Interior floor finish in exit enclosures and exit access corridors and spaces not separated from them by walls complying with 30.3.6 shall be not less than Class II.

**30.3.3.3.3** Interior floor finish shall comply with 10.2.7.1 or 10.2.7.2, as applicable.

### 30.3.4 Detection, Alarm, and Communications Systems.

**30.3.4.1 General.**

**30.3.4.1.1** Apartment buildings four or more stories in height or with more than 11 dwelling units, other than those meeting the requirements of 30.3.4.1.2, shall be provided with a fire alarm system in accordance with Section 9.6, except as modified by 30.3.4.2 through 30.3.4.6.

**30.3.4.1.2** A fire alarm system shall not be required in buildings where each dwelling unit is separated from other contiguous dwelling units by fire barriers *(see Section 8.3)* having a minimum 1-hour fire resistance rating, and where each dwelling unit has either its own independent exit or its own independent stairway or ramp discharging at the finished ground level.

CHAPTER 31 • Existing

**31.3.3.3 Interior Floor Finish.** In buildings utilizing Option 1 or Option 2, newly installed interior floor finish in exits and exit access corridors shall be not less than Class II in accordance with 10.2.7.

### 31.3.4 Detection, Alarm, and Communications Systems.

**31.3.4.1 General.**

**31.3.4.1.1** Apartment buildings four or more stories in height or with more than 11 dwelling units, other than those meeting the requirements of 31.3.4.1.2, shall be provided with a fire alarm system in accordance with Section 9.6, except as modified by 31.3.4.2 through 31.3.4.6.

**31.3.4.1.2** A fire alarm system shall not be required where each dwelling unit is separated from other contiguous dwelling units by fire barriers *(see Section 8.3)* having a minimum ½-hour fire resistance rating, and where each dwelling unit has either its own independent exit or its own independent stairway or ramp discharging at the finished ground level.

The intent of 30/31.3.4.1.2 is to exempt town house–type apartment buildings from the requirement for a fire alarm system, because, during a fire, each apartment unit retains safe egress routes for longer than is typical of standard apartment buildings with interior exit access corridors. The safe egress route helps to ensure that any delay in occupant notification resulting from the absence of an alarm system can be tolerated without undue risk.

CHAPTER 30 • New

**30.3.4.2 Initiation.**

**30.3.4.2.1** Initiation of the required fire alarm system shall be by manual means in accordance with 9.6.2, unless the building complies with 30.3.4.2.2.

**30.3.4.2.2** Initiation of the required fire alarm system by manual means shall not be required in buildings four or fewer stories in height, containing not more than 16 dwelling units, and protected throughout by an approved, supervised automatic sprinkler system installed in accordance with 30.3.5.1.

**30.3.4.2.3** In buildings protected throughout by an approved, supervised automatic sprinkler system in accordance with 30.3.5, required fire alarm systems shall be initiated upon operation of the automatic sprinkler system.

CHAPTER 31 • Existing

**31.3.4.2 Initiation.**

**31.3.4.2.1** Initiation of the required fire alarm system shall be by manual means in accordance with 9.6.2, unless the building complies with 31.3.4.2.2.

**31.3.4.2.2** Initiation of the required fire alarm system by manual means shall not be required in buildings four or fewer stories in height, containing not more than 16 dwelling units, and protected throughout by an approved, supervised automatic sprinkler system installed in accordance with 31.3.5.3.

**31.3.4.2.3** In buildings using Option 2, the required fire alarm system shall be initiated by the automatic fire detection system in addition to the manual initiation means of 31.3.4.2.1.

CHAPTER 30 • New

CHAPTER 31 • Existing

**31.3.4.2.4** In buildings using Option 3, the required fire alarm system shall be initiated upon operation of the automatic sprinkler system in addition to the manual initiation means of 31.3.4.2.1.

**31.3.4.2.5** In buildings using Option 4, the required fire alarm system shall be initiated upon operation of the automatic sprinkler system in addition to the manual initiation means of 31.3.4.2.1.

**30.3.4.3 Notification.**

**30.3.4.3.1** Occupant notification shall be provided automatically in accordance with Section 9.6, and the following shall also apply:

(1) Visible signals shall be installed in units designed for the hearing impaired.
(2) Positive alarm sequence in accordance with 9.6.3.4 shall be permitted.

**30.3.4.3.2** Annunciation, and annunciation zoning, in accordance with 9.6.7 shall be provided, unless the building complies with either 30.3.4.3.3 or 30.3.4.3.4. Annunciation shall be provided at a location readily accessible from the primary point of entry for emergency response personnel.

**30.3.4.3.3** Annunciation, and annunciation zoning, shall not be required in buildings two or fewer stories in height and having not more than 50 dwelling units.

**30.3.4.3.4** Annunciation, and annunciation zoning, shall not be required in buildings four or fewer stories in height containing not more than 16 dwelling units and protected throughout by an approved, supervised automatic sprinkler system installed in accordance with 30.3.5.1.

**30.3.4.3.5** Fire department notification shall be accomplished in accordance with 9.6.4.

**31.3.4.3 Notification.**

**31.3.4.3.1** Occupant notification shall be provided automatically in accordance with Section 9.6, and the following shall also apply:

(1) Visible signals shall be installed in units designed for the hearing impaired.
(2) Positive alarm sequence in accordance with 9.6.3.4 shall be permitted.
(3) Existing approved presignal systems shall be permitted in accordance with 9.6.3.3.

**31.3.4.3.2** An annunciator panel, whose location shall be approved by the authority having jurisdiction, connected with the required fire alarm system shall be provided, unless the building meets the requirements of 31.3.4.3.3 or 31.3.4.3.4.

**31.3.4.3.3** Annunciation shall not be required in buildings two or fewer stories in height and having not more than 50 rooms.

**31.3.4.3.4** Annunciation shall not be required in buildings four or fewer stories in height containing not more than 16 dwelling units and protected throughout by an approved, supervised automatic sprinkler system installed in accordance with 31.3.5.3.

**31.3.4.3.5** Fire department notification shall be accomplished in accordance with 9.6.4.

If a fire alarm system is required in an apartment building, then it must provide notification to the fire department using one of the four methods described in 9.6.4.2 (i.e., auxiliary fire alarm system, central station fire alarm system, proprietary supervising station fire alarm system, or remote supervising station fire alarm system). This requirement, which first appeared in the 2003 edition of the *Code*, applies to both new and existing buildings.

Note that 9.6.4.3 recognizes that some existing fire alarm systems are not readily adaptable to provide automatic fire department notification. In such cases, the authority having jurisdiction (AHJ) can approve an alternative plan to ensure a prompt fire department response. With the proliferation of personal cellular phones in recent years, the AHJ might consider approving the installation of signs located at the manual fire alarm boxes that read "Local Alarm Only — In Case of Fire Call 911," or similar verbiage, in lieu of requiring automatic notification. In all cases where a supervised automatic sprinkler system is required by the *Code*, a sprinkler waterflow condition must automatically provide alarm notification to the fire department (see 9.7.2.2).

CHAPTER 30 • New

30.3.4.4 Detection. (Reserved)

30.3.4.5* Smoke Alarms. Smoke alarms shall be installed in accordance with 9.6.2.10 in every sleeping area, outside every sleeping area in the immediate vicinity of the bedrooms, and on all levels of the dwelling unit, including basements.

A.30.3.4.5 Previous editions of the *Code* permitted the single-station smoke alarm required by 30.3.4.5 to be omitted from each apartment where a complete automatic smoke detection system was installed throughout the building. With such a system, when one detector is activated, an alarm is sounded throughout the building. Experience with complete smoke detection systems in apartment buildings has shown that numerous nuisance alarms are likely to occur. Where there is a problem with frequent nuisance alarms, occupants ignore the alarm, or the system is either disconnected or otherwise rendered inoperative.

CHAPTER 31 • Existing

31.3.4.4 Detection.

31.3.4.4.1* In buildings using Option 2, a complete automatic fire detection system in accordance with 9.6.1.3 and 31.3.4.4.2 shall be required.

A.31.3.4.4.1 It is intended that a building compliant with Option 2 function as described in the paragraph that follows.

Occupants within a living unit become aware of a fire emergency, either through personal awareness or through being alerted by the smoke alarm(s) installed within the living unit. Other building occupants are alerted to the fire emergency by the building fire alarm system that is initiated by manual fire alarm boxes adjacent to the exits, heat detection within the living unit where the fire emergency exists, smoke detection in the common areas outside the living unit, or a combination thereof. The installation of system heat detectors versus smoke detectors within the living unit is intended to eliminate nuisance-type alarms and reduce occupant complacency from frequent false alarms. The installation of smoke detection within the living unit should only be contemplated after a careful analysis of the goals and with the approval of the authority having jurisdiction.

31.3.4.4.2 Automatic fire detection devices shall be installed as follows:

(1) Smoke detectors shall be installed in all common areas and work spaces outside the living unit, such as exit stairs, egress corridors, lobbies, storage rooms, equipment rooms, and other tenantless spaces in environments that are suitable for proper smoke detector operation.
(2) Heat detectors shall be located within each room of the living unit.

31.3.4.5 Smoke Alarms.

31.3.4.5.1* In buildings other than those equipped throughout with an existing, complete automatic smoke detection system, smoke alarms shall be installed in accordance with 9.6.2.10, as modified by 31.3.4.5.2, outside every sleeping area in the immediate vicinity of the bedrooms and on all levels of the dwelling unit, including basements.

A.31.3.4.5.1 NFPA *101* provides adequate, balanced fire protection and takes into consideration the passive and active systems required in a given occupancy. The level of protection prescribed by *NFPA 72, National Fire Alarm Code*, which includes smoke alarms in all sleeping rooms, without exception, does not necessarily take into consideration the complete protection package mandated by NFPA *101*.

31.3.4.5.2 Smoke alarms required by 31.3.4.5.1 shall not be required to be provided with a secondary (standby) power source.

CHAPTER 30 • New

CHAPTER 31 • Existing

**31.3.4.5.3** In buildings other than those equipped throughout with an existing, complete automatic smoke detection system or a complete, supervised automatic sprinkler system in accordance with 31.3.5, smoke alarms shall be installed in every sleeping area in accordance with 9.6.2.10, as modified by 31.3.4.5.4.

**31.3.4.5.4** Smoke alarms required by 31.3.4.5.3 shall be permitted to be battery powered.

**30.3.4.6* Protection of Fire Alarm System.** The provision of 9.6.1.8.1.3 shall not apply to the smoke detection required at each fire alarm control unit by 9.6.1.8.1(1).

**A.30.3.4.6** It is the intent that smoke detection be provided at each fire alarm control unit, regardless of the presence of sprinkler systems.

**31.3.4.6* Protection of Fire Alarm System.** The provision of 9.6.1.8.1.3 shall not apply to the smoke detection required at each fire alarm control unit by 9.6.1.8.1(1).

**A.31.3.4.6** It is the intent that smoke detection be provided at each fire alarm control unit, regardless of the presence of sprinkler protection.

Existing apartment buildings using Option 2 are protected throughout by a fire detection system (see 31.3.4.4). The increased travel distance permitted in an Option 2 apartment building (see 31.2.6.1 and 31.2.6.2) is based on early occupant notification of fire. Therefore, the detectors must initiate the alarm system in addition to the initiation provided by manual fire alarm boxes.

Sprinkler systems protect the corridors of existing apartment buildings using Option 3 (see 31.3.5.9). The activation of the sprinkler system must initiate the alarm system in addition to the initiation provided by manual fire alarm boxes.

Existing apartment buildings using Option 4 are protected throughout by automatic sprinkler systems (see 31.3.5.10). The activation of the sprinkler system must initiate the alarm system in addition to the initiation provided by manual fire alarm boxes.

Automatic fire alarm annunciation is exempted by 30/31.3.4.3.4, based on the presence of automatic sprinklers and small building size. Given the additional limitation on building height and number of units, it is believed that fire in a fully sprinklered building can be controlled to a level that allows a delay by responding emergency forces in locating a fire.

In existing apartment buildings using Option 2, a total automatic fire detection system is required and must be interconnected with the building fire alarm system in accordance with 31.3.4.2.3. This system is required in addition to the smoke alarms required by 31.3.4.5. Note that 31.3.4.4 does not require the fire detection system to be comprised solely of smoke detectors but, instead, permits the use of either heat or smoke detectors, or combinations of the two. Heat detectors are permitted by 31.3.4.4, because they are used as part of a system that is separate from the smoke alarms addressed in 31.3.4.5. The smoke alarms will alert occupants within an apartment of a fire originating within that unit. When an occupant leaves the apartment, the door closes and latches behind the occupant (see 31.3.6.2.3), and the occupant pulls a manual fire alarm box. If the occupant fails to sound the alarm manually and the fire continues to develop in the apartment, the heat detectors will initiate the building fire alarm system prior to the fire becoming a threat to other apartment units. Fire detection systems have proved very effective where used. In addition, because the system is required to be tied into the building fire alarm system, the use of heat detectors instead of system smoke detectors would eliminate many nuisance alarms that might occur because of cooking or smoking.

The smoke alarm(s) required by 30.3.4.5 and 31.3.4.5.1 should be located in the hall area(s) that provides access to rooms used for sleeping. New apartment buildings are also required to provide smoke alarms in sleeping rooms, regardless of sprinkler protection; this requirement is new to the 2009 edition of the *Code*. In multilevel apartment units, the smoke alarm covering the upper level should normally be located at the top of the stairs. The smoke alarm(s) should be mounted on the ceiling or on the wall; those mounted on the wall should be within 12 in. (305 mm) of, but not closer than 4 in. (100 mm) from, the ceiling. The smoke alarm should be remotely located from the cooking area. Where unusual factors such as room configuration, air movement, or stagnant air pockets must be considered, the authority having jurisdiction (AHJ) and the designer should determine the place-

CHAPTER 30 • New

ment of the smoke alarms. See *NFPA 72®, National Fire Alarm Code®*,[2] for additional details.

Note that 9.6.2.10.2 requires smoke alarms to be powered as required by *NFPA 72; NFPA 72* requires smoke alarms to be powered by the building's electrical system, which is achieved by using directly wired or plug-in-type smoke alarms. Battery-powered units do not meet the requirements of 9.6.2.10.2.

**30.3.5 Extinguishment Requirements.**

**30.3.5.1** All buildings shall be protected throughout by an approved, supervised automatic sprinkler system installed in accordance with 30.3.5.2.

**30.3.5.2** Where an automatic sprinkler system is installed, either for total or partial building coverage, the system shall be installed in accordance with Section 9.7, as modified by 30.3.5.3 and 30.3.5.4. In buildings four or fewer stories above grade plane, systems in accordance with NFPA 13R, *Standard for the Installation of Sprinkler Systems in Residential Occupancies up to and Including Four Stories in Height*, shall be permitted.

**30.3.5.3** In buildings sprinklered in accordance with NFPA 13, *Standard for the Installation of Sprinkler Systems*, closets less than 12 ft² (1.1 m²) in area in individual dwelling units shall not be required to be sprinklered. Closets that contain equipment such as washers, dryers, furnaces, or water heaters shall be sprinklered, regardless of size.

Paragraph 30.3.5.3 exempts small closets from being sprinklered because of the limited fuel load characteristic of apartment unit closets. The closets exempted are limited to those within a living unit; closets in common building areas are not exempted. Also, any closet that contains HVAC equipment or washers and dryers is not permitted to take advantage of the sprinkler exemption due to the inherent ignition sources and combustible fuel load.

In the 1997 edition of the *Code*, it was the intent that 30.3.5.3 override the requirements in both NFPA 13, *Standard for the Installation of Sprinkler Systems*, and

CHAPTER 31 • Existing

It is not the *Code*'s intent to prohibit interconnecting smoke alarms within a single apartment. If an apartment unit needs more than one smoke alarm, interconnection will probably be required to meet the performance criterion for audibility detailed in 9.6.2.10.3.

**31.3.5 Extinguishment Requirements.**

**31.3.5.1 Reserved.**

**31.3.5.2 Reserved.**

**31.3.5.3*** Where an automatic sprinkler system is installed, either for total or partial building coverage, the system shall be installed in accordance with Section 9.7, as modified by 31.3.5.4 and 31.3.5.5. In buildings four or fewer stories above grade plane, systems in accordance with NFPA 13R, *Standard for the Installation of Sprinkler Systems in Residential Occupancies up to and Including Four Stories in Height*, shall be permitted.

**A.31.3.5.3** Although not required by the *Code*, the use of residential sprinklers or quick-response sprinklers is encouraged for new installations of sprinkler systems within dwelling units, apartments, and guest rooms. Caution should be exercised, because the system needs to be designed for the sprinkler being used.

**31.3.5.4** In individual dwelling units, sprinkler installation shall not be required in closets not exceeding 24 ft² (2.2 m²) and in bathrooms not exceeding 55 ft² (5.1 m²). Closets that contain equipment such as washers, dryers, furnaces, or water heaters shall be sprinklered, regardless of size.

CHAPTER 30 • New

NFPA 13R, *Standard for the Installation of Sprinkler Systems in Residential Occupancies up to and Including Four Stories in Height*.[3] As a result of subsequent changes to NFPA 13R, the provision now applies only where the sprinkler system is designed in accordance with NFPA 13, which only permits the omission of sprinklers from closets not greater than 24 ft² (2.2 m²) in hotels and motels. It is not the intent of 30.3.5.3 to be more restrictive than NFPA 13R, which permits the omission of sprinklers from closets in any residential occupancy having an area of not greater than 24 ft² (2.2 m²), with the least dimension of the closet not exceeding 36 in. (915 mm) and the walls and ceilings of the closet surfaced with noncombustible or limited-combustible material (such as gypsum wallboard).

**30.3.5.4** The draft stop and closely spaced sprinkler requirements of NFPA 13, *Standard for the Installation of Sprinkler Systems*, shall not be required for convenience openings complying with 8.6.8.2 where the convenience opening is within the dwelling unit.

The *Code* permits NFPA 13R, *Standard for the Installation of Sprinkler Systems in Residential Occupancies up to and Including Four Stories in Height*, to be used, within its scope, in place of NFPA 13, *Standard for the Installation of Sprinkler Systems*. However, the provision of 30.3.5.5, which requires the use of listed quick-response sprinklers or listed residential sprinklers within dwelling units of new apartment buildings, supersedes any sprinkler options permitted by NFPA 13R or NFPA 13.

**30.3.5.5** Listed quick-response or listed residential sprinklers shall be used throughout all dwelling units.

**30.3.5.6** Open parking structures complying with NFPA 88A, *Standard for Parking Structures*, that are contiguous with apartment buildings shall be exempt from the sprinkler requirements of 30.3.5.1.

**30.3.5.7** Buildings with unprotected openings in accordance with 8.6.6 shall be protected throughout by an approved, supervised automatic sprinkler system in accordance with 30.3.5.

**30.3.5.8 Reserved.**

CHAPTER 31 • Existing

**31.3.5.5** The draft stop and closely spaced sprinkler requirements of NFPA 13, *Standard for the Installation of Sprinkler Systems*, shall not be required for convenience openings complying with 8.6.8.2 where the convenience opening is within the dwelling unit.

**31.3.5.6 Reserved.**

**31.3.5.7 Reserved.**

**31.3.5.8 Reserved.**

**31.3.5.9** Buildings using Option 3 shall be provided with automatic sprinkler protection installed in accordance with 31.3.5.9.1 through 31.3.5.9.4.

**31.3.5.9.1** Automatic sprinklers shall be installed in the corridor, along the corridor ceiling, utilizing the maximum spacing requirements of the standards referenced by Section 9.7.

**31.3.5.9.2** An automatic sprinkler shall be installed within every dwelling unit that has a door opening to the corridor, with such sprinkler positioned over the center of the door, unless the door to the dwelling unit has not less than a 20-minute fire protection rating and is self-closing.

**31.3.5.9.3** The workmanship and materials of the sprinkler installation specified in 31.3.5.9 shall meet the requirements of Section 9.7.

**31.3.5.9.4** Where Option 3 is being used to permit the use of $1^3/_4$ in. (44 mm) thick, solid-bonded wood-core doors in accordance with 31.2.2.1.3, sprinklers shall be provided within the exit enclosures in accordance with NFPA 13, *Standard for the Installation of Sprinkler Systems*.

**30.3.5.9 Reserved.**

**31.3.5.10** Buildings using Option 4 shall be protected throughout by an approved automatic sprinkler system in accordance with 31.3.5.3 and meeting the requirements of Section 9.7 for supervision for buildings seven or more stories in height.

**30.3.5.10 Reserved.**

**31.3.5.11*** Where sprinklers are being used as an option to any requirement in this *Code*, the sprinklers shall be installed throughout the space in accordance with the requirements of that option.

**A.31.3.5.11** For example, if an Option 3 sprinkler system were being used to justify use of Class C wall finish in an exit enclosure, the sprinkler system would need to be extended into the exit enclosure, even if the rest of the requirements for Option 3 did not require the sprinklers in the exit enclosure.

**30.3.5.11 Reserved.**

**31.3.5.12 High-Rise Building Sprinklers.**

**31.3.5.12.1** All high-rise buildings, other than those meeting 31.3.5.12.2 or 31.3.5.12.3 shall be protected throughout by an approved, supervised automatic sprinkler system in accordance with 31.3.5.3.

**31.3.5.12.2** An automatic sprinkler system shall not be required where every dwelling unit has exterior exit access in accordance with 7.5.3.

**31.3.5.12.3*** An automatic sprinkler system shall not be required in buildings having an approved, engineered life safety system in accordance with 31.3.5.12.4.

**A.31.3.5.12.3** This system might consist of a combination of any or all of the following systems:

(1) Partial automatic sprinkler protection
(2) Smoke detection alarms
(3) Smoke control
(4) Compartmentation or other approved systems, or both

**31.3.5.12.4** Where required by 31.3.5.12.3, an engineered life safety system shall be developed by a registered professional engineer experienced in fire and life safety system design, shall be approved by the authority having jurisdiction, and shall include any or all of the following:

(1) Partial automatic sprinkler protection
(2) Smoke detection systems
(3) Smoke control systems
(4) Compartmentation
(5) Other approved systems

CHAPTER 30 • New

**30.3.5.12** Portable fire extinguishers in accordance with 9.7.4.1 shall be provided in hazardous areas addressed by 30.3.2.1, unless the building is protected throughout with an approved, supervised automatic sprinkler system in accordance with 30.3.5.2.

CHAPTER 31 • Existing

**31.3.5.13** Portable fire extinguishers in accordance with 9.7.4.1 shall be provided in hazardous areas addressed by 31.3.2.1, unless the building is protected throughout with an approved, supervised automatic sprinkler system in accordance with 31.3.5.3.

For existing apartment buildings, Option 3 and Option 4 require the installation of automatic sprinklers. Exhibit 30/31.9 illustrates the sprinkler location requirements for an Option 3 existing apartment building. A 20-minute fire protection–rated, self-closing corridor door is permitted by 31.3.5.9.2 to serve in lieu of the sprinklers positioned inside each apartment unit in the vicinity of the corridor door; however, the corridor sprinklers must still be provided.

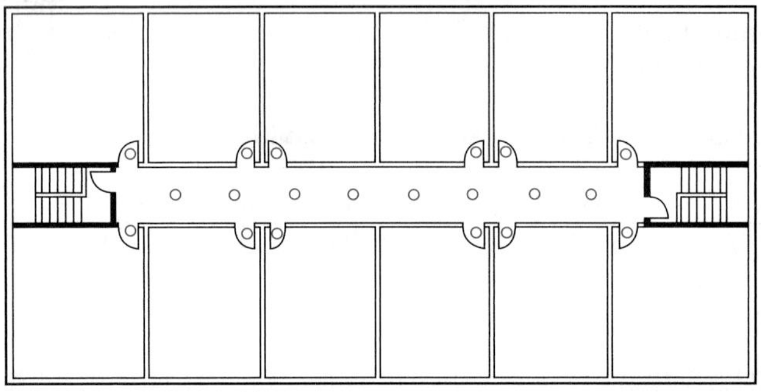


***Exhibit 30/31.9** Option 3 sprinkler protection for existing apartment buildings.*

The *Code* provides numerous incentives for existing apartment buildings to use Option 4 (complete sprinkler protection), as detailed in 31.3.5.10. Some of the more significant incentives that apply to existing apartment buildings are provided in 31.2.4.3 (single exit), 31.2.6 (increased permitted travel distances), 31.2.11.1 (elimination of smokeproof enclosure requirement for high-rise buildings), 31.3.6.2.2 (elimination of corridor door fire protection rating requirement), and 31.3.7.1 (elimination of smoke compartmentation).

One of the objectives of the *Code* is to provide a structure that will protect occupants who are not intimate with the initial fire development for the time needed to evacuate (see 4.1.1). Given that objective, new apartment buildings are required to use quick-response or residential sprinklers throughout apartment dwelling units. The use of approved residential or quick-response sprinklers within dwelling units of existing apartment buildings is encouraged by A.31.3.5.3. The *Code*'s intent is to obtain the quick response provided by these sprinklers as well as the high-spray pattern provided by residential sprinklers. The technology associated with quick-response and residential sprinklers helps to maintain tenability within the room of fire origin.

Designers of sprinkler systems must use caution, as residential and quick-response sprinklers cannot always be installed in a system that was originally designed for standard sprinklers. Situations also exist where residential or quick-response sprinklers might not be listed for use, such as an area with vaulted ceilings. In such cases, the designer could provide the best alternative sprinkler.

Approved supervised sprinkler systems are required throughout existing high-rise apartment buildings per 31.3.5.12. See the definition of *high-rise building* in 3.3.32.7. However, the *Code* does provide two alternatives. The first exempts sprinklers throughout if each living unit has direct exterior exit access. The *Code* also permits the application of an approved engineered life safety system in lieu of installing sprinklers throughout. Although not required, A.31.3.5.12.2 recommends that this engineered life safety system include some combination of automatic sprinkler protection, detection, smoke control, and compartmentation. The *Code* further requires that the authority having jurisdiction (AHJ) approve an alternative approach. During the planning phase, the designer should meet with the AHJ to determine whether a system is acceptable in lieu of automatic sprinklers.

### 30.3.6 Corridors.

**30.3.6.1 Walls.** Exit access corridor walls shall comply with 30.3.6.1.1 or 30.3.6.1.2.

### 31.3.6 Corridors.

**31.3.6.1* Walls.** Exit access corridor walls shall consist of fire barriers in accordance with Section 8.3 having a minimum $\frac{1}{2}$-hour fire resistance rating.

CHAPTER 30 • New

30.3.6.1.1 In buildings not complying with 30.3.6.1.1, exit access corridor walls shall consist of fire barriers in accordance with Section 8.3 that have not less than a 1-hour fire resistance rating.

30.3.6.1.2 In buildings protected throughout by an approved, supervised automatic sprinkler system in accordance with 30.3.5.2, corridor walls shall have a minimum ½-hour fire resistance rating.

**30.3.6.2 Doors.**

**30.3.6.2.1** Doors that open onto exit access corridors shall have not less than a 20-minute fire protection rating in accordance with Section 8.3.

**30.3.6.2.2 Reserved.**

**30.3.6.2.3** Doors that open onto exit access corridors shall be self-closing and self-latching.

**30.3.6.3 Unprotected Openings.**

**30.3.6.3.1** Unprotected openings, other than those from spaces complying with 30.3.6.3.2, shall be prohibited in exit access corridor walls and doors.

**30.3.6.3.2** Spaces shall be permitted to be unlimited in area and open to the corridor, provided that the following criteria are met:

(1) The space is not used for guest rooms or guest suites or hazardous areas.
(2) The building is protected throughout by an approved, supervised automatic sprinkler system in accordance with 30.3.5.
(3) The space does not obstruct access to required exits.

**30.3.6.4 Transoms, Louvers, or Transfer Grilles.** Transoms, louvers, or transfer grilles shall be prohibited in walls or doors of exit access corridors.

CHAPTER 31 • Existing

**A.31.3.6.1** The intent is to recognize that existing partitions of sound wood lath and plaster, wire lath and plaster, or gypsum lath and plaster construction have demonstrated the ability to contain most room fires. Recent data on archaic construction methods have established the fire resistance rating of such construction at about 20 minutes. Such construction meets the intent of 31.3.6.1.

**31.3.6.2 Doors.**

**31.3.6.2.1** Doors that open onto exit access corridors, other than those complying with 8.3.4 or in buildings meeting the requirement of 31.3.6.2.2, shall have not less than a 20-minute fire protection rating in accordance with Section 8.3.

**31.3.6.2.2** In buildings using Option 3 or Option 4, doors shall be constructed to resist the passage of smoke.

**31.3.6.2.3** Doors that open onto exit access corridors shall be self-closing and self-latching.

**31.3.6.3 Unprotected Openings.**

**31.3.6.3.1** Unprotected openings, other than those from spaces complying with 31.3.6.3.2, shall be prohibited in exit access corridor walls and doors.

**31.3.6.3.2** Spaces shall be permitted to be unlimited in area and open to the corridor, provided that the following criteria are met:

(1) The space is not used for guest rooms or guest suites or hazardous areas.
(2) The building is protected throughout by an approved, supervised automatic sprinkler system in accordance with 31.3.5.3.
(3) The space does not obstruct access to required exits.

**31.3.6.4 Transoms, Louvers, or Transfer Grilles.** Transoms, louvers, or transfer grilles shall be prohibited in walls or doors of exit access corridors.

The provisions of 30/31.3.6 reflect concern for providing safety for occupants in their apartments during a fire. The minimum 1-hour fire resistance rating required for corridor wall construction in new nonsprinklered apartment buildings is intended to prevent fire from moving from the corridor to an apartment or from an apartment to the corridor.

The minimum ½-hour fire resistance rating required for corridor wall construction in existing apartment buildings recognizes that most existing lath and plaster walls provide a 30-minute fire resistance rating.

The provision of 30.3.6.1.2 also permits a reduction to a ½-hour fire resistance rating in new sprinklered apartment buildings. Although this reduction would result in little savings in new construction, it could be useful in the rehabilitation of existing structures that are required to meet the provisions for new construction (see 4.6.8 and Chapter 43). If automatic sprinkler protection is provided throughout the building, the existing corridor walls should not have to be replaced.

The installation and proper maintenance of the required self-closing device on the door between an apartment and the common corridor could lead to a

CHAPTER 30 • New

significant reduction in fatalities caused by fire in apartment buildings. Studies of typical apartment fires indicate that fire spreads beyond the apartment of origin because doors are left open as occupants escape.

In other cases, fatalities occur when occupants who suspect a fire open the door to a room fully involved with fire or cause full fire involvement of the room by introducing oxygen through the open door. Spring-loaded hinges or closers will cause these doors to close and latch, preventing smoke or fire from spreading into the corridor and exposing other occupants.

The doors required by 30/31.3.6.2 provide a level of protection commensurate with the expected fuel load in the apartment unit and the fire resistance of the corridor wall construction. The purpose is to box a fire out of or within an apartment unit by means of corridor wall and door construction. Fuel load studies conducted by the former National Bureau of Standards (now the National Institute of Standards and Technology) demonstrated that residential occupancies typically have fuel loads capable of sustaining a fire for approximately 20 minutes to 30 minutes.

Exhibit 30/31.10 and Exhibit 30/31.11 detail the corridor wall construction and opening protection requirements of 30.3.6 and 31.3.6, respectively.

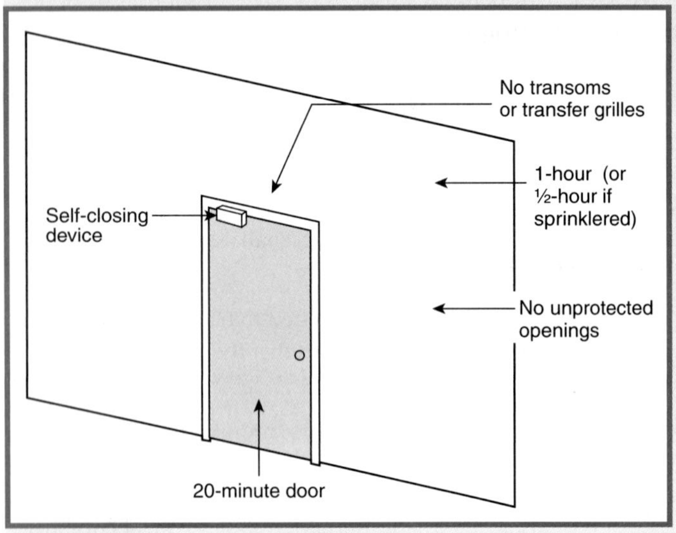


*Exhibit 30/31.10 Corridor wall construction in new apartment building.*

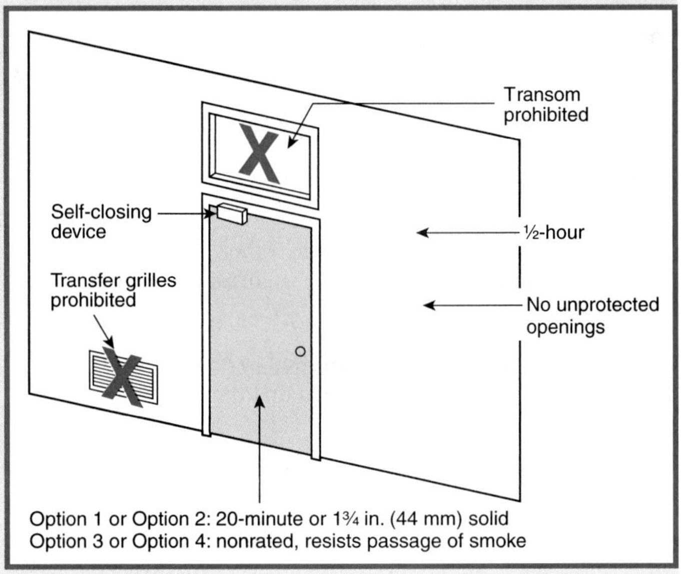


*Exhibit 30/31.11 Corridor wall construction in existing apartment building.*

### 30.3.7 Subdivisions of Building Spaces.

Buildings shall be subdivided in accordance with 30.3.7.1 or 30.3.7.2.

**30.3.7.1** In buildings not meeting the requirement of 30.3.7.2, dwelling units shall be separated from each other by walls and floors constructed as fire barriers having a minimum 1-hour fire resistance rating.

CHAPTER 31 • Existing

### 31.3.7 Subdivision of Building Spaces — Smoke Partitions.

In buildings other than those meeting the requirements of 31.3.7.1, 31.3.7.2, 31.3.7.3, 31.3.7.4, or 31.3.7.5, the following criteria shall be met:

(1) Smoke partitions in accordance with Section 8.4 shall be provided in exit access corridors to establish not less than two compartments of approximately equal size.
(2) The length of each smoke compartment, measured along the corridor, shall not exceed 200 ft (61 m).

**31.3.7.1** Smoke partitions shall not be required in buildings using Option 4.

CHAPTER 30 • New

30.3.7.2 In buildings protected throughout by an approved, supervised, automatic sprinkler system, dwelling units shall be separated from each other by walls and floors constructed as fire barriers having a minimum ½-hour fire resistance rating.

CHAPTER 31 • Existing

**31.3.7.2** Smoke partitions shall not be required in buildings having exterior exit access in accordance with 7.5.3 that provides access to two exits.

**31.3.7.3** Smoke partitions shall not be required in buildings complying with 31.2.4.2, 31.2.4.3, 31.2.4.4, or 31.2.4.5.

**31.3.7.4** Smoke partitions shall not be required in buildings with exits not more than 50 ft (15 m) apart.

**31.3.7.5** Smoke partitions shall not be required where each dwelling unit has direct access to the exterior at the finished ground level.

The smoke partitions required by 31.3.7 for existing apartment buildings are relatively easy to provide, because no fire resistance rating is required and smoke dampers are not required at duct penetrations. In most cases, installing a set of cross-corridor doors with smoke-actuated automatic closers will meet the requirement. Exemptions to the smoke partition requirement are provided for sprinklered buildings (31.3.7.1), buildings with a single exit (31.3.7.3), and buildings that do not use corridors as required exit access (31.3.7.2 and 31.3.7.5).

The provision of 31.3.7.4 exempts smoke partitions from being located on a floor where the exit stairs are spaced not farther than 50 ft (15 m) apart, measured along the corridor.

### 30.3.8 Special Protection Features. (Reserved)

### 31.3.8 Special Protection Features. (Reserved)

## 30.4 Special Provisions

### 30.4.1 High-Rise Buildings.

**30.4.1.1** High-rise buildings shall comply with Section 11.8. The provisions of 30.3.5.3 and 30.3.5.4 shall be permitted.

**30.4.1.2*** Emergency plans in accordance with Section 4.8 shall be provided and shall include the following:

(1) Egress procedures
(2) Methods
(3) Preferred evacuation routes for each event, including appropriate use of elevators

**A.30.4.1.2** See 4.8.2.1(4).

## 31.4 Special Provisions

### 31.4.1 High-Rise Buildings.

**31.4.1.1** High-rise buildings shall comply with 31.2.11.1 and 31.3.5.12.

**31.4.1.2*** Emergency plans in accordance with Section 4.8 shall be provided and shall include the following:

(1) Egress procedures
(2) Methods
(3) Preferred evacuation routes for each event, including appropriate use of elevators

**A.31.4.1.2** See 4.8.2.1(4).

In response to recommendations from the NFPA High-Rise Building Safety Advisory Committee following the September 11, 2001, terrorist attacks on the World Trade Center in New York City and the Pentagon in Arlington, Virginia, the provisions of 30/31.4.1.2, which are new to the 2009 edition of the *Code*, require both new and existing high-rise apartment buildings to be provided with emergency plans. See the extensive provisions of A.4.8.2.1 and A.4.8.2.1(3) and the associated commentary, which are also new to the 2009 edition, for details on the items that should be included in the emergency plan and a primer on the development of evacuation strategies for specific buildings.

CHAPTER 30 • New

**30.4.2 Reserved.**

## 30.5 Building Services

### 30.5.1 Utilities.

Utilities shall comply with the provisions of Section 9.1.

### 30.5.2 Heating, Ventilating, and Air-Conditioning.

**30.5.2.1** Heating, ventilating, and air-conditioning equipment shall comply with the provisions of Section 9.2.

NFPA 90A, *Standard for the Installation of Air-Conditioning and Ventilating Systems,*[4] as referenced in Section 9.2, prohibits the use of public corridors in residential occupancies as part of the system for supply, return, or exhaust air. This prohibition is intended to limit the transfer of heat and smoke between apartment units and the corridor via the air-handling system. In addition, NFPA 90A requires automatic shutdown of the air-handling system upon detection of smoke in the system if it exceeds specified capacities.

**30.5.2.2** Unvented fuel-fired heaters, other than gas space heaters in compliance with NFPA 54, *National Fuel Gas Code*, shall not be used.

### 30.5.3 Elevators, Escalators, and Conveyors.

Elevators, escalators, and conveyors shall comply with the provisions of Section 9.4.

### 30.5.4 Rubbish Chutes, Incinerators, and Laundry Chutes.

Rubbish chutes, incinerators, and laundry chutes shall comply with the provisions of Section 9.5.

## 30.6 Reserved

## 30.7 Operating Features

### 30.7.1 Emergency Instructions for Residents of Apartment Buildings.

Emergency instructions shall be provided annually to each dwelling unit to indicate the location of alarms, egress paths, and actions to be taken, both in response to a fire in the dwelling unit and in response to the sounding of the alarm system.

CHAPTER 31 • Existing

**31.4.2 Reserved.**

## 31.5 Building Services

### 31.5.1 Utilities.

Utilities shall comply with the provisions of Section 9.1.

### 31.5.2 Heating, Ventilating, and Air-Conditioning.

**31.5.2.1** Heating, ventilating, and air-conditioning equipment shall comply with the provisions of Section 9.2.

**31.5.2.2** Unvented fuel-fired heaters, other than gas space heaters in compliance with NFPA 54, *National Fuel Gas Code*, shall not be used.

### 31.5.3 Elevators, Escalators, and Conveyors.

Elevators, escalators, and conveyors shall comply with the provisions of Section 9.4.

### 31.5.4 Rubbish Chutes, Incinerators, and Laundry Chutes.

Rubbish chutes, incinerators, and laundry chutes shall comply with the provisions of Section 9.5.

## 31.6 Reserved

## 31.7 Operating Features

### 31.7.1 Emergency Instructions for Residents of Apartment Buildings.

Emergency instructions shall be provided annually to each dwelling unit to indicate the location of alarms, egress paths, and actions to be taken, both in response to a fire in the dwelling unit and in response to the sounding of the alarm system.

The manner in which the information required by Section 30/31.7.1 is provided to the residents, and the nature of its contents, are at the discretion of the authority having jurisdiction (AHJ) and depend on the building, its layout, and the protection provided. For example, the instructions could be provided to residents when they sign their lease and move into their apartment and every year thereafter when the lease is renewed. The building's management should review the instructions periodically so they can be updated with any needed revisions resulting from changes to the building's configuration or protection systems.

### 30.7.2 Contents and Furnishings.

**30.7.2.1** Contents and furnishings shall not be required to comply with Section 10.3.

**30.7.2.2** Furnishings or decorations of an explosive or highly flammable character shall not be used outside of dwelling units.

**30.7.2.3** Fire-retardant coatings shall be maintained to retain the effectiveness of the treatment under service conditions encountered in actual use.

### 31.7.2 Contents and Furnishings.

**31.7.2.1** Contents and furnishings shall not be required to comply with Section 10.3.

**31.7.2.2** Furnishings or decorations of an explosive or highly flammable character shall not be used outside of dwelling units.

**31.7.2.3** Fire-retardant coatings shall be maintained to retain the effectiveness of the treatment under service conditions encountered in actual use.

## References Cited in Commentary


1. NFPA 13, *Standard for the Installation of Sprinkler Systems*, 2007 edition, National Fire Protection Association, Quincy, MA.
2. *NFPA 72®, National Fire Alarm Code®*, 2007 edition, National Fire Protection Association, Quincy, MA.
3. NFPA 13R, *Standard for the Installation of Sprinkler Systems in Residential Occupancies up to and Including Four Stories in Height*, 2007 edition, National Fire Protection Association, Quincy, MA.
4. NFPA 90A, *Standard for the Installation of Air-Conditioning and Ventilating Systems*, 2009 edition, National Fire Protection Association, Quincy, MA.

## CHAPTERS 32 AND 33

# New and Existing Residential Board and Care Occupancies

The primary characteristics that differentiate residential board and care occupancies from other residential occupancies is the assumed ability (or lack thereof) of occupants to evacuate the building in the event of a fire or similar emergency and the availability or level of personal care services. *Personal care*, as defined in 3.3.192, includes assistance with many of the activities of daily living. Personal care services might include assisting residents with bathing and dressing and helping residents with bill payment and similar household maintenance–related tasks. Personal care does not include nursing home–type care; nor does it include medical care.

Prior to the 2003 edition of the *Code*, application of the requirements for both new and existing residential board and care facilities required the determination of the occupants' evacuation capability — that is, the occupants' ability to move, as a group, to a point of safety in the event of a fire. Evacuation capability was broken down into three subclasses — prompt, slow, and impractical. Ongoing evaluation by the authority having jurisdiction (AHJ) was required to ensure the facility was not being used outside the limitations of its design (e.g., a facility designed and constructed using the provisions for slow evacuation capability actually having an impractical evacuation capability). When tasked with the development of provisions for residential board and care facilities to be included in *NFPA 5000®, Building Construction and Safety Code®*,[1] the NFPA Technical Committee on Board and Care Facilities recognized that, because a facility's population is expected to change over time, a facility's evacuation capability will likely change over time as well. It was not, then, practical to simply insert the requirements from this *Code* into *NFPA 5000*. As such, the committee modified the requirements for new board and care facilities so as not to depend on the evacuation capability of the occupants of the facility.

For consistency with *NFPA 5000*, the committee also revised the provisions of Chapter 32 of this *Code*, which address new facilities, so they no longer depend on the determination of evacuation capability. Chapter 33, which addresses existing facilities, retains the evacuation capability provisions so as to not place existing facilities out of compliance. Since new board and care facilities might contain occupants who do not have the ability to evacuate without assistance, they must be designed and constructed to facilitate the "defend-in-place" occupant protection strategy, much like health care occupancies. To utilize the defend-in-place strategy, the building must be able to withstand the effects of fire for the time necessary to either evacuate the occupants or relocate them to a safe location within the building.

Chapters 32 and 33 classify residential board and care occupancies based on the number of residents. For this purpose, the chapters are further subdivided to address requirements for small (16 or fewer residents) and large (more than 16 residents) facilities. As the number of residents put at risk by fire increases, the requirements naturally become stricter.

Of the determinations that must be made to classify a residential board and care occupancy (i.e., availability of personal care, number of residents, and, in the case of existing facilities, evacuation capability), the most difficult is evacuation capability. Evacuation capability is established on the basis of the occupants' (i.e., residents and staff working together) ability to move to a safe location, such as an enclosed exit stair or a point outside of the structure. The term *evacuation capability* is defined in 3.3.70; A.3.3.70 provides guidance on classifying evacuation capability.

Where an existing facility does not comply with the requirements for new facilities in Chapter 32, Chapter 33 requires facility management to furnish the AHJ with an evacuation capability determination conducted using a procedure acceptable to the AHJ. If such documentation is not furnished, the evacuation capability is considered, by default, as impractical.

Protection features for residential board and care occupancies range from regulating the allowable types of construction, to mandating alarm and detection systems, to mandating automatic sprinkler protection for all new facilities.

Another difference between board and care occupancies and other residential occupancies is highlighted in Section 32/33.4, which addresses the location of a residential board and care occupancy within an apartment building. The apartment building itself is evaluated on its suitability to house the residential board and care occupancy. The apartment units used as a residential board and care occupancy are judged individually, based on the requirements of Section 32/33.2, which applies to small residential board and care occupancies.

As in the case of other occupancy chapters that address occupants with limited self-preservation capability, Chapters 32 and 33 rely on staff intervention and staff support to assist the residents during fire and similar emergencies. It is the responsibility of the staff to understand and implement the emergency plan for the facility. The plan must include a method for familiarizing residents with the procedures to be followed during a fire.

## 32.1 General Requirements

### 32.1.1 Application.

**32.1.1.1 General.** The requirements of this chapter shall apply to new buildings or portions thereof used as residential board and care occupancies. *(See 1.3.1.)*

**32.1.1.2 Reserved.**

## 33.1 General Requirements

### 33.1.1* Application.

**A.33.1.1** The requirements of Chapter 33 are designed to accommodate typical changes in the capabilities of the resident, such as those due to accidents, temporary illness, cyclical variations in capabilities, and gradual aging. This approach is based on the assumption that the capabilities of the resident will be evaluated not less than annually, and for residents with geriatric problems or degenerative diseases, not less than every 6 months. Also, residents should be re-evaluated after each accident or illness that requires hospitalization.

The requirements of Chapter 33 were developed on the assumption that the occupants will normally evacuate the building in fire emergencies. During fire exit drills, all occupants should evacuate the building with staff assistance, as needed. Exceptions can be made in facilities with an evacuation capability rating of impractical. Managers of board and care homes with nursing home backgrounds sometimes are not aware of the differences between the requirements of 19.7.1 and 33.7.3.

**33.1.1.1 General.** The requirements of this chapter shall apply to existing buildings or portions thereof currently occupied as residential board and care occupancies.

**33.1.1.2* Chapter 32 Compliance.** Any facility meeting the requirements of Chapter 32 shall not be required to meet those of Chapter 33.

**A.33.1.1.2** The provision of 33.1.1.2 was added after Chapter 32 was revised in its entirety to avoid potential conflicts between the two chapters. Occupancies meeting Chapter 32 requirements are deemed to comply with Chapter 33.

The provisions for new board and care facilities are addressed in Chapter 32; the provisions for existing board and care facilities (i.e., existing conditions in board and care facilities) are addressed in Chapter 33.

Prior to the 2006 edition of the *Code*, renovations, additions, and changes of occupancy were required to comply with the requirements for new construction. For residential board and care facilities, such renovations, additions, and changes of occupancy were required to meet the provisions of Chapter 32, while existing conditions were subject to the provisions of Chapter 33. For the 2006 edition of the *Code*, Chapter 43, Building Rehabilitation, was added. Chapter 43 promotes the adaptive reuse of existing buildings without sacrificing the needed level of life safety. The provisions of Chapter 43 blend the requirements for new construction with those for existing conditions, so as to require additional life safety features as the rehabilitation work category increases in complexity. The rehabilitation work categories are repair, renovation, modification, reconstruction, change of use or occupancy classification, and addition. See 4.6.8, 4.6.12, and Chapter 43.

**32.1.1.3 Chapter Sections.** This chapter is divided into five sections as follows:

(1) Section 32.1 — General Requirements
(2) Section 32.2 — Small Facilities (that is, sleeping accommodations for not more than 16 residents)
(3) Section 32.3 — Large Facilities (that is, sleeping accommodations for more than 16 residents)
(4) Section 32.4 — Suitability of an Apartment Building to House a Board and Care Occupancy *(Sections 32.5 and 32.6 are reserved.)*
(5) Section 32.7 — Operating Features

**32.1.1.4 Conversion.** For the purposes of this chapter, exceptions for conversions shall apply only for a change of occupancy from an existing residential or health care occupancy to a residential board and care occupancy.

**33.1.1.3 Chapter Sections.** This chapter is divided into five sections as follows:

(1) Section 33.1 — General Requirements
(2) Section 33.2 — Small Facilities (that is, sleeping accommodations for not more than 16 residents)
(3) Section 33.3 — Large Facilities (that is, sleeping accommodations for more than 16 residents)
(4) Section 33.4 — Suitability of an Apartment Building to House a Board and Care Occupancy *(Sections 33.5 and 33.6 are reserved.)*
(5) Section 33.7 — Operating Features

**33.1.1.4 Conversion.** For the purposes of this chapter, exceptions for conversions shall apply only for a change of occupancy from an existing residential or health care occupancy to a residential board and care occupancy.

Residential board and care occupancies take many forms: assisted living facilities, halfway houses, retirement homes, rooming houses, and community living centers, among others. Regardless of the label, the level of care that is provided is the key to identifying a residential board and care facility.

In recent years, the number of retirement community facilities has grown. These facilities might provide different living arrangements for the elderly within the same building or a group of buildings. They also might offer any combination of independent living facilities (apartments), board and care facilities, and full nursing facilities. It is important that the occupancy classification for each building or area is properly identified and that proper separation between the occupancies is provided as necessary. See 32/33.1.2 for details on multiple occupancies involving board and care facilities.

From 1990 to 2006, NFPA documented multiple-death (defined as three or more fatalities) fires in 26 board and care occupancies resulting in 141 deaths. Commentary Table 32/33.1 provides a list of those fires, including those for which NFPA prepared fire investigation reports.

The following were major contributing factors to the loss of life in those fires investigated by NFPA:

1. Lack of automatic sprinklers
2. Doors open to the room of fire origin
3. Doors open to stairs or unprotected vertical openings
4. Ineffective staff or resident training or response

Chapters 32 and 33 address basic fire protection features for board and care facilities while maintaining the ability to operate such a facility in a noninstitutional environment. The requirements for small board and care facilities are similar to the provisions for one- and two-family dwellings and lodging or rooming houses. The requirements for existing large facilities, other than those in which residents are classified as impractical to evacuate, are similar to the requirements

***Commentary Table 32/33.1 Residential Board and Care Multiple-Death Fires***

| Year | Location | Fatalities |
|---|---|---|
| 1990 | Georgia | 4 |
| 1990 | Texas | 4 |
| 1990 | Bessemer, AL[1] | 4 |
| 1990 | Wisconsin | 3 |
| 1991 | Colorado Springs, CO[1] | 10 |
| 1992 | Detroit, MI[1] | 10 |
| 1993 | Texas | 3 |
| 1994 | Alabama | 6 |
| 1994 | Broward County, FL[1] | 6 |
| 1995 | Mississauga, Ontario[1] | 8 |
| 1995 | Oregon | 4 |
| 1995 | California | 3 |
| 1995 | Michigan | 3 |
| 1996 | Connecticut | 3 |
| 1996 | California | 3 |
| 1996 | Laurinberg, NC[1] | 8 |
| 1996 | Shelby County, TN[1] | 4 |
| 1996 | Ste. Genevieve, Quebec[1] | 7 |
| 1996 | Pennsylvania | 4 |
| 1997 | Harveys Lake, PA[1] | 10 |
| 1998 | Arlington, WA[1] | 8 |
| 2000 | Pennsylvania | 3 |
| 2003 | California | 4 |
| 2004 | Pennsylvania | 3 |
| 2004 | Tennessee | 5 |
| 2006 | Missouri | 11 |

[1]NFPA fire investigation report.

*Source:* NFPA, Fire Incident Data Organization (FIDO).

for new hotels; the requirements for new large facilities are similar to those for health care facilities because of the potential for occupants who are unable to evacuate themselves in the event of a fire. Existing large facilities in which residents are classified as impractical to evacuate must comply with the requirements of Chapter 19 or Chapter 32 (see 33.1.1.2 and 33.3.1.2.2). Although the provisions of Chapters 32 and 33 might be similar to those of other residential occupancies, certain requirements differ due to the unique characteristics of board and care facilities — such as the varying degrees to which occupants are able to respond to a fire emergency.

The requirements of Chapters 32 and 33 are based on two main concepts, as follows:

1. Larger buildings are more difficult to evacuate than smaller buildings and require more built-in fire protection.
2. Occupants who are more difficult to evacuate require more built-in fire protection than occupants who are easier to evacuate.

Chapter 32 essentially assumes impractical evacuation capability, while Chapter 33 requires ongoing evaluation to determine evacuation capability.

It is anticipated that a small facility typically will be located in a structure that has the appearance of, and that operates in a manner similar to, a dwelling. The operation and size of a small facility demand unique consideration with respect to the fire protection features provided. Certain fire protection features that are appropriate for large facilities, such as smoke barriers, might not be appropriate and might not provide adequate protection in small facilities. For this reason, 33.2.1.2.1.2, which permits small facilities to comply with the requirements for large facilities, applies only to those facilities that have previously met the criteria for the exemption. The 1985 edition of the *Code* permitted small facilities to comply with the requirements for large facilities in lieu of the provisions for small facilities. As stated in 33.2.1.2.1.2, a small facility that has previously been approved, based on the requirements for a large facility, is permitted to continue to be evaluated as a large facility. However, any other small facility must meet the provisions for a small facility and is not permitted to meet the provisions for a large facility as an alternative.

Several requirements in Chapter 32 are exempted for conversions. Where a building previously occupied as another type of residential occupancy or a health care occupancy is converted to a board and care facility, such change of use must comply with the requirements for new construction or Chapter 43 in accordance with 4.6.12. This requirement would apply where a hotel, an apartment building, a lodging or rooming house, a dwelling, a hospital, a nursing home, or a limited care facility is converted to a residential board and care facility. However, certain provisions of Chapter 32 are intended to eliminate undue hardship while maintaining a reasonable degree of life safety. In such cases, the specific wording of Chapter 32 exempts the existing building from meeting a requirement that would otherwise apply to a new board and care facility. For example, 32.2.2.5.1.2 permits existing 28 in. (710 mm) wide doors in converted facilities to remain in use rather than being replaced with the 32 in. (810 mm) wide doors normally required in new board and care facilities.

CHAPTER 32 • New

## 32.1.2 Multiple Occupancies.

**32.1.2.1** Multiple occupancies shall comply with 6.1.14 and 32.1.2 in buildings other than those meeting the requirement of 32.1.2.2.

**32.1.2.2** The requirement of 32.1.2.1 shall not apply to apartment buildings housing residential board and care occupancies in conformance with Section 32.4. In such facilities, any safeguards required by Section 32.4 that are more restrictive than those for other housed occupancies shall apply only to the extent prescribed by Section 32.4.

**32.1.2.3** No board and care occupancy shall have its sole means of egress or means of escape pass through any nonresidential or non-health care occupancy in the same building.

**32.1.2.4** No board and care occupancy shall be located above a nonresidential or non-health care occupancy, unless the board and care occupancy and exits therefrom are separated from the nonresidential or non-health care occupancy by construction having a minimum 2-hour fire resistance rating.

CHAPTER 33 • Existing

## 33.1.2 Multiple Occupancies.

**33.1.2.1** Multiple occupancies shall comply with 6.1.14 in buildings other than those meeting the requirement of 33.1.2.2.

**33.1.2.2** The requirement of 33.1.2.1 shall not apply to apartment buildings housing residential board and care occupancies in conformance with Section 33.4. In such facilities, any safeguards required by Section 33.4 that are more restrictive than those for other housed occupancies shall apply only to the extent prescribed by Section 33.4.

**33.1.2.3** No board and care occupancy shall have its sole means of egress or means of escape pass through any nonresidential or non-health care occupancy in the same building.

**33.1.2.4** No board and care occupancy shall be located above a nonresidential or non-health care occupancy, unless one of the following conditions is met:

(1) The board and care occupancy and exits therefrom are separated from the nonresidential or non-health care occupancy by construction having a minimum 2-hour fire resistance rating.
(2) The nonresidential or non-health care occupancy is protected throughout by an approved, supervised automatic sprinkler system in accordance with Section 9.7 and is separated therefrom by construction having a minimum 1-hour fire resistance rating.

The location of a board and care occupancy in a multiple occupancy building presents a life safety challenge for the occupants of the board and care occupancy. The typical configuration of such buildings creates the potential for significant time to elapse before occupants of the board and care occupancy become aware of an emergency in another part of the building and take the necessary action. The requirements of 32/33.1.2 help to ensure that it is safe to locate board and care occupancies within these multiple occupancy buildings by providing the necessary protection and separation. (See 6.1.14 for details on multiple occupancies.)

The requirements in 32/33.1.2.4 mandate that where a residential board and care facility is located above another type of occupancy, that board and care facility and its exit system must be separated from the other occupancy. Therefore, if a new residential board and care occupancy is located on the second floor, the exit stair must have a 2-hour fire-rated enclosure, even though 7.1.3.2 permits a 1-hour fire-rated enclosure. Where the separation requirements in Chapters 32 and 33 differ from those in Table 6.1.14.4.1(a) and Table 6.1.14.4.1(b), the more restrictive requirements apply — that is, those provisions requiring the higher fire resistance rating. Note that the requirements of 32/33.1.2.4 requiring rated separations supersede the option provided by Chapter 6 for mixed occupancies.

The provision of 33.1.2.2 clarifies that existing board and care facilities located within an apartment building need not comply with the requirements for a mixed apartment/board and care occupancy. The provisions of Section 33.4 apply to the entire building and supplement the provisions of Chapter 31 for apartment buildings. In addition, the apartment unit housing a board and care facility must comply with the provisions of Section 33.2 (see 33.4.1.2). Where a new board and care facility is constructed as part of a new apartment building or opens in an existing apartment building, it must comply with the requirements of

Chapter 6 for multiple occupancies, as well as those of Section 32.4.

The provisions of 32/33.1.2.3 and 32/33.1.2.4 are intended to provide added protection for the board and care occupancy during evacuation. They apply wherever a mixture of board and care and nonresidential or non-health care occupancies exists, whether in a new or existing building.

### 32.1.3 Special Definitions.

A list of special terms used in this chapter follows:

(1) **Personal Care.** See 3.3.192.
(2) **Point of Safety.** See 3.3.197.
(3) **Residential Board and Care Occupancy.** See 3.3.178.12.
(4) **Residential Board and Care Resident.** See 3.3.215.
(5) **Staff (Residential Board and Care).** See 3.3.245.
(6) **Thermal Barrier.** See 3.3.27.3.

### 33.1.3 Special Definitions.

A list of special terms used in this chapter follows:

(1) **Evacuation Capability.** See 3.3.70.
(2) **Impractical Evacuation Capability.** See 3.3.70.1.
(3) **Personal Care.** See 3.3.192.
(4) **Point of Safety.** See 3.3.197.
(5) **Prompt Evacuation Capability.** See 3.3.70.2.
(6) **Residential Board and Care Occupancy.** See 3.3.178.12.
(7) **Residential Board and Care Resident.** See 3.3.215.
(8) **Slow Evacuation Capability.** See 3.3.70.3.
(9) **Staff (Residential Board and Care).** See 3.3.245.
(10) **Thermal Barrier.** See 3.3.27.3.

A number of key terms, such as *evacuation capability*, *personal care*, and *point of safety*, are referenced in 32/33.1.3. The user needs to understand these terms to make effective use of the requirements for board and care facilities.

Evacuation capability (see definition in 3.3.70) is an underlying factor for the Chapter 33 provisions for existing facilities. However, in most occupancy chapters, the *Code* assumes that the building occupants have an evacuation capability similar to that of others within that occupancy, and the requirements are based on the ability of occupants to reach safety by means of exits. In Chapter 32 and the institutional occupancy chapters (health care and detention and correctional), the *Code* assumes that many of the building occupants will be incapable of evacuating the building, and the protection of life from fire is achieved by the defend-in-place method. In large residential buildings (hotels and apartment buildings), where evacuation capability might be affected due to the large size of the building, substantial, built-in fire protection is required.

In Chapter 33, evacuation capability must be determined before proceeding to identify applicable requirements. The numerous and diverse types of facilities that are included in residential board and care facilities preclude all occupants from having the same evacuation capability. For example, the occupants in an orphanage, a shelter for battered spouses, a group home for highly functioning mentally handicapped persons, or a halfway house for prison parolees might have normal, that is, prompt evacuation capability. In facilities housing elderly physically or mentally impaired persons, occupants might be slow moving or might need assistance in recognizing the need for evacuation. In some facilities, evacuation of the building might not be practical at all.

Evacuation capability for an entire facility is not determined based on the resident who is least capable. A facility that houses one impaired resident might have excellent evacuation capability if the staff or an assigned resident "buddy" is able to provide the assistance needed to effect a prompt evacuation of the entire group. Evacuation capability is based on the ability to relocate to a point of safety that is not necessarily a public way (see the definition of *point of safety* in 3.3.197). The protection features required by Chapter 33 are intended to coordinate with the evacuation capability of the occupants. As such, the fire endurance of the structure, the interior finish materials, and the types and arrangement of means of escape and exits, as well as the corridor enclosure provisions, vary, depending on whether a facility houses occupants who are prompt, slow, or impractical to evacuate. Facilities that are impractical to evacuate use the defend-in-place concept. In small facilities, this concept is achieved by improving the protection of vertical openings. In large facilities, the concept is achieved by mandating the use of the health care provisions of

Chapters 18 and 19. In all cases, an existing facility is permitted to meet the requirements for new facilities in Chapter 32 in lieu of those of Chapter 33 (see 33.1.1.2).

Personal care (see definition in 3.3.192) is significant, because the occupants of a board and care facility require care. Personal care is not medical care, as might be provided in a hospital or nursing home, but, rather, a form of assistance in meeting the demands of daily living. The term *transient medical care,* as used in A.3.3.192, refers to the kind of medical care that is normally provided in the home by one family member for another. Transient medical care does not refer to skilled nursing or acute medical care.

The term *point of safety* (see definition in 3.3.197) is another term that is specifically used in Chapters 32 and 33. It is well recognized that there are many buildings from which evacuation of all occupants to the outside cannot be achieved within a reasonable amount of time. Chapters 32 and 33 establish the criteria for a point of safety within the building. Essentially, a point of safety is an area where residents can remain in safety until the fire is extinguished or until outside assistance can arrive to complete evacuation to the exterior.

Several sections of the *Code* published in the 1980s referred to a finish rating of 15 minutes or 20 minutes. The term *finish rating* is similar to, but not as widely used as, the term *thermal barrier* (see definition in 3.3.27.3). For this reason, Chapters 32 and 33 use the term *thermal barrier* in lieu of *finish rating* in specifying the protection of structural elements and the separation of areas where automatic sprinkler protection is omitted. As noted in A.3.3.27.3, finish ratings might be used to determine a material's acceptability as a thermal barrier.

### 32.1.4 Acceptability of Means of Egress or Escape.

No means of escape or means of egress shall be considered as complying with the minimum criteria for acceptance, unless emergency evacuation drills are regularly conducted using that route in accordance with the requirements of 32.7.3.

### 32.1.5* Fire Resistance–Rated Assemblies.

Fire resistance–rated assemblies shall comply with Section 8.3.

**A.32.1.5** The provisions of 8.3.1(4) address a $^1/_2$-hour fire resistance rating. The information in A.8.3.1(4) addresses common materials used in barriers having a minimum $^1/_2$-hour fire resistance rating.

### 32.1.6 Reserved.

### 32.1.7 Reserved.



### 33.1.4 Acceptability of Means of Egress or Escape.

No means of escape or means of egress shall be considered as complying with the minimum criteria for acceptance, unless emergency evacuation drills are regularly conducted using that route in accordance with the requirements of 33.7.3.

### 33.1.5* Fire Resistance–Rated Assemblies.

Fire resistance–rated assemblies shall comply with Section 8.3.

**A.33.1.5** The provisions of 8.3.1(4) address a $^1/_2$-hour fire resistance rating. The information in A.8.3.1(4) addresses common materials used in barriers having a minimum $^1/_2$-hour fire resistance rating.

### 33.1.6 Changes in Facility Size.

A change in facility size from small to large shall be considered a change in occupancy subclassification and shall require compliance with the provisions applicable to new construction.

### 33.1.7* Changes in Group Evacuation Capability.

A change in evacuation capability to a slower level shall be permitted where the facility conforms to the requirements applicable to new construction, conversions, and the new evacuation capability.

**A.33.1.7** When the group evacuation capability changes to a level of greater risk, the owner/operator of the facility needs to take such action as is necessary, within a reasonable time frame, to restore the evacuation capability of the facility to that for which it was approved. If subsequent evaluations indicate that the original evacuation capability of the facility cannot or is not being maintained at the original level of risk, the facility would be considered as having changed the occupancy subclassification to one of greater risk, and the safeguards required for the level of greater risk would apply. If a facility improves its original evacuation capability to one of less risk, a re-evaluation and upgrading to the requirements for new construction is not needed.

The acceptability of the means of egress or escape is addressed by 32/33.1.4. Exits and means of escape are worthless unless residents are familiar with them and are comfortable using them. An exit or means of escape that is never used in drills will probably not be used during an emergency evacuation. This does not mean that, if windows serve as secondary means of escape, a resident must practice escaping out the window during a drill. However, during drills, it would be important to identify the appropriate windows and ensure that residents are familiar with their operation and their proper use during escape.

Subsections 33.1.6 and 33.1.7 address changes that might occur over the life of an existing board and care occupancy. Physical/structural growth will be easily identified, since permits would normally be required for such changes. Changes in evacuation capability might be subtler and will require a close review of the facility's fire drill records. Note that the requirements of 33.1.6 and 33.1.7 supersede those of Chapter 43 for change of use (see Section 43.7).

## 32.2 Small Facilities

### 32.2.1 General.

**32.2.1.1 Scope.**

**32.2.1.1.1** Section 32.2 shall apply to residential board and care occupancies providing sleeping accommodations for not more than 16 residents.

**32.2.1.1.2** Where there are sleeping accommodations for more than 16 residents, the occupancy shall be classified as a large facility in accordance with Section 32.3.

**32.2.1.2 Reserved.**

## 33.2 Small Facilities

### 33.2.1 General.

**33.2.1.1 Scope.**

**33.2.1.1.1** Section 33.2 shall apply to residential board and care occupancies providing sleeping accommodations for not more than 16 residents.

**33.2.1.1.2** Where there are sleeping accommodations for more than 16 residents, the occupancy shall be classified as a large facility in accordance with Section 33.3.

**33.2.1.2 Requirements Based on Evacuation Capability.**

**33.2.1.2.1** Small facilities, other than those meeting the requirement of 33.2.1.2.1.1 or 33.2.1.2.1.2, shall comply with the requirements of Section 33.2, as indicated for the appropriate evacuation capability; the ability of all occupants, residents, staff, and family members shall be considered in determining evacuation capability.

**33.2.1.2.1.1*** Facilities where the authority having jurisdiction has determined equivalent safety is provided in accordance with Section 1.4 shall not be required to comply with Section 33.2.

**A.33.2.1.2.1.1** In determining equivalency for existing buildings, conversions, modernizations, renovations, or unusual design concepts, the authority having jurisdiction might permit evaluations based on the residential board and care occupancies fire safety evaluation system (FSES) of NFPA 101A, *Guide on Alternative Approaches to Life Safety*.

**33.2.1.2.1.2** Facilities that were previously approved as complying with the requirements for a large facility having the same evacuation capability shall not be required to comply with Section 33.2.

**33.2.1.2.2** Facility management shall furnish to the authority having jurisdiction, upon request, an evacuation capability determination using a procedure acceptable to the authority having jurisdiction; where such documentation is not furnished, the evacuation capability shall be classified as impractical.

The importance of an accurate evaluation of evacuation capabilities in existing facilities cannot be overstated. Ineffective resident or staff response was a contributing factor in many of the multiple-death fires listed in Commentary Table 32/33.1.

Determining a facility's evacuation capability is not simply a matter of timing a fire drill in the middle of the day. Many variables affect a resident's capability to evacuate, and these variables must be carefully considered and factored into the documentation presented to the authority having jurisdiction (AHJ) for approval. Some variables that should be considered follow.

*Time of Day.* An occupant's ability to evacuate might be slowed dramatically when the occupant must be awakened. In such a situation, the occupant must process the information that evacuation is necessary and then begin evacuating.

*Medication.* Many individuals in board and care occupancies take various medications for behavior control or as sleeping aids. If an individual is medicated, he or she might need additional assistance in responding and evacuating.

*Mobility and Location of Occupants.* Once individuals become aware of an emergency and take action, their ability to move through the building must be considered. Individuals using wheelchairs, walkers, or canes are further slowed when using stairs or ramps or when opening doors.

*Staff Assistance.* Though the *Code* does not specify minimum staffing levels, staffing levels should be considered, especially where high resident-to-staff ratios exist. Given the additional needs mentioned in the first three variables, the staff will be limited in their ability to affect evacuation time where multiple residents need assistance.

The evacuation capability of the population of a board and care occupancy might vary over time. The required documentation should be reviewed regularly to ensure that it accurately represents the current evacuation capability of the residents and staff.

When determining equivalency in accordance with 33.2.1.2.1.1, it is important to note that the equivalency measurement systems of the 2007 edition of NFPA 101A, *Guide on Alternative Approaches to Life Safety*,[2] were calibrated against the requirements of the 2006 edition of NFPA *101* and might not accurately evaluate equivalency with the requirements of the 2009 edition of the *Life Safety Code*. At the time this handbook went to press, the 2010 edition of NFPA 101A was being prepared. Once issued, the 2010 edition of NFPA 101A can be used to measure equivalency against the requirements of the 2009 edition of the *Code*.

The provision of 33.2.1.2.1.2 continues to recognize an existing situation that resulted from compliance with a provision of the 1985 edition of the *Code* that permitted small board and care facilities to comply with the requirements for large facilities. The protection features applicable to large facilities might not necessarily provide adequate protection for small facilities. See the commentary following 32/33.1.1.4.

CHAPTER 32 • New

**32.2.1.3 Minimum Construction Requirements.** (No requirements.)

CHAPTER 33 • Existing

**33.2.1.3 Minimum Construction Requirements.**

**33.2.1.3.1 Prompt Evacuation Capability.** (No special requirements.)

**33.2.1.3.2 Slow Evacuation Capability.**

**33.2.1.3.2.1** The facility shall be housed in a building where the interior is fully sheathed with lath and plaster or other material providing a minimum 15-minute thermal barrier, as modified by 33.2.1.3.2.3 through 33.2.1.3.2.7, including all portions of bearing walls, bearing partitions, floor construction, and roofs.

**33.2.1.3.2.2** All columns, beams, girders, and trusses shall be encased or otherwise protected with construction having a minimum $^1/_2$-hour fire resistance rating.

**33.2.1.3.2.3** Exposed steel or wood columns, girders, and beams (but not joists) located in the basement shall be permitted.

**33.2.1.3.2.4** Buildings of Type I, Type II(222), Type II(111), Type III(211), Type IV, or Type V(111) construction shall not be required to meet the requirements of 33.2.1.3.2. *(See 8.2.1.)*

**33.2.1.3.2.5** Areas protected by approved automatic sprinkler systems in accordance with 33.2.3.5 shall not be required to meet the requirements of 33.2.1.3.2.

**33.2.1.3.2.6** Unfinished, unused, and essentially inaccessible loft, attic, or crawl spaces shall not be required to meet the requirements of 33.2.1.3.2.

**33.2.1.3.2.7** Where the facility has demonstrated to the authority having jurisdiction that the group is capable of evacuating the building in 8 minutes or less, or where the group achieves an E-score of 3 or less using the board and care occupancies evacuation capability determination methodology of NFPA 101A, *Guide on Alternative Approaches to Life Safety*, the requirements of 33.2.1.3.2 shall not apply.

**33.2.1.3.3 Impractical Evacuation Capability.** Nonsprinklered buildings shall be of any construction type in accordance with 8.2.1, other than Type II(000), Type III(200), or Type V(000) construction. Buildings protected throughout by an approved, supervised automatic sprinkler system in accordance with 33.2.3.5 shall be permitted to be of any type of construction.

Because 32.2.3.5.1 requires new small board and care facilities to be sprinklered, no additional requirements with respect to minimum building construction types apply for new construction. However, no sprinkler mandate is specified for existing small board and care facilities. Therefore, 33.2.1.3.2 and 33.2.1.3.3 establish minimum construction requirements to provide an adequate level of safety for existing small facilities with slow or impractical evacuation capability.

Exhibit 32/33.1 illustrates the concept of sheathing

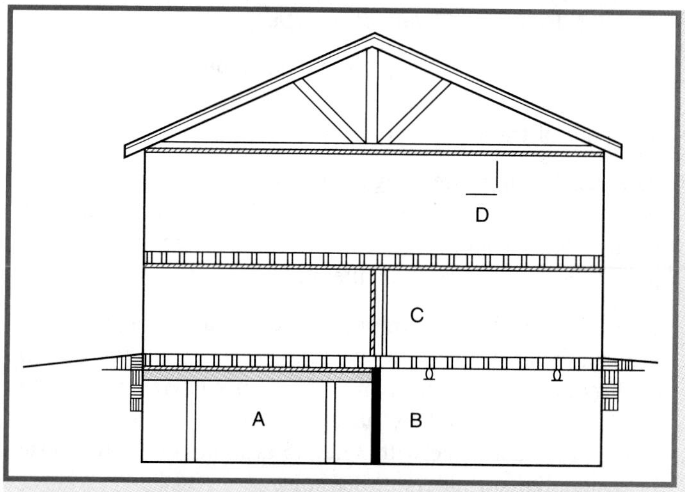


***Exhibit 32/33.1*** *Sheathing requirements in a small facility with slow evacuation capability.*

the interior of a small board and care facility building with a slow evacuation capability to achieve the 15-minute thermal barrier that is required by 33.2.1.3.2.



The nonsprinklered areas (A, C, and D) are required to have sheathing to protect bearing walls, floor construction, and roofs. The heavy timber columns and beams in area A do not require sheathing but must provide a minimum fire resistance rating of 30 minutes. As permitted by 33.2.1.3.2.5, the sprinklered areas of the building are exempt from the sheathing requirement.

The provision of 33.2.1.3.2.7 is intended to permit unsheathed, unsprinklered wood frame construction in facilities that house groups capable of evacuation to a point of safety within 8 minutes. For such groups, the additional evacuation time provided by fire-resistant sheathing is not necessary.

All existing small facilities with impractical evacuation capability must be protected with a supervised automatic sprinkler system per 33.2.3.5.3. The provision of 33.2.1.3.3 permitting any construction type is applicable if the entire building, not only the residential board and care facility, is protected with a supervised automatic sprinkler system.

**32.2.2 Means of Escape.**

Designated means of escape shall be continuously maintained free of all obstructions or impediments to full instant use in the case of fire or emergency.

**32.2.2.1 Reserved.**

**33.2.2 Means of Escape.**

Designated means of escape shall be continuously maintained free of all obstructions or impediments to full instant use in the case of fire or emergency.

**33.2.2.1 Number of Means of Escape.**

**33.2.2.1.1** Each normally occupied story of the facility shall have not less than two remotely located means of escape that do not involve using windows, unless the facility meets the requirement of 33.2.2.1.4 or 33.2.2.1.5.

**33.2.2.1.2** Not less than one of the means of escape required by 33.2.2.1.1 shall be in accordance with 33.2.2.2.

**33.2.2.1.3** The provisions of Chapter 7 shall not apply to means of escape, unless specifically referenced in this chapter.

**33.2.2.1.4** In prompt evacuation capability facilities, one means of escape shall be permitted to involve windows complying with 33.2.2.3.1(3).

**33.2.2.1.5** A second means of escape from each story shall not be required where the entire building is protected throughout by an approved automatic sprinkler system complying with 33.2.3.5 and the facility has two means of escape; this provision shall not be permitted to be used in conjunction with 33.2.2.3.3.

CHAPTER 32 • New

**32.2.2.2 Primary Means of Escape.**

**32.2.2.2.1** Every sleeping room and living area shall have access to a primary means of escape located to provide a safe path of travel to the outside.

**32.2.2.2.2** Where sleeping rooms or living areas are above or below the level of exit discharge, the primary means of escape shall be an interior stair in accordance with 32.2.2.4, an exterior stair, a horizontal exit, or a fire escape stair.

**32.2.2.3 Secondary Means of Escape.**

**32.2.2.3.1** Sleeping rooms, other than those complying with 32.2.2.3.2, and living areas in facilities without a sprinkler system installed in accordance with 32.2.3.5 shall have a second means of escape consisting of one of the following:

(1) Door, stairway, passage, or hall providing a way of unobstructed travel to the outside of the dwelling at street or the finished ground level that is independent of, and remotely located from, the primary means of escape
(2) Passage through an adjacent nonlockable space independent of, and remotely located from, the primary means of escape to any approved means of escape
(3)* Outside window or door operable from the inside, without the use of tools, keys, or special effort, that provides a clear opening of not less than 5.7 $ft^2$ (0.53 $m^2$), with the width not less than 20 in. (510 mm), the height not less than 24 in. (610 mm), and the bottom of the opening not more than 44 in. (1120 mm) above the floor, with such means of escape acceptable, provided that one of the following criteria is met:
   (a) The window is within 20 ft (6100 mm) of the finished ground level.
   (b) The window is directly accessible to fire department rescue apparatus, as approved by the authority having jurisdiction.
   (c) The window or door opens onto an exterior balcony.

**A.32.2.2.3.1(3)** A window with dimensions of 20 in. × 24 in. (510 mm × 610 mm) has an opening of 3.3 $ft^2$ (0.31 $m^2$), which is less than the required 5.7 $ft^2$ (0.53 $m^2$). Therefore, either the height or width needs to exceed the minimum requirement to provide the required clear area.

CHAPTER 33 • Existing

**33.2.2.2 Primary Means of Escape.**

**33.2.2.2.1** Every sleeping room and living area shall have access to a primary means of escape located to provide a safe path of travel to the outside.

**33.2.2.2.2** Where sleeping rooms or living areas are above or below the level of exit discharge, the primary means of escape shall be an interior stair in accordance with 33.2.2.4, an exterior stair, a horizontal exit, or a fire escape stair.

**33.2.2.2.3** In slow and impractical evacuation capability facilities, the primary means of escape for each sleeping room shall not be exposed to living areas and kitchens, unless the building is protected by an approved automatic sprinkler system in accordance with 33.2.3.5 utilizing quick-response or residential sprinklers throughout.

**33.2.2.2.4** Standard-response sprinklers shall be permitted for use in hazardous areas in accordance with 33.2.3.2.

**33.2.2.3 Secondary Means of Escape.**

**33.2.2.3.1** In addition to the primary route, each sleeping room shall have a second means of escape consisting of one of the following, unless the provisions of 33.2.2.3.2, 33.2.2.3.3, or 33.2.2.3.4 are met:

(1) Door, stairway, passage, or hall providing a way of unobstructed travel to the outside of the dwelling at street or the finished ground level that is independent of, and remotely located from, the primary means of escape
(2) Passage through an adjacent nonlockable space independent of, and remotely located from, the primary means of escape to any approved means of escape
(3)* Outside window or door operable from the inside, without the use of tools, keys, or special effort, that provides a clear opening of not less than 5.7 $ft^2$ (0.53 $m^2$), with the width not less than 20 in. (510 mm), the height not less than 24 in. (610 mm), and the bottom of the opening not more than 44 in. (1120 mm) above the floor, with such means of escape acceptable, provided that one of the following criteria is met:
   (a) The window is within 20 ft (6100 mm) of the finished ground level.
   (b) The window is directly accessible to fire department rescue apparatus, as approved by the authority having jurisdiction.
   (c) The window or door opens onto an exterior balcony.

**A.33.2.2.3.1(3)** A window with dimensions of 20 in. × 24 in. (510 mm × 610 mm) has an opening of 3.3 $ft^2$ (0.31 $m^2$), which is less than the required 5.7 $ft^2$ (0.53 $m^2$). Therefore, either the height or width needs to exceed the minimum requirement to provide the required clear area.

(4) Windows having a sill height below the adjacent finished ground level that are provided with a window well meeting the following criteria:
   (a) The window well has horizontal dimensions that allow the window to be fully opened.
   (b) The window well has an accessible net clear opening of not less than 9 $ft^2$ (0.84 $m^2$), with a length and width of not less than 36 in. (915 mm).
   (c) A window well with a vertical depth of more than 44 in. (1120 mm) is equipped with an approved permanently affixed ladder or with steps meeting the following criteria:
      i. The ladder or steps do not encroach more than 6 in. (150 mm) into the required dimensions of the window well.
      ii. The ladder or steps are not obstructed by the window.

**32.2.2.3.2** Sleeping rooms that have a door leading directly to the outside of the building with access to the finished ground level or to an exterior stairway meeting the requirements of 32.2.2.6.3 shall be considered as meeting all the requirements for a second means of escape.



(4) Windows having a sill height below the adjacent finished ground level that are provided with a window well meeting the following criteria:
   (a) The window well has horizontal dimensions that allow the window to be fully opened.
   (b) The window well has an accessible net clear opening of not less than 9 $ft^2$ (0.84 $m^2$), with a length and width of not less than 36 in. (915 mm).
   (c) A window well with a vertical depth of more than 44 in. (1120 mm) is equipped with an approved permanently affixed ladder or with steps meeting the following criteria:
      i. The ladder or steps do not encroach more than 6 in. (150 mm) into the required dimensions of the window well.
      ii. The ladder or steps are not obstructed by the window.

**33.2.2.3.2** Sleeping rooms that have a door leading directly to the outside of the building with access to the finished ground level or to a stairway that meets the requirements of exterior stairs in 33.2.2.2.2 shall be considered as meeting all the requirements for a second means of escape.

**33.2.2.3.3** A second means of escape from each sleeping room shall not be required where the facility is protected throughout by an approved automatic sprinkler system in accordance with 33.2.3.5.

**33.2.2.3.4** Existing approved means of escape shall be permitted to continue to be used.

The provisions of 33.2.2.1, 32/33.2.2.2, and 32/33.2.2.3 establish the criteria for acceptable means of escape in small board and care facilities. In new facilities, every sleeping room and living area must be provided with access to a primary and secondary means of escape per 32.2.2.2 and 32.2.2.3, much like the other residential occupancies. Note, however, that the requirement for a secondary means of escape is exempted when the building is sprinklered per 32.2.2.3.1. In existing facilities, 33.2.2.1 requires each story of the facility to be provided with at least two means of escape. Only one of the means of escape must meet the provisions for a primary means of escape. The second means of escape is permitted to be a window, provided that the window complies with 33.2.2.3.1(3) and the facility evacuation capability is prompt (see 33.2.2.1.4).

In existing facilities, the second means of escape from each floor is not required if the entire building housing the residential board and care facility is protected throughout by an automatic sprinkler system in accordance with 33.2.3.5. In this instance, the single means of escape must meet the criteria for a primary means of escape specified in 33.2.2.2. However, the facility itself must have at least two means of escape.

Where a window is considered as a secondary means of escape within a sleeping room, the window must meet the criteria detailed in 33.2.2.3.1(3), but use of the window is not limited to any specific evacuation capability. Windows are not permitted to serve as primary means of escape.

The provisions of 32/33.2.2.2 specify a primary means of escape that is arranged so that an occupant can travel safely to the outside at grade level. The intent of the requirement is to ensure that use of the primary means of escape will not be lost due to fire on another floor. Exhibit 32/33.2 depicts an exterior stair (A) that serves as the primary means of escape for the second floor. Occupants of the second floor can travel safely to the outside at grade, because the interior stair

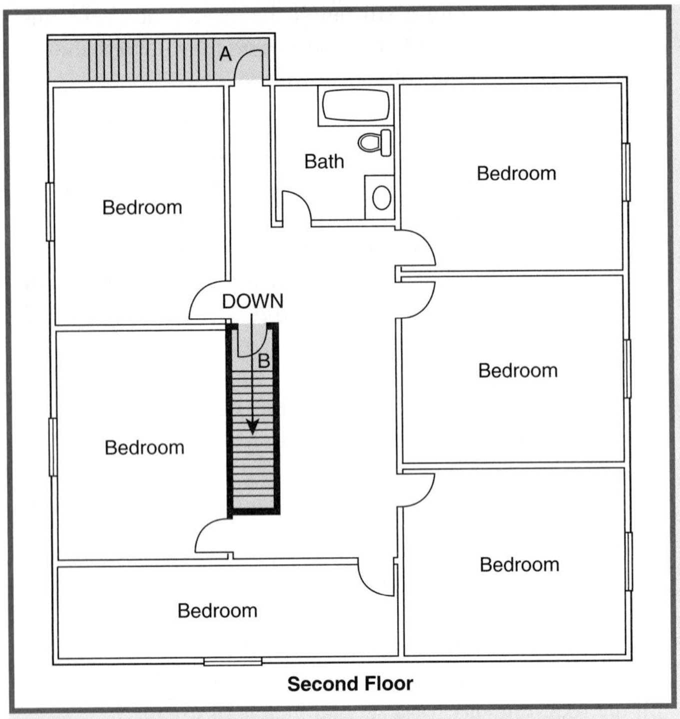


***Exhibit 32/33.2** Exterior stair used as primary means of escape.*

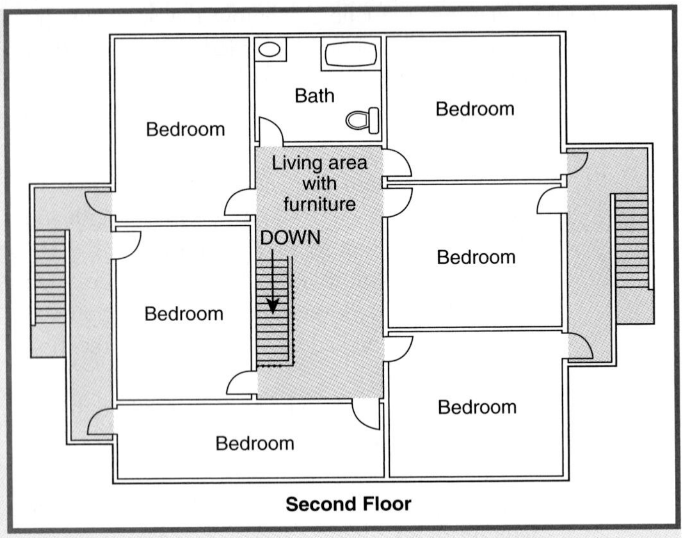


***Exhibit 32/33.3** Alternate arrangement for exterior stairs used as primary means of escape in existing facilities.*

(B) is separated from the second floor by enclosing construction on the second floor.

The primary means of escape from rooms above or below grade level will involve vertical travel, such as stairs. For this reason, the *Code* establishes a higher level of reliability by requiring the primary means of escape to be an enclosed interior stair, an exterior stair, a horizontal exit, or an existing fire escape stair. In Exhibit 32/33.2, this requirement is met by using the exterior stair as the primary means of escape from the second floor, even if the partially enclosed interior stair (second floor only) is used for day-to-day travel between floors.

In existing board and care occupancies with slow and impractical evacuation capability, and without quick-response or residential sprinklers throughout, 33.2.2.2.3 prohibits the primary means of escape from being exposed to common living spaces and kitchens. Therefore, the primary means of escape from a sleeping room is not permitted to include travel through a day room, a common use space, or a space that is open to a common living space. Exhibit 32/33.3 depicts an example meeting this requirement. By using the outside balconies and exterior stairs as the primary means of escape, the means of escape can be used by occupants of the second floor without exposing them to a fire involving the contents of a common living area.

The objective of 33.2.2.2.3 is to reduce the probability that smoke and heat from a fire involving the contents of a common living area will adversely affect the use of the primary means of escape. The requirement is based, in part, on historical fire experience, which indicates that fires in residential board and care facilities frequently originate in the furniture and contents of common living spaces.

In recognition of the fact that an automatic sprinkler system using quick-response or residential sprinklers provides a high level of protection, 33.2.2.2.3 permits the primary means of escape to be exposed to common living areas where such sprinkler protection is provided. Furthermore, 33.2.2.2.4 permits standard-response sprinklers to be used, in lieu of quick-response or residential sprinklers, in hazardous areas that are required to be separated from other parts of the building per 33.2.3.2. The provision for standard-response sprinklers is permitted because sleeping residents do not occupy hazardous areas.

A secondary means of escape from each sleeping and living area is required for existing small board and care facilities and new nonsprinklered small board and care facilities (as permitted for conversions by 32.2.3.5.2). The main purpose for the secondary means of escape is to provide the occupants with a reasonable escape alternative when fire or smoke blocks the primary means of escape. Four acceptable methods for providing a secondary means of escape are outlined by 32/33.2.2.3.1(1) through (4). Exhibit 32/33.4 illustrates several methods for providing secondary means of escape.

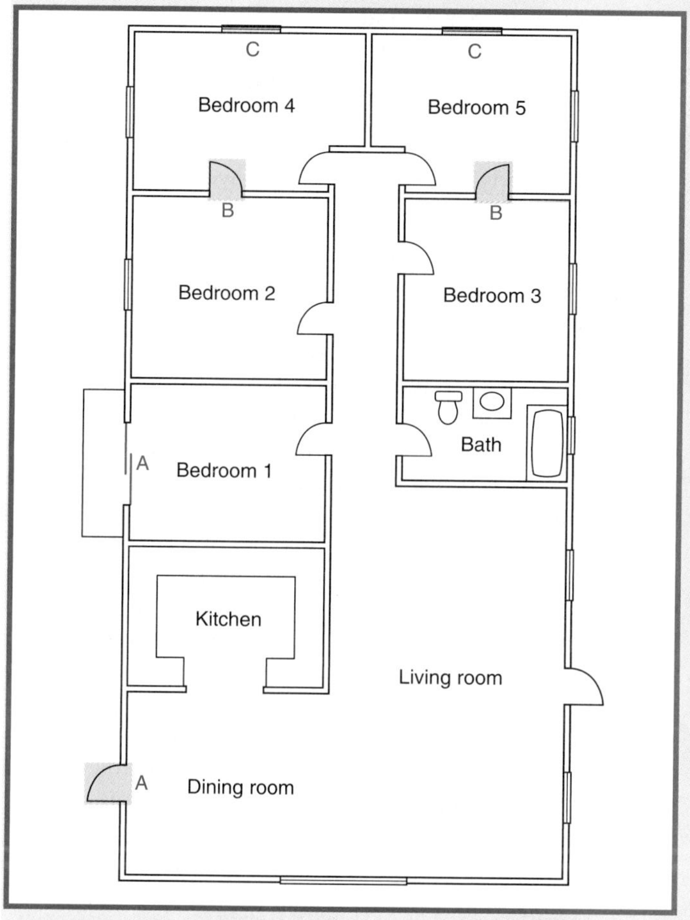


***Exhibit 32/33.4*** *Secondary means of escape options.*

The doors marked A in Exhibit 32/33.4 meet the intent of 32/33.2.2.3.1(1), because they are independent of, and remotely located from, the primary means of escape required by 32/33.2.2.2. If the sleeping room has a second door that leads to the same hallway as the door serving as a primary means of escape, little additional protection is provided, because fire or smoke could affect use of both doors at approximately the same time. If the corridor within the facility into which a sleeping room door opens is separated from all common living spaces, it might be determined that the arrangement is acceptable, provided that the corridor does actually lead to two separate independent and remote means of escape. This arrangement is similar to that permitted in other occupancies in which protected corridors are provided. In this case, requiring two doors from the sleeping room to the corridor would provide little additional safety.

The doors marked B in Exhibit 32/33.4 provide a secondary means of escape that passes through an adjacent space, such as another sleeping room. The unlocked doors that lead from bedroom 2 into bedroom 4, and from bedroom 3 into bedroom 5, provide free and unobstructed access in accordance with 32/33.2.2.3.1(2). Once a resident reaches bedroom 4 or bedroom 5, the secondary means of escape is window C, in accordance with 32/33.2.2.3.1(3) or 32/33.2.2.3.1(4).

The windows that are marked C in Exhibit 32/33.4 comply with the minimum dimensions specified in 32/33.2.2.3.1(3) and are permitted as a second means of escape from a story of an existing small facility only if the evacuation capability is prompt (see 33.2.2.1.4). However, the use of an operable window of the minimum dimensions specified in 32/33.2.2.3.1(3) is permitted as a secondary means of escape from sleeping rooms and living areas, regardless of the residents' evacuation capability.

The arrangement for providing secondary means of escape described in 32/33.2.2.3.1(4) recognizes the increasing trend of developing or converting basements into living space or sleeping areas. Fire in these areas or the areas above them could easily block the primary means of escape, which is usually a single stair to the upper level. This option provides requirements for the size of the window well, in addition to the window size, to provide sufficient space to operate the window and move up to grade level. For additional guidance, see Figure A.24.2.2.3.3, which applies to window wells in one- and two-family dwellings, the requirements for which are identical to those for small board and care facilities.

Exhibit 32/33.5 illustrates the minimum dimensions required for secondary means of escape windows. Note that the minimum width dimension cannot be simultaneously used with the minimum height dimension, because the minimum area requirement will not be satisfied. If either the minimum height or minimum width dimension is used, the other dimension must be increased to yield the required opening area.

In addition to the minimum size of the window, the utility of the window must be ensured by one of the following three alternatives:

1. The window must be within 20 ft (6100 mm) of grade so that dropping from the open window is possible.

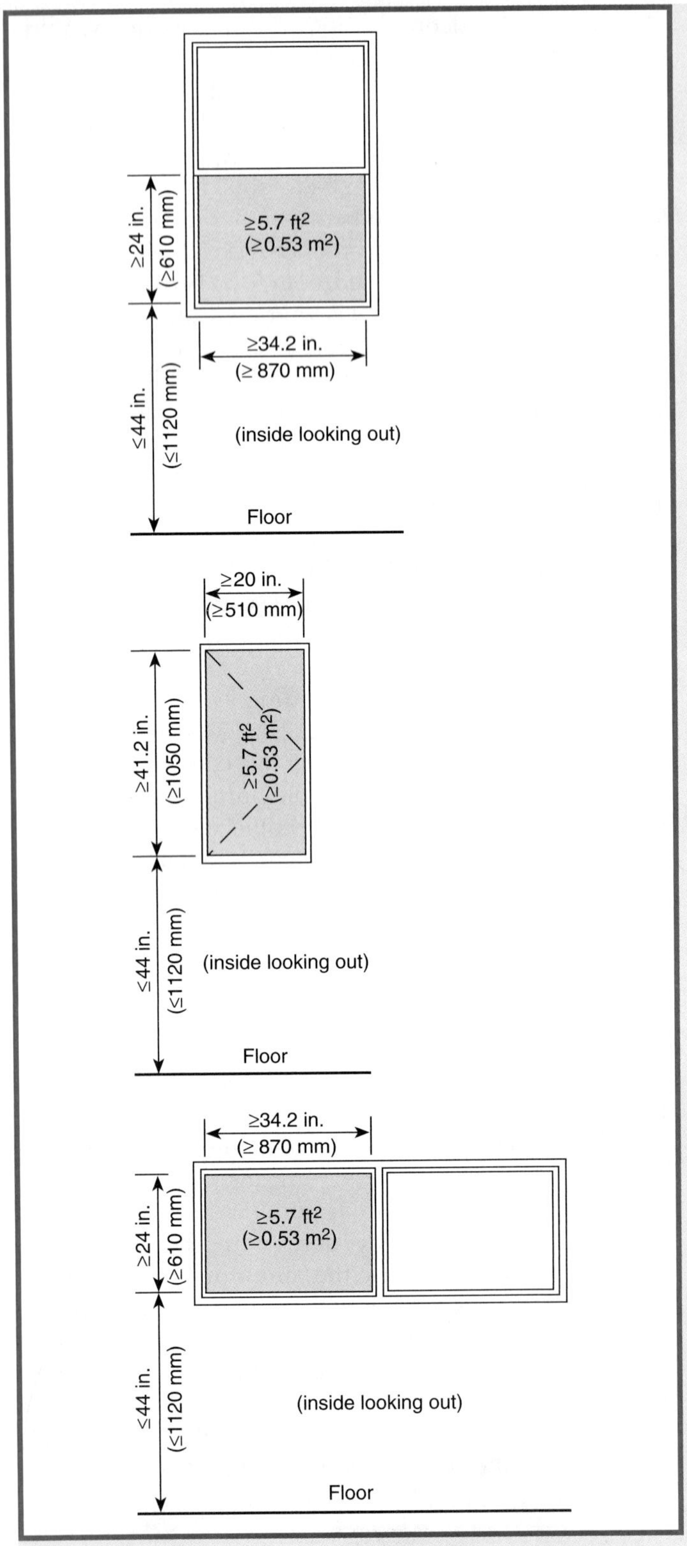


***Exhibit 32/33.5*** *Minimum dimensions for escape windows.*

2. The fire department must be capable of rescuing the occupant from the window. [The authority having jurisdiction (AHJ) must determine acceptable means of fire department rescue, such as by means of aerial ladder apparatus or ground ladders, and additional criteria necessary for approval, such as fire department vehicle accessibility.]
3. The occupant must be capable of reaching an exterior balcony to breathe fresh air while awaiting either rescue or fire extinguishment.

A facility is exempted from providing secondary means of escape from sleeping rooms if it meets one of three conditions that follow. First, 32/33.2.2.3.2 permits such an exemption if the sleeping room has a door leading directly to the outside of the building, with access to grade. In this case, the door to the outside serves as the equivalent of both the primary and secondary means of escape. Exhibit 32/33.3 illustrates such an arrangement.

Second, the secondary means of escape is exempted where a residential board and care facility is protected throughout with an automatic sprinkler system in accordance with 32/33.2.3.5. However, 33.2.2.3.3 is not permitted to be used in conjunction with 33.2.2.1.5, because the result would be a single means of escape from each room and each floor. Therefore, in existing facilities, the secondary means of escape from a sleeping room is exempted only if a second means of escape is provided from each floor and the facility is protected by an automatic sprinkler system.

Third, the secondary means of escape is exempted where an existing board and care facility is provided with a means of escape arrangement that has been approved by the AHJ per 33.2.2.3.4.

CHAPTER 32 • New

**32.2.2.4 Interior Stairs Used for Primary Means of Escape.** Interior stairs shall be protected in accordance with 32.2.2.4.1 through 32.2.2.4.4, unless they meet the requirement of 32.2.2.4.5, 32.2.2.4.6, or 32.2.2.4.7.

**32.2.2.4.1** Interior stairs shall be enclosed with fire barriers in accordance with Section 8.3 having a minimum $^1/_2$-hour resistance rating.

**32.2.2.4.2** Stairs shall comply with 7.2.2.5.3.

**32.2.2.4.3** The entire primary means of escape shall be arranged so that occupants are not required to pass through a portion of a lower story, unless that route is separated from all spaces on that story by construction having a minimum $^1/_2$-hour fire resistance rating.

**32.2.2.4.4** In buildings of construction other than Type II(000), Type III(200), or Type V(000), the supporting construction shall be protected to afford the required fire resistance rating of the supported wall.

**32.2.2.4.5** Stairs that connect a story at street level to only one other story shall be permitted to be open to the story that is not at street level.

**32.2.2.4.6** In buildings three or fewer stories in height and protected by an approved automatic sprinkler system in accordance with 32.2.3.5, stair enclosures shall not be required, provided that there still remains a primary means of escape from each sleeping area that does not require occupants to pass through a portion of a lower floor, unless that route is separated from all spaces on that floor by construction having a minimum $^1/_2$-hour fire resistance rating.

**32.2.2.4.7** Stairs serving a maximum of two stories in buildings protected with an approved automatic sprinkler system in accordance with 32.2.3.5 shall be permitted to be unenclosed.

CHAPTER 33 • Existing

**33.2.2.4 Interior Stairs Used for Primary Means of Escape.** Interior stairs used for primary means of escape shall comply with 33.2.2.4.1 through 33.2.2.4.9.

**33.2.2.4.1** Interior stairs shall be enclosed with fire barriers in accordance with Section 8.3 having a minimum $^1/_2$-hour fire resistance rating and shall comply with 7.2.2.5.3.

**33.2.2.4.2 Reserved.**

**33.2.2.4.3** The entire primary means of escape shall be arranged so that it is not necessary for occupants to pass through a portion of a lower story, unless that route is separated from all spaces on that story by construction having a minimum $^1/_2$-hour fire resistance rating.

**33.2.2.4.4** In buildings of construction other than Type II(000), Type III(200), or Type V(000), the supporting construction shall be protected to afford the required fire resistance rating of the supported wall.

**33.2.2.4.5** Stairs that connect a story at street level to only one other story shall be permitted to be open to the story that is not at street level.

**33.2.2.4.6** Stair enclosures shall not be required in buildings three or fewer stories in height that house prompt or slow evacuation capability facilities, provided that both of the following criteria are met:

(1) The building is protected by an approved automatic sprinkler system in accordance with 33.2.3.5 that uses quick-response or residential sprinklers.
(2) A primary means of escape from each sleeping area exists that does not pass through a portion of a lower floor, unless that route is separated from all spaces on that floor by construction having a minimum $^1/_2$-hour fire resistance rating.

**33.2.2.4.7** Stair enclosures shall not be required in buildings that are two or fewer stories in height, that house prompt evacuation capability facilities with not more than eight residents, and that are protected by an approved automatic sprinkler system in accordance with 33.2.3.5 that uses quick-response or residential sprinklers.

**33.2.2.4.8** The provisions of 33.2.2.3.3, 33.2.3.4.3.6, or 33.2.3.4.3.7 shall not be used in conjunction with 33.2.2.4.7.

**33.2.2.4.9** Stairs shall be permitted to be open at the topmost story only where all of the following criteria are met:

(1) The building is three or fewer stories in height.
(2) The building houses prompt or slow evacuation capability facilities.

(3) The building is protected by an approved automatic sprinkler system in accordance with 33.2.3.5.
(4) The entire primary means of escape of which the stairs are a part is separated from all portions of lower stories.

The intent of 32/33.2.2.4 is to require that an interior stair serving as a primary means of escape be enclosed. It does not mandate that an interior stair used for day-to-day use, but not considered a primary means of escape, be enclosed. However, the stair might require separation from the floor to prevent exposure of occupants to unsafe conditions while they travel through the primary means of escape (see 32/33.2.2.2, 32/33.2.3.1, and Exhibit 32/33.2 and its associated commentary).

If the interior stair serves as primary means of escape, it must be arranged so that occupants are not required to pass through occupied or furnished portions of lower floors. Passage through unfurnished vestibule-like areas on lower floors is permitted if such vestibules are separated from occupied and furnished areas by walls and doors. These vestibules provide safety equivalent to that provided by a stair enclosure.

It is the intent of the *Code* that interior stairs in accordance with 32.2.2.4 and 33.2.2.4, and all their associated exemptions (32.2.2.4.5 through 32.2.2.4.7 and 33.2.2.4.5 through 33.2.2.4.9), qualify as enclosed interior stairs permitted by 32/33.2.2.2 to serve as the primary means of escape.

The intent of 32/33.2.2.4.5 is to permit a stair that connects the first floor to the second floor to be open to the second floor but separated from the effects of fire on the first floor. This provision also permits a stair that connects the basement level to the first floor to be open to the basement level but separated from the effects of fire on the first floor. This partially enclosed interior stair can serve as a primary means of escape in accordance with 32/33.2.2.2.

Exhibit 32/33.6 illustrates a partially enclosed interior stair (separated from ground floor) in accordance with 32/33.2.2.4.5 that serves as the primary means of escape for the second floor. This partially enclosed interior stair is considered to be the equivalent of an enclosed interior stair. The separating walls and doors on the first floor serve the dual purposes of enclosing the stair on that floor and providing a route that does not expose occupants to occupied or furnished areas of the first floor. Thus, the first-floor stair "lobby" cannot be used as a lounge and cannot contain furniture or furnishings.

The intent of 32/33.2.2.4.6 is to permit an unenclosed interior stair to serve as the equivalent of an enclosed interior stair in new small facilities and existing small facilities with prompt or slow evacuation capability. However, the buildings must be of three or fewer stories and must be protected throughout with an automatic sprinkler system using quick-response or residential sprinklers. Exhibit 32/33.6 can also be used to illustrate the provisions of 32/33.2.2.4.6. Although

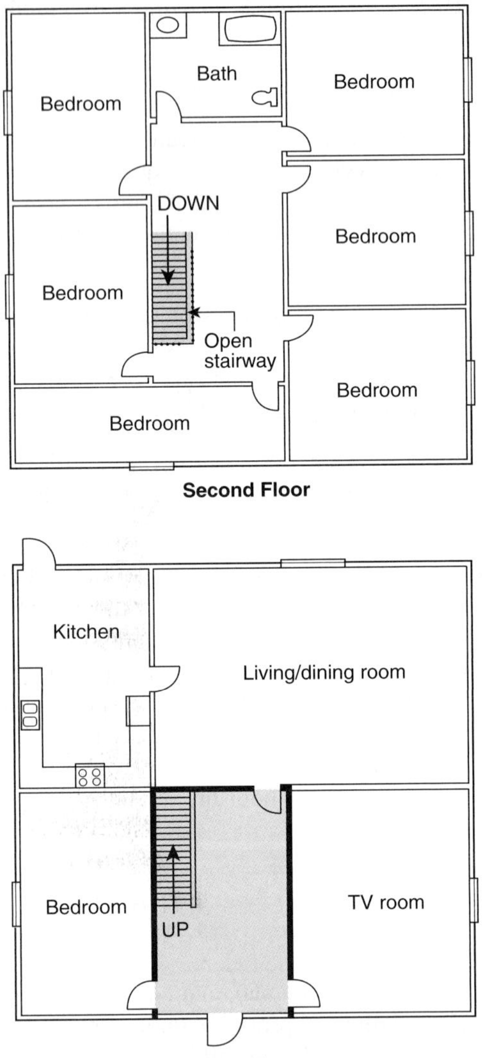


**Exhibit 32/33.6** *Partially enclosed interior stair.*

CHAPTER 32 • New

CHAPTER 33 • Existing

the enclosing walls around the vestibule on the first floor serve as the stair enclosure on that floor in accordance with 32/33.2.2.4.5, the same enclosing walls serve to protect the escape path from the areas that are occupied or furnished on the first floor in accordance with 32/33.2.2.4.6. Additionally, given the presence of sprinklers and other criteria of 32/33.2.2.4.6, the open stair can extend to a third level.

The provisions of 32/33.2.2.4.7 permit a two-story open stair (and its associated exposure to the areas that are occupied or furnished, or both, on the ground floor) to serve as primary means of escape for new small facilities and existing small facilities (not more than eight residents) with prompt evacuation capability, provided that the facility is sprinklered using quick-response or residential sprinklers. This provision, in effect, equates such a board and care facility with a one- or two-family dwelling. An unenclosed interior stair meeting the criteria of this provision is considered the equivalent of an enclosed interior stair.

For existing facilities, the *Code* prohibits the use of the following provisions in conjunction with 33.2.2.4.7 (see 33.2.2.4.8):

1. Paragraph 33.2.2.3.3, which exempts bedrooms from a required secondary means of escape if the building is sprinklered
2. Paragraphs 33.2.3.4.3.6 and 33.2.3.4.3.7, which exempt common space smoke detectors where the building is sprinklered and the bedrooms are provided with smoke alarms

Multiple use of the provisions specified in items 1 and 2, which are intended for application to sprinklered buildings, could result in a level of life safety less than that required by Chapters 32 and 33.

In existing buildings, 33.2.2.4.9 permits stairs to be open at the topmost story only where the entire primary means of escape associated with the stairs is separated from all portions of lower stories. In addition, this provision requires the following:

1. Buildings are to be of three or fewer stories.
2. Buildings are to house facilities with prompt or slow evacuation capability.
3. Buildings are to be protected by an approved automatic sprinkler system in accordance with 33.2.3.5.

**32.2.2.5 Doors.**

**32.2.2.5.1** Doors, other than those meeting the requirements of 32.2.2.5.1.1 and 32.2.2.5.1.2, and paths of travel to a means of escape shall be not less than 32 in. (810 mm) wide.

**32.2.2.5.1.1** Bathroom doors shall be not less than 24 in. (610 mm) wide.

**32.2.2.5.1.2** In conversions *(see 32.1.1.4)*, 28 in. (710 mm) doors shall be permitted.

**32.2.2.5.2** Doors shall be swinging or sliding.

**32.2.2.5.3** Every closet door latch shall be readily opened from the inside.

**32.2.2.5.4** Every bathroom door shall be designed to allow opening from the outside during an emergency when locked.

**32.2.2.5.5** No door in any means of escape, other than those meeting the requirement of 32.2.2.5.5.1 or 32.2.2.5.5.2, shall be locked against egress when the building is occupied.

**32.2.2.5.5.1** Delayed-egress locks complying with 7.2.1.6.1 shall be permitted on exterior doors only.

**32.2.2.5.5.2** Access-controlled egress locks complying with 7.2.1.6.2 shall be permitted.

**33.2.2.5 Doors.**

**33.2.2.5.1** Doors, other than bathroom doors addressed in 33.2.2.5.1.1, and paths of travel to a means of escape shall be not less than 28 in. (710 mm) wide.

**33.2.2.5.1.1** Bathroom doors shall be not less than 24 in. (610 mm) wide.

**33.2.2.5.1.2 Reserved.**

**33.2.2.5.2** Doors shall be swinging or sliding.

**33.2.2.5.3** Every closet door latch shall be readily opened from the inside.

**33.2.2.5.4** Every bathroom door shall be designed to allow opening from the outside during an emergency when locked.

**33.2.2.5.5** No door in any means of escape, other than those meeting the requirement of 33.2.2.5.5.1 or 33.2.2.5.5.2, shall be locked against egress when the building is occupied.

**33.2.2.5.5.1** Delayed-egress locks complying with 7.2.1.6.1 shall be permitted on exterior doors only.

**33.2.2.5.5.2** Access-controlled egress locks complying with 7.2.1.6.2 shall be permitted.

CHAPTER 32 • New

**32.2.2.5.6** Forces to open doors shall comply with 7.2.1.4.5.

**32.2.2.5.7** Door-latching devices shall comply with 7.2.1.5.9.

**32.2.2.5.8** Floor levels at doors shall comply with 7.2.1.3.

If an existing dwelling is converted to a small board and care facility, the provisions of 4.6.12 require that such a change of occupancy is to meet the requirements of 4.6.8, which, in turn, references Chapter 43 for building rehabilitation. Chapter 43 requires such a change of occupancy to a higher hazard category to meet the requirements for new board and care facilities (see 43.7.2.2). The provision of 32.2.2.5.1.2 recognizes the hardship and minor improvement that would be realized if existing 28 in. (710 mm) wide doors were required to be replaced by 32 in. (810 mm) wide doors.

Residential board and care facilities are prohibited from having any door in the means of escape locked against egress while the building is occupied in accordance with 32/33.2.2.5.5. This prohibition is consistent with a fundamental means of egress provision of Chapter 7. Chapter 7 permits a door to have a locking device that allows the door to be easily opened from within the facility for the purpose of egress but does not allow the door to be opened from outside the facility. Ordinary double-cylinder locks and chain locks do not meet these provisions.

Although resident sleeping room doors are located in the means of escape, it is the intent of 32/33.2.2.5.7 that the multiple latching/locking devices addressed by 7.2.1.5.9.3 and 7.2.1.5.9.4 be permitted.

**32.2.2.6 Stairs.**

**32.2.2.6.1** Stairs shall comply with 7.2.2, unless otherwise specified in this chapter.

**32.2.2.6.2** Winders complying with 7.2.2.2.4 shall be permitted only in conversions.

**32.2.2.6.3*** Exterior stairs shall be protected against blockage caused by fire within the building.

**A.32.2.2.6.3** Exterior stair protection can be accomplished through separation by physical distance, arrangement of the stairs, protection of the openings exposing the stairs, or other means acceptable to the authority having jurisdiction.

### 32.2.3 Protection.

**32.2.3.1 Protection of Vertical Openings.**

**32.2.3.1.1 Reserved.**

**32.2.3.1.2** Vertical openings, other than those meeting the requirement of 32.2.3.1.4, shall be separated by smoke partitions in accordance with Section 8.4 having a minimum $^1/_2$-hour fire resistance rating.

**32.2.3.1.3 Reserved.**

**32.2.3.1.4** Stairs shall be permitted to be open where complying with 32.2.2.4.6 or 32.2.2.4.7.

CHAPTER 33 • Existing

**33.2.2.5.6** Forces to open doors shall comply with 7.2.1.4.5.

**33.2.2.5.7** Door-latching devices shall comply with 7.2.1.5.9.

**33.2.2.6 Stairs.**

**33.2.2.6.1** Stairs shall comply with 7.2.2, unless otherwise specified in this chapter.

**33.2.2.6.2** Winders complying with 7.2.2.2.4 shall be permitted.

**33.2.2.6.3*** Exterior stairs shall be protected against blockage caused by fire within the building.

**A.33.2.2.6.3** Exterior stair protection can be accomplished through separation by physical distance, arrangement of the stairs, protection of the openings exposing the stairs, or other means acceptable to the authority having jurisdiction.

### 33.2.3 Protection.

**33.2.3.1 Protection of Vertical Openings.**

**33.2.3.1.1** Vertical openings, other than stairs complying with 33.2.2.4.5, 33.2.2.4.6, or 33.2.2.4.7, shall be protected so as not to expose a primary means of escape.

**33.2.3.1.2** Vertical openings required to be protected by 33.2.3.1.1 shall be considered protected where separated by smoke partitions in accordance with Section 8.4 that resist the passage of smoke from one story to any primary means of escape on another story.

**33.2.3.1.3** Smoke partitions used to protect vertical openings shall have a minimum $^1/_2$-hour fire resistance rating.

**33.2.3.1.4** Any doors or openings to the protected vertical opening shall be capable of resisting fire for a minimum of 20 minutes.

CHAPTER 32 • New

Exterior stairs do not have to meet the Chapter 7 requirements for outside stairs per 32/33.2.2.6.3. However, if the exterior stair is to be used as a primary means of escape, protection must be provided to reduce the likelihood that a fire within the facility will render the stair useless. Although this provision applies to small board and care facilities, note that 7.2.2.6.3.1(2) exempts outside stairs that serve a two-story building from the protection requirements of 7.2.2.6.3 if a remotely located second exit is provided. In such a case, the presence of an additional remote means of escape might be judged as adequate to eliminate the need to protect the exterior stair from a fire within the building. The text of A.32/A.33.2.2.6.3 provides additional guidance on protecting exterior stairs in small board and care facilities.

For new small board and care facilities, 32.2.3.1 mandates the enclosure of vertical openings with smoke partitions having a minimum ½-hour fire resistance rating in accordance with Section 8.4. See the definition of *smoke partition* in 3.3.238.

A smoke partition that limits the transfer of smoke is different from a smoke barrier that restricts smoke movement from one side of a barrier to the other. A smoke partition should be thought of as a barrier that reasonably limits, but doesn't necessarily prevent, smoke transfer. As such, suspended ceiling systems and monolithic surfaced ceilings are available that provide resistance to smoke transfer that is approximately equal to the traditional nonrated corridor wall or partition. See Section 8.4 and its commentary for details on smoke partitions.

Per 32.2.3.1.4, stairs are permitted to be open if they meet one of the options provided by 32.2.2.4.6 or 32.2.2.4.7. The two open-stair options for new small facilities are summarized as follows:

1. Paragraph 32.2.2.4.6 permits open stairs in sprinklered buildings not exceeding three stories in height, as long as each story is provided with a primary means of escape that is arranged so that occupants are not required to pass through a lower floor, unless that path is separated from all spaces on the lower floors by ½-hour-rated fire barriers.
2. Paragraph 32.2.2.4.7 permits completely open stairs in sprinklered buildings, provided that the stair serves (connects) not more than two stories.

CHAPTER 33 • Existing

In existing small board and care facilities, vertical openings are permitted to be unenclosed, except in cases where, by leaving the vertical opening unenclosed, the primary means of escape route is exposed to the unprotected vertical opening. Exhibit 32/33.7 illustrates an interior stair that, if it were not enclosed, would create an unprotected vertical opening. The interior stair is not part of the primary means of escape, but the vertical opening it creates must be enclosed, so that the route to the exterior stair (which serves as the primary means of escape for the second floor) is not exposed to an unprotected vertical opening. The enclosure around the vertical opening must be, at a minimum, a smoke partition.

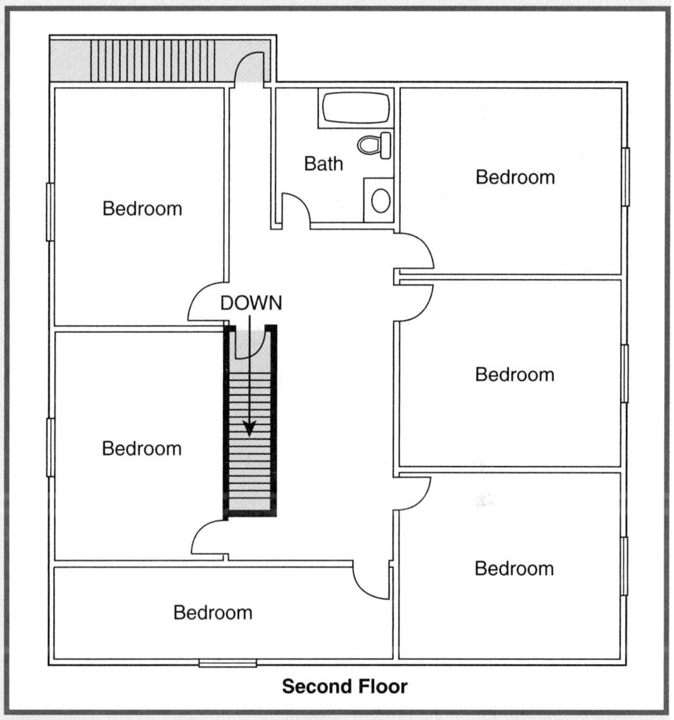


***Exhibit 32/33.7*** *Vertical opening protected so as not to expose the primary means of escape.*

In Exhibit 32/33.8, the vertical opening created by the interior stair does not expose the primary means of escape, which is the direct route from each bedroom to the exterior balconies and stairs.

**32.2.3.2 Hazardous Areas.**

**32.2.3.2.1*** Any space where there is storage or activity having fuel conditions exceeding those of a one- or two-

**33.2.3.2 Hazardous Areas.**

**33.2.3.2.1** Any space where there is storage or activity having fuel conditions exceeding those of a one- or two-family

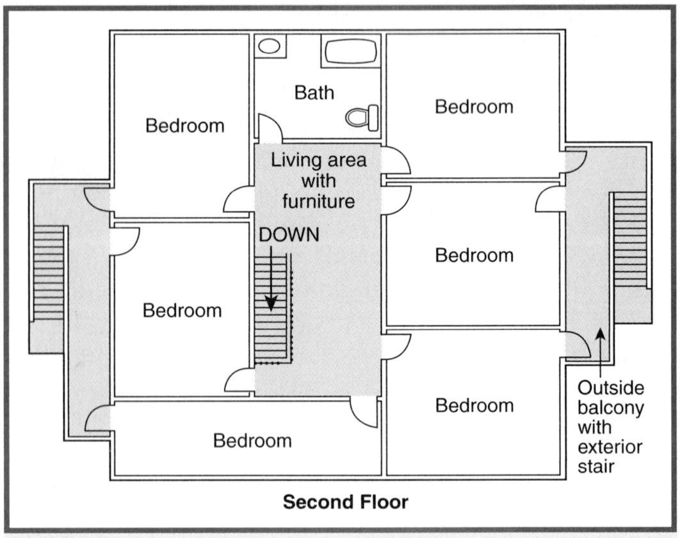


***Exhibit 32/33.8*** *Vertical opening not exposing the primary means of escape.*

family dwelling and that possesses the potential for a fully involved fire shall be protected in accordance with 32.2.3.2.4 and 32.2.3.2.5.

**A.32.2.3.2.1** Spaces containing approved, properly installed and maintained furnaces and heating equipment, furnace rooms, and cooking and laundry facilities should not be classified as hazardous areas solely on the basis of such equipment.

**32.2.3.2.2** Spaces requiring protection in accordance with 32.2.3.2.1 shall include, but shall not be limited to, areas for cartoned storage, food or household maintenance items in wholesale or institutional-type quantities and concentrations, or mass storage of residents' belongings.

**32.2.3.2.3 Reserved.**

**32.2.3.2.4** Any hazardous area that is on the same floor as, and is in or abuts, a primary means of escape or a sleeping room shall be protected by one of the following means:

(1) Protection shall be an enclosure having a minimum 1-hour fire resistance rating, in accordance with 8.2.3, and an automatic fire detection system connected to the fire alarm system provided in 32.2.3.4.1.
(2) Protection shall be automatic sprinkler protection, in accordance with 32.2.3.5, and a smoke partition, in accordance with Section 8.4, located between the hazardous area and the sleeping area or primary escape

dwelling and that possesses the potential for a fully involved fire shall be protected in accordance with 33.2.3.2.4 and 33.2.3.2.5.

**33.2.3.2.2** Spaces requiring protection in accordance with 33.2.3.2.1 shall include, but shall not be limited to, areas for cartoned storage, food or household maintenance items in wholesale or institutional-type quantities and concentrations, or mass storage of residents' belongings.

**33.2.3.2.3** Areas containing approved, properly installed and maintained furnaces and heating equipment, furnace rooms, and cooking and laundry facilities shall not be classified as hazardous areas solely on the basis of such equipment.

**33.2.3.2.4** Any hazardous area that is on the same floor as, and is in or abuts, a primary means of escape or a sleeping room shall be protected by one of the following means:

(1) Protection shall be an enclosure having a minimum 1-hour fire resistance rating, with self-closing or automatic-closing fire doors in accordance with 7.2.1.8 having a minimum $^{3}/_{4}$-hour fire protection rating.
(2) Protection shall be automatic sprinkler protection, in accordance with 33.2.3.5, and a smoke partition, in accordance with Section 8.4, located between the hazardous area and the sleeping area or primary escape

CHAPTER 32 • New

route, with any doors in such separation self-closing or automatic-closing in accordance with 7.2.1.8.

**32.2.3.2.5** Other hazardous areas shall be protected by one of the following:

(1) Enclosure having a minimum ½-hour fire resistance rating, with a self-closing or automatic-closing door in accordance with 7.2.1.8 that is equivalent to minimum 1¾ in. (44 mm) thick, solid-bonded wood-core construction, and protected by an automatic fire detection system connected to the fire alarm system provided in 32.2.3.4.1
(2) Automatic sprinkler protection in accordance with 32.2.3.5, regardless of enclosure

CHAPTER 33 • Existing

route, with any doors in such separation self-closing or automatic-closing in accordance with 7.2.1.8.

**33.2.3.2.5** Other hazardous areas shall be protected by one of the following:

(1) Enclosure having a minimum ½-hour fire resistance rating, with self-closing or automatic-closing doors in accordance with 7.2.1.8 equivalent to minimum 1¾ in. (44 mm) thick, solid-bonded wood-core construction
(2) Automatic sprinkler protection in accordance with 33.2.3.5, regardless of enclosure

It is recognized that small board and care facilities closely resemble one- and two-family dwellings. However, one of the most notable differences between the two is the type of hazards that might be present. In a small board and care facility, greater quantities of household maintenance and cleaning products, cartoned food, and mass storage of residents' belongings result in areas where a fire could quickly grow to full room involvement. These are the areas that 32/33.2.3.2.1 and 32/33.2.3.2.2 intend to be separated in accordance with 32/33.2.3.2.4 and 32/33.2.3.2.5.

The protection of hazardous contents areas is based on the potential impact that a fire in the hazardous contents would have on a primary means of escape or on sleeping rooms. If the hazardous area is located on the same floor as sleeping rooms or a primary means of escape, and if a sleeping room or means of escape is exposed to the hazardous area, one of the following two protection options is permitted:

1. The hazardous contents room must be separated from the remainder of the floor by construction with at least a 1-hour fire resistance rating, and automatic fire detection connected to the alarm system must be provided.
2. Automatic sprinkler protection must be provided within the hazardous contents room, and the separating construction must meet the requirements for smoke partitions in Section 8.4 but is not required to be fire rated.

If the hazardous area is located on a different floor or does not abut a primary means of escape or sleeping rooms, the hazard is considered less severe and can be protected using one of the following two methods:

1. The hazardous contents room must be separated from the remainder of the floor by construction with at least a ½-hour fire rating, and automatic fire detection connected to the alarm system must be provided.
2. Automatic sprinkler protection must be provided within the hazardous contents room; however, no smoke-resisting separation is required.

For example, consider a basement in a wood frame building housing a small board and care facility. The basement, which is used only for the storage of combustible materials, is not a required means of escape. If the basement storage area does not abut a sleeping area on the same floor and is sprinklered, sheathing the ceiling to provide fire resistance separation is not required. In applying the provisions of 32.2.3.2, note that the sprinkler protection required in nearly all new small board and care facilities by 32.2.3.5.1 should make the protection of hazardous contents areas relatively easy.

**32.2.3.3 Interior Finish.**

**32.2.3.3.1 General.** Interior finish shall be in accordance with Section 10.2.

**32.2.3.3.2 Interior Wall and Ceiling Finish.** Interior wall and ceiling finish materials complying with Section 10.2 shall be Class A, Class B, or Class C.

**33.2.3.3 Interior Finish.**

**33.2.3.3.1 General.** Interior finish shall be in accordance with Section 10.2.

**33.2.3.3.2 Interior Wall and Ceiling Finish.** Interior wall and ceiling finish materials complying with Section 10.2 shall be as follows:

CHAPTER 32 • New

32.2.3.3.3 **Interior Floor Finish.**

**32.2.3.3.3.1** Interior floor finish shall comply with Section 10.2.

**32.2.3.3.3.2** Interior floor finish shall comply with 10.2.7.1 or 10.2.7.2, as applicable.

**32.2.3.4 Detection, Alarm, and Communications Systems.**

**32.2.3.4.1 Fire Alarm Systems.** A manual fire alarm system shall be provided in accordance with Section 9.6.

**32.2.3.4.2 Occupant Notification.** Occupant notification shall be provided automatically, without delay, in accordance with 9.6.3.

**32.2.3.4.3 Smoke Alarms.**

**32.2.3.4.3.1** Approved smoke alarms shall be provided in accordance with 9.6.2.10.

**32.2.3.4.3.2** Smoke alarms shall be installed on all levels, including basements but excluding crawl spaces and unfinished attics.

CHAPTER 33 • Existing

(1) Class A or Class B in facilities other than those having prompt evacuation capability
(2) Class A, Class B, or Class C in facilities having prompt evacuation capability

**33.2.3.3.3 Interior Floor Finish.** (No requirements.)

**33.2.3.4 Detection, Alarm, and Communications Systems.**

**33.2.3.4.1 Fire Alarm Systems.** A manual fire alarm system shall be provided in accordance with Section 9.6, unless the provisions of 33.2.3.4.1.1 or 33.2.3.4.1.2 are met.

**33.2.3.4.1.1** A fire alarm system shall not be required where interconnected smoke alarms complying with 33.2.3.4.3 and not less than one manual fire alarm box per floor arranged to continuously sound the smoke detector alarms are provided.

**33.2.3.4.1.2** Other manually activated continuously sounding alarms acceptable to the authority having jurisdiction shall be permitted in lieu of a fire alarm system.

**33.2.3.4.2 Occupant Notification.** Occupant notification shall be in accordance with 9.6.3.

**33.2.3.4.3* Smoke Alarms.**

**A.33.2.3.4.3** Most often, smoke alarms sounding an alarm at 85 dBA or greater, installed outside the bedroom area, will meet the intent of this requirement. Smoke alarms remotely located from the bedroom might not be loud enough to awaken the average person. In such cases, it is recommended that smoke alarms be interconnected so that the activation of any smoke alarm will cause all smoke alarms to activate.

NFPA *101* provides adequate, balanced fire protection and takes into consideration the passive and active systems required in a given occupancy. The level of protection prescribed by *NFPA 72*, *National Fire Alarm Code*, which includes smoke alarms in all sleeping rooms, without exception, does not necessarily take into consideration the complete protection package prescribed by NFPA *101*.

**33.2.3.4.3.1** Approved smoke alarms shall be provided in accordance with 9.6.2.10, unless otherwise indicated in 33.2.3.4.3.6 and 33.2.3.4.3.7.

**33.2.3.4.3.2** Smoke alarms shall be installed on all levels, including basements but excluding crawl spaces and unfinished attics.

CHAPTER 32 • New

32.2.3.4.3.3 Additional smoke alarms shall be installed in all living areas, as defined in 3.3.19.5.

32.2.3.4.3.4 Each sleeping room shall be provided with an approved smoke alarm in accordance with 9.6.2.10.

32.2.3.4.4* **Protection of Fire Alarm System.** The provision of 9.6.1.8.1.3 shall not apply to the smoke detection required at each fire alarm control unit by 9.6.1.8.1(1).

A.32.2.3.4.4 It is the intent that smoke detection be provided at each fire alarm control unit, regardless of the presence of sprinkler protection.

CHAPTER 33 • Existing

33.2.3.4.3.3 Additional smoke alarms shall be installed for living rooms, dens, day rooms, and similar spaces.

33.2.3.4.3.4 **Reserved.**

33.2.3.4.3.5 Smoke alarms shall be powered from the building electrical system and, when activated, shall initiate an alarm that is audible in all sleeping areas.

33.2.3.4.3.6 Smoke alarms in accordance with 33.2.3.4.3.1 shall not be required where buildings are protected throughout by an approved automatic sprinkler system, in accordance with 33.2.3.5, that uses quick-response or residential sprinklers, and are protected with approved smoke alarms installed in each sleeping room, in accordance with 9.6.2.10, that are powered by the building electrical system.

33.2.3.4.3.7 Smoke alarms in accordance with 33.2.3.4.3.1 shall not be required where buildings are protected throughout by an approved automatic sprinkler system, in accordance with 33.2.3.5, that uses quick-response or residential sprinklers, with existing battery-powered smoke alarms in each sleeping room, and where, in the opinion of the authority having jurisdiction, the facility has demonstrated that testing, maintenance, and a battery replacement program ensure the reliability of power to the smoke alarms.

33.2.3.4.4* **Protection of Fire Alarm System.** The provision of 9.6.1.8.1.3 shall not apply to the smoke detection required at each fire alarm control unit by 9.6.1.8.1(1).

A.33.2.3.4.4 It is the intent that smoke detection be provided at each fire alarm control unit, regardless of the presence of sprinkler protection.

In both new and existing board and care facilities, a means of manually initiating the fire alarm system is required. However, 33.2.3.4.1 contains two provisions for existing facilities. The use of a "system" of interconnected multiple-station smoke alarms is permitted by 33.2.3.4.1.1 to meet the fire alarm requirement by providing one manual fire alarm box that is integrated with the smoke alarms on each floor. In addition, 33.2.3.4.1.2 recognizes that, in a small existing building, a sophisticated fire alarm system that employs components listed for use in fire alarm systems might not be necessary. The requirements can be satisfied by the installation of alternative means of notifying the occupants, such as electric bells activated by a clearly identified switch on each floor where approved by the authority having jurisdiction (AHJ).

The requirement of 32.2.3.4.3.1 does not mandate a system of smoke detectors in a small facility. If the building is small enough, single-station smoke alarms might meet the criterion of audibility in all sleeping areas. However, if the building is of significant size or consists of multiple levels, interconnected multiple-station smoke alarms will probably be needed. Additional smoke alarms are required in living rooms and day rooms.

Prior to the 2003 edition of the *Code*, several provisions permitted the omission of smoke alarms from small board and care facilities. However, given the wider acceptance of unprotected vertical openings permitted by 32.2.3.1, the smoke alarm exemptions are no longer permitted for new facilities. Several conditions for exempting smoke alarms from existing small board and care facilities, however, are provided. To exempt the requirement for common space smoke alarms, as permitted by 33.2.3.4.3.6 and 33.2.3.4.3.7, the entire building must be protected with an automatic sprinkler system using quick-response or residential sprinklers in accordance with 33.2.3.5, and the bedrooms must be provided with smoke alarms. If the existing smoke alarms in the bedrooms are powered

**32.2.3.5* Extinguishment Requirements.**

**A.32.2.3.5** All sprinkler systems installed in accordance with NFPA 13, *Standard for the Installation of Sprinkler Systems*, and NFPA 13R, *Standard for the Installation of Sprinkler Systems in Residential Occupancies up to and Including Four Stories in Height*, are required to be inspected, tested, and maintained in accordance with NFPA 25, *Standard for the Inspection, Testing, and Maintenance of Water-Based Fire Protection Systems*. However, systems installed in accordance with NFPA 13D, *Standard for the Installation of Sprinkler Systems in One- and Two-Family Dwellings and Manufactured Homes*, are historically exempt from applying NFPA 25. While there is a great deal of information in NFPA 25 that is not appropriate for NFPA 13D sprinkler systems, there are some basic concepts of inspection, testing, and maintenance that are critical to system performance and must be performed when an NFPA 13D sprinkler system is installed in a board and care occupancy. The frequencies mandated by this *Code* are slightly different from those required by NFPA 25. It is the intent of this *Code* to utilize the frequencies stated in Chapter 32, but to reference the purpose and the procedures for running the inspections, tests, and maintenance from NFPA 25.

**32.2.3.5.1*** All facilities, other than those meeting the requirement of 32.2.3.5.2, shall be protected throughout by an approved automatic sprinkler system, installed in accordance with 32.2.3.5.3, using quick-response or residential sprinklers.

**A.32.2.3.5.1** Where any provision requires the use of an automatic sprinkler system in accordance with 32.2.3.5, the provision of 32.2.3.5.2 is not permitted to be used.

**32.2.3.5.2*** In conversions, sprinklers shall not be required in small board and care homes serving eight or fewer residents when all occupants have the ability as a group to move reliably to a point of safety within 3 minutes.

**A.32.2.3.5.2** Where a facility utilizing the provision of 32.2.3.5.2 contains residents who can no longer comply with the 3-minute evacuation response, 33.1.7 requires the facility to comply with the requirements for new construction, including automatic sprinkler protection. *(See also A.33.1.7.)*



solely by batteries, they do not need to be replaced with electrically powered smoke alarms if the AHJ judges that the facility has an adequate testing, maintenance, and battery replacement program.

**33.2.3.5* Extinguishment Requirements.**

**A.33.2.3.5** All sprinkler systems installed in accordance with NFPA 13, *Standard for the Installation of Sprinkler Systems*, and NFPA 13R, *Standard for the Installation of Sprinkler Systems in Residential Occupancies up to and Including Four Stories in Height*, are required to be inspected, tested, and maintained in accordance with NFPA 25, *Standard for the Inspection, Testing, and Maintenance of Water-Based Fire Protection Systems*. However, systems installed in accordance with NFPA 13D, *Standard for the Installation of Sprinkler Systems in One- and Two-Family Dwellings and Manufactured Homes*, are historically exempt from applying NFPA 25. While there is a great deal of information in NFPA 25 that is not appropriate for NFPA 13D sprinkler systems, there are some basic concepts of inspection, testing, and maintenance that are critical to system performance and must be performed when an NFPA 13D sprinkler system is installed in a board and care occupancy. The frequencies mandated by this *Code* are slightly different from those required by NFPA 25. It is the intent of this *Code* to utilize the frequencies stated in Chapter 32, but to reference the purpose and the procedures for running the inspections, tests, and maintenance from NFPA 25.

**33.2.3.5.1 Reserved.**

**33.2.3.5.2** Where an automatic sprinkler system is installed, for either total or partial building coverage, the following requirements shall be met:

(1) The system shall be in accordance with Section 9.7 and shall initiate the fire alarm system in accordance with 33.2.3.4.1, as modified by 33.2.3.5.2.1 through 33.2.3.5.2.6.
(2) The adequacy of the water supply shall be documented to the authority having jurisdiction.

**33.2.3.5.2.1*** In prompt evacuation capability facilities, the following shall apply:

CHAPTER 32 • New

CHAPTER 33 • Existing

(1) An automatic sprinkler system in accordance with NFPA 13D, *Standard for the Installation of Sprinkler Systems in One- and Two-Family Dwellings and Manufactured Homes*, shall be permitted.
(2) Automatic sprinklers shall not be required in closets not exceeding 24 $ft^2$ (2.2 $m^2$) and in bathrooms not exceeding 55 $ft^2$ (5.1 $m^2$), provided that such spaces are finished with lath and plaster or materials providing a 15-minute thermal barrier.

**A.33.2.3.5.2.1** The decision to permit the use of the criteria from NFPA 13D, *Standard for the Installation of Sprinkler Systems in One- and Two-Family Dwellings and Manufactured Homes*, in these occupancies is based on the following:

(1) The desire to obtain a level of fire suppression and control approximately equivalent to that delivered by residential facilities protected by such systems *(see A.1.1 in NFPA 13D)*
(2) The fact that potential fire exposure and challenge to the suppression system in a small board and care facility are of the same nature and are no more severe than those found in residences

Chapter 33 permits the use of NFPA 13D and NFPA 13R, *Standard for the Installation of Sprinkler Systems in Residential Occupancies up to and Including Four Stories in Height*, outside of their scopes. This permission is based on a review of the occupancy and a recognition that the fires in board and care facilities are similar to those of other residential occupancies and that the level of protection is appropriate. In some circumstances, such as those for impractical evacuation capabilities, the requirements of NFPA 13D and NFPA 13R have been supplemented with requirements for additional water supplies to compensate for the special needs of the board and care occupancy.

**33.2.3.5.2.2** In slow and impractical evacuation capability facilities, the following shall apply:

(1) An automatic sprinkler system in accordance with NFPA 13D, *Standard for the Installation of Sprinkler Systems in One- and Two-Family Dwellings and Manufactured Homes*, with a 30-minute water supply, shall be permitted.
(2) All habitable areas and closets shall be sprinklered.
(3) Automatic sprinklers shall not be required in bathrooms not exceeding 55 $ft^2$ (5.1 $m^2$), provided that such spaces are finished with lath and plaster or materials providing a 15-minute thermal barrier.

**33.2.3.5.2.3** In prompt and slow evacuation facilities, where an automatic sprinkler system is in accordance with NFPA

CHAPTER 32 • New

CHAPTER 33 • Existing

13, *Standard for the Installation of Sprinkler Systems*, sprinklers shall not be required in closets not exceeding 24 $ft^2$ (2.2 $m^2$) and in bathrooms not exceeding 55 $ft^2$ (5.1 $m^2$), provided that such spaces are finished with lath and plaster or materials providing a 15-minute thermal barrier.

**33.2.3.5.2.4** In prompt and slow evacuation capability facilities in buildings four or fewer stories, above grade plane systems in accordance with NFPA 13R, *Standard for the Installation of Sprinkler Systems in Residential Occupancies up to and Including Four Stories in Height*, shall be permitted.

**33.2.3.5.2.5** In impractical evacuation capability facilities in buildings four or fewer stories above grade plane, systems in accordance with NFPA 13R, *Standard for the Installation of Sprinkler Systems in Residential Occupancies up to and Including Four Stories in Height*, shall be permitted. All habitable areas and closets shall be sprinklered. Automatic sprinklers shall not be required in bathrooms not exceeding 55 $ft^2$ (5.1 $m^2$), provided that such spaces are finished with lath and plaster or materials providing a 15-minute thermal barrier.

**33.2.3.5.2.6** Initiation of the fire alarm system shall not be required for existing installations in accordance with 33.2.3.5.6.

**32.2.3.5.3** Where an automatic sprinkler system is installed, for either total or partial building coverage, the following requirements shall be met:

(1) The system shall be in accordance with NFPA 13, *Standard for the Installation of Sprinkler Systems*, and shall initiate the fire alarm system in accordance with 32.2.3.4.1.
(2) The adequacy of the water supply shall be documented to the authority having jurisdiction.

**32.2.3.5.3.1** In buildings four or fewer stories above grade plane, systems in accordance with NFPA 13R, *Standard for the Installation of Sprinkler Systems in Residential Occupancies up to and Including Four Stories in Height*, shall be permitted. All habitable areas and closets shall be sprinklered.

**32.2.3.5.3.2*** An automatic sprinkler system with a 30-minute water supply, and complying with the following requirements and with NFPA 13D, *Standard for the Installation of Sprinkler Systems in One- and Two-Family Dwellings and Manufactured Homes*, shall be permitted:

(1) All habitable areas and closets shall be sprinklered.
(2) Facilities with more than eight residents shall be treated as two-family dwellings with regard to water supply.

**33.2.3.5.3** All impractical evacuation capability facilities shall be protected throughout by an approved, supervised automatic sprinkler system in accordance with 33.2.3.5.2.

**A.32.2.3.5.3.2** The decision to permit the use of the criteria from NFPA 13D, *Standard for the Installation of Sprinkler Systems in One- and Two-Family Dwellings and Manufactured Homes*, in these occupancies is based on the following:

(1) The desire to obtain a level of fire suppression and control approximately equivalent to that delivered by residential facilities protected by such systems (*see A.1.1 in NFPA 13D*)
(2) The fact that potential fire exposure and challenge to the suppression system in a small board and care facility are of the same nature and are no more severe than those found in residences

Chapter 32 permits the use of NFPA 13D, and NFPA 13R, *Standard for the Installation of Sprinkler Systems in Residential Occupancies up to and Including Four Stories in Height*, outside of their scopes. This permission is based on a review of the occupancy and a recognition that the fires in board and care facilities are similar to those of other residential occupancies and that the level of protection is appropriate. The requirements of NFPA 13D and NFPA 13R have been supplemented with requirements for additional water supplies to compensate for the special needs of the board and care occupancy.

NFPA 13D contains additional requirements for a piping system serving both sprinkler and domestic needs.

**32.2.3.5.4** Automatic sprinkler systems installed in accordance with NFPA 13, *Standard for the Installation of Sprinkler Systems*, and NFPA 13R, *Standard for the Installation of Sprinkler Systems in Residential Occupancies up to and Including Four Stories in Height*, shall be provided with electrical supervision in accordance with 9.7.2.

**33.2.3.5.4 Reserved.**

**32.2.3.5.5** Automatic sprinkler systems installed in accordance with NFPA 13D, *Standard for the Installation of Sprinkler Systems in One- and Two-Family Dwellings and Manufactured Homes*, shall be provided with valve supervision by one of the following methods:

(1) Single listed control valve that shuts off both domestic and sprinkler systems and separate shutoff for the domestic system only
(2) Electrical supervision in accordance with 9.7.2
(3) Valve closure that causes the sounding of an audible signal in the facility

**33.2.3.5.5 Reserved.**

**32.2.3.5.6** Sprinkler piping serving not more than six sprinklers for any isolated hazardous area shall be permitted to be installed in accordance with 9.7.1.2 and shall meet the following requirements:

(1) In new installations, where more than two sprinklers are installed in a single area, waterflow detection shall be

**33.2.3.5.6** Sprinkler piping serving not more than six sprinklers for any isolated hazardous area shall be permitted to be installed in accordance with 9.7.1.2 and shall meet the following requirements:

(1) In new installations, where more than two sprinklers are installed in a single area, waterflow detection shall be

provided to initiate the fire alarm system required by 32.2.3.4.1.

(2) The duration of water supplies shall be as required by 32.2.3.5.3.2.

**32.2.3.5.7** Systems installed in accordance with NFPA 13D, *Standard for the Installation of Sprinkler Systems in One- and Two-Family Dwellings and Manufactured Homes*, shall be inspected, tested, and maintained in accordance with 32.2.3.5.7.1 through 32.2.3.5.7.15, which reference specific sections of NFPA 25, *Standard for the Inspection, Testing, and Maintenance of Water-Based Fire Protection Systems*. The frequency of the inspection, test, or maintenance shall be in accordance with this *Code*, whereas the purpose and procedure shall be from NFPA 25.

**32.2.3.5.7.1** Control valves shall be inspected monthly in accordance with 13.3.2 of NFPA 25, *Standard for the Inspection, Testing, and Maintenance of Water-Based Fire Protection Systems*.

**32.2.3.5.7.2** Gages shall be inspected monthly in accordance with 13.2.7.1 of NFPA 25, *Standard for the Inspection, Testing, and Maintenance of Water-Based Fire Protection Systems*.

**32.2.3.5.7.3** Alarm devices shall be inspected quarterly in accordance with 5.2.6 of NFPA 25, *Standard for the Inspection, Testing, and Maintenance of Water-Based Fire Protection Systems*.

**32.2.3.5.7.4** Alarm devices shall be tested semiannually in accordance with 5.3.3 of NFPA 25, *Standard for the Inspection, Testing, and Maintenance of Water-Based Fire Protection Systems*.

**32.2.3.5.7.5** Valve supervisory switches shall be tested semiannually in accordance with 13.3.3.5 of NFPA 25, *Standard for the Inspection, Testing, and Maintenance of Water-Based Fire Protection Systems*.

**32.2.3.5.7.6** Visible sprinklers shall be inspected annually in accordance with 5.2.1 of NFPA 25, *Standard for the Inspection, Testing, and Maintenance of Water-Based Fire Protection Systems*.

**32.2.3.5.7.7** Visible pipe shall be inspected annually in accordance with 5.2.2 of NFPA 25, *Standard for the Inspection, Testing, and Maintenance of Water-Based Fire Protection Systems*.

**32.2.3.5.7.8** Visible pipe hangers shall be inspected annually in accordance with 5.2.3 of NFPA 25, *Standard for the Inspection, Testing, and Maintenance of Water-Based Fire Protection Systems*.



provided to initiate the fire alarm system required by 33.2.3.4.1.

(2) The duration of water supplies shall be as required for the sprinkler systems addressed in 33.2.3.5.2.

**33.2.3.5.7** Systems installed in accordance with NFPA 13D, *Standard for the Installation of Sprinkler Systems in One- and Two-Family Dwellings and Manufactured Homes*, shall be inspected, tested, and maintained in accordance with 33.2.3.5.7.1 through 33.2.3.5.7.15, which reference specific sections of NFPA 25, *Standard for the Inspection, Testing, and Maintenance of Water-Based Fire Protection Systems*. The frequency of the inspection, test, or maintenance shall be in accordance with this *Code*, whereas the purpose and procedure shall be from NFPA 25.

**33.2.3.5.7.1** Control valves shall be inspected monthly in accordance with 13.3.2 of NFPA 25, *Standard for the Inspection, Testing, and Maintenance of Water-Based Fire Protection Systems*.

**33.2.3.5.7.2** Gages shall be inspected monthly in accordance with 13.2.7.1 of NFPA 25, *Standard for the Inspection, Testing, and Maintenance of Water-Based Fire Protection Systems*.

**33.2.3.5.7.3** Alarm devices shall be inspected quarterly in accordance with 5.2.6 of NFPA 25, *Standard for the Inspection, Testing, and Maintenance of Water-Based Fire Protection Systems*.

**33.2.3.5.7.4** Alarm devices shall be tested semiannually in accordance with 5.3.3 of NFPA 25, *Standard for the Inspection, Testing, and Maintenance of Water-Based Fire Protection Systems*.

**33.2.3.5.7.5** Valve supervisory switches shall be tested semiannually in accordance with 13.3.3.5 of NFPA 25, *Standard for the Inspection, Testing, and Maintenance of Water-Based Fire Protection Systems*.

**33.2.3.5.7.6** Visible sprinklers shall be inspected annually in accordance with 5.2.1 of NFPA 25, *Standard for the Inspection, Testing, and Maintenance of Water-Based Fire Protection Systems*.

**33.2.3.5.7.7** Visible pipe shall be inspected annually in accordance with 5.2.2 of NFPA 25, *Standard for the Inspection, Testing, and Maintenance of Water-Based Fire Protection Systems*.

**33.2.3.5.7.8** Visible pipe hangers shall be inspected annually in accordance with 5.2.3 of NFPA 25, *Standard for the Inspection, Testing, and Maintenance of Water-Based Fire Protection Systems*.

CHAPTER 32 • New

**32.2.3.5.7.9** Buildings shall be inspected annually prior to the onset of freezing weather to ensure that there is adequate heat wherever water-filled piping is run in accordance with 5.2.5 of NFPA 25, *Standard for the Inspection, Testing, and Maintenance of Water-Based Fire Protection Systems.*

**32.2.3.5.7.10** A representative sample of fast-response sprinklers shall be tested once the sprinklers in the system are 20 years old in accordance with 5.3.1.1.1.2 of NFPA 25, *Standard for the Inspection, Testing, and Maintenance of Water-Based Fire Protection Systems.* If the sample fails the test, all of the sprinklers represented by that sample shall be replaced. If the sprinklers pass the test, the test shall be repeated every 10 years thereafter.

**32.2.3.5.7.11** A representative sample of dry-pendent sprinklers shall be tested once the sprinklers in the system are 10 years old in accordance with 5.3.1.1.1.5 of NFPA 25, *Standard for the Inspection, Testing, and Maintenance of Water-Based Fire Protection Systems.* If the sample fails the test, all of the sprinklers represented by that sample shall be replaced. If the sprinklers pass the test, the test shall be repeated every 10 years thereafter.

**32.2.3.5.7.12** Antifreeze solutions shall be tested annually in accordance with 5.3.4 of NFPA 25, *Standard for the Inspection, Testing, and Maintenance of Water-Based Fire Protection Systems.*

**32.2.3.5.7.13** Control valves shall be operated through their full range and returned to normal annually in accordance with 13.3.3.1 of NFPA 25, *Standard for the Inspection, Testing, and Maintenance of Water-Based Fire Protection Systems.*

**32.2.3.5.7.14** Operating stems of OS&Y valves shall be lubricated annually in accordance with 13.3.4 of NFPA 25, *Standard for the Inspection, Testing, and Maintenance of Water-Based Fire Protection Systems.*

**32.2.3.5.7.15** Dry-pipe systems that extend into the unheated portions of the building shall be inspected, tested, and maintained in accordance with 13.4.4 of NFPA 25, *Standard for the Inspection, Testing, and Maintenance of Water-Based Fire Protection Systems.*

CHAPTER 33 • Existing

**33.2.3.5.7.9** Buildings shall be inspected annually prior to the onset of freezing weather to ensure that there is adequate heat wherever water-filled piping is run in accordance with 5.2.5 of NFPA 25, *Standard for the Inspection, Testing, and Maintenance of Water-Based Fire Protection Systems.*

**33.2.3.5.7.10** A representative sample of fast-response sprinklers shall be tested once the sprinklers in the system are 20 years old in accordance with 5.3.1.1.1.2 of NFPA 25, *Standard for the Inspection, Testing, and Maintenance of Water-Based Fire Protection Systems.* If the sample fails the test, all of the sprinklers represented by that sample shall be replaced. If the sprinklers pass the test, the test shall be repeated every 10 years thereafter.

**33.2.3.5.7.11** A representative sample of dry-pendent sprinklers shall be tested once the sprinklers in the system are 10 years old in accordance with 5.3.1.1.1.5 of NFPA 25, *Standard for the Inspection, Testing, and Maintenance of Water-Based Fire Protection Systems.* If the sample fails the test, all of the sprinklers represented by that sample shall be replaced. If the sprinklers pass the test, the test shall be repeated every 10 years thereafter.

**33.2.3.5.7.12** Antifreeze solutions shall be tested annually in accordance with 5.3.4 of NFPA 25, *Standard for the Inspection, Testing, and Maintenance of Water-Based Fire Protection Systems.*

**33.2.3.5.7.13** Control valves shall be operated through their full range and returned to normal annually in accordance with 13.3.3.1 of NFPA 25, *Standard for the Inspection, Testing, and Maintenance of Water-Based Fire Protection Systems.*

**33.2.3.5.7.14** Operating stems of OS&Y valves shall be lubricated annually in accordance with 13.3.4 of NFPA 25, *Standard for the Inspection, Testing, and Maintenance of Water-Based Fire Protection Systems.*

**33.2.3.5.7.15** Dry-pipe systems that extend into the unheated portions of the building shall be inspected, tested, and maintained in accordance with 13.4.4 of NFPA 25, *Standard for the Inspection, Testing, and Maintenance of Water-Based Fire Protection Systems.*

New small board and care facilities must be protected by an automatic sprinkler system using quick-response or residential sprinklers in accordance with 32.2.3.5.1. This requirement recognizes the ability of quick-response and residential sprinklers to maintain tenability in the room of origin during most fire scenarios.

The provision of 32.2.3.5.2 recognizes the difficulties in retrofitting buildings that are converted to small board and care facilities and provides some relief in these situations.

The provision of 33.2.3.5.2 does not require the installation of automatic sprinkler systems in existing small board and care facilities. Rather, it establishes the criteria for installing automatic sprinkler systems that are provided voluntarily for the purpose of applying modifications to other *Code* requirements based on the presence of such systems.

Although a small board and care facility is of a different occupancy classification than a dwelling or mobile home, 32.2.3.5.3.2 and 33.2.3.5.2.1 permit the use of residential sprinkler systems installed in accordance with NFPA 13D, *Standard for the Installation of Sprinkler Systems in One- and Two-Family Dwellings and Manufactured Homes*,[3] for the reasons explained in A.32.2.3.5.3.2 and A.33.2.3.5.2.1. In new facilities and existing facilities with slow or impractical evacuation capability, occupants might not be immediately evacuated; therefore, the normal 10-minute water supply duration specified in NFPA 13D is required to be increased to 30 minutes. Also, in new facilities and existing facilities with slow or impractical evacuation capability, sprinklers are required in closets and all habitable areas.

The exemption for sprinklers in the bathrooms and closets of existing facilities, as permitted by 33.2.3.5.2.3, supplements the requirements of NFPA 13, *Standard for the Installation of Sprinkler Systems*.[4] In addition to meeting the size limitation requirements, the walls and ceilings of bathroom and closet spaces must have a 15-minute thermal barrier rating to qualify for the sprinkler exemption. The 15-minute thermal barrier rating includes walls and ceilings behind fixtures, such as prefabricated tub and shower enclosures.

The use of sprinkler systems installed in accordance with NFPA 13R, *Standard for the Installation of Sprinkler Systems in Residential Occupancies up to and Including Four Stories in Height*,[5] is recognized by 32.2.3.5.3.1, 33.2.3.5.2.4, and 33.2.3.5.2.5. In all new facilities and existing facilities with impractical evacuation capability, closets and habitable areas (other than existing small bathrooms) must be sprinklered.

In existing facilities with prompt and slow evacuation capability, the sprinkler systems might need to be supervised, depending on the requirements of the installation standard used. For new small board and care facilities, 32.2.3.5.4 requires electrical supervision of automatic sprinkler systems installed in accordance with NFPA 13 and NFPA 13R. Paragraph 32.2.3.5.5 requires supervision of NFPA 13D systems by one of three methods: a single valve controlling both the domestic and sprinkler water supply, electrical supervision in accordance with 9.7.2, or an audible alarm device that sounds when the sprinkler water supply valve is closed.

All existing small facilities with impractical evacuation capability must be sprinklered per 33.2.3.5.3. In a multiple occupancy, if sprinkler protection is provided only in the board and care facility, and not throughout the building, any modifications to requirements predicated on complete building sprinkler coverage are not permitted to be used.

The importance of the role of the sprinkler system in protecting occupants who cannot readily evacuate the building (defend-in-place strategy) requires that sprinkler systems in all new facilities and existing facilities with impractical evacuation capability be supervised in accordance with 9.7.2 or as specified in 32.2.3.5.5 for new small facilities with NFPA 13D systems. Note that 9.7.2 requires electrical supervision of control valves and the transmission of waterflow alarms to the fire department. NFPA 13D and NFPA 13R permit the sprinkler systems to be installed with the domestic water supply valve as the only means to shut off the sprinklers; no valves control only the sprinkler system.

The provisions of 32/33.2.3.5.6 that require water supply duration to be in accordance with 32.2.3.5.3.2 and 33.2.3.5.2 affect facilities where unlimited public water is not available and captive sources such as tanks are used. Either a 10-minute or 30-minute water supply duration is needed, depending on whether the facility is new or existing, and, if existing, depending on whether it is of prompt, slow, or impractical evacuation capability. Because 9.7.1.2 requires a capacity of 0.15 gpm/ft$^2$ (6.1 mm/min) for up to six sprinklers protecting an isolated hazardous area, a significant water reserve might be necessary.

Because there are very minimal maintenance requirements for sprinkler systems installed in accordance with NFPA 13D, and because the scope of NFPA 25, *Standard for the Inspection, Testing, and Maintenance of Water-Based Fire Protection Systems*,[6] excludes NFPA 13D sprinkler systems, 32/33.2.3.5.7 specifies a series of testing and maintenance requirements for such systems when installed in small board and care occupancies. Where NFPA 13D is utilized outside its originally intended scope (one- and two-family dwellings and manufactured homes), the *Code* supplements the requirements of NFPA 13D to ensure a high level of reliability, because the system is either a mandatory system or it is being used to modify some other *Code* requirement. The testing and maintenance require-

CHAPTER 32 • New

ments of 32/33.2.3.5.7 are not onerous. Several of the provisions, such as monthly visual inspection of control valves per 32/33.2.3.5.7.1, can be accomplished by the facility's owner or operator. Such routine visual inspection will help to ensure a control valve is not inadvertently closed, which could lead to the system's failure in the event of a fire.

**32.2.3.6 Construction of Corridor Walls.**

**32.2.3.6.1** Corridor walls, other than those meeting the provisions of 32.2.3.6.2, shall meet the following requirements:

(1) The walls separating sleeping rooms shall have a minimum $^1/_2$-hour fire resistance rating. The minimum $^1/_2$-hour fire resistance rating shall be considered to be achieved if the partitioning is finished on both sides with lath and plaster or materials providing a 15-minute thermal barrier.
(2) Sleeping room doors shall be substantial doors, such as those of $1^3/_4$ in. (44 mm) thick, solid-bonded wood-core construction or of other construction of equal or greater stability and fire integrity.
(3) Any vision panels shall be fixed fire window assemblies in accordance with 8.3.4 or shall be wired glass not exceeding 9 $ft^2$ (0.84 $m^2$) each in area and installed in approved frames.

CHAPTER 33 • Existing

**33.2.3.6 Construction of Corridor Walls.**

**33.2.3.6.1** Unless otherwise indicated in 33.2.3.6.1.1 through 33.2.3.6.1.4, corridor walls shall meet all of the following requirements:

(1) Walls separating sleeping rooms shall have a minimum $^1/_2$-hour fire resistance rating. The minimum $^1/_2$-hour fire resistance rating shall be considered to be achieved if the partitioning is finished on both sides with lath and plaster or materials providing a 15-minute thermal barrier.
(2) Sleeping room doors shall be substantial doors, such as those of $1^3/_4$ in. (44 mm) thick, solid-bonded wood-core construction or of other construction of equal or greater stability and fire integrity.
(3) Any vision panels shall be fixed fire window assemblies in accordance with 8.3.4 or shall be wired glass not exceeding 9 $ft^2$ (0.84 $m^2$) each in area and installed in approved frames.

**33.2.3.6.1.1** In prompt evacuation capability facilities, all sleeping rooms shall be separated from the escape route by smoke partitions in accordance with Section 8.4, and door closing shall be regulated by 33.2.3.6.4.

**33.2.3.6.1.2** The requirement of 33.2.3.6.1 shall not apply to corridor walls that are smoke partitions in accordance with Section 8.4 and that are protected by automatic sprinklers in accordance with 33.2.3.5 on both sides of the wall and door, and the following shall also apply:

(1) In such instances, there shall be no limitation on the type or size of glass panels.
(2) Door closing shall comply with 33.2.3.6.4.

**33.2.3.6.1.3** Sleeping arrangements that are not located in sleeping rooms shall be permitted for nonresident staff members, provided that the audibility of the alarm in the sleeping area is sufficient to awaken staff who might be sleeping.

**33.2.3.6.1.4** In previously approved facilities, where the facility has demonstrated to the authority having jurisdiction that the group is capable of evacuating the building in 8 minutes or less, or where the group achieves an E-score of 3 or less using the board and care occupancies evacuation capability determination methodology of NFPA 101A, *Guide on Alternative Approaches to Life Safety*, sleeping rooms shall be separated from escape routes by walls and doors that are smoke resistant.

CHAPTER 32 • New

**32.2.3.6.2** The requirements of 32.2.3.6.1 shall not apply to corridor walls that are smoke partitions in accordance with Section 8.4 where the facility is protected in accordance with 32.2.3.5, and the following shall also apply:

(1) In such instances, there shall be no limitation on the type or size of glass panels.
(2) Door closing shall comply with 32.2.3.6.4.

**32.2.3.6.3** No louvers, operable transoms, or other air passages shall penetrate the wall, except properly installed heating and utility installations other than transfer grilles, which shall be prohibited.

**32.2.3.6.4** Doors shall meet the following requirements:

(1) Doors shall be provided with latches or other mechanisms suitable for keeping the doors closed.
(2) No doors shall be arranged to prevent the occupant from closing the door.
(3) Doors shall be self-closing or automatic-closing in accordance with 7.2.1.8 in buildings other than those protected throughout by an approved automatic sprinkler system in accordance with 32.2.3.5.

CHAPTER 33 • Existing

**33.2.3.6.2 Reserved.**

**33.2.3.6.3** No louvers, operable transoms, or other air passages shall penetrate the wall, except properly installed heating and utility installations other than transfer grilles, which shall be prohibited.

**33.2.3.6.4** Doors shall meet the following requirements:

(1) Doors shall be provided with latches or other mechanisms suitable for keeping the doors closed.
(2) No doors shall be arranged to prevent the occupant from closing the door.
(3) Doors shall be self-closing or automatic-closing in accordance with 7.2.1.8 in buildings other than those protected throughout by an approved automatic sprinkler system in accordance with 33.2.3.5.2.

The intent of 32/33.2.3.6.1 in requiring corridor walls to have a ½-hour fire resistance rating is to require a nominal resistance to burn-through, particularly where the fire rating of existing partitions cannot be documented. Examples of acceptable partition assemblies include, but are not limited to, ½ in. (13 mm) thick gypsum board, wood lath and plaster, or metal lath and plaster.

Per 32.2.3.6.2 and 33.2.3.6.1.2, fire resistance–rated materials are not required where sprinkler protection is provided on both sides of the corridor wall and door. Complete sprinkler protection, as required for new construction by 32.2.3.5.1 and permitted for existing facilities by 33.2.3.5, would clearly meet this criterion. Therefore, this provision represents the most typical case where corridor walls and doors are required only to meet the requirements for smoke partitions (see Section 8.4).

There are many existing board and care facilities that employ sleep-in staff. Placing a staff cot in the supervisor's station, living room, or other room does not reclassify that room as a sleeping room. The provision in 33.2.3.6.1.3 is intended to permit staff members to sleep in locations that are not separated from the corridors.

Paragraph 33.2.3.6.1.4 permits a previously approved situation to continue to be recognized in existing small facilities with residents who perform in the faster half of the overall slow evacuation capability category. This provision cannot be used for a first-time evaluation of the adequacy of smoke-resisting corridor walls.

Doors in corridor walls are required by 32/33.2.3.6.4(3) to be self-closing or automatic-closing, unless the entire building is protected throughout by an approved automatic sprinkler system.

CHAPTER 32 • New

**32.2.4 Reserved.**

**32.2.5 Building Services.**

**32.2.5.1 Utilities.** Utilities shall comply with Section 9.1.

**32.2.5.2 Heating, Ventilating, and Air-Conditioning.**

**32.2.5.2.1** Heating, ventilating, and air-conditioning equipment shall comply with 9.2.1 and 9.2.2, unless otherwise required in this chapter.

CHAPTER 33 • Existing

**33.2.4 Reserved.**

**33.2.5 Building Services.**

**33.2.5.1 Utilities.** Utilities shall comply with Section 9.1.

**33.2.5.2 Heating, Ventilating, and Air-Conditioning.**

**33.2.5.2.1** Heating, ventilating, and air-conditioning equipment shall comply with the provisions of 9.2.1 and 9.2.2, except as otherwise required in this chapter.

**32.2.5.2.2** No stove or combustion heater shall be located to block escape in case of fire caused by the malfunction of the stove or heater.

**32.2.5.2.3** Unvented fuel-fired heaters shall not be used in any residential board and care facility.

**32.2.5.3 Elevators, Escalators, and Conveyors.** Elevators, escalators, and conveyors shall comply with Section 9.4.



**33.2.5.2.2** No stove or combustion heater shall be located to block escape in case of fire caused by the malfunction of the stove or heater.

**33.2.5.2.3** Unvented fuel-fired heaters shall not be used in any residential board and care facility.

The provision of 32/33.2.5.2.2 does not require a kitchen containing a stove to be completely separated by smoke partitions, only that the stove be located so that a malfunction does not result in a blockage of the means of escape. If, in the opinion of the authority having jurisdiction (AHJ), the location of the stove would cause the means of escape to be blocked in the event of a malfunction, the application of 32/33.2.3.2 might be appropriate for mitigating the hazard.

The use of a typical kerosene portable heater, as well as other fuel-fired, unvented heaters, is prohibited by 32/33.2.5.2.3.

## 32.3 Large Facilities

### 32.3.1 General.

**32.3.1.1 Scope.**

**32.3.1.1.1** Section 32.3 shall apply to residential board and care occupancies providing sleeping accommodations for more than 16 residents.

**32.3.1.1.2** Facilities having sleeping accommodations for not more than 16 residents shall comply with Section 32.2.

**32.3.1.2 Reserved.**

## 33.3 Large Facilities

### 33.3.1 General.

**33.3.1.1 Scope.**

**33.3.1.1.1** Section 33.3 shall apply to residential board and care occupancies providing sleeping accommodations for more than 16 residents.

**33.3.1.1.2** Facilities having sleeping accommodations for not more than 16 residents shall be evaluated in accordance with Section 33.2.

**33.3.1.1.3** Facilities meeting the requirements of Section 33.3 shall be considered to have met the requirements of Section 33.2 for prompt evacuation capability or slow evacuation capability.

**33.3.1.2 Requirements Based on Evacuation Capability.**

**33.3.1.2.1 Prompt and Slow.** Large facilities classified as prompt or slow evacuation capability, other than those meeting the requirement of 33.3.1.2.1.1 or 33.3.1.2.1.2, shall comply with the requirements of Section 33.3, as indicated for the appropriate evacuation capability.

**33.3.1.2.1.1*** Facilities where the authority having jurisdiction has determined equivalent safety is provided in accordance with Section 1.4 shall not be required to comply with the requirements of Section 33.3, as indicated for the appropriate evacuation capability.

**A.33.3.1.2.1.1** In determining equivalency for existing buildings, conversions, modernizations, renovations, or unusual design concepts, the authority having jurisdiction might permit evaluations based on the residential board and care occupancies fire safety evaluation system (FSES) of NFPA 101A, *Guide on Alternative Approaches to Life Safety*.

**33.3.1.2.1.2** Facilities that were previously approved as complying with 33.3.1.2.2 shall not be required to comply with the requirements of Section 33.3, as indicated for the appropriate evacuation capability.

**33.3.1.2.2* Impractical.** Large facilities classified as impractical evacuation capability shall meet the requirements for limited care facilities in Chapter 19, unless the authority having jurisdiction has determined equivalent safety is provided in accordance with Section 1.4.

**A.33.3.1.2.2** In determining equivalency for existing buildings, the authority having jurisdiction might permit evaluations based on the health care occupancies fire safety evaluation system (FSES) of NFPA 101A, *Guide on Alternative Approaches to Life Safety*, substituting the mandatory safety requirements values of Table A.33.3.1.2.2 for those contained in NFPA 101A.

***Table A.33.3.1.2.2 Substitute Mandatory Safety Requirements Values***

| Zone Location | Containment ($S_a$) | Extinguishment ($S_b$) | People Movement ($S_c$) |
|---|---|---|---|
| First floor | 5 | 6 | 3 |
| Above or below first floor | 9 | 8 | 5 |
| Over 75 ft (23 m) in height | 9 | 8 | 5 |

**33.3.1.2.3 Evacuation Capability Determination.**

**33.3.1.2.3.1** Facility management shall furnish to the authority having jurisdiction, upon request, an evacuation capability determination using a procedure acceptable to the authority having jurisdiction.

**33.3.1.2.3.2** Where the documentation required by 33.3.1.2.3.1 is not furnished, the evacuation capability shall be classified as impractical.

The importance of an accurate evaluation of evacuation capabilities in existing facilities cannot be overstated. Ineffective resident or staff response was a contributing factor in many of the multiple-death fires listed in Commentary Table 32/33.1.

Determining a facility's evacuation capability is not simply a matter of timing a fire drill in the middle of the day. Many variables affect a resident's capability to evacuate, and these variables must be carefully considered and factored into the documentation presented

CHAPTER 32 • New

to the authority having jurisdiction (AHJ) for approval. Some variables that should be considered follow.

*Time of Day.* An occupant's ability to evacuate might be slowed dramatically when the occupant must be awakened. In such a situation, the occupant must process the information that evacuation is necessary and then begin evacuating.

*Medication.* Many individuals in board and care occupancies take various medications for behavior control or as sleeping aids. If an individual is medicated, he or she might need additional assistance in responding and evacuating.

*Mobility and Location of Occupants.* Once individuals become aware of an emergency and take action, their ability to move through the building must be considered. Individuals using wheelchairs, walkers, or canes are further slowed when using stairs or ramps or when opening doors.

*Staff Assistance.* Though the *Code* does not specify minimum staffing levels, staffing levels should be considered, especially where high resident-to-staff ratios exist. Given the additional needs mentioned in the first three variables, the staff will be limited in their ability to affect evacuation time where multiple residents need assistance.

The evacuation capability of the population of a board and care occupancy might vary over time. The required documentation should be reviewed regularly to ensure that it accurately represents the current evacuation capability of the residents and staff.

When determining equivalency in accordance with 33.3.1.2.1.1 or 33.3.1.2.2, it is important to note that the equivalency measurement systems of the 2007 edition of NFPA 101A, *Guide on Alternative Approaches to Life Safety,* were calibrated against the requirements of the 2006 edition of NFPA *101* and might not accurately evaluate equivalency with the requirements of the 2009 edition of the *Life Safety Code*. At the time this handbook went to press, the 2010 edition of NFPA 101A was being prepared. Once issued, the 2010 edition of NFPA 101A can be used to measure equivalency against the requirements of the 2009 edition of the *Code*.

The difficulty in moving occupants to the outside of a facility with an impractical evacuation capability is comparable to that of doing so in a health care facility. Therefore, 33.3.1.2.2 mandates that existing large board and care facilities with impractical evacuation capability are subject to the requirements of Chapter 19, rather than those of Chapter 33. Chapter 19 employs a detailed defend-in-place strategy. If the equivalency methodologies of NFPA 101A are to be applied to a large board and care facility with impractical evacuation capability, the health care fire safety evaluation system (FSES) must be used instead of the board and care FSES.

The requirements in Section 32.3 for new large board and care facilities, which were significantly revised for the 2003 edition of the *Code*, are predicated on the assumption the facility might be occupied by residents classified as having impractical evacuation capability. Since the requirements are based on an assumed worst-case scenario, no evaluation of evacuation capability is required in facilities meeting the requirements of Chapter 32.

**32.3.1.3 Minimum Construction Requirements.** Large board and care facilities shall be limited to the building construction types specified in Table 32.3.1.3 *(see 8.2.1)*, based on the number of stories in height as defined in 4.6.3.

CHAPTER 33 • Existing

**33.3.1.3 Minimum Construction Requirements.** Large facilities shall be limited to the building construction types specified in Table 33.3.1.3. *(See 8.2.1.)*

Because evacuation strategies might be limited to moving residents to a point of safety, the *Code* regulates construction type to ensure building stability if the residents are to remain inside. The stability of the building is maintained either by the use of an automatic sprinkler system (as required for new construction by 32.3.3.5.1) or by the use of fire-resistant construction. Although Table 32.3.1.3 and Table 33.3.1.3 are new to the 2009 edition of the *Code*, it is not their intent to change any technical construction requirement from the previous edition. Rather, the tables summarize the new construction requirements that were previously contained in *NFPA 5000, Building Construction and Safety Code,* and the construction requirements for existing large board and care facilities that were previously spread across numerous paragraphs. The addition of the new tables is intended to make the *Code* more user friendly.

*Table 32.3.1.3 Construction Type Limitations*

| Construction Type | Sprinklered[b] | Stories in Height[a] | | | | |
|---|---|---|---|---|---|---|
| | | 1 | 2 | 3 | 4–12 | >12 |
| I (442)[c, d] | Yes | X | X | X | X | X |
| | No | NP | NP | NP | NP | NP |
| I (332)[c, d] | Yes | X | X | X | X | X |
| | No | NP | NP | NP | NP | NP |
| II (222)[c, d] | Yes | X | X | X | X | NP |
| | No | NP | NP | NP | NP | NP |
| II (111)[c, d] | Yes | X | X | X | NP | NP |
| | No | NP | NP | NP | NP | NP |
| II (000) | Yes | X | X | NP | NP | NP |
| | No | NP | NP | NP | NP | NP |
| III (211) | Yes | X | X | NP | NP | NP |
| | No | NP | NP | NP | NP | NP |
| III (200) | Yes | X | NP | NP | NP | NP |
| | No | NP | NP | NP | NP | NP |
| IV (2HH) | Yes | X | X | NP | NP | NP |
| | No | NP | NP | NP | NP | NP |
| V (111) | Yes | X | X | NP | NP | NP |
| | No | NP | NP | NP | NP | NP |
| V (000) | Yes | X | NP | NP | NP | NP |
| | No | NP | NP | NP | NP | NP |

X: Permitted. NP: Not permitted.

[a]See 4.6.3.

[b]Building protected throughout by an approved automatic sprinkler system installed in accordance with 9.7.1.1(1), and provided with quick-response or residential sprinklers throughout. (*See 32.3.3.5.*)

[c]Any building of Type I, Type II(222), or Type II(111) construction is permitted to include roofing systems involving combustible supports, decking, or roofing, provided that all of the following are met:

(1) The roof covering meets Class A requirements in accordance with NFPA 256, *Standard Methods of Fire Tests of Roof Coverings*.

(2) The roof is separated from all occupied portions of the building by a noncombustible floor assembly having not less than a 2-hour fire resistance rating that includes not less than $2^1/_2$ in. (63 mm) of concrete or gypsum fill.

(3) The structural elements supporting the 2-hour fire resistance–rated floor assembly specified in item (2) is required to have only the fire resistance rating required of the building.

[d]Any building of Type I, Type II(222), or Type II(111) construction is permitted to include roofing systems involving combustible supports, decking, or roofing, provided that all of the following criteria are met:

(1) The roof covering meets Class A requirements in accordance with NFPA 256, *Standard Methods of Fire Tests of Roof Coverings*.

(2) The roof/ceiling assembly is constructed with fire-retardant-treated wood meeting the requirements of NFPA 220, *Standard on Types of Building Construction*.

(3) The roof/ceiling assembly has the required fire resistance rating for the type of construction.

*Table 33.3.1.3 Construction Type Limitations*

| Construction Type | Sprinklered[b] | Stories in Height[a] 1[c] | 2 | 3 | 4 | 5 | 6 | >6 |
|---|---|---|---|---|---|---|---|---|
| I (442)[d, e] | Yes | X | X | X | X | X | X | X |
| | No | X | X | X | X | X | X | X |
| I (332)[d, e] | Yes | X | X | X | X | X | X | X |
| | No | X | X | X | X | X | X | X |
| II (222)[d, e] | Yes | X | X | X | X | X | X | X |
| | No | X | X | X | X | X | X | X |
| II (111)[d, e] | Yes | X | X | X | X | X | X | X |
| | No | X | X | X | X | X | X | NP |
| II (000) | Yes | X | X | X2 | X2 | X2 | X2 | NP |
| | No | X1 | X1 | NP | NP | NP | NP | NP |
| III (211) | Yes | X | X | X | X | X | X | X |
| | No | X | X | X | X | X | X | NP |
| III (200) | Yes | X | X | X2 | X2 | X2 | X2 | NP |
| | No | X1 | X1 | NP | NP | NP | NP | NP |
| IV (2HH) | Yes | X | X | X | X | X | X | X |
| | No | X | X | NP | NP | NP | NP | NP |
| V (111) | Yes | X | X | X2 | X2 | X2 | X2 | NP |
| | No | X | X | NP | NP | NP | NP | NP |
| V (000) | Yes | X | X | X2 | X2 | NP | NP | NP |
| | No | X1 | X1 | NP | NP | NP | NP | NP |

NP: Not permitted.

X: Permitted.

X1: Permitted if the interior walls are covered with lath and plaster or materials providing a 15-minute thermal barrier.

X2: Permitted if the interior walls are covered with lath and plaster or materials providing a 15-minute thermal barrier, and protected throughout by an approved automatic sprinkler system installed in accordance with 33.3.3.5.

[a]See 4.6.3.

[b]Building protected throughout by an approved, supervised automatic sprinkler system installed in accordance with Section 9.7. (*See 33.3.3.5.*)

[c]One-story prompt evacuation capability facilities having 30 or fewer residents with egress directly to the exterior at the finished ground level is permitted to be of any construction type.

[d]Any building of Type I, Type II(222), or Type II(111) construction is permitted to include roofing systems involving combustible supports, decking, or roofing, provided that all of the following are met:

(1) The roof covering meets Class A requirements in accordance with NFPA 256, *Standard Methods of Fire Tests of Roof Coverings.*

(2) The roof is separated from all occupied portions of the building by a noncombustible floor assembly having not less than a 2-hour fire resistance rating that includes not less than $2^1/_2$ in. (63 mm) of concrete or gypsum fill, and the attic or other space so developed is either unused or protected throughout by an approved automatic sprinkler system in accordance with 33.3.3.5.1.

[e]Any building of Type I, Type II(222), or Type II(111) construction is permitted to include roofing systems involving combustible supports, decking, or roofing, provided that all of the following are met:

(1) The roof covering meets Class A requirements in accordance with NFPA 256, *Standard Methods of Fire Tests of Roof Coverings.*

(2) The roof/ceiling assembly is constructed with fire-retardant-treated wood meeting the requirements of NFPA 220, *Standard on Types of Building Construction.*

(3) The roof/ceiling assembly has the required fire resistance rating for the type of construction.

CHAPTER 32 • New

**32.3.1.4 Occupant Load.** The occupant load, in number of persons for whom means of egress and other provisions are required, shall be determined on the basis of the occupant load factors of Table 7.3.1.2 that are characteristic of the use of the space, or shall be determined as the maximum probable population of the space under consideration, whichever is greater.

The determination of actual occupant load is based on the total number of residents, staff, and visitors. If the actual occupant load of the facility exceeds the occupant load calculated on the basis of one person per 200 $ft^2$ (18.6 $m^2$), as stipulated in Table 7.3.1.2, the egress capacity must be designed to meet the actual (larger) occupant load. However, if the actual occupant load is smaller than the calculated occupant load, the minimum egress capacity must not be less than that required for the calculated (larger) occupant load.

### 32.3.2 Means of Egress.

**32.3.2.1 General.**

**32.3.2.1.1** Means of egress from resident rooms and resident dwelling units to the outside of the building shall be in accordance with Chapter 7 and this chapter.

**32.3.2.1.2** Means of escape within the resident room or resident dwelling unit shall comply with Section 24.2 for one- and two-family dwellings.

**32.3.2.2 Means of Egress Components.**

**32.3.2.2.1 Components Permitted.** Components of means of egress shall be limited to the types described in 32.3.2.2.2 through 32.3.2.2.10.

**32.3.2.2.2 Doors.** Doors in means of egress shall be as follows:

(1) Doors complying with 7.2.1 shall be permitted.
(2) Doors within individual rooms and suites of rooms shall be permitted to be swinging or sliding.
(3) No door, other than those meeting the requirement of 32.3.2.2.2(4) or (5), shall be equipped with a lock or latch that requires the use of a tool or key from the egress side.
(4) Delayed-egress locks in accordance with 7.2.1.6.1 shall be permitted, provided that not more than one device is located in any egress path.
(5) Access-controlled egress doors in accordance with 7.2.1.6.2 shall be permitted.
(6) Doors located in the means of egress that are permitted to be locked under other provisions of Chapter 32, other than those meeting the requirement of 32.3.2.2.2(4) or (5), shall have adequate provisions made for the rapid removal of occupants by means such as remote control of locks, keying of all locks to keys carried by staff at all times, or other such reliable means available to staff at all times.

CHAPTER 33 • Existing

**33.3.1.4 Occupant Load.** The occupant load, in number of persons for whom means of egress and other provisions are required, shall be determined on the basis of the occupant load factors of Table 7.3.1.2 that are characteristic of the use of the space, or shall be determined as the maximum probable population of the space under consideration, whichever is greater.

### 33.3.2 Means of Egress.

**33.3.2.1 General.**

**33.3.2.1.1** Means of egress from resident rooms and resident dwelling units to the outside of the building shall be in accordance with Chapter 7 and this chapter.

**33.3.2.1.2** Means of escape within the resident room or resident dwelling unit shall comply with Section 24.2 for one- and two-family dwellings.

**33.3.2.2 Means of Egress Components.**

**33.3.2.2.1 Components Permitted.** Components of means of egress shall be limited to the types described in 33.3.2.2.2 through 33.3.2.2.10.

**33.3.2.2.2 Doors.** Doors in means of egress shall be as follows:

(1) Doors complying with 7.2.1 shall be permitted.
(2) Doors within individual rooms and suites of rooms shall be permitted to be swinging or sliding.
(3) No door in any means of egress, other than those meeting the requirement of 33.3.2.2.2(4) or (5), shall be locked against egress when the building is occupied.
(4) Delayed-egress locks in accordance with 7.2.1.6.1 shall be permitted, provided that not more than one device exists in a means of egress.
(5) Access-controlled egress doors in accordance with 7.2.1.6.2 shall be permitted.
(6) Revolving doors complying with 7.2.1.10 shall be permitted.

(7) Only one such locking device, as described in 32.3.2.2.2(6), shall be permitted on each door.

**32.3.2.2.3 Stairs.** Stairs complying with 7.2.2 shall be permitted.

**32.3.2.2.4 Smokeproof Enclosures.** Smokeproof enclosures complying with 7.2.3 shall be permitted.

**32.3.2.2.5 Horizontal Exits.** Horizontal exits complying with 7.2.4 shall be permitted.

**32.3.2.2.6 Ramps.** Ramps complying with 7.2.5 shall be permitted.

**32.3.2.2.7 Exit Passageways.** Exit passageways complying with 7.2.6 shall be permitted.

**32.3.2.2.8 Fire Escape Ladders.** Fire escape ladders complying with 7.2.9 shall be permitted.

**32.3.2.2.9 Alternating Tread Devices.** Alternating tread devices complying with 7.2.11 shall be permitted.

**32.3.2.2.10 Areas of Refuge.** Areas of refuge complying with 7.2.12 shall be permitted.



**33.3.2.2.3 Stairs.** Stairs complying with 7.2.2 shall be permitted.

**33.3.2.2.4 Smokeproof Enclosures.** Smokeproof enclosures complying with 7.2.3 shall be permitted.

**33.3.2.2.5 Horizontal Exits.** Horizontal exits complying with 7.2.4 shall be permitted.

**33.3.2.2.6 Ramps.** Ramps complying with 7.2.5 shall be permitted.

**33.3.2.2.7 Exit Passageways.** Exit passageways complying with 7.2.6 shall be permitted.

**33.3.2.2.8 Fire Escape Ladders.** Fire escape ladders complying with 7.2.9 shall be permitted.

**33.3.2.2.9 Alternating Tread Devices.** Alternating tread devices complying with 7.2.11 shall be permitted.

**33.3.2.2.10 Areas of Refuge.** Areas of refuge complying with 7.2.12 shall be permitted.

A general reference to Chapter 7 is made in 32/33.3.2.1 rather than repeating specific provisions. Many of the requirements contained in 32/33.3.2 are Chapter 7 provisions that require occupancy chapter permission, such as in 32/33.3.2.2.2(4), which permits the use of delayed-egress locks in accordance with 7.2.1.6.1. The limits placed on travel distance in 32/33.3.2.6 are examples of provisions for which the occupancy chapters are permitted to establish restrictions.

Facilities are prohibited from having any door locked against egress while the building is occupied per 32/33.3.2.2.2(3). This is consistent with a fundamental means of egress provision of Chapter 7. This requirement permits a door to have a locking device that allows the door to be opened from within the facility for the purpose of egress but does not allow the door to be opened from outside the facility. Ordinary double-cylinder locks and chain locks do not meet these provisions.

The use of delayed-egress locks that comply with 7.2.1.6.1 is permitted by 32/33.3.2.2.2(4), provided that not more than one delayed-egress device is encountered in any means of egress path. This provision requires that the building be either protected throughout by automatic sprinklers or equipped throughout with an automatic fire detection system. The 15-second or 30-second delay permitted by 7.2.1.6.1 does not affect the immediate release of the lock upon activation of the sprinklers or detectors or upon loss of power to the lock. The delayed-egress device helps provide security for infrequently used doors in board and care facilities, while doors remain available for emergency use. Chains and padlocks do not provide this feature.

**32.3.2.3 Capacity of Means of Egress.**

**32.3.2.3.1** The capacity of means of egress shall be in accordance with Section 7.3.

**32.3.2.3.2** Street floor exits shall be sufficient for the occupant load of the street floor plus the required capacity of stairs and ramps discharging onto the street floor.

**32.3.2.3.3** The width of corridors shall be sufficient for the occupant load served but shall be not less than 60 in. (1525 mm).

**33.3.2.3 Capacity of Means of Egress.**

**33.3.2.3.1** The capacity of means of egress shall be in accordance with Section 7.3.

**33.3.2.3.2** Street floor exits shall be sufficient for the occupant load of the street floor plus the required capacity of stairs and ramps discharging onto the street floor.

**33.3.2.3.3** The width of corridors serving an occupant load of 50 or more shall be sufficient for the occupant load served but shall be not less than 44 in. (1120 mm).

CHAPTER 32 • New

**32.3.2.4 Number of Exits.** The minimum number of exits as required by Section 7.4 shall be provided on every story.

**32.3.2.5 Arrangement of Means of Egress.**

**32.3.2.5.1** Access to all required exits shall be in accordance with Section 7.5.

**32.3.2.5.2** Common paths of travel shall not exceed 75 ft (23 m).

**32.3.2.5.3 Reserved.**

**32.3.2.5.4** Dead-end corridors shall not exceed 30 ft (9.1 mm).

**32.3.2.5.5** Any room, or any suite of rooms, exceeding 2000 $ft^2$ (185 $m^2$) shall be provided with not less than two exit access doors located remotely from each other.

**32.3.2.6 Travel Distance to Exits.** Travel distance from any point in a room to the nearest exit, measured in accordance with Section 7.6, shall not exceed 250 ft (76 m).

CHAPTER 33 • Existing

**33.3.2.3.4** Corridors serving an occupant load fewer than 50 shall be not less than 36 in. (915 mm) wide.

**33.3.2.4 Number of Exits.** The minimum number of exits as required by Section 7.4 shall be provided on every story.

**33.3.2.5 Arrangement of Means of Egress.**

**33.3.2.5.1** Access to all required exits shall be in accordance with Section 7.5.

**33.3.2.5.2** Common paths of travel shall not exceed 110 ft (33.5 m) in buildings not protected throughout by an automatic sprinkler system in accordance with 33.3.3.5.

**33.3.2.5.3** In buildings protected throughout by automatic sprinkler systems in accordance with 33.3.3.5, common paths of travel shall not exceed 160 ft (48.8 m).

**33.3.2.5.4** Dead-end corridors shall not exceed 50 ft (15 m).

**33.3.2.6 Travel Distance to Exits.**

**33.3.2.6.1** Travel distance from the door within a room, suite, or living unit to a corridor door shall not exceed 75 ft (23 m) in buildings not protected throughout by an approved automatic sprinkler system in accordance with 33.3.3.5.

**33.3.2.6.2** Travel distance from the door within a room, suite, or living unit to a corridor door shall not exceed 125 ft (38 m) in buildings protected throughout by an approved automatic sprinkler system in accordance with 33.3.3.5.

**33.3.2.6.3** Travel distance from the corridor door of any room to the nearest exit shall be in accordance with 33.3.2.6.3.1, 33.3.2.6.3.2, or 33.3.2.6.3.3.

**33.3.2.6.3.1** Travel distance from the corridor door of any room to the nearest exit, measured in accordance with Section 7.6, shall not exceed 100 ft (30 m).

**33.3.2.6.3.2** Travel distance to exits shall not exceed 200 ft (61 m) for exterior ways of exit access arranged in accordance with 7.5.3.

**33.3.2.6.3.3** Travel distance to exits shall not exceed 200 ft (61 m) if the exit access and any portion of the building that is tributary to the exit access are protected throughout by approved automatic sprinkler systems in accordance with 33.3.3.5. In addition, the portion of the building in which 200 ft (61 m) travel distance is permitted shall be separated from the remainder of the building by construction having a minimum 1-hour fire resistance rating, for buildings three or fewer stories in height, and a minimum 2-hour fire resistance rating for buildings four or more stories in height.

CHAPTER 32 • New

**32.3.2.7 Discharge from Exits.** Exit discharge shall comply with Section 7.7.

**32.3.2.8 Illumination of Means of Egress.** Means of egress shall be illuminated in accordance with Section 7.8.

**32.3.2.9 Emergency Lighting.** Emergency lighting in accordance with Section 7.9 shall be provided, unless each sleeping room has a direct exit to the outside at the finished ground level.

**32.3.2.10 Marking of Means of Egress.** Means of egress shall be marked in accordance with Section 7.10.

**32.3.2.11 Special Means of Egress Features.**

**32.3.2.11.1 Reserved.**

**32.3.2.11.2 Lockups.** Lockups in residential board and care occupancies shall comply with the requirements of 22.4.5.

CHAPTER 33 • Existing

**33.3.2.7 Discharge from Exits.** Exit discharge shall comply with Section 7.7.

**33.3.2.8 Illumination of Means of Egress.** Means of egress shall be illuminated in accordance with Section 7.8.

**33.3.2.9 Emergency Lighting.** Emergency lighting in accordance with Section 7.9 shall be provided in all buildings with more than 25 rooms, unless each sleeping room has a direct exit to the outside of the building at the finished ground level.

**33.3.2.10 Marking of Means of Egress.** Means of egress shall be marked in accordance with Section 7.10.

**33.3.2.11 Special Means of Egress Features.**

**33.3.2.11.1 Reserved.**

**33.3.2.11.2 Lockups.** Lockups in residential board and care occupancies, other than approved existing lockups, shall comply with the requirements of 23.4.5.

Street-floor egress capacity must be provided in accordance with 32/33.3.2.3.2, such that it is sufficient to accommodate the convergence of first-floor occupants with occupants leaving exit enclosures from the upper and lower floors and traversing areas of the first floor. This concept is common in hotel, apartment, business, and mercantile occupancies. See the commentary following 28/29.2.3.2 and Exhibit 28/29.3.

The provisions of 32/33.3.2.4 are similar to those for hotels. No building or story is permitted to have a single exit. Note that 7.4.1.2 requires at least three exits for floors with more than 500 people; at least four exits are required for those with more than 1000 people. This requirement will probably have minimal impact on board and care facilities, because such large floors would probably need additional exits to meet travel distance limitations.

Common path of travel in board and care facilities is measured in the usual manner outlined in A.7.5.1.5. Prior to the mid-1990s, the board and care occupancy chapters used a modified corridor common path of travel similar to that currently used in the hotel and apartment occupancy chapters.

Travel distance to exits is addressed in 32/33.3.2.6. For new large board and care facilities, the travel distance limitation is straightforward: 250 ft (76 m) from any point to the nearest exit. For existing large board and care facilities, the travel distance limitations of 33.3.2.6 are divided into two segments — within a room or suite and within the common corridor system or along the exterior exit access balcony.

Exhibit 32/33.9 illustrates an existing large board and care facility with three separate sections, or wings. Wings B and C are nonsprinklered portions of the building, and Wing A is protected by an automatic sprinkler system. In the nonsprinklered areas (B and C), 33.3.2.6.1 limits the travel distance within the room/suite to 75 ft (23 m). In the sprinklered area (A), the permitted travel distance within the room/suite is 125 ft (38 m) per 33.3.2.6.2. Once outside the room/suite, 33.3.2.6.3.1 limits the travel distance within a nonsprinklered interior corridor to an exit to 100 ft (30 m), as in area B of the building. However, the distance is permitted to be increased to 200 ft (61 m) if the travel is by way of exterior exit access (area C) or if the building is protected by an automatic sprinkler system (area A), per 33.3.2.6.3.2 and 33.3.2.6.3.3, respectively. Note that, where the increased travel distance is utilized in a partially sprinklered building, the sprinklered and nonsprinklered areas must be separated by a 1-hour fire barrier if the building is three stories or fewer in height or a 2-hour fire barrier if the building is more than three stories in height.

The provision of 32/33.3.2.9 that permits the omission of emergency lighting does not apply to facilities with exterior balconies that require travel on stairs to reach ground level; it applies only to facilities having doors opening directly at ground level.

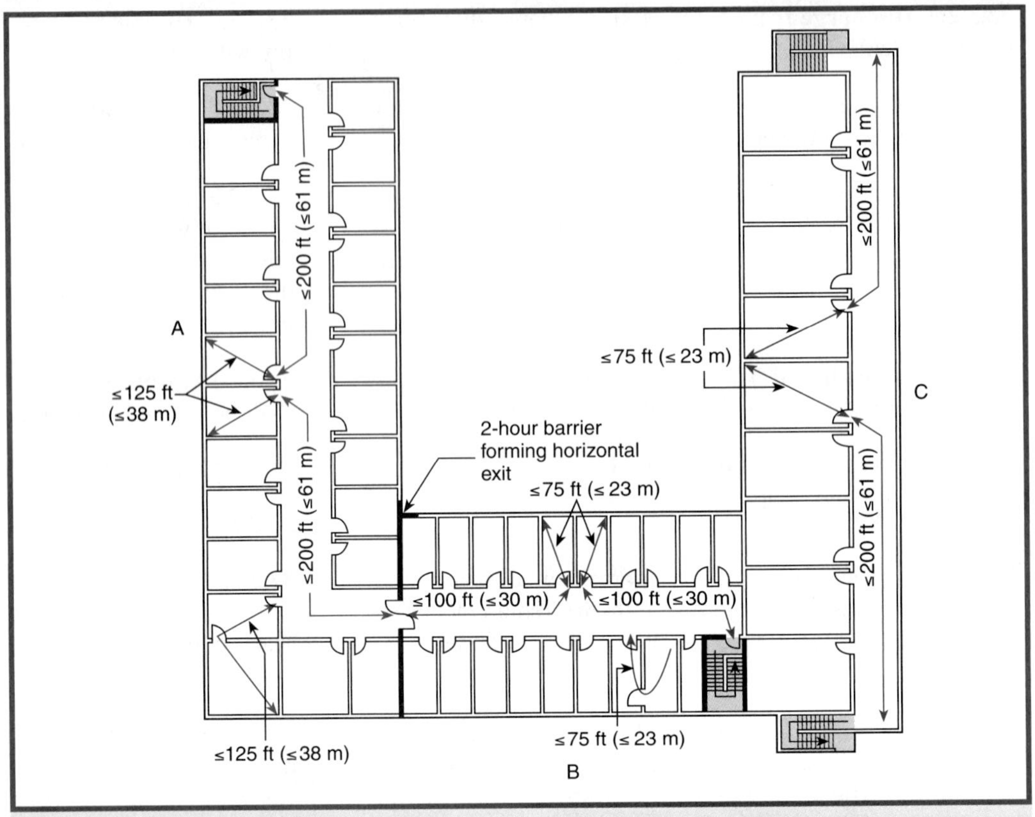


***Exhibit 32/33.9*** *Travel distance limitations.*

### 32.3.3 Protection.

**32.3.3.1 Protection of Vertical Openings.**

**32.3.3.1.1** Vertical openings shall be enclosed or protected in accordance with Section 8.6.

### 33.3.3 Protection.

**33.3.3.1 Protection of Vertical Openings.**

**33.3.3.1.1** Vertical openings shall comply with 33.3.3.1.1.1, 33.3.3.1.1.2, or 33.3.3.1.1.3.

**33.3.3.1.1.1** Vertical openings shall be enclosed or protected in accordance with Section 8.6.

**33.3.3.1.1.2** Unprotected vertical openings not part of required egress shall be permitted by the authority having jurisdiction where such openings do not endanger required means of egress, provided that the building is protected throughout by an approved automatic sprinkler system in accordance with 33.3.3.5, and the exits and required ways of travel thereto are adequately safeguarded against fire and smoke within the building, or where every individual room has direct access to an exterior exit without passing through a public corridor.

**33.3.3.1.1.3** In buildings two or fewer stories in height, unprotected vertical openings shall be permitted by the authority having jurisdiction, provided that the building is protected throughout by an approved automatic sprinkler system in accordance with 33.3.3.5.

CHAPTER 32 • New

**32.3.3.1.2** Unenclosed vertical openings in accordance with 8.6.8.2 shall be permitted.

**32.3.3.1.3** No floor below the level of exit discharge used only for storage, heating equipment, or purposes other than residential occupancy shall have unprotected openings to floors used for residential occupancy.

Because 32.3.3.5.1 requires an automatic sprinkler system in all new large board and care facilities, a communicating space is permitted to be separated from the remainder of the building by a smoke barrier in accordance with 8.6.6(4), rather than by a 1-hour fire barrier.

**32.3.3.2 Protection from Hazards.**

**32.3.3.2.1** Hazardous areas shall be protected in accordance with Section 8.7.

**32.3.3.2.2** The areas described in Table 32.3.3.2.2 shall be protected as indicated.

*Table 32.3.3.2.2 Hazardous Area Protection*

| Hazardous Area Description | Separation/Protection† |
|---|---|
| Boiler and fuel-fired heater rooms | 1 hour |
| Central/bulk laundries larger than 100 $ft^2$ (9.3 $m^2$) | 1 hour |
| Paint shops employing hazardous substances and materials in quantities less than those that would be classified as a severe hazard | 1 hour |
| Physical plant maintenance shops | 1 hour |
| Soiled linen rooms | 1 hour |
| Storage rooms larger than 50 $ft^2$ (4.6 $m^2$), but not exceeding 100 $ft^2$ (9.3 $m^2$), storing combustible material | Smoke partition |
| Storage rooms larger than 100 $ft^2$ (9.3 $m^2$) storing combustible material | 1 hour |
| Trash collection rooms | 1 hour |

†Minimum fire resistance rating.

CHAPTER 33 • Existing

**33.3.3.1.2 Reserved.**

**33.3.3.1.3** No floor below the level of exit discharge and used only for storage, heating equipment, or purposes other than residential occupancy shall have unprotected openings to floors used for residential occupancy.

Automatic sprinklers are not required in existing board and care facilities. However, if automatic sprinklers are installed, 33.3.3.1.1.2 and 33.3.3.1.1.3 permit the authority having jurisdiction (AHJ) to exempt the requirements for protection of vertical openings in certain circumstances.

**33.3.3.2 Protection from Hazards.**

**33.3.3.2.1** Rooms containing high-pressure boilers, refrigerating machinery, transformers, or other service equipment subject to possible explosion shall not be located directly under or adjacent to exits, and such rooms shall be effectively separated from other parts of the building as specified in Section 8.7.

**33.3.3.2.2** Hazardous areas, which shall include, but shall not be limited to, the following, shall be separated from other parts of the building by construction having a minimum 1-hour fire resistance rating, with communicating openings protected by approved self-closing fire doors, or such areas shall be equipped with automatic fire-extinguishing systems:

(1) Boiler and heater rooms
(2) Laundries
(3) Repair shops
(4) Rooms or spaces used for storage of combustible supplies and equipment in quantities deemed hazardous by the authority having jurisdiction

CHAPTER 32 • New | CHAPTER 33 • Existing

The lists that appear in Table 32.3.3.2.2 and in 33.3.3.2.2 are not all-inclusive. Hazardous areas are those that contain materials that, because of their basic nature or the quantity of combustible materials involved, represent a significantly higher fire hazard than would otherwise be typical of the contents of a residential board and care facility.

Prior to the 2003 edition of the *Code*, most hazardous areas in new large board and care facilities were permitted to be enclosed by only smoke partitions due to the mandatory requirement for automatic sprinklers. However, due to the revisions to Chapter 32 for the 2003 edition of the *Code*, which eliminated the requirement for evaluation of evacuation capability in new facilities, it must be assumed that facilities might contain occupants classified as having impractical evacuation capability. Therefore, the hazardous area protection requirements for new large board and care facilities closely mirror those in Chapter 18 for new health care occupancies (see 18.3.2.1). Other than small storage rooms, hazardous areas must be enclosed by 1-hour-rated fire barriers in addition to being protected by the automatic sprinkler system mandated by 32.3.3.5.1.

**32.3.3.3* Interior Finish.**

**A.32.3.3.3** The provisions in 10.2.8 to allow modifications to interior finish requirements where automatic sprinklers are provided are permitted.

**32.3.3.3.1 General.** Interior finish shall be in accordance with Section 10.2.

**32.3.3.3.2 Interior Wall and Ceiling Finish.** Interior wall and ceiling finish materials complying with Section 10.2 shall be in accordance with the following:

(1) Exit enclosures — Class A
(2) Lobbies and corridors — Class B
(3) Rooms and enclosed spaces — Class B

**32.3.3.3.3 Interior Floor Finish.**

**32.3.3.3.3.1** Interior floor finish shall comply with Section 10.2.

**32.3.3.3.3.2** Interior floor finish in exit enclosures and exit access corridors and spaces not separated from them by walls complying with 32.3.3.6 shall be not less than Class II.

**32.3.3.3.3.3** Interior floor finish shall comply with 10.2.7.1 or 10.2.7.2, as applicable.

**32.3.3.4 Detection, Alarm, and Communications Systems.**

**32.3.3.4.1 General.** A fire alarm system shall be provided in accordance with Section 9.6.

**32.3.3.4.2 Initiation.** The required fire alarm system shall be initiated by all of the following:

(1) Manual means in accordance with 9.6.2

**33.3.3.3 Interior Finish.**

**33.3.3.3.1 General.** Interior finish shall be in accordance with Section 10.2.

**33.3.3.3.2 Interior Wall and Ceiling Finish.** Interior wall and ceiling finish materials complying with Section 10.2 shall be Class A or Class B.

**33.3.3.3.3 Interior Floor Finish.** Interior floor finish, other than approved existing floor coverings, shall be Class I or Class II in corridors or exits.

**33.3.3.4 Detection, Alarm, and Communications Systems.**

**33.3.3.4.1 General.** A fire alarm system in accordance with Section 9.6 shall be provided, unless each sleeping room has exterior exit access in accordance with 7.5.3, and the building is three or fewer stories in height.

**33.3.3.4.2 Initiation.** The required fire alarm system shall be initiated by all of the following means:

(1) Manual means in accordance with 9.6.2, unless there are other effective means (such as a complete automatic sprinkler or automatic detection system) for notification of fire as required

CHAPTER 32 • New

(2) Manual fire alarm box located at a convenient central control point under continuous supervision of responsible employees
(3) Required automatic sprinkler system
(4) Required detection system

**32.3.3.4.3 Annunciator Panel.** An annunciator panel, connected to the fire alarm system, shall be provided at a location readily accessible from the primary point of entry for emergency response personnel.

**32.3.3.4.4 Occupant Notification.** Occupant notification shall be provided automatically, without delay, in accordance with 9.6.3.

**32.3.3.4.5 High-Rise Buildings.** High-rise buildings shall be provided with an approved emergency voice communication/alarm system in accordance with 11.8.4.

**32.3.3.4.6* Emergency Forces Notification.** Emergency forces notification shall meet the following requirements:

(1) Fire department notification shall be accomplished in accordance with 9.6.4.
(2) Smoke detection devices or smoke detection systems shall be permitted to initiate a positive alarm sequence in accordance with 9.6.3.4 for not more than 120 seconds.

**A.32.3.3.4.6** Positive alarm sequence applies only to emergency forces notification. Occupant notification is required to occur immediately upon activation of the detection device or system.

**32.3.3.4.7 Smoke Alarms.** Approved smoke alarms shall be installed in accordance with 9.6.2.10 inside every sleeping room, outside every sleeping area in the immediate vicinity of the bedrooms, and on all levels within a resident unit.

CHAPTER 33 • Existing

(2) Manual fire alarm box located at a convenient central control point under continuous supervision of responsible employees
(3) Automatic sprinkler system, other than that not required by another section of this *Code*
(4) Required detection system, other than sleeping room smoke alarms

**33.3.3.4.3 Reserved.**

**33.3.3.4.4 Occupant Notification.** Occupant notification shall be provided automatically, without delay, by internal audible alarm in accordance with 9.6.3.

**33.3.3.4.5 Reserved.**

**33.3.3.4.6* Emergency Forces Notification.** In case of a fire, provisions shall be made for the immediate notification of the public fire department, by either telephone or other means, or, where there is no public fire department, this notification shall be made to the private fire brigade.

**A.33.3.3.4.6** See A.29.3.4.3.6.

**33.3.3.4.7 Smoke Alarms.** Smoke alarms shall be provided in accordance with 33.3.3.4.7.1, 33.3.3.4.7.2, or 33.3.3.4.7.3.

**33.3.3.4.7.1** Each sleeping room shall be provided with an approved smoke alarm in accordance with 9.6.2.10 that is powered from the building electrical system.

**33.3.3.4.7.2** Existing battery-powered smoke alarms, rather than building electrical service–powered smoke alarms, shall be accepted where, in the opinion of the authority having jurisdiction, the facility has demonstrated that testing, maintenance, and battery replacement programs ensure the reliability of power to the smoke alarms.

**33.3.3.4.7.3** Sleeping room smoke alarms shall not be required in facilities having an existing corridor smoke detection system that complies with Section 9.6 and is connected to the building fire alarm system.

CHAPTER 32 • New

**32.3.3.4.8 Smoke Detection Systems.**

**32.3.3.4.8.1** Corridors and spaces open to the corridors, other than those meeting the requirement of 32.3.3.4.8.3, shall be provided with smoke detectors that comply with *NFPA 72, National Fire Alarm Code*, and are arranged to initiate an alarm that is audible in all sleeping areas.

**32.3.3.4.8.2 Reserved.**

**32.3.3.4.8.3** Smoke detection systems shall not be required in unenclosed corridors, passageways, balconies, colonnades, or other arrangements with one or more sides along the long dimension fully or extensively open to the exterior at all times.

**32.3.3.4.9* Protection of Fire Alarm System.** The provision of 9.6.1.8.1.3 shall not apply to the smoke detection required at each fire alarm control unit by 9.6.1.8.1(1).

**A.32.3.3.4.9** It is the intent that smoke detection be provided at each fire alarm control unit, regardless of the presence of sprinkler protection.

CHAPTER 33 • Existing

**33.3.3.4.8 Smoke Detection Systems.**

**33.3.3.4.8.1** All living areas, as defined in 3.3.19.5, and all corridors shall be provided with smoke detectors that comply with *NFPA 72, National Fire Alarm Code*, and are arranged to initiate an alarm that is audible in all sleeping areas, as modified by 33.3.3.4.8.2 and 33.3.3.4.8.3.

**33.3.3.4.8.2** Smoke detection systems shall not be required in living areas in facilities protected throughout by an approved automatic sprinkler system installed in accordance with 33.3.3.5.

**33.3.3.4.8.3** Smoke detection systems shall not be required in unenclosed corridors, passageways, balconies, colonnades, or other arrangements with one or more sides along the long dimension fully or extensively open to the exterior at all times.

**33.3.3.4.9* Protection of Fire Alarm System.** The provision of 9.6.1.8.1.3 shall not apply to the smoke detection required at each fire alarm control unit by 9.6.1.8.1(1).

**A.33.3.3.4.9** It is the intent that smoke detection be provided at each fire alarm control unit, regardless of the presence of sprinkler protection.

In addition to the normal distribution of manual fire alarm boxes (see 9.6.2), 32/33.3.3.4.2(2) requires locations such as that of the telephone operator to be equipped with a manual fire alarm box. The intent is that a manual fire alarm box is to be available at the location where a report of an emergency phoned in by residents or staff would be received.

Sleeping room smoke alarms are exempt from activating the building fire alarm system. The detection devices installed in the sleeping rooms are usually single-station or multiple-station smoke alarms and are not part of a required automatic detection system. Therefore, such smoke alarms are intended to notify the occupants of the room of a smoke condition. The provision of 33.3.3.4.2(4) emphasizes this intent. The *Code*, in fact, prohibits sleeping room smoke alarms from activating the fire alarm system, as stated in 9.6.2.10.4, to prevent numerous nuisance alarms, which could pose a particular problem in large board and care facilities. Because the purpose of the sleeping room smoke alarms is to warn the occupants of an individual room, the notification of the management and other occupants is the occupant's responsibility. Therefore, manual alarm initiation should be emphasized in the required training for residents. See 32/33.7.2 for resident training requirements.

The location of audible alarm notification devices in residential board and care facilities affects their audibility. In most new construction, corridor walls are of such sound insulating character that a sounding device would be needed in each room to meet the performance criterion for alarm audibility throughout the building. If sounding devices are installed only in the corridor, they might have to operate at dangerous sound levels to awaken residents in their rooms.

New large board and care facilities must be provided with means to automatically notify the fire department of an alarm condition (see 9.6.4) per 32.3.3.4.6. In existing facilities, automatic emergency forces notification is not required by 33.3.3.4.6; however, means must be provided for staff to call the fire department at a minimum. Although direct fire alarm connection to the fire department is not required, such connection is the preferable method of providing fire department notification. If a telephone is provided, the telephone must be equipped for direct outside dial without going through a switchboard; the telephone is not permitted to be a pay phone.

The purpose of placing smoke alarms in each sleeping room, as required by 32/33.3.3.4.7, is to alert the occupants of a room to the presence of smoke within that room. The alarms are not permitted to be

CHAPTER 32 • New

connected to the building fire alarm system as previously discussed. When an occupant leaves a room, the door automatically closes behind the occupant, and the occupant is expected to pull a manual fire alarm box. If the occupant fails to sound the alarm manually, compensation is provided by corridor smoke detectors or by automatic sprinklers. See 32/33.3.3.4.8 and 32/33.3.3.5.

In existing board and care facilities, 33.3.3.4.7.2 applies only to existing battery-powered alarms — not to newly installed alarms in existing facilities. Battery-powered alarms are permitted only if they already exist and the facility can document that they are properly maintained and tested to ensure their reliability.

The provision of 33.3.3.4.7.3 recognizes that the installation of corridor smoke detection systems, rather than sleeping room smoke alarms, was a *Code* requirement in earlier editions. Note that the installation of a new corridor smoke detection system does not waive the need for single-station smoke alarms in each room.

However, if an existing facility already has a corridor smoke detection system, single-station smoke alarms in bedrooms are not required.

New large board and care facilities must be provided with a corridor smoke detection system in accordance with 32.3.3.4.8.1. In existing facilities, 33.3.3.4.8 requires a system of smoke detectors in the corridors and living areas where the facilities are not fully sprinklered. Note that 33.3.3.4.8.2 does not exempt the requirement of 33.3.3.4.7 for the provision of smoke alarms in each sleeping room even when automatic sprinklers are installed. The *Code* is not equating sprinklers with smoke detectors but establishes that a fully sprinklered existing building is an adequate alternative to smoke detection in common spaces. If the facility uses exterior access corridors in the motel style, smoke detection is not required in the exterior corridors in accordance with 32/33.3.3.4.8.3.

**32.3.3.5 Extinguishment Requirements.**

**32.3.3.5.1 General.** All buildings shall be protected throughout by an approved automatic sprinkler system installed in accordance with 9.7.1.1(1) and provided with quick-response or residential sprinklers throughout.

CHAPTER 33 • Existing

**33.3.3.5 Extinguishment Requirements.**

**33.3.3.5.1* General.** Where an automatic sprinkler system is installed, for either total or partial building coverage, the system shall be installed in accordance with Section 9.7, as modified by 33.3.3.5.1.1, 33.3.3.5.1.2, and 33.3.3.5.1.3.

**A.33.3.3.5.1** It is intended that this requirement apply to existing small facilities that are converted to large facilities.

Chapter 33 permits the use of NFPA 13D, *Standard for the Installation of Sprinkler Systems in One- and Two-Family Dwellings and Manufactured Homes*, and NFPA 13R, *Standard for the Installation of Sprinkler Systems in Residential Occupancies up to and Including Four Stories in Height*, outside of their scopes. This permission is based on a review of the occupancy and a recognition that the fires in board and care facilities are similar to those of other residential occupancies and that the level of protection is appropriate. In some circumstances, such as those for impractical evacuation capabilities, the requirements of NFPA 13D and NFPA 13R have been supplemented with requirements for additional water supplies to compensate for the special needs of the board and care occupancy.

**33.3.3.5.1.1** In buildings four or fewer stories above grade plane, systems in accordance with NFPA 13R, *Standard for the Installation of Sprinkler Systems in Residential Occupancies up to and Including Four Stories in Height*, shall be permitted.

**33.3.3.5.1.2** Automatic sprinklers shall not be required in closets not exceeding 24 $ft^2$ (2.2 $m^2$) and in bathrooms not

CHAPTER 32 • New

CHAPTER 33 • Existing

exceeding 55 ft$^2$ (5.1 m$^2$), provided that such spaces are finished with lath and plaster or materials with a 15-minute thermal barrier.

**33.3.3.5.1.3** Initiation of the fire alarm system shall not be required for existing installations in accordance with 33.3.3.5.5.

**32.3.3.5.2 Reserved.**

**33.3.3.5.2 High-Rise Buildings.** All high-rise buildings shall be protected throughout by an approved, supervised automatic sprinkler system in accordance with 33.3.3.5, as modified by 33.3.3.5.3. Such systems shall initiate the fire alarm system in accordance with Section 9.6.

**32.3.3.5.3 Reserved.**

**33.3.3.5.3 Closets and Bathrooms.** Automatic sprinklers shall not be required in small clothes closets where the smallest dimension does not exceed 36 in. (915 mm), the area does not exceed 24 ft$^2$ (2.2 m$^2$), and the walls and ceiling are finished with noncombustible or limited-combustible materials.

**32.3.3.5.4 Supervision.** Automatic sprinkler systems shall be provided with electrical supervision in accordance with 9.7.2.

**33.3.3.5.4 Supervision.** Automatic sprinkler systems shall be supervised in accordance with Section 9.7; waterflow alarms shall not be required to be transmitted off-site.

**32.3.3.5.5 Reserved.**

**33.3.3.5.5 Domestic Water Supply Option.** Sprinkler piping serving not more than six sprinklers for any isolated hazardous area in accordance with 9.7.1.2 shall be permitted; in new installations where more than two sprinklers are installed in a single area, waterflow detection shall be provided to initiate the fire alarm system required by 33.3.3.4.1.

**32.3.3.5.6 Portable Fire Extinguishers.** Portable fire extinguishers shall be provided in accordance with 9.7.4.1.

**33.3.3.5.6 Portable Fire Extinguishers.** Portable fire extinguishers in accordance with 9.7.4.1 shall be provided near hazardous areas.

Automatic sprinklers are required in all new large residential board and care facilities. Although not required, there are incentives for installing sprinklers in existing facilities. In new large facilities, sprinkler systems must meet NFPA 13, *Standard for the Installation of Sprinkler Systems*. In existing facilities having not more than four stories, 33.3.3.5.1.1 permits sprinkler systems in accordance with NFPA 13R, *Standard for the Installation of Sprinkler Systems in Residential Occupancies up to and Including Four Stories in Height*.

Prior to the 2003 edition of the *Code*, new large facilities were also permitted to be sprinklered in accordance with NFPA 13R. However, the *Code* now assumes new facilities might house residents not having the ability to evacuate or relocate without assistance. Given the potential need to use the defend-in-place strategy of occupant protection, complete automatic sprinkler protection must be provided in accordance with NFPA 13, with quick-response or residential sprinklers throughout. This requirement recognizes the ability of quick-response and residential sprinklers to maintain tenability in the room of origin for most fire scenarios.

The provision of 33.3.3.5.1.2 applies to sprinkler systems installed in accordance with NFPA 13R and NFPA 13 in existing facilities. The requirement for wall and ceiling surfaces to provide a 15-minute thermal barrier where sprinklers are omitted includes the wall and ceiling sections behind prefabricated tub and shower enclosures. This provision helps to confine a fire that originates in a bathroom.

For existing facilities, 33.3.3.5.1 does not require quick-response or residential sprinklers. However, NFPA 13R and NFPA 13 require quick-response sprinklers if a sprinkler system is installed in the areas of a board and care facility designated as light hazard by these standards.

CHAPTER 32 • New

**32.3.3.6* Corridors and Separation of Sleeping Rooms.**

**A.32.3.3.6** It is not the intent to prohibit furniture in corridors and spaces open to corridors, provided that the minimum required width is maintained. Storage is not permitted in corridors or spaces open to corridors.

**32.3.3.6.1** Access shall be provided from every resident use area to at least one means of egress that is separated from all sleeping rooms by walls complying with 32.3.3.6.3 through 32.3.3.6.6.

**32.3.3.6.2** Sleeping rooms shall be separated from corridors, living areas, and kitchens by walls complying with 32.3.3.6.3 through 32.3.3.6.6.

**32.3.3.6.3** Walls required by 32.3.3.6.1 or 32.3.3.6.2 shall be smoke partitions in accordance with Section 8.4 having a minimum $^1/_2$-hour fire resistance rating.

**32.3.3.6.4** Doors protecting corridor openings shall not be required to have a fire protection rating, but shall be constructed to resist the passage of smoke.

CHAPTER 33 • Existing

**33.3.3.6 Corridors and Separation of Sleeping Rooms.**

**33.3.3.6.1** Access shall be provided from every resident use area to not less than one means of egress that is separated from all other rooms or spaces by walls complying with 33.3.3.6.3 through 33.3.3.6.6.3, unless otherwise indicated in 33.3.3.6.1.1 through 33.3.3.6.1.3.

**33.3.3.6.1.1** Rooms or spaces, other than sleeping rooms, protected throughout by an approved automatic sprinkler system in accordance with 33.3.3.5 shall not be required to comply with 33.3.3.6.1.

**33.3.3.6.1.2** Prompt evacuation capability facilities in buildings two or fewer stories in height, where not less than one required means of egress from each sleeping room provides a path of travel to the outside without traversing any corridor or other spaces exposed to unprotected vertical openings, living areas, and kitchens, shall not be required to comply with 33.3.3.6.1.

**33.3.3.6.1.3** Rooms or spaces, other than sleeping rooms, provided with a smoke detection and alarm system connected to activate the building evacuation alarm shall not be required to comply with 33.3.3.6.1. Furnishings, finishes, and furniture, in combination with all other combustibles within the spaces, shall be of minimum quantity and arranged so that a fully developed fire is unlikely to occur.

**33.3.3.6.2** Sleeping rooms shall be separated from corridors, living areas, and kitchens by walls complying with 33.3.3.6.3 through 33.3.3.6.6.3.

**33.3.3.6.3** Walls required by 33.3.3.6.1 or 33.3.3.6.2 shall comply with 33.3.3.6.3.1, 33.3.3.6.3.2, or 33.3.3.6.3.3.

**33.3.3.6.3.1** Walls shall have a minimum $^1/_2$-hour fire resistance rating.

**33.3.3.6.3.2** In buildings protected throughout by an approved automatic sprinkler system in accordance with 33.3.3.5, walls shall be smoke partitions in accordance with Section 8.4, and the provisions of 8.4.3.5 shall not apply.

**33.3.3.6.3.3** In buildings two or fewer stories in height that are classified as prompt evacuation capability and that house not more than 30 residents, walls shall be smoke partitions in accordance with Section 8.4, and the provisions of 8.4.3.5 shall not apply.

**33.3.3.6.4** Doors in walls required by 33.3.3.6.1 or 33.3.3.6.2 shall comply with 33.3.3.6.4.1, 33.3.3.6.4.2, 33.3.3.6.4.3, or 33.3.3.6.4.4.

CHAPTER 32 • New

CHAPTER 33 • Existing

**33.3.3.6.4.1** Doors shall have a minimum 20-minute fire protection rating.

**33.3.3.6.4.2** Solid-bonded wood-core doors of not less than $1^{3}/_{4}$ in. (44 mm) thickness shall be permitted to continue in use.

**33.3.3.6.4.3** In buildings protected throughout by an approved automatic sprinkler system in accordance with 33.3.3.5, doors that are nonrated shall be permitted to continue in use.

**33.3.3.6.4.4** Where automatic sprinkler protection is provided in the corridor in accordance with 31.3.5.9, the following requirements shall be met:

(1) Doors shall not be required to have a fire protection rating, but shall be in accordance with 8.4.3.
(2) The provisions of 8.4.3.5 shall not apply.
(3) Doors shall be equipped with latches for keeping the doors tightly closed.

**32.3.3.6.5** Door-closing devices shall not be required on doors in corridor wall openings, other than those serving exit enclosures, smoke barriers, enclosures of vertical openings, and hazardous areas.

**33.3.3.6.5** Where walls and doors are required by 33.3.3.6.1 and 33.3.3.6.2, the following requirements shall be met:

(1) Such walls and doors shall be constructed as smoke partitions in accordance with Section 8.4.
(2) The provisions of 8.4.3.5 shall not apply.
(3) No louvers, transfer grilles, operable transoms, or other air passages shall penetrate such walls or doors, except properly installed heating and utility installations.

**32.3.3.6.6** No louvers, transfer grilles, operable transoms, or other air passages, other than properly installed heating and utility installations, shall penetrate the walls or doors specified in 32.3.3.6.

**33.3.3.6.6** Doors in walls required by 33.3.3.6.1 and 33.3.3.6.2 shall comply with 33.3.3.6.6.1, 33.3.3.6.6.2, or 33.3.3.6.6.3.

**33.3.3.6.6.1** Doors shall be self-closing or automatic-closing in accordance with 7.2.1.8, and doors in walls separating sleeping rooms from corridors shall be automatic-closing in accordance with 7.2.1.8.2.

**33.3.3.6.6.2** Doors to sleeping rooms that have occupant-control locks such that access is normally restricted to the occupants or staff personnel shall be permitted to be self-closing.

**33.3.3.6.6.3** In buildings protected throughout by an approved automatic sprinkler system installed in accordance with 33.3.3.5, doors, other than doors to hazardous areas, vertical openings, and exit enclosures, shall not be required to be self-closing or automatic-closing.

Access to at least one exit that is separate from sleeping rooms must be provided per 32/33.3.3.6.1. For existing board and care facilities, 33.3.3.6.1 contains three provisions that address special circumstances for an access to an exit that passes through a sitting room, television room, living room, or other common use space. See 33.3.3.6.1.1 through 33.3.3.6.1.3.

Exhibit 32/33.10 illustrates arrangements requir-

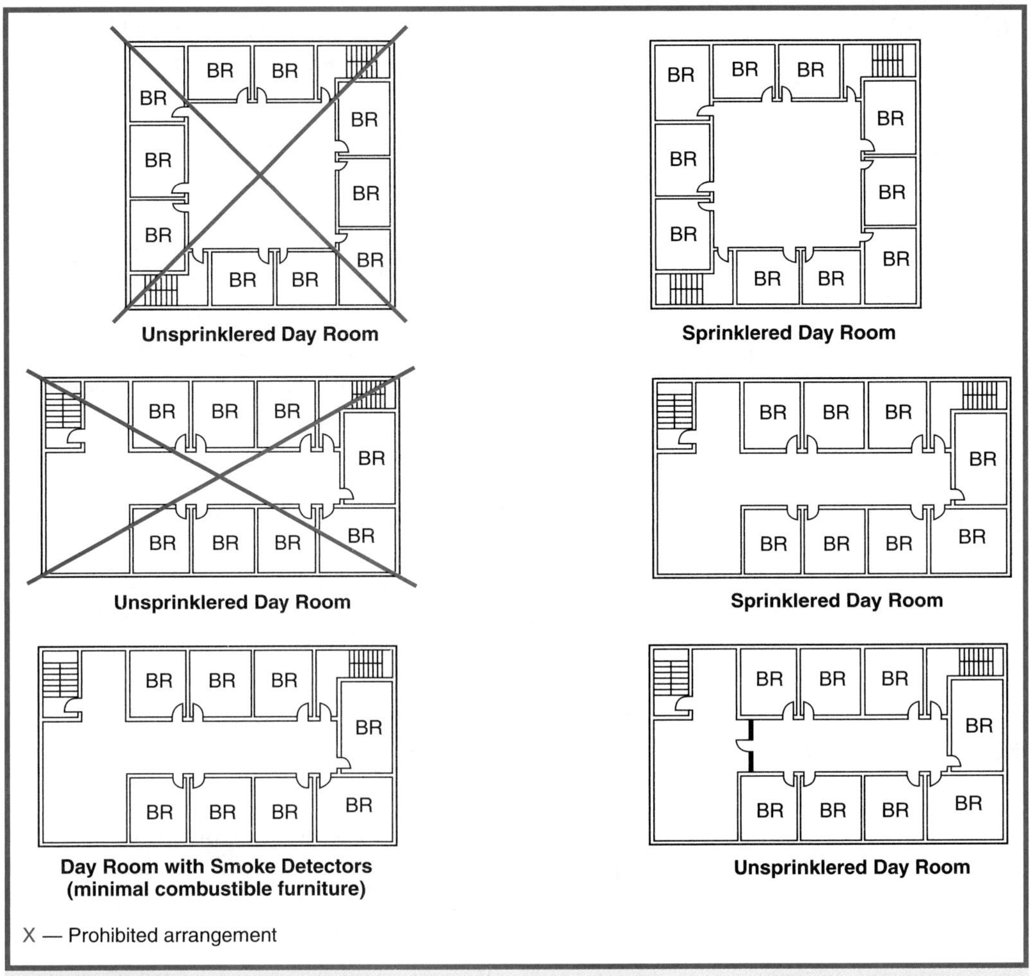


***Exhibit 32/33.10*** *Alternate egress arrangements.*

ing egress travel through furnished day rooms that would be prohibited in existing board and care facilities, unless the space is sprinklered or provided with a combination of a smoke detection and alarm system and the combustibility of furnishings is controlled.

Sleeping rooms in new large board and care facilities must be separated from corridors by smoke partitions, in accordance with 32.3.3.6.3, that have a fire resistance rating of ½ hour (see Section 8.4). Doors in corridor walls to spaces other than exits, smoke barriers, or vertical opening or hazardous area enclosures must be smoke resistant; however, no fire protection rating is required per 32.3.3.6.4, and the doors are not required to be self-closing or automatic-closing per 32.3.3.6.5. The provision to omit self-closers on corridor doors mirrors the provisions for health care occupancies in Chapters 18 and 19.

In nonsprinklered existing buildings, the corridor walls must have a fire resistance rating of ½ hour. The walls are permitted to be smoke partitions with no fire resistance rating if the building is protected throughout by an automatic sprinkler system (see 33.3.3.6.3.2) or if the facility is moderately sized with prompt evacuation capability (see 33.3.3.6.3.3).

The intent of 33.3.3.6.4.2 is to minimize the impact of converting a health care facility or hotel to a board and care facility by permitting existing doors to remain in use under a variety of conditions.

Existing sleeping room doors are required to be automatic-closing in accordance with 33.3.3.6.6.1 if the building is not protected by an automatic sprinkler system. In nonsprinklered facilities in which the residents control the privacy lock on their own sleeping room doors, a self-closer (such as spring hinges or a

CHAPTER 32 • New

hydraulic door check) is acceptable. Such a device is permitted because, in practice, such doors are usually kept closed. Therefore, the likelihood that the door will be chocked or held open is minimal. If the building is sprinklered, doors to spaces other than exits, smoke barriers, or vertical opening or hazardous area enclosures do not require self-closers. In such cases, staff should be trained to close doors in the event of a fire.

**32.3.3.7 Subdivision of Building Spaces.** Buildings shall be subdivided by smoke barriers in accordance with 32.3.3.7.1 through 32.3.3.7.21.

**32.3.3.7.1** Every story shall be divided into not less than two smoke compartments, unless it meets the requirement of 32.3.3.7.4, 32.3.3.7.5, 32.3.3.7.6, or 32.3.3.7.7.

**32.3.3.7.2** Each smoke compartment shall have an area not exceeding 22,500 $ft^2$ (2100 $m^2$).

**32.3.3.7.3** The travel distance from any point to reach a door in the required smoke barrier shall be limited to a distance of 200 ft (61 m).

**32.3.3.7.4** Smoke barriers shall not be required on stories that do not contain a board and care occupancy located above the board and care occupancy.

**32.3.3.7.5** Smoke barriers shall not be required in areas that do not contain a board and care occupancy and that are separated from the board and care occupancy by a fire barrier complying with Section 8.3.

**32.3.3.7.6** Smoke barriers shall not be required on stories that do not contain a board and care occupancy and that are more than one story below the board and care occupancy.

**32.3.3.7.7** Smoke barriers shall not be required in open parking structures protected throughout by an approved, supervised automatic sprinkler system in accordance with 32.3.3.5.

**32.3.3.7.8** Smoke barriers shall be constructed in accordance with Section 8.5 and shall have a minimum 1-hour fire resistance rating, unless they meet the requirement of 32.3.3.7.9 or 32.3.3.7.10.

**32.3.3.7.9** Where an atrium is used, smoke barriers shall be permitted to terminate at an atrium wall constructed in accordance with 8.6.7(1)(c), in which case not less than two separate smoke compartments shall be provided on each floor.

**32.3.3.7.10*** Dampers shall not be required in duct penetrations of smoke barriers in fully ducted heating, ventilating, and air-conditioning systems.

CHAPTER 33 • Existing

**33.3.3.7 Subdivision of Building Spaces.** The requirements of 33.3.3.7.1 through 33.3.3.7.6 shall be met for all sleeping floors.

**33.3.3.7.1** Every sleeping room floor shall be divided into not less than two smoke compartments of approximately the same size, with smoke barriers in accordance with Section 8.5, unless otherwise indicated in 33.3.3.7.4, 33.3.3.7.5, and 33.3.3.7.6.

**33.3.3.7.2** Smoke dampers shall not be required.

**33.3.3.7.3** Additional smoke barriers shall be provided such that the travel distance from a sleeping room corridor door to a smoke barrier shall not exceed 150 ft (46 m).

**33.3.3.7.4** Smoke barriers shall not be required in buildings protected throughout by an approved automatic sprinkler system installed in accordance with 33.3.3.5.

**33.3.3.7.5** Smoke barriers shall not be required where each sleeping room is provided with exterior ways of exit access arranged in accordance with 7.5.3.

**33.3.3.7.6** Smoke barriers shall not be required where the aggregate corridor length on each floor is not more than 150 ft (46 m).

**A.32.3.3.7.10** Where the smoke control system design requires dampers in order that the system functions effectively, it is not the intent of 32.3.3.7.10 to permit the damper to be omitted.

The term *fully ducted* means the supply and return-air systems are provided with continuous ducts from all air registers to the air-handling unit.

**32.3.3.7.11** Not less than 15 net $ft^2$ (1.4 net $m^2$) per resident shall be provided within the aggregate area of corridors, lounge or dining areas, and other low hazard areas on each side of the smoke barrier.

**32.3.3.7.12** On stories not housing residents, not less than 6 net $ft^2$ (0.56 net $m^2$) per occupant shall be provided on each side of the smoke barrier for the total number of occupants in adjoining compartments.

**32.3.3.7.13*** Doors in smoke barriers shall be substantial doors, such as $1^3/_4$ in. (44 mm) thick, solid-bonded wood-core doors, or shall be of construction that resists fire for a minimum of 20 minutes.

**A.32.3.3.7.13** Smoke barrier doors are intended to provide access to adjacent zones. The pair of cross-corridor doors are required to be opposite swinging. Access to both zones is required.

**32.3.3.7.14** Nonrated factory- or field-applied protective plates extending not more than 48 in. (1220 mm) above the bottom of the door shall be permitted.

**32.3.3.7.15** Cross-corridor openings in smoke barriers shall be protected by a pair of swinging doors or a horizontal-sliding door complying with 7.2.1.14.

**32.3.3.7.16** Swinging doors shall be arranged so that each door swings in a direction opposite from the other.

**32.3.3.7.17*** Doors in smoke barriers shall comply with 8.5.4 and shall be self-closing or automatic-closing in accordance with 7.2.1.8.

**A.32.3.3.7.17** Smoke barriers might include walls having door openings other than cross-corridor doors. There is no restriction in the *Code* regarding which doors or how many doors form part of a smoke barrier. For example, doors from the corridor to individual rooms are permitted to form part of a smoke barrier.

**32.3.3.7.18*** Vision panels consisting of fire-rated glazing or wired glass panels in approved frames shall be provided in each cross-corridor swinging door and in each cross-corridor horizontal-sliding door in a smoke barrier.

**A.32.3.3.7.18** It is not the intent to require the frame to be a listed assembly.

CHAPTER 32 • New

**32.3.3.7.19** Rabbets, bevels, or astragals shall be required at the meeting edges, and stops shall be required at the head and sides of door frames in smoke barriers.

**32.3.3.7.20** Positive latching hardware shall not be required.

**32.3.3.7.21** Center mullions shall be prohibited.

Smoke barriers are required in new large residential board and care facilities due to the potential for occupancy by residents who might not be able to be readily evacuated to the outside. The smoke barrier provisions of 32.3.3.7 are nearly identical to those for health care occupancies, which also use the defend-in-place protection strategy for occupants. See 18.3.7 and its associated commentary for additional details.

The smoke barrier required by 33.3.3.7 for nonsprinklered existing facilities provides for horizontal movement of occupants and limits the number of rooms and, therefore, the number of occupants exposed to a single fire that might block a corridor. Because no fire rating is required for the barrier, and because smoke dampers are not required, the provision of smoke barriers is not overly burdensome.

A horizontal exit is permitted to be used to comply with 33.3.3.7 and, therefore, might serve more than one function. In addition, the smoke compartment is permitted to be considered a point of safety (see definition of *point of safety* in 3.3.197) for the purpose of determining evacuation capability under the following conditions:

1. The smoke barrier has at least a ½-hour fire resistance rating.
2. Protection is provided by an automatic sprinkler system throughout the building.
3. The smoke compartment has access to an exit that does not require return to the fire area.

**32.3.3.8* Cooking Facilities.** Cooking facilities, other than those within individual residential units, shall be protected in accordance with 9.2.3.

**A.32.3.3.8** The scope of NFPA 96, *Standard for Ventilation Control and Fire Protection of Commercial Cooking Operations*, is limited to appliances that produce grease-laden vapors and does not apply to domestic cooking equipment used for food warming or limited cooking.

**32.3.3.9 Standpipes.**

**32.3.3.9.1 General.** Where required, standpipe and hose systems shall be installed and maintained in accordance with 9.7.4.2.

**32.3.3.9.2 In High-Rise Buildings.** Class I standpipe systems shall be installed throughout all high-rise buildings.

**32.3.3.9.3 Roof Outlets.** Roof outlets shall not be required on roofs having a slope of 3 in 12 or greater.

### 32.3.4 Special Provisions.

**32.3.4.1 High-Rise Buildings.** High-rise buildings shall comply with Section 11.8.

**32.3.4.2 Reserved.**

CHAPTER 33 • Existing

### 33.3.4 Special Provisions.

**(Reserved)**

CHAPTER 32 • New

32.3.5 Reserved.

32.3.6 Building Services.

**32.3.6.1 Utilities.** Utilities shall comply with Section 9.1.

**32.3.6.2 Heating, Ventilating, and Air-Conditioning.**

**32.3.6.2.1** Heating, ventilating, and air-conditioning equipment shall comply with Section 9.2.

**32.3.6.2.2** No stove or combustion heater shall be located such that it blocks escape in case of fire caused by the malfunction of the stove or heater.

**32.3.6.2.3** Unvented fuel-fired heaters shall not be used in any board and care occupancy.

**32.3.6.3 Elevators, Dumbwaiters, and Vertical Conveyors.**

**32.3.6.3.1** Elevators, dumbwaiters, and vertical conveyors shall comply with Section 9.4.

**32.3.6.3.2*** In high-rise buildings, one elevator shall be provided with a protected power supply and shall be available for use by the fire department in case of emergency.

**A.32.3.6.3.2** "Protected power supply" means a source of electrical energy of sufficient capacity to allow proper operation of the elevator and its associated control and communications systems. The power supply's point of origin, system of distribution, type and size of overcurrent protection, degree of isolation from other portions of the building electrical system, and degree of mechanical protection should be such that it is unlikely that the supply would be disrupted at any but the advanced stages of building fire involvement or by structural collapse.

A protected power supply might consist of, and should provide, not less than the level of reliability associated with an electrical distribution system with service equipment located and installed in accordance with 230.72(B) and 230.82(5) of *NFPA 70, National Electrical Code*. The distribution system is not to have any other connection to the building electrical distribution system. A protected power supply is not required to incorporate two sources of energy or automatic transfer capability from a normal to an emergency source; for example, an alternate set of service conductors.

The number and type of elevators to be connected to a protected power supply should be limited, or the characteristics of the protected power supply should be selected to ensure conformance with 230.95 of *NFPA 70*, without the provision of ground fault protection for the supply.

An elevator installation supplied by a protected power supply should comply with Article 620 of *NFPA 70*, except

CHAPTER 33 • Existing

33.3.5 Reserved.

33.3.6 Building Services.

**33.3.6.1 Utilities.** Utilities shall comply with the provisions of Section 9.1.

**33.3.6.2 Heating, Ventilating, and Air-Conditioning.**

**33.3.6.2.1** Heating, ventilating, and air-conditioning equipment shall comply with the provisions of Section 9.2.

**33.3.6.2.2** No stove or combustion heater shall be located such that it blocks escape in case of fire caused by the malfunction of the stove or heater.

**33.3.6.2.3** Unvented fuel-fired heaters shall not be used in any board and care occupancy.

**33.3.6.3 Elevators, Dumbwaiters, and Vertical Conveyors.** Elevators, dumbwaiters, and vertical conveyors shall comply with Section 9.4.

that the energy absorption means required by 620.91 of *NFPA 70* should always be connected on the load side of the disconnecting means. The energy absorption means should not consist of loads likely to become inoperative or disconnected under the conditions assumed to exist when the elevator is under the control of fire department personnel. Examples of such loads include light and power loads external to the elevator equipment room.

**32.3.6.4 Rubbish Chutes, Incinerators, and Laundry Chutes.** Rubbish chutes, incinerators, and laundry chutes shall comply with Section 9.5.

## 32.4* Suitability of an Apartment Building to House a Board and Care Occupancy

**A.32.4** Board and care occupancies in apartment buildings will usually be small facilities housing 16 or fewer residents. It is intended that the board and care occupancy conform to the requirements of Section 32.2 for small board and care facilities. In the unusual case where an apartment houses a large board and care facility, it would be reasonable for the authority having jurisdiction, using the requirement of 4.6.1, to apply the provisions of Section 32.3 to the apartment. In addition, the apartment building in which the facility is housed needs to comply with the requirements for apartment buildings in Chapters 30 and 31 and the additional criteria presented in Section 32.4.

A board and care facility located within an apartment building is usually a small facility housing 16 or fewer residents. It is intended that the board and care facility within the apartment building conform to the requirements of Section 32/33.2 for small board and care facilities. In the unusual case where an apartment building houses a large board and care facility, it is reasonable for the authority having jurisdiction (AHJ), in accordance with Section 1.4, to apply the provisions of Section 32/33.3 to the apartment unit. In addition, the apartment building in which the facility is housed is required to comply with the requirements for apartment buildings in Chapters 30 and 31 and the additional criteria provided in Section 32/33.4.

### 32.4.1 General.

**32.4.1.1 Scope.**

**32.4.1.1.1** Section 32.4 shall apply to apartment buildings that have one or more individual apartments used as a board and care occupancy. *(See 32.1.2.2.)*

**32.4.1.1.2** The provisions of Section 32.4 shall be used to determine the suitability of apartment buildings, other than those complying with 32.4.1.1.4, to house a residential board and care facility.



**33.3.6.4 Rubbish Chutes, Incinerators, and Laundry Chutes.** Rubbish chutes, incinerators, and laundry chutes shall comply with the provisions of Section 9.5.

## 33.4* Suitability of an Apartment Building to House a Board and Care Occupancy

**A.33.4** Board and care occupancies in apartment buildings will usually be small facilities housing 16 or fewer residents. It is intended that the board and care occupancy conform to the requirements of Section 33.2 for small board and care facilities. In the unusual case where an apartment houses a large board and care facility, it would be reasonable for the authority having jurisdiction, using the requirement of 4.6.1, to apply the provisions of Section 33.3 to the apartment. In addition, the apartment building in which the facility is housed needs to comply with the requirements for apartment buildings in Chapters 30 and 31 and the additional criteria presented in Section 33.4.

### 33.4.1 General.

**33.4.1.1 Scope.**

**33.4.1.1.1** Section 33.4 shall apply to apartment buildings that have one or more individual apartments used as a board and care occupancy. *(See 33.1.2.2.)*

**33.4.1.1.2** The provisions of Section 33.4 shall be used to determine the suitability of apartment buildings to house a residential board and care facility.

CHAPTER 32 • New

**32.4.1.1.3** The suitability of apartment buildings not used for board and care occupancies shall be determined in accordance with Chapter 30.

**32.4.1.1.4** If a new board and care occupancy is created in an existing apartment building, the suitability of such buildings for apartments not used for board and care occupancies shall be determined in accordance with Chapter 31.

**32.4.1.2 Requirements for Individual Apartments.** Requirements for individual apartments used as residential board and care occupancies shall be as specified in Section 32.2. Egress from the apartment into the common building corridor shall be considered acceptable egress from the board and care facility.

**32.4.1.3* Additional Requirements.** Apartment buildings housing board and care facilities shall comply with the requirements of Chapter 30 and the additional requirements of Section 32.4, unless the authority having jurisdiction has determined that equivalent safety for housing a residential board and care facility is provided in accordance with Section 1.4.

**A.32.4.1.3** In determining equivalency for conversions, modernizations, renovations, or unusual design concepts, the authority having jurisdiction might permit evaluations based on the residential board and care occupancies fire safety evaluation system (FSES) of NFPA 101A, *Guide on Alternative Approaches to Life Safety*.

**32.4.1.4 Minimum Construction Requirements.**

**32.4.1.4.1** In addition to the requirements of Chapter 30, apartment buildings, other than those complying with 32.4.1.4.2, housing residential board and care facilities shall meet the construction requirements of 32.3.1.3.

**32.4.1.4.2** If a new board and care occupancy is created in an existing apartment building, the construction requirements of 19.1.6 shall apply.

### 32.4.2 Means of Egress.

**32.4.2.1** The requirements of Section 30.2 shall apply only to the parts of means of egress serving the apartment(s) used as a residential board and care occupancy, as modified by 32.4.2.2.

**32.4.2.2** If a new board and care occupancy is created in an existing apartment building, the requirements of Section 31.2 shall apply to the parts of the means of egress serving the apartment(s) used as a residential board and care occupancy.

CHAPTER 33 • Existing

**33.4.1.1.3** The suitability of existing apartment buildings not used for board and care occupancies shall be determined in accordance with Chapter 31.

**33.4.1.2 Requirements for Individual Apartments.** Requirements for individual apartments used as residential board and care occupancies shall be as specified in Section 33.2. Egress from the apartment into the common building corridor shall be considered acceptable egress from the board and care facility.

**33.4.1.3 Additional Requirements.**

**33.4.1.3.1*** Apartment buildings housing board and care facilities shall comply with the requirements of Section 33.4, unless the authority having jurisdiction has determined that equivalent safety for housing a residential board and care facility is provided in accordance with Section 1.4.

**A.33.4.1.3.1** In determining equivalency for existing buildings, conversions, modernizations, renovations, or unusual design concepts, the authority having jurisdiction might permit evaluations based on the residential board and care occupancies fire safety evaluation system (FSES) of NFPA 101A, *Guide on Alternative Approaches to Life Safety*.

**33.4.1.3.2** All facilities shall meet the requirements of Chapter 31 and the additional requirements of Section 33.4.

**33.4.1.4 Minimum Construction Requirements.** In addition to the requirements of Chapter 31, apartment buildings housing residential board and care facilities for groups classified as prompt or slow evacuation capability shall meet the construction requirements of 33.3.1.3, and those for groups classified as impractical evacuation capability shall meet the construction requirements of 19.1.6.

### 33.4.2 Means of Egress.

The requirements of Section 31.2 shall apply only to the parts of means of egress serving the apartment(s) used as a residential board and care occupancy.

CHAPTER 32 • New

### 32.4.3 Protection.

**32.4.3.1 Interior Finish.**

**32.4.3.1.1** The requirements of 30.3.3 shall apply only to the parts of means of egress serving the apartment(s) used as a residential board and care occupancy, as modified by 32.4.3.1.2.

**32.4.3.1.2** If a new board and care occupancy is created in an existing apartment building, the requirements of 31.3.3 shall apply to the parts of the means of egress serving the apartment(s) used as a residential board and care occupancy.

**32.4.3.2 Construction of Corridor Walls.**

**32.4.3.2.1** The requirements of 30.3.6 shall apply only to corridors serving the residential board and care facility, including that portion of the corridor wall separating the residential board and care facility from the common corridor, as modified by 32.4.3.2.2.

**32.4.3.2.2** If a new board and care occupancy is created in an existing apartment building, the requirements of 31.3.6 shall apply to the corridor serving the residential board and care facility.

**32.4.3.3 Subdivision of Building Spaces. (Reserved)**

## 32.5 Reserved

## 32.6 Reserved

## 32.7 Operating Features

### 32.7.1 Emergency Plan.

**32.7.1.1** The administration of every residential board and care facility shall have, in effect and available to all supervisory personnel, written copies of a plan for protecting all persons in the event of fire, for keeping persons in place, for evacuating persons to areas of refuge, and for evacuating persons from the building when necessary.

**32.7.1.2** The emergency plan shall include special staff response, including the fire protection procedures needed to ensure the safety of any resident, and shall be amended or revised whenever any resident with unusual needs is admitted to the home.

CHAPTER 33 • Existing

### 33.4.3 Protection.

**33.4.3.1 Interior Finish.** The requirements of 31.3.3 shall apply only to the parts of means of egress serving the apartment(s) used as a residential board and care occupancy.

**33.4.3.2 Construction of Corridor Walls.** The requirements of 31.3.6 shall apply only to corridors serving the residential board and care facility, including that portion of the corridor wall separating the residential board and care facility from the common corridor.

**33.4.3.3 Subdivision of Building Spaces.** The requirements of 31.3.7 shall apply to those stories with an apartment(s) used as a residential board and care occupancy.

## 33.5 Reserved

## 33.6 Reserved

## 33.7 Operating Features

### 33.7.1 Emergency Plan.

**33.7.1.1** The administration of every residential board and care facility shall have, in effect and available to all supervisory personnel, written copies of a plan for protecting all persons in the event of fire, for keeping persons in place, for evacuating persons to areas of refuge, and for evacuating persons from the building when necessary.

**33.7.1.2** The emergency plan shall include special staff response, including the fire protection procedures needed to ensure the safety of any resident, and shall be amended or revised whenever any resident with unusual needs is admitted to the home.

CHAPTER 32 • New

32.7.1.3 All employees shall be periodically instructed and kept informed with respect to their duties and responsibilities under the plan, and such instruction shall be reviewed by the staff not less than every 2 months.

32.7.1.4 A copy of the plan shall be readily available at all times within the facility.

### 32.7.2 Resident Training.

32.7.2.1 All residents participating in the emergency plan shall be trained in the proper actions to be taken in the event of fire.

32.7.2.2 The training required by 32.7.2.1 shall include actions to be taken if the primary escape route is blocked.

32.7.2.3 If a resident is given rehabilitation or habilitation training, training in fire prevention and the actions to be taken in the event of a fire shall be a part of the training program.

32.7.2.4 Residents shall be trained to assist each other in case of fire to the extent that their physical and mental abilities permit them to do so without additional personal risk.

### 32.7.3 Emergency Egress and Relocation Drills.

Emergency egress and relocation drills shall be conducted in accordance with 32.7.3.1 through 32.7.3.6.

32.7.3.1 Emergency egress and relocation drills shall be conducted not less than six times per year on a bimonthly basis, with not less than two drills conducted during the night when residents are sleeping, as modified by 32.7.3.5 and 32.7.3.6.

32.7.3.2 The emergency drills shall be permitted to be announced to the residents in advance.

32.7.3.3 The drills shall involve the actual evacuation of all residents to an assembly point, as specified in the emergency plan, and shall provide residents with experience in egressing through all exits and means of escape required by the *Code*.

32.7.3.4 Exits and means of escape not used in any drill shall not be credited in meeting the requirements of this *Code* for board and care facilities.

32.7.3.5 Actual exiting from windows shall not be required to comply with 32.7.3; opening the window and signaling for help shall be an acceptable alternative.

32.7.3.6 Residents who cannot meaningfully assist in their own evacuation or who have special health problems shall not be required to actively participate in the drill. Section 18.7 shall apply in such instances.

CHAPTER 33 • Existing

33.7.1.3 All employees shall be periodically instructed and kept informed with respect to their duties and responsibilities under the plan, and such instruction shall be reviewed by the staff not less than every 2 months.

33.7.1.4 A copy of the plan shall be readily available at all times within the facility.

### 33.7.2 Resident Training.

33.7.2.1 All residents participating in the emergency plan shall be trained in the proper actions to be taken in the event of fire.

33.7.2.2 The training required by 32.7.2.1 shall include actions to be taken if the primary escape route is blocked.

33.7.2.3 If the resident is given rehabilitation or habilitation training, training in fire prevention and the actions to be taken in the event of a fire shall be a part of the training program.

33.7.2.4 Residents shall be trained to assist each other in case of fire to the extent that their physical and mental abilities permit them to do so without additional personal risk.

### 33.7.3 Emergency Egress and Relocation Drills.

Emergency egress and relocation drills shall be conducted in accordance with 33.7.3.1 through 33.7.3.6.

33.7.3.1 Emergency egress and relocation drills shall be conducted not less than six times per year on a bimonthly basis, with not less than two drills conducted during the night when residents are sleeping, as modified by 33.7.3.5 and 33.7.3.6.

33.7.3.2 The emergency drills shall be permitted to be announced to the residents in advance.

33.7.3.3 The drills shall involve the actual evacuation of all residents to an assembly point, as specified in the emergency plan, and shall provide residents with experience in egressing through all exits and means of escape required by this *Code*.

33.7.3.4 Exits and means of escape not used in any drill shall not be credited in meeting the requirements of this *Code* for board and care facilities.

33.7.3.5 Actual exiting from windows shall not be required to comply with 33.7.3; opening the window and signaling for help shall be an acceptable alternative.

33.7.3.6 If the board and care facility has an evacuation capability classification of impractical, those residents who cannot meaningfully assist in their own evacuation or who have special health problems shall not be required to actively participate in the drill. Section 19.7 shall apply in such instances.

CHAPTER 32 • New

### 32.7.4 Smoking.

**32.7.4.1*** Smoking regulations shall be adopted by the administration of board and care occupancies.

**A.32.7.4.1** Smoking regulations should include the following:

(1) Smoking should be prohibited in any room, compartment, or area where flammable or combustible liquids, combustible gases, or oxygen is used or stored and in any other hazardous location, and the following also should apply:
  (a) Such areas should be posted with signs that read NO SMOKING or the international symbol for no smoking.
  (b) In residential board and care facilities where smoking is totally prohibited and signs so indicating are placed at all major entrances, secondary signs with language that prohibits smoking are not required.
(2) Smoking by residents classified as not responsible with regard to their ability to safely use and dispose of smoking materials should be prohibited.
(3) Where a resident, as specified in A.32.7.4.1(2), is under direct supervision by staff or by a person approved by the administration, smoking might be permitted.
(4) Smoking materials should not be provided to residents or maintained by residents without the approval of the administration.
(5) Areas where smoking is permitted should be clearly identified.
(6) Ashtrays of noncombustible material and safe design should be provided and required to be used in all areas where smoking is permitted.
(7) Self-closing cover devices into which ashtrays can be emptied should be made available to all areas where smoking is permitted and should be required to be used.

**32.7.4.2** Where smoking is permitted, noncombustible safety-type ashtrays or receptacles shall be provided in convenient locations.

### 32.7.5* Furnishings, Mattresses, and Decorations.

**A.32.7.5** The requirements applicable to draperies/curtains, upholstered furniture, and mattresses apply only to new draperies/curtains, new upholstered furniture, and new mattresses. The term *new* means unused, normally via procurement from the marketplace, either by purchase or donation, of items not previously used. Many board and care facilities allow residents to bring into the board and care home upholstered furniture items from the resident's previous residence. Such items are not new and, thus, are not regulated. On the other hand, some of the larger board and care homes

CHAPTER 33 • Existing

### 33.7.4 Smoking.

**33.7.4.1*** Smoking regulations shall be adopted by the administration of board and care occupancies.

**A.33.7.4.1** Smoking regulations should include the following:

(1) Smoking should be prohibited in any room, compartment, or area where flammable or combustible liquids, combustible gases, or oxygen is used or stored and in any other hazardous location, and the following also should apply:
  (a) Such areas should be posted with signs that read NO SMOKING or the international symbol for no smoking.
  (b) In residential board and care facilities where smoking is totally prohibited and signs so indicating are placed at all major entrances, secondary signs with language that prohibits smoking are not required.
(2) Smoking by residents classified as not responsible with regard to their ability to safely use and dispose of smoking materials should be prohibited.
(3) Where a resident, as specified in A.33.7.4.1(2), is under direct supervision by staff or by a person approved by the administration, smoking might be permitted.
(4) Smoking materials should not be provided to residents or maintained by residents without the approval of the administration.
(5) Areas where smoking is permitted should be clearly identified.
(6) Ashtrays of noncombustible material and safe design should be provided and required to be used in all areas where smoking is permitted.
(7) Self-closing cover devices into which ashtrays can be emptied should be made available to all areas where smoking is permitted and should be required to be used.

**33.7.4.2** Where smoking is permitted, noncombustible safety-type ashtrays or receptacles shall be provided in convenient locations.

### 33.7.5* Furnishings, Mattresses, and Decorations.

**A.33.7.5** The requirements applicable to draperies/curtains, upholstered furniture, and mattresses apply only to new draperies/curtains, new upholstered furniture, and new mattresses. The term *new* means unused, normally via procurement from the marketplace, either by purchase or donation, of items not previously used. Many board and care facilities allow residents to bring into the board and care home upholstered furniture items from the resident's previous residence. Such items are not new and, thus, are not regulated. On the other hand, some of the larger board and care homes

CHAPTER 32 • New

purchase contract furniture, as is done in hotels. Such new, unused furniture, whether purchased or received as a donation, is regulated by the requirements of 32.7.5.2. By federal law, mattresses manufactured and sold within the United States must pass testing per 16 CFR 1632, "Standard for the Flammability of Mattresses and Mattress Pads" (FF4-72).

**32.7.5.1** New draperies, curtains, and other similar loosely hanging furnishings and decorations in board and care facilities shall be in accordance with the provisions of 10.3.1.

**32.7.5.2*** New upholstered furniture within board and care facilities shall comply with 32.7.5.2.1 or 32.7.5.2.2.

**A.32.7.5.2** New upholstered furniture within board and care homes should be tested for rates of heat release in accordance with 10.3.3.

**32.7.5.2.1** New upholstered furniture shall be tested in accordance with the provisions of 10.3.2.1(1) and 10.3.3.

**32.7.5.2.2** Upholstered furniture belonging to residents in sleeping rooms shall not be required to be tested, provided that a smoke alarm is installed in such rooms; battery-powered single-station smoke alarms shall be permitted in such rooms.

**32.7.5.3*** Newly introduced mattresses within board and care facilities shall comply with 32.7.5.3.1 or 32.7.5.3.2.

**A.32.7.5.3** New mattresses within board and care homes should be tested for rates of heat release in accordance with 10.3.4.

**32.7.5.3.1** Newly introduced mattresses shall be tested in accordance with the provisions of 10.3.2.2 and 10.3.4.

**32.7.5.3.2** Mattresses belonging to residents in sleeping rooms shall not be required to be tested, provided that a smoke alarm is installed in such rooms; battery-powered single-station smoke alarms shall be permitted in such rooms.

CHAPTER 33 • Existing

purchase contract furniture, as is done in hotels. Such new, unused furniture, whether purchased or received as a donation, is regulated by the requirements of 33.7.5.2. By federal law, mattresses manufactured and sold within the United States must pass testing per 16 CFR 1632, "Standard for the Flammability of Mattresses and Mattress Pads" (FF 4-72).

**33.7.5.1** New draperies, curtains, and other similar loosely hanging furnishings and decorations in board and care facilities shall be in accordance with the provisions of 10.3.1.

**33.7.5.2*** New upholstered furniture within board and care facilities shall comply with 33.7.5.2.1 or 33.7.5.2.2.

**A.33.7.5.2** New upholstered furniture within board and care homes should be tested for rates of heat release in accordance with 10.3.3.

**33.7.5.2.1** New upholstered furniture shall be tested in accordance with the provisions of 10.3.2.1(1) and 10.3.3.

**33.7.5.2.2** Upholstered furniture belonging to residents in sleeping rooms shall not be required to be tested, provided that a smoke alarm is installed in such rooms; battery-powered single-station smoke alarms shall be permitted in such rooms.

**33.7.5.3*** Newly introduced mattresses within board and care facilities shall comply with 33.7.5.3.1 or 33.7.5.3.2.

**A.33.7.5.3** New mattresses within board and care homes should be tested for rates of heat release in accordance with 10.3.4.

**33.7.5.3.1** Newly introduced mattresses shall be tested in accordance with the provisions of 10.3.2.2 and 10.3.4.

**33.7.5.3.2** Mattresses belonging to residents in sleeping rooms shall not be required to be tested, provided that a smoke alarm is installed in such rooms; battery-powered single-station smoke alarms shall be permitted in such rooms.

The provisions of 32/33.7.5 extend the level of life safety provided to a residential board and care facility by further attempting to prevent room flashover. However, rather than impose these requirements retroactively on existing facilities, the requirement applies to new upholstered furniture and mattresses. The text of A.32/A.33.7.5 sufficiently details the meaning of the term *new* in this context.

Draperies must be flame resistant in accordance with 10.3.1. Newly introduced upholstered furniture and mattresses must be resistant to cigarette ignition in accordance with 10.3.2. Newly introduced upholstered furniture and mattresses must have limited rates of heat release in accordance with 10.3.3 and 10.3.4, unless the building is sprinklered. See the commentary on Section 10.3.

### 32.7.6 Staff.

Staff shall be on duty and in the facility at all times when residents requiring evacuation assistance are present.

### 33.7.6 Staff.

Staff shall be on duty and in the facility at all times when residents requiring evacuation assistance are present.

CHAPTER 32 • New

### 32.7.7 Inspection of Door Openings.

Door assemblies for which the door leaf is required to swing in the direction of egress travel shall be inspected and tested not less than annually in accordance with 7.2.1.15.

CHAPTER 33 • Existing

### 33.7.7 Inspection of Door Openings.

Door assemblies for which the door leaf is required to swing in the direction of egress travel shall be inspected and tested not less than annually in accordance with 7.2.1.15.

Doors in board and care facilities that are required to swing in the direction of egress travel must be annually inspected using the criteria specified in 7.2.1.15, which are new to the 2009 edition of the *Code*, as required by 32/33.7.7. Such doors include those that serve areas with occupant loads of 50 or more and those that serve exit enclosures. The inspection criteria are intended to ensure that such doors will function as needed during a fire emergency. See 7.2.1.15 and the associated commentary for additional details.

## References Cited in Commentary


1. *NFPA 5000®, Building Construction and Safety Code®*, 2009 edition, National Fire Protection Association, Quincy, MA.
2. NFPA 101A, *Guide on Alternative Approaches to Life Safety*, 2007 edition, National Fire Protection Association, Quincy, MA. (The edition of NFPA 101A that corresponds with the 2009 edition of NFPA *101®, Life Safety Code®*, will be published in 2010.)
3. NFPA 13D, *Standard for the Installation of Sprinkler Systems in One- and Two-Family Dwellings and Manufactured Homes*, 2007 edition, National Fire Protection Association, Quincy, MA.
4. NFPA 13, *Standard for the Installation of Sprinkler Systems*, 2007 edition, National Fire Protection Association, Quincy, MA.
5. NFPA 13R, *Standard for the Installation of Sprinkler Systems in Residential Occupancies up to and Including Four Stories in Height*, 2007 edition, National Fire Protection Association, Quincy, MA.
6. NFPA 25, *Standard for the Inspection, Testing, and Maintenance of Water-Based Fire Protection Systems*, 2008 edition, National Fire Protection Association, Quincy, MA.

CHAPTER 34

# Reserved

In the 2009 edition, Chapter 34 has been reserved for future use.

CHAPTER 35

# Reserved

In the 2009 edition, Chapter 35 has been reserved for future use.

## CHAPTERS 36 AND 37

# New and Existing Mercantile Occupancies

Mercantile occupancies include stores, markets, and other rooms, buildings, or structures used for the display and sale of merchandise. This occupancy classification includes, but is not limited to, the following:

1. Supermarkets
2. Convenience stores
3. Department stores
4. Hardware stores
5. Video sales/rental stores
6. Pharmacies
7. Rental equipment centers
8. Automobile sales showrooms
9. Flea markets and craft centers
10. Building materials/supplies centers
11. Shopping centers/malls
12. Office supply stores
13. Computer and electronics stores
14. Sporting goods stores
15. Warehouse club stores

Minor merchandising operations in buildings that house other predominant occupancies, such as a newsstand in an office building, are typically classified as incidental uses and must, therefore, meet the *Code* requirements of the predominant occupancy (see 6.1.14.1.3).

The life safety provisions for mercantile occupancies are based on their characteristic of displaying merchandise for sales purposes, which introduces significant quantities of fuel in sales areas occupied by persons who are mostly unfamiliar with the building. Mercantile occupancies are also characterized by the use of layouts of merchandise displays and store fixtures that can confuse the egress path. Fires in department stores, mall buildings, and similar mercantile occupancies that resulted in occupant fatalities have been practically unheard of in the United States over the past two decades. Although some serious fires have occurred in such properties, the established *Code* provisions have served the life safety needs of the occupants very well.

As marketing techniques change to meet consumer demands — beginning in the 1960s when the first covered shopping malls were built — store design and layout also change. Consumers are offered choices that include everything from one-stop shopping to unique specialty stores. As the hypermarket, or big-box store, concept became popular in the early 1980s, the general public found itself shopping in warehouse-type surroundings. The *Code* provisions that apply to mercantile occupancies have recognized these challenges to providing adequate life safety via a combination of flexible general requirements and specialized provisions, such as those contained in 36/37.4.4 for mall buildings and 36/37.4.5 for bulk merchandising retail buildings.

The life safety measures needed for mercantile occupancies are as diverse as the types of mercantile facilities. Although the nature of the actual store design — as well as the merchandise that is found in the stores — drives much of the *Code* criteria, the ongoing need to prevent the theft of merchandise also affects the protection requirements.

The features of a mercantile occupancy that determine the needed protection include the items for sale, the location of the areas occupied by the public with respect to the level of exit discharge, and the size (i.e., gross area) of the facility. Guidance on establishing the appropriate subclassification for mercantile occupancies is provided by 36/37.1.4.2.

Establishing and controlling the widths of aisles that lead to exits is an important consideration. For example, 36/37.2.5.5 establishes minimum widths, which are based on the clear width, to prevent boxed

CHAPTER 36 • New

or loose merchandise from obstructing the egress path. In certain larger stores, minimum 60 in. (1525 mm) aisles might be the norm to accommodate shopping carts as well as large numbers of occupants. Automatic sprinkler protection and a manual fire alarm system complement the major features of the protection package for the larger Class A stores.

The requirements for bulk merchandising retail buildings found in 36/37.4.5 establish criteria that meet the special needs of such stores. The typical bulk merchandising retail store includes display and storage racks that are often more than 20 ft (6100 mm) high. Display merchandise is typically maintained at the lower levels, while the excess inventory of merchandise is stored on the upper tiers of the rack systems. In such cases, the range of materials in the occupancies is extensive and can include building materials, paint, electrical equipment, and indoor/outdoor power equipment and appliances. In some cases, the store inventory might consist of foodstuffs as well as household goods. Due to the crossover nature of such occupancies — which are part warehouse and part retail store — 36/37.4.5.2 and 36/37.4.5.3 establish requirements for providing the egress measures needed for an occupancy with a large occupant load and the fire protection measures needed for a warehouse.

## 36.1 General Requirements

### 36.1.1 Application.

**36.1.1.1** The requirements of this chapter shall apply to new buildings or portions thereof used as mercantile occupancies. *(See 1.3.1.)*

**36.1.1.2** The provisions of this chapter shall apply to life safety requirements for all new mercantile buildings. Specific requirements shall apply to suboccupancy groups, such as Class A, Class B, and Class C mercantile occupancies; covered malls; and bulk merchandising retail buildings, and are contained in paragraphs pertaining thereto.

**36.1.1.3** Additions to existing buildings shall comply with 36.1.1.3.1, 36.1.1.3.2, and 36.1.1.3.3.

**36.1.1.3.1** Additions to existing buildings shall conform to the requirements of 4.6.8.

**36.1.1.3.2** Existing portions of the structure shall not be required to be modified, provided that the new construction has not diminished the fire safety features of the facility.

**36.1.1.3.3** Existing portions shall be upgraded if the addition results in a change of mercantile subclassification. *(See 36.1.4.2.)*

**36.1.1.4** When a mercantile occupancy changes from Class C to Class A or Class B, or from Class B to Class A, the provisions of this chapter shall apply.

CHAPTER 37 • Existing

## 37.1 General Requirements

### 37.1.1 Application.

**37.1.1.1** The requirements of this chapter shall apply to existing buildings or portions thereof currently occupied as mercantile occupancies.

**37.1.1.2** The provisions of this chapter shall apply to life safety requirements for all existing mercantile buildings. Specific requirements shall apply to suboccupancy groups, such as Class A, Class B, and Class C mercantile occupancies; covered malls; and bulk merchandising retail buildings, and are contained in paragraphs pertaining thereto.

**37.1.1.3** Additions to existing buildings shall comply with 37.1.1.3.1, 37.1.1.3.2, and 37.1.1.3.3.

**37.1.1.3.1** Additions to existing buildings shall conform to the requirements of 4.6.8.

**37.1.1.3.2** Existing portions of the structure shall not be required to be modified, provided that the new construction has not diminished the fire safety features of the facility.

**37.1.1.3.3** Existing portions shall be upgraded if the addition results in a change of mercantile subclassification. *(See 37.1.4.2.)*

**37.1.1.4** When a change in mercantile occupancy sub-classification occurs, the following requirements shall be met:

(1) When a mercantile occupancy changes from Class A to Class B or Class C, or from Class B to Class C, the provisions of this chapter shall apply.
(2) When a mercantile occupancy changes from Class C to Class A or Class B, or from Class B to Class A, the provisions of Chapter 36 shall apply.

CHAPTER 36 • New

CHAPTER 37 • Existing

The provisions for new mercantile occupancies are addressed in Chapter 36; the provisions for existing mercantile occupancies (i.e., existing conditions in mercantile occupancies) are addressed in Chapter 37.

In prior editions of the *Code*, renovations, additions, and changes of occupancy were required to comply with the requirements for new construction. For mercantile occupancies, such renovations, additions, and changes of occupancy were required to meet the provisions of Chapter 36, while existing conditions were subject to the provisions of Chapter 37. Chapter 43, Building Rehabilitation, was added for the 2006 edition of the *Code*. Chapter 43 was written to promote the adaptive reuse of existing buildings without sacrificing the needed level of life safety. The provisions of Chapter 43 blend the requirements for new construction with those for existing conditions, so as to require additional life safety features as the rehabilitation work category increases in complexity. The rehabilitation work categories are repair, renovation, modification, reconstruction, change of use, change of occupancy classification, and addition. See 4.6.8, 4.6.12, and Chapter 43.

To understand the full intent and scope of 37.1.1.1, it is necessary to review it concurrently with Sections 1.2 and 1.3. Although a building code might permit existing buildings to be excluded from coverage under some form of a grandfather clause, the *Life Safety Code*, by virtue of its interest in safety to life, requires that existing building arrangements comply with the *Code* requirements that apply to existing buildings. The requirements applicable to existing mercantile occupancies are contained in Chapter 37.

If a building complies with an earlier edition of the *Code*, it is not grandfathered and, thereby, exempted from compliance with a more current edition that has been adopted as law in the building's jurisdiction. The NFPA technical committees on safety to life are especially careful to avoid adopting requirements for existing buildings that become more stringent from one edition of the *Code* to the next, unless the change is absolutely necessary to meet the level of safety to life intended. Thus, the old adage of "once in compliance, always in compliance" does not hold.

Commentary Table 36/37.1 summarizes the definitions of Class A, Class B, and Class C mercantile occupancies presented in 36/37.1.4.2.1 and further explained in its associated commentary.

Additions to existing mercantile occupancies must conform to the requirements for new construction in accordance with 36/37.1.1.3. However, the existing portion of the occupancy generally is permitted to continue in use if it complies with the provisions of Chapter 37. If, however, the addition results in a change in the mercantile occupancy subclassification (see 36/37.1.4.2) — such as a change from Class C to Class B or from Class B to Class A — the existing portion of the enlarged overall facility must be upgraded to meet the provisions that apply to new construction. The provisions of 36/37.1.1.3 are illustrated in the paragraphs that follow and in Exhibit 36/37.1.

***Commentary Table 36/37.1 Subclassification of Mercantile Occupancies***

| Store Class | Height | Aggregate Gross Area[1] ft² (m²) |
|---|---|---|
| A | >3 stories[2] | >30,000 (>2800) |
| B | ≤3 stories[2] | >3000 (>280) and ≤30,000 (≤2800) |
| C | One story only[3] | ≤3000 (≤280) |

[1]Sections of floors not used for sales purposes are not counted in the area classification.

[2]Stories not used for sales above or below sales floor are not counted in the height classification.

[3]A mezzanine ≤ $\frac{1}{3}$ the area (new) or ≤ $\frac{1}{2}$ the area (existing) of the floor below is permitted (see 8.6.9 and 36/37.1.4.2.3).

In Exhibit 36/37.1, Part (a), the new construction, which includes 10,000 ft² (930 m²) of additional sales area and approximately 2000 ft² (186 m²) of new storage area, is added to an existing Class B mercantile occupancy with 5000 ft² (465 m²) of existing sales area. The size and placement of the new addition neither change the Class B mercantile subclassification of the enlarged overall facility nor diminish the fire safety features of the existing portion of the facility. Therefore, the addition is constructed in accordance with the requirements of Chapter 36, and the existing portion of the building is permitted to continue to be used, without upgrade, if it meets the requirements of Chapter 37. If the existing portion of the building does not meet the requirements of Chapter 37, it must be upgraded to meet those requirements.

Exhibit 36/37.1, Part (b), depicts new construction, identical to that of Part (a), that is added to an existing Class B mercantile occupancy with 14,000 ft² (1300 m²) of existing sales area. Although the size of the addition does not change the Class B mercantile subclassification of the overall facility, the placement of the new

 

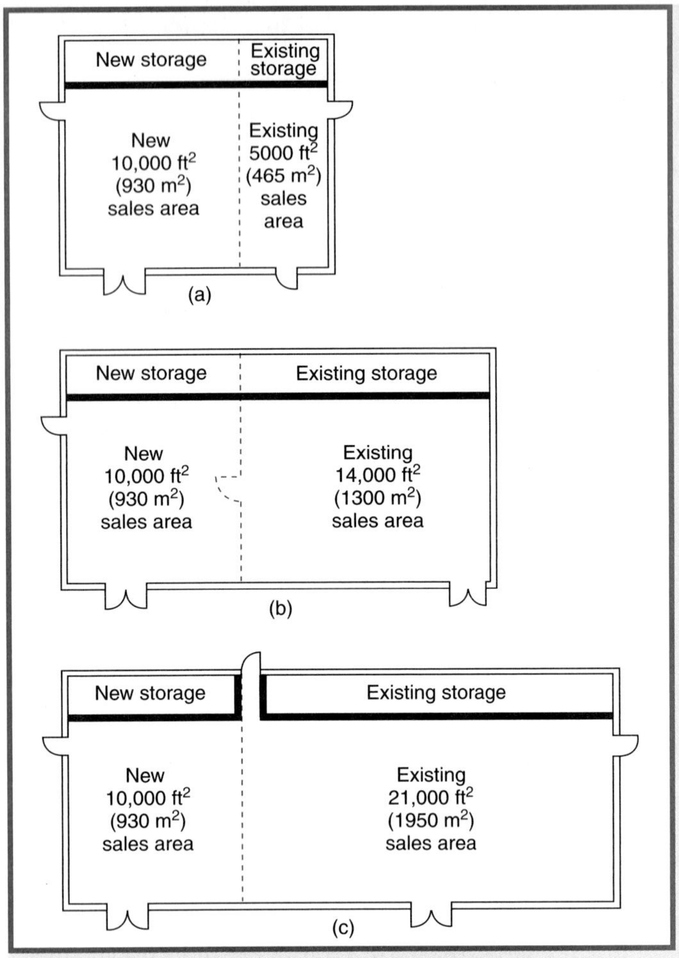


***Exhibit 36/37.1*** *Additions to existing mercantile occupancies.*

addition appears to have diminished the fire safety of the existing portion of the building with respect to travel distance. The broken line in Part (b) represents what had been an exterior wall and exit door in the existing mercantile occupancy prior to construction of the addition. The door allowed occupants in the upper left portion of the existing building to reach an exit within the allowable 150 ft (46 m) travel distance specified for existing nonsprinklered mercantile occupancies in accordance with 37.2.6.2. Without the exit door, occupants of the existing portion of the building must be able to reach an exit — one of the three doors in the perimeter of the enlarged facility — within the same 150 ft (46 m) travel distance limitation. If this is not possible, an additional exit within that distance must be constructed, or the building must be sprinklered to increase the allowable travel distance to 250 ft (76 m). Because the new construction must meet the provisions of Chapter 36, the entire building — new and existing portions — must be sprinklered in accordance with 36.3.5.1(2), because the building exceeds 12,000 ft² (1115 m²) in gross area.

Exhibit 36/37.1, Part (c), depicts new construction, identical to that of Part (a) and Part (b), that is added to an existing Class B mercantile occupancy with 21,000 ft² (1950 m²) of existing sales area. The size of the new sales area, when added to that of the existing mercantile occupancy, exceeds 30,000 ft² (2800 m²) and results in a change in mercantile subclassification from Class B to Class A [see 36/37.1.4.2.1(1)]. In accordance with the provisions of 36/37.1.1.3 and the clarification of intent offered in 36/37.1.1.4, the entire building — new and existing portions — must meet the requirements for new mercantile occupancies as detailed in Chapter 36.

## 36.1.2 Multiple Occupancies.

### 36.1.2.1 General.

**36.1.2.1.1** All multiple occupancies shall be in accordance with 6.1.14 and 36.1.2.

**36.1.2.1.2** Where there are differences in the specific requirements in this chapter and provisions for mixed occupancies or separated occupancies as specified in 6.1.14.3 and 6.1.14.4, the requirements of this chapter shall apply.

### 36.1.2.2 Combined Mercantile Occupancies and Parking Structures.

**36.1.2.2.1** The fire barrier separating parking structures from a building classified as a mercantile occupancy shall be a fire barrier having a minimum 2-hour fire resistance rating.

## 37.1.2 Multiple Occupancies.

### 37.1.2.1 General.

**37.1.2.1.1** All multiple occupancies shall be in accordance with 6.1.14 and 37.1.2.

**37.1.2.1.2** Where there are differences in the specific requirements in this chapter and provisions for mixed occupancies or separated occupancies as specified in 6.1.14.3 and 6.1.14.4, the requirements of this chapter shall apply.

### 37.1.2.2 Combined Mercantile Occupancies and Parking Structures.

**37.1.2.2.1** The fire barrier separating parking structures from a building classified as a mercantile occupancy shall be a fire barrier having a minimum 2-hour fire resistance rating.

CHAPTER 36 • New

**36.1.2.2.2** Openings in the fire barrier required by 36.1.2.2.1 shall not be required to be protected with fire protection–rated opening protectives in enclosed parking structures that are protected throughout by an approved, supervised automatic sprinkler system in accordance with 9.7.1.1(1), or in open parking structures, provided that all of the following conditions are met:

(1) The openings do not exceed 25 percent of the area of the fire barrier in which they are located.
(2) The openings are used as a public entrance and for associated sidelight functions.
(3) The building containing the mercantile occupancy is protected throughout by an approved, supervised automatic sprinkler system in accordance with 9.7.1.1(1).
(4)* Means are provided to prevent spilled fuel from accumulating adjacent to the openings and entering the building.

**A.36.1.2.2.2(4)** Means to prevent spilled fuel from accumulating and entering the mercantile occupancy building can be by curbs, scuppers, special drainage systems, sloping the floor away from the door openings, or floor elevation differences of not less than 4 in. (100 mm).

(5) Physical means are provided to prevent vehicles from being parked or driven within 10 ft (3050 mm) of the openings.
(6) The openings are protected as a smoke partition in accordance with Section 8.4, with no minimum fire protection rating required.

CHAPTER 37 • Existing

**37.1.2.2.2** Openings in the fire barrier required by 37.1.2.2.1 shall not be required to be protected with fire protection–rated opening protectives in enclosed parking structures that are protected throughout by an approved, supervised automatic sprinkler system in accordance with 9.7.1.1(1), or in open parking structures, provided that all of the following conditions are met:

(1) The openings do not exceed 25 percent of the area of the fire barrier in which they are located.
(2) The openings are used as a public entrance and for associated sidelight functions.
(3) The building containing the mercantile occupancy is protected throughout by an approved, supervised automatic sprinkler system in accordance with 9.7.1.1(1).
(4)* Means are provided to prevent spilled fuel from accumulating adjacent to the openings and entering the building.

**A.37.1.2.2.2(4)** Means to prevent spilled fuel from accumulating and entering the mercantile occupancy building can be by curbs, scuppers, special drainage systems, sloping the floor away from the door openings, or elevation differences of not less than 4 in. (100 mm).

(5) Physical means are provided to prevent vehicles from being parked or driven within 10 ft (3050 mm) of the openings.
(6) The openings are protected as a smoke partition in accordance with Section 8.4, with no minimum fire protection rating required.

The provisions of 36/37.1.2.2 address combined mercantile occupancies and parking structures and are very similar to the requirements of 38/39.1.2.2, which address combined business occupancies and parking structures. It is common for multistory mercantile occupancies (such as department stores and shopping mall buildings) and multistory business occupancies (such as office buildings) to be attached to multistory parking garages. Such garages provide access to the mercantile or business occupancy at multiple levels. To allow flexibility in the number and types of openings and in the degree of stringency required for opening protectives, such as fire doors and fire windows, the criteria in 36/37.1.2.2.2 outline a set of provisions that, where applied in total, will safely permit a reduction in the 2-hour fire resistance rating required by 36/37.1.2.2.1. The reduction permits the use of nonrated glazing and opening protectives. This reduction permits the use of glass doors and sidelights in the barrier between the mercantile occupancy and the garage, which increases security in the garage, because customers and staff can view the parking area through the glass doors or sidelights.

Note that all seven requirements mandated by 36/37.1.2.2.2 — the sprinkler requirement for enclosed garages in the base paragraph and the six requirements of 36/37.1.2.2.2(1) through (6) — must be met as a whole to apply the exemption. Otherwise, a continuous 2-hour fire resistance–rated separation with properly protected openings between the mercantile occupancy and the parking structure is required.

### 36.1.3 Special Definitions.

A list of special terms used in this chapter follows:

(1) **Anchor Building.** See 3.3.32.2.
(2) **Bulk Merchandising Retail Building.** See 3.3.32.4.

### 37.1.3 Special Definitions.

A list of special terms used in this chapter follows:

(1) **Anchor Building.** See 3.3.32.2.
(2) **Bulk Merchandising Retail Building.** See 3.3.32.4.

(3) **Gross Leasable Area.** See 3.3.19.3.
(4) **Major Tenant.** See 3.3.157.
(5) **Mall.** See 3.3.158.
(6) **Mall Building.** See 3.3.32.9.
(7) **Open-Air Mercantile Operation.** See 3.3.187.

(3) **Gross Leasable Area.** See 3.3.19.3.
(4) **Major Tenant.** See 3.3.157.
(5) **Mall.** See 3.3.158.
(6) **Mall Building.** See 3.3.32.9.
(7) **Open-Air Mercantile Operation.** See 3.3.187.

In the 2003 edition of the *Code*, the term *anchor store* was replaced with the term *anchor building*, as defined in 3.3.32.2, recognizing that such a structure might contain other than mercantile occupancies. From a merchandising viewpoint, a shopping mall developer or operator might refer to any of the large tenants that have vast expanses of floor space and instant name recognition — and that are often positioned at the ends and corners of the mall building — as anchor buildings. However, the *Code* reserves the use of the term *anchor building* for those perimeter buildings with means of egress independent from the mall.

See Exhibit 36/37.2, which illustrates the difference between an anchor building and a store that, while large, is not an anchor building. Required egress from an anchor building is not permitted to pass through the mall. The store at the left of the exhibit satisfies this requirement and, therefore, is an anchor building. The opening between the anchor building and the mall is permitted over and above the egress width satisfied by the store's required means of egress. The store at the right of the exhibit relies on exits from the mall as part of its required egress capacity and, therefore, is not an anchor building.

The term *bulk merchandising retail building* (see definition in 3.3.32.4) applies to the special provisions of 36/37.4.5 for mercantile occupancies characterized by warehouse-type sales areas where merchandise is stored on pallets, in solid piles, or in racks extending far above head height. The storage arrangement and quantities of combustible materials pose challenges that differ from those typically found in department stores and supermarkets and, therefore, warrant special protection criteria.

The 2009 edition of the *Code* introduces the term *major tenant* (see definition in 3.3.157), which is a tenant space that has at least one main entrance from the outside that also serves as an exit. The intent of this definition and the corresponding provision in 36/37.4.4.3.6 is to avoid needlessly oversizing the means of egress from the mall, given that some occupants of the major tenants will egress directly to the outside. Note, however, that means of egress from the mall is based on the occupant load calculated in accordance with Figure 7.3.1.2(a) and Figure 7.3.1.2(b). The occupant load of the mall for which means of egress must be provided is based on the gross leasable area of the mall building, excluding anchor buildings; no provision is made for major tenants. As a result, the new definition and provisions have no effect on the required means of egress from malls as intended. The concept will require further development for a future edition of the *Code*.

The terms *mall* (see definition in 3.3.158) and *mall building* (see definition in 3.3.32.9) differ from each other so that certain requirements apply only to the

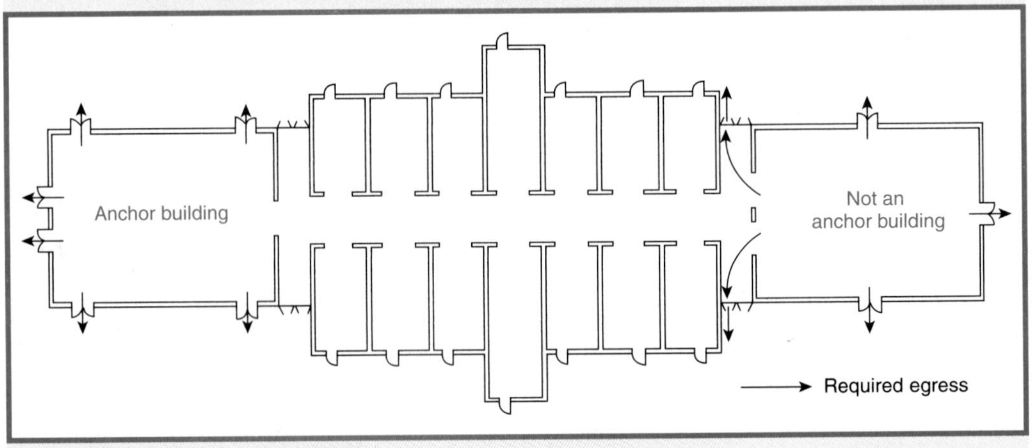


***Exhibit 36/37.2** Anchor building and non-anchor building.*

covered pedestrian way (the mall), while other requirements apply to the entire building, including all tenant spaces and common areas (the mall building). For example, the provisions of 36/37.4.4 require automatic sprinkler protection throughout the mall building but require an alarm system — and, under certain conditions, a smoke control system — only within the mall.

### 36.1.4 Classification of Occupancy.

**36.1.4.1 General.** Mercantile occupancies shall include all buildings and structures or parts thereof with occupancy as defined in 6.1.10.

**36.1.4.2 Subclassification of Occupancy.**

**36.1.4.2.1** Mercantile occupancies shall be subclassified as follows:

(1) Class A, all mercantile occupancies having an aggregate gross area of more than 30,000 $ft^2$ (2800 $m^2$) or occupying more than three stories for sales purposes
(2) Class B, as follows:
   (a) All mercantile occupancies of more than 3000 $ft^2$ (280 $m^2$), but not more than 30,000 $ft^2$ (2800 $m^2$), aggregate gross area and occupying not more than three stories for sales purposes
   (b) All mercantile occupancies of not more than 3000 $ft^2$ (280 $m^2$) gross area and occupying two or three stories for sales purposes
(3) Class C, all mercantile occupancies of not more than 3000 $ft^2$ (280 $m^2$) gross area and used for sales purposes occupying one story only

**36.1.4.2.2** For the purpose of the classification required in 36.1.4.2.1, the requirements of 36.1.4.2.2.1, 36.1.4.2.2.2, and 36.1.4.2.2.3 shall be met.

**36.1.4.2.2.1** The aggregate gross area shall be the total gross area of all floors used for mercantile purposes.

**36.1.4.2.2.2** Where a mercantile occupancy is divided into sections, regardless of fire separation, the aggregate gross area shall include the area of all sections used for sales purposes.

**36.1.4.2.2.3** Areas of floors not used for sales purposes, such as an area used only for storage and not open to the public, shall not be counted for the purposes of the classifications in 36.1.4.2.1(1), (2), and (3), but means of egress shall be provided for such nonsales areas in accordance with their occupancy, as specified by other chapters of this *Code*.



The term *gross leasable area* is defined (see 3.3.19.3) to provide a criterion under which an occupant load can be calculated for use in sizing the means of egress system for the mall only. See 7.3.1.2 for details on calculating occupant load for determining required egress capacity.

Open-air mercantile operations (see definition in 3.3.187) are addressed in 36/37.4.3.

### 37.1.4 Classification of Occupancy.

**37.1.4.1 General.** Mercantile occupancies shall include all buildings and structures or parts thereof with occupancy as defined in 6.1.10.

**37.1.4.2 Subclassification of Occupancy.**

**37.1.4.2.1** Mercantile occupancies shall be subclassified as follows:

(1) Class A, all mercantile occupancies having an aggregate gross area of more than 30,000 $ft^2$ (2800 $m^2$) or occupying more than three stories for sales purposes
(2) Class B, as follows:
   (a) All mercantile occupancies of more than 3000 $ft^2$ (280 $m^2$), but not more than 30,000 $ft^2$ (2800 $m^2$), aggregate gross area and occupying not more than three stories for sales purposes
   (b) All mercantile occupancies of not more than 3000 $ft^2$ (280 $m^2$) gross area and occupying two or three stories for sales purposes
(3) Class C, all mercantile occupancies of not more than 3000 $ft^2$ (280 $m^2$) gross area used for sales purposes and occupying one story only, excluding mezzanines

**37.1.4.2.2** For the purpose of the classification required in 37.1.4.2.1, the requirements of 37.1.4.2.2.1, 37.1.4.2.2.2, and 37.1.4.2.2.3 shall be met.

**37.1.4.2.2.1** The aggregate gross area shall be the total gross area of all floors used for mercantile purposes.

**37.1.4.2.2.2** Where a mercantile occupancy is divided into sections, regardless of fire separation, the aggregate gross area shall include the area of all sections used for sales purposes.

**37.1.4.2.2.3** Areas of floors not used for sales purposes, such as an area used only for storage and not open to the public, shall not be counted for the purposes of the classifications in 37.1.4.2.1(1), (2), and (3), but means of egress shall be provided for such nonsales areas in accordance with their occupancy, as specified by other chapters of this *Code*.

CHAPTER 36 • New

**36.1.4.2.3** Mezzanines shall comply with 8.6.9.

**36.1.4.2.4** Where a number of tenant spaces under different management are located in the same building, the aggregate gross area for subclassification shall be one of the following:

(1) Where tenant spaces are not separated, the aggregate gross floor area of all such tenant spaces shall be used in determining classification per 36.1.4.2.1.
(2) Where individual tenant spaces are separated by fire barriers with a 2-hour fire resistance rating, each tenant space shall be individually classified.
(3) Where tenant spaces are separated by fire barriers with a 1-hour fire resistance rating, and the building is protected throughout by an approved, supervised automatic sprinkler system in accordance with 9.7.1.1(1), each tenant space shall be individually classified.
(4) The tenant spaces in a mall building in accordance with 36.4.4 shall be classified individually.

CHAPTER 37 • Existing

**37.1.4.2.3** The floor area of a mezzanine, or the aggregate floor area of multiple mezzanines, shall not exceed one-half of the floor area of the room or story in which the mezzanines are located; otherwise, such mezzanine or aggregated mezzanines shall be treated as floors.

**37.1.4.2.4** Where a number of tenant spaces under different management are located in the same building, the aggregate gross area for subclassification shall be one of the following:

(1) Where tenant spaces are not separated, the aggregate gross floor area of all such tenant spaces shall be used in determining classification per 37.1.4.2.1.
(2) Where individual tenant spaces are separated by fire barriers with a 1-hour fire resistance rating, each tenant space shall be individually classified.
(3) The tenant spaces in a mall building in accordance with 37.4.4 shall be classified individually.

As noted in 36/37.1.4.1, guidance on the classification of a mercantile occupancy is provided by the definition in 6.1.10. Note that, per 6.1.14.1.3, minor merchandising operations in buildings that house other predominant occupancies are subject to the requirements of the predominant occupancy. For example, a newsstand located in an office building would be treated under the same business occupancy requirements (Chapters 38 and 39) as the office building.

Further clarification of the subclassification of stores as Class A, Class B, or Class C is provided by 36/37.1.4.2.1 through 36/37.1.4.2.4. Most of these provisions are included in the footnotes to Commentary Table 36/37.1. The user should also note the following:

1. The aggregate gross area is the sum of the gross areas of all floors used for mercantile (sales) purposes.
2. If the store is divided so that some portions are not used for sales purposes, such as shipping/receiving/storage areas, only the sales areas are included in the aggregate gross area.
3. With the exception of mall buildings (see 36/37.4.4), the aggregate gross area of stores must be used in subclassifying a mercantile occupancy in accordance with 36/37.1.4.2.1 under the following conditions:
   a. If stores are contiguous to one another (even if under different ownership or management and occupying numerous buildings)
   b. If sections or floors used for sales within any building are considered as separate stores (e.g., because they are under different management)
   c. If the contiguous or intermixed stores described in items 3(a) and (b) are not separated from each other by the 2-hour or 1-hour fire barriers specified in 36/37.1.4.2.4

Mezzanines are addressed by the one-third area rule of 36.1.4.2.3 and 8.6.9 for new construction and the one-half area rule of 37.1.4.2.3 for existing mercantile occupancies. A mezzanine with an area that does not exceed the applicable one-third or one-half area rule does not constitute a story and, therefore, is not a factor in determining mercantile occupancy subclassification based on the number of floors used for sales purposes. The area of such mezzanines used for sales purposes (see 36/37.1.4.2.2) is, however, a factor in determining occupancy subclassification based on floor area devoted to sales purposes. For example, a new mercantile occupancy with a 2100 $ft^2$ (195 $m^2$) main sales floor and a 700 $ft^2$ (65 $m^2$) sales mezzanine has a gross area of 2800 $ft^2$ (260 $m^2$) and is, therefore, a Class C mercantile occupancy. A store with a 2400 $ft^2$ (225 m²) main sales floor and an 800 ft² (75 m²) sales mezzanine has a gross area of 3200 ft² (300 m²) and, so, is a Class B mercantile occupancy. In each case, the mezzanine meets the maximum one-third area rule and is not treated as a story.

Mezzanines with areas in excess of the maximum one-third area rule (or one-half area rule for existing mercantile occupancies) constitute stories and, thus, sales levels. Therefore, such mezzanines must be considered when determining mercantile occupancy subclassification. For example, a set of plans might show a proposed store with three floor levels of 8000 ft² (740 m²) each that are used for sales purposes and a single 4000 ft² (370 m²) sales mezzanine. Because the so-called mezzanine is not a mezzanine based on the maximum one-third area rule of 8.6.9 referenced by 36.1.4.2.3, the store will actually use four floor levels for sales purposes. Although its 28,000 ft² (2590 m²) sales area would seem to indicate the store is a Class B occupancy, the four floor levels used for sales purposes result in a Class A subclassification in accordance with the definition in 36/37.1.4.2.1(1).

To qualify as a Class A, Class B, or Class C mercantile occupancy, a store must meet the requirements of 36/37.1.4.2.1, which are summarized in Commentary Table 36/37.1. The classification process is important, because specific life safety requirements vary in degree of stringency for each mercantile class. A store's classification, while based directly on the size of the sales areas, is indirectly a measure of the number of occupants at risk from any given fire.

Some mercantile occupancies locate their sales and storage areas together (e.g., furniture warehouse sales areas). In such cases, the mercantile occupancy subclassification is determined using the total aggregate gross area that is open to public use. The same procedure should be followed for bulk merchandising retail buildings.

The mezzanine measurement provisions of 37.1.4.2.3 for existing mercantile occupancies use a one-half area rule, as opposed to the one-third area rule for new mercantile occupancies. The one-third rule for new mercantile occupancy mezzanines correlates with the requirements in 8.6.9.2. Because the one-half area rule was applied to mercantile occupancies long before the general provisions for mezzanines were added to Chapter 8, it has been retained only for existing (but not new) mercantile occupancies. Mezzanines in existing mercantile occupancies continue to be evaluated on the basis of the previously applicable one-half area criterion to prevent the abrupt noncompliance of existing buildings due to an issue that does not significantly lower the level of safety to life.

Examples of mezzanine arrangements to which the maximum one-third area rule can be applied are depicted in Exhibit 36/37.3. Exhibit 36/37.4 shows examples of mezzanine arrangements to which the maximum one-half area rule of 37.1.4.2.3 for existing mercantile occupancies can be applied. For purpose of illustration, assume that all the mezzanines, as well as the entire main floor level, are used for sales purposes. Part (a) through Part (d) of Exhibit 36/37.3 depict a new single story or single floor level with mezzanine, because the aggregate areas of the mezzanines [3000 ft² (280 m²)] do not exceed one-third of the floor area [10,000 ft² (930 m²)] of the room or story in which the

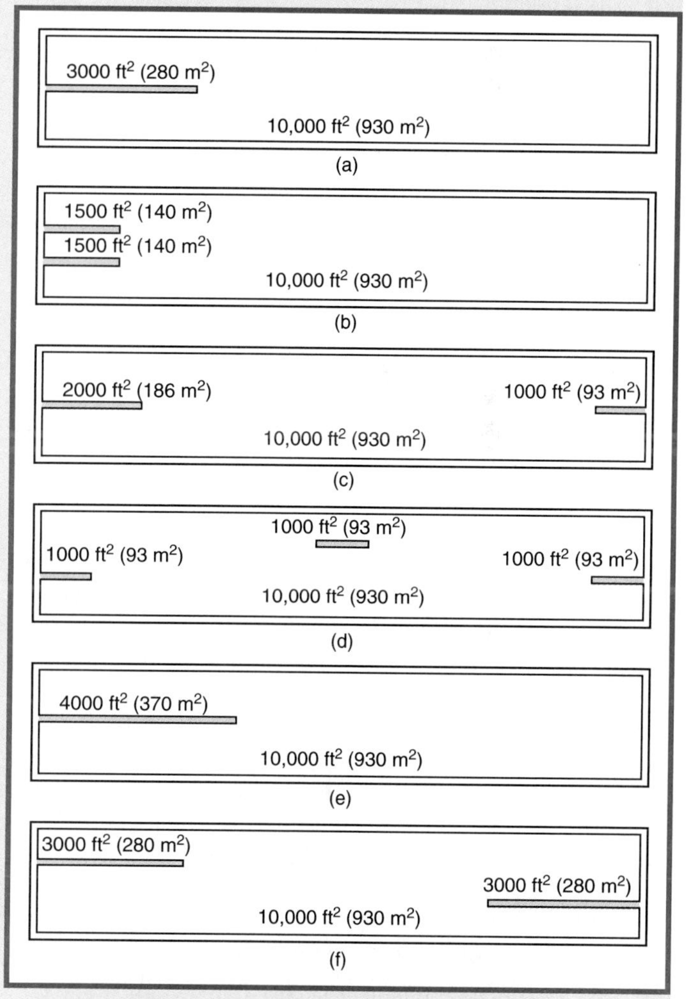


***Exhibit 36/37.3*** *Elevation views of new mercantile occupancy mezzanine arrangements.*

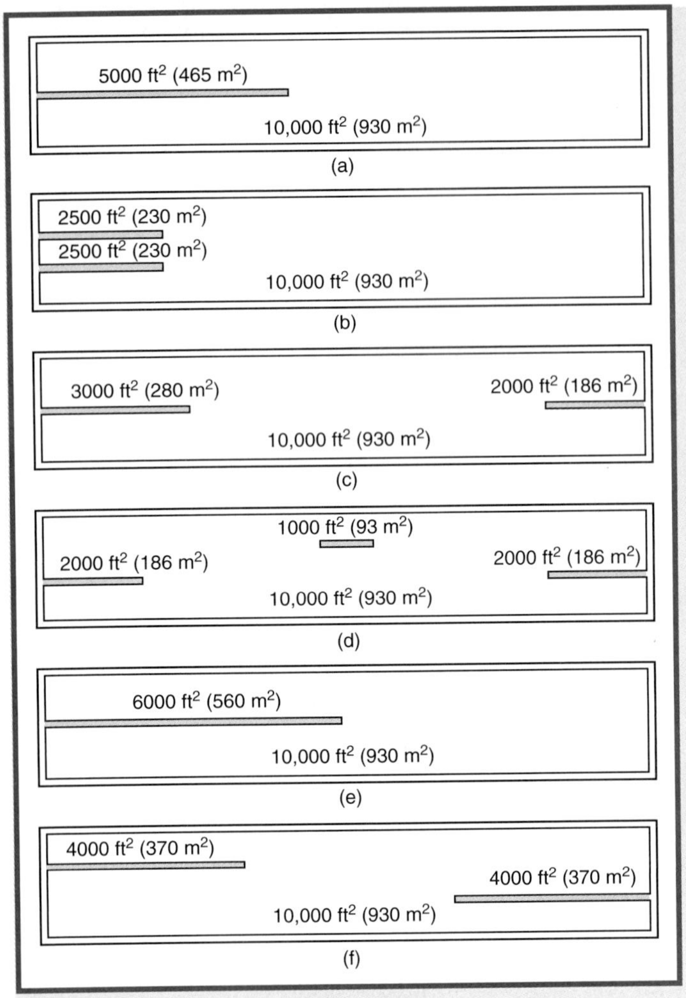


***Exhibit 36/37.4** Elevation views of existing mercantile occupancy mezzanine arrangements.*

mezzanine is located. Similarly, Part (a) through Part (d) of Exhibit 36/37.4 depict an existing single story or single floor level with mezzanine, because the aggregate areas of the mezzanines [5000 ft² (465 m²)] do not exceed one-half of the floor area [10,000 ft² (930 m²)] of the room or story in which the mezzanine is located.

In Part (e) of Exhibit 36/37.3, the new single 4000 ft² (370 m²) intermediate level referred to by occupants as a mezzanine exceeds the one-third area rule. Similarly, in Part (e) of Exhibit 36/37.4, the existing single 6000 ft² (560 m²) intermediate level referred to by occupants as a mezzanine exceeds the one-half area rule. Therefore, in both cases, the intermediate level is not a mezzanine for *Life Safety Code* purposes but is a story by itself. Part (e) of Exhibit 36/37.3 and Part (e) of Exhibit 36/37.4, therefore, depict two-story mercantile occupancies.

In Part (f) of Exhibit 36/37.3, one of the 3000 ft² (280 m²) mezzanines fits within the maximum one-third area allowance for new mezzanines and can be called a mezzanine without constituting a floor level. Similarly, in Part (f) of Exhibit 36/37.4, one of the 4000 ft² (370 m²) mezzanines fits within the maximum one-half area allowance for existing mercantile occupancies and can be called a mezzanine without constituting a floor level. In both cases, however, the other mezzanine, although of the same size and thus, by itself, not in excess of the one-third or one-half area rule, does create a story, because the sum of the areas of the two mezzanines [6000 ft² (560 m²) in Exhibit 36/37.3 and 8000 ft² (740 m²) in Exhibit 36/37.4] exceeds one-third and one-half, respectively, of the 10,000 ft² (930 m²) lower floor level. Thus, Part (f) of Exhibit 36/37.3 and Part (f) of Exhibit 36/37.4 each depict a two-story mercantile occupancy with a mezzanine.

Although the mezzanines in Part (a) through Part (d) of Exhibit 36/37.3 and Part (a) through Part (d) of Exhibit 36/37.4 do not establish separate stories, their areas, because they are used for sales, are included in the total gross sales area used to establish mercantile occupancy subclassification in accordance with 36/37.1.4.2.1. Part (a) through Part (d) of Exhibit 36/37.3 show 13,000 ft² (1200 m²) of sales area and would be classified as Class B mercantile occupancies. Similarly, Part (a) through Part (d) of Exhibit 36/37.4 show 15,000 ft² (1400 m²) of sales area and would be classified as Class B mercantile occupancies.

In addition to the maximum one-third and one-half area limitations of 36/37.1.4.2.3, the provisions of 8.6.9 also apply to mezzanines. For example, a mezzanine used for sales purposes that meets the one-third or one-half area rule would not affect the mercantile occupancy subclassification with respect to number of stories used for sales purposes; however, the mezzanine would be required to be sufficiently open, in accordance with 8.6.9.3, to avoid treatment as a separate floor in terms of number of means of egress (see 36/37.2.4) and the other egress arrangement requirements that apply to floors or stories.

Note that, for existing mercantile occupancies [see 37.1.4.2.4(2)], the fire barrier separation required to waive aggregate gross area is 1 hour, rather than the 2-hour rating required for new mercantile occupancies via the provision of 36.1.4.2.4(2). The same 1-hour rating applies to new construction only if the building is sprinklered [see 36.1.4.2.4(3)].

CHAPTER 36 • New

### 36.1.5 Classification of Hazard of Contents.

**36.1.5.1** The contents of mercantile occupancies shall be classified in accordance with Section 6.2.

**36.1.5.2** Mercantile occupancies classified as high hazard in accordance with Section 6.2 shall meet the following additional requirements:

(1) Exits shall be located so that not more than 75 ft (23 m) of travel from any point is needed to reach the nearest exit.
(2) From every point, there shall be not less than two exits accessible by travel in different directions (no common path of travel).
(3) All vertical openings shall be enclosed.

### 36.1.6 Minimum Construction Requirements.

(No special requirements.)

### 36.1.7 Occupant Load.

The occupant load, in number of persons for whom means of egress and other provisions are required, shall be determined on the basis of the occupant load factors of Table 7.3.1.2 that are characteristic of the use of the space, or shall be determined as the maximum probable population of the space under consideration, whichever is greater.

CHAPTER 37 • Existing

### 37.1.5 Classification of Hazard of Contents.

**37.1.5.1** The contents of mercantile occupancies shall be classified in accordance with Section 6.2.

**37.1.5.2** Mercantile occupancies classified as high hazard in accordance with Section 6.2 shall meet the following additional requirements:

(1) Exits shall be located so that not more than 75 ft (23 m) of travel from any point is needed to reach the nearest exit.
(2) From every point, there shall be not less than two exits accessible by travel in different directions (no common path of travel).
(3) All vertical openings shall be enclosed.

### 37.1.6 Minimum Construction Requirements.

(No special requirements.)

### 37.1.7 Occupant Load.

The occupant load, in number of persons for whom means of egress and other provisions are required, shall be determined on the basis of the occupant load factors of Table 7.3.1.2 that are characteristic of the use of the space, or shall be determined as the maximum probable population of the space under consideration, whichever is greater.

Hazard of contents is addressed in 36/37.1.5, which refers to Section 6.2 for classification. Typically, unless an unusually hazardous situation exists, the contents of mercantile occupancies are classified as ordinary hazard.

Because the total package of life safety provided by the requirements of Chapters 36 and 37 anticipates the display of significant quantities of combustibles, it provides an acceptable level of safety without making it necessary to classify the typical mercantile occupancy environment as highly hazardous. Specifically, the requirements of Chapters 36 and 37 are adequate without imposing the stringent high hazard contents requirements of 36/37.1.5.2 on all but the most hazardous of mercantile occupancies.

Operations that would require classification of a mercantile occupancy as high hazard include dispensing gunpowder or other explosives in bulk or dispensing gasoline or flammable solvents by pouring them into open containers. NFPA 30, *Flammable and Combustible Liquids Code,*[1] regulates the sale of flammable liquids, such as camp stove fuel and rubbing alcohol, with regard to display configuration, total amount, and separation from ignition sources.

Exhibit 36/37.5 illustrates an egress arrangement from a high hazard area of a mercantile occupancy that meets the requirements of 36/37.1.5.2(1) and (2), which address limited travel distance and the exclusion of common path of travel. Doors 1 and 2 lead to remote corridor segments that provide access to independent and remote exits. Travel in two independent directions is possible from any point within the high hazard contents room. Travel distance from any point within the high hazard contents room to the nearest exit does not exceed 75 ft (23 m). Although mercantile occupancy requirements are generally lenient in permitting unprotected vertical openings (see 36/37.3.1), all vertical openings in high hazard mercantile occupancies are required to be fully enclosed (see Section 8.6) in accordance with 36/37.1.5.2(3).

The term *minimum construction,* as used in 36/37.1.6, describes the construction of the building housing the occupancy. Some occupancy chapters, such as Chapters 18 and 19, which address the life safety needs of nonambulatory occupants of health care occupancies, require a minimum building construction type to help ensure structural integrity for a prolonged evacuation or for safe refuge within the

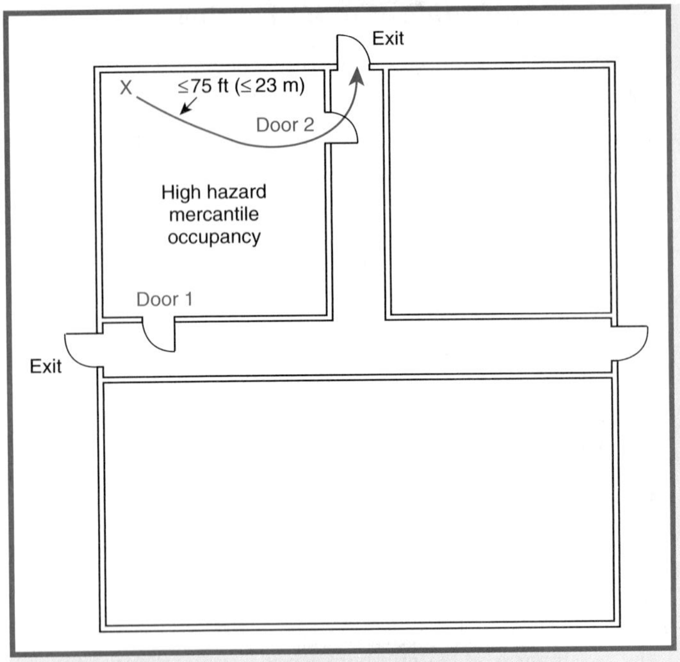


***Exhibit 36/37.5*** *Egress arrangement from area of mercantile occupancy classified as high hazard.*

building. Because mercantile occupancies characteristically are used by ambulatory customers and employees (note that mobility-impaired occupants are not necessarily nonambulatory or incapable of self-preservation) and do not provide sleeping accommodations, no minimum construction requirements are imposed.

The occupant load factors for mercantile uses specified in Table 7.3.1.2 are based on the observation that, during the normal use of a mercantile occupancy, the largest number of customers usually occupies the street floor or a basement sales area. In assigning a higher occupant load to the street floor, the *Code* recognizes merchandising techniques that arrange merchandise to take advantage of the heavy flow of traffic on the street floor. Customers are attracted to merchandise displays as they walk through portions of the street floor to reach escalators, elevators, and stairs to other floors. Thus, larger numbers of occupants are expected to occupy the street floor.

The street floor, as distinguished from other sales floors, is any floor that has an entrance/exit that is directly accessible from the street with not more than three risers of ascent or descent. The term *street floor* is defined in 3.3.253. If differences in the ground level on different sides of a store create several floors of this nature, the *Code* treats them all as street floors; however, a slightly different occupant load factor is used in accordance with footnote b to Table 7.3.1.2. If the only access to a store from the street is by means of stairs or escalators, the principal sales floor, rather than the street level, must be considered the street floor for the purpose of choosing an occupant load factor and calculating the occupant load.

The terms *mall* and *mall building* have different meanings [see commentary following 36/37.1.3(7)]. Therefore, the intent of footnote e to Table 7.3.1.2 is that the egress capacity of the overall mall building is to be sized to handle an occupant load that is calculated in two steps. First, the occupant load is calculated individually for each store and tenant space using the occupant load factors of Table 7.3.1.2. Second, the required egress capacity for the mall itself (the covered pedestrian way) is calculated using the occupant load factors shown in Figure 7.3.1.2(a) and Figure 7.3.1.2(b). Each store or tenant space must have sufficient egress capacity for its occupant load. The egress capacity of the mall must be based on Figure 7.3.1.2(a) and Figure 7.3.1.2(b), which, in effect, automatically accounts for those persons who are in the mall (the covered pedestrian way) and those persons who discharge from stores into the mall as part of the stores' means of egress.

For example, consider a mall building with 21 tenant stores located on the street floor. Each store uses 6000 $ft^2$ (560 $m^2$) of the 7500 $ft^2$ (700 $m^2$) of gross leasable area as sales area [assume that the other 1500 $ft^2$ (140 $m^2$) is storage area]. Using an occupant load factor of 30 $ft^2$ (2.8 $m^2$) per person for the sales areas and 300 $ft^2$ (27.9 $m^2$) for the storage areas, in accordance with Table 7.3.1.2, each store must size its means of egress system to handle 205 persons [6000/30 + 1500/300 (560/2.8 + 140/27.9) = 205]. Store occupants use the mall as part of the required means of egress from each store. With 21 tenant stores, each with 7500 $ft^2$ (700 $m^2$) of gross leasable area, the mall has a gross leasable area of 157,500 $ft^2$ (14,700 $m^2$), which is the basis on which the means of egress from the mall must be sized. Figure 7.3.1.2(a) and Figure 7.3.1.2(b) indicate that, for a gross leasable area of 157,500 $ft^2$ (14,700 $m^2$), the occupant load factor is 36 $ft^2$ (3.34 $m^2$) per person. The mall must, therefore, provide a means of egress system for 157,500 $ft^2$ / 36 $ft^2$ per person (14,700 $m^2$ / 3.34 $m^2$ per person), or 4375 persons (or 4400 persons if using SI units, due to rounding).

## 36.2 Means of Egress Requirements

### 36.2.1 General.

**36.2.1.1** All means of egress shall be in accordance with Chapter 7 and this chapter.

**36.2.1.2** No inside open stairway or inside open ramp shall be permitted to serve as a component of the required means of egress system for more than one floor.

**36.2.1.3** Where there are two or more floors below the street floor, the same stairway or other exit shall be permitted to serve all floors, but all required exits from such areas shall be independent of any open stairways between the street floor and the floor below it.

**36.2.1.4** Where exits from the upper floor also serve as an entrance from a principal street, the upper floor shall be classified as a street floor in accordance with the definition of street floor in 3.3.253 and shall be subject to the requirements of this chapter for street floors.

**36.2.1.5** High hazard mercantile occupancies shall be arranged in accordance with 36.1.5.2.

## 37.2 Means of Egress Requirements

### 37.2.1 General.

**37.2.1.1** All means of egress shall be in accordance with Chapter 7 and this chapter.

**37.2.1.2** No inside open stairway, inside open escalator, or inside open ramp shall be permitted to serve as a component of the required means of egress system for more than one floor.

**37.2.1.3** Where there are two or more floors below the street floor, the same stairway or other exit shall be permitted to serve all floors, but all required exits from such areas shall be independent of any open stairways between the street floor and the floor below it.

**37.2.1.4** Where exits from the upper floor also serve as an entrance from a principal street, the upper floor shall be classified as a street floor in accordance with the definition of street floor in 3.3.253 and shall be subject to the requirements of this chapter for street floors.

**37.2.1.5** High hazard mercantile occupancies shall be arranged in accordance with 37.1.5.2.

Even where unenclosed interior stairs or ramps are permitted by 36/37.3.1, the use of such stairs or ramps as exit access for more than one floor is prohibited by 36/37.2.1.2.

Street floors are addressed by 36/37.2.1.4. Exhibit 36/37.6 illustrates a case where two floors qualify as street floors because each has one side located at a ground level. Note, however, that each street floor has its other sides located either above or below the building's other ground level. As a result, these floors must have their exits arranged to allow horizontal travel to the exterior at one end of the floor and vertical travel (either up or down to ground level) at the other end of the floor. The egress capacity of the doors to the exterior on floor 1 must accommodate that portion of the occupant load from an upper floor that is expected to travel down to and through the exits to the exterior from floor 1. This egress capacity is in addition to the assigned portion of the floor 1 occupant load. The reverse is true for floor 2, which must increase the size of its exterior exit door capacity to accommodate occupants traveling up from floor 1, as well as those traveling down to and through the exterior exits on floor 2. The provisions of 7.3.1.5, 7.3.1.6, and 36/37.2.3.2 explain how to add egress capacity based on the number of occupants expected to discharge from floors above and below the street floor. Exhibit 36/37.10, which accompanies the commentary that follows 36/37.2.3.2, provides an example of how to calculate exit capacity for a street floor similar to that illustrated by floor 2 in Exhibit 36/37.6.

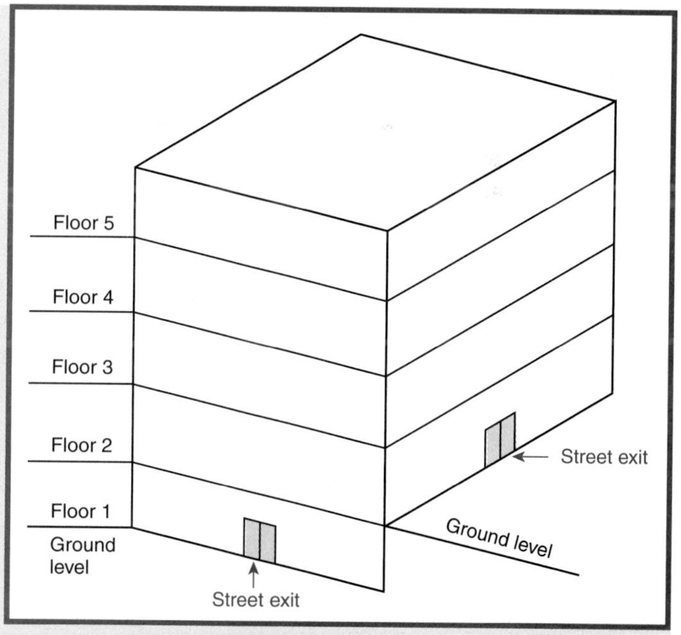


***Exhibit 36/37.6** Mercantile occupancy with two street floors.*

CHAPTER 36 • New

## 36.2.2 Means of Egress Components.

**36.2.2.1 Components Permitted.** Components of means of egress shall be limited to the types described in 36.2.2.2 through 36.2.2.12.

**36.2.2.2 Doors.**

**36.2.2.2.1** Doors complying with 7.2.1 shall be permitted.

**36.2.2.2.2*** Locks complying with 7.2.1.5.4 shall be permitted only on principal entrance/exit doors.

**A.36.2.2.2.2** The words "principal entrance/exit doors" describe doors that the authority having jurisdiction can reasonably expect to be unlocked in order for the facility to do business.

**36.2.2.2.3** Elevator lobby exit access door-locking arrangements in accordance with 7.2.1.6.3 shall be permitted.

**36.2.2.2.4 Reserved.**

**36.2.2.2.5** Delayed-egress locks complying with 7.2.1.6.1 shall be permitted.

**36.2.2.2.6** Access-controlled egress doors complying with 7.2.1.6.2 shall be permitted in buildings protected throughout by an approved, supervised fire detection system in accordance with Section 9.6 or an approved automatic sprinkler system in accordance with 9.7.1.1(1).

**36.2.2.2.7** Horizontal or vertical security grilles or doors complying with 7.2.1.4.1(3) shall be permitted to be used as a part of the required means of egress from a tenant space.

**36.2.2.2.8** All doors at the foot of stairs from upper floors or at the head of stairs leading to floors below the street floor shall swing in the direction of egress travel.

**36.2.2.2.9** Revolving doors complying with 7.2.1.10 shall be permitted.

**36.2.2.3 Stairs.**

**36.2.2.3.1** Stairs complying with 7.2.2 shall be permitted.

**36.2.2.3.2** Spiral stairs complying with 7.2.2.2.3 shall be permitted.

**36.2.2.4 Smokeproof Enclosures.** Smokeproof enclosures complying with 7.2.3 shall be permitted.

CHAPTER 37 • Existing

## 37.2.2 Means of Egress Components.

**37.2.2.1 Components Permitted.** Components of means of egress shall be limited to the types described in 37.2.2.2 through 37.2.2.12.

**37.2.2.2 Doors.**

**37.2.2.2.1** Doors complying with 7.2.1 shall be permitted.

**37.2.2.2.2*** Locks complying with 7.2.1.5.4 shall be permitted only on principal entrance/exit doors.

**A.37.2.2.2.2** The words "principal entrance/exit doors" describe doors that the authority having jurisdiction can reasonably expect to be unlocked in order for the facility to do business.

**37.2.2.2.3** Elevator lobby exit access door-locking arrangements in accordance with 7.2.1.6.3 shall be permitted.

**37.2.2.2.4** The re-entry provisions of 7.2.1.5.7 shall not apply. *[See 7.2.1.5.7.2(1).]*

**37.2.2.2.5** Delayed-egress locks complying with 7.2.1.6.1 shall be permitted.

**37.2.2.2.6** Access-controlled egress doors complying with 7.2.1.6.2 shall be permitted in buildings protected throughout by an approved, supervised fire detection system in accordance with Section 9.6 or an approved automatic sprinkler system in accordance with 9.7.1.1(1).

**37.2.2.2.7** Horizontal or vertical security grilles or doors complying with 7.2.1.4.1(3) shall be permitted to be used as part of the required means of egress from a tenant space.

**37.2.2.2.8** All doors at the foot of stairs from upper floors or at the head of stairs leading to floors below the street floor shall swing in the direction of egress travel.

**37.2.2.2.9** Revolving doors complying with 7.2.1.10 shall be permitted.

**37.2.2.2.10** In Class C mercantile occupancies, doors shall be permitted to swing inward against the direction of egress travel where such doors serve only the street floor area.

**37.2.2.3 Stairs.**

**37.2.2.3.1** Stairs complying with 7.2.2 shall be permitted.

**37.2.2.3.2** Spiral stairs complying with 7.2.2.2.3 shall be permitted.

**37.2.2.3.3** Winders complying with 7.2.2.2.4 shall be permitted.

**37.2.2.4 Smokeproof Enclosures.** Smokeproof enclosures complying with 7.2.3 shall be permitted.

CHAPTER 36 • New

**36.2.2.5 Horizontal Exits.** Horizontal exits complying with 7.2.4 shall be permitted.

**36.2.2.6 Ramps.** Ramps complying with 7.2.5 shall be permitted.

**36.2.2.7 Exit Passageways.**

**36.2.2.7.1** Exit passageways complying with 7.2.6 shall be permitted.

**36.2.2.7.2*** Exit passageways in a mall building shall be permitted to accommodate the following occupant loads independently:

(1) Portion of the occupant load assigned to the exit passageway from only the mall/pedestrian way
(2) Largest occupant load assigned to the exit passageway from a single tenant space

**A.36.2.2.7.2** Egress from a mall building should be designed as follows:

(1) The mall/pedestrian way has been assigned no occupant load, but it is required to be provided with means of egress sized to accommodate the total occupant load of the mall building based on the gross leasable area.
(2) The exits for the mall/pedestrian way are permitted to be provided by a combination of exterior exit doors and exit passageways.
(3) After completion of A.36.2.2.7.2(1), each tenant space is to be judged individually for occupant load and egress capacity, and the following also apply:
    (a) The step specified in A.36.2.2.7.2(3) normally sends a portion or all (per 36.4.4.3.4) of the tenant space's occupant load into the mall.
    (b) Any remaining occupants are sent through the back of the tenant space into an exit passageway that might serve multiple tenant spaces and the mall.
(4) The width of the exit passageway is required to be sized for the most restrictive of the following:
    (a) Width of not less than 66 in. (1675 mm) per 36.4.4.2.2(3)
    (b) Portion of the egress capacity from the largest single tenant space being served by the exit passageway
    (c) Portion of the egress capacity from the mall being provided by the exit passageway

The concepts used in A.36.2.2.7.2(4)(a) through (c) include the following:

(1) After proper egress capacity is provided for the mall/pedestrian way, each tenant space is then required to independently provide egress capacity for its occupants.

CHAPTER 37 • Existing

**37.2.2.5 Horizontal Exits.** Horizontal exits complying with 7.2.4 shall be permitted.

**37.2.2.6 Ramps.** Ramps complying with 7.2.5 shall be permitted.

**37.2.2.7 Exit Passageways.**

**37.2.2.7.1** Exit passageways complying with 7.2.6 shall be permitted.

**37.2.2.7.2*** Exit passageways in a mall building shall be permitted to accommodate the following occupant loads independently:

(1) Portion of the occupant load assigned to the exit passageway from only the mall/pedestrian way
(2) Largest occupant load assigned to the exit passageway from a single tenant space

**A.37.2.2.7.2** Egress from a mall building should be designed as follows:

(1) The mall/pedestrian way has been assigned no occupant load, but it is required to be provided with means of egress sized to accommodate the total occupant load of the mall building based on the gross leasable area.
(2) The exits for the mall/pedestrian way are permitted to be provided by a combination of exterior exit doors and exit passageways.
(3) After completion of A.37.2.2.7.2(1), each tenant space is to be judged individually for occupant load and egress capacity, and the following also apply:
    (a) The step specified in A.37.2.2.7.2(3) normally sends a portion or all (per 37.4.4.3.4) of the tenant space's occupant load into the mall.
    (b) Any remaining occupants are sent through the back of the tenant space into an exit passageway that might serve multiple tenant spaces and the mall.
(4) The width of the exit passageway is required to be sized for the most restrictive of the following:
    (a) Width of not less than 66 in. (1675 mm) per 37.4.4.2.2(3)
    (b) Portion of the egress capacity from the largest single tenant space being served by the exit passageway
    (c) Portion of the egress capacity from the mall being provided by the exit passageway

The concepts used in A.37.2.2.7.2(4)(a) through (c) include the following:

(1) After proper egress capacity is provided for the mall/pedestrian way, each tenant space is then required to independently provide egress capacity for its occupants.

CHAPTER 36 • New

(2) The mall required exit passageway width and the tenant space required exit passageway width are not required to be added together.
(3) The required exit passageway width for a tenant space is not required to be added to that of other tenant spaces using the same exit passageway.

**36.2.2.8 Reserved.**

**36.2.2.9 Reserved.**

**36.2.2.10 Fire Escape Ladders.** Fire escape ladders complying with 7.2.9 shall be permitted.

**36.2.2.11 Alternating Tread Devices.** Alternating tread devices complying with 7.2.11 shall be permitted.

**36.2.2.12 Areas of Refuge.**

**36.2.2.12.1** Areas of refuge complying with 7.2.12 shall be permitted.

**36.2.2.12.2** In buildings protected throughout by an approved, supervised automatic sprinkler system in accordance with 9.7.1.1(1), two rooms or spaces separated from each other by smoke-resistant partitions in accordance with the definition of area of refuge in 3.3.20 shall not be required.

CHAPTER 37 • Existing

(2) The mall required exit passageway width and the tenant space required exit passageway width are not required to be added together.
(3) The required exit passageway width for a tenant space is not required to be added to that of other tenant spaces using the same exit passageway.

**37.2.2.8 Escalators and Moving Walks.** Escalators and moving walks complying with 7.2.7 shall be permitted.

**37.2.2.9 Fire Escape Stairs.** Fire escape stairs complying with 7.2.8 shall be permitted.

**37.2.2.10 Fire Escape Ladders.** Fire escape ladders complying with 7.2.9 shall be permitted.

**37.2.2.11 Alternating Tread Devices.** Alternating tread devices complying with 7.2.11 shall be permitted.

**37.2.2.12 Areas of Refuge.**

**37.2.2.12.1** Areas of refuge complying with 7.2.12 shall be permitted.

**37.2.2.12.2** In buildings protected throughout by an approved, supervised automatic sprinkler system in accordance with 9.7.1.1(1), two rooms or spaces separated from each other by smoke-resistant partitions in accordance with the definition of area of refuge in 3.3.20 shall not be required.

Only the principal entrance/exit doors of a mercantile occupancy are permitted to be equipped with the special key-operated dead bolt lock described by 7.2.1.5.4, per 36/37.2.2.2.2. See Exhibit 36/37.7. It must be easy to determine that the device is locked by using means such as a flag indicator that can be seen at a distance from the door. Other doors along the perimeter of the building are prohibited from being equipped with a key-operated dead bolt lock, because the probability is low that these doors will be consistently unlocked when the principal entrance/exit door is unlocked each day when the occupancy opens to the public for business. Locked egress doors have contributed to many fire deaths; the criteria in 7.2.1.5.4 and 36/37.2.2.2.2 provide for building security but ensure that occupants will be able to open required egress doors and leave the building in the event of a fire.

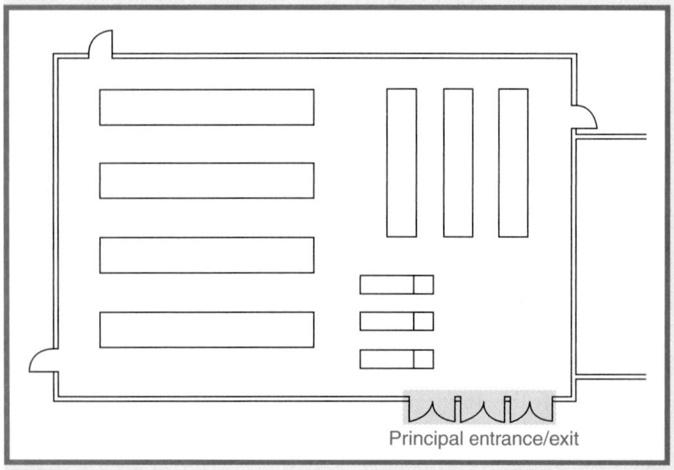


***Exhibit 36/37.7** Principal entrance/exit.*

Although Chapter 36 does not address stairwell re-entry, the re-entry provisions of 7.2.1.5.7 apply to new mercantile occupancies. Stairs connecting five or more stories must provide either re-entry from the stairwell back onto all floors at any time or similar re-entry following automatic release of locking devices initiated by the building fire alarm system per 7.2.1.5.7(2). Some stairwell doors are permitted by 7.2.1.5.7.1 to remain locked from the stairwell side of the door to provide building security, while other doors must allow re-entry. The location and number of re-entry points provide the same overall level of life safety for this type of occupancy as that intended by the base provisions of 7.2.1.5.7. Paragraph 37.2.2.2.4 exempts existing mercantile occupancies from the stairwell re-entry provisions.

In recognition of the security needs of a mercantile occupancy, 36/37.2.2.2.5 permits the use of the delayed-egress locking device covered by 7.2.1.6.1 on any door, provided that the building is protected throughout by an approved, supervised automatic sprinkler system or an approved, supervised automatic fire detection system. In effect, the allowable 15-second or 30-second delay will be experienced only under non-fire conditions or very early in a fire's growth, because the door must be usable immediately upon sprinkler operation, smoke or heat detection, or loss of power that controls the locking mechanism.

In mercantile occupancies with either complete sprinkler or fire detection systems, 36/37.2.2.2.6 recognizes access-controlled egress doors as security measures that do not compromise the use of the means of egress system.

Although 7.2.1.4.1(3) establishes provisions for the arrangement and use of security grilles or doors, it requires that an occupancy chapter specifically permit the use of such measures. For mercantile occupancies, 36/37.2.2.2.7 provides that recognition.

The provision of 36/37.2.2.2.8 supplements the door provisions of 7.2.1.4 by requiring doors that otherwise would not have to swing in the direction of egress travel to do so, based on their location. The queuing and accumulation of people at doors in locations such as at the foot of stairs from upper floors makes it difficult for occupants to step back to allow the door to swing inward.

Revolving doors are addressed by 36/37.2.2.2.9. The provisions of 7.2.1.10 specify that the use of a revolving door, regardless of whether it is permitted as part of the required means of egress, requires a conforming side-hinged swinging door to be positioned and usable within the same wall as, and to be located within 10 ft (3050 mm) of, the revolving door. This requirement helps to ensure that, once people move toward the door, if the collapsibility and other safety features of the door fail and render it unusable, egress from the vicinity would still be possible without retracing steps and traveling toward the fire. Existing revolving doors are permitted to continue to be used without having to meet some of the more stringent requirements that apply to new revolving doors. See the provisions of 7.2.1.10.1.

Paragraph 36/37.2.2.4 does not mandate the use of smokeproof enclosures in a mercantile occupancy, but it does recognize a smokeproof enclosure as part of the means of egress system, provided that the smokeproof enclosure meets the requirements of 7.2.3. For an example of an occupancy requiring a smokeproof enclosure, see 31.2.11.1, in which existing nonsprinklered or partially sprinklered high-rise apartment buildings are required to be provided with smokeproof enclosures in accordance with 7.2.3.

Exit passageways are addressed in 36/37.2.2.7. Exit passageways are frequently used within the means of egress system of mall buildings as a way of meeting the travel distance limitations or avoiding numerous exit doors along exterior walls located at the rear of tenant spaces. In effect, the exit passageway labeled A in Exhibit 36/37.8 moves the exit closer to the occupants to create a building arrangement that would otherwise require occupants to travel farther than allowable to reach an exit door in an exterior wall. The exit passageway labeled B in Exhibit 36/37.8 runs along the rear of multiple-tenant spaces and provides access to the exterior only at each end of the exit passageway for security reasons. In both cases, the exit passageway is a *Code*-complying exit in accordance with 7.2.6 and provides the same degree of safety that an exit stair enclosure would provide an occupant of an upper floor in a multistory building. Because an exit passageway might not be readily recognized as an exit, it must be maintained clear of storage or anything else that might impede its use as an exit. While signage indicating the prohibition of such storage is not required, it can help improve the probability that exit passageways will be maintained clear and unobstructed.

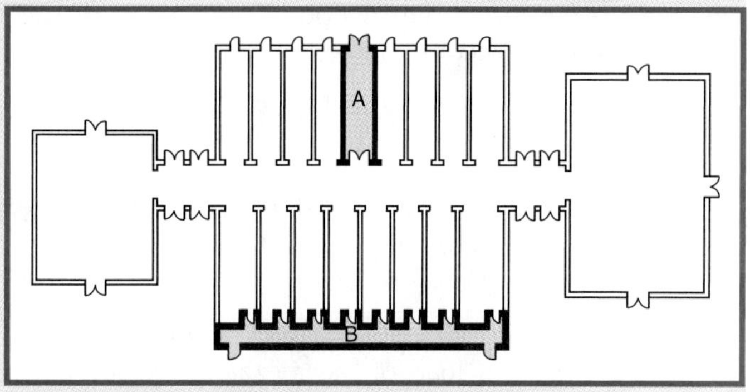


***Exhibit 36/37.8*** *Typical uses of exit passageways in mall buildings.*

Although the provisions of 7.2.6.4 require an exit passageway to be sized to accommodate the aggregate required capacity of all exits discharging through the exit passageway, 36/37.2.2.7.2 permits some reduction in the required width of exit passageways in mall buildings. The provision recognizes that the sizing of the means of egress from the mall — calculated in accordance with the provisions of Figure 7.3.1.2(a) and Figure 7.3.1.2(b) — provides egress capacity for occupants of the mall and occupants of the adjoining tenant spaces within the mall building. Requiring an exit passageway in a mall building to be of sufficient size to accommodate both its assigned mall occupant load and the occupant load of all tenant spaces discharging through the exit passageway would be equivalent to counting a portion of the building's occupants twice and, thereby, needlessly oversizing the means of egress system.

Existing escalators and moving walks are recognized by 37.2.2.8 as part of the means of egress in accordance with 7.2.7. To qualify as exits, existing escalators and moving walks must also meet the requirements of 7.2.2.5 that address enclosure.

Existing fire escape stairs are recognized by 37.2.2.9 as part of the means of egress. Note that 7.2.8.1.2 permits only those occupancy chapters that apply to existing buildings to locate a fire escape stair within the required means of egress. Furthermore, 7.2.8.1.2.1 permits existing buildings to use fire escape stairs for not more than 50 percent of the building's required egress capacity.

In accordance with the provisions of 36/37.2.2.10 and 36/37.2.2.11, both fire escape ladders and alternating tread devices are permitted within the means of egress of mercantile occupancies, but only as permitted by the relatively narrow provisions of 7.2.9 and 7.2.11. The provisions of 7.2.11, in effect, restrict the use of alternating tread devices to locations where the *Code* recognizes the use of fire escape ladders.

### 36.2.3 Capacity of Means of Egress.

**36.2.3.1** The capacity of means of egress shall be in accordance with Section 7.3.

**36.2.3.2** In Class A and Class B mercantile occupancies, street floor exits shall be sufficient for the occupant load of the street floor plus the required capacity of stairs and ramps discharging through the street floor.



### 37.2.3 Capacity of Means of Egress.

**37.2.3.1** The capacity of means of egress shall be in accordance with Section 7.3.

**37.2.3.2** In Class A and Class B mercantile occupancies, street floor exits shall be sufficient for the occupant load of the street floor plus the required capacity of stairs, ramps, escalators, and moving walks discharging through the street floor.

The provisions of 7.3.1.6 mandate that any required egress capacity from a mezzanine that passes through the room below must be added to the required egress capacity of the room through which the egress passes.

Exhibit 36/37.9 illustrates a case in which a mezzanine is open to the street floor. The exits from the street floor must accommodate the following:

1. Occupant load of the street floor
2. Occupant load of the mezzanine in accordance with 7.3.1.6
3. Required capacity provided by the stairs from other floors discharging through the street floor in accordance with 36/37.2.3.2

To determine the egress capacity for the street floor, the occupant load of the mezzanine (1000 persons) is added to the occupant load of the street floor (2000 persons). In addition, because one-half of the

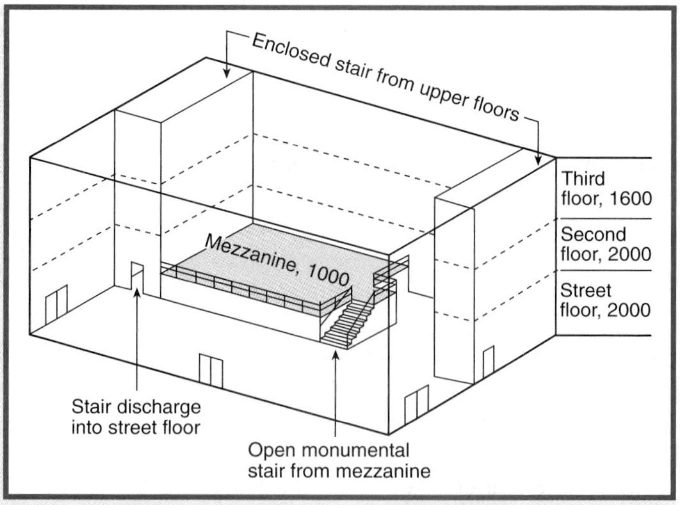


***Exhibit 36/37.9*** *Mercantile occupancy with mezzanine open to the street floor.*

exits from the upper floors discharge through the street floor, the egress capacity of the street floor must accommodate the capacity of the exit stair enclosure that discharges through that floor. The maximum occupant load on any upper floor is 2000 (second floor), and 36/37.2.7.2 permits a maximum of one-half of the exits (and one-half of the egress capacity in new mercantile occupancies) to discharge through the street floor, provided that the building is sprinklered. Therefore, the street floor must be provided with egress capacity for 4000 persons (2000 for street floor + 1000 for mezzanine + 1000 for upper floors = 4000) or 800 in. [66 ft 8 in. (20 m)] of exit width using the factor of 0.2 in. (5 mm) per person for level egress components found in Table 7.3.3.1.

The provisions of 36/37.2.3.2 require that the exits for the street floor of a Class A or Class B mercantile occupancy have sufficient capacity to handle the occupant load of the street floor and the capacity of the exits discharging through the street floor, such as an enclosed exit stair that accommodates occupants who, when exiting the building during an emergency, must travel up from the basement sales area or down from the upper sales floors and mix with the customers already occupying the street floor.

Because people move more quickly in the horizontal direction than in the vertical direction, it is permissible to provide less door width than stair width for a given number of occupants within any given egress path. For example, in mercantile occupancies, in accordance with the egress capacity factors of Table 7.3.3.1, level components and ramps require only 0.2 in. (5 mm) of width per person, whereas stairs require 0.3 in. (7.6 mm) of width per person. As a rough approximation, for every 44 in. (1120 mm) of stair discharging through the street floor, an additional 30 in. (760 mm) of door width opening to the outside must be added to the street floor. Exhibit 36/37.10 illustrates an example of the calculation method for determining the required exit capacity for the street floor, which follows.

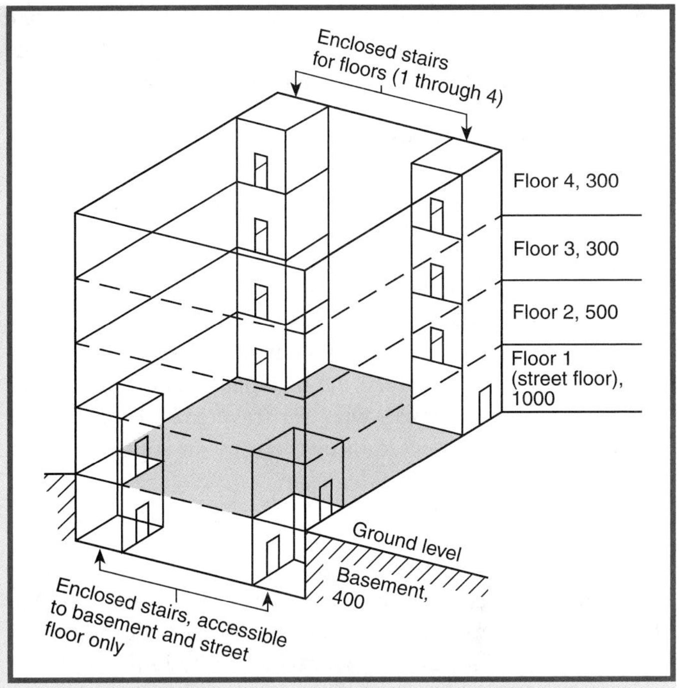


***Exhibit 36/37.10*** *Calculation of exit capacity required for a street floor in accordance with 36/37.2.3.2.*

| | |
|---|---|
| Street floor occupant load alone | 1000 |
| Maximum upper floor occupant load discharging back through street floor (500/2) | + 250 |
| Basement occupant load discharging back through street floor (400/2) | + 200 |
| Total occupant load | 1450 |

1450 persons × 0.2 in. (5 mm) per person for level exit components per Table 7.3.3.1 = 290 in., or 24 ft 2 in. (7250 mm) of exit width required from the street floor egress system

### 36.2.4 Number of Exits.

**36.2.4.1** Exits shall comply with the following, except as otherwise permitted by 36.2.4.2 through 36.2.4.5:

(1) The number of means of egress shall be in accordance with Section 7.4.
(2) Not less than two separate exits shall be provided on every story.
(3) Not less than two separate exits shall be accessible from every part of every story.

### 37.2.4 Number of Exits.

**37.2.4.1** Exits shall comply with the following, except as otherwise permitted by 37.2.4.2 through 37.2.4.5:

(1) The number of means of egress shall be in accordance with Section 7.4.
(2) Not less than two separate exits shall be provided on every story.
(3) Not less than two separate exits shall be accessible from every part of every story.

**CHAPTER 36 • New**

**36.2.4.2** Exit access, as required by 36.2.4.1(3), shall be permitted to include a single exit access path for the distances permitted as common paths of travel by 36.2.5.3.

**36.2.4.3** A single means of egress shall be permitted in a Class C mercantile occupancy, provided that the travel distance to the exit or to a mall pedestrian way (*see 36.4.4.2*) does not exceed 75 ft (23 m).

**36.2.4.4** A single means of egress shall be permitted in a Class C mercantile occupancy, provided that the travel distance to the exit or to a mall does not exceed 100 ft (30 m), and the story on which the occupancy is located, and all communicating levels that are traversed to reach the exit or mall, are protected throughout by an approved, supervised automatic sprinkler system in accordance with 9.7.1.1(1).

**36.2.4.5** A single means of egress to an exit or to a mall shall be permitted from a mezzanine within any Class A, Class B, or Class C mercantile occupancy, provided that the common path of travel does not exceed 75 ft (23 m), or does not exceed 100 ft (30 m) if protected throughout by an approved, supervised automatic sprinkler system in accordance with 9.7.1.1(1).

**CHAPTER 37 • Existing**

**37.2.4.2** Exit access as required by 37.2.4.1(3) shall be permitted to include a single exit access path for the distances permitted as common paths of travel by 37.2.5.3.

**37.2.4.3** A single means of egress shall be permitted in a Class C mercantile occupancy, provided that the travel distance to the exit or to a mall pedestrian way (*see 37.4.4.2*) does not exceed 75 ft (23 m).

**37.2.4.4** A single means of egress shall be permitted in a Class C mercantile occupancy, provided that the travel distance to the exit or to a mall does not exceed 100 ft (30 m), and the story on which the occupancy is located, and all communicating levels that are traversed to reach the exit or mall, are protected throughout by an approved, supervised automatic sprinkler system in accordance with 9.7.1.1(1).

**37.2.4.5** A single means of egress to an exit or to a mall shall be permitted from a mezzanine within any Class A, Class B, or Class C mercantile occupancy, provided that the common path of travel does not exceed 75 ft (23 m), or does not exceed 100 ft (30 m) if protected throughout by an approved, supervised automatic sprinkler system in accordance with 9.7.1.1(1).

The provisions of 36/37.2.4, which apply to the required number of exits for mercantile occupancies, clarify that any level that constitutes a story must have at least two exits located on that story. This means that the occupants of the story must be able to enter two exits (such as an enclosed exit stair on an upper floor of a multistory building) without having to travel to another story to reach the entrances to the exits. Because a mezzanine that meets the maximum one-third or one-half area rule of 36/37.1.4.2.3 does not constitute a story [see the commentary following 36.1.4.2.4(4) and 37.1.4.2.4(3)], two exits are not required on the mezzanine, but the criteria of 36/37.2.4.1(3) must be met with respect to providing access to two separate exits, or the single means of egress provisions of 36/37.2.4.3, 36/37.2.4.4, or 36/37.2.4.5 must be met.

The provision of 36/37.2.5.3 allows the occupant to travel in one direction for a maximum distance (the common path allowance) before requiring exit access in two separate directions. Therefore, although the story or mezzanine must eventually provide access to two exits in accordance with 36/37.2.4.1(3), the access is required to be available only at the point where the allowable common path is expended. (See 36/37.2.5.3 for permitted common path of travel distances.)

Although the basic requirement of 36/37.2.4 mandates that a mercantile occupancy is to be provided with at least two remotely located exits, 36/37.2.4.3 permits a single means of egress for Class C mercantile occupancies, such as small convenience stores. If the travel distance from any point in such a store to an exit is 75 ft (23 m) or less, the likelihood that a fire might surprise and overcome the customers before they could escape is low (see Exhibit 36/37.11). The provision of 36/37.2.4.4 permits a single exit in small, sprinklered mercantile occupancies if travel to an exit is not more than 100 ft (30 m). Furthermore, a single exit is permitted in Class C occupancies where travel distance to a mall that qualifies as a pedestrian way in accordance with 36/37.4.4.2 does not exceed 100 ft (30 m). The provisions of 36/37.4.4.2 include an automatic sprinkler system requirement for the entire mall building. Additional flexibility and a potential increase in security is provided by 36/37.2.4.4 for those small stores protected by means of automatic sprinkler installations within the store and for those portions of the overall building that occupants must traverse to reach an exit or pedestrian way.

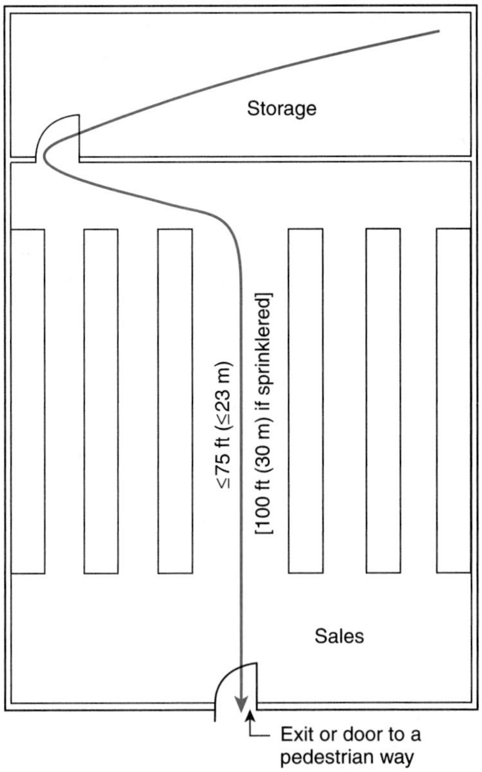


***Exhibit 36/37.11*** *Single exit permitted in a Class C mercantile occupancy if travel distance is limited.*

### 36.2.5 Arrangement of Means of Egress.

**36.2.5.1** Means of egress shall be arranged in accordance with Section 7.5.

**36.2.5.2** Dead-end corridors shall comply with 36.2.5.2.1 or 36.2.5.2.2.

**36.2.5.2.1** In buildings protected throughout by an approved, supervised automatic sprinkler system in accordance with 9.7.1.1(1), dead-end corridors shall not exceed 50 ft (15 m).

**36.2.5.2.2** In all buildings not complying with 36.2.5.2.1, dead-end corridors shall not exceed 20 ft (6100 mm).

**36.2.5.3** Common paths of travel shall be limited as follows:

(1) Common paths of travel shall not exceed 75 ft (23 m) in mercantile occupancies classified as low or ordinary hazard.



### 37.2.5 Arrangement of Means of Egress.

**37.2.5.1** Means of egress shall be arranged in accordance with Section 7.5.

**37.2.5.2*** Dead-end corridors shall not exceed 50 ft (15 m).

**A.37.2.5.2** The purpose of 37.2.5.2 is to avoid pockets or dead ends of such size that they pose an undue danger of persons becoming trapped in case of fire.

It is recognized that dead ends exceeding the permitted limits exist and, in some cases, are impractical to eliminate. The authority having jurisdiction might permit such dead ends to continue to exist, taking into consideration any or all of the following:

(1) Tenant arrangement
(2) Automatic sprinkler protection
(3) Smoke detection
(4) Exit remoteness

**37.2.5.3*** Common paths of travel shall be limited in accordance with 37.2.5.3.1 or 37.2.5.3.2.

**A.37.2.5.3** It is recognized that common paths of travel exceeding the permitted limits exist and, in some cases, are

CHAPTER 36 • New

(2) Common paths of travel shall not exceed 100 ft (30 m) in mercantile occupancies classified as low or ordinary hazard where the building is protected throughout by an approved, supervised automatic sprinkler system in accordance with 9.7.1.1(1).
(3) Common paths of travel shall not be permitted in mercantile occupancies classified as high hazard.

**36.2.5.4** Aisles leading to each exit shall be required, and the aggregate width of such aisles shall be not less than the required width of the exit.

**36.2.5.5** Required aisles shall be not less than 36 in. (915 mm) in clear width.

**36.2.5.6** In Class A mercantile occupancies, not less than one aisle of a 60 in. (1525 mm) minimum width shall lead directly to an exit.

**36.2.5.7** In mercantile occupancies other than bulk merchandising retail buildings, if the only means of customer entrance is through one exterior wall of the building, one-half of the required egress width from the street floor shall be located in such wall. Means of egress from floors above or below the street floor shall be arranged in accordance with Section 7.5.

**36.2.5.8** Not less than one-half of the required exits shall be located so as to be reached without passing through checkout stands.

**36.2.5.9** Checkout stands or associated railings or barriers shall not obstruct exits, required aisles, or approaches thereto.

**36.2.5.10*** Where wheeled carts or buggies are used by customers, adequate provision shall be made for the transit and parking of such carts to minimize the possibility that they might obstruct means of egress.

**A.36.2.5.10** To eliminate the obstruction to the means of egress of the interior exit access and the exterior exit discharge, it is the intent to provide adequate area for transit and parking of wheeled carts or buggies used by customers. This area includes corral areas adjacent to exits that are constructed to restrict the movement of wheeled carts or buggies therefrom.

CHAPTER 37 • Existing

impractical to eliminate. The authority having jurisdiction might permit such paths of travel to continue to exist, taking into consideration any or all of the following:

(1) Tenant arrangement
(2) Automatic sprinkler protection
(3) Smoke detection
(4) Exit remoteness

**37.2.5.3.1** In buildings protected throughout by an approved, supervised automatic sprinkler system in accordance with 9.7.1.1(1), common paths of travel shall not exceed 100 ft (30 m).

**37.2.5.3.2** In buildings not complying with 37.2.5.3.1, common paths of travel shall not exceed 75 ft (23 m).

**37.2.5.4** Aisles leading to each exit shall be required, and the aggregate width of such aisles shall be not less than the required width of the exit.

**37.2.5.5** Required aisles shall be not less than 28 in. (710 mm) in clear width.

**37.2.5.6** In Class A mercantile occupancies, not less than one aisle of a 60 in. (1525 mm) minimum width shall lead directly to an exit.

**37.2.5.7** In mercantile occupancies other than bulk merchandising retail buildings, if the only means of customer entrance is through one exterior wall of the building, one-half of the required egress width from the street floor shall be located in such wall. Means of egress from floors above or below the street floor shall be arranged in accordance with Section 7.5.

**37.2.5.8** Not less than one-half of the required exits shall be located so as to be reached without passing through checkout stands.

**37.2.5.9** Checkout stands or associated railings or barriers shall not obstruct exits, required aisles, or approaches thereto.

**37.2.5.10*** Where wheeled carts or buggies are used by customers, adequate provision shall be made for the transit and parking of such carts to minimize the possibility that they might obstruct means of egress.

**A.37.2.5.10** To eliminate the obstruction to the means of egress of the interior exit access and the exterior exit discharge, it is the intent to provide adequate area for transit and parking of wheeled carts or buggies used by customers. This area includes corral areas adjacent to exits that are constructed to restrict the movement of wheeled carts or buggies therefrom.

**CHAPTER 36 • New**

**36.2.5.11** Exit access in Class A and Class B mercantile occupancies that are protected throughout by an approved, supervised automatic sprinkler system in accordance with 9.7.1.1(1), and exit access in all Class C mercantile occupancies, shall be permitted to pass through storerooms, provided that the following conditions are met:

(1) Not more than 50 percent of exit access shall be provided through the storeroom.
(2) The storeroom shall not be subject to locking.
(3) The main aisle through the storeroom shall be not less than 44 in. (1120 mm) wide.
(4) The path of travel through the storeroom shall be defined, direct, and continuously maintained in an unobstructed condition.

**CHAPTER 37 • Existing**

**37.2.5.11** Exit access in Class A mercantile occupancies that are protected throughout by an approved, supervised automatic sprinkler system in accordance with 9.7.1.1(1), and exit access in all Class B and Class C mercantile occupancies, shall be permitted to pass through storerooms, provided that the following conditions are met:

(1) Not more than 50 percent of exit access shall be provided through the storeroom.
(2) The storeroom shall not be subject to locking.
(3) The main aisle through the storeroom shall be not less than 44 in. (1120 mm) wide.
(4) The path of travel through the storeroom shall be defined, direct, and continuously maintained in an unobstructed condition.

The provision of 36.2.5.2.1 recognizes the additional level of safety to life provided by a complete automatic sprinkler system and allows added flexibility when designing the location of corridors and exits in buildings where approved sprinkler systems are installed. The provision allows dead-end corridor pockets in new sprinklered mercantile occupancies to be as long as 50 ft (15 m). Dead-end corridor pockets in existing mercantile occupancies are allowed to be 50 ft (15 m) long without any requirement for sprinklers.

Common path of travel limits are provided in 36/37.2.5.3. See the commentary following A.7.5.1.5 for a detailed discussion on common path of travel. Also see 36/37.2.4.2, which permits the access to a single exit or a portion of the access to multiple exits to be common.

The provisions of 36/37.2.5.4 are intended to prevent constrictions in the means of egress system that would delay the egress of building occupants. The aggregate width of aisles leading to an exit is required to provide egress width equal to that required of the exit to which they lead. Without this provision, occupants could be forced to squeeze through a relatively narrow aisle or similar constriction before reaching, for example, an expansive bank of doors to the outside. The egress capacity at the doors, rather than providing simultaneous egress for the large number of occupants assigned to that exit, would not be fully utilized. Occupants would move through the doors a few at a time as they passed slowly through the constriction. The requirement of 36/37.2.5.4 is illustrated in Exhibit 36/37.12 in the upper left and right corners of the floor plan of the mercantile occupancy.

The minimum 36 in. (915 mm) aisle width required for new mercantile occupancies by 36.2.5.5, and

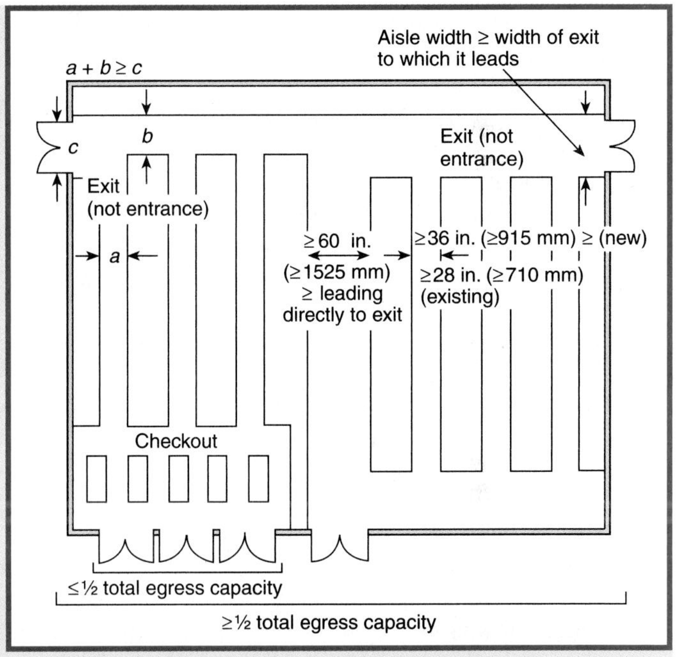


***Exhibit 36/37.12** Means of egress arrangement in a Class A mercantile occupancy.*

the minimum 28 in. (710 mm) aisle width required for existing mercantile occupancies by 37.2.5.5, are illustrated in Exhibit 36/37.12. These minimum widths are consistent with those prescribed by 7.3.4.1(2) and 7.3.4.1.2.

The intent of 36/37.2.5.4 through 36/37.2.5.6 is to ensure that the interior arrangement of counters, racks, and displays of merchandise does not block or obscure access to an exit. The arrangement illustrated in Exhibit 36/37.12 meets the requirements for a Class A store. Essentially, the width of the exit determines the minimum widths of the aisles, with the added proviso that one of the aisles must be at least 60 in. (1525 mm) wide and lead directly to an exit.

In establishing the requirements of 36/37.2.5.7, the *Code* demonstrates its concern regarding the arrangement of many discount and variety stores that have one large main exit/entrance located in the front of the store and the other exits (which cannot be used as entrances) situated at points unfamiliar to the public. In these mercantile occupancy arrangements, the wall containing the main exit/entrance must be sized to handle one-half of the required egress capacity of the store, because the public is familiar with this entrance/exit and most customers will use it as an exit under emergency conditions. This requirement is illustrated in the lower portion of Exhibit 36/37.12. Note that, prior to the 2006 edition, the *Code* required two-thirds of the required egress capacity to be provided via the wall containing the main exit/entrance. This requirement was deemed to be onerous given the overall good life safety record associated with mercantile occupancies and was, thus, revised to the current one-half criteria.

One of the most frequently violated provisions of Chapter 36/37 is contained in 36/37.2.5.8. In many supermarkets and discount and variety stores, it is necessary to pass through checkout counters, around shopping carts, and through turnstiles to exit the facility. This process causes congestion or blockage during an emergency. The *Code* requires at least one-half of all exits to be located so that occupants can avoid passing through or around these impediments to egress. See Exhibit 36/37.12.

The potential encroachment on egress width by shopping carts is addressed by 36/37.2.5.10. In jurisdictions where returnable beverage bottle legislation has been enacted, stores and markets have had to create space for collecting empty bottles and refunding deposit charges. An area commonly used is located near the entrance/exit where wheeled shopping carts were formerly stored to be clear of the path of egress travel. The displaced carts are now sometimes stored so that they obstruct the means of egress. This example illustrates a situation where a properly designed, installed, and complying means of egress might be compromised abruptly by unexpected changes.

The provisions of 36/37.2.5.11 address egress paths through storerooms in the following occupancies:

1. All Class C mercantile occupancies
2. Existing Class B mercantile occupancies
3. New Class B mercantile occupancies protected throughout by an approved, supervised automatic sprinkler system
4. All Class A mercantile occupancies protected throughout by an approved, supervised automatic sprinkler system

The storeroom is limited by 36/37.2.5.11(1) to providing a maximum of 50 percent of the store's exit access in number of exits and exit capacity. Therefore, because two exits are required, neither of the following limits can be exceeded:

1. Only one of the two required exits can be reached by exit access travel through the storeroom.
2. A maximum of one-half of the store's occupant load is permitted to egress through the storeroom.

Exhibit 36/37.13 and Exhibit 36/37.14 illustrate the application of the provisions of 36/37.2.5.11. The exit access path through the storeroom must be defined. Prior to the 2009 edition, the *Code* required fixed barriers, such as guardrails, to define the aisle. It was found, however, that the rails were sometimes used to

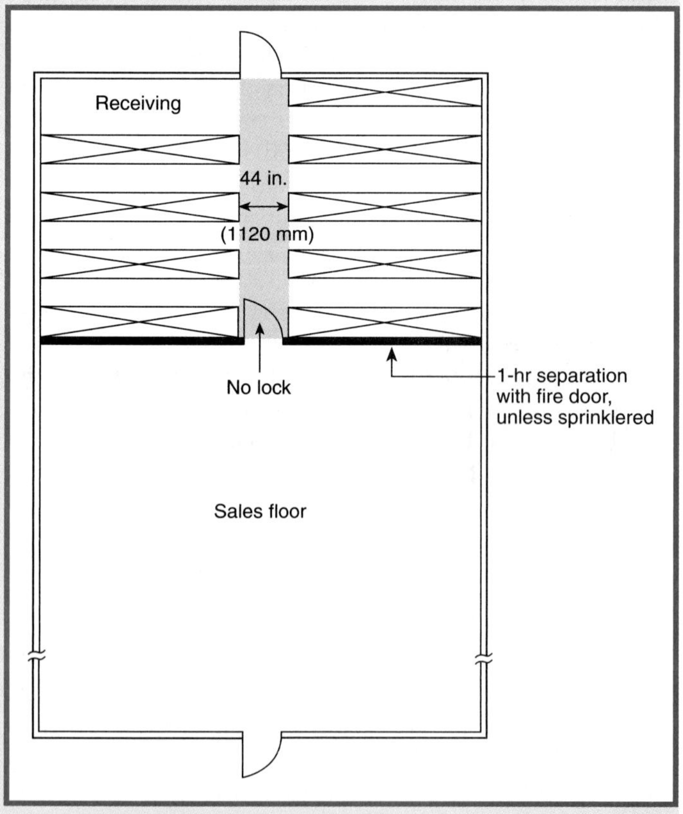


***Exhibit 36/37.13*** *Exit access through a storeroom as permitted by 36/37.2.5.11.*

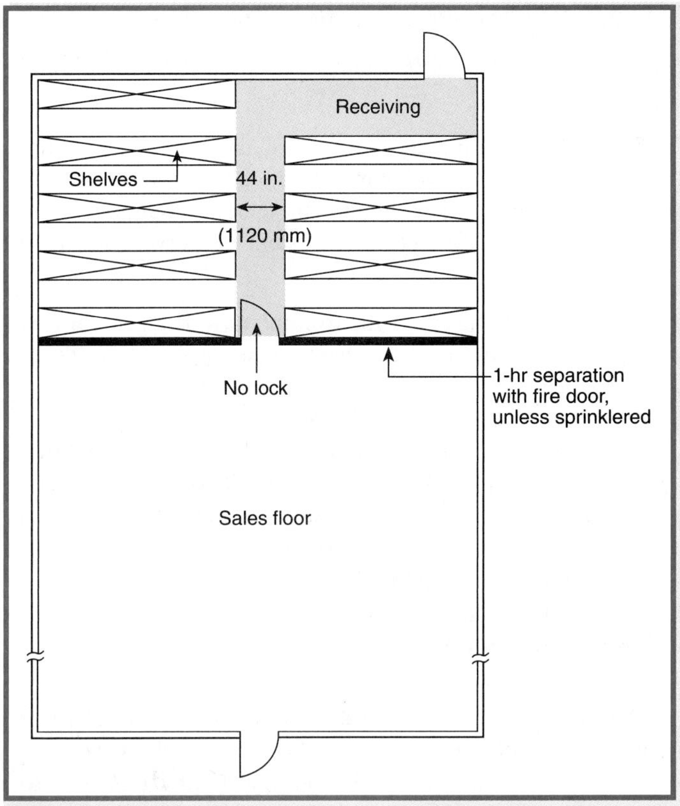


*Exhibit 36/37.14 Exit access through a storeroom that is problematic because it passes through receiving area.*

support merchandise and other storage, thus rendering the aisle useless. Maintenance of the required exit access path depends on the education of store employees. Aisles can be defined by painting stripes on the floor and providing signage; however, if such means prove to be ineffective, the authority having jurisdiction (AHJ) has the authority to require whatever is necessary to maintain the means of egress unobstructed.

### 36.2.6 Travel Distance to Exits.

Travel distance shall be as specified in 36.2.6.1, 36.2.6.2, and 36.2.6.3 and shall be measured in accordance with Section 7.6.

**36.2.6.1** In mercantile occupancies classified as ordinary hazard, travel distance shall not exceed 150 ft (46 m).

**36.2.6.2** In mercantile occupancies classified as ordinary hazard in buildings protected throughout by an approved, supervised automatic sprinkler system in accordance with 9.7.1.1(1), travel distance shall not exceed 250 ft (76 m).

**36.2.6.3** In mercantile occupancies classified as high hazard, travel distance shall not exceed 75 ft (23 m).

### 37.2.6 Travel Distance to Exits.

Travel distance shall be as specified in 37.2.6.1 and 37.2.6.2 and shall be measured in accordance with Section 7.6.

**37.2.6.1** In buildings protected throughout by an approved, supervised automatic sprinkler system in accordance with 9.7.1.1(1), travel distance shall not exceed 250 ft (76 m).

**37.2.6.2** In buildings not complying with 37.2.6.1, the travel distance shall not exceed 150 ft (46 m).

In accordance with Section 7.6, travel distance limitations apply to only the first (or nearest) exit from a given point in the building. In other words, the 150 ft (46 m) travel distance limit for nonsprinklered mercantile occupancies [250 ft (76 m) for sprinklered occupancies] requires that at least one exit must be located within 150 ft (46 m) [250 ft (76 m) if sprinklered] of a point in the building; it does not require that all exits must be within the prescribed travel distance limitations from any point. Note that these travel distance limitations were increased from those found prior to the 2003 edition of the *Code*, recognizing the good life safety history associated with mercantile occupancies.

CHAPTER 36 • New

## 36.2.7 Discharge from Exits.

**36.2.7.1** Exit discharge shall comply with Section 7.7 and 36.2.7.2.

**36.2.7.2*** Fifty percent of the exits shall be permitted to discharge through the level of exit discharge in accordance with 7.7.2 only where the building is protected throughout by an approved, supervised automatic sprinkler system in accordance with 9.7.1.1(1).

**A.36.2.7.2** The basis for the exemption to the general rule on complete enclosure of exits up to their point of discharge to the outside of the building is that, with the specified safeguards, reasonable safety is maintained.

A stairway is not considered to discharge through the street floor area if it leads to the street through a fire resistance–rated enclosure (exit passageway) separating it from the main area, even though there are doors between the first-floor stairway landing and the main area.

The provisions of 36.2.7.2 should not be confused with those for open stairways, as permitted by 36.3.1(1).

CHAPTER 37 • Existing

## 37.2.7 Discharge from Exits.

**37.2.7.1** Exit discharge shall comply with Section 7.7 and 37.2.7.2.

**37.2.7.2*** Fifty percent of the exits shall be permitted to discharge through the level of exit discharge in accordance with 7.7.2 only where the building is protected throughout by an approved automatic sprinkler system in accordance with 9.7.1.1(1).

**A.37.2.7.2** The basis for the exemption to the general rule on complete enclosure of exits up to their point of discharge to the outside of the building is that, with the specified safeguards, reasonable safety is maintained.

A stairway is not considered to discharge through the street floor area if it leads to the street through a fire resistance–rated enclosure (exit passageway) separating it from the main area, even though there are doors between the first floor stairway landing and the main area.

The provisions of 37.2.7.2 should not be confused with those for open stairways, as permitted by 37.3.1(1) and (2).

The restriction imposed by 36/37.2.7.2 is intended to prevent more than 50 percent of the exits from any floor from discharging through the street floor. Furthermore, such exit discharge is permitted only where the building is sprinklered throughout. The remaining 50 percent of the exits must discharge directly to the exterior. The requirements of 36/37.2.7.2 are more stringent than those of 7.7.2, as they mandate automatic sprinkler protection throughout the building in recognition of the potentially high combustible fuel load of merchandise on display characteristic of mercantile occupancies. Previous editions of the *Code* also limited the path of travel from the stair discharge to the exit to 50 ft (15 m); this travel distance limit was deleted for the 2009 edition based on the good life safety record associated with mercantile occupancies and the significant restriction in design flexibility caused by such a limit. The provisions of 7.7.2 adequately address the path of travel to the exit.

CHAPTER 36 • New

## 36.2.8 Illumination of Means of Egress.

Means of egress shall be illuminated in accordance with Section 7.8.

## 36.2.9 Emergency Lighting.

Class A and Class B mercantile occupancies and mall buildings shall have emergency lighting facilities in accordance with Section 7.9.

## 36.2.10 Marking of Means of Egress.

Where an exit is not immediately apparent from all portions of the sales area, means of egress shall have signs in accordance with Section 7.10.

## 36.2.11 Special Means of Egress Features.

**36.2.11.1 Reserved.**

CHAPTER 37 • Existing

## 37.2.8 Illumination of Means of Egress.

Means of egress shall be illuminated in accordance with Section 7.8.

## 37.2.9 Emergency Lighting.

Class A and Class B mercantile occupancies and mall buildings shall have emergency lighting facilities in accordance with Section 7.9.

## 37.2.10 Marking of Means of Egress.

Where an exit is not immediately apparent from all portions of the sales area, means of egress shall have signs in accordance with Section 7.10.

## 37.2.11 Special Means of Egress Features.

**37.2.11.1 Reserved.**

CHAPTER 36 • New

**36.2.11.2 Lockups.** Lockups in mercantile occupancies shall comply with the requirements of 22.4.5.

CHAPTER 37 • Existing

**37.2.11.2 Lockups.** Lockups in mercantile occupancies, other than approved existing lockups, shall comply with the requirements of 23.4.5.

Illumination for the means of egress, addressed in 36/37.2.8, is not the same as emergency lighting. Failure of the building power supply might cause failure of the means of egress illumination system, which is not required to have a backup, auxiliary, or secondary power supply unless mandated by 36/37.2.9, which addresses emergency lighting. Due to their small size and small occupant load, Class C mercantile occupancies are not required by the *Code* to be provided with emergency lighting.

The intent of 36/37.2.10 is to avoid requiring exit signs in small areas where the exit is readily apparent. For example, exit signs should not be required in the office of a service station, the purchase and dining areas of a small fast-food restaurant, or in a Class C store where size and arrangement comply with the single-exit provisions of 36/37.2.4.3 or 36/37.2.4.4.

If a mercantile occupancy is provided with a lockup for detaining suspected shoplifters, it must meet the provisions of 22/23.4.5, as specified in 36/37.2.11.2. The lockup criteria require the application of some of the concepts of detention and correctional occupancies to other occupancies where persons might be detained for security purposes, without classifying the lockup as a detention and correctional occupancy. See 22/23.4.5 and related commentary for details on the lockup provisions.

## 36.3 Protection

### 36.3.1 Protection of Vertical Openings.

Any vertical opening shall be protected in accordance with Section 8.6, except under the following conditions:

(1) In Class A or Class B mercantile occupancies protected throughout by an approved, supervised automatic sprinkler system in accordance with 9.7.1.1(1), unprotected vertical openings shall be permitted at one of the following locations:
    (a) Between any two floors
    (b) Among the street floor, the first adjacent floor below, and the adjacent floor (or mezzanine) above
(2) In Class C mercantile occupancies, unprotected openings shall be permitted between the street floor and the mezzanine.
(3) The draft stop and closely spaced sprinkler requirements of NFPA 13, *Standard for the Installation of Sprinkler Systems*, shall not be required for unenclosed vertical openings permitted in 36.3.1(1) and (2).

### 36.3.2 Protection from Hazards.

**36.3.2.1* General.** Hazardous areas shall be protected in accordance with 36.3.2.1.1 or 36.3.2.1.2.

**A.36.3.2.1** It is the intent to permit a suspended natural gas–fired unit heater that complies with the requirements of 9.2.2 to be installed and used in a mercantile occupancy

## 37.3 Protection

### 37.3.1 Protection of Vertical Openings.

Any vertical opening shall be protected in accordance with Section 8.6, except under the following conditions:

(1) In Class A or Class B mercantile occupancies protected throughout by an approved, supervised automatic sprinkler system in accordance with 9.7.1.1(1), unprotected vertical openings shall be permitted at one of the following locations:
    (a) Between any two floors
    (b) Among the street floor, the first adjacent floor below, and the adjacent floor (or mezzanine) above
(2) In Class C mercantile occupancies, unprotected openings shall be permitted between the street floor and the mezzanine.
(3) The draft stop and closely spaced sprinkler requirements of NFPA 13, *Standard for the Installation of Sprinkler Systems*, shall not be required for unenclosed vertical openings permitted in 37.3.1(1) and (2).

### 37.3.2 Protection from Hazards.

**37.3.2.1* General.** Hazardous areas shall be protected in accordance with 37.3.2.1.1 or 37.3.2.1.2.

**A.37.3.2.1** It is the intent to permit a suspended natural gas–fired unit heater that complies with the requirements of 9.2.2 to be installed and used in a mercantile occupancy

## CHAPTER 36 • New

without classifying the area in which it is located as hazardous.

**36.3.2.1.1*** Hazardous areas shall be protected in accordance with Section 8.7.

**A.36.3.2.1.1** These areas can include, but are not limited to, areas used for general storage, boiler or furnace rooms, and maintenance shops that include woodworking and painting areas.

**36.3.2.1.2** In general storage and stock areas protected by an automatic extinguishing system in accordance with 9.7.1.1(1) or 9.7.1.2, an enclosure shall be exempt from the provisions of 8.7.1.2.

**36.3.2.2* High Hazard Contents Areas.** High hazard contents areas, as classified in Section 6.2, shall meet all of the following criteria:

(1) The area shall be separated from other parts of the building by fire barriers having a minimum 1-hour fire resistance rating, with all openings therein protected by self-closing fire door assemblies having a minimum $^3/_4$-hour fire protection rating.
(2) The area shall be protected by an automatic extinguishing system in accordance with 9.7.1.1(1) or 9.7.1.2.
(3) In high hazard areas, all vertical openings shall be enclosed.

**A.36.3.2.2** The requirement for separating high hazard contents areas from other parts of the building is intended to isolate the hazard, and 8.2.3.3 is applicable.

**36.3.2.3 Cooking Equipment.** Cooking equipment shall be protected in accordance with 9.2.3, unless the cooking equipment is one of the following types:

(1) Outdoor equipment
(2) Portable equipment not flue-connected
(3) Equipment used only for food warming

### 36.3.3 Interior Finish.

**36.3.3.1 General.** Interior finish shall be in accordance with Section 10.2.

**36.3.3.2 Interior Wall and Ceiling Finish.** Interior wall and ceiling finish materials complying with Section 10.2 shall be Class A or Class B.

**36.3.3.3 Interior Floor Finish.**

## CHAPTER 37 • Existing

without classifying the area in which it is located as hazardous.

**37.3.2.1.1*** Hazardous areas shall be protected in accordance with Section 8.7.

**A.37.3.2.1.1** These areas can include, but are not limited to, areas used for general storage, boiler or furnace rooms, and maintenance shops that include woodworking and painting areas.

**37.3.2.1.2** In general storage and stock areas protected by an automatic extinguishing system in accordance with 9.7.1.1(1) or 9.7.1.2, an enclosure shall be exempt from the provisions of 8.7.1.2.

**37.3.2.2* High Hazard Contents Areas.** High hazard contents areas, as classified in Section 6.2, shall meet the following criteria:

(1) The area shall be separated from other parts of the building by fire barriers having a minimum 1-hour fire resistance rating, with all openings therein protected by self-closing fire door assemblies having a minimum $^3/_4$-hour fire protection rating.
(2) The area shall be protected by an automatic extinguishing system in accordance with 9.7.1.1(1) or 9.7.1.2.

**A.37.3.2.2** The requirement for separating high hazard contents areas from other parts of the building is intended to isolate the hazard, and 8.2.3.3 is applicable.

**37.3.2.3 Cooking Equipment.** Cooking equipment shall be protected in accordance with 9.2.3, unless the cooking equipment is one of the following types:

(1) Outdoor equipment
(2) Portable equipment not flue-connected
(3) Equipment used only for food warming

### 37.3.3 Interior Finish.

**37.3.3.1 General.** Interior finish shall be in accordance with Section 10.2.

**37.3.3.2 Interior Wall and Ceiling Finish.**

**37.3.3.2.1** Interior wall and ceiling finish materials complying with Section 10.2 shall be Class A or Class B.

**37.3.3.2.2** Existing Class C interior wall and ceiling finish shall be permitted as follows:

(1) On walls
(2) Throughout Class C stores

**37.3.3.3 Interior Floor Finish.** (No requirements.)

CHAPTER 36 • New

**36.3.3.3.1** Interior floor finish shall comply with Section 10.2.

**36.3.3.3.2** Interior floor finish in exit enclosures shall be Class I or Class II.

**36.3.3.3.3** Interior floor finish shall comply with 10.2.7.1 or 10.2.7.2, as applicable.

Paragraph 36/37.3.1 addresses vertical openings. The criteria in 36/37.3.1(1) specify conditions under which such openings are permitted in sprinklered Class A and Class B mercantile occupancies.

Paragraph 36/37.3.2 addresses the protection of hazardous areas. The requirements in 8.7.1.2 normally mandate that a hazardous area protected by automatic sprinklers, rather than by enclosure with fire barriers with a 1-hour fire resistance rating and doors with a 45-minute fire protection rating, is to be enclosed by walls and doors that are at least smoke resisting. Hazardous areas composed of general storage and stock areas in a mercantile occupancy are permitted to be protected by automatic sprinklers without the need for a smoke-resisting enclosure per 36/37.3.2.1.2. In a shoe store, for example, where the shoe storage area is sprinklered, no door would be required on the opening between the sales floor and the storage area.

Section 8.7, as referenced by 36/37.3.2.1.1, requires one of the following:

1. Separation of a hazardous contents area from the remainder of the occupancy by means of suitable construction
2. Installation of an automatic sprinkler system in a hazardous area
3. Both items 1 and 2 where the hazard is severe

Paragraph 36/37.3.3 addresses interior finish. The provision of 37.3.3.2.2 states that, in existing Class C stores only, all interior finish (walls and ceilings) is permitted to be rated as Class C (flame spread index as high as 200). Existing Class A and Class B stores are permitted to use Class C interior finish on the walls, but such finish is prohibited on the ceiling.

### 36.3.4 Detection, Alarm, and Communications Systems.

**36.3.4.1 General.** Class A mercantile occupancies shall be provided with a fire alarm system in accordance with Section 9.6.

**36.3.4.2 Initiation.** Initiation of the required fire alarm system shall be by any one of the following means:

(1) Manual means in accordance with 9.6.2.1(1)
(2) Approved automatic fire detection system that complies with 9.6.2.1(2) and provides protection throughout the building, plus a minimum of one manual fire alarm box in accordance with 9.6.2.6
(3) Approved automatic sprinkler system that complies with 9.6.2.1(3) and provides protection throughout the building, plus a minimum of one manual fire alarm box in accordance with 9.6.2.6

**36.3.4.3 Notification.**

**36.3.4.3.1 Occupant Notification.** During all times that the mercantile occupancy is occupied, the required fire alarm system, once initiated, shall activate an alarm in accordance with 9.6.3 throughout the mercantile occupancy,

CHAPTER 37 • Existing

### 37.3.4 Detection, Alarm, and Communications Systems.

**37.3.4.1 General.** Class A mercantile occupancies shall be provided with a fire alarm system in accordance with Section 9.6.

**37.3.4.2 Initiation.** Initiation of the required fire alarm system shall be by one of the following means:

(1) Manual means per 9.6.2.1(1)
(2) Approved automatic fire detection system that complies with 9.6.2.1(2) and provides protection throughout the building, plus a minimum of one manual fire alarm box in accordance with 9.6.2.6
(3) Approved automatic sprinkler system that complies with 9.6.2.1(3) and provides protection throughout the building, plus a minimum of one manual fire alarm box in accordance with 9.6.2.6

**37.3.4.3 Notification.**

**37.3.4.3.1 Occupant Notification.** During all times that the mercantile occupancy is occupied, the required fire alarm system, once initiated, shall perform one of the following functions:

CHAPTER 36 • New

and positive alarm sequence in accordance with 9.6.3.4 shall be permitted.

**36.3.4.3.2 Emergency Forces Notification.** Emergency forces notification shall be provided and shall include notifying the following:

(1) Fire department in accordance with 9.6.4
(2) Local emergency organization, if provided

CHAPTER 37 • Existing

(1) It shall activate an alarm in accordance with 9.6.3 throughout the mercantile occupancy, and positive alarm sequence in accordance with 9.6.3.4 or a presignal system in accordance with 9.6.3.3 shall be permitted.
(2) Occupant notification shall be permitted to be made via a voice communication or public address system in accordance with 9.6.3.9.2.

**37.3.4.3.2 Emergency Forces Notification.** Emergency forces notification shall be provided and shall include notifying the following:

(1) Fire department in accordance with 9.6.4
(2) Local emergency organization, if provided

Neither Class B nor Class C mercantile occupancies are required to have a fire alarm system.

Because all new Class A stores and most existing Class A stores must be sprinklered based on gross floor area (see 36/37.3.5.1), it is logical that the sprinkler system waterflow method described in 36/37.3.4.2(3) will be used most commonly to activate the fire alarm system. The requirement for manual fire alarm boxes is waived if the sprinkler waterflow activates the fire alarm system. Eliminating the manual fire alarm boxes and satisfying the initiation requirements by means of waterflow through the sprinkler system may reduce the number of nuisance alarms. However, in accordance with 9.6.2.6, at least one manual fire alarm box must be provided at a location acceptable to the authority having jurisdiction (AHJ).

Positive alarm sequence, which is an updated form of a presignal system for which numerous safeguards must be provided, is recognized by 36/37.3.4.3.1. Presignal systems, as recognized by 37.3.4.3.1(1), are only permitted in existing mercantile occupancies.

Note that 37.3.4.3.1 provides a choice between two methods of notification for existing mercantile occupancies only. Many Class A stores are provided with a continuously attended location; 37.3.4.3.1(2) can, therefore, be used. If such a location is not provided or not considered reliable by the AHJ, 37.3.4.3.1(1) must be applied to provide an automatic general alarm in accordance with 9.6.3. In all new mercantile occupancies, other than mall buildings, occupant notification must be provided automatically in accordance with 9.6.3.

If a fire alarm system is required, emergency forces notification must also be provided, as specified by 36/37.3.4.3.2. Several different methods of automatically notifying the fire department are permitted by 9.6.4.

### 36.3.5 Extinguishment Requirements.

**36.3.5.1** Mercantile occupancies shall be protected by an approved automatic sprinkler system in accordance with 9.7.1.1(1) as follows:

(1) Throughout all mercantile occupancies three or more stories in height
(2) Throughout all mercantile occupancies exceeding 12,000 ft$^2$ (1115 m$^2$) in gross area
(3) Throughout stories below the level of exit discharge where such stories have an area exceeding 2500 ft$^2$ (232 m$^2$) and are used for the sale, storage, or handling of combustible goods and merchandise
(4) Throughout multiple occupancies protected as mixed occupancies in accordance with 6.1.14 where the con-

### 37.3.5 Extinguishment Requirements.

**37.3.5.1** Mercantile occupancies, other than one-story buildings that meet the requirements of a street floor, as defined in 3.3.253, shall be protected by an approved automatic sprinkler system in accordance with 9.7.1.1(1) as follows:

(1) Throughout all mercantile occupancies with a story over 15,000 ft$^2$ (1400 m$^2$) in area
(2) Throughout all mercantile occupancies exceeding 30,000 ft$^2$ (2800 m$^2$) in gross area
(3) Throughout stories below the level of exit discharge where such stories have an area exceeding 2500 ft$^2$ (232 m$^2$) and are used for the sale, storage, or handling of combustible goods and merchandise
(4) Throughout multiple occupancies protected as mixed occupancies in accordance with 6.1.14 where the con-

CHAPTER 36 • New

ditions of 36.3.5.1(1), (2), or (3) apply to the mercantile occupancy

**36.3.5.2** Automatic sprinkler systems in Class A mercantile occupancies shall be supervised in accordance with 9.7.2.

**36.3.5.3** Portable fire extinguishers shall be provided in all mercantile occupancies in accordance with 9.7.4.1.

CHAPTER 37 • Existing

ditions of 37.3.5.1(1), (2), or (3) apply to the mercantile occupancy

**37.3.5.2 Reserved.**

**37.3.5.3** Portable fire extinguishers shall be provided in all mercantile occupancies in accordance with 9.7.4.1.

For information on the proper criteria for an approved automatic sprinkler system, refer to the following:

1. NFPA 13, *Standard for the Installation of Sprinkler Systems*[2]
2. NFPA 25, *Standard for the Inspection, Testing, and Maintenance of Water-Based Fire Protection Systems*[3]
3. *Automatic Sprinkler and Standpipe Systems*[4]

All basement areas larger than 2500 $ft^2$ (232 $m^2$) and used for the sales, storage, or handling of combustible merchandise must be sprinklered per 36/37.3.5.1(3) to avoid the potential threat to occupants of the floors above. Studies have shown that there is a higher rate of fire incidence in basements than in other areas of stores. Because smoke and heat rise, a fire in a basement can quickly render exits and exit discharges located on the street floor unusable. This danger is especially acute in mercantile occupancies, where allowances for various vertical openings in accordance with the provisions of 36/37.3.1 are more lenient than those for many other occupancies.

The sprinkler exemption in 37.3.5.1 applies to existing buildings only. It is believed that, in existing, one-story street-floor buildings that comply with all other provisions of the *Code*, including exit travel distance limitations, adequate life safety is provided. Therefore, requiring a building to be sprinklered retroactively is unnecessary. The term *street floor* is defined in 3.3.253 and includes a maximum of three risers of ascent or descent to reach the ground level.

The portable fire extinguishers required by 36/37.3.5.3 are to be used by properly trained employees of the mercantile occupancy as required by 36/37.7.3.

### 36.3.6 Corridors.

**36.3.6.1*** Where access to exits is provided by corridors, such corridors shall be separated from use areas by fire barriers in accordance with Section 8.3 having a minimum 1-hour fire resistance rating, except under any of the following conditions:

(1) Where exits are available from an open floor area
(2) Within a space occupied by a single tenant
(3) Within buildings protected throughout by an approved, supervised automatic sprinkler system in accordance with 9.7.1.1(1)

**A.36.3.6.1** The intent of 36.3.6.1(2) and (3) is to permit spaces within single tenant spaces, or within buildings protected throughout by an approved, supervised automatic sprinkler system, to be open to the exit access corridor without separation.

**36.3.6.2** Openings in corridor walls required by 36.3.6.1 to have a fire resistance rating shall be protected in accordance with Section 8.3.

### 37.3.6 Corridors.

(No requirements.)

### 36.3.7 Subdivision of Building Spaces.

(No special requirements.)

### 37.3.7 Subdivision of Building Spaces.

(No special requirements.)

CHAPTER 36 • New

## 36.4 Special Provisions

### 36.4.1 Limited Access or Underground Buildings.

See Section 11.7.

### 36.4.2 High-Rise Buildings.

High-rise buildings shall comply with the automatic sprinkler requirements of 11.8.3.1.

### 36.4.3 Open-Air Mercantile Operations.

**36.4.3.1** Open-air mercantile operations, such as open-air markets, gasoline filling stations, roadside stands for the sale of farm produce, and other outdoor mercantile operations shall be arranged and conducted to maintain free and unobstructed ways of travel at all times.

**36.4.3.2** Ways of travel shall allow prompt escape from any point of danger in case of fire or other emergency, with no dead ends in which persons might be trapped due to display stands, adjoining buildings, fences, vehicles, or other obstructions.

**36.4.3.3** Mercantile operations that are conducted in roofed-over areas shall be treated as mercantile buildings, provided that canopies over individual small stands to protect merchandise from the weather are not construed as constituting buildings for the purpose of this *Code*.

CHAPTER 37 • Existing

## 37.4 Special Provisions

### 37.4.1 Limited Access or Underground Buildings.

See Section 11.7.

### 37.4.2 High-Rise Buildings.

(No additional requirements.)

### 37.4.3 Open-Air Mercantile Operations.

**37.4.3.1** Open-air mercantile operations, such as open-air markets, gasoline filling stations, roadside stands for the sale of farm produce, and other outdoor mercantile operations shall be arranged and conducted to maintain free and unobstructed ways of travel at all times.

**37.4.3.2** Ways of travel shall allow prompt escape from any point of danger in case of fire or other emergency, with no dead ends in which persons might be trapped due to display stands, adjoining buildings, fences, vehicles, or other obstructions.

**37.4.3.3** Mercantile operations that are conducted in roofed-over areas shall be treated as mercantile buildings, provided that canopies over individual small stands to protect merchandise from the weather are not construed as constituting buildings for the purpose of this *Code*.

The provisions of Section 11.8 for high rise buildings, whether applied singly, in various combinations, or in total, must be mandated by specific occupancy chapter requirements. In new high-rise mercantile occupancies, 36.4.2 requires only the provisions of 11.8.3.1 — an approved, supervised, automatic sprinkler system with a sprinkler control valve and waterflow device on each floor. The new high-rise mercantile occupancy must have a sprinkler system in accordance with 36.3.5.1 and the associated system supervision requirement of 36.3.5.2 for Class A stores, regardless of the reference to 11.8.3.1.

The performance requirements of 36/37.4.3.1 and 36/37.4.3.2 are virtually open-ended provisions that provide guidance for the arrangement, use, and display of merchandise for sale in open-air mercantile operations. The phrase "ways of travel" is purposely used to avoid confusion with means of egress. The term *means of egress* (see definition in 3.3.161) is strictly defined, and its use implies the application of the minimum requirements of Chapter 7. The phrase "ways of travel" is not defined and implies no specific minimum *Code* provisions. Most open-air mercantile operations have unlimited means of entering and evacuating the areas used to display goods. For this reason, it is not necessary to provide specific *Code* requirements beyond the precautionary measures expressed in these paragraphs.

The intent of 36/37.4.3.3 is to exempt small merchandise stands with canopies from classification as mercantile buildings. All other roofed-over areas should be treated as buildings classified by area and height as Class A, Class B, or Class C mercantile occupancies and subject to the appropriate provisions of Chapters 36 and 37.

### 36.4.4 Mall Buildings.

The provisions of 36.4.4 shall apply to mall buildings three or fewer stories in height and any number of anchor buildings. *(See 3.3.32.9.)*

### 37.4.4 Mall Buildings.

The provisions of 37.4.4 shall apply to mall buildings and any number of anchor buildings. *(See 3.3.32.9.)*

CHAPTER 36 • New

**36.4.4.1 General.** The mall building shall be treated as a single building for the purpose of calculation of means of egress and shall be subject to the requirements for appropriate occupancies, except as modified by the provisions of 36.4.4; and the mall shall be of a clear width not less than that needed to accommodate egress requirements as set forth in other sections of this *Code*.

**36.4.4.2 Pedestrian Way.** The mall shall be permitted to be considered a pedestrian way, provided that the criteria of 36.4.4.2.1 and 36.4.4.2.2 are met.

**36.4.4.2.1** The travel distance within a tenant space to an exit or to the mall shall not exceed the maximum travel distance permitted by the occupancy chapter.

**36.4.4.2.2** An additional 200 ft (61 m) shall be permitted for travel through the mall space, provided that all the following requirements are met:

(1) The mall shall be of a clear width not less than that needed to accommodate egress requirements, as set forth in other sections of this chapter, but shall be not less than 20 ft (6100 mm) wide in its narrowest dimension.
(2) On each side of the mall floor area, the mall shall be provided with an unobstructed exit access of not less than 10 ft (3050 mm) in clear width parallel to, and adjacent to, the mall tenant front.
(3)* The exit access specified in 36.4.4.2.2(2) shall lead to an exit having a width of not less than 66 in. (1675 mm).

**A.36.4.4.2.2(3)** The minimum requirement for terminating mall exit access in not less than 66 in. (1675 mm) of egress width relates to the minimum requirement for not less than one aisle in Class A mercantile occupancies with 30,000 ft$^2$ (2800 m$^2$) or greater sales area to be 60 in. (1525 mm) in width.

(4) The mall, and all buildings connected thereto, except open parking structures, shall be protected throughout by an approved, supervised automatic sprinkler system in accordance with 9.7.1.1(1), which shall be installed in such a manner that any portion of the system serving tenant spaces can be taken out of service without affecting the operation of the portion of the system serving the mall.
(5)* Walls dividing tenant spaces from each other shall have a fire resistance rating of not less than 1 hour, and the following also shall apply:
   (a) The partition shall extend to the underside of the ceiling or to the roof or floor above.
   (b) No separation shall be required between a tenant space and the mall.

CHAPTER 37 • Existing

**37.4.4.1 General.** The mall building shall be treated as a single building for the purpose of calculation of means of egress and shall be subject to the requirements for appropriate occupancies, except as modified by the provisions of 37.4.4; and the mall shall be of a clear width not less than that needed to accommodate egress requirements as set forth in other sections of this *Code*.

**37.4.4.2 Pedestrian Way.** The mall shall be permitted to be considered a pedestrian way, provided that the criteria of 37.4.4.2.1 and 37.4.4.2.2 are met.

**37.4.4.2.1** The travel distance within a tenant space to an exit or to the mall shall not exceed the maximum travel distance permitted by the occupancy chapter.

**37.4.4.2.2** An additional 200 ft (61 m) shall be permitted for travel through the mall space, provided that all the following requirements are met:

(1) The mall shall be of a clear width not less than that needed to accommodate egress requirements as set forth in other sections of this chapter, but shall be not less than 20 ft (6100 mm) wide in it narrowest dimension.
(2) On each side of the mall floor area, the mall shall be provided with an unobstructed exit access of not less than 10 ft (3050 mm) in clear width parallel to, and adjacent to, the mall tenant front.
(3)* The exit access specified in 37.4.4.2.2(2) shall lead to an exit having a width of not less than 66 in. (1675 mm).

**A.37.4.4.2.2(3)** The minimum requirement for terminating mall exit access in not less than 66 in. (1675 mm) of egress width relates to the minimum requirement for not less than one aisle in Class A mercantile occupancies with 30,000 ft$^2$ (2800 m$^2$) or greater sales area to be 60 in. (1525 mm) in width.

(4) The mall, and all buildings connected thereto, except open parking structures, shall be protected throughout by an approved, supervised automatic sprinkler system in accordance with 9.7.1.1(1).
(5) Walls dividing tenant spaces from each other shall extend from the floor to the underside of the roof deck, to the floor deck above, or to the ceiling where the ceiling is constructed to limit the transfer of smoke, and the following also shall apply:
   (a) Where the tenant areas are provided with an engineered smoke control system, walls shall not be required to divide tenant spaces from each other.

CHAPTER 36 • New

**A.36.4.4.2.2(5)** Walls providing tenant separations are only required to extend to the underside of the ceiling assembly, regardless of the ceiling's fire-resistive rating. If a ceiling is not provided in either of the tenant spaces, then the wall should extend to the underside of the roof or floor above.

(6)* Malls with a floor opening connecting more than two levels shall be provided with a smoke control system.

**A.36.4.4.2.2(6)** Fire experience in mall shopping centers indicates that the most likely place of fire origin is in the tenant space, where the combustible fire load is far greater than in the mall. Furthermore, any fires resulting from the comparatively low fire load in the mall are more likely to be detected and extinguished in their incipient stages. Early detection is likely due to the nature of the mall as a high-traffic pedestrian way. Such fires produce less smoke development in a greater volume of space than fires in the more confined adjacent tenant space. Smoke control systems that address fire experience in malls are necessary to ensure the integrity of the mall as a pedestrian way by maintaining it reasonably free of the products of combustion for a duration not less than that required to evacuate the area of the building that is affected by the fire. Secondary considerations should include the following:

(1) Confinement of the products of combustion to the area of origin
(2) Removal of the products of combustion, with a minimum of migration of such products of combustion from one tenant space to another
(3) Achievement of evacuation without the need for smoke control in one- and two-level mall buildings protected by automatic sprinklers

Systems, or combinations of systems, that can be engineered to address fires in malls of three or more levels include the following:

(1) Separate mechanical exhaust or control systems
(2) Mechanical exhaust or control systems in conjunction with heating, ventilating, and air-conditioning systems
(3) Automatically or manually released gravity roof vent devices, such as skylights, relief dampers, or smoke vents
(4) Combinations of items (1), (2), and (3) in this list, or any other engineered system designed to accomplish the purpose of this section

**36.4.4.3 Means of Egress Details.**

**36.4.4.3.1** Dead ends not exceeding a length equal to twice the width of the mall, measured at the narrowest location within the dead-end portion of the mall, shall be permitted.

CHAPTER 37 • Existing

(b) No separation shall be required between a tenant space and the mall.

(6)* Malls with a floor opening connecting more than two levels shall be provided with a smoke control system.

**A.37.4.4.2.2(6)** Fire experience in mall shopping centers indicates that the most likely place of fire origin is in the tenant space, where the combustible fire load is far greater than in the mall. Furthermore, any fires resulting from the comparatively low fire load in the mall are more likely to be detected and extinguished in their incipient stages. Early detection is likely due to the nature of the mall as a high-traffic pedestrian way. Such fires produce less smoke development in a greater volume of space than fires in the more confined adjacent tenant space. Smoke control systems that address fire experience in malls are necessary to ensure the integrity of the mall as a pedestrian way by maintaining it reasonably free of the products of combustion for a duration not less than that required to evacuate the area of the building that is affected by the fire. Secondary considerations should include the following:

(1) Confinement of the products of combustion to the area of origin
(2) Removal of the products of combustion, with a minimum of migration of such products of combustion from one tenant space to another
(3) Achievement of evacuation without the need for smoke control in one- and two-level mall buildings protected by automatic sprinklers

Systems, or combinations of systems, that can be engineered to address fires in malls of three or more levels include the following:

(1) Separate mechanical exhaust or control systems
(2) Mechanical exhaust or control systems in conjunction with heating, ventilating, and air-conditioning systems
(3) Automatically or manually released gravity roof vent devices, such as skylights, relief dampers, or smoke vents
(4) Combinations of items (1), (2), and (3) in this list, or any other engineered system designed to accomplish the purpose of this section

**37.4.4.3 Means of Egress Details.**

**37.4.4.3.1** Dead ends not exceeding a length equal to twice the width of the mall, measured at the narrowest location within the dead-end portion of the mall, shall be permitted.

CHAPTER 36 • New

**36.4.4.3.2** Every story of a mall building shall be provided with the number of means of egress specified by Section 7.4 and as modified by 36.4.4.3.2.1 or 36.4.4.3.2.2.

**36.4.4.3.2.1** Exit access travel shall be permitted to be common for the distances permitted as common paths of travel by 36.2.5.3.

**36.4.4.3.2.2** A single means of egress shall be permitted in a Class C mercantile occupancy or a business occupancy, provided that the travel distance to the exit or to a mall pedestrian way (*see 36.4.4.2*) does not exceed 100 ft (30 m).

**36.4.4.3.3** Every floor of a mall shall be provided with the number of means of egress specified by Section 7.4, with not less than two means of egress remotely located from each other.

**36.4.4.3.4** Class A and Class B mercantile occupancies connected to a mall shall be provided with the number of means of egress required by Section 7.4, with not less than two means of egress remotely located from one another.

**36.4.4.3.5*** Each individual anchor building shall have means of egress independent of the mall.

**A.36.4.4.3.5** It is not the intent of 36.4.4.3.5 to require that large tenant spaces be considered anchor stores. A tenant space not considered in determining the occupant load of the mall is required to be arranged so that all of its means of egress will be independent of the mall.

**36.4.4.3.6** Each individual major tenant of a mall building shall be permitted to have a maximum of one-half of its means of egress independent of the mall.

**36.4.4.3.7** Every mall shall be provided with unobstructed exit access parallel to, and adjacent to, the mall tenant fronts and extending to each mall exit.

**36.4.4.3.8** Each assembly occupancy with an occupant load of 500 or more shall have not less than one-half of its required means of egress independent of the mall.

**36.4.4.3.9** Emergency lighting shall be provided in accordance with 36.2.9.

**36.4.4.4 Detection, Alarm, and Communications Systems.**

**36.4.4.4.1 General.** Malls shall be provided with a fire alarm system in accordance with Section 9.6.

**36.4.4.4.2 Initiation.** Initiation of the required fire alarm system shall be by means of the required automatic sprinkler system in accordance with 9.6.2.1(3).

**36.4.4.4.3 Notification.**

CHAPTER 37 • Existing

**37.4.4.3.2** Every story of a covered mall building shall be provided with the number of means of egress specified by Section 7.4 and as modified by 37.4.4.3.2.1 or 37.4.4.3.2.2.

**37.4.4.3.2.1** Exit access travel shall be permitted to be common for the distances permitted as common paths of travel by 37.2.5.3.

**37.4.4.3.2.2** A single means of egress shall be permitted in a Class C mercantile occupancy or a business occupancy, provided that the travel distance to the exit or to a mall pedestrian way (*see 37.4.4.2*) does not exceed 100 ft (30 m).

**37.4.4.3.3** Every floor of a mall shall be provided with the number of means of egress specified by Section 7.4, with not less than two means of egress remotely located from each other.

**37.4.4.3.4** Class A and Class B mercantile occupancies connected to a mall shall be provided with the number of means of egress required by Section 7.4, with not less than two means of egress remotely located from one another.

**37.4.4.3.5*** Each individual anchor building shall have means of egress independent of the mall.

**A.37.4.4.3.5** It is not the intent of 37.4.4.3.5 to require that large tenant spaces be considered anchor stores. A tenant space not considered in determining the occupant load of the mall is required to be arranged so that all of its means of egress will be independent of the mall.

**37.4.4.3.6** Each individual major tenant of a mall building shall be permitted to have a maximum of one-half of its means of egress independent of the mall.

**37.4.4.3.7** Every mall shall be provided with unobstructed exit access parallel to, and adjacent to, the mall tenant fronts and extending to each mall exit.

**37.4.4.3.8 Reserved.**

**37.4.4.3.9** Emergency lighting shall be provided in accordance with 37.2.9.

**37.4.4.4 Detection, Alarm, and Communications Systems.**

**37.4.4.4.1 General.** Malls shall be provided with a fire alarm system in accordance with Section 9.6.

**37.4.4.4.2 Initiation.** Initiation of the required fire alarm system shall be by means of the required automatic sprinkler system in accordance with 9.6.2.1(3).

**37.4.4.4.3 Notification.**

CHAPTER 36 • New

**36.4.4.4.3.1 Occupant Notification.** During all times that the mall is occupied, the required fire alarm system, once initiated, shall perform one of the following functions:

(1) It shall activate a general alarm in accordance with 9.6.3 throughout the mall.
(2) Positive alarm sequence in accordance with 9.6.3.4 shall be permitted.
(3) Occupant notification shall be permitted to be made via a voice communication or public address system in accordance with 9.6.3.9.2.

**36.4.4.4.3.2*** Visible signals shall not be required in malls. *(See 9.6.3.5.7 and 9.6.3.5.8.)*

**A.36.4.4.4.3.2** It is the intent to permit the omission of visible alarm notification appliances from the mall or pedestrian way in mall buildings. It is anticipated that occupants with hearing impairments will receive cues from other building occupants and respond accordingly. Visible signals should be provided in public restrooms and other adjunct spaces in the mall subject to occupancy solely by persons with hearing impairments.

**36.4.4.4.3.3 Emergency Forces Notification.** Emergency forces notification shall be provided and shall include notifying the following:

(1) Fire department in accordance with 9.6.4
(2) Local emergency organization, if provided

**36.4.4.4.4 Emergency Control.** The fire alarm system shall be arranged to automatically actuate smoke management or smoke control systems in accordance with 9.6.5.2(3).

**36.4.4.5 Tenant Spaces.** Each individual tenant space shall have means of egress to the outside or to the mall, based on occupant load calculated by using Table 7.3.1.2.

**36.4.4.6 Exit Passageways.** Exit passageways shall comply with 36.4.4.6.1 and 36.4.4.6.2.

**36.4.4.6.1** Exit passageways in a mall building shall be permitted to accommodate the following occupant loads independently:

(1) Portion of the occupant load assigned to the exit passageway from only the mall
(2) Largest occupant load assigned to the exit passageway from a single tenant space

**36.4.4.6.2*** Rooms housing building service equipment, janitor closets, and service elevators shall be permitted to open directly onto exit passageways, provided that the following criteria are met:

CHAPTER 37 • Existing

**37.4.4.4.3.1 Occupant Notification.** During all times that the mall is occupied, the required fire alarm system, once initiated, shall perform one of the following functions:

(1) It shall activate an alarm in accordance with 9.6.3 throughout the mall.
(2) Positive alarm sequence in accordance with 9.6.3.4 shall be permitted.
(3) Occupant notification shall be permitted to be made via a voice communication or public address system in accordance with 9.6.3.9.2.

**37.4.4.4.3.2 Emergency Forces Notification.** Emergency forces notification shall be provided and shall include notifying the following:

(1) Fire department in accordance with 9.6.4
(2) Local emergency organization, if provided

**37.4.4.4.4 Emergency Control.** The fire alarm system shall be arranged to automatically actuate smoke management or smoke control systems in accordance with 9.6.5.2(3).

**37.4.4.5 Tenant Spaces.** Each individual tenant space shall have means of egress to the outside or to the mall based on occupant load calculated by using Table 7.3.1.2.

**37.4.4.6 Exit Passageways.** Exit passageways shall comply with 37.4.4.6.1 and 37.4.4.6.2.

**37.4.4.6.1** Exit passageways in a mall building shall be permitted to accommodate the following occupant loads independently:

(1) Portion of the occupant load assigned to the exit passageway from only the mall
(2) Largest occupant load assigned to the exit passageway from a single tenant space

**37.4.4.6.2*** Rooms housing building service equipment, janitor closets, and service elevators shall be permitted to open directly onto exit passageways, provided that the following criteria are met:

CHAPTER 36 • New

(1) The required fire resistance rating between such rooms or areas and the exit passageway shall be maintained in accordance with 7.1.3.2.
(2) Such rooms or areas shall be protected by an approved, supervised automatic sprinkler system in accordance with 9.7.1.1(1), but the exceptions in NFPA 13, *Standard for the Installation of Sprinkler Systems*, allowing the omission of sprinklers from such rooms shall not be permitted.
(3) Service elevators opening into the exit passageway shall not open into areas other than exit passageways.
(4) Where exit stair enclosures discharge into the exit passageway, the provisions of 7.2.1.5.7 shall apply, regardless of the number of stories served.

**A.36.4.4.6.2** Rooms opening onto the exit passageway are intended to include building service elevators, elevator machine rooms, electrical rooms, telephone rooms, janitor closets, restrooms, and similar normally unoccupied spaces not requiring hazardous area protection in accordance with Section 8.7.

**36.4.4.7 Plastic Signs.** Within every store or level, and from sidewall to sidewall of each tenant space facing the mall, plastic signs shall be limited as follows:

(1) Plastic signs shall not exceed 20 percent of the wall area facing the mall.
(2) Plastic signs shall not exceed a height of 36 in. (915 mm), except if the sign is vertical, in which case the height shall not exceed 8 ft (2440 mm) and the width shall not exceed 36 in. (915 mm).
(3) Plastic signs shall be located a minimum distance of 18 in. (455 mm) from adjacent tenants.
(4) Plastics, other than foamed plastics, shall meet one of the following criteria:
    (a) They shall be light-transmitting plastics.
    (b) They shall have a self-ignition temperature of 650°F (343°C) or greater when tested in accordance with ASTM D 1929, *Standard Test Method for Determining Ignition Temperatures of Plastic*, and a flame spread index not greater than 75 and a smoke developed index not greater than 450 when tested in the manner intended for use in accordance with ASTM E 84, *Standard Test Method for Surface Burning Characteristics of Building Materials*, or ANSI/UL 723, *Standard for Test for Surface Burning Characteristics of Building Materials*.
(5) The edges and backs of plastic signs in the mall shall be fully encased in metal.
(6) Foamed plastics shall have a maximum heat release rate of 150 kW when tested in accordance with ANSI/UL 1975, *Standard for Fire Tests for Foamed Plastics Used*

CHAPTER 37 • Existing

(1) The required fire resistance rating between such rooms or areas and the exit passageway shall be maintained in accordance with 7.1.3.2.
(2) Such rooms or areas shall be protected by an approved automatic sprinkler system in accordance with 9.7.1.1(1), but the exceptions in NFPA 13, *Standard for the Installation of Sprinkler Systems*, allowing the omission of sprinklers from such rooms shall not be permitted.
(3) Service elevators opening into the exit passageway shall not open into areas other than exit passageways.
(4) Where exit stair enclosures discharge into the exit passageway, the provisions of 7.2.1.5.7 shall apply, regardless of the number of stories served.

**A.37.4.4.6.2** Rooms opening onto the exit passageway are intended to include building service elevators, elevator machine rooms, electrical rooms, telephone rooms, janitor closets, restrooms, and similar normally unoccupied spaces not requiring hazardous area protection in accordance with Section 8.7.

**37.4.4.7 Plastic Signs.** Within every store or level, and from sidewall to sidewall of each tenant space facing the mall, plastic signs shall be limited as follows:

(1) Plastic signs shall not exceed 20 percent of the wall area facing the mall.
(2) Plastic signs shall not exceed a height of 36 in. (915 mm), except if the sign is vertical, in which case the height shall not exceed 8 ft (2440 mm) and the width shall not exceed 36 in. (915 mm).
(3) Plastic signs shall be located a minimum distance of 18 in. (455 mm) from adjacent tenants.
(4) Plastics, other than foamed plastics, shall meet one of the following criteria:
    (a) They shall be light-transmitting plastics.
    (b) They shall have a self-ignition temperature of 650°F (343°C) or greater when tested in accordance with ASTM D 1929, *Standard Test Method for Determining Ignition Temperatures of Plastic*, and a flame spread index not greater than 75 and a smoke developed index not greater than 450 when tested in the manner intended for use in accordance with ASTM E 84, *Standard Test Method for Surface Burning Characteristics of Building Materials*, or ANSI/UL 723, *Standard for Test for Surface Burning Characteristics of Building Materials*.
(5) The edges and backs of plastic signs in the mall shall be fully encased in metal.
(6) Foamed plastics shall have a maximum heat release rate of 150 kW when tested in accordance with ANSI/UL 1975, *Standard for Fire Tests for Foamed Plastics Used*

CHAPTER 36 • New

*for Decorative Purposes*, and shall have physical characteristics in accordance with the following:

(a) The minimum density of foamed plastic signs shall be not less than 20 lb/ft$^3$ (320 kg/m$^3$).
(b) The thickness of foamed plastic signs shall be not greater than $\frac{1}{2}$ in. (13 mm).

**36.4.4.8 Kiosks.** Kiosks and similar structures (temporary or permanent) shall not be considered as tenant spaces and shall meet the following requirements:

(1) Combustible kiosks and similar structures shall be constructed of any of the following materials:
  (a) Fire-retardant-treated wood complying with the requirements for fire-retardant-impregnated wood in NFPA 703, *Standard for Fire Retardant–Treated Wood and Fire-Retardant Coatings for Building Materials*
  (b) Light-transmitting plastics complying with Chapter 47 of *NFPA 5000, Building Construction and Safety Code*
  (c) Foamed plastics having a maximum heat release rate not greater than 100 kW when tested in accordance with ANSI/UL 1975, *Standard for Fire Tests for Foamed Plastics Used for Decorative Purposes*
  (d) Aluminum composite material (ACM) having a Class A rating, as specified in Section 10.2, when tested as an assembly in the maximum thickness intended for use
  (e) Textiles and films meeting the flame propagation performance criteria contained in NFPA 701, *Standard Methods of Fire Tests for Flame Propagation of Textiles and Films*
(2) Kiosks or similar structures located within the mall shall be protected with approved fire suppression and detection devices.
(3) The minimum horizontal separation between kiosks, or groups of kiosks, and other structures within the mall shall be 20 ft (6100 mm).
(4) Each kiosk, or group of kiosks, or similar structure shall have a maximum area of 300 ft$^2$ (27.8 m$^2$).

**36.4.4.9* Smoke Control.** Smoke control in accordance with Section 9.3 and complying with 8.6.7(5) shall be provided in a mall with floor openings connecting more than two levels.

**A.36.4.4.9** Fire experience in mall shopping centers indicates that the most likely place of fire origin is in the tenant space where the combustible fire load is far greater than in the mall.

Furthermore, any fires resulting from the comparatively low fire load in the mall are more likely to be detected and

CHAPTER 37 • Existing

*for Decorative Purposes*, and shall have physical characteristics in accordance with the following:

(a) The minimum density of foamed plastic signs shall be not less than 20 lb/ft$^3$ (320 kg/m$^3$).
(b) The thickness of foamed plastic signs shall be not greater than $\frac{1}{2}$ in. (13 mm).

**37.4.4.8 Kiosks.** Kiosks and similar structures (temporary or permanent) shall not be considered as tenant spaces and shall meet the following requirements:

(1) Combustible kiosks and similar structures shall be constructed of any of the following materials:
  (a) Fire-retardant-treated wood complying with the requirements for fire-retardant-impregnated wood in NFPA 703, *Standard for Fire Retardant–Treated Wood and Fire-Retardant Coatings for Building Materials*
  (b) Light-transmitting plastics complying with Chapter 47 of *NFPA 5000, Building Construction and Safety Code*
  (c) Foamed plastics having a maximum heat release rate not greater than 100 kW when tested in accordance with ANSI/UL 1975, *Standard for Fire Tests for Foamed Plastics Used for Decorative Purposes*
  (d) Aluminum composite material (ACM) having a Class A rating, as specified in Section 10.2, when tested as an assembly in the maximum thickness intended for use
  (e) Textiles and films meeting the flame propagation performance criteria contained in NFPA 701, *Standard Methods of Fire Tests for Flame Propagation of Textiles and Films*
(2) Kiosks or similar structures located within the mall shall be protected with approved fire suppression and detection devices.
(3) The minimum horizontal separation between kiosks, or groups of kiosks, and other structures within the mall shall be 20 ft (6100 mm).
(4) Each kiosk, or group of kiosks, or similar structure shall have a maximum area of 300 ft$^2$ (27.8 m$^2$).

extinguished in their incipient stages. Early detection is likely due to the nature of the mall as a high-traffic pedestrian way. Such fires produce less smoke development in a greater volume of space than fires in the more confined adjacent tenant space.

Smoke control systems that address fire experience in malls are necessary in order to achieve the following:

(1) Ensure the integrity of the mall as a pedestrian way by maintaining it reasonably free of the products of combustion for a duration not less than that required to evacuate the building
(2) Confine the products of combustion to the area of origin
(3) Remove the products of combustion with a minimum of migration of such products of combustion from one tenant to another

Systems, or combinations of systems, that can be engineered to address fires in malls include the following:

(1) Separate mechanical exhaust or control systems
(2) Mechanical exhaust or control systems in conjunction with heating, ventilating, and air-conditioning systems
(3) Automatically or manually released gravity roof vent devices, such as skylights, relief dampers, or smoke vents
(4) Combinations of items (1), (2), and (3) in this list, or any other engineered system designed to accomplish the purpose of this section

**36.4.4.10 Automatic Extinguishing Systems.**

**36.4.4.10.1** The mall building and all anchor buildings shall be protected throughout by an approved, supervised automatic sprinkler system in accordance with 9.7.1.1(1) and 36.4.4.10.2.

**36.4.4.10.2** The system shall be installed in such a manner that any portion of the system serving tenant spaces can be taken out of service without affecting the operation of the portion of the system serving the mall.

The provisions for new mall buildings in 36.4.4 apply only to buildings up to three stories in height. For new mall buildings with more than three stories, the equivalency concept of Section 1.4 or performance-based design option of Chapter 5 should be used to engineer a unique life safety system that meets the goals and objectives of the *Code* (see Chapter 4). For existing mall buildings, the provisions of 37.4.4 apply, regardless of number of stories.

It is common for mall buildings to have food courts and areas for live performances. Such spaces with occupant loads of 50 or more are considered assembly occupancies. The provision of 36/37.4.4.1 clarifies that the requirements for the applicable occupancies need to be followed, except as modified by 36/37.4.4. One of the modifications relates to sizing the means of egress from the mall using a calculation based on gross leasable area (GLA). The use of the gross leasable area concept for sizing the means of egress for the mall typically will result in adequate capacity, even where large assembly occupancies are located in part of the mall building.

Consider the examples that follow. (In these examples, it is noted that using SI values will sometimes yield results that differ from those using the traditional inch-pound values, due to rounding. Use of either the SI or inch-pound values is deemed acceptable per Section 1.5.)

*Example 1*

A 5000-seat cinema complex (i.e., a large assembly occupancy) is to be housed within a new mall building. The cinema seating area, lobby, and circulation space will occupy 100,000 ft$^2$ (9290 m$^2$). The mall building will have 550,000 ft$^2$ (51,100 m$^2$) of GLA [450,000 ft$^2$ (41,800 m$^2$) for mercantile use and 100,000 ft$^2$ (9290 m$^2$) for the cinema complex].

Using Figure 7.3.1.2(a) and Figure 7.3.1.2(b), the GLA of the cinema will require that the mall have sufficient egress capacity to accommodate 2000 persons from the 5000-seat cinema. This is based on a calculation in which 100,000 ft$^2$ (9290 m$^2$) is divided by 55 ft$^2$ (5.1 m$^2$) per person, because the mall building's GLA exceeds 400,000 ft$^2$ (37,160 m$^2$). Also, the mall must have adequate egress capacity for another 8180 persons due to the GLA associated with the mercantile areas. This additional capacity is based on a calculation in which 450,000 ft$^2$ (41,800 m$^2$) is divided by 55 ft$^2$ (5.1 m$^2$) per person. Given the main entrance/exit requirement of Chapters 12 and 13, egress for half the cinema occupant load (i.e., 2500 persons) will be provided through doors leading directly to the outside or through exit passageways. If the cinema were occupied to 100 percent capacity, the other 2500 persons would be expected to use the mall as exit access. Note that 36.4.4.3.8, which applies to new malls, permits not more than 50 percent of the occupant load of an assembly occupancy with an occupant load of 500 or more to egress through the mall; the remaining 50 percent of the occupant load must egress independent of the mall. Although there might appear to be a capacity deficiency of 500 persons, the system provides safeguards that follow in paragraphs 1 through 3.

**1.** Cinemas do not normally operate at 100 percent capacity. Management typically stops selling tickets at 80 percent capacity, because the larger crowds make for inefficient access to the highly profitable concession stands, thus reducing revenue. Yet, the occupant load is established by counting all seats.

**2.** The mall, not the mall building, is required to have a fire alarm system. This requirement considers that it is very unusual to evacuate the entire mall building due to a fire in either the mall or one of the tenant spaces. Thus, the mall egress capacity is not fully used simultaneously, although the mall has excess capacity that easily absorbs the cinema occupants not otherwise considered.

**3.** If the number of persons entering the mall from the tenant space — for emergency egress — is greater than that for which the mall's egress system was sized, it doesn't mean that the additional persons are unable to leave the building. Rather, it means that it takes longer to discharge all occupants to the outside. The requirements for sprinkler protection throughout the mall building, and for smoke control within the mall, help to maintain tenable conditions to allow a longer egress time. The mall provides for safe exit access similar to that provided within an atrium.

*Example 2*

A restaurant with an occupant load of 300 persons is to be located within a new mall building that has GLA of 200,000 ft$^2$ (18,580 m$^2$). The restaurant's 300-person occupant load is derived by dividing the 4500 ft$^2$ (418 m$^2$) of net area usable for patron standing and seating by the 15 ft$^2$ (1.4 m$^2$) per person occupant load factor characteristic of the assembly use. However, the restaurant occupies a total GLA of 6000 ft$^2$ (557 m$^2$).

Using Figure 7.3.1.2(a) and Figure 7.3.1.2(b), the GLA of the restaurant requires the mall to provide sufficient egress capacity to accommodate 150 persons from the 300-person restaurant. This egress capacity is based on a calculation in which 6000 ft$^2$ (557 m$^2$) is divided by 40 ft$^2$ (3.7 m$^2$) per person, because the mall building's GLA is 200,000 ft$^2$ (18,580 m$^2$). Also, the mall must have adequate egress capacity for another 4850 persons due to the GLA associated with the mercantile areas. This additional capacity is based on a calculation in which 194,000 ft$^2$ (18,020 m$^2$) is divided by 40 ft$^2$ (3.7 m$^2$) per person. Given the main entrance/exit requirement of Chapters 12 and 13, egress for one-half the restaurant occupant load (i.e., 150 persons) will be provided through doors leading directly to the outside or through exit passageways. The other 150 persons would be expected to use the mall as exit access. This results in a perfect match between the 150 persons who egress from the restaurant into the mall and the 150-person egress capacity imposed on the mall based on the GLA of the restaurant.

In recent years, mall shopping areas have increased in both number and size. Two approaches in addressing the life safety aspects of these complexes were developed. The first approach (described in the base paragraph of 36/37.4.4.1) treats the mall and the attached stores essentially as one large Class A store subject to all the provisions of Chapters 36 and 37. If viewed in this way, the mall would be treated as an aisle of a store.

The second approach allows the mall to be considered as a pedestrian way through which occupants of the attached stores are permitted to egress during a fire. The phrase "pedestrian way" is intended to convey the meaning of the term *exit access* (defined in 3.3.76).

The provisions of 36/37.4.4.2 recognize that, if the mall and all the buildings attached to the mall are protected by automatic sprinklers, occupants fleeing into the mall from a fire in a store are then moving into a space whose volume, size, and arrangement affords most of the benefits provided by an enclosed stair or a horizontal exit, as well as providing many of the benefits of an outdoor area. This criterion considers the mall to be a safe area for the occupants of the tenant spaces attached to it, despite the fact that the mall is not separated from these attached spaces by the type of construction normally provided for an exit as required by 7.1.3.2.

If a mall is considered as a pedestrian way, the maximum travel distance to an exit or to the mall from any point within a tenant space attached to the mall is that permitted by the applicable occupancy chapter. The reasoning behind this provision is that use of the mall for egress is as acceptable as the use of an exit. A travel distance of up to 200 ft (61 m), in addition to the travel distance allowed within the tenant space, is permitted within the mall if the conditions of 1 through 6, which follow, are met.

**1.** The mall building (the mall and all tenant spaces and attached buildings) is sprinklered. The sprinkler system must be electrically supervised. Note that, if the shopping complex is considered as one building, rather than as a mall building with a complying pedestrian way, sprinkler protection most likely is also required under the 12,000 $ft^2$ (1115 $m^2$) gross area criterion of 36.3.5.1(2).

**2.** The clear width of the mall is at least 20 ft (6100 mm) or wider if mandated by the egress capacity. Note that, where the mall is considered as a pedestrian way, an occupant load is not calculated for the mall based on its area. The required capacity of the means of egress for the mall is calculated on the basis of the aggregate gross leasable area of the attached stores (excluding anchor buildings), including kiosks and similar sales areas.

**3.** At least 10 ft (3050 mm) of clear, unobstructed space is available for exit access in front of all store fronts. This requirement is designed to prohibit displays of merchandise, kiosks, or small sales stands from being located directly in front of the store fronts and ensures that the mall will have a minimum clear width of 20 ft (6100 mm).

**4.** Each exit access terminates at an exit with a minimum width of 66 in. (1675 mm).

**5.** Walls separating stores have a fire resistance rating of at least 1 hour. Such walls are permitted to terminate at the underside of a nonrated ceiling. If the tenant space has no finished ceiling, the wall must terminate at the underside of the floor or roof above. The store front is permitted to be open to the mall; no separating construction is required.

**6.** A smoke control system is provided in the mall if it has a floor opening connecting two or more stories. Since the tenant spaces are generally open to the mall, this requirement is essential if the mall is to be used as a safe means of egress. For detailed requirements on the design, installation, and maintenance of smoke control systems in malls, see NFPA 92B, *Standard for Smoke Management Systems in Malls, Atria, and Large Spaces.*[5]

If the conditions of 1 through 6 are not met, the mall is still permitted to be used as part of the exit access from the mall building, but the additional travel distance to an exit would not be permitted. Therefore, from any point within the overall mall building, which includes the stores and the mall, travel distance would be limited to 150 ft (46 m) for nonsprinklered buildings or 250 ft (76 m) for sprinklered mercantile occupancies (see 36/37.2.6), or as otherwise required by the applicable occupancy chapter, depending on the use of the tenant space. In the majority of configurations, this restriction would preclude the use of the mall as an exit access.

Exhibit 36/37.15 illustrates many of the requirements necessary to qualify a mall as a pedestrian way.

Paragraph 36/37.4.4.3.2 reaffirms the fundamental *Code* requirement for providing at least two independent means of egress — more if the occupant load exceeds 500 persons, in accordance with 7.4.1.2.

Note that, in larger stores (Class A and Class B mercantile occupancies), the second exit must be

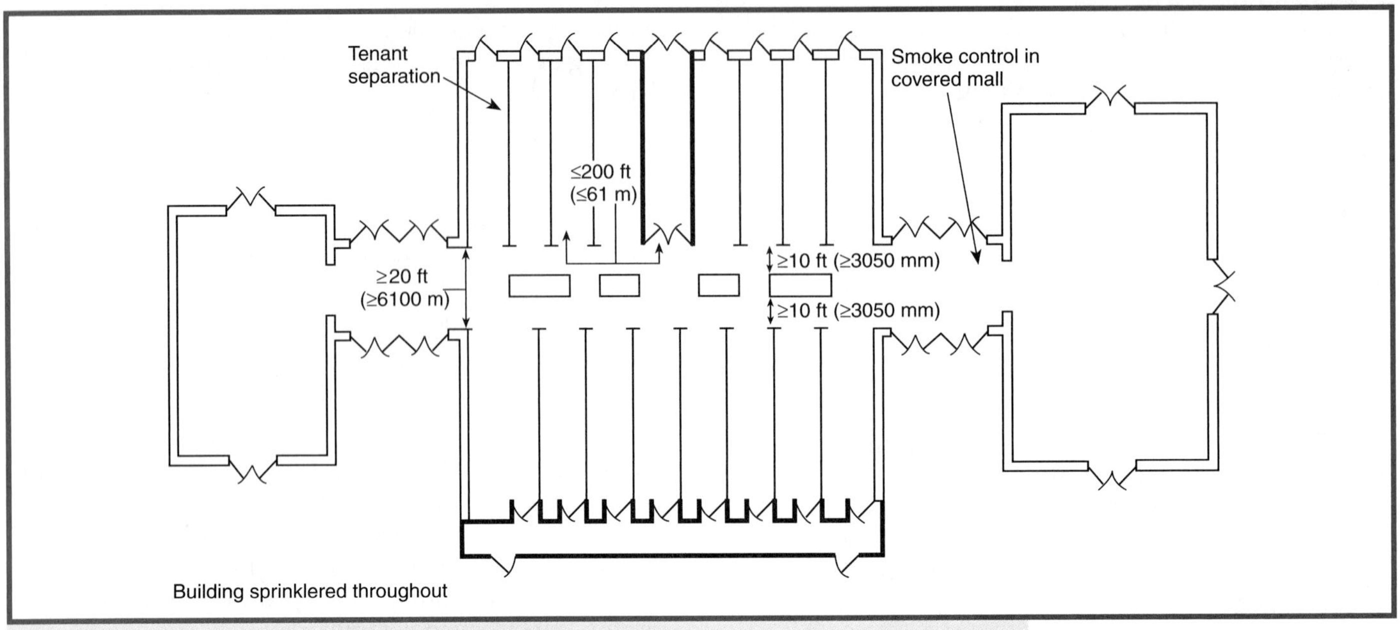


***Exhibit 36/37.15*** *Mall meeting the requirements of a pedestrian way.*

remote from the first exit. This requirement is usually met by evacuating occupants directly from the store to the outside or directly into an exit passageway without entering the mall.

The provision of 36/37.4.4.3.6 for a *major tenant* (see definition in 3.3.157), which is new to the 2009 edition of the *Code,* was intended to prevent oversizing the means of egress from the mall where such major tenant spaces have means of egress directly to the outside but don't meet the criteria for an *anchor building* (see definition in 3.3.32.2). For this edition of the *Code,* the concept does not affect the required egress capacity from the mall, because such determination is made based on the gross leasable area of the mall building, excluding the aggregate area of anchor buildings as specified in Table 7.3.1.2, with no allowance for major tenants. The major tenant concept will require further development for a future edition of the *Code.*

The provisions of 36/37.4.4.2.2(2) and (3) are echoed by 36/37.4.4.3.7, though specific measurements are not provided.

Although the provisions of 36/37.4.4 address the overall mall building, the provisions of 36/37.4.4.4.1, which apply to alarm systems, require only that the alarm system be provided for the mall (the covered pedestrian way). In addition, the provisions of 36/37.3.4.1 require that any Class A mercantile occupancy within the mall building also be provided with an alarm system. Therefore, Class B and Class C mercantile occupancies within the mall building are not required to have alarm systems.

Note that, per 36/37.4.4.4.2, manual fire alarm boxes are not required, but the sprinkler system must have a waterflow device that initiates the fire alarm system. However, in accordance with the provisions of 9.6.2.6, at least one manual fire alarm box must be provided at a location acceptable to the authority having jurisdiction (AHJ).

Note that 36/37.4.4.4.3.1 provides a choice between two methods of notification. Many large shopping malls do have a continuously attended location, and 36/37.4.4.4.3.1(3), which permits the use of a voice communication or public address system meeting 9.6.3.9.2, can be used. If such a location is not provided or the AHJ does not consider the location reliable, 36/37.4.4.4.3.1(1) must be applied. If the general alarm option is used, positive alarm sequence is permitted by 36/37.4.4.4.3.1(2). In either case, the notification must be provided to the occupants of the mall but is not required to be provided within the individual tenant spaces.

Visible alarm notification appliances are not required in malls per 36.4.4.4.3.2, which is new to the 2009 edition of the *Code.* The effectiveness of visible notification appliances in large-volume spaces such as malls is questionable. It is reasonable to assume that, in the event of a fire, hearing-impaired occupants will follow the cues of other occupants in the process of evacuating. While the omission of visible signals in malls is permitted, they should be provided in adjunct mall spaces, such as public restrooms.

Paragraph 9.6.4 permits several different methods of automatically notifying the fire department, as required by 36.4.4.4.3.3 and 37.4.4.4.3.2.

Although the requirements of Chapter 7 prohibit normally unoccupied rooms from having doors open directly into an exit enclosure, 36/37.4.4.6.2 specifically permits rooms housing building service equipment, janitor closets, and service elevators to open directly into exit passageways in mall buildings, provided that the additional criteria specified in 36/37.4.4.6.2(1) through (4) are met. The *Code* permits this allowance in recognition of operational needs and the incorporation of current design criteria in mall buildings. The conditions that are unique to this type of facility include the following:

1. Limitation on the number of floors (not more than three for new construction)
2. Main concourse for occupant movement, with specific requirements for size and smoke control, that leads to multiple points of egress
3. Facilities required to be fully protected by an automatic sprinkler system

The provision of 36/37.4.4.6.2(1) states that the exit passageway with door openings from support spaces is not to be treated as a corridor but as an exit passageway meeting the fire-rated separation requirements of 7.1.3.2.

All areas that open onto the exit passageway must be protected by an automatic sprinkler system per 36/37.4.4.6.2(2). This requirement is restated to prevent use of the provisions in NFPA 13, *Standard for the Installation of Sprinkler Systems*, which permit the omission of sprinkler protection if certain conditions are met.

Paragraph 36/37.4.4.6.2(3) addresses communication among floors by elevator shafts and their associated openings. This requirement permits only those openings associated with an elevator that opens onto an exit passageway. This limitation would prohibit an elevator from opening to another use area, such as a storage or loading area, thereby limiting the exposure from the effects of fire from areas other than exit passageways.

The provision of 36/37.4.4.6.2(4) requires that stairwell re-entry is maintained in continuous occupant control in accordance with 7.2.1.5.7. It prohibits the use of the exemption in 7.2.1.5.7, which permits doors to be locked from the stairwell side if the building does not exceed four stories.

The text of A.36/A.37.4.4.6.2 clarifies the types of spaces that are permitted to have doors that open directly onto the exit passageway. Such spaces include rooms with contents that are no more hazardous than those typically found in a mall building. These spaces are usually small and are associated with limited amounts of combustibles.

In a mall building, it is necessary to provide for services to the tenant spaces that are maintained by the mall management (e.g., water, electricity, telephone, fire protection). These services must be located in a common space controlled by the mall management and, therefore, cannot be located within the tenant spaces. Frequently, these services are logically located with direct access to service corridors or exit passageways/corridors at the rear of the tenant spaces.

This common design practice has prompted many designers to seek specific approval of such designs from local authorities to permit numerous buildings to be built in this manner. There is a long history of mall buildings built in this manner with no adverse experience.

Smoke control systems meeting Section 9.3 are required in all new mall buildings with floor openings connecting more than two levels, regardless of the mall's use as a pedestrian way, per 36.4.4.9. In addition, electrically supervised automatic sprinkler systems are required in all new mall buildings per 36.4.4.10. Sprinkler systems must be arranged with control valves to allow the sprinklers serving the tenant spaces to be taken out of service without affecting the sprinklers serving the mall, because the tenant spaces are expected to undergo relatively frequent renovations over the life of the building.

### 36.4.5 Bulk Merchandising Retail Buildings.

New bulk merchandising retail buildings exceeding 12,000 ft$^2$ (1115 m$^2$) in area shall comply with the requirements of this chapter, as modified by 36.4.5.1 through 36.4.5.6.2.

### 37.4.5 Bulk Merchandising Retail Buildings.

Existing bulk merchandising retail buildings exceeding 15,000 ft$^2$ (1400 m$^2$) in area shall comply with the requirements of this chapter, as modified by 37.4.5.1 through 37.4.5.6.2.

CHAPTER 36 • New

**36.4.5.1 Minimum Construction Requirements.** Bulk merchandising retail buildings shall have a distance of not less than 16 ft (4875 mm) from the floor to the ceiling, from the floor to the floor above, or from the floor to the roof of any story.

**36.4.5.2 Means of Egress Requirements.**

**36.4.5.2.1** All means of egress shall be in accordance with Chapter 7 and this chapter.

**36.4.5.2.2** Not less than 50 percent of the required egress capacity shall be located independent of the main entrance/exit doors.

**36.4.5.3 Storage, Arrangement, Protection, and Quantities of Hazardous Commodities.** The storage, arrangement, protection, and quantities of hazardous commodities shall be in accordance with the applicable provisions of the following:

(1) NFPA 1, *Fire Code*
(2) NFPA 13, *Standard for the Installation of Sprinkler Systems*
(3) NFPA 30, *Flammable and Combustible Liquids Code*
(4) NFPA 30B, *Code for the Manufacture and Storage of Aerosol Products*
(5) NFPA 430, *Code for the Storage of Liquid and Solid Oxidizers*
(6) NFPA 432, *Code for the Storage of Organic Peroxide Formulations*
(7) NFPA 434, *Code for the Storage of Pesticides*
(8) NFPA 1124, *Code for the Manufacture, Transportation, Storage, and Retail Sales of Fireworks and Pyrotechnic Articles*

**36.4.5.4 Detection, Alarm, and Communications Systems.**

**36.4.5.4.1 General.** Bulk merchandising retail buildings shall be provided with a fire alarm system in accordance with Section 9.6.

**36.4.5.4.2 Initiation.** Initiation of the required fire alarm system shall be by means of the required approved automatic sprinkler system *(see 36.4.5.5)* in accordance with 9.6.2.1(3).

**36.4.5.4.3 Occupant Notification.** During all times that the mercantile occupancy is occupied, the required fire alarm system, once initiated, shall activate an alarm in accordance with 9.6.3 throughout the mercantile occupancy, and positive alarm sequence in accordance with 9.6.3.4 shall be permitted.

CHAPTER 37 • Existing

**37.4.5.1 Minimum Construction Requirements.** (No requirements.)

**37.4.5.2 Means of Egress Requirements.**

**37.4.5.2.1** All means of egress shall be in accordance with Chapter 7 and this chapter.

**37.4.5.2.2** Not less than 50 percent of the required egress capacity shall be located independent of the main entrance/exit doors.

**37.4.5.3 Storage, Arrangement, Protection, and Quantities of Hazardous Commodities.** The storage, arrangement, protection, and quantities of hazardous commodities shall be in accordance with the applicable provisions of the following:

(1) NFPA 1, *Fire Code*
(2) NFPA 13, *Standard for the Installation of Sprinkler Systems*
(3) NFPA 30, *Flammable and Combustible Liquids Code*
(4) NFPA 30B, *Code for the Manufacture and Storage of Aerosol Products*
(5) NFPA 430, *Code for the Storage of Liquid and Solid Oxidizers*
(6) NFPA 432, *Code for the Storage of Organic Peroxide Formulations*
(7) NFPA 434, *Code for the Storage of Pesticides*
(8) NFPA 1124, *Code for the Manufacture, Transportation, Storage, and Retail Sales of Fireworks and Pyrotechnic Articles*

**37.4.5.4 Detection, Alarm, and Communications Systems.**

**37.4.5.4.1 General.** Bulk merchandising retail buildings shall be provided with a fire alarm system in accordance with Section 9.6.

**37.4.5.4.2 Initiation.** Initiation of the required fire alarm system shall be by means of the required approved automatic sprinkler system *(see 37.4.5.5)* in accordance with 9.6.2.1(3).

**37.4.5.4.3 Occupant Notification.** During all times that the mercantile occupancy is occupied, the required fire alarm system, once initiated, shall perform one of the following functions:

(1) It shall activate an alarm in accordance with 9.6.3 throughout the mercantile occupancy, and positive alarm sequence in accordance with 9.6.3.4 shall be permitted.

CHAPTER 36 • New

36.4.5.4.4 **Emergency Forces Notification.** Emergency forces notification shall be provided and shall include notifying the following:

(1) Fire department in accordance with 9.6.4
(2) Local emergency organization, if provided

**36.4.5.5 Extinguishing Requirements.** Bulk merchandising retail buildings shall be protected throughout by an approved, supervised automatic sprinkler system in accordance with 9.7.1.1(1) and the applicable provisions of the following:

(1) NFPA 1, *Fire Code*
(2) NFPA 13, *Standard for the Installation of Sprinkler Systems*
(3) NFPA 30, *Flammable and Combustible Liquids Code*
(4) NFPA 30B, *Code for the Manufacture and Storage of Aerosol Products*

**36.4.5.6 Emergency Plan and Employee Training.**

**36.4.5.6.1** There shall be in effect an approved written plan for the emergency egress and relocation of occupants.

**36.4.5.6.2** All employees shall be instructed and periodically drilled with respect to their duties under the plan.

CHAPTER 37 • Existing

(2) Occupant notification shall be permitted to be made via a voice communication or public address system in accordance with 9.6.3.9.2.

**37.4.5.4.4 Emergency Forces Notification.** Emergency forces notification shall be provided and shall include notifying the following:

(1) Fire department in accordance with 9.6.4
(2) Local emergency organization, if provided

**37.4.5.5 Extinguishing Requirements.** Bulk merchandising retail buildings shall be protected throughout by an approved, supervised automatic sprinkler system in accordance with 9.7.1.1(1) and the applicable provisions of the following:

(1) NFPA 1, *Fire Code*
(2) NFPA 13, *Standard for the Installation of Sprinkler Systems*
(3) NFPA 30, *Flammable and Combustible Liquids Code*
(4) NFPA 30B, *Code for the Manufacture and Storage of Aerosol Products*

**37.4.5.6 Emergency Plan and Employee Training.**

**37.4.5.6.1** There shall be in effect an approved written plan for the emergency egress and relocation of occupants.

**37.4.5.6.2** All employees shall be instructed and periodically drilled with respect to their duties under the plan.

Bulk merchandising retail buildings provide life safety challenges that differ from typical mercantile occupancies. Fires in bulk merchandising retail buildings demonstrate the need for specific requirements to help ensure the adequate life safety of building occupants. The provisions of 36/37.4.5 apply to new bulk merchandising retail buildings exceeding 12,000 ft$^2$ (1115 m$^2$) and existing facilities exceeding 15,000 ft$^2$ (1400 m$^2$).

The term *bulk merchandising retail building* (see definition in 3.3.32.4) refers to occupancies with storage height in excess of 12 ft (3660 mm), which differentiates such a building from typical mercantile occupancies. If the storage and display of combustible materials exceeds 12 ft (3660 mm) in height, the requirements of 36/37.4.5 are to be applied.

The minimum 16 ft (4875 mm) ceiling height requirement for new construction (see 36.4.5.1) is intended to provide a full 10 ft (3050 mm) of clearance above the heads of building occupants to allow for smoke accumulation early in the fire while building evacuation takes place.

The requirement that not less than 50 percent of the required egress capacity be located independent of the main entrance/exit doors (see 36/37.4.5.2.2) will help provide better distribution of egress capacity around the perimeter of the building, thus providing occupants with multiple, independent routes for egress.

Bulk merchandising retail buildings are characterized by the storage and display of significant quantities of hazardous commodities. Thus, reference is made to numerous NFPA documents that address hazardous materials (see 36/37.4.5.3). Some of the documents include specific requirements that address the display of such materials.

The extinguishing requirements refer to Section 9.7 (see 36/37.4.5.5) and, therefore, adopt the requirements of NFPA 13, *Standard for the Installation of Sprinkler Systems*. In addition, the companion specialized storage standards are mandatorily referenced.

As the history of fires in bulk merchandising retail buildings has shown, it is important to have an approved, written emergency evacuation plan with employees instructed and periodically drilled in their duties (see 36/37.4.5.6).

CHAPTER 36 • New

### 36.4.6 Retail Sales of Consumer Fireworks, 1.4G.

Mercantile occupancies in which the retail sale of consumer fireworks, 1.4G, is conducted shall comply with NFPA 1124, *Code for the Manufacture, Transportation, Storage, and Retail Sales of Fireworks and Pyrotechnic Articles*.

## 36.5 Building Services

### 36.5.1 Utilities.

Utilities shall comply with the provisions of Section 9.1.

### 36.5.2 Heating, Ventilating, and Air-Conditioning.

Heating, ventilating, and air-conditioning equipment shall comply with the provisions of Section 9.2.

### 36.5.3 Elevators, Escalators, and Conveyors.

Elevators, escalators, and conveyors shall comply with the provisions of Section 9.4.

### 36.5.4 Rubbish Chutes, Incinerators, and Laundry Chutes.

Rubbish chutes, incinerators, and laundry chutes shall comply with the provisions of Section 9.5.

## 36.6 Reserved

## 36.7 Operating Features

### 36.7.1 Emergency Plans.

Emergency plans complying with Section 4.8 shall be provided in high-rise buildings.

### 36.7.2 Drills.

In every Class A or Class B mercantile occupancy, employees shall be periodically trained in accordance with Section 4.7.

### 36.7.3 Extinguisher Training.

Employees of mercantile occupancies shall be periodically instructed in the use of portable fire extinguishers.

### 36.7.4 Food Service Operations.

Food service operations shall comply with 12.7.2.

CHAPTER 37 • Existing

### 37.4.6 Retail Sales of Consumer Fireworks, 1.4G.

Mercantile occupancies in which the retail sale of consumer fireworks, 1.4G, is conducted, other than approved existing facilities, shall comply with NFPA 1124, *Code for the Manufacture, Transportation, Storage, and Retail Sales of Fireworks and Pyrotechnic Articles*.

## 37.5 Building Services

### 37.5.1 Utilities.

Utilities shall comply with the provisions of Section 9.1.

### 37.5.2 Heating, Ventilating, and Air-Conditioning.

Heating, ventilating, and air-conditioning equipment shall comply with the provisions of Section 9.2.

### 37.5.3 Elevators, Escalators, and Conveyors.

Elevators, escalators, and conveyors shall comply with the provisions of Section 9.4.

### 37.5.4 Rubbish Chutes, Incinerators, and Laundry Chutes.

Rubbish chutes, incinerators, and laundry chutes shall comply with the provisions of Section 9.5.

## 37.6 Reserved

## 37.7 Operating Features

### 37.7.1 Emergency Plans.

Emergency plans complying with Section 4.8 shall be provided in high-rise buildings.

### 37.7.2 Drills.

In every Class A or Class B mercantile occupancy, employees shall be periodically trained in accordance with Section 4.7.

### 37.7.3 Extinguisher Training.

Employees of mercantile occupancies shall be periodically instructed in the use of portable fire extinguishers.

### 37.7.4 Food Service Operations.

Food service operations shall comply with 13.7.2.

**36.7.5 Upholstered Furniture and Mattresses.**

The provisions of 10.3.2 shall not apply to upholstered furniture and mattresses.

**37.7.5 Upholstered Furniture and Mattresses.**

The provisions of 10.3.2 shall not apply to upholstered furniture and mattresses.

The authority having jurisdiction (AHJ) determines the extent of the extinguisher training required by 36/37.7.3 (e.g., instruction only or instruction and hands-on use).

## References Cited in Commentary


1. NFPA 30, *Flammable and Combustible Liquids Code,* 2008 edition, National Fire Protection Association, Quincy, MA.
2. NFPA 13, *Standard for the Installation of Sprinkler Systems,* 2007 edition, National Fire Protection Association, Quincy, MA.
3. NFPA 25, *Standard for the Inspection, Testing, and Maintenance of Water-Based Fire Protection Systems,* 2008 edition, National Fire Protection Association, Quincy, MA.
4. Bryan, J. L., *Automatic Sprinkler and Standpipe Systems,* 3d edition, National Fire Protection Association, Quincy, MA, 1997.
5. NFPA 92B, *Standard for Smoke Management Systems in Malls, Atria, and Large Spaces,* 2009 edition, National Fire Protection Association, Quincy, MA.

CHAPTERS 38 AND 39

# New and Existing Business Occupancies

Persons who are awake and ready to begin emergency egress or relocation, with little or no staff assistance, as soon as they become aware of a fire typically occupy business occupancies. Historical evidence validates that the package of life safety features imposed on business occupancies by the *Code* doesn't need to be very extensive. Nonetheless, several notable multiple-death fires have occurred in business occupancies in the United States in recent years. (The term *multiple-death* means three or more fatalities for the purpose of fire data analysis.)

On October 17, 2003, a fire broke out on the twelfth floor of the 37-story, nonsprinklered Cook County Administration Building in Chicago, Illinois. Six occupants perished after becoming trapped in an exit stair. On February 9, 2000, a fire took place in a 3-story (with a basement), partially sprinklered building in Newton, Massachusetts, and resulted in five deaths. The fire, of undetermined cause, started in a second-floor nonsprinklered office. Smoke spread quickly throughout the building, making escape impossible for those victims who perished. Another noteworthy fire resulting in five deaths took place in an Atlanta, Georgia, high-rise office building in 1989. One of the fire victims was intimate with the fire source in an electrical vault; the other four victims were occupying their areas on the same floor when the fire began. This was the first office building fire in 17 years to result in more than three fatalities.

The bombing of the Alfred Murrah Federal Office Building in Oklahoma City, Oklahoma, in 1995 killed 168 people and injured 475. The bomb caused about one-third of the floor area of the nine-story building to collapse. The September 11, 2001, attacks on the World Trade Center in New York City and the Pentagon in Arlington, Virginia, killed some 2800 and 125 building occupants, respectively. Thousands more were injured. The *Code* cannot protect against the effects of terrorist attacks, such as the bombing of a building, or the intentional collision of a commercial airliner into a building. Such incidents will, however, continue to be discussed by code-development organizations for many years to come.

It is common for business occupancies to occupy high-rise buildings. Where business occupancies are located in new high-rise buildings, the complete protection package detailed in Section 11.8 is mandated; for existing business occupancies in high-rise buildings, either sprinkler protection or an engineered life safety system that provides protection equivalent to that of sprinklers is required.

The life safety features in Chapters 38 and 39 center on arrangement of the means of egress as well as alarm and occupant notification provisions. The travel distance and common path of travel allowances are generous. Fire resistance–rated corridor walls or other mitigating features, such as sprinkler protection, are required in an effort to keep the means of egress system usable.

## 38.1 General Requirements

### 38.1.1 Application.

**38.1.1.1** The requirements of this chapter shall apply to new buildings or portions thereof used as business occupancies. *(See 1.3.1.)*

## 39.1 General Requirements

### 39.1.1 Application.

**39.1.1.1** The requirements of this chapter shall apply to existing buildings or portions thereof currently occupied as business occupancies.

CHAPTER 38 • New

**38.1.1.2** The provisions of this chapter shall apply to life safety requirements for all new business buildings.

**38.1.1.3** Additions to existing buildings shall conform to the requirements of 4.6.8. Existing portions of the structure shall not be required to be modified, provided that the new construction has not diminished the fire safety features of the facility.

CHAPTER 39 • Existing

**39.1.1.2** The provisions of this chapter shall apply to life safety requirements for existing business buildings. Specific requirements shall apply to high-rise buildings *(see definition in 3.3.32.7)* and are contained in paragraphs pertaining thereto.

The provisions for new business occupancies are addressed in Chapter 38; the provisions for existing business occupancies (i.e., existing conditions in business occupancies) are addressed in Chapter 39.

In prior editions of the *Code*, renovations, additions, and changes of occupancy were required to comply with the requirements for new construction. For business occupancies, such renovations, additions, and changes of occupancy were required to meet the provisions of Chapter 38, while existing conditions were subject to the provisions of Chapter 39. Chapter 43, Building Rehabilitation, was added for the 2006 edition of the *Code*. Chapter 43 was written to promote the adaptive reuse of existing buildings without sacrificing the needed level of life safety. The provisions of Chapter 43 blend the requirements for new construction with those for existing conditions, so as to require additional life safety features as the rehabilitation work category increases in complexity. The rehabilitation work categories are repair, renovation, modification, reconstruction, change of use or occupancy classification, and addition. See 4.6.8, 4.6.12, and Chapter 43.

To understand the full intent and scope of 39.1.1.1 for existing buildings, it is necessary to review it concurrently with Sections 1.2 and 1.3. Although a building code might exclude existing buildings from coverage under some form of a grandfather clause, the *Life Safety Code*, by virtue of its interest in safety to life, does not condone existing building arrangements that do not comply with the *Code* requirements that apply to existing buildings. The requirements that apply to existing business occupancies are contained in Chapter 39.

If a building complies with an earlier edition of the *Code*, it is not grandfathered and, thereby, exempted from compliance with a more current edition of the *Code* that has been adopted as law in the building's jurisdiction. The NFPA technical committees on safety to life are especially careful to avoid adopting requirements for existing buildings that become more stringent from one edition of the *Code* to the next, unless the change is absolutely necessary to enhance the overall package of safety to life intended by the *Code*. Thus, the old adage of "once in compliance, always in compliance" does not hold.

The provisions of Chapter 39 are intended to be applied retroactively. Due consideration has been given to the practical difficulties of making alterations in existing functioning facilities. The specified provisions, viewed as a whole, establish minimum, acceptable criteria for safety to life that reasonably minimize the likelihood of a life-threatening fire.

The requirements of Chapter 39 are permitted to be modified in instances where compliance is impractical or where alternate but equal provisions are proposed. The modifications must provide a level of protection equivalent to that achieved by compliance with the corresponding *Code* provisions. Note that Section 1.4 permits alternatives to literal *Code* compliance that maintain a building design as *Code* conforming. However, the authority having jurisdiction (AHJ) ultimately determines whether equivalent safety has been provided.

The *Code* does not limit the methods that an AHJ might use to determine equivalency. However, NFPA 101A, *Guide on Alternative Approaches to Life Safety,*[1] provides an equivalency system that uses numerical values to analyze the fire safety effectiveness of a building design. This system, known as the Fire Safety Evaluation System (FSES), provides a method by which alternative designs can be evaluated as options to literal *Code* compliance.

The 2010 edition of NFPA 101A, although published one year after the 2009 edition of the *Life Safety Code,* is the proper edition of NFPA 101A to consult for one potential equivalency system for business occupancies. Its measurement system has been calibrated against the requirements of the 2009 edition of the *Code*, whereas the fire safety evaluation systems contained in the 2007 edition of NFPA 101A were calibrated against the requirements of the 2006 edition of the *Code*.

In providing the equivalency concept, the *Code* does not limit equivalency evaluations to those based solely on the system presented for business occupancies in NFPA 101A. The AHJ retains the power to evaluate and approve alternative designs on the basis of appropriate supporting data. The FSES is permitted to be used to aid in this evaluation. Use of the FSES is in no way mandated, nor is the AHJ required to accept the results of an evaluation using the NFPA 101A equivalency system.

Although the FSES was primarily developed to evaluate alternative designs in existing buildings, it is particularly useful for determining equivalency for conversions, modernizations, renovations, or unusual design concepts. However, the FSES is only a tool to help determine equivalency — it should not be used to circumvent *Code* requirements. *Code* requirements must be met, or equivalent safety must be provided by alternative means approved by the AHJ.

Additions to existing buildings are addressed by 38.1.1.3. Although construction of an addition generally does not require existing portions of the building to be modified, Exhibit 38/39.1 illustrates a case where the planned new construction would diminish the fire safety features of the existing building and, thus, necessitate corrective action within the existing portion of the building. The location of new room A creates an excessively long dead-end corridor, B, which must be corrected.

In Exhibit 38/39.1, in addition to creating an unacceptable dead-end corridor, the construction of room A diminishes the fire safety features in two other ways; however, both are negligible and do not warrant correction. The door from corridor B into room A was formerly an exit door to the outside. Thus, with the new addition, the number of exits has been decreased from three to two; also, the travel distance for occupants in some of the rooms off corridor B has been increased, because the nearest exit for those occupants becomes the pair of doors at the front of the building (i.e., at the bottom of the exhibit). If the occupant load of the floor doesn't exceed 500 persons, only two exits are required (see 7.4.1.2), and the loss of one of the three exits is permitted without further correction. Also, if the maximum allowable travel distance [200 ft (61 m) where the building is not sprinklered or 300 ft (91 m) where the building is sprinklered, in accordance with 38/39.2.6] is not exceeded, the travel distance increase caused by the addition of room A is permitted without further correction. Thus, only the newly created, excessively long dead-end corridor needs to be corrected.

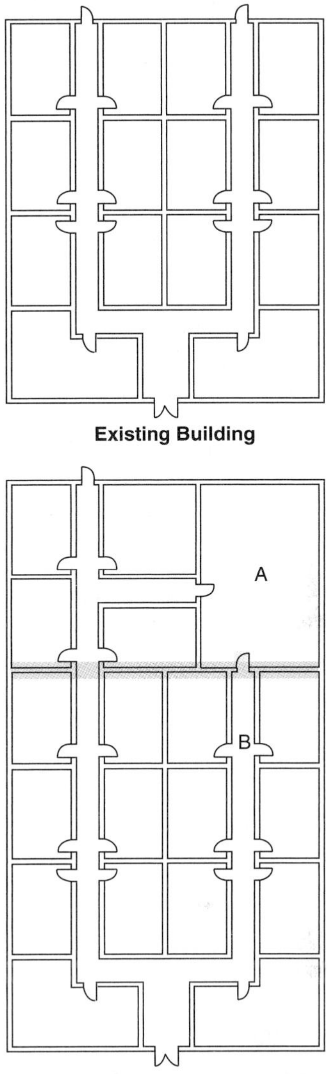


***Exhibit 38/39.1*** *An addition that diminishes existing life safety features.*

### 38.1.2 Multiple Occupancies.

#### 38.1.2.1 General.

**38.1.2.1.1** All multiple occupancies shall be in accordance with 6.1.14 and 38.1.2.

### 39.1.2 Multiple Occupancies.

#### 39.1.2.1 General.

**39.1.2.1.1** All multiple occupancies shall be in accordance with 6.1.14 and 39.1.2.

CHAPTER 38 • New

**38.1.2.1.2** Where there are differences in the specific requirements in this chapter and provisions for mixed occupancies or separated occupancies as specified in 6.1.14.3 and 6.1.14.4, the requirements of this chapter shall apply.

**38.1.2.2 Combined Business Occupancies and Parking Structures.**

**38.1.2.2.1** The fire barrier separating parking structures from a building classified as a business occupancy shall be a fire barrier having a minimum 2-hour fire resistance rating.

**38.1.2.2.2** Openings in the fire barrier required by 38.1.2.2.1 shall not be required to be protected with fire protection–rated opening protectives in enclosed parking structures that are protected throughout by an approved, supervised automatic sprinkler system in accordance with 9.7.1.1(1), or in open parking structures, provided that all of the following conditions are met:

(1) The openings do not exceed 25 percent of the area of the fire barrier in which they are located.
(2) The openings are used as a public entrance and for associated sidelight functions.
(3) The building containing the business occupancy is protected throughout by an approved, supervised automatic sprinkler system in accordance with 9.7.1.1(1).
(4)* Means are provided to prevent spilled fuel from accumulating adjacent to the openings and entering the building.

**A.38.1.2.2.2(4)** Means to prevent spilled fuel from accumulating and entering the business occupancy building can be by curbs, scuppers, special drainage systems, sloping the floor away from the door openings, or elevation differences not less than 4 in. (100 mm).

(5) Physical means are provided to prevent vehicles from being parked or driven within 10 ft (3050 mm) of the openings.
(6) The openings are protected as a smoke partition in accordance with Section 8.4, with no minimum fire protection rating required.

CHAPTER 39 • Existing

**39.1.2.1.2** Where there are differences in the specific requirements in this chapter and provisions for mixed occupancies or separated occupancies as specified in 6.1.14.3 and 6.1.14.4, the requirements of this chapter shall apply.

**39.1.2.2 Combined Business Occupancies and Parking Structures.**

**39.1.2.2.1** The fire barrier separating parking structures from a building classified as a business occupancy shall be a fire barrier having a minimum 2-hour fire resistance rating.

**39.1.2.2.2** Openings in the fire barrier required by 39.1.2.2.1 shall not be required to be protected with fire protection–rated opening protectives in enclosed parking structures that are protected throughout by an approved, supervised automatic sprinkler system in accordance with 9.7.1.1(1), or in open parking structures, provided that all of the following conditions are met:

(1) The openings do not exceed 25 percent of the area of the fire barrier in which they are located.
(2) The openings are used as a public entrance and for associated sidelight functions.
(3) The building containing the business occupancy is protected throughout by an approved, supervised automatic sprinkler system in accordance with 9.7.1.1(1).
(4)* Means are provided to prevent spilled fuel from accumulating adjacent to the openings and entering the building.

**A.39.1.2.2.2(4)** Means to prevent spilled fuel from accumulating and entering the business occupancy building can be by curbs, scuppers, special drainage systems, sloping the floor away from the door openings, or elevation differences not less than 4 in. (100 mm).

(5) Physical means are provided to prevent vehicles from being parked or driven within 10 ft (3050 mm) of the openings.
(6) The openings are protected as a smoke partition in accordance with Section 8.4, with no minimum fire protection rating required.

Minor office occupancies that are incidental to operations in another occupancy are considered incidental to the predominant occupancy, rather than part of a mixed occupancy, and are subject to the *Code* provisions that apply to the predominant occupancy. The commentary associated with 38/39.1.4, which follows 38/39.1.7, discusses classification of business occupancies in more detail.

The determination of those criteria that constitute a minor or incidental office area cannot be based solely on percentage of business area in comparison to overall building area. For example, a 200 $ft^2$ (19 $m^2$) office area in a 4000 $ft^2$ (370 $m^2$) warehouse can reasonably be judged as incidental to the storage operations and result in the building being classified as a storage occupancy. However, a 20,000 $ft^2$ (1860 $m^2$) office area in a 400,000 $ft^2$ (37,200 $m^2$) distribution warehouse represents the same proportion of business use but cannot be judged as incidental (see Exhibit 38/39.2). The 20,000 $ft^2$ (1860 $m^2$) office area probably has an occu-

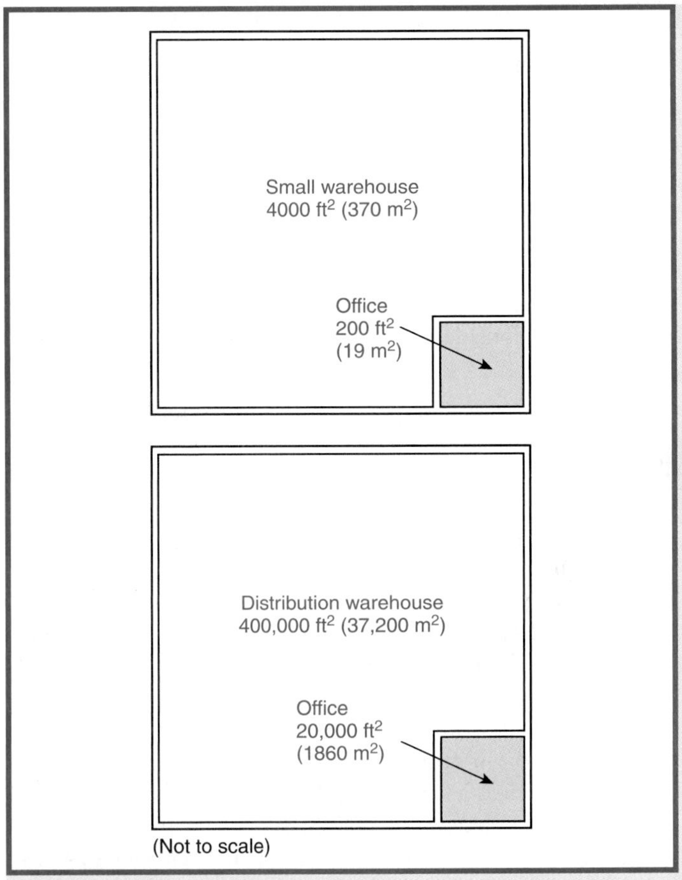


***Exhibit 38/39.2*** *Incidental and nonincidental office use.*

pant load of approximately 200 persons. The *Code* requirements that apply to business occupancies, which are more stringent than those that apply to storage occupancies, are needed to protect the occupants of the office area adequately. The distribution warehouse is classified as a multiple occupancy that is part storage occupancy and part business occupancy. If packaging operations take place in the warehouse, it might also be classified as part industrial occupancy. Consequently, the requirements of 6.1.14 for either mixed or separated multiple occupancies apply.

The provisions of 38/39.1.2.2 address combined business occupancies and parking structures and are very similar to the requirements of 36/37.1.2.2, which address combined mercantile occupancies and parking structures. It is very common for multistory business occupancies, such as office buildings, and multistory mercantile occupancies, such as department stores and shopping mall buildings, to be attached to multistory parking garages. These garages provide access to the business or mercantile occupancy at multiple levels. The provisions of 38/39.1.2.2.2 outline a set of provisions that, if applied in total, will safely permit a reduction in the 2-hour fire resistance–rated separation requirement of 38/39.1.2.2.1. This reduction allows flexibility in the number and types of openings and considers the stringent requirements for opening protectives, such as fire doors and windows. The reduction also permits the use of nonrated glazing and opening protectives, which permits the use of glass doors and sidelights in the barrier between the business occupancy and the garage. Security in the garage is thereby increased, because occupants can view the area through the glass doors or sidelights. This feature, in turn, helps to meet the security concerns of office building managers and tenants.

Note that all seven requirements mandated by 38/39.1.2.2.2 — the sprinkler requirement for enclosed garages per the base paragraph and its six subparts — must be met as a whole to apply the exemption. Otherwise, a 2-hour fire resistance–rated separation between the business occupancy and the parking structure is required.

### 38.1.3 Special Definitions.

Special terms applicable to this chapter are defined in Chapter 3.

### 38.1.4 Classification of Occupancy.

Business occupancies shall include all buildings and structures or parts thereof with occupancy as defined in 6.1.11.

### 38.1.5 Classification of Hazard of Contents.

The contents of business occupancies shall be classified as ordinary hazard in accordance with Section 6.2.

### 39.1.3 Special Definitions.

Special terms applicable to this chapter are defined in Chapter 3.

### 39.1.4 Classification of Occupancy.

Business occupancies shall include all buildings and structures or parts thereof with occupancy as defined in 6.1.11.

### 39.1.5 Classification of Hazard of Contents.

The contents of business occupancies shall be classified as ordinary hazard in accordance with Section 6.2.

CHAPTER 38 • New

### 38.1.6 Minimum Construction Requirements.

(No requirements.)

### 38.1.7 Occupant Load.

The occupant load, in number of persons for whom means of egress and other provisions are required, shall be determined on the basis of the occupant load factors of Table 7.3.1.2 that are characteristic of the use of the space, or shall be determined as the maximum probable population of the space under consideration, whichever is greater.

CHAPTER 39 • Existing

### 39.1.6 Minimum Construction Requirements.

(No requirements.)

### 39.1.7 Occupant Load.

The occupant load, in number of persons for whom means of egress and other provisions are required, shall be determined on the basis of the occupant load factors of Table 7.3.1.2 that are characteristic of the use of the space, or shall be determined as the maximum probable population of the space under consideration, whichever is greater.

Paragraph 38/39.1.4 addresses classification of occupancy.

Per the *Code*'s definition of a business occupancy (see 6.1.11.1), an occupancy used for the transaction of business (other than that classified as a mercantile occupancy) is covered by the provisions of Chapters 38 and 39.

Business occupancies include doctors' offices, dentists' offices (see Chapters 20 and 21 for ambulatory health care occupancies), and general offices, as well as city halls, town halls, and courthouses, all of which have areas for keeping books and records and transacting business. Other occupancies included under the definition of business occupancies are service facilities common to office buildings, such as newsstands, lunch counters (with seating areas for fewer than 50 people), barber shops, and beauty parlors.

Birth centers occupied by fewer than four patients, not including infants, at any one time are classified as business occupancies in accordance with the guidelines of A.6.1.11.1 and the definition of the term *birth center* in 3.3.29 and its corresponding annex text in A.3.3.29.

Note that the *Code*'s definition of a business occupancy does not include types of stores that, although considered businesses, are covered under the provisions of Chapters 36 and 37. For example, supermarkets, department stores, and other occupancies that display and sell merchandise would not be considered business occupancies. Neither would the assembly portions of city halls, town halls, and courthouses with seating for 50 or more people, which are covered by Chapters 12 and 13.

Classification of hazard of contents is addressed in 38/39.1.5. Most occupancy chapters refer to Section 6.2 for classification of hazard of contents. However, the requirement of 38/39.1.5 emphasizes that, unless an extraordinarily hazardous situation exists, the contents of business occupancies are to be classified as ordinary hazard. This requirement is intended to prevent the user from classifying the hazard of contents as high hazard, except where a combustible load far in excess of the usual, yet considerable, quantity of boxed records and paper files exists. Isolated hazardous contents areas within the overall ordinary hazard business occupancy, such as storage rooms, must be protected or separated in accordance with the requirements of 38/39.3.2.

Building contents classified by the *Code* as ordinary hazard for the purpose of life safety are not always classified as ordinary hazard by other codes or standards, such as NFPA 13, *Standard for the Installation of Sprinkler Systems*.[2] For purposes of sprinkler system design, the anticipated fuel load of business occupancies is classified as light hazard.

There are no construction requirements for business occupancies; therefore, 38/39.1.6 serves as a placeholder. Some occupancy chapters, such as Chapters 18 and 19, which address the life safety needs of nonambulatory health care occupants, require a minimum building construction type to help ensure the structural integrity required for a lengthy evacuation or for safe refuge within the building. Because business occupancies are normally occupied by those who are ambulatory, and because they do not typically provide sleeping accommodations, no minimum construction requirements are imposed.

Subsection 38/39.1.7 references Table 7.3.1.2 for determining the occupant load factors that apply to the use areas of a business occupancy. Because the number of people expected to occupy certain types of office buildings can be determined with a great degree of accuracy (such as by means of a company's detailed account of its office space), it might be beneficial to compare such an occupant load with an occupant load calculated on the basis of one person per 100 $ft^2$ (9.3 $m^2$) of gross floor area (see Table 7.3.1.2). In office occupancies where people work in highly concentrated groups (such as a customer service call center or secretarial pool area), the actual number of people occupying a space might exceed the figure calculated by gross area. As emphasized in Section 7.3, where such a situation exists, the egress capacity must be designed to accommodate the actual (larger) occupant load. Note that the converse is not true; that is, if the actual occupant load is less than the gross area calculation, the *Code* still requires that the gross area calculation (i.e., the larger occupant load) be used to determine the occupant load for which the egress capacity must be provided.

## 38.2 Means of Egress Requirements

### 38.2.1 General.

**38.2.1.1** All means of egress shall be in accordance with Chapter 7 and this chapter.

**38.2.1.2** If, owing to differences in grade, any street floor exits are at points above or below the street or the finished ground level, such exits shall comply with the provisions for exits from upper floors or floors below the street floor.

**38.2.1.3** Stairs and ramps serving two or more floors below a street floor occupied for business use shall be permitted in accordance with 38.2.1.3.1 and 38.2.1.3.2.

**38.2.1.3.1** Where two or more floors below the street floor are occupied for business use, the same stairs or ramps shall be permitted to serve each.

**38.2.1.3.2** An inside open stairway or inside open ramp shall be permitted to serve as a required egress facility from not more than one floor level below the street floor.

**38.2.1.4** Floor levels that are below the street floor; are used only for storage, heating, and other service equipment; and are not subject to business occupancy shall have means of egress in accordance with Chapter 42.



## 39.2 Means of Egress Requirements

### 39.2.1 General.

**39.2.1.1** All means of egress shall be in accordance with Chapter 7 and this chapter.

**39.2.1.2** If, owing to differences in grade, any street floor exits are at points above or below the street or the finished ground level, such exits shall comply with the provisions for exits from upper floors or floors below the street floor.

**39.2.1.3** Stairs and ramps serving two or more floors below a street floor occupied for business use shall be permitted in accordance with 39.2.1.3.1 and 39.2.1.3.2.

**39.2.1.3.1** Where two or more floors below the street floor are occupied for business use, the same stairs, escalators, or ramps shall be permitted to serve each.

**39.2.1.3.2** An inside open stairway, inside open escalator, or inside open ramp shall be permitted to serve as a required egress facility from not more than one floor level below the street floor.

**39.2.1.4** Floor levels that are below the street floor; are used only for storage, heating, and other service equipment; and are not subject to business occupancy shall have means of egress in accordance with Chapter 42.

Exhibit 38/39.3 illustrates a case where two floors qualify as street floors in accordance with 38/39.2.1.2, because each floor has one side located at a ground level. Note, however, that each of the two floors has its other sides located either above or below the building's other ground level. As a result, floors 1 and 2 must have their exits arranged to allow horizontal travel to the exterior at one end of the floor and vertical travel (either up or down to ground level) at the other end of the floor. The egress capacity of the doors to the exterior on floor 1 must accommodate that portion of the occupant load from an upper floor that is expected to travel down to and through the exits to the exterior from floor 1. This portion of the occupant load is to be added to the portion of the floor 1 occupant load assigned to a given exit. The reverse is true for floor 2, which must increase the size of its exterior exit capacity to accommodate occupants traveling up from floor 1, as well as those traveling down to and through the exterior exits on floor 2. The provisions of 7.3.1.5, 7.3.1.6, and 38/39.2.3.3 explain how to add egress capacity based on the number of occupants expected to discharge from floors above and below the street floor.

Paragraph 38/39.2.1.3.2 prohibits the use of unenclosed interior stairs or unenclosed interior ramps as exit access for more than one floor below the street

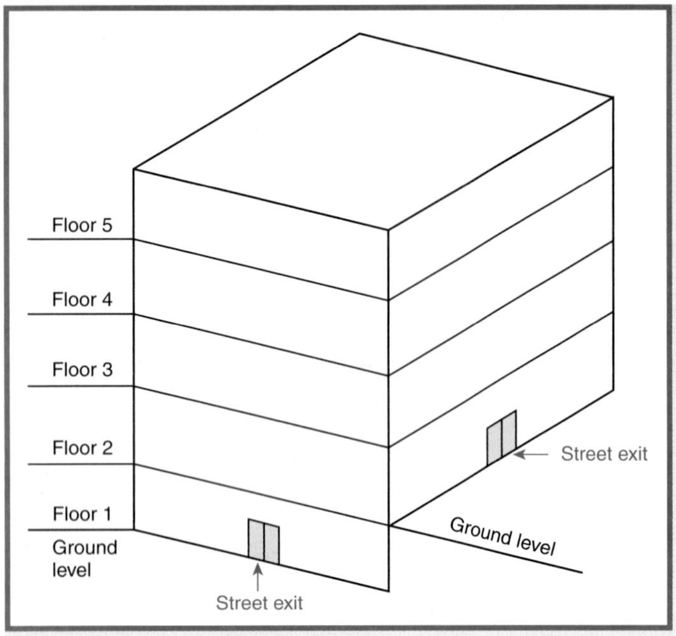


***Exhibit 38/39.3** Business occupancy with two street floors.*

floor; it does not establish permission for the presence of an open stairway or open ramp. See 38/39.3.1, which addresses the protection of vertical openings in business occupancies, to determine if the stair or ramp is permitted to be unenclosed. The floor with the largest occupant load is used to determine the required width of the stair or ramp serving multiple floors. This requirement ensures that a stair or other component of a means of egress will accommodate its assigned portion of the population of any floor it serves.

The implementation of 38/39.2.1.4 results in a significant reduction in the number and size of exits for floors located below the street floor that are used only for storage or for heating and service equipment and that are not subject to business occupancy use. These reductions are permitted, because the expected population of such floors will be well below that of a floor used as a typical business occupancy. Also see Section 7.12, which specifically regulates means of egress from boiler rooms and similar spaces.

### 38.2.2 Means of Egress Components.

**38.2.2.1 Components Permitted.** Means of egress components shall be limited to the types described in 38.2.2.2 through 38.2.2.12.

**38.2.2.2 Doors.**

**38.2.2.2.1** Doors complying with 7.2.1 shall be permitted.

**38.2.2.2.2*** Locks complying with 7.2.1.5.4 shall be permitted only on principal entrance/exit doors.

**A.38.2.2.2.2** The words "principal entrance/exit doors" describe doors that the authority having jurisdiction can reasonably expect to be unlocked in order for the facility to do business.

**38.2.2.2.3** Elevator lobby exit access door-locking arrangements in accordance with 7.2.1.6.3 shall be permitted.

**38.2.2.2.4 Reserved.**

### 39.2.2 Means of Egress Components.

**39.2.2.1 Components Permitted.** Means of egress components shall be limited to the types described in 39.2.2.2 through 39.2.2.12.

**39.2.2.2 Doors.**

**39.2.2.2.1** Doors complying with 7.2.1 shall be permitted.

**39.2.2.2.2*** Locks complying with 7.2.1.5.4 shall be permitted only on principal entrance/exit doors.

**A.39.2.2.2.2** The words "principal entrance/exit doors" describe doors that the authority having jurisdiction can reasonably expect to be unlocked in order for the facility to do business.

**39.2.2.2.3** Elevator lobby exit access door-locking arrangements in accordance with 7.2.1.6.3 shall be permitted.

**39.2.2.2.4** The re-entry provisions of 7.2.1.5.7 shall not apply to the following:

(1) Existing business occupancies that are not high-rise buildings
(2) Existing high-rise business occupancy buildings that are protected throughout by an approved automatic sprinkler system in accordance with 9.7.1.1(1)
(3) Existing high-rise business occupancy buildings having approved existing means for providing stair re-entry

CHAPTER 38 • New

**38.2.2.2.5** Delayed-egress locks complying with 7.2.1.6.1 shall be permitted.

**38.2.2.2.6** Access-controlled egress doors complying with 7.2.1.6.2 shall be permitted.

**38.2.2.2.7** Horizontal or vertical security grilles or doors complying with 7.2.1.4.1(3) shall be permitted to be used as part of the required means of egress from a tenant space.

**38.2.2.2.8 Reserved.**

**38.2.2.2.9** Revolving doors complying with 7.2.1.10 shall be permitted.

CHAPTER 39 • Existing

**39.2.2.2.5** Delayed-egress locks complying with 7.2.1.6.1 shall be permitted.

**39.2.2.2.6** Access-controlled egress doors complying with 7.2.1.6.2 shall be permitted.

**39.2.2.2.7** Horizontal or vertical security grilles or doors complying with 7.2.1.4(3) shall be permitted to be used as part of the required means of egress from a tenant space.

**39.2.2.2.8** Approved existing horizontal-sliding or vertical-rolling fire doors shall be permitted in means of egress under the following conditions:

(1) They are held open by fusible links.
(2) The fusible links are rated at not less than 165°F (74°C).
(3) The fusible links are located not more than 10 ft (3050 mm) above the floor.
(4) The fusible links are in immediate proximity to the door opening.
(5) The fusible links are not located above a ceiling.
(6) The door is not credited with providing any protection under this *Code*.

**39.2.2.2.9** Revolving doors complying with 7.2.1.10 shall be permitted.

Only the principal entrance/exit doors of a business occupancy are permitted by 38/39.2.2.2.2 to be equipped with the special key-operated lock described by the provisions of 7.2.1.5.4. It must be easy to determine that the device is locked by using means such as a flag indicator that can be seen at a distance from the door. Other doors along the perimeter of the building are prohibited from being equipped with a key-operated lock, because it cannot be guaranteed that these doors will be unlocked when the principal entrance/exit door is unlocked each day when the occupancy opens to the public for business. See Exhibit 38/39.4 for an example of the principal entrance/exit in a business occupancy.

Prior to the 2009 edition of the *Code*, all elevator lobbies were required to provide direct access to not less than one exit (typically a stair) without requiring occupants to pass through any space subject to locking. The 2009 edition introduces the concept of elevator lobby exit access door-locking arrangements in 7.2.1.6.3. The new criteria permit elevators to open to lobbies that are secured from the remainder of the floor; to reach an exit, occupants in the elevator lobby are required to go through the secured area. The requirements of 7.2.1.6.3, which include the installation of an approved, supervised automatic sprinkler system throughout the building, ensure that the doors will unlock to allow occupants to reach an exit in the event of a fire. The provisions of 7.2.1.6.3 are permitted to be used only where specifically referenced by the applicable occupancy chapter; such arrangement is

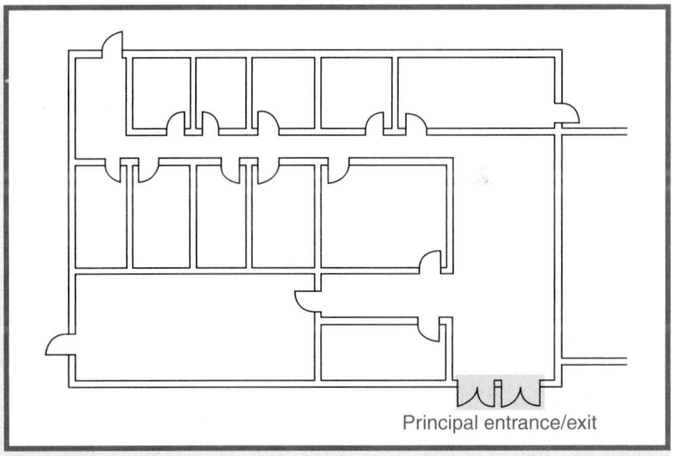


***Exhibit 38/39.4*** *Principal entrance/exit.*

permitted in business occupancies by 38/39.2.2.2.3. See 7.2.1.6.3 and its associated commentary for additional details on elevator lobby exit access door-locking arrangements.

Note that, per 39.2.2.2.4, existing business occupancies that are not high-rise buildings are exempt from the re-entry provisions of 7.2.1.5.7, which apply to exit stair enclosure doors. Existing high-rise business occupancies are required to be provided with stairway re-entry in accordance with 7.2.1.5.7, unless the building is sprinklered or the building is provided with an approved existing means for providing re-entry. The criteria applicable to existing high-rise business occupancies are new to the 2009 edition of the *Code* and were added in direct response to the 2003 Cook County Administration Building fire in Chicago that resulted in six deaths. The fire occurred on the twelfth floor of the 37-story, nonsprinklered high-rise building. The exit stairs were provided with no means for re-entry to the building — an arrangement previously permitted by the *Code* for all existing business occupancies. The six victims all perished when they became trapped in an exit stair and encountered heavy smoke. The subsequent fire investigation determined that the fatalities could have been prevented if the building had been sprinklered or if stairway re-entry had been provided; thus, 39.2.2.2.4 requires existing high-rise business occupancies to be provided with sprinkler protection or stairway re-entry. It is noted that this requirement is intended to be provided retroactively; existing buildings without such provision are not grandfathered. See 4.6.6 for details on the time allowed for compliance for existing buildings. All new business occupancies must meet the re-entry provisions of 7.2.1.5.7; thus, 38.2.2.2.4 is reserved as a placeholder.

The use of the delayed-egress lock covered by 7.2.1.6.1 is permitted on any door by 38/39.2.2.2.5 in recognition of the security needs of a business occupancy. Per 7.2.1.6.1, the building must be protected throughout by an approved, supervised automatic sprinkler system or an approved, supervised automatic fire detection system. In effect, the allowable 15-second or 30-second delay will be experienced only under non-fire conditions or very early in a fire's growth, because the door must be usable immediately upon sprinkler operation, smoke or heat detection, or loss of power that controls the locking mechanism.

Access-controlled egress doors in business occupancies are recognized by 38/39.2.2.2.6 as security measures that do not compromise the use of the means of egress system, provided that they meet the criteria specified in 7.2.1.6.2.

Paragraph 7.2.1.4.1(3) establishes provisions for the arrangement and use of horizontal or vertical security grilles or doors if such features are specifically recognized by an occupancy chapter. For business occupancies, such recognition is provided by 38/39.2.2.2.7.

Horizontal-sliding or vertical-rolling fire doors exist in many business occupancies for purposes of property protection. Although the *Code* normally does not recognize these doors within the required means of egress, 39.2.2.2.8 provides a special exemption for existing horizontal-sliding or vertical-rolling fire doors. By requiring the fusible link to be positioned in immediate proximity to the door opening, rated 165°F (74°C) or higher, and located not more than 10 ft (3050 mm) above the floor, the *Code* helps to ensure that the door will remain open until rising temperatures make it unsafe to pass through the door opening. The door will not close early in the fire development; therefore, it cannot be credited as a fire door for life safety purposes. However, the door might serve for property protection. See Exhibit 38/39.5 for an example of an existing vertical-rolling fire door as permitted by 39.2.2.2.8.

Paragraph 38/39.2.2.2.9 addresses revolving doors. The provisions of 7.2.1.10 specify that the use of a revolving door, regardless of whether it is permitted as part of the required means of egress, requires a con-

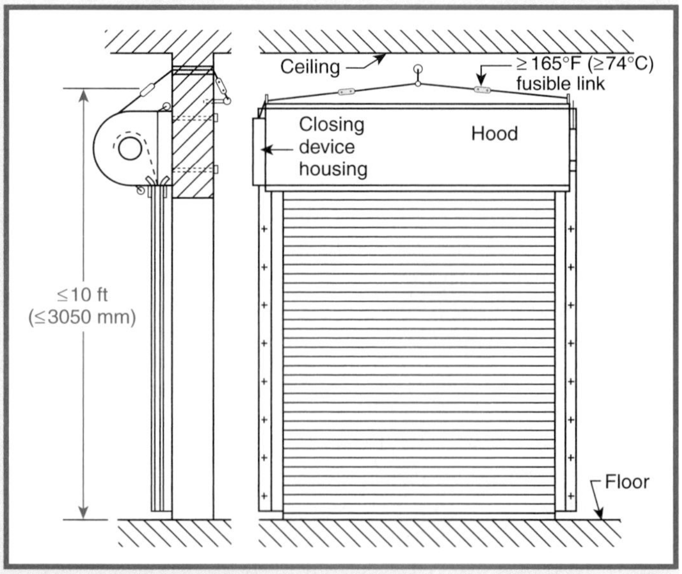


***Exhibit 38/39.5*** *Existing vertical-rolling fire door in accordance with 39.2.2.2.7.*

CHAPTER 38 • New

forming side-hinged swinging door to be positioned and usable within the same wall as, and to be located within 10 ft (3050 mm) of, the revolving door. This requirement helps to ensure that, once people move toward the door, if the collapsibility and other safety features of the door fail and render it unusable, egress from the vicinity would still be possible without retracing steps and requiring travel toward the fire.

**38.2.2.3 Stairs.**

**38.2.2.3.1** Stairs complying with 7.2.2 shall be permitted.

**38.2.2.3.2** Spiral stairs complying with 7.2.2.2.3 shall be permitted.

**38.2.2.4 Smokeproof Enclosures.** Smokeproof enclosures complying with 7.2.3 shall be permitted.

**38.2.2.5 Horizontal Exits.** Horizontal exits complying with 7.2.4 shall be permitted.

**38.2.2.6 Ramps.** Ramps complying with 7.2.5 shall be permitted.

**38.2.2.7 Exit Passageways.** Exit passageways complying with 7.2.6 shall be permitted.

**38.2.2.8 Reserved.**

**38.2.2.9 Reserved.**

**38.2.2.10 Fire Escape Ladders.** Fire escape ladders complying with 7.2.9 shall be permitted.

**38.2.2.11 Alternating Tread Devices.** Alternating tread devices complying with 7.2.11 shall be permitted.

**38.2.2.12 Areas of Refuge.**

**38.2.2.12.1** Areas of refuge complying with 7.2.12 shall be permitted.

**38.2.2.12.2** In buildings protected throughout by an approved, supervised automatic sprinkler system in accordance with 9.7.1.1(1), two rooms or spaces separated from each other by smoke-resistant partitions in accordance with the definition of area of refuge in 3.3.20 shall not be required.

CHAPTER 39 • Existing

**39.2.2.3 Stairs.**

**39.2.2.3.1** Stairs complying with 7.2.2 shall be permitted.

**39.2.2.3.2** Spiral stairs complying with 7.2.2.2.3 shall be permitted.

**39.2.2.3.3** Winders complying with 7.2.2.2.4 shall be permitted.

**39.2.2.4 Smokeproof Enclosures.** Smokeproof enclosures complying with 7.2.3 shall be permitted.

**39.2.2.5 Horizontal Exits.** Horizontal exits complying with 7.2.4 shall be permitted.

**39.2.2.6 Ramps.** Ramps complying with 7.2.5 shall be permitted.

**39.2.2.7 Exit Passageways.** Exit passageways complying with 7.2.6 shall be permitted.

**39.2.2.8 Escalators and Moving Walks.** Escalators and moving walks complying with 7.2.7 shall be permitted.

**39.2.2.9 Fire Escape Stairs.** Fire escape stairs complying with 7.2.8 shall be permitted.

**39.2.2.10 Fire Escape Ladders.** Fire escape ladders complying with 7.2.9 shall be permitted.

**39.2.2.11 Alternating Tread Devices.** Alternating tread devices complying with 7.2.11 shall be permitted.

**39.2.2.12 Areas of Refuge.**

**39.2.2.12.1** Areas of refuge complying with 7.2.12 shall be permitted.

**39.2.2.12.2** In buildings protected throughout by an approved, supervised automatic sprinkler system in accordance with 9.7.1.1(1), two rooms or spaces separated from each other by smoke-resistant partitions in accordance with the definition of area of refuge in 3.3.20 shall not be required.

Paragraph 38/39.2.2.4 does not mandate smokeproof enclosures. However, smokeproof enclosures are recognized as part of the means of egress system in business occupancies if they meet the requirements of 7.2.3. For an example of an occupancy requiring a smokeproof enclosure, see 31.2.11.1, which specifies that existing nonsprinklered or partially sprinklered high-rise apartment buildings are required to be provided with smokeproof enclosures in accordance with 7.2.3.

Existing escalators and moving walks are permitted to serve within the means of egress of existing business occupancies per 39.2.2.8. Note that 7.2.7 permits escalators and moving walks to continue to be located within the required means of egress if permitted by an occupancy chapter. In earlier editions of the *Code*, such escalators and moving walks might have been permitted and credited with providing egress capacity for 75 persons. To qualify as exits, existing escalators and moving walks must also meet the requirements of 7.1.3.2, which address exit enclosures. Escalators protected using the sprinkler-vent, spray nozzle, rolling shutter, or partial enclosure method do not constitute acceptable exits but could continue to serve as exit access if previously approved as such.

Existing fire escape stairs are permitted to serve within the means of egress of existing business occupancies per 39.2.2.9. Note that 7.2.8.1.2.1 permits existing buildings to continue to use fire escape stairs for not more than 50 percent of their required egress capacity.

Paragraph 38/39.2.2.11 addresses alternating tread devices. The provisions of 7.2.11, in effect, restrict the use of alternating tread devices to locations where the *Code* recognizes the use of fire escape ladders. See 38/39.2.2.10, 7.2.9, and 7.2.11.

Paragraph 38/39.2.2.12 addresses areas of refuge. Areas accessible to persons with severe mobility impairment in new buildings must be provided with accessible means of egress in accordance with 7.5.4.1. Existing business occupancies are exempt from the provisions of 7.5.4.1. For the stories above the level of exit discharge, where providing ramps is usually not feasible, areas of refuge (see 7.2.12) will typically be used to meet the requirements for accessible means of egress in new construction. The provision of 38/39.2.2.12.2 permits a sprinklered story of a business occupancy to be considered an area of refuge, even if an occupant does not have access to any of the tenant spaces. The effectiveness of sprinkler systems should allow an occupant with mobility impairment to remain on the floor of fire origin without experiencing untenable conditions. Doors to tenant spaces that are locked create inaccessibility to spaces other than the corridor, so the corridor effectively serves as the area of refuge.

### 38.2.3 Capacity of Means of Egress.

**38.2.3.1** The capacity of means of egress shall be in accordance with Section 7.3.

**38.2.3.2*** The clear width of any corridor or passageway serving an occupant load of 50 or more shall be not less than 44 in. (1120 mm).

**A.38.2.3.2** It is not the intent that this provision apply to noncorridor or nonpassageway areas of exit access, such as the spaces between rows of desks created by office layout or low-height partitions.

**38.2.3.3** Street floor exits shall be sufficient for the occupant load of the street floor plus the required capacity of open stairs and ramps discharging through the street floor.



### 39.2.3 Capacity of Means of Egress.

**39.2.3.1** The capacity of means of egress shall be in accordance with Section 7.3.

**39.2.3.2** The clear width of any corridor or passageway serving an occupant load of 50 or more shall be not less than 44 in. (1120 mm).

**39.2.3.3** Street floor exits shall be sufficient for the occupant load of the street floor plus the required capacity of open stairs, ramps, escalators, and moving walks discharging through the street floor.

Chapter 7 mandates that any required egress capacity from a mezzanine that passes through the room below must be added to the required egress capacity of the room through which the egress passes.

Exhibit 38/39.6 illustrates a case in which a mezzanine is open to the street floor. The exits from the street floor must accommodate the following:

1. Occupant load of the street floor
2. Occupant load of the mezzanine in accordance with 7.3.1.6
3. Required capacity provided by open stairs from other floors discharging through the street floor in accordance with 38/39.2.3.3

The exits for the street floor of a business occupancy must have sufficient capacity to handle the occupant load of the street floor and the capacity of any open stairs or ramps discharging through the street floor per 38/39.2.3.3. This provision represents a change from previous editions of the *Code*, prior to the 2009 edition, which formerly required the capacity of

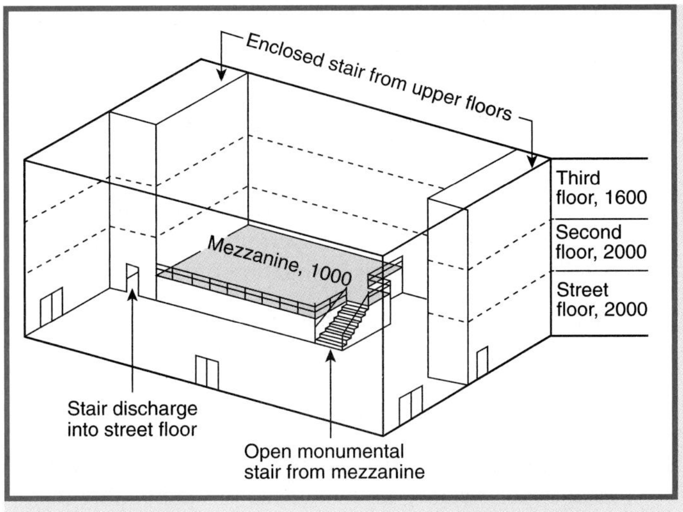


***Exhibit 38/39.6*** *Business occupancy with a mezzanine open to the street floor.*

enclosed exit stairs to be added to the occupant load of the level of exit discharge.

Corridors in business occupancies must have a clear width of at least 44 in. (1120 mm) only if serving an occupant load of 50 or more persons per 38/39.2.3.2. If a corridor serves fewer than 50 persons, the minimum 36 in. (915 mm) width — mandated by 7.3.4.1 for egress components in general — would apply.

A corridor with the minimum 44 in. (1120 mm) width required by 38/39.2.3.2 has sufficient egress capacity, where calculated using the 0.2 in. (5 mm) per person capacity factor of Table 7.3.3.1 for level components, for approximately 220 persons; that is, 44 in./0.2 in. per person (1120 mm/5 mm per person). For example, in a corridor that runs from one end of a building to the other end with an exit stair located at each end, 220 persons can travel from the midpoint of that corridor to the exit enclosure at one end. Another 220 persons can travel to the exit enclosure at the other end. Therefore, in this example, the occupant load of the floor would have to exceed 440 persons before the minimum 44 in. (1120 mm) corridor width must be increased.

Because people move more quickly in the horizontal direction than in the vertical direction, it is permissible to provide less door width than stair width within any given egress path for a given number of occupants. For example, in business occupancies, in accordance with the egress capacity factors of Table 7.3.3.1, level components and ramps require only 0.2 in. (5 mm) of width per person, whereas stairs require 0.3 in. (7.6 mm) of width per person. As a rough approximation, for every 44 in. (1120 mm) of stair discharging through the street floor, an additional 30 in. (760 mm) of door width opening to the outside must be added for the street floor.

### 38.2.4 Number of Exits.

**38.2.4.1** Exits shall comply with the following, except as otherwise permitted by 38.2.4.2 through 38.2.4.6:

(1) The number of means of egress shall be in accordance with Section 7.4.
(2) Not less than two separate exits shall be provided on every story.
(3) Not less than two separate exits shall be accessible from every part of every story.

**38.2.4.2** Exit access, as required by 38.2.4.1(3), shall be permitted to include a single exit access path for the distances permitted as common paths of travel by 38.2.5.3.

**38.2.4.3** A single exit shall be permitted for a room or area with a total occupant load of fewer than 100 persons, provided that the following criteria are met:

(1) The exit shall discharge directly to the outside at the level of exit discharge for the building.
(2) The total distance of travel from any point, including travel within the exit, shall not exceed 100 ft (30 m).

### 39.2.4 Number of Exits.

**39.2.4.1** Exits shall comply with the following, except as otherwise permitted by 39.2.4.2 through 39.2.4.6:

(1) The number of means of egress shall be in accordance with 7.4.1.1 and 7.4.1.3 through 7.4.1.6.
(2) Not less than two separate exits shall be provided on every story.
(3) Not less than two separate exits shall be accessible from every part of every story.

**39.2.4.2** Exit access, as required by 39.2.4.1(3), shall be permitted to include a single exit access path for the distances permitted as common paths of travel by 39.2.5.3.

**39.2.4.3** A single exit shall be permitted for a room or area with a total occupant load of fewer than 100 persons, provided that the following criteria are met:

(1) The exit shall discharge directly to the outside at the level of exit discharge for the building.
(2) The total distance of travel from any point, including travel within the exit, shall not exceed 100 ft (30 m).

CHAPTER 38 • New

(3) The total distance of travel specified in 38.2.4.3(2) shall be on the same floor level or, if traversing of stairs is necessary, such stairs shall not exceed 15 ft (4570 mm) in height, and the stairs shall be provided with complete enclosures to separate them from any other part of the building, with no door openings therein.
(4) A single outside stair in accordance with 7.2.2 shall be permitted to serve all floors permitted within the 15 ft (4570 mm) vertical travel limitation.

**38.2.4.4** Any business occupancy three or fewer stories in height, and not exceeding an occupant load of 30 people per floor, shall be permitted a single separate exit to each floor, provided that the following criteria are met:

(1) This arrangement shall be permitted only where the total travel distance to the outside of the building does not exceed 100 ft (30 m) and where the exit is enclosed in accordance with 7.1.3.2, serves as an exit from no other levels, and discharges directly to the outside.
(2) A single outside stair in accordance with 7.2.2 shall be permitted to serve all floors.

**38.2.4.5** A single means of egress shall be permitted from a mezzanine within a business occupancy, provided that the common path of travel does not exceed 75 ft (23 m), or 100 ft (30 m) if protected throughout by an approved, supervised automatic sprinkler system in accordance with 9.7.1.1(1).

**38.2.4.6** A single exit shall be permitted for a single-tenant space/building two or fewer stories in height, provided that both of the following criteria are met:

(1) The building is protected throughout by an approved, supervised automatic sprinkler system in accordance with 9.7.1.1(1).
(2) The total travel to the outside does not exceed 100 ft (30 m).

CHAPTER 39 • Existing

(3) The total distance of travel specified in 39.2.4.3(2) shall be on the same floor level or, if traversing of stairs is necessary, such stairs shall not exceed 15 ft (4570 mm) in height, and the stairs shall be provided with complete enclosures to separate them from any other part of the building, with no door openings therein.
(4) A single outside stair in accordance with 7.2.2 shall be permitted to serve all floors permitted within the 15 ft (4570 mm) vertical travel limitation.

**39.2.4.4** Any business occupancy three or fewer stories in height, and not exceeding an occupant load of 30 people per floor, shall be permitted a single separate exit to each floor, provided that the following criteria are met:

(1) This arrangement shall be permitted only where the total travel distance to the outside of the building does not exceed 100 ft (30 m) and where the exit is enclosed in accordance with 7.1.3.2, serves as an exit from no other levels, and discharges directly to the outside.
(2) A single outside stair in accordance with 7.2.2 shall be permitted to serve all floors.

**39.2.4.5** A single means of egress shall be permitted from a mezzanine within a business occupancy, provided that the common path of travel does not exceed 75 ft (23 m), or 100 ft (30 m) if protected throughout by an approved automatic sprinkler system in accordance with 9.7.1.1(1).

**39.2.4.6** A single exit shall be permitted for a single-tenant space/building two or fewer stories in height, provided that both of the following criteria are met:

(1) The building is protected throughout by an approved, supervised automatic sprinkler system in accordance with 9.7.1.1(1).
(2) The total travel to the outside does not exceed 100 ft (30 m).

Paragraph 38/39.2.4.1 requires a minimum of two exits. For new business occupancies, see 7.4.1.2, which requires a minimum of three means of egress or a minimum of four means of egress where the occupant load exceeds 500 and 1000, respectively.

The provisions of 38/39.2.4.1(2), which apply to the required number of exits for business occupancies, clarify that any level that constitutes a story must have at least two exits located on that story. The occupants of the story must be able to enter an exit (such as an enclosed exit stair on an upper floor of a multistory building) without having to travel to another story to reach the entrance to the exit. Because a mezzanine that meets the maximum one-third area rule of 8.6.9 does not constitute a story (see 8.6.9.2.1), two exits are not required on the mezzanine. However, the criteria of 38/39.2.4.1(3) must be met with respect to providing access to two separate exits, or the provisions for common path of travel in 38/39.2.4.2 or 38/39.2.4.5 must be met.

The provision for common path of travel in 38/39.2.4.2 applies only to 38/39.2.4.1(3), which requires access to two separate exits from every part of every level (story or mezzanine). Occupants are allowed to travel in one direction for a maximum distance (the common path allowance) before requiring access in two separate directions. Therefore, although the story or mezzanine must eventually provide access to two exits in accordance with 38/39.2.4.1(3), that access is required to be available only at the point where the allowable common path is expended.

Exhibit 38/39.7 and Exhibit 38/39.8 illustrate two cases where a single exit from a room or area in a business occupancy is permitted in accordance with 38/39.2.4.3. In the first case, the travel distance from the area is located on the same floor level as the exit. In the second case, stairs must be traversed.

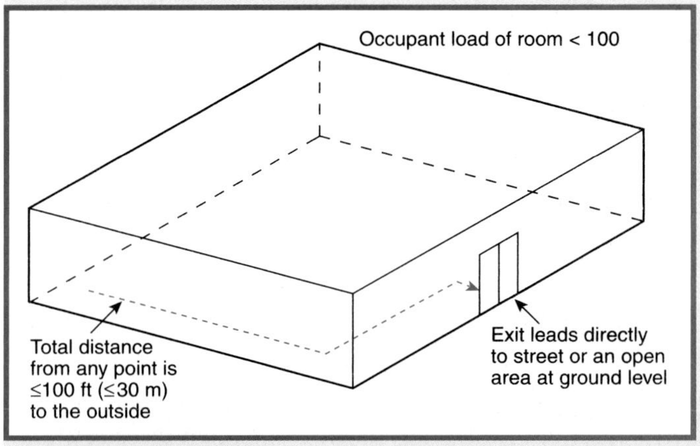


***Exhibit 38/39.7*** *Single exit from area or room in business occupancy in accordance with 38/39.2.4.3 — travel from area to exit without stairs.*

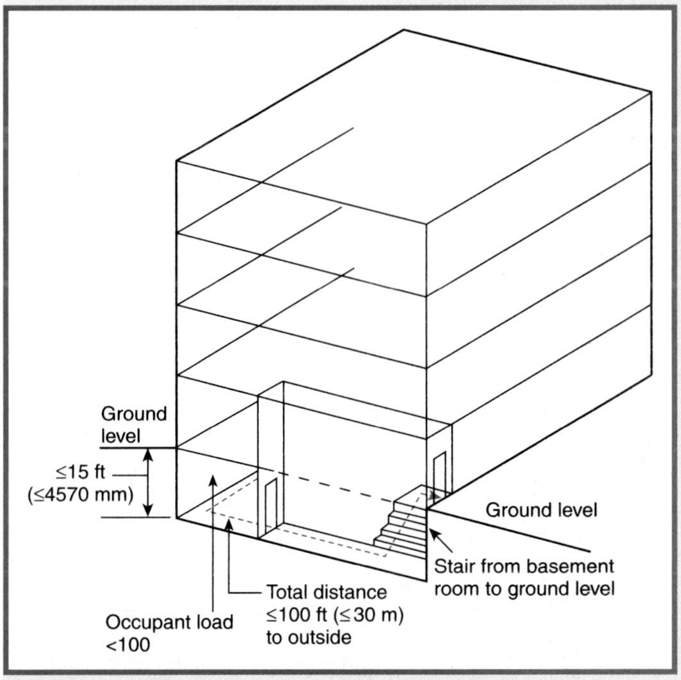


***Exhibit 38/39.8*** *Single exit from area or room in business occupancy in accordance with 38/39.2.4.3 — stairs traversed in traveling from the area to the exit.*

To use the single-exit provision of 38/39.2.4.3, all five of the following criteria must be met:

1. Occupant load fewer than 100 persons
2. Direct exit to a street or to an open exterior area at ground level
3. Total distance of not more than 100 ft (30 m) from any point in the room to the exterior [note that this is total distance from any point to the exterior, not travel distance as measured in Section 7.6; therefore, total distance includes the distance traveled on enclosed stairs (exit)]
4. Stairs not more than 15 ft (4570 mm) in height
5. Stairs completely enclosed with no door openings between the stair enclosure and the rest of the building, or stairs meeting requirements applicable to outside stairs (see 7.2.2.6.3)

Exhibit 38/39.9 illustrates a single exit from the third floor of a business occupancy in accordance with 38/39.2.4.4. The stair is totally enclosed, has an opening onto a building floor only at the third floor, and discharges directly to the street with no communication at the second and first floors. A similar, but separate, arrangement could be provided for the second floor of the same building.

To use the single-exit provision of 38/39.2.4.4, all five of the following criteria must be met:

1. Building height not more than three stories
2. Occupant load of each floor not more than 30

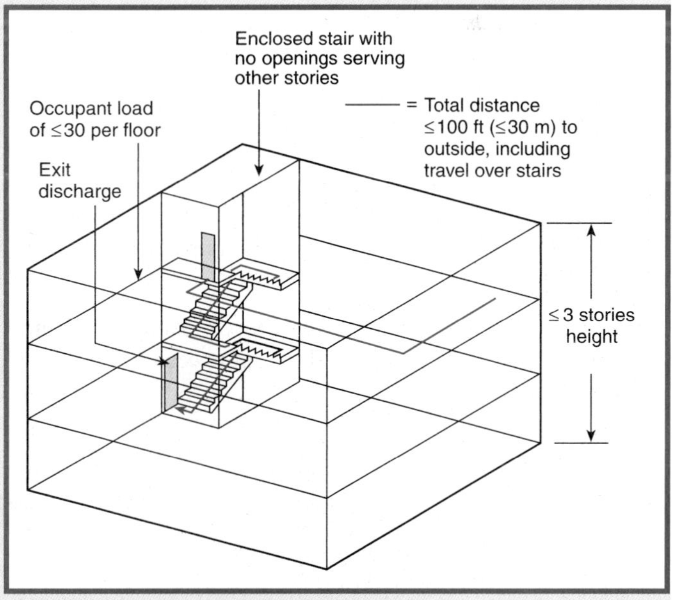


***Exhibit 38/39.9*** *Single exit from third floor of a business occupancy in accordance with 38/39.2.4.4.*

3. Total distance from any point on any floor to exterior at ground level not more than 100 ft (30 m), including travel over stairs [note that this is total distance from any point to the exterior, not travel distance as measured in Section 7.6; therefore, total distance includes the distance traveled on enclosed stairs (exit)]
4. Stair not used by, nor open to, any other floor
5. Stair totally enclosed or meeting requirements applicable to outside stairs (see 7.2.2.6.3)

It is noted that, when referring to the single-exit stair, 38/39.2.4.3(3) uses the words "with no door openings therein," and 38/39.2.4.4(1) uses the words "serves as an exit from no other levels." While the two provisions use different language, the intent is the same: no openings to other levels are permitted in the single exit stair enclosure, regardless of whether it serves as an exit from the other levels or it is intended to be used for convenience only. The presence of doors in the enclosure, even if properly rated, introduces the potential for the single exit to be rendered unusable by a fire on another floor, thus trapping the occupants for which the single exit is intended. The language discrepancy in 38/39.2.4.3(3) and 38/39.2.4.4(1) was unintentional and has been identified for correlation in a future edition of the *Code*.

Although 38/39.2.4.2 permits common access to the two required means of egress for limited distances, 38/39.2.4.5 exempts a mezzanine in a business occupancy from providing a point where access to two exits is available if the single means of egress leads to an exit within the same limited distances as those allowed for common path of travel.

The provision of 38/39.2.4.6 provides some relief from the requirement that mandates two separate exits on every story, which affects town house–type, sprinklered business occupancies. These town house–type business occupancies typically have two stories with an open interior stair and are of such limited size that, if a second stair were added, little usable space would remain, and the two stairs would, in effect, be located side by side. The provision offers any single-tenant space in a fully sprinklered building with a maximum of two stories, or any sprinklered single-tenant building with a maximum of two stories, the option of providing only one exit if the total travel distance to the outside does not exceed 100 ft (30 m). Note that a companion provision in 38/39.3.1.1(2) that addresses vertical opening protection permits the open interior stair in town house–style business occupancies.

### 38.2.5 Arrangement of Means of Egress.

**38.2.5.1** Means of egress shall be arranged in accordance with Section 7.5.

**38.2.5.2** Dead-end corridors shall be permitted in accordance with 38.2.5.2.1 or 38.2.5.2.2.

**38.2.5.2.1** In buildings protected throughout by an approved, supervised automatic sprinkler system in accordance with 9.7.1.1(1), dead-end corridors shall not exceed 50 ft (15 m).

**38.2.5.2.2** In buildings other than those complying with 38.2.5.2.1, dead-end corridors shall not exceed 20 ft (6100 mm).

**38.2.5.3** Limitations on common path of travel shall be in accordance with 38.2.5.3.1, 38.2.5.3.2, and 38.2.5.3.3.

### 39.2.5 Arrangement of Means of Egress.

**39.2.5.1** Means of egress shall be arranged in accordance with Section 7.5.

**39.2.5.2*** Dead-end corridors shall not exceed 50 ft (15 m).

**A.39.2.5.2** It is recognized that dead ends exceeding the permitted limits exist and, in some cases, are impractical to eliminate. The authority having jurisdiction might permit such dead ends to continue to exist, taking into consideration any or all of the following:

(1) Tenant arrangement
(2) Automatic sprinkler protection
(3) Smoke detection
(4) Exit remoteness

**39.2.5.3*** Limitation on common path of travel shall be in accordance with 39.2.5.3.1, 39.2.5.3.2, and 39.2.5.3.3.

**A.39.2.5.3** It is recognized that common paths of travel exceeding the permitted limits exist and, in some cases, are impractical to eliminate. The authority having jurisdiction might permit such common paths of travel to continue to exist, taking into consideration any or all of the following:

CHAPTER 38 • New | CHAPTER 39 • Existing

(1) Tenant arrangement
(2) Automatic sprinkler protection
(3) Smoke detection
(4) Exit remoteness

**38.2.5.3.1** Common path of travel shall not exceed 100 ft (30 m) in a building protected throughout by an approved, supervised automatic sprinkler system in accordance with 9.7.1.1(1).

**38.2.5.3.2** Common path of travel shall not exceed 100 ft (30 m) within a single tenant space having an occupant load not exceeding 30 persons.

**38.2.5.3.3** In buildings other than those complying with 38.2.5.3.1 or 38.2.5.3.2, common path of travel shall not exceed 75 ft (23 m).

**39.2.5.3.1** Common path of travel shall not exceed 100 ft (30 m) on a story protected throughout by an approved automatic sprinkler system in accordance with 9.7.1.1(1).

**39.2.5.3.2** Common path of travel shall not be limited in a single-tenant space with an occupant load not exceeding 30 people.

**39.2.5.3.3** In buildings other than those complying with 39.2.5.3.1 or 39.2.5.3.2, common path of travel shall not exceed 75 ft (23 m).

Because they have separate and distinct requirements, the *Code* separates dead-end corridors and common path of travel into distinct and separate subsections. Dead-end corridors are limited to 20 ft (6100 mm) in new business occupancies that are not protected throughout by an approved, supervised automatic sprinkler system. The provision of 38.2.5.2.1 recognizes the additional level of safety to life that a complete automatic sprinkler system provides; it, therefore, allows added flexibility when designing the location of corridors and exits in buildings where approved sprinkler systems are installed by permitting the dead-end corridor pocket to be as long as 50 ft (15 m). Existing business occupancies are permitted a 50 ft (15 m) dead-end corridor, regardless of the presence of sprinklers.

Three typical dead-end corridors are illustrated in Exhibit 38/39.10. Dead-end pockets are located in the corridor between points B and C, F and G, and H and I. They are limited to a maximum length of 20 ft (6100 mm) [50 ft (15 m) for existing business occupancies or sprinklered new business occupancies].

See the commentary associated with A.7.5.1.5 for a detailed discussion on common path of travel. Also see the commentary associated with 38/39.2.4.2, following 38/39.2.4.6, which permits a portion of the access to a single exit or multiple exits to be common.

The restriction on common path of travel is separate and distinct from the restriction on dead-end corridors. A common path of travel might sometimes involve a dead-end corridor, and dead ends might involve common path of travel, but not in every case. For example, the elevator lobby shown in Exhibit 38/39.10 is a dead-end corridor but not a common path of travel.

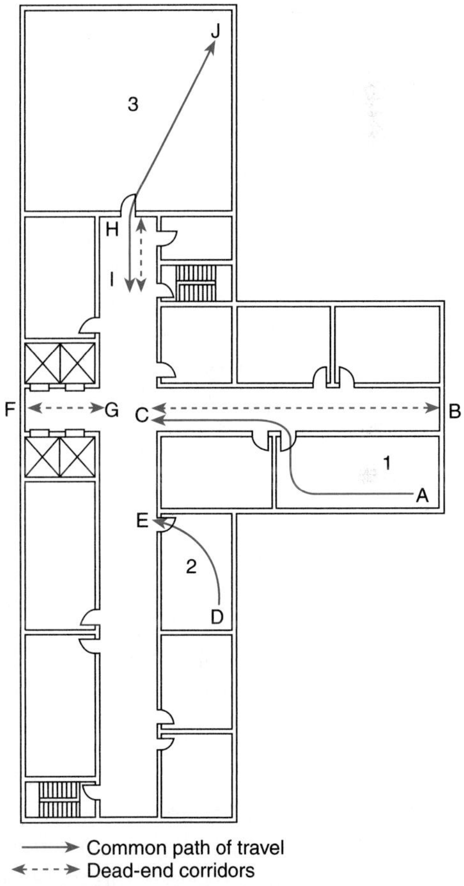


***Exhibit 38/39.10** Dead-end corridor pockets and common paths of travel.*

The method for measuring common path of travel is similar to that for measuring travel distance (see Section 7.6). The starting point for measurement of common path of travel is the same as the starting point for travel distance measurement — the most remote point. The difference is that, instead of terminating at the entrance to an exit, common path of travel measurement often ends before the exit's entrance, because it terminates at the point where the occupant has a choice of two distinct and separate paths to an exit (see the definition of the term *common path of travel* in 3.3.42). See rooms 1, 2, and 3 in Exhibit 38/39.10, where common paths of travel occur between points A and C, D and E, and J and I.

The provision of 38/39.2.5.3.1 permits the common path of travel to be extended from 75 ft (23 m) to 100 ft (30 m) if sprinklers are provided. For new business occupancies, the building must be protected throughout by an approved, supervised automatic sprinkler system to utilize the provision for increased common path of travel; for existing business occupancies, the sprinkler system is not required to be supervised and is not required to protect the entire building but only the floor on which the increased common path is located. This provision recognizes the additional level of safety to life that automatic sprinkler protection provides and allows added flexibility when designing the location of corridors and exits in buildings where approved sprinkler systems are installed.

The provision of 38.2.5.3.2 permits common path of travel in a new business occupancy to be extended from 75 ft (23 m) to 100 ft (30 m), without requiring the sprinkler protection addressed in 38.2.5.3.1, if the common path of travel occurs wholly within a maximum 30-person [normally, approximately 3000 $ft^2$ (279 $m^2$), based on the business occupant load factor of 100 $ft^2$ (9.3 $m^2$) per person] single-tenant space, with no additional common path encountered once the common space, such as the corridor, is reached. In Exhibit 38/39.10, 38.2.5.3.2 could be applied to room 2 but not to room 1 or room 3, because, upon leaving those rooms, additional common path of travel is encountered within the corridor.

The criteria addressed by 38.2.5.3.2 are not included in Chapter 39, because an existing business occupancy is offered the 25 ft (7620 mm) increase in allowable common path of travel — an increase to 100 ft (30 m) as specified in 39.2.5.3.1 — which is easier to meet. The criterion in 39.2.5.3.2 exempts a single-tenant space with a maximum occupant load of not more than 30 people from the common path of travel requirement. The tenant space would normally have an area of approximately 3000 $ft^2$ (279 $m^2$), based on the business occupant load factor of 100 $ft^2$ (9.3 $m^2$) per person. This provision can be used only if the single door from that tenant space leads to a corridor that does not have a dead end in excess of 50 ft (15 m). For an existing business occupancy, 39.2.5.3.2 might permit the common path of travel indicated between points J and I in Exhibit 38/39.10.

Exhibit 38/39.11 shows additional examples of common paths of travel in a business occupancy. Also see the commentary associated with Section 7.5 on arrangement of means of egress.

In suite A of Exhibit 38/39.11, the travel from point X to point A is a common path of travel; although there are two routes to reach the main corridor, they both merge at common point A. In suite B, the travel from point X to point B is common path of travel and does not appear to exceed the 75 ft (23 m) maximum; if it were in excess of 75 ft (23 m) but not more than 100 ft (30 m), it would be permitted by either 38/39.2.5.3.1 (involving sprinkler protection) or 38/39.2.5.3.2 (involving single-tenant space). Although suites C and D do not have common paths of travel, the remoteness of

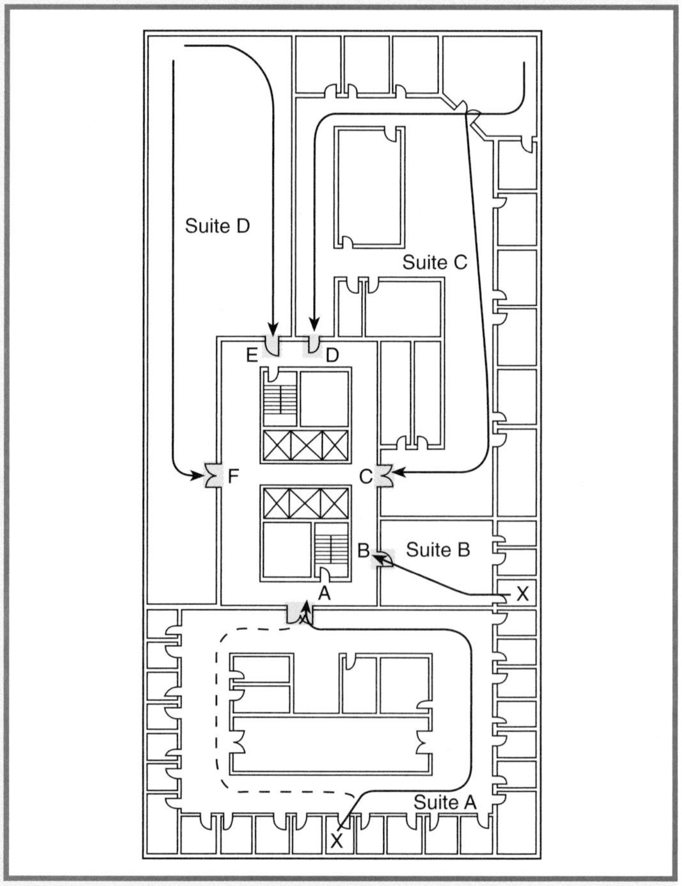


***Exhibit 38/39.11*** *Common path of travel.*

the two exit access doors from each suite is questionable. See 7.5.1.3 for details on means of egress remoteness.

The common path of travel restriction regulates where an office space requires two exit access doors. If the common path of travel is exceeded, a second door from the office space is required. The door must be positioned so that any resulting common path of travel complies with the allowable distances. In addition, the second door must be remotely located from the first door (see 7.5.1.3), and each door must lead to remote exits by means of remote paths. Therefore, in a single requirement, the *Code* regulates not only the number of exit access doors required from an office area but also the arrangement of those doors.

### 38.2.6 Travel Distance to Exits.

Travel distance shall comply with 38.2.6.1 through 38.2.6.3.

**38.2.6.1** Travel distance shall be measured in accordance with Section 7.6.

**38.2.6.2** Travel distance to an exit shall not exceed 200 ft (61 m) from any point in a building, unless otherwise permitted by 38.2.6.3.

**38.2.6.3** Travel distance shall not exceed 300 ft (91 m) in business occupancies protected throughout by an approved, supervised automatic sprinkler system in accordance with Section 9.7.

### 38.2.7 Discharge from Exits.

Exit discharge shall comply with Section 7.7.

### 38.2.8 Illumination of Means of Egress.

Means of egress shall be illuminated in accordance with Section 7.8.

### 38.2.9 Emergency Lighting.

**38.2.9.1** Emergency lighting shall be provided in accordance with Section 7.9 in any building where any one of the following conditions exists:

(1) The building is three or more stories in height.
(2) The occupancy is subject to 50 or more occupants above or below the level of exit discharge.
(3) The occupancy is subject to 300 or more total occupants.

**38.2.9.2** Emergency lighting in accordance with Section 7.9 shall be provided for all underground and limited access structures, as defined in 3.3.254.11 and 3.3.254.3.

### 38.2.10 Marking of Means of Egress.

Means of egress shall have signs in accordance with Section 7.10.



### 39.2.6 Travel Distance to Exits.

Travel distance shall comply with 39.2.6.1 through 39.2.6.3.

**39.2.6.1** Travel distance shall be measured in accordance with Section 7.6.

**39.2.6.2** Travel distance to an exit shall not exceed 200 ft (61 m) from any point in a building, unless otherwise permitted by 39.2.6.3.

**39.2.6.3** Travel distance shall not exceed 300 ft (91 m) in business occupancies protected throughout by an approved, supervised automatic sprinkler system in accordance with Section 9.7.

### 39.2.7 Discharge from Exits.

Exit discharge shall comply with Section 7.7.

### 39.2.8 Illumination of Means of Egress.

Means of egress shall be illuminated in accordance with Section 7.8.

### 39.2.9 Emergency Lighting.

**39.2.9.1** Emergency lighting shall be provided in accordance with Section 7.9 in any building where any one of the following conditions exists:

(1) The building is three or more stories in height.
(2) The occupancy is subject to 100 or more occupants above or below the level of exit discharge.
(3) The occupancy is subject to 1000 or more total occupants.

**39.2.9.2** Emergency lighting in accordance with Section 7.9 shall be provided for all underground and limited access structures, as defined in 3.3.254.11 and 3.3.254.3.

### 39.2.10 Marking of Means of Egress.

Means of egress shall have signs in accordance with Section 7.10.

CHAPTER 38 • New

38.2.11 Special Means of Egress Features.

38.2.11.1 Reserved.

**38.2.11.2 Lockups.** Lockups in business occupancies shall comply with the requirements of 22.4.5.

CHAPTER 39 • Existing

39.2.11 Special Means of Egress Features.

39.2.11.1 Reserved.

**39.2.11.2 Lockups.** Lockups in business occupancies, other than approved existing lockups, shall comply with the requirements of 23.4.5.

Subsection 38/39.2.6 addresses travel distance. In accordance with Section 7.6, travel distance requirements apply to only the first (or nearest) exit from a given point in a building. In other words, the 200 ft (61 m) travel distance limit requires that at least one exit is to be located within 200 ft (61 m) of any point in the building; it does not require that all exits be within 200 ft (61 m) of any point in the building.

The provision of 38/39.2.6.3 permits the travel distance to be increased to 300 ft (91 m) if the building is protected throughout by an approved, electrically supervised automatic sprinkler system. This provision recognizes the additional level of safety to life that a complete automatic sprinkler system provides and allows added flexibility in the design and arrangement of the means of egress.

If any of the three conditions of 38/39.2.9.1 exists, emergency lighting as specified in Section 7.9 is required for the business occupancy. Note that 38/39.2.9.1(1) previously referred to buildings with two or more stories located above the level of exit discharge; the provision was editorially revised for the 2009 edition to refer to buildings a minimum of three stories in height. Note that the thresholds for fire alarm systems in business occupancies are the same as those for emergency lighting (see 38/39.3.4.1). If a business occupancy is required to be provided with emergency lighting, a fire alarm system is also required.

If a business occupancy is provided with a lockup for security purposes, it must meet the provisions of 22/23.4.5, as specified in 38/39.2.11.2. The lockup criteria require the application of some of the concepts of detention and correctional occupancies to other occupancies where persons might be detained for security purposes, without classifying the lockup as a detention and correctional occupancy. See 22/23.4.5 and related commentary for details on the lockup provisions.

## 38.3 Protection

### 38.3.1 Protection of Vertical Openings.

**38.3.1.1** Vertical openings shall be enclosed or protected in accordance with Section 8.6, unless otherwise permitted by one of the following:

(1) Unenclosed vertical openings in accordance with 8.6.8.2 shall be permitted.
(2) Exit access stairs in accordance with 38.2.4.6 shall be permitted to be unenclosed.

## 39.3 Protection

### 39.3.1 Protection of Vertical Openings.

**39.3.1.1** Vertical openings shall be enclosed or protected in accordance with Section 8.6, unless otherwise permitted by the following:

(1) Unenclosed vertical openings in accordance with 8.6.8.2 shall be permitted.
(2) Exit access stairs in accordance with 39.2.4.6 shall be permitted to be unenclosed.
(3) Unprotected vertical openings shall be permitted in buildings complying with all of the following:
    (a) Where protected throughout by an approved automatic sprinkler system in accordance with 9.7.1.1(1)
    (b) Where no unprotected vertical opening serves as any part of any required means of egress
    (c) Where required exits consist of exit doors that discharge directly to the finished ground level in accordance with 7.2.1, outside stairs in accordance with 7.2.2, smokeproof enclosures in accordance with 7.2.3, or horizontal exits in accordance with 7.2.4

CHAPTER 38 • New

38.3.1.2 Floors that are below the street floor and are used for storage or other than a business occupancy shall have no unprotected openings to business occupancy floors.

The provisions for vertical openings in 38/39.3.1.1 reference Section 8.6. Paragraph 8.6.6 permits the three-story communicating space (sometimes referred to as a "mini-atrium"), unless there is a prohibition on such use in the applicable occupancy chapter. Neither Chapter 38 nor Chapter 39 prohibits the use of 8.6.6. Note that 8.6.6 requires that, if the communicating space (the vertical opening and all areas open to it) contains ordinary hazard contents, it must be protected by automatic sprinklers. In accordance with 38/39.1.5, contents within business occupancies are typically classified as ordinary hazard.

The provision of 38/39.3.1.1(1) — via its reference to 8.6.8.2 — permits, for example, a two-level office or a reference library in an office building to have an unenclosed convenience stair.

The provision of 38/39.3.1.1(2) completes the single exit package for town house–type and similarly arranged business occupancies by permitting the single means of egress to include an unenclosed stair. See the commentary that follows 38/39.2.4.6.

### 38.3.2 Protection from Hazards.

**38.3.2.1* General.** Hazardous areas including, but not limited to, areas used for general storage, boiler or furnace rooms, and maintenance shops that include woodworking and painting areas shall be protected in accordance with Section 8.7.

**A.38.3.2.1** It is not the intent of this provision that rooms inside individual tenant spaces that are used to store routine office supplies for that tenant be required to be either separated or sprinklered.

**38.3.2.2* High Hazard Contents Areas.** High hazard contents areas, as classified in Section 6.2, shall meet the following criteria:

(1) The area shall be separated from other parts of the building by fire barriers having a minimum 1-hour fire resistance rating, with all openings therein protected by self-closing fire door assemblies having a minimum $^3/_4$-hour fire protection rating.
(2) The area shall be protected by an automatic extinguishing system in accordance with 9.7.1.1(1) or 9.7.1.2.

**A.38.3.2.2** The requirement for separating high hazard contents areas from other parts of the building is intended to isolate the hazard, and 8.2.3.3 is applicable.

CHAPTER 39 • Existing

39.3.1.2 Floors that are below the street floor and are used for storage or other than a business occupancy shall have no unprotected openings to business occupancy floors.

Application of 39.3.1.1(3) requires not only that the building housing the existing business occupancy be protected with complete automatic sprinkler protection, but also that all building exits be either smokeproof enclosures, outside stairs, horizontal exits, or doors leading directly to the outside at ground level. Otherwise, the unprotected vertical openings must be suitably enclosed.

The separation requirement of 38/39.3.1.2 prevents the possibility that a fire in a basement housing a hazardous area with a high fuel load (such as areas used for workshops, repairs, or storage of maintenance supplies, files, and records) might directly expose the floor of exit discharge through an unprotected vertical opening. A fire in a basement can quickly cause exits and exit discharges located on the street floor to become unusable when smoke and heat rise.

### 39.3.2 Protection from Hazards.

**39.3.2.1* General.** Hazardous areas including, but not limited to, areas used for general storage, boiler or furnace rooms, and maintenance shops that include woodworking and painting areas shall be protected in accordance with Section 8.7.

**A.39.3.2.1** It is not the intent of this provision that rooms inside individual tenant spaces that are used to store routine office supplies for that tenant be required to be separated or sprinklered.

**39.3.2.2* High Hazard Contents Areas.** High hazard contents areas, as classified in Section 6.2, shall meet the following criteria:

(1) The area shall be separated from other parts of the building by fire barriers having a minimum 1-hour fire resistance rating, with all openings therein protected by self-closing fire door assemblies having a minimum $^3/_4$-hour fire protection rating.
(2) The area shall be protected by an automatic extinguishing system in accordance with 9.7.1.1(1) or 9.7.1.2.

**A.39.3.2.2** The requirement for separating high hazard contents areas from other parts of the building is intended to isolate the hazard, and 8.2.3.3 is applicable.

CHAPTER 38 • New

**38.3.2.3 Cooking Equipment.** Cooking equipment shall be protected in accordance with 9.2.3, unless the cooking equipment is one of the following types:

(1) Outdoor equipment
(2) Portable equipment not flue-connected
(3) Equipment used only for food warming

CHAPTER 39 • Existing

**39.3.2.3 Cooking Equipment.** Cooking equipment shall be protected in accordance with 9.2.3, unless the cooking equipment is one of the following types:

(1) Outdoor equipment
(2) Portable equipment not flue-connected
(3) Equipment used only for food warming

The provisions of 38/39.3.2 reflect the intent of Section 8.4, which requires one of the following:

1. Separation of a hazardous area from the remainder of the occupancy by means of fire-rated construction
2. Installation of automatic sprinklers in the hazardous area
3. Protection by both items 1 and 2 where the hazard is severe

Where a hazardous area in a new business occupancy is protected by automatic sprinklers, that area is required to be enclosed by walls and doors meeting the requirements for smoke partitions in Section 8.4. See 8.7.1.2.

### 38.3.3 Interior Finish.

**38.3.3.1 General.** Interior finish shall be in accordance with Section 10.2.

**38.3.3.2 Interior Wall and Ceiling Finish.**

**38.3.3.2.1** Interior wall and ceiling finish material complying with Section 10.2 shall be Class A or Class B in exits and in exit access corridors.

**38.3.3.2.2** Interior wall and ceiling finishes shall be Class A, Class B, or Class C in areas other than those specified in 38.3.3.2.1.

**38.3.3.3 Interior Floor Finish.**

**38.3.3.3.1** Interior floor finish shall comply with Section 10.2.

**38.3.3.3.2** Interior floor finish in exit enclosures shall be Class I or Class II.

**38.3.3.3.3** Interior floor finish shall comply with 10.2.7.1 or 10.2.7.2, as applicable.

### 39.3.3 Interior Finish.

**39.3.3.1 General.** Interior finish shall be in accordance with Section 10.2.

**39.3.3.2 Interior Wall and Ceiling Finish.**

**39.3.3.2.1** Interior wall and ceiling finish materials complying with Section 10.2 shall be Class A or Class B in exits and in exit access corridors.

**39.3.3.2.2** Interior wall and ceiling finishes shall be Class A, Class B, or Class C in areas other than those specified in 39.3.3.2.1.

**39.3.3.3 Interior Floor Finish.** (No requirements.)

The requirement that interior floor finish be Class I or Class II (see Section 10.2) applies only to exits, such as enclosed stairs, in new business occupancies. The intent is that the interior floor finish materials used in exits are to resist the spread of fire if exposed to the radiant energy from a fully developed room fire by means of an open door. The provision of 10.2.8.2 permits a reduction of one class of interior floor finish (i.e., from Class I to Class II, or from Class II to no classification required) in sprinklered buildings.

In all cases, regardless of sprinkler protection, new carpet and carpetlike floor finishes must comply with ASTM D 2859, *Standard Test Method for Ignition Characteristics of Finished Textile Floor Covering Materials*,[3] as referenced in 10.2.7.1 via 38.3.3.3.3. Other floor finish materials must have a minimum critical radiant flux of 0.1 W/cm$^2$ per 10.2.7.2. Existing business occupancies have no interior floor finish requirements (see 39.3.3.3).

CHAPTER 38 • New

### 38.3.4 Detection, Alarm, and Communications Systems.

**38.3.4.1 General.** A fire alarm system in accordance with Section 9.6 shall be provided in all business occupancies where any one of the following conditions exists:

(1) The building is three or more stories in height.
(2) The occupancy is subject to 50 or more occupants above or below the level of exit discharge.
(3) The occupancy is subject to 300 or more total occupants.

**38.3.4.2 Initiation.** Initiation of the required fire alarm system shall be by one of the following means:

(1) Manual means in accordance with 9.6.2.1(1)
(2) Means of an approved automatic fire detection system that complies with 9.6.2.1(2) and provides protection throughout the building
(3) Means of an approved automatic sprinkler system that complies with 9.6.2.1(3) and provides protection throughout the building

**38.3.4.3 Occupant Notification.** During all times that the building is occupied, the required fire alarm system, once initiated, shall activate a general alarm in accordance with 9.6.3 throughout the building, and positive alarm sequence in accordance with 9.6.3.4 shall be permitted.

**38.3.4.4 Emergency Forces Notification.** Emergency forces notification shall be provided and shall include notifying the following:

(1) Fire department in accordance with 9.6.4
(2) Local emergency organization, if provided

CHAPTER 39 • Existing

### 39.3.4 Detection, Alarm, and Communications Systems.

**39.3.4.1 General.** A fire alarm system in accordance with Section 9.6 shall be provided in all business occupancies where any one of the following conditions exists:

(1) The building is three or more stories in height.
(2) The occupancy is subject to 100 or more occupants above or below the level of exit discharge.
(3) The occupancy is subject to 1000 or more total occupants.

**39.3.4.2 Initiation.** Initiation of the required fire alarm system shall be by one of the following means:

(1) Manual means in accordance with 9.6.2.1(1)
(2) Means of an approved automatic fire detection system that complies with 9.6.2.1(2) and provides protection throughout the building
(3) Means of an approved automatic sprinkler system that complies with 9.6.2.1(3) and provides protection throughout the building

**39.3.4.3 Occupant Notification.** During all times that the building is occupied *(see 7.2.1.1.3),* the required fire alarm system, once initiated, shall perform one of the following functions:

(1) It shall activate a general alarm in accordance with 9.6.3 throughout the building, and the following also shall apply:
    (a) Positive alarm sequence in accordance with 9.6.3.4 shall be permitted.
    (b) A presignal system in accordance with 9.6.3.3 shall be permitted.
(2) Occupant notification shall be permitted to be made via a voice communication or public address system in accordance with 9.6.3.9.2.

A fire alarm system is required in a business occupancy under the same conditions as those under which emergency lighting is required (see 38/39.2.9.1). If any one of the three conditions of 38/39.3.4.1 exists, a fire alarm system must be provided. In previous editions of the *Code,* 38/39.3.4.1(1) referred to buildings with two or more stories in height above the level of exit discharge; the provision was editorially revised for the 2009 edition to refer to buildings three or more stories in height.

A required fire alarm system must have initiation means per 38/39.3.4.2, but the requirement for manual

CHAPTER 38 • New

CHAPTER 39 • Existing

fire alarm boxes is waived if the system is initiated by either an automatic fire detection system providing protection throughout the building or an automatic sprinkler system providing protection throughout the building. This waiver does not exempt the fire alarm system but only the manual fire alarm boxes. Note that 9.6.2.6 requires at least one manual fire alarm box to be provided at a location acceptable to the authority having jurisdiction (AHJ).

When the required fire alarm system is initiated by one of the means specified in 38/39.3.4.2, the system must automatically sound a general alarm throughout the building. In existing business occupancies, if a continuously attended location is provided (as is often the case in high-rise or other large office buildings), the alarm is permitted to sound at that location only, with the appropriate emergency action initiated at that location by using a voice communication or public address system (see 9.6.3.9.2). See 38/39.3.4.3 for details on occupant notification requirements.

Note that only existing presignal systems are permitted in existing business occupancies [see 39.3.4.3(1)(b)]; where presignal systems are used, the fire department must be notified automatically without delay in case of a delay in notifying, or failure to notify, the building occupants. The better, fail-safe system — positive alarm sequence — is permitted for both new and existing business occupancies. See 9.6.3.3, 9.6.3.4, and *NFPA 72®, National Fire Alarm Code®*,[4] for details on presignal and positive alarm sequence systems.

The provision of 38.3.4.4, which is new to the 2009 edition of the *Code,* requires automatic emergency forces notification in accordance with 9.6.4 for all new business occupancies that are required to be provided with a fire alarm system.

### 38.3.5 Extinguishment Requirements.

Portable fire extinguishers shall be provided in every business occupancy in accordance with 9.7.4.1.

### 39.3.5 Extinguishment Requirements.

Portable fire extinguishers shall be provided in every business occupancy in accordance with 9.7.4.1.

Although no requirements for automatic sprinkler systems are provided in 38/39.3.5, 38.4.2 has the effect of requiring new high-rise office buildings to be protected by automatic sprinklers, because the referenced provisions of Section 11.8 require sprinklers. Also, if the atrium provisions of 8.6.7 are used, a sprinkler system is required throughout the building. The following features provide additional incentives to encourage sprinkler installation:

1. Nonrated openings to attached parking structures (38/39.1.2.2)
2. Elevator lobby exit access door locking (38/39.2.2.2.3)
3. Delayed-egress locks (38/39.2.2.2.5)
4. Stories constituting areas of refuge (38/39.2.2.12)
5. Number of exits (38/39.2.4)
6. Dead-end corridors (38/39.2.5.2)
7. Common path of travel (38/39.2.5.3)
8. Travel distance to exits (38/39.2.6)
9. Discharge of exits through the level of exit discharge (38/39.2.7 per Section 7.7)
10. Protection from hazards (38/39.3.2)
11. Interior finish (38/39.3.3 per Section 10.2)
12. Elimination of manual fire alarm boxes (38/39.3.4.2)
13. Nonrated corridors (38.3.6.1)

### 38.3.6 Corridors.

**38.3.6.1*** Where access to exits is provided by corridors, such corridors shall be separated from use areas by fire barriers in accordance with Section 8.3 having a minimum 1-hour fire resistance rating, unless one of the following conditions exists:

(1)* Where exits are available from an open floor area
(2)* Within a space occupied by a single tenant
(3) Within buildings protected throughout by an approved, supervised automatic sprinkler system in accordance with 9.7.1.1(1)

### 39.3.6 Corridors.

(No requirements.)

CHAPTER 38 • New

CHAPTER 39 • Existing

**A.38.3.6.1** The intent of 38.3.6(1) through (3) is to permit spaces to be open to the exit access corridor without separation.

**A.38.3.6.1(1)** Where exits are available from an open floor area, such as open plan buildings, corridors are not required to be separated. An example of an open plan building is a building in which the work spaces and accesses to exits are delineated by the use of tables, desks, bookcases, or counters, or by partitions that are less than floor-to-ceiling height.

**A.38.3.6.1(2)** It is the intent of this provision that a single tenant be limited to an area occupied under a single management and work the same hours. The concept is that people under the same employ working the same hours would likely be familiar with their entire tenant space. It is not the intent to apply this provision simply because tenants are owned by the same organization. For example, in a government-owned office building, the offices of different federal agencies would be considered multiple tenants because an employee normally works for one agency. The agencies might work various hours. Another example of multiple tenancy would be a classroom building of a university, because some classrooms might be in use at times when other classrooms are not being used.

**38.3.6.2** Openings in corridor walls required by 38.3.6.1 to have a fire resistance rating shall be protected in accordance with Section 8.3.

Corridors in new business occupancies are addressed in 38.3.6; no corridor requirements are specified for existing business occupancies.

The provision of 38.3.6.1(1) provides for the popular "office landscape" or "open office" arrangement. If there is direct access to exits from the open area, it is not necessary to provide corridors. This provision recognizes that a fire in an open space is subject to more rapid observation and response than a fire in an enclosed room or office.

The provision of 38.3.6.1(2) recognizes that, in areas occupied by a single tenant, there is a high level of familiarity with the area, and the same people occupy the partitioned offices or spaces on a regular basis. Such spaces are exempt from corridor requirements.

The provision of 38.3.6.1(3) recognizes the value of automatic sprinklers as a life safety feature that helps to control fire growth and, thus, maintains the exit access usable for a longer time. Such sprinklered buildings are exempt from all corridor requirements.

If any of the exemptions for rated corridors in business occupancies are utilized, there is no need to provide a smoke-resistant barrier between the corridor and the adjoining rooms, as is required for some other occupancies (see, for example, health care, 18/19.3.6).

### 38.3.7 Subdivision of Building Spaces.

(No special requirements.)

### 39.3.7 Subdivision of Building Spaces.

(No special requirements.)

CHAPTER 38 • New

## 38.4 Special Provisions

### 38.4.1 Limited Access or Underground Buildings.

See Section 11.7.

### 38.4.2* High-Rise Buildings.

High-rise buildings shall comply with Section 11.8.

**A.38.4.2** In the design of high-rise buildings, special consideration should also be given to a life safety system including, but not limited to, the following features:

(1) Movement of occupants to safety
(2) Control of fire and smoke
(3) Psychological features
(4) Communications systems
(5) Elevators
(6) Emergency planning
(7) Overall system reliability

### 38.4.3 Air Traffic Control Towers.

**38.4.3.1** Air traffic control towers shall comply with the requirements of this chapter and Section 11.3.

**38.4.3.2** The requirements of Section 11.8 shall not apply to air traffic control towers.

CHAPTER 39 • Existing

## 39.4 Special Provisions

### 39.4.1 Limited Access or Underground Buildings.

See Section 11.7.

### 39.4.2 High-Rise Buildings.

**39.4.2.1** All high-rise business occupancy buildings shall be provided with a reasonable degree of safety from fire, and such degree of safety shall be accomplished by one of the following means:

(1) Installation of a complete, approved, supervised automatic sprinkler system in accordance with 9.7.1.1(1)
(2) Installation of an engineered life safety system complying with the following:
   (a) The engineered life safety system shall be developed by a registered professional engineer experienced in fire and life safety systems design.
   (b) The life safety system shall be approved by the authority having jurisdiction and shall be permitted to include any or all of the following systems:
      i. Partial automatic sprinkler protection
      ii. Smoke detection alarms
      iii. Smoke control
      iv. Compartmentation
      v. Other approved systems

**39.4.2.2*** A limited, but reasonable, time shall be permitted for compliance with any part of 39.4.2.1, commensurate with the magnitude of expenditure and the disruption of services.

**A.39.4.2.2** In some cases, appreciable cost might be involved in bringing an existing occupancy into compliance. Where this is true, it would be appropriate for the authority having jurisdiction to prescribe a schedule determined jointly with the facility, allowing suitable periods of time for the correction of the various deficiencies and giving due weight to the ability of the owner to secure the necessary funds.

**39.4.2.3** In addition to the requirements of 39.4.2.1 and 39.4.2.2, all buildings, regardless of height, shall comply with all other applicable provisions of this chapter.

### 39.4.3 Air Traffic Control Towers.

**39.4.3.1** Air traffic control towers shall comply with the requirements of this chapter and Section 11.3.

**39.4.3.2** The requirements of Section 11.8 shall not apply to air traffic control towers.

## 38.5 Building Services

### 38.5.1 Utilities.

Utilities shall comply with the provisions of Section 9.1.

### 38.5.2 Heating, Ventilating, and Air-Conditioning.

Heating, ventilating, and air-conditioning equipment shall comply with the provisions of Section 9.2.

### 38.5.3 Elevators, Escalators, and Conveyors.

Elevators, escalators, and conveyors shall comply with the provisions of Section 9.4.

### 38.5.4 Rubbish Chutes, Incinerators, and Laundry Chutes.

Rubbish chutes, incinerators, and laundry chutes shall comply with the provisions of Section 9.5.

## 38.6 Reserved

## 38.7 Operating Features

### 38.7.1 Emergency Plans.

Emergency plans complying with Section 4.8 shall be provided in high-rise buildings.

### 38.7.2 Drills.

In all business occupancy buildings occupied by more than 500 persons, or by more than 100 persons above or below the street level, employees and supervisory personnel shall be periodically instructed in accordance with Section 4.7 and shall hold drills periodically where practicable.

### 38.7.3 Extinguisher Training.

Designated employees of business occupancies shall be periodically instructed in the use of portable fire extinguishers.

### 38.7.4 Food Service Operations.

Food service operations shall comply with 12.7.2.

### 38.7.5 Upholstered Furniture and Mattresses.

The provisions of 10.3.2 shall not apply to upholstered furniture and mattresses.



## 39.5 Building Services

### 39.5.1 Utilities.

Utilities shall comply with the provisions of Section 9.1.

### 39.5.2 Heating, Ventilating, and Air-Conditioning.

Heating, ventilating, and air-conditioning equipment shall comply with the provisions of Section 9.2.

### 39.5.3 Elevators, Escalators, and Conveyors.

Elevators, escalators, and conveyors shall comply with the provisions of Section 9.4.

### 39.5.4 Rubbish Chutes, Incinerators, and Laundry Chutes.

Rubbish chutes, incinerators, and laundry chutes shall comply with the provisions of Section 9.5.

## 39.6 Reserved

## 39.7 Operating Features

### 39.7.1 Emergency Plans.

Emergency plans complying with Section 4.8 shall be provided in high-rise buildings.

### 39.7.2 Drills.

In all business occupancy buildings occupied by more than 500 persons, or by more than 100 persons above or below the street level, employees and supervisory personnel shall be periodically instructed in accordance with Section 4.7 and shall hold drills periodically where practicable.

### 39.7.3 Extinguisher Training.

Designated employees of business occupancies shall be periodically instructed in the use of portable fire extinguishers.

### 39.7.4 Food Service Operations.

Food service operations shall comply with 13.7.2.

### 39.7.5 Upholstered Furniture and Mattresses.

The provisions of 10.3.2 shall not apply to upholstered furniture and mattresses.

Emergency plans must be provided for both new and existing high-rise business occupancies per 38/39.7.1, a new requirement for the 2009 edition of the *Code*. This requirement, and the companion requirements of Section 4.8 and associated Annex A language, were developed and revised, respectively, in response to recommendations by the NFPA High Rise Building Safety Advisory Committee, which was appointed following the collapse of the World Trade Center towers on September 11, 2001. See Section 4.8 and its associated commentary for details on the contents of the required emergency plan.

The authority having jurisdiction (AHJ) determines the extent of the portable fire extinguisher training required by 38/39.7.3 (e.g., instruction only or instruction and hands-on use).

## References Cited in Commentary

1. NFPA 101A, *Guide on Alternative Approaches to Life Safety*, 2007 edition, National Fire Protection Association, Quincy, MA. (The edition of NFPA 101A that corresponds with the 2009 edition of NFPA *101®*, *Life Safety Code®*, will be the 2010 edition.)
2. NFPA 13, *Standard for the Installation of Sprinkler Systems*, 2007 edition, National Fire Protection Association, Quincy, MA.
3. ASTM D 2859, *Standard Test Method for Ignition Characteristics of Finished Textile Floor Covering Materials*, 2004 edition, ASTM International, 100 Barr Harbor Drive, P.O. Box C700, West Conshohocken, PA 19428-2959.
4. *NFPA 72®*, *National Fire Alarm Code®*, 2007 edition, National Fire Protection Association, Quincy, MA.

CHAPTER 40

# Industrial Occupancies

The industrial occupancy classification is broad in its scope and application. The following are examples of industrial occupancies:

1. Factories of all kinds
2. Pumping stations
3. Telephone exchanges
4. Gas plants
5. Laundries
6. Laboratories
7. Recycling plants
8. Refineries
9. Food processing plants
10. Drycleaning plants
11. Auto body and repair shops
12. Sawmills
13. Hangars (for servicing aircraft)
14. Power plants
15. Post office central sorting/maintenance facilities

The range of facilities that are classified as industrial occupancies is diverse. Industrial occupancies comprise a wide variety of building configurations, uses, and equipment types. Some industrial occupancies might be considered innocuous with respect to the threat of fire hazard, such as a factory that manufactures concrete blocks. An industrial occupancy subject to the threat of serious fire hazard might be a petroleum processing and refining plant, where the threat of explosion is always present. The subclassification system used in 40.1.4.1 is intended to assist the user in establishing the level of hazard to the occupants of an industrial occupancy.

The requirements of Chapter 40 were written to provide adequate life safety without unduly restricting the functional operations of a facility. For example, 40.2.2.10 and 40.2.2.11 permit fire escape ladders and slide escapes as part of an occupant protection package that balances the need for rapid escape from platforms and other industrial structures with the ability of the occupants to use such egress devices. By permitting the use of fire escape ladders and slide escapes, Chapter 40 recognizes that functional requirements necessitate occupant access to unusual spaces within the industrial facility and that efficient egress from these spaces is important.

A unique life safety consideration addressed in Chapter 40 involves egress for occupants of ancillary facilities. Paragraph 40.2.5.1 recognizes that some types of industrial processes and equipment cannot be immediately abandoned if the building fire alarm sounds. If workers do not remain in the building long enough to effect orderly equipment shutdown during a fire emergency, dangers greater than fire might result. The protection measures required by 40.2.5.1 provide for the safety of occupants who must remain while others leave the building.

Another unique feature that the *Code* addresses for industrial occupancies is the equipment access dimensional criteria of Table 40.2.5.2.1. These dimensional criteria, although more lenient than those of Chapter 7, provide adequate egress paths for the small number of occupants using any of those routes to reach major aisles that lead to exits.

The statistics provided by the national fire incident databases demonstrate that the potential loss of life from fire in an industrial occupancy is directly related to the hazard of the industrial operation or process. Most multiple-death industrial fires are the result of flash fires caused by highly combustible material or explosions involving combustible dusts, flammable liquids, or gases.

Until recently, industrial fire losses have constituted a high percentage of the annual property loss from fire; however, such fires have not, as a general rule, resulted in extensive loss of life. With most rules, however, there are exceptions. In 2002 and 2003, a total of 18 people died in fires or explosions in three separate incidents — all involving the processing of combustible particles or dust.

In the first incident, which occurred in May 2002, five workers were killed in an explosion at a rubber reclaiming plant located in Vicksburg, Mississippi. The fire, which originated in the rubber dryer system, ignited the building's roof and spread to the bagging room, where rubber dust ignited and exploded. In the second incident, which occurred in January 2003, six workers were killed in a dust explosion at a pharmaceutical plant in Kinston, North Carolina. The accumulation of dust above a suspended ceiling led to the blast, which could be felt 25 miles (40 kilometers) away. In the third incident, which occurred in February 2003, seven workers were killed when insulation particles inside an oven ignited and exploded at an automobile insulation manufacturing plant in Corbin, Kentucky. Although it is not mandatorially referenced by the *Code*, NFPA 654, *Standard for the Prevention of Fire and Dust Explosions from the Manufacturing, Processing, and Handling of Combustible Particulate Solids*,[1] should be applied where industrial processes involve combustible dusts to reduce the likelihood of such catastrophic fires and explosions.

In March 2005, an explosion at a Texas City, Texas, oil refinery — an example of a high hazard industrial occupancy — killed 15 workers and injured more than 170. The explosion occurred in the refinery's isomerization unit — the location of equipment used to boost the octane in gasoline — when the system was being restarted following maintenance a few days earlier. Although the *Code* does not directly address the hazards associated with handling flammable liquids, it does reference NFPA 30, *Flammable and Combustible Liquids Code*,[2] which provides requirements for such operations to minimize the probability of fires and explosions (see 8.7.3.1). Other industry standards, such as those published by the American Petroleum Institute (API), directly address the hazards associated with refineries.

One of the major features to be considered in the design of an industrial occupancy's life safety system is the use of automatic sprinkler protection. Originally developed for industrial property protection, the automatic sprinkler has also been largely responsible for an excellent life safety record in industrial occupancies — limiting the size of a fire by means of sprinklers provides sufficient time for the safe evacuation of occupants. This record has been recognized by the fire protection community, as evidenced by the widespread use of automatic sprinkler systems in buildings with significant hazards to life. The contribution of the automatic sprinkler to safety to life can be fully appreciated only when the wide range of fire risks associated with the many processes used in an industrial facility are recognized.

Employees and other occupants of industrial buildings are generally ambulatory and capable of quick response to fires. They are also able to exit rapidly once properly alerted. To capitalize on this employee capability, many industrial facilities include life safety measures in their emergency preplanning. A well-conceived plan provides a valuable tool in preventing loss of life. Provisions that should be part of the emergency preplan include the following:

1. Measures for alerting employees
2. Identification and posting of exit access routes
3. Establishment of group assembly areas for occupants once they have evacuated the building
4. Procedures for determining that all employees have safely evacuated

Responsibilities are usually established and assigned in the preplan to ensure that the tasks necessary to facilitate safe evacuation of the building are performed. The preplan should routinely be evaluated through simulated fire exercises and drills. Only through the execution of such drills can flaws in the preplan be recognized and modified.

Although the life safety record in industrial occupancies has been good, the trend toward constructing large industrial plants that house hazardous operations might prove problematic. The introduction of combustible materials, such as extensive quantities of plastics, has increased the need for additional measures to help protect workers from fire. Compared with the industrial buildings of the early twentieth century, the modern industrial complex has placed a larger number of employees in a more complex and increasingly hazardous environment. This trend has increased the need for facility managers to concentrate on life safety principles not only during the design stage but also during day-to-day plant operations.

As part of their employee training programs, most industrial firms include education in the use of first aid fire-fighting equipment, such as in-plant standpipes, hose, and portable fire extinguishers. Although first aid fire-fighting measures are primarily a property protection measure, they also provide a significant life safety benefit when utilized correctly by trained individuals. Industrial training of this type, where fully utilized, has resulted in a major reduction in loss of property and life.

## 40.1 General Requirements

### 40.1.1 Application.

**40.1.1.1** The requirements of this chapter shall apply to both new and existing industrial occupancies.

**40.1.1.2** Industrial occupancies shall include factories making products of all kinds and properties used for operations such as processing, assembling, mixing, packaging, finishing or decorating, repairing, and similar operations.

**40.1.1.3** Incidental high hazard operations protected in accordance with Section 8.7 and 40.3.2 in occupancies containing low or ordinary hazard contents shall not be the basis for high hazard industrial occupancy classification.

Unlike most occupancies addressed by the *Code*, both new and existing industrial occupancies are covered in one chapter. Where requirements vary, exemptions that apply to existing industrial occupancies are often provided, or additional requirements that are limited to new industrial occupancies are specified.

### 40.1.2 Multiple Occupancies.

All multiple occupancies shall be in accordance with 6.1.14.

Subsection 40.1.2 directs the user to the multiple occupancies provisions of 6.1.14, which permit protecting multiple occupancies either as mixed or as separated. If a multiple occupancy building is protected via the provisions of 6.1.14.4 for separated uses, the required separation, in terms of fire resistance rating, is specified by Table 6.1.14.4.1(a) and Table 6.1.14.4.1(b).

### 40.1.3 Special Definitions.

Special terms applicable to this chapter are defined in Chapter 3.

Although no definitions are listed in 40.1.3, industrial occupancies are subclassified and defined in 40.1.4.1 under the labels *general industrial occupancy, special-purpose industrial occupancy,* and *high hazard industrial occupancy.* See also 3.3.178.8, 3.3.178.8.1, 3.3.178.8.2, and 3.3.178.8.3.

### 40.1.4 Classification of Occupancy.

Classification of occupancy shall be in accordance with 6.1.12.

The method for determining the degree of hazard to life safety posed by an industrial occupancy is often a matter of personal judgment and not science. The authority having jurisdiction (AHJ) must use judgment based on past experience, review of reference materials and engineering analyses, and full discussion with third parties to evaluate the life safety measures in an industrial occupancy. The *Code* establishes broad categories of occupancy classification so that the relative risks to life safety posed by various types of buildings can be assessed.

A common error made when classifying industrial occupancies is the use of hazard categories for automatic sprinklers contained in NFPA 13, *Standard for the Installation of Sprinkler Systems,*[3] to determine the hazard to life safety. While the guidelines in NFPA 13 might not differ greatly from those of the *Life Safety Code* where classifying occupancies with high hazards, the remaining categories specified in NFPA 13 are usually not suitable for the general industrial occupancy classification of the *Code.* (The use of NFPA 13 is particularly inappropriate where classifying low hazard occupancies, which are classified as light hazard by NFPA 13.) The distinction is that the life safety industrial occupancy classification is concerned with determining the overall hazard to occupants in a manufacturing building for purposes of implementing an adequate means of egress system, while the NFPA 13 classification system is concerned with defining the hazard so that a sprinkler system can be designed to meet the challenge of the hazard.

To examine the conflicts between life safety occupancy classification and classifications in other fire codes, consider a metalworking plant using a flammable solvent in a dip tank coating operation. From a life safety standpoint, the normally ordinary hazard classification of the metalworking plant should not be changed to high hazard solely because of the presence of a dip tank coater. An adequate means of safe egress leading away from the coater is required to ensure the safety of the occupants. However, additional exits and a reduction in travel distance to an exit, as specified for a high hazard contents area, are not required. Nevertheless, if the coater is the principal piece of equipment in a separately enclosed area, that area might be considered as a high hazard industrial occupancy.

When determining the life safety hazard classification for an industrial occupancy, the AHJ should carefully analyze the nature of that industrial operation to ensure an accurate evaluation of the hazard to occupants. A number of resources are available for properly determining the degree of risk to life safety. One resource that should not be overlooked is the expertise of the industrial plant operator, who can provide a wealth of hazard information, although some such information might be treated as confidential to prevent competitors from learning the details of an industrial process. In such a case, the enforcing authority must handle that information with discretion; once an enforcing authority is known to be an outside source of data on industrial secrets, further cooperation will be difficult to obtain. Likewise, facility operators should be forthcoming with process information having an effect on emergency response operations.

Another resource is the engineering department of the company responsible for a facility's insurance coverage. In addition, discussions with officials who oversee jurisdictions where similar facilities exist and a review of available literature, such as the NFPA *Fire Protection Handbook*[4]; the NFPA *Industrial Fire Protection Handbook*[5]; and *Industrial Fire Protection Engineering*,[6] will provide further information on a particular process and its associated hazards.

To assess the risk to life safety in an industrial occupancy, a number of factors should be considered. It should be determined if the manufacturing process includes the handling of flammable, reactive, or explosive materials in quantities that could directly expose occupants to a fire or explosion. If so, the occupancy is a strong candidate for a high hazard classification. See 40.1.4.1.3.

It should also be determined whether the manufacturing process requires a large number of people or whether it is basically a large collection of machines or equipment occasionally attended by operators. In some instances, operators might be clustered in one location, such as a control room. If a building predominantly houses machinery or equipment and is occupied by few employees, the building can be classified as a special-purpose industrial occupancy. See 40.1.4.1.2.

If an industrial building is used mostly for storage of materials (such as preparatory stock for assembly or finished goods), it might meet the requirements for classification as a storage occupancy. See Chapter 42.

Hazard classification is based on the burning and explosive characteristics of the materials contained in a building, not on the quantity of combustibles. For example, there is no reason to classify a building as high hazard simply because it is associated with a manufacturing process that requires extensive quantities of ordinary combustible materials to be distributed in such a manner that the process involves a high combustible fuel load.

The classification of an industrial occupancy, for life safety purposes, is not based on the type of structure housing the industrial process. The basic purpose of the hazard classification in Section 6.2 is to evaluate the risk posed to occupants by the burning characteristics of the building's contents. The classification is determined by an evaluation of the contents and other factors in a fire's development that affect the time available for safe evacuation of the occupants. Once employees are evacuated to a safe location, the extent of fire spread in the structure becomes a threat to property. As long as life safety measures are met, the threat of heavy fire damage to a building is beyond the scope of the *Life Safety Code*.

**40.1.4.1 Subclassification of Occupancy.** Each industrial occupancy shall be subclassified according to its use as described in 40.1.4.1.1, 40.1.4.1.2, and 40.1.4.1.3.

**40.1.4.1.1 General Industrial Occupancy.** General industrial occupancies shall include the following:

(1) Industrial occupancies that conduct ordinary and low hazard industrial operations in buildings of conventional design that are usable for various types of industrial processes
(2) Industrial occupancies that include multistory buildings where floors are occupied by different tenants, or buildings that are usable for such occupancy and, therefore, are subject to possible use for types of industrial processes with a high density of employee population

**40.1.4.1.2 Special-Purpose Industrial Occupancy.** Special-purpose industrial occupancies shall include the following:

(1) Industrial occupancies that conduct ordinary and low hazard industrial operations in buildings designed for, and that are usable only for, particular types of operations
(2) Industrial occupancies that are characterized by a relatively low density of employee population, with much of the area occupied by machinery or equipment

It can be difficult to determine if a building qualifies as a special-purpose industrial occupancy. For example, a structure is often erected to protect a large machine or equipment from weather. Once constructed, authorities might try to impose means of egress requirements applicable to a general industrial occupancy, despite the fact that only a handful of personnel are expected to occupy the building. Steel mills, paper plants, power-generating plants, and other operations with large machines are examples of the types of industrial occupancies requiring massive structures for process control and weather protection. These structures often represent minimum hazards to life safety and are typically classified as special-purpose industrial occupancies. In many of the more modern operations, all process control is conducted from a control room by remote means, which further reduces the number of occupants likely to be exposed to a fire in the equipment areas.

The special-purpose industrial occupancy classification must not be applied to a building simply to reduce egress requirements. Economic considerations, or staffing limitations that result in occupancy by fewer employees than usual, cannot be used as justification for reducing life safety features; the full number and arrangement of exits required for a general industrial occupancy must be maintained. A reduction in aisles, doors, stairways, and other components of the means of egress cannot be justified by the temporary classification of a building as a special-purpose industrial occupancy.

**40.1.4.1.3* High Hazard Industrial Occupancy.** High hazard industrial occupancies shall include the following:

(1) Industrial occupancies that conduct industrial operations that use high hazard materials or processes or house high hazard contents
(2) Industrial occupancies in which incidental high hazard operations in low or ordinary hazard occupancies that are protected in accordance with Section 8.7 and 40.3.2 are not required to be the basis for overall occupancy classification

**A.40.1.4.1.3** Additional information on the definition of high hazard industrial occupancy can be found in A.3.3.178.8.2.

A high hazard industrial occupancy classification is limited to those industrial buildings housing extremely hazardous operations. Incidental use of restricted quantities of flammable liquids in a building does not constitute a high hazard, although some additional life safety precautions might be required during the limited period of use. Refer to NFPA 30, *Flammable and Combustible Liquids Code*, for guidance. Storage of flammable liquids, such as paint, in sealed containers does not require a high hazard occupancy classification, unless the operation includes mixing or blending operations that require the containers to be opened. Mixing and blending of flammable liquids is permitted to be conducted in a separate room with a fire barrier between the storage and mixing areas. The mixing and blending room would be considered a high hazard industrial occupancy, while the adjacent, fire-separated storage area would be considered a general purpose industrial occupancy or possibly a storage occupancy subject to the requirements of Chapter 42.

Combustible dusts released from an industrial or manufacturing process constitute a significant threat to life safety, as demonstrated by the three incidents described in the commentary following the title of this chapter, and might justify a high hazard classification. Major loss of life has occurred in industrial occupancies that release extensive quantities of combustible dusts. Opportunity for the rapid escape of employees who work in operations that release combustible dust should be provided to prevent injury or loss of life if a dust explosion occurs. In high hazard occupancies that are subject to explosions, the provisions of 40.3.2 require special consideration of the techniques for explosion suppression or venting to ensure the life safety of occupants. Full use of fire protection engineering techniques should be employed in these occupancies to minimize the risk to life safety.

The industrial occupancies that clearly require classification as high hazard are those associated with the production of explosives or highly reactive chemicals. In some especially hazardous operations, additional exits will be necessary to ensure rapid egress to prevent loss of life in the event of an explosion or fire. Where the installation of the preventive or protective measures specified in 40.3.2 is not possible due to the nature of the industrial operation, consideration should be given to operating procedures that restrict access to a limited number of people during the hazardous portion of the operation. The operating procedures would limit the potential threat to those trained personnel who are fully aware of the extent of the hazard. Procedures should also include a record of personnel who have signed in or out. This procedure ensures prompt determination of the number of personnel exposed to a hazardous operation and, thus, the number who might require rescue.

**40.1.4.2 Change of Industrial Occupancy Subclassification.** Changing from one subclassification of industrial occupancy to another shall be permitted only if the structure, building, or portion thereof conforms to the requirements of this chapter that apply to new construction for the new use.

Although 40.1.4.2 states changes in industrial occupancy subclassification are permitted only if the building meets the new construction requirements for the new subclassification, it is noted that the *Code* includes Chapter 43, Building Rehabilitation, which makes provisions for changes in occupancy classification and requirements depend on the relative change in hazard category (see Section 43.7). The provisions of 40.1.4.2 will need to be coordinated with 4.6.8 and Chapter 43 for a future edition; until such time, it is appropriate to apply Chapter 43 where there is a change in industrial occupancy subclassification. In some cases, Chapter 43 permits a building to meet less restrictive requirements where there is a change in use or occupancy classification to promote adaptive reuse of existing building stock. In other cases, such as where a general industrial occupancy changes to a high hazard industrial occupancy, the building must meet the more restrictive new construction requirements. See Chapter 43 and the commentary therein for additional details on building rehabilitation.

### 40.1.5 Classification of Hazard of Contents.

Classification of hazard of contents shall be in accordance with Section 6.2.

### 40.1.6 Minimum Construction Requirements.

(No requirements.)

Some occupancy chapters, such as Chapters 18 and 19, which address the life safety needs of nonambulatory health care occupants, specify minimum building construction type requirements to ensure structural integrity for the time needed for a lengthy evacuation or for safe refuge within the building. No minimum construction requirements are imposed by Chapter 40, because industrial occupancies characteristically have ambulatory occupants and do not provide sleeping accommodations. Occupants will likely have the ability to egress the building quickly before the fire-resisting qualities of the building construction become an issue.

### 40.1.7* Occupant Load.

The occupant load, in number of persons for whom means of egress and other provisions are required, shall be determined on the basis of the occupant load factors of Table 7.3.1.2 that are characteristic of the use of the space, or shall be determined as the maximum probable population of the space under consideration, whichever is greater.

**A.40.1.7** In most cases, the requirements for maximum travel distance to exits will be the determining factor, rather than numbers of occupants, because exits provided to satisfy travel distance requirements will be sufficient to provide egress capacity for all occupants, except in cases of an unusual arrangement of buildings or the high occupant load of a general manufacturing occupancy.

The occupant load of an industrial building is based on an average of 100 $ft^2$ (9.3 $m^2$) of gross floor area per occupant in accordance with Table 7.3.1.2. Many industrial users of the *Code* confuse this concept with the actual number of employees who use the facility. The usual complaint is that the number of potential employees calculated for egress purposes in accordance with the 100 $ft^2$ (9.3 $m^2$) criterion far exceeds the anticipated or actual number of employees. Many industrial managers argue that using the larger number as a basis for egress design requires more exits, wider doors, and more passageways than are needed for emergency egress purposes, reducing productive work space and resulting in increased cost.

The concept of determining occupant load by using an occupant load factor is useful, although it does not necessarily relate directly to the actual number of building occupants. The occupant load factor is used as a means of calculating the minimum egress requirements, based on the needs of an average industrial occupancy. Although actual conditions might vary in an individual location, the egress width determined by the occupant load calculation will normally provide the necessary, adequate, and required means of egress for a typical industrial building with little or no penalty to the building's owner/operator.

See Exhibit 40.1 for examples of occupant load determination using the occupant load factor for a general industrial occupancy and using the probable number of occupants for a special-purpose industrial occupancy.

In Exhibit 40.1, Part (a), the general industrial occupancy must provide a means of egress for at least 2000 persons, based on use of an occupant load factor of 1 person per 100 $ft^2$ (9.3 $m^2$).

In Exhibit 40.1, Part (b), a special-purpose industrial occupancy can size its means of egress for the maximum 20 persons (actual anticipated employee population) who are expected to occupy the facility under any probable condition.

In Exhibit 40.1, Part (c), the 200-person tour groups that visit this special-purpose industrial occupancy on the first Monday of each month must be added to the 45 employees (actual employee population) who are normally present, for a total occupant load of 245 persons.

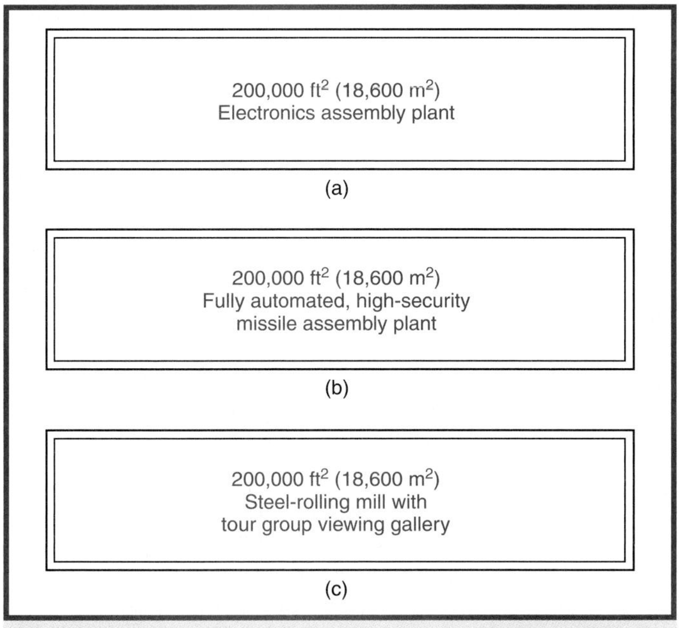


***Exhibit 40.1*** *Determination of occupant load of industrial occupancies.*

## 40.2 Means of Egress Requirements

### 40.2.1 General.

**40.2.1.1** Each required means of egress shall be in accordance with the applicable portions of Chapter 7.

**40.2.1.2*** Normally unoccupied utility chases that are secured from unauthorized access and are used exclusively for routing of electrical, mechanical, or plumbing equipment shall not be required to comply with the provisions of Chapter 7.

**A.40.2.1.2** Horizontal and vertical utility chases in large industrial buildings used for routing of piping, ducts, and wiring must provide a reasonable level of access for occasional maintenance workers but do not warrant compliance with the comprehensive egress requirements of Chapter 7. Minimum access in these cases is governed by electrical and mechanical codes; 40.2.5.2, Industrial Equipment Access; and the Occupational Safety and Health Administration (OSHA) for facilities in the United States. Utility chases governed by this paragraph might involve tunnels or large open spaces located above or below occupied floors; however, such spaces differ from mechanical equipment rooms, boiler rooms, and furnace rooms, based on the anticipated frequency of use by maintenance workers. Portions of utility chases where the anticipated presence of maintenance workers is routine are not intended to be included by this paragraph.

### 40.2.2 Means of Egress Components.

**40.2.2.1 Components Permitted.** Components of means of egress shall be limited to the types described in 40.2.2.2 through 40.2.2.13.

**40.2.2.2 Doors.**

**40.2.2.2.1** Doors complying with 7.2.1 shall be permitted.

**40.2.2.2.2** Delayed-egress locks complying with 7.2.1.6.1 shall be permitted.

Use of the delayed-egress locking device covered by 7.2.1.6.1 is permitted on any door in recognition of the security needs of some industrial occupancies. In effect, the allowable 15-second or 30-second delay will be experienced only under non-fire conditions or very early in a fire's growth, because the door must be usable immediately upon sprinkler operation, smoke or heat detection, or loss of power that controls the locking mechanism. The building must be protected throughout by an approved, supervised automatic sprinkler system or an approved, supervised automatic fire detection system to permit the use of delayed-egress locks per 7.2.1.6.1.

**40.2.2.2.3** Access-controlled egress doors complying with 7.2.1.6.2 shall be permitted.

Paragraph 40.2.2.2.3 permits the installation of access-controlled egress doors in industrial occupancies, provided that they meet the provisions of 7.2.1.6.2. Access-controlled egress doors are frequently confused with so-called "mag lock" doors, whereby an occupant must swipe a card or enter a code on a keypad, for example, to unlock the door in the direction of egress travel. The *Code* prohibits such locking arrangements on required means of egress doors, even if they are provided with an emergency release button and are arranged to unlock upon activation of the fire alarm system. To comply with the *Code*, access-controlled egress doors must be provided with all of the features described in 7.2.1.6.2(1) through (8). The motion sensor arranged to detect approaching occupants and unlock the door described in 7.2.1.6.2(1) is perhaps the most frequently overlooked requirement.

**40.2.2.2.4** Approved existing horizontal-sliding fire doors shall be permitted in the means of egress under the following conditions:

(1) They are held open by fusible links.
(2) The fusible links are rated at not less than 165°F (74°C).

(3) The fusible links are located not more than 10 ft (3050 mm) above the floor.
(4) The fusible links are in immediate proximity to the door opening.
(5) The fusible links are not located above a ceiling.
(6) The door is not credited with providing any protection under this *Code*.

Horizontal-sliding fire doors exist in many industrial occupancies for property protection purposes. Although the *Code* normally does not recognize these doors within the required means of egress, 40.2.2.2.4 makes a special exemption for existing horizontal-sliding fire doors. By requiring the fusible link to be positioned in immediate proximity to the door opening, rated 165°F (74°C) or higher, and located not more than 10 ft (3050 mm) above the floor, the *Code* helps to ensure that the door will remain open until rising temperatures make it unsafe to pass through the door opening. Because the door will not close early in the fire development, the door cannot be credited as a fire door for life safety purposes. However, the door might serve as a means of property protection. See Exhibit 40.2.

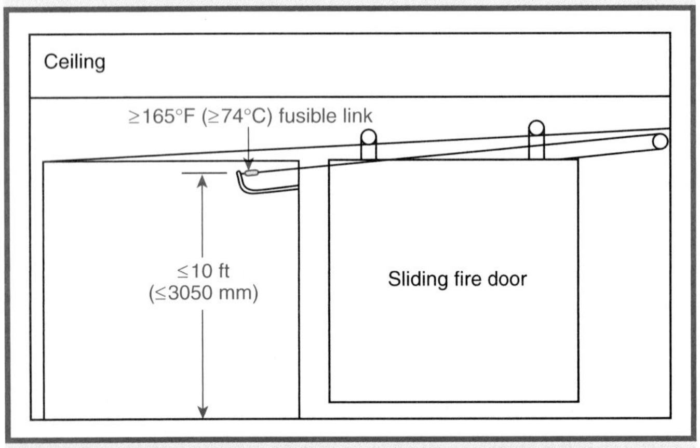


***Exhibit 40.2** Existing horizontal-sliding fire door in accordance with 40.2.2.2.4.*

**40.2.2.3 Stairs.**

**40.2.2.3.1** Stairs shall comply with 7.2.2 and shall be permitted to be modified as follows:

(1) Noncombustible grated stair treads and noncombustible grated landing floors shall be permitted.
(2) Industrial equipment access stairs in accordance with 40.2.5.2 shall be permitted.

**40.2.2.3.2** Spiral stairs complying with 7.2.2.2.3 shall be permitted.

**40.2.2.3.3** Existing winders complying with 7.2.2.2.4 shall be permitted.

Paragraph 40.2.2.3.1(1) exempts stair treads and landings in industrial occupancies from the provisions of 7.2.2.3.3.1, which would otherwise require that all stair treads and stair landing floors be solid. Although the requirement for solid treads and landing floors is intended to prevent occupants from avoiding the use of the stairs because they become afraid when they are able to see through the openings to the floor or ground below, occupants of industrial occupancies are usually more familiar, and thus more comfortable, with grated or expanded metal treads and landings. There is also a high degree of certainty that occupants will be wearing shoes appropriate for the environment, and not high heels that could get stuck in the grate openings. The grated walking surfaces provide slip resistance in what are sometimes greasy and slippery surroundings. For consistency, 7.2.2.3.3.4(3) alerts the user that industrial occupancies, in accordance with Chapter 40, are exempt from the solid tread and landing provisions.

Paragraph 40.2.2.3.1(2) serves to remind the user that 40.2.5.2 has special provisions for industrial equipment access stairs that differ from the requirements of Chapter 7. See the commentary following 40.2.5.2.2.

**40.2.2.4 Smokeproof Enclosures.** Smokeproof enclosures complying with 7.2.3 shall be permitted.

Paragraph 40.2.2.4 does not mandate the use of smokeproof enclosures. It does, however, recognize such an enclosure as part of the means of egress system in an industrial occupancy only if that enclosure meets the requirements of 7.2.3. For an example of an occupancy requiring a smokeproof enclosure, see 31.2.11.1, which specifies that existing nonsprinklered or partially sprinklered high-rise apartment buildings are required to be provided with smokeproof enclosures in accordance with 7.2.3.

**40.2.2.5 Horizontal Exits.**

**40.2.2.5.1** Horizontal exits complying with 7.2.4 shall be permitted.

**40.2.2.5.2*** In horizontal exits where the opening is protected by a fire door assembly on each side of the wall in which it is located, one fire door shall be of the swinging type, as provided in 7.2.4.3.7, and the other shall be permitted to be an automatic-sliding fire door that shall be kept open whenever the building is occupied.

**A.40.2.2.5.2** The customary building code requirement for fire doors on both sides of an opening in a fire wall is permitted to be met by having an automatic-sliding fire door on one side and a self-closing fire door swinging out from the other side of the wall. This arrangement qualifies only as a horizontal exit from the sliding door side. For further information, see A.7.2.4.3.10.

Paragraph 40.2.2.5.1 does not mandate the use of horizontal exits. It does, however, recognize a horizontal exit as part of the means of egress system in an industrial occupancy if that exit meets the requirements of 7.2.4, as modified by 40.2.2.5.2.

Paragraphs 40.2.2.5.2 and A.40.2.2.5.2 recognize the common practice of combining a horizontal exit that is used for life safety with a fire barrier having a significant fire resistance rating that is used for property protection. Opening protectives for such a fire barrier can require the use of a set of doors to achieve the required fire protection rating. It is impractical for both doors to swing in the same direction without interfering with each other; yet, operation of two doors that swing in opposite directions is cumbersome for daily or frequent use. The use of a combination of swinging and sliding doors, as shown in Exhibit 40.3, provides an acceptable arrangement for day-to-day functioning of the building. The normally open sliding door does not compromise life safety, because by the time its fusible link mechanism releases the door and allows it to close, temperatures in the vicinity of the door opening render use of the door impractical. See also the commentary following 40.2.2.2.4(6). The provisions of 40.2.2.2.4 also permit an existing horizontal-sliding door (as depicted in Exhibit 40.2) to serve within the means of egress.

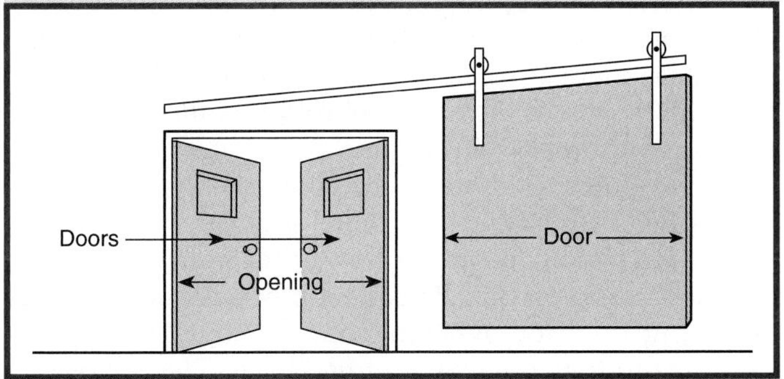


*Exhibit 40.3 Combination swinging and sliding doors permitted by 40.2.2.5.2.*

**40.2.2.6 Ramps.** Ramps shall comply with 7.2.5, except that industrial equipment access ramps shall be permitted to be in accordance with 40.2.5.2.

Paragraph 40.2.2.6 does not mandate the use of ramps in industrial occupancies. It does, however, recognize a ramp as part of the means of egress system if that ramp meets the requirements of 7.2.5. Paragraph 40.2.2.6 also serves to remind the user that 40.2.5.2 has special provisions for industrial equipment access ramps that differ from the requirements of Chapter 7. See the commentary following 40.2.5.2.2.

**40.2.2.7 Exit Passageways.** Exit passageways complying with 7.2.6 shall be permitted.

Paragraph 40.2.2.7 does not mandate the use of exit passageways in industrial occupancies. It does, however, recognize an exit passageway as part of the means of egress system if that exit passageway meets the requirements of 7.2.6.

**40.2.2.8 Escalators and Moving Walks.** Existing previously approved escalators and moving walks complying with 7.2.7 and located within the required means of egress shall be permitted.

Note that 7.2.7 permits existing escalators and moving walks to continue to be recognized within the required means of egress if permitted by an occupancy chapter. In earlier editions of the *Code*, such escalators and moving walks were recognized as providing egress capacity for 75 persons. To qualify as exits (as opposed to exit access), escalators and moving walks must also meet the requirements of 7.1.3.2, which address exit enclosures.

Note that escalators protected in accordance with the sprinkler-vent, spray nozzle, rolling shutter, or partial enclosure method do not constitute acceptable exits but can continue to serve as exit access if previously approved as such.

**40.2.2.9 Fire Escape Stairs.** Existing fire escape stairs complying with 7.2.8 shall be permitted.

**40.2.2.10 Fire Escape Ladders.**

**40.2.2.10.1** Fire escape ladders complying with 7.2.9 shall be permitted.

**40.2.2.10.2** Fixed industrial stairs in accordance with the minimum requirements for fixed stairs in ANSI A1264.1, *Safety Requirements for Workplace Floor and Wall Openings, Stairs and Railing Systems*, shall be permitted where fire escape ladders are permitted in accordance with 7.2.9.1.

The geometry associated with the incline angle and the size and shape of surfaces intended for foot placement on fire escape ladders falls within the range permitted for fixed industrial stairs. However, most fixed industrial stairs meet criteria that result in a safer arrangement than that provided by the fire escape ladder detailed in 7.2.9. Therefore, 40.2.2.10.2 recognizes fixed industrial stairs as a substitute for fire escape ladders.

**40.2.2.11 Slide Escapes.**

**40.2.2.11.1** Approved slide escapes complying with 7.2.10 shall be permitted as components in 100 percent of the required means of egress for both new and existing high hazard industrial occupancies.

**40.2.2.11.2** Slide escapes permitted by 40.2.2.11.1 shall be counted as means of egress only where regularly used in emergency egress drills to ensure that occupants are familiar with their use through practice.

The intent of 40.2.2.11 is to permit the use of slide escapes, which are commonly used components for means of egress from areas that house explosives or other highly hazardous materials in chemical industry buildings. This provision allows consideration of slide escapes as part of the required means of egress from both new and existing high hazard industrial occupancies. In many high hazard industrial occupancies, slide escapes are the only practical means of ensuring safe egress prior to an explosion or flash fire. As required by 40.2.2.11.2, occupants must be drilled in the use of the slide escapes to help ensure sufficient familiarity for quick egress under emergency conditions.

**40.2.2.12 Alternating Tread Devices.** Alternating tread devices complying with 7.2.11 shall be permitted.

The provisions of 7.2.11, in effect, limit the use of alternating tread devices to those locations where the *Code* recognizes the use of fire escape ladders (and fixed industrial stairs). See 40.2.2.10.1, 40.2.2.10.2, 7.2.9, and 7.2.11.

**40.2.2.13 Areas of Refuge.** Areas of refuge complying with 7.2.12 shall be permitted.

### 40.2.3 Capacity of Means of Egress.

Capacity of means of egress shall comply with either 40.2.3.1 or 40.2.3.2.

**40.2.3.1** The capacity of means of egress shall be in accordance with Section 7.3.

**40.2.3.2** In industrial occupancies, means of egress shall be sized to accommodate the occupant load as determined in accordance with 40.1.7; spaces not subject to human occupancy because of the presence of machinery or equipment shall not be included in the computation.

Prior to the 1991 edition, the *Code* required a minimum 44 in. (1120 mm) width for corridors and passageways within the required means of egress of industrial occupancies. A corridor or passageway of that minimum width would have provided egress capacity for 220 persons [i.e., 44 in./0.2 in. per person (approximately 1120 mm/5 mm per person) in accordance with Table 7.3.3.1 for level egress components]. That minimum requirement produced unnecessarily large egress systems, relative to the occupant load, in many industrial occupancies. Therefore, the requirement was eliminated, and the minimum 36 in. (915 mm) width requirement of 7.3.4.1(2), which addresses the minimum width of any exit access, was made applicable to industrial occupancies. Exit access is required to be wider than 36 in. (915 mm) only if a corridor or passageway in an industrial occupancy is to provide capacity for more than 180 persons [i.e., 36 in./0.2 in. per person (approximately 915 mm/5 mm per person)]. See the commentary following A.40.1.7 for details on the determination of occupant load in an industrial occupancy.

Paragraph 40.2.3.2 imposes practical limits on the number of required means of egress and on the arrangement of the means of egress in industrial occupancies. No life safety purpose is served by providing exits from the center of a large machine or equipment installation that is unoccupied under normal operating conditions. A number of industries provide weather shelter for large processes and equipment. Typical examples include steel-rolling mills, paper extruders, and metalworking machines, all of which occupy a majority of the floor space in the sheltered building. In many of the more sophisticated operations, full process control is conducted from a remotely located control room. Personnel normally occupy the building only for maintenance and adjustment purposes, and then only on a limited basis. The provision of exits from these special-purpose industrial occupancies serves no useful purpose and could unjustly impose an economic penalty in the name of safety.

The large areas normally enclosed by special-purpose structures would require excessive egress width if the occupant load were calculated on the basis of the 100 ft$^2$ (9.3 m$^2$) per person specified for general industrial occupancies. Such arrangements might actually require exits from the interior of machinery and equipment installations, which would be incompatible with the equipment's design. In many cases, these exits would originate from locations that, even under normal operating conditions, would be considered dangerous for humans. Poorly conceived exit facilities serve no life safety purpose and detract from an otherwise well-designed egress system.

### 40.2.4 Number of Means of Egress.

See also Section 7.4.

**40.2.4.1** The number of means of egress shall comply with either 40.2.4.1.1 or 40.2.4.1.2.

**40.2.4.1.1** Not less than two means of egress shall be provided from every story or section, and not less than one exit shall be reached without traversing another story.

**40.2.4.1.2** A single means of egress shall be permitted from any story or section in low and ordinary hazard industrial occupancies, provided that the exit can be reached within the distance permitted as a common path of travel.

**40.2.4.2** In new buildings, floors or portions thereof with an occupant load of more than 500 shall have the minimum number of separate and remote means of egress specified by 7.4.1.2.

**40.2.4.3** Areas with high hazard contents shall comply with Section 7.11.

The provisions of 40.2.4.1.1, which apply to the minimum required number of means of egress for industrial occupancies, clarify that, in addition to providing every story or section with access to at least two means of egress, one of the exits must be located on each floor, so that the entrance to that exit (e.g., a door that opens into an enclosed exit stair) can be reached without traveling to another floor.

Paragraph 40.2.4.1.2 recognizes that there are small floors or areas in low and ordinary hazard industrial occupancies that, if provided with access to only a single exit, are no less safe than larger areas of a building that have access to two exits where an occupant must first travel through the maximum allowable common path. Where a single exit is provided, the occupant travels the 50 ft (15 m) [or 100 ft (30 m) in sprinklered buildings] of common path allowed by Table 40.2.5, enters the exit, and is judged to have reached a point of safety (see Exhibit 40.4). In larger buildings and larger building areas that do not meet the limited travel distance for a single exit, a minimum of two exits must be provided. By traveling to the nearer of the two exits, the occupant is permitted to travel the same 50 ft (15 m) [or 100 ft (30 m) in sprinklered buildings] of common path that the occupant of the single exit building traveled to reach the one exit before reaching the point where travel to the two exits in different directions is possible. Although the occupant of the single exit building has reached an exit by this point, the occupant of the multiple exit building is then allowed an additional 150 ft (46 m) [200 ft (61 m) if building is sprinklered] of exit access travel before the safety of an exit must be reached. Therefore, the single exit exemption provides a level of life safety that is at least equivalent to that of the multiple exit building.

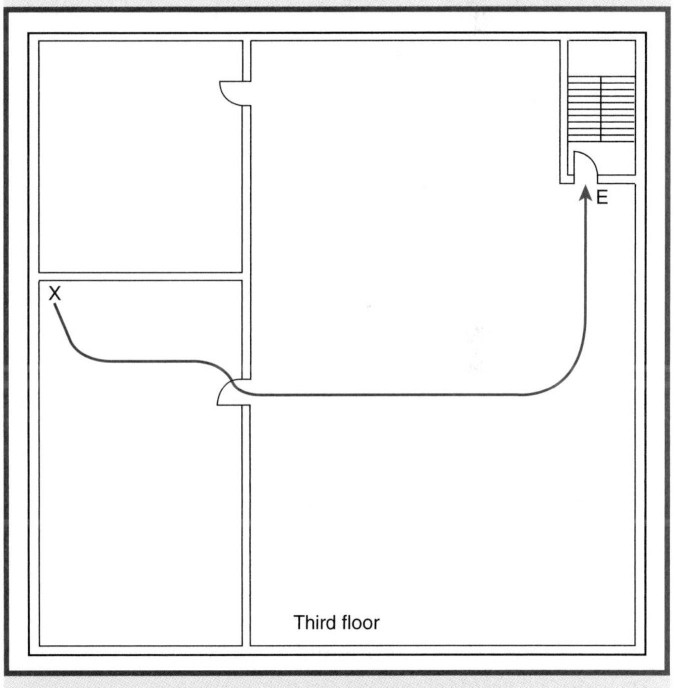


***Exhibit 40.4** Single means of egress from story of low or ordinary hazard industrial occupancy.*

In older editions, the *Code* required more than two exits based on occupant load for assembly occupancies only. Third, fourth, and subsequent exits were provided in industrial occupancies to meet travel distance requirements or as a convenience for day-to-day use. Paragraph 7.4.1.2 expands the concept of requiring three or four exits based on occupant load to apply to all occupancies. Paragraph 40.2.4.2, in compliance with the option offered by 7.4.1.2, exempts existing buildings from the requirement for third and fourth exits to avoid unnecessarily forcing existing, previously complying means of egress systems into noncompliance.

Section 7.11 includes an adequate set of provisions for high hazard areas and is referenced by 40.2.4.3 to provide commensurate protection to industrial occupancies that contain high hazard areas. The provisions of Section 7.11 are vital to life safety in high hazard occupancies. The requirement for two means of egress for all high hazard occupancies recognizes the possibility that a fire or explosion might block or destroy one of the two exits. Two separate and equal means of egress from high hazard areas provide a necessary redundancy to ensure the evacuation of occupants under fire or explosion conditions and to minimize the potential for injury or loss of life. Subsection 7.11.4 recognizes that it is not necessary to require two means of egress from very small high hazard areas [maximum 200 $ft^2$ (18.6 $m^2$)] with limited occupant load (maximum three persons) if the room door can be reached within 25 ft (7620 mm) of travel.

## 40.2.5 Arrangement of Means of Egress.

Means of egress, arranged in accordance with Section 7.5, shall not exceed that provided by Table 40.2.5.

See the discussion of dead-end corridor pockets and common path of travel in A.7.5.1.5 and its associated commentary.

### 40.2.5.1 Ancillary Facilities.

**40.2.5.1.1*** New ancillary facilities shall be arranged to allow travel in independent directions after leaving the ancillary facility so that both means of egress paths do not become compromised by the same fire or similar emergency.

**A.40.2.5.1.1** Ancillary facilities located within industrial occupancies might include administrative office, laboratory, control, and employee service facilities that are incidental to the predominant industrial function and are of such size that separate occupancy classification is not warranted.

**40.2.5.1.2*** New ancillary facilities in special-purpose industrial occupancies where delayed evacuation is anticipated shall have not less than a 2-hour fire resistance–rated separation from the predominant industrial occupancy, and shall have one means of egress that is separated from the predominant industrial occupancy by 2-hour fire resistance–rated construction.

**A.40.2.5.1.2** Occupants of ancillary facilities located within special-purpose industrial occupancies might be required by administrative controls to remain in the facility when a fire occurs in the predominant industrial area, so that they can perform an orderly shutdown of process equipment to control the spread of the fire and minimize damage to important equipment.

The presence of ancillary facilities within an industrial occupancy can create unusual challenges to life safety. For example, the means of egress for factory office workers, who might have little knowledge of the industrial processes and operations and their respective hazards, might require leaving the safety of an office area and traveling across the factory production floor.

*Table 40.2.5 Arrangement of Means of Egress*

| Level of Protection | General Industrial Occupancy | | Special-Purpose Industrial Occupancy | | High Hazard Industrial Occupancy |
|---|---|---|---|---|---|
| | ft | m | ft | m | |
| **Dead-End Corridor** | | | | | |
| Protected throughout by an approved, supervised automatic sprinkler system in accordance with 9.7.1.1(1) | 50 | 15 | 50 | 15 | Prohibited, except as permitted by 7.11.4 |
| Not protected throughout by an approved, supervised automatic sprinkler system in accordance with 9.7.1.1(1) | 50 | 15 | 50 | 15 | Prohibited, except as permitted by 7.11.4 |
| **Common Path of Travel** | | | | | |
| Protected throughout by an approved, supervised automatic sprinkler system in accordance with 9.7.1.1(1) | 100 | 30 | 100 | 30 | Prohibited, except as permitted by 7.11.4 |
| Not protected throughout by an approved, supervised automatic sprinkler system in accordance with 9.7.1.1(1) | 50 | 15 | 50 | 15 | Prohibited, except as permitted by 7.11.4 |

In other cases, safe egress is not ensured for employees assigned to a control room who might have to perform orderly shutdown of certain processes to control the spread of fire before evacuating a building. The requirements of 40.2.5.1.1 and 40.2.5.1.2 are illustrated in Exhibit 40.5.

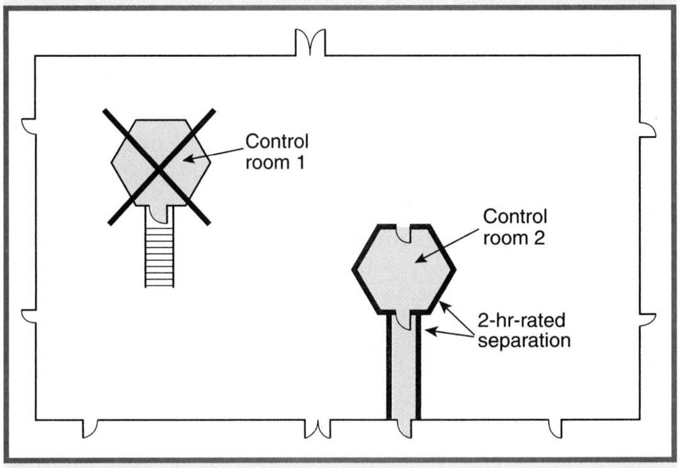


***Exhibit 40.5*** *Ancillary facilities.*

In Exhibit 40.5, an occupant of control room 1, which is elevated and has a single means of egress via a stair leading down to the main production floor, is forced to travel in one direction only into the open manufacturing area. This arrangement does not meet the requirement of 40.2.5.1.1, which mandates that egress be arranged to allow travel in independent directions after leaving the ancillary facility, so that both means of egress paths are not compromised by the same fire or similar emergency. Control room 1 requires a second exit access door and stair remotely located from the first.

Control room 2 in Exhibit 40.5 meets the requirements of both 40.2.5.1.1 and 40.2.5.1.2. Control room 2 permits egress travel in independent directions, so that both means of egress paths are not compromised by the same fire or similar emergency. Further, it provides one of the two means of egress via an exit passageway–like arrangement separated from the predominant industrial occupancy by 2-hour fire resistance–rated construction. Also, control room 2 is surrounded by 2-hour fire resistance–rated construction. This protection allows occupants charged with special emergency duties to delay their egress and still be afforded adequate life safety.

The requirements of 40.2.5.1 for ancillary facilities were added to the *Code* for the 1997 edition and are not required to be applied retroactively to existing facilities.

**40.2.5.2 Industrial Equipment Access.**

**40.2.5.2.1** Industrial equipment access doors, walkways, platforms, ramps, and stairs that serve as a component of the means of egress from the involved equipment shall be permitted in accordance with the applicable provisions of Chapter 7, as modified by Table 40.2.5.2.1.

***Table 40.2.5.2.1 Industrial Equipment Access Dimensional Criteria***

| Feature | Dimensional Criteria |
|---|---|
| Minimum horizontal dimension of any walkway, landing, or platform | 22 in. (560 mm) clear |
| Minimum stair or ramp width | 22 in. (560 mm) clear between rails |
| Minimum tread width | 22 in. (560 mm) clear |
| Minimum tread depth | 10 in. (255 mm) |
| Maximum riser height | 9 in. (230 mm) |
| Handrails are permitted to terminate, at the required height, at a point directly above the top and bottom risers. | |
| Maximum height between landings | 12 ft (3660 mm) |
| Minimum headroom | 6 ft 8 in. (2030 mm) |
| Minimum width of door openings | 22 in. (560 mm) clear |

**40.2.5.2.2** Any means of egress component permitted by 40.2.5.2.1 shall serve not more than 20 people.

Paragraph 40.2.5.2 permits industrial equipment access walkways, platforms, ramps, stairs, and doors serving not more than 20 persons to deviate from some of the usual dimensional criteria specified by Chapter 7. The dimensional criteria detailed in Table 40.2.5.2.1 are illustrated in Exhibit 40.6.

## 40.2.6 Travel Distance to Exits.

Travel distance, measured in accordance with Section 7.6, shall not exceed that provided by Table 40.2.6.

The travel distance exemption permitted by the footnote to Table 40.2.6 is meant to provide flexibility in determining the layout of the means of egress system in a single-story industrial building with a large floor area that houses a low or ordinary hazard general industrial occupancy. The exemption is limited to use in one-story buildings. Any stairs or other impediments to the rapid movement of occupants would result in

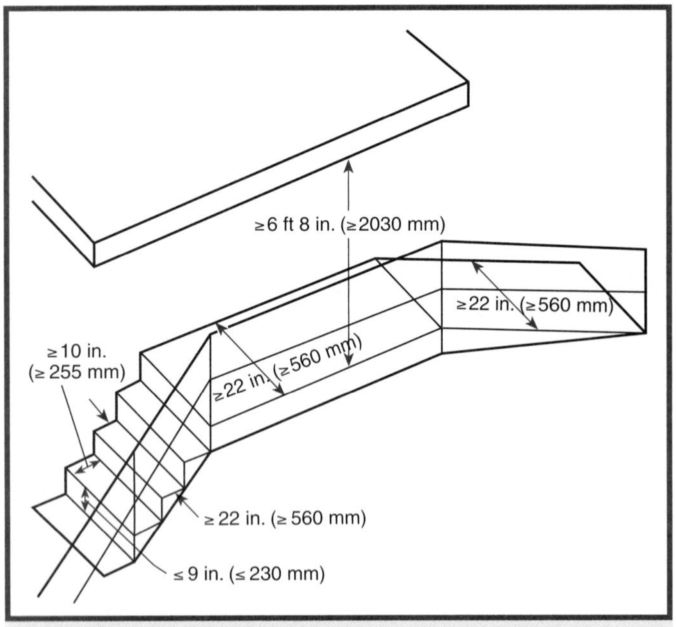


***Exhibit 40.6*** *Industrial equipment access dimensional criteria.*

slower evacuation of the building and increase the possibility of exposure to smoke or fire. The exemption requires a performance-based analysis to demonstrate that safe egress can be accomplished. NFPA 204, *Standard for Smoke and Heat Venting*,[7] might be of assistance. In addition, NFPA 92B, *Standard for Smoke Management Systems in Malls, Atria, and Large Spaces*,[8] can be consulted where designing buildings with ceilings of heights that approximate those of mall buildings and atria. Also see Chapter 5 for details on performance-based designs.

The construction of tunnels and elevated means of egress that originate from the center of an industrial building with an extensive floor area is rarely attempted. Only a handful of buildings have ever been provided with such egress facilities, and most were World War II era airframe manufacturing buildings of massive size. In most industrial buildings, it is not practicable or economical to construct exit tunnels or overhead passageways. These special types of means of egress are not easily altered if modifications are necessary to adjust to changes in the layout of the facility. In addition, the construction costs for tunnels and elevated passageways are high due to the special design features required to ensure their safety, including fire resistance–rated supports for the elevated passageways, waterproofing, and other features necessary to maintain the integrity of underground tunnels. Another negative factor in such construction is the confining nature of a tunnel or elevated passage, which tends to discourage the use of these means of egress.

The use of horizontal exits that pass through fire walls is common in many industrial occupancies. The provisions in Chapter 7 are required to be fully considered to ensure the safe use of horizontal exits. A common violation of the provisions of Chapter 7 is the failure to provide the proper type of fire door in a horizontal exit fire barrier. A horizontal-sliding fire door is not an acceptable life safety feature. Such a door is permitted in existing installations in accordance with 40.2.2.2.4, but, even then, the door is not credited with protecting the opening for the purposes of this *Code*. If the horizontal exit is to be used from both sides of a fire wall, careful consideration of the direction of door swing is necessary to ensure that the *Code* will recognize this use. In many instances, two doors swinging in opposite directions will be required, so that the exit is permitted to be used as a means of egress from both sides of the fire wall. See 7.2.1.4, 7.2.4.3.6, and 40.2.2.5.

Low and ordinary hazard special-purpose industrial occupancies, which are characterized by large, specialized equipment and low occupant load, are permitted an increase in travel distance beyond that al-

***Table 40.2.6 Maximum Travel Distance to Exits***

| | General Industrial Occupancy | | Special-Purpose Industrial Occupancy | | High Hazard Industrial Occupancy | |
|---|---|---|---|---|---|---|
| **Level of Protection** | **ft** | **m** | **ft** | **m** | **ft** | **m** |
| Protected throughout by an approved, supervised automatic sprinkler system in accordance with 9.7.1.1(1) | 250 | 76† | 400 | 122 | 75 | 23 |
| Not protected throughout by an approved, supervised automatic sprinkler system in accordance with 9.7.1.1(1) | 200 | 61 | 300 | 91 | NP | NP |

NP: Not permitted.

†In one-story buildings, a travel distance of 400 ft (122 m) is permitted, provided that a performance-based analysis demonstrates that safe egress can be accomplished.

lowed for low and ordinary general industrial occupancies. Table 40.2.6 permits an increase to 300 ft (91 m) if the building is not sprinklered, and an increase to 400 ft (122 m) if the building is protected throughout by a supervised sprinkler system.

For a summary of the various travel distance allowances for industrial occupancies, see Exhibit 40.7.

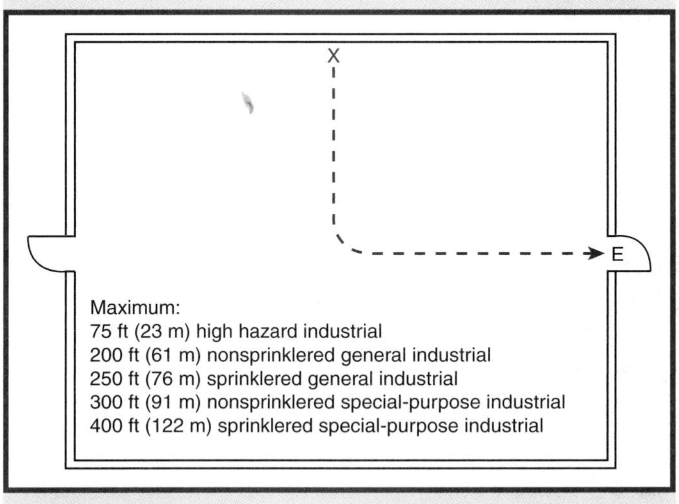


***Exhibit 40.7** Summary of industrial occupancy travel distance options permitted by Table 40.2.6.*

### 40.2.7 Discharge from Exits.

Discharge from exits shall be in accordance with Section 7.7.

### 40.2.8 Illumination of Means of Egress.

Means of egress shall be illuminated in accordance with Section 7.8 or with natural lighting that provides the required level of illumination in structures occupied only during daylight hours.

### 40.2.9* Emergency Lighting.

**A.40.2.9** The authority having jurisdiction should review the facility and designate the stairs, aisles, corridors, ramps, and passageways that should be required to be provided with emergency lighting. In large locker rooms or laboratories using hazardous chemicals, for example, the authority having jurisdiction should determine that emergency lighting is needed in the major aisles leading through those spaces.

**40.2.9.1** Emergency lighting shall be provided in accordance with Section 7.9, except as otherwise exempted by 40.2.9.2.

**40.2.9.2** Emergency lighting shall not be required for the following:

(1) Special-purpose industrial occupancies without routine human habitation
(2) Structures occupied only during daylight hours, with skylights or windows arranged to provide the required level of illumination on all portions of the means of egress during such hours

The intent of 40.2.8 is not to require the installation of extensive and unneeded illumination systems in industrial occupancies. Illumination is required for the exit access, which is limited to designated aisles, corridors, and passageways that lead to an exit. No requirement is specified for the provision of illumination throughout the building, which in many industrial occupancies would involve lighting an extensive floor area. The purpose of the lighting system is to ensure that occupants are able to see the means of egress, not to illuminate the operation of production facilities.

In addition, the *Code* does not require illumination of the means of egress if the building is occupied during daylight hours only and the building, including stairways, has sufficient windows and skylights to ensure natural illumination. The authority having jurisdiction (AHJ) should make certain that the building is not occupied after daylight hours.

The exemptions of 40.2.9.2 for emergency lighting are included for the same reasons that illumination of the means of egress is not required (see 40.2.8). Paragraph 40.2.9.2(1) addresses special-purpose industrial occupancies that are not routinely occupied. There is no need to install an extensive and costly emergency lighting system in a normally unoccupied building.

### 40.2.10 Marking of Means of Egress.

Means of egress shall have signs in accordance with Section 7.10.

### 40.2.11 Special Means of Egress Features.

**40.2.11.1 Reserved.**

**40.2.11.2 Lockups.**

**40.2.11.2.1** Lockups in new industrial occupancies shall comply with the requirements of 22.4.5.

**40.2.11.2.2** Lockups in existing industrial occupancies, other than approved existing lockups, shall comply with the requirements of 23.4.5.

Where an industrial occupancy is provided with a lockup for security purposes, it must meet the provisions of 22/23.4.5, as specified in 40.2.11.2. The lockup criteria require the application of some of the concepts of detention and correctional occupancies to other occupancies where persons might be detained for security purposes, without classifying the lockup as a detention and correctional occupancy. See 22/23.4.5 and related commentary for details on the lockup provisions.

## 40.3 Protection

### 40.3.1 Protection of Vertical Openings.

Any vertical opening shall be protected in accordance with Section 8.6, unless otherwise permitted by one of the following:

(1) In special-purpose industrial and high hazard industrial occupancies where unprotected vertical openings exist and are necessary to manufacturing operations, such openings shall be permitted beyond the specified limits, provided that every floor level has direct access to one or more enclosed stairs or other exits protected against obstruction by any fire or smoke in the open areas connected by the unprotected vertical openings.

(2) Approved existing open stairs, existing open ramps, and existing escalators shall be permitted where connecting only two floor levels.

(3) Approved, existing unprotected vertical openings in buildings with low or ordinary hazard contents that are protected throughout by an approved automatic sprinkler system in accordance with 9.7.1.1(1) shall be permitted, provided that the following conditions exist:

  (a) The vertical opening does not serve as a required exit.

  (b) All required exits consist of outside stairs in accordance with 7.2.2, smokeproof enclosures in accordance with 7.2.3, or horizontal exits in accordance with 7.2.4.

(4) Vertical openings in accordance with 8.6.8.2 shall be permitted.

Paragraph 40.3.1(1) strictly limits the use of unprotected vertical openings in high hazard and special-purpose industrial occupancies. Direct access to one or more enclosed stairways or to other exits is required from any areas connected by unprotected vertical openings. This provision recognizes that many high hazard and special-purpose industrial occupancies require openings between floor levels to accommodate piping, conveyors, and other devices and equipment essential to the orderly operation of the facility. In most of these situations, full enclosure is not practical or feasible. In high hazard occupancies, the provision of two means of egress will, in most situations, be sufficient to comply with this exemption. In special-purpose industrial occupancies, additional exits or other special arrangements will normally be required for compliance with the provision that stairways and exits be protected against obstruction from fire and smoke in open areas connected by unprotected vertical openings.

Paragraph 40.3.1(2) limits the use of existing open stairways, existing open ramps, and existing escalators that are unenclosed or unprotected by permitting them to connect only two floors. An existing open stairway connecting three floors would have to be enclosed, protected, or permitted by another of the exemptions to 40.3.1.

Paragraph 40.3.1(3) recognizes that an existing industrial occupancy might contain unprotected vertical openings and still provide a reasonable level of safety to life if the building houses only low or ordinary hazard contents and is protected by a complete automatic sprinkler system. Smokeproof enclosures and outside stairways (the only types of vertical exits permitted by this exemption) must be fully enclosed or protected against vertical fire spread and must meet the requirements of Chapter 7. The unenclosed vertical openings are not permitted to serve as part of the means of egress, although they can remain as convenience openings and stairways to be used for normal operations.

### 40.3.2* Protection from Hazards.

**A.40.3.2** Emergency lighting should be considered where operations require lighting to perform orderly manual emergency operation or shutdown, maintain critical services, or provide safe start-up after a power failure.

**40.3.2.1** All high hazard industrial occupancies, operations, or processes shall have approved, supervised automatic extinguishing systems in accordance with Section 9.7 or other protection appropriate to the particular hazard, such as explosion venting or suppression.

**40.3.2.2** Protection in accordance with 40.3.2.1 shall be provided for any area subject to an explosion hazard in order to minimize danger to occupants in case of fire or other emergency before they have time to use exits to escape.

**40.3.2.3** Activation of the fire-extinguishing or suppression system required by 40.3.2.1 shall initiate the required building fire alarm system in accordance with 40.3.4.3.4.

**40.3.2.4** Hazardous areas in industrial occupancies protected by approved automatic extinguishing systems in accordance with Section 9.7 shall be exempt from the smoke-resisting enclosure requirement of 8.7.1.2.

The intent of 40.3.2 is to provide for the life safety of the occupants of industrial buildings by controlling the risk associated with hazardous operations. The alternatives offered in 40.3.2 are not all-inclusive, and a proper fire protection engineering solution might not incorporate the listed provisions. The *Code* intends to allow for engineering judgment in a wide range of potentially hazardous situations, including some where protection might be limited. The intent of 40.3.2 is also broad in application, because, in many highly hazardous operations, an explosion might be immediately preceded by a fire or other emergency, such as an overheated reactor vessel, an exothermic reaction, or increased pressure. Because such conditions might initiate an explosion, depending on the process and arrangement of the equipment, immediate egress from the facility might be necessary. If fire or other emergencies are likely to develop rapidly into an explosion, adequate precautions are necessary for life safety. Where a sprinkler system is used to provide the protection required by 40.3.2.1, it must be electrically supervised.

In many modern facilities, provisions that prove adequate for the life safety of occupants might already be included for process control and property protection, and any additional measures will not increase the life safety of operators to an appreciable degree.

The NFPA *Fire Protection Handbook* discusses the basic principles of explosion prevention, venting, and suppression. The applicable chapters also contain an extensive bibliography on the subject. Requirements for the design and use of vents to limit pressures developed by explosions are specified in NFPA 68, *Standard on Explosion Protection by Deflagration Venting*.[9] Standards for explosion prevention systems are found in NFPA 69, *Standard on Explosion Prevention Systems*.[10]

Paragraph 8.7.1.2 requires that, where a hazardous area is protected by automatic sprinklers, the hazardous area must be enclosed by smoke partitions rather than with fire barriers with a 1-hour fire resistance rating and doors with a 45-minute fire protection rating. Paragraph 40.3.2.4 exempts hazardous areas in industrial occupancies from the requirement for smoke partitions if those areas are protected by automatic sprinklers. For consistency, similar wording appears in 8.7.1.2(2).

### 40.3.3 Interior Finish.

**40.3.3.1 General.** Interior finish shall be in accordance with Section 10.2.

**40.3.3.2 Interior Wall and Ceiling Finish.** Interior wall and ceiling finish materials complying with Section 10.2 shall be Class A, Class B, or Class C in operating areas and shall be as required by 7.1.4 in exit enclosures.

**40.3.3.3 Interior Floor Finish.**

**40.3.3.3.1** Interior floor finish in exit enclosures and in exit access corridors shall be not less than Class II.

**40.3.3.3.2** Interior floor finish in areas other than those specified in 40.3.3.3.1 shall not be required to comply with Section 10.2.

### 40.3.4 Detection, Alarm, and Communications Systems.

**40.3.4.1 General.** A fire alarm system shall be required in accordance with Section 9.6 for industrial occupancies, unless the total occupant load of the building is under 100 persons and unless, of these, fewer than 25 persons are above or below the level of exit discharge.

**40.3.4.2 Initiation.** Initiation of the required fire alarm system shall be by any of the following means:

(1) Manual means in accordance with 9.6.2.1(1)
(2) Approved automatic fire detection system in accordance with 9.6.2.1(2) throughout the building, plus a minimum of one manual fire alarm box in accordance with 9.6.2.6
(3) Approved, supervised automatic sprinkler system in accordance with 9.6.2.1(3) throughout the building, plus a minimum of one manual fire alarm box in accordance with 9.6.2.6

**40.3.4.3 Notification.**

**40.3.4.3.1** The required fire alarm system shall meet one of the following criteria:

(1) It shall provide occupant notification in accordance with 9.6.3.
(2) It shall sound an audible and visible signal in a constantly attended location for the purposes of initiating emergency action.

**40.3.4.3.2** Positive alarm sequence in accordance with 9.6.3.4 shall be permitted.

**40.3.4.3.3** Existing presignal systems in accordance with 9.6.3.3 shall be permitted.

**40.3.4.3.4** In high hazard industrial occupancies, as described in 40.1.4.1.3, the required fire alarm system shall automatically initiate an occupant evacuation alarm signal in accordance with 9.6.3.

The requirements of 40.3.4.3.1 and 40.3.4.3.4 specify two separate and distinct provisions for audible alarms activated by the fire alarm system required by 40.3.4.1. In low and ordinary hazard industrial occupancies, the system is permitted to activate an evacuation alarm or to sound an alarm at a constantly attended location for the purpose of initiating emergency action (see 40.3.4.3.1). This provision permits an interface between the alarm system and the plant's emergency organization. The alarm system is permitted to be controlled from a central security console or a similar location. The key feature is that the location from which the alarm sounds must be constantly staffed. This requirement is not intended to mandate the installation of supervisory service, such as that connected to a central station, but the location must be fully attended at all times when the building is occupied.

In high hazard occupancies, the alarm must be arranged to automatically provide evacuation signals (see 40.3.4.3.4), because the safety of the occupants of these areas depends on their immediate notification of a fire.

Note that 40.3.4.3.3 recognizes existing presignal systems but not new presignal systems. If an automatic form of delay is desired for an existing alarm system that does not already have a presignal feature, or for a new alarm system, the more reliable system feature known as *positive alarm sequence* is permitted by 40.3.4.3.2. The positive alarm sequence option might be applied to the high hazard industrial occupancies addressed in 40.3.4.3.4 for which an automatic form of occupant notification is needed. Also, positive alarm sequence might be used in industrial occupancies, other than those that are high hazard, where the provisions of 40.3.4.3.1(1) are used instead of those of 40.3.4.3.1(2).

### 40.3.5 Extinguishment Requirements.

(No requirements.)

### 40.3.6 Corridors.

The provisions of 7.1.3.1 shall not apply.

Without the exemption to the requirements of 7.1.3.1 provided by 40.3.6, all new industrial occupancy corridors serving more than 30 persons would be required to have a 1-hour fire resistance rating, with openings protected by 20-minute fire protection–rated door assemblies. The exemption to 7.1.3.1 is provided because of the ambulatory nature of occupants of industrial occupancies and the operational need for openings, even where corridors are provided.

## 40.4 Special Provisions — High-Rise Buildings

The automatic sprinkler requirements of 11.8.3.1 shall be required for new high-rise industrial occupancies, except for general low hazard or special-purpose industrial occupancies.

Section 40.4 references a portion of the high-rise building provisions of Section 11.8 that were written to allow an occupancy chapter to mandate their use. New, high-rise, general purpose industrial occupancy buildings that are classified as ordinary hazard and new high-rise industrial occupancy buildings that are classified as high hazard are required to be protected throughout by an approved, supervised automatic sprinkler system in accordance with 11.8.3.1. The remainder of Section 11.8 is not mandated for high-rise industrial occupancy buildings.

## 40.5 Building Services

### 40.5.1 Utilities.

Utilities shall comply with the provisions of Section 9.1.

### 40.5.2 Heating, Ventilating, and Air-Conditioning.

Heating, ventilating, and air-conditioning equipment shall comply with the provisions of Section 9.2.

### 40.5.3 Elevators, Escalators, and Conveyors.

Elevators, escalators, and conveyors shall comply with the provisions of Section 9.4.

### 40.5.4 Rubbish Chutes, Incinerators, and Laundry Chutes.

Rubbish chutes, incinerators, and laundry chutes shall comply with the provisions of Section 9.5.

## 40.6* Special Provisions for Aircraft Servicing Hangars

**A.40.6** For further information on aircraft hangars, see NFPA 409, *Standard on Aircraft Hangars*.

**40.6.1** The requirements of Sections 40.1 through 40.5 shall be met, except as modified by 40.6.1.1 through 40.6.1.4.

**40.6.1.1** There shall be not less than two means of egress from each aircraft servicing area.

**40.6.1.2** Exits from aircraft servicing areas shall be provided at intervals not exceeding 150 ft (46 m) on all exterior walls.

**40.6.1.3** Where horizontal exits are provided, doors shall be provided in the horizontal exit fire barrier at intervals not exceeding 100 ft (30 m).

**40.6.1.4** Where dwarf, or "smash," doors are provided in doors that accommodate aircraft, such doors shall be permitted for compliance with 40.6.1.1 through 40.6.1.3.

**40.6.2** Means of egress from mezzanine floors in aircraft servicing areas shall be arranged so that the travel distance to the nearest exit from any point on the mezzanine does not exceed 75 ft (23 m), and such means of egress shall lead directly to a properly enclosed stair discharging directly to the exterior, to a suitable cutoff area, or to outside stairs.

**40.6.3** Dead ends shall not exceed 50 ft (15 m) for other than high hazard contents areas and shall not be permitted for high hazard contents areas.

Section 40.6, which addresses aircraft servicing hangars, is nearly identical to Section 42.6, which addresses aircraft storage hangars. Because aircraft hangars are used for both storage and repair, corresponding requirements can be found in both Chapters 40 and 42.

## 40.7 Operating Features — Upholstered Furniture and Mattresses

The provisions of 10.3.2 shall not apply to upholstered furniture and mattresses.

### References Cited in Commentary


1. NFPA 654, *Standard for the Prevention of Fire and Dust Explosions from the Manufacturing, Processing, and Handling of Combustible Particulate Solids,* 2006 edition, National Fire Protection Association, Quincy, MA.
2. NFPA 30, *Flammable and Combustible Liquids Code,* 2008 edition, National Fire Protection Association, Quincy, MA.
3. NFPA 13, *Standard for the Installation of Sprinkler Systems,* 2007 edition, National Fire Protection Association, Quincy, MA.
4. NFPA *Fire Protection Handbook,* 20th edition, National Fire Protection Association, Quincy, MA, 2008.
5. Schroll, R. C., *Industrial Fire Protection Handbook,* 2nd edition, CRC Press, Boca Raton, FL, 2002.
6. Zalosh, R. G., *Industrial Fire Protection Engineering,* John Wiley and Sons, Hoboken, NJ, 2003.
7. NFPA 204, *Standard for Smoke and Heat Venting,* 2007 edition, National Fire Protection Association, Quincy, MA.
8. NFPA 92B, *Standard for Smoke Management Systems in Malls, Atria, and Large Spaces,* 2009 edition, National Fire Protection Association, Quincy, MA.
9. NFPA 68, *Standard on Explosion Protection by Deflagration Venting,* 2007 edition, National Fire Protection Association, Quincy, MA.
10. NFPA 69, *Standard on Explosion Prevention Systems,* 2008 edition, National Fire Protection Association, Quincy, MA.

# CHAPTER 41

# Reserved

Typically, the occupancy chapters are paired so that the even-numbered chapter in the pair addresses new facilities of the occupancy type and the odd-numbered chapter addresses existing facilities of the occupancy type. Chapter 40, which precedes this chapter, addresses both new and existing industrial occupancies in a single chapter. Chapter 41 has been reserved to permit the chapter on new storage occupancies to be assigned an even number (i.e., Chapter 42). The reserved chapter number might be used at a future date if the requirements for industrial occupancies are split into a pair of chapters — one for new construction and one for existing buildings.

CHAPTER 42

# Storage Occupancies

Storage occupancies include all buildings or structures used primarily for the storage or sheltering of goods, merchandise, products, or vehicles. The following are examples of storage occupancies:

1. Barns
2. Hangars (for aircraft storage only)
3. Freight terminals
4. Bulk oil storage
5. Truck and marine terminals
6. Parking garages
7. Cold storage
8. Grain elevators
9. Warehouses

Chapter 42 covers a range of facilities used for storage of a wide variety of commodities. While the same life safety philosophy that prevails in the other occupancy chapters applies to storage occupancies, the protection scheme is less complicated, given the relatively small number of people who characteristically occupy a storage occupancy. Although some warehouse facilities are substantially larger than buildings housing other occupancies, few people typically occupy them.

Once the basic characteristics of a given storage occupancy are determined, the general protection measures of Sections 42.2 and 42.3 can be applied. In addition to these measures, the supplementary provisions that are specific to a particular type of storage occupancy can be applied. These provisions include those for aircraft storage hangars (Section 42.6), grain and other bulk storage elevators (Section 42.7), and parking structures (Section 42.8).

## 42.1 General Requirements

### 42.1.1 Application.

**42.1.1.1** The requirements of this chapter shall apply to both new and existing storage occupancies.

**42.1.1.2** Storage occupancies shall include all buildings or structures used primarily for the storage or sheltering of goods, merchandise, products, vehicles, or animals.

Note that Chapter 42 applies to both new and existing storage occupancies. Where the requirements vary, exemptions that apply to existing storage occupancies are often provided, or additional requirements that are limited to new storage occupancies are specified.

Minor storage that is incidental to another occupancy is treated as part of the other occupancy. See 6.1.14.1.3.

### 42.1.2 Multiple Occupancies.

All multiple occupancies shall be in accordance with 6.1.14.

Subsection 42.1.2 directs the user to the multiple occupancies provisions of 6.1.14, which permit protecting the multiple occupancies either as mixed or as separated. If the multiple occupancy building is protected via the provisions of 6.1.14.4 for separated uses, the required separation, in terms of fire resistance rating, is specified by Table 6.1.14.4.1(a) and Table 6.1.14.4.1(b).

### 42.1.3 Special Definitions.

Special terms applicable to this chapter are defined in Chapter 3.

Life safety provisions for storage locations are not extensive, because the number of occupants is generally low, and many of those who occupy such a structure are present for only short periods of time. Furthermore, employees of storage occupancies normally do not remain in one location; instead, their assignments require that they move about and perform activities of a short-term nature.

Due to the special characteristics of storage occupancies, a number of provisions are included in the *Code* to modify, as required, those provisions that normally apply to occupancies with larger populations.

### 42.1.4 Classification of Occupancy.

**42.1.4.1** Storage occupancies shall include all buildings and structures or parts thereof with occupancy as defined in 6.1.13.

**42.1.4.2** Incidental storage in another occupancy shall not be the basis for overall occupancy classification.

**42.1.4.3** Storage occupancies or areas of storage occupancies that are used for the purpose of packaging, labeling, sorting, special handling, or other operations requiring an occupant load greater than that normally contemplated for storage shall be classified as industrial occupancies. *(See Chapter 40.)*

The purpose of 42.1.4.3 is to provide suitable egress facilities for storage occupancies, or portions of storage occupancies, with a population greater than normally expected. It is common practice to employ large numbers of people in a storage building for industrial types of operations, such as labeling, sorting, or packaging. Such operations require additional egress in accordance with the provisions of Chapter 40 for industrial occupancies.

### 42.1.5 Classification of Hazard of Contents.

Contents of storage occupancies shall be classified as low hazard, ordinary hazard, or high hazard in accordance with Section 6.2, depending on the character of the materials stored, their packaging, and other factors.

No basis for comparison exists between the hazard categories for storage facilities in NFPA 13, *Standard for the Installation of Sprinkler Systems*,[1] and those of the *Life Safety Code*. The hazard categories for storage facilities contained in NFPA 13 are established for the design of automatic sprinkler systems.

There is a strong inclination to use the potential for rapid fire growth associated with high-piled or racked storage as justification for establishing strict life safety provisions. However, the arrangement of buildings typical for this type of storage is adequate to allow safe and rapid egress at the first notification or discovery of fire. If a building is not protected by automatic sprinklers, the *Code* provides adequate provisions — such as those for travel distance to an exit — to help ensure the safety of the occupants.

### 42.1.6 Minimum Construction Requirements.

(No requirements.)

Some occupancy chapters, such as Chapters 18 and 19, which address the life safety needs of nonambulatory health care occupants, specify minimum building construction type requirements to ensure structural integrity for the time needed for a lengthy evacuation or for safe refuge within the building. No minimum construction requirements are imposed by Chapter 42, because, characteristically, storage occupancies have few occupants, and those few occupants are ambulatory.

### 42.1.7* Occupant Load.

The occupant load, in number of persons for whom means of egress and other provisions are required, shall be determined on the basis of the maximum probable population of the space under consideration.

**A.42.1.7** There is no occupant load factor specified for storage occupancies. Rather, the probable maximum number of persons present needs to be considered in determining the occupant load.

Although 42.1.7 and Table 7.3.1.2 do not provide a required occupant load factor for calculating a minimum occupant load to size a means of egress system in a storage occupancy, it is necessary to establish an occupant load. The occupant load is determined on the basis of the maximum number of persons expected to occupy the storage occupancy under any anticipated facility operation. Due to the low occupant load characteristic of storage occupancies, compliance with other *Code* provisions — such as minimum widths for doors, corridors, or passageways; minimum number of exits; and travel distance allowances — generally provides a means of egress system capable of handling the actual occupant load, without specifically considering the occupant load when the means of egress is designed.

## 42.2 Means of Egress Requirements

### 42.2.1 General.

**42.2.1.1** Each required means of egress shall be in accordance with the applicable portions of Chapter 7.

**42.2.1.2*** Normally unoccupied utility chases that are secured from unauthorized access and are used exclusively for routing of electrical, mechanical, or plumbing equipment shall not be required to comply with the provisions of Chapter 7.

**A.42.2.1.2** Horizontal and vertical utility chases in large industrial buildings used for routing of piping, ducts, and wiring must provide a reasonable level of access for occasional maintenance workers but do not warrant compliance with the comprehensive egress requirements of Chapter 7. Minimum access in these cases is governed by the electrical and mechanical code; 40.2.5.2, Industrial Equipment Access; and the Occupational Safety and Health Administration (OSHA) for facilities in the United States. Utility chases governed by this paragraph might involve tunnels or large open spaces located above or below occupied floors; however, such spaces differ from mechanical equipment rooms, boiler rooms, and furnace rooms, based on the anticipated frequency of use by maintenance workers. Portions of utility chases where the anticipated presence of maintenance workers is routine are not intended to be included by this paragraph.

### 42.2.2 Means of Egress Components.

**42.2.2.1 Components Permitted.** Components of means of egress shall be limited to the types described in 42.2.2.2 through 42.2.2.12.

**42.2.2.2 Doors.**

**42.2.2.2.1** Doors complying with 7.2.1 shall be permitted.

**42.2.2.2.2** Delayed-egress locks complying with 7.2.1.6.1 shall be permitted.

**42.2.2.2.3** Access-controlled egress doors complying with 7.2.1.6.2 shall be permitted.

**42.2.2.2.4** Approved existing horizontal-sliding fire doors shall be permitted in the means of egress under the following conditions:

(1) They are held open by fusible links.
(2) The fusible links are rated at not less than 165°F (74°C).
(3) The fusible links are located not more than 10 ft (3050 mm) above the floor.
(4) The fusible links are in immediate proximity to the door opening.
(5) The fusible links are not located above a ceiling.
(6) The door is not credited with providing any protection under this *Code*.

Use of the delayed-egress locking device in accordance with all criteria of 7.2.1.6.1 is permitted on any door in recognition of the security needs of some storage occupancies. In effect, the allowable 15-second or 30-second delay will be experienced only under non-fire conditions or very early in a fire's growth, because the door must be usable immediately upon sprinkler operation, smoke or heat detection, and loss of power that controls the locking mechanism. The building must be protected throughout by an approved, supervised automatic sprinkler system or an approved, supervised automatic fire detection system.

Paragraph 42.2.2.2.3 recognizes the use of access-controlled egress doors in storage occupancies as a security measure that does not compromise the use of the means of egress.

Horizontal-sliding doors exist in many storage occupancies for property protection purposes. Although the *Code* normally does not recognize these doors within the required means of egress, 42.2.2.2.4 makes an exemption for existing horizontal-sliding fire doors. See Exhibit 42.1. By requiring the fusible link to be positioned in immediate proximity to the door opening, rated 165°F (74°C) or higher, and located not more than 10 ft (3050 mm) above the floor, the *Code* helps to ensure that the door will remain open until rising temperatures make it unsafe to pass through the door opening. Because the door will not close early in the

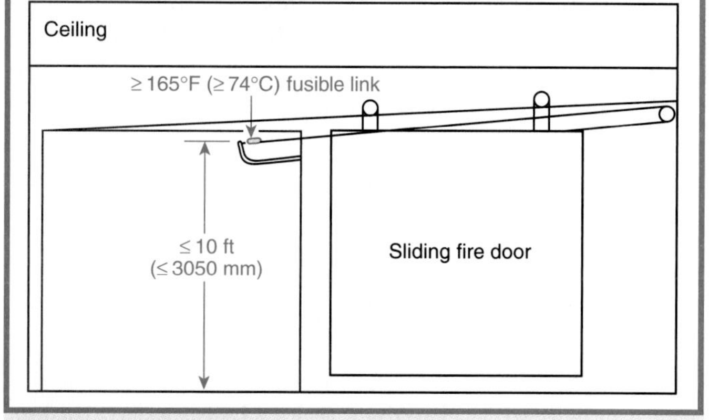


***Exhibit 42.1** Existing horizontal-sliding fire door in accordance with 42.2.2.2.4.*

fire development, the door cannot be credited as a fire door for life safety purposes. However, the door might serve as a means of property protection; for example, to create separate fire areas to limit the maximum foreseeable loss for insurance purposes.

**42.2.2.3 Stairs.**

**42.2.2.3.1** Stairs shall comply with 7.2.2 and shall be permitted to be modified as follows:

(1) Noncombustible grated stair treads and noncombustible grated landing floors shall be permitted.
(2) Industrial equipment access stairs in accordance with 40.2.5.2 shall be permitted.

**42.2.2.3.2** Spiral stairs complying with 7.2.2.2.3 shall be permitted.

**42.2.2.3.3** Existing winders complying with 7.2.2.2.4 shall be permitted.

Paragraph 42.2.2.3.1(1) exempts stair treads and landings in storage occupancies from the provisions of 7.2.2.3.3.1, which would otherwise require that all stair treads and stair landings be solid. Although the requirement for solid treads and landings is intended to prevent occupants from avoiding the use of the stairs because they become afraid when they are able to see through the openings to the floor or ground below, occupants of storage occupancies are usually more familiar, and thus more comfortable, with grated or expanded metal treads and landings. There is also a high degree of certainty that occupants will be wearing shoes appropriate for the environment, and not high heels that could get stuck in the grate openings. The grated walking surfaces provide slip resistance in what are sometimes greasy and slippery surroundings.

Paragraph 42.2.2.3.1(2) serves to remind the user that the special provisions for industrial equipment access stairs in 40.2.5.2 are permitted to be used in storage occupancies. The provisions of 40.2.5.2 differ from the requirements of Chapter 7. See the commentary following 40.2.5.2.2.

**42.2.2.4 Smokeproof Enclosures.** Smokeproof enclosures complying with 7.2.3 shall be permitted.

Paragraph 42.2.2.4 does not mandate the use of smokeproof enclosures. However, it does recognize a smokeproof enclosure as part of the means of egress system in a storage occupancy if that smokeproof enclosure meets the requirements of 7.2.3. For an example of an occupancy requiring a smokeproof enclosure, see 31.2.11.1, which specifies that existing nonsprinklered and partially sprinklered high-rise apartment buildings are required to be provided with smokeproof enclosures in accordance with 7.2.3.

**42.2.2.5 Horizontal Exits.**

**42.2.2.5.1** Horizontal exits complying with 7.2.4 shall be permitted.

**42.2.2.5.2*** In horizontal exits where the opening is protected by a fire door assembly on each side of the wall in which it is located, one fire door shall be of the swinging type, as provided in 7.2.4.3.7, and the other shall be permitted to be an automatic-sliding fire door that shall be kept open whenever the building is occupied.

**A.42.2.2.5.2** The customary building code requirement for fire doors on both sides of an opening in a fire wall is permitted to be met by having an automatic-sliding fire door on one side and a self-closing fire door swinging out from the other side of the wall. This arrangement qualifies only as a horizontal exit from the sliding door side. For further information, see A.7.2.4.3.10.

Paragraph 42.2.2.5.1 does not mandate the use of horizontal exits. However, it does recognize a horizontal exit as part of the means of egress system in a storage occupancy if that horizontal exit meets the requirements of 7.2.4, as modified by 42.2.2.5.2.

Paragraphs 42.2.2.5.2 and A.42.2.2.5.2 recognize the common practice of combining a horizontal exit that is used for life safety with a fire barrier of a significant fire resistance rating that is used for property protection. Opening protectives for such a fire barrier can require the use of a set of two doors to achieve the required fire protection rating. It is impractical for both doors to swing in the same direction without interfering with each other; yet, operation of two doors that swing in opposite directions is cumbersome for daily or frequent use. One swinging and one sliding door, as shown in Exhibit 42.2, provide an acceptable arrangement for day-to-day functioning of the building. The open sliding door does not compromise life safety, because by the time its fusible link mechanism releases the door and allows it to close, temperatures in the vicinity of the door opening render use of the door impractical.

**42.2.2.6 Ramps.**

**42.2.2.6.1** Ramps complying with 7.2.5 shall be permitted.

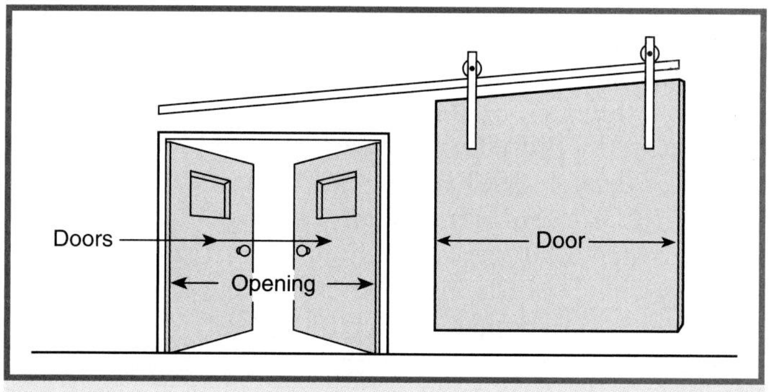


*Exhibit 42.2 Combination swinging and sliding doors permitted by 42.2.2.5.2.*

**42.2.2.6.2** Industrial equipment access ramps in accordance with 40.2.5.2 shall be permitted.

Paragraph 42.2.2.6.1 does not mandate the use of ramps in storage occupancies. However, it does recognize a ramp as part of the means of egress system if that ramp meets the requirements of 7.2.5.

Paragraph 42.2.2.6.2 recognizes the industrial access ramp provisions of 40.2.5.2, which are a relaxation of the ramp provisions of 7.2.5. For example, Table 40.2.5.2.1 permits a minimum ramp width of 22 in. (560 mm) instead of the 44 in. (1120 mm) minimum of Table 7.2.5.2(a). However, the industrial equipment access provisions of 40.2.5.2 include the restriction that the egress component, in this case a ramp, is to serve not more than 20 persons.

**42.2.2.7 Exit Passageways.** Exit passageways complying with 7.2.6 shall be permitted.

Paragraph 42.2.2.7 does not mandate the use of exit passageways in storage occupancies. However, it does recognize an exit passageway as part of the means of egress system if that exit passageway meets the requirements of 7.2.6.

**42.2.2.8 Fire Escape Stairs.** Existing fire escape stairs complying with 7.2.8 shall be permitted.

**42.2.2.9 Fire Escape Ladders.**

**42.2.2.9.1** Fire escape ladders complying with 7.2.9 shall be permitted.

**42.2.2.9.2** Fixed industrial stairs in accordance with the minimum requirements for fixed stairs in ANSI A1264.1, *Safety Requirements for Workplace Floor and Wall Openings, Stairs and Railing Systems,* shall be permitted where fire escape ladders are permitted in accordance with 7.2.9.1.

The geometry associated with the incline angle and the size and shape of surfaces intended for foot placement on fire escape ladders falls within the range permitted for fixed industrial stairs. However, most fixed industrial stairs meet criteria that result in a safer arrangement than that provided by the fire escape ladder detailed in 7.2.9. Therefore, 42.2.2.9.2 recognizes fixed industrial stairs as a substitute for fire escape ladders.

**42.2.2.10 Slide Escapes.** Existing slide escapes complying with 7.2.10 shall be permitted.

The intent of 42.2.2.10 is to permit the continued use of existing slide escapes, which are a common means of egress from areas that house explosives or other highly hazardous materials in warehouses associated with the chemical industry. The provision permits slide escapes to be considered as part of the required means of egress from existing storage occupancies only if the slide escape meets the requirements of 7.2.10.

**42.2.2.11 Alternating Tread Devices.** Alternating tread devices complying with 7.2.11 shall be permitted.

The provisions of 7.2.11, in effect, limit the use of alternating tread devices to those locations where the *Code* recognizes the use of fire escape ladders. See 42.2.2.9.1, 7.2.9, and 7.2.11.

**42.2.2.12 Areas of Refuge.** Areas of refuge complying with 7.2.12 shall be permitted.

### 42.2.3 Capacity of Means of Egress.

The capacity of means of egress shall be in accordance with Section 7.3.

Prior to the 1991 edition, the *Code* required a minimum 44 in. (1120 mm) width for corridors and passageways within the required means of egress of storage occupancies. A corridor or passageway of that minimum width would have provided egress capacity for 220 persons [i.e., 44 in./0.2 in. per person (approximately 1120 mm/5 mm per person) in accordance with Table 7.3.3.1 for level egress components]. That requirement produced artificially large egress systems, relative to the occupant load, in many storage occupancies. The requirement was eliminated, and the minimum 36 in. (915 mm) width requirement of 7.3.4.1(2), which addresses the minimum width of any exit access, was made applicable to storage occupancies. Exit access is required to be wider than 36 in. (915 mm) only if a corridor or passageway in a storage occupancy is to provide capacity for more than 180 persons [i.e., 36 in./0.2 in. per person (approximately 915 mm/5 mm per person)].

See the commentary following A.42.1.7 for details on the determination of occupant load in a storage occupancy.

### 42.2.4 Number of Means of Egress.

See also Section 7.4.

**42.2.4.1** The number of means of egress shall be as follows:

(1) In low hazard storage occupancies, a single means of egress shall be permitted from any story or section.
(2) In ordinary hazard storage occupancies, a single means of egress shall be permitted from any story or section, provided that the exit can be reached within the distance permitted as a common path of travel.
(3) All buildings or structures not complying with 42.2.4.1(1) or (2) and used for storage, and every section thereof considered separately, shall have not less than two separate means of egress as remotely located from each other as practicable.

**42.2.4.2** In new buildings, floors or portions thereof with an occupant load of more than 500 persons shall have the minimum number of separate and remote means of egress specified by 7.4.1.2.

**42.2.4.3** Areas with high hazard contents shall comply with Section 7.11.

Paragraphs 42.2.4.1(1) and (2) modify the requirement for two, separate, remotely located means of egress, due, in part, to the small number of employees typically found in a storage occupancy and the exemplary life safety fire record of such facilities. Paragraph 42.2.4.1(1) recognizes that a low hazard storage occupancy is not subject to a self-propagating fire, and, therefore, considers a single means of egress to be safe. Paragraph 42.2.4.1(2) permits a single means of egress in an ordinary hazard storage occupancy if the total travel distance to the single exit does not exceed the 50 ft (15 m) or 100 ft (30 m) common path of travel allowance for nonsprinklered and sprinklered buildings, respectively (see Table 42.2.5). This allowance is made because such a single exit arrangement is equivalent or superior to a two-exit arrangement that applies the maximum common path of travel allowance and subsequently requires additional travel distance to reach an exit.

In Exhibit 42.3, a single exit is depicted in Part (a). It is located within the distance permitted for common path of travel (see Table 42.2.5), as addressed by 42.2.4.1(2) for ordinary hazard storage occupancies, and creates a situation no more dangerous than the common path of travel shown as X1 to C1 in the two-exit building depicted in Part (b).

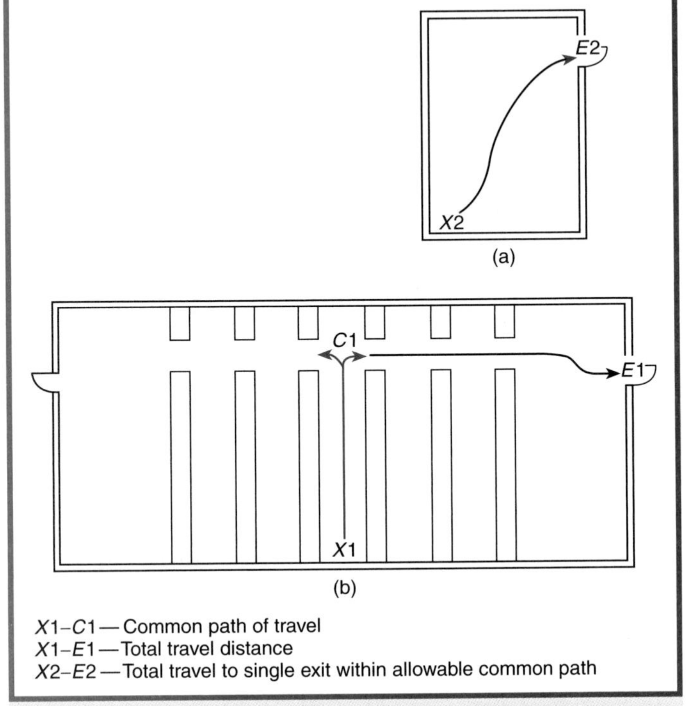


***Exhibit 42.3*** *Common path of travel in single exit building compared to that in two-exit building.*

### 42.2.5 Arrangement of Means of Egress.

Means of egress, arranged in accordance with Section 7.5, shall not exceed that provided by Table 42.2.5.

By definition, no self-propagating fire can occur in low hazard contents. If a fire will not spread or continue to burn, building occupants will not be subject to an emergent need to egress the building by means of paths that avoid the fire. Therefore, the *Code* establishes no maximum dead-end corridor and no maximum common path of travel for storage occupancies with low hazard contents. See Section 6.2.

An ordinary hazard storage occupancy, despite its characteristically low occupant load, is not permitted to provide a common path of travel that forces an oc-

*Table 42.2.5 Arrangements of Means of Egress*

| Level of Protection | Low Hazard Storage Occupancy | Ordinary Hazard Storage Occupancy | | High Hazard Storage Occupancy |
|---|---|---|---|---|
| | | ft | m | |
| **Dead-End Corridor** | | | | |
| Protected throughout by an approved, supervised automatic sprinkler system in accordance with 9.7.1.1(1) | NL | 100 | 30 | Prohibited, except as permitted by 7.11.4 |
| Not protected throughout by an approved, supervised automatic sprinkler system in accordance with 9.7.1.1(1) | NL | 50 | 15 | Prohibited, except as permitted by 7.11.4 |
| **Common Path of Travel** | | | | |
| Protected throughout by an approved, supervised automatic sprinkler system in accordance with 9.7.1.1(1) | NL | 100 | 30 | Prohibited, except as permitted by 7.11.4 |
| Not protected throughout by an approved, supervised automatic sprinkler system in accordance with 9.7.1.1(1) | NL | 50 | 15 | Prohibited, except as permitted by 7.11.4 |

NL: Not limited.

cupant to travel in only one direction for more than 50 ft (15 m) [100 ft (30 m) in a sprinklered building] without providing a route to a second, remotely located exit.

By definition, the potential for an extremely rapid-developing fire or an explosion is a characteristic of high hazard contents. If a fire spreads with extreme rapidity, building occupants will have an emergent need to egress the building by means of paths that avoid the fire. Therefore, the *Code* permits no dead-end corridors and no common path of travel for storage occupancies with high hazard contents, except as permitted by 7.11.4. See Section 6.2 and 7.11.4.

### 42.2.6* Travel Distance to Exits.

Travel distance, measured in accordance with Section 7.6, shall not exceed that provided by Table 42.2.6.

**A.42.2.6** The travel distance to exits specified recognizes a low population density. Consideration should be given to locating areas that have a relatively high population, such as lunchrooms, meeting rooms, packaging areas, and offices, near the outside wall of the building to keep the travel distance to a minimum.

Subsection 42.2.6 establishes limitations on travel distance for storage occupancies. Note that the provisions create a direct relationship between the level of hazard of contents housed within a building and its life safety requirements. Therefore, in low hazard storage occupancies, no limitation is imposed on travel distance.

The absence of travel distance restrictions for low hazard storage occupancies is reasonable, because the small fire risk posed by low hazard materials, coupled with the low number of occupants, provides a minimal

*Table 42.2.6 Maximum Travel Distance to Exits*

| Level of Protection | Low Hazard Storage Occupancy | Ordinary Hazard Storage Occupancy | | High Hazard Storage Occupancy | |
|---|---|---|---|---|---|
| | | ft | m | ft | m |
| Protected throughout by an approved, supervised automatic sprinkler system in accordance with 9.7.1.1(1) | NL | 400 | 122 | 100 | 30 |
| Not protected throughout by an approved, supervised automatic sprinkler system in accordance with 9.7.1.1(1) | NL | 200 | 61 | 75 | 23 |
| Flammable and combustible liquid products stored and protected in accordance with NFPA 30, *Flammable and Combustible Liquids Code* | NA | NA | NA | 150 | 46 |

NL: Not limited. NA: Not applicable.

risk to life safety. The imposition of restrictive provisions would not be consistent with good fire protection and reasonable life safety requirements, because the probability of fire is relatively low, and occupants are not expected to experience difficulty in evacuating the building. See Section 6.2 for guidelines on the classification of low hazard contents.

As the level of hazard of contents increases, travel distance limitations are imposed. Storage buildings housing ordinary hazards and lacking sprinkler protection are limited to 200 ft (61 m) of travel distance to the nearest exit. A distance of 400 ft (122 m) is permitted if complete automatic sprinkler protection is provided. In high hazard storage occupancies, travel distance is restricted to a maximum of 75 ft (23 m) in nonsprinklered buildings and 100 ft (30 m) if the building is equipped with a complete automatic sprinkler system.

The last entry in Table 42.2.6 addresses an increase in travel distance for storage occupancies where flammable and combustible liquid products are stored and protected in accordance with NFPA 30, *Flammable and Combustible Liquids Code*.[2] Since the 1996 edition, NFPA 30 has provided adequate safeguards to permit increasing the travel distance allowance from 75 ft (23 m) to 150 ft (46 m). Flammable and combustible liquids storage facilities not in compliance with the 1996, 2000, 2003, or 2008 edition of NFPA 30 should not make use of the travel distance increase.

### 42.2.7 Discharge from Exits.

Discharge from exits shall be in accordance with Section 7.7.

### 42.2.8 Illumination of Means of Egress.

**42.2.8.1** Means of egress shall be illuminated in accordance with Section 7.8.

**42.2.8.2** In structures occupied only during daylight hours, means of egress shall be permitted to be illuminated with windows arranged to provide the required level of illumination on all portions of the means of egress during such hours, when approved by the authority having jurisdiction.

The intent of 42.2.8 is not to require the installation of extensive and unneeded exit illumination systems in storage occupancies. Illumination is required for the exit and for the exit access, which is limited to designated aisles, corridors, and passageways that lead to an exit. Limiting the extent of the lighting system to egress areas eliminates the necessity for installing specialized lighting systems throughout storage areas, a practice that might be extremely costly while providing little or no return in safety to life.

Paragraph 42.2.8.2 waives the requirement for illumination systems if a building, including the stairways, is sufficiently lit during periods of occupancy by means of natural lighting. The term *windows*, as used in the text of the exemption, should not be interpreted literally. The term is meant to include skylights, open wall sections, and similar means of illumination by natural sources. The provisions are based on the fact that there is no need for a lighting system if the building is unoccupied during non-daylight hours.

### 42.2.9 Emergency Lighting.

Emergency lighting shall be provided in normally occupied storage occupancies in accordance with Section 7.9, except for spaces occupied only during daylight hours with natural illumination in accordance with 42.2.8.2.

Emergency lighting is exempted in storage occupancies that are naturally illuminated when occupied for the reasons stated in the commentary following 42.2.8.2. The exemption permits circuit arrangements that disconnect power from emergency lighting systems when the building is unoccupied. In many warehouses, power is turned off during periods when the building is unoccupied. This power disconnection serves fire prevention, energy conservation, and security purposes.

### 42.2.10 Marking of Means of Egress.

Means of egress shall have signs in accordance with Section 7.10.

### 42.2.11 Special Means of Egress Features.

**42.2.11.1 Reserved.**

**42.2.11.2 Lockups.**

**42.2.11.2.1** Lockups in new storage occupancies shall comply with the requirements of 22.4.5.

**42.2.11.2.2** Lockups in existing storage occupancies, other than approved existing lockups, shall comply with the requirements of 23.4.5.

If a storage occupancy is provided with a lockup for security purposes, it must meet the provisions of 22/23.4.5, as specified in 42.2.11.2. The lockup criteria require the application of some of the concepts of detention and correctional occupancies to other occupancies where persons might be detained for security purposes, without classifying the lockup as a detention and correctional occupancy. See 22/23.4.5 and related commentary for details on the lockup provisions.

## 42.3 Protection

### 42.3.1 Protection of Vertical Openings.

Any vertical opening shall be protected in accordance with Section 8.6, unless otherwise permitted by one of the following:

(1) Existing open stairs, existing open ramps, and existing open escalators shall be permitted where connecting only two floor levels.
(2) Existing unprotected vertical openings in buildings with low or ordinary hazard contents, and protected throughout by an approved automatic sprinkler system in accordance with 9.7.1.1(1), shall be permitted where they do not serve as required exits, and where all required exits consist of outside stairs in accordance with 7.2.2, smokeproof enclosures in accordance with 7.2.3, or horizontal exits in accordance with 7.2.4.

Paragraph 42.3.1(2) recognizes that an existing storage occupancy might contain unprotected vertical openings and still provide a reasonable level of safety to life if the building houses only low or ordinary hazard contents and is protected by a complete automatic sprinkler system. Smokeproof enclosures and outside stairs (the only types of vertical exits permitted by this exemption) must be fully enclosed or protected against vertical fire spread and must meet the requirements of Chapter 7. The unenclosed vertical openings are not permitted to serve as part of the means of egress, although they can remain as convenience openings and stairways to be used for normal operations.

### 42.3.2 Protection from Hazards.

(No requirements.) *(See also Section 8.7.)*

### 42.3.3 Interior Finish.

**42.3.3.1 General.** Interior finish shall be in accordance with Section 10.2.

**42.3.3.2 Interior Wall and Ceiling Finish.** Interior wall and ceiling finish materials complying with Section 10.2 shall be Class A, Class B, or Class C in storage areas and shall be as required by 7.1.4 in exit enclosures.

**42.3.3.3 Interior Floor Finish.**

**42.3.3.3.1** Interior floor finish in exit enclosures shall be not less than Class II.

**42.3.3.3.2** Interior floor finish in areas other than those specified in 42.3.3.3.1 shall not be required to comply with Section 10.2.

### 42.3.4 Detection, Alarm, and Communications Systems.

**42.3.4.1 General.** A fire alarm system shall be required in accordance with Section 9.6 for storage occupancies, except as modified by 42.3.4.1.1, 42.3.4.1.2, and 42.3.4.1.3.

**42.3.4.1.1** Storage occupancies limited to low hazard contents shall not be required to have a fire alarm system.

**42.3.4.1.2** Storage occupancies with ordinary or high hazard contents not exceeding an aggregate floor area of 100,000 ft$^2$ (9300 m$^2$) shall not be required to have a fire alarm system.

**42.3.4.1.3** Storage occupancies protected throughout by an approved automatic sprinkler system in accordance with Section 9.7 shall not be required to have a fire alarm system.

**42.3.4.2 Initiation.** Initiation of the required fire alarm system shall be by any of the following means:

(1) Manual means in accordance with 9.6.2.1(1)
(2) Approved automatic fire detection system in accordance with 9.6.2.1(2) throughout the building, plus a minimum of one manual fire alarm box in accordance with 9.6.2.6
(3) Approved, supervised automatic sprinkler system in accordance with 9.6.2.1(3) throughout the building, plus a minimum of one manual fire alarm box in accordance with 9.6.2.6

**42.3.4.3 Notification.**

**42.3.4.3.1** The required fire alarm system shall meet one of the following criteria:

(1) It shall provide occupant notification in accordance with 9.6.3.
(2) It shall sound an audible and visible signal in a constantly attended location for the purposes of initiating emergency action.

**42.3.4.3.2** Positive alarm sequence in accordance with 9.6.3.4 shall be permitted.

**42.3.4.3.3** Existing presignal systems in accordance with 9.6.3.3 shall be permitted.

**42.3.4.3.4** In high hazard storage occupancies, the required fire alarm system shall automatically initiate an occupant evacuation alarm signal in accordance with 9.6.3.

Subsection 42.3.4 requires the installation of a fire alarm system in nonsprinklered storage occupancies with an aggregate floor area of over 100,000 $ft^2$ (9300 $m^2$). An alarm system is not required in a storage occupancy limited to housing low hazard contents, regardless of its size, nor is one required in a sprinklered storage occupancy, regardless of size. Storage placement limits visibility in buildings with large floor areas. As a result, personnel who work in storage areas might be unaware of the occurrence of fire for a long period. If fire spreads, which is highly possible in an unprotected storage building, means of exit access could be blocked. An alarm system provides a means of alerting all occupants to the presence of fire and allows for timely egress.

The requirements of 42.3.4.3.1 and 42.3.4.3.4 specify two separate and distinct provisions for audible alarms activated by the fire alarm system required by 42.3.4.1. In low and ordinary hazard storage occupancies (see 42.3.4.3.1), the system is permitted to activate an evacuation alarm or sound an alarm at a constantly attended location for the purpose of initiating emergency action. This provision permits an interface between the alarm system and the building's emergency organization. The alarm system is permitted to be controlled from a central security console or a similar location. The key feature is that the location from which the alarm sounds must be constantly staffed. This requirement is not intended to mandate the installation of supervisory service, such as that connected to a central station, but the location must be fully attended at all times when the building is occupied.

In high hazard storage occupancies (see 42.3.4.3.4), the alarm must be arranged to automatically provide evacuation signals, because the safety of the occupants of these areas depends on their immediate notification of a fire.

Note that 42.3.4.3.3 recognizes existing presignal systems but not new presignal systems. If an automatic form of delay is desired for an existing alarm system that doesn't already have a presignal feature, or for a new alarm system, the more reliable system feature known as *positive alarm sequence* is permitted. The positive alarm sequence option permitted by 42.3.4.3.2 might be applied to the high hazard storage occupancies addressed in 42.3.4.3.4 for which an automatic form of occupant notification is needed. Also, positive alarm sequence might be used in storage occupancies, other than those that are high hazard, where the provisions of 42.3.4.3.1(1) are used instead of those of 42.3.4.3.1(2).

The *Code* does not specify an alarm system as a property protection requirement, although the probability of property loss is reduced in any occupancy where an alarm system is installed.

### 42.3.5 Extinguishment Requirements.

(No requirements.)

### 42.3.6 Corridors.

The provisions of 7.1.3.1 shall not apply.

Without the exemption to the requirements of 7.1.3.1 provided by 42.3.6, all new storage occupancy corridors serving more than 30 persons would be required to have a 1-hour fire resistance rating, with openings protected by 20-minute fire protection–rated door assemblies. The exemption to 7.1.3.1 is provided because of the ambulatory nature of occupants of storage occupancies; the operational need for openings, even where corridors are provided; and the functional need served by open floor areas.

## 42.4 Special Provisions — High-Rise Buildings

The automatic sprinkler requirements of 11.8.3.1 shall be required for new high-rise storage occupancies, except for low hazard storage occupancies.

The provisions of Section 42.4, which apply to high-rise storage occupancy buildings, reference a portion of the high-rise building provisions of Section 11.8 that were written to allow an occupancy chapter to mandate their use. New high-rise storage occupancy buildings that are classified as ordinary hazard or high hazard are required to be protected throughout by an approved, supervised automatic sprinkler system in accordance with 11.8.3.1. The remainder of Section 11.8 is not mandated for high-rise storage occupancy buildings.

## 42.5 Building Services

### 42.5.1 Utilities.

Utilities shall comply with the provisions of Section 9.1.

### 42.5.2 Heating, Ventilating, and Air-Conditioning.

Heating, ventilating, and air-conditioning equipment shall comply with the provisions of Section 9.2.

### 42.5.3 Elevators, Escalators, and Conveyors.

Elevators, escalators, and conveyors shall comply with the provisions of Section 9.4.

### 42.5.4 Rubbish Chutes, Incinerators, and Laundry Chutes.

Rubbish chutes, incinerators, and laundry chutes shall comply with the provisions of Section 9.5.

## 42.6* Special Provisions for Aircraft Storage Hangars

**A.42.6** For further information on aircraft hangars, see NFPA 409, *Standard on Aircraft Hangars.*

**42.6.1** The requirements of Sections 42.1 through 42.5 shall be met, except as modified by 42.6.1.1 through 42.6.3.

**42.6.1.1** There shall be not less than two means of egress from each aircraft storage area.

**42.6.1.2** Exits from aircraft storage areas shall be provided at intervals not exceeding 150 ft (46 m) on all exterior walls.

**42.6.1.3** Where horizontal exits are provided, doors shall be provided in the horizontal exit fire barrier at intervals not exceeding 100 ft (30 m).

**42.6.1.4** Where dwarf, or "smash," doors are provided in doors that accommodate aircraft, such doors shall be permitted for compliance with 42.6.1.1, 42.6.1.2, and 42.6.1.3.

**42.6.2** Means of egress from mezzanine floors in aircraft storage areas shall be arranged so that the travel distance to the nearest exit from any point on the mezzanine does not exceed 75 ft (23 m), and such means of egress shall lead directly to a properly enclosed stair discharging directly to the exterior, to a suitable cutoff area, or to outside stairs.

**42.6.3** Dead ends shall not exceed 50 ft (15 m) for other than high hazard contents areas and shall not be permitted for high hazard contents areas.

For provisions that apply to aircraft servicing hangars, see Section 40.6.

Section 42.6 specifies two alternate methods of providing egress from aircraft storage hangars. Where egress is possible through the outside wall, a distance of 150 ft (46 m) between exit doors is adequate. In larger hangars, the storage bay might have offices and other rooms located along one or more sides, with the walls constructed of fire resistance–rated materials. In those cases where the wall has a fire resistance rating so as to qualify as a horizontal exit, exit spacing of up to 100 ft (30 m) is specified. If the wall is nonrated, access to the outside is required. During inclement weather, large hangar doors are typically closed, so it is common procedure to provide small access doors for personnel in the larger aircraft hangar door. The small door can be considered a normal means of egress from an aircraft hangar. If possible, the door should swing in the direction of egress; however, this might not be possible due to the design of the aircraft door. For further information on aircraft hangars, see NFPA 409, *Standard on Aircraft Hangars.*[3]

## 42.7* Special Provisions for Grain Handling, Processing, Milling, or Other Bulk Storage Facilities

**A.42.7** For further information, see NFPA 61, *Standard for the Prevention of Fires and Dust Explosions in Agricultural and Food Processing Facilities.* The egress requirements for storage elevators are based on the possibility of fire and are not based on the possibility of grain dust explosions.

### 42.7.1 General.

The requirements of Sections 42.1 through 42.5 shall be met, except as modified by 42.7.2 through 42.7.4.2.

### 42.7.2 Number of Means of Egress.

There shall be not less than two means of egress from all working levels of the head house, as modified by 42.7.2.1, 42.7.2.2, and 42.7.2.3.

**42.7.2.1** One of the two means of egress shall be a stair to the level of exit discharge, and, if this means of egress is interior to the structure, it shall be enclosed by a dust-resistant, 1-hour fire resistance–rated enclosure in accordance with 7.1.3.2. Exterior stair means of egress shall be protected from the structure by a 1-hour fire resistance–rated wall that extends at least 10 ft (3050 mm) beyond the stair.

**42.7.2.2** The second means of egress shall be one of the following:

(1) Exterior stair or basket ladder–type fire escape that is accessible from all working levels of the structure and provides a passage to the finished ground level

(2) Exterior stair or basket ladder–type fire escape that is accessible from all working levels of the structure, provides access to adjoining structures, and provides a continuous path to the means of egress described in 42.7.3

**42.7.2.3** Stair enclosures in existing structures shall be permitted to have non-fire-rated dust-resistant enclosures.

### 42.7.3 Fire Escapes.

An exterior stair or basket ladder–type fire escape shall provide passage to the finished ground level from the top of the end of an adjoining structure, such as a silo, conveyor, gallery, or gantry.

It is not the intent of 42.7.2.1 to require a fully dust-tight shaft, because the door will allow passage of limited amounts of dust during the normal course of daily operations. However, the shaft should be separated from the operating areas by fire resistance–rated construction and should be as free of dust as possible. Stairs that are exterior to the structure are not required to be enclosed; however, they must be separated from the structure by a 1-hour fire barrier that extends 10 ft (3050 mm) beyond the stair in all directions.

Subsection 42.7.2 requires that one means of egress from the head house must be an enclosed stair if it is interior to the structure. The alternate means of egress can be either an outside stair or a basket ladder–type fire escape connecting all working levels and leading to either the ground or the top of an adjoining structure that complies with 42.7.3.

The principal hazard of elevator storage structures that handle combustible materials is the potential for a dust explosion. A dust explosion can be violent enough to damage or destroy the primary means of egress required in 42.7.2.

### 42.7.4 Underground Spaces.

**42.7.4.1 Number of Means of Egress.**

**42.7.4.1.1** Underground spaces shall have not less than two means of egress, one of which shall be permitted to be a means of escape, except as permitted in 42.7.4.1.2.

**42.7.4.1.2** Where the horizontal travel distance to the means of egress is less than 50 ft (15 m) in normally unoccupied spaces, a single means of egress shall be permitted.

**42.7.4.2 Travel Distance to Exits.** Travel distance, measured in accordance with Section 7.6, shall not exceed that provided by Table 42.7.4.2.

## 42.8 Special Provisions for Parking Structures

### 42.8.1 General Requirements.

**42.8.1.1 Application.** The provisions of 42.8.1 through 42.8.5.4 shall apply to parking structures of the closed or open type, above or below grade plane, but shall not apply to mechanical or exclusively attendant-type parking facilities that are not occupied by customers. The requirements of Sections 42.1 through 42.7 shall not apply.

The intent of the special provisions for parking structures is to provide adequate life safety for the patrons, who probably will be unfamiliar with the parking structure and its arrangement. Where parking attendants are the only occupants who enter the parking area, the *Code*'s intent is to provide exits in accordance with the previous sections of Chapter 42. In such instances, the provisions for ordinary hazard contents storage occupancies apply.

Section 42.8 is self-contained and, therefore, independent of Sections 42.1 through 42.7, which apply to other storage occupancies. However, Section 42.8 does

*Table 42.7.4.2 Maximum Travel Distance to Means of Escape or Exits*

| Level of Protection | Travel Distance ft | Travel Distance m |
|---|---|---|
| Protected throughout by an approved, supervised automatic sprinkler system in accordance with 9.7.1.1(1) | 400 | 122 |
| Not protected throughout by an approved, supervised automatic sprinkler system in accordance with 9.7.1.1(1) | 200 | 61 |
| Existing structures | Unlimited | |

reference other portions of the *Code*, mainly the core Chapters 1 through 7.

For further information on garages, see NFPA 88A, *Standard for Parking Structures*.[4]

**42.8.1.2 Multiple Occupancies.**

**42.8.1.2.1** Where both parking and repair operations are conducted in the same building, the entire building shall comply with Chapter 40, except as modified by 42.8.1.2.2.

**42.8.1.2.2** Where the parking and repair sections are separated by not less than 1-hour fire-rated construction, the parking and repair sections shall be permitted to be treated separately.

**42.8.1.2.3** In areas where repair operations are conducted, the means of egress shall comply with Chapter 40.

Paragraph 42.8.1.2.2 permits a building to house parking and repair operations simultaneously and permits such operations to be treated independently if they are separated by 1-hour fire resistance–rated construction. The provisions of Chapter 40 would govern the repair operations, and Section 42.8 would cover the parking facilities.

**42.8.1.3 Definition — Open Parking Structure.** See 3.3.254.6.

The definition of the term *open parking structure* (see 3.3.254.6) specifies the degree to which the structure's exterior walls must have openings. Parking structures that meet the definition of the term *open parking structure* provide sufficient area in exterior walls to vent the products of combustion to a greater degree than an enclosed parking structure. Open parking structures — as contrasted with enclosed parking structures — are permitted to use vehicle ramps as a second means of egress [42.8.2.2.6.1(2)], have longer travel distance allowances (Table 42.8.2.6.1), and are exempt from the alarm system requirement (42.8.3.4.1.2).

**42.8.1.4 Classification of Occupancy.** Incidental vehicle parking in another occupancy shall not be the basis for overall occupancy classification.

**42.8.1.5 Classification of Hazard of Contents.** Parking structures used only for the storage of vehicles shall be classified as ordinary hazard in accordance with Section 6.2.

Paragraph 42.8.1.5 appropriately classifies the hazard of contents as ordinary hazard for garages used only for the storage of vehicles. With the increased use of combustible materials in vehicle bodies and interiors, a garage presents a hazard greater than that of low hazard contents, as defined by the hazard of contents classifications specified in Section 6.2. The presence of gasoline and diesel fuel in closed automobile fuel tanks does not warrant a high hazard classification.

**42.8.1.6 Minimum Construction Requirements.** (No requirements.)

**42.8.1.7 Occupant Load.** (No requirements.)

### 42.8.2 Means of Egress Requirements.

**42.8.2.1 General.** Means of egress shall be in accordance with Chapter 7 and 42.8.2.

**42.8.2.2 Means of Egress Components.**

**42.8.2.2.1 Components Permitted.** Components of means of egress shall be limited to the types described in 42.8.2.2.2 through 42.8.2.2.9.

**42.8.2.2.2 Doors.**

**42.8.2.2.2.1** Doors complying with 7.2.1 shall be permitted.

**42.8.2.2.2.2** Special locking arrangements complying with 7.2.1.6 shall be permitted.

**42.8.2.2.2.3** An opening for the passage of automobiles shall be permitted to serve as an exit from a street floor, provided that no door or shutter is installed therein.

**42.8.2.2.3 Stairs.**

**42.8.2.2.3.1** Stairs complying with 7.2.2 shall be permitted, unless otherwise permitted by 42.8.2.2.3.2.

**42.8.2.2.3.2** In open-air parking structures, stairs complying with 7.2.2.5.1 shall not be required.

Stairs in open parking structures are not required to be enclosed to be considered as pseudo-exits; this provision is new to the 2009 edition of the *Code*. Companion revisions to the travel distance provisions in 42.8.2.6 indicate that travel distance in open parking structures is measured to either an exit, as is typically required, or to an open stair, and the travel distance along the open stair is unlimited. This provision recognizes the low incidence of loss of life from fire in open parking structures and the personal crime issues associated with stair enclosures.

**42.8.2.2.3.3** Existing winders complying with 7.2.2.2.4 shall be permitted.

**42.8.2.2.3.4** Paragraph 7.2.2.4.5.3(2) shall not apply to guards for parking garages that are accessible to the general public.

**42.8.2.2.4 Smokeproof Enclosures.** Smokeproof enclosures complying with 7.2.3 shall be permitted.

**42.8.2.2.5 Horizontal Exits.** Horizontal exits complying with 7.2.4 shall be permitted.

**42.8.2.2.6 Ramps.**

**42.8.2.2.6.1** Ramps shall be permitted in accordance with any of the following conditions:

(1) Ramps complying with 7.2.5 shall be permitted and shall not be subject to normal vehicular traffic where used as an exit.
(2) In a ramp-type open parking structure with open vehicle ramps not subject to closure, the ramp shall be permitted to serve in lieu of the second means of egress from floors above the level of exit discharge, provided that the ramp discharges directly outside at the street level.
(3) For parking structures extending only one floor level below the level of exit discharge, a vehicle ramp leading directly to the outside shall be permitted to serve in lieu of the second means of egress, provided that no door or shutter is installed therein.

**42.8.2.2.6.2** Paragraph 7.2.2.4.5.3(2) shall not apply to guards for parking garages that are accessible to the general public.

Paragraphs 42.8.2.2.6.1(2) and (3) permit the use of vehicle ramps as part of the means of egress. Properly arranged ramps can facilitate safe egress to a degree well in excess of that required for the given number of occupants.

Paragraph 42.8.2.2.6.1(2) allows consideration of ramps in open-air parking structures as a secondary means of egress from floors located above the street level where they are arranged to provide clear and unobstructed discharge to the street level. Ramps from floors located above the street level are required to be open and must not be enclosed by walls or other means that will confine smoke and heat in the ramp structure. Ramps located in enclosed garages — except those addressed by 42.8.2.2.6.1(3) — cannot be considered as part of the egress system, and normal means of egress (specified in 42.8.2.2) needs to be provided.

Paragraph 42.8.2.2.6.1(3) permits a ramp to be used as a secondary means of egress in a garage that extends not more than one floor level below the level of exit discharge. The ramp must not have a door or a shutter and must lead directly outside.

**42.8.2.2.7 Exit Passageways.** Exit passageways complying with 7.2.6 shall be permitted.

**42.8.2.2.8 Fire Escape Stairs.** Fire escape stairs complying with 7.2.8 shall be permitted for existing parking structures only.

**42.8.2.2.9 Areas of Refuge.**

**42.8.2.2.9.1** Areas of refuge complying with 7.2.12 shall be permitted, as modified by 42.8.2.2.9.2.

**42.8.2.2.9.2** In open-air parking structures, the area of refuge requirements of 7.2.12.1.2(2) shall not apply.

**42.8.2.3 Capacity of Means of Egress.** See also 42.8.2.4 and 42.8.2.5.

**42.8.2.4 Number of Means of Egress.** See also Section 7.4.

**42.8.2.4.1** Not less than two means of egress shall be provided from every floor or section of every parking structure.

**42.8.2.4.2** In new buildings, floors or portions thereof with an occupant load of more than 500 persons shall have the minimum number of separate and remote means of egress specified by 7.4.1.2.

Note that there is no single exit exemption to the two-exit rule for parking garages.

**42.8.2.5 Arrangement of Means of Egress.** See also Section 7.5.

**42.8.2.5.1** A common path of travel shall be permitted for the first 50 ft (15 m) from any point in the parking structure.

**42.8.2.5.2** Dead ends shall not exceed 50 ft (15 m).

**42.8.2.5.3** Where fuel-dispensing devices are located within a parking structure, 42.8.2.5.3.1 and 42.8.2.5.3.2 shall apply.

**42.8.2.5.3.1** Travel away from the fuel-dispensing device in any direction shall lead to an exit with no dead end in which occupants might be trapped by fire.

**42.8.2.5.3.2** Within closed parking structures containing fuel-dispensing devices, exits shall be arranged and located to meet the following additional requirements:

(1) Exits shall lead to the outside of the building on the same level or to stairs, with no upward travel permitted, unless direct outside exits are available from that floor.

(2) Any story below the story at which fuel is being dispensed shall have exits leading directly to the outside via outside stairs or doors at the finished ground level.

Paragraph 42.8.2.5.3 specifies the conditions required for protection of the occupants of parking garages from fires that might be caused by fuel-dispensing operations located inside the building. Additional provisions apply where fuel dispensing takes place in enclosed parking structures. Paragraph 42.8.2.5.3.2(2) requires that direct access to the outside be provided from floors located below those on which gasoline is dispensed. This requirement prevents gasoline vapors, which are heavier than air, from accumulating in enclosed portions of a means of egress, such as inside exit stairs.

The hazards associated with dispensing gasoline inside buildings are avoided by dispensing fuel outdoors, as in the case of ordinary gasoline filling stations. See NFPA 30A, *Code for Motor Fuel Dispensing Facilities and Repair Garages*,[5] for requirements on dispensing fuel indoors.

**42.8.2.6 Travel Distance to Exits.**

**42.8.2.6.1** Travel distance, measured in accordance with Section 7.6, shall not exceed that provided by Table 42.8.2.6.1, except as otherwise permitted in 42.8.2.6.2.

**42.8.2.6.2** In open parking structures, travel distance shall comply with one of the following:

(1) The travel distance to an exit shall not exceed the travel distance specified in Table 42.8.2.6.1.
(2) The travel distance to a stair that does not meet the provisions for an exit enclosure shall not exceed the travel distance specified in Table 42.8.2.6.1, and travel along the stair shall not be limited.

The provisions of 42.8.2.6.2(2), which are new to the 2009 edition of the *Code*, permit open stairs in open parking structures to be equivalent to enclosed exits for the purpose of measuring travel distance to an exit. These criteria were added to the *Code* for consistency with NFPA 88A, *Standard for Parking Structures*, and recognize the good life safety record associated with open parking structures. Further, these criteria are intended to improve crime safety in open parking structures by eliminating hiding locations for would-be assailants. See the companion provision of 42.8.2.2.3.2, which exempts the requirement for enclosure of exit stairs in open parking structures.

**42.8.2.7 Discharge from Exits.** Exit discharge shall comply with Section 7.7.

**42.8.2.8 Illumination of Means of Egress.** Means of egress shall be illuminated in accordance with Section 7.8 or with natural lighting that provides the required level of illumination in structures occupied only during daylight hours.

**42.8.2.9 Emergency Lighting.** Parking structures shall be provided with emergency lighting in accordance with Section 7.9, except for structures occupied only during daylight hours and arranged to provide the required level of illumination of all portions of the means of egress by natural means.

**42.8.2.10 Marking of Means of Egress.** Means of egress shall have signs in accordance with Section 7.10.

**42.8.2.11 Special Means of Egress Features. (Reserved)**

### 42.8.3 Protection.

**42.8.3.1 Protection of Vertical Openings.**

**42.8.3.1.1 Vertical Openings in Enclosed Parking Structures.**

**42.8.3.1.1.1** Vertical openings through floors in buildings four or more stories in height shall be enclosed with walls or partitions having a minimum 2-hour fire resistance rating.

**42.8.3.1.1.2** For buildings three or fewer stories in height, the walls or partitions required by 42.8.3.1.1.1 shall have a minimum 1-hour fire resistance rating.

***Table 42.8.2.6.1 Maximum Travel Distance to Exits***

| | Enclosed Parking Structure | | Open Parking Structure | | Parking Structure Open Not Less than 50% on All Sides | |
|---|---|---|---|---|---|---|
| **Level of Protection** | **ft** | **m** | **ft** | **m** | **ft** | **m** |
| Protected throughout by an approved, supervised automatic sprinkler system in accordance with 9.7.1.1(1) | 200 | 61 | 400 | 122 | 400 | 122 |
| Not protected throughout by an approved, supervised automatic sprinkler system in accordance with 9.7.1.1(1) | 150 | 46 | 300 | 91 | 400 | 122 |

**42.8.3.1.1.3** Ramps in enclosed parking structures shall not be required to be enclosed when one of the following safeguards is provided:

(1) An approved, automatic sprinkler system fully protecting the enclosed parking structure
(2) An approved, automatic, supervised fire detection system installed throughout the enclosed parking structure, and a mechanical ventilation system capable of providing a minimum of 1 $ft^3$/min per $ft^2$ of floor area (300 L/min per $m^2$ of floor area) during hours of normal operation
(3)* Where a parking structure consists of sprinklered enclosed parking levels, and sprinklered or nonsprinklered open parking levels

**A.42.8.3.1.1.3(3)** It is common practice to construct a parking structure that consists of open parking levels above grade plane meeting the opening requirements for an open parking structure, but that also has enclosed parking levels below grade plane that need to comply with the requirements for an enclosed parking structure. It is impractical to have enclosed ramps between the enclosed level(s) and the open level(s) of such a parking structure.

**42.8.3.1.1.4** Sprinkler systems provided in accordance with 42.8.3.1.1.3(1) or (3) shall be supervised in accordance with 9.7.2.

**42.8.3.1.2 Open Parking Structures.** Unprotected vertical openings through floors in open parking structures shall be permitted. [**88A:**4.7.5]

Requirements for the protection of vertical openings in parking structures, which are largely extracted from NFPA 88A, *Standard for Parking Structures,* are provided in 42.8.3.1. These provisions permit ramps to be unenclosed under the following conditions:

1. The parking garage is enclosed and is protected by an approved, electrically supervised automatic sprinkler system.
2. The parking garage is enclosed and is protected by a fire detection system and mechanical ventilation.
3. The parking garage meets the definition of the term *open parking structure* in 3.3.254.6.

**42.8.3.2 Protection from Hazards.** (No requirements.)

**42.8.3.3 Interior Finish.**

**42.8.3.3.1 General.** Interior finish shall be in accordance with Section 10.2.

**42.8.3.3.2 Interior Wall and Ceiling Finish.** Interior wall and ceiling finish materials complying with Section 10.2 shall be Class A, Class B, or Class C in parking structures and shall be as required by 7.1.4 in exit enclosures.

**42.8.3.3.3 Interior Floor Finish.**

**42.8.3.3.3.1** Interior floor finish in exit enclosures shall be not less than Class II.

**42.8.3.3.3.2** Interior floor finish in areas other than those specified in 42.8.3.3.3.1 shall not be required to comply with Section 10.2.

**42.8.3.4 Detection, Alarm, and Communications Systems.**

**42.8.3.4.1 General.** A fire alarm system shall be required in accordance with Section 9.6 for parking structures, except as modified by 42.3.4.1.1, 42.3.4.1.2, and 42.3.4.1.3.

**42.8.3.4.1.1** Parking structures not exceeding an aggregate floor area of 100,000 $ft^2$ (9300 $m^2$) shall not be required to have a fire alarm system.

**42.8.3.4.1.2** Open parking structures shall not be required to have a fire alarm system.

**42.8.3.4.1.3** Parking structures protected throughout by an approved automatic sprinkler system in accordance with Section 9.7 shall not be required to have a fire alarm system.

**42.8.3.4.2 Initiation.** Initiation of the required fire alarm system shall be by one of the following means:

(1) Manual means in accordance with 9.6.2.1(1)
(2) Approved automatic fire detection system in accordance with 9.6.2.1(2) throughout the building, plus a minimum of one manual fire alarm box in accordance with 9.6.2.6
(3) Approved supervised automatic sprinkler system in accordance with 9.6.2.1(3) throughout the building, plus a minimum of one manual fire alarm box in accordance with 9.6.2.6

**42.8.3.4.3 Notification.**

**42.8.3.4.3.1** The required fire alarm system shall sound an audible alarm in a continuously attended location for purposes of initiating emergency action.

**42.8.3.4.3.2** Positive alarm sequence in accordance with 9.6.3.4 shall be permitted.

**42.8.3.4.3.3** Existing presignal systems in accordance with 9.6.3.3 shall be permitted.

**42.8.3.5 Extinguishing Requirements.** (No requirements.)

**42.8.3.6 Corridors.** The provisions of 7.1.3.1 shall not apply.

### 42.8.4 Special Provisions — High-Rise Buildings.

(No requirements.)

### 42.8.5 Building Services.

**42.8.5.1 Utilities.** Utilities shall comply with the provisions of Section 9.1.

**42.8.5.2 Heating, Ventilating, and Air-Conditioning.** Heating, ventilating, and air-conditioning equipment shall comply with the provisions of Section 9.2.

**42.8.5.3 Elevators, Escalators, and Conveyors.** Elevators, escalators, and conveyors shall comply with the provisions of Section 9.4.

**42.8.5.4 Rubbish Chutes, Incinerators, and Laundry Chutes.** Rubbish chutes, incinerators, and laundry chutes shall comply with the provisions of Section 9.5.

## 42.9 Operating Features — Upholstered Furniture and Mattresses

The provisions of 10.3.2 shall not apply to upholstered furniture and mattresses.

## References Cited in Commentary

1. NFPA 13, *Standard for the Installation of Sprinkler Systems,* 2007 edition, National Fire Protection Association, Quincy, MA.
2. NFPA 30, *Flammable and Combustible Liquids Code,* 2008 edition, National Fire Protection Association, Quincy, MA.
3. NFPA 409, *Standard on Aircraft Hangars,* 2004 edition, National Fire Protection Association, Quincy, MA.
4. NFPA 88A, *Standard for Parking Structures,* 2007 edition, National Fire Protection Association, Quincy, MA.
5. NFPA 30A, *Code for Motor Fuel Dispensing Facilities and Repair Garages,* 2008 edition, National Fire Protection Association, Quincy, MA.

CHAPTER 43

# Building Rehabilitation

Chapter 43 first appeared in the 2006 edition of the *Code*. In editions prior to 2006, any alteration or any installation of new equipment was required to meet, as nearly as practicable, the requirements for new construction. Paragraph 4.6.8 on building rehabilitation directs the user to Chapter 43. Chapter 43 presents provisions based on a set of concepts that differ from those of the 2003 and earlier editions, including those specified in paragraphs 1 through 4, which follow.

**1.** During a rehabilitation project, a building must meet the base level of life safety required by the *Code* chapter applicable to the existing occupancy. For example, an assembly occupancy undergoing rehabilitation must meet the requirements of Chapter 13 for existing assembly occupancies. See 4.6.8.3, 43.1.2.1(1), and 43.7.1.1.

**2.** The rehabilitation work must maintain or increase the level of *Code* compliance.

**3.** Rehabilitation work in existing construction elements or building features is held to a lower standard than rehabilitation work in new elements or features.

**4.** Upgrades (other than those required for compliance with the existing occupancy chapter) are typically required only in the rehabilitation work areas, not throughout the occupancy or building.

The requirements of this chapter strive to maintain or improve the existing level of life safety without requiring all rehabilitation work to comply with the provisions applicable to new construction. The goal of this approach is to encourage the continued use or adaptive reuse of existing buildings. Often building rehabilitation is not undertaken because of the perception that unwanted or unwarranted upgrades will be forced on the building owner. This chapter establishes the level of acceptable *Code* compliance.

The level of *Code* compliance established by this chapter uses a stepped approach to mandate requirements. Minor levels of rehabilitation must meet minimal requirements; major rehabilitation projects must meet more significant requirements.

NFPA did not originate the concept of a building rehabilitation code or a code chapter on rehabilitation. In 1997, the U.S. Department of Housing and Urban Development (HUD) published *Nationally Applicable Recommended Rehabilitation Provisions (NARRP)*.[1] NARRP was devised to provide a basis for developing local and model codes that promote the continued use of existing building stock. NFPA first addressed the subject in 2001–2002 when its building code committees developed Chapter 15, Building Rehabilitation, for *NFPA 5000®, Building Construction and Safety Code®*.[2] Chapter 43 of NFPA *101* addresses only the life safety subset of the building rehabilitation provisions from *NFPA 5000*.

The organization of this chapter differs from that of the other chapters of this *Code*. Section 43.1 contains the general or administrative provisions, while Section 43.2 contains the definitions. The provisions of the two sections lead the user to classifying the rehabilitation work category as repair, renovation, modification, reconstruction, change of use or occupancy classification, or addition. The user then moves directly to the applicable provisions — Sections 43.3 through 43.6, respectively, for repair, renovation, modification, and reconstruction; Section 43.7 for change of use or occupancy classification; or Section 43.8 for addition. Sections 43.3 through 43.8 provide options for treating historic building rehabilitation via the special provisions contained in Section 43.10, Historic Buildings.

## 43.1 General

### 43.1.1 Classification of Rehabilitation Work Categories.

Rehabilitation work on existing buildings shall be classified as one of the following work categories:

(1) Repair
(2) Renovation
(3) Modification
(4) Reconstruction
(5) Change of use or occupancy classification
(6) Addition

See 43.2.2.1 for definitions of the six categories of rehabilitation work — repair, renovation, modification, reconstruction, change of use or occupancy classification, and addition. The six categories are a key concept of this chapter for achieving the objective of proportionality of work. That is, the more work that is proposed for the rehabilitation project, the more work that might be required by the *Code* in terms of upgrading existing conditions.

For example, the provisions of Section 43.6 for reconstruction require more work than is required by Section 43.5 for modification, which, in turn, requires more work than is required by Section 43.4 for renovation. Section 43.5 does not repeat the provisions of Section 43.4 but mandatorily references their use and provides only the incremental features not contained in Section 43.4. See 43.5.1.1, which requires modification to meet the provisions of Section 43.5, as well as the provisions of Section 43.4, applicable to renovation. Similarly, 43.6.1.1 requires that reconstruction meet the provisions of Section 43.6, as well as those of Section 43.5, applicable to modification, and Section 43.4, applicable to renovation.

### 43.1.2 Applicable Requirements.

**43.1.2.1** Any building undergoing repair, renovation, modification, or reconstruction *(see 43.2.2.1.1 through 43.2.2.1.4)* shall comply with both of the following:

(1) Requirements of the applicable existing occupancy chapters *(see Chapters 13, 15, 17, 19, 21, 23, 24, 26, 29, 31, 33, 37, 39, 40, and 42)*
(2) Requirements of the applicable section of this chapter *(see Sections 43.3, 43.4, 43.5, and 43.6)*

Chapter 43 does not mandate improvements or set minimum acceptable standards for spaces that are not undergoing rehabilitation. Such improvements or standards are left to other chapters to require, as the *Code* applies both to new construction and to existing situations. It is the intent of 1.3.1, 4.4.2.1, and 4.6.10.1 that an existing situation, even if not undergoing rehabilitation, needs to comply with the *Code* provisions detailed in the applicable existing occupancy chapter. For example, an existing theater must meet the provisions of Chapter 13 for existing assembly occupancies, even where no rehabilitation is taking place. Yet, due to inadequate enforcement or waivers, not all existing buildings (i.e., existing situations) are *Code* compliant. Therefore, 43.1.2.1 establishes that any building undergoing repair, renovation, modification, or reconstruction be in compliance with the applicable existing occupancy chapter — even for features and systems not related to the rehabilitation project — before the user proceeds to implement the criteria of Sections 43.3 through 43.6. A similar provision, generalized to have applicability to all rehabilitation work categories, appears in 4.6.8.3.

Two examples of the effect of the requirements of 43.1.2.1 follow.

***Example 1***

An existing two-story business occupancy building will undergo a modification involving the reconfiguration of the second-floor tenant space. The second floor is served by only a single exit. If 39.2.4 requires the second floor to have a minimum of two exits, a second exit needs to be added as a condition for proceeding with the rehabilitation project. The reconfiguration of the second-floor space (but not the addition of the second exit) must meet the modification provisions of Section 43.5. See 43.1.4.5 and its commentary.

***Example 2***

An existing two-story business occupancy building will undergo a reconstruction involving the reconfiguration of the second-floor corridor shared by multiple occupant spaces. The second floor has an occupant load of 400 (which will not be changed by the rehabilitation project) and is served by two exits with a combined capacity of 300 persons. Subsection 39.2.3 requires egress capacity for the existing business occupancy to be in compliance with Section 7.3. It would appear that 43.1.2.1(1) requires that egress capacity for an additional 100 persons be added as a condition for proceeding with the rehabilitation project. However, 43.4.2 (which is positioned within Section 43.4 for renovations but has applicability to reconstruction because 43.6.1.1 requires compliance with Sections 43.4, 43.5, and 43.6) offers the two possible exemptions specified in paragraphs 1 and 2, which follow.

**1.** The authority having jurisdiction (AHJ) is permitted to establish the occupant load as the 300 persons for whom the existing means of egress is adequate, provided that measures are established to prevent occupancy by more than 300 persons. Such measures would have the effect of making the egress capacity sufficient for the occupant load, so as to preclude having to add additional egress capacity.

**2.** If the existing 300-person egress capacity was *previously approved* as being adequate for the 400-person occupant load, the egress system need not be upgraded. See 3.3.198 for a definition of the term *previously approved*.

In Example 2, where the existing 300-person egress capacity was not previously approved and the current AHJ does not permit its continued use, elements must be added to the egress system to increase the egress capacity to 400 persons. The reconstruction of the second-floor corridor (but not the addition of egress elements to increase the egress capacity) must meet the reconstruction provisions of Section 43.6. See the commentary following 43.1.4.5.

The point of Example 2 is that, although 43.1.2.1 requires buildings undergoing repair, renovation, modification, or reconstruction to meet the provisions of the applicable existing occupancy chapter, the user needs to check for any applicable exemptions within other sections of Chapter 43.

**43.1.2.2** Any building undergoing change of use or change of occupancy classification *(see 43.2.2.1.5 and 43.2.2.1.6)* shall comply with the requirements of Section 43.7.

**43.1.2.3** Any building undergoing addition *(see 43.2.2.1.7)* shall comply with the requirements of Section 43.8.

**43.1.2.4** Historic buildings undergoing rehabilitation shall comply with the requirements of Section 43.10.

The provisions of 43.1.2.2 through 43.1.2.4 supplement those of 43.1.2.1 to complete the road map directing the user to the appropriate section of Chapter 43, based on the rehabilitation work category assigned to the project. See 43.2.2.1 for definitions of the six categories of rehabilitation work — repair, renovation, modification, reconstruction, change of use or occupancy classification, and addition.

**43.1.2.5** Nothing in this chapter shall be interpreted as excluding the use of the performance-based option of Chapter 5.

The performance-based option of Chapter 5 is a rigorous and formalized method of equivalency. See 43.1.4.2 and the commentary that follows 43.1.4.2 for more information.

### 43.1.3 Multiple Rehabilitation Work Categories.

**43.1.3.1** Work of more than one rehabilitation work category shall be permitted to be part of a single work project.

**43.1.3.2** Where a project includes one category of rehabilitation work in one building area and another category of rehabilitation work in a separate area of the building, each project area shall comply with the requirements of the respective category of rehabilitation work.

**43.1.3.3** Where a project consisting of modification and reconstruction is performed in the same work area, or in contiguous work areas, the project shall comply with the requirements applicable to reconstruction, unless otherwise specified in 43.1.3.4.

**43.1.3.4** Where the reconstruction work area is less than 10 percent of the modification work area, the two shall be considered as independent work areas, and the respective requirements shall apply.

It is the intent of 43.1.3 to permit multiple categories of work on a single rehabilitation project. For example, a bathroom is being rehabilitated by relocating the water closet and wallpapering the walls. These two projects, whether performed separately or at the same time, would be treated in the same manner (i.e., the water closet relocation is a modification and the wallpapering is a renovation). Each project must comply with the requirements for its level of work.

Paragraph 43.1.3.2 addresses the situation where a rehabilitation project includes one category of rehabilitation work in one building area and another category of rehabilitation work in a separate area of the building. The provision permits each project to comply with its respective category of rehabilitation work. Exhibit 43.1 depicts such a situation. The floor plan shown is that of the second floor of a multistory building. The second floor is a business occupancy with multiple occupant spaces. The two rooms at the top of the exhibit are undergoing a rehabilitation that will involve reconfiguration of the space so as to be classified as a modification. The corridor in the lower portion of the exhibit serves more than a single occupant space, and

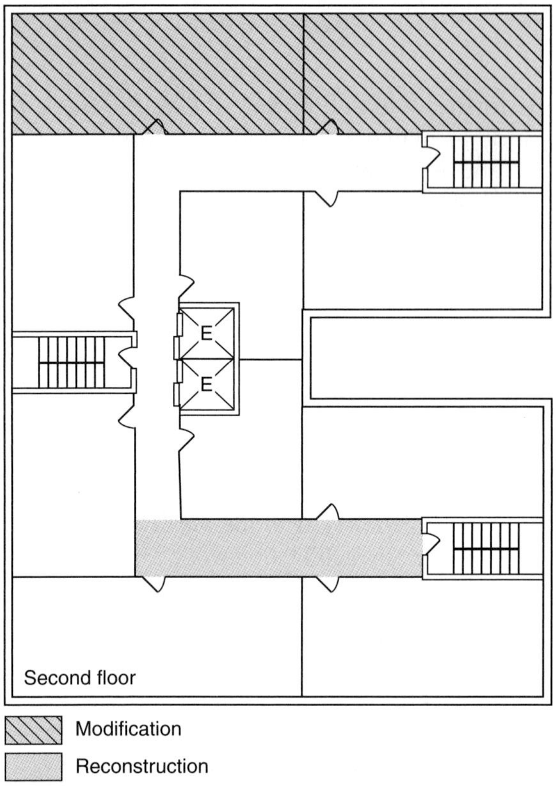


***Exhibit 43.1*** *Modification area treated independently of reconstruction area.*

its reconfiguration is classified as a reconstruction. Provided that the authority having jurisdiction (AHJ) judges that the areas are separate areas (note that 43.1.3.2 uses the term *separate area* and not *separated area*, so as to suggest that separation distance might be used to establish separate areas), the modification is permitted to comply independently with the provisions for modification, and the reconstruction is permitted to comply independently with the provisions for reconstruction. If the modification area were on a different floor than the reconstruction, the requirement for a separate area would also be met.

Per 43.1.3.3 and 43.1.3.4, for projects that involve modification and reconstruction in the same work area or in contiguous work areas, and where the reconstruction area is at least 10 percent of the modification area, the entire project must comply with reconstruction requirements. This requirement prevents a major rehabilitation project from being classified as a combination of a modification project (e.g., an occupant space reconfiguration) and a reconstruction project (e.g., rehabilitation work performed in a corridor shared by multiple occupant spaces, including the tenant occupying the space being reconfigured). Without the safeguard provided by 43.1.3.3, an entire floor could be rehabilitated without mandating some of the upgrades associated with reconstruction. An example of such an upgrade can be found in 43.6.4.2, which mandates compliance with the sprinkler provisions applicable to new construction for the occupancy on any story where the rehabilitation work area exceeds 50 percent of the area of that story.

Exhibit 43.2 illustrates the provisions of 43.1.3.3 and 43.1.3.4. The floor plan shown is that of the second floor of a multistory building. The second floor is a business occupancy with multiple occupant spaces. The two rooms at the top of the exhibit are undergoing a rehabilitation that involves reconfiguration of the space so as to be classified as a modification. The corridor in the vicinity of the two rooms undergoing rehabilitation serves more than a single occupant space, and its reconfiguration is classified as a reconstruction. The corridor reconstruction project exceeds 10 percent of the modification work area. Per 43.1.3.3, the overall project must comply with the requirements applicable to reconstruction.

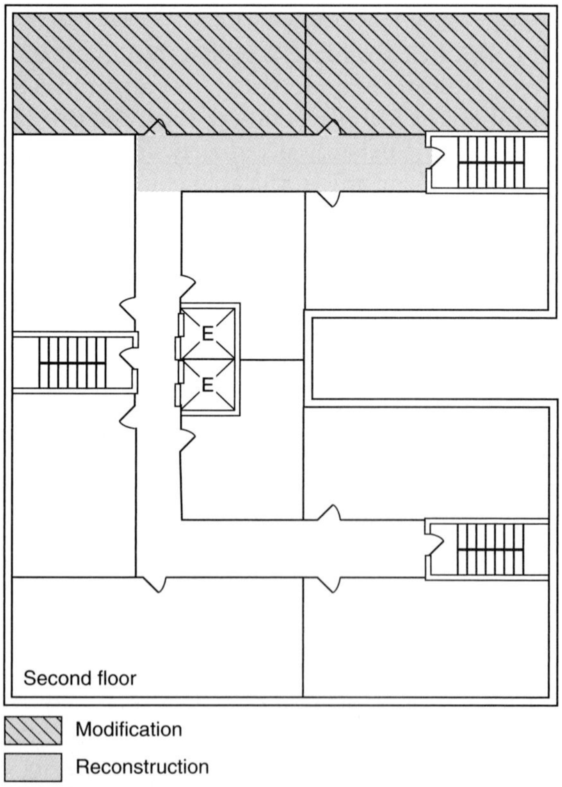


***Exhibit 43.2*** *Reconstruction provisions required for modification area and reconstruction area.*

### 43.1.4 Compliance.

**43.1.4.1** Repairs, renovations, modifications, reconstruction, changes of use or occupancy classification, and additions shall conform to the specific requirements for each category in other sections of this chapter.

**43.1.4.2** This chapter shall not prevent the use of any alternative material, alternative design, or alternative method of construction not specifically prescribed herein, provided that the alternative has been deemed to be equivalent and its use authorized by the authority having jurisdiction in accordance with Section 1.4.

Paragraph 43.1.4.2 provides an equivalency allowance for all projects. This provision might seem redundant with those of Section 1.4 but is included in this chapter to emphasize that the traditional methods of equivalent compliance are permitted to be used in addition to the special provision addressed in 43.1.4.3.

**43.1.4.3** Where compliance with this chapter, or with any provision required by this chapter, is technically infeasible or would impose undue hardship because of structural, construction, or dimensional difficulties, the authority having jurisdiction shall be authorized to accept alternative materials, design features, or operational features.

Paragraph 43.1.4.3 permits the authority having jurisdiction (AHJ) to accept alternatives that might not be fully equivalent to *Code* requirements where the applicant demonstrates that full compliance would be technically infeasible or would impose an undue hardship.

The term *technically infeasible* is defined in 43.2.2.5.

One of the source documents for this chapter, *Nationally Applicable Recommended Rehabilitation Provisions (NARRP)*, addresses the concept of *disproportionate cost*.[3] While not specifically discussed in the *Code*, disproportionate cost might be a consideration for undue hardship. One jurisdiction that participated in the development of *NARRP* indicated that the following three tests are necessary to determine such an economic hardship:

1. Cost of compliance in an existing building versus the cost of new construction
2. Cost of compliance as a proportion of the cost of the proposed project
3. Cost of the proposed project versus the replacement cost of the building

It is important that the AHJ and the building owner maintain records of all approved compliance alternatives. These records might be needed in the future to document compliance with the wording of 43.4.1.4 ("The work shall not make the building less conforming with . . . any previous approved alternative arrangements . . ."). The AHJ might require peer review of the proposed alternatives to judge their acceptability under 43.1.4.3 and the general equivalency provision of 43.1.4.2.

**43.1.4.4** Elements, components, and systems of existing buildings with features that exceed the requirements of this *Code* for new construction, and not otherwise required as part of previously documented, approved alternative arrangements, shall not be prevented by this chapter from being modified, provided that such elements, components, and systems remain in compliance with the applicable *Code* provisions for new construction.

As noted in the commentary following the title of this chapter, Chapter 43 was developed using the concept that rehabilitation work should not reduce the existing level of *Code* compliance. However, 43.1.4.4 establishes that, if the existing condition exceeds that required for new construction, the condition is permitted to be altered, provided that the resulting feature meets the requirements for new construction. For example, if a rehabilitation project in an existing hospital involves reconstruction, the corridor width requirements for the reconstruction would be as specified in paragraphs 1 and 2, which follow.

**1.** Per 43.1.2.1(2), the hospital must meet the requirements of Chapter 19 for existing health care occupancies. Paragraph 19.2.3.4 requires the corridor to be not less than 48 in. (1220 mm) in width.

**2.** Per 43.6.1.1(2) and 43.5.1.3, any newly constructed corridors must meet the width requirement for new construction, typically an 8 ft (2440 mm) width in patient care areas per 18.2.3.4. If the existing corridor were 10 ft (3050 mm) wide, 43.1.4.4 permits the corridor width to be reduced to 8 ft (2440 mm) during the reconstruction project. This provision is consistent with 4.6.8.4. See also A.4.6.8.5.

**43.1.4.5** Work mandated by any accessibility, property, housing, or fire code; mandated by the existing building requirements of this *Code*; or mandated by any licensing rule or ordinance, adopted pursuant to law, shall conform only to the requirements of that code, rule, or ordinance and shall not be required to conform to this chapter, unless the code requiring such work so provides.

Work of the type listed in 43.1.4.5 is not considered a rehabilitation project. Accordingly, such work need not comply with the provisions of Chapter 43. The work required by such retrospective regulation needs to comply only with the provisions of the *Code* requiring that the work be performed. For example, if an existing building undergoing repair, renovation, modification, or reconstruction is determined to have an inadequate egress system, based on the requirements of the applicable existing occupancy chapter of this *Code*, 4.6.8.3 requires that improvements to the egress system be made to bring the building into compliance with the existing occupancy chapter [see also 43.1.2.1(1)]. The fact that work is being done on the egress system to comply with 4.6.8.3 would not also impose the requirements of Sections 43.3 through 43.6.

Example 1, which appears in the commentary following 43.1.2.1(2), illustrates the provision of 43.1.4.5. An existing two-story business occupancy building will undergo a modification involving the reconfiguration of the second-floor tenant space. The second floor is served by only a single exit. If 39.2.4 requires the second floor to have a minimum of two exits, a second exit needs to be added as a condition for proceeding with the rehabilitation project. The work associated with adding the second exit is to be performed without classifying it as one of the rehabilitation work categories, and the work is not subject to the provisions of Chapter 43. The reconfiguration of the second-floor space (but not the addition of a second exit) must meet the modification provisions of Section 43.5.

## 43.2 Special Definitions

### 43.2.1 General.

The words and terms used in Chapter 43 shall be defined as detailed in 43.2.2, unless the context clearly indicates otherwise.

### 43.2.2 Special Definitions.

**43.2.2.1 Categories of Rehabilitation Work.** The nature and extent of rehabilitation work undertaken in an existing building.

**43.2.2.1.1 Repair.** The patching, restoration, or painting of materials, elements, equipment, or fixtures for the purpose of maintaining such materials, elements, equipment, or fixtures in good or sound condition.

*Repair* is the first category of the repair/renovation/modification/reconstruction continuum that establishes the amount of rehabilitation work permitted. Examples of rehabilitation work that might meet the definition of repair are provided in paragraphs 1 through 4, which follow.

**1.** A 24 in. (610 mm) wide by 24 in. (610 mm) high piece of wallpaper, vandalized with graffiti, is cut and peeled away from an existing corridor wall and replaced with a similarly sized piece of wallpaper in a theater. [The combustibility of the replacement patch of wallpaper is not germane to classifying the rehabilitation work category. Once the category is established as that of repair, the provisions of Section 43.3 apply, and 43.3.1.3 requires that the repair be done using like materials (such as wallpaper retained from the original installation, provided that the use of such material is not prohibited by some other *Code* provision) or materials permitted by other sections of the *Code* — typically the interior finish provisions of the ___.3.3 subsection of the applicable existing occupancy chapter.]

**2.** Four 24 in. × 24 in. (610 mm × 610 mm) lay-in ceiling tiles, damaged by water from a roof leak, are replaced in an existing office.

**3.** A portion of an existing plaster-on-lath wall, where plaster has been disengaged from the lath after being impacted by a wheeled cart, is patched with gypsum wallboard compound, sanded, and painted to match the wall section in an existing hospital.

**4.** Chipped paint areas on doors and door frames in an existing detention and correctional occupancy building are touched up by brushing new paint over the chipped areas.

**43.2.2.1.2 Renovation.** The replacement in kind or strengthening of load-bearing elements; or the refinishing, replacement, bracing, strengthening, or upgrading of existing materials, elements, equipment, or fixtures, without involving the reconfiguration of spaces.

*Renovation* is the second category of the repair/renovation/modification/reconstruction continuum that establishes the amount of rehabilitation work permitted. Examples of rehabilitation work that might meet the definition of renovation are provided in paragraphs 1 through 5, which follow.

**1.** An existing corridor wall in an apartment building is wallpapered, regardless of whether it had been papered before.

2. A lay-in tile ceiling is removed and replaced to modernize the décor in an existing office.

3. The existing walls, ceilings, doors, window casings and door casings, and other trim materials are repainted (i.e., refinished) in a tenanted office space to freshen the interior décor prior to a new tenant occupying the space.

4. The existing lavatories and water closets in a school building, which are badly stained with mineral deposits, are replaced (i.e., swapped out on a one-to-one basis without any relocation) for aesthetic reasons.

5. The existing shelving for the display of merchandise in a bulk merchandising retail building is replaced (i.e., swapped out on a one-to-one basis without any relocation) with heavy-duty shelving, so as to provide support for heavy items that the existing shelving could not.

**43.2.2.1.3 Modification.** The reconfiguration of any space; the addition, relocation, or elimination of any door or window; the addition or elimination of load-bearing elements; the reconfiguration or extension of any system; or the installation of any additional equipment.

*Modification* is the third category of the repair/renovation/modification/reconstruction continuum that establishes the amount of rehabilitation work permitted. Examples of rehabilitation work that might meet the definition of modification are provided in paragraphs 1 through 4, which follow.

1. A second door is installed — for the convenience of occupants — in the corridor wall that separates an existing tenanted office space from the common corridor serving multiple tenants. (If the door is added to correct a *Code* deficiency by shortening an excessive common path of travel to the length permitted by 39.2.5.3 for existing business occupancies, the work is not to be considered a rehabilitation project and is not subject to the provisions of Chapter 43. This is further explained in the commentary following 43.1.4.5.)

2. Two existing hotel guest rooms are combined into one larger room by removing the wall between the two rooms. All work occurs exclusively within the envelope of the guest rooms and does not affect the common corridor serving the guest rooms on that floor.

3. Ten percent of the shelving for the display of merchandise in a grocery store is removed, and the remaining 90 percent of the shelving is relocated so as to create wider aisles for the convenience of patrons.

4. A sprinkler system is voluntarily (i.e., not statutorily) installed throughout a warehouse building so the owner can qualify for a savings on the building's property insurance premium. (For modification work involving the entire building, the extensive modifications provisions of 43.5.2.1 would normally have the effect of requiring the rehabilitation work category to be changed from modification to reconstruction, but 43.5.2.2 permits modification work that is exclusively fire protection system work to retain its original classification of modification.)

As introduced in the example in paragraph 4, extensive modifications, as addressed in 43.5.2, might force a change in rehabilitation work category from modification to reconstruction. For example, per 43.5.2.1, the modification of an entire building or an entire occupancy within a building is required (with exemptions) to be classified as reconstruction rather than modification. Similarly, per 43.5.2.3, where the total area of all the rehabilitation work areas included in a modification exceeds 50 percent of the area of the building, the rehabilitation work category is required (with exemptions) to be classified as reconstruction rather than modification. See 43.5.2.

**43.2.2.1.4* Reconstruction.** The reconfiguration of a space that affects an exit or a corridor shared by more than one occupant space; or the reconfiguration of a space such that the rehabilitation work area is not permitted to be occupied because existing means of egress and fire protection systems, or their equivalent, are not in place or continuously maintained.

*Reconstruction* is the final category of the repair/renovation/modification/reconstruction continuum that establishes the amount of rehabilitation work permitted. Examples of rehabilitation work that might meet the definition of reconstruction are provided in paragraphs 1 through 4, which follow.

1. The corridor serving the multiple occupant spaces on a floor of an existing jewelry retail sales building is relocated to unite two sales spaces occupied by one of the tenants (i.e., the tenant's space was formerly divided into two sales areas by the existing corridor so as to require travel across the common corridor to move between the two areas) while continuing to provide all occupant spaces on the floor with access to the two exits required by 37.2.4.1.

**2.** A floor in an existing hotel building is gutted to the columns and exterior walls, and hotel guest suites are constructed in the space formerly occupied as individual guest rooms.

**3.** A wing in an existing hospital is closed to occupancy and isolated from the remainder of the building by temporary fire resistance–rated barriers while the required smoke barriers and corridor walls are relocated, and a new elevator and associated hoistway are added to facilitate day-to-day operations; the other wing of the hospital building remains occupied during the rehabilitation, as it is served by an exit at its far end and another exit at the central core of the building where the two wings are joined.

**4.** An exit passageway, serving as the discharge for an enclosed exit stair located within the core of a multistory, multi-occupant space, existing office building, is extended so as to discharge to the outside at a new location along an exterior wall, because an addition will be constructed to abut the building at the location where the exit passageway formerly discharged through the exterior wall.

The definition of the term *reconstruction* addresses work that affects an exit or corridor shared by more than one occupant space. The following situations are considered to involve more than one occupant space:

1. Work affecting a corridor on a hotel guest room floor
2. Work affecting a corridor on a hospital patient floor
3. Work affecting a corridor on an elementary school floor

Extensive modifications, as addressed in 43.5.2, might force a change in rehabilitation work category from modification to reconstruction. For example, per 43.5.2.1, the modification of an entire building or an entire occupancy within a building is required (with exemptions) to be classified as reconstruction rather than modification. Similarly, per 43.5.2.3, where the total area of all the rehabilitation work areas included in a modification exceeds 50 percent of the area of the building, the rehabilitation work category is required (with exemptions) to be classified as reconstruction rather than modification. See 43.5.2.

**A.43.2.2.1.4** It is not the intent that a corridor, aisle, or circulation space within a suite be considered as a corridor that is shared by more than one occupant space. The suite should be considered as only one occupant space. The following situations should be considered to involve more than one occupant space:

(1) Work affecting a corridor that is common to multiple guest rooms on a floor of a hotel occupancy
(2) Work affecting a corridor that is common to multiple living units on a floor of an apartment building occupancy
(3) Work affecting a corridor that is common to multiple tenants on a floor of a business occupancy

**43.2.2.1.5 Change of Use.** A change in the purpose or level of activity within a structure that involves a change in application of the requirements of the *Code*.

The term *change of use* is meant to address any change in the purpose or level of activity that, although it does not create a change of occupancy, does result in one or more differences in *Code* provisions applicable to the uses before and after the change. For example, although the provisions of Chapter 29 for emergency egress drills in hotels and dormitories are similar, such drills are required in dormitories for occupants and staff, but, in hotels, the provisions apply only to employees, as the other occupants change from night to night. Examples of rehabilitation work that might meet the definition of change of use include the following:

1. A family day-care home is changed to a day-care occupancy when the number of clients is increased from 12 to 15, resulting in having to comply with the requirements of Sections 17.1 through 17.5 rather than Section 17.6.
2. A small board and care occupancy is changed to a large board and care occupancy when a living room is converted to a bedroom, so that the number of sleeping accommodations for clients increases from 16 to 18, resulting in having to comply with the requirements of Section 33.3 rather than Section 33.2.
3. The contents and processes in an existing general purpose industrial occupancy building are changed so as to become more hazardous, and, therefore, the occupancy requires reclassification as a high hazard industrial occupancy and compliance with the special requirements for such.
4. The furniture is removed from a patient sleeping room in a hospital, and medical supplies are stored in the room, creating a hazardous area subject to the requirements for the protection from hazards.
5. Large dining tables are removed from an assembly occupancy restaurant with an occupant load of 280 persons and replaced by small cocktail tables increasing the occupant load to 320 persons, resulting in the requirement for a fire alarm system.

Other examples of change of use are presented in the commentary following 43.7.1.

The applicable occupancy chapter might further supplement the definition of the term *change of use* for purposes of applying the provisions of 43.7.1 to that occupancy. For example, 18/19.1.1.4.2 exempts some changes from one health care occupancy subclassification to another from being considered a change of use. Users are cautioned to consult the applicable occupancy chapters in addition to the provisions of Chapter 43.

**43.2.2.1.6 Change of Occupancy Classification.** The change in the occupancy classification of a structure or portion of a structure.

See the commentary following 43.7.2.

**43.2.2.1.7 Addition.** An increase in the building area, aggregate floor area, building height, or number of stories of a structure.

See the commentary following Section 43.8 title.

**43.2.2.2* Equipment or Fixture.** Any plumbing, heating, electrical, ventilating, air-conditioning, refrigerating, and fire protection equipment; and elevators, dumbwaiters, escalators, boilers, pressure vessels, or other mechanical facilities or installations related to building services.

**A.43.2.2.2** Equipment or fixtures do not include manufacturing, production, or process equipment, but do include connections from building service to process equipment.

**43.2.2.3 Load-Bearing Element.** Any column, girder, beam, joist, truss, rafter, wall, floor, or roof sheathing that supports any vertical load in addition to its own weight, or any lateral load.

**43.2.2.4 Rehabilitation Work Area.** That portion of a building affected by any renovation, modification, or reconstruction work as initially intended by the owner, and indicated as such in the permit, but excluding other portions of the building where incidental work entailed by the intended work must be performed, and excluding portions of the building where work not initially intended by the owner is specifically required.

The definition of the term *rehabilitation work area* clarifies that if a provision of this chapter requires work in an area of the building not initially intended by the rehabilitation plan, such additional work does not increase the size of the rehabilitation work area. This concept is illustrated in Exhibit 43.3, which depicts a two-story dormitory. Reconstruction on the second floor exceeds 50 percent of the floor area and mandates the requirement of 43.6.2.2.2 for illumination and emergency lighting to be provided throughout the second floor in accordance with the requirements applicable to new construction for the applicable occupancy (in this case, Chapter 28 for new hotels and dormitories). The installation of illumination and emergency lighting throughout the second floor does not increase the size of the rehabilitation work area. If this exemption were not provided, the rehabilitation work area would have been increased to include the entire second floor, and because the second floor exceeds 50 percent of the entire building area, 43.6.4.1 would have required that automatic sprinklers be installed on both floors in accordance with 28.3.5.1. Instead, per the requirement of 43.6.4.2, the initial rehabilitation work area exceeding 50 percent of the area of the second floor mandates a requirement for the sprinklering of that floor only.

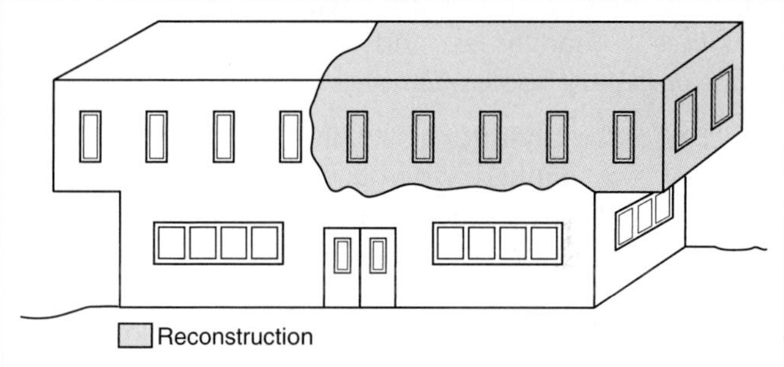


***Exhibit 43.3** Rehabilitation work area is not to be increased by work required in other areas.*

As another example of work area size concept, a sprinkler system is voluntarily installed as a modification involving the entire area of the third floor of an office building. Piping associated with the riser that supplies water to the sprinkler system is installed on the first and second floors. The work associated with the installation of the riser on the first and second floors is considered incidental. The rehabilitation work area is established as being the third floor only.

**43.2.2.5 Technically Infeasible.** A change to a building that has little likelihood of being accomplished because the existing structural conditions require the removal or alteration of a load-bearing member that is an essential part of the structural frame, or because other existing physical or site constraints prohibit modification or addition of elements, spaces, or features that are in full and strict compliance with applicable requirements.

The term *technically infeasible* is used in the compliance provisions of 43.1.4.3.

## 43.3 Repairs

The basic provisions of the repair requirements of Section 43.3 are as follows:

1. Perform the repair with like materials, unless the material is currently prohibited, or materials permitted by other sections of the *Code*. See 43.3.1.3.
2. Do not reduce the level of *Code* compliance. See 43.3.1.4.
3. Ensure that the building undergoing repair meets the requirements of the applicable existing occupancy chapter. See 43.1.2.1(1) and 4.6.8.3.

The difference between the terms *repair* and *renovation*, as defined in 43.2.2.1.1 and 43.2.2.1.2, respectively, is mostly one of quantity. An extensive repair becomes a renovation, and a minor renovation becomes a repair. Some examples are as follows:

1. The replacement of a section of corridor carpeting that was stained when a bottle of liquid bleach was spilled is typically a repair. The replacement of the corridor carpeting is typically a renovation.
2. The replacement of a few ceiling tiles is typically a repair. The replacement of a ceiling is typically a renovation.
3. The patching of a hole in a wall is typically a repair. The removal and replacement of a wall is typically a renovation. However, the removal, replacement, and relocation of a wall is a modification.
4. The replacement of a door closer that is not functioning is typically a repair. The replacement of a door is typically a renovation.

See the examples of repair, renovation, and modification in the commentary following 43.2.2.1.1, 43.2.2.1.2, and 43.2.2.1.3.

### 43.3.1 General Requirements.

**43.3.1.1** A repair, as defined in 43.2.2.1.1, in other than historic buildings shall comply with the requirements of Section 43.3.

**43.3.1.2** Repairs in historic buildings shall comply with the requirements of one of the following:

(1) Section 43.3
(2) Section 43.3, as modified by Section 43.10

**43.3.1.3** The work shall be done using like materials or materials permitted by other sections of this *Code*.

The general requirement of 43.3.1.3 for the work to be done using like materials or materials permitted in other parts of this *Code* represents a distinct difference between rehabilitation work classified as repair and that classified as renovation. Repair projects permit the use of materials similar to those that existed before the repair work was done, provided that the use of such material is not prohibited by another *Code* provision. Therefore, the repair to a stained section of carpeting might be done with a piece of carpeting retained from the original installation. On the other hand, renovation requires the use of materials that are permitted by other sections of the *Code* that apply to existing buildings (see 43.4.1.3). In some cases, such as a renovation involving the replacement of corridor carpeting or any other interior finish material, the materials used must comply with the requirements for new construction (see 43.4.3).

The provision of 43.3.1.3 can be illustrated by an example. The existing interior wall finish in the corridor of a nonsprinklered office building is a *previously approved* (see definition in 3.3.198) Class A textile wall covering. A piece of the textile wall covering, vandalized with graffiti, is cut and peeled away from the existing corridor wall and is replaced with Class A textile wall covering retained from the original installation. Although 10.2.4.1(1) would not permit new Class A textile wall covering to be installed in a nonsprinklered corridor, 10.2.4.1(4) permits previously approved existing Class A textile wall covering to be continued in use. The repair is permitted to be made using the original material.

**43.3.1.4** The work shall not make the building less conforming with the other sections of this *Code*, or with any previously approved alternative arrangements, than it was before the repair was undertaken.

The requirement in 43.3.1.4 that repairs must not make a building less conforming with other *Code* requirements is a basic premise throughout this chapter. Additionally, per 43.1.2.1(1) and 4.6.8.3, the building that undergoes repair must meet the requirements of the applicable existing occupancy chapter. See the commentary following 43.1.2.1(2).

## 43.4 Renovations

The basic provisions of the renovation requirements of Section 43.4 are as follows:

1. The renovation work, other than that involving new interior finish materials, must be performed in compliance with the *Code* provisions applicable to existing buildings. See 43.4.1.3. (New interior finish materials must meet the requirements for new construction. See 43.4.3.)
2. The renovation work must not reduce the level of *Code* compliance. See 43.4.1.4.
3. The building undergoing renovation must meet the requirements of the applicable existing occupancy chapter. See 43.1.2.1(1) and 4.6.8.3.

### 43.4.1 General Requirements.

**43.4.1.1** A renovation, as defined in 43.2.2.1.2, in other than historic buildings shall comply with the requirements of Section 43.4.

**43.4.1.2** Renovations in historic buildings shall comply with the requirements of one of the following:

(1) Section 43.4
(2) Section 43.4, as modified by Section 43.10

**43.4.1.3** All new work shall comply with the requirements of this *Code* applicable to existing buildings.

**43.4.1.4** The work shall not make the building less conforming with other sections of this *Code*, or with any previous approved alternative arrangements, than it was before the renovation was undertaken, unless otherwise specified in 43.4.1.5.

**43.4.1.5** Minor reductions in the clear opening dimensions of replacement doors and windows that result from the use of different materials shall be permitted, unless such reductions are prohibited.

The exemption permitted by 43.4.1.5 for areas undergoing renovation is meant to permit *minor* or inconsequential reductions in the clear width of openings of doors or windows that are caused by using replacement materials. It is not uncommon for a door replacement project to result in a slightly narrower opening than had been provided before the renovation, due to the use of different materials or products manufactured in accordance with current product standards. The *Code* intentionally allows the authority having jurisdiction (AHJ) to determine how much deviation to permit. For example, a reduction of 2 in. (51 mm) in the clear width previously provided by a 36 in. (915 mm) wide door leaf resulting in 32 in. (815 mm) of clear width might be considered minor, because the door opening provides the minimum clear width required by 7.2.1.2.3 for the purpose of accommodating a wheelchair user. A similar 2 in. (51 mm) reduction in the clear width previously provided by a 34 in. (865 mm) wide door leaf resulting in 30 in. (760 mm) of clear width should not be considered minor or inconsequential, because the door opening would no longer ensure passage by a wheelchair user.

### 43.4.2 Capacity of Means of Egress.

The capacity of means of egress, determined in accordance with Section 7.3, shall be sufficient for the occupant load thereof, unless one of the following conditions exists:

(1) The authority having jurisdiction shall be permitted to establish the occupant load as the number of persons for which existing means of egress is adequate, provided that measures are established to prevent occupancy by a greater number of persons.
(2)* The egress capacity shall have been previously approved as being adequate.

The provisions of 43.4.2 were relocated for the 2009 edition of the *Code*. The text had previously been positioned within Section 43.6 so as to have application only to reconstruction. Its former placement had the effect of requiring rehabilitation projects undergoing less work than that of reconstruction (i.e., repair, renovation, or modification) to meet stricter criteria related to egress capacity than required for rehabilitation projects categorized as reconstruction. The provisions of 43.4.2 can be applied to rehabilitation projects involving renovation, modification, or reconstruction, as Section 43.5 for modification requires compliance with Section 43.4, as does Section 43.6 for reconstruction. See the commentary following 43.1.1(6).

**A.43.4.2(2)** Some building codes have permitted an increase in egress capacity in buildings protected throughout by an approved automatic sprinkler system. The intent of 43.4.2(2) is that, during a renovation project, egress capacity is permitted to continue to be evaluated using the previously approved method.

### 43.4.3 Interior Finish Requirements.

New interior finish materials shall meet the requirements for new construction.

Paragraph 43.4.3 requires that the *Code* provisions applicable to new construction be applied to the installation of new interior finish materials. This provision is stricter than that in 43.4.1.3, which permits other renovation work to be done per the *Code* requirements applicable to existing buildings.

An example of the application of 43.4.3 follows. The corridor walls in a nonsprinklered day-care occupancy building are being refinished by installing plastic laminate paneling over the existing painted gypsum board. The paneling is required to meet the *Code* provisions applicable to new construction. Paragraph 16.3.3.2, applicable to interior wall finish in new day-care occupancies, requires Class A material in corridors. Had the normal provision of 43.4.1.3 applied, so as to permit the material to comply with the *Code* provisions for existing buildings, 17.3.3.2 would have permitted the use of Class A or Class B interior finish materials.

### 43.4.4 Other Requirements.

The reconfiguration or extension of any system, or the installation of any additional equipment, shall comply with Section 43.5.

Paragraph 43.4.4 has the effect of expanding the definition of *modification* and limiting the definition of *renovation*. The reconfiguration or extension of any system, or the installation of any additional equipment, must be classified as a modification, not as a renovation. The effect of this requirement is that such reconfiguration, extension, or installation is required to comply with the requirements of other *Code* sections applicable to new construction. Had this provision not appeared, the reconfiguration, extension, or installation would have been permitted to be done per the *Code* requirements applicable to existing buildings, as 43.4.1.3 directs.

## 43.5 Modifications

The basic provisions of the modification requirements of Section 43.5 are as follows:

1. Newly constructed elements, components, and systems are required to comply with the requirements of other *Code* sections applicable to new construction.
2. Work must also meet the renovation provisions of Section 43.4.
3. The modification work must not reduce the level of *Code* compliance. See 43.4.1.4, applicable per 43.5.1.1(2).
4. The building undergoing modification must meet the requirements of the applicable existing occupancy chapter. See 43.1.2.1(1) and 4.6.8.3.

### 43.5.1 General Requirements.

**43.5.1.1** A modification, as defined in 43.2.2.1.3, in other than historic buildings shall comply with both of the following:

(1) Section 43.5
(2) Section 43.4

**43.5.1.2** Modifications in historic buildings shall comply with the requirements of one of the following:

(1) 43.5.1.1(1) and (2)
(2) 43.5.1.1(1) and (2), as modified by Section 43.10

**43.5.1.3** Newly constructed elements, components, and systems shall comply with the requirements of other sections of this *Code* applicable to new construction.

Paragraph 43.5.1.3 requires that the *Code* provisions applicable to new construction be applied to newly constructed elements, components, and systems. This is the requirement that is mainly responsible for making the provisions for modification stricter than those for renovation. Paragraph 43.4.1.3 permits rehabilitation work classified as renovation (other than that involving the installation of interior finish materials) to be done per the *Code* requirements applicable to existing buildings.

### 43.5.2 Extensive Modifications.

Subsection 43.5.2 has the effect of expanding the definition of the term *reconstruction*, and limiting the definition of the term *modification*, via the introduction of criteria for judging a modification to be an extensive modification subject to the reconstruction provisions of Section 43.6.

**43.5.2.1** The modification of an entire building or an entire occupancy within a building shall be considered as a reconstruction and shall comply with the requirements of Section 43.6 for the applicable occupancy, unless otherwise specified in 43.5.2.2.

**43.5.2.2** Modification work that is exclusively electrical, plumbing, mechanical, fire protection system, or structural work shall not be considered a reconstruction, regardless of its extent.

**43.5.2.3** Where the total area of all the rehabilitation work areas included in a modification exceeds 50 percent of the area of the building, the work shall be considered as a reconstruction and shall comply with the requirements of Section 43.6 for the applicable occupancy, unless otherwise specified in 43.5.2.4.

**43.5.2.4** Rehabilitation work areas in which the modification work is exclusively plumbing, mechanical, fire protection system, or electrical work shall not be included in the computation of total area of all rehabilitation work areas.

Two examples related to extensive modifications follow.

*Example 1*

Exhibit 43.4 illustrates an existing two-story hotel undergoing modification throughout the second floor. The modification includes cutting through the roof to add skylight windows along the length of the interior corridor; installing skylight windows in each guest room; and reconfiguring the bathroom in each guest room by removing the bathtub and installing a glass-enclosed shower. Paragraph 43.5.2.3 requires that the modification of more than 50 percent of the area of the building be reclassified as a reconstruction and meet the requirements of Section 43.6. Paragraph 43.6.4.1 requires that the rehabilitation work area involving reconstruction (see 43.6.1.3) of more than 50 percent of the aggregate building area be sprinklered (on floor 2 and floor 1) if sprinklers are required for new construction by the occupancy chapter. Paragraph 28.3.5.1, applicable to new hotels, requires sprinklers for the building arrangement shown in Exhibit 43.4. Thus, as part of the rehabilitation, floor 2 and floor 1

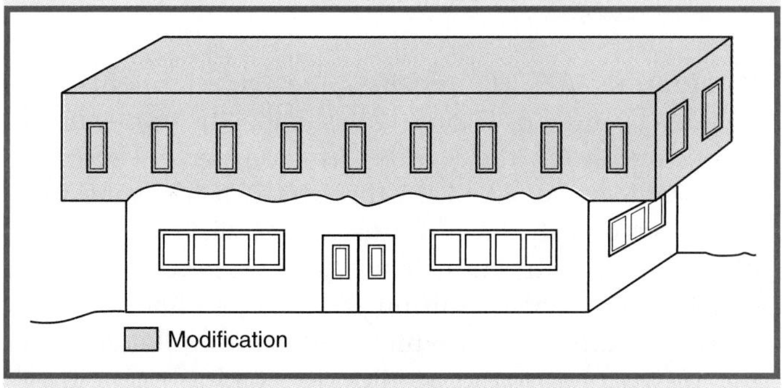


***Exhibit 43.4** Extensive modification might require reclassification to reconstruction.*

must be sprinklered. The effect of having to reclassify the rehabilitation work from modification to reconstruction is significant in raising the required level of life safety above that which existed prior to the rehabilitation project.

*Example 2*

Exhibit 43.4 illustrates an existing two-story hotel undergoing modification throughout the second floor. The modification is limited to the voluntary addition of a sprinkler system throughout the floor, as automatic sprinkler systems are not required by this *Code* for existing hotels that are not in high-rise buildings. The system installation will make extensive use of sidewall sprinklers to preclude the need for removing the ceiling or requiring guests to vacate the area while the work is being done. The modification is not required to be reclassified as reconstruction, because 43.5.2.4 exempts modification work that is exclusively plumbing, mechanical, fire protection system, or electrical work from having to be included in the computational area for purposes of applying the 50 percent criterion of 43.5.2.3. The installation of a sprinkler system is fire protection system work. The rehabilitation project remains a modification that must comply with the provisions of 43.5.1.

## 43.6 Reconstruction

The basic provisions of the reconstruction requirements of Section 43.6 are as follows:

1. Newly constructed elements, components, and systems are required to comply with the requirements of other *Code* sections applicable to new construction.
2. Work must also meet the renovation provisions of Section 43.4 and the modification provisions of Section 43.5.
3. The reconstruction work must not reduce the level of *Code* compliance. See 43.4.1.4, applicable per 43.6.1.1(3).
4. The building undergoing modification must meet the requirements of the applicable existing occupancy chapter. See 43.1.2.1(1) and 4.6.8.3.

As explained in the commentary following the title of this chapter, NFPA first addressed the subject of special provisions for existing building rehabilitation when its building code committees developed Chapter 15, Building Rehabilitation, for *NFPA 5000, Building*

*Construction and Safety Code*. In Chapter 15 of *NFPA 5000*, an existing building is required to meet progressively more stringent requirements as the rehabilitation work changes (from repair to renovation to modification to reconstruction), but the building itself is not required to meet a minimum prescribed level of performance as a condition for proceeding with the rehabilitation. The direction taken by *NFPA 5000* is consistent with that traditionally assumed by model building codes. Building codes typically do not require existing buildings that are simply being occupied, but for which there is no rehabilitation project, to be upgraded to the level of life safety required by NFPA *101* for existing buildings. For example, NFPA *101* requires existing business occupancy buildings to be in compliance with the provisions of Chapter 39, Existing Business Occupancies.

The reconstruction section of Chapter 15 of *NFPA 5000* is where the rehabilitation project becomes sufficiently complex so as to mandate requirements for work in a variety of elements and systems that are not part of the original rehabilitation work plan. Section 43.6 of this *Code* is modeled after the reconstruction section of Chapter 15 of *NFPA 5000*, but Section 43.6 addresses only the life safety subset of the building rehabilitation provisions from *NFPA 5000*. Section 43.6 has less effect than its counterpart in *NFPA 5000*, because 43.1.2.1(1) and 4.6.8.3 require compliance with the applicable existing occupancy chapters as a condition for using Chapter 43 for repair, renovation, modification, or reconstruction. The requirement of 43.1.2.1(1) ensures that the building being rehabilitated has many of the incremental features required by Section 43.6, albeit such features will often be in compliance with the provisions for existing buildings and might not meet all the requirements for new construction exactly. For example, 43.1.2.1(1) has the effect of requiring the building undergoing rehabilitation to meet the illumination requirements applicable to existing buildings, which means that stairs might not have the 10 ft-candle (108 lux) illumination level required of new stairs by 7.8.1.3(1). See 43.6.2.2.3, which requires some reconstruction to be provided with illumination in accordance with the requirements applicable to new construction.

Section 43.6 has its biggest effect in 43.6.4, where sprinklers are required for the floor containing the rehabilitation work area (in some cases, sprinklers also are required on all floors below) if the work area is large, but only if sprinklers are required by the section of the *Code* applicable to new construction for the occupancy. For example, if the rehabilitation work area in an existing hotel building is large enough to mandate the sprinkler requirement of 43.6.4.1 or 43.6.4.2, sprinklers are required, because 28.3.5.1, applicable to new hotels, requires sprinklers. On the other hand, if the rehabilitation work area in an existing, non-high-rise business occupancy building is large enough to mandate the sprinkler requirement of 43.6.4.1 or 43.6.4.2, sprinklers are not required, because the provisions of 38.3.5 and 38.4.2, applicable to new business occupancies, do not require sprinklers if the building is not a high-rise building.

### 43.6.1 General Requirements.

**43.6.1.1** A reconstruction, as defined in 43.2.2.1.4, in other than historic buildings shall comply with all of the following:

(1) Section 43.6
(2) Section 43.5, except that any stairway replacing an existing stairway shall be permitted to comply with 7.2.2.2.1.1(3)
(3) Section 43.4

**43.6.1.2** Reconstruction work in historic buildings shall comply with the requirements of one of the following:

(1) 43.6.1.1(1), (2), and (3)
(2) 43.6.1.1(1), (2), and (3), as modified by Section 43.10

**43.6.1.3** Wherever the term *rehabilitation work area* is used in Section 43.6, it shall include only the area affected by reconstruction work and areas covered by 43.5.2.

**43.6.1.4** Other rehabilitation work areas affected exclusively by renovation or modification work shall not be included in the rehabilitation work area required to comply with Section 43.6.

### 43.6.2 Means of Egress.

**43.6.2.1 General.** The means of egress shall comply with the requirements applicable to the existing occupancy *[see 43.1.2.1(1)]*, as modified by 43.6.2.

Paragraph 43.6.2.1 repeats the requirements of 43.1.2.1(1) and 4.6.8.3 but makes it specific to means of egress and adds the words "as modified by 43.6.2." The provisions of 43.6.2.2.1 through 43.6.2.2.3 mandate compliance with the illumination provisions applicable to new construction. They have limited additional effect over that resulting from compliance with 43.1.2.1(1) and 4.6.8.3, which require compliance with the provisions of the applicable existing occupancy chapter. For each occupancy classification, the chapter applicable to existing buildings applies the same illumination requirement as the chapter for new construction (i.e., compliance with Section 7.8). One effect of 43.6.2.2 that would not result from compliance with only 43.1.2.1(1) is the requirement for a minimum 10 ft-candle (108 lux) illumination level on new stairs, as required by 7.8.1.3(1). For example, 43.6.2.2.3 establishes a rehabilitation threshold at which illumination of the exit stairs serving the rehabilitation area is required. Such illumination of new stairs must provide the 10 ft-candle (108 lux) illumination level detailed in 7.8.1.3(1). Compliance with only 43.1.2.1(1) or 4.6.8.3 would provide a minimum illumination level of 1 ft-candle (10.8 lux) for other than new stairs.

**43.6.2.2 Illumination and Emergency Lighting of Means of Egress.**

**43.6.2.2.1** Means of egress in rehabilitation work areas shall be provided with illumination and emergency lighting in accordance with the requirements of other sections of this *Code* applicable to new construction for the occupancy.

**43.6.2.2.2** Where the reconstruction rehabilitation work area on any floor exceeds 50 percent of that floor area, means of egress throughout the floor shall be provided with illumination and emergency lighting in accordance with the requirements of other sections of this *Code* applicable to new construction for the occupancy, unless otherwise specified in 43.6.2.2.4.

**43.6.2.2.3** In a building with rehabilitation work areas involving more than 50 percent of the aggregate floor area within the building, the means of egress within the rehabilitation work area and the means of egress, including the exit and exit discharge paths, serving the rehabilitation work area shall be provided with illumination and emergency lighting in accordance with the requirements of other sections of this *Code* applicable to new construction for the occupancy, unless otherwise specified in 43.6.2.2.4.

**43.6.2.2.4** Means of egress within a tenant space that is entirely outside the rehabilitation work area shall be permitted to comply with the requirements for illumination and emergency lighting applicable to the existing occupancy in lieu of the requirements for illumination and emergency lighting applicable to new construction required by 43.6.2.2.2 and 43.6.2.2.3.

### 43.6.3 Fire Barriers and Smoke Barriers.

**43.6.3.1** In small residential board and care occupancies and one- and two-family dwellings where the rehabilitation work area is in any attached dwelling unit, walls separating the dwelling units, where such walls are not continuous from the foundation to the underside of the roof sheathing, shall be constructed to provide a continuous fire separation using construction materials that are consistent with the existing wall or that comply with the requirements for new buildings of the occupancy involved.

**43.6.3.2** The following shall apply to work required by 43.6.3.1:

(1) It shall be performed on the side of the wall of the dwelling unit that is part of the rehabilitation work area.
(2) It shall not be required to be continuous through concealed floor spaces.

The provisions of 43.6.3 have applicability only to small residential board and care occupancies and one- and two-family dwellings. Paragraph 43.6.3.1 has the effect of requiring that there be fire separations between the dwelling unit undergoing reconstruction and any adjacent dwelling units. This provision will, in some cases, involve an upgrade that would not be required by 43.1.2.1(1) or 4.6.8.3.

Paragraph 43.6.3.2 approaches the fire separation installation required by 43.6.3.1 in a practical way. Paragraph 43.6.3.2(1) permits the work needed for compliance to be done on the side of the wall in the dwelling unit that is part of the rehabilitation work area. In many cases, access is not readily available to the other side of the wall, because it is in a dwelling unit that is not part of the rehabilitation work area. Paragraph 43.6.3.2(2) recognizes the difficulty and disruptive effects of performing work in the portion of the wall sandwiched between the ceiling and the floor or roof above.

### 43.6.4 Extinguishing Systems.

Section 43.6 on reconstruction has its most profound effect in 43.6.4, where some degree of sprinklering is required (if the applicable occupancy chapter requires new construction to be sprinklered) if the rehabilitation work area exceeds a threshold expressed as a percentage of aggregate building area or a percentage of the area of the floor undergoing rehabilitation.

**43.6.4.1** In a building with rehabilitation work areas involving over 50 percent of the aggregate building area, automatic sprinkler systems shall be provided on the highest floor containing a rehabilitation work area and on all floors below in accordance with the requirements of other sections of this *Code* applicable to new construction for the occupancy.

**43.6.4.2** On any story with rehabilitation work areas involving over 50 percent of the area of the story, a sprinkler system shall be provided throughout the story in accordance with the requirements of other sections of this *Code* applicable to new construction for the occupancy.

Paragraphs 43.6.4.1 and 43.6.4.2 are the two provisions of Section 43.6 that do the most to raise the level of life safety above that required for rehabilitation projects by earlier editions of the *Code*. In earlier editions, any alteration or any installation of new equipment was required to meet, as nearly as practicable, the requirements for new construction. However, only the altered, renovated, or modernized portion of an existing building, system, or individual component was required to meet the provisions of the *Code* that are applicable to new construction. An extensive rehabilitation project that did not include sprinklering was not required to be sprinklered (in other than health care occupancies, which have specialized requirements for installing sprinklers in the smoke compartment undergoing major rehabilitation — see, for example, 18.1.1.4.3.3 and 18.1.1.4.3.4). The provisions of 43.6.4.1 and 43.6.4.2 require sprinklers for major reconstruction, even where the plan for the rehabilitation project does not involve sprinklers.

The application of 43.6.4.1 is illustrated in Exhibit 43.5. The existing, three-story, nonsprinklered hotel building is undergoing reconstruction. The rehabilitation work area is comprised of all of the second floor and portions of the first floor, so that the rehabilitation work area exceeds 50 percent of the aggregate building area. The threshold of 43.6.4.1 is exceeded; therefore, sprinklers are required to be provided on the highest floor containing a rehabilitation work area (i.e., the second floor) and on all floors below (i.e., the first floor) if sprinklers are required by other sections of the *Code* applicable to new construction for the occupancy. New hotels are addressed in Chapter 28, and 28.3.5.1 requires new hotels to be sprinklered. Thus, the major reconstruction mandates the sprinklering of the first and second floors, but sprinklers are not required on the third floor.

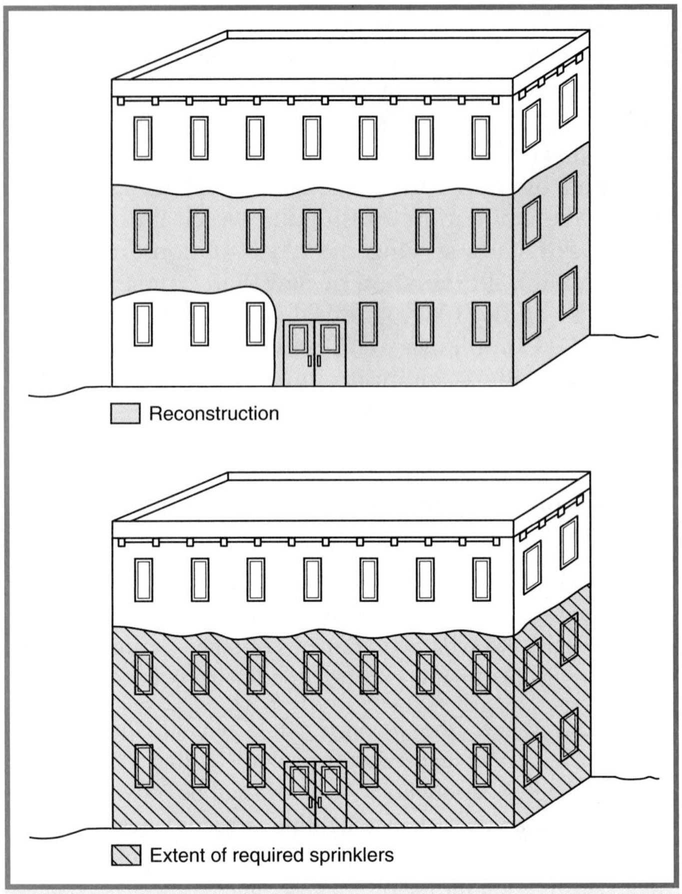


***Exhibit 43.5*** *Rehabilitation work area is large enough to require sprinklering of the first and second floors.*

The application of 43.6.4.2 is illustrated in Exhibit 43.6. The existing, three-story, nonsprinklered hotel building is undergoing reconstruction. The rehabilitation work area is comprised of two-thirds of the second floor, so that the rehabilitation work area exceeds 50 percent of the area of the story. The threshold of 43.6.4.2 is exceeded; therefore, sprinklers are required to be provided throughout the story containing the rehabilitation work area (i.e., the second floor) if sprinklers are required by other sections of the *Code* applicable to new construction for the occupancy. New hotels are addressed in Chapter 28, and 28.3.5.1 requires new hotels to be sprinklered. Thus, the major reconstruction mandates the sprinklering of the second floor, but sprinklers are not required on the first and third floors.

**43.6.4.3** Where sprinklers are installed in an elevator hoistway or elevator machine room as part of the rehabilitation work, the elevators shall comply with the fire fighters' emergency operations requirements of ASME A17.1/CSA B44, *Safety Code for Elevators and Escalators*.

The intent of 43.6.4.3 is more easily understood by first understanding the effect of 9.4.3.2. Paragraph 9.4.3.2 mandates compliance with the fire fighters' emergency operations requirements of ASME A17.3, *Safety Code for Existing Elevators and Escalators*,[4] not with the requirements of ASME A17.1/CSA B44, *Safety Code for Elevators and Escalators*.[5] ASME A17.3 requires existing elevators to meet the Phase I Emergency Operation (i.e., elevator recall) and Phase II Emergency Operation (i.e., fire fighters' service) provisions of the 1987

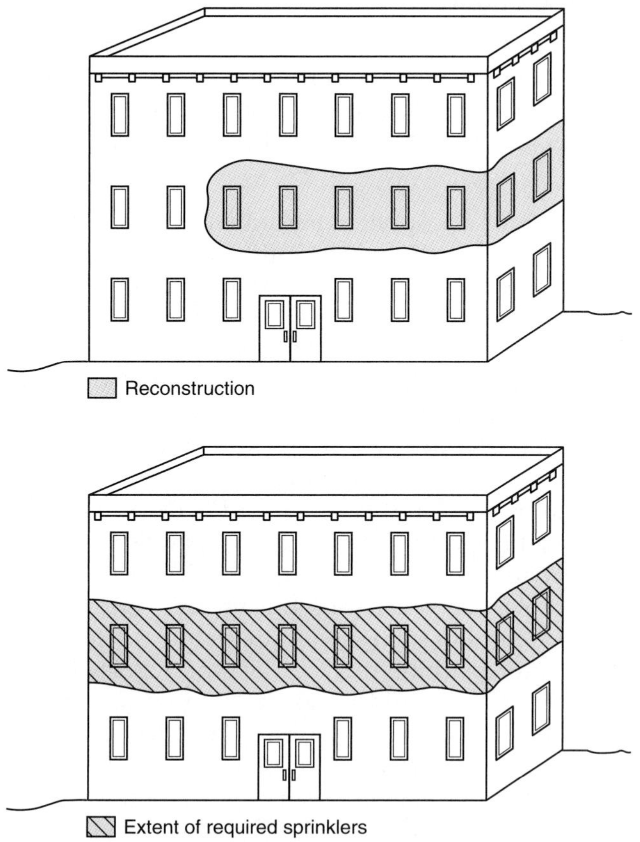


*Exhibit 43.6 Rehabilitation work area is large enough to require sprinklering of the second floor.*

edition of ASME A17.1,[6] unless the elevator was required to comply with a later edition of ASME A17.1 at the time of installation or alteration. Therefore, the emergency operations features provided for existing elevators might not be as robust as the emergency operations features required for new elevators by the current edition of ASME A17.1/CSA B44.

In 43.6.4.3, the issue is that of installing sprinklers in elevator hoistways or elevator machine rooms. Water discharging from sprinklers in such areas has the potential to adversely affect the operation of the elevator. The more recent editions of ASME A17.1 require a shunt-trip feature that calls the elevator out of service prior to sprinkler system waterflow. Paragraph 43.6.4.3 requires compliance with ASME A17.1/CSA B44, as an added provision to that required by 9.4.3.2, to ensure that the shunt-trip feature is provided where sprinklers are installed in existing elevator hoistways or elevator machine rooms.

**43.6.4.4** Any rehabilitation work areas in a building that is required to be provided with a standpipe system by other sections of this *Code* shall be provided with standpipes up to and including the highest rehabilitation work area floor.

Paragraph 43.6.4.4 has the potential to be misinterpreted.

First, the intent of 43.6.4.4 is to require the standpipe only if such standpipe is required by the provisions of the applicable existing occupancy chapter. More than one occupancy chapter applicable to new construction requires high-rise buildings to comply with Section 11.8, which, in turn, requires standpipes. If the corresponding occupancy chapter for existing buildings does not reference Section 11.8 (or otherwise require the building to have standpipes), it is not the intent of 43.6.4.4 to require the existing building that is undergoing reconstruction to be provided with standpipes. For example, 28.4.1, which applies to new high-rise hotels, requires compliance with Section 11.8, which requires standpipes, but 29.4.1 and 29.3.5.1, which apply to existing high-rise hotels, requires sprinklers but not compliance with Section 11.8. If an existing high-rise hotel building is undergoing reconstruction, standpipes are not required to be added as part of the rehabilitation project. As an example of the corollary condition, 17.4.2, which applies to existing day-care occupancies located in the high-rise portion of a building, requires compliance with Section 11.8, which, in turn, requires standpipes. If a floor housing an existing day-care occupancy is located in the high-rise portion of a building and that floor is undergoing reconstruction, standpipes are required to be added as part of the rehabilitation project for compliance with 43.6.4.4.

Second, it is not the intent of 43.6.4.4 to require standpipes to be installed in portions of the building not required by the applicable occupancy chapter to be provided with standpipes. For example, 13.4.5.12, which applies to existing assembly occupancy stages, requires standpipes on the stage. The requirement for standpipes on the stage is not meant to mandate a requirement for standpipes to be installed "up to and including the highest rehabilitation work area floor," as specified in 43.6.4.4. Note that the stage standpipes are required for compliance with 43.1.2.1(1) and 4.6.8.3, which has the effect of mandating the provisions of 13.4.5.12 and is unrelated to the provision of 43.6.4.4.

**43.6.4.5** The standpipes required by 43.6.4.4 shall be located and installed in accordance with NFPA 14, *Standard for the Installation of Standpipe and Hose Systems*, unless otherwise provided in 43.6.4.6 and 43.6.4.7.

**43.6.4.6** No pump shall be required, provided that the following criteria are met:

(1) The standpipes are capable of accepting delivery by fire department apparatus of a minimum of 250 gpm at 65 psi (945 L/min at 4.5 bar) to the topmost floor in buildings equipped throughout with an automatic sprinkler system or a minimum of 500 gpm at 65 psi (1890 L/min at 4.5 bar) to the topmost floor in other buildings.
(2) Where the standpipe terminates below the topmost floor, the standpipe is designed to meet the flow/pressure requirements of 43.6.4.6(1) for possible future extension of the standpipe.

**43.6.4.7** In other than high-rise buildings, the required interconnection of the standpipes for a wet system shall be permitted at the lowest level of the rehabilitation work area.

Paragraphs 43.6.4.6 and 43.6.4.7 offer some relief from the criteria of NFPA 14, *Standard for the Installation of Standpipe and Hose Systems*.[7] These provisions are consistent with the intent of the NARRP document on which this chapter is based. See the commentary following the chapter title. A rehabilitation chapter should promote the continued use and adaptive reuse of existing structures without burdening the facility with unreasonable expense while still ensuring adequate life safety.

Note that 43.6.4.6(2) might have the effect of requiring the standpipe being installed as part of a rehabilitation project to be designed for more than its immediate need, so that it can accommodate future rehabilitation work on floors above that undergoing reconstruction. It would be false economy to design the standpipe system to meet only its current need and then have to replace it, or otherwise supplement it, during future rehabilitation projects.

### 43.6.5 Fire Alarm Systems — Smoke Alarms.

**43.6.5.1** In lodging or rooming houses, hotels and dormitories, and apartment buildings, individual sleeping rooms, guest rooms, and dwelling units within any rehabilitation work area shall be provided with smoke alarms complying with the requirements of other sections of this *Code* applicable to new construction for the occupancy.

**43.6.5.2** Where the rehabilitation work area is located in residential board and care occupancies or one- and two-family dwelling units, smoke alarms complying with the requirements of other sections of this *Code* applicable to new construction for the occupancy shall be provided.

### 43.6.6 Elevators.

In high-rise buildings, where the rehabilitation work area is one entire floor, or where the rehabilitation work area is 20 percent or more of the occupied floor area of the building, all floors shall be accessible by at least one elevator.

Paragraph 43.6.6 applies only in high-rise buildings, and only where the rehabilitation work area encompasses at least one entire floor or at least 20 percent of the occupied floor area of the building. Those thresholds are judged to have created a reconstruction project of sufficient size to justify requiring that all floors be accessible by at least one elevator. Paragraph 9.4.3.2 requires the elevator, if existing, to have emergency operations features in accordance with ASME A17.3. Paragraphs 43.6.1.1(2), 43.5.1.3, and 9.4.3.1 require the elevator, if new, to have emergency operations features in accordance with ASME A17.1/CSA B44. The elevator recall provisions of Phase I Emergency Operation remove the elevator from service upon smoke detection in the elevator machine room or landing lobbies to prevent misuse that could injure building occupants. The fire fighters' service provisions of Phase II Emergency Operation permit the elevator to be placed back in service under the command of trained emergency forces personnel who might use the elevator to shuttle firefighting equipment to floors in the vicinity of the fire floor or to rescue persons unable to use the exit stairs.

## 43.7 Change of Use or Occupancy Classification

Section 43.7 addresses, in individual subsections, change of use that does not involve a change of occupancy (hereafter referred to as *change of use*) and change of use that does involve a change of occupancy (hereafter referred to as *change of occupancy*).

### 43.7.1 Change of Use.

*Change of use* is defined in 43.2.2.1.5 as a change in the purpose or level of activity within a structure that involves a change in application of the requirements of the *Code*. Examples of change of use include the following:

1. An assembly occupancy restaurant that is not required to be sprinklered by the provisions of Chapter 13 is rehabilitated for use as an assembly occupancy nightclub with an occupant load ex-

ceeding 100. The resulting change in application of the requirements of the *Code* is that the building is required to be sprinklered in accordance with 13.3.5.1(4).

2. A 280-person assembly occupancy restaurant, with large dining tables, that is not required to have a fire alarm system by the provisions of Chapter 13 is rehabilitated by replacing the large tables with smaller tables so as to increase the occupant load to 320 persons. The resulting change in application of the requirements of the *Code* is that the building is required to have a fire alarm system in accordance with 13.3.4.1.1.
3. An educational occupancy classroom is rehabilitated for use as an educational occupancy science laboratory using chemicals. The resulting change in application of the requirements of the *Code* is that the laboratory must be protected in accordance with 14.3.2.5, as 43.7.1.2 mandates compliance with the requirements applicable to new hazardous areas.
4. A health care occupancy patient sleeping room is rehabilitated for use as a health care occupancy soiled linen storage room by removing the furniture. [Note that, per 6.1.14.1.3(1), storage use is permitted to be considered incidental to the predominant health care occupancy, rather than being classified as a storage occupancy. Thus, there is no change of occupancy.] The resulting change in application of the requirements of the *Code* is that the room is required to be protected as a new hazardous area in accordance with 18.3.2.1, as 43.7.1.2 mandates compliance with the requirements applicable to new hazardous areas.
5. A mercantile occupancy department store is rehabilitated for use as mercantile occupancy bulk merchandising retail building. The resulting change in application of the requirements of the *Code* is that the building is required to meet the special criteria of 37.4.5 for bulk merchandising retail buildings.

**43.7.1.1** A change of use that does not involve a change of occupancy classification shall comply with the requirements applicable to the new use in accordance with the applicable existing occupancy chapter, unless the change of use creates a hazardous contents area as addressed in 43.7.1.2.

**43.7.1.2** A change of use that does not involve a change of occupancy classification but that creates a hazardous area shall comply with the requirements applicable to the new use in accordance with the applicable occupancy chapter for new construction.

**43.7.1.3** Any repair, renovation, modification, or reconstruction work undertaken in connection with a change of use that does not involve a change of occupancy classification shall comply with the requirements of Sections 43.3, 43.4, 43.5, and 43.6, respectively.

A change of use might occur without any repair, renovation, modification, or reconstruction work. For example, consider the assembly occupancy change of use described in item 2 of the commentary following the title of 43.7.1. Large tables are replaced with small tables, permitting the occupant load to be increased from 280 to 320 persons. Provided that the new use does not create a hazardous contents area, 43.7.1.1 requires compliance with the requirements applicable to the new use in accordance with the applicable existing occupancy chapter. In this case, the requirements of Chapter 13 are applied, and, although the restaurant did not formerly require a fire alarm system, a fire alarm system is required in accordance with 13.3.4.1.1.

Another example of a change of use that might occur without any repair, renovation, modification, or reconstruction work is the health care occupancy change of use described in item 4 of the commentary following the title of 43.7.1. Furniture is moved out of a patient room and soiled linen is placed in storage in the room. The provision of 43.7.1.2 mandates that the newly created hazardous area be protected in accordance with the applicable occupancy chapter for new construction. In this case, the requirements of 18.3.2.1 are applied, so that the room is sprinklered and separated from the remainder of the floor by 1-hour fire resistance–rated barriers.

A change of use might occur in conjunction with repair, renovation, modification, or reconstruction work. For example, consider the educational occupancy change of use described in item 3 of the commentary following the title of 43.7.1. In creating the science laboratory that employs the use of chemicals, rehabilitation work is undertaken to install laboratory benches with related water piping, gas piping, fume hoods, and exhaust fans. The rehabilitation work is categorized as modification. The provision of 43.7.1.3 requires compliance with the provisions of Section 43.5 for modification. Additionally, the provision of 43.7.1.2 requires the laboratory to be protected in accordance with 14.3.2.5.

### 43.7.2 Change of Occupancy Classification.

Where the occupancy classification of an existing building or portion of an existing building is changed in other than historic buildings, the building shall meet the requirements of 43.7.2.1 or 43.7.2.2.

The term *change of occupancy classification* is defined in 43.2.2.1.6 as the change in the occupancy classification of a structure or portion of a structure. The definition is simple, because the term itself is almost self-explanatory. The definition clarifies that the change might apply to a portion of a structure and, not necessarily, to a structure as a whole. Examples of change of occupancy classification include the following:

1. A restaurant with an occupant load of fewer than 50 is rehabilitated for use as a restaurant with an occupant load of 60. The occupancy is reclassified from a mercantile occupancy (or business occupancy) to an assembly occupancy.
2. A bed and breakfast with sleeping accommodations for 16 is rehabilitated for use as a bed and breakfast with sleeping accommodations for 20. The occupancy is reclassified from a lodging or rooming house to a hotel.
3. A doctor's office for patient examination is rehabilitated for use as a dialysis clinic for eight patients. The occupancy is reclassified from a business occupancy to an ambulatory health care occupancy.
4. A high school is rehabilitated for use as 10 condominium living units. The occupancy is reclassified from an educational occupancy to an apartment building.
5. A department store is rehabilitated for use as a telemarketing call center. The occupancy is reclassified from a mercantile occupancy to a business occupancy.

Compliance with the provisions of an occupancy chapter that applied to the occupancy prior to a change of occupancy classification does not ensure life safety in the newly created occupancy. As a minimum, the new occupancy is required to meet the provisions of the applicable existing occupancy chapter for the occupancy created by the change [see 43.7.2.1(1)] and the sprinkler, alarm system, and hazardous area requirements of the applicable new occupancy chapter for the occupancy created by the change [see 43.7.2.1(2)]. If the change of occupancy classification is such that the new occupancy has a higher hazard classification category (as addressed in Table 43.7.3) than that of the prior occupancy, the new occupancy is required to meet the provisions of the applicable new occupancy chapter (see 43.7.2.2). The process for handling change of occupancy is addressed in more detail in the commentary following A.43.7.2.1(2) and the commentary following 43.7.2.2.

**43.7.2.1** Where a change of occupancy classification occurs within the same hazard classification category or to an occupancy classification of a lesser hazard classification category (that is, a higher hazard category number), as addressed by Table 43.7.3, the building shall meet both of the following:

(1) Requirements of the applicable existing occupancy chapters for the occupancy created by the change *(see Chapters 13, 15, 17, 19, 21, 23, 24, 26, 29, 31, 33, 37, 39, 40, and 42)*
(2)* Automatic sprinkler and detection, alarm, and communications system requirements and the requirements for hazardous areas applicable to new construction for the occupancy created by the change *(see Chapters 12, 14, 16, 18, 20, 22, 24, 26, 28, 30, 32, 36, 38, 40, and 42)*

**A.43.7.2.1(2)** It is not the intent of 43.7.2.1(2) to supersede the provision of 32.2.3.5.2 that exempts automatic sprinklers from small board and care facility conversions serving eight or fewer residents when all occupants have the ability as a group to move reliably to a point of safety within 3 minutes.

Paragraph 43.7.2.1 addresses change of occupancy classification where the new occupancy has the same or lower hazard classification category (as addressed in Table 43.7.3) than that of the prior occupancy. Note that, for purposes of applying the hazard category classifications of Table 43.7.3, a higher hazard category number (e.g., 4) designates a lower hazard or challenge to life safety than does a lower hazard category number (e.g., 1). The term *lower hazard* means that the occupancy and occupant characteristics are such that adequate life safety can be provided using a less extensive mix of life safety features than would be required to protect an occupancy with a higher hazard category.

The process of establishing whether the new occupancy has the same or a lower hazard classification category than the prior occupancy is illustrated by the examples in paragraphs 1 through 3, which follow.

**1.** A business occupancy office building (hazard category 3 per Table 43.7.3) is rehabilitated to become a residential occupancy apartment building (hazard category 3). The hazard category after the change of occupancy is the same as before the change. The applicable provisions are those of 43.7.2.1(1) and (2).

**2.** A health care occupancy hospital (hazard category 2) is rehabilitated to become an ambulatory health care occupancy outpatient surgical center (hazard category 3). The hazard category after the change of occupancy is lower (i.e., it presents less hazard or challenge to life safety) than that which existed before the change. The applicable provisions are those of 43.7.2.1(1) and (2).

**3.** A residential occupancy apartment building for the elderly (hazard category 3) is rehabilitated to become a residential board and care occupancy (hazard category 2). The hazard category after the change of occupancy is not the same or lower than that before the change, and the provisions of 43.7.2.1 do not apply. Rather, the hazard category after the change of occupancy is higher than that before the change, and the provisions of 43.7.2.2 apply. See the commentary following 43.7.2.2.

Use of the provisions of 43.7.2.1 is illustrated by the examples in paragraphs 1 and 2, which follow.

**1.** A four-story business occupancy office building (hazard category 3) is rehabilitated to become a residential occupancy hotel (hazard category 3) where guest rooms are accessed from an interior corridor system. Per 43.7.2.1(1), the new hotel must meet the requirements of Chapter 29 for existing hotels and dormitories. Per 43.7.2.1(2), the new hotel must also meet the automatic sprinkler, detection, alarm, and communications systems, and hazardous areas requirements of Chapter 28 for new hotels and dormitories, which have the effect of mandating some features not required by Chapter 29. For example, 28.3.5.1 requires that the hotel building be sprinklered. With respect to the detection, alarm, and communications systems, the following requirements are a result of having to comply with 28.3.4:

- **a.** The hotel is not permitted to have a presignal system (see 28/29.3.4.3.2 and 9.6.3.3).
- **b.** A visible notification appliance (i.e., a strobe) must be provided in guest rooms and guest suites specifically required and equipped to accommodate hearing-impaired individuals (see 28.3.4.3.3).
- **c.** Visible notification appliances must be provided in occupiable areas, other than guest rooms and guest suites (see 28.3.4.3.4).
- **d.** Alarm annunciation must be provided (see 28.3.4.3.5).
- **e.** Emergency forces (i.e., fire department) notification must be provided in accordance with 9.6.4 (see 28.3.4.3.6).
- **f.** The smoke alarms, which are required in every guest room and every living area and sleeping room within a guest suite, must be in compliance with 9.6.2.10, so as to be provided with secondary power and interconnected within each guest suite (see 28.3.4.5 and the exemptions, offered only for existing hotels, in 29.3.4.5.1 and 29.3.4.5.2).

Also, with respect to the protection of hazardous areas, Table 28.3.2.2.2 requires some new hazardous areas, such as guest laundries, to be protected by sprinklers and isolated from the remainder of the floor by 1-hour fire resistance–rated barriers. Table 29.3.2.2.2 requires guest laundries to be protected by sprinklers or isolated from the remainder of the floor by 1-hour fire resistance–rated barriers.

**2.** A two-story residential occupancy hotel (hazard category 3) is rehabilitated to become a business occupancy office building (hazard category 3) with an occupant load on each floor of fewer than 50. Per 43.7.2.1(1), the new office building must meet the requirements of Chapter 39 for existing business occupancies. Per 43.7.2.1(2), the new office building must also meet the automatic sprinkler, detection, alarm, and communications systems, and hazardous areas requirements, of Chapter 38 for new business occupancies, which have no additional effect. Neither Chapter 38 nor Chapter 39 requires non-high-rise business occupancy buildings to be sprinklered. Although the threshold for requiring a fire alarm system differs for new and existing business occupancies (see 38/39.3.4.1), the new business occupancy does not exceed either threshold and is not required to be provided with a fire alarm system. The provisions for the protection of hazardous areas of 38.3.2 are identical to those of 39.3.2, so as not to require any protection in excess of that mandated for an existing hazardous area in a business occupancy.

**43.7.2.2** Where a change of occupancy classification occurs to an occupancy classification of a higher hazard classification category (i.e., a lower hazard category number), as addressed by Table 43.7.3, the building shall comply with the requirements of the occupancy chapters applicable to new construction for the occupancy created by the change *(see Chapters 12, 14, 16, 18, 20, 22, 24, 26, 28, 30, 32, 36, 38, 40, and 42).*

See the commentary following A.43.7.2.1(2) on the subject of comparing the hazard classification category of the new occupancy against that of the occupancy that existed prior to the change of occupancy classification.

Use of the provision of 43.7.2.2 is illustrated by the examples in paragraphs 1 and 2, which follow.

**1.** A residential occupancy apartment building for the elderly (hazard category 3) is rehabilitated to become a residential board and care occupancy (hazard category 2). The hazard category after the change of occupancy is not the same as or lower than that before the change, and the provisions of 43.7.2.1 do not apply. Rather, the hazard category after the change of occupancy is higher than that before the change, and the provisions of 43.7.2.2 apply. Per 43.7.2.2, the new board and care facility must meet the requirements of Chapter 32 for new residential board and care occupancies.

**2.** An ambulatory health care occupancy outpatient surgical center (hazard category 3) is rehabilitated to become a health care occupancy surgical and inpatient sleeping facility (hazard category 2) where four or more surgical patients can remain for more than 24 hours. The hazard category after the change of occupancy is not the same as or lower than that before the change, and the provisions of 43.7.2.1 do not apply. Rather, the hazard category after the change of occupancy is higher than that before the change, and the provisions of 43.7.2.2 apply. Per 43.7.2.2, the new inpatient surgical care facility must meet the hospital requirements of Chapter 18 for new health care occupancies.

**43.7.2.3** In historic buildings where a change of occupancy classification occurs within the same hazard classification category or to an occupancy classification in a lesser hazard classification category (i.e., a higher hazard category number), as addressed by Table 43.7.3, the building shall meet the requirements of one of the following:

(1) 43.7.2.1(1) and (2)
(2) 43.7.2.1(1) and (2), as modified by Section 43.10

**43.7.2.4** In historic buildings where a change of occupancy classification occurs to an occupancy classification in a higher hazard classification category (that is, a lower hazard category number), as addressed by Table 43.7.3, the building shall meet the requirements of one of the following:

(1) 43.7.2.2
(2) 43.7.2.2, as modified by Section 43.10

The 2006 edition of the *Code* included a provision, 43.7.2.5, that was deleted for the 2009 edition. The provision permitted any portion of the building in which the occupancy classification is not changed to comply with the requirements of the applicable existing occupancy chapter, provided that the existing occupancy was adequately separated from the new occupancy, as might occur through compliance with the occupancy separation requirements of 6.1.14.4. The provision had the unintended effect of permitting, for example, the portion of the building housing the existing occupancy to remain unsprinklered, even where the requirements applicable to the new occupancy mandated that the entire building (i.e., not just the occupancy) be sprinklered. With the deletion of former 43.7.2.5, the provisions of 43.7.2.2 require that the entire building comply with the requirements of the occupancy chapter applicable to new construction for the occupancy created by the change.

The provisions of 43.7.2.2 are further illustrated by the example that follows. The illustration in Part (a) of Exhibit 43.7 depicts a one-story ambulatory health care occupancy outpatient surgical center (hazard category 3) before a rehabilitation project changes the occupancy of a portion of the building. The ambulatory health care occupancy complies with Chapter 21 for existing ambulatory health care occupancies, including the features that follow:

1. The building is of Type V(000) construction, as permitted by 21.1.6.1.
2. The portion of the corridor system running along the wing at the left of the exhibit is 44 in. (1120 mm) wide, as required by 21.2.3.2.
3. The portion of the corridor system along the wing at the right of the exhibit exceeds the minimum width required by 21.2.3.2 and is 8 ft (2440 mm) wide.
4. The interior wall and ceiling finish in rooms and spaces separated from the corridor is Class C, as permitted by 21.3.3 and 39.3.3.2.2.
5. The interior wall and ceiling finish in the corridor is Class B, as permitted by 21.3.3 and 39.3.3.2.1.
6. The building is nonsprinklered, as 21.3.5 and 39.3.5 do not require sprinklers.
7. The corridor walls have no fire resistance rating, the corridor doors have no fire protection rating, and some use areas are left open to the corridor, as 21.3.6 and 39.3.6 (see 21.1.1.1.2) have no corridor separation requirements.

The illustration in Part (b) of Exhibit 43.7 depicts the one-story building (previously addressed in this commentary) after the rehabilitation project. A portion of the wing at the right of the illustration has undergone a change of occupancy to a health care occupancy inpatient sleeping facility (hazard category 2) where four or more surgical patients from other portions of the building can remain for more than 24 hours. All other portions of the building were not affected by the rehabilitation project and remain an ambulatory health care occupancy outpatient surgical center (hazard category 3). The rehabilitation project created a change of occupancy for the portion of the building that now houses the inpatient sleeping facility. The new health care occupancy has a hazard category (i.e., hazard category 2) that is higher than that of the ambulatory health care occupancy (i.e., hazard category 3) and must comply with the requirements of 43.7.2.2 rather than 43.7.2.1.

The provisions of 43.7.2.2 have the effect of requiring the building to comply with the requirements of Chapter 18 for new health care (HC) occupancies. The provisions of 18.1.2.2 permit the ambulatory health care (AHC) occupancy portion of the building to retain its classification as an AHC occupancy, without having to meet the requirements of Chapter 18 for HC occupancies, where the AHC occupancy is separated from the HC occupancy by minimum 2-hour fire resistance–rated barriers and the AHC occupancy does not house, treat, or provide customary access for occupants of the HC occupancy who are incapable of self-preservation. In this case, the health care occupancy inpatients are patients who received their surgical services as outpatients but were kept overnight in the adjacent health care occupancy inpatient area. The patients were not initially admitted as inpatients and were then moved to the ambulatory health care occupancy to receive their surgical procedures.

The separation between the existing AHC occupancy and the new HC occupancy, as depicted in Part (b) of Exhibit 43.7, is required to be a minimum 2-hour fire resistance–rated barrier in accordance with 18.1.2.2(2). Further, the barrier must be a horizontal exit in accordance with 18.2.2.5 and 7.2.4, because 18.1.2.4 requires all means of egress from the health care occupancy inpatient area that traverse the ambulatory health care space to meet the provisions of Chapter 18, unless otherwise permitted by 18.1.2.5. Paragraph 18.1.2.5 permits, as an exemption to the requirement of 18.1.2.4, a horizontal exit to serve as the necessary separation where the horizontal exit is in compliance with 18.2.2.5.

For compliance with all applicable provisions related to the required fire resistance rating of the separation between the new health care occupancy inpatient sleeping area and the existing ambulatory health care occupancy surgical center, a horizontal exit is provided. The horizontal exit is constructed to have a 2-hour fire resistance rating for compliance with 18.2.2.5 and 7.2.4.3.1.

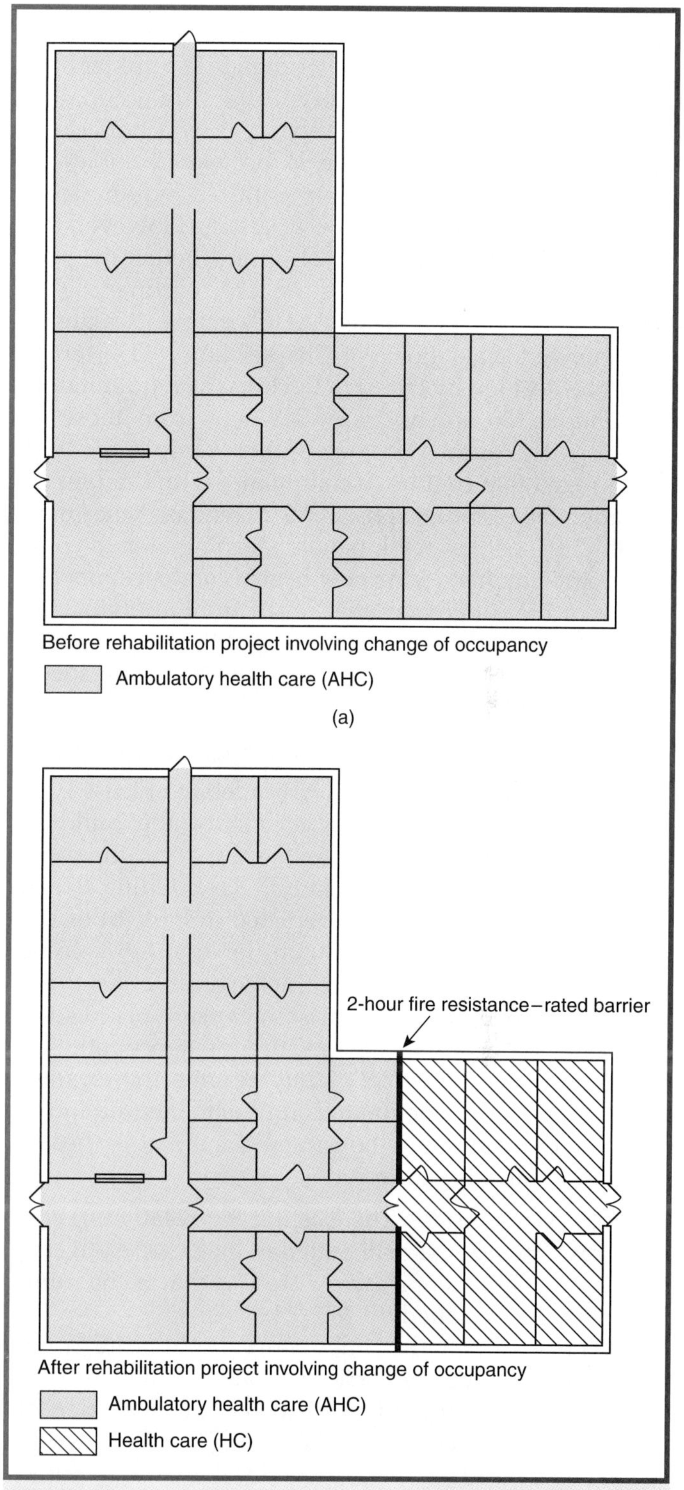


***Exhibit 43.7*** *Change of occupancy made to a portion of the building.*

The entire building depicted in Exhibit 43.7 must be sprinklered for compliance with 18.3.5.1, which requires that the building containing the health care occupancy (not just the health care occupancy) be protected throughout by an approved, supervised automatic sprinkler system. Other than the sprinkler provision, the existing ambulatory health care occupancy surgical center — which is separated by a horizontal exit from the new health care occupancy inpatient sleeping area — must comply with the requirements for ambulatory health care occupancies. However, the requirement of 43.7.2.2 is not clear on whether the provisions of Chapter 21 for existing AHC occupancies or those of Chapter 20 for new AHC occupancies are to be followed. The choice of Chapter 20 or Chapter 21 must be decided by the AHJ. Luckily, the requirements of Chapter 20 are not very different from those of Chapter 21. For the purposes of this example, the AHJ has judged that continued compliance with Chapter 21 is adequate. Paragraph 43.7.2.2 requires the new health care occupancy inpatient sleeping area to comply with Chapter 18 for new health care occupancies. Some of the differences that result from applying the requirements of Chapter 18 to part of the building and those of Chapter 21 to the remaining areas are specified in the paragraphs that follow.

**1.** *Building construction type.* The existing Type V(000) construction must be upgraded to at least Type V(111) construction in the portion of the building housing the new health care occupancy inpatient sleeping area (i.e., the portion of the building to the right of the horizontal exit depicted in Part (b) of Exhibit 43.7) for compliance with Table 18.1.6.1. Type V(111) construction might be achieved by sheathing the Type V(000) construction with gypsum board so as to provide the requisite 1-hour fire resistance rating.

The provision of 18.1.2.2(4) permits the existing Type V(000) construction to continue to be used in the portion of the building housing the ambulatory health care occupancy surgical center.

**2.** *Corridor width.* The existing 8 ft (2440 mm) corridor width must be maintained in the new health care occupancy inpatient sleeping area, as that is the minimum width specified by 18.2.3.4.

The width of the ambulatory health care occupancy surgical center corridor located immediately to the left of the horizontal exit in the lower portion of Exhibit 43.7 is greater than the 44 in. (1120 mm) width required by 21.2.3.2. It is also wider than that required by 20.2.3.2 for new ambulatory health care occupancies; therefore, per 4.6.8.4 and 18.1.2.5, the width could be decreased to 44 in. (1120 mm), and such change would create new rehabilitation work categorized as a modification. Any modification is subject to the provisions of Section 43.5. Per 43.5.1.3, the provisions of 20.2.3.2 are made applicable, and the result is the same as just described — the corridor width is permitted to be decreased to 44 in. (1120 mm).

Paragraph 21.2.3.2 permits the existing 44 in. (1120 mm) width corridor running along the wing at the left of Exhibit 43.7 to continue to be used, just as it was prior to the rehabilitation project.

**3.** *Interior wall and ceiling finish.* The existing Class C interior wall and ceiling finish in the rooms of the new health care occupancy inpatient sleeping area is permitted to continue to be used in each of those rooms that individually has a capacity not exceeding four persons via the combined effect of the exemption provided in 18.3.3.2.1 and that of 10.2.8.1, which applies because the building is sprinklered throughout for compliance with 18.3.5.1, as previously addressed.

Paragraphs 21.3.3 and 39.3.3.2.2 permit the ambulatory health care occupancy surgical center Class C interior wall and ceiling finish in the rooms and spaces separated from the corridor to continue to be used, just as it was prior to the rehabilitation project.

The existing Class B interior wall and ceiling finish in the corridor of the ambulatory health care surgical center could be changed to a Class C material if the change were treated as new rehabilitation work categorized as a renovation. Any renovation is subject to the provisions of Section 43.4. Per 43.4.3, new interior finish material must meet the requirements for new construction. Where 38.3.3.2.1 requires either Class A or Class B material in corridors, the presence of the new sprinkler system makes the provision of 10.2.8.1 applicable, which has the effect of permitting the new interior wall and ceiling finish in the surgical center corridor to be Class C material.

**4.** *Corridor walls and doors.* The existing nonrated corridor walls and doors in the new health care occupancy inpatient sleeping area are permitted to remain in place if they resist the passage of smoke as required by 18.3.6.2 and 18.3.6.3, because the rehabilitation project includes sprinklering the building for compliance with 18.3.5.1.

The existing nonrated corridor walls and doors, and the unprotected openings between use areas and the corridor, in the ambulatory health care surgical center are permitted to remain in place, just as they were prior to the rehabilitation project, as 21.3.6 and 39.3.6 (see 21.1.1.1.2) have no corridor separation requirements.

### 43.7.3* Hazard Category Classifications.

The relative degree of hazard between different occupancy classifications shall be as set forth in the hazard category classifications of Table 43.7.3.

*Table 43.7.3 Hazard Categories and Classifications*

| Hazard Category | Occupancy Classification |
|---|---|
| 1 (highest hazard) | Industrial or storage occupancies with high hazard contents |
| 2 | Health care, detention and correctional, residential board and care |
| 3 | Assembly, educational, day care, ambulatory health care, residential, mercantile, business, general and special-purpose industrial, ordinary hazard storage |
| 4 (lowest hazard) | Industrial or storage occupancies with low hazard contents |

**A.43.7.3** Table 43.7.3 groups all the residential occupancy classifications into the general category of residential. The category of residential includes one- or two-family dwellings, lodging or rooming houses, hotels and dormitories, and apartment buildings.

Table 43.7.3 provides the hazard category classifications for each occupancy classification addressed in the *Code*. Hazard category classification is used in the requirements of 43.7.2 on change of occupancy and has been applied in the examples in the commentary following A.43.7.2.1(2), 43.7.2.2, and 43.7.2.4(2). Hazard category classification is not used in 43.7.1, as it does not apply to a change of use that does not involve a change of occupancy.

The column at the right of Table 43.7.3 carries the heading "occupancy classification." The user of Table 43.7.3 locates the occupancy classification before the change of occupancy, looks to the left column of that row and notes the associated hazard category, locates the occupancy classification of the new occupancy, and similarly notes its hazard category. The occupancy classifications in Table 43.7.3 are limited to assembly, educational, day care, health care, ambulatory health care, detention and correctional, residential, residential board and care, mercantile, business, industrial, and storage. The table combines all residential occupancy classifications into one (i.e., *residential*), but, officially, the residential occupancy classifications are one- and two-family dwellings, lodging or rooming houses, hotels and dormitories, and apartment buildings.

Table 43.7.3 does not apply to a change from an industrial occupancy to another subclassification of an industrial occupancy (e.g., from an industrial occupancy with low hazard contents to an industrial occupancy with ordinary hazard contents), because such a change is a change of use and not a change of occupancy. Similarly, Table 43.7.3 does not apply to a change from a storage occupancy to another subclassification of a storage occupancy (e.g., from a storage occupancy with low hazard contents to a storage occupancy with ordinary hazard contents), because such a change is a change of use and not a change of occupancy. The row of the table for hazard category 4 might be used, for example, if an industrial occupancy with low hazard contents is changed to any occupancy other than an industrial occupancy, or if an occupancy other than an industrial occupancy is changed to an industrial occupancy with low hazard contents. Similarly, the row of the table for hazard category 1 might be used, for example, if an industrial occupancy with high hazard contents is changed to any occupancy other than an industrial occupancy, or if an occupancy other than an industrial occupancy is changed to an industrial occupancy with high hazard contents.

## 43.8 Additions

The term *addition* is defined in 43.2.2.1.7 as an increase in the building area, aggregate floor area, height, or number of stories of a structure. In other words, an addition affects a structure by creating an increase in at least one of the four categories that follow:

1. Building area
2. Aggregate floor area
3. Height
4. Number of stories

Typically, an addition affects a structure by creating an increase in more than one of the four categories listed in the previous paragraph. For example, Exhibit 43.8 depicts an existing three-story building to which a six-story addition has been constructed. Prior to construction of the addition, the building is considered to be the existing three-story structure. After the addition is built, the original building and the addition are considered to be a single building. The addition affects the building by creating an increase in each of the four categories listed in the previous paragraph as follows:

1. *Increase in building area.* The building area (i.e., the footprint or ground area comprising the space within the perimeter of the exterior building walls) is double that which existed prior to the addition.
2. *Increase in aggregate floor area.* The aggregate floor area is triple that which existed prior to the addition.

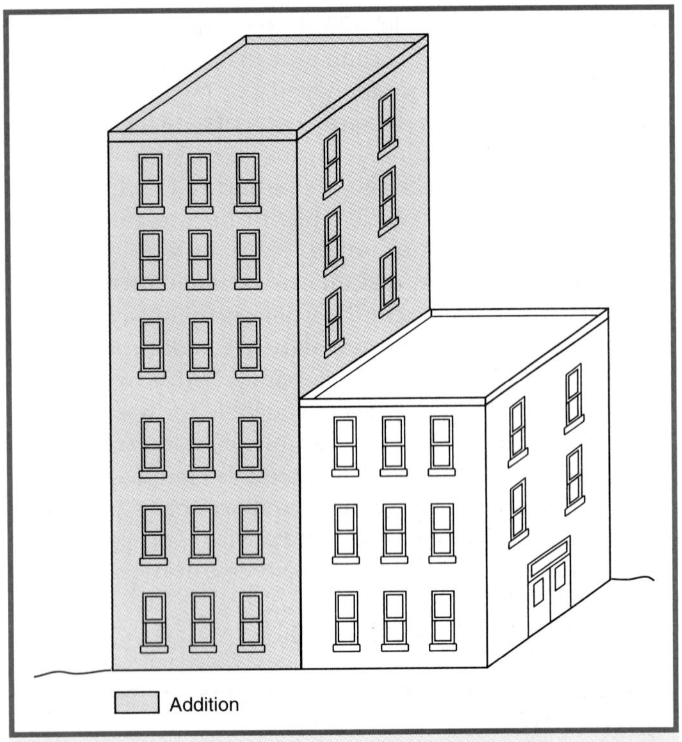


*Exhibit 43.8 Addition to an existing building.*

3. *Increase in height*. The height of the building is double that which existed prior to the addition.
4. *Increase in number of stories*. The number of stories is double that which existed prior to the addition.

Note that it is possible that an addition would not be visible or obvious to observers stationed outside the perimeter of the building. For example, a multistory building with an open-air court at its center core might undergo a rehabilitation project that extends the floors at each story to cover the space formerly occupied by the court. Such a rehabilitation project is considered an addition, because it has the effect of increasing the building area and the aggregate floor area. Similarly, an intermediate floor or multiple intermediate floors might be added within a high-ceiling space of an existing building, and such rehabilitation project would constitute an addition that is subject to the requirements of Section 43.8.

### 43.8.1 General Requirements.

**43.8.1.1** Where an addition, as defined in 43.2.2.1.7, is made to a building, both of the following criteria shall be met:

(1) The addition shall comply with other sections of this *Code* applicable to new construction for the occupancy.

(2) The existing portion of the building shall comply with the requirements of this *Code* applicable to existing buildings for the occupancy.

In earlier sections of the chapter, modification was defined as the step along the repair/renovation/modification/reconstruction continuum at which newly constructed elements, components, and systems are required to comply with the provisions of other sections of the *Code* applicable to new construction (see 43.5.1.3). The requirement for compliance with the provisions for new construction also applies to the rehabilitation work category of reconstruction, via the mandate of 43.6.1.1(2), and to any change of occupancy classification where the new occupancy has a higher hazard classification category than the prior occupancy (see 43.7.2.2). Paragraph 43.8.1.1(1) carries the requirement for compliance with the provisions for new construction to the rehabilitation work category of addition.

Paragraph 43.8.1.1(2), applicable to any existing building involved with the rehabilitation work category of addition, serves the same purpose as 4.6.8.3 and 43.1.2.1(1) for the rehabilitation work categories of repair, renovation, modification, and reconstruction. Per 43.8.1.1(2), an existing building to which an addition is being constructed is required to be subject to the requirements of the *Code* applicable to existing buildings for the occupancy, even if the existing building is not undergoing repair, renovation, modification, or reconstruction. This provision is consistent with 1.3.1, 4.4.2.1, and 4.6.10.1.

**43.8.1.2** An addition shall not create or extend any nonconformity with regard to fire safety or the means of egress in the existing building for which the addition is constructed.

The rehabilitation work category of addition introduces the potential for creating nonconformities, with other *Code* provisions, in the existing building for which the addition is constructed. The existing building might be wholly compliant with the applicable occupancy chapters for existing buildings before the addition is constructed. The addition might, for example, have the effect of increasing the travel distance for the existing building to an excessive, noncompliant length if the addition abuts the existing building where a door in its exterior wall formerly served as an exit. Paragraph 43.8.1.2 requires the user to address such issues in the existing building to avoid focusing solely on the addition.

**43.8.1.3** Any repair, renovation, alteration, or reconstruction work within an existing building to which an addition is being made shall comply with the requirements of Sections 43.3, 43.4, 43.5, and 43.6.

The work involved with the rehabilitation work category of addition will most often necessitate rehabilitation work within the existing building. For example, where an addition abuts the exterior wall of an existing building at a point where an exit door discharges to the outside, the door might need to be removed, relocated, or otherwise addressed for continued *Code* compliance. Such work will generally fall into the rehabilitation work category of modification or reconstruction. Paragraph 43.8.1.3 requires compliance with the provisions for the applicable work category, as detailed in Sections 43.3, 43.4, 43.5, or 43.6.

### 43.8.2 Heights.

No addition shall increase the height of an existing building beyond that permitted under the applicable provisions for new building construction.

Chapter 43 is based on *NFPA 5000, Building Construction and Safety Code,* Chapter 15, Building Rehabilitation, as addressed in the commentary that follows the chapter title. The subject of building height is addressed in *NFPA 5000* in the height and area limitations of Chapter 7. The subject of height is not directly addressed in this *Code,* so 43.8.2 has limited application. One might proffer that 43.8.2 serves to help enforce the building construction requirements detailed in the ___1.6 subsection of the applicable occupancy chapter. For example, a second story is planned to be constructed as an addition to an existing single-story nursing home of Type II(000) construction. Table 19.1.6.1, applicable to building construction types for existing health care occupancies, permits an existing, two-story Type II(000) nursing home to be continued in use if sprinklered. Table 18.1.6.1, applicable to building construction types for new health care occupancies, does not permit a two-story Type II(000) nursing home. The addition can be constructed only if the building construction type is upgraded to at least that provided by Type II(111) construction. The same criteria would need to be met where complying with 43.8.1.1(1), which requires that the addition meet the provisions of other sections of the *Code* applicable to new construction for the occupancy.

### 43.8.3 Fire Protection Systems.

In other than one- and two-family dwellings, existing compartment areas without an approved separation from the addition shall be protected by an approved automatic sprinkler system where the combined areas would be required to be sprinklered by the provisions applicable to new construction for the occupancy.

Paragraph 43.8.3 was revised for the 2009 edition of the *Code,* as the text that appeared in the 2006 edition was subject to misinterpretation. The current text clearly states that sprinklering of the existing area is required only if the combined (i.e., unseparated) areas are required to be sprinklered by the provisions applicable to new construction. For example, in applying the provisions of 43.8.3 to an existing, low-rise business occupancy building undergoing a rehabilitation project categorized as addition, sprinklers would not be required, because Chapter 38, applicable to new business occupancies, has no sprinkler system mandate for business occupancy buildings that are not high-rise (see 38.3.5).

Paragraph 43.8.3 requires automatic sprinklers under either of the situations that follow in paragraph 1 or paragraph 2.

**1.** The addition is required by the applicable new occupancy chapter to be sprinklered, and the sprinkler system must be extended into the nonseparated portion of the existing building, so as not to have a fire compartment that is partially sprinklered.

**2.** The combined area of the nonseparated spaces (i.e., the space in the original building and the space from the addition that is left open to the original building or is otherwise improperly separated from the original building) exceeds an area-based sprinkler threshold in the applicable occupancy chapter. For example, 36.3.5.1(2), applicable to new mercantile occupancies, requires automatic sprinklers throughout mercantile occupancies exceeding 12,000 $ft^2$ (1115 $m^2$). The 12,000 $ft^2$ (1115 $m^2$) threshold should be applied to the combined, nonseparated area if the area of the addition, by itself, is below the sprinkler threshold.

Note that the provision of 43.8.3 does not apply to one- and two-family dwellings. Existing one- and two-family dwellings are not required to be sprinklered; new one- and two-family dwellings are required to be sprinklered (see 24.3.5.1). If one- and two-family dwellings were not exempted from the provision of 43.8.3, the addition of a garage to an existing nonsprinklered dwelling would require the retroactive sprinklering of the dwelling and the new garage.

### 43.8.4 Smoke Alarms.

Where an addition is made to a one- or two-family dwelling or a small residential board and care occupancy, interconnected smoke alarms, powered by the electrical system, meeting the requirements of the other sections of this *Code* shall be installed and maintained in the addition.

Paragraph 43.8.4 does not require an upgrade of the protection offered by the smoke alarms in the existing portion of the building. Compliance with 43.8.1.1(2) would require the existing dwelling to meet the existing smoke alarm provisions of 24.3.4. Compliance with 43.8.4 would also require hardwired, interconnected smoke alarms (i.e., smoke alarms in compliance with the provisions of 9.6.2.9 for new smoke alarm installations) in the addition, not in the existing portion of the building.

## 43.9 Reserved

In *NFPA 5000, Building Construction and Safety Code*, Chapter 15, Building Rehabilitation, Section 15.9 addresses damaged or unsafe buildings — a subject germane to building codes. There is no text for Section 43.9 in this *Code*, because the subject of damaged or unsafe buildings is not directly applicable to the scope of the *Code*. The section numbering in Chapter 43 of this *Code* and Chapter 15 of *NFPA 5000* has been made consistent to assist users who work with both documents. Thus, Section 43.9 is shown as having been reserved.

## 43.10 Historic Buildings

The term *historic building* is defined in 3.3.32.8 as "a building or facility deemed to have historical, architectural, or cultural significance by a local, regional, or national jurisdiction." Historic buildings might be protected by government statute in jurisdictions that also enforce this *Code*. The preceding sections of this chapter have the effect of requiring compliance with provisions of this *Code* that — while increasing the level of life safety — might adversely affect the historic nature of a building. Even minor repairs can cause substantial damage to what preservationists call the historic fabric of a historic building. NFPA 914, *Code for Fire Protection of Historic Structures*,[8] includes definitions of the terms *historic fabric* and *preservation* that are helpful in putting the provisions of Section 43.10 into perspective with those of the remainder of the chapter. The definitions read as follows:

> *Historic Fabric.* Original or added building or construction materials, features, and finishes that existed during the period that is deemed to be most architecturally or historically significant, or both.
>
> *Preservation.* The act or process of applying measures necessary to sustain the existing form, integrity, and materials of a historic building or structure.

### 43.10.1 General Requirements.

Historic buildings undergoing rehabilitation shall comply with the requirements of one of the following:

(1) Section 43.10
(2) Sections 43.3, 43.4, 43.5, 43.6, and 43.7, as they relate, respectively, to repair, renovation, modification, reconstruction, and change of use or occupancy classification
(3) NFPA 914, *Code for Fire Protection of Historic Structures*

Paragraph 43.10.1 offers three options for *Code* compliance for historic buildings undergoing rehabilitation. The three options are specified in paragraphs 1 through 3, which follow.

**1.** The historic building is permitted to comply with Section 43.10 (i.e., 43.10.2 through 43.10.5). Section 43.10 requires compliance with the sections of Chapter 43 appropriate to the rehabilitation work category but offers relief in 43.10.4 from specific *Code* provisions that might adversely affect the historic fabric where the detailed evaluation report required by 43.10.2 justifies an exemption. The provisions of 43.10.4 permit exemptions where compensating features are provided, so that life safety is not reduced to an unacceptable level. The compensating features might not provide strict compliance with the applicable occupancy chapter. For example, 43.10.4.4 allows the authority having jurisdiction (AHJ) to permit existing front doors to swing in the opposite direction of egress travel, provided that other exits have sufficient egress capacity to serve the total occupant load. In an assembly occupancy, the AHJ might base permission to use the exemption on compliance with all of the following:

**a.** The written evaluation required by 43.10.2 supports the need to retain the existing direction of door swing.

**b.** Trained staff is provided to direct occupants to the other exits to help avoid the situation where large numbers of occupants "rush" the door that swings back into the building.
**c.** Normal building operation is such that the front door is not used as the main entrance, because occupants will tend to try to exit via the door they used to enter the building.

**2.** The historic building is permitted to comply with the sections of Chapter 43 appropriate to the rehabilitation work category without using any of the provisions of 43.10.2 through 43.10.5. In other words, the historic building rehabilitation must be accomplished by the requirements applicable to any building, historic or not.

**3.** The historic building is permitted to comply with NFPA 914, *Code for Fire Protection of Historic Structures,* which has the effect of sending the user to NFPA 914. The decision to permit compliance with NFPA 914 in lieu of the provisions of this *Code* was made with the knowledge that NFPA 914 requires that fire safety issues be evaluated in accordance with the provisions of NFPA *101*. In other words, compliance with NFPA 914 helps to ensure that adequate life safety is provided in historic buildings.

### 43.10.2 Evaluation.

A historic building undergoing modification, reconstruction, or change of occupancy classification in accordance with the requirements of Chapter 43 shall be investigated and evaluated as follows:

(1) A written report shall be prepared for such a building and filed with the authority having jurisdiction by a registered design professional.
(2) If the subject matter of the report does not require an evaluation by a registered design professional, the authority having jurisdiction shall be permitted to allow the report to be prepared by a licensed building contractor, electrician, plumber, or mechanical contractor responsible for the work.
(3) The licensed person preparing the report shall be knowledgeable in historic preservation, or the report shall be coauthored by a preservation professional.
(4) The report shall identify each required safety feature in compliance with Chapter 43 and where compliance with other chapters of this *Code* would be damaging to the contributing historic features.
(5) The report shall describe each feature not in compliance with this *Code* and demonstrate how the intent of this *Code* is met in providing an equivalent level of safety.
(6) The local preservation official shall be permitted to review and comment on the written report or shall be permitted to request review comments on the report from the historic preservation officer.
(7) Unless it is determined by the authority having jurisdiction that a report is required to protect the health and safety of the public, the submission of a report shall not be required for a building that is being rehabilitated for the personal use of the owner or a member of the owner's immediate family and is not intended for any use or occupancy by the public.

### 43.10.3 Repairs.

Repairs to any portion of a historic building shall be permitted to be made with original or like materials and original methods of construction, except as otherwise provided in Section 43.10.

### 43.10.4 Repair, Renovation, Modification, or Reconstruction.

**43.10.4.1 General.** Historic buildings undergoing repair, renovation, modification, or reconstruction shall comply with the applicable requirements of Sections 43.3, 43.4, 43.5, and 43.6, except as specifically permitted in 43.10.4.

**43.10.4.2 Replacement.** Replacements shall meet the following criteria:

(1) Replacement of existing or missing features using original or like materials shall be permitted.
(2) Partial replacement for repairs that match the original in configuration, height, and size shall be permitted.
(3) Replacements shall not be required to meet the requirements of this *Code* that specify material standards, details of installation and connection, joints, or penetrations; or continuity of any element, component, or system in the building.

**43.10.4.3 Means of Egress.** Existing door openings, window openings intended for emergency egress, and corridor and stairway widths narrower than those required for nonhistoric buildings under this *Code* shall be permitted, provided that one of the following criteria is met:

(1) In the opinion of the authority having jurisdiction, sufficient width and height exists for a person to pass through the opening or traverse the exit, and the capacity of the egress system is adequate for the occupant load.
(2) Other operational controls to limit the number of occupants are approved by the authority having jurisdiction.

**43.10.4.4 Door Swing.** Where approved by the authority having jurisdiction, existing front doors shall not be required to swing in the direction of egress travel, provided that other approved exits have sufficient egress capacity to serve the total occupant load.

**43.10.4.5 Transoms.** In fully sprinklered buildings of hotel and dormitory occupancies, apartment occupancies, and residential board and care occupancies, existing transoms in corridors and other fire resistance–rated walls shall be permitted to remain in use, provided that the transoms are fixed in the closed position.

**43.10.4.6 Interior Finishes.**

**43.10.4.6.1** Existing interior wall and ceiling finishes, in other than exits, shall be permitted to remain in place where it is demonstrated that such finishes are the historic finish.

**43.10.4.6.2** Interior wall and ceiling finishes in exits, other than in one- and two-family dwellings, shall meet one of the following criteria:

(1) The material shall have a flame spread classification of Class C or better.
(2) Existing materials not meeting the minimum Class C flame spread criteria shall be surfaced with an approved fire-retardant paint or finish.
(3) Existing materials not meeting the minimum Class C flame spread criteria shall be permitted to be continued in use, provided that the building is protected throughout by an approved automatic sprinkler system.

**43.10.4.7 Stairway Enclosure.**

**43.10.4.7.1** Stairways shall be permitted to be unenclosed in a historic building where such stairways serve only one adjacent floor.

**43.10.4.7.2** In buildings of three or fewer stories in height, exit enclosure construction shall limit the spread of smoke by the use of tight-fitting doors and solid elements; however, such elements shall not be required to have a fire rating.

**43.10.4.8 One-Hour Fire-Rated Assemblies.** Existing walls and ceilings shall be exempt from the minimum 1-hour fire resistance–rated construction requirements of other sections of this *Code* where the existing wall and ceiling are of wood lath and plaster construction in good condition.

**43.10.4.9 Stairway Handrails and Guards.**

**43.10.4.9.1** Existing grand stairways shall be exempt from the handrail and guard requirements of other sections of this *Code*.

**43.10.4.9.2** Existing handrails and guards on grand staircases shall be permitted to remain in use, provided that they are not structurally dangerous.

**43.10.4.10 Exit Signs.** The authority having jurisdiction shall be permitted to accept alternative exit sign or directional exit sign location, provided that signs installed in compliance with other sections of this *Code* would have an adverse effect on the historic character and such alternative signs identify the exits and egress path.

**43.10.4.11 Sprinkler Systems.**

**43.10.4.11.1** Historic buildings that do not conform to the construction requirements specified in other chapters of this *Code* for the applicable occupancy or use and that, in the opinion of the authority having jurisdiction, constitute a fire safety hazard shall be protected throughout by an approved automatic sprinkler system.

**43.10.4.11.2** The automatic sprinkler system required by 43.10.4.11.1 shall not be used as a substitute for, or serve as an alternative to, the required number of exits from the facility.

### 43.10.5 Change of Occupancy.

**43.10.5.1 General.** Historic buildings undergoing a change of occupancy shall comply with the applicable provisions of Section 43.7, except as otherwise permitted by 43.10.5.

**43.10.5.2 Means of Egress.** Existing door openings, window openings intended for emergency egress, and corridor and stairway widths narrower than those required for nonhistoric buildings under this *Code* shall be permitted, provided that one of the following criteria is met:

(1) In the opinion of the authority having jurisdiction, sufficient width and height exists for a person to pass through the opening or traverse the exit, and the capacity of the egress system is adequate for the occupant load.
(2) Other operational controls to limit the number of occupants are approved by the authority having jurisdiction.

**43.10.5.3 Door Swing.** Where approved by the authority having jurisdiction, existing front doors shall not be required to swing in the direction of egress travel, provided that other approved exits have sufficient capacity to serve the total occupant load.

**43.10.5.4 Transoms.** In corridor walls required to be fire rated by this *Code*, existing transoms shall be permitted to remain in use, provided that the transoms are fixed in the closed position and one of the following criteria is met:

(1) An automatic sprinkler shall be installed on each side of the transom.
(2) Fixed wired glass set in a steel frame or other approved glazing shall be installed on one side of the transom.

**43.10.5.5 Interior Finishes.** Existing interior wall and ceiling finishes shall meet one of the following criteria:

(1) The material shall comply with the flame spread classification of other sections of this *Code* applicable to the occupancy.
(2) Materials not complying with 43.10.5.5(1) shall be permitted to be surfaced with an approved fire-retardant paint or finish.
(3) Materials not complying with 43.10.5.5(1) shall be permitted to be continued in use, provided that the building is protected throughout by an approved automatic sprinkler system, and the nonconforming materials are substantiated as being historic in character.

**43.10.5.6 One-Hour Fire-Rated Assemblies.** Existing walls and ceilings shall be exempt from the minimum 1-hour fire resistance–rated construction requirements of other sections of this *Code* where the existing wall and ceiling are of wood lath and plaster construction in good condition.

**43.10.5.7 Stairs and Handrails.**

**43.10.5.7.1** Existing stairs and handrails shall comply with the requirements of this *Code*, unless otherwise specified in 43.10.5.7.2.

**43.10.5.7.2** The authority having jurisdiction shall be permitted to accept alternatives for grand stairways and associated handrails where the alternatives are approved as meeting the intent of this *Code*.

**43.10.5.8 Exit Signs.** The authority having jurisdiction shall be permitted to accept alternative exit sign or directional exit sign location, provided that signs installed in compliance with other sections of this *Code* would have an adverse effect on the historic character and such alternative signs identify the exits and egress path.

**43.10.5.9 Exit Stair Live Load.** Existing historic stairways in buildings changed to hotel and dormitory occupancies and apartment occupancies shall be permitted to be continued in use, provided that the stairway can support a 75 lb/ft$^2$ (3600 N/m$^2$) live load.

## References Cited in Commentary


1. *Nationally Applicable Recommended Rehabilitation Provisions (NARRP),* 1997, U.S. Department of Housing and Urban Development, Washington, DC.
2. *NFPA 5000®, Building Construction and Safety Code®*, 2009 edition, National Fire Protection Association, Quincy, MA.
3. See note 1.
4. ASME A17.3, *Safety Code for Existing Elevators and Escalators*, 2005 edition, American Society of Mechanical Engineers, Three Park Avenue, New York, NY 10016-5990.
5. ASME A17.1/CSA B44, *Safety Code for Elevators and Escalators*, 2007 edition, American Society of Mechanical Engineers, Three Park Avenue, New York, NY 10016-5990.
6. ASME A17.1, *Safety Code for Elevators and Escalators*, 1987 edition, American Society of Mechanical Engineers, Three Park Avenue, New York, NY 10016-5990.
7. NFPA 14, *Standard for the Installation of Standpipe and Hose Systems*, 2007 edition, National Fire Protection Association, Quincy, MA.
8. NFPA 914, *Code for Fire Protection of Historic Structures*, 2007 edition, National Fire Protection Association, Quincy, MA.

ANNEX A

# Explanatory Material

*Annex A is not a part of the requirements of this NFPA document but is included for informational purposes only. This annex contains explanatory material, numbered to correspond with the applicable text paragraphs.*

The material contained in Annex A of the 2009 edition of the *Life Safety Code* is not a part of the requirements of the *Code* but is included with the *Code* for informational purposes only. For the convenience of readers, in this handbook, the Annex A material is interspersed among the text of Chapters 1 through 43 and, therefore, is not repeated here.



ANNEX B

# Elevators for Occupant-Controlled Evacuation Prior to Phase I Emergency Recall Operations

Annex B provides guidance on the design, installation, and use of elevators for occupant-controlled evacuation prior to Phase I Emergency Recall Operations mandated by the Firefighters' Emergency Operations provisions of ASME A17.1/CSA B44, *Safety Code for Elevators and Escalators*.[1] As with the other annexes to the *Code*, Annex B provides the *Code* user with information that is not contained in the body of the *Code* (i.e., Chapters 1 through 43). Annex B differs from Annex A, Explanatory Material, in that its provisions are formatted as mandates, using the word *shall*, that can be enforced by an authority having jurisdiction (AHJ). Annex B can become an enforceable document if specifically adopted by a regulatory authority, but is otherwise advisory, even though its provisions are formatted as mandates. As indicated in the definition of the term *authority having jurisdiction* in 3.2.2, the AHJ might be a person outside the governmental bodies that typically adopt the *Code*. A building developer might adopt Annex B as a mandatory reference in the construction documents for a new building in which the elevators are to be used for occupant-controlled evacuation. An owner of an existing building might reference Annex B as part of the specifications for the retrofitting of an elevator in the building for occupant-controlled evacuation. A design professional might consult Annex B for guidance in providing services, even where Annex B is not specifically adopted or referenced.

The content of Annex B had its genesis following the September 11, 2001, attacks on the World Trade Center towers when Richard Bukowski of the National Institute of Standards and Technology (NIST) requested that the standards-development organizations with interests in elevators, fire and life safety codes, and fire fighter operations work together to develop a framework under which elevators could be used for occupant evacuation and fire-fighting operations. The request was consistent with Recommendation 20 of the NIST Final Report on the Collapse of the World Trade Center Towers, which states:

> Recommendation 20: NIST recommends that the full range of current and next generation evacuation technologies should be evaluated for future use, including protected/hardened elevators, . . . which may allow all occupants an equal opportunity for evacuation and facilitate emergency response access.[2]

In response to the NIST request, the American Society of Mechanical Engineers (ASME), which publishes ASME A17.1/CSA B44, sponsored the ASME Workshop on Use of Elevators in Fires and Other Emergencies in Atlanta, Georgia, in March 2004. Cosponsors of the workshop included NIST, NFPA, the International Code Council (ICC), the US Access Board, the International Association of Fire Fighters (IAFF), and Elevator World.

Recommendations developed during the ASME workshop were assigned to two ASME task groups for study. The task groups, one on the use of elevators for occupant egress, and the other on the use of elevators by fire fighters, began the work of developing hazard analyses on the respective subjects in October 2004. At the time this commentary was prepared in the second half of 2008, the task groups continued to work diligently. The completed documentation for the hazard analyses exceeded one hundred pages, and the task group reports remained internal working documents not available for public distribution.

Annex B was developed by the NFPA Technical Committee on Means of Egress. Members of the technical committee have actively participated in the

ASME task groups, particularly on the task group related to the use of elevators for occupant egress, so as to be aware of the issues studied and the progress made to date. Annex B was written to utilize current elevator technology, strengthen building construction elements in the area of the elevators, and enhance information dissemination for building occupants. It is expected that the ASME task group work will lead to significant future improvements in Annex B to utilize new technology for elevator construction, controls, and operations — a new elevator emergency operations procedure that has tentatively been named "emergency evacuation operation" (EEO).

*This annex is not a part of the requirements of this NFPA document but is included for informational purposes only. Information in this annex is intended to be adopted by the jurisdiction at the discretion of the adopting jurisdiction. Additionally, information in this annex is intended to be incorporated on a voluntary basis by building owners and developers who might have a desire to include occupant evacuation elevators in their design projects.*

*Although this annex is written in mandatory language, it is not intended to be enforced or applied unless specifically adopted by the jurisdiction or, if it is being applied on a voluntary basis, by the building owner or developer.*

*The provisions of this annex are applicable where elevators are intended to be used for general building occupant evacuation during alarm conditions prior to Phase I Emergency Recall Operation.*

*It is not the intent to require application of these requirements where limited or supervised use of elevators for evacuation is part of a formal or informal evacuation strategy, including, but not limited to, relocation or evacuation of patients in health care occupancies and relocation or evacuation by occupants with disabilities in other occupancies.*

The fourth paragraph of the italicized introductory text that follows the title of Annex B provides important information relative to the intended scope of Annex B. It is not the intent that a health care occupancy, like the hospital described in the paragraph that follows, be required to comply with the provisions of Annex B in order to utilize elevators as part of the emergency plan to evacuate or relocate patients under fire or similar emergency.

Exhibit B.1 depicts a patient sleeping floor on the fifth story of an existing five-story hospital. The partitions delineating the sleeping rooms are not shown for purposes of simplifying the exhibit. The smoke barrier divides the floor into two smoke compartments, A and B. Similar smoke barriers are provided on the other four stories at the same relative location as on the fifth story, so that the smoke barriers are vertically aligned throughout the building height, creating two smoke compartments per floor, A and B. The written emergency plan provides for patients to be moved by the elevator located in the smoke compartment not involved in the fire. For example, if the fire is in compartment A of the fifth story, the elevators are not used in compartment A of any of the stories. The elevator in compartment B is used to evacuate or relocate patients, as it is on the safe side of the smoke barrier. The emergency plan employed should not be subjected to the requirements of Annex B.

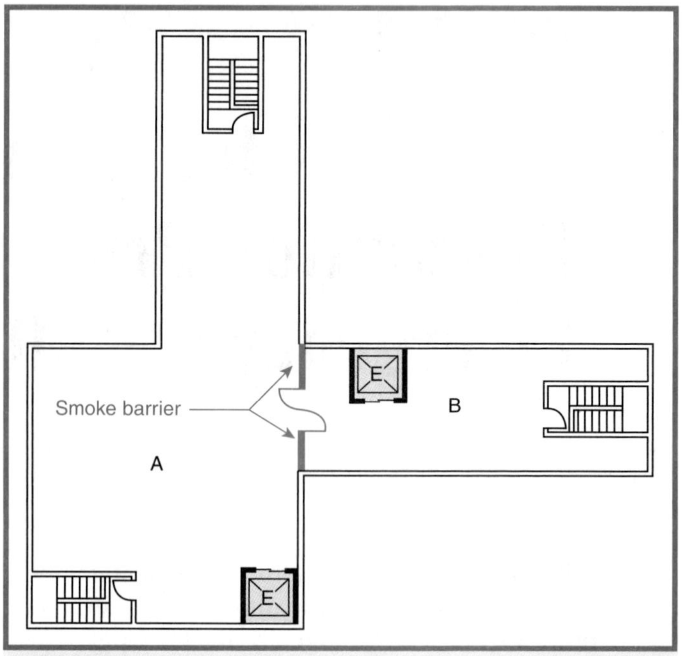


***Exhibit B.1.*** *Elevator use for patient evacuation or relocation not subject to the requirements of Annex B.*

## B.1 General

**B.1.1** Elevators that are installed in new buildings in compliance with the provisions of Annex B shall be permitted to be used for occupant-controlled evacuation prior to Phase I Emergency Recall Operation mandated by the Firefighters' Emergency Operation provisions of ASME A17.1/CSA B44, *Safety Code for Elevators and Escalators.*

Note: The Phase I Emergency Recall Operation mandated by the Firefighters' Emergency Operation provisions of ASME A17.1/CSA B 44, *Safety Code for Elevators and Escalators*, recalls elevators upon detection of smoke by smoke detectors installed in the following locations:

(1) At each floor served by the elevator in the lobby (landing) adjacent to the hoistway doors
(2) In the associated elevator machine room
(3) In the elevator hoistway where sprinklers are located in the hoistway

Where smoke from a fire remote from the elevator lobby (landing), elevator machine room, and elevator hoistway can be kept from reaching the elevator lobby (landing), elevator machine room, and elevator hoistway, the associated elevators can continue to operate in a fire emergency. The provisions of Annex B address the features that need to be provided to make such elevator operation safe for evacuation.

The commentary for Annex B is relatively brief, as the annex includes extensive notes (i.e., text that begins with the word "Note") that provide clarification and explain intent in much the same way that handbook commentary does. For example, the note that follows B.1.1 provides information from which the user learns that smoke detectors (other than those at the elevator lobby/landing, elevator machine room, and elevator hoistway) are not permitted by ASME A17.1/CSA B44 to recall elevators. The provisions of Annex B are intended to help keep smoke from reaching the smoke detectors that do recall the elevators and help ensure that it is safe for those elevators to continue to run during a fire emergency. Smoke that reaches other smoke detectors on the floor should not affect the continued operation of the occupant evacuation elevators.

**B.1.2** Occupant evacuation elevators in accordance with Annex B shall not be permitted to satisfy requirements of this *Code* applicable to the following:

(1) Number of means of egress
(2) Capacity of means of egress
(3) Arrangement of means of egress

The provision of B.1.2 specifically directs that occupant evacuation elevators in accordance with Annex B are not permitted to satisfy any of the means of egress requirements of the *Code* related to number, capacity, or arrangement. For example, a floor that is provided with two enclosed exit stairs and one occupant evacuation elevator is credited with having two exits, not three. Where each of the two exit stairs has capacity for 150 persons, the floor's total egress capacity is 300 persons, as the elevator is not credited with providing any egress capacity. Where one exit stair is at one end of the floor, the second exit stair is at the other end of the floor, and the occupant evacuation elevator is located at the midpoint of the length of the floor, occupants in the vicinity of the elevator must be able to reach one of the exit stairs within the allowable travel distance, as travel distance measurement ends at an exit, and the elevator is not an exit.

The effect of the provision of B.1.2 is that there is no *Code*-driven incentive to provide occupant evacuation elevators. It is expected that, as Annex B matures over future editions to include true EEO (see the last paragraph of the commentary that follows the title of the annex), occupant evacuation elevators that satisfy some of the means of egress requirements will be mandated for new building construction. The technology needed to make an elevator that is an equivalent to an exit stair is in an infant stage. Current interest and development activity suggest that this stage will advance quickly.

## B.2 Occupant Information Features

**B.2.1** An evacuation plan approved by the authority having jurisdiction shall be implemented, specifically including the procedures for occupant evacuation using the exit stairs and the occupant evacuation elevators.

Note: Building occupants have traditionally been taught not to use elevators in fire or similar emergencies. The evacuation plan should include more than notification that the elevators can be used for emergency evacuation. The plan should include training to make occupants aware that the elevators will be available only for the period of time prior to elevator recall via smoke detection in the elevator lobby, machine room, or hoistway. Occupants should be prepared to use the exit stairs (which are required to be directly accessible from the elevator lobby by B.8.3) where the elevator has been called out of service.

A typical evacuation plan needs to include emergency evacuation or relocation procedures and instructions, specific to the building, in an easy to comprehend format. The evacuation plan required by B.2.1 is atypical in that, in addition to including the provisions of a typical plan, it must undo the occupants' lifelong belief that elevators are not to be used in fire and similar emergencies. The message that the evacuation plan needs to convey is that use of elevators is encouraged for occupant evacuation, but, if the elevators are called out of service before occupants can board them, occupants must be prepared to use the stairs. Note that B.8.1 requires the occupant evacuation elevators to be within an occupant evacuation shaft system that provides direct access from the elevator lobby to an enclosed exit stair. It would be unsafe to rely on a system that encourages occupants to wait in an elevator lobby for an elevator and then forces them to re-enter other portions of the floor (e.g., a common exit access corridor) in order to reach an exit stair once elevators have been called out of service due to smoke breaching the occupant evacuation shaft system.

**B.2.2** Occupant evacuation elevators shall be marked with signage indicating the elevators are suitable for use by building occupants for evacuation during fires.

The signage required by B.2.2 is to be present on a day-to-day basis, rather than just under fire emergency, so as to inform occupants that the building elevator system differs from that in the majority of buildings; that is, those elevator systems for which the message has been ingrained by years of training that elevators are not to be used in fire emergencies. The required signage serves to help disseminate the information that B.2.1 requires to be part of the evacuation plan. It replaces the signage currently required by ASME A17.1/CSA B44 that directs occupants to use stairs, and not elevators, in fire emergencies.

**B.2.3** Conditions necessary for the continued safe operation of the occupant evacuation elevators and the associated elevator lobbies and elevator machine rooms shall be continuously monitored and displayed at the building emergency command center by a standard emergency service interface system meeting the requirements of *NFPA 72, National Fire Alarm Code*, and NEMA SB 30, *Fire Service Annunciator and Interface.*

**B.2.4** The building emergency command center location specified in B.2.3 shall be provided with a means to override normal elevator operation and to initiate manually a Phase I Emergency Recall Operation of the occupant-controlled elevators in accordance with ASME A17.1/CSA B44, *Safety Code for Elevators and Escalators.*

As explained in the commentary that follows the annex title, Annex B was written before completion of the ASME hazard analyses that are expected to lead to an enhanced occupant evacuation elevator system employing emergency evacuation operation (EEO). Also, Annex B was written to include only technologies that are currently available. The technology needed to comply with the requirements of B.2.3 and B.2.4 exists.

The standard emergency service interface system required by B.2.3 is addressed in Annex F of *NFPA 72®*, *National Fire Alarm Code®*,[3] which reprints in its entirety NEMA SB 30, *Fire Service Annunciator and Interface.*[4]

The provision of B.2.3 does not enumerate the conditions that must be monitored for the continued safe operation of the occupant evacuation elevators. Once occupant evacuation elevator systems are installed in more than a few buildings, a set of typical conditions to be monitored will become apparent. In the interim, the AHJ will be asked to approve the designer's choice of conditions and, perhaps, require additional conditions to be monitored. For example, the status of air-conditioning equipment that maintains proper temperature in the elevator machine room to ensure that controllers continue to operate might be monitored and displayed at the building emergency command center (i.e., the same emergency command center required by 11.8.6 for high-rise buildings).

The provision of B.2.4 helps to ensure that the emergency response personnel in the emergency command center can manually override normal elevator operation once the conditions necessary for the continued safe operation of the occupant evacuation elevators no longer exist. If the requirement of B.2.4 were not part of Annex B, emergency response personnel would have to go to the street level elevator lobby to recall the elevators manually by using a special emergency services key.

**B.2.5** Occupant evacuation elevator lobbies shall be equipped with a status indicator arranged to display the following:

(1) Illuminated green light and the message "Elevators available for occupant evacuation" while the elevators are operating under emergency conditions but before Phase I Emergency Recall Operation in accordance with the Fire Fighters' Emergency Operation requirements of ASME A17.1/CSA B44, *Safety Code for Elevators and Escalators*
(2) Illuminated red light and the message "Elevators out of service, use exit stairs" once the elevators are under Phase I Emergency Recall Operation
(3) No illuminated light but the message "Elevators are operating normally" while the elevators are operating under nonemergency conditions

The status indicators, which are required by B.2.5 to be positioned within the elevator lobbies served by the occupant evacuation elevators, provide occupants with information about the operating status of the elevators. The message required by B.2.5(3), that elevators are operating normally, is the message building occupants will see on a normal day-to-day basis under nonemergency conditions. Together with the signage required by B.2.2, the message informs occupants that the elevator system in the building differs from that in most buildings. Because the message required by B.2.5(3) is meant to be the norm, no illuminated light is required to accompany the message.

The messages required by B.2.5(1) and (2) advise occupants of elevator operating status under emergency conditions. As such, each requires an illuminated light to accompany the message — a green light is to be illuminated while it is safe to use the elevators for emergency evacuation, and a red light is to be illuminated once the elevators have been called out of service so as not to be available for occupant use.

Given that B.2.5 requires that the occupant evacuation elevator system be capable of providing a different message for each of the three elevator operating conditions specified, a fixed placard will not suffice. The sign or message board will need to be electrically or electronically operated. The equipment technology needed to meet the requirements of B.2.5 exists.

## B.3 Fire Detection, Alarm, and Communication

**B.3.1** The building shall be protected throughout by an approved fire alarm system in accordance with Section 9.6.

### B.3.2 Smoke Detectors.

**B.3.2.1** Smoke detectors shall be installed in all occupiable areas within the building in accordance with the requirements of *NFPA 72, National Fire Alarm Code*, except as otherwise provided in B.3.2.2.

Note: The occupant evacuation elevator will function only until Phase I Emergency Recall Operation. The required smoke detection system in occupiable areas is intended to provide building occupants with the early warning needed to permit elevator use early in the fire.

**B.3.2.2** Smoke detectors shall not be required to be installed in all occupiable areas where all of the following conditions are met:

(1) The building is protected throughout by an approved, supervised automatic sprinkler system in accordance with Section B.4.
(2) The sprinkler system is provided with a sprinkler control valve and waterflow device on each floor.
(3) The sprinkler control valves and waterflow devices required by B.3.2.2(2) are monitored by the building fire alarm system.

Note: The exemption permitted by B.3.2.2 eliminates the need to install smoke detectors in all occupied areas of the building where the elevator evacuation protocol can be initiated by the sprinkler system that is arranged to indicate the floor of fire origin when a sprinkler flows water.

The note that follows B.3.2.1 explains that the requirement for smoke detectors to be installed in all occupiable areas is intended to provide occupants with early warning to permit elevator use early in the fire. Early use of elevators is important if a significant number of persons are to be evacuated via elevator, as there is no guarantee that the elevators will continue to be in service long into the fire emergency. As soon as smoke is detected in an elevator lobby, machine room, or hoistway, the elevators will be called out of service. See the note that follows B.1.1.

The provision of B.3.2.2, which exempts smoke detectors from occupiable areas in sprinklered buildings, relies on waterflow through the sprinkler system to initiate the fire alarm system that notifies occupants to evacuate. For other than fast-developing fires, the initiation of the alarm system via sprinkler system waterflow will be slower than that by smoke detection, resulting in a delay in the start of occupant evacuation. The option provided to sprinklered buildings by B.3.2.2 is a compromise that was established during the Report on Comments phase of the *Code*-development process that produced Annex B. Proponents of the option argued than an alternative to the smoke detection of all occupiable areas was needed in order to make the system viable from a daily operations standpoint. It is particularly important that the building features required by Annex B be rigorously maintained to help keep smoke from reaching elevator lobbies, machine rooms, or hoistways and to prevent recalling the elevators before occupants complete their evacuation via elevator.

**B.3.3** The fire alarm system shall include an emergency voice/alarm communication system in accordance with *NFPA 72, National Fire Alarm Code*, with the ability to provide voice directions on a selective basis to any building floor.

Note: The emergency voice/alarm communication system with the ability to provide voice directions on a selective basis to any building floor might be used to instruct occupants of the fire floor who are able to use stairs to relocate to a floor level below. The selective voice notification feature might be used to provide occupants of a given elevator lobby with a status report or supplemental instructions.

**B.3.4** The emergency voice/alarm communication system shall be arranged so that intelligible voice instructions are audible in the elevator lobbies under conditions where the elevator lobby doors are in the closed position.

Note: An audible notification appliance will need to be positioned in the elevator lobby in order to meet the requirement of B.3.4. The continued use of the occupant evacuation elevator system is predicated on elevator lobby doors that are closed to keep smoke from reaching the elevator lobby smoke detector that is arranged to initiate the Phase I Emergency Recall Operation.

See the notes that follow B.3.3 and B.3.4 for guidance and examples on the use of emergency voice/alarm communication systems.

## B.4 Sprinklers

**B.4.1** The building shall be protected throughout by an approved, supervised automatic sprinkler system in accordance with 9.7.1.1(1), except as otherwise specified in B.4.2.

**B.4.2** Sprinklers shall not be installed in elevator machine rooms serving occupant evacuation elevators, and such prohibition shall not cause an otherwise fully sprinklered building to be classified as nonsprinklered.

Note: The presence of sprinklers in the elevator machine room would necessitate the installation of a shunt trip for automatically disconnecting the main line power for compliance with ASME A17.1/CSA B44, *Safety Code for Elevators and Escalators*, as it is unsafe to operate elevators while sprinkler water is being discharged in the elevator machine room. The presence of a shunt trip conflicts with the needs of the occupant evacuation elevator, as it disconnects the power without ensuring that the elevator is first returned to a safe floor so as to prevent trapping occupants. The provision of B.4.2, prohibiting the sprinklering of elevator machine rooms, deviates from the requirements of NFPA 13, *Standard for the Installation of Sprinkler Systems*, which permits no such exemption. However, NFPA 13 permits a similar exemption for electrical equipment rooms where the room is dedicated to electrical equipment only; the equipment is installed in a 2-hour fire-rated enclosure, including protection for penetrations; and no combustible storage is stored in the room. Similar safeguards are imposed on the occupant evacuation elevator by B.6.1 and B.6.2.

**B.4.3** Where a hoistway serves occupant evacuation elevators, sprinklers shall not be installed at the top of the elevator hoistway or at other points in the hoistway more than 24 in. (610 mm) above the pit floor, and such prohibition shall not cause this building to be classified as nonsprinklered.

Note: NFPA 13, *Standard for the Installation of Sprinkler Systems*, permits sprinklers to be omitted from the top of the elevator hoistway where the hoistway for passenger elevators is noncombustible and the car enclosure materials meet the requirements of ASME A17.1/CSA B44, *Safety Code for Elevators and Escalators*. The provision of B.5.3 restricts occupant evacuation elevators to passenger elevators that are in noncombustible hoistways and for which the car enclosure materials meet the requirements of ASME A17.1/CSA B 44. *(See B.5.3.)*

The presence of the sprinkler system required by B.4.1 is a fundamental premise on which Annex B is based. If the building were not sprinklered, it would not be safe for occupants to wait in elevator lobbies to evacuate via elevators.

The note that follows B.4.2 fully explains the rationale for prohibiting sprinklers from elevator machine rooms. The note that follows B.4.3 explains how the provisions of NFPA 13, *Standard for the Installation of Sprinkler Systems*,[5] and ASME A17.1/CSA B44 work together to permit the omission of sprinklers in the hoistway, except near the pit floor.

## B.5 Elevator Installation

**B.5.1** Except as modified by B.5.2, occupant evacuation elevators shall be installed in accordance with ASME A17.1/CSA B44, *Safety Code for Elevators and Escalators*.

**B.5.2** Shunt breakers shall not be installed on elevator systems used for occupant evacuation.

Note: Elevator shunt breakers are intended to disconnect the electric power to an elevator prior to sprinkler system waterflow impairing the functioning of the elevator. The provision of B.4.2 prohibits the installation of sprinklers in the elevator machine room and at the top of the elevator hoistway, obviating the need for shunt breakers. The provision of B.5.2 is not actually an exemption to the provisions of ASME A17.1/CSA B44, *Safety Code for Elevators and Escalators*, as ASME A17.1/CSA B44 requires the automatic main line power disconnect (shunt trip) only where sprinklers are located in the elevator machine room or in the hoistway more than 24 in. (610 mm) above the pit floor. The provision of B.4.2 prohibits sprinklers in the elevator machine room. The provision of B.4.3 prohibits sprinklers at the top of the hoistway and at other points in the hoistway more than 24 in. (610 mm) above the pit floor in recognition of the limitations on combustibility established by B.5.3.

**B.5.3** Occupant evacuation elevators shall be limited to passenger elevators that are in noncombustible hoistways and for which the car enclosure materials meet the requirements of ASME A17.1/CSA B44, *Safety Code for Elevators and Escalators*.

The elevator technology required for compliance with Annex B exists in the 2007 edition of ASME A17.1/CSA B44. Future editions of ASME A17.1/CSA B44 are expected to include criteria to permit Annex B to be expanded to include a new elevator emergency operations procedure (EEO), as addressed in the commentary following the annex title.

The note that follows B.5.2 fully explains the rationale for prohibiting shunt breakers on elevator systems used for occupant evacuation.

The provision of B.5.3 works with that of B.4.3 to make it safe to permit the omission of sprinklers in the hoistway, except near the pit floor.

## B.6 Elevator Machine Rooms

**B.6.1** Elevator machine rooms associated with occupant evacuation elevators shall be separated from all building areas, other than elevator hoistways, by minimum 2-hour fire resistance–rated construction.

Note: The minimum 2-hour fire resistance–rated separation is based on the omission of sprinklers from the elevator machine room in accordance with B.4.2.

**B.6.2** Elevator machine rooms associated with occupant evacuation elevators shall be used for no purpose other than as elevator machine rooms.

Note: The requirement of B.6.2 is consistent with that in ASME A17.1/CSA B44, *Safety Code for Elevators and Escalators*, which permits only machinery and equipment used in conjunction with the function or use of the elevator to be in the elevator machine room. An inspection program should be implemented to ensure that the elevator machine room is kept free of storage.

The provision of B.6.1 works with that of B.4.2 to ensure that the nonsprinklered elevator machine room is separated from all building areas, other than the elevator hoistway, by minimum 2-hour fire resistance–rated construction. The allowance for the elevator machine room to be open to the hoistway recognizes the functional need for cables to be connected between the motorized driver in the machine room and the elevator car in the hoistway. The minimum 2-hour fire resistance–rated separation required for the elevator machine room by B.6.1 is consistent with that of 8.6.5(1) for the protection of vertical openings created by elevator hoistways that connect four or more stories in new construction.

The provision of B.6.2 repeats a requirement of ASME A17.1/CSA B44, as it is important to remind the user not to store materials in the nonsprinklered elevator machine room. See B.4.2 and its associated note.

## B.7 Electrical Power and Control Wiring

**B.7.1** The following features associated with occupant evacuation elevators shall be supplied by both normal power and Type 60, Class 2, Level 1 standby power:

(1) Elevator equipment
(2) Elevator machine room ventilation and cooling equipment
(3) Elevator controller cooling equipment

**B.7.2** Wiring for power of the elevators shall meet one of the following criteria:

(1) The wiring shall utilize type CI cable with a minimum 1-hour fire resistance rating.
(2) The wiring shall be enclosed in a minimum 1-hour fire resistance construction.

Standby power is further addressed by NFPA 110, *Standard for Emergency and Standby Power Systems*.[6] A Type 60 emergency power supply system (EPSS) must restore power within 60 seconds of the failure of the primary power source. A Class 2 EPSS must be capable of operating at its rated load without being refueled for a minimum of 2 hours. Level 1 performance is specified based on the technical committee's judgment that failure of the EPSS is critical to human life and safety. See NFPA 110.

The provision of B.7.2 protects the elevator power wiring from a fire originating in any building area through which the wiring runs. Without such protection, a fire that is remote from the elevator hoistway and elevator lobbies might disable the power supply, preventing the elevators from being used for occupant evacuation.

## B.8 Occupant Evacuation Shaft System

**B.8.1** Occupant evacuation elevators shall be provided with an occupant evacuation shaft system consisting of all of the following:

(1) Elevator hoistway
(2) Enclosed elevator lobby outside the bank or group of hoistway doors on each floor served by the elevators

*Exception: Elevator lobbies are not required to be enclosed when located either on the street floor or level of exit discharge.*

(3) Enclosed exit stair with doors to all floors, at and above grade level, served by the elevators

**B.8.2** Occupant evacuation elevator lobbies shall have minimum floor area as follows:

(1) The elevator lobby floor area shall accommodate, at 3 $ft^2$ (0.28 $m^2$) per person, a minimum of 25 percent of the occupant load of the floor area served by the lobby.
(2) The elevator lobby floor area also shall accommodate one wheelchair space of 30 in. × 48 in. (760 mm × 1220 mm) for each 50 persons, or portion thereof, of the occupant load of the floor area served by the lobby.

Note: Elevator lobbies provide a safe place for building occupants to await the elevators and extend the time available for such use by providing a barrier to smoke and heat that might threaten the elevator car or hoistway. Smoke detectors within the elevator lobbies are arranged to initiate a Phase I Emergency Recall Operation if the lobby is breached by smoke.

**B.8.3** Access to the exit stair required by B.8.1(3) shall be directly from the enclosed elevator lobby on each floor.

**B.8.4** The occupant evacuation shaft system shall be enclosed and separated from the remainder of the building by walls complying with the following:

(1) The shaft system walls shall be smoke barriers in accordance with Section 8.5.
(2) The shaft system walls separating the elevator lobby from the remainder of the building shall have a minimum 1-hour fire resistance rating and minimum $^3/_4$-hour fire protection–rated opening protectives.
(3) The shaft system walls separating the elevator hoistway from the remainder of the building shall have a minimum 2-hour fire resistance rating and minimum $1^1/_2$-hour fire protection–rated opening protectives.
(4) The shaft system walls separating the enclosed exit stair from the remainder of the building shall have a minimum 2-hour fire resistance rating and minimum $1^1/_2$-hour fire protection–rated opening protectives.

The occupant evacuation shaft system, as addressed in Section B.8, provides the building construction features that support the occupant evacuation elevator system. The concepts on which the requirements for the occupant evacuation shaft system are based include the following:

1. The elevator hoistway must be served at each floor by an elevator lobby where building occupants can wait in safety for elevators.
2. An enclosed exit stair needs to be located immediately adjacent to, and directly accessible from, each elevator lobby to provide a means for occupant evacuation once elevators are called out of service.
3. The elevator hoistway, elevator lobby, and associated enclosed exit stair (i.e., the areas that comprise the occupant evacuation shaft system) need to be protected from fire originating outside the occupant evacuation shaft system.
4. Smoke from fire outside the occupant evacuation shaft system must not enter the occupant evacuation shaft system in sufficient quantity to initiate elevator recall via the smoke detectors in the elevator lobbies and hoistway.
5. Fire must not breach the occupant evacuation shaft system for the period of time that the elevators can be used effectively for occupant evacuation.
6. Each elevator lobby must be sized to accommodate the number of persons expected to need, or benefit from, the occupant elevator evacuation system.
7. Water from discharging sprinklers and fire fighter hose needs to be kept out of the hoistway to permit elevator equipment to continue operating safely.

Exhibit B.2 illustrates the occupant evacuation shaft system required by Section B.8. The shaft system is the combined area of the hoistway, elevator lobby, and associated enclosed exit stair. Note that occupants of the elevator lobby have direct access to an enclosed exit stair without having to enter the corridor.

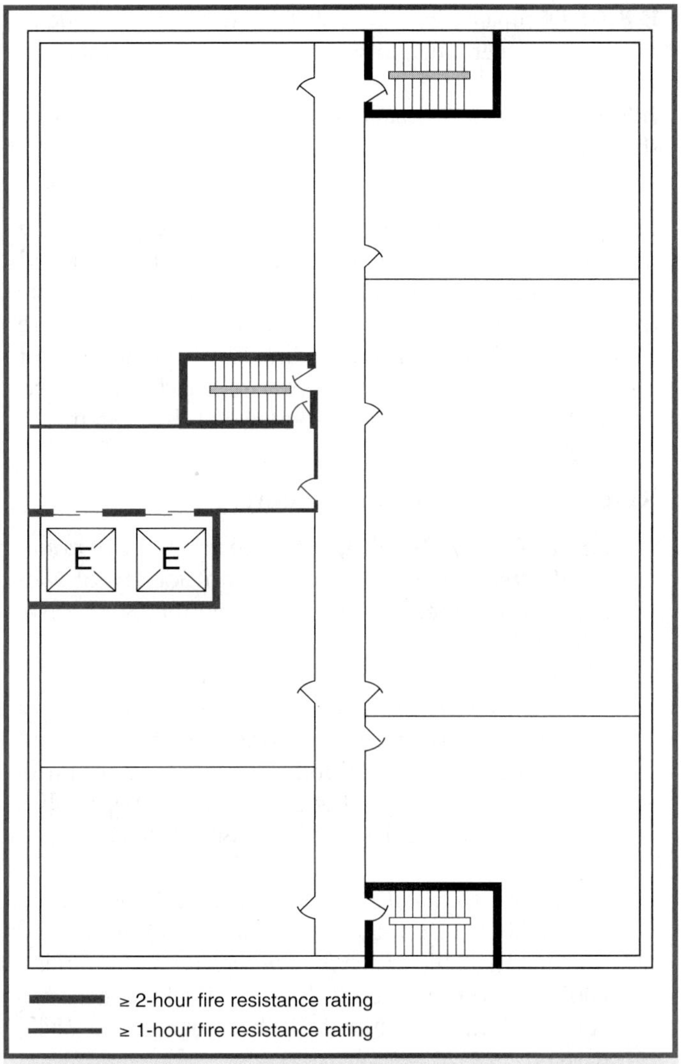


***Exhibit B.2.*** *Occupant evacuation shaft system separated from remainder of floor.*

**B.8.5** Occupant evacuation shaft system enclosures shall be constructed to provide a minimum of classification Level 2 in accordance with ASTM C 1629/C 1629M, *Standard Classification for Abuse-Resistant Nondecorated Interior Gypsum Panel Products and Fiber-Reinforced Cement Panels.*

The provision of B.8.5 helps to ensure that the barriers separating the occupant evacuation shaft system from the remainder of the floor include the impact resistance needed to withstand the challenges of day-to-day wear and tear. The test method cited, ASTM C 1629/C 1629M, *Standard Classification for Abuse-Resistant Nondecorated Interior Gypsum Panel Products and Fiber-Reinforced Cement Panels,*[7] was developed for gypsum panel products and fiber-reinforced cement products but can be applied to wall assemblies of any construction material. The standard directs that tests be run to demonstrate that the wall assembly has resistance to surface abrasion and indentation, including impact by soft and hard bodies.

**B.8.6** The occupant evacuation shaft system shall be protected from water infiltration by one of the following methods:

(1) The shaft system perimeter walls and opening protectives, other than the elevator lobby doors, shall be constructed such that an accumulation of water to a depth of 2 in. (51 mm) on the side of the wall not within the occupant evacuation shaft system shall be prevented from entering the shaft system.
(2) Drains shall be installed to manage the flow of two fire department hoses and three fire sprinklers concurrently discharging such that water does not enter the shaft system.

The elevator hoistway must be protected from water infiltration at all sides, not just at the elevator hoistway door opening. Water from discharging sprinklers and fire fighter hose needs to be kept out of the hoistway to permit elevator equipment to continue operating safely.

**B.8.7** Occupant evacuation shaft system elevator lobby doors shall have all of the following features:

(1) The doors shall have a fire protection rating of not less than $\frac{3}{4}$ hour.
(2) The doors shall be smoke leakage–rated assemblies in accordance with NFPA 105, *Standard for the Installation of Smoke Door Assemblies and Other Opening Protectives.*
(3) The doors shall have an automatic-positioning bottom seal to resist the passage of water at floor level from outside the shaft system.

Note: The elevator lobby doors addressed in B.8.7 do not include the elevator hoistway doors. The elevator hoistway doors serving fire-rated hoistway enclosures in accordance with 8.6.5 must meet the criteria of Table 8.3.4.2.

The elevator lobby doors have a greater potential than the other elements of the occupant evacuation shaft system to permit smoke infiltration into the occupant evacuation shaft system, which would cause recall of the elevators via smoke detection in the elevator lobby.

The elevator lobby doors on the fire floor will be opened and closed repeatedly as occupants move into the elevator lobby. However, when the doors are in the closed position, they are expected to properly retard the passage of smoke, as they must be smoke leakage–rated assemblies in accordance with NFPA 105, *Standard for the Installation of Smoke Door Assemblies and Other Opening Protectives*.[8]

The requirement of B.8.7(3) for an automatic-positioning bottom seal on elevator lobby doors introduces a door element not typically required by fire and life safety codes. The intent of the provision is explained via its performance-based requirement that the seal must resist the passage of water at floor level from outside the occupant evacuation shaft system.

**B.8.8** Occupant evacuation shaft system elevator lobby doors shall have the following features:

(1) Each door shall be automatic-closing in accordance with 7.2.1.8.2, as modified by B.8.8(2).
(2) In addition to the automatic-closing means addressed by 7.2.1.8.2, the elevator lobby door on any floor shall also close in response to any alarm signal initiated on that floor.
(3) Each door shall be provided with a vision panel arranged to allow people within the lobby to view conditions on the other side of the door.

Elevator lobby doors are permitted to remain open on a normal, day-to-day basis but must be arranged to close automatically in accordance with 7.2.1.8.2 upon detection of smoke at the door opening and upon loss of electrical power. Furthermore, B.8.8(2) includes a requirement in addition to those of 7.2.1.8.2 by requiring that the door be released from its open position, so as to become self-closing, in response to any alarm signal initiated on that floor. The requirement is consistent with the intent of many of the provisions of Section B.8, which is to maintain the elevators in service by keeping smoke away from the elevator lobby smoke detectors.

**B.8.9** Each occupant evacuation shaft system exit stair enclosure door shall be provided with a vision panel arranged to allow people on either side of the door to view conditions on the other side of the door.

**B.8.10** Occupant evacuation shaft system exit stair enclosures shall be permitted to serve as occupant egress stairs.

**B.8.11** Occupant evacuation shaft system elevator lobbies shall be permitted to serve as areas of refuge.

The provisions of B.8.10 and B.8.11 help to emphasize that elevator systems, elevator landings, and enclosed exit stairs, as addressed by Annex B, are permitted to be used on a normal, day-to-day basis as well as under fire emergencies. The familiarity gained by repeated use of these components in nonemergency conditions is expected to enhance the emergency use of the system.

## References Cited in Commentary

1. ASME A17.1/CSA B44, *Safety Code for Elevators and Escalators*, 2007 edition, American Society of Mechanical Engineers, Three Park Avenue, New York, NY 10016-5990.
2. Final Report on the Collapse of the World Trade Center Towers, Federal Building and Fire Safety Investigation of the World Trade Center Disaster, NIST NCSTAR 1, National Institute of Standards and Technology, Gaithersburg, MD, September 2005, http://wtc.nist.gov/NISTNCSTAR1CollapseofTowers.pdf
3. *NFPA 72®, National Fire Alarm Code®*, 2007 edition, National Fire Protection Association, Quincy, MA.
4. NEMA SB 30, *Fire Service Annunciator and Interface*, 2005 edition, National Electrical Manufacturers Association, 1300 North 17th Street, Suite 1847, Rosslyn, VA 22209.
5. NFPA 13, *Standard for the Installation of Sprinkler Systems*, 2007 edition, National Fire Protection Association, Quincy, MA.
6. NFPA 110, *Standard for Emergency and Standby Power Systems*, 2005 edition, National Fire Protection Association, Quincy, MA.
7. ASTM C 1629/C 1629M, *Standard Classification for Abuse-Resistant Nondecorated Interior Gypsum Panel Products and Fiber-Reinforced Cement Panels*, 2005 edition, ASTM International, 100 Barr Harbor Drive, P.O. Box C700, West Conshohocken, PA 19428-2959.
8. NFPA 105, *Standard for the Installation of Smoke Door Assemblies and Other Opening Protectives*, 2007 edition, National Fire Protection Association, Quincy, MA.

ANNEX C

# Supplemental Evacuation Equipment

Annex C provides guidance on the installation, maintenance, and use of supplemental evacuation equipment of the platform rescue systems type and the controlled descent devices type. The terms *supplemental evacuation equipment*, *platform rescue system*, and *controlled descent device* are defined in C.1.1.4, C.1.1.2, and C.1.1.1, respectively. As with the other annexes to the *Code*, Annex C provides the *Code* user with information that is not contained in the body of the *Code* (i.e., Chapters 1 through 43). Annex C differs from Annex A, Explanatory Material, in that its provisions are formatted as mandates, using the word *shall*, that can be enforced by an authority having jurisdiction (AHJ). Annex C can become an enforceable document if specifically adopted by a regulatory authority but is otherwise advisory, even though its provisions are formatted as mandates. As indicated in the definition of the term *authority having jurisdiction* in 3.2.2, the AHJ might be a person outside the governmental bodies that typically adopt the *Code*. A building developer might adopt Annex C as a mandatory reference in the construction documents for a new building in which supplemental evacuation equipment is to be installed. An owner of an existing building might reference Annex C as part of the specifications for the retrofitting of supplemental evacuation equipment in the building. A design professional might consult Annex C for guidance in providing services, even where Annex C is not specifically adopted or referenced.

*This annex is not a part of the requirements of this NFPA document but is included for informational purposes only. Information in this annex is intended to be adopted by the jurisdiction at the discretion of the adopting jurisdiction. Additionally, information in this annex is intended to be incorporated on a voluntary basis by building owners and developers who might have a desire to include supplemental evacuation equipment in their projects.*

*Although this annex is written in mandatory language, it is not intended to be enforced or applied unless specifically adopted by the jurisdiction or, if it is being applied on a voluntary basis, by the building owner or developer.*

Note: Traditionally, supplemental evacuation equipment has not been regulated or recognized by the *Code*. Until recently, such equipment was considered to include only items such as chain ladders and rope fire escape ladders for use in single-family homes. The criteria specified in Annex C also provides no regulation or recognition for the private installation and use of such equipment by an owner and family, while providing a framework of regulations for the use of controlled descent devices and platform rescue systems in commercial and residential multistory buildings. The broader term *supplemental evacuation equipment* provides for subsets of equipment to be added as further technologies develop.

The numerous fatalities in the September 11, 2001, attack on the World Trade Center in New York City prompted responses on many levels, including challenges to the fundamental concepts of egress systems for tall buildings. One long-held principle in high-rise building design was that most emergency incidents require only partial evacuation or relocation of building occupants. In the September 11 incident, the exit stair enclosures were penetrated and stairs destroyed or severely compromised on the floors of aircraft impact. These floors were many stories above the reach of even the highest fire department ladders. There were hundreds of people on the floors above those directly impacted by the aircraft who could not evacuate.

While official investigations into the incident were being conducted, inventors and engineers began work on means to evacuate occupants of tall buildings in situations where exit stairs are not available. The need to consider such alternatives was identified in the NIST Final Report on the Collapse of the World Trade Center Towers, which states:

> Recommendation 20: NIST recommends that the full range of current and next generation evacuation technologies should be evaluated for future use, including protected/hardened elevators, exterior escape devices, and stairwell descent devices, which may allow all occupants an equal opportunity for evacuation and facilitate emergency response access.[1]

The work in developing supplemental evacuation equipment identified a variety of technologies, including group evacuation platform systems, cable-supported descent devices, flexible chutes, personal helicopters, parachutes, and helium balloon vests. Some of the technologies existed and others were adaptations of equipment already being used, while others were entirely novel in concept and design.

In 2003, several interested parties submitted a proposed framework for regulating supplemental evacuation equipment within the *Code* as a new section in Chapter 7, Means of Egress. The proposal was considered by the Technical Committee on Means of Egress, which determined that the equipment should not be credited with satisfying any of the requirements for number of means of egress, egress capacity, travel distance, common path of travel, or dead-end corridors. Additionally, the technical committee identified several principles it considered important. The following principles were identified:

1. Any equipment installed as supplemental evacuation equipment should not adversely affect the use of required egress systems.
2. The equipment should meet the requirements of a suitable product standard.
3. The equipment should be mechanically sound and reliable for use under the expected conditions.
4. The equipment should be simple to use with little or no training required for the user.
5. The equipment should provide a suitable level of protection for the user.
6. The equipment should be reasonably safe for other users and persons on the ground.
7. The equipment should be usable by persons with physical impairments.
8. The equipment should only be used if the required egress systems are not accessible and only as directed by authorized building personnel or emergency responders.

Some of the supplemental evacuation equipment that was conceptualized or underwent initial development cannot meet the principles enumerated in items 1 through 8, primarily because of safety issues or complexity in use of the equipment. For example, even a skilled user of parachutes might lose control of a parachute and plummet to the ground in adverse wind conditions. Two technologies showed potential to evacuate occupants while meeting the prescribed principles — the controlled descent device and the platform rescue system. While leaving open the possibility for other technologies to be recognized for a future edition of the *Code*, the technical committee codified the requirements for the controlled descent device and the platform rescue system for inclusion in Annex C, as they were the only equipment that met the needed criteria for manufacture, certification, installation, and safe use.

## C.1 General

### C.1.1 Definitions.

**C.1.1.1 Controlled Descent Device.** A system operating on the exterior of a building or structure that lowers one or two people per descent, each wearing a rescue harness, at a controlled rate from an upper level to the ground or other safe location.

The controlled descent device (CDD) had its origin in equipment that has been in use for several decades by window washers and others who need to access vertical faces of buildings and other structures via a boatswain's chair. In the 1970s, this equipment and concept were adapted for use as an escape device from construction cranes and offshore oil drilling platforms. The design has since been refined and adapted for multistory building use and is available commercially from several manufacturers.

Most forms of CDD are intended for use by one, or possibly two, persons per descent, as shown in Exhibit C.1 and Exhibit C.2. The CDD equipment typically consists of a cable that can be anchored to the building, a harness or other means for securing the user, and a speed governor, as shown in Exhibit C.3. The operation of a CDD is based on gravity acting on the user,

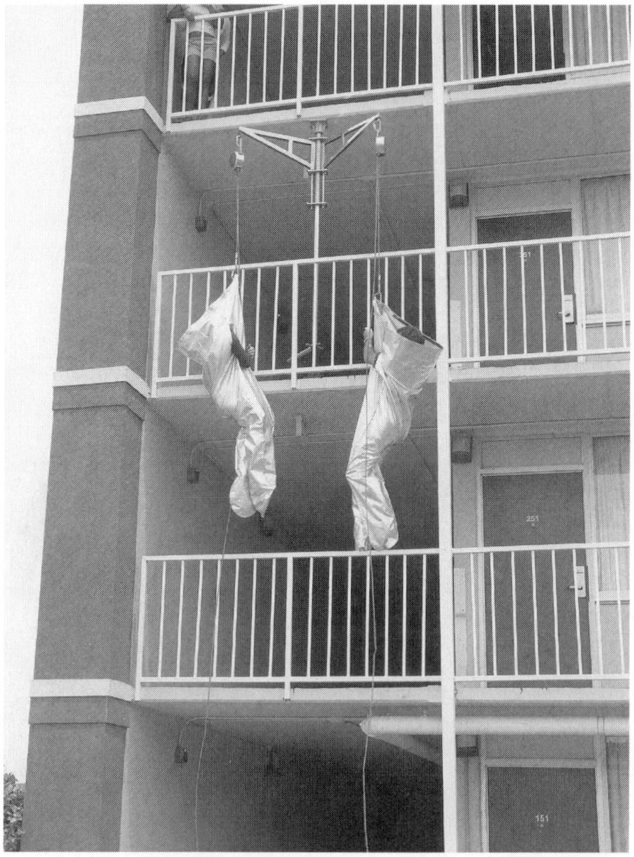

**Exhibit C.1** *Dual controlled descent device in use from apartment building balcony. (Photo courtesy of High-Rise Escape Systems, Inc.)*

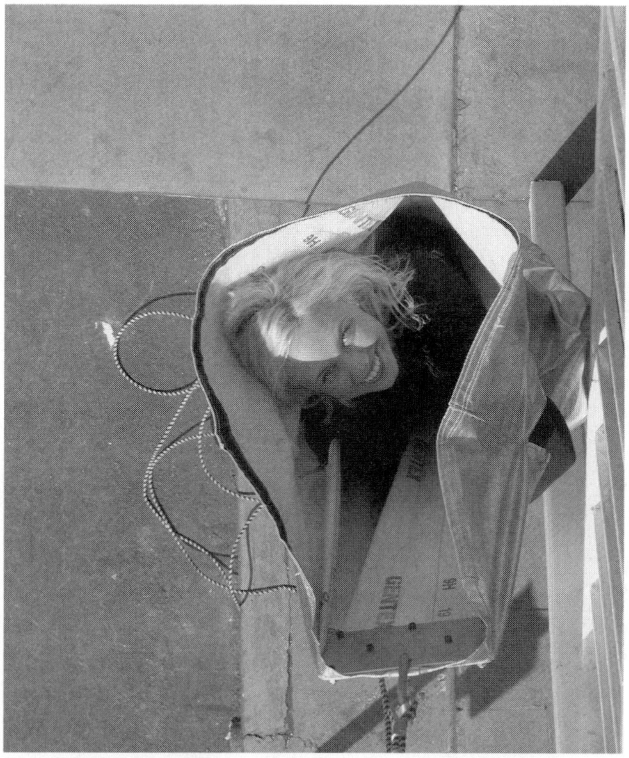

**Exhibit C.2** *Evacuee inside protective suit while using controlled descent device. (Photo courtesy of High-Rise Escape Systems, Inc.)*

while the device limits the rate of descent. A generally constant velocity is achieved once the user steps free of the building, but the speed is limited by the product specification standard (which uses metric units as its primary units; see C.4(1) for the reference) to 2.0 m/s (6.7 ft/s), which is equivalent to the rate experienced by a person jumping to the ground from a height of approximately 200 mm (8 in.). Most products allow the user to move laterally while descending by pressing hands or feet against the building face and pushing sideways. Some products are one-use devices, while others can be used repeatedly by various means of multiple cables and harnesses, or by retrieving and redeploying the cable and the harness.

**C.1.1.2 Platform Rescue System.** An enclosed platform or set of enclosed platforms, moving vertically along guides or other means on the exterior of a building or structure, intended for the evacuation of multiple occupants from an upper level or levels to the ground or other safe location that has the capability of transporting emergency responders to upper levels of a building.

A platform rescue system bears conceptual similarity to a lifeboat on a ship and to a window washer's platform. A platform rescue system consists of one or more enclosed cabins, each with a rigid platform that can transport multiple building occupants per descent. The rigid platforms with enclosed cabins travel vertically on one or more guideways at the exterior of a building wall. By the nature of its operation, the platform rescue system includes a source of mechanical power for raising, as well as lowering, the platforms. At the time this commentary was prepared, two forms of platform rescue systems appeared to have commercial potential: one system is permanently installed at, and structurally supported from, the roof of the building, such as that shown in Exhibit C.4, and the other is portable, arrives at the building on a truck, and then is supported and controlled from

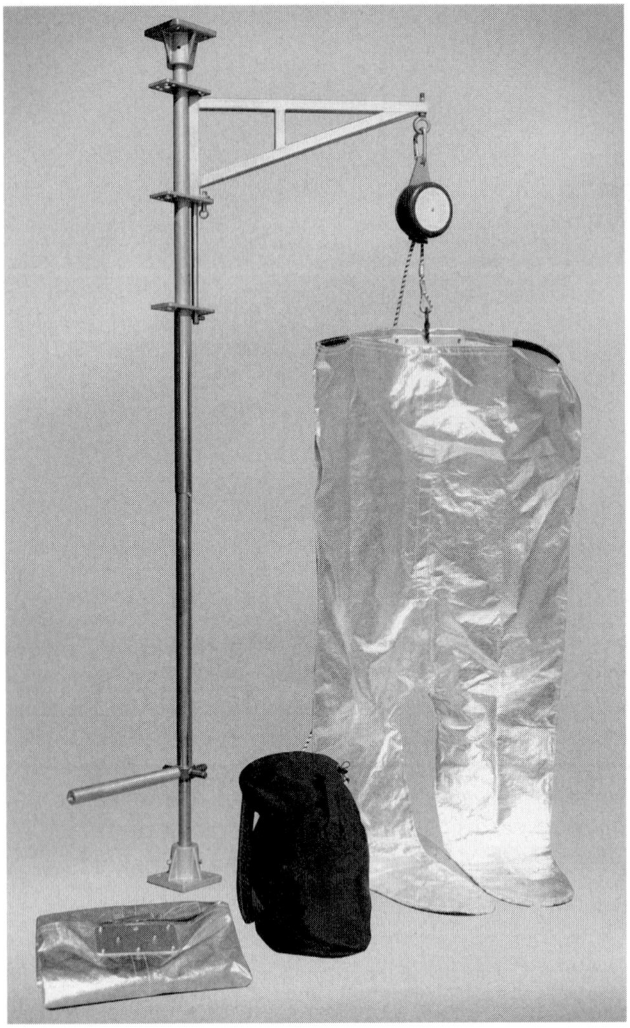

**Exhibit C.3** *Controlled descent equipment, consisting of the anchor assembly, cable, protective suit, and speed governor. (Photo courtesy of High-Rise Escape Systems, Inc.)*

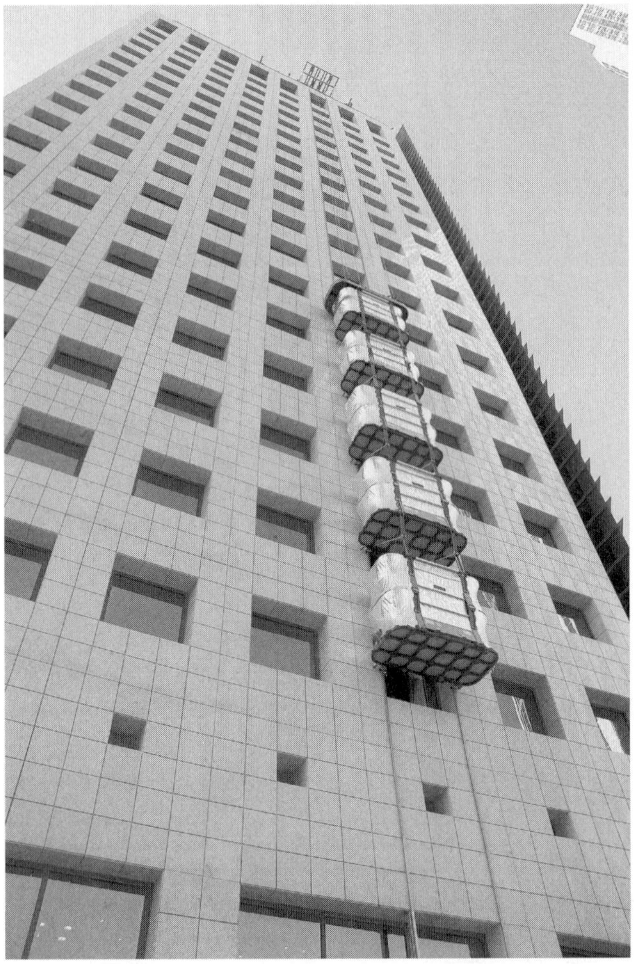

**Exhibit C.4** *Roof-supported platform rescue system with multiple platforms as installed on high-rise building. (Photo courtesy of Escape Rescue Systems, Ltd.)*

ground level. The roof-supported system depicted in Exhibit C.4 is equipped with five platforms and can be used to evacuate approximately 200 people per trip. Exhibit C.5 depicts occupants as they leave the cabin enclosure and move away from the building. The cabin enclosure is made to collapse and store against the platform to permit the next platform to descend to ground level and discharge its occupants. The process repeats until the topmost platform reaches ground level and discharges its occupants.

Because the platform systems can ascend with a load, as well as descend, they have the capability to transport equipment and emergency responders to upper floors of the building on each return trip.

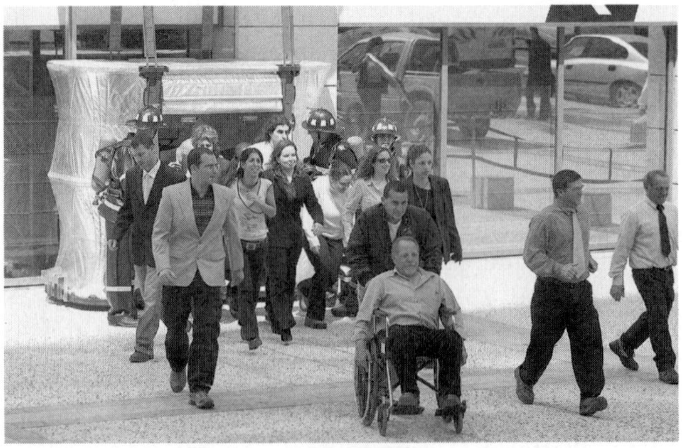

**Exhibit C.5** *Ground level discharge of evacuees from cabin of roof-supported platform rescue system. (Photo courtesy of Escape Rescue Systems, Ltd.)*

**C.1.1.3 Supplemental Escape Device or System.** Dedicated equipment that supplements the means of egress or means of escape for exiting a building or structure.

Note: Supplemental escape devices and systems are not a substitute for the required means of egress or means of escape. If properly installed, maintained, and used, controlled descent devices and platform rescue systems might provide an added means of escape for the occupants where the required means of egress or means of escape is not usable or accessible, and where the event that has caused failure of the required system has not also impaired the functionality of the device or system itself.

**C.1.1.4 Supplemental Evacuation Equipment.** Devices or systems that are not a part of the required means of egress or escape, but that might enhance use of the means of egress or escape, or provide an alternate to the means of egress or escape.

### C.1.2 Reserved.

## C.2 Supplemental Escape Devices or Systems

The fundamental requirements for the installation, maintenance, and use of supplemental escape devices and systems are found in Section C.2. These requirements apply, regardless of the technology involved, including application to any new technologies developed subsequent to the publication of the 2009 edition of the *Code*.

Annex C is not intended to limit or regulate the personal use of escape devices, such as chain ladders in a single-family home, where the equipment is selected, installed, and used by the homeowner and family. See the first paragraph of the note that follows the first paragraph of Section C.2. This exclusion should also extend to an individual apartment owner/occupant, where intended for personal use by the owner/occupant and family. Conversely, where a multistory building developer, owner, or manager proposes installation of multiple devices and systems for use by occupants, Annex C would apply.

Although Annex C is not intended to regulate equipment like chain ladders, there is a product standard, ASTM F 2175, *Standard Specification for Portable and Permanent Emergency Escape Ladders for Residential Use*,[2] for chain ladders of the type illustrated in Exhibit C.6. At least one manufacturer's product has been evaluated and certified as being compliant with the standard.

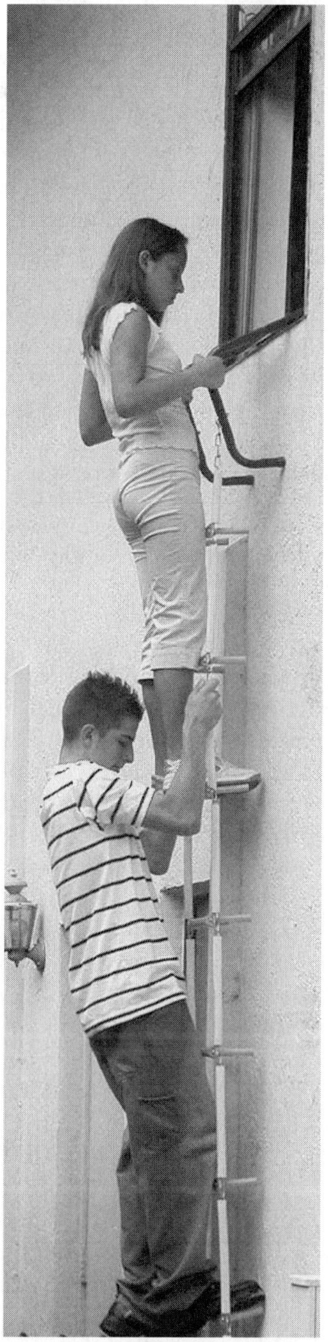

***Exhibit C.6*** *Portable escape ladder in use on a single-family dwelling. The portable escape ladder depicted is for use by the home owner and family and is not addressed by Annex C. (Photo courtesy of Bold Industries)*

A supplemental escape device or system, other than that provided or installed for use by the owner and owner's family, and the installation of such device or system, shall comply with Sections C.3 or C.4, as appropriate, and the following criteria:

Note: The provisions of Section C.2 are not intended to preclude the installation of supplemental escape devices or systems that do not meet these requirements where intended for personal use, such as by an owner and family.

It should be recognized that supplemental escape devices or systems addressed by these requirements are intended to be used only when all other means of egress are unusable and remaining in place to await the restoration of the means of egress is considered untenable.

Generally, fire departments have the capability of providing external rescue of building occupants within reach of their portable ladders, aerial ladders, and aerial platform devices. Where a fire department responds to a building emergency and has the capability to provide timely assistance with external rescue, that assistance should be used instead of the supplemental escape devices or systems.

(1) Each supplemental escape device or system shall be of an approved type and shall comply with an approved product safety standard.

The detailed specifications and performance requirements for a particular type of product are best suited for placement in a product standard. The provision of C.2(1) requires that supplemental escape devices and systems comply with an approved product standard. Annex C recognizes two acceptable standards for supplemental escape devices and systems: ASTM E 2484, *Standard Specification for High-Rise Building External Evacuation Controlled Descent Devices*,[3] and ASTM E 2513, *Standard Specification for Multi-Story Building External Evacuation Platform Rescue Systems*,[4] for controlled descent devices and platform rescue systems, respectively. Other standards might be used for this purpose if acceptable to the AHJ as indicated in the definition of the term *approved* in 3.2.1. For example, a manufacturer might propose using ASME A17.7/CSA B 44.7, *Performance-Based Safety Code for Elevators and Escalators*,[5] as the approved product safety standard required by C.2(1). If the use of ASME A17.7/CSA B 44.7 is approved by the AHJ, then ASME A17.7/CSA B 44.7 would apply instead of ASTM E 2513.

ASTM E 2484 for controlled descent devices, referenced in the preceding paragraph and cited in Annex D, Informational References, is the 2006 edition. Subsequent to its inclusion in the committee work that produced Annex C, the standard was revised and published as ASTM E 2484, *Standard Specification for Multi-Story Building External Evacuation Controlled Descent Devices*.[6] Based on comments received during the ASTM revision process, the term *multi-story* replaced the term *high-rise*, which has a specific definition in the *Code* (see 3.3.32.7). The former title of ASTM E 2484 incorrectly suggested that the equipment was not suitable for use on buildings lower in height than a high-rise building. Several substantive changes regarding test procedures, as well as some editorial changes, were also made for the 2008 edition of ASTM E 2484.

Based on the current structure and language of Annex C, it is likely that future technologies will be incorporated into the annex only after a product standard specific to that technology has been developed and published.

(2) The installation of escape devices or systems shall be approved.

Annex C grants the AHJ the authority to approve the product, the product standard, the installation, and the evacuation plan, where one is required.

Note: Use of a supplemental escape device or system typically requires that a window or exterior door be opened. The window or door should be closed, except when it is in use for escape. Where the design of the building does not provide exterior doors or operable windows and a window must be broken to use the device or system, consideration should be given to the probable effect of that action, such as showering the emergency response personnel and equipment below with sharp pieces of glass. In such a situation, to obtain approval, it might be appropriate to require tempered safety glass on windows that must be broken to deploy the supplemental escape device and access the system.

(3) The supplemental escape device or system shall be installed, inspected, tested, maintained, and used in accordance with the manufacturer's instructions.

(4) The location of each supplemental escape system access point shall be identified with a readily visible sign complying with the following:

(a) The sign shall be in plainly legible letters that read SUPPLEMENTAL ESCAPE DEVICE.

(b) The minimum height of the lettering shall be $^3/_4$ in. (19 mm), with a stroke width of $^1/_8$ in. (3 mm).

Since supplemental devices and systems will only be used on rare occasions, it is important that signage and instructions be provided where the equipment is located and that the signage be readily understandable to the user.

(5) Each sign required by C.2(4) shall comply with the following:

(a) The sign shall include the following in plainly legible letters: "Use only when exits are not accessible and building evacuation is imperative, as directed by authorized building personnel or emergency responders."
(b) The minimum height of the lettering shall be $^1/_2$ in. (13 mm).

(6) A sign with instructions for use of the escape device or system shall be provided and shall comply with the following:

(a) The sign shall be posted at the equipment and the equipment's access location.
(b) The minimum height of lettering on the instructions shall be $^1/_2$ in. (13 mm).
(c) Pictographs demonstrating use of the escape device or system shall be provided.

Note: Given the nature of the probable circumstances surrounding its deployment, the proper use of the supplemental escape device or system should be readily apparent to the user or trained operator.

(7) The signs and instructions specified in C.2(4), (5), and (6) shall be illuminated as follows:

(a) The signs shall be continuously illuminated while the building is occupied.
(b) The level of illumination provided shall be in accordance with 7.10.6.3, 7.10.7.2, or an approved equivalent.

(8) Where emergency lighting is required by Chapters 11 through 43, it shall be provided as follows:

(a) The illumination shall be in accordance with 7.9.1.
(b) The level of illumination required by 7.9.2.1 shall be provided to illuminate the supplemental escape device or system at its access location and the required signage.

(9) The supplemental escape device or system and its installation shall accommodate persons with various disabilities and of all ages.

Providing access to new buildings for persons with severe mobility impairment (see 3.3.228) triggers a need to provide accessible means of egress in accordance with 7.5.4. Ongoing technological development of elevators that are suitable for use during an emergency evacuation supplements the current requirements for accessible means of egress, so as to provide persons with mobility impairment with an egress system that is nearly equivalent to that which enclosed exit stairs provide to persons capable of using the stairs. However, any new elevator technology might not be implemented readily in existing buildings. Addressing the needs of persons with mobility impairment in existing buildings remains a challenge. Where building stairs can accommodate a stair descent device [see 7.2.12.2.3(2) and the extensive advisory text of A.7.2.12.2.3(2)], such equipment might be used to evacuate persons with mobility impairment. The external supplemental devices and systems addressed by Annex C offer an alternative that can enhance the safety of persons who cannot use the stairs, even if stairs are available for evacuation. Where external supplemental devices and systems are to be used for evacuating persons with mobility impairment while exit stairs are still in service, such procedure needs to be incorporated into the facility's evacuation plan.

Note: It is not the intent of C.2(9) that access ramps, doorways, controls, signage, and other features of the supplemental escape device or system meet all requirements for accessibility for persons with disabilities. The equipment is supplemental in nature and is not recognized as part of the required means of egress. A number of other occupants should be trained to assist persons with disabilities to access the equipment. In selecting the equipment and approving the installation, consideration should be given to how persons with mobility impairments will access the equipment.

Even when exit stairs are usable, elevators might not be able to be used. Use of a supplemental escape device or system to evacuate persons with mobility impairments might be desirable. Such circumstances should be considered and incorporated into the facility's evacuation plan, which should also identify the trained operators authorized to deploy the equipment for such use.

(10) The installation shall be approved such that use of the supplemental escape device or system shall not cause any harm or injury to the user, operator, or others who might be in the vicinity of the equipment when in use.

Evaluating and approving an installation that is safe for the user, the operator, and others requires experienced judgment. There is no expectation that all risk can be eliminated from an installation of supplemental devices and systems. The evaluation of the risk should be analogous to an evaluation of the use of stairs that provide a significant level of protection to evacuees within the stairwell but that still have the potential for an enclosure door to fail to latch, allowing smoke and heat to enter the stair enclosure, or for evacuees to stumble and fall, causing injury to themselves and others on the stairs.

(11) Where an evacuation plan is required by Chapters 11 through 43, or by other regulation, an approved, written evacuation plan shall be provided as follows:

(a) The plan shall be in accordance with 4.8.2.
(b) The plan shall not rely on the use of supplemental escape devices and systems but shall accommodate the use of such a system by specifying the following:
   i. Role of the supplemental escape device or system in the overall plan
   ii. Role and authority of emergency response personnel with respect to the supplemental escape device or system
   iii. Person or persons authorized to direct the deployment of, and to operate, the escape device or system
   iv. Special considerations, if any, that affect the usability of the supplemental escape device or system
   v. Training required for operators and users

Annex C does not require that a building have an evacuation plan. An evacuation plan is a component of an emergency plan, as addressed by Section 4.8 [see 4.8.2.1(3)]. The provisions of Section 4.8 apply where required by other chapters of the *Code*. Evacuation plans are required by the *Code* provisions for emergency plans in assembly, educational, day-care, health care, ambulatory health care, detention and correctional, hotel and dormitory, residential board and care, mercantile, and business occupancies. For an example of an occupancy that requires an emergency plan and the related paper trail that leads to the requirement for an evacuation plan, see 12/13.7.13.1 and 4.8.2.1(3). The provision of C.2(11) specifies that, in those occupancies where supplemental escape devices or systems are installed, and in which an evacuation plan is required, the required evacuation plan must include criteria related to the use of the supplemental escape devices or systems. Note the criteria that are to be addressed specifically, as detailed in C.2(11)(b)i. through v.

Note: An evacuation plan can be a highly effective tool in determining who should be evacuated under various scenarios and how that evacuation will be accomplished. Even where none is required, an evacuation plan is recommended to identify, among other things, those persons who are authorized to deploy supplemental escape devices and systems.

The more sophisticated the equipment and the greater the number of potential evacuees, the greater is the need to have a trained and authorized person decide which equipment to deploy and when it should be deployed, based on the circumstances at the time. Such a person would be the incident commander, typically the emergency response officer in charge, whether from a private brigade or public service.

Even where a building or facility is not required to have an approved evacuation plan by the *Code*, the supplemental escape device or system operating procedures should be integrated into the building evacuation and emergency procedures to the extent provided.

(12) User and operator training shall be provided in conjunction with the installation of the supplemental escape device or system, and periodically thereafter. Where an approved evacuation plan is required, training shall be provided in accordance with the approved plan.

This text of C.2(12) does not specify a frequency for periodic training. The frequency should be tailored to the individual building and situation. Conducting training in conjunction with periodic evacuation drills will help to refresh the knowledge of potential users of the supplemental escape devices or systems.

(13) The supplemental escape device or system shall be inspected and tested in accordance with the manufacturer's instructions but not less frequently than annually. Notification of testing shall be provided to building occupants or the authority having jurisdiction, as appropriate. Written records of the inspection and testing shall be maintained by the owner for a minimum of 1 year after the next scheduled inspection and testing.

Although C.2(13) requires that inspection, testing, and maintenance be performed not less frequently than once per year, the manufacturer's instructions might mandate that such activities be conducted more frequently for some of the functions, components, or subsystems of the supplemental escape device or system. Any manufacturer's requirement that inspection, testing, and maintenance be conducted more frequently than once per year needs to take precedence over the frequency specified by C.2(12).

The testing of supplemental escape devices or systems provides an opportunity for the AHJ and building personnel to familiarize themselves with the equipment and its operation. Advance notification of testing, where provided to the AHJ and building personnel, can help to ensure a participation level that serves multiple educational needs. The testing activities might be done in conjunction with demonstrations and other training for the occupants who might have to use the equipment under emergency conditions.

Note: It is important that the supplemental escape device or system does not remain idle for many years in order to help ensure that it will be functional if it does need to be used. The manufacturer's instructions for the particular model of equipment involved should be followed.

(14) Supplemental escape devices and systems shall be listed, certified, or approved to operate as intended over the prevalent climatic conditions for the location in which they are installed.

ASTM E 2513 and ASTM E 2484 [see the commentary that follows C.2(1)] specify that the equipment must perform as intended under a range of temperature, wind, rain, snow, and ice conditions. These specifications are typical for climates similar to much of the temperate zones of the world. Where climatic conditions different from those addressed by the standard are likely to exist, the AHJ should request documentation from the manufacturer that the equipment listing is applicable for the expected climatic conditions.

## C.3 Platform Rescue Systems

Where platform rescue systems are installed or provided, they shall comply with the following:

(1) The platform rescue system shall comply with ASTM E 2513, *Standard Specification for Multi-Story Building External Evacuation Platform Rescue Systems*, or an approved, equivalent product safety standard.
(2) The platform rescue system shall be deployed with trained operators to assist with evacuation of occupants.

Installations of platform rescue systems are more complex technologically and will, by their nature, involve the evacuation of more building occupants. Consequently, emergency responders are needed who have been trained in the use of the equipment, who are available to assist evacuees at the time the equipment is deployed, and who are proficient in maintaining communication with the incident commander. ASTM E 2513 requires voice communication between the platform rescue system operator, who typically is the incident commander, and the platform operator and occupants at all times. The required communication can be accomplished either by fixed equipment installed on the platform or by portable equipment carried by the platform operator, such as the two-way radios typically used by emergency responders.

(3) Where a fixed installation of electrical or other type power is required to operate the platform rescue system, a redundant source of power shall be provided.
(4) The installation shall be designed such that the vertical distance to be traversed by the platform rescue system shall not exceed the limit specified in the product's listing, certification, or approved installation.
(5) The platform access from within buildings shall be by ramps or stairs, and the following also shall apply:
    (a) Portable ramps and stairs shall be permitted.
    (b) The maximum slope of a ramp shall be as low as practical.
    (c) The maximum riser height of stairs shall be 9 in. (230 mm).
    (d) The minimum tread depth of stairs shall be 9 in. (230 mm).
(6) The platform access opening shall be sized in accordance with the following:
    (a) For installations in new construction, the platform access opening shall be a minimum 32 in. (810 mm) in width and a minimum 48 in. (1220 mm) in height.
    (b) For installations in existing construction, the platform access opening shall be as large as practical but shall not be required to exceed 32 in. (810 mm) in width and 48 in. (1220 mm) in height.

The dimensions required for openings to access the platform rescue system in new buildings were specified so as to be large enough to accommodate a person using a wheelchair without having to leave the wheelchair but with the assistance of another person. In existing construction, building construction elements and existing window openings might make it infeasible to create an opening as large as that required for new construction, but the openings provided should be as close as practical to the size required for installations in new construction. The provision of C.3(6)(b), for existing construction, was written in anticipation that persons who use wheelchairs might have to enter the cabin with the assistance of others but without their wheelchairs, followed by the loading of the wheelchairs. Where such procedure is anticipated, it needs to be documented in the facility's evacuation plan.

(7) The platform access and egress shall not be by ladders.
(8) Rooftop operating equipment and systems shall be protected from accumulations of climatic ice or snow and fire suppression ice.

## C.4 Controlled Descent Devices

Where controlled descent devices are installed or provided, they shall comply with the following:

(1) The controlled descent device shall comply with ASTM E 2484, *Standard Specification for High-Rise Building External Evacuation Controlled Descent Devices*, or an approved, equivalent product safety standard.
(2) The installation shall be designed such that the vertical distance to be traversed by the controlled descent device shall not exceed the limit specified in the product's listing, certification, or approved installation.
(3) Where a fixed installation of electrical or other type power is required to operate the controlled descent device, a redundant source of power shall be provided.
(4) Rooftop operating equipment and systems shall be protected from accumulations of climatic ice or snow and fire suppression ice.
(5) Controlled descent device building access openings in new building installations shall be a minimum of 32 in. (810 mm) wide and 42 in. (1065 mm) high.
(6) Controlled descent device building access openings in existing buildings shall be a minimum of 20 in. (510 mm) wide and 24 in. (610 mm) high and shall provide a clear opening of not less than 5.7 $ft^2$ (0.53 $m^2$).
(7) The approved occupant load and weight limits shall be posted adjacent to the controlled descent device installation or building access opening in minimum $^1/_2$ in. (13 mm) letters, with a minimum $^1/_{16}$ in. (1.6 mm) stroke.
(8) The occupant load and weight limits shall not be exceeded in use.

The minimum access opening dimensions specified by C.4(6) for existing buildings are the same as specified for windows for rescue in educational occupancies (see 14/15.2.11.1.1) and for secondary means of escape for residential occupancies (see 24.2.2.3.3). The opening size criteria had their advent with the provisions for educational occupancies rescue window openings of sufficient size to permit an emergency responder equipped with self-breathing apparatus to move through the opening. Such openings were chosen, as they are large enough to permit the use of the controlled descent device. Larger openings, which further facilitate use of the controlled descent device, are required by C.4(5) for installations in new buildings.

### References Cited in Commentary

1. Final Report on the Collapse of the World Trade Center Towers, Federal Building and Fire Safety Investigation of the World Trade Center Disaster, NIST NCSTAR 1, National Institute of Standards and Technology, Gaithersburg, MD, September 2005, http://wtc.nist.gov/NISTNCSTAR1CollapseofTowers.pdf
2. ASTM F 2175, *Standard Specification for Portable and Permanent Emergency Escape Ladders for Residential Use*, 2002 edition, ASTM International, 100 Barr Harbor Drive, P.O. Box C700, West Conshohocken, PA 19428-2959.
3. ASTM E 2484, *Standard Specification for High-Rise Building External Evacuation Controlled Descent Devices*, 2006 edition, ASTM International, 100 Barr Harbor Drive, P.O. Box C700, West Conshohocken, PA 19428-2959.
4. ASTM E 2513, *Standard Specification for Multi-Story Building External Evacuation Platform Rescue Systems*, 2007 edition, ASTM International, 100 Barr Harbor Drive, P.O. Box C700, West Conshohocken, PA 19428-2959.
5. ASME A17.7/CSA B 44.7, *Performance-Based Safety Code for Elevators and Escalators*, 2007 edition, American Society of Mechanical Engineers, Three Park Avenue, New York, NY 10016-5990.
6. ASTM E 2484, *Standard Specification for Multi-Story Building External Evacuation Controlled Descent Devices*, 2008 edition, ASTM International, 100 Barr Harbor Drive, P.O. Box C700, West Conshohocken, PA 19428-2959.

ANNEX D

# Informational References

## D.1 Referenced Publications

The documents or portions thereof listed in this annex are referenced within the informational sections of this code and are not part of the requirements of this document unless also listed in Chapter 2 for other reasons.

Note that mandatory referenced publications appear in Chapter 2. Many of the documents shown in Annex D also appear in Chapter 2, and, although shown here for advisory purposes, they remain mandatory in the body of the *Code* (Chapters 1 through 43).

### D.1.1 NFPA Publications.

National Fire Protection Association, 1 Batterymarch Park, Quincy, MA 02169-7471.

NFPA 1, *Fire Code*, 2009 edition.

NFPA 10, *Standard for Portable Fire Extinguishers*, 2007 edition.

NFPA 13, *Standard for the Installation of Sprinkler Systems*, 2007 edition.

NFPA 13D, *Standard for the Installation of Sprinkler Systems in One- and Two-Family Dwellings and Manufactured Homes*, 2007 edition.

NFPA 13R, *Standard for the Installation of Sprinkler Systems in Residential Occupancies up to and Including Four Stories in Height*, 2007 edition.

NFPA 14, *Standard for the Installation of Standpipe and Hose Systems*, 2007 edition.

NFPA 22, *Standard for Water Tanks for Private Fire Protection*, 2008 edition.

NFPA 25, *Standard for the Inspection, Testing, and Maintenance of Water-Based Fire Protection Systems*, 2008 edition.

NFPA 30, *Flammable and Combustible Liquids Code*, 2008 edition.

NFPA 58, *Liquefied Petroleum Gas Code*, 2008 edition.

NFPA 61, *Standard for the Prevention of Fires and Dust Explosions in Agricultural and Food Processing Facilities*, 2008 edition.

NFPA 68, *Standard on Explosion Protection by Deflagration Venting*, 2007 edition.

*NFPA 70®*, *National Electrical Code®*, 2008 edition.

*NFPA 72®*, *National Fire Alarm Code®*, 2007 edition.

NFPA 80, *Standard for Fire Doors and Other Opening Protectives*, 2007 edition.

NFPA 82, *Standard on Incinerators and Waste and Linen Handling Systems and Equipment*, 2004 edition.

NFPA 90A, *Standard for the Installation of Air-Conditioning and Ventilating Systems*, 2009 edition.

NFPA 92A, *Standard for Smoke-Control Systems Utilizing Barriers and Pressure Differences*, 2009 edition.

NFPA 92B, *Standard for Smoke Management Systems in Malls, Atria, and Large Spaces*, 2009 edition.

NFPA 96, *Standard for Ventilation Control and Fire Protection of Commercial Cooking Operations*, 2008 edition.

NFPA 99, *Standard for Health Care Facilities*, 2005 edition.

NFPA 101A, *Guide on Alternative Approaches to Life Safety*, 2007 edition.

NFPA 105, *Standard for the Installation of Smoke Door Assemblies and Other Opening Protectives*, 2007 edition.

NFPA 110, *Standard for Emergency and Standby Power Systems*, 2005 edition.

NFPA 170, *Standard for Fire Safety and Emergency Symbols*, 2006 edition.

NFPA 204, *Standard for Smoke and Heat Venting*, 2007 edition.

NFPA 211, *Standard for Chimneys, Fireplaces, Vents, and Solid Fuel–Burning Appliances*, 2006 edition.

NFPA 220, *Standard on Types of Building Construction*, 2009 edition.

NFPA 241, *Standard for Safeguarding Construction, Alteration, and Demolition Operations*, 2004 edition.

NFPA 251, *Standard Methods of Tests of Fire Resistance of Building Construction and Materials*, 2006 edition.

NFPA 253, *Standard Method of Test for Critical Radiant Flux of Floor Covering Systems Using a Radiant Heat Energy Source*, 2006 edition.

NFPA 255, *Standard Method of Test of Surface Burning Characteristics of Building Materials*, 2006 edition.

NFPA 259, *Standard Test Method for Potential Heat of Building Materials*, 2008 edition.

NFPA 260, *Standard Methods of Tests and Classification System for Cigarette Ignition Resistance of Components of Upholstered Furniture*, 2009 edition.

NFPA 261, *Standard Method of Test for Determining Resistance of Mock-Up Upholstered Furniture Material Assemblies to Ignition by Smoldering Cigarettes*, 2009 edition.

NFPA 265, *Standard Methods of Fire Tests for Evaluating Room Fire Growth Contribution of Textile Coverings on Full Height Panels and Walls*, 2007 edition.

NFPA 269, *Standard Test Method for Developing Toxic Potency Data for Use in Fire Hazard Modeling*, 2007 edition.

NFPA 286, *Standard Methods of Fire Tests for Evaluating Contribution of Wall and Ceiling Interior Finish to Room Fire Growth*, 2006 edition.

NFPA 307, *Standard for the Construction and Fire Protection of Marine Terminals, Piers, and Wharves*, 2006 edition.

NFPA 409, *Standard on Aircraft Hangars*, 2004 edition.

NFPA 501A, *Standard for Fire Safety Criteria for Manufactured Home Installations, Sites, and Communities*, 2005 edition.

NFPA 551, *Guide for the Evaluation of Fire Risk Assessments*, 2007 edition.

NFPA 601, *Standard for Security Services in Fire Loss Prevention*, 2005 edition.

NFPA 701, *Standard Methods of Fire Tests for Flame Propagation of Textiles and Films*, 2004 edition.

NFPA 703, *Standard for Fire Retardant–Treated Wood and Fire-Retardant Coatings for Building Materials*, 2009 edition.

NFPA 914, *Code for Fire Protection of Historic Structures*, 2007 edition.

NFPA 1124, *Code for the Manufacture, Transportation, Storage, and Retail Sales of Fireworks and Pyrotechnic Articles*, 2006 edition.

NFPA 1221, *Standard for the Installation, Maintenance, and Use of Emergency Services Communications Systems*, 2007 edition.

NFPA 1600, *Standard on Disaster/Emergency Management and Business Continuity Programs*, 2007 edition.

*NFPA 5000®, Building Construction and Safety Code®*, 2009 edition.

NFPA *Fire Protection Handbook*, 19th edition, 2003.

NFPA *Fire Protection Handbook*, 20th edition, 2008.

Waksman, D. and J. B. Ferguson. August 1974. Fire Tests of Building Interior Covering Systems. In *Fire Technology* 10:211–220.

*SFPE Handbook of Fire Protection Engineering*, 3rd edition, National Fire Protection Association, 1 Batterymarch Park, P. O. Box 9101, Quincy, MA 02269-9101.

### D.1.2 Other Publications.

**D.1.2.1 ACI Publication.** American Concrete Institute, P.O. Box 9094, Farmington Hills, MI 48333. www.concrete.org

ACI 216.1/TMS 0216.1, *Standard Method for Determining Fire Resistance of Concrete and Masonry Assemblies*, 1997.

**D.1.2.2 ANSI Publications.** American National Standards Institute, Inc., 25 West 43rd Street, 4th floor, New York, NY 10036. www.ansi.org

ANSI/BHMA A156.10, *American National Standard for Power Operated Pedestrian Doors*, 1999.

ANSI/BHMA A156.19, *American National Standard for Power Assist and Low Energy Power Operated Doors*, 2002.

ICC/ANSI A117.1, *American National Standard for Accessible and Usable Buildings and Facilities*, 2003.

**D.1.2.3 ASCE Publications.** American Society of Civil Engineers, 1801 Alexander Bell Drive, Reston, VA 20191-4400. www.asce.org

ASCE/SFPE 29, *Standard Calculation Methods for Structural Fire Protection*, 1999.

**D.1.2.4 ASHRAE Publications.** American Society of Heating, Refrigerating and Air Conditioning Engineers, Inc., 1791 Tullie Circle, NE, Atlanta, GA 30329-2305. www.ashrae.org

ASHRAE *Handbook and Product Directory — Fundamentals*, 2001.

Klote, J.H., and Milke, J.A., *Principles of Smoke Management*, 2002.

**D.1.2.5 ASME Publications.** American Society of Mechanical Engineers, Three Park Avenue, New York, NY 10016-5990. www.asme.org

ASME A17.1/CSA B44, *Safety Code for Elevators and Escalators*, 2006.

ASME A17.3, *Safety Code for Existing Elevators and Escalators*, 2005.

**D.1.2.6 ASTM Publications.** ASTM International, 100 Barr Harbor Drive, P.O. Box C700, West Conshohocken, PA 19428-2959. www.astm.org

ASTM C 1629/C 1629M, *Standard Classification for Abuse-Resistant Nondecorated Interior Gypsum Panel Products and Fiber-Reinforced Cement Panels*, 2005.

ASTM D 2859, *Standard Test Method for Ignition Characteristics of Finished Textile Floor Covering Materials*, 2004.

ASTM E 84, *Standard Test Method for Surface Burning Characteristics of Building Materials,* 2004.

ASTM E 119, *Standard Test Methods for Fire Tests of Building Construction and Materials*, 2007a.

ASTM E 814, *Standard Test Method for Fire Tests of Through-Penetration Fire Stops*, 2002.

ASTM E 1352, *Standard Test Method for Cigarette Ignition Resistance of Mock-Up Upholstered Furniture Assemblies*, 2002.

ASTM E 1353, *Standard Test Methods for Cigarette Ignition Resistance of Components of Upholstered Furniture*, 2002.

ASTM E 1355, *Standard Guide for Evaluating the Predictive Capability of Deterministic Fire Models*, 2004.

ASTM E 1472, *Standard Guide for Documenting Computer Software for Fire Models*, 2003.

ASTM E 1537, *Standard Test Method for Fire Testing of Upholstered Furniture*, 2002.

ASTM E 1590, *Standard Test Method for Fire Testing of Mattresses*, 2002.

ASTM E 1996, *Standard Test Method for Fire-Resistive Joint Systems*, 2001.

ASTM E 2030, *Guide for Recommended Uses of Photoluminescent (Phosphorescent) Safety Markings*, 2002.

ASTM E 2174, *Standard Practice for On-Site Inspection of Installed Fire Stops*, 2001.

ASTM E 2238, *Standard Guide for Evacuation Route Diagrams*, 2002.

ASTM E 2280, *Standard Guide for Fire Hazard Assessment of the Effect of Upholstered Seating Furniture Within Patient Rooms of Health Care Facilities*, 2003.

ASTM E 2307, *Standard Test Method for Determining Fire Resistance of Perimeter Fire Barrier Systems Using Intermediate-Scale, Multi-Story Test Apparatus*, 2004e1.

ASTM E 2393, *Standard Practice for On-Site Inspection of Installed Fire Resistive Joint Systems and Perimeter Fire Barriers*, 2004.

ASTM E 2484, *Standard Specification for High-Rise Building External Evacuation Controlled Descent Devices*, 2006.

ASTM E 2513, *Standard Specification for Multi-Story Building External Evacuation Platform Rescue Systems*, 2007.

ASTM F 1637, *Standard Practice for Safe Walking Surfaces*, 2004.

ASTM F 1870, *Standard Guide for Selection of Fire Test Methods for the Assessment of Upholstered Furnishings in Detention and Correctional Facilities*, 2005.

**D.1.2.7 FMGR Publications.** FM Global Research, FM Global, 1301 Atwood Avenue, P.O. Box 7500, Johnston, RI 02919. www.fmglobal.com

FM 4880, *Approval Standard for Class I Insulated Wall or Wall and Roof/Ceiling Panels; Plastic Interior Finish Materials; Plastic Exterior Building Panels; Wall/Ceiling Coating Systems; Interior or Exterior Finish Systems*, 1994.

**D.1.2.8 NEMA Publications.** National Electrical Manufacturers Association, 1300 North 17th Street, Suite 1847, Rosslyn, VA 22209.

NEMA SB 30, *Fire Service Annunciator and Interface*, 2005.

ANSI/NEMA Z535.1, *Standard for Safety Colors*, 2006.

**D.1.2.9 NIST Publications.** National Institute of Standards and Technology, 100 Bureau Drive, Gaithersburg, MD 20899-1070. www.nist.gov

NISTIR 5445, *Feasibility of Fire Evacuation by Elevators at FAA Control Towers*, 1994.

**D.1.2.10 SFPE Publications.** Society of Fire Protection Engineers, 7315 Wisconsin Avenue, Suite 1225 W, Bethesda, MD 20814. www.sfpe.org

*SFPE Computer Software Directory.*

*SFPE Enforcer's Guide to Performance-Based Design Review.*

*SFPE Engineering Guide — Evaluation of the Computer Fire Model DETACT-QS.*

*SFPE Engineering Guide to Human Behavior in Fire.*

*SFPE Engineering Guide to Performance-Based Fire Protection Analysis and Design of Buildings*, 1998.

*SFPE Guidelines for Peer Review in the Fire Protection Design Process.*

**D.1.2.11 UL Publications.** Underwriters Laboratories Inc., 333 Pfingsten Road, Northbrook, IL 60062-2096. www.ul.com

UL *Fire Resistance Directory*, 2007.

ANSI/UL 263, *Standard for Fire Tests of Building Construction and Materials*, 2003.

ANSI/UL 723, *Standard for Test for Surface Burning Characteristics of Building Materials,* 2003, Revised 2005.

ANSI/UL 1040, *Standard for Fire Test of Insulated Wall Construction*, 1996, Revised 2001.

ANSI/UL 1479, *Standard for Fire Tests of Through-Penetration Firestops*, 2003, Revised 2007.

ANSI/UL 1715, *Standard for Fire Test of Interior Finish Material*, 1997, Revised 2004.

UL Subject 1724, *Outline of Investigation for Fire Tests for Electrical Circuit Protective Systems*, 1991.

UL 1975, *Standard for Fire Tests for Foamed Plastics Used for Decorative Purposes*, 2006.

ANSI/UL 2079, *Standard for Tests for Fire Resistance of Building Joint Systems*, 2004, Revised 2006.

UL 2196, *Tests of Fire Resistive Cables*, 2001.

**D.1.2.12 U.S. Government Publications.** U.S. Government Printing Office, Washington, DC 20402. www.access.gpo.gov/

Title 16, *Code of Federal Regulations*, Part 1630, "Standard for the Surface Flammability of Carpets and Rugs" (FF 1-70).

Title 16, *Code of Federal Regulations*, Part 1632, "Standard for the Flammability of Mattresses and Mattress Pads" (FF 4-72).

Title 28, *Code of Federal Regulations*, Part 36, Appendix A, "Americans with Disabilities Act Accessibility Guidelines for Buildings and Facilities."

Title 29, *Code of Federal Regulations*, Part 1910, Subparts E and L, "OSHA Regulations for Emergency Procedures and Fire Brigades."

Title 29, *Code of Federal Regulations*, Part 1910.146, "Permit-Required Confined Spaces."

## D.2 Informational References

The following documents or portions thereof are listed here as informational resources only. They are not a part of the requirements of this document.

*Australian Fire Engineering Guidelines*. 1996. Sydney, Australia: Fire Code Perform Centre, Ltd.

*British Standard Firesafety Engineering in Buildings*, DD240: Part 1. 1997. London, England: British Standards Institution.

Endsley, Bolte, and Jones. *Designing for Situation Awareness: An approach to user-centered design*. 2003. Boca Raton, FL: CRC Press, Taylor and Francis.

Freeman, J. R. 1889. Experiments relating to hydraulics of fire streams. Paper No. 426, *Transactions*, American Society of Civil Engineers, XXI:380–83.

Gann, R. G., V. Babrauskas, R. D. Peacock, and J. R. Hall. 1994. Fire conditions for smoke toxicity measurement. *Fire and Materials* 18(193): 193–99.

Groner, N. E., and M. L. Levin. 1992. Human factor considerations in the potential for using elevators in building emergency evacuation plans, NIST-GCR-92-615. Gaithersburg, MD: National Institute of Standards and Technology.

Kaplan, H. L., and G. E. Hartzell. 1984. Modeling of toxicological effects of fire gases: I. Incapacitation effects of narcotic fire gases. *Journal of Fire Sciences* 2:286–305.

Klote, J. H., B. M. Levin, and N. E. Groner. 1994. Feasibility of fire evacuations by elevators at FAA control towers, NISTIR 5445. Gaithersburg, MD: National Institute of Standards and Technology.

Klote, J. H., B. M. Levin, and N. E Groner. "Feasibility of Fire Evacuation by Elevators at FAA Control Towers," National Institute of Standards and Technology, NISTIR 5443, 1994.

Levin, B. M., and N. E. Groner. 1992. Human behavior aspects of staging areas for fire safety in GSA buildings, NIST-GCR-92-606. Gaithersburg, MD: National Institute of Standards and Technology.

Levin, B. M., and N. E. Groner. 1994. Human factor considerations for the potential use of elevators for fire evacuation of FAA air traffic control towers, NIST-GCR-94-656. Gaithersburg, MD: National Institute of Standards and Technology.

Olenick, S., and D. Carpenter. 2003. An updated international survey of computer models for fire and smoke. *Journal of Fire Protection Engineering* 3(2):87–110.

Seigel, L. G. 1969. The protection of flames from burning buildings. *Fire Technology* 5(1):43–51.

Templer, J. A. 1992. *The Staircase: Studies of Hazards, Falls, and Safer Design*. Cambridge, MA: MIT Press.

Tu, K.-M., and S. Davis. 1976. Flame spread of carpet systems involved in room fires, NFSIR 76-1013. Washington, DC: Center for Fire Research, National Bureau of Standards.

## D.3 References for Extracts in Informational Sections

*NFPA 5000®, Building Construction and Safety Code®*, 2009 edition.

**PART TWO**

# Supplements

The four supplements collected in Part Two of this handbook were written by recognized experts in the fields they cover. Printed in black within a green box, these supplements are not part of the *Code* or the commentary. They present additional, useful information about specialized subjects in more depth than is allowed by the *Code*-and-commentary format of this handbook. The supplements give case histories of fires that influenced the *Life Safety Code*; give detailed information on elevator emergency operation; provide an overview of how fire test requirements interact with the requirements found in NFPA *101*; and bring the reader up to date on the changes in the *Code* since the 2006 edition. Much like the commentary, the supplements are intended to provide useful guidance for *Code* users. For further supplemental material, visit http://www.nfpa.org/101handbook.

SUPPLEMENT 1

# Case Histories: Fires Influencing the *Life Safety Code*

Paul E. Teague, M.A.
Updated by Chief Ronald R. Farr

*Editor's Note: This supplement illustrates how historically significant fires have led to improvements in the Life Safety Code.*

*Paul E. Teague, former editor of Fire Journal magazine, is a veteran award-winning engineering journalist. Currently, he is the national editor and supplements director for Design News magazine, the largest mechanical engineering magazine in the United States.*

*Ronald Farr is the Fire Chief of Kalamazoo Township Fire Department in Kalamazoo, Michigan.*

Codes and standards are living documents. Born of the efforts of men and women to make their environment safer, codes and standards grow into maturity based on fire experience and the observations and research of those responsible for them. The best codes and standards, such as those produced by NFPA, never age, as they are continually updated with new information that allows them to adapt to an ever-changing world.

Such is the case with NFPA *101*®, *Life Safety Code*®. Originally known as the *Building Exits Code*, it had its origins in the effort to make factories safer for workers in the early days of the twentieth century. Its first focus was on the hazards of stairways and fire escapes, the need for fire drills in various occupancies, and the construction and arrangement of exits.

However, as American society changed, technology blossomed, and fire experience accumulated, the *Code* grew in scope. It began to include provisions for sprinklers, alarm and detection systems, protection of interior finish, and other important features. Of the thousands of fires whose lessons are reflected in the latest edition of the *Code*, probably none has had a bigger impact than the Triangle Shirtwaist fire of March 25, 1911. It was the Triangle Shirtwaist fire that prompted creation of NFPA's Committee on Safety to Life and, ultimately, development of the *Code* itself.

## TRIANGLE SHIRTWAIST FIRE

Since its founding in 1896, NFPA has always placed special importance on its life safety work. NFPA's original objectives, "establishing proper safeguards against loss of life and property by fire," placed life safety ahead of property protection. Yet, until the Triangle Shirtwaist fire, there was not one technical committee devoted exclusively to life safety concerns.

The Triangle Shirtwaist Company was located on the eighth, ninth, and tenth floors of the Asch Building at the intersection of Washington Place and Green Street in New York City's Washington Square. The building was a "loft," typical of many in its day. The Triangle Company, with more than 500 employees, was reportedly the largest business of its kind in the city. Most of the employees were young women, many of them recent immigrants, who worked six days a week in cramped and dirty quarters.

### Numerous Fire Hazards

New York City law at the time required buildings 11 stories and higher to have stone floors and metal window frames. The Asch Building was only 10 stories high and was constructed with wood floors, wood trim, and wood window frames. Unsafe as they were, these features of the building's construction were only part of the fire danger that workers unwittingly faced every day.

Buildings with 10,000 $ft^2$ of floor space per floor were required to have three staircases per floor. The Asch Building had two. The building's architect had pleaded for approval of two staircases, because there was also an outside fire escape that could be reached by windows on each floor. The fire escape terminated at the second floor, not at the ground.

Labor laws in effect at the time required that factory doors open outward, *if practical.* The architect claimed this design was not practical in the Asch Building, because each landing was only one stair width from the door. All doors had to open inward.

Those same labor laws required that factory doors be kept unlocked during the workday. Doors at the Triangle Company reportedly were usually locked during the workday to keep track of the workers and prevent them from stealing material.

Rags consisting of cutaway cloth materials regularly accumulated on the floors. When last collected, an accumulation of 2252 pounds of rags had been removed. At the time of the fire, the rags had not been removed for about two months.

The Triangle workers were crowded together on the top three floors of the Asch Building. Aisles leading to exits were narrow and obstructed. Partitions were placed in front of doors and elevators. A fire insurance inspector had recommended in 1909 that the company keep the doors unlocked during the workday and conduct fire drills. The owners took no action on those recommendations.

**Fire Begins in the Rags.** No NFPA investigative report was written on the Triangle Shirtwaist fire, but two books describe the horror that took place: *The Triangle Shirtwaist Fire*, by Corinne Naden (Franklin Watts, Inc., 1971); and *The Triangle Fire*, by Leon Stein (J. B. Lippincott, 1962). The descriptions of the building and the fire reported here are summarized from these two books.

It was near quitting time on March 25, 1911, when one of the workers on the eighth floor noticed smoke coming from one of the rag bins. A fire in a rag bin was reportedly not unusual, but this fire spread with astonishing speed, despite the attempts of supervisors to extinguish it using pails of water. The fire spread from the rags to cutting tables and then to cloth patterns hanging on wire above the tables. In no time, flames consumed the wood floor trim, the sewing tables, and the partitions, and then spread to the ceiling.

Workers on the eighth floor rushed for the doors. One door was locked. When workers finally got it unlocked, it opened inward. The panicked workers piled up against the door, making it difficult for those who arrived first to open it. Eventually, they were able to open the door, and workers rushed into the stairway. However, some fell at the seventh floor level, and those behind piled up until there was no more room in the stairway. A policeman, who had seen the fire from the street, saw the pile-up as he ran up the stairs to help. He untangled the pile-up, and about 125 workers escaped down that stairway.

Someone used a telephone connection to the tenth-floor executive offices to report the fire. Other workers frantically rang for the elevators. Because the elevators had been summoned to the tenth floor, at first they didn't stop on the eighth floor. When they did stop, workers crowded into them, one on top of another. The elevators made so many trips to save workers on the eighth and tenth floors that the operators were overcome by smoke and exhaustion.

Some workers on the eighth floor climbed out the windows to the narrow fire escape. At least one worker fell down the fire escape to the courtyard below. Others climbed down to the sixth floor, went back into the building through a window, and walked down the inside staircase.

Many of the workers on the tenth floor escaped to the roof of the building, where law students from an adjacent building rescued them. Of the approximately 70 workers on the tenth floor, only one died. That death occurred because the victim jumped from a window.

The only telephone communication to the ninth floor was through the tenth-floor switchboard. No one on the tenth floor notified the ninth-floor workers of the fire.

**Ninth-Floor Workers Were the Last to Be Informed.** There were about 260 workers on the ninth floor. There were also eight double rows of sewing machines on 75-ft-long tables that took up nearly the entire floor. The only way to leave the tables was to walk to the north end of the building. Workers sitting at the south end had to walk the entire length of the rows of tables to reach the area where the exits were located. Along the way, they had to negotiate around chairs, wicker baskets, and other items that obstructed the passageways.

When the quitting bell rang, one worker walked down one of the stairways to go home. When he reached the eighth floor, he saw it was in flames. He was the first ninth-floor worker to learn of the fire. Confused, he simply continued moving. By the time he thought of running back up the stairs to warn his coworkers, it was too late. He was unable to get back up the stairway.

The rest of the workers on the ninth floor learned of the fire when flames leaped through the windows. About 150 people raced for the Green Street exit, and more than 100 of them made it down to the sidewalk. Others ran to the Washington Place exit, but it was locked. Some rushed for the fire escape. Jammed with people and hot from the fire, the fire escape pulled away from the building and partially collapsed, sending bodies flying to the courtyard below.

Many workers, including those who found the Washington Place exit locked, congregated at the elevators and summoned them. However, the elevators were already packed with people from the eighth and tenth floors. Some of the workers jumped or were pushed into the elevator shafts. A few slid down the cables, some landing on the roofs of the elevators.

To escape the searing heat and suffocating smoke, many of the workers climbed out to the window ledge and jumped to their deaths. The impact of their bodies was so great that it not only broke the fire department nets, but also smashed holes in the concrete and glass pavement.

The fire department arrived at the scene early, but could do little except cool the exterior of the building. The department's equipment was good for fighting fires only up to seven stories. In total, about 147 people died in the Triangle Shirtwaist fire.

### Move for Reform

The Asch Building was a firetrap, but it was not the worst one in the city. In 1910, a public agency investigated conditions in 1243 coat and suit shops. Nine days before the Triangle Shirtwaist fire, a local New York City newspaper published excerpts from the agency's report. The report stated that 99 percent of the shops were deficient in safety. Many had only one exit, many others had locked doors during the workday, and 94 percent had doors that opened inward rather than outward.

Whether that report by itself would have generated remedial action is open to question. The dismal record of previous attempts by unions and others to mobilize action indicates that improvements would not likely have been made. The Triangle Shirtwaist fire, however, illustrated more than a report ever could the dangers lurking in lofts and other types of buildings.

In fact, the Triangle Shirtwaist fire aroused the nation and eventually revolutionized an industry. Unions, particularly the garment workers' union, intensified their activities to bring about improvements in working conditions for their members. Citizens of all economic classes in New York City banded together to work for safer factories, and politicians passed new laws to protect workers.

Almost immediately after the fire, New York City residents formed the Committee on Safety. Among its members was Frances Perkins, who later became U.S. Secretary of Labor. The chairman was Henry Stimson, who soon left that position to become Secretary of War. He was succeeded as chairman by Henry Morgenthau. The committee became a focal point for efforts to pass laws mandating improvements in factories and other buildings.

In June 1911, New York Governor John Alden Dix created the New York State Factory Investigating Commission to look into conditions in all factories and allocated the commission a $10,000 budget. Chairman of the commission was Robert Wagner, Sr., then a state senator. Samuel Gompers was also on the commission.

In October of the same year, the Sullivan-Hoey Law was passed. It established the New York City Fire Prevention Bureau, the first in the country, and expanded the powers of the fire commissioner.

**NFPA Broadens Its Focus to Include Life Safety.** NFPA members were shocked but not surprised by the fire. For years, they had warned of many of the dangers present in buildings like the Asch Building, in particular fire escapes. The April 1911 *NFPA Quarterly* stated that fire escapes had long been recognized as a "delusion." For a quarter of a century, the article continued, fire escapes had "contributed the principal element of tragedy to all fires where panic resulted. Iron is quickly heated and expansion of the bolts, stays, and fastenings soon pulls the frame loose so that the weight of a single body may precipitate it into a street or alley."

At the NFPA Annual Meeting in May 1911, R. H. Newbern presented a paper on private fire departments and fire drills, declaring the value of drills in educating factory workers in procedures to help avoid panic and promote survival. A year later, Mr. Newbern's recommendations were published in a pamphlet titled "Exit Drills in Factories, Schools, Department Stores, and Theatres." This was the first safety-to-life publication produced by NFPA. However, there was still no specific NFPA committee devoted exclusively to life safety.

**Formation of the Safety to Life Committee.** At the 1913 NFPA Annual Meeting, President H. L. Phillips suggested to members that they could include "a section or committee having for its object the consideration of safety of life against accidents of every description." Later during that meeting, members listened to a speech titled "The Social and Human Cost of Fire" by Frances Perkins of the New York Committee on Safety. She urged them to study hazardous industries, publish the results, and publish rules that would help keep people in factories safe.

Perkins had witnessed the Triangle Shirtwaist fire. She had seen workers leap from the ninth floor to the street below and had been horrified. She told NFPA members that when she counted the social, human, and economic cost of that fire, she found it was enormous. "We lost not only those workers in the Triangle Shirtwaist fire," Perkins said, "we lost their valuable services to society as economic factors. . . . It is because that social and human loss is to the entire community that this problem of fire deserves the closest attention of all people who are interested in the general progress and welfare of humanity. . . . Nothing is so important as human health and happiness . . . and if it costs dollars and cents to procure . . . then we must pay . . . and if it reduces profits we must reduce those profits. . . . You who are more or less technical . . . must help us by giving . . . the correct information . . . which we will be only too glad to use."

On June 23, 1913, NFPA's Executive Committee formed the Committee on Safety to Life and entrusted this new committee to suggest the scope of its work. The July 1913 *Quarterly* stated that the formation of the committee was "the crystalization of a latent feeling which has for some time existed in the membership" for focusing attention on life safety.

The new committee, headed by H. W. Forster, spent the first few years studying fires involving loss of life and attempting to analyze the cause of that loss of life. At the 1914 Annual Meeting, the committee delivered its first report, which included a special section on egress, a statement that sprinklers can save lives, and preliminary specifications for outside fire escapes.

According to the report, the committee's studies showed that existing laws "are exceedingly deficient in this very important matter of egress. A number of states report frankly that they have no real legislation upon the subject."

The preliminary specifications for outside fire escapes were controversial and received a great deal of attention from the membership. The committee members did not like outside fire escapes, and many felt they were a delusion, as stated in the 1911 *Quarterly*. Nevertheless, the committee felt they had to face the fact that fire escapes existed and would be used.

The committee wrote, "Admitting . . . that a fire escape on a building is usually an admission that life is not safe in it, the fact remains that the outside fire escape is the commonest special provision for escape . . . [and] this Association should determine upon proper precautions for such escapes, and use its influence to have them adopted and enforced."

At the 1915 Annual Meeting, NFPA adopted revised specifications for fire escapes. In 1916, the committee's work was published in a pamphlet, "Outside Stairs for Fire Exits." In 1918, another committee report was published in a pamphlet titled "Safeguarding Factory Workers from Fire." The pamphlets were widely circulated, put into general use, and, with other documents, form the basis of the present *Life Safety Code*.

In 1921, the Committee on Safety to Life was enlarged to include representation from interested groups not previously participating in its work. Work was started on the further development and integration of previous committee publications to provide a comprehensive guide to exits and related features of life safety from fires in all classes of occupancy. This work resulted in the publication in 1927 of the first edition of NFPA's *Building Exits Code*.

## COCOANUT GROVE FIRE

As anyone involved in any safety endeavor will attest, it often takes a tragedy to alert society to dangers that must be addressed. The Triangle Shirtwaist fire moved the nation toward the prevention of many fire hazards. However, as time passes, the public forgets the lessons it learned and is forced to learn them once again through another tragedy. Thirty-one years after the Triangle Shirtwaist fire, in which locked exits trapped and doomed many workers, the United States witnessed another major fire in a building with locked exits.

The fire occurred in 1942 at the Cocoanut Grove, one of the most popular nightclubs in Boston. It was a one-story-and-basement structure built in 1916. The original property was of reinforced concrete construction. Several additions had been made to the building, and a rolling roof had been installed over the dance floor.

### State of Fire Protection: 1911 to 1942

There are many differences between the fire at the Triangle Shirtwaist Company and that of the Cocoanut

Grove. One building was a high-rise factory, and the other was a single-story nightclub. The biggest difference lies in the state of the art of fire protection at the time. In 1911, when the Triangle Shirtwaist fire erupted, there were no universally recognized standards for exits. In 1942, when the Cocoanut Grove burned, those standards existed and were part of NFPA's *Building Exits Code*. Evidently, they were ignored. As a result, 492 people died.

Virtually all the hazards at the Cocoanut Grove were covered by the 1942 edition of the *Building Exits Code*. The main problems appear to have been the chaotic condition of Boston's building regulations and lax enforcement.

As the *Christian Science Monitor* said in an editorial after the fire, "action will be taken to prevent another Cocoanut Grove, and somebody could have taken action to prevent this one."

The late Robert S. Moulton, long-time NFPA Technical Secretary and Secretary to the Committee on Safety to Life, wrote a report on the fire that was widely circulated. Much of the information that follows comes from that report.

### Fire Hazards in the Popular Night Spot

In 1942, the Broadway Cocktail Lounge was added to the Cocoanut Grove nightclub. The lounge was installed in a group of old brick-joisted buildings varying in height from two stories to three and one-half stories and was connected to the main property by a passageway with doorways leading to dressing rooms for entertainers.

The basement of the original structure contained the Melody Lounge, another cocktail area. The Melody Lounge had false walls made of light wooden frame covered with light wallboard. Decorations in the lounge included colorful fabrics, artificial leather on the walls, and cloth on the ceiling. In addition, there were imitation coconut palm trees in the lounge and in the main dining/dancing hall. Light fixtures were made from coconut shells, with the wiring concealed in the "foliage." These decorations had reportedly been flame-proofed.

**No Easy Way Out.** The only obvious exit from the Melody Lounge was a door at the top of the stairway leading to a narrow hallway on the first floor, then to a foyer and the main entrance. Another door, this one leading to an outside alley, was concealed behind the false walls of the lounge. It was locked. A door leading to the street from the narrow hallway at the head of the stairs was equipped with panic hardware. However, this door was locked.

According to writer Paul Benzaquin in his book, *Holocaust* (Henry Holt and Company, 1959), there was also a passageway from the Melody Lounge to the kitchen, but it seems that only employees knew of this passageway. Its door was painted and draped and unlikely to be seen by those who didn't know it was there. Nevertheless, the door was counted as an exit by the city's fire commissioner in his post-fire report.

Many other doors were locked as well, and some opened inward. The false walls obscured many of the windows, and the main doorway of the Cocoanut Grove was blocked by a revolving door.

**A Capacity Crowd That Kept Getting Bigger.** The official seating capacity of the nightclub was about 600 persons. No one knows exactly how many patrons were there on the night of November 28, 1942, but unofficial estimates indicate that there were about 1000 people. Benzaquin reports that waiters were setting up more tables to accommodate additional patrons.

Overcrowding was not (and probably is still not) unusual in nightclubs. Nightclubs are businesses established to make a profit, and the more patrons they serve, the greater their profit. NFPA's Moulton said he was told the club was often congested, particularly on Saturday evenings.

According to Benzaquin, the club's application for a new license requested permission to install an additional 30 fixed stools for the new cocktail lounge. He writes that the stools were installed *before* permission was granted, on the assumption that there would be no objection.

That was probably a reasonable assumption. A member of the city's licensing board testified at the fire commissioner's hearing that the Cocoanut Grove got its original license and several renewals without any hearings to determine whether it complied with regulations.

**The 12-Minute Fire.** Benzaquin states in his book that the fire lasted about 12 minutes. It started in the Melody Lounge and was possibly ignited accidentally by a busboy who was holding a match while replacing a light bulb in one of the fake palm trees. As Moulton reported, however, the exact source of ignition was of less importance than the inadequacy of the exits and the extensive use of combustible decorations.

According to the fire commissioner's report, the fire immediately spread throughout the Melody Lounge along the underside of the false ceiling. Feeding on the combustible decorations, the fire reached and ascended the stairway and passed through the connecting passageway into the foyer, past the main entrance, and into the dining room and other areas of the club.

When the fire began to spread rapidly, panic ensued. Most of the patrons in the Melody Lounge raced for the stairway, their only obvious exit. Many died on those stairs. Those who escaped the basement lounge through the stairway piled up in the corridor while attempting to reach the main entrance. If the door from that corridor to the outside had been unlocked, many might have been saved.

Led by a few quick-thinking employees, a few patrons made their escape from the lounge by going through the concealed door to the kitchen area, and some of them escaped through a door to an alley outside. Others tried to get to the main floor but could not because of the heat. A few escaped through a basement window into a courtyard, and a few others survived the fire by seeking refuge in a large refrigerator.

Moulton wrote that about 100 people died at the Broadway entrance to the club, more than 190 ft from the stairway leading from the Melody Lounge, where the fire started. He reported that about 200 were trapped behind the revolving door at the main entrance. That revolving door, which under the best of conditions would slow exit travel, jammed and blocked the exit.

### Lessons Learned

There were few "new" lessons to be learned from the Cocoanut Grove fire. Even before the Triangle Shirtwaist fire in 1911, the danger of locked, blocked, and concealed exits was known. After the Triangle Shirtwaist fire NFPA had publicized its views on exits and means of egress in pamphlet form.

The 1942 *Building Exits Code* prohibited revolving doors as exits in places of assembly and required that other occupancies that used revolving doors must also have swinging doors immediately adjacent or within 20 ft.

That same edition of the *Code* required that "decorations of theatres and assembly halls shall be of fire resistive or nonflammable materials. Fabrics and papers used for such purposes shall be treated with an effective flame-proofing material." A cautionary note warned, "Paper and cloth decorative materials should be kept to a minimum in places of assembly since such flimsy materials increase the hazard of the kindling and spread of fire."

The decorative materials in the Cocoanut Grove were supposedly flame-proofed, but, if this was true, the flame-proofing was ineffective. The fire did demonstrate, once again, that "fireproof" buildings — the Cocoanut Grove building was "fireproof" when first erected — can still be death traps due to their contents. It also proved that fire inspections should be conducted when facilities are in operation. According to Moulton, the Boston building inspector reported that he had inspected the building and found the exits adequate. This might have been true when the doors were unlocked and the building was not crowded with 1000 people.

"There is a real danger in attempting to remedy conditions such as were responsible for the Cocoanut Grove tragedy by the enactment of more laws," wrote Moulton. "In our opinion, building and fire officials can now do practically everything that is necessary to assure public safety from fire without any more laws."

Six months after the fire, at the 1943 NFPA Annual Meeting, Moulton reported to the membership that, due to the war, the Safety to Life Committee had been unable to meet. The committee members did exchange correspondence, however, and Moulton said they believed "our existing recommendations, that date back to 1913, are adequate."

**Code Changes.** There was one change involving the *Building Exits Code* that did come about immediately after and as a direct result of the Cocoanut Grove fire: The *Code* was adopted by many more jurisdictions across the country, due in large part to the efforts of the fire service. The Committee on Safety to Life reported on that increased usage at the 1945 NFPA Annual Meeting.

It was during the 1945 NFPA Annual Meeting that the Committee recommended a change in the method of exit measurement, clarification of the need for stairway enclosure, provisions covering loose chairs in nightclubs, and changes in lighting and signs. These changes were incorporated into the 1946 edition of the *Code*, as was a special note on interior finish.

**Interior Finish.** Combustible decorations were a factor in the Cocoanut Grove fire. Nevertheless, interior finish continued to be a major fire problem in the 1940s. In 1946, the nation witnessed the LaSalle and Winecoff hotel fires. The latter, with 119 fatalities, was the largest multiple-death hotel fire of the twentieth century.

The Committee on Safety to Life was concerned about the dangers of combustible interior finish. Therefore, it recommended, and the full membership approved, a caution in the 1946 *Code*, which stated, "where interior finish materials are used having a higher combustibility, greater rate of fire spread, or potentialities of greater generation of smoke or fumes than wood, the exits specified in the *Code* may not be sufficient to provide adequate life safety from fire."

The lack of a standard way to measure the combustibility of interior finish hampered the committee. In the July 1943 *Quarterly*, A. J. Steiner of Underwriters Laboratories described a new method he was developing to test the combustibility of interior finish. The Steiner Tunnel Test was recommended for adoption at the 1953 NFPA Annual Meeting by the NFPA Building Construction Committee. It was eventually incorporated into the *Building Exits Code.*

## OUR LADY OF ANGELS SCHOOL FIRE

Combustible interior finish was one of the factors that led to fire spread at the Our Lady of Angels School in Chicago in December 1958. Wood trim in one corridor and combustible ceiling tile in classrooms in one wing (and perhaps in other areas of the building) provided fuel for this fire.

### Avoidable Problem

The primary cause of loss of life, according to the NFPA investigative report of the fire, was *the inadequacy of the exit facilities.* As a result of this completely avoidable problem, 90 pupils and three nuns died.

Adequacy of exits, as determined by proper enclosure; provision of at least two exits remote from each other; and sufficient exit capacity were well-established fundamentals of fire protection by 1958. The Triangle Shirtwaist fire, the Cocoanut Grove fire, and hundreds of other fires had demonstrated the consequences of neglected exits. The 1958 edition of the *Building Exits Code* specified exact requirements for adequate exits and for other elements of school fire safety.

Chester I. Babcock, then manager of the NFPA fire records department, and Rex Wilson, then an NFPA engineer and later a consultant, investigated the Our Lady of Angels fire for NFPA. A year later, Babcock wrote, "We know now and have known since before most of today's schools were built how to design and protect a school so that the lives of the pupils and teachers will be safe from fire. Refinements and improvements are needed and undoubtedly will come, but this does not mean that fire protection engineering has been groping for an answer. Practical methods of assuring life safety from fire that have stood the test of time and are based on sound fire protection engineering principles have been available for years."

**One Fire Area.** In 1953, the two-story school building was connected to another old, two-story, brick, wood-joisted building by a two-story, brick-joisted annex. The NFPA report of the fire stated that the building constituted one fire area, due to open stairways and the fact that the masonry division wall between the north wing and the annex had substandard doorway protection.

The stairways in the school were open except for two located in the front of the north wing. Those stairs were enclosed at the second-story level by substandard doors that were held open at the time of the fire. Because the three stairways from the second floor corridor of the north wing were connected through a common corridor, pupils in second-story classrooms, in effect, had no way out.

**Origin of the Fire.** About 2:25 P.M., one half-hour before school was normally dismissed, fire broke out in combustible materials at the bottom of the rear stairway of the north wing. Pupils from one of the second-floor classrooms had taken trash to the boiler room incinerator, as was their routine. The students returned to the classroom at 2:30 P.M. and reported that they had smelled smoke. Their teacher informed a teacher in a nearby room, who went to find the principal. When the principal could not be found, both teachers led their classes out of the building to the parish church. Smoke was already at head level in the second-floor corridor. Only after they had their classes settled in the church did one of the teachers run back to the school and operate the fire alarm signal.

The school's janitor noticed smoke and ran to the parish house to tell the housekeeper to call the fire department. Apparently, the housekeeper waited a few minutes before placing the call. The fire department reported that at about 2:42 P.M., it received the first of some 15 calls reporting the fire.

Hot fire gases and smoke billowed up the chimney-like stairwell and mushroomed through the second-story corridor. Eventually the hot gases and combustible interior finish in the corridor ignited. The heat broke the large glass transoms over the classroom doors, and the hot gases and flames entered the rooms.

**Those Who Escaped and Those Who Did Not.** As soon as the fire alarm rang, occupants of the first floor left the building by means of the five available stairways, according to the NFPA report. The evacuation of pupils in the second-floor annex and south wing was hampered by smoke that came through an open door in the division wall at that level. Either the janitor or a fire fighter closed the door.

Pupils in the second-floor north wing did not escape as easily. Their travel through the corridor to the stairways was blocked by heavy smoke and heat. Some jumped from their classroom windows. Others were taken down fire department ladders. Many died in their classrooms, some at their desks.

### Aftermath of the Fire

One immediate effect of the Our Lady of Angels fire was a public awakening to the hazards in the nation's schools. According to Babcock's followup report, within a year after the fire, hazardous conditions had been eliminated in thousands of schools across the country.

Throughout this country's history, major improvements in safety have been made after terrible fires. The Iroquois Theater fire brought about improvements in theater safety; the Triangle Shirtwaist fire brought about improvements in factories; the Cocoanut Grove fire resulted in improvements in nightclubs; and the LaSalle, Winecoff, MGM Grand, Stouffer's, and DuPont Plaza fires resulted in improvements in hotels.

In 1959, NFPA sampled more than 2000 fire departments to analyze the level of improvements made in school safety. Many improvements had been made. Nearly every community had acted on such issues as frequent and improved exit drills, tighter control of waste disposal, inspections, and proper storage of combustible supplies. However, that same survey revealed that needed improvements had not been made in about 30,000 schools.

NFPA conducted an informal telephone survey in 1978, 20 years after the Our Lady of Angels fire. The consensus from that informal survey was that schools were safer. (Indeed, one respondent said they couldn't help but be safer than they had been in 1958, when they were the "lousiest-constructed buildings in existence!") Unfortunately, schools in 1978 were not as safe as fire professionals had hoped. The passage of time and the growing concern with vandalism and security had blocked out the memories of the Our Lady of Angels tragedy.

**Los Angeles School Fire Tests.** The most publicized result of the fire was the fire test program conducted by the Los Angeles Fire Department. The tests, conducted in 1959 and 1960 under the direction of then Los Angeles Fire Marshal Raymond M. Hill, were designed to investigate methods of protecting multistory, open-stairway school buildings. One of the conclusions drawn from the tests was that complete automatic sprinkler protection offered the best chance for escape.

The 1958 edition of the *Building Exits Code* provided for sprinklers in schools. The 1960 edition retained those provisions and totally reorganized the section of the *Code* covering educational occupancies. That edition classified schools as follows:

*Group A:* One-story buildings with exterior or interior access, or multistory buildings with access only by exterior balconies and outside stairs

*Group B:* Buildings of two stories or more with egress through corridors and interior stairways

*Group C:* Sprinklered buildings

*Group D:* Open-plan schools

*Group E:* Existing buildings

There were somewhat different requirements for each group.

A great deal of discussion took place among members of the Committee on Safety to Life in 1960 regarding whether they should recommend permitting open stairways in two-story sprinklered schools. The committee decided not to make this recommendation that year. The 1961 edition of the *Code,* however, did permit open stairs in sprinklered two-story schools. One reason for this decision was that committee members noted that, in two-story buildings, pupils constantly pass through the doors anyway.

In 1966, the year the *Building Exits Code* was reorganized and renamed the *Life Safety Code,* a provision was added that required all parts of school buildings below grade to be sprinklered. In addition, the allowable travel distance to the nearest exit was increased from 100 ft to 150 ft, under normal conditions, and up to 200 ft in sprinklered school buildings.

## BEVERLY HILLS SUPPER CLUB FIRE

Those who study fires can't help but have a feeling of *déjà vu.* It seems that the same fire problems return to haunt us time and again. Inadequate means of egress, lack of employee preparedness and training, and a general noncompliance with proven provisions of the *Life Safety Code* were all factors in the Triangle, Cocoanut Grove, and Our Lady of Angels fires, as well as in countless others.

These problems were critical factors again on May 28, 1977, at the Beverly Hills Supper Club. In a fire at the club, a public assembly occupancy that billed itself as the "Showplace of the Nation," 164 people died. NFPA conducted an in-depth investigation of the fire, and much of what follows was taken from the investigative report prepared by Richard L. Best.

### Fire Conditions in the Showplace of the Nation

The Beverly Hills Supper Club was a glamorous nightclub in Southgate, Kentucky, just outside Cincinnati, Ohio. Banquets, dinner dances, balls, floor shows, fashion shows, weddings, wedding receptions, and business meetings were all held in the club's "18" function rooms.

The quotation marks around the number 18 represent the advertised number of function rooms. There were actually five main dining rooms, the large "Cabaret Room," a small function room called the

"Zebra Room," and the main bar. Three of the large dining rooms could be subdivided into smaller rooms by folding partitions.

There had been a wedding reception in the Zebra Room on the day of the fire. The wedding party had left at approximately 8 P.M. Performers were scheduled to entertain guests in the Cabaret Room around 8:30 P.M. There were an estimated 1200 to 1300 guests in the Cabaret Room, about triple the number that could be accommodated safely. Numerous patrons later said that tables were squeezed together and the narrow aisles were obstructed with chairs. There were about 2400 to 2800 patrons in the club altogether.

**Delayed Notification.** Employees discovered the fire between 8:45 and 8:50 P.M. in the empty Zebra Room. It had started in a concealed space, and the origin was presumed by investigators to have been electrical in nature.

Some employees alerted the club's hostess, while other employees ran around looking for the management. Two managers tried to fight the fire with portable fire extinguishers — with the help of busboys and waiters — but their efforts were to no avail. One of the managers eventually ran to the hostess and told her to evacuate the patrons. By that time, it was about 9:00. Someone notified the fire department about a minute later.

As this general description of events indicates, about 15 minutes might have elapsed between discovery of the fire and notification of employees. That delay was a critical factor in evacuation efforts. Also, it seems that there was some degree of staff confusion regarding evacuation procedures, since employees had not been trained in them.

Once notification of patrons started, an interesting phenomenon took place. According to interviews conducted by the Kentucky State Police after the fire, waiters and waitresses instinctively took responsibility for the safety of the patrons they were serving. They went directly to those guests and to other guests in those rooms and told them to leave. They did not, however, necessarily take responsibility for guests they were not serving or guests in different parts of the building.

The Cabaret Room was isolated from the rest of the club once the show was in progress. There were no waiters, waitresses, busboys, or hostesses traveling to and from the kitchen or standing in the service halls between dining room seatings. This indicates that employees serving the Cabaret Room did not see other employees rushing around notifying patrons and the management of the fire, so they were totally unaware of the danger. However, one busboy, who had just left the Cabaret Room to work in another room, learned of the fire and decided to take action.

**Quick Thinking.** In a display of courage, calmness, and good sense, the busboy took upon himself the responsibility of evacuating patrons from the Cabaret Room. He was walking down one of the main corridors from the Cabaret Room to the Viennese Room when he learned of the fire. He looked toward the Zebra Room and saw smoke coming through the top edge of the closed doors. He quickly told a bartender to leave, then spun around and ran back to the Cabaret Room.

When he arrived there, he told the host to open the doors of the room. The host also moved the rope divider and reservations stand from the corridor and instructed people waiting in line to walk toward the Garden Room area in another part of the building.

The busboy then walked into the Cabaret Room, calmly climbed up onto the stage where a performance was taking place, took the microphone, and spoke to the guests in the room. This is what he told the post-fire investigators:

> The first thing I did was . . . ask them to look at the exit sign . . . "I want you to all notice that exit sign and I want you to look at the other corner of the room and there will be another exit sign . . . I want the left side of my room to go out of the exit sign behind that I'm pointing to now . . . I want my right half of the room to go out of the other exit sign . . . There is a fire in the small room on the other side of the building . . . I don't think there is any reason to panic or rush . . . you should leave."

Although he later said that some people looked at him as if he were crazy, people did begin to leave. Of the 164 fatalities in the fire, most occurred in the Cabaret Room. There is no way of knowing how many more would have died if the busboy had not taken charge.

Once he was back in the hallway, the busboy saw smoke billowing toward him so he went to an exit. "There were just three doors, and one was locked," he said. "I tried to bang it open with my shoulder [but] I couldn't."

**The Human Factor.** Post-fire interviews showed, not surprisingly, that people in general did not take the fire threat too seriously at first. Much of the evacuation in the early stages of the fire was without difficulty, partly because people proceeded calmly and deliberately, some perhaps not even believing there was a serious fire in the making.

When heavy smoke and intense heat descended on patrons trying to leave the Cabaret Room, those people suddenly realized the seriousness of the situation.

Some began to rush and push, and some stumbled and fell, blocking exits with their bodies. One fire fighter reported seeing people stacked two and three high.

One bartender told of a young woman who had fallen near an exit. Other people fell on top of her. The bartender and one of his coworkers tried to pull her out, but they were unable to move her. "And there was a man that was on top," the bartender said. "He was a heavy guy and he was reaching up his arms and so I thought he was all right . . . the first thought was to get him off the top so you can do something with the bottom ones . . . I had him wrap his arms around my neck and I pushed up against this door as hard as I could . . . and I didn't have enough strength to lift him and he just looked at me and shook his head . . . there was nothing I could do."

### Familiar Factors Contributed to Deaths

The rapid fire spread along the main corridor of the club, delay in notifying patrons in the Cabaret Room, insufficient exit capacity, and an excessive number of people in the Cabaret Room were all major factors that resulted in employees and guests having insufficient time to escape this fire. Virtually all of these factors were covered in the *Life Safety Code* in existence at that time. Some other specific factors covered in the *Code* are examined in the following sections.

**Construction.** Previous editions of the *Code* defined Class A places of assembly as those having a capacity of 1000 people or more. The Beverly Hills Supper Club's total occupant load was 2375. Unprotected, noncombustible construction such as that of the Beverly Hills Supper Club was not permitted for Class A assembly occupancies. That construction was permitted for Class C occupancies, which were restricted to 300 people or less. (It is now permitted for Class A occupancies, but only if the building is fully sprinklered.)

**Number of Exits.** The number of exits, based on 100 persons per unit of exit width and on square footage, should have been 27.5 exit units. The actual number was 16.5. The second floor had no exits with components permitted by the *Code*. (The Melody Lounge at the Cocoanut Grove was also overcrowded.) The Cabaret Room should have had four exits, since it was itself a Class A place of assembly. It had only three. (The Cocoanut Grove's Melody Lounge had only one obvious exit.) There was evidence of locked doors and chains and locks on panic hardware. (The same was true at the Cocoanut Grove.) Exits were not well marked. A door to the corridor, for example, appeared to be part of the wall paneling, and it was not marked as an exit. (The Cocoanut Grove's Melody Lounge had a door that was painted and draped and not likely to be seen by patrons. In addition, false walls concealed some windows.)

**Obstructions.** There was seating in the aisles in the Cabaret Room. Tables were placed too close together, and there were too many chairs and other items restricting the aisles. There also were chairs and tables stored on the platform outside the Viennese Room that led to steps to double doors. (Chairs and tables also blocked aisles at the Cocoanut Grove.)

**Enclosures.** Vertical openings should be enclosed. The curved stairway in the club's Hallway of Mirrors was neither enclosed nor protected.

**Interior Finish.** The 1976 *Code* required interior finish in all means of egress in all places of assembly to be Class A — that is, with a flame spread rating of 0–25. The interior finish in the Hallway of Mirrors and the main north-south corridor had a flame spread rating greater than 25. It is interesting to note how many of these factors were also present in the Cocoanut Grove fire 35 years before.

**Alarm Systems.** One of the factors that made it difficult for patrons to escape was a delay in notification of the fire. An alarm system would have eliminated that delay. The *Code* required alarm systems in all occupancies except storage facilities and places of assembly. Committee members had discussed the importance of alarm systems for a long time, but many felt an alarm system could cause panic. The Beverly Hills Supper Club fire demonstrated the need for an alarm system, however, and so the requirement was added for public assembly occupancies in the next edition of the *Code*, which was published in 1981. Still concerned with the potential for panic and aware of tests showing the value of voice alarms, the committee added an important provision to its alarm requirements.

Manual fire alarm boxes were required to alert occupants. The fire alarm boxes send an alarm to a central office or other location on the property that is continuously staffed while the occupancy is in use. The central office must have a way of then notifying occupants, either through a voice alarm over a public address system or a vocal fire alarm system. The alarm notification requirement was made retroactive to apply to both new and existing buildings.

**Sprinklers.** Historically, the *Code* had required sprinklers in assembly occupancies used as exhibit halls. Cost was a perceived prohibitive factor in efforts to spread that requirement to other public assembly occupancies. After the Beverly Hills Supper Club fire, however, the committee realized that the life-saving potential of sprinklers outweighed their cost.

The committee approached sprinkler requirements in the following two ways. Members reassessed construction requirements for all classes of assembly occupancies, consolidated them, and required sprinklers based on construction type and location of assembly occupancy within the building. It was decided that even fire-resistive buildings having four or more stories above the exit discharge should be sprinklered. These provisions applied to new buildings, and some were made retroactive for existing buildings.

In addition, every Class A and Class B occupancy was required to be sprinklered throughout. This requirement applied only to new construction. There were some exceptions, but none that applied to facilities such as the Beverly Hills Supper Club.

Discussion of the value of sprinklering all places of assembly was ongoing after the Beverly Hills Supper Club fire. Numerous fires — including the Gulliver's Discotheque fire in New York and the Upstairs Lounge fire in New Orleans, both of which took place during the 1970s and involved a fire blocking a means of egress — highlighted similar problems and emphasized the need for sprinklers.

## RHODE ISLAND NIGHTCLUB FIRE

Tragedy struck again on the night of February 20, 2003, as fans gathered at The Station nightclub in West Warwick, Rhode Island, to see Great White, a 1980s heavy metal band. Within seconds after the band started to perform, sparks from a pyrotechnics display ignited expanded foam plastic insulation that surrounded the stage area. As a result of this tragic fire in which 100 occupants perished, changes would be made to fire and life safety codes in an effort to make public assembly occupancies safer.

### Recap of That Night

Published reports (*The Providence Journal*) indicated that more than 400 fans had crowded into the single-story, wood frame building for Great White's late night show. At approximately 11:00 P.M. the band started to play their opening number. The band's manager ignited a "gerb," a pyrotechnic canister that releases a fountain of sparks, as part of the opening. Within seconds, the walls and the ceiling around the stage (covered with the foam) caught fire. Confused as to whether or not the fire was a part of the band's act, many patrons delayed heading for the exits during the initial seconds of the fire. This decision proved fatal in many cases.

The fire quickly spread across the ceiling toward the front doors. The lights didn't go out initially, but the thick smoke limited visibility, and commotion ensued. As patrons began to rush toward exit doorways and windows, people fell and were trampled. As occupants were trying to leave by the main exit, falling patrons jammed it, preventing many from reaching safety. In the confusion, others fled in different directions, some to the bathrooms, which offered no escape. Within four minutes, the club was engulfed in flames.

In the end, the fire claimed 100 lives, injured more than 200, and ranked as the fourth deadliest nightclub fire in U.S. history.

**The Building.** The single-story, unprotected wood frame building was constructed in 1946. The nonsprinklered structure had a floor area of approximately 6275 ft$^2$. Between 1946 and 2000, the building changed ownership eight times and had various uses, including meeting house (1964), restaurant (1974), and pub (1985). In 1991, the building reopened as a nightclub and was eventually renamed "The Station" in 2000. In response to complaints from neighbors about loud music and noise, expanded foam plastic material had been installed on the walls and ceiling at the raised platform.

**The Hazards.** Interior finish played a significant role in the rapid spread of the fire. According to the *Life Safety Code*, the interior finish is required to be Class A or B for general assembly areas with occupant loads of more than 300. Class C interior finish is permitted if the occupant load is 300 or less. In addition, the foam attached to the walls and ceiling at the raised platform would be subject to the provisions for cellular or foamed plastic, which prohibits the use of this particular material as interior finish unless it is in extremely insignificant amounts or the material has been subjected to fire testing that substantiates the combustibility characteristics for the use intended under actual fire conditions.

**Exits.** The means of egress arrangement leading to the main entrance doors made it difficult for people to escape. The arrangement of the front entrance corridor made occupants negotiate their way through an intermediate door that opened into a small foyer through which they could then reach the main doors leading directly to the outside. The corridor and foyer contained openings into both the club portion of the facility and the bar area. The small foyer was reportedly designed as a control point to prevent occupants from getting into the club without a ticket, but this arrangement proved to be disastrous when the large crowd rushed to the main entrance, from two directions, to escape the blaze.

Even though there were three other exits from the building, most patrons were unaware of them. The exit in the main bar never became available to occupants in the show area as the fire and heavy black smoke spread through the nightclub. Several occupants familiar with the building and staff managed to escape through the kitchen exit, but most occupants did not realize the kitchen exit was there despite the exit signs marking its location. The exit door near the raised platform was quickly eliminated as an option once the fire spread around the door, preventing escape.

### Codes

Three weeks after the Rhode Island nightclub fire, NFPA sponsored a public forum and special meeting of the Technical Committee on Assembly Occupancies in Boston, Massachusetts. The meeting was held in response to the Rhode Island fire. Fire officials and those who lost family and/or friends testified before the Technical Committee. A subsequent meeting of the committee was held on July 8–9, 2003, at NFPA headquarters. As a result of input from members of the Technical Committee and fire service members, a number of Tentative Interim Amendments (TIAs) to the relevant Codes were proposed in an effort to prevent similar tragedies in the future.

On July 25, 2003, the Standards Council reviewed and issued the technical committee's recommended TIAs for NFPA *101*®, *Life Safety Code*®, 2003 edition, and *NFPA 5000*®, *Building Construction and Safety Code*®, 2003 edition. The TIAs, which went into effect August 14, 2003, required the following:

- Fire sprinklers must be installed in new nightclubs and similar assembly occupancies regardless of occupant load and in existing facilities that accommodate more than 100.
- Building owners must inspect exits to ensure they are free of obstructions and must maintain records of each inspection.
- At least one trained crowd manager must be present for all gatherings of more than 50 except religious services. (For gatherings of more than 250, additional crowd managers are required at a ratio of 1:250.)
- Festival seating is prohibited for crowds of more than 250 unless a life-safety evaluation approved by the authority having jurisdiction has been performed. (Festival seating, according to NFPA *101*, is a form of audience/spectator accommodation in which no seating, other than a floor or ground surface, is provided for the audience to gather and observe a performance.)

### What's to Come

The TIAs issued by the Standards Council were again reviewed. After modifications were made, they were incorporated into the 2006 edition of NFPA *101* and *NFPA 5000*.

In February 2003, the National Institute of Standards and Technology (NIST) launched an investigation into the tragic nightclub fire. At the conclusion of its investigation, the National Construction Safety Team (NCST) led by NIST recommended specific improvements to building standards, codes, and practices based on its findings and recommended research and other appropriate actions needed to improve the structural fire safety of buildings and evacuation procedures.

## ONGOING CHALLENGE

The story of fire protection is one that continues. Fire protection professionals study history and conduct research to determine code requirements needed to protect lives. They continuously use their influence to ensure that those requirements are adopted and enforced. Unfortunately it often takes a tragedy to bolster their efforts, and even then, if action isn't taken immediately, people forget.

In Nevada, momentum toward tighter codes had slowed down a year after the 1980 MGM Grand fire. Subsequent fires brought back memories of that tragedy. Today, the Ballys Las Vegas (formerly the MGM Grand) has installed about 30,000 sprinklers, 8000 loudspeakers, and other fire protection equipment. In addition, the American Automobile Association (AAA) now includes fire protection among the factors it considers when rating hotels in its travel guides.

Sometimes fires demonstrate the wisdom of committee members. For example, the 1987 Dupont Plaza Hotel fire illustrated that the Committee on Safety to Life was correct in requiring corridors and lobbies to be separated from assembly areas by 1-hour rated walls, unless the building is sprinklered or 50 percent of the egress is independent of the lobby.

The Las Vegas Hilton fire in 1981, which resulted in eight deaths, illustrated that committee members were correct in restricting carpeting on walls. That fire saw flames leapfrogging up the side of the building, entering windows, and spreading along carpeting on the walls and ceilings. The committee had been convinced of the dangers of carpeting on walls through fire tests sponsored by the carpeting industry, which had pushed for regulation of its own products.

It is always tempting to concentrate on the tragedies, because they are so obvious. However, there are positive results to consider, even if they are not as well documented. It is impossible to know the number of lives that have been saved because vertical openings were enclosed; exits were adequate and unlocked; and alarm, detection, and sprinkler systems were in place.

The key, once requirements are put into codes and the codes are adopted, is enforcement. The challenge for everyone who reads this handbook is to make certain that the codes, which contain the accumulated fire protection knowledge of generations, are enforced. To paraphrase Frances Perkins' speech to the 1913 NFPA Annual Meeting, People are not always their own masters. "It is necessary for organizations like yours . . . to insist on safety for them." That is our job.

## REFERENCES

NFPA 1126, *Standard for the Use of Pyrotechnics before a Proximate Audience*, 2006 edition.

*NFPA 5000®, Building Construction and Safety Code®*, 2006 edition.

Benzaquin, Paul, *Holocaust*, Henry Holt and Company, 1959.

Naden, Corinne, *The Triangle Shirtwaist Fire*, Franklin Watts, Inc., 1971.

Stein, Leon, *The Triangle Fire*, J.B. Lippincott, 1962.

SUPPLEMENT 2

# Extracts from ASME *Elevator Code and Handbook*

*Editor's Note: This supplement provides the reader with detailed information on elevator emergency operation and signaling devices. It consists of extracted material from ASME A17.1, Safety Code for Elevators and Escalators, 2007, and its accompanying handbook.*

## EXTRACTS FROM ASME A17.1, SECTION 2.27 EMERGENCY OPERATION AND SIGNALING DEVICES*

NOTE (2.27): Additional requirements, including those for firefighters' communications systems, may be found in the building code.

### 2.27.1 Car Emergency Signaling Devices

**2.27.1.1 Emergency Communications**

*2.27.1.1.1* A two-way communications means between the car and a location staffed by authorized personnel shall be provided.

*2.27.1.1.2* When the two-way communications location is not staffed 24 h a day, by authorized personnel who can take appropriate action, the means of two-way communications shall automatically be directed within 30 s to an additional on- or off-site location, staffed by authorized personnel, where an appropriate response can be taken.

*2.27.1.1.3* The two-way communication means within the car shall comply with the following requirements:

(a) In jurisdictions enforcing NBCC, Appendix E of CSA B44, or in jurisdictions not enforcing NBCC, ICC/ANSI A117.1.

(b) A push button to actuate the two-way communication means shall be provided in or adjacent to a car operating panel. The push button shall be visible and permanently identified as "HELP". The identification shall be on or adjacent to the "HELP" button. When the push button is actuated, the emergency two-way communication means shall initiate a call for help and establish two-way communications.

(c) A visual indication on the same panel as the "HELP" push button shall be provided, that is activated by authorized personnel, to acknowledge that two-way communications link has been established. The visual indication shall be extinguished when the two-way communication link is terminated.

(d) The two-way communication means shall provide on demand to authorized personnel, information that identifies the building location and elevator number and that assistance is required.

(e) After the call acknowledgement signals are sent [2.27.1.1.3(c)], the two-way voice communications shall be available between the car and authorized personnel.

(f) The two-way communications, once established, shall be disconnected only when authorized personnel outside the car terminate the call.

(g) The two-way communication means shall not use a handset in the car.

(h) The two-way communications shall not be transmitted to an automated answering system. The call for help shall be answered by authorized personnel.

(i) Operating instructions shall be incorporated with or adjacent to the "HELP" button.

*2.27.1.1.4* Where the elevator rise is 18 m (60 ft) or more, a two-way voice communication means within the building accessible to emergency personnel shall be provided and comply with the following requirements:

(a) The means shall enable emergency personnel within the building to establish two-way voice communications to each car individually. Two-way voice communication shall be established without any intentional delay and shall not require intervention by a person within the car. The means shall override communications to outside of the building.
(b) Two-way voice communications, once established, shall be disconnected only when emergency personnel outside the car terminates the call.
(c) Once the two-way voice communication has been established, the visual indication [see 2.27.1.1.3(c)] within the car shall illuminate. The visual indication shall be extinguished when the two-way communication is terminated.
(d) Operating instructions shall be incorporated with or adjacent to the two-way voice communication outside the car. Instructions shall conform to 2.27.7.3.

*2.27.1.1.5* If the emergency communication means is normally connected to the building's main power supply, it shall automatically transfer to an alternate source(s) of power when the normal power supply fails. The alternate source(s) of power (standby, emergency, etc.) shall be capable of providing power for illumination of the visual indication [see 2.27.1.1.3(c)] within the car, and the means of emergency communications for at least 4 h; and the audible signaling device (see 2.27.1.2) for at least 1 h.

**2.27.1.2 Emergency Stop Switch Audible Signal.** When an emergency stop switch (2.26.2.5) is provided, an audible signaling device shall be provided. The audible signaling device shall

(a) have a rated sound pressure rating of not less than 80 dBA nor greater than 90 dBA at 3 m (10 ft)
(b) respond without delay after the switch has been activated
(c) be located inside the building and audible inside the car and outside the hoistway
(d) for elevators with a rise greater than 30 m (100 ft), be duplicated as follows:
   (1) one device shall be mounted on the car
   (2) a second device shall be placed at the designated level

### 2.27.2 Emergency or Standby Power System

Where an emergency or standby power system is provided to operate an elevator in the event of normal power supply failure, the requirements of 2.27.2.1 through 2.27.2.5 shall be complied with.

**2.27.2.1** The emergency or standby power system shall be capable of operating the elevator(s) with rated load (see 2.16.8), at least one at a time, unless otherwise required by the building code.

**2.27.2.2** The transfer between the normal and the emergency or standby power system shall be automatic.

**2.27.2.3** An illuminated signal marked "ELEVATOR EMERGENCY POWER" shall be provided in the elevator lobby at the designated level to indicate that the normal power supply has failed and the emergency or standby power is in effect.

**2.27.2.4** Where the emergency or standby power system is not capable of operating all elevators simultaneously, requirements of 2.27.2.4.1 through 2.27.2.4.5 shall be conformed to.

*2.27.2.4.1* A selector switch(es) marked "ELEVATOR EMERGENCY POWER" in red lettering a minimum of 5 mm (0.25 in.) in height, that is key-operated or under a locked cover (see 2.27.8), shall be provided to permit the selection of the elevator(s) to operate on the emergency or standby power system. The key shall be Group 3 Security (see 8.1).

*2.27.2.4.2* The selector switch(es) positions shall be marked to correspond with the elevator identification number (see 2.29) and a position marked "AUTO."

*2.27.2.4.3* The selector switch(es) shall be located at the designated level in view of all elevator entrances, or if located elsewhere means shall be provided adjacent to the selector switch(es) to indicate that the elevator is at the designated level with the doors in the normally open position.

*2.27.2.4.4* When the selector switch is in the "AUTO" position, automatic power selection shall be provided, that will return each elevator that is not on designated attendant operation, inspection operation, or Phase II In-Car Emergency Operation, one or more at a time, to the recall level. Failure of the selected car to move shall cause power to be transferred to another car.

*2.27.2.4.5* The selector switch(es) positions corresponding to the elevator identification numbers (see 2.29.1) shall override the automatic power selection. Operation of the selector switch(es) shall not cause power to be removed from any elevator until the elevator is stopped.

NOTE (2.27.2.4): The selector switch(es) should normally be placed in the "AUTO" position.

**2.27.2.5** When the emergency or standby power system is designed to operate only one elevator at a time, the energy absorption means (if required) shall be permitted to be located on the supply side of the elevator power disconnecting means, provided all other requirements of 2.26.10 are conformed to when operating any of the elevators the power might serve. Other building loads, such as power and lights that can be supplied by the emergency or standby power system, shall not be considered as a means of absorbing the regenerated energy for the purposes of conforming to 2.26.10, unless such loads are normally powered by the emergency or standby power system.

### 2.27.3 Firefighters' Emergency Operation: Automatic Elevators

Firefighters' Emergency Operation shall apply to all automatic elevators except where the hoistway or a portion thereof is not required to be fire-resistive construction (see 2.1.1.1), the rise does not exceed 2 000 mm (80 in.), and the hoistway does not penetrate a floor.

NOTE (2.27.3): When the structure (building, etc.) is located in a flood hazard area, the alternate and designated levels (see 8.12.1) should be above the base flood elevation.

**2.27.3.1 Phase I Emergency Recall Operation**

*2.27.3.1.1* A three-position key-operated switch that will not change position without a deliberate action by the user, shall be

(a) provided only at the designated level for each single elevator or for each group of elevators.
(b) labeled "FIRE RECALL" and its positions marked "RESET," "OFF," and "ON" (in that order), with the "OFF" position as the center position. The "FIRE RECALL" letters shall be a minimum of 5 mm (0.25 in.) high in red or a color contrasting with a red background.
(c) located in the lobby within sight of the elevator or all elevators in that group and shall be readily accessible.

*2.27.3.1.2* An additional key-operated "FIRE RECALL" switch, with two positions that will not change position without a deliberate action by the user, marked "OFF" and "ON" (in that order), shall be permitted only at the building fire control station.

*2.27.3.1.3* The switch(es) shall be rotated clockwise to go from the "RESET" (designated level switch only), to "OFF" to "ON" positions. Keys shall be removable only in the "OFF" and "ON" positions.

*2.27.3.1.4* Only the "FIRE RECALL" switch(es) or fire alarm initiating device located at floors that are served by the elevator, or in the hoistway, or in an elevator machine room, or a control space, or a control room (see 2.27.3.2) shall initiate Phase I Emergency Recall Operation.

*2.27.3.1.5* All "FIRE RECALL" switches shall be provided with an illuminated visual signal to indicate when Phase I Emergency Recall Operation is in effect.

*2.27.3.1.6* When a "FIRE RECALL" switch is in the "ON" position all cars controlled by the switch shall operate as follows:

(a) A car traveling towards the designated level shall continue nonstop to the designated level and power-operated doors shall open and remain open.

    On cars with two entrances, if both entrances can be opened at the designated level, only the doors serving the lobby where the "FIRE RECALL" switch is located shall open and remain open.
(b) A car traveling away from the designated level shall reverse at or before the next available landing without opening its doors and proceed to designated level.
(c) A stopped car shall have the in-car stop switch (see 2.26.2.21) and the emergency stop switch in the car (see 2.26.2.5) when provided, rendered inoperative as soon as the car moves away from the landing. A moving car shall have the in-car stop switch and the emergency stop switch in the car when provided, rendered inoperative without delay. Once the emergency stop switch in the car and the in-car stop switch have been rendered inoperative, they shall remain inoperative while the car is on Phase I Emergency Recall Operation. All other stop switches required by 2.26.2 shall remain operative.
(d) A car standing at a landing other than the designated level, with the doors open and the in-car stop switch and the emergency stop switch in the car when provided, in the run position, shall conform to the following:
    (1) Elevators having automatic power-operated horizontally sliding doors shall close the doors without delay and proceed to the designated level.
    (2) Elevators having power-operated vertically sliding doors provided with automatic or

momentary pressure closing operation per 2.13.3.4 shall have the closing sequence initiated without delay in accordance with 2.13.3.4.1, 2.13.3.4.2, 2.13.3.4.3, and 2.13.3.4.5, and the car shall proceed to the designated level.

(3) Elevators having power-operated doors provided with continuous pressure closing operation (see 2.13.3.2), or elevators having manual doors, shall be provided with a visual and audible signal system [see 2.27.3.1.6(h)] to alert an operator to close the doors and shall, when the doors are closed, proceed to the designated level. Sequence operation, if provided, shall remain effective.

(e) Door reopening devices for power-operated doors that are sensitive to smoke or flame shall be rendered inoperative without delay. Door reopening devices not sensitive to smoke or flame (e.g., mechanically actuated devices) are permitted to remain operative. Door closing for power-operated doors shall conform to 2.13.5.

(f) All car and corridor call buttons shall be rendered inoperative. All call-registered lights and directional lanterns shall be extinguished and remain inoperative. Car position indicators, where provided, shall remain operative. Where provided, landing position indicators shall be extinguished and remain inoperative, except at the designated level and the building fire control station, where they shall remain operative.

(g) Where provided on elevators with vertically sliding doors, corridor door open and door close buttons shall remain operative.

(h) An illuminated visual and audible signal system shall be activated. The visual signal shall be one of the symbols shown in Exhibit S2.1 and located on the car-operating panel. The entire circular or square area or the outline of the hat, or the outline of the area shown in Exhibit S2.1 shall be illuminated. The visual signal shall remain activated until the car is restored to automatic operation. When the door is open, the audible signal shall remain active until the door is closed. When the door is closed, the audible signal shall remain active for a minimum of 5 s. The audible signal shall not be active when the car is at the recall level.

(i) A car stopped at a landing shall have the in-car door open button rendered inoperative as soon as the car moves away from the landing. The in-car door open button shall remain inoperative when a car stops to reverse direction. Once the in-car door open button has been rendered inoperative, it shall remain inoperative until the car has returned to the designated level.

(j) Where an additional "FIRE RECALL" switch is provided, both "FIRE RECALL" switches shall be in the "ON" position to recall the elevator to the designated level if the elevator was recalled to the alternate level (see 2.27.3.2.4).

(k) To remove the elevator(s) from Phase I Emergency Recall Operation, the "FIRE RECALL" switch shall be rotated first to the "RESET," and then to the "OFF" position, provided that

(1) the additional two-position "FIRE RECALL" switch, where provided, is in the "OFF" position

(2) no fire alarm initiating device is activated (see 2.27.3.2).

(l) Means used to remove elevators from normal operation shall not prevent Phase I Emergency Recall Operation, except

(1) as specified in this Code

(2) as controlled by elevator personnel

(m) No device, that measures load, shall prevent operation of the elevator at or below the capacity and loading required in 2.16.

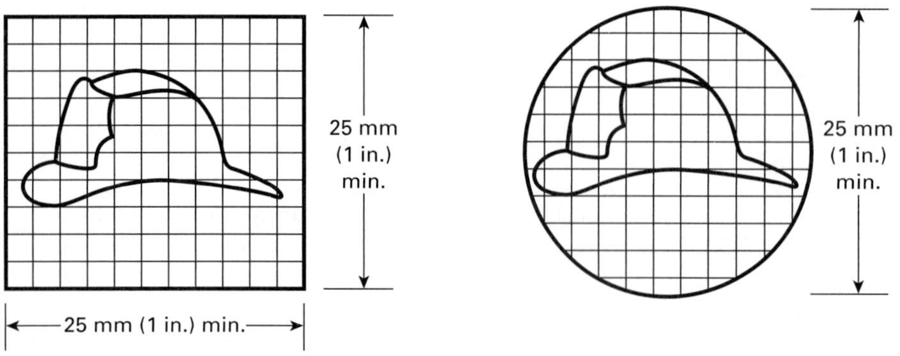


GENERAL NOTE: Grid is for scaling purposes only.

***Exhibit S2.1*** *Visual Signal. [From ASME A17.1, Section 2.27, Fig. 2.27.3.1.6(h)]*

(n) If the normal power supply, emergency power supply, and standby power supply are not available and the elevator is equipped with an alternate source of power that is insufficient to move the car to the recall level, the following requirements shall apply:

(1) The visual signal [2.27.3.1.6(h)] shall extinguish.
(2) A car that is not at a landing shall move to the closest landing it is capable of reaching.
(3) A car that has automatic power-operated horizontally sliding doors or power-operated vertically sliding doors provided with automatic closing operation and is stopped at a landing, shall open the doors, and then within 15 s, initiate reclosing.
(4) A car that is stopped at a landing shall have its door open button operative.
(5) A car stopped at a landing shall not move until normal power, emergency power, or standby power becomes available.

**2.27.3.2 Phase I Emergency Recall Operation by Fire Alarm Initiating Devices**

*2.27.3.2.1* In jurisdictions not enforcing the NBCC, fire alarm initiating devices used to initiate Phase I Emergency Recall Operation shall be installed in conformance with the requirements of NFPA 72, and shall be located

(a) at each floor served by the elevator
(b) in the associated elevator machine room, control space, or control room
(c) in the elevator hoistway, when sprinklers are located in those hoistways

*2.27.3.2.2* In jurisdictions enforcing the NBCC, smoke detectors, or, if applicable, the building fire alarm system (fire alarm initiating devices), used to initiate Phase I Emergency Recall Operation, shall be installed in conformance with the requirements of the NBCC, and shall be located in

(a) each elevator lobby
(b) the machine room

NOTE (2.27.3.2.2): Fire alarm initiating devices are referred to as fire detectors in the NBCC.

*2.27.3.2.3* Phase I Emergency Recall Operation to the designated level shall conform to the following:

(a) The activation of a fire alarm initiating device specified in 2.27.3.2.1 or 2.27.3.2.2(a) at any floor, other than at the designated level, shall cause all elevators that serve that floor, and any associated elevator of a group automatic operation, to be returned nonstop to the designated level.
(b) The activation of a fire alarm initiating device specified in 2.27.3.2.1(b) or 2.27.3.2.2(b) shall cause all elevators having any equipment located in that machine room, and any associated elevators of a group automatic operation, to be returned nonstop to the designated level. If the machine room is located at the designated level, the elevator(s) shall be returned nonstop to the alternate level.
(c) In jurisdictions not enforcing NBCC, the activation of a fire alarm initiating device specified in 2.27.3.2.1(c) or in jurisdictions enforcing NBCC, the initiation of a fire detector in the hoistway shall cause all elevators having any equipment in that hoistway, and any associated elevators of a group automatic operation, to be returned nonstop to the designated level, except that initiating device(s) installed at or below the lowest landing of recall shall cause the car to be sent to the upper recall level.
(d) The Phase I Emergency Recall Operation to the designated level shall conform to 2.27.3.1.6(a) through (n).

*2.27.3.2.4* Phase I Emergency Recall Operation to an alternate level (see 1.3) shall conform to the following:

(a) the activation of a fire alarm initiating device specified in 2.27.3.2.1(a) or 2.27.3.2.2(b) that is located at the designated level, shall cause all elevators serving that level to be recalled to an alternate level, unless Phase I Emergency Recall is in effect
(b) the requirements of 2.27.3.1.6(f), (j), (m), and (n)
(c) the requirements of 2.27.3.1.6(a), (b), (c), (d), (e), (g), (h), (i), (k), and (l), except that all references to the "designated level" shall be replaced with "alternate level"

*2.27.3.2.5* The recall level shall be determined by the first activated fire alarm initiating device for that group (see 2.27.3.2.1 or 2.27.3.2.2).

If the car(s) is recalled to the designated level by the "FIRE RECALL" switch(es) [see also 2.27.3.1.6(j)], the recall level shall remain the designated level.

*2.27.3.2.6* When a fire alarm initiating device in the machine room, control space, control room, or hoistway initiates Phase I Emergency Recall Operation, as required by 2.27.3.2.3 or 2.27.3.2.4, the visual signal [see 2.27.3.1.6(h) and Exhibit S2.1] shall illuminate intermittently only in a car(s) with equipment in that machine room, control space, control room, or hoistway. When activated, a heat detector [2.27.3.2.1(d)] in the machine room, control space, or control room shall cause the visual signal [see 2.27.3.1.6(h) and Exhibit S2.1] to illuminate intermittently only in a car(s) with equipment in that machine room, control space, or control room.

**2.27.3.3 Phase II Emergency In-Car Operation.** A three-position ("OFF," "HOLD," and "ON," in that order) key-operated switch that will not change position without a deliberate action by the user, shall be labeled "FIRE OPERATION"; provided in an operating panel in each car; and shall be readily accessible. The label "FIRE OPERATION" lettering shall be a minimum of 5 mm (0.25 in.) high in red or a color contrasting with a red background. It shall become effective only when Phase I Emergency Recall Operation is in effect and the car has been returned to the recall level. The switch shall be rotated clockwise to go from "OFF" to "HOLD" to "ON."

The key shall only be removable in the "OFF" and "HOLD" position. For elevators with power-operated doors, the "OFF," "HOLD," and "ON" positions shall not change the mode of operation within Phase II Emergency In-Car Operation until the car is at a landing with the doors in the normal open position, except as required by 2.27.3.3.4 and 2.27.3.4. The three modes of operation within Phase II In-Car Operation ("OFF," "HOLD," and "ON") are specified by 2.27.3.3.1 through 2.27.3.3.4.

For elevators with manual doors, after the car and hoistway doors have been opened at least once at the recall level, the "OFF," "HOLD," and "ON" positions shall then change the mode of operation in accordance with 2.27.3.3.1 through 2.27.3.3.4.

*2.27.3.3.1* When the "FIRE OPERATION" switch is in the "ON" position, the elevator shall be on Phase II Emergency In-Car Operation, for use by emergency personnel only, and the elevator shall operate as follows:

(a) The elevator shall be operable only by a person in the car.
(b) The car shall not respond to landing calls. Directional lanterns, where provided, shall remain inoperative. Car position indicators, where provided, shall remain operative. Landing position indicators, where provided, shall remain inoperative, except at the designated level and the building fire control station, where they shall remain operative.
(c) Door open and close buttons shall be provided for power-operated doors and located as required by 2.27.3.3.7. Buttons shall be a minimum of 19 mm (0.75 in.) in the smallest dimension. The door open and door close buttons shall be labeled "OPEN" and "CLOSE." The door open and close buttons shall be operative when the elevator is stopped within an unlocking zone.
(d) The opening of power-operated doors shall be controlled only by a continuous-pressure door open button. If the button is released prior to the doors reaching the normal open position, the doors shall automatically reclose. Requirements 2.13.3.3, 2.13.3.4, 2.13.4.2.1(b)(2), and 2.13.4.2.1(c) do not apply.

    On cars with multiple entrances, if more than one entrance can be opened at the same landing, separate door open buttons shall be provided for each entrance.
(e) Open power-operated doors shall be closed only by continuous pressure on the door close button. If the button is released prior to the doors reaching the fully closed position, horizontally sliding doors shall automatically reopen, and vertically sliding doors shall automatically stop or stop and reopen.

    On cars with multiple entrances, if more than one entrance can be opened at the same landing, a separate door close button shall be provided for each entrance.
(f) Opening and closing of power-operated car doors or gates that are opposite manual swing or manual slide hoistway doors shall conform to 2.27.3.3.1(d) and (e).
(g) All door reopening devices, except the door open button, shall be rendered inoperative. Full-speed closing shall be permitted.

    Landing door opening and closing buttons, where provided, shall be rendered inoperative.
(h) Every car shall be provided with a button labeled "CALL CANCEL," located as required in 2.27.3.3.7, that shall be effective during Phase II Emergency In-Car Operation. When activated, all registered calls shall be canceled and a traveling car shall stop at or before the next available landing. The button shall be a minimum of 19 mm (0.75 in.) in the smallest dimension.
(i) Floor selection means shall be provided in the car to permit travel to all landings served by the car, and shall be operative at all times, except as in 2.27.3.3.2 and 8.12.1. Means to prevent the operation of the floor selection means or door-operating buttons shall be rendered inoperative. The floor selection means shall be operable without the use of keys, cards, tools, or special knowledge. The floor selection means shall be permitted to be located behind the locked cover specified in 2.27.3.3.7, only if floor selection means for all landings served are included behind the locked cover. Where buttons not accessible to the public are provided they shall be a minimum of 19 mm (0.75 in.) in the smallest dimension.

(j) A traveling car shall stop at the next available landing for which a car call was registered. When a car stops at a landing, all registered car calls shall be canceled.

(k) Means used to remove elevators from normal operation shall not prevent Phase II Emergency In-Car Operation, except

(1) as specified in this Code
(2) as controlled by elevator personnel

(l) No device, that measures load, shall prevent operation of the elevator at or below the capacity and loading required in 2.16.

(m) Every car shall be provided with a switch, conforming to the requirements of 2.26.2.33 and located as required in 2.27.3.3.7. When the switch is in the "STOP" position, all registered calls shall be canceled and power shall be removed from the elevator driving-machine motor and brake. When the switch is moved to the "RUN" position from the "STOP" position, the car shall not move, except for leveling, until a call is entered. If the type of switch used is a button, it shall be a minimum of 19 mm (0.75 in.) in the smallest dimension.

NOTE [2.27.3.3.1(m)]: This requirement does not limit the firefighters' stop switch to a specific style of switch. Toggle switches and push/pull buttons are two possible styles. A switch, if provided, should be operable to the "STOP" position by a firefighter wearing protective gloves (see NFPA 1971).

(n) If the normal power supply, emergency power supply, and standby power supply are not available and the elevator is equipped with an alternate source of power that is insufficient to move the car to all landings, the requirements of 2.27.3.1.6(n)(1) through (5) shall apply.

*2.27.3.3.2* For elevators with power-operated doors, when the car is at a landing, with the doors open, and the "FIRE OPERATION" switch is in the "HOLD" position, the car shall remain at the landing with the doors open. The door close buttons shall be inoperative, and car calls shall not be registered.

For elevators with manual doors, when the car is at a landing and the "FIRE OPERATION" switch is in the "HOLD" position, the car shall remain at the landing and car calls shall not be registered.

*2.27.3.3.3* When the car is at a landing other than the recall level, with the doors in the normal open position, and the "FIRE OPERATION" switch is in the "OFF" position, power-operated doors shall operate as follows:

(a) Horizontal sliding doors shall close automatically. All door reopening devices shall remain inoperative. Door open buttons shall remain operative. Full-speed closing is permitted. If the "FIRE OPERATION" switch is turned to the "ON" or "HOLD" position prior to the completion of door closing, the doors shall reopen.

(b) Elevators having vertically sliding doors shall have corridor "DOOR OPEN" and "DOOR CLOSE" buttons rendered operative. All door reopening devices shall remain inoperative. Door closing shall be in accordance with 2.27.3.3.1(e). Full-speed closing is permitted. If the "FIRE OPERATION" switch is turned to the "ON" or "HOLD" position prior to the completion of door closing, the doors shall reopen.

*2.27.3.3.4* When the doors are in the closed position and the "FIRE OPERATION" switch is placed in the "OFF" position, the car shall return to the recall level in conformance with 2.27.3.1.6(a) through (n) and 2.27.3.2.5.

*2.27.3.3.5* Elevators shall be removed from Phase II Emergency In-Car Operation only when the "FIRE OPERATION" switch is in the "OFF" position and the car is at the designated level and the doors are in the normal open position.

*2.27.3.3.6* The occurrence of an accidental ground or short circuit in elevator electrical equipment located on the landing side of the hoistway enclosure and in associated wiring, as a result of exposure to water, shall not disable Phase II Emergency In-Car Operation once it has been activated.

*2.27.3.3.7* The "FIRE OPERATION" switch (2.27.3.3), the "CALL CANCEL" button [2.27.3.3.1(h)], the "STOP" switch [2.27.3.3.1(m)], the door open button(s), the door close button(s), the additional visual signal (2.27.3.3.8), and the operating instructions shown in Exhibit S2.4 shall be grouped together at the top of a main car operating panel behind a locked cover.

The firefighters' operation panel cover shall be openable by the same key that operates the "FIRE OPERATION" switch. The cover shall be permitted to open automatically when the car is on Phase I Emergency Recall Operation and at the recall level. When the key is in the "FIRE OPERATION" switch, the cover shall not be capable of being closed. When closed, the cover shall be self-locking.

Where rear doors are provided, buttons for both the front and rear doors shall be provided in the firefighters' operation panel. The door open and door close buttons for the rear entrance shall be labeled "OPEN REAR" and "CLOSE REAR."

All buttons and switches shall be readily accessible, located not more than 1 800 mm (72 in.) above the floor and shall be arranged as shown in Exhibit S2.2. Requirement 2.26.12 does not apply to these buttons and switches. The front of the cover shall contain the words "FIREFIGHTERS' OPERATION" in red letters at least 10 mm (0.4 in.) high.

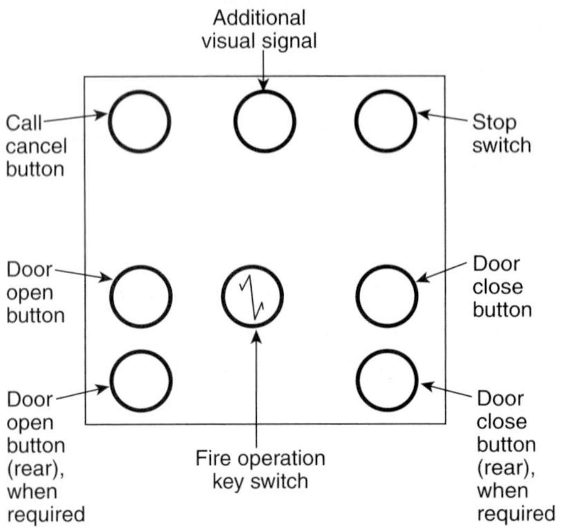


GENERAL NOTES:
(a) Switches and buttons show only the location not the labeling.
(b) When manually operated doors are provided, door open and close buttons and instructions for their use are not required.
(c) Not to scale.

***Exhibit S2.2*** *Panel Layout. (From ASME A17.1 Section 2.27, Fig. 2.27.3.3.7)*

*2.27.3.3.8* An additional visual signal shall be provided and located as required by 2.27.3.3.7. The additional visual signal shall be one of the symbols shown in Exhibit S2.1. The entire circular or square area shown in Exhibit S2.1 shall be illuminated. This additional visual signal shall be activated whenever the visual signal in 2.27.3.1.6(h) is activated.

**2.27.3.4 Interruption of Power.** Upon the resumption of power (normal, emergency, or standby), the car shall be permitted to move to reestablish absolute car position. Restoration of electrical power following a power interruption shall not cause any elevator to be removed from Phase I Emergency Recall Operation or Phase II Emergency In-Car Operation.

The failure and subsequent restoration of electrical power (normal, emergency, or standby) shall not cause any elevator to be removed from Phase I Emergency Operation or Phase II Emergency In-Car Operation.

(a) Elevators on Phase I Emergency Operation shall be permitted to move only to the next floor in the direction of the recall level to reestablish absolute car position prior to conforming to 2.27.3.1 and 2.27.3.2.
(b) Elevators on Phase II Emergency In-Car Operation with the key in the "OFF" position shall be permitted to move only to the next floor in the direction of the recall level to reestablish absolute car position prior to conforming to 2.27.3.3.3 and 2.27.3.3.4. If the key is moved to the "ON" or "HOLD" position before the doors are fully closed, 2.27.3.4(c) or (d) shall apply, and automatic power-operated doors shall open if in a level zone.
(c) Elevators on Phase II Emergency In-Car Operation with the key in the "HOLD" position shall not move, except for leveling within a leveling zone. Automatic power-operated doors shall open if the doors are not fully closed and the car is in a level zone.
(d) Elevators on Phase II Emergency In-Car Operation with the key in the "ON" position shall not move, except for leveling within a leveling zone, until a car call is entered. Automatic power-operated doors shall not move until a door open or close button is pressed; after which they shall conform to 2.27.3.3.1(d) and (e). After a car call is entered, the car shall be permitted to move only to the next floor in the direction of the recall level to reestablish absolute car position prior to answering car calls.

**2.27.3.5 Multicompartment Elevators.** Multicompartment elevators shall also conform to 2.27.3.5.1 and 2.27.3.5.7.

*2.27.3.5.1* The "FIRE RECALL" switch (2.27.3.1) shall be located at the designated level served by the upper compartment.

*2.27.3.5.2* The "FIRE OPERATION" switch (see 2.27.3.3) shall be located in the upper compartment.

*2.27.3.5.3* A means to display the entire floor area in the lower compartment shall be located in the upper compartment. The means shall display the lower compartment only when Phase I and Phase II is in effect.

*2.27.3.5.4* A switch labeled "LOWER CAR LOCKOUT" with two positions marked "OFF" and "ON" shall be located behind the firefighters' operation panel cover (see 2.27.3.3.7).

NOTE (2.27.3.5.4): The switch should be operable by a firefighter wearing protective gloves (see NFPA 1971).

(a) The "LOWER CAR LOCKOUT" switch shall only be functional when Phase II is in effect.
(b) When placed in the "ON" position, the "LOWER CAR LOCKOUT" switch shall

(1) disable all door reopening devices in the lower compartment, and
(2) initiate closing of the lower compartment doors in accordance with 2.13.4.2.1(c).

(c) When the car is stopped at a landing and the "LOWER CAR LOCKOUT" switch is in the "OFF" position, the lower compartment doors shall be opened.

**2.27.4 Firefighters' Emergency Operation: Nonautomatic Elevators**

Firefighters' Emergency Operation shall apply to all nonautomatic elevators, except as follows:

(a) where the hoistway or a portion thereof is not required to be fire-resistive construction (see 2.1.1.1), the rise does not exceed 2 000 mm (80 in.), and the hoistway does not penetrate a floor
(b) in jurisdictions enforcing the NBCC where the NBCC does not require Firefighters' Emergency Operation
(c) where Firefighters' Emergency Operation is provided voluntarily these requirements shall also apply

**2.27.4.1 Phase I Emergency Recall Operation.** A three-position key-operated switch shall be provided at the designated level for each single elevator or for each group of elevators. The three-position switch shall be labeled "FIRE RECALL" and its positions marked "RESET," "OFF," and "ON" (in that order), with the "OFF" position as the center position. The "FIRE RECALL" letters shall be a minimum of 5 mm (0.25 in.) high in red or a color contrasting with a red background. The three-position switch shall be located in the lobby within sight of the elevator or all elevators in that group and shall be readily accessible.

An additional "FIRE RECALL" switch with two positions, "OFF" and "ON" (in that order), shall be permitted only at the building fire control station.

The switch(es) shall be rotated clockwise to go from the "RESET" (designated level switch only), to the "OFF" and to the "ON" positions.

All keys shall be removable only in the "OFF" and "ON" positions.

Only the "FIRE RECALL" switch(es) or fire alarm initiating devices located at floors that are served by the elevator, in the hoistway, or in an elevator machine room, or a control space, or a control room (see 2.27.3.2) shall initiate Phase I Emergency Recall Operation.

All "FIRE RECALL" switches shall be provided with an illuminated visual signal to indicate when Phase I Emergency Recall Operation is in effect.

When all switches are in the "OFF" position, normal elevator service shall be in effect and the fire alarm initiating devices required by 2.27.4.2 shall be operative.

When a "FIRE RECALL" switch is in the "ON" position, a visual and audible signal shall be provided to alert the attendant to return nonstop to the designated or alternate level. The visual signal shall read "FIRE RECALL — RETURN TO _____" [insert level to which the car should be returned (the designated or alternate level)]. The signal system shall be activated when Phase I Emergency Recall Operation is in effect.

Where an additional "FIRE RECALL" switch is provided, both "FIRE RECALL" switches must be in the "ON" position to recall the elevator to the designated level if the elevator was recalled to the alternate level.

Where an additional "FIRE RECALL" switch is provided, it shall not affect the visual signal if the designated level fire alarm initiating device (see 2.27.3.2.4) has been activated.

To extinguish the audible and visual signals, the "FIRE RECALL" switch shall be rotated first to the "RESET" and then to the "OFF" position, provided that:

(a) the additional two-position "FIRE RECALL" switch, where provided, is in the "OFF" position
(b) no fire alarm initiating device is activated (see also 2.27.3.2.4)

No device, that measures load, shall prevent operation of the elevator at or below the capacity and loading required in 2.16.

**2.27.4.2 Phase I Emergency Recall Operation by Fire Alarm Initiating Devices.** Fire alarm initiating devices shall be installed at each floor served by the elevator, and in the associated machine room, control space, or control room, and elevator hoistway, in compliance with the requirements in NFPA 72 or NBCC, whichever is applicable (see Part 9). In jurisdictions enforcing the NBCC, compliance with 2.27.4.2 is not required where the NBCC specifies manual Emergency Recall operations only.

Phase I Emergency Recall Operation, conforming to 2.27.4.1, shall be initiated when any Phase I Emergency Recall Operation fire alarm initiating device at the elevator lobbies, machine room, control space, control room, or hoistway is activated.

Phase I Emergency Recall Operation, when initiated by a Phase I Emergency Recall Operation fire alarm initiating device, shall be maintained until canceled by moving the "FIRE RECALL" switch to the "RESET" position.

When a fire alarm initiating device in the machine room, control space, control room, or hoistway initiates

Phase I Emergency Recall Operation as required by 2.27.3.2.3 or 2.27.3.2.4, the visual signal [see 2.27.3.1.6(h) and Exhibit S2.1] shall illuminate intermittently only in a car(s) with equipment in that machine room, control space, control room, or hoistway. When activated, a heat detector [2.27.3.2.1(d)] in the machine room, control space, or control room shall cause the visual signal [see 2.27.3.1.6(h) and Exhibit S2.1] to illuminate intermittently only in a car(s) with equipment in that machine room, control space, or control room.

### 2.27.5 Firefighters' Emergency Operation: Automatic Elevators with Designated-Attendant Operation

**2.27.5.1** When designated-attendant operation is not in effect, elevators shall conform to 2.27.3.

**2.27.5.2** When operated by a designated attendant in the car, except hospital service:

(a) elevators parked at the recall level shall conform to 2.27.3 without delay; elevators parked at a floor other than the recall level shall conform to 2.27.3.1.6(h). At the completion of a time delay of not less than 10 s and not more than 30 s, elevators parked at a floor away from the recall level shall conform to 2.27.3.

(b) A moving car shall conform to 2.27.3.

**2.27.5.3** When an elevator that is provided with firefighters' emergency operation is on hospital service, a visual signal as shown in Fig. 2.27.3.1.6(h) shall illuminate and a continuous audible signal, audible within the car, shall sound when the "FIRE RECALL" switch(es) (see 2.27.3.1) is in the "ON" position, or when a fire alarm initiating device (see 2.27.3.2) is activated to alert the operator of an emergency. A means located in the car shall be permitted for manually silencing the audible signal, after the signal has been active for at least 5 s. The signal shall be automatically reactivated when the doors open.

The car shall remain under control of the operator until removed from hospital service. An elevator on firefighters' emergency operation shall not be placed on hospital service.

### 2.27.6 Firefighters' Emergency Operation: Inspection Operation

When an elevator that is provided with firefighters' service is on inspection operation (see 2.26.1.4 and 2.26.1.5) or when the hoistway access switch(es) has been enabled [see 2.12.7.3.3(a)], a continuous audible signal, audible at the location where the operation is activated shall sound when the "FIRE RECALL" switch(es) (see 2.27.3.1) is in the "ON" position or when the fire alarm initiating device (see 2.27.3.2) is activated to alert the operator of an emergency. The car shall remain under the control of the operator until removed from inspection operation or hoistway access operation. Inspection operation or hoistway access operation shall take precedence over Phase I Emergency Recall Operation and Phase II Emergency In-Car Operation.

### 2.27.7 Firefighters' Emergency Operation: Operating Procedures

**2.27.7.1** Instructions for operation of elevators under Phase I Emergency Recall Operation shall be incorporated with or adjacent to the "FIRE RECALL" switch at the designated level. The instructions shall include only the wording shown in Exhibit S2.3.

**FIREFIGHTERS' OPERATION**

**To recall elevators**
**Insert fire key and turn to "ON"**

***Exhibit S2.3*** *Phase I Emergency Recall Operation Instructions. (From ASME A17.1 Section 2.27, Fig. 2.27.7.1)*

**2.27.7.2** A sign containing instructions for operation of elevators under Phase II Emergency In-Car Operation shall be incorporated with or adjacent to the switch in each car and shall be visible only when the cover (2.27.3.3.7) is open. The sign shall include only the wording and graphics shown in Exhibit S2.4, except

(a) for elevators with manually operated doors, the instructions for opening and closing the doors shall be permitted to be replaced with short phrases such as "PUSH DOOR" or "PULL DOOR UP"

(b) for elevators with vertically sliding doors, the instructions for returning the car to the recall floor shall be permitted to be expanded to include instructions for closing the door

**2.27.7.3** Instructions shall be in letters not less than 3 mm (0.125 in.) in height and shall be permanently installed and protected against removal or defacement.

**2.27.7.4** In jurisdictions that enforce the NBCC, a symbol showing a red firefighters' hat on a contrasting background, as shown in Exhibit S2.1 (figure not to

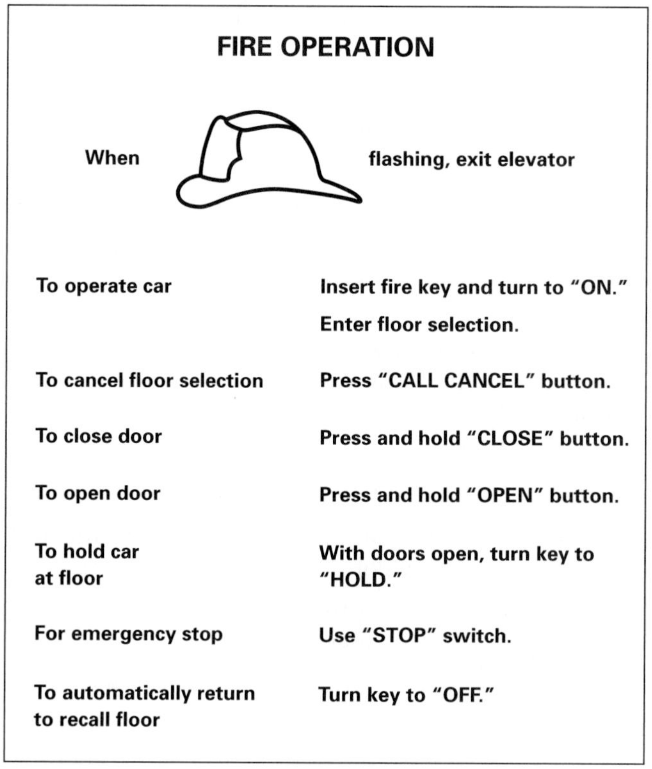


***Exhibit S2.4*** *Phase II Emergency In-Car Operation. (From ASME A177.1 Section 2.27, Fig. 2.27.7.2)*

scale), shall be used exclusively to identify elevators that comply with 2.27.3 and additional NBCC requirements. This identification shall be located on the elevator entrance frame or adjacent to it at each emergency recall level. The identification on the entrance frame, or adjacent to it, shall be a minimum of 50 mm (2 in.) in height.

### 2.27.8 Switch Keys

The key switches required by 2.27.2 through 2.27.5 for all elevators in a building shall be operable by the same key. The keys shall be Group 3 Security (see 8.1). There shall be a key for each switch provided.

These keys shall be kept on the premises in a location readily accessible to firefighters and emergency personnel, but not where they are available to the public. This key shall be of a tubular, 7 pin, style 137 construction and shall have a bitting code of 6143521. The key shall be coded "FEO-K1." The possession of the "FEO-K1" key shall be limited to elevator personnel, emergency personnel, and elevator equipment manufacturers.

Where provided, a lock box, including its lock and other components, shall conform to the requirements of UL 1037 (see Part 9).

NOTE (2.27.8): Local authorities may specify additional requirements for a uniform keyed lock box and its location to contain the necessary keys.

### 2.27.9 Elevator Corridor Call Station Pictograph

When the building code requires a sign be posted adjacent to hall call fixtures instructing occupants not to use the elevator in case of fire, the sign shown in Exhibit S2.5 shall be provided. The sign shall include only the wording and graphics shown in Exhibit S2.5. When the building code specifies a different design, 2.27.9 shall not apply.

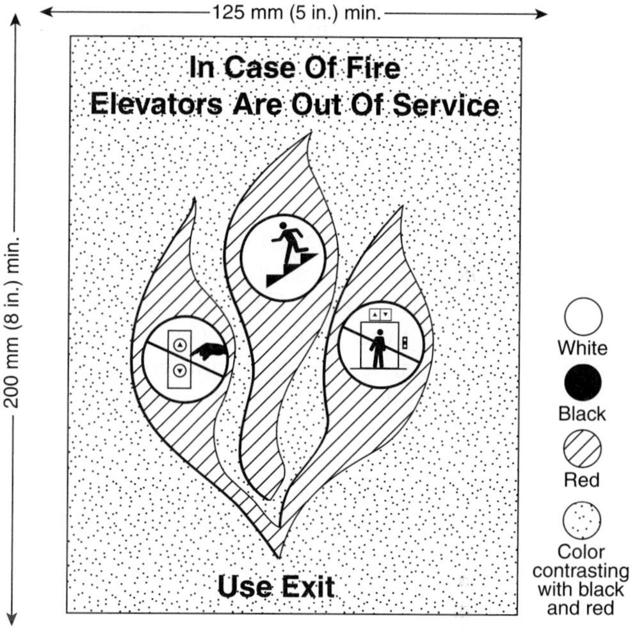


***Exhibit S2.5*** *Elevator Corridor Call Station Pictograph. (From ASME A17.1 Section 2.27, Fig. 2.27.9)*

## EXTRACTS FROM *ASME A17.1 HANDBOOK*, SECTION 2.27 EMERGENCY OPERATION AND SIGNALING DEVICES**

A note was added in ASME A17.1-2000/CSA B44-00 to recognize that additional requirements may be found in the building codes. For example, IBC requires fire department communication system in high-rise buildings (IBC Section 907.2.12.3).

ASME A17.1a-2002/CSA B44-02 Update No. 1 made major revisions to car emergency signaling requirements. The Code requires a means for all passengers, both able-bodied and disabled, to communicate

**Reprinted from *ASME A17.1 Handbook* — 2007, by Edward A. Donoghue, by permission of The American Society of Mechanical Engineers. All rights reserved.

in an emergency. Requirements were prepared to address the following reported concerns:

(a) reports of passengers being trapped overnight, weekends, and holidays
(b) alarm bells being ignored
(c) alarm bells not working
(d) no one accepting responsibility or accountability for providing assistance
(e) deficiencies with new technology being utilized at this time
(f) needs of all elevator passengers

In addition to these requirements, building codes require that all elevators in high-rise buildings (see building code for definition) have a communication system from the elevator lobby, car, machine room, control room, machinery space, and control space outside the hoistway to the building's central control station. See commentary on car lighting in 2.14.7.1.

*2.27.1.1.1* In all buildings, a means of two-way communications is required that allows a trapped passenger to call for help and reach someone trained to respond to the call for help. Call routing may be different at different times of the day (for example, normal business hours, versus nights and weekends), but a call for help should always reach a trained person, permitting action to be taken in a timely manner.

*2.27.1.1.3(a)* Requirements ensure there is no conflict with accessibility requirements (ICC/ANSI A117.1 and ASME A17.1/CSA B44, Appendix E, ADAAG and ADA/ABA AG).

*2.27.1.1.3(b)* Provides a recognizable means accessible to the passenger to initiate a call for help and establish two-way communications. The term "HELP" describes the passenger's immediate need. Historically the alarm button has always been visible and thus the help button should be visible.

*2.27.1.1.3(c)* Provides an indication, for hearing-impaired passengers, that the call for help has been received and acknowledged by authorized personnel.

*2.27.1.1.3(d)* Provides a means for authorized personnel to identify the location of the elevators independent of the passenger having to provide this information.

*2.27.1.1.3(e)* Provides a means to communicate to the passenger that help is being sent.

*2.27.1.1.3(f)* The person who receives the call is in the best position to decide how long to continue the conversation. Communications must not cut off after a pre-determined time limit, etc.

*2.27.1.1.3(g)* Prohibits the use of handsets since they are easily subject to vandalism.

*2.27.1.1.3(h)* The passenger needs help when a call is placed, not days later when someone listens to voice mail.

*2.27.1.1.4* Provides arriving rescuers with the means to communicate with the passenger in high-rise buildings where direct voice communication may not be practical.

*2.27.1.1.4(a)* Establishes a reasonable time frame in which communications are to be established. Requires the capability for two-way communication with a single car at a time.

*2.27.1.1.4(b)* See Commentary to 2.27.1.1.3(f).

*2.27.1.1.4(c)* Provides a visual indication to the passenger that two-way communications is activated.

*2.27.1.1.4(d)* Provides authorized or "emergency" personnel with operating instructions.

*2.27.1.1.5* Provides an alternate power source if normal power fails. The visual signal is part of the emergency communications system and should have the same minimum time standard as the two-way communications means. Duration requirements for the audible signal was changed to 1 hr as it was previously, unintentionally included in the 4 hr requirement.

**2.27.1.2** This discourages the use of an emergency stop switch to hold a car at a floor, etc.

### 2.27.2 Emergency or Standby Power System

Emergency or standby power for an elevator is not required by the ASME A17.1/CSA B44 Code. If provided, then it must comply with 2.27.2. Building codes typically require standby power for at least one elevator able to travel to each floor in a high-rise building (see definition of building code in 1.3). This elevator does not have to stop at every floor, but every floor must be served by at least one elevator supplied with standby power. As an example, in a 20-story building elevator group A serves floors 1 through 10 and elevator group B serves floors 1 and 11 through 20. Standby power would have to be supplied to one elevator in group A and one elevator in group B. If the same 20-story building had an elevator that served all floors 1 through 20, then standby power could be supplied to that elevator only.

Building codes in the United States address the need to provide accessible means of egress during a fire. Accessible means of egress include elevators, operating on Phase II Emergency Operation. When accessible means of egress include elevators, they shall be provided with standby power.

The National Electrical Code (NEC®) has requirements for both legally required standby power systems (Article 701) and optional standby power systems (Article 702). Legally required standby power systems provide electric power when normal power is interrupted to aid fire fighting, rescue operations, control of health hazards, and similar operations. Optional standby power systems provide electric power when normal power is interrupted to eliminate physical discomfort, interruption of an industrial process, damage to equipment, or disruption of business.

Emergency power systems are those essential for safety to human life and must conform to requirements of NEC® Article 700. For additional information, see the NFPA 110 standard for emergency and standby power systems.

Legally required standby power systems have requirements that are very similar to emergency power systems. Upon loss of normal power, the legally required standby power system must be able to supply power within 60 s, whereas emergency power system must be able to supply power within 10 s. Wiring for legally required standby power systems can be installed in the same raceway, cables, or boxes used for other general wiring. In contrast, emergency power system wiring must be entirely independent of all other wiring.

Elevators are normally connected to legally required standby power systems and not emergency power systems. Some hospital elevators are hooked into emergency power systems.

Requirement 2.27.2.1 facilitates availability of power for an elevator system. Power transfer and selection speeds up the evacuation process, minimizes entrapments, and allows use of an elevator by firefighters.

Requirement 2.27.2.4 requires automatic sequence operation. When the switch is left in the AUTO position, each car in turn will move to the recall floor and open their door(s). Automatic sequencing must be arranged that it can be overridden by the manual selection switch. This provides arriving firefighters with ability to select which elevator will receive power. Changing the car selected by the switch must not cause an emergency stop; power will be transferred only after the elevator makes a normal stop at a floor.

See also the commentary on 2.26.10 and Section 620-101 of the National Electrical Code®.

### 2.27.3 Firefighters' Emergency Operations — Automatic Elevators

In 2005, the National Fire Protection Association reported 1,602,000 fires resulting in 3,675 fire deaths in the United States. There was a civilian fire fatality every 143 min and a civilian fire injury every 29 min. Since 1980, the NFPA has recorded 254 fatal fires in high-rise buildings (over 7 stories) in the United States and Canada. These fires resulted in 3,567 deaths of the public and included 383 firefighters. The last available set of figures showing a comparison between two countries is from 2002. Combined figures covering office buildings, hotels, apartment buildings, and hospitals are 7,300 reported structure fires with 15 civilian deaths, 300 civilian injuries, and $26 million dollars in direct property damage. If extrapolated to all property uses, these figures suggest a total of 10,200 high rise fires in 2002, civilian deaths of approximately 28, injuries of 350 and direct property damage at $143 million. The total building fire incidents in the United States were 1,734,500 with 6,196 deaths not including those lost on September 11, 2001 at the World Trade Center attack. In Canada, the comparative figures available for 2001 were 55,300 fire incidents, resulting in 337 deaths. An equally important set of figures is the total number of injuries, in both the United States (21,100) and Canada (1,754). Only through an examination of the data does a true picture of the fire problem that we are facing today emerge. Between both countries, it is estimated that in the past 25 years, there have been thousands of new high-rise buildings built.

The building codes define a high-rise building as a building more than (23 m) 75 ft in height measured from the lowest level of fire department vehicle access to the highest occupiable floor. For a short period after the events of September 11, 2001, there was a period of indecision about the potential future of high-rise construction around the world. All one has to do today is look at the skyline in any major city in North America to recognize the high-rise building boom is back in full swing. In the past, office occupancies had been classified as a low-risk fire hazard. This was true in older, compartmentalized high-rise buildings, with no multifloor HVAC systems, and office furnishings made of wood or metal. However, the modern high-rise building is different. Fire and smoke spreading to other floors of the structure (i.e., World Trade Center bombings of 2001, 2003 Chicago Cook County Building fire etc.) are the true nightmare facing the firefighting forces of both countries. A factor in this fire problem is the furnishings. The vast majority of today's building interiors use various forms of plastic. Firefighters commonly refer to plastic as frozen gasoline. As plastic is heated from exposure to fire, it goes through a decomposition process that emits toxic, disabling gases (e.g., hydrogen chloride) and flammable hydrocarbon gases, which rapidly spread and cause immediate propagation of the fire across large areas. The smoke from these products of combustion is dense and black, causing trapped occupants to have little or no visibility, encounter choking smoke, and face heat of temperatures well above what a human being can endure.

Today's high-rise buildings present new and different problems to fire suppression personnel and techniques. The cause of fires in high-rise buildings and the materials used in them, including furniture and fixtures, are not any different from those used in conventional low-rise structures. However, if a fire breaks out in the top story of a high rise, the fire service must transport their firefighters and equipment to the upper floors via elevators operating on Phase II Firefighters' In-Car Operation. In some fires, firefighters had to use stairs to reach the fire floor. Keep in mind that the firefighters, while wearing all of their protective gear weigh an additional 65 lb (29.5 kg). Firefighters also carry long lengths of hose and attachments weighing an additional 50 lb (22.6 kg) to 65 lb (29.5 kg). Using the stairs to gain access to upper floors in a high-rise structure is the last resort. However, firefighters' will use stairs where there is no other choice, as was the case during the World Trade Center attacks on September 11, 2001. After reaching the fire floor, the firefighters will be subjected to high heat [temperatures above 200°F (93°C)]. Their protective clothing will only provide a limited amount of protection, taking into account the "pre-heating" of the gear, depending on the amount of heat exposure, etc. Elevators must be a reliable tool to be utilized by the firefighters in the performance of their duties; however, elevators cannot be relied upon during a fire in a building.

A firefighting commander prefers a fire that is located on the top floor of a building over a fire on a lower floor. Why? Because the life hazard is on the fire floor (top floor), where only the roof and the sky are being exposed. In contrast, a fire on the 10th floor of a 34-story building has a life hazard on all floors above the fire, as well as the fire floor, requiring additional staffing to accomplish the tasks of search, rescue, and fire extinguishment. Recent improvements to the National Fire Incident Reporting System (NFIRS) Version 5.0 now allows the exact floor of fire origin to be indicated, revealing the fact that in high-rise fires reported, the fire floor was on floor 6 or below. Usually the lower floors of any high-rise building will locate the service areas such as maintenance, heating, coffee shops, restaurants, cleaners and other support functions on those floors, with the resulting fires. Many fires do start on higher floors, but the average is floor 6 or below.

Firefighters have immediate concerns relating to smoke and heat spread, stack effect, and uncontrolled evacuation of building occupants down the same stairways that firefighters are trying to use to move up to locate, surround, and extinguish the fire. A few points to keep in mind: At the Meridian Plaza fire in Philadelphia, there was a total failure of all building systems early in the fire, and secondly, the World Trade Center explosion and resulting fire was below grade, and it took 11 h to complete the evacuation. The events of September 11, 2001 provided terrible reminders of the life hazard that we all must face during a fire in a high-rise building.

Let's review some of the reasons that led to the Code requirements for firefighters' emergency operation. Elevators are unsafe in a fire because:

(a) person may push a corridor button and have to wait for an elevator that may never respond; valuable time to escape is lost.
(b) elevators respond to car and corridor calls; one of these may be at the fire floor.
(c) elevators cannot start until the car and hoistway doors are closed. This could lead to overcrowding of an elevator and the blockage of the doors, and thus prevent closing.
(d) power failure during a fire can happen at any time and thus lead to passenger entrapment.

Fatal delivery of the elevator to the fire floor can be caused by any of the following:

(1) an elevator passenger pressing the car button for the fire floor
(2) one or both of the corridor call buttons may be pushed on the fire floor
(3) heat may melt or deform the corridor push button or its wiring at the fire floor
(4) normal functioning of the elevator, such as high or low reversal, may occur at the fire floor
(5) heat from the fire or loss of air conditioning in the machinery space, machine room, control space, or control room may have a detrimental effect on solid-state control equipment, resulting in erratic elevator operation

The ASME A17.1/CSA B44 Code recognized all of these conditions and has reacted by mandating Phase I Emergency Recall Operation. The building code also requires a sign in elevator lobbies to advise building occupants not to use elevators in a fire. See Handbook Commentary on 2.27.9.

Firefighters' Emergency Operation (FEO) is also known as Firefighters' Service or special emergency service [SES] features. The ASME A17 and CSA B44 Committees have strived to standardize the operation to eliminate variations amongst different elevator equipment that may confuse firefighters' during an emergency. The automatic or manual return of elevators to the designated level (see 1.3 for definition) is referred to as Phase I Emergency Recall Operation. Phase II Emergency In-Car operation refers to provisions allowing emergency personnel to operate the elevator from within the car.

**2.27.3.1 Phase I Emergency Recall Operation.** ASME A17.1b-1989 through ASME A17.1b-1992 required Phase I for an elevator with a rise of 7.62 m (25 ft) or more. Under earlier editions of the Code, an elevator could have nearly 15.24 m (50 ft) of rise [just less than 7.62 m (25 ft) above and below the designated landing], and still not have been required to have Phase I and Phase II operation. The term "designated level" (see 1.3) refers to the main floor or other level that best serves the needs of emergency personnel for firefighting and rescue purposes. The term "alternate landing" (see 1.3) refers to a floor level identified by the building code or fire authority, other than the designated landing. The term "recall level" (see 1.3) refers to the designated or alternate level that the car returns to when Phase I Emergency Recall Operation is activated. These requirements apply for all automatic elevators except when the hoistway or a portion thereof is not required to be constructed of fire-resistive construction (2.1.1.1), the rise does not exceed 2 000 mm or 80 in., and the hoistway does not penetrate a floor. An example of this would be an elevator that only traveled from one level in a lobby to a second level in the same lobby and not penetrating a fire barrier. This arrangement can be seen in department stores or malls.

A three-position key-operated switch must be provided in the designated level lobby for each single elevator or for a group of elevators. The location of the three-position Phase I Emergency Recall switch has been standardized so that the switch will be located where all of the elevators are within sight and readily accessible. The key is to be removable only in the "ON" and "OFF" positions. The specified key positions standardize around a clockwise rotation to reach the "ON" position similar to the requirements for the Phase II Emergency In-Car Operation switch. Prior to the ASME A17.1-2000/CSA B44-00, the three-position Phase I key switch included the "BYPASS" position in jurisdictions not enforcing NBCC. Bypass allowed building or emergency personnel to return elevators to normal service without clearing an activated (alarmed) fire alarm initiating device (e.g., smoke detector). However, the entire automatic Phase I Emergency Recall system would be disabled when the key was in the "BYPASS" position. The fire alarm initiating devices that are used today are far superior to the ones that were first used. Today's systems can be monitored, maintained, and cleared from their control panel.

Beginning with ASME A17.1-1996, the expertise of NFPA 72 was recognized as the proper authority to determine the number, type, and location of fire alarm initiating devices in a building. In continuing with this transition, in ASME A17.1-2000/CSA B44-00 the "BYPASS" position was replaced with the "RESET" position on the three-position Phase I Emergency Recall Operation switch. The "RESET" feature will be utilized by emergency personnel (1.3) to reset the elevators returning them to normal service, after Phase I Emergency Recall Operation has been activated. If the fire alarm initiating device has not been cleared before using the "RESET" feature, then the Phase I Emergency Recall Operation will continue in effect until the device has been replaced, repaired, or bypassed by the fire alarm system. The Phase I switch shall be labeled "FIRE RECALL" and its positions marked as "RESET," "OFF," and "ON" (in that order), with the "OFF" position as the center position. An additional key-operated "FIRE RECALL" switch, with two positions, marked "OFF" and "ON" (in that order), is permitted only at the building fire control station. Keys shall be removable in the "OFF" and "ON" positions only. The switches cannot be spring loaded.

During Phase I operation the elevator is not available to the general public as automatic elevator use may be hazardous during a fire emergency. When an elevator is out of service during a fire, the public is unable to use it as a means of exiting from the building. Depending on the building fire plan, occupants will be directed to either the stairwells, places of refuge, or to be active participants in the emergency plan developed for their safety by the building owners/operators.

Earlier editions of the ASME A17.1/CSA B44 Code addressed only automatic door operations. The 1981 and later editions of the Code cover operation of vertically sliding doors, doors controlled by constant pressure buttons, and manual doors. The only time an automatic elevator will not return upon activation of Phase I is when that car is at a landing with its door(s) open and the in-car stop switch, emergency stop switch (in-car, top-of-car, pit, etc.), or some other electrical protective device is activated.

Requirement 2.27.3.1.6(b) recognizes that an elevator at a landing with the in-car stop switch or emergency stop switch in the "STOP" position should not be recalled, as this is not a normal condition. The stop switch may have been activated to facilitate an inspection or maintenance and recalling the elevator could be a hazard to elevator personnel. Once the car moves, the in-car stop switch is disabled, just like the emergency stop switch, and the elevator cannot be stopped using the switch. This feature prevents a person (such as building cleaning personnel) with access to the in-car stop switch key from activating the in-car stop switch, after the doors are closed and the elevators is being recalled. This would create an unsafe condition, as the firefighters would have to search for the car immediately. Moreover, the occupant may be putting himself or herself in great danger.

For passenger safety, 2.27.3.1.6(e) requires elevators doors to close at a slower speed when a door-reopening device is rendered inoperative. Mechanically actuated door-reopening devices are not sensitive to smoke or flame and can remain operative. Flame is the glowing, gaseous, visible part of a fire. Smoke or flame can register a signal, whereas a direct flame fire will destroy. Unless the fire was inside the car, the cars would all have responded to the recall level well in advance of fire directly impinging on the hoistway door reversal device. The reference to 2.13.5 recognizes "nudging" and, therefore, it is not unsafe to disconnect mechanically actuated door-reopening devices.

Requirements 2.27.3.1.6(f) and (g) allow full control of those doors that may have to be closed from the corridor. Also, the automatic closing of vertical slide doors requires an active "OPEN" or "STOP" button on the corridor. An active corridor "DOOR OPEN" button allows the user to open a closed hoistway door to access a car with a manual gate that is in an open position. A firefighter may need the "DOOR OPEN" button to open the door to see if anyone is in the car.

Operating hall position indicators [2.27.3.1.6(f)] may convey a message that the elevators may be used. Only where elevator location is important to firefighters, such as the designated level and the building fire control station, may hall position indicators remain in operation. Car position indicators are always required by the firefighters utilizing the elevators, thus these devices are to remain operative.

As the car will not be called to the fire floor, and the recall level elevator landing is free of smoke, it is safe to keep the doors open. Arriving firefighting forces will be able to immediately determine if all cars have answered the recall, and passengers are not trapped in cars within the hoistway. If the Incident Commander (IC) of the firefighting forces cannot account for and verify where the elevators are, then firefighters will have to be diverted from other critical duties of rescue and suppression to search for and establish control over those elevators and their occupants.

The visible and audible signals [2.27.3.1.6(h)] alert passengers in an automatically operated elevator of the emergency and can minimize any apprehension that the passengers may have while the elevator is returning to the main floor. In an attendant-operated elevator, this signal alerts the attendant of the emergency and signals them to return immediately to the designated level. When on inspection operation, the inspector or maintenance personnel are also alerted to the emergency by this signal.

Requirement 2.27.3.1.6(j) recognized that if the smoke detector at the designated level is activated, turning only the additional Phase I switch to the "ON" position will not override the fire alarm initiating device sending the car to the alternate level. Where an additional "FIRE RECALL" switch is provided, both "FIRE RECALL" switches must be in the "ON" position to recall the elevator to the designated level if the elevator was recalled to the alternate level (2.27.3.2.4). This is because the additional switch may be at a location where the condition of the designated level lobby cannot be determined. This also prevents a melted Phase I switch from recalling the cars from the alternate to the designated level.

To remove the elevators from Phase I, the "FIRE RECALL" switch shall first be rotated to the "RESET" position, and then to the "OFF" position. If a second recall switch is provided, it must be in the "OFF" position to remove the elevator from Phase I Emergency Recall Operation. Means used to remove elevators from normal operation, other than as specified in this code, shall not prevent Phase I Emergency Recall Operation. This requirement gives firefighters priority over elevator use by service personnel, movers, security lock out, etc. This feature was included at the request of the fire service community, who often arrived at a fire, only to find that most of the elevators were not accessible for their use.

On the other hand, changes in the ASME A17.1/CSA B44-2007 Code recognize that cars shut down for safety reasons in accordance with other code requirements (such as an earthquake or flood) should not respond to Firefighters' Emergency Operation. The ASME A17.1/CSA B44-2007 edition also recognizes the existence of battery operated devices used to move an elevator during a power failure. Without knowing where the fire is, these devices can move the elevator to let the passengers out as soon as possible, while the fire is still in its early stages, so they can exit the building.

**2.27.3.2 Phase I Emergency Recall Operation by Fire Alarm Initiations Device.** An initiation device is defined by NFPA 72 as a system component that originates transmission of a change-of-state condition, such as in a smoke detector, etc.

*2.27.3.2.1* The reference to the National Fire Alarm Code®, NFPA 72 is to a standard with expertise to specify the type and installation of automatic initiating devices. NFPA 72 has been revised, at the request of the ASME A17 Committee, to address fire alarm systems in all building types. Members of the National Fire Alarm Code®, NFPA 72 Committee have the expertise to determine when fire conditions require automatic elevator recall. See Chart 2.27.3.2.1(a) for excerpts from the NFPA Fire Alarm Code® Handbook. Beginning with ASME A17.1b-1997 a fire alarm initiating device must be provided at all floors. ASME A17.1 recognizes that devices other than smoke detectors may be more appropriate under some conditions. Those conditions are specified within NFPA 72. See Chart 2.27.3.2.1(b).

*Editor's Note: Please refer to the ASME A17.1 Handbook for Charts 2.27.3.2.1(a) and (b).*

*2.27.3.2.2* To harmonize with the requirements in NBCC the term "smoke detector" substitutes for "fire-alarm initiating device" and "elevator lobby" for elevator landing."

*2.27.3.2.4* The following is the basis for alternate floor recall. It is not preordained that the designated level has the lowest fuel load of any other floor in the buildings. This may be the case in some major, high-rise office buildings, but it certainly is not applicable to many other buildings, such as apartments, hotels, showrooms, or buildings with elaborate reception areas. However, even if it were a fact, a firebomb can suddenly provide an enormous fuel load on an otherwise fire-resistant floor.

Most of buildings have elevators without an express zone. In buildings with express zones, it is safer to park elevators away from any potential fire floor. It is feared that if the mandatory alternate floor requirement is repealed and made permissive, then many buildings would revert to the early Code requirements requiring return to the designated level. This would be a step backwards in protecting the riding public from arriving at a fire floor.

When elevators are returned to an alternate level, firefighters have not lost control. If conditions dictate that the designated level is safe, firefighters can call the elevators to the designated level by turning the required three-position keyed switch to the "ON" position. The key switch overrides alternate floor recall operation and returns all elevators to the designated level, even though the elevators may be parked at a floor above an express zone. ASME A17.1a-2005/CSA B44-04 Update 1-05 made a change so that once this happens, the designated level remains the recall level, even if the key switch is reset.

Typically, the designated level is also the location of the central command station. It would be difficult to effectively utilize a designated level central command station if the designated level is engulfed in a rapidly spreading fire such as the one that destroyed the main floor of the MGM Hotel. Elevators that are returned to, or parked at, the main floor are of no value if the result is loss of life.

While sprinklers will reduce the probability of a large fire, smoke in dangerous quantities may be produced. Sprinkler manufacturers argue for the effectiveness of sprinklers in stopping fire in a large number of buildings, but as smoke control advocates note, it is smoke, and not the flames themselves cause the majority of fire deaths. Smoke control advocates believe that sprinklers allow too much smoke to develop before sprinklers activate.

Use of smoke detectors for the recall function has also been questioned because of the possibility that smoke may be present on floors above and/or below the fire floor. The Code has addressed this in 2.27.3.2.5 by indicating that the first smoke detector activation determines the recall level (see 1.3). It is highly improbable that smoke detectors on floors other than the fire floor would activate beforehand.

As a corollary to smoke detectors required to initiate elevator recall, others argue that the water flow switch associated with the on-floor sprinkler system is more positive. Smoke detectors can initiate elevator recall when the smoke reaches the elevators and threatens passengers; but smoke or water flow in a remote part of the building should not trigger a recall.

*2.27.3.2.5* This requirement states that the elevator only needs to respond to the first detector, activated. The likelihood of two simultaneous fires is infinitesimal. It is assumed that the smoke detector at the fire floor will be the first one that is activated. Subsequent alarms would most likely occur due to smoke migration and would not affect the choice of the recall floor. Revisions made in ASME A17.1a-2005/CSA B44-04 Update 1-05 clarified the cars should never move to the alternate floor after being recalled to the designated level.

Connecting smoke detectors to the elevator system appropriately positions the elevators while the fire department is still on the way. This feature prevents building occupants from being delivered to a fire floor, and permits the firefighters to quickly assess if all elevators have been recalled. Detectors at the designated level prevent the passengers from being delivered to a fire at that floor. The detectors no longer serve a purpose once the passengers are out and the firefighters have arrived. The detectors are still useful for tracking smoke spread at the fire alarm panel. Once the firefighters decide it is safe to return the cars to the designated level there is no reason to return the cars to the alternate again.

**2.27.3.3 Phase II Emergency In-Car Operation.** Beginning with the 1981 edition of ASME A17.1, Phase II operation is required whenever Phase I operation is provided. Previously the requirement was predicated on the needs of emergency personnel. The current requirement takes into account the need by firefighters during an emergency including evacuating the disabled. Disabled persons are always a concern, but the term "handicapped" in the normal context is not applicable. In a fire, even a firefighter can be considered disabled, especially when near exhaustion or if his/her compressed air supply is gone. Further, able-bodied occupants can become disabled from smoke, from walking up or down steps, or from shock. Therefore, when you hear that provisions must be made for the disabled during a fire, expand your overall picture, because even normal ambulatory persons can suddenly become nonambulatory.

Phase II firefighters' operation is for firefighters. Some of the input received from firefighters is as follows:

Firefighters need the elevator for their use. The Fire Services have long complained of elevators not being available to them upon arrival at the fire building. Elevators operating on Phase II are "firefighters' tools" and firefighters want the maximum number of elevators available. Firefighters will take command during a fire, and they will determine whether and how many elevators are to be used. Firefighters are willing to accept the risks that are associated with running elevators during a fire. It is standard operating procedure for the firefighters to use the elevators not only to carry equipment for firefighting or evacuation purposes, but to also disperse fire personnel to non-fire-involved floors. The presence of a firefighter reduces occupant fears, and firefighters can direct occupant movement strategy since they are in constant communication with the fire command post.

Many firefighters stated that there are times when they cannot afford the luxury of using personnel to operate an elevator on a return trip to the main floor. They requested placing the Phase II switch in the elevator to the "OFF" position to automatically cause the elevator to return to the main floor for use by later arriving firefighters. However, Standard Operating Guidelines (SOG) dictate that whenever staffing does permit, a firefighter with a radio should be dedicated as the "taxi" operator of any car being placed onto Phase II operation. That firefighter would be responsible for the shuttling of firefighters and their equipment to the discharge floor, usually a minimum of two stories below the fire floor. This would be their task until relieved by another firefighter assigned that position. There also is a requirement that when the car is on Phase II operation, turning the switch in the car to the "HOLD" position at a floor will permit the firefighter to remove the key, and leave the car without the danger of an unauthorized person taking the car to another floor.

The ASME A17 Code Committee was aware of the need to evacuate the disabled during a fire. ASME A17.1a-1992 and later editions require firefighters' service on all elevators. Building codes, Life Safety Code (NFPA 101), American with Disabilities Act Accessibility Guidelines (ADAAG), and Americans with Disabilities Act/Architectural Barriers Act Accessibility Guidelines (ADA/ABA AG) envision the use of elevators operating on Phase II as a principal means of evacuating the disabled during a fire. Phase II is a major step forward by providing firefighters with the necessary tools to accomplish this task. However, the elevator industry must continue its research and development into making the elevator reliable for evacuation during a fire. Firefighters need access to all floors that the elevator serves, so security systems, etc. must be overridden. ASME A17.1/CSA B44-2007 recognized that modern elevators do not always have traditional car call buttons, provided they give firefighters access without causing unnecessary delay and/or confusion.

ASME A17.1-2004/CSA B44-04 incorporated a number of new requirements. The FIRE OPERATION switch (2.27.3.3), the CALL CANCEL button [2.27.3.3.1(h)], the stop switch [2.27.3.3.1(m)], the door open button(s), the door close button(s), the additional visual signal (2.27.3.3.8), and the operating instructions shown in Exhibit S2.4 are required to be grouped together at the top of a main car operating panel behind a locked cover. This panel came about for a number of reasons. To eliminate confusion, firefighters wanted all of the components that they would be using in one area.

A STOP SWITCH, which will be accessible only to the firefighters is required in the fire operation panel. The firefighter operation panel cover must be operable by the same key that operates the FIRE OPERATION switch. The cover shall be permitted to open automatically when the car is on Phase I Emergency Recall Operation and at the recall level. When closed, the cover shall be self-locking. Where rear doors are provided, buttons for both the front and rear doors are required to be provided in the firefighters' operation panel. The door open and close buttons for the rear entrance must be labeled "OPEN REAR" and "CLOSE REAR."

All buttons and switches must be readily accessible, located not more than 1 800 mm or 72 in. above the floor and shall be arranged as shown in Exhibit S2.2. Requirement 2.26.12 does not apply to these buttons and switches. These controls are not required to comply with ADAAG, ADA/ABA AG, ICC/ANSI A117.1 or ASME A17/CSA B44 Appendix E, thus the ASME A17.1/CSA B44 Code specifies minimum sizes to ensure that a firefighter wearing gloves can operate them. The front of the cover must contain the words "FIREFIGHTERS OPERATION" in red letters at least 10 mm or 0.4 in. high.

The key-operated switch is called the "FIRE OPERATION" switch, labeled "OFF," "HOLD," and "ON," in that order. It shall be rotated clockwise, to go from "OFF" to "HOLD" to "ON." Removable only in the "OFF" and "HOLD" position, it shall not change the mode of operation within Phase II Emergency In-Car Operation until the car is at a landing with its doors in the normal open position. By preventing the key from being removed from the fire operation switch, when in the "ON" position, reduces the potential of leaving a car stranded after a fire emergency. It also reduces the possibility of unauthorized personnel entering an empty car, and taking it to another floor, as it is unlikely a firefighter would not remove their fire operations key when exiting a car.

As requested, firefighters may reverse the elevator direction at the next available landing by turning Phase II switch to "OFF" (2.27.3.3.4). The car shall remain on Phase II operation, and, without going through a door open and close sequence, will return to the designated level. This provides the firefighter with a means of aborting an upward flight when conditions warrant their return to the designated level options.

Means used to remove elevators from normal operation, other than as specified in this Code, shall not prevent Phase II Emergency In-Car Operation. Appropriate requirements for cars with more than one entrance are established [2.27.3.3.1(d)]. Requirement 2.27.3.3.1(e) recognizes that reopening large vertically sliding doors with continuous pressure closing is impractical and may introduce a delay factor impeding safety. Requirement 2.27.3.3.1(g) recognizes that door-reopening devices are not necessary since constant pressure operation is required.

At the request of firefighters, 2.27.3.3.2 was revised in ASME A17.1/CSA B44-2007 to address elevators with power operated or manually operated doors.

For standardization, 2.27.3.3.3 and 2.27.3.3.4 define Phase II operation in the "OFF" position and the car is not at the recall level, so that turning the key "OFF" returns the car to the floor where the firefighter started.

Requirement 2.27.3.3.4 was revised in ASME A17.1/CSA B44-2007 to clarify elevator operation when the Phase II switch is placed in the "OFF" position. If Phase I had been activated by the fire alarm initiating device at the designated lever, the car will return to the alternate level unless it was overridden by the Phase I switch.

*2.27.3.3.6* Water from automatic sprinklers and/or fire department hose streams may cause an accidental ground or short circuit in elevator electrical equipment that is located on the landing side of the hoistway enclosure. Equipment such as hall lanterns and corridor call buttons must not shut down a car operating on Phase II.

**2.27.3.4 Interruption of Power.** This requirement clarifies that during power interruption, Phase I or Phase II must remain in effect upon restoration of power. The elevator must be designed to recover from the power failure without further endangering the firefighters or other passengers. Firefighters normally use elevators to move between the recall floor and a staging floor typically two floors below the fire. Firefighters typically do not move the elevator past the fire floor. If the elevator control system needs to move the car to re-establish its position, movement should only occur when the firefighters are ready, and not take the car past the fire floor.

**2.27.3.5 Multicompartment Elevators.** Prior to ASME A17.1/CSA B44-2007, designers developed operational steps for double-deck elevators on Phase II. This led to some complex processes that differed from building to building. To provide consistency for firefighters, the code defines a method allowing a firefighter in the upper deck to verify that lower deck is vacant and to control the doors on the lower deck. To respect the privacy of passengers in nonemergency situations the viewing means is disabled during normal operation.

### 2.27.4 Firefighters' Emergency Operation — Nonautomatic Elevators

This requirement establishes the operation requirements of elevators, which are not covered by 2.27.3. A standard sign alerts the operator as to which floor the elevator should be returned to. See Handbook commentary on 2.27.3.

### 2.27.5 Firefighters' Emergency Operation — Automatic Elevators With Designated Attendant Operation

A "designated attendant" (see 1.3) is where the elevator is controlled solely by authorized personnel (see

1.3) such as attendant service, independent service, hospital service, and similar operations.

A car could be left at the fire floor, exposing the hoistway to fire, when it could be recalled. The delay gives ample warning prior to recall. ASME A17.1/CSA B44-2007 eliminated the time delay if the car was parked at the recall level, since an arriving firefighter could ride the car up into the building thinking that the elevator was operating on Phase II, and then be put in danger when the doors open automatically.

"Hospital Service" (see 1.3) is a special case of operation by a designated attendant (see 1.3) used only for medical emergencies. Hospital service elevators, are used for transporting critical patients — not food or laundry. Bringing a patient to the lobby instead of an operating room, etc. could be life threatening. Firefighters can use another elevator until the car is released from hospital service. The code beginning with ASME A17.1a-2005/CSA B44-04 Update 1-05 allows the operator to temporarily silence the audible signal, since noise may inhibit patient care.

### 2.27.6 Firefighters' Emergency Operation — Inspection Operation

This requirement recognizes that taking the elevator control away from elevator personnel may be hazardous. This requirement provides for notification of an emergency in the building.

### 2.27.7 Firefighters' Emergency Operation — Operating Procedures

Operating procedures must be incorporated with or be adjacent to the Phase I and Phase II key-operated switches. This assures that, during an emergency, emergency personnel have quick access to the procedures. Since firefighters' service is now standardized, the Code specifies signs with simple and clear wording that explain the operation of the elevators. Signs must not deviate from the required text in ASME A17.1/CSA B44. However, the requirement allows the instructions to be modified for manual doors. An explanation of the "RESET" position is not necessary on the Phase I sign because this is a building function, not a firefighters' operation.

Requirement 2.27.7.4 recognizes a requirement in NBCC.

### 2.27.8 Switch Keys

ASME A17.1/CSA B44-2007 incorporated a requirement for a single specific key coded "FEO-K1" to be used on all elevators to eliminate the confusion and delay that occurs when hunting for keys during a response to an emergency. Some jurisdictions may adopt their own standard key while accomplishing the same goal. The distribution of the uniform key should be controlled through laws and training.

The required switch keys for Phase I and Phase II operation must be the same to assure a speedy response to the emergency situation. To allow for simultaneous operation of all key switches a key is required for all Phase I and Phase II key switches.

A Note is included to suggest that local jurisdictions may legislate uniform keyed lock box requirements to assure the availability of emergency keys when building personnel are not available. It is not within the jurisdiction of ASME A17.1/CSA B44 to mandate a uniform keyed lock box.

### 2.27.9 Elevator Car Call Station Pictograph

If the building code requires a sign, but does not specify its appearance, then the sign in ASME A17.1/CSA B44 Exhibit S2.5 must be used. Previously, designers were free to provide any sign, resulting in inconsistency and possible confusion. ASME A17.1/CSA B44-2007 clarifies that the figure background may to be the base material of the sign, but that the circles must be filled in with white.

SUPPLEMENT 3

# Fire Tests for *Life Safety Code* Users


## Marcelo M. Hirschler


*Editor's Note: This supplement is written to assist the reader in determining the applicability of fire test standards, especially those found in the Life Safety Code.*

*Dr. Marcelo M. Hirschler is a fire safety consultant with GBH International. He chairs the NFPA Technical Committee on Hazard and Risk of Contents and Furnishings and the Advisory Committee on the Glossary on Terminology and is a member of various other NFPA technical committees, including the Technical Committee on Fire Tests. He is also active in the ASTM committee E05 on Fire Standards and in a number of other codes and standards arenas.*

## FIRE PROPERTIES

Fire test standards typically relate to two types of fire properties: fire resistance and reaction-to-fire. Fire resistance is associated with fire barriers and opening protection. Thus, fire resistance tests are concerned with preventing fire from penetrating into a compartment. Reaction-to-fire is associated with materials and products, including interior finishes, furnishings and contents. Reaction-to-fire tests are concerned with preventing the fire from causing damage, by minimizing or eliminating the release of heat, smoke, and combustion products or the spread of flame. Performance-based provisions related to fire modeling use primarily results of reaction-to-fire tests.

Evaluating the level of performance or prescribed function offered by tested materials or assemblies requires an understanding of both the mechanics of a particular test and its limitations. Every test standard contains, in its scope and applicability, information explaining what it is supposed to do (namely what properties it measures) and for what type of materials it should be used. This is very important because it is a common error to use a test for the wrong material or to test for the wrong issue. A test that is commonly specified for an incorrect use is ASTM E 84, *Standard Test Method for Surface Burning Characteristics of Building Materials*, originally identical to NFPA 255, *Standard Method of Test of Surface Burning Characteristics of Building Materials*. This is a test that is so extensively used in many codes (including the *Life Safety Code*®) that it is often specified for assessing fire properties it cannot measure or for testing materials that it should not be used with. ASTM E 84 is a reaction-to-fire test that is suitable to determine the flame spread index and smoke developed index of materials. Moreover, in order for a material to be suitable for this test, the material must, by its own structural quality or the manner in which it is applied, be capable of supporting itself in position or of being supported in the test apparatus. This test has often been specified, incorrectly, to obtain results on properties like fire resistance (which should be measured using NFPA 251, *Standard Methods of Tests of Fire Resistance of Building Construction and Materials*), or to determine whether a material is noncombustible (which should be assessed with a test like ASTM E 136, *Standard Test Method for Behavior of Materials in a Vertical Tube Furnace at 750°C)*, or whether it is limited combustible (which is determined by testing in accordance with NFPA 259, *Standard Test Method for Potential Heat of Building Materials*). See also the discussion on combustibility fire testing below. Other misapplications include using the test for products, such as furniture, that cannot be physically placed in the apparatus, or for materials that cannot be supported in the apparatus throughout the test.

Many of the tests referred to in the *Life Safety Code* have equivalent counterparts administered by other standards-writing organizations such as the American Society for Testing and Materials (ASTM) and Underwriters Laboratories (UL). In recent years all three organizations have withdrawn some of their standards for harmonization purposes. Section 1.4 of the *Life Safety Code* permits the application or use of equivalent alternatives. Alternatives could include fire test documents different from those specified, or different test protocols if the proper technical documentation is provided to demonstrate equivalency between the tests and verify that the alternative approach fulfills the intended purpose of the applicable code requirement. The 2009 edition of the *Life Safety Code* officially recognizes the technical equivalence of ASTM and UL standard test methods to the corresponding NFPA test methods: ASTM E 119 and UL 263 for NFPA 251, ASTM E 2074 and UL 10B for NFPA 252 (both sets of fire resistance tests) and ASTM E 84 and UL 723 for the uses where NFPA 255 was previously required, ASTM E 648 for NFPA 253, ASTM E 108 and UL 790 for NFPA 256, ASTM E 1352 for NFPA 261, and ASTM E 1353 for NFPA 260 (all sets of reaction-to-fire tests). See Table S3.1.

***Table S3.1*** *Fire Test Standards*

| NFPA | ASTM | UL |
|---|---|---|
| 251, *Standard Methods of Tests of Fire Resistance of Building Construction and Materials* | E 119, *Standard Test Methods for Fire Tests of Building Construction and Materials1* | 263, *Standard for Fire Tests of Building Construction and Materials* |
| 252, *Standard Methods of Fire Tests of Door Assemblies* | E 2074, *Standard Test Method for Fire Tests of Door Assemblies, Including Positive Pressure Testing of Side-Hinged and Pivoted Swinging Door Assemblies* (replaced ASTM E 152, withdrawn) | 10B, *Standard for Fire Tests of Door Assemblies* |
| 253, *Standard Method of Test for Critical Radiant Flux of Floor Covering Systems Using a Radiant Heat Energy Source* | E 648, *Standard Test Method for Critical Radiant Flux of Floor-Covering Systems Using a Radiant Heat Energy Source* | |
| 255, *Standard Method of Test of Surface Burning Characteristics of Building Materials* (proposed for withdrawal) | E 84, *Standard Test Method for Surface Burning Characteristics of Building Materials* | 723, *Standard for Test for Surface Burning Characteristics of Building Materials* |
| 256, *Standard Methods of Fire Tests of Roof Coverings* (withdrawn) | E 108, *Standard Test Methods for Fire Tests of Roof Coverings* | 790, *Standard for Standard Test Methods for Fire Tests of Roof Coverings* |
| 257, *Standard on Fire Test for Window and Glass Block Assemblies* | E 2010, *Standard Test Method for Positive Pressure Fire Tests of Window Assemblies* (replaced ASTM E 163, withdrawn) | 9, *Standard for Fire Tests of Window Assemblies* |
| 258, *Recommended Practice for Determining Smoke Generation of Solid Materials* (withdrawn) | E 662, *Standard Test Method for Specific Optical Density of Smoke Generated by Solid Materials* | |
| 259, *Standard Test Method for Potential Heat of Building Materials* | | |
| 260, *Standard Methods of Tests and Classification System for Cigarette Ignition Resistance of Components of Upholstered Furniture* | E 1353, *Standard Test Methods for Cigarette Ignition Resistance of Components of Upholstered Furniture* | |
| 261, *Standard Method of Test for Determining Resistance of Mock-Up Upholstered Furniture Material Assemblies to Ignition by Smoldering Cigarettes* | E 1352, *Standard Test Method for Cigarette Ignition Resistance of Mock-Up Upholstered Furniture Assemblies* | |

*Table S3.1* Continued

| NFPA | ASTM | UL |
|---|---|---|
| 262, *Standard Method of Test for Flame Travel and Smoke of Wires and Cables for Use in Air-Handling Spaces* | | 910, *Standard for Safety Test for Flame-Propagation and Smoke-Density Values for Electrical and Optical-Fiber Cables Used in Spaces Transporting Environmental Air* (withdrawn) |
| 263, *Standard Method of Test for Heat and Visible Smoke Release Rates for Materials and Products* (withdrawn) | E 906, *Standard Test Method for Heat and Visible Smoke Release Rates for Materials and Products* | |
| 265, *Standard Methods of Fire Tests for Evaluating Room Fire Growth Contribution of Textile Coverings on Full Height Panels and Walls* | | 1715*, *Standard for Fire Test of Interior Finish Material* |
| 266, *Standard Method of Test for Fire Characteristics of Upholstered Furniture Exposed to Flaming Ignition Source* (withdrawn) | E 1537, *Standard Test Method for Fire Testing of Upholstered Furniture* | 1056, *Standard for Safety Fire Test of Upholstered Furniture* (withdrawn) |
| 267, *Standard Method of Test for Fire Characteristics of Mattresses and Bedding Assemblies Exposed to Flaming Ignition Source* (withdrawn) | E 1590, *Standard Test Method for Fire Testing of Mattresses* | 1895, *Standard for Safety Fire Test of Mattresses* (withdrawn) |
| 268, *Standard Test Method for Determining Ignitibility of Exterior Wall Assemblies Using a Radiant Heat Energy Source* | | |
| 269, *Standard Test Method for Developing Toxic Potency Data for Use in Fire Hazard Modeling* | E 1678, *Standard Test Method for Measuring Smoke Toxicity for Use in Fire Hazard Analysis*<br>E 1822, *Standard Test Method for Fire Testing of Stacked Chairs* | |
| 270, *Standard Test Method for Measurement of Smoke Obscuration Using a Conical Radiant Source in a Single Closed Chamber* | E 1995, *Standard Test Method for Measurement of Smoke Obscuration Using a Conical Radiant Source in a Single Closed Chamber, with the Test Specimen Oriented Horizontally* | |
| 271, *Standard Method of Test for Heat and Visible Smoke Release Rates for Materials and Products Using an Oxygen Consumption Calorimeter* | E 1354, *Standard Test Method for Heat and Visible Smoke Release Rates for Materials and Products Using an Oxygen Consumption Calorimeter* | |
| 272, *Standard Method of Test for Heat and Visible Smoke Release Rates for Upholstered Furniture Components or Composites and Mattresses Using an Oxygen Consumption Calorimeter (withdrawn)* | | |
| 285, *Standard Fire Test Method for Evaluation of Fire Propagation Characteristics of Exterior Non-Load-Bearing Wall Assemblies Containing Combustible Components* | | |

*(continues)*

*Table S3.1 Continued*

| NFPA | ASTM | UL |
|---|---|---|
| 286, *Standard Methods of Fire Tests for Evaluating Contribution of Wall and Ceiling Interior Finish to Room Fire Growth* | | 1715*, *Standard for Fire Test of Interior Finish Material* |
| 287, *Standard Test Methods for Measurement of Flammability of Materials in Cleanrooms Using a Fire Propagation Apparatus (FPA)* | E 2058, *Standard Test Methods for Measurement of Synthetic Polymer Material Flammability Using a Fire Propagation Apparatus (FPA)* | |
| 288, *Standard Methods of Fire Tests of Floor Fire Door Assemblies Installed Horizontally in Fire Resistance–Rated Floor Systems* | | |
| 289, *Standard Method of Fire Test for Individual Fuel Packages* | | 1975, *Standard for Fire Tests for Foamed Plastics Used for Decorative Purposes* |
| 701, *Standard Methods of Fire Tests for Flame Propagation of Textiles and Films* | D 568, *Standard Test Method for Rate of Burning and/or Extent and Time of Burning of Flexible Plastics in a Vertical Position)* (withdrawn) | 214, *Standard for Safety Tests for Flame-Propagation of Fabrics and Films* (withdrawn) |
| 705, *Recommended Practice for a Field Flame Test for Textiles and Films* | D 1929, *Standard Test Method for Ignition Properties of Plastics* | |
| | D 2859, *Standard Test Method for Ignition Characteristics of Finished Textile Floor Covering Materials* | |
| | E 136, Standard Test Method for Behavior of Materials in a Vertical Tube Furnace at 750°C | |
| | E 162, Test Method for Surface Flammability of Materials Using a Radiant Heat Energy Source | |
| | E 814, Standard Test Method for Fire Tests of Through-Penetration Fire Stops | 1479, Standard for Fire Tests of Through-Penetration Firestops |
| | E 1529, Standard Test Methods for Determining Effects of Large Hydrocarbon Pool Fires on Structural Members and Assemblies | 1709, Standard for Rapid Rise Fire Tests of Protection Materials for Structural Steel |
| | E 1623, Test Method for Determination of Fire and Thermal Parameters of Materials, Products, and Systems Using an Intermediate Scale Calorimeter (ICAL) | |
| | E 1966, Standard Test Method for Fire-Resistive Joint Systems | 2079, Standard for Tests for Fire Resistance of Building Joint Systems |
| | E 2257, Standard Test Method for Room Fire Test of Wall and Ceiling Materials and Assemblies | |

Note: This table contains NFPA fire test standards and those fire test standards from other organizations, ASTM and UL, that are either similar to NFPA fire test standards or relevant to the *Life Safety Code.*

*UL 1715 is different from both NFPA 265 and NFPA 286, but is a room-corner fire test, normally used for the same purposes as those other tests. That is, it assesses the fire behavior of an interior finish material in a full-scale scenario. See the section on interior wall and ceiling finish later in this supplement. UL 1975 is similar but not identical to NFPA 289 but can be used for the same applications.

## FIRE RESISTANCE TESTING

Buildings or structures occupied or used in accordance with the individual occupancy chapters of the *Life Safety Code* (Chapters 11 through 43) are required to meet the minimum construction requirements of those chapters. NFPA 220, *Standard on Types of Building Construction*,[1] is referenced in Chapter 8 of the *Life Safety Code*. It describes the types of building construction (that is, construction classifications) and the fire resistance ratings applicable to each construction element for each type of building. The fire test to be used to assess fire resistance ratings of elements of building construction is NFPA 251, *Standard Methods of Tests of Fire Resistance of Building Construction and Materials*. See also Table S3.1 for alternative similar fire test methods. NFPA 251 (also referenced primarily in Chapter 8) applies to assemblies of masonry units, composite assemblies of structural materials for buildings (including interior and exterior bearing and other walls and partitions, columns, girders, beams, slabs, and composite slab and beam assemblies for floors and roofs), as well as other assemblies and structural units that constitute permanent integral parts of a finished building. The fire test has specific testing criteria for each type of assembly. Fire barriers, or fire barrier assemblies, are intended to be used as separation barriers or to provide protection of building elements from the effects of fire for a given time as required by Chapter 8, Features of Fire Protection. It is important to note that a fire resistance rating applies to the entire assembly as tested. A fire resistance rating is never assigned to an individual material or product; rather it represents the composite performance of an assembly including all of the components and the specific construction details of the rated assembly.

NFPA 251 exposes one side of an assembly (construction element), except for columns and beams, to a standard time-temperature curve (as shown in Exhibit S3.1) inside a furnace leaving the other side unexposed. This is known as a time-temperature curve because the test method specifies the temperature that needs to be measured in the furnace at each point in time. The furnace used must be capable of providing the prescribed temperatures over a given period of time, by following the time-temperature curve shown in Exhibit S3.1. The test method provides criteria for assessing how long (in hours or minutes) it takes for heat to penetrate each assembly and reach an unacceptable temperature rise on the unexposed side or protected element, and how long it takes for the flame or hot gases penetrating through the assembly to ignite cotton waste placed on the unexposed side, during the test. The fire resistance rating will be the time at which the first of the failure criteria is reached, as assessed either by the transmission of heat, the passage of hot gases sufficient to ignite cotton waste, or by structural collapse of the test specimen assembly. The temperature rise failure criterion on the unexposed side is 250°F (140°C) above the test specimen's initial temperature for walls and partitions. For load bearing elements, the test also monitors the load carrying capability of the test specimen during the test exposure. When required, the fire exposure is followed by the application of a specified standard fire hose stream.

If the assembly to be evaluated will be used as a load-bearing element, the test is conducted with a load placed on the assembly, to evaluate the load-bearing capacity of the assembly. Some construction assemblies are simply intended to limit the transmission or temperature and/or flames to the unexposed surface. On the other hand, many construction assemblies, such as beams and columns, and floor and roof assemblies, must also sustain an applied load for a pe-

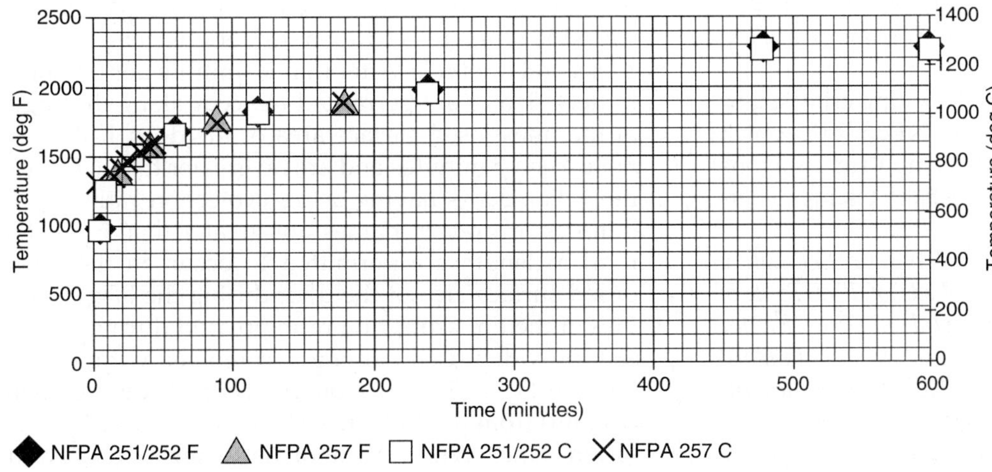


***Exhibit S3.1*** *Standard time-temperature curves for NFPA 251/252 and for NFPA 257.*

riod of time equal to the desired fire resistance rating, and must therefore be tested under the relevant applied load. Walls and partitions are thus permitted to be tested either with load or without.

Depending on the structural design of the assembly, certain levels of temperature must not be exceeded at any one point, or an average temperature cannot be exceeded, with temperature limitations ranging from 800°F to 1300°F (427°C to 704°C). An alternative test exists for structural steel columns, whereby the column is not loaded during the test. The test measures the ability of the added protection to control the transmission of heat through the specimen during the specified period of fire exposure. The average temperature of the steel in such columns must not rise above 1000°F (538°C), and the temperature in any one of the measured points cannot exceed 1200°F (649°C).

In many cases, the assembly is also subjected to a hose stream test. The use of such a test was inspired by the interest in simulating the effect of water hoses used by emergency personnel to fight fires; in fact, however, the hose stream test itself is not intended to simulate that effect. If required to pass a hose stream test, an assembly with a fire rating of 1 hour or more would have to survive exposure to a hose stream test for half the period of its fire resistance rating, but not for more than 1 hour. When the condition of acceptance requires a hose stream test, after the fire resistance rating has been established, a duplicate assembly is exposed in the furnace to the time-temperature curve for the period required by the hose stream test conditions, then removed from the furnace and immediately subjected to the hose stream test. The hose stream is delivered under pre-set conditions (based on a certain hose, play pipe nozzle, distance from the test specimen, nozzle pressure, and test duration). The hose stream is applied in a specific pattern to fully develop the effects of impact, cooling, and erosion on the entire test specimen. The specimen must withstand the hose stream test such that no openings are created that would permit projection of water from the hose stream beyond the unexposed surface.

Further information on specific testing criteria and testing limitations can be found in NFPA 251, which should be consulted before making any firm decisions about the applicability of certain tests, or testing of certain assemblies.

Other fire resistance tests used by the *Life Safety Code* are NFPA 252, *Standard Methods of Fire Tests of Door Assemblies*; NFPA 257, *Standard on Fire Test for Window and Glass Block Assemblies*; NFPA 288, *Standard Methods of Fire Tests of Floor Fire Door Assemblies Installed Horizontally in Fire Resistance–Rated Floor Systems*; and ASTM E 814, *Standard Test Method for Fire Tests of Through-Penetration Fire Stops*. All of these tests use basically the same standard time-temperature curve that NFPA 251 uses (except that the curve in NFPA 257 includes more detail over the short initial time periods; see Exhibit S3.1). However, there are also some differentiating characteristics, which are related to the products being tested. NFPA 80, *Standard for Fire Doors and Other Opening Protectives*,[2] contains installation requirements for all types of fire doors and windows, and thereby regulates the installation and maintenance of assemblies and devices used to protect openings in walls, floors, and ceilings against the spread of fire and smoke within, into, or out of buildings. NFPA 80 is extensively referenced in the *Life Safety Code*, especially in Chapter 7 (Means of Egress) and Chapter 8 (Features of Fire Protection).

### Building Products

**Fire Doors.** Door assemblies in fire barriers must be tested according to NFPA 252, *Standard Methods of Fire Tests of Door Assemblies* (see also Table S3.1 for alternative similar fire test methods). NFPA 252 provides methods for measuring the relative performance of fire door assemblies where subjected to a prescribed fire test exposure followed by a prescribed hose stream application, using the same time-temperature curve as NFPA 251 (see Exhibit S3.1). The fire door assembly must be tested as a complete assembly, because the effectiveness of the opening protective depends on a satisfactory performance of the entire door assembly, which consists of the door, door frame, and associated hardware. In NFPA 252, the fire door assembly specimen is mounted in a furnace wall and exposed to the standard time-temperature curve. The door assembly is not permitted to develop gaps or openings through the assembly, nor is flaming permitted to occur on the unexposed surface of a door assembly during the first 30 minutes of the fire resistance-rating period, although some intermittent light flames no greater than 6 in. (150 mm) are permitted for periods not exceeding 10-second intervals. After that 30-minute period, intermittent flames are permitted to occur along the edges of the unexposed surface area of the door, if they do not exceed 5 minutes and are no greater than 6 in. (150 mm). For doors having a fire protection rating of 45 minutes or greater, flames not greater than 6 in. (150 mm) in length are permitted to occur on the unexposed surface area of the door during the last 15 minutes of the fire protection rating period during the fire test, provided such flaming is contained within a distance of 1½ in. (38 mm) from the vertical edge and 3 in. (76 mm) from the top edge of the door or frame of the vision panel. When the door hardware is also evaluated for use on fire doors, it must keep the door in a closed position for an exposure period of 3 hours. The latch bolt must remain projected and be intact after the fire exposure test. Note the absence of any criterion addressing temperature transmission to the unexposed side. The fire doors must usually also be exposed to a hose stream test, which subjects the test assembly to the impact, erosion, and cooling effects of the hose stream, immediately following the fire resistance test. The hose stream is directed at the middle and then at all parts of the exposed surface, slowly making changes in direction. However, certain provisions within the *Life Safety Code* provide for the installation of door assemblies having a fire protection rating of 20 minutes without the hose stream test. One must carefully evaluate the particular requirements associated with the opening protective so that it satisfies the minimum acceptable criteria.

A modern trend within code-writing organizations is to require certain applications of fire door assemblies (typically side-hinged and swinging doors) to be tested under a positive pressure scenario. This provision requires that the door assemblies be tested with a neutral pressure plane located 40 in. (1015 mm) above the finished floor. NFPA 252 does not stipulate the height of the neutral plane but records the height in the test results. This permits the test standard to accommodate the many gradients of pressure planes at which a furnace can be operated. The test report document issued following a classification test records the location of the neutral pressure plane to which the door assembly has been tested. The *Life Safety Code* does not stipulate the minimum required height of the neutral pressure plane for testing the door. If a neutral plane is not established along the height of the test specimen, then it is assumed that the door will be tested under normal testing procedures, which is running the furnace at near atmospheric pressure. This would establish the neutral pressure plane at the top of the door assembly. It is generally recognized that, if a lower neutral pressure plane is established on the door assembly within the furnace, then the test could be considered to be more severe. A door tested under a positive pressure should be accepted as meeting the requirements established for a door tested at atmospheric pressure. Listing agencies have different approaches on how to list and label doors being tested under positive pressure. Additional information associated with these criteria can be found in NFPA 80, *Standard for Fire Doors and Other Opening Protectives*, which should be consulted for the installation requirements associated with all types of fire doors.

*Fire protection rating* is the appropriate term for the fire resistance associated with an opening protective as detailed in NFPA 252 (for fire doors) and in NFPA 257 (for fire window assemblies). *Fire resistance rating* is the appropriate term for use with a fire barrier, such as used in walls or floors. In the *Life Safety Code* and *NFPA 5000*®, *Building Construction and Safety Code*®[3], the technical committees have been very careful to use each term appropriately and consistently. However, there are fire doors and glazing assemblies that have a fire resistance rating by virtue of the fact that they were tested using NFPA 251; in that case the code does not consider them to be opening protectives.

**Fire Window Assemblies.** Fire window assemblies are permitted to be used in fire barriers having a fire resistance rating of one hour or less if they have a fire protection rating of 45 minutes and represent up to 25 percent of the fire barrier. Fire windows must be tested in accordance with NFPA 257, *Standard on Fire Test for Window and Glass Block Assemblies* (see also Table S3.1 for alternative similar fire test methods and Exhibit S3.1 for the time-temperature curve). The NFPA 257 test method is intended to evaluate the ability of a window or other light-transmitting assembly to remain in an opening during a predetermined test exposure period. Recent editions of NFPA 257 have no references to a particular time limit for testing, and time-temperature guidelines are included for up to 3 hours. Earlier editions limited testing to 45 minutes, but now the test is permitted to be run for the length of time a test sponsor requests. The period of time is then recorded on the appropriate test records. A testing time limit is no longer relevant because new materials and technology exist for window assemblies that will permit increased exposure times and maintain the integrity of the fire barriers in which they are installed. Note that, just as in NFPA 252, there is no criterion addressing temperature transmission to the unexposed side. Discussions are continuing on the amount of radiant heat permitted to transfer through the window assembly to the unexposed side of the window. Currently, the radiant heat transferred is not required to be recorded. A test procedure is available to measure this radiant heat flux and is detailed in Annex C of NFPA 257, with some additional information on radiant heat transmissions in Annex B. The conditions associated with radiant energy could be considered as a factor in the application of a fire-modeling program that might have an occupant passing by such opening protectives, or could, in principle, be used as pass/fail criteria. All considerations and applications for a material's particular use should be reviewed with the limitations of the test results in mind.

In NFPA 257, the test specimen is mounted in a furnace wall and exposed to the standard time-temperature curve. A window assembly is considered to have met the requirements for acceptable performance if it remains in the opening during the fire resistance and hose stream tests, within the following five criteria:

1. No flaming shall occur on the unexposed surface of the assembly.
2. There shall be no separation of the glazing material edges from the glazing frame that creates openings.
3. At the perimeter of operable components, movement from the initial closed position shall not exceed the thickness of the frame member at any point.
4. The window assembly shall not move away from the wall to the extent that an opening is created.
5. There shall be no openings in the window assembly.

Exhibits S3.2 and S3.3 represent two views of an assembly that has been exposed to both the fire resistance and the hose stream tests. As with fire doors, fire windows are installed in accordance with the provisions of NFPA 80, *Standard for Fire Doors and Other Opening Protectives*, which should be consulted for the installation requirements associated with all types of fire windows. NFPA 80 includes limitations on the size and total area permitted for the glazing material installed in fire window assemblies, and also requires that each individual glazing unit have a label that is visible after installation. Also, in NFPA 80, fire window assemblies having a rating of 20 minutes or 30 minutes are limited to the size that has been tested. A window protection of 45 minutes is limited to the maximum area tested and must have no exposed area of individual glazing material exceeding 1296 in.$^2$ (0.84 m$^2$) and no dimension exceeding 54 in. (1370 mm), unless it has been specifically tested with dimensions in excess of those values. Glazing is currently available that has been tested with dimensions exceeding that size limitation. One should review the appropriate listing associated with the protection rating given to a fire window assembly.

Many types of glazing materials are being introduced into the market, and several types of fire-rated glazing products (including wired glass) can satisfy the acceptance criteria of NFPA 257. Nonsymmetrical fire protection–rated glazing systems are tested with each face exposed to the furnace, and the assigned fire protection rating is that of the shortest duration obtained from the two tests conducted. It is important that the installation and testing limitations be reviewed for the particular installation.

Technological advances within the glazing industry have provided systems using fire-resistant glazing

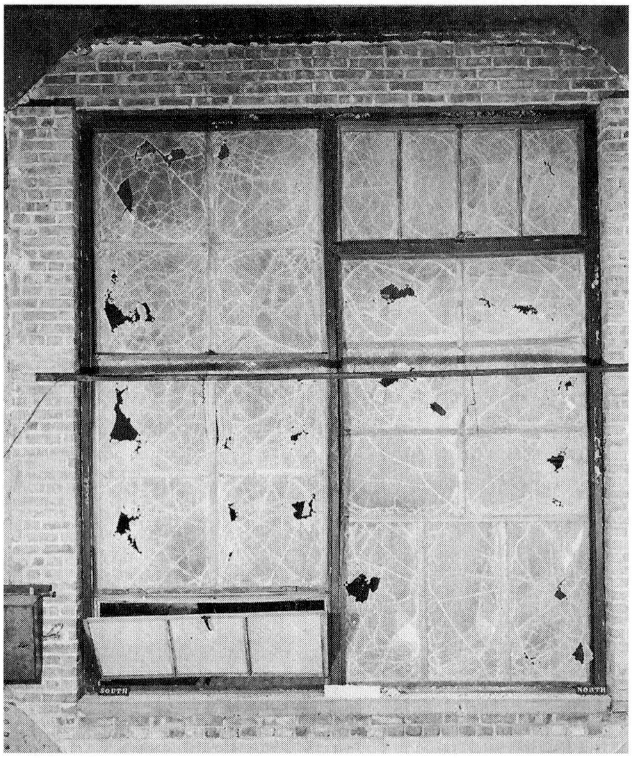

**Exhibit S3.2** *Unexposed side of window assembly after fire exposure and hose stream application.*

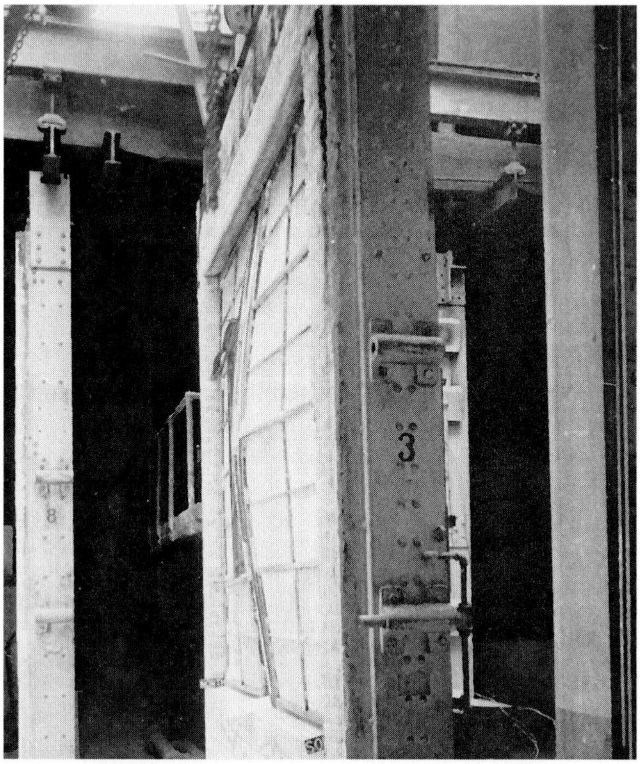

**Exhibit S3.3** *Exposed side of window assembly after fire exposure and hose stream application.*

materials that are actually fire barrier walls. These glazing walls would have been tested in accordance with NFPA 251 and satisfy the particular pass/fail criteria for fire barriers. The pass/fail criteria include a limitation in the temperature rise on the unexposed side of the test specimen, and a successful hose stream application. The installation requirements and limitations for these glazing wall assemblies would be highlighted in the applicable listing requirements and the manufacturers' specifications. This type of glazing would not be required to comply with the installation requirements, because it is not considered an opening protective device.

**Through-Penetrations.** Generally, when fire barriers are tested for a particular hourly rating, these assemblies are tested without any penetrations. It is recognized that within a building these fire barriers will have various penetrations for building services, utilities, and other applications. Penetrations of fire barriers require the appropriate protection by devices or materials that have been tested and listed for that particular application to maintain the fire barrier's integrity. In this edition of the *Life Safety Code* (see 8.3.5.1 and 8.3.5.6), through-penetration and membrane penetrations — for cables, cable trays, conduits, pipes, tubes, combustion vents, exhaust vents, wires, and similar items to accommodate electrical, mechanical, plumbing, and communications systems that pass through a wall, floor, or floor/ceiling assembly constructed as a fire barrier — are required (rather than recommended) to be protected by a firestop system or device, and must be tested in accordance with ASTM E 814, *Standard Method for Fire Tests of Through-Penetration Fire Stops*, which establishes the testing protocols for through-penetrations.

Penetrations of a rated assembly that require special consideration are usually tested using a recognized test procedure based on the standard time-temperature curve, normally that contained within ASTM E 814. Additional information can be found in documents published by the individual listing agencies for assemblies that have been tested for specific fire ratings.

The ASTM E 814 test protocol establishes F and T ratings as one part of the acceptance criteria for through-penetration systems. The F rating signifies the ability of the penetrating firestop system to withstand a prescribed fire test for a period of time without permitting the passage of flame through the opening or the occurrence of flaming on any element of the unexposed side of the penetrating firestop system. The T rating relates to the transmission of heat through the penetrating firestop system for a given period of time. An acceptable T rating is one that limits the rise of the temperature on the unexposed surface of the penetrating firestop system or penetrating item to no more than 325°F (181°C) above the initial temperature, and for which there is no flame occurrence on the unexposed side. The penetrating firestop is exposed to the same fire test conditions created by the time-temperature curve in NFPA 251, *Standard Methods of Tests of Fire Resistance of Building Construction and Materials.* The *Life Safety Code; NFPA 5000, Building Construction and Safety Code;* NFPA 221, *Standard for High-Challenge Fire Walls, and Fire Barrier Walls;*[4] and other codes require that the penetrating firestop be under a minimum positive pressure differential of 0.01 in. of water (2.5 Pa) at the location of the penetrating item. This positive pressure must be maintained for the duration of the time for which it is being tested. The penetrating firestop system must be tested for the same time period as that of the fire barrier in which it is installed. The penetrating firestop system must also be subjected to the effects of an applied hose stream test.

**Joints.** Joints used in the construction of fire barriers can include expansion, seismic, and control joints. These joints are tested at their maximum joint width in accordance with NFPA 251. The test includes joints to their full height or length of the test assembly. The fire-resistive joint system tested must include a splice or a method of connecting two or more lengths of the joint system. The test must be conducted so that the joint system is tested under a minimum positive pressure differential of 0.01 in. of water (2.5 Pa) for the total time of the test. There is an exception for expansion or seismic joints designed to prevent the penetration of fire and shown to have a fire resistance rating of not less than the required fire resistance rating of the floor when tested in accordance with ANSI/UL 2079, *Test of Fire Resistance of Building Joint Systems* (see 8.6.3 of NFPA *101*). Fire-resistive joint systems that are designed to accommodate movement must be preconditioned by cycling under the conditions of ASTM E 1399, *Standard Test Method for Cyclic Movement and Measuring the Minimum and Maximum Joint Widths of Architectural Joint Systems.*[5]

**Fire Dampers.** Chapter 7, Means of Egress, states that fire barriers forming horizontal exits shall not be penetrated by ducts, unless such ducts are existing penetrations protected by fire dampers approved and listed for the particular application. Fire dampers are tested either for static systems, where the HVAC system is automatically shut down in the event of a fire, or for dynamic systems, where the HVAC system does not shut down. Fire dampers used in dynamic systems are investigated for closure under their maximum recommended airflow. Fire dampers are tested in accordance with ANSI/UL 555, *Standard for Fire Dampers*. Fire dampers used in rated fire-resistive floor-ceiling and roof-ceiling assemblies are tested in accordance with ANSI/UL 555C, *Standard for Ceiling Dampers*. The fire dampers are tested in assemblies under the conditions of the fire exposure of the same time-temperature curve as in NFPA 251. The ANSI/UL standards provide the acceptance criteria in regard to the flaming on the unexposed side, closing time of the damper, air leakage, if applicable, and hose stream application. It should be noted that fire dampers are not tested for the limitation of heat transmission through the fire damper assembly. This particular condition is recognized in the requirements of NFPA 90A, *Standard for the Installation of Air-Conditioning and Ventilating Systems*,[6] associated with the limitation on the number of fire dampers permitted to be installed in a vertical duct that has multiple floor penetrations.

**Smoke Dampers.** Paragraph 8.5.5.2 discusses the use of smoke dampers. Where a smoke barrier is penetrated by a duct or air transfer opening, a smoke damper designed and tested in accordance with the requirements of ANSI/UL 555S, *Standard for Leakage Rated Dampers for Use in Smoke Control Systems*, must be installed. Where a smoke barrier is also constructed as a fire barrier, a combination fire/smoke damper designed and tested in accordance with the requirements of both ANSI/UL 555S and ANSI/UL 555 must be installed.

**Floor Fire Doors.** Paragraph 8.3.3.4 regulates floor fire doors. It states that floor fire door assemblies shall be tested in accordance with NFPA 288, *Standard Methods of Fire Tests of Floor Fire Door Assemblies Installed Horizontally in Fire Resistance–Rated Floor Systems,* and shall achieve a fire resistance rating not less than the assembly being penetrated. It also states that floor fire door assemblies shall be listed and labeled for the application. The time-temperature curve in NFPA 288 is the same as that in NFPA 251, but there is no required hose stream test. The transmission of heat through the specimen during the fire resistance rating period shall not raise the average temperature on its unexposed surface more than 250°F (139°C) above its initial temperature. Additionally, a temperature rise of 325°F (181°C) shall not be exceeded at any one point.

### Critical Test Limitations of Fire Resistance Tests

Although test assemblies have been rated for a specific period using a fire resistance test, it must be recognized that the test is only intended to be a comparative test. Therefore, under actual field conditions, some assemblies fail prematurely and others remain in place longer than expected. The simulated test exposure used in the test protocol was established around 1920; it represents one level of fire severity considered to be a "typical office building" scenario of that era. Research continues to determine whether the varying types of fuel loads found in more modern occupancies would require a different type of time-temperature curve. Such research is always ongoing and differing opinions are expressed by various investigators. It is worth mentioning, however, that the time-temperature curve from the test used by European countries for assessing fire resistance, namely ISO 834, *Fire-resistance tests — Elements of building construction*,[7] is very similar to that in NFPA 251.

Currently, discussions are ongoing regarding the application of particular fire modeling programs to predict the results of testing of assemblies, as well as what the pass/fail criteria should be. An ASTM standard guide, ASTM E 2032, *Standard Guide for Extension of Data from Fire Resistance Tests Conducted in Accordance with ASTM E 119*, has been issued to address the extension of fire resistance results obtained from fire tests performed in accordance with NFPA 251 or ASTM E 119 to constructions that have not been tested. The guide is based on principles involving the extension of test data using simple considerations. The acceptance of these principles and their application is on a worst-case scenario.

It is always important to remember that new materials may present unforeseen issues that will need to be resolved. A good example is the recent understanding that high-strength concrete can cause explosive spalling to occur at relatively low temperatures. This finding could have an adverse effect on the fire protection properties assumed for a construction element using such materials.

Another area of concern for the fire resistance of a test assembly is its integrity, or the protection of through-penetrations. The test criteria in NFPA 251 do not address conventional openings found in assemblies, such as those needed for incorporation of electrical receptacles, or penetrations by electrical wires, cables or raceways, plumbing pipes, utility services, and construction joints, unless they have been specifically tested as part of the assembly. All penetrations require special review and consideration. A source for evaluating certain penetrations permitted in rated assemblies is found in the introduction of the UL *Fire Resistance Directory*.[8] This document addresses the hourly ratings for beams, floors, roofs, columns, walls, and partitions. Its design information section provides information pertaining to the different penetrations found in rated assemblies and the required protection or limitations.

The publication "Guideline on Fire Ratings of Archaic Materials and Assemblies," by Robert Brady Williamson, Cecile Grant, Joseph Zicherman, Fred Fisher, Harry Hasegawa, Herman Spaeth, Harriet Watson, Vytenis Babrauskas, and Norman Kornsand, for the National Institute of Building Sciences for the Department of Housing and Urban Development, contains information on construction materials typical of an earlier time, generally prior to 1950. It contains data on fire resistance and reaction-to-fire, including flame spread, smoke production, and degree of combustibility. The information has also been included in NFPA 914, *Code for Fire Protection of Historic Structures*,[9] as Annex O.

## REACTION-TO-FIRE TESTING

### Major Properties and Products

Interior finish as it relates to the *Life Safety Code* refers to the exposed interior wall surfaces, exposed interior ceiling finishes, and exposed interior floor finishes. The reaction-to-fire properties associated with the regulation of interior wall and ceiling finish are flame spread and smoke development in a traditional standard test (ASTM E 84, *Standard Test Method for Surface Burning Characteristics of Building Materials*; see also Table S3.1 for alternative similar fire test methods). Alternatively, in a room-corner test or in a specialized large-scale test, the reaction-to-fire properties associated with wall and ceiling finish are heat and smoke release and flame propagation (potentially leading to flashover). The reaction-to-fire properties associated with interior floor finish are ignition characteristics (in accordance with ASTM D 2859, *Standard Test Method for Ignition Characteristics of Finished Textile Floor Covering Materials*) and critical radiant flux (in accordance with NFPA 253, *Standard Method of Test for Critical Radiant Flux of Floor Covering Systems Using a Radiant Heat Energy Source*; see also Table S3.1 for alternative similar fire test methods). These provisions should not be associated or confused with fire resistance ratings. As discussed above, the properties associated with interior finish are reaction-to-fire properties and not fire resistance properties. They refer to the ability of a material to contribute to overall fire and smoke growth and spread. An interior finish classification should also not be compared or confused with a material's combustibility or the degrees of combustibility.

**Interior Wall and Ceiling Finish.** There are two types of approaches being used to evaluate interior wall and ceiling finishes. Each use of a material for a particular application of interior finish needs to be coordinated with the appropriate testing procedure, and each interior finish testing method has a specific scope and application. There is a possibility that a single product could be used in different applications and be tested using different fire test methods. The end use application must be identified, because that knowledge stipulates the appropriate test method and applicable results.

*Steiner Tunnel Test.* The traditional approach to testing interior wall and ceiling finish for use within a code involves ASTM E 84, *Standard Test Method for Surface Burning Characteristics of Building Materials*, a test conducted in a piece of equipment known as the Steiner tunnel. Depending on occupancy and use within the occupancy, the *Life Safety Code* limits the use of interior wall and ceiling finish materials to minimize flame propagation and smoke development on the exposed wall and ceiling surfaces. This approach consists of evaluating the flame spread over the surface of a material, and the smoke developed, when the material is exposed to a prescribed gas-fed fire. The *Life Safety Code* provides, in 10.2.3, three classifications for interior finish, based on a flame spread index (FSI) and a smoke development index (SDI), as tested in accordance with ASTM E 84 (see also Table S3.1 for alternative similar fire test methods). The classifications (with their corresponding flame spread index and smoke development index values) are shown in Table S3.2. The flame spread index and the smoke development index both reflect the comparative fire-test response of a material when compared with two established benchmarks: a $\frac{1}{4}$ in. (6.3 mm) thick inorganic reinforced cement board (assigned both an FSI and an SDI of 0) and a nominal $\frac{25}{32}$ in. (19.8 mm) select grade red oak flooring board (assigned both an FSI and an SDI of 100). The FSI is a comparative nondimensional figure and does not directly represent a flame speed, flame velocity, or flame propagation. The SDI is also a comparative nondimensional figure and does not directly represent optical density or smoke release rate.

***Table S3.2 Flame Spread Index (FSI) and Smoke Development Index (SDI) Values for Interior Wall and Ceiling Finish Classifications***

| Class | FSI | SDI |
|---|---|---|
| Class A | 0–25 | 0–450 |
| Class B | 26–75 | 0–450 |
| Class C | 76–200 | 0–450 |

The testing apparatus used in ASTM E 84 is shown in Exhibits S3.4 and S3.5. The specimens are required to be at least 20 in. (508 mm) wide by 24 ft (7.3 m) long

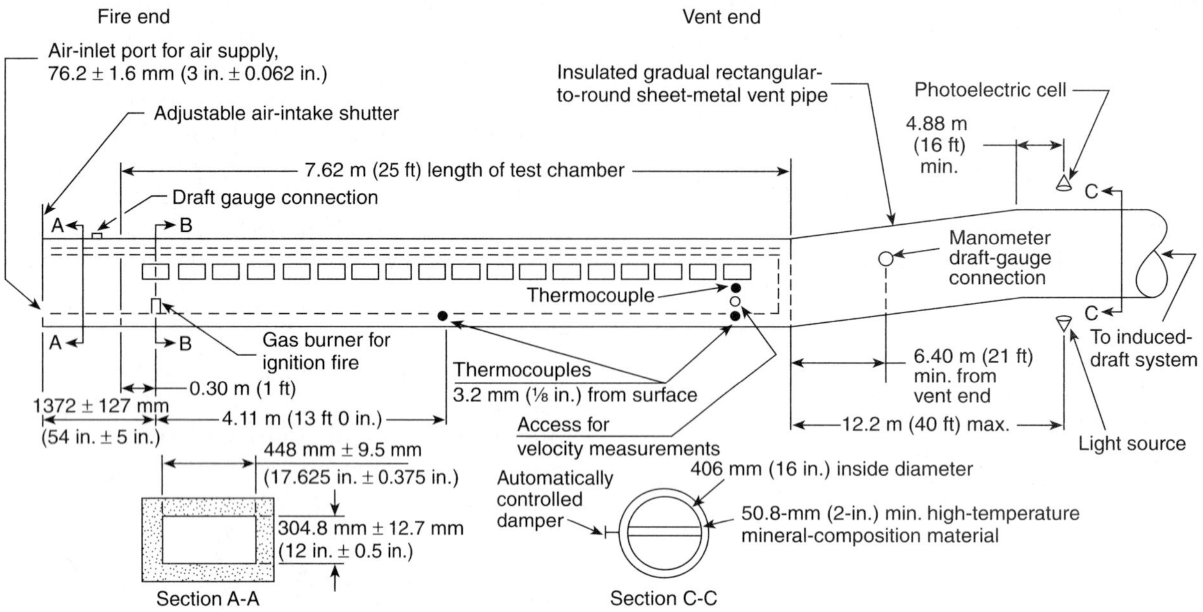


***Exhibit S3.4*** *Schematic diagram of tunnel test apparatus used to characterize the surface burning of materials.*

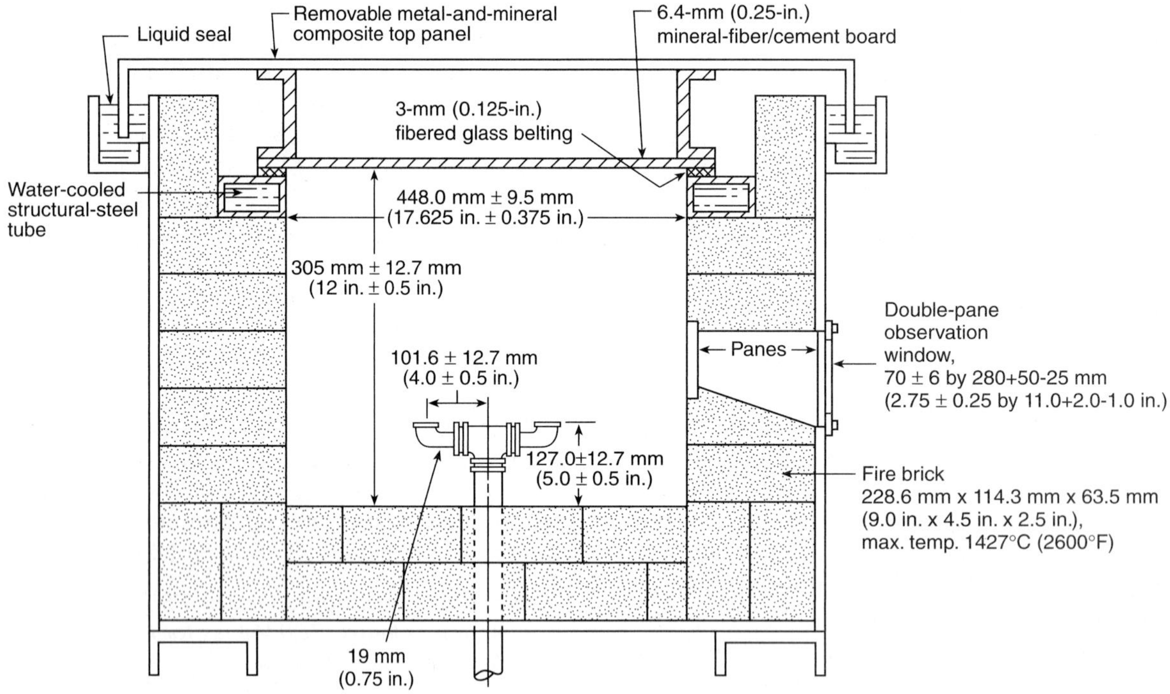


***Exhibit S3.5*** *Cross-sectional view of the tunnel test apparatus.*

and are placed within the test apparatus. A gas flame of approximately 300,000 Btu/sec (89 kW) is applied at one end of the tunnel, and a regulated constant draft is applied through the tunnel from the flame end. The progress of the flame front is observed through side windows for 10 minutes. The FSI is a relative indication of flame propagation, but is not in any way an indication of fire resistance or of combustibility — only of the ability of the material to resist propagation of flame spread across its surface. It is possible that a material with a low ability to spread flame (for example, bare sheet metal) could also exhibit little or no fire resistance when exposed to the testing criteria of NFPA 251. The smoke development represents a degree of obscuration and is measured by a photoelectric cell mounted in the test chamber's exhaust outlet, opposite a light source. A reduction in the light transmitted, due to the smoke particulates that pass by the photoelectric cell, is recorded and used to calculate the SDI. It should be noted that there is no direct relationship between the flame spread and smoke development values. It is possible that a material having a low flame spread index could also exhibit a very high smoke development index. Specimens tested in the Steiner tunnel test must be representative of the material for which test results are desired. When specific materials and products are considered for use or are reviewed for compliance with a provision of the *Life Safety Code,* it is critical that the intended end use correspond with the tested configuration. If the material or product differs in composition or is mounted or applied in a manner that deviates from the tested specimen, it could have an adverse effect. The actual FSI and SDI are likely to be different from those established in the original test results. It is very important therefore, to follow the manufacturer or listing instructions when installing or applying the interior finish material. Section 6.8 of ASTM E 84 discusses the mandatory methods for specimen preparation and mounting for testing some materials, as discussed below. The Appendix of ASTM E 84 provides guidance on the different mounting configurations for some other types of building materials when tested in the Steiner tunnel. This appendix is provided as a guide and cannot be used as a requirement, and so caution should be used when applying it to particular materials.

As stated above, information on the mandatory required procedures for mounting and testing some materials in the Steiner tunnel test has been developed and incorporated into ASTM E 84, in Section 6.8, and more of them are under development (see Table S3.3). The ASTM committee on Fire Standards, ASTM E05, is working on such mounting methods and is developing further standard practices. Not all of them are critical in the *Life Safety Code.*

Some materials that cannot support themselves in the tunnel and that are artificially supported by a wire mesh have been demonstrated to have FSI characteristics that are significantly different from those found in actual field installations. Therefore, the permitted use of wire mesh to support test specimens has been limited in recent editions of ASTM E 84. It has also been established that the ASTM E 84 test method is not suitable for certain building materials. Included are those that, due to their own structural quality or the manner in which they are applied, are not capable of supporting themselves in position or of being supported in the test furnace at a thickness comparable to their recommended use. When using these materials as interior finishes, a different test protocol might be required. An appropriate test for these types of materials would be NFPA 286, *Standard Methods of Fire Tests for Evaluating Contribution of Wall and Ceiling Interior Finish to Room Fire Growth.*

***Table S3.3*** *Steiner Tunnel Specimen Preparation and Mounting Practices to Assess Surface Burning Characteristics of Specific Materials*

| Designation | Application |
|---|---|
| E 2231 | Pipe and Duct Insulation Systems |
| E 2404 | Textile, Paper and Vinyl Wall and Ceiling Coverings |
| E 2573 | Site-Fabricated Stretch Systems |
| E 2579 | Wood Products |
| E XXXX | Reflective Insulation Materials and Radiant Barrier Materials for Building Applications |
| In progress | Plastic Pipe and Tubing for Building Applications |
| In progress | Floor Covers |
| In progress | Vapor Barriers |

Table A.10.2.2 provides a compilation of the interior finish requirements of the occupancy chapters (Chapters 11 through 43) of the *Life Safety Code,* based on ASTM E 84. Wherever the use of Class C interior wall and ceiling finish is required, Class A or Class B is permitted, and wherever Class B interior wall and ceiling finish is required, Class A is also permitted.

*Room-Corner Test.* As an alternative to the Steiner tunnel test, 10.2.3.2 explains that interior wall and ceiling finish materials can be tested in accordance with a room-corner test, namely NFPA 286, *Standard Methods of Fire Tests for Evaluating Contribution of Wall and Ceiling Interior Finish to Room Fire Growth,* and, if they meet the appropriate conditions (from 10.2.3.7.2), they can be used anywhere a material is required to meet Class A, Class B, or Class C finish requirements in accordance with ASTM E 84, as explained above. This is a critical difference in approach, since a room-corner test exposes an interior wall or ceiling finish material when applied to walls (or walls and ceilings) of a room, and it measures heat and smoke release. Historically, codes have regulated materials on walls and ceilings using ASTM E 84. Full-scale room-corner fire test research has shown that flame spread indices produced by ASTM E 84 may not reliably predict all aspects of the fire behavior of textile wall and ceiling coverings. NFPA 286, known as a room-corner test, was developed for assessing the fire and smoke obscuration performance of interior wall and ceiling finish materials. As long as an interior wall or ceiling finish material is tested by NFPA 286 using a mounting system, substrate, and adhesive (if appropriate) that are representative of actual use, the room-corner test provides an adequate evaluation of a product's flammability and smoke obscuration behavior. Manufacturers, installers, and specifiers should be encouraged to use NFPA 286, because this standard fire test has the ability to characterize actual product behavior, as opposed to data generated by tests using ASTM E 84, which only allow comparisons of one product's performance with that of another. If a manufacturer or installer chooses to test a wall finish in accordance with NFPA 286, additional testing in accordance with ASTM E 84 is not necessary. The test results from ASTM E 84 are suitable for classification purposes but should not be used as input for fire models, because they are not generated in units suitable for engineering calculations. Actual test results for heat, smoke, and combustion product release from NFPA 286 are suitable for use as input for fire models for performance-based design.

In NFPA 286, the test compartment is a "standard" room, with dimensions of 8 ft × 12 ft × 8 ft high (2.4 m × 3.7 m × 2.4 m high), including a 30 in. × 80 in. (0.76 m × 2.03 m) doorway in the center of the 8 ft × 8 ft (2.4 m × 2.4 m) wall. (See Exhibit S3.6.) The test material is installed completely covering the three walls of the "standard" room (all except for the wall containing the doorway), as well as the entire ceiling (if appropriate). If a ceiling covering only is being tested, the test material covers the ceiling only.

The ignition source for NFPA 286 is a gas burner with a nominal 12 in. × 12 in. (305 mm × 305 mm) porous top surface of a refractory material, as shown in Exhibit S3.7, which produces a diffusion flame that will expose the walls in the corner of the room where the specimens are mounted to a predetermined energy source. The gas burner is located flush against the two back walls and is used at a net heat output of 40 kW ± 1 kW for the first 5 minutes, followed by a net heat output of 160 kW ± 5 kW for the next 10 minutes. The combustion products from the test room are collected in a hood that is fed into a 3 ft × 3 ft (0.91 m × 0.91 m) plenum just outside the doorway connected to an exhaust duct. Within this exhaust duct, measurements of gas velocity, temperature, and concentrations of selected gases are made. The hood is designed to develop a minimum flow rate, sufficient to capture all the products of combustion being expelled from the fire test room. The canopy hood and exhaust duct are shown in Exhibit S3.8. All the measuring instrumentation is placed in that exhaust duct. The room-corner test method assesses heat release (by the principle of oxygen consumption calorimetry), smoke release into the duct, and the release of combustion products. It is understood that heat release rate is the most critical reaction-to-fire property, as it parallels the intensity of

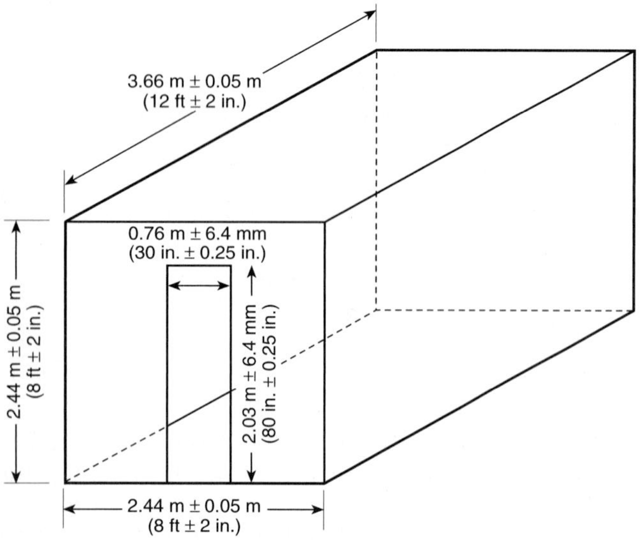


***Exhibit S3.6*** *Interior fire test room dimensions and interior doorway dimensions for the NFPA 286 test.*

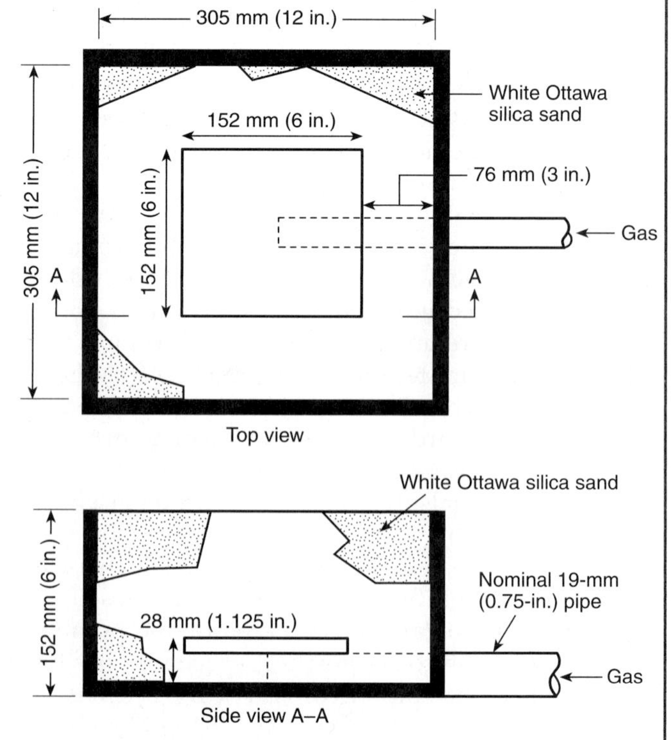


***Exhibit S3.7*** *Gas burner for the NFPA 286 test.*

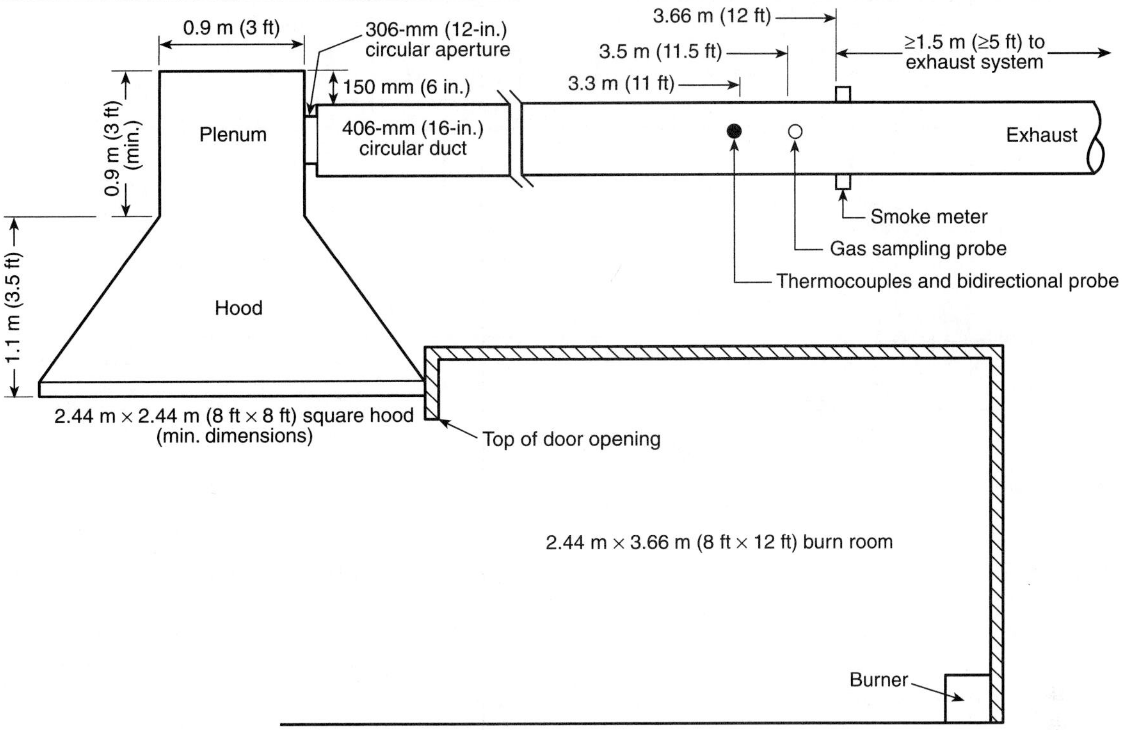


***Exhibit S3.8*** *Canopy hood and exhaust duct for the NFPA 286 test.*

the fire. The *Life Safety Code*, like most other codes, requires that an interior finish material in this test meet the following conditions:

1. Flames shall not spread to the ceiling during the 40 kW exposure.
2. During the 160 kW exposure, the following criteria shall be met:
   a. Flames shall not spread to the outer extremities of the sample on the 8 ft × 12 ft (2.4 m × 3.7 m) wall.
   b. Flashover shall not occur.
3. The peak heat release rate throughout the test shall not exceed 800 kW.
4. For new installations, the total smoke released throughout the test shall not exceed 1000 m$^2$. Values derived from NFPA 286 are in SI units; there is no straightforward inch-pound equivalent.

Flashover is determined to have occurred in the test chamber when any two of the following conditions have been attained:

1. A heat flux at the floor reaches 25 kW/m$^2$.
2. The average upper air temperature exceeds 1200°F (650°C).
3. Flames exit the doorway.
4. A paper target on the floor ignites spontaneously.

The pass/fail criterion for smoke release was determined following an assessment of smoke released in a room-corner test and in the Steiner tunnel test by a number of interior finish materials, which suggested that a material with a total smoke released value exceeding 1000 m$^2$ in a room-corner test would be likely also to exceed an SDI of 450 in the Steiner tunnel test. (See Exhibit S3.9.) It should be noted that the requirement for smoke release within the *Life Safety Code* does not apply to existing installations. The technical committee determined that this new requirement should not be applied retroactively.

A separate room-corner test had been developed earlier for use with textile materials that are used as wall coverings: NFPA 265, *Standard Methods of Fire Tests for Evaluating Room Fire Growth Contribution of Textile Coverings on Full Height Panels and Walls.* The room, burner, and instrumentation are identical to those in NFPA 286. However, NFPA 265 differs from NFPA 286 in two ways:

1. The exposure after 5 minutes at 40 kW increases only to 150 kW for 10 minutes.
2. The gas burner is recessed slightly [approximately 2 in. (51 mm) in each direction] from the walls.

This is a critical difference in that the flames from the burner itself in the NFPA 265 test do not reach the

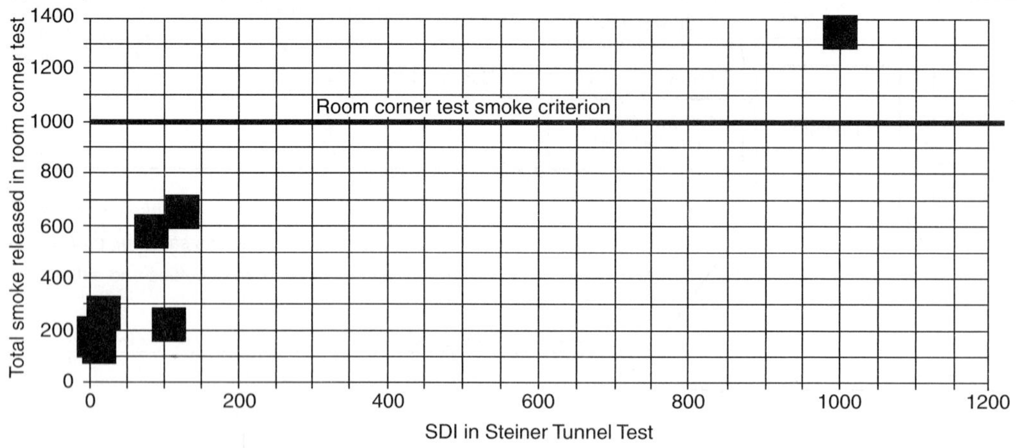


***Exhibit S3.9*** *Comparison of smoke values in different test methods.*

ceiling during the initial test period (i.e., at 150 kW), while those from the NFPA 286 burner do have direct flame impingement on the ceiling even during the initial test period. Therefore, the *Life Safety Code* and other codes limit the application of NFPA 265 only to textile wall coverings (and to expanded vinyl wall covering materials).

Interior finishes that are classified as textile materials require special consideration and appropriate testing, due primarily to their very low thickness. Textile wall covering materials can include napped, tufted, looped, woven, and nonwoven or similar materials. The NFPA 265 test procedure was developed because fire research had shown that a Class A flame spread index in a textile material does not accurately predict the overall burning characteristic behavior of this material in this particular end use.

Two test protocols, Method A and Method B, used to be approved for testing a textile material in accordance with NFPA 265. Method A uses a corner-test exposure and mounts the test specimen on only sections of two walls of the test compartment. The test specimens are mounted only on the rear wall and on the left side wall and extend 2 ft (0.6 m) down from the ceiling. Method B uses the same test compartment configuration but requires that the test specimens be mounted so that they fully cover the three complete walls (not the wall containing the doorway) with the test specimen. Since the 2006 edition of the *Life Safety Code,* Method B of NFPA 265 has been eliminated from the permitted test methods. The test compartment is identical to that in NFPA 286, as is the gas burner (but not its intensity or location, as described above). (See Exhibit S3.10.) Interestingly, when a textile wall covering is tested in accordance with Method A of NFPA 265 (a frequent occurrence), the corresponding results used to be suitable for code approval, but have never been considered suitable for computer modeling of the fire hazard.

For a textile wall covering material to be considered acceptable by the *Life Safety Code* when tested in accordance with NFPA 265, flames must not spread to the ceiling during the 40 kW exposure, flames must not spread to the outer extremity of the test specimen during the 150 kW exposure, and the test specimen in the room cannot reach flashover.

Fire research involving the full-scale room-corner fire test scenarios has documented that textile materials found to be Class A via the Steiner tunnel test can have a burning behavior that is unsatisfactory. So, the fire safety conclusions drawn from the two test methods can be different. It was decided that the conclusions drawn from the more realistic room-corner tests were more likely to be correct. Thus, the *Life Safety Code* now requires that textile wall covering materials be tested in accordance with NFPA 265 and pass the requirements of 10.2.3.7.1, or be tested in accordance with NFPA 286 and pass the requirements of 10.2.3.7.2, or be tested in accordance with ASTM E 84 and obtain a Class A rating and be installed in an occupancy that is fully sprinklered if it extends from the floor to the ceiling (see 10.2.4.1). It is important to note that the pass/fail criteria associated with NFPA 265 are similar to those associated with NFPA 286, with two exceptions: the measurement of smoke release is not a requirement, and the added requirement for a peak heat release rate of 800 kW is not included.

Expanded vinyl wall and ceiling covering materials can be tested in the same way as textile wall covering materials, namely using ASTM E 84 or NFPA 265, but with the same limitations of use. Alternatively, they can be tested as other interior finish materials, namely using NFPA 286, without limitations of use. Foam plastic insulation cannot be used exposed as an

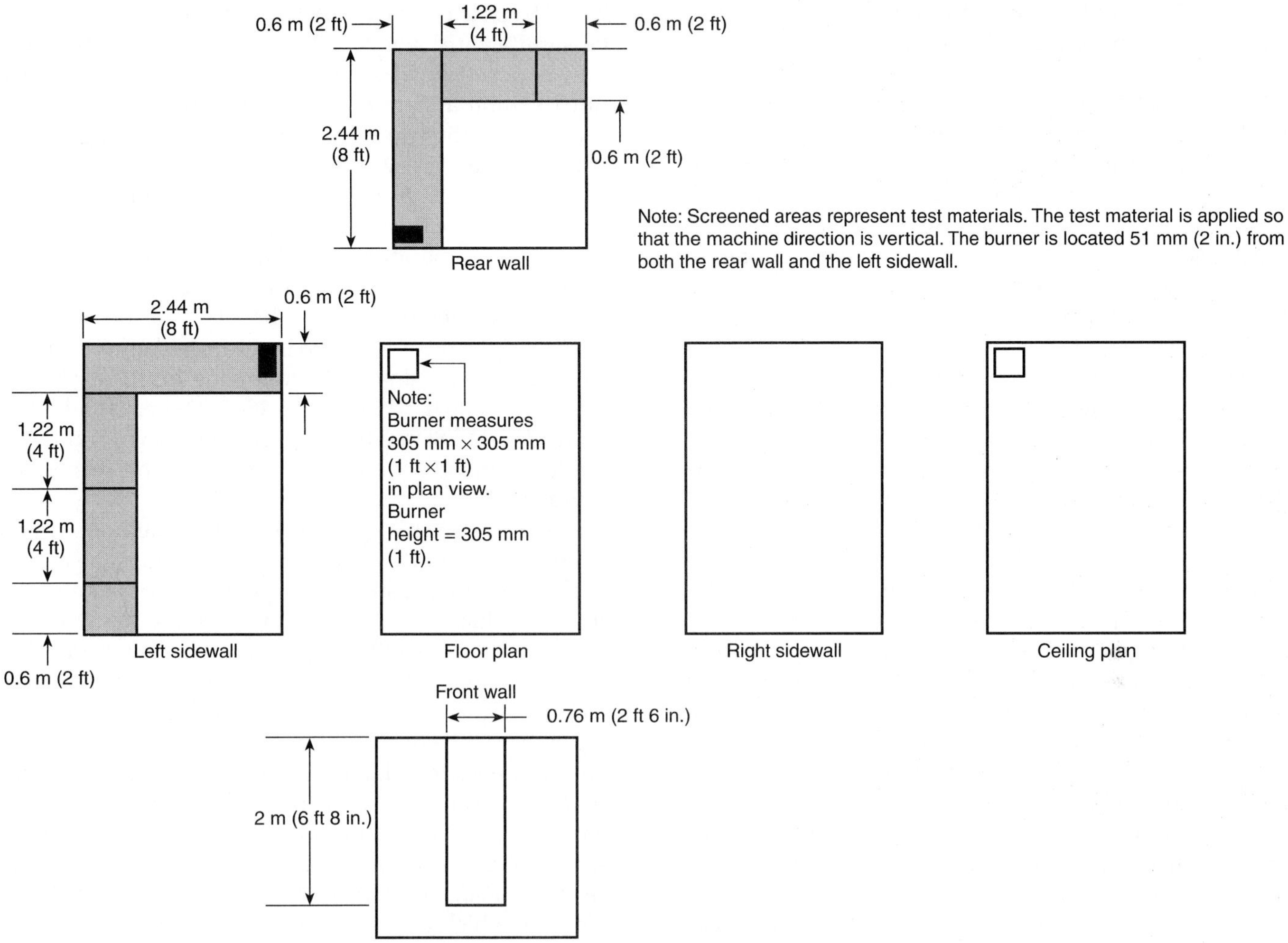


***Exhibit S3.10*** *Specimen mounting for Method A test protocol of NFPA 265.*

interior finish material, except as tested using NFPA 286. Alternatively, foam plastic insulation can be protected from the occupied interior of the building by being covered with a thermal barrier.

Another widely used room-corner test, not used in the *Life Safety Code*, is ASTM E 2257, *Standard Test Method for Room Fire Test of Wall and Ceiling Materials and Assemblies* (similar to ISO 9705, *Fire Tests — Full Scale Room Fire Tests for Surface Products*[10]). It is used by the European Union for regulation of building products; by NFPA 301, *Code for Safety to Life from Fire on Merchant Vessels*,[11] for case furniture; and by the *High Speed Craft Code*[12] of the International Maritime Organization (IMO) for regulation of interior finish "fire restricting materials." The test is basically the same as NFPA 286 (see Exhibits S3.5 through S3.7, which describe the room, ignition burner, and instrumentation), except that the ignition source is a gas burner, which has an output of 100 kW for the first 10 minutes, followed by an output of 300 kW for a subsequent 10 minutes. Just like NFPA 286, this test assesses heat and smoke release and the development of flashover. Tested materials can be required to meet different sets of pass/fail criteria or classifications into categories.

UL 1715, *Standard for Fire Test of Interior Finish Material*, is an early version of a room-corner test, which is widely used in codes, including the *Life Safety Code*, for assessing the fire performance of cellular or foamed plastic materials (foam plastics) used as interior finish. It uses a 30 lb (13.6 kg) wood crib in a corner of the same basic room as NFPA 265 or NFPA 286. In the test, the specimen, the interior finish material, is mounted on the back wall of the room and on 8 ft (2.4 m) of one of the side walls. Measurements are based on temperature and visual observations of extent of flame spread within the room (i.e., whether the flame reaches the extremities and whether it exits the room and indicates flashover). Of course, optional measurements of heat and smoke release are also possible. It has been shown that UL 1715 is less severe than NFPA 286.

FM 4880, *Approval Standard for Class 1 Insulated Wall or Wall and Roof/Ceiling Panels; Plastic Interior Finish Materials; Plastic Exterior Building Panels; Wall/Ceiling Coating Systems; Interior or Exterior Finish Systems,*[13] is a fire test suitable for assessing the fire performance (heat release or flame spread) of cellular or foamed plastic materials (foam plastics) used as interior finish. It requires that the assembly tested not support a self-propagating fire when subjected to a 25 ft (7.6 m) high corner test, as evidenced by flaming or material damage, after exposure to a 750 lb (340 kg) wood crib fire. Other test options exist within the standard, depending on the application of the product tested: the FM equivalent to NFPA 287/ASTM E 2058, a 50 ft (15.2 m) high corner test, and a room corner test (such as NFPA 265, NFPA 286, or ISO 9705). No smoke measurements are made. UL 1040, *Standard for Fire Test of Insulated Wall Construction,* is similar to FM 4880 in that it uses a 764 lb (347 kg) wood crib ignition source in a corner configuration and assesses whether surface burning extends beyond 19 ft (5.5 m) from the intersection of the two walls. Smoke release is not assessed.

UL 1040, UL 1715, and FM 4880 are all used, together with NFPA 286, for assessing the fire performance (but not the smoke release) of foam plastics as interior finish. The tests are also widely used in codes for assessing the suitability of a material as a thermal barrier separating foam plastics and/or metal composite materials (MCMs) from the interior of the building or from plenums.

The 2009 edition of the *Life Safety Code* added the requirements that new installations of cellular or foamed plastic materials for use as interior finish tested in accordance with UL 1040 or FM 4880, tests which do not include a smoke component, must also be tested for smoke release. It explains further that suitable smoke release tests include the following:

1. Additional measurements of smoke release into the duct that demonstrate that the total smoke released throughout the test does not exceed 1000 $m^2$
2. NFPA 286, with the acceptance criterion of 10.2.3.7.2 (4)
3. ASTM E 84, with a smoke developed index not exceeding 450

A new test was developed for 2009: NFPA 275, *Standard Method of Fire Tests for the Evaluation of Thermal Barriers Used Over Foam Plastic Insulation,* which consists of two parts: (a) a fire resistance test and (b) an integrity fire test. The fire resistance test can be conducted using the time-temperature curve of NFPA 251, ASTM E 119, or UL 263, but the test specimen can be significantly smaller (31.5 × 31.5 in. or 800 × 800 mm exposed surface area), and the thermal barrier must exhibit a 15-minute fire resistance rating so that during the 15-minute test period, the average measured temperature rise above the average temperature at the start of the fire test for the thermocouples on the unexposed side does not exceed 250°F (139°C), and the measured temperature rise of any such single thermocouple does not exceed 325°F (181°C). The integrity fire test exposes the thermal barrier and the underlying foam plastic or MCM to be protected, and it can be conducted using any of the following four tests: NFPA 286, UL 1040, UL 1715, or FM 4880. The pass-fail criteria for NFPA 286 are those discussed above, and those for the other tests are as specified in the respective standards.

A common misapplication of test methods needs to be pointed out here: textile materials normally used as floor coverings, such as carpets or carpet-like materials, that have achieved a Class I or a Class II rating (see details in the following section) are not permitted to be installed as interior wall or ceiling finish. In other words, carpets cannot be used to cover walls or ceilings where an interior wall or ceiling finish rating is required unless they have been tested as wall or ceiling coverings. The reason for this is that a classification is obtained by testing with NFPA 253, *Standard Method of Test for Critical Radiant Flux of Floor Covering Systems Using a Radiant Heat Energy Source,* and this test method, which generates a critical radiant flux and not a flame spread or heat release, is applicable only when the material is installed as a floor covering or as an interior floor finish.

Another common misapplication of test methods is one whereby a textile material is tested by means of NFPA 701, *Standard Methods of Fire Tests for Flame Propagation of Textiles and Films* (see more details later in this supplement), and then installed as interior finish on walls, ceilings, or floors. NFPA 701 is intended to apply to fabrics or other materials used in curtains, draperies, or other window treatments. It is also suitable, in Test 1, to a number of materials having an area density not greater than 21 oz/$yd^2$ (700 g/$m^2$), and, in Test 2, to fabrics and films, with or without reinforcement or backing, with area densities greater than 21 oz/$yd^2$ (700 g/$m^2$). NFPA 701 assesses vertical flame propagation performance criteria, which are suitable for draperies, curtains, and other similar loosely hanging furnishings and decorations (see 10.3.1 of the *Life Safety Code*). However, NFPA 701 is an unsuitable test for assessing the fire problem potentially associated with textiles applied to a solid backing and used as wall linings or textiles installed horizontally on floors or ceilings. This is explained in Annex A of the *Life Safety Code*. It has recently also been understood that the fire performance of site-fabricated stretch systems (which often have a textile cover) is not properly assessed using NFPA 701 but needs to be assessed using ASTM E 84, with the test specimen preparation and mounting procedure specified in ASTM E 2573.

As stated above, it is critical that every material be assessed using the tests appropriate to the end-use application. Thus, if the same type of material is employed in different end-use applications, it may require testing via various test methods to be qualified for all applications.

**Interior Floor Finish.** Interior floor finish is defined in the *Life Safety Code* as the interior finish of floors, ramps, stair treads and risers, and other walking surfaces. Interior floor finish needs to meet the requirements of two different fire tests: an ignition test and a critical radiant flux test.

The United States Flammable Fabrics Act requires that all carpets and rugs manufactured, imported, distributed, or marketed in the United States must comply with the requirements of 16 CFR 1630, "Standard for the Surface Flammability of Carpets and Rugs" (FF 1–70).[14] Because the *Life Safety Code* is applicable outside of the United States, it references (in 10.2.2.2 and 10.2.7.1) a standard test method that is substantially similar to 16 CFR 1630: ASTM D 2859. (The *Code* does explain that the two are basically equivalent.) In the test method, a No. 1588 methenamine timed burning tablet (commonly known as methenamine pill) weighing 0.0052 oz (0.149 g) is placed flat on a test specimen consisting of a section of carpet and ignited with a lighted match (ensuring that the match does not ignite the carpet). If the charred portion of the test specimen does not exceed 3 in. (76 mm) in length, the test specimen passes the test. This test method is only applicable to interior floor finish that is a textile, because most hard surface flooring materials are known to meet the test requirements.

Interior floor finish materials used in regulated environments, as determined by the *Life Safety Code* or where the authority having jurisdiction determines that their particular burning characteristics are unknown, often must also meet a minimum critical radiant flux when tested in accordance with NFPA 253 (see also Table S3.1 for alternative similar fire test methods). Paragraph 10.2.2.2 of the *Life Safety Code* specifies when interior floor finishes are required to have a fire safety classification rating, and 10.2.7 describes the criteria needed. Interior floor finishes are grouped in two classes in accordance with their critical radiant flux ratings:

1. Class I Interior Floor Finish: critical radiant flux not less than 0.45 $W/cm^2$
2. Class II Interior Floor Finish: critical radiant flux not less than 0.22 $W/cm^2$ but less than 0.45 $W/cm^2$

The *Life Safety Code* also states (10.2.7.2) that a critical radiant flux of 0.1 $W/cm^2$ (which is basically considered to be equivalent to a "pass" in the ASTM D 2859 test) is minimally required for floor coverings other than carpets. This applies to floor coverings with unknown fire performance, and is discussed in more detail in A.10.2.7.2 and A.10.2.7.3.

The NFPA 253 test method measures the critical radiant flux (CRF) behavior of a horizontally mounted floor covering system exposed to a radiant heater, inside a test chamber (see Exhibits S3.11 through S3.13, which show the apparatus used to test the floor covering specimens in this test method). A gas-fired panel serving as a radiant heat energy source is installed at one end of the test chamber, on an incline (at a 30° angle) so that it extends over the test specimen. The radiant heater applies a graded heat flux that ranges between approximately 0.1 and 1.1 $W/cm^2$ close to the two ends of the test specimen. The test specimen is ignited by a pilot flaming ignition source at the end of the test chamber where the heat flux applied is highest.

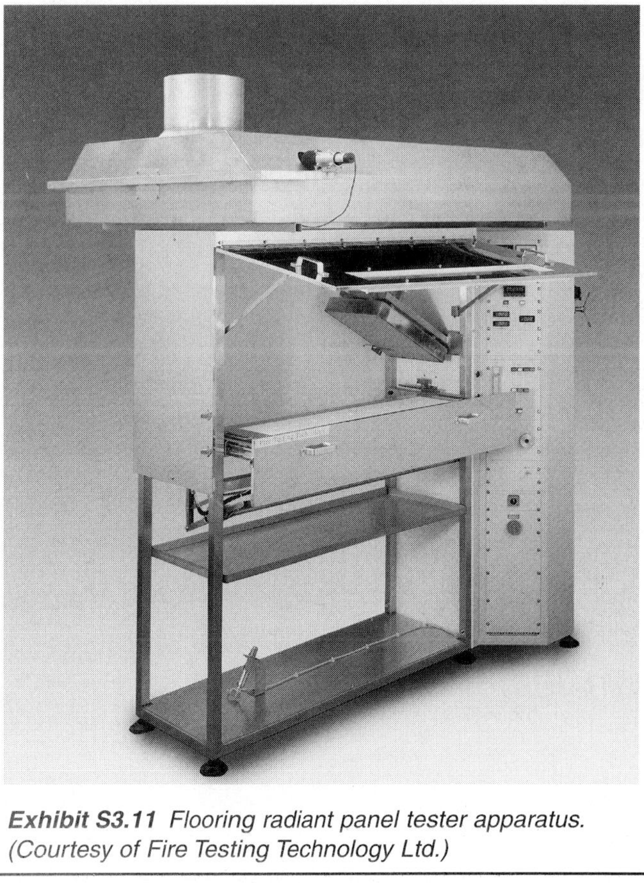

***Exhibit S3.11*** *Flooring radiant panel tester apparatus. (Courtesy of Fire Testing Technology Ltd.)*

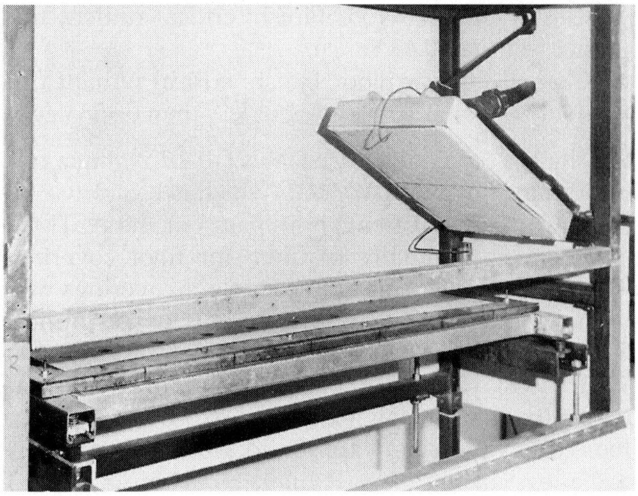

***Exhibit S3.12*** *Flooring radiant panel test showing carpet specimen and gas-fueled panel.*

The test chamber is calibrated by assigning a heat flux to each position along the length of the test chamber.

Thus, the test method measures the heat flux at the point of flame out, which is when the material does not continue to support flaming, and that value is considered the CRF. The test specimens are required, to the extent possible, to simulate actual field installation practices. For example, if a carpet is to be mounted with a pad and/or an underlayment, it must be tested in that same way. The CRF provides a basis for estimating a critical aspect of fire exposure behavior for floor covering systems. It should be noted that this test is intended primarily for regulating floor coverings installed in building corridors, exits, and exit access corridors, which often have little or no combustible wall or ceiling finish. An occupancy with combustible finishes would be expected to contribute much more to fire hazard.

The CRF is determined by measuring the distance that has burned. The test specimen is tested for 10 minutes following the exposure to a radiant energy source to a maximum of 1 W/cm$^2$. The distance burned is converted to a CRF value by plotting the distance on the standard radiant heat energy flux profile, as shown in Exhibit S3.14, which shows the calibration curve

***Exhibit S3.13*** *Flooring radiant panel schematic side elevation.*

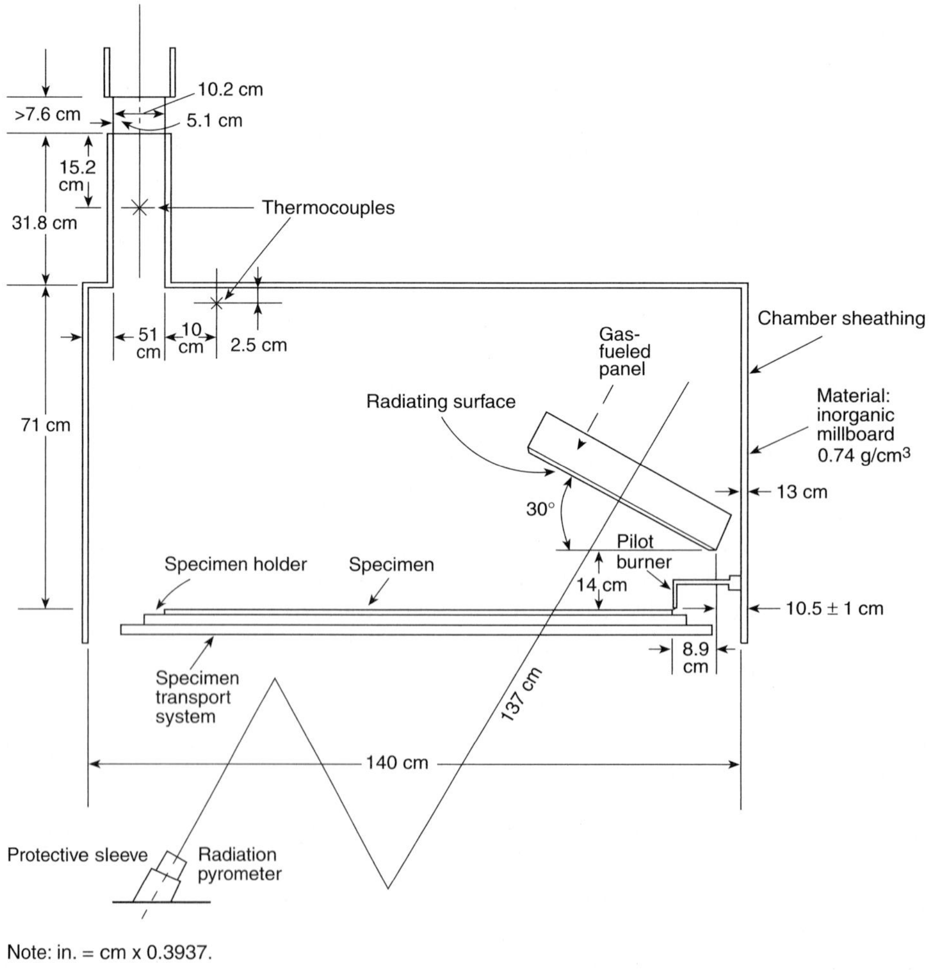

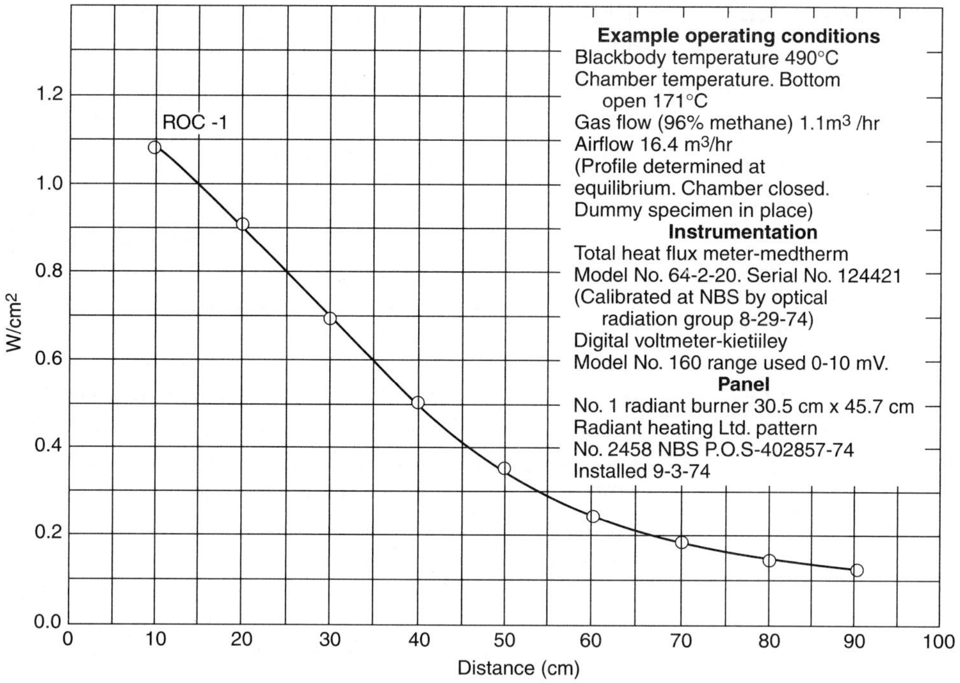


***Exhibit S3.14*** *Standard radiant heat energy flux profile.*

used. The CRF is the level of incident radiant heat energy at the time the test specimen ceases flaming or glowing activities. The higher the CRF, the more resistant to the radiant exposure the material is and, subsequently, flame propagation across the surface, than materials with a lower CRF.

As discussed above, it is important to point out that carpet-like materials, when used in applications other than as floor coverings, must be tested using the fire test method appropriate for the application. Thus, if a carpet-like material is used as wall or ceiling finish, it must be tested using the Steiner tunnel test (ASTM E 84, *Standard Method of Test of Surface Burning Characteristics of Building Materials,* or equivalent, with the appropriate mounting method) or a room-corner test (NFPA 286, *Standard Methods of Fire Tests for Evaluating Contribution of Wall and Ceiling Interior Finish to Room Fire Growth*; NFPA 265, *Standard Methods of Fire Tests for Evaluating Room Fire Growth Contribution of Textile Coverings on Full Height Panels and Walls*; or their equivalents). Similarly, if a carpet-like material is used as a curtain or a drape, it must be tested using a vertical flame propagation test (NFPA 701, *Standard Methods of Fire Tests for Flame Propagation of Textiles and Films*). In neither case is it acceptable to test via NFPA 253, *Standard Method of Test for Critical Radiant Flux of Floor Covering Systems Using a Radiant Heat Energy Source,* or equivalent.

Cellulose loose fill insulation and other exposed insulation materials installed on attic floors are required by codes, even if not specifically discussed in the *Life Safety Code,* to have a critical radiant flux of not less than 0.12 W/cm$^2$ when tested in accordance with ASTM E 970, *Standard Test Method for Critical Radiant Flux of Exposed Attic Floor Insulation Using a Radiant Heat Energy Source*. In *NFPA 5000* this applies to: (a) cellulose loose fill insulation, which must also meet the requirements of CPSC 16 CFR, Part 1209, "Interim Safety Standard for Cellulose Insulation,"[15] and CPSC 16 CFR, Part 1404, "Cellulose Insulation,"[16] and to (b) thermoplastic exposed insulation materials that melt or shrink away when exposed to radiant heat, which must also meet the following criteria:

1. Exhibit a flame spread index and a smoke developed index when tested in accordance with CAN/ULC S102.2, *Standard Method of Test for Surface Burning Characteristics of Floor Coverings and Miscellaneous Materials and Assemblies,*[17] which is the Steiner tunnel test, with floor mounting
2. No ignition when tested in accordance with ASTM E 970
3. A self-ignition temperature of 752°F (400°C) or greater where tested in accordance with ASTM D 1929, *Standard Test Method for Determining Ignition Temperature of Plastics*

The 2009 edition of the *Life Safety Code* added a feature that will make it easier for users of the code to understand the subtleties of the use of each interior finish fire test: Table A.10.2 shows the fire test methods and classification criteria that apply to each of the individual types of interior finish materials.

**Interior Contents and Furnishings.** Beyond interior finish, compartments tend to have a number of combustibles brought in by the occupier. Such contents and furnishings need to be considered for fire involvement. They include furnishings such as upholstered furniture, mattresses, curtains, draperies, and other similar loosely hanging materials and decorations. Certain occupancies in the *Life Safety Code* require that these particular elements possess a certain appropriate degree of fire performance and do not propagate or assist in flame spread. Test requirements (if applicable) are found in Section 10.3. The overall fire growth in certain fires has been related directly to the types of furnishings and decorations found within the facility.

*Upholstered Furniture.* The *Life Safety Code* contains provisions for upholstered furniture to comply with requirements for smoldering ignition (similar to cigarette ignition) and flaming ignition, if applicable according to the occupancy chapters (Chapters 11 through 43). The applicable provisions of the *Life Safety Code* that address the requirement for upholstered furniture to resist cigarette ignition are found in subsection 10.3.2.1. There are two relevant fire test methods: NFPA 260, *Standard Methods of Tests and Classification System for Cigarette Ignition Resistance of Components of Upholstered Furniture*, and NFPA 261, *Standard Method of Test for Determining Resistance of Mock-Up Upholstered Furniture Material Assemblies to Ignition by Smoldering Cigarettes* (see Table S3.1 for alternative similar fire test methods). The major difference between the two test methods is that NFPA 260 addresses individual components that will be used to make an upholstered furniture item, and NFPA 261 addresses small mock-ups of the various composites used for the upholstered furniture item. In both tests, a lit cigarette covered by a layer of sheeting material is placed on the test item, and the resulting char (or flame) is assessed visually. The char length is the distance, to the nearest 0.2 in. (5 mm), from the center of the original location of the lit cigarette. Both tests are permitted to be used for testing of upholstered furniture.

NFPA 260 contains tests for assessing components such as cover fabrics, welt cords, decking materials, interior fabrics, and filling and padding materials. The Upholstered Furniture Action Council (UFAC) originally developed this test method. Compliance with the method for residential upholstered furniture, on a voluntary basis, is managed by UFAC itself. The test method establishes a classification system for determining the resistance of upholstered furniture components to ignition by a smoldering cigarette. A Class 1 designation is given to materials that are considered resistant to cigarette ignition, in that the material does not show evidence of flaming ignition on any part of the test assembly and the resulting char length does not exceed 1.5 in. (38 mm).

NFPA 261 provides test methods to evaluate the resistance of upholstered furniture assemblies to smoldering ignition, when exposed to a lit cigarette under specific conditions in a mock-up test assembly. The National Bureau of Standards (now the National Institute of Standards and Technology) initially developed this test. The individual materials assessed include cover fabrics, filling materials, and welt tapes. In this test, the results are not identified in Classes, such as in NFPA 260, but a material will fail if flaming ignition occurs or if the maximum char length exceeds 1.5 in. (38 mm).

The occupancy chapters in the *Life Safety Code* are entitled to choose whether they will apply the smoldering requirements. In fact, some occupancy chapters have opted out of testing upholstered furniture for smoldering — principally day-care homes (with 12 or fewer clients) — and mercantile, business, and storage occupancies. Both of the American trade associations for manufacturers of residential upholstered furniture (UFAC or its sister organization, the American Furniture Manufacturers Association) and the American trade association for manufacturers of institutional and contract upholstered furniture (BIFMA, Business and Institutional Furniture Manufacturers Association) have been demanding that all their members comply with the smoldering resistance test since the 1970s. UFAC requires NFPA 260 (equivalent to ASTM E 1353 and the UFAC test), and BIFMA requires NFPA 261 (equivalent to ASTM E 1352). It should also be noted that sprinklers have no effect on controlling smoldering ignition (ignition by cigarettes), since they require an increase in room temperature to operate, and there will be no increase in room temperature until well after the upholstered furniture item that fails the cigarette test has erupted into flames.

Two California documents are referenced by some state agencies for investigating the effect of smoldering cigarettes on upholstered furniture components: California Technical Bulletin 116, *Cigarette Test of Upholstered Furniture*;[18] and California Technical Bulletin 117, *Flame and Smoldering Resistance of Furniture Components*.[19] California Technical Bulletin 116 requires that three cigarettes (each covered by a layer of sheeting material) be placed at each of a number of locations on an actual full-scale item of upholstered furniture, such as smooth surfaces, decking, welts, quilted locations, tufted locations, crevices, and tops of arms and backs. In each case, the test item fails if there is ignition or if the char length exceeds 2 in. (51 mm). In California Technical Bulletin 117 (which also contains flaming ignition tests), individual upholstery items are tested, and the test item fails if there is ignition or if the char length exceeds 2 in. (51 mm). There are some differences in the pass/fail criteria of each of these tests, which is critical if a comparison is made between the test results. These California Technical Bulletin test methods are not used in the *Life Safety Code* for assessing resistance to smoldering ignition. The most important requirement that addresses the fire hazard of upholstered furniture is testing that assesses the heat released. The *Life Safety Code* recognizes, in 10.3.3, ASTM E 1537, *Standard Test Method for Fire Testing of Upholstered Furniture*, as the relevant test method for assessing heat release of upholstered furniture. This test is substantially similar to NFPA 266, *Standard Method of Test for Fire Characteristics of Upholstered Furniture Exposed to Flaming Ignition Source*, which was withdrawn to avoid duplication. In this test method, a full-scale upholstered furniture item (or a full-scale mock-up) is ignited with a gas burner to assess the heat release, smoke obscuration, mass loss, and generation of toxic gases. These fire properties are important when developing certain fire hazard considerations during fire modeling. The test item is placed in a standard room (which could be the same room as that used for NFPA 265 or NFPA 286, or a slightly different room, known as the "California room") or in a furniture calorimeter. The test scenarios can be used interchangeably because it has been demonstrated that they provide comparable results for test specimens having heat release rates of 600 kW or less (and those providing higher heat release rates would not be considered safe anyway). The test specimen is ignited with a square gas burner. The burner applies a volume flow rate of 13 L/min ± 0.5 L/min of propane (approximately 19.3 kW) for 80 seconds. See Exhibit S3.15 for the application of the gas burner in this test. Generally, the requirements are waived if suitable active fire protection measures such as sprinklers are present. If applicable (depending on the occupancy), the pass/fail criteria are the following:

1. The peak rate of heat release for the single upholstered furniture item shall not exceed 80 kW.
2. The total energy released by the single upholstered furniture item during the first 10 minutes of the test shall not exceed 25 MJ.

California Technical Bulletin 133, *Flammability Test Procedures for Seating Furniture and Use in Public Occupancies*,[20] is technically equivalent to ASTM E 1537, except that it uses only the California room for testing

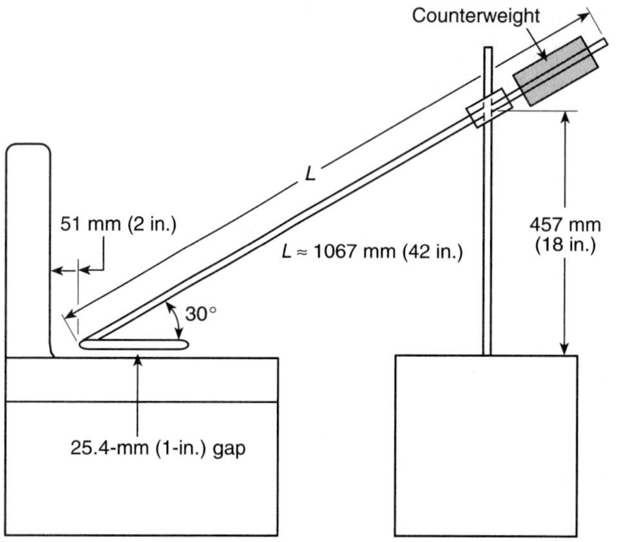


***Exhibit S3.15*** *Positioning of square gas burner on the upholstered furniture item.*

the furniture items and that it includes the same severe pass/fail test criteria used in the 2009 edition of the *Life Safety Code* (as well as additional test criteria related to smoke obscuration and carbon monoxide emission).

Another test procedure used to evaluate the properties of upholstered furniture is ASTM E 1474, *Standard Test Method for Determining the Heat Release Rate of Upholstered Furniture and Mattress Components or Composites Using a Bench Scale Oxygen Consumption Calorimeter* (see also Table S3.1 for alternative similar fire test methods). This test is an application of the cone calorimeter (this test is explained later, in the discussion of NFPA 271, *Standard Method of Test for Heat and Visible Smoke Release Rates for Materials and Products Using an Oxygen Consumption Calorimeter*), and uses an oxygen consumption calorimeter to assess ignitability, heat release, smoke obscuration, mass loss, and generation of toxic products from a small section of an upholstered furniture component or composite. Test specimens are 100 mm × 100 mm × ≤ 51 mm thick. In the test method, the samples are exposed to a controlled level of radiant energy from a conical electric heater, 35 kW/m$^2$. Data from this test has been shown to be useful in predicting the fire performance of the actual full-scale item (or of the full-scale test methods discussed above). However, issues such as product design and minor components affect the results.

*Mattresses.* The *Life Safety Code* contains provisions for mattresses to comply with requirements for smoldering ignition (that is, cigarette ignition) and flaming ignition, if applicable according to the occupancy chapters (Chapters 11 through 43). The requirements for mattresses are very similar to those for upholstered furniture. The applicable provisions of the *Life Safety Code* that address the requirement for a mattress to resist cigarette ignition are found in 10.3.2. There is one relevant fire test method, which is actually a federal requirement in the United States: the cigarette ignition of mattresses, mattress tickings, and mattress pads must comply with Department of Commerce (DOC) FF 4-72 or CFR 1632[21]. In the test, a lit cigarette is placed on the test item and the resulting char (or flame) assessed visually. The test item fails if there is ignition or if the char length exceeds 2 in. (51 mm).

The occupancy chapters in the *Life Safety* Code are entitled to choose whether they will apply the smoldering requirements for mattresses. In fact, the same occupancies have opted out of testing mattresses as upholstered furniture.

The most important requirement that addresses the fire hazard of mattresses is (as with upholstered furniture) testing that assesses the heat released. The *Life Safety Code* recognizes, in 10.3.4, ASTM E 1590, *Standard Test Method for Fire Testing of Mattresses*, as the relevant test method for assessing heat release of upholstered furniture. This test is substantially similar to NFPA 267, *Standard Method of Test for Fire Characteristics of Mattresses and Bedding Assemblies Exposed to Flaming Ignition Source*, which was withdrawn to avoid duplication. In this test method, a full-scale mattress is ignited with a gas burner to assess the heat release, smoke obscuration, mass loss, and generation of toxic gases. These fire properties are important when developing certain fire hazard considerations during fire modeling. The test item is placed in a standard room (which could be the same room as that used for NFPA 265 or NFPA 286, or the California room) or in a furniture calorimeter. The test scenarios can be used interchangeably because it has been demonstrated that they provide comparable results for test specimens having heat release rates of 600 kW or less (and those providing higher heat release rates would not be considered safe anyway). The test specimen is ignited with a T-shaped gas burner, which applies a volume flow rate of 12 L/min ± 0.5 L/min of propane (approximately 17.8 kW) for 180 seconds. See Exhibit S3.16 for the application of the gas burner in this test. Generally, the requirements are waived if suitable active fire protection measures such as sprinklers are present. If applicable, the pass/fail criteria are the following:

1. The peak rate of heat release for the single mattress shall not exceed 250 kW.
2. The total energy released by the single mattress during the first 5 minutes of the test shall not exceed 40 MJ.

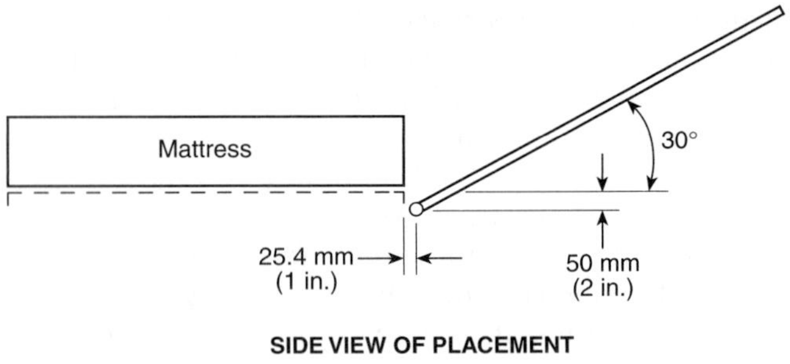


***Exhibit S3.16*** *Positioning of T-shaped gas burner on the mattress.*

California Technical Bulletin 129, *Flammability Test Procedures for Mattresses for Use in Public Buildings*,[22] is technically equivalent to ASTM E 1590 except that it uses only the California room for testing the furniture items and that it includes the same severe pass/fail test criteria used in the 2009 edition of the *Life Safety Code* (as well as an additional test criterion related to mass loss).

The cone calorimeter application standard, ASTM E 1474, can also be used for mattress composites or components, in a similar fashion to the use for upholstered furniture test specimens.

*Curtains, Draperies, and Decorations.* NFPA 701, *Standard Methods of Fire Tests for Flame Propagation of Textiles and Films*, is mandated for testing of curtains, drapes, or similar loosely hanging furnishings or decorations. NFPA 701 provides the means to evaluate the vertical propagation of a small flame beyond the area exposed to the source of ignition. NFPA 701 includes two methods of assessing flame propagation propensity. The test method to be used depends on the areal density of the test specimen (weight per unit surface) and some other characteristics. Test Method 1 is used for fabrics that weigh up to 21 oz/yd$^2$ (700 g/m$^2$), and in particular for single-layer fabrics and multilayer curtain and drapery assemblies, but is not permitted to be used for vinyl-coated fabric blackout linings (because it has been shown that these linings produce erroneous results with this method). In relation to NFPA 701, Test Method 1, curtains and drapes also include the following items, if they weigh up to 21 oz/yd$^2$ (700 g/m$^2$): window curtains, stage or theater curtains, vertical folding shades, roll-type window shades, hospital privacy curtains, window draperies, fabric vertical shades or blinds, horizontal folding shades, swags, and fabric horizontal shades or blinds. Test Method 1 also applies to the following textile items, if they weigh up to 21 oz/yd$^2$ (700 g/m$^2$): table skirts, table linens, display booth separators, and textile wall hangings. Test Method 2 is to be used for the heavier fabrics and films (with or without reinforcement or backing), weighing over 21 oz/yd$^2$ (700 g/m$^2$) and for fabrics used in awnings and tents and for vinyl-coated fabric blackout linings and lined draperies using a vinyl-coated fabric blackout lining.

The test methods in the 1999 edition of NFPA 701, and in more recent ones, were introduced in the revisions between the 1989 and 1996 editions, which eliminated the "small-scale test," because it was found that a "pass" in that test was not indicative of a good fire performance. The difference between the NFPA 701 Test Method 1 and the small-scale test previously included in the standard is that the test specimen is now larger and the overall time exposure to the flame is increased. Test Method 1 employs 10 specimens of material, each 2.9 in. × 15.75 in. (150 mm × 400 mm), which are exposed to a Bunsen gas burner for 45 seconds. The pass/fail criterion, addressing vertical flame propagation performance, requires that there be no flaming for more than 2 seconds after the test flame is removed and that the average weight loss of the test specimen not be greater than 40 percent. Test Method 2 of NFPA 701 is similar to the previous "large-scale test" in specimen size and test protocol, but differs somewhat in the test enclosure. Test Method 2 employs test specimens that are tested in a folded or flat configuration, and that have sizes 24 in. × 46.25 in. (610 mm × 1.2 m) or 5 in. × 46.25 in. (125 mm × 1.2 m), respectively. Each test specimen is then exposed to a Bunsen gas burner for 2 minutes. The pass/fail criterion, addressing (vertical) flame propagation performance, also requires that there be no flaming for more than 2 seconds after the test flame is removed. Additionally, it requires that the length of char on an individual folded test specimen not exceed 41.3 in. (1050 mm), and that the length of char on any flat test specimen not exceed 40.7 in. (1035 mm). Both test methods require that, if any portions or residues of the test specimen drip or fall to the test chamber floor during or after application of the test flame, flaming will not continue. The results of the two tests contained in NFPA 701 should not be compared to each other, as they use different types of pass/fail criteria. However, it can be assumed that Test Method 2 represents a more severe condition than Test Method 1.

NFPA 701 stipulates that each fabric is also to be subjected to exposures applicable to its intended use, such as laundering, dry cleaning, weathering, and other exposure to water. It is believed that the accelerated exposure tests detailed in NFPA 701 (akin to weathering or aging, to some extent) provide sufficient conditioning to permit a reasonable appraisal of the durability of the fire retardant treatment for the useful life of the fabric. Procedures on how to provide accelerated dry cleaning, laundering, weathering, and water leaching for the fabrics are also provided in NFPA 701.

NFPA 701 is also used in the *Life Safety Code* for assessing the fire performance of (a) membrane structure fabrics of temporary and permanent membrane structures, (b) tent fabrics, (c) combustible scenery of cloth, film, vegetation (dry), and similar materials in assembly occupancies, (d) materials in exhibit booths in assembly occupancies, and (e) textiles and films in mercantile occupancy kiosks (malls).

The text of NFPA 705, *Recommended Practice for a Field Flame Test for Textiles and Films*, was originally contained in Chapter 10 of the 1989 edition of NFPA 701. It was developed as a stand-alone document during the revision leading to the 1996 edition of NFPA 701. NFPA 705 is a recommended practice that provides guidance to enforcement officials confronted with the assessment of products already installed. Thus, officials can use this test for the field application of an open-flame ignition source to textiles and films that have been in use in the field or for which reliable laboratory data are not available. This recommended practice provides the authority having jurisdiction with a field procedure for determining the tendency of textiles and films to sustain burning subsequent to the application of a relatively small open flame. There is no correlation between the testing provisions found in NFPA 705 and the testing methods of NFPA 701. Field application of the NFPA 705 testing procedures is somewhat useful, but must be used with good judgment and within limitations. Field tests should not be relied on as a sole means for ensuring adequate fire performance of decorative materials, but they can be used to augment a comprehensive regulatory program. This test is not actually used in the *Life Safety Code* but is used by code officials and inspectors as a preliminary test to determine whether further testing is warranted.

*Unprotected Foam Plastics.* Furnishings and contents made with foamed plastic materials that are unprotected from ignition are required to have a heat release rate not exceeding 100 kW when tested in accordance with UL 1975, *Standard for Fire Tests for Foamed Plastics Used for Decorative Purposes* (see 10.3.7 of the *Life Safety Code*). The same test method also applies to other foam displays, as follows:

1. In theaters, motion picture theaters, and television stage settings, with or without horizontal projections, to decorative packages of foamed plastic (see 12.4.5.11.4)

2. Exposed foamed plastic materials and unprotected materials containing foamed plastic used for decorative purposes or stage scenery (see 12.7.4.3 and 13.7.4.3)
3. Foam plastic materials of construction of exhibit booths in assembly occupancies (see 12.7.5.3.4 and 13.7.5.3.4)
4. Foam plastic materials of construction of kiosks in malls (see 36.4.4.8 and 37.4.4.8)

In every case, any single fuel package cannot have a heat release rate exceeding 100 kW. There are some other fuel packages that are also tested by means of UL 1975 and that are required to have a heat release rate not to exceed 150 kW:

1. Cardboard, honeycombed paper, and other similar combustible materials used for construction of exhibit booths in places of assembly (see 12.7.5.3.4 and 13.7.5.3.4)
2. Foamed plastics and materials containing foamed plastics on stages (see 12.7.5.3.6.2 and 13.7.5.3.6.2)
3. Foam plastics used in plastic signs in malls (see 36.4.4.7 and 37.4.4.7)

UL 1975 is a "furniture calorimeter" test method, in which the fuel package under test is exposed to a wood crib ignition source (340 g) and where all relevant fire properties are measured, with the critical property being the rate of heat release.

Another new test was developed in 2009, namely NFPA 289, *Standard Method of Fire Test for Individual Fuel Packages*. It consists of a furniture calorimeter, with six basic ignition sources: 20, 40, 70, 100, 160, and 300 kW, using the same gas burner as in NFPA 286. A series of ad hoc tests conducted with the gas burner located at 1.2 m from the floor, and 1.2 m below the bottom of the hood (with the top of the hood at 3.0 m from the floor), showed approximate flow rates and flame heights associated with each ignition source (Table S3.4). The ignition sources chosen correspond to the following concepts:

***Table S3.4** Approximate Flow Rates and Flame Heights for Various Heat Release Rates (HRR)*

| HRR (kW) | Flow Rate (L/sec) | Flame Height (mm) |
|---|---|---|
| 20 | 16.5 | 380 |
| 40 | 30.7 | 610 |
| 60 | 47.2 | 815 |
| 70 | 54.8 | 920 |
| 100 | 77.9 | 1120 |
| 160 | 122.7 | 1525 |
| 300 | 226.5 | 2085 |

1. A 20 kW ignition source is similar to the peak heat release rate of the wood crib ignition source used in UL 1975, *Standard for Fire Tests for Foamed Plastics Used for Decorative Purposes*.
2. A 40 kW ignition source can be used as a more severe approach to testing the same products otherwise tested using the 20 kW ignition source if additional fire safety is required. Moreover, a 40 kW ignition source also corresponds to the heat output from a small wastebasket fire. Finally, a 40 kW ignition source is also the minimum ignition source used for testing of interior finish materials with NFPA 286, *Standard Methods of Fire Tests for Evaluating Contribution of Wall and Ceiling Interior Finish to Room Fire Growth*.
3. A 70 kW ignition source offers an intermediate range between the 40 kW and 100 kW ignition sources.
4. A 100 kW source is the lower ignition source used for testing of interior finish materials either with ASTM E 2257, *Standard Test Method for Room Fire Test of Wall and Ceiling Materials or Assemblies*, or with ISO 9705, *Fire Tests — Full Scale Room Fire Tests for Surface Products*. It is used to initially differentiate interior finish materials on their likelihood of leading to flashover.
5. A 160 kW ignition source is the higher ignition source used for testing of interior finish materials with NFPA 286. It is used to assess whether such interior finish materials are likely to lead to flashover.
6. A 300 kW ignition source is the higher ignition source used for testing of interior finish materials with either ASTM E 2257 or ISO 9705. It is used to differentiate interior finish materials with very low levels of heat release and very low likelihood of leading to flashover.

**Fire Retardant–Treated Wood.** The *Life Safety Code* requires that some uses of wood be restricted to fire retardant-treated wood. It defines this material as "a wood product impregnated with chemical by a pressure process or other means during manufacture, which is tested in accordance with ASTM E 84, has a listed flame spread of 25 or less, and shows no evidence of significant progressive combustion when the test is continued for an additional 20-minute period; nor does the flame front progress more than 10.5 ft (3200 mm) beyond the centerline of the burners at any time during the test." So, this product is required to meet a more severe test than the normal test contained within ASTM E 84. The test is discussed in NFPA 703, *Standard for Fire Retardant–Treated Wood and Fire-Retardant Coatings for Building Materials*. Requirements for fire retardant-treated wood can be found in the chapters on assembly occupancies, when dealing with grandstands (see 12.4.8 and 13.4.8) and when dealing with exhibit booths (see 12.7.5.3.4 and 13.4.7.5.3.4). The requirements are also found in 19.1.6.8, which deals with wood studs within non–load-bearing partitions for existing health care occupancies. Finally they are found when dealing with the materials of construction of kiosks and similar structures in malls (see 36.4.4.8 and 37.4.4.8).

**Fire-Retardant Coatings.** The *Life Safety Code* requires that fire-retardant coatings meet specific fire tests. Paragraph 10.2.6.1, dealing with interior finish, specifically allows existing interior finish surfaces to be upgraded to a higher level of fire performance using fire-retardant coatings, but only if the coatings have been specifically designed and approved for the application. The language states, "The required flame spread or smoke development classification of existing surfaces of walls, partitions, columns, and ceilings shall be permitted to be secured by applying approved fire-retardant coatings to surfaces having higher flame spread ratings than permitted. Such treatments shall be tested, or shall be listed and labeled for application to the material to which they are applied, and shall comply with the requirements of NFPA 703, *Standard for Fire Retardant–Treated Wood and Fire-Retardant Coatings for Building Materials.*" In this case, the coating must have been tested using the normal ASTM E 84 test (rather than the longer test method used for fire retardant–treated wood) with the specific material (typically with the actual type of wood) intended to be used and listed for the application by a recognized listing agency. The reason for this requirement is that coatings may exhibit different fire behavior when different substrates (including different species of wood) are treated with the same coating. Also, in tests, multiple coatings can lead to paint delamination and bubbling or blistering of paint. Testing has also shown that thin coatings generally take on the characteristics of the substrate. In a fire, delamination, bubbling and blistering of paint can generate an accelerated rate of flame spread.

**Roof Coverings.** The *Life Safety Code* requires that some roof coverings meet a classification based on NFPA 256, *Standard Methods of Fire Tests of Roof Coverings.* In the standard roof coverings are classified into three classes, depending on their characteristics:

1. Class A roof coverings are intended to be effective against severe fire exposure, to afford a high degree of fire protection to the roof deck, not to slip from position, and not to present a flying brand hazard.
2. Class B roof coverings are intended to be effective against moderate fire exposure, to afford a moderate degree of fire protection to the roof deck, not to slip from position, and not to present a flying brand hazard.
3. Class C roof coverings are intended to be effective against light fire exposure, to afford a light degree of fire protection to the roof deck, not to slip from position, and not to present a flying brand hazard.

NFPA 256 includes six tests: intermittent flame, spread of flame, burning brand, flying brand, rain, and weathering. In the intermittent flame test, a luminous gas flame is applied for a number of cycles (flame on/flame off) and observations are made for the following:

1. Appearance of sustained flaming on the underside of the test deck
2. Production of flaming or glowing brands
3. Displacement of portions of the test sample
4. Exposure or falling away of portions of the roof deck

Acceptance is based on there being no sustained flaming on the underside of the deck. In the spread of flame test, a gas flame is applied continuously to the roof assembly. Acceptance is based on there being no flame spread beyond 6 ft (1820 mm, Class A), 8 ft (2440 mm, Class B), or 13 ft (3960 mm, Class C). In the burning brand test, burning brands are placed on the surface of each test deck at the location considered most vulnerable (the point of minimum coverage over the deck joint) with respect to ignition of the deck. Acceptance is based on there being no sustained flaming on the underside of the deck. In the flying brand test, a gas flame is applied to the roof deck in the presence of an air current. Acceptance is based on there being no flying, flaming brands or particles that continue to glow after reaching the floor. Details of the tests required for each classification are described in Table S3.5.

Roof membranes in permanent or temporary membrane structures (see Sections 11.9 and 11.10) need to have some classification, meaning that they can be Class C. Roof coverings are regulated in the following cases:

1. Buildings of Type I(443), Type I(332), Type II(222), or Type II(111) construction for new and existing health care occupancies: Roof coverings need to be Class A (sections 18.1.6.5 and 19.1.6.5).
2. Buildings of Type I, Type II(222), or Type II(111) construction for existing detention occupancies: Roof coverings need to be Class C (section 23.1.6.5).

***Table S3.5** Tests and Test Assemblies Required for Roof Covering Classification by NFPA 256*

| Material to be Tested | Intermittent Flame Test | Spread of Flame Test | Burning Brand Test | Flying Brand Test[1] | Rain Test[2] | Weathering Test[3] |
|---|---|---|---|---|---|---|
| Other than wood shakes or shingles, for installation on combustible decks | | | | | | |
| Class A | 2 | 2 | 4 | None | None | None |
| Class B | 2 | 2 | 2 | None | None | None |
| Noncombustible decks only | None | 2 | None | When required | When required | When required |
| Wood shakes and shingles[4] | | | | | | |
| Class A | 3 (2) [5] | 3 | 6 (2) [5] | 3 (2) [5] | 6 | 15 |
| Class B or Class C | 3 (2) [5] | 3 | 3 (2) [5] | 3 (2) [5] | 6 | 15 |

[1] Test is performed where there is a possibility that during the test exposure the roof covering will break into flaming particles that support combustion on the floor.

[2] Test is conducted where the fire-retardant characteristics of the roof covering are adversely affected by water.

[3] Test is conducted with materials or constructions where the fire-retardant characteristics of the roof covering are adversely affected by weather.

[4] Number in parentheses is the number of samples from the rain test to be tested. Number in square brackets is the number of samples from the weathering test to be tested.

3. Buildings of Type I, Type II(222), or Type II(111) construction for existing residential board and care occupancies: Roof coverings need to be Class A (section 33.3.1.3.4).

## Tests for Other Fire Properties

**Combustibility — Noncombustible and Limited Combustible.** Many codes, including the *Life Safety Code*, require that certain materials (particularly materials of construction) be classified as "noncombustible." Noncombustibility is assessed by testing a specimen of a material that is 1.5 in. × 1.5 in. × 2 in. (38 mm × 38 mm × 51 mm) in a vertical tube furnace heated to 1382°F (750°C) and waiting for temperature rises. A material is classified as noncombustible if, when tested in accordance with ASTM E 136, *Test Method for Behavior of Materials in a Vertical Tube Furnace at 750°C*, it meets the following three criteria:

1. The recorded temperature of the surface and interior thermocouples does not at any time during the test rise more than 54°F (30°C) above the furnace temperature at the beginning of the test.
2. There is no flaming from the specimen after the first 30 seconds of test.
3. If the weight loss of the specimen during testing exceeds 50 percent of the initial weight, the recorded temperature of the surface and interior thermocouples does not, at any time during the test, rise above the furnace air temperature at the beginning of the test, and there is no flaming of the specimen.

Another test is often also used to assess whether a material is classified as noncombustible, namely ISO 1182, *Reaction to fire tests for building products — Noncombustibility test*.[23] This test is used in the European Union and in the marine world, both internationally by the International Maritime Organization (IMO) and in the United States by the Coast Guard.

There are many instances in the *Life Safety Code* where the concept of "limited combustible" is used, almost exclusively for materials of construction, as a test criterion that is exclusive to NFPA codes and standards. A material is "limited combustible" if it is "a building construction material not complying with the definition of noncombustible material that, in the form in which it is used, has a potential heat value not exceeding 3500 Btu/lb (8141 kJ/kg), where tested in accordance with NFPA 259, *Standard Test Method for Potential Heat of Building Materials*, and complies with (a) or (b): (a) materials having a structural base of noncombustible material, with a surfacing not exceeding a thickness of $^1/_8$ in. (3.2 mm) that has a flame spread index not greater than 50; and (b) materials, in the form and thickness used, other than as described in (a), having neither a flame spread index greater than 25 nor evidence of continued progressive combustion and of such composition that surfaces that would be exposed by cutting through the material on any plane would have neither a flame spread index greater than 25 nor evidence of continued progressive combustion. (Materials subject to increase in combustibility or flame spread index beyond the limits herein established through the effects of age, moisture, or other atmospheric condition shall be considered combustible.)" Note that the "flame spread index" associated with this definition is based on testing in accordance with ASTM E 84, *Standard Method of Test of Surface Burning Characteristics of Building Materials* (see also Table S3.1 for alternative similar fire test methods). Testing in accordance with NFPA 259 requires that a small piece of the material be pulverized and combusted by a combination of tests in an oxygen bomb calorimeter (at very high pressure and in an atmosphere of pure oxygen) to assess the gross (or complete) heat of combustion and in the vertical tube furnace at 1382°F (750°C). The final result is a "potential heat content." Materials classified as "limited combustible" can be used as replacements for noncombustible materials in a number of applications, albeit only in NFPA codes and standards.

It is important to understand that there is a fundamental difference between the concepts of "gross heat of combustion" (which is the theoretical amount of heat released if a material is completely combusted to its final products — such as carbon dioxide and water — and is measured by oxygen bomb calorimeters) and "effective heat of combustion" (which is the actual amount of heat released in a realistic fire scenario, and is assessed by oxygen consumption, or heat release, calorimeters). Oxygen consumption calorimetry is used in tests of various scales, starting at bench-scale (with 100 mm × 100 mm, or almost 4 in. × 4 in. test specimens). Calorimetry is based on the empirical observation that there is a direct relationship between the mass of oxygen consumed during combustion and the heat released. The relationship is that approximately $13.1 \times 10^3$ kJ of heat are released per 1 kg of oxygen consumed.

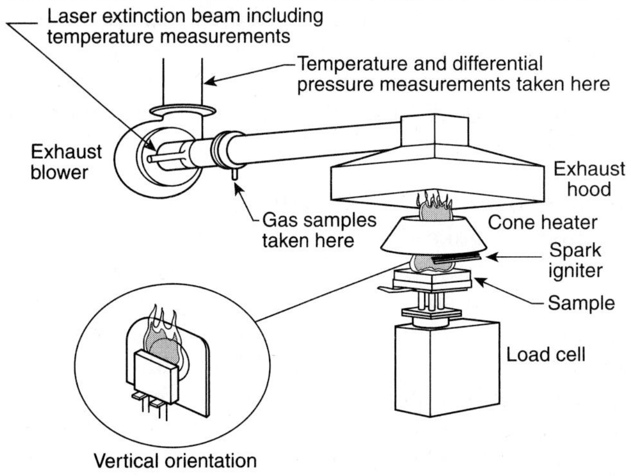


***Exhibit S3.17*** *Schematic diagram of the cone calorimeter.*

**Heat Release Rate: Cone Calorimeter Testing.** NFPA 271, *Standard Method of Test for Heat and Visible Smoke Release Rates for Materials and Products Using an Oxygen Consumption Calorimeter* (or ASTM E 1354, which is equivalent), is a small-scale test procedure for determining the ignitibility, heat release rate, mass loss rate, smoke obscuration, effective heat of combustion, and toxic gas release from burning of materials and products. The test procedure uses a cone calorimeter apparatus that exposes a test specimen to a controlled constant level of radiant heating ranging up to 100 kW/m² (see Exhibit S3.17). The test results are useful in the evaluation of materials, mathematical modeling, and product research and development. They are also very useful for predictions of heat release results from larger-scale tests, such as many of the tests discussed earlier, including room-corner tests (NFPA 286 and 265), furniture tests (ASTM E 1537 and E 1590), furniture calorimeter tests (UL 1975), and so on. Application standards exist for this cone calorimeter test method, such as NFPA 272, discussed earlier for upholstered furniture or mattress composites or components. Test specimens are roughly 4 in. × 4 in. (100 mm × 100 mm) with a maximum thickness of 2 in. (50 mm), and they can be exposed horizontally or vertically. However, test samples are most meaningfully exposed horizontally — irrespective of the application that the test is intended to investigate — due to the configuration of the ignition source. Interestingly, this test is not used much for regulatory purposes, but the test itself is an upgrade of the Ohio State University heat release rate calorimeter (ASTM E 906, *Standard Test Method for Heat and Visible Smoke Release Rates for Materials and Products*, which is equivalent to NFPA 263, *Standard Method of Test for Heat and Visible Smoke Release Rates for Materials and Products*, withdrawn to avoid duplication). The Ohio State heat release test is used by the United States Federal Aviation Administration for aircraft regulation. The main use of the cone calorimeter test in the *Life Safety Code* is to obtain input values for use in the performance calculations contained in Chapter 5. NFPA 1, *Fire Code*,[24] now requires that nonmetallic rubbish containers exceeding a capacity of 40 gallons (0.15 ml³) be manufactured of materials having a peak rate of heat release not exceeding 300 kW/m² at a flux of 50 kW/m² when tested in the horizontal orientation. The tested materials should be a thickness as used in the container but not less than of 0.25 in. (6 mm), in accordance with ASTM E 1354, *Standard Test Method for Heat and Visible Smoke Release Rates for Materials and Products Using an Oxygen Consumption Calorimeter*. The 2009 edition of NFPA 1 also requires that plastic materials used to construct rigid components of soft contained play equipment structures (such as tubes, windows, panels, junction boxes, pipes, slides, and decks) exhibit a peak rate of heat release not exceeding 400 kW/$m^2$ when tested in accordance with ASTM E 1354 at an incident heat flux of 50 kW/$m^2$ in the horizontal orientation at a thickness of 6 mm.

**Smoke Obscuration — Small- and Large-Scale Test Methods.** Smoke obscuration is a critical fire property, since victims of a fire must be able to see their way to the exits (or rescuers must be able to see the way in) so that they can escape or be rescued. Thus, smoke obscuration is particularly critical in full-scale tests. However, it is important to recognize that the values being developed for smoke obscuration from small-scale tests might not have application or correlation to the particular base performance fire scenarios or other end-use applications, since smoke obscuration is a less easily scalable property than heat release. Activities are ongoing to address some of these concerns.

Small-scale tests that address smoke obscuration measurements can be subdivided into static and dynamic test methods. There are two static test methods: NFPA 258, *Recommended Practice for Determining Smoke Generation of Solid Materials* (now withdrawn to avoid duplication), and NFPA 270, *Standard Test Method for Measurement of Smoke Obscuration Using a Conical Radiant Source in a Single Closed Chamber*, and their equivalents (ASTM E 662 and ASTM E 1995; see Table S3.1). Dynamic test methods for smoke obscuration are almost invariably associated with the measurement of other fire properties, typically heat release. In fact, every test method mentioned here regarding heat release measurements can be used for assessing smoke obscuration, both on a small scale and on a large scale.

**Smoke Toxicity.** Smoke toxicity is not a critical fire property, since the toxic potency of the smoke from most materials or properties is very similar. Thus, although victims of a fire often die after having been overcome by smoke inhalation, the effect is normally a consequence of the fire having become big (i.e., of having reached a very high heat release rate). Annex A of the *Life Safety Code* does discuss a smoke toxicity test, NFPA 269, *Standard Test Method for Developing Toxic Potency Data for Use in Fire Hazard Modeling*, when considering a fractional effective dose (FED) calculation approach for assessing untenability for a performance evaluation. The FED is evaluated based on concentrations of carbon monoxide, hydrogen cyanide, carbon dioxide, hydrogen chloride, hydrogen bromide, and anoxia effects (low oxygen concentration). It is possible to use the test data, combined with laboratory experience, to estimate the FED value that leads to the survival of virtually all people.

Finally, ASTM E 84 (see the earlier discussion of interior finish and Table S3.1) is used for assessing both flame spread and smoke obscuration. NFPA 258, *Recommended Practice for Determining Smoke Generation of Solid Materials*, has long been the most popular test method for assessing the smoke obscuration tendency of materials or products. It uses a small radiant furnace (at an incident heat flux of 25 kW/$m^2$) with a gas igniter to expose a 3 in. × 3 in. (75 mm × 75 mm) vertical test specimen — in a closed chamber where a vertical light beam impinges on a photocell. Smoke obscuration is assessed by the reduction of light reaching the photocell.

The Technical Committee on Fire Tests decided that the test results of this procedure were being used as a regulatory tool and were incorrectly finding their way into fire modeling applications. As a result, NFPA 258 was first revised to become a recommended practice and then withdrawn. The scope of ASTM E 662 indicates that the measurement of smoke obscuration with this test method should be used as a research and development tool only and should not be used as a basis for determining ratings for building codes or other regulatory purposes. To provide a potential regulatory tool, the committee developed NFPA 270, *Standard Test Method for Measurement of Smoke Obscuration Using a Conical Radiant Source in a Single Closed Chamber*, a test in which smoke obscuration is assessed using a conical radiant source (instead of the original radiant source) on horizontal test specimens at two incident heat fluxes (25 and 50 kW/$m^2$) in the same closed chamber. There remain observations that the measurement of smoke obscuration in small-scale tests is not sufficiently well correlated with the lack of visibility during open burning of the same combustible material in an actual product.

Section D2.3 of NFPA 270 provides some additional information on comparisons of smoke obscuration measurements with different test methods. This section notes that little information exists on the correlation (or lack thereof) between the different test methods that measure smoke obscuration. This is important when evaluating the behavior of a material for input into performance criteria associated with a particular fire modeling scenario or code requirement. In fact, only a few test methods generate smoke obscuration data in units that are suitable for such fire modeling calculations, and even then comparisons of numbers with similar units can be misleading. Sound judgment and experience with additional large-scale testing are usually essential when using the smoke obscuration values developed from any small-scale smoke obscuration test for particular real-life applications.

In fact, it is important that the results of any test

procedure — especially from those that use a small sample for testing — are used with caution in their final application. Tests that use only a small test specimen exposed to a controlled energy source are not likely to truly reflect the end use and the open burning characteristics exhibited by a product.

## TESTING LABORATORIES

It is not the intent of the *Life Safety Code* to require the use of any specific testing laboratory. The *Code* leaves the evaluation of laboratories to the authority having jurisdiction. The *Code* provides the minimum standards that dictate the testing methods, and leaves the decision of who will perform this testing procedure and the details of how it will be performed to the appropriate responsible individuals. NFPA does not approve, inspect, or certify installations, procedures, materials, or equipment, or approve or evaluate testing laboratories. Obtaining information on testing labs is seldom a simple task. There are a few directories that provide some categories or listings of fire testing labs by the characteristics of what they do and which fire tests they perform.

There are six commercial fire testing laboratories in the United States associated with the North American Fire Testing Laboratories Consortium (NAFTL). The purpose of the NAFTL Consortium is to provide a forum for the exchange of technical information, conduct studies, and develop industry consensus positions relating to the full range of fire tests (i.e., reaction to fire, fire suppression, fire resistance and fire detection). Membership in NAFTL is open to any accredited North American-based, independent commercial laboratory engaged in fire testing or research. The labs are, in alphabetical order: FM Approvals (Norwood, MA), Intertek Testing Services (multiple locations), NGC Testing Services (Buffalo, NY), Southwest Research Institute (San Antonio, TX), Underwriters Laboratories (multiple locations), and Western Fire Center (Kelso, WA). There are also other independent testing labs that can perform tests to meet the criteria of the referenced standards in the *Life Safety Code*.

## ADDITIONAL READINGS


*ASTM International Directory of Testing Labs,* ASTM International, 100 Barr Harbor Drive, West Conshohocken, PA 19428-2959. Date of latest edition: 2003.

American Council of Independent Laboratories Inc., 1629 K Street, NW, Suite 400, Washington, DC 20006-1633. http://www.acil.org/.

National Voluntary Laboratory Accreditation Program, National Institute of Standards and Technology, *Directory of Accredited Laboratories,* Standards Services Division, 100 Bureau Drive, Gaithersburg, MD 20899-2140. http://ts.nist.gov/Standards/scopes/programs.htm. Latest edition updated: July 3, 2008.

North American Fire Testing Laboratories Consortium, 1629 K Street, NW, Suite 400, Washington, DC 20006-1633. www.naftl.org.


## REFERENCES (EXCLUDING NFPA, ASTM AND UL FIRE TEST STANDARDS)


1. NFPA 220, *Standard on Types of Building Construction,* 2006 edition, National Fire Protection Association.
2. NFPA 80, *Standard for Fire Doors and Other Opening Protectives,* 2007 edition, National Fire Protection Association.
3. *NFPA 5000®, Building Construction and Safety Code®,* 2009 edition, National Fire Protection Association.
4. NFPA 221, *Standard for High Challenge Fire Walls, Fire Walls, and Fire Barrier Walls,* 2009 edition, National Fire Protection Association.
5. ASTM E 1399, *Standard Test Method for Cyclic Movement and Measuring the Minimum and Maximum Joint Widths of Architectural Joint Systems,* 2005.
6. NFPA 90A, *Standard for the Installation of Air-Conditioning and Ventilating Systems,* 2009 edition, National Fire Protection Association.
7. ISO 834, *Fire-resistance tests — Elements of building construction,* International Organization for Standardization, 1 rue de Varembé, Case postale 56, CH-1211, Geneva 20, Switzerland.
8. UL *Fire Resistance Directory,* 2006.
9. NFPA 914, *Code for Fire Protection of Historic Structures,* 2007 edition, National Fire Protection Association.
10. ISO 9705, *Fire Tests — Full Scale Room Fire Tests for Surface Products* International Organization for Standardization, 1 rue de Varembé, Case postale 56, CH-1211, Geneva 20, Switzerland.
11. NFPA 301, *Code for Safety to Life from Fire on Merchant Vessels,* 2008 edition, National Fire Protection Association.
12. *International Code of Safety for High Speed Craft,* International Maritime Organization 4 Albert Embankment, London, SE1 7SR, United Kingdom, 2000.
13. FM 4880, *Approval Standard for Class 1 Insulated Wall or Wall and Roof/Ceiling Panels; Plastic Interior Finish Materials; Plastic Exterior Building Panels; Wall/Ceiling Coating Systems; Interior or Exterior Finish Systems,* FM Global, Norwood, MA, 2004.

14. 16 CFR 1630, "Standard for the Surface Flammability of Carpets and Rugs" (FF 1-70).
15. 16 CFR, Part 1209, "Interim Safety Standard for Cellulose Insulation."
16. 16 CFR, Part 1404, "Cellulose Insulation."
17. CAN/ULC S102.2, *Standard Method of Test for Surface Burning Characteristics of Floor Coverings and Miscellaneous Materials and Assemblies,* Underwriters Laboratories of Canada, Scarborough, Ontario, Canada.
18. California Technical Bulletin 116, *Cigarette Test of Upholstered Furniture,* California Bureau of Home Furnishings and Thermal Insulation, 3485 Orange Grove Ave., North Highlands, CA, 1980.
19. California Technical Bulletin 117, *Flame and Smoldering Resistance of Furniture Components,* California Bureau of Home Furnishings and Thermal Insulation, 3485 Orange Grove Ave., North Highlands, CA, 2000.
20. California Technical Bulletin 133, *Flammability Test Procedures for Seating Furniture and Use in Public Occupancies,* California Bureau of Home Furnishings and Thermal Insulation, 3485 Orange Grove Ave., North Highlands, CA, 1991.
21. 16 CFR 1632, "Standard for the Flammability of Mattresses and Mattress Pads" (FF 4-72).
22. California Technical Bulletin 129, *Flammability Test Procedures for Mattresses for Use in Public Buildings,* California Bureau of Home Furnishings and Thermal Insulation, 3485 Orange Grove Ave., North Highlands, CA, 1992.
23. ISO 1182, *Reaction to fire tests for building products — Non-combustibility test,* International Organization for Standardization, 1 rue de Varembé, Case postale 56, CH-1211, Geneva 20, Switzerland.
24. NFPA 1, *Fire Code,* 2009 edition, National Fire Protection Association.

### NFPA Fire Test Standards Referenced

The following publications are available from the National Fire Protection Association, 1 Batterymarch Park, Quincy, MA 02169-7471.

NFPA 251, *Standard Methods of Tests of Fire Resistance of Building Construction and Materials,* 2006 edition.

NFPA 252, *Standard Methods of Fire Tests of Door Assemblies,* 2008 edition.

NFPA 253, *Standard Method of Test for Critical Radiant Flux of Floor Covering Systems Using a Radiant Heat Energy Source,* 2006 edition.

NFPA 255, *Standard Method of Test of Surface Burning Characteristics of Building Materials,* 2006 edition.

NFPA 256, *Standard Methods of Fire Tests of Roof Coverings,* withdrawn, last edition 2003.

NFPA 257, *Standard on Fire Test for Window and Glass Block Assemblies,* 2007 edition.

NFPA 258, *Recommended Practice for Determining Smoke Generation of Solid Materials,* withdrawn, last edition 2003.

NFPA 259, *Standard Test Method for Potential Heat of Building Materials,* 2008 edition.

NFPA 260, *Standard Methods of Tests and Classification System for Cigarette Ignition Resistance of Components of Upholstered Furniture,* 2009 edition.

NFPA 261, *Standard Method of Test for Determining Resistance of Mock-Up Upholstered Furniture Material Assemblies to Ignition by Smoldering Cigarettes,* 2009 edition.

NFPA 262, *Standard Method of Test for Flame Travel and Smoke of Wires and Cables for Use in Air-Handling Spaces,* 2007 edition.

NFPA 263, *Standard Method of Test for Heat and Visible Smoke Release Rates for Materials and Products,* withdrawn, last edition 1995.

NFPA 265, *Standard Methods of Fire Tests for Evaluating Room Fire Growth Contribution of Textile Coverings on Full Height Panels and Walls,* 2007 edition.

NFPA 266, *Standard Method of Test for Fire Characteristics of Upholstered Furniture Exposed to Flaming Ignition Source,* withdrawn, last edition 1999.

NFPA 267, *Standard Method of Test for Fire Characteristics of Mattresses and Bedding Assemblies Exposed to Flaming Ignition Source,* withdrawn, last edition 2000.

NFPA 268, *Standard Test Method for Determining Ignitability of Exterior Wall Assemblies Using a Radiant Heat Energy Source,* 2007 edition.

NFPA 269, *Standard Test Method for Developing Toxic Potency Data for Use in Fire Hazard Modeling,* 2007 edition.

NFPA 270, *Standard Test Method for Measurement of Smoke Obscuration Using a Conical Radiant Source in a Single Closed Chamber,* 2008 edition.

NFPA 271, *Standard Method of Test for Heat and Visible Smoke Release Rates for Materials and Products Using an Oxygen Consumption Calorimeter,* 2004 edition.

NFPA 272, *Standard Method of Test for Heat and Visible Smoke Release Rates for Upholstered Furniture Components or Composites and Mattresses Using an*

*Oxygen Consumption Calorimeter*, withdrawn, last edition 2004.

NFPA 274, *Standard Test Method to Evaluate Fire Performance Characteristics of Pipe Insulation*, 2009 edition.

NFPA 275, *Standard Method of Fire Tests for the Evaluation of Thermal Barriers Used Over Foam Plastic Insulation*, 2009 edition.

NFPA 285, *Standard Fire Test Method for Evaluation of Fire Propagation Characteristics of Exterior Non-Load-Bearing Wall Assemblies Containing Combustible Components*, 2006 edition.

NFPA 286, *Standard Methods of Fire Tests for Evaluating Contribution of Wall and Ceiling Interior Finish to Room Fire Growth*, 2006 edition.

NFPA 287, *Standard Test Methods for Measurement of Flammability of Materials in Cleanrooms Using a Fire Propagation Apparatus (FPA)*, 2007 edition.

NFPA 288, *Standard Methods of Fire Tests of Floor Fire Door Assemblies Installed Horizontally in Fire Resistance–Rated Floor Systems*, 2007 edition.

NFPA 289, *Standard Method of Fire Test for Individual Fuel Packages*, 2009 edition.

NFPA 290, *Standard for Fire Testing of Passive Protection Materials for Use on LP-Gas Containers*, 2009 edition.

NFPA 701, *Standard Methods of Fire Tests for Flame Propagation of Textiles and Films*, 2004 edition.

NFPA 703, *Standard for Fire Retardant–Treated Wood and Fire-Retardant Coatings for Building Materials*, 2009 edition.

NFPA 705, *Recommended Practice for a Field Flame Test for Textiles and Films*, 2009 edition.


### ASTM Fire Test Standards Referenced

The following publications are available from ASTM International, 100 Bar Harbor Drive, P.O. Box C700, West Conshohocken, PA, 19428-2959.


ASTM D 1929, *Standard Test Method for Determining Ignition Temperature of Plastics*, 2001.

ASTM D 2859, *Standard Test Method for Flammability of Finished Textile Floor Covering Materials*, 2006.

ASTM D 2863, *Standard Test Method for Measuring the Minimum Oxygen Concentration to Support Candle-Like Combustion of Plastics (Oxygen Index)*, 2006a.

ASTM E 84, *Standard Test Method for Surface Burning Characteristics of Building Materials*, 2008a.

ASTM E 108, *Standard Test Methods for Fire Tests of Roof Coverings*, 2007a.

ASTM E 119, *Standard Test Methods for Fire Tests of Building Construction and Materials*, 2008a.

ASTM E 136, *Standard Test Method for Behavior of Materials in a Vertical Tube Furnace at 750°C*, 2004.

ASTM E 162, *Standard Test Method for Surface Flammability of Materials Using a Radiant Heat Energy Source*, 2008.

ASTM E 648, *Standard Test Method for Critical Radiant Flux of Floor-Covering Systems Using a Radiant Heat Energy Source*, 2008.

ASTM E 662, *Standard Test Method for Specific Optical Density of Smoke Generated by Solid Materials*, 2006.

ASTM E 814, *Standard Test Method for Fire Tests of Through-Penetration Fire Stops*, 2008.

ASTM E 906, *Standard Test Method for Heat and Visible Smoke Release Rates for Materials and Products*, 2007.

ASTM E 970, *Standard Test Method for Critical Radiant Flux of Exposed Attic Floor Insulation Using a Radiant Heat Energy Source*, 2007.

ASTM E 1352, *Standard Test Method for Cigarette Ignition Resistance of Mock-Upholstered Furniture Assemblies*, 2008a.

ASTM E 1353, *Standard Test Methods for Cigarette Ignition Resistance of Components of Upholstered Furniture*, 2008a.

ASTM E 1354, *Standard Test Method for Heat and Visible Smoke Release Rates for Materials and Products Using an Oxygen Consumption Calorimeter*, 2008.

ASTM E 1474, *Standard Test Method for Determining the Heat Release Rate of Upholstered Furniture and Mattress Components or Composites Using a Bench Scale Oxygen Consumption Calorimeter*, 2007.

ASTM E 1529, *Standard Test Methods for Determining Effects of Large Hydrocarbon Pool Fires on Structural Members and Assemblies*, 2006.

ASTM E 1537, *Standard Test Method for Fire Testing of Upholstered Furniture*, 2007.

ASTM E 1590, *Standard Test Method for Fire Testing of Mattresses*, 2007.

ASTM E 1623, *Standard Test Method for Determination of Fire and Thermal Parameters of Materials, Products, and Systems Using an Intermediate Scale Calorimeter (ICAL)*, 2004.

ASTM E 1678, *Standard Test Method for Measuring Smoke Toxicity for Use in Fire Hazard Analysis*, 2007.

ASTM E 1822, *Standard Test Method for Fire Testing of Stacked Chairs*, 2007.

ASTM E 1966, *Standard Test Method for Fire-Resistive Joint Systems*, 2007.

ASTM E 1995, *Standard Test Method for Measurement of Smoke Obscuration Using a Conical Radiant Source in a Single Closed Chamber, With the Test Specimen Oriented Horizontally*, 2008.

ASTM E 2010, *Standard Test Method for Positive Pressure Fire Tests of Window Assemblies*, withdrawn, last edition 2001.

ASTM E 2032, *Standard Guide for Extension of Data from Fire Resistance Tests Conducted in Accordance with ASTM E 119*, 2008.

ASTM E 2058, *Standard Test Methods for Measurement of Synthetic Polymer Material Flammability Using a Fire Propagation Apparatus (FPA)*, 2006.

ASTM E 2074, *Standard Test Method for Positive Pressure Fire Tests of Window Assemblies*, withdrawn, last edition 2000.

ASTM E 2231, *Standard Practice for Specimen Preparation and Mounting of Pipe and Duct Insulation Materials to Assess Surface Burning Characteristics*, 2007a.

ASTM E 2257, *Standard Test Method for Room Fire Test of Wall and Ceiling Materials and Assemblies*, 2008.

ASTM E 2404, *Standard Practice for Specimen Preparation and Mounting of Textile, Paper or Vinyl Wall or Ceiling Coverings to Assess Surface Burning Characteristics*, 2007a.

ASTM E 2573, *Standard Practice for Specimen Preparation and Mounting of Site-Fabricated Stretch Systems to Assess Surface Burning Characteristics*, 2007a.

ASTM E 2579, *Standard Practice for Specimen Preparation and Mounting of Wood Products to Assess Surface Burning Characteristics*, 2007.

ASTM E XXXX, *Standard Practice for Specimen Preparation and Mounting of Reflective Insulation and Sheet Radiant Barriers for Building Applications.*

## UL Fire Test Standards Referenced

The following publications are available from Underwriters Laboratories Inc., 333 Pfingsten Road, Northbrook, IL 60062-2096.

UL 9, *Standard for Fire Tests of Window Assemblies*, revised 2005.

UL 10B, *Standard for Fire Tests of Door Assemblies*, 2008.

UL 214, *Standard for Safety Tests for Flame-Propagation of Fabrics and Films*, withdrawn.

UL 263, *Standard for Fire Tests of Building Construction and Materials*, 2003.

UL 555, *Standard for Fire Dampers*, 2006.

UL 555C, *Standard for Ceiling Dampers*, 2006.

UL 555S, *Standard for Leakage Rated Dampers for Use in Smoke Control Systems*, revised 2006.

UL 723, *Standard for Test for Surface Burning Characteristics of Building Materials*, 2003.

UL 790, *Standard for Standard Test Methods for Fire Tests of Roof Coverings*, 2004.

UL 910, *Standard for Safety Test for Flame-Propagation and Smoke-Density Values for Electrical and Optical-Fiber Cables Used in Spaces Transporting Environmental Air*, withdrawn.

UL 1040, *Standard for Fire Test of Insulated Wall Construction*, revised 2001.

UL 1479, *Standard for Fire Tests of Through-Penetration Firestops*, 2003.

UL 1056, *Standard for Safety Fire Test of Upholstered Furniture*, withdrawn.

UL 1715, *Standard for Fire Test of Interior Finish Material*, 1997.

UL 1895, *Standard for Safety Fire Test of Mattresses*, withdrawn.

UL 1975, *Standard for Fire Tests for Foamed Plastics Used for Decorative Purposes*, 2006.

UL 2079, *Standard for Tests for Fire Resistance of Building Joint Systems*, 2004.

SUPPLEMENT 4

# Technical/Substantive Changes 2006–2009 Editions

| Subject / 2009 Edition Text | Notes |
|---|---|
| **Chapter 1 Administration** | No changes |
| **Chapter 2 Referenced Publications** | Edition date for numerous references updated |
| **2.2 NFPA Publications.** National Fire Protection Association, 1 Batterymarch Park, Quincy, MA 02169-7471.<br>NFPA 170, *Standard for Fire Safety and Emergency Symbols*, 2006 edition. | New reference, see 7.10.3.2 |
| **2.3.6 ASTM Publications.** ASTM International, 100 Barr Harbor Drive, P.O. Box C700, West Conshohocken, PA 19428-2959. www.astm.org. | |
| ASTM E 648, *Standard Test Method for Critical Radiant Flux of Floor Covering Systems Using a Radiant Heat Energy Source*, 2006. | New reference, see 10.2.7.3 |
| ASTM E 2073, *Standard Test Method for Photopic Luminance of Photoluminescent (Phosphorescent) Markings*, 2007. | New reference, see 7.2.2.5.5.10 |
| **2.3.8 UL Publications.** Underwriters Laboratories Inc., 333 Pfingsten Road, Northbrook, IL 60062-2096. www.ul.com | |
| UL 294, *Standard for Access Control System Units*, 2004. | New reference, see 7.2.1.6.3(1) |
| **2.3.10 Other Publication.**<br>*Webster's Third New International Dictionary of the English Language, Unabridged*, Merriam-Webster, Inc., Springfield, MA, 2002. | Replaces previous dictionary cited |
| **Chapter 3 Definitions** | |
| **3.3.3 Accessible Route.** A continuous unobstructed path that complies with this *Code* and ICC/ANSI A117.1, *American National Standard for Accessible and Usable Buildings and Facilities*. | New definition for term used in 7.5.4 |
| **(3.3.19 Area)**<br>**3.3.19.6** ***Occupiable Area.*** An area of a facility occupied by people on a regular basis. | New definition for term used in various locations, for example: 9.6.2.9 and 28.3.4.3.4 |
| **(3.3.21 Assembly)**<br>**3.3.21.1** ***Door Assembly.*** Any combination of a door, frame, hardware, and other accessories that is placed in an opening in a wall that is intended primarily for access or for human entrance or exit. [**252,** 2008] | New definition for term used throughout 7.2.1 |
| **3.3.25* Attic.** The space located between the ceiling of a story and the roof directly above that habitable story. | New definition for term used various locations, for example: 8.6.10.1(2) |
| **3.3.28 Basement.** Any story of a building wholly or partly below grade plane that is not considered the first story above grade plane. *(See also 3.3.115.1, First Story Above Grade Plane.)* | New definition for term used in definition of first story above grade plane |

| Subject / 2009 Edition Text | Notes |
|---|---|
| **3.3.65 Elevator Lobby.** A landing from which occupants directly enter an elevator car(s) and into which occupants directly enter upon leaving an elevator car(s). | New definition for term used in 7.2.1.6.3 |
| **(3.3.77 Exit Discharge)**<br>**3.3.77.1*** ***Level of Exit Discharge.*** The story that is either (1) the lowest story from which not less than 50 percent of the required number of exits and not less than 50 percent of the required egress capacity from such a story discharge directly outside at the finished ground level; or (2) where no story meets the conditions of item (1), the story that is provided with one or more exits that discharge directly to the outside to the finished ground level via the smallest elevation change. | Definition revised to reference finished ground level |
| **3.3.85 Finished Ground Level (Grade).** The level of the finished ground (earth or other surface on ground). *(See also 3.3.115, Grade Plane.)* | New definition for term used in definition of level of exit discharge |
| **3.3.115 Grade Plane.** A reference plane representing the average of the finished ground level adjoining the building at all exterior walls. When the finished ground level slopes down from the exterior walls, the grade plane is established by the lowest points within the area between the building and the lot line or, when the lot line is more than 6 ft (1830 mm) from the building, between the building and a point 6 ft (1830 mm) from the building. | New definition associated with terms finished ground level (grade) and first story above grade plane |
| **3.3.115.1** ***First Story Above Grade Plane.*** Any story having its finished floor surface entirely above grade plane, except that a basement is to be considered as a first story above grade plane where the finished surface of the floor above the basement is (1) more than 6 ft (1830 mm) above grade plane or (2) more than 12 ft (3660 mm) above the finished ground level at any point. | New definition associated with terms finished ground level (grade) and grade plane |
| **3.3.155 Lock-Up.** An incidental use area in other than a detention and correctional occupancy where occupants are restrained and such occupants are mostly incapable of self preservation because of security measures not under the occupants' control. | Definition revised to include words "incidental use" |
| **3.3.157 Major Tenant.** A tenant space, in a mall building, with one or more main entrances from the exterior that also serve as exits and are independent of the mall. | New definition for term used in 36/37.4.4.3.6 |
| **(3.3.178 Occupancy)**<br>**3.3.178.7*** ***Health Care Occupancy.*** An occupancy used to provide medical or other treatment or care simultaneously to four or more patients on an inpatient basis, where such patients are mostly incapable of self-preservation due to age, physical or mental disability, or because of security measures not under the occupants' control. | Definition revised to apply only to inpatient form of health care – see 3.3.178.1 for outpatient form of health care |
| **(3.3.178 Occupancy)**<br>**3.3.178.15*** ***Storage Occupancy.*** An occupancy used primarily for the storage or sheltering of goods, merchandise, products, or vehicles. | Definition revised to delete reference to animals |
| **3.3.207* Reconstruction.** The reconfiguration of a space that affects an exit or a corridor shared by more than one occupant space; or the reconfiguration of a space such that the rehabilitation work area is not permitted to be occupied because existing means of egress and fire protection systems, or their equivalent, are not in place or continuously maintained. | Definition revised "shared by more than a single tenant" to "shared by more than one occupant space" |
| **3.3.230* Situation Awareness.** The perception of the elements in the environment within a volume of time and space, the comprehension of their meaning, and the projection of their status in the near future. | New definition for term used in 4.5.5 |
| **3.3.239* Smokeproof Enclosure.** An enclosure designed to limit the movement of products of combustion produced by a fire. | Definition revised to include components in addition to stairs |
| **3.3.250* Stories in Height.** The story count starting with the level of exit discharge and ending with the highest occupiable story containing the occupancy considered. | New definition for term used in 4.6.3 |
| **(3.3.262 Tower)**<br>**3.3.262.1** ***Air Traffic Control Tower.*** An enclosed structure or building at airports with elevated levels for support of equipment and occupied for observation, control, operation, and signaling of aircraft in flight and on the ground. | New definition for term used 11.3.4 |

| Subject / 2009 Edition Text | Notes |
|---|---|
| **Chapter 4 General** | |
| **4.1.1* Fire.** A goal of this *Code* is to provide an environment for the occupants that is reasonably safe from fire by the following means:<br>(1)*Protection of occupants not intimate with the initial fire development<br>(2) Improvement of the survivability of occupants intimate with the initial fire development<br>**4.1.2* Comparable Emergencies.** An additional goal is to provide life safety during emergencies that can be mitigated using methods comparable to those used in case of fire. | 4.1.1 revised to delete "similar emergencies" and 4.1.2 added to address "comparable emergencies" |
| **4.3.1* General.** The protection methods of this *Code* are based on the hazards associated with fire and other events that have comparable impact on a building and its occupancy.<br>**4.3.2 Single Fire Source.** The fire protection methods of this *Code* assume a single fire source. | 4.3.1 is new provision<br>4.3.2 reformatted existing text |
| **4.5.5* Situation Awareness.** Systems used to achieve the goals of Section 4.1 shall be effective in facilitating and enhancing situation awareness, as appropriate, by building management, other occupants and emergency responders of the functionality or state of critical building systems, the conditions that might warrant emergency response, and the appropriate nature and timing of such responses. | New provision |
| **4.6.3 Stories in Height.** Unless otherwise specified in another provision of this *Code*, the stories in height of a building for locating an occupancy shall be determined as follows:<br>(1) The stories in height shall be counted starting with the level of exit discharge and ending with the highest occupiable story containing the occupancy considered.<br>(2) Stories below the level of exit discharge shall not be counted as stories.<br>(3) Interstitial spaces used solely for building or process systems directly related to the level above or below shall not be considered a separate story.<br>(4) A mezzanine shall not be counted as a story for the purpose of determining the allowable stories in height.<br>(5) Where a maximum one-story above grade parking structure, enclosed, open, or a combination thereof, of Type I or Type II (222) construction or open Type IV construction, with grade entrance, is provided under a building of occupancies other than assembly, health care, detention and correctional, and ambulatory health care occupancies, the number of stories shall be permitted to be measured from the floor above such a parking area. | New subsection with application to the construction type limitations tables in the __1.6 subsection of various occupancy chapters |
| **4.8.2.1*** Emergency plans shall include the following:<br>. . .<br>(3)* Evacuation procedures appropriate to the building, its occupancy, and emergencies *(see Section 4.3)*<br>(4) Appropriateness of the use of elevators<br>. . . | Items (3) and (4) are new |
| **Chapter 5 Performance-Based Option** | |
| **5.4.2.1** Each assumption and design specification used in the design shall be accurately translated into input data specifications, as appropriate for the method or model. | Revised to replace "calculation method" with "method" |
| **5.4.4* Operational Status and Effectiveness of Building Features and Systems.** The performance of fire protection systems, building features, and emergency procedures shall reflect the documented performance and reliability of the components of those systems or features, unless design specifications are incorporated to modify the expected performance. | Revised to add "emergency procedures" |
| **Chapter 6** | |
| [former] ~~**6.1.2.2. Small Assembly Uses . . .**~~ | Text on small assembly uses moved to Annex A as there is no occupancy classification of small assembly |
| **6.1.5.1* Definition — Health Care Occupancy.** An occupancy used to provide medical or other treatment or care simultaneously to four or more patients on an inpatient basis, where | Definition revised to apply only to inpatient form of health care — see |

| Subject / 2009 Edition Text | Notes |
|---|---|
| such patients are mostly incapable of self-preservation due to age, physical or mental disability, or because of security measures not under the occupants' control. | 3.3.178.1 for outpatient form of health care |
| **6.1.13.1* Definition — Storage Occupancy.** An occupancy used primarily for the storage or sheltering of goods, merchandise, products, or vehicles. | Definition revised to delete reference to animals |
| **Chapter 7 Means of Egress**<br>**7.1.3.2.1** Where this *Code* requires an exit to be separated from other parts of the building, the separating construction shall meet the requirements of Section 8.2 and the following:<br>. . .<br>(5)* Structural elements, or portions thereof, that support exit components and either penetrate into a fire resistance–rated assembly or are installed within a fire resistance–rated wall assembly shall be protected, as a minimum to the fire resistance rating required by 7.1.3.2.1(1) or (2).<br>. . .<br>(9) Penetrations into, and openings through, an exit enclosure assembly shall be limited to the following:<br>(a) . . .<br>(b)* Electrical conduit serving the exit enclosure<br>. . . | Item (5) is new<br><br>Item (9)(b) revised "stairway" to "exit enclosure" |
| **7.1.5.1** Means of egress shall be designed and maintained to provide headroom in accordance with other sections of this *Code*, and such headroom shall be not less than 7 ft 6 in. (2285 mm), with projections from the ceiling not less than 6 ft 8 in. (2030 mm) with a tolerance of $-\frac{3}{4}$ in. ($-19$ mm), above the finished floor, unless otherwise specified by the following:<br>(1) . . .<br>(2) . . . | Revised to include tolerance of $-\frac{3}{4}$ in. ($-19$ mm) |
| **7.2.1.1.3.2** Where means of egress doors are locked in a building that is not considered occupied, occupants shall not be locked beyond their control in buildings or building spaces, except for lockups in accordance with 22.4.5 and 23.4.5, detention and correctional occupancies, and health care occupancies. | Text moved from advisory annex provision to a mandatory requirement |
| **7.2.1.2 Door Leaf Width.**<br>. . .<br>**7.2.1.2.3.2** | Provisions of 7.2.1.2 through 7.2.1.2.3.2 are a reformatting/repositioning of former 7.2.1.2 through 7.2.1.2.4, and includes changing "door" to "door assembly," "door leaf," and "door opening," as appropriate, with no technical change |
| **7.2.1.4.1* Swinging-Type Door Assembly Requirement.** Any door assembly in a means of egress shall be of the side-hinged or pivoted-swinging type, and shall be installed to be capable of swinging from any position to the full required width of the opening in which it is installed, unless otherwise specified as follows:<br>. . .<br>(4) Horizontal-sliding door assemblies shall be permitted under any of the following conditions:<br>(a) . . .<br>(b) . . .<br>(c) Unless prohibited by Chapters 11 through 43, horizontal-sliding door assemblies serving a room or area with an occupant load of fewer than 10 shall be permitted, provided that all of the following criteria are met:<br>i. The area served by the door assembly has no high hazard contents.<br>ii. The door assembly is readily operable from either side without special knowledge or effort. | Item (c) is new and is modeled after a similar provision added in 2006 to the health care occupancies chapters |

| **Subject / 2009 Edition Text** | **Notes** |
|---|---|
| iii. The force required to operate the door assembly in the direction of door leaf travel is not more than 30 lbf (133 N) to set the door leaf in motion and is not more than 15 lbf (67 N) to close the door assembly or open it to the minimum required width.<br>iv. The door assembly complies with any required fire protection rating, and, where rated, is self-closing or automatic-closing by means of smoke detection in accordance with 7.2.1.8 and is installed in accordance with NFPA 80, *Standard for Fire Doors and Other Opening Protectives*.<br>v. Corridor door assemblies required to be self-latching shall have a latch or other mechanism that ensures that the door leaf will not rebound into a partially open position if forcefully closed. | |
| **7.2.1.4.3.2** Surface-mounted latch release hardware on the door leaf shall be exempt from being included in the maximum 7 in. (180 mm) projection requirement of 7.2.1.4.3.1, provided that both of the following criteria are met:<br>(1) The hardware is mounted to the side of the door leaf that faces the aisle, corridor, passageway, or landing when the door leaf is in the open position.<br>(2) The hardware is mounted not less than 34 in. (865 mm), and not more than 48 in. (1220 mm), above the floor. | New provision |
| **7.2.1.5.5 Electrically Controlled Egress Door Assemblies.** Door assemblies in the means of egress shall be permitted to be electrically locked if equipped with approved, listed hardware that incorporates a built-in switch, provided that the following conditions are met:<br>(1) The hardware for occupant release of the lock is affixed to the door leaf.<br>(2) The hardware has an obvious method of operation that is readily operated in the direction of egress.<br>(3) The hardware is capable of being operated with one hand in the direction of egress.<br>(4) Operation of the hardware interrupts the power supply directly to the electric lock and unlocks the door assembly in the direction of egress.<br>(5) Loss of power to the hardware automatically unlocks the door assembly in the direction of egress. | New provision |
| **7.2.1.5.7.2** The requirements of 7.2.1.5.7, except as provided in 7.2.1.5.7.3, shall not apply to the following:<br>(1) . . .<br>(2) Existing installations in high-rise buildings as permitted in Chapters 11 through 43 where the occupancy is within a building protected throughout by an approved, supervised automatic sprinkler system in accordance with 9.7.1<br>(3) Existing approved stairwell re-entry installations as permitted by Chapters 11 through 43<br>(4) . . .<br>(5) . . . | Items (2) and (3) are new |
| **7.2.1.5.7.3** When the provisions of 7.2.1.5.7.2 are used, signage on the stair door leaves shall be required as follows;<br>(1) Door assemblies allowing re-entry shall be identified as such on the stair side of the door leaf.<br>(2) Door assemblies not allowing re-entry shall be provided with a sign on the stair side indicating the location of the nearest door opening, in each direction of travel, that allows re-entry or exit. | New provision |
| **7.2.1.6.3 Elevator Lobby Exit Access Door Assemblies Locking.** Where permitted in Chapters 11 through 43, door assemblies separating the elevator lobby from the exit access required by 7.4.1.6.1 shall be permitted to be electronically locked, provided that all the following criteria are met:<br>(1) The electronic switch for releasing the lock is listed in accordance with UL 294, *Standard for Access Control System Units*<br>(2) The building is protected throughout by a fire alarm system in accordance with Section 9.6. | New Provision |

| Subject / 2009 Edition Text | Notes |
|---|---|
| (3) The building is protected throughout by an approved, supervised automatic sprinkler system in accordance with Section 9.7.<br>(4) Waterflow in the sprinkler system required by 7.2.1.6.3(3) is arranged to initiate the building fire alarm system.<br>(5) The elevator lobby is protected by an approved, supervised smoke detection system in accordance with Section 9.6.<br>(6) Detection of smoke by the detection system required by 7.2.1.6.3(5) is arranged to initiate the building fire alarm system.<br>(7) Initiation of the building fire alarm system by other than manual fire alarm boxes unlocks the elevator lobby door assembly.<br>(8) Loss of power to the elevator lobby electronic lock system unlocks the elevator lobby door assemblies.<br>(9) The elevator lobby electronic lock system is not supplied with emergency or standby electrical power.<br>(10) Once unlocked, the elevator lobby door assemblies remain unlocked until the building fire alarm system has been manually reset.<br>(11) Where the elevator lobby door assemblies remain latched after being unlocked, latch-releasing hardware in accordance with 7.2.1.5.9 is affixed to the door leaves.<br>(12) A two-way communication system is provided for communication between the elevator lobby and a central control point that is constantly staffed.<br>(13) The central control point staff required by 7.2.1.6.3(12) is capable, trained, and authorized to provide emergency assistance.<br>(14) The provisions of 7.2.1.6.1 for delayed-egress locking systems are not applied to the elevator lobby door assemblies.<br>(15)*The provisions of 7.2.1.6.2 for access-controlled egress door assemblies are not applied to the elevator lobby door assemblies. | |
| **7.2.1.9.2 Self-Closing or Self-Latching Door Leaf Operation.** Where door leaves are required to be self-closing or self-latching and are operated by power upon the approach of a person, or are provided with power-assisted manual operation, they shall be permitted in the means of egress where they meet the following criteria: | Provision expanded to have application to doors that are self-latching, not only to doors that are self-closing |
| **7.2.1.15 Inspection of Door Openings.**<br>**7.2.1.15.1** Where required by Chapters 11 through 43, door assemblies for which the door leaf is required to swing in the direction of egress travel shall be inspected and tested not less than annually in accordance with 7.2.1.15.2 through 7.2.1.15.8.<br>**7.2.1.15.2** Fire-rated door assemblies shall be inspected and tested in accordance with NFPA 80, *Standard for Fire Doors and Other Opening Protectives*.<br>**7.2.1.15.3** The inspection and testing interval for fire-rated and nonrated door assemblies shall be permitted to exceed 12 months under a written performance-based program in accordance with 5.2.2 of NFPA 80, *Standard for Fire Doors and Other Opening Protectives*.<br>**7.2.1.15.4** A written record of the inspections and testing shall be signed and kept for inspection by the authority having jurisdiction.<br>**7.2.1.15.5** Functional testing of door assemblies shall be performed by individuals who can demonstrate knowledge and understanding of the operating components of the type of door being subjected to testing.<br>**7.2.1.15.6** Door assemblies shall be visually inspected from both sides of the opening to assess the overall condition of the assembly.<br>**7.2.1.15.7** As a minimum, the following items shall be verified:<br>(1) Floor space on both sides of the openings is clear of obstructions, and door leaves open fully and close freely.<br>(2) Forces required to set door leaves in motion and move to the fully open position do not exceed the requirements in 7.2.1.4.5.<br>(3) Latching and locking devices comply with 7.2.1.5.<br>(4) Releasing hardware devices are installed in accordance with 7.2.1.5.9.1.<br>(5) Door leaves of paired openings are installed in accordance with 7.2.1.5.10.<br>(6) Door closers are adjusted properly to control the closing speed of door leaves in accordance with accessibility requirements. | New provision |

| Subject / 2009 Edition Text | Notes |
|---|---|
| (7) Projection of door leaves into the path of egress does not exceed the encroachment permitted by 7.2.1.4.3.<br>(8) Powered door openings operate in accordance with 7.2.1.9.<br>(9) Signage required by 7.2.1.4.1(3), 7.2.1.5.4, 7.2.1.6, and 7.2.1.9 is intact and legible.<br>(10) Door openings with special locking arrangements function in accordance with 7.2.1.6<br>(11) Security devices that impede egress are not installed on openings, as required by 7.2.1.5.11.<br>**7.2.1.15.8** Door openings not in proper operating condition shall be repaired or replaced without delay. | |
| **7.2.2.2.1.2 Minimum New Stair Width.**<br>. . .<br>**(F)** The clear width of door openings discharging from stairways required to be a minimum of 56 in. (1420 mm) wide in accordance with 7.2.2.2.1.2(B) shall be in accordance with 7.2.1.2.3.2(9). | Item (F) reworded for clarity without technical change |
| **7.2.2.3.2.5** In existing buildings, a door assembly at the top of a stair shall be permitted to open directly to the stair, provided that the door leaf does not swing over the stair and the door opening serves an area with an occupant load of fewer than 50 persons. | Provision revised to delete application to dwellings |
| **7.2.2.3.3.4** The requirement of 7.2.2.3.3.1 shall not apply to noncombustible grated stair treads and landings in the following occupancies:<br>. . .<br>(4) Storage occupancies as otherwise provided in Chapter 42 | Item (4) is new for completeness but is not a technical change |
| **7.2.2.3.6.3** Where the bottom or top riser adjoins a sloping public way, walk, or driveway having an established finished ground level and serves as a landing, the bottom or top riser shall be permitted to have a variation in height of not more than 1 in. in every 12 in. (25 mm in every 305 mm) of stairway width. | Provision revised to add "or top" in two places |
| **7.2.2.3.6.4*** All tread nosings of stairs utilizing the provision of 7.2.2.3.6.3 shall be marked in accordance with 7.2.2.5.4.3. Those portions of the marking stripe at locations where the riser height below the nosing is inconsistent by more than $^{3}/_{16}$ in. (4.8 mm), relative to other risers in the stair flight, shall be distinctively colored or patterned, incorporating safety yellow, to warn descending users of the inconsistent geometry relative to other steps in the flight. | New provision |
| **7.2.2.4.1.2** In addition to the handrails required at the sides of stairs by 7.2.2.4.1.1, the following provisions shall apply:<br>(1) For new stairs, handrails shall be provided within 30 in. (760 mm) of all portions of the required egress width.<br>(2) For existing stairs, handrails shall meet the following criteria:<br>(a) They shall be provided within 44 in. (1120 mm) of all portions of the required egress width.<br>(b) Such stairs shall not have their egress capacity adjusted to a higher occupant load than permitted by the capacity factor in Table 7.3.3.1 if the stair's clear width between handrails exceeds 60 in. (1525 mm). | Item (1) revised as it formerly had application only where stair width exceeded 6 ft 3 in. (1905 mm)<br><br>Item (2)(b) is new |
| **7.2.2.5.4* Stairway Identification.**<br>**7.2.2.5.4.1** New enclosed stairs serving three or more stories and existing enclosed stairs serving five or more stories shall comply with 7.2.2.5.4.1(A) through (M).<br>. . .<br>**(K)*** Signage that reads NO ROOF ACCESS and is located under the stairway identification letter shall designate stairways that do not provide roof access. Lettering shall be a minimum of 1 in. (25 mm) high and shall be in accordance with 7.10.8.2. | Item (K) revised so that a sign is required only if stairway does not provide roof access |

| Subject / 2009 Edition Text | Notes |
|---|---|
| **7.2.2.5.4.4*** Where new contrast marking is provided for stairway handrails, it shall be applied to, or be part of, at least the upper surface of the handrail; have a minimum width of $^1/_2$ in. (13 mm); and extend the full length of each handrail. After marking, the handrail shall comply with 7.2.2.4.4.<br>[former] ~~7.2.2.5.4.8* Where new contrasting marking is applied to stairs, such marking shall comply with the following:~~<br>~~(1) The marking shall include a continuous strip as a coating on, or as a material integral with, the full width of the leading edge of each tread.~~<br>~~(2) The marking shall include a continuous strip as a coating on, or as a material integral with, the full width of the leading edge of each landing nosing.~~<br>~~(3) The marking strip width, measured horizontally from the leading vertical edge of the nosing, shall be consistent at all nosings.~~<br>~~(4) The marking strip width shall be 1 in. to 2 in. (25 mm to 51 mm).~~ | Provision replaces 7.2.2.5.4.8 |
| **7.2.2.5.5 Exit Stair Path Markings.**<br>. . .<br>**7.2.2.5.5.1 Exit Stair Treads.**<br>. . .<br>**7.2.2.5.5.2 Exit Stair Landings.**<br>. . .<br>**7.2.2.5.5.3 Exit Stair Handrails.**<br>. . .<br>**7.2.2.5.5.4 Perimeter Demarcation Marking.**<br>. . .<br>**7.2.2.5.5.5* Obstacles.**<br>. . .<br>**7.2.2.5.5.6 Doors Serving Exit Enclosure.**<br>. . .<br>**7.2.2.5.5.7 Door Hardware Marking.**<br>. . .<br>**7.2.2.5.5.8 Emergency Exit Symbol.**<br>. . .<br>**7.2.2.5.5.9 Uniformity.**<br>. . .<br>**7.2.2.5.5.10 Materials.**<br>. . .<br>**7.2.2.5.5.11 Exit Stair Illumination.**<br>. . . | New provisions |
| **7.2.2.6.2* Visual Protection.** Outside stairs shall be arranged to avoid any impediments to their use by persons having a fear of high places. Outside stairs more than 36 ft (11 m) above the finished ground level, other than previously approved existing stairs, shall be provided with an opaque visual obstruction not less than 48. in. (1220 mm) in height. | Provision revised from "more than 3 stories" to "more than 36 ft (11 m) above the finished ground level" |
| **7.2.2.6.4 Protection of Openings.** All openings below an outside stair shall be protected with an assembly having a minimum $^3/_4$-hour fire protection rating as follows:<br>(1) Where located in an enclosed court *(see 3.3.46.1)*, the smallest dimension of which does not exceed one-third its height<br>(2) . . . | Item (1) revised to have application to enclosed courts, not to any court |
| **7.2.3.7 Natural Ventilation.** Smokeproof enclosures using natural ventilation shall comply with 7.2.3.3 and the following:<br>(1) Where access to the enclosure is by means of an open exterior balcony, the door assembly to the enclosure shall have a minimum $1^1/_2$-hour fire protection rating and shall be self-closing or shall be automatic-closing by actuation of a smoke detector.<br>. . . | Item (1) revised to apply to an enclosure and not only to a stair |

| Subject / 2009 Edition Text | Notes |
|---|---|
| **7.2.3.9 Enclosure Pressurization.** | Title revised to apply to an enclosure and not only to a stair |
| **7.2.3.10.1** For both mechanical ventilation and pressurized enclosure systems, the activation of the systems shall be initiated by a smoke detector installed in an approved location within 10 ft (3050 mm) of each entrance to the smokeproof enclosure. | Provision revised to apply to "each entrance" and not only to the entrance |
| **7.2.4.1.2*** Horizontal exits shall be permitted to be substituted for other exits where the total egress capacity and the total number of the other exits (stairs, ramps, door openings leading outside the building) is not less than half that required for the entire area of the building or connected buildings, and provided that none of the other exits is a horizontal exit, unless otherwise permitted by 7.2.4.1.3. | Provision revised so as to apply to the total number of exits and not only to the total egress capacity |
| **7.2.4.3.1** Fire barriers separating buildings or areas between which there are horizontal exits shall have a minimum 2-hour fire resistance rating, unless otherwise provided in 7.2.4.4.1, and shall provide a separation that is continuous to the finished ground level. *(See also Section 8.3.)* | Provision revised from "barriers separating building areas" to "barriers separating buildings or areas" |
| **7.2.4.4 Bridges Serving Horizontal Exits Between Buildings.** The provisions of 7.2.4.4 shall apply to bridges serving horizontal exits between buildings and to the associated horizontal exit fire barrier.<br>**7.2.4.4.1** The minimum 2-hour fire resistance–rated barrier required by 7.2.4.3.1 shall extend as follows:<br>(1) Vertically from the ground to a point 10 ft (3050 mm) above the bridge or to the roofline, whichever is lower<br>(2) Horizontally for not less than 10 ft (3050 mm) to each side of the bridge | Reformatting and repositioning of former 7.2.4.4.7 to keep related items together |
| **7.2.5.6.1* Visual Protection.** Outside ramps shall be arranged to avoid any impediments to their use by persons having a fear of high places. Outside ramps more than 36 ft (11 m) above the finished ground level shall be provided with an opaque visual obstruction not less than 48. in. (1220 mm) in height. | Provision revised from "more than 3 stories" to "more than 36 ft (11 m) above the finished ground level" |
| **7.2.6.4.2** In new construction, the minimum width of any exit passageway into which an exit stair discharges, or that serves as a horizontal transfer within an exit stair system, shall meet the following criteria:<br>(1) The minimum width of the exit passageway shall be not less than two-thirds of the width of the exit stair.<br>(2) Where stairs are credited with egress capacity in accordance with 7.3.3.2, the exit passageway width shall be sized to accommodate the same capacity as the stair, with such capacity determined by use of the capacity factors in Table 7.3.3.1. | New provision |
| **7.2.8.5.2** Replacement fire escape stairs in occupancies serving more than 10 occupants shall have visual enclosures to avoid any impediments to their use by persons having a fear of high places. Fire escape stairs more than 36 ft (11 m) above the finished ground level shall be provided with an opaque visual obstruction not less than 48 in. (1220 mm) in height. | Provision revised from "more than 3 stories" to "more than 36 ft (11 m) above the finished ground level" |
| **7.2.10.2.1** Slide escapes, where permitted as a required means of egress, shall be rated at a capacity of 60 persons. | Revised from "shall have" to "shall be rated" — no technical change |
| **7.2.11.3** Handrails of alternating tread devices shall comply with the following:<br>(1) The handrail height of alternating tread devices, measured above tread nosings, shall be uniform, not less than 30 in. (760 mm), and not more than 34 in. (865 mm).<br>(2) Handrails for alternating tread devices shall be permitted to terminate at a location vertically above the top and bottom risers.<br>(3) Handrails for alternating tread devices shall not be required to be continuous between flights or to extend beyond the top or bottom risers.<br>(4) Alternating tread device guards, with a top rail that also serves as a handrail, shall have a | New provision |

| Subject / 2009 Edition Text | Notes |
|---|---|
| height of not less than 30 in. (760 mm), and not more than 34 in. (865 mm), measured vertically from the leading edge of the device tread nosing.<br>(5) Open guards of alternating tread devices shall have rails such that a sphere 21 in. (535 mm) in diameter is not able to pass through any opening. | |
| **7.2.12.1.1** An area of refuge used as part of a required accessible means of egress in accordance with 7.5.4; consisting of a story in a building that is protected throughout by an approved, supervised automatic sprinkler system in accordance with Section 9.7; and having an accessible story that is one or more stories above or below a story of exit discharge shall meet the following criteria:<br>(1) Each elevator landing shall be provided with a two-way communication system for communication between the elevator landing and the fire command center or a central control point approved by the authority having jurisdiction.<br>(2) Directions for the use of the two-way communication system, instructions for summoning assistance via the two-way communication system, and written identification of the location shall be posted adjacent to the two-way communication system.<br>(3) The two-way communication system shall include both audible and visible signals.<br>**7.2.12.1.2** An area of refuge used as part of a required accessible means of egress in accordance with 7.5.4 in other than a building that is protected throughout by an approved, supervised automatic sprinkler system in accordance with Section 9.7 shall meet the following criteria:<br>(1) The area of refuge shall meet the general requirements of Section 7.1.<br>(2) The area of refuge shall meet the requirements of 7.2.12.2 and 7.2.12.3. | Provision revised so that areas of refuge in sprinklered buildings are required to have two-way communication system at each elevator landing; areas of refuge in nonsprinklered buildings are required to meet multiple provisions as in earlier editions |
| **7.3.1.1.2** For other than existing means of egress, where more than one means of egress is required, the means of egress shall be of such width and capacity that the loss of any one means of egress leaves available not less than 50 percent of the required capacity. | New provision |
| **Table 7.3.1.2 Occupant Load Factor** | Occupant load factor added for air traffic control tower observation levels |
| **7.3.2.2** Projections within the means of egress of not more than $4\frac{1}{2}$ in. (114 mm) on each side shall be permitted at a height of 38 in. (965 mm) and below. In the case of stair and landing handrails forming part of a guard, in accordance with 7.2.2.4.4.3, such projections shall be permitted at a height of 42 in. (1065 mm) and below. | Provision expanded to include new second sentence |
| **7.3.3.1** Egress capacity for approved components of means of egress shall be based on the capacity factors shown in Table 7.3.3.1, unless otherwise provided in 7.3.3.2. | Provision revised to recognize new 7.3.3.2 |
| **7.3.3.2*** For stairways wider than 44 in. (1120 mm) and subject to the 0.3 in. (7.6 mm) width per person capacity factor, the capacity shall be permitted to be increased using the following equation:<br>$C = 146.7 + \left[\frac{(Wn - 44)}{0.218}\right]$<br>where:<br>$C$ = capacity, in persons, rounded to the nearest integer<br>$Wn$ = nominal width of the stair as permitted by 7.3.2.2 (in.) | New provision |
| **7.4.1.6.3** Doors separating the elevator lobby from the exit access required by 7.4.1.6.1 shall be permitted to be electronically locked in accordance with 7.2.1.6.3. | New provision |
| **7.4.2 Spaces About Electrical Equipment.**<br>**7.4.2.1 600 Volts, Nominal, or Less.** The minimum number of means of egress for working space about electrical equipment, other than existing electrical equipment, shall be in accordance with *NFPA 70, National Electrical Code*, Article 110.26(C).<br>**7.4.2.2 Over 600 Volts, Nominal.** The minimum number of means of egress for working space about electrical equipment, other than existing electrical equipment, shall be in accordance with *NFPA 70, National Electrical Code*, Article 110.33(A). | New provision |

| Subject / 2009 Edition Text | Notes |
|---|---|
| **7.5.1.3** Remoteness shall be provided in accordance with 7.5.1.3.1 through 7.5.1.3.7.<br>**7.5.1.3.1** Where more than one exit, exit access, or exit discharge is required from a building or portion thereof, such exits, exit accesses, or exit discharges shall be remotely located from each other and be arranged to minimize the possibility that more than one has the potential to be blocked by any one fire or other emergency condition.<br>**7.5.1.3.2*** Where two exits, exit accesses, or exit discharges are required, they shall be located at a distance from one another not less than one-half the length of the maximum overall diagonal dimension of the building or area to be served, measured in a straight line between the nearest edge of the exits, exit accesses, or exit discharges, unless otherwise provided in 7.5.1.3.3 through 7.5.1.3.5.<br>**7.5.1.3.3** In buildings protected throughout by an approved, supervised automatic sprinkler system in accordance with Section 9.7, the minimum separation distance between two exits, exit accesses, or exit discharges, measured in accordance with 7.5.1.3.2, shall be not less than one-third the length of the maximum overall diagonal dimension of the building or area to be served.<br>**7.5.1.3.4*** In other than high-rise buildings, where exit enclosures are provided as the required exits specified in 7.5.1.3.2 or 7.5.1.3.3 and are interconnected by not less than a 1-hour fire resistance–rated corridor, exit separation shall be measured along the shortest line of travel within the corridor.<br>**7.5.1.3.5** In existing buildings, where more than one exit, exit access, or exit discharge is required, such exits, exit accesses, or exit discharges shall be exempt from the diagonal measurement separation distance criteria of 7.5.1.3.2 and 7.5.1.3.3, provided that such exits, exit accesses, or exit discharges are remotely located in accordance with 7.5.1.3.1.<br>**7.5.1.3.6** In other than existing buildings, where more than two exits, exit accesses, or exit discharges are required, at least two of the required exits, exit accesses, or exit discharges shall be arranged to comply with the minimum separation distance requirement.<br>**7.5.1.3.7** The balance of the exits, exit accesses, or exit discharges specified in 7.5.1.3.6 shall be located so that, if one becomes blocked, the others are available. | Provisions of 7.5.1.3 expanded to require remoteness for exit accesses, exits, and exit discharges<br>Provision permitting remoteness distance to be measured along 1-hr corridor revised so as not to apply in high-rise buildings<br>Provision reworded to clarify that existing installations are subject only to the qualitative remoteness requirement of 7.5.1.3.1 and not to the quantitative remoteness requirement 7.5.1.3.2 or 7.5.1.3.3<br>Provision revised to clarify that it does not apply to existing installations for consistency with 7.5.1.3.5 |
| **7.7.3.1** Where more than one exit discharge is required, exit discharges shall be arranged to meet the remoteness criteria of 7.5.1.3. | Provision revised for consistency with 7.5.1.3 |
| **7.8.1.3*** The floors and other walking surfaces within an exit and within the portions of the exit access and exit discharge designated in 7.8.1.1 shall be illuminated as follows:<br>. . .<br>(3) In assembly occupancies, the illumination of the walking surfaces of exit access shall be at least 0.2 ft-candle (2.2 lux) during periods of performances or projections involving directed light.<br>. . . | Item (3) revised from "floors" to "walking surfaces" |
| **7.9.2.4** Emergency generators providing power to emergency lighting systems shall be installed, tested, and maintained in accordance with NFPA 110, *Standard for Emergency and Standby Power Systems*. Stored electrical energy systems, where required in this *Code*, other than battery systems for emergency luminaires in accordance with 7.9.2.5, shall be installed and tested in accordance with NFPA 111, *Standard on Stored Electrical Energy Emergency and Standby Power Systems*. | Provision revised so as not to apply to battery systems for emergency luminaires in accordance with 7.9.2.5 |
| **7.9.3.1.1** Testing of required emergency lighting systems shall be permitted to be conducted as follows:<br>(1) Functional testing shall be conducted monthly with a minimum of 3 weeks and a maximum of 5 weeks between tests, for not less than 30 seconds, except as otherwise permitted by 7.9.3.1.1(2).<br>(2)* The test interval shall be permitted to be extended beyond 30 days with the approval of the authority having jurisdiction.<br>. . . | Item (1) revised from "30-day intervals" to "monthly with a minimum of 3 weeks and a maximum of 5 weeks between tests"<br>Item (2) is new |

| Subject / 2009 Edition Text | Notes |
|---|---|
| **7.10.1.2.2*** Horizontal components of the egress path within an exit enclosure shall be marked by approved exit or directional exit signs where the continuation of the egress path is not obvious. | New provision |
| **7.10.1.6* Floor Proximity Exit Signs.** Where floor proximity exit signs are required in Chapters 11 through 43, such signs shall comply with 7.10.3, 7.10.4, 7.10.5, and 7.10.6 for externally illuminated signs and 7.10.7 for internally illuminated signs. Such signs shall be located near the floor level in addition to those signs required for doors or corridors. The bottom of the sign shall be not less than 6 in. (150 mm), but not more than 18 in. (455 mm), above the floor. For exit doors, the sign shall be mounted on the door or adjacent to the door, with the nearest edge of the sign within 4 in. (100 mm) of the door frame. | Provision revised to require compliance with 7.10.3, 7.10.4, 7.10.5, and 7.10.6 for externally illuminated signs and 7.10.7 for internally illuminated signs |
| **7.10.1.7* Floor Proximity Egress Path Marking.** Where floor proximity egress path marking is required in Chapters 11 through 43, an approved floor proximity egress path marking system that is internally illuminated shall be installed within 18 in. (455 mm) of the floor. Floor proximity egress path marking systems shall be listed in accordance with ANSI/UL 1994, *Standard for Luminous Egress Path Marking Systems*. The system shall provide a visible delineation of the path of travel along the designated exit access and shall be essentially continuous, except as interrupted by doorways, hallways, corridors, or other such architectural features. The system shall operate continuously or at any time the building fire alarm system is activated. The activation, duration, and continuity of operation of the system shall be in accordance with 7.9.2. The system shall be maintained in accordance with the product manufacturing listing. | Provision revised to require compliance with ANSI/UL 1994 |
| **7.10.2.2** Directional exit signs shall be provided within horizontal components of the egress path within exit enclosures as required by 7.10.1.2.2. | New provision |
| **7.10.3.2*** Where approved by the authority having jurisdiction, pictograms in compliance with NFPA 170, *Standard for Fire Safety and Emergency Symbols*, shall be permitted. | Provision revised to reference NFPA 170 |
| **7.10.8.5* Evacuation Diagram.** Where a posted floor evacuation diagram is required in Chapters 11 through 43, floor evacuation diagrams reflecting the actual floor arrangement and exit locations shall be posted and oriented in a location and manner acceptable to the authority having jurisdiction. | New provision |
| **Chapter 8 Features of Fire Protection**<br>**8.2.2.5** Where door assemblies are required elsewhere in this *Code* to be smoke leakage–rated in accordance with 8.2.2.5, door assemblies shall comply with the following:<br>. . . | Provision revised to clarify its application to "smoke leakage–rated" door assemblies |
| **8.3.3.7** Fire resistance–rated glazing complying with 8.3.2.1.1 shall be permitted in fire doors and fire window assemblies in accordance with their listings. | New provision |
| **8.3.3.11.1** Fire protection–rated glazing used in doors shall bear a four-part identification in the form of D — H (or NH) — T (or NT) — XXX, with the component parts defined as follows:<br>(1) D, which indicates that the glazing is to be used in fire door assemblies and that the glazing meets the fire protection requirements of NFPA 252, *Standard Methods of Fire Tests of Door Assemblies*<br>. . . | Item (1) revised to reference NFPA 252 |
| **Table 8.3.4.2 Minimum Fire Protection Ratings for Opening Protectives in Fire Resistance–Rated Assemblies** | Table expanded to include entry for horizontal exits served by bridges between buildings for consistency with 7.2.4.4 |

| Subject / 2009 Edition Text | Notes |
|---|---|
| **8.3.5.1.1** The requirements of 8.3.5.1 shall not apply where otherwise permitted by any one of the following:<br>. . .<br>(4) Where firestopping materials are used with the following penetrating items, the penetration is limited to one floor, and the firestopping material is capable of preventing the passage of flame and hot gases sufficient to ignite cotton waste when subjected to the time–temperature fire conditions of NFPA 251 under a minimum positive pressure differential of 0.01 in. water column (2.5 Pa) at the location of the penetration for the time period equivalent to the required fire resistance rating of the assembly penetrated:<br>(a) Steel, ferrous, or copper cables<br>(b) Cable or wire with steel jackets<br>(c) Cast-iron, steel, or copper pipes<br>(d) Steel conduit or tubing | Item (4) is new |
| **8.3.5.1.2** The maximum nominal diameter of the penetrating item, as indicated in 8.3.5.1.1(4)(a) through (d), shall not be greater than 4 in. (100 mm) and shall not exceed an aggregate 100 in.$^2$ (64,520 mm$^2$) opening in any 100 ft$^2$ (9.3 m$^2$) of floor or wall area. | New provision |
| **8.3.6.7* Exterior Curtain Walls and Perimeter Joints.**<br>**8.3.6.7.1** Voids created between the fire resistance–rated floor assembly and the exterior curtain wall shall be protected with a perimeter joint system that is designed and tested in accordance with ASTM E 2307, *Standard Test Method for Fire Resistance of Perimeter Fire Barriers Using Intermediate-Scale, Multistory Apparatus*.<br>**8.3.6.7.2** The perimeter joint system shall have an F rating equal to the fire resistance rating of the floor assembly. | New provision |
| **8.5.5.4 Installation, Testing, and Maintenance.**<br>**8.5.5.4.1** Air-conditioning, heating, ventilating ductwork, and related equipment, including smoke dampers and combination fire and smoke dampers, shall be installed in accordance with NFPA 90A, *Standard for the Installation of Air-Conditioning and Ventilating Systems*, and NFPA 105, *Standard for the Installation of Smoke Door Assemblies and Other Opening Protectives*.<br>**8.5.5.4.2** Smoke dampers and combination fire and smoke dampers shall be inspected, tested, and maintained in accordance with NFPA 105, *Standard for the Installation of Smoke Door Assemblies and Other Opening Protectives*. | Provision expanded to include testing and maintenance, not only installation<br><br>Reference added to NFPA 105<br><br>Reference added to NFPA 105 |
| **8.6.7* Atriums.** Unless prohibited by Chapters 11 through 43, an atrium shall be permitted, provided that the following conditions are met:<br>(1) The atrium is separated from the adjacent spaces by fire barriers with not less than a 1-hour fire resistance rating with opening protectives for corridor walls, unless one of the following is met:<br>. . .<br>(c)* Glass walls and inoperable windows shall be permitted in lieu of the fire barriers where all the following are met:<br>. . .<br>vii. The glass is continuous vertically, without horizontal mullions, window treatments, or other obstructions that would interfere with the wetting of the entire glass surface. | Item (1)(c)vii is new |
| **8.6.8.2** Where permitted by Chapters 11 through 43, unenclosed vertical openings not concealed within the building construction shall be permitted as follows:<br>. . .<br>(4) In new construction, the convenience opening shall be separated from the corridor referenced in 8.6.8.2(3) by a smoke partition, unless Chapters 11 through 43 require the corridor to have a fire resistance rating.<br>. . . | Item (4) is new |

| Subject / 2009 Edition Text | Notes |
|---|---|
| **8.6.9.1 Mezzanines.**<br>[former] ~~8.6.9.1.1 A mezzanine shall not be included as a story for the purpose of determining the allowable number of stories in a building.~~ | Former 8.6.9.1.1 deleted as subject is addressed by new 4.6.3 |
| **Chapter 9 Building service and Fire Protection Equipment**<br>**9.1.3.2** New generator controllers shall be monitored by the fire alarm system, where provided, or at an attended location, for the following conditions:<br>(1) Generator running<br>(2) Generator fault<br>(3) Generator switch in nonautomatic position | New provision |
| **9.3.1** Where required by the provisions of another section of this *Code*, smoke control systems shall be installed, inspected, tested, and maintained in accordance with NFPA 92A, *Standard for Smoke-Control Systems Utilizing Barriers and Pressure Differences*; NFPA 92B, *Standard for Smoke Management Systems in Malls, Atria, and Large Spaces*; NFPA 204, *Standard for Smoke and Heat Venting*; or nationally recognized standards, engineering guides, or recommended practices, as approved by the authority having jurisdiction. | Provision revised to reference NFPA 92A and NFPA 92B |
| **9.4.6.3** The elevator inspections and tests required by 9.4.6.1 shall be performed at frequencies complying with one of the following:<br>(1) Inspection and test frequencies specified in Appendix N of ASME A17.1/CSA B44, *Safety Code for Elevators and Escalators*<br>(2) Inspection and test frequencies specified by the authority having jurisdiction | New provision |
| **9.4.7 Openings to Exit Enclosures.** Conveyors, elevators, dumbwaiters, and pneumatic conveyors serving various stories of a building shall not open to an exit enclosure. | Provision revised to have application to "exit enclosures" and not to all exits |
| **9.6.1.8 Protection of Fire Alarm System.**<br>**9.6.1.8.1*** In areas that are not continuously occupied, and unless otherwise permitted by 9.6.1.8.1.1, 9.6.1.8.1.2, or 9.6.1.8.1.3, automatic smoke detection shall be installed to provide notification of fire at the following locations:<br>(1) Each fire alarm control unit<br>(2) Notification appliance circuit power extenders<br>(3) Supervising station transmitting equipment<br>**9.6.1.8.1.1** The provisions of 9.6.1.8.1(2) and 9.6.1.8.1(3) shall not apply to existing alarm systems.<br>**9.6.1.8.1.2** Where ambient conditions prohibit installation of a smoke detector, a heat detector shall be used.<br>**9.6.1.8.1.3** Automatic smoke detection shall not be required where buildings are protected throughout by an approved, supervised automatic sprinkler system in accordance with Section 9.7 and the area containing the fire alarm control unit is sprinklered. | New provision |
| **9.6.2.3** A manual fire alarm box shall be provided as follows, unless modified by another section of this *Code*:<br>(1) For new alarm system installations, the manual fire alarm box shall be located within 5 ft (1.5 m) of exit doorways.<br>(2) For existing alarm system installations, the manual fire alarm box either shall be provided in the natural exit access path near each required exit or within 5 ft (1.5 m) of exit doorways. | Provision revised from "in natural path of travel" to "within 5 ft (1.5 m) of exit doorways" for new installations |
| **9.6.2.4** Manual fire alarm boxes shall be mounted on both sides of grouped openings over 40 ft (12.2 m) in width, and within 5 ft (1.5 m) of each side of the opening. | New provision |
| **9.6.2.10.1.2** The installation of smoke alarms in sleeping rooms shall be required where required by Chapters 11 through 43. | New provision |

| Subject / 2009 Edition Text | Notes |
|---|---|
| **9.6.2.10.2** Smoke alarms, other than existing battery operated smoke alarms as permitted by other sections of this *Code*, shall be powered in accordance with the requirements of *NFPA 72, National Fire Alarm Code.* | Provision revised to require smoke alarm power to be in compliance with NFPA 72 for new installations |
| **9.6.3.5.7*** Public mode visual notification appliances in accordance with *NFPA 72* shall not be required in designated areas as permitted by Chapters 11 through 43, provided that they are replaced with approved alternative visible means.<br>**9.6.3.5.8*** Where visible signals are not required, as permitted by 9.6.3.5.7, documentation of such omission shall be maintained in accordance with 9.7.7. | New provisions |
| [former] ~~**9.6.3.6.4** In mall buildings in accordance with Chapter 36 and Chapter 37, notification within the mall shall be permitted in accordance with 36.4.4.4.3.1(3) and 37.4.4.4.3.1(3).~~ | Provision deleted for correlation with new 9.6.3.9.2 |
| **9.6.3.9.1** Automatically transmitted or live voice evacuation or relocation instructions shall be in accordance with *NFPA 72, National Fire Alarm Code.*<br>**9.6.3.9.2*** Where permitted by Chapters 11 through 43, automatically transmitted or live voice announcements shall be permitted to be made via a voice communication or public address system that complies with the following:<br>(1) Occupant notification, either live or recorded, shall be initiated at a constantly attended receiving station by personnel trained to respond to an emergency.<br>(2) An approved secondary power supply shall be provided for other than existing, previously approved systems.<br>(3) The system shall be audible above the expected ambient noise level.<br>(4) Emergency announcements shall take precedence over any other use. | Provision revised to make compliance with NFPA 72 the norm, and 9.6.3.9.2 (new) an alternate that must be permitted by the occupancy chapter in order to use it |
| **9.6.3.10.2** Emergency voice/alarm communication systems shall be permitted to be used for other purposes, subject to the approval of the authority having jurisdiction, if the fire alarm system takes precedence over all other signals, with the exception of mass notification inputs. | Provision revised from "voice communication" to "emergency voice/alarm communication" for correlation with NFPA 72; exemption added for mass notification inputs |
| **9.6.7.4.3** Unless otherwise prohibited elsewhere in this *Code*, where a building not exceeding four stories in height is protected by an automatic sprinkler system in accordance with 9.7.1.1(1), the sprinkler system shall be permitted to be annunciated on the fire alarm system as a single zone. | New provision |
| **Chapter 10 Interior Finish, Contents, and Furnishings**<br>**10.2.3.4*** Products required to be tested in accordance with ASTM E 84, *Standard Test Method for Surface Burning Characteristics of Building Materials*, or ANSI/UL 723, *Standard for Test for Surface Burning Characteristics of Building Materials*, shall be classified as follows in accordance with their flame spread and smoke development, except as indicated in 10.2.3.4(4):<br>(1) Class A interior wall and ceiling finish shall be characterized by the following:<br>(a) Flame spread index, 0–25<br>(b) Smoke developed index, 0–450<br>. . . | Item (1) revised to delete reference to continued propagation of fire |
| **10.2.4.3.1.2** New installations of cellular or foamed plastic materials tested in accordance with ANSI/UL 1040, *Standard for Fire Test of Insulated Wall Construction*, or FM 4880, *Approval Standard for Class 1 Insulated Wall or Wall and Roof/Ceiling Panels; Plastic Interior Finish Materials; Plastic Exterior Building Panels; Wall/Ceiling Coating Systems; Interior or Exterior Finish Systems*, shall also be tested for smoke release. Suitable smoke release tests include the following:<br>(1) Additional measurements of smoke release into the duct that demonstrate that the total smoke released throughout the test does not exceed 1000 $m^2$ | New provision |

| Subject / 2009 Edition Text | Notes |
|---|---|
| (2) NFPA 286, *Standard Methods of Fire Tests for Evaluating Contribution of Wall and Ceiling Interior Finish to Room Fire Growth*, with the acceptance criterion of 10.2.3.7.2(4)<br>(3) ASTM E 84, *Standard Test Method for Surface Burning Characteristics of Building Materials;* or ANSI/UL 723, *Standard for Test for Surface Burning Characteristics for Building Materials;* with a smoke developed index not exceeding 450 | |
| **10.2.7.3*** Interior floor finishes shall be classified in accordance with 10.2.7.4, based on test results from NFPA 253, *Standard Method of Test for Critical Radiant Flux of Floor Covering Systems Using a Radiant Heat Energy Source*, or ASTM E 648, *Standard Test Method for Critical Radiant Flux of Floor Covering Systems Using a Radiant Heat Energy Source.* | Provision revised to recognize ASTM E 648 |
| **10.3.3*** Where required by the applicable provisions of this *Code*, upholstered furniture, unless the furniture is located in a building protected throughout by an approved automatic sprinkler system, shall have limited rates of heat release when tested in accordance with ASTM E 1537, *Standard Test Method for Fire Testing of Upholstered Furniture*, as follows:<br>(1) The peak rate of heat release for the single upholstered furniture item shall not exceed 80 kW.<br>(2) The total energy released by the single upholstered furniture item during the first 10 minutes of the test shall not exceed 25 MJ. | Item (1) revised from 250 kW to 80 kW<br>Item (2) revised from 5 minutes and 40 MJ to 10 minutes and 25 MJ |
| **10.3.4*** Where required by the applicable provisions of this *Code*, mattresses, unless the mattress is located in a building protected throughout by an approved automatic sprinkler system, shall have limited rates of heat release when tested in accordance with ASTM E 1590, *Standard Test Method for Fire Testing of Mattresses*, as follows:<br>(1) The peak rate of heat release for the mattress shall not exceed 100 kW.<br>(2) The total energy released by the mattress during the first 10 minutes of the test shall not exceed 25 MJ. | Item (1) revised from 250 kW to 100 kW<br>Item (2) revised from 5 minutes and 40 MJ to 10 minutes and 25 MJ |
| **Chapter 11 Special Structures and High-Rise Buildings**<br>**11.3.4 Additional Requirements for Air Traffic Control Towers.**<br>**11.3.4.1 Definition — Air Traffic Control Tower.**<br>. . .<br>**11.3.4.2 Use of Accessory Levels.**<br>. . .<br>**11.3.4.3 Minimum Construction Requirements.**<br>. . .<br>**11.3.4.4 Means of Egress.**<br>**11.3.4.4.1 Number of Means of Egress.**<br>. . .<br>**11.3.4.4.2 Egress for Occupant Load.**<br>. . .<br>**11.3.4.4.3 Areas Excluded from Occupant Load.**<br>. . .<br>**11.3.4.4.4 Single Means of Egress.**<br>. . .<br>**11.3.4.4.5 Smokeproof Enclosures.**<br>. . .<br>**11.3.4.4.6 Discharge from Exits.**<br>. . .<br>**11.3.4.5 Protection.**<br>**11.3.4.5.1 Detection, Alarm, and Communications Systems.**<br>. . .<br>**11.3.4.5.2 Extinguishing Requirements.**<br>. . .<br>**11.3.4.6 Contents and Furnishings.**<br>. . .<br>**11.3.4.7 Uses.**<br>. . . | New provisions |

| Subject / 2009 Edition Text | Notes |
|---|---|
| **11.5.2.2** Buildings on piers not meeting the requirements of 11.5.2.1 and occupied for other than cargo handling and storage shall be in accordance with both of the following:<br>(1) Means of egress shall be arranged in accordance with Chapters 12 through 43<br>(2) One of the following measures shall be provided on piers extending over 150 ft (46 m) from shore to minimize the possibility that fire under or on the pier blocks the escape of occupants to shore:<br>. . . | Provision revised to require compliance with both (1) and (2) |
| **11.7.4.3** Exits from underground structures with an occupant load of more than 100 persons in the underground portions of the structure and having a floor used for human occupancy located more than 30 ft (9140 mm) below the lowest level of exit discharge, or having more than one level located below the lowest level of exit discharge, shall be provided with outside smoke-venting facilities or other means to prevent the exits from becoming charged with smoke from any fire in the areas served by the exits. | Provision revised to delete requirement that exits be cut off from level of exit discharge |
| **11.8.2.2 Elevator Lobby Exit Access Door Locking.** In other than newly constructed high-rise buildings, locks in accordance with 7.2.1.6.3 shall be permitted. | New provision |
| **11.8.6.2** The emergency command center shall contain the following:<br>. . .<br>(5) Elevator fire recall switch in accordance with ASME A17.1/CSA B44, *Safety Code for Elevators and Escalators*<br>(6) Elevator emergency power selector switch(es) where provided in accordance with ASME A17.1/CSA B44.<br>. . . | Items (5) and (6) are new |
| **11.8.7 Emergency Plans.** Emergency plans shall be provided in accordance with 4.8.2. | New provision |
| **11.9.5.2.2** Electric heaters, their placement, and their installation shall be approved by the authority having jurisdiction. | New provision |
| **Chapter 12 New Assembly Occupancies**<br>**12.1.6 Minimum Construction Requirements.** Assembly occupancies shall be limited to the building construction types specified in Table 12.1.6, based on the number of stories in height as defined in 4.6.3, unless otherwise permitted by the following *(see 8.2.1)*:<br>. . .<br>**Table 12.1.6 Construction Type Limitations** | Provision, and associated Table 12.1.6, revised so that it is applied based on number of stories in height — no technical change intended |
| **12.2.2.2.7** Elevator lobby exit access door locking in accordance with 7.2.1.6.3 shall be permitted. | New provision |
| **12.2.5.6.4* Aisle Stairs and Ramps.** The following shall apply to aisle stairs and ramps:<br>. . .<br>[former] ~~(3) The marking stripe exemption of 12.2.5.6.9.3 shall not be permitted for aisle stairs.~~<br>. . . | Former item (3) deleted |
| **12.2.6.1** Travel distance shall be measured in accordance with Section 7.6. | New provision — no technical change |
| **12.2.10.3** Evacuation diagrams in accordance with 7.10.8.5 shall be provided. | New provision |
| [former 12.3.4.1(2)] ~~(2) Voice communication or public address systems complying with 12.3.4.3.4 shall not be required to comply with 9.6.1.~~ | Provision deleted for correlation with new 12.3.4.3.3 through 12.3.4.3.7 and new 9.6.3.9.2 |

| Subject / 2009 Edition Text | Notes |
|---|---|
| **12.3.4.2.1** Initiation of the required fire alarm system shall be by both of the following means:<br>(1) Manual means . . .<br>(a) . . .<br>(b) . . .<br>(2) Where automatic sprinklers are provided, sprinkler system waterflow shall initiate the fire alarm system, even where manual fire alarm boxes are provided in accordance with 12.3.4.2.1(1). | Provision revised so as to require compliance with BOTH (1) and (2)<br><br>Item (2) is new |
| **12.3.4.3.3** Occupant notification shall be by means of voice announcements in accordance with 9.6.3.9, initiated by the person in the constantly attended receiving station.<br>**12.3.4.3.4** Occupant notification shall be by means of visible signals in accordance with 9.6.3.5, initiated by the person in the constantly attended receiving station, unless otherwise permitted by 12.3.4.3.5.<br>**12.3.4.3.5*** Visible signals shall not be required in the assembly seating area, or the floor area used for the contest, performance, or entertainment, where the occupant load exceeds 1000 and an approved, alternative visible means of occupant notification is provided. *(See 9.6.3.5.7.)*<br>**12.3.4.3.6** The announcement shall be permitted to be made via a voice communication or public address system in accordance with 9.6.3.9.2.<br>**12.3.4.3.7** Where the authority having jurisdiction determines that a constantly attended receiving station is impractical, both of the following shall be provided:<br>(1) Automatically transmitted evacuation or relocation instructions shall be provided in accordance with *NFPA 72, National Fire Alarm Code.*<br>(2) The system shall be monitored by a supervising station in accordance with *NFPA 72, National Fire Alarm Code.* | Provisions of 12.3.4.3.3 through 12.3.4.3.7 are new for correlation with new 9.6.3.9.2 |
| **12.3.5.2** Any building containing one or more assembly occupancies where the aggregate occupant load of the assembly occupancies exceeds 300 shall be protected by an approved, supervised automatic sprinkler system in accordance with Section 9.7 as follows *(see also 12.1.6, 12.2.6, 12.3.2, and 12.3.6)*:<br>(1) . . .<br>(2) . . .<br>(3) . . . | Provision revised so threshold for sprinklers is based on the aggregate occupant load of the assembly occupancies present in the building |
| **12.4.2.1** To be considered smoke protected, an assembly seating facility shall comply with the following:<br>(1) All enclosed . . . by the following:<br>(a) . . .<br>(b)* . . .<br>(2) All means of egress serving a smoke-protected assembly seating area shall be provided with smoke-actuated ventilation facilities or natural ventilation designed as follows:<br>(a) The ventilation system shall be designed to maintain the level of smoke at not less than 6 ft (1830 mm) above the floor of the means of egress.<br>(b) The ventilation system shall be in accordance with NFPA 92B, *Standard for Smoke Management Systems in Malls, Atria, and Large Spaces*, or, where applicable, NFPA 92A, *Standard for Smoke-Control Systems Utilizing Barriers and Pressure Differences.* | Mandatory references to NFPA 92B and NFPA 92A are new |
| **12.4.3.3.3** Each smoke compartment shall have an independent air supply and exhaust system capable of smoke control or smoke exhaust functions. The system shall be in accordance with NFPA 92A, *Standard for Smoke-Control Systems Utilizing Barriers and Pressure Differences*, or NFPA 92B, *Standard for Smoke Management Systems in Malls, Atria, and Large Spaces.* | Mandatory references to NFPA 92B and NFPA 92A are new, replacing former requirement to provide six air changes per hour |
| **12.4.5.5.1.2** Smoke control systems used for compliance with 12.4.5.5.1.1 shall be in accordance with NFPA 92B, *Standard for Smoke Management Systems in Malls, Atria, and Large Spaces*, or, where applicable, NFPA 92A, *Standard for Smoke-Control Systems Utilizing Barriers and Pressure Differences.* | New provision |

| Subject / 2009 Edition Text | Notes |
|---|---|
| **12.4.5.6.3** The main proscenium opening used for viewing performances shall be provided with proscenium opening protection as described in 12.4.5.7. | Provision revised to replace "curtain" with "proscenium opening protection" |
| **12.4.5.7 Proscenium Opening Protection**<br>**12.4.5.7.1** Where required by 12.4.5.6, the proscenium opening shall be protected by a listed, minimum 20-minute opening protective assembly, a fire curtain complying with NFPA 80, *Standard for Fire Doors and Other Opening Protectives*, or an approved water curtain complying with NFPA 13, *Standard for the Installation of Sprinkler Systems*.<br>**12.4.5.7.2** Proscenium opening protection provided by other than a fire curtain shall activate upon automatic detection of a fire and upon manual activation. | Provisions revised to offer the third option of using a listed opening protective assembly as described in 2007 edition of NFPA 80 |
| **12.7.1.3 Inspection of Door Openings.** Door openings shall be inspected in accordance with 7.2.1.15. | New provision |
| [former] ~~12.7.4.5 The provision of 10.3.2 for cigarette ignition resistance of newly introduced upholstered furniture and mattresses shall not apply to assembly occupancies.~~ | Provision deleted |
| **12.7.9.1.1** Seats in assembly occupancies accommodating more than 200 persons shall be securely fastened to the floor, except where fastened together in groups of not less than three and as permitted by 12.7.9.2. | Provision revised by deleting maximum 7 chair grouping |
| **12.7.12 Clothing.** Clothing and personal effects shall not be stored in corridors, and spaces not separated from corridors, unless otherwise permitted by the following:<br>(1) This requirement shall not apply to corridors, and spaces not separated from corridors, that are protected by an approved, supervised automatic sprinkler system in accordance with Section 9.7.<br>(2) This requirement shall not apply to corridors, and spaces not separated from corridors, that are protected by a smoke detection system in accordance with Section 9.6. | Provision revised to apply to "spaces not separated from corridors," as well as to corridors |
| **12.7.13 Emergency Plans.**<br>**12.7.13.1** Emergency plans shall be provided in accordance with Section 4.8.<br>**12.7.13.2** Where assembly occupancies are located in the high-rise portion of a building, the emergency plan shall include egress procedures, methods, and preferred evacuation routes for each event considered to be a life safety hazard that could impact the building, including the appropriateness of the use of elevators. | Provisions are new |
| **Chapter 13 Existing Assembly Occupancies**<br>**13.1.6 Minimum Construction Requirements.** Assembly occupancies shall be limited to the building construction types specified in Table 13.1.6, based on the number of stories in height as defined in 4.6.3, unless otherwise permitted by the following *(see 8.2.1)*:<br>. . .<br>**Table 13.1.6 Construction Type Limitations** | Provision, and associated Table 13.1.6, revised so that it is applied based on number of stories in height — no technical change intended. |
| **13.2.2.2.7** Elevator lobby exit access door locking in accordance with 7.2.1.6.3 shall be permitted. | New provision |
| **13.2.5.6.4* Aisle Stairs and Ramps.** The following shall apply to aisle stairs and ramps:<br>. . .<br>[former] ~~(3) The marking stripe exemption of 13.2.5.6.9.3 shall not be permitted for aisle stairs~~<br>. . . | Former item (3) deleted |
| **13.2.6.1** Travel distance shall be measured in accordance with Section 7.6. | New provision — no technical change |
| **13.2.10.3** Evacuation diagrams in accordance with 7.10.8.5 shall be provided. | New provision |

| **Subject / 2009 Edition Text** | **Notes** |
|---|---|
| **13.3.4.2.1** Initiation of the required fire alarm system shall be by both of the following means, and the system shall be provided with an emergency power source:<br>(1) Manual means . . .<br>(a) . . .<br>(b) . . .<br>(2) Where automatic sprinklers are provided, sprinkler system waterflow shall initiate the fire alarm system, even where manual fire alarm boxes are provided in accordance with 13.3.4.2.1(1). | Provision revised so as to require compliance with BOTH (1) and (2)<br><br>Item (2) is new |
| **13.3.4.3.3** Occupant notification shall be by means of voice announcements in accordance with 9.6.3.9 initiated by the person in the constantly attended receiving station. | Provision revised to require compliance with 9.6.3.9 |
| **13.3.4.3.6** The announcement shall be permitted to be made via a voice communication or public address system in accordance with 9.6.3.9.2. | Provision revised to permit occupant notification by voice communication or public address system in compliance with 9.6.3.9.2 |
| **13.3.4.3.7** Where the authority having jurisdiction determines that a constantly attended receiving station is impractical, automatically transmitted evacuation or relocation instructions shall be provided in accordance with *NFPA 72, National Fire Alarm Code.* | Provision revised to require compliance with NFPA 72 |
| **13.4.5.7.1** On every legitimate stage, the main proscenium opening used for viewing performances shall be provided with proscenium opening protection as follows:<br>(1) The proscenium opening protection shall comply with 12.4.5.7.<br>(2) Asbestos shall be permitted in lieu of a listed fabric.<br>(3) Manual curtains of any size shall be permitted. | Provision revised to recognize protection per new requirements in Chapter 12, and retain former options; outdated requirements inconsistent with new treatment in Chapter 12 deleted |
| **13.4.5.7.3** Proscenium opening protection provided by other than a fire curtain in accordance with 12.4.5.7 *[see 13.4.5.7.1(1)]* shall activate upon automatic detection of a fire and upon manual activation. | Existing provisions restated |
| **13.7.1.3 Inspection of Door Openings.** Door openings shall be inspected in accordance with 7.2.1.15. | New provision |
| [former] ~~13.7.4.5 The provision of 10.3.2 for cigarette ignition resistance of newly introduced upholstered furniture and mattresses shall not apply to assembly occupancies.~~ | Provision deleted |
| **13.7.9.1.1** Seats in assembly occupancies accommodating more than 200 persons shall be securely fastened to the floor, except where fastened together in groups of not less than three and as permitted by 13.7.9.2. | Provision revised by deleting maximum 7 chair grouping |
| **13.7.12 Clothing.** Clothing and personal effects shall not be stored in corridors, and spaces not separated from corridors, unless otherwise permitted by the following:<br>(1) This requirement shall not apply to corridors, and spaces not separated from corridors, that are protected by an approved automatic sprinkler system in accordance with Section 9.7.<br>(2) This requirement shall not apply to corridors, and spaces not separated from corridors, that are protected by a smoke detection system in accordance with Section 9.6.<br>(3) This requirement shall not apply to storage in metal lockers, provided that the required egress width is maintained. | Provision revised to apply to "spaces not separated from corridors," as well as to corridors |
| **13.7.13 Emergency Plans.**<br>**13.7.13.1** Emergency plans shall be provided in accordance with Section 4.8.<br>**13.7.13.2** Where assembly occupancies are located in the high-rise portion of a building, the emergency plan shall include egress procedures, methods, and preferred evacuation routes for each event considered to be a life safety hazard that could impact the building, including the appropriateness of the use of elevators. | Provisions are new |

| Subject / 2009 Edition Text | Notes |
|---|---|
| **Chapter 14 New Educational Occupancies** | |
| **14.2.2.2.4** Elevator lobby exit access door locking in accordance with 7.2.1.6.3 shall be permitted. | New provision |
| **14.2.6.1** Travel distance shall be measured in accordance with Section 7.6. | New provision — no technical change |
| **14.3.2.3** Stages and platforms shall be protected in accordance with Chapter 12. | Provision expanded to require protection of platforms |
| **14.3.2.4 Alcohol-Based Hand-Rub Dispensers.** Alcohol-based hand-rub dispensers shall be protected in accordance with 8.7.3, unless all of the following conditions are met:<br>(1) Dispensers shall be installed in rooms or spaces separated from corridors and exits.<br>(2) The maximum individual dispenser fluid capacity shall be as follows:<br>(a) 0.32 gal (1.2 L) for dispensers in rooms<br>(b) 0.53 gal (2.0 L) for dispensers in suites of rooms<br>(3) The dispensers shall be separated from each other by horizontal spacing of not less than 48 in. (1220 mm).<br>(4) Storage of quantities greater than 5 gal (18.9 L) in a single fire compartment shall meet the requirements of NFPA 30, *Flammable and Combustible Liquids Code.*<br>(5) The dispensers shall not be installed over or directly adjacent to an ignition source.<br>(6) Dispensers installed directly over carpeted floors shall be permitted only in sprinklered rooms or spaces. | New provision |
| **14.3.2.5** Educational occupancy laboratories using chemicals shall be in accordance with 8.7.4. | New provision |
| **14.3.5 Extinguishment Requirements**<br>**14.3.5.1*** Educational occupancy buildings exceeding 20,000 $ft^2$ (1860 $m^2$) shall be protected throughout by an approved, supervised automatic sprinkler system in accordance with Section 9.7.<br>**14.3.5.2** Educational occupancy buildings four or more stories in height shall be protected throughout by an approved, supervised automatic sprinkler system in accordance with Section 9.7.<br>. . . | New provision<br><br>New provision |
| **14.3.6 Corridors.** Corridors shall be separated from other parts of the story by walls having a 1-hour fire resistance rating in accordance with Section 8.3, unless otherwise permitted by the following:<br>(1) . . .<br>(2) The following shall apply to buildings protected throughout by an approved, supervised automatic sprinkler system in accordance with Section 9.7:<br>(a) Corridor walls shall not be required to be rated, provided that such walls form smoke partitions in accordance with Section 8.4.<br>(b) The provisions of 8.4.3.5 shall not apply to normally occupied classrooms.<br>. . . | Item (2)(b) is new and exempts classroom door closers in sprinklered building |
| **14.7.2.2** Approved training programs designed for education and training and for the practice of emergency egress to familiarize occupants with the drill procedure, and to establish conduct of the emergency egress as a matter of routine, shall be permitted to receive credit on a one-for-one basis for not more than four of the emergency egress drills required by 14.7.2.3, provided that a minimum of four emergency egress drills are completed prior to the conduct of the first such training and practice program. | New provision |
| **14.7.3.3 Inspection of Door Openings.** Door openings shall be inspected in accordance with 7.2.1.15. | New provision |

| Subject / 2009 Edition Text | Notes |
|---|---|
| [former] ~~**14.7.4.4** The provision of 10.3.2 for cigarette ignition resistance of newly introduced upholstered furniture and mattresses shall not apply to educational occupancies protected throughout by an approved, supervised automatic sprinkler system in accordance with Section 9.7.~~ | Provision deleted |
| **Chapter 15 Existing Educational Occupancies** | |
| **15.2.2.2.4** Elevator lobby exit access door locking in accordance with 7.2.1.6.3 shall be permitted. | New provision |
| **15.2.6.1** Travel distance shall be measured in accordance with Section 7.6 | New provision — no technical change |
| **15.3.2.3** Stages and platforms shall be protected in accordance with Chapter 13. | Provision expanded to require protection of platforms |
| **15.3.2.4 Alcohol-Based Hand-Rub Dispensers.** Alcohol-based hand-rub dispensers shall be protected in accordance with 8.7.3, unless all of the following conditions are met:<br>(1) Dispensers shall be installed in rooms or spaces separated from corridors and exits.<br>(2) The maximum individual dispenser fluid capacity shall be as follows:<br>(a) 0.32 gal (1.2 L) for dispensers in rooms<br>(b) 0.53 gal (2.0 L) for dispensers in suites of rooms<br>(3) The dispensers shall be separated from each other by horizontal spacing of not less than 48 in. (1220 mm).<br>(4) Storage of quantities greater than 5 gal (18.9 L) in a single fire compartment shall meet the requirements of NFPA 30, *Flammable and Combustible Liquids Code.*<br>(5) The dispensers shall not be installed over or directly adjacent to an ignition source.<br>(6) Dispensers installed directly over carpeted floors shall be permitted only in sprinklered rooms or spaces. | New provision |
| **15.3.2.5** Educational occupancy laboratories using chemicals shall be in accordance with 8.7.4. | New provision |
| **15.3.6 Corridors.** Corridors shall be separated from other parts of the story by walls having a minimum $^1/_2$-hour fire resistance rating in accordance with Section 8.3, unless otherwise permitted by the following:<br>(1) . . .<br>(2)* The following shall apply to buildings protected throughout by an approved automatic sprinkler system with valve supervision in accordance with Section 9.7:<br>(a) Corridor walls shall not be required to be rated, provided that such walls form smoke partitions in accordance with Section 8.4.<br>(b) The provisions of 8.4.3.5 shall not apply to normally occupied classrooms.<br>. . . | Item (2)(b) is new and exempts classroom door closers in sprinklered building |
| **15.7.2.2** Approved training programs designed for education and training and for the practice of emergency egress to familiarize occupants with the drill procedure, and to establish conduct of the emergency egress as a matter of routine, shall be permitted to receive credit on a one-for-one basis for not more than four of the emergency egress drills required by 15.7.2.3, provided that a minimum of four emergency egress drills are completed prior to the conduct of the first such training and practice program. | New provision |
| **15.7.3.3 Inspection of Door Openings.** Door openings shall be inspected in accordance with 7.2.1.15. | New provision |
| [former] ~~**15.7.4.4** The provision of 10.3.2 for cigarette ignition resistance of newly introduced upholstered furniture and mattresses shall not apply to educational occupancies protected throughout by an approved automatic sprinkler system in accordance with Section 9.7.~~ | Provision deleted |

| Subject / 2009 Edition Text | Notes |
|---|---|
| **Chapter 16 New Day-Care Occupancies**<br>**16.1.6 Minimum Construction Requirements.**<br>**16.1.6.1** Day-care occupancies, other than day-care homes, shall be limited to the building construction types specified in Table 16.1.6.1 based on the number of stories in height as defined in 4.6.3. *(See 8.2.1.)*<br>**Table 16.1.6.1 Construction Type Limitations** | Provision, and associated Table 16.1.6.1, revised so that it is applied based on number of stories in height — no technical change intended |
| **16.2.2.2.4 Elevator Lobby Exit Access Door Locking.** Elevator lobby exit access door locking in accordance with 7.2.1.6.3 shall be permitted. | New provision |
| **16.3.2.6 Alcohol-Based Hand-Rub Dispensers.** Alcohol-based hand-rub dispensers shall be protected in accordance with 8.7.3, unless all of the following conditions are met:<br>(1) Dispensers shall be installed in rooms or spaces separated from corridors and exits.<br>(2) The maximum individual dispenser fluid capacity shall be as follows:<br>(a) 0.32 gal (1.2 L) for dispensers in rooms<br>(b) 0.53 gal (2.0 L) for dispensers in suites of rooms<br>(3) Dispensers shall be separated from each other by horizontal spacing of not less than 48 in. (1220 mm).<br>(4) Storage of quantities greater than 5 gal (18.9 L) in a single fire compartment shall meet the requirements of NFPA 30, *Flammable and Combustible Liquids Code.*<br>(5) Dispensers shall not be installed over or directly adjacent to an ignition source.<br>(6) Dispensers installed directly over carpeted floors shall be permitted only in sprinklered rooms or spaces. | New provision |
| **16.3.4.1 General.** Day-care occupancies, other than day-care occupancies housed in one room having at least one door opening directly to the outside at grade plane or to an exterior exit access balcony in accordance with 7.5.3, shall be provided with a fire alarm system in accordance with Section 9.6. | Provision revised so room must have door directly to outside to be exempted from fire alarm system requirement |
| **16.3.4.5 Detection.** A smoke detection system in accordance with Section 9.6 shall be installed in day-care occupancies, other than those housed in one room having at least one door opening directly to the outside at grade plane or to an exterior exit access balcony in accordance with 7.5.3, and such system shall comply with both of the following: | Provision revised so room must have door directly to outside to be exempted from smoke detection system requirement |
| **16.6.1.1.5** Places of religious worship shall not be required to meet the provisions of Section 16.6 where operating a day-care home while services are being held in the building. | Provision corrected from "nursery" to "day-care home" |
| **16.6.2.6.1** Travel distance shall be measured in accordance with Section 7.6. | New provision — no technical change |
| **16.6.3.2.1 Alcohol-Based Hand-Rub Dispensers.** Alcohol based hand-rub dispensers shall be protected in accordance with 8.7.3, unless all of the following conditions are met:<br>(1) Dispensers shall be installed in rooms or spaces separated from corridors and exits.<br>(2) The maximum individual dispenser fluid capacity shall be as follows:<br>(a) 0.32 gal (1.2 L) for dispensers in rooms<br>(b) 0.53 gal (2.0 L) for dispensers in suites of rooms<br>(3) Dispensers shall be separated from each other by horizontal spacing of not less than 48 in. (1220 mm).<br>(4) Storage of quantities greater than 5 gal (18.9 L) in a single fire compartment shall meet the requirements of NFPA 30, *Flammable and Combustible Liquids Code.*<br>(5) Dispensers shall not be installed over or directly adjacent to an ignition source.<br>(6) Dispensers installed directly over carpeted floors shall be permitted only in sprinklered rooms or spaces. | New provision |
| **16.6.3.4.3** Single-station or multiple-station smoke alarms or smoke detectors shall be provided in all rooms used for sleeping in accordance with 9.6.2.10. | New provision |

| Subject / 2009 Edition Text | Notes |
|---|---|
| **16.7.3.4 Inspection of Door Openings.** Door openings shall be inspected in accordance with 7.2.1.15. | New provision |
| **16.7.4.4** The provision of 10.3.2 for cigarette ignition resistance of newly introduced upholstered furniture and mattresses shall not apply to day-care homes. | Provision revised so only day-care homes are exempted, not day-care occupancies |
| **16.7.5* Day-Care Staff.** Adequate adult staff shall be on duty in the facility and alert at all times where clients are present. | Provision revised to delete reference to "awake" |
| **Chapter 17 Existing Day-Care Occupancies**<br>**17.1.6 Minimum Construction Requirements.**<br>**17.1.6.1** Day-care occupancies, other than day-care homes, shall be limited to the building construction types specified in Table 17.1.6.1 based on the number of stories in height as defined in 4.6.3. *(See 8.2.1.)*<br>**Table 17.1.6.1 Construction Type Limitations** | Provision, and associated Table 17.1.6.1, revised so that it is applied based on number of stories in height — no technical change intended. |
| **17.2.2.2.4 Elevator Lobby Exit Access Door Locking.** Elevator lobby exit access door locking in accordance with 7.2.1.6.3 shall be permitted. | New provision |
| **17.3.2.6 Alcohol-Based Hand-Rub Dispensers** Alcohol-based hand-rub dispensers shall be protected in accordance with 8.7.3, unless all of the following conditions are met:<br>(1) Dispensers shall be installed in rooms or spaces separated from corridors and exits.<br>(2) The maximum individual dispenser fluid capacity shall be as follows:<br>(a) 0.32 gal (1.2 L) for dispensers in rooms<br>(b) 0.53 gal (2.0 L) for dispensers in suites of rooms<br>(3) Dispensers shall be separated from each other by horizontal spacing of not less than 48 in. (1220 mm).<br>(4) Storage of quantities greater than 5 gal (18.9 L) in a single fire compartment shall meet the requirements of NFPA 30, *Flammable and Combustible Liquids Code.*<br>(5) Dispensers shall not be installed over or directly adjacent to an ignition source.<br>(6) Dispensers installed directly over carpeted floors shall be permitted only in sprinklered rooms or spaces. | New provision |
| **17.6.2.6.1** Travel distance shall be measured in accordance with Section 7.6. | New provision — no technical change |
| **17.6.3.2.1 Alcohol-Based Hand-Rub Dispensers.** Alcohol based hand-rub dispensers shall be protected in accordance with 8.7.3, unless all of the following conditions are met:<br>(1) Dispensers shall be installed in rooms or spaces separated from corridors and exits.<br>(2) The maximum individual dispenser fluid capacity shall be as follows:<br>(a) 0.32 gal (1.2 L) for dispensers in rooms<br>(b) 0.53 gal (2.0 L) for dispensers in suites of rooms<br>(3) Dispensers shall be separated from each other by horizontal spacing of not less than 48 in. (1220 mm).<br>(4) Storage of quantities greater than 5 gal (18.9 L) in a single fire compartment shall meet the requirements of NFPA 30, *Flammable and Combustible Liquids Code.*<br>(5) Dispensers shall not be installed over or directly adjacent to an ignition source.<br>(6) Dispensers installed directly over carpeted floors shall be permitted only in sprinklered rooms or spaces. | New provision |
| **17.6.3.4.3** Single-station or multiple-station smoke alarms or smoke detectors shall be provided in all rooms used for sleeping in accordance with 9.6.2.10, other than as permitted by 17.6.3.4.4. | New provision |
| **17.7.3.4 Inspection of Door Openings.** Door openings shall be inspected in accordance with 7.2.1.15. | New provision |

| Subject / 2009 Edition Text | Notes |
|---|---|
| **17.7.4.4** The provision of 10.3.2 for cigarette ignition resistance of newly introduced upholstered furniture and mattresses shall not apply to day-care homes. | Provision revised so only day-care homes are exempted, not day-care occupancies |
| **17.7.5* Day-Care Staff.** Adequate adult staff shall be on duty in the facility and alert at all times where clients are present. | Provision revised to delete reference to "awake" |
| **Chapter 18 New Health Care Occupancies**<br>**18.1.1.1.5*** It shall be recognized that, in buildings housing certain patients, it might be necessary to lock doors and bar windows to confine and protect building inhabitants. | Provision simplified for correlation with 18.2.2.2.4 through 18.2.2.2.5.2 |
| **18.1.1.4.2 Changes of Use or Occupancy Classification.** Changes of use or occupancy classification shall comply with 4.6.12, unless otherwise permitted by the following:<br>(1) A change from a hospital to a nursing home or from a nursing home to a hospital shall not be considered a change in occupancy classification or a change in use.<br>(2) A change from a hospital or nursing home to a limited care facility shall not be considered a change in occupancy classification or a change in use.<br>(3) A change from a hospital or nursing home to an ambulatory health care facility shall not be considered a change in occupancy classification or a change in use. | Former item (1) deleted ~~[(1) A change from one health care occupancy subclassification to another shall require compliance with the requirements for new construction]~~ for correlation with Chapter 43<br>Remainder revised to have application to change of use, as well as change of occupancy classification |
| **18.1.2.2*** Sections of health care facilities shall be permitted to be classified as other occupancies, provided that they meet all of the following conditions:<br>(1) They are not intended to serve health care occupants for purposes of housing, treatment, or customary access by patients incapable of self-preservation.<br>(2) They are separated from areas of health care occupancies by construction having a minimum 2-hour fire resistance rating in accordance with 8.2.1.3.<br>(3) The construction type and supporting construction of the health care occupancy is based on the story on which it is located in the building in accordance with the provisions of 18.1.6 and Table 18.1.6.1.<br>(4) The construction type of the areas of the building enclosing the other occupancies is based on the applicable occupancy chapters of this *Code*. | Item (2) revised, via reference to 8.2.1.3, to require separating barrier to be vertically aligned (i.e., not a floor/ceiling assembly, but a wall)<br>Items (3) and (4) are new |
| **18.1.6 Minimum Construction Requirements.** | Former 18.1.6.1 through 18.1.6.4 deleted, related to counting stories and primary level of exit discharge (LED) — per 3.3.77.1, building can have only one LED |
| **Table 18.1.6.1 Construction Type Limitations** | Table reformatted, but no technical change |
| **18.2.2.2.2** Locks shall not be permitted on patient sleeping room doors, unless otherwise permitted by the following:<br>(1) Key-locking devices that restrict access to the room from the corridor and that are operable only by staff from the corridor side shall be permitted, provided that such devices do not restrict egress from the room.<br>(2) Locks complying with 18.2.2.2.5 shall be permitted. | Item (2) is new |
| **18.2.2.2.4** Doors within a required means of egress shall not be equipped with a latch or lock that requires the use of a tool or key from the egress side, unless otherwise permitted by the following:<br>(1) Locks complying with 18.2.2.2.5 shall be permitted.<br>(2)*Delayed-egress locks complying with 7.2.1.6.1 shall be permitted.<br>(3)*Access-controlled egress doors complying with 7.2.1.6.2 shall be permitted.<br>(4) Elevator lobby exit access door locking in accordance with 7.2.1.6.3 shall be permitted. | Provisions on door locking expanded to include locking for specialized protective measures for patient safety (e.g., infant abduction concerns); delayed egress locking provision revised to remove former limitation of one such device per egress path |

| Subject / 2009 Edition Text | Notes |
|---|---|
| **18.2.2.2.5** Door-locking arrangements shall be permitted in accordance with either 18.2.2.2.5.1 or 18.2.2.2.5.2.<br>**18.2.2.2.5.1*** Door-locking arrangements shall be permitted where the clinical needs of patients require specialized security measures or where patients pose a security threat, provided that one of the following criteria is met:<br>(1) Staff can readily unlock doors at all times in accordance with 18.2.2.2.6.<br>(2) The provisions of 18.2.2.2.5.2 are met.<br>**18.2.2.2.5.2** Door-locking arrangements shall be permitted where patient special needs require specialized protective measures for their safety, provided that all of the following criteria are met:<br>(1) Staff can readily unlock doors at all times in accordance with 18.2.2.2.6.<br>(2) A total (complete) smoke detection system is provided throughout the locked space in accordance with 9.6.2.9, or locked doors can be remotely unlocked at an approved, constantly attended location within the locked space.<br>(3)*The building is protected throughout by an approved, supervised automatic sprinkler system in accordance with 18.3.5.1.<br>(4) The locks are electrical locks that fail safely so as to release upon loss of power to the device.<br>(5) The locks release by independent activation of each of the following:<br>(a) Activation of the smoke detection system required by 18.2.2.2.5.2(2)<br>(b) Waterflow in the automatic sprinkler system required by 18.2.2.2.5.2(3) | |
| **18.2.2.2.10.2** Horizontal-sliding doors serving an occupant load of fewer than 10 shall be permitted, provided that all of the following criteria are met:<br>. . .<br>(5) Where corridor doors are required to latch, the doors are equipped with a latch or other mechanism that ensures that the doors will not rebound into a partially open position if forcefully closed. | Item (5) revised to have application only where corridor doors are required to latch |
| **18.2.4.1** Not less than two exits shall be provided on every story.<br>**18.2.4.2** Not less than two separate exits shall be accessible from every part of every story. | New provisions |
| **18.2.5.3 Common Path of Travel.** Common path of travel shall not exceed 100 ft (30 m). | New provision |
| **18.2.5.5.2** Non-sleeping rooms of more than 2500 ft$^2$ (230 m$^2$) shall have not less than two exit access doors remotely located from each other. | Reinsertion of provision inadvertently removed for 2006 edition |
| **18.2.5.7.1.2* Suite Separation.** Suites shall be separated from the remainder of the building, and from other suites, by walls and doors meeting the requirements of 18.3.6.2 through 18.3.6.5. | Provision expanded to require separation from adjacent suites, not just non-suite spaces |
| **18.2.5.7.2 Sleeping Suites.** Sleeping suites shall be in accordance with the following:<br>(1) Sleeping suites for patient care shall comply with the provisions of 18.2.5.7.2.1 through 18.2.5.7.2.4.<br>(2) Sleeping suites not for patient care shall comply with the provisions of 18.2.5.7.4. | New roadmap to steer user to correct subsection depending on whether sleeping suite is for patient care |
| **18.2.5.7.2.3 Sleeping Suite Maximum Size.**<br>**(A)** . . .<br>**(B)** Sleeping suites greater than 5000 ft$^2$ (460 m$^2$) and not exceeding 7500 ft$^2$ (700 m$^2$) shall be permitted where both of the following are provided in the suite:<br>(1)* Direct visual supervision in accordance with 18.2.5.7.2.1(C)(1)(a)<br>(2) Total coverage (complete) automatic smoke detection in accordance with 9.6.2.9 and 18.3.4 | Item (B)(1) revised to reference supervision requirement without permitting exemption for spaces protected by smoke detection |

| Subject / 2009 Edition Text | Notes |
|---|---|
| **18.2.5.7.3 Non-Sleeping Suites.** Non-sleeping suites shall be in accordance with the following:<br>(1) Non-sleeping suites for patient care shall comply with the provisions of 18.2.5.7.3.1 through 18.2.5.7.3.4.<br>(2) Non-sleeping suites not for patient care shall comply with the provisions of 18.2.5.7.4. | New roadmap to steer user to correct subsection depending on whether non-sleeping suite is for patient care |
| **18.2.5.7.4 Non-Patient-Care Suites.** The egress provisions for non-patient-care suites shall be in accordance with the primary use and occupancy of the space, except that in no case shall the maximum travel distance to an exit from within the suite exceed 200 ft (61 m). | New provision |
| **18.2.6 Travel Distance.**<br>[former] ~~18.2.6.2.1 The travel distance between any room door required as an exit access and an exit shall not exceed 150 ft (46 m).~~ | Provision deleted |
| **Table 18.3.2.1 Hazardous Area Protection** | Entries for soiled linen and collected trash revised to include volume threshold for protection as a hazardous area |
| **18.3.2.6* Alcohol-Based Hand-Rub Dispensers.** Alcohol-based hand-rub dispensers shall be protected in accordance with 8.7.3, unless all of the following conditions are met:<br>(1) Where dispensers are installed in a corridor, the corridor shall have a minimum width of 6 ft (1830 mm).<br>(2) The maximum individual dispenser fluid capacity shall be as follows:<br>(a) 0.32 gal (1.2 L) for dispensers in rooms, corridors, and areas open to corridors<br>(b) 0.53 gal (2.0 L) for dispensers in suites of rooms<br>(3) Where aerosol containers are used, the maximum capacity of the aerosol dispenser shall be 18 oz. (0.51 kg) and shall be limited to Level 1 aerosols as defined in NFPA 30B, *Code for the Manufacture and Storage of Aerosol Products*.<br>(4) Dispensers shall be separated from each other by horizontal spacing of not less than 48 in. (1220 mm).<br>(5) Not more than an aggregate 10 gal (37.8 L) of alcohol based hand-rub solution or 1135 oz (32.2 kg) of Level 1 aerosols, or a combination of liquids and Level 1 aerosols not to exceed, in total, the equivalent of 10 gal (37.8 L) or 1135 oz (32.2 kg,) shall be in use outside of a storage cabinet in a single smoke compartment.<br>(6) Storage of quantities greater than 5 gal (18.9 L) in a single smoke compartment shall meet the requirements of NFPA 30, *Flammable and Combustible Liquids Code*.<br>(7) Dispensers shall not be installed in the following locations:<br>(a) Above an ignition source for a horizontal distance of 1 in. (25 mm) to each side of the ignition source<br>(b) To the side of an ignition source within a 1 in. (25 mm) horizontal distance from the ignition source<br>(c) Beneath an ignition source within a 1 in. (25 mm) vertical distance from the ignition source<br>(8) Dispensers installed directly over carpeted floors shall be permitted only in sprinklered smoke compartments. | Item (3) is new and recognizes aerosol dispensers<br><br>Item (5) revised to set maximum quantity for aerosol products<br><br>Item (7) replaces former requirement that dispensers not be installed over or directly adjacent to an ignition source |
| **18.3.4.3.3.3** The provision of 9.6.7.4.3, which permits sprinkler system waterflow to be annunciated as a single building zone, shall be prohibited. | New provision |
| **18.3.6.3.5** Doors shall be self-latching and provided with positive latching hardware. | Provision expanded to require self-latching, not only positive latching |
| **18.3.6.3.6** Doors to toilet rooms, bathrooms, shower rooms, sink closets, and similar auxiliary spaces that do not contain flammable or combustible materials shall not be required to meet the latching requirements of 18.3.6.3.5. | Provision revised to clarify that exemption applies to both the self-latching and positive latching requirement of 18.3.6.3.5 |

| Subject / 2009 Edition Text | Notes |
|---|---|
| **18.3.6.3.7** Powered doors that comply with the requirements of 7.2.1.9 shall not be required to meet the latching requirements of 18.3.6.3.5, provided that:<br>(1) The door is equipped with a means for keeping the door closed that is acceptable to the authority having jurisdiction<br>(2) The device used is capable of keeping the door fully closed if a force of 5 lbf (22N) is applied at the latch edge of a swinging door and applied in any direction to a sliding or folding door. | New provision |
| **18.3.6.3.8** Corridor doors utilizing an inactive leaf shall have automatic flush bolts on the inactive leaf to provide positive latching. | New provision |
| [former] ~~18.3.7.3 Smoke barriers shall be provided on stories that are usable but unoccupied.~~ | Provision deleted |
| **18.3.8 Special Protection Features. (Reserved)**<br>[former] ~~**18.3.8* Special Protection Features — Outside Window or Door.**~~<br>~~**18.3.8.1** Every patient sleeping room shall have an outside window or outside door, unless otherwise permitted by the following:~~<br>~~(1) This requirement shall not apply to newborn nurseries and rooms intended for occupancy for less than 24 hours, such as those housing obstetrical labor beds, recovery beds, and observation beds in the emergency department.~~<br>~~(2) Windows in atrium walls shall be considered outside windows for the purposes of this requirement.~~<br>~~**18.3.8.2** Where windows are required by 18.3.8.1, the allowable sill height shall not exceed 36 in. (915 mm) above the floor, unless otherwise permitted by the following~~<br>~~(1) The window sill in special nursing care areas, such as those housing ICU, CCU, hemodialysis, and neonatal patients, shall not exceed 60 in. (1525 mm) above the floor.~~<br>~~(2) The window sill in limited care facilities shall not exceed 44 in. (1120 mm) above the floor.~~ | Provision deleted |
| **18.4.3 Nonsprinklered Existing Smoke Compartment Rehabilitation.**<br>**Table 18.4.3.2 Construction Type Limitations (Nonsprinklered Buildings)** | Table reformatted, but no technical change |
| **18.5.4 Rubbish Chutes, Incinerators, and Laundry Chutes.**<br>. . .<br>**18.5.4.2*** The fire resistance rating of chute charging rooms and chute discharging rooms shall not be required to exceed 1 hour. | New provision |
| **18.7.4* Smoking.** Smoking regulations shall be adopted and shall include not less than the following provisions:<br>(1) Smoking shall be prohibited in any room, ward, or individual enclosed space where flammable liquids, combustible gases, or oxygen is used or stored and in any other hazardous location, and such areas shall be posted with signs that read NO SMOKING or shall be posted with the international symbol for no smoking.<br>. . . | Item (1) revised to apply to an individual enclosed space |
| **18.7.7 Engineered Smoke Control Systems.**<br>**18.7.7.1** New engineered smoke control systems shall be designed, installed, tested, and maintained in accordance with NFPA 92A, *Standard for Smoke-Control Systems Utilizing Barriers and Pressure Differences*, and NFPA 92B, *Standard for Smoke Management Systems in Malls, Atria, and Large Spaces*, as applicable. | Provision revised to require compliance with NFPA 92A and NFPA 92B |
| **Chapter 19 Existing Health Care Occupancies**<br>**19.1.1.1.5*** It shall be recognized that, in buildings housing certain patients, it might be necessary to lock doors and bar windows to confine and protect building inhabitants. | Provision simplified for correlation with 19.2.2.2.4 through 19.2.2.2.5.2 |

| Subject / 2009 Edition Text | Notes |
|---|---|
| **19.1.1.4.2 Changes of Use or Occupancy Classification.** Changes of use or occupancy classification shall comply with 4.6.12, unless otherwise permitted by the following:<br>(1) A change from a hospital to a nursing home or from a nursing home to a hospital shall not be considered a change in occupancy classification or a change in use.<br>(2) A change from a hospital or nursing home to a limited care facility shall not be considered a change in occupancy classification or a change in use.<br>(3) A change from a hospital or nursing home to an ambulatory health care facility shall not be considered a change in occupancy classification or a change in use. | Former item (1) deleted ~~[(1) A change from one health care occupancy subclassification to another shall require compliance with the requirements for new construction]~~ for correlation with Chapter 43<br>Remainder revised to have application to change of use, as well as change of occupancy classification |
| **19.1.2.2*** Sections of health care facilities shall be permitted to be classified as other occupancies, provided that they meet all of the following conditions:<br>(1) They are not intended to serve health care occupants for purposes of housing, treatment, or customary access by patients incapable of self-preservation.<br>(2) They are separated from areas of health care occupancies by construction having a minimum 2-hour fire resistance rating in accordance with 8.2.1.3.<br>(3) The construction type and supporting construction of the health care occupancy is based on the story on which it is located in the building in accordance with the provisions of 19.1.6 and Table 19.1.6.1.<br>(4) The construction type of the areas of the building enclosing the other occupancies is based on the applicable occupancy chapters of this *Code*.<br>(5) For other than previously approved occupancy separation arrangements, the entire building is protected throughout by an approved, supervised automatic sprinkler system in accordance with Section 9.7. | Item (2) revised, via reference to 8.2.1.3, to require separating barrier to be vertically aligned (i.e., not a floor/ceiling assembly, but a wall)<br>Items (3) through (5) are new |
| **19.1.6 Minimum Construction Requirements.** | Former 19.1.6.1 through 19.1.6.4 deleted, related to counting stories and primary level of exit discharge (LED) — per 3.3.77.1, building can have only one LED |
| **Table 19.1.6.1 Construction Type Limitations** | Table reformatted, but no technical change |
| **19.2.2.2.2** Locks shall not be permitted on patient sleeping room doors, unless otherwise permitted by the following:<br>(1) Key-locking devices that restrict access to the room from the corridor and that are operable only by staff from the corridor side shall be permitted, provided that such devices do not restrict egress from the room.<br>(2) Locks complying with 19.2.2.2.5 shall be permitted. | Item (2) is new |
| **19.2.2.2.4** Doors within a required means of egress shall not be equipped with a latch or lock that requires the use of a tool or key from the egress side, unless otherwise permitted by the following:<br>(1) Locks complying with 19.2.2.2.5 shall be permitted.<br>(2)* Delayed-egress locks complying with 7.2.1.6.1 shall be permitted.<br>(3)* Access-controlled egress doors complying with 7.2.1.6.2 shall be permitted.<br>(4) Elevator lobby exit access door locking in accordance with 7.2.1.6.3 shall be permitted.<br>(5) Approved existing door-locking installations shall be permitted.<br>**19.2.2.2.5** Door-locking arrangements shall be permitted in accordance with either 19.2.2.2.5.1 or 19.2.2.2.5.2.<br>**19.2.2.2.5.1*** Door-locking arrangements shall be permitted where the clinical needs of patients require specialized security measures or where patients pose a security threat, provided that one of the following criteria is met:<br>(1) Staff can readily unlock doors at all times in accordance with 19.2.2.2.6.<br>(2) The provisions of 19.2.2.2.5.2 are met. | Provisions on door locking expanded to include locking for specialized protective measures for patient safety (e.g., infant abduction concerns); delayed egress locking provision revised to remove former limitation of one such device per egress path |

| Subject / 2009 Edition Text | Notes |
|---|---|
| **19.2.2.2.5.2*** Door-locking arrangements shall be permitted where patient special needs require specialized protective measures for their safety, provided that all of the following are met:<br>(1) Staff can readily unlock doors at all times in accordance with 19.2.2.2.6.<br>(2) A total (complete) smoke detection system is provided throughout the locked space in accordance with 9.6.2.9, or locked doors can be remotely unlocked at an approved, constantly attended location within the locked space.<br>(3)* The building is protected throughout by an approved, supervised automatic sprinkler system in accordance with 19.3.5.1.<br>(4) The locks are electrical locks that fail safely so as to release upon loss of power to the device.<br>(5) The locks release by independent activation of each of the following:<br>(a) Activation of the smoke detection system required by 19.2.2.2.5.2(2)<br>(b) Waterflow in the automatic sprinkler system required by 19.2.2.2.5.2(3) | |
| **19.2.2.2.10.2** Horizontal-sliding doors serving an occupant load of fewer than 10 shall be permitted, provided that all of the following criteria are met:<br>. . .<br>(5) Where corridor doors are required to latch, the doors are equipped with a latch or other mechanism that ensures that the doors will not rebound into a partially open position if forcefully closed. | Item (5) revised to have application only where corridor doors are required to latch |
| **19.2.4.1** Not less than two exits shall be provided on every story.<br>**19.2.4.2** Not less than two separate exits shall be accessible from every part of every story. | New provisions |
| **19.2.5.2* Dead-End Corridors.** Existing dead-end corridors not exceeding 30 ft (9.1 m) shall be permitted. Existing dead-end corridors exceeding 30 ft (9.1 m) shall be permitted to continue in use if it is impractical and unfeasible to alter them. | Provision revised to permit existing dead-end corridors not exceeding that permitted for new construction to remain in use |
| **19.2.5.5.2** Non-sleeping rooms of more than 2500 $ft^2$ (230 $m^2$) shall have not less than two exit access doors remotely located from each other. | Reinsertion of provision inadvertently removed for 2006 edition |
| **19.2.5.7.1.2* Suite Separation.** Suites shall be separated from the remainder of the building, and from other suites, by one of the following: | Provision expanded to require separation from adjacent suites, not just non-suite spaces |
| **19.2.5.7.2 Sleeping Suites.** Sleeping suites shall be in accordance with the following:<br>(1) Sleeping suites for patient care shall comply with the provisions of 19.2.5.7.2.1 through 19.2.5.7.2.4.<br>(2) Sleeping suites not for patient care shall comply with the provisions of 19.2.5.7.4. | New roadmap to steer user to correct subsection depending on whether sleeping suite is for patient care |
| **19.2.5.7.3 Non-Sleeping Suites.** Non-sleeping suites shall be in accordance with the following:<br>(1) Non-sleeping suites for patient care shall comply with the provisions of 19.2.5.7.3.1 through 19.2.5.7.3.4.<br>(2) Non-sleeping suites not for patient care shall comply with the provisions of 19.2.5.7.4 | New roadmap to steer user to correct subsection depending on whether non-sleeping suite is for patient care |
| **19.2.5.7.4 Non-Patient-Care Suites.** The egress provisions for non-patient-care suites shall be in accordance with the primary use and occupancy of the space, except that in no case shall the maximum travel distance to an exit from within the suite exceed 200 ft (61 m). | New provision |
| **19.2.6 Travel Distance.**<br>[former] ~~**19.2.6.2.1** The travel distance between any room door required as an exit access and an exit shall not exceed 100 ft (30 m), unless otherwise permitted by 19.2.6.2.2.~~<br>~~**19.2.6.2.2** The maximum travel distance specified in 19.2.6.2.1 shall be permitted to be increased by 50 ft (15 m) in buildings protected throughout by an approved, supervised automatic sprinkler system in accordance with 19.3.5.6.~~ | Provisions deleted |

| Subject / 2009 Edition Text | Notes |
|---|---|
| **19.3.2.1.5** Hazardous areas shall include, but shall not be restricted to, the following:<br>. . .<br>(5) Rooms with soiled linen in volume exceeding 64 gal (242 L)<br>(6) Rooms with collected trash in volume exceeding 64 gal (242 L) | Items (5) and (6) for soiled linen and collected trash revised to include volume threshold for protection as a hazardous area |
| **19.3.2.6* Alcohol-Based Hand-Rub Dispensers.** Alcohol-based hand-rub dispensers shall be protected in accordance with 8.7.3, unless all of the following conditions are met:<br>(1) Where dispensers are installed in a corridor, the corridor shall have a minimum width of 6 ft (1830 mm).<br>(2) The maximum individual dispenser fluid capacity shall be as follows:<br>(a) 0.32 gal (1.2 L) for dispensers in rooms, corridors, and areas open to corridors<br>(b) 0.53 gal (2.0 L) for dispensers in suites of rooms<br>(3) Where aerosol containers are used, the maximum capacity of the aerosol dispenser shall be 18 oz. (0.51 kg) and shall be limited to Level 1 aerosols as defined in NFPA 30B, *Code for the Manufacture and Storage of Aerosol Products*.<br>(4) Dispensers shall be separated from each other by horizontal spacing of not less than 48 in. (1220 mm).<br>(5) Not more than an aggregate 10 gal (37.8 L) of alcohol-based hand-rub solution or 1135 oz (32.2 kg) of Level 1 aerosols, or a combination of liquids and Level 1 aerosols not to exceed, in total, the equivalent of 10 gal (37.8 L) or 1135 oz (32.2 kg,) shall be in use outside of a storage cabinet in a single smoke compartment.<br>(6) Storage of quantities greater than 5 gal (18.9 L) in a single smoke compartment shall meet the requirements of NFPA 30, *Flammable and Combustible Liquids Code*.<br>(7) Dispensers shall not be installed in the following locations:<br>(a) Above an ignition source for a horizontal distance of 1 in. (25 mm) to each side of the ignition source<br>(b) To the side of an ignition source within a 1 in. (25 mm) horizontal distance from the ignition source<br>(c) Beneath an ignition source within a 1 in. (25 mm) vertical distance from the ignition source<br>(8) Dispensers installed directly over carpeted floors shall be permitted only in sprinklered smoke compartments. | Item (3) is new and recognizes aerosol dispensers<br><br>Item (5) revised to set maximum quantity for aerosol products<br><br>Item (7) replaces former requirement that dispensers not be installed over or directly adjacent to an ignition source |
| **19.3.5.2** High-rise buildings shall comply with 19.4.2. | New provision |
| **19.3.6.3.7** Powered doors that comply with the requirements of 7.2.1.9 shall be considered as complying with the requirements of 19.3.6.3.5 provided the door is equipped with a means for keeping the door closed that is acceptable to the authority having jurisdiction and the device used is capable of keeping the door fully closed if a force of 5 lbf (22N) is applied at the latch edge of a swinging door and applied in any direction to a sliding or folding door. | New provision |
| **19.3.8 Special Protection Features. (Reserved)**<br>[former] ~~**19.3.8* Special Protection Features — Outside Window or Door.** Every patient sleeping room shall have an outside window or outside door, unless otherwise permitted by the following:~~<br>~~(1) This requirement shall not apply to newborn nurseries and rooms intended for occupancy for less than 24 hours, such as those housing obstetrical labor beds, recovery beds, and observation beds in the emergency department.~~<br>~~(2) Windows in atrium walls shall be considered outside windows for the purposes of this requirement.~~ | Provision deleted |
| **19.4.2 High-Rise Buildings.** All high-rise buildings containing health care occupancies shall be protected throughout by an approved, supervised automatic sprinkler system installed in accordance with Section 9.7 within 12 years of the adoption of this *Code*. | New provision |

| Subject / 2009 Edition Text | Notes |
|---|---|
| **19.7.4* Smoking.** Smoking regulations shall be adopted and shall include not less than the following provisions:<br>(1) Smoking shall be prohibited in any room, ward, or individual enclosed space where flammable liquids, combustible gases, or oxygen is used or stored and in any other hazardous location, and such areas shall be posted with signs that read NO SMOKING or shall be posted with the international symbol for no smoking.<br>. . . | Item (1) revised to apply to an individual enclosed space |
| **Chapter 20 New Ambulatory Health Care Occupancies**<br>**20.1.6.1** Ambulatory health care occupancies shall be limited to the building construction types specified in Table 20.1.6.1, unless otherwise permitted by 20.1.6.6. *(See 8.2.1.)*<br>. . .<br>**Table 20.1.6.1 Construction Type Limitations** | Provision, and associated Table 20.1.6.1, revised so that it is applied based on number of stories in height — no technical change intended |
| **20.2.2.3** Elevator lobby exit access door locking in accordance with 7.2.1.6.3 shall be permitted. | New provision |
| **20.3.2.6* Alcohol-Based Hand-Rub Dispensers.** Alcohol-based hand-rub dispensers shall be protected in accordance with 8.7.3, unless all of the following conditions are met:<br>(1) Where dispensers are installed in a corridor, the corridor shall have a minimum width of 6 ft (1830 mm).<br>(2) The maximum individual dispenser fluid capacity shall be as follows:<br>(a) 0.32 gal (1.2 L) for dispensers in rooms, corridors, and areas open to corridors<br>(b) 0.53 gal (2.0 L) for dispensers in suites of rooms<br>(3) Dispensers shall be separated from one another by horizontal spacing of not less than 48 in. (1220 mm).<br>(4) Not more than an aggregate 10 gal (37.8 L) of alcohol-based hand-rub solution shall be in use outside of a storage cabinet in a single smoke compartment.<br>(5) Storage of quantities greater than 5 gal (18.9 L) in a single smoke compartment shall meet the requirements of NFPA 30, *Flammable and Combustible Liquids Code.*<br>(6) Dispensers shall not be installed in the following locations:<br>(a) Above an ignition source for a horizontal distance of 1 in. (25 mm) to each side of the ignition source<br>(b) To the side of an ignition source within a 1 in. (25 mm) horizontal distance from the ignition source<br>(c) Beneath an ignition source within a 1 in. (25 mm) vertical distance from the ignition source<br>. . . | Item (6) replaces former requirement that dispensers not be installed over or directly adjacent to an ignition source |
| **20.3.7.12** Vision panels in doors in smoke barriers, if provided, shall be of fire-rated glazing or wired glass in approved frames. | Provision revised to remove requirement that vision panels be provided |
| **20.7.5.2** Newly introduced upholstered furniture shall comply with 10.3.2.1 and one of the following provisions:<br>. . .<br>**20.7.5.3** Newly introduced mattresses shall comply with 10.3.2.2 and one of the following provisions:<br>. . . | Provisions revised to require cigarette ignition resistance testing |
| **Chapter 21 Existing Ambulatory Health Care Occupancies**<br>**21.1.6.1** Ambulatory health care occupancies shall be limited to the building construction types specified in Table 21.1.6.1, unless otherwise permitted by 21.1.6.6. *(See 8.2.1.)*<br>**Table 21.1.6.1 Construction Type Limitations** | Provision, and associated Table 21.1.6.1, revised so that it is applied based on number of stories in height — no technical change intended |

| Subject / 2009 Edition Text | Notes |
|---|---|
| **21.2.2.3** Elevator lobby exit access door locking in accordance with 7.2.1.6.3 shall be permitted. | New provision |
| **21.3.2.6* Alcohol-Based Hand-Rub Dispensers.** Alcohol-based hand-rub dispensers shall be protected in accordance with 8.7.3, unless all of the following conditions are met:<br>(1) Where dispensers are installed in a corridor, the corridor shall have a minimum width of 6 ft (1830 mm).<br>(2) The maximum individual dispenser fluid capacity shall be as follows:<br>(a) 0.32 gal (1.2 L) for dispensers in rooms, corridors, and areas open to corridors<br>(b) 0.53 gal (2.0 L) for dispensers in suites of rooms<br>(3) Dispensers shall be separated from one another by horizontal spacing of not less than 48 in. (1220 mm).<br>(4) Not more than an aggregate 10 gal (37.8 L) of alcohol-based hand-rub solution shall be in use outside of a storage cabinet in a single smoke compartment.<br>(5) Storage of quantities greater then 5 gal (18.9 L) in a single smoke compartment shall meet the requirements of NFPA 30, *Flammable and Combustible Liquids Code*.<br>(6) Dispensers shall not be installed in the following locations:<br>(a) Above an ignition source for a horizontal distance of 1 in. (25 mm) to each side of the ignition source<br>(b) To the side of an ignition source within a 1 in. (25 mm) horizontal distance from the ignition source<br>(c) Beneath an ignition source within a 1 in. (25 mm) vertical distance from the ignition source<br>. . . | Item (6) replaces requirement that dispensers not be installed over or directly adjacent to an ignition source |
| [former] ~~**21.3.7.11** A vision panel of fire-rated glazing or wired glass panels shall be required in smoke barrier cross-corridor doors.~~ | Provision deleted |
| **21.7.5.2** Newly introduced upholstered furniture shall comply with 10.3.2.1 and one of the following provisions:<br>. . .<br>**21.7.5.3** Newly introduced mattresses shall comply with 10.3.2.2 and one of the following provisions:<br>. . . | Provisions revised to require cigarette ignition resistance testing |
| **Chapter 22 New Detention and Correctional Occupancies**<br>**22.1.6 Minimum Construction Requirements.**<br>**22.1.6.1** Detention and correctional occupancies shall be limited to the building construction types specified in Table 22.1.6.1. *(See 8.2.1.)*<br>. . .<br>**Table 22.1.6.1 Construction Type Limitations** | Former 22.1.6.1 through 22.1.6.3 deleted, related to counting stories and primary level of exit discharge (LED) — per 3.3.77.1, building can have only one LED<br>Table 22.1.6.1, revised so that it is applied based on number of stories in height — no technical change intended |
| **22.2.6.1** Travel distance shall be measured in accordance with Section 7.6. | New provision — no technical change |
| **22.3.4.2.2*** Use of the provision of 9.6.1.8.1.3 shall be permitted only as an exemption to 9.6.1.8.1(2) and (3). | New provision |
| **22.4.4 Nonsprinklered Existing Building Renovations.**<br>. . .<br>**Table 22.4.4.2.1 Construction Type Limitations — Nonsprinklered Buildings** | Table 22.4.4.2.1, revised so that it is applied based on number of stories in height — no technical change intended |

| Subject / 2009 Edition Text | Notes |
|---|---|
| **22.7.4.2** Newly introduced upholstered furniture within detention and correctional occupancies shall be tested in accordance with the provisions of 10.3.2.1(2).<br>**22.7.4.3** Newly introduced mattresses within detention and correctional occupancies shall be tested in accordance with the provisions of 10.3.2.2. | Provisions revised to require cigarette ignition resistance testing |
| **Chapter 23 Existing Detention and Correctional Occupancies** | |
| **23.1.6 Minimum Construction Requirements.**<br>**23.1.6.1** Detention and correctional occupancies shall be limited to the building construction types specified in Table 23.1.6.1. *(See 8.2.1.)*<br>. . . | Former 23.1.6.1 through 23.1.6.4 deleted, related to counting stories and primary level of exit discharge (LED) — per 3.3.77.1, building can have only one LED |
| **Table 23.1.6.1 Construction Type Limitations** | Table 23.1.6.1, revised so that it is applied based on number of stories in height — no technical change intended |
| **23.2.6.1** Travel distance shall be measured in accordance with Section 7.6. | New provision — no technical change |
| [former] ~~**23.3.4.1.2** Existing systems lacking the monitoring of wiring required by 9.6.1.5 shall be permitted to be continued in use in buildings protected by a complete automatic extinguishing system.~~ | Provision deleted |
| **23.3.4.2.2*** Use of the provision of 9.6.1.8.1.3 shall be permitted only as an exemption to 9.6.1.8.1(2) and (3). | New Provision |
| **Chapter 24 One- and Two-Family Dwellings** | |
| **24.2.4.8** Floor levels at doors in the primary means of escape shall comply with 7.2.1.3, unless otherwise permitted by the following: | |
| (1) In existing buildings, where the door discharges to the outside or to an exterior balcony or exterior exit access, the floor level outside the door shall be permitted to be one step lower than the inside, but shall not be in excess of 8 in. (205 mm). | Item (1) revised to be limited to existing buildings |
| (2) In new buildings, where the door discharges to the outside or to an exterior exit access, an exterior landing with not more than a 7 in. (180 mm) drop below the door threshold and a minimum dimension of 36 in. (915 mm) or the width of the door leaf, whichever is smaller, shall be permitted. | Item (2) is new and addresses landings at doors in new buildings |
| (3) A door at the top of an interior stair shall be permitted to open directly at a stair, provided that the door does not swing over the stair and the door serves an area with an occupant load of fewer than 50 persons. | Item (3) revised to be limited to doors at interior stair |
| **24.3.4.1*** Smoke alarms shall be installed in accordance with 9.6.2.10 in the following locations:<br>(1) All sleeping rooms<br>. . . | Item (1) is new |
| **Chapter 26 Lodging or Rooming Houses** | |
| **26.3.4.5.2** In other than existing buildings, the smoke alarms required by 26.3.4.5.1 shall be interconnected in accordance with 9.6.2.10.3. | Provision revised to require interconnection only in new buildings |
| **26.3.4.6* Protection of Fire Alarm System.** The provision of 9.6.1.8.1.3 shall not apply to the smoke detection required at each fire alarm control unit by 9.6.1.8.1(1). | New provision |
| **Chapter 28 New Hotels and Dormitories** | |
| **28.2.2.2.2.4** Elevator lobby exit access door locking in accordance with 7.2.1.6.3 shall be permitted. | New provision |

| Subject / 2009 Edition Text | Notes |
|---|---|
| **28.2.6.3.3.2** Where the building is not protected throughout by an approved, supervised automatic sprinkler system, the 200 ft (61 m) travel distance shall be permitted within any portion of the building that is protected by an approved, supervised automatic sprinkler system, provided that the sprinklered portion of the building is separated from any nonsprinklered portion by fire barriers having a fire resistance rating as follows:<br>(1) Minimum 1-hour fire resistance rating for buildings three or fewer stories in height<br>(2) Minimum 2-hour fire resistance rating for buildings four or more stories in height | Provision reworded for clarification — no technical change |
| **28.3.4.3.6** Emergency forces notification shall be provided in accordance with 9.6.4. | Provision revised to require compliance with 9.6.4 |
| **28.3.4.6* Protection of Fire Alarm System.** The provision of 9.6.1.8.1.3 shall not apply to the smoke detection required at each fire alarm control unit by 9.6.1.8.1(1). | New provision |
| **28.3.7.3** Doors in the barriers required by 28.3.7.1 and 28.3.7.2 shall have a fire protection rating of not less than 20 minutes and shall not be required to be self-closing. | New provision |
| **28.4.1.2*** Emergency plans in accordance with Section 4.8 shall be provided and shall include the following:<br>(1) Egress procedures<br>(2) Methods<br>(3) Preferred evacuation routes for each event, including appropriate use of elevators | New provision |
| **28.7.5 Emergency Plans.** Emergency plans in accordance with Section 4.8 shall be provided. | New provision |
| **28.7.6 Contents and Furnishings.**<br>[former] ~~**28.3.3.4.1** Contents and furnishings shall not be required to comply with Section 10.3.~~<br>. . .<br>**28.7.6.2 Upholstered Furniture and Mattresses.**<br>**28.7.6.2.1** Newly introduced upholstered furniture shall meet the criteria specified in 10.3.2.1 and 10.3.3.<br>**28.7.6.2.2** Newly introduced mattresses shall meet the criteria specified in 10.3.2.2 and 10.3.4. | Provision deleted; associated material relocated to 28.7.6<br><br>New provisions |
| **Chapter 29 Existing Hotels and Dormitories**<br>**29.2.2.2.2.4** Elevator lobby exit access door locking in accordance with 7.2.1.6.3 shall be permitted. | New provision |
| **29.2.6.3.3.2** Where the building is not protected throughout by an approved, supervised automatic sprinkler system, the 200 ft (61 m) travel distance shall be permitted within any portion of the building that is protected by an approved, supervised automatic sprinkler system, provided that the sprinklered portion of the building is separated from any nonsprinklered portion by fire barriers having a fire resistance rating as follows:<br>(1) Minimum 1-hour fire resistance rating for buildings three or fewer stories in height<br>(2) Minimum 2-hour fire resistance rating for buildings four or more stories in height | Provision reworded for clarification — no technical change |
| **29.3.4.6* Protection of Fire Alarm System.** The provision of 9.6.1.8.1.3 shall not apply to the smoke detection required at each fire alarm control unit by 9.6.1.8.1(1). | New provision |
| **29.3.7 Subdivision of Building Spaces.** In buildings other than those meeting the requirements of 29.3.7.1, 29.3.7.2, or 29.3.7.3, every guest room floor shall be divided into not less than two smoke compartments of approximately the same size by smoke partitions in accordance with Section 8.4.<br>**29.3.7.1** Smoke partitions shall not be required in buildings protected throughout by an approved automatic sprinkler system in accordance with 29.3.5 or a corridor sprinkler system conforming to 31.3.5.9 through 31.3.5.10. | Provisions revised to require smoke partitions rather than smoke barriers |

| Subject / 2009 Edition Text | Notes |
| --- | --- |
| **29.3.7.2** Smoke partitions shall not be required where each guest room is provided with exterior ways of exit access arranged in accordance with 7.5.3.<br>**29.3.7.3** Smoke partitions shall not be required where the aggregate corridor length on each floor is not more than 150 ft (46 m).<br>**29.3.7.4** Additional smoke partitions shall be provided so that the travel distance from a guest room corridor door to a smoke partition shall not exceed 150 ft (46 m). | |
| **29.4.1.2*** Emergency plans in accordance with Section 4.8 shall be provided and shall include the following:<br>(1) Egress procedures<br>(2) Methods<br>(3) Preferred evacuation routes for each event, including appropriate use of elevators | New provision |
| **29.7.5 Emergency Plans.** Emergency plans in accordance with Section 4.8 shall be provided. | New provision |
| **29.7.6 Contents and Furnishings.**<br>[former] ~~**29.3.3.4.1** Contents and furnishings shall not be required to comply with Section 10.3.~~ | Provision deleted; associated material relocated to 29.7.6 |
| . . .<br>**29.7.6.2 Upholstered Furniture and Mattresses.**<br>**29.7.6.2.1** Newly introduced upholstered furniture shall meet the criteria specified in 10.3.2.1 and 10.3.3.<br>**29.7.6.2.2** Newly introduced mattresses shall meet the criteria specified in 10.3.2.2 and 10.3.4. | New provisions |
| **Chapter 30 New Apartment Buildings** | |
| **30.2.2.2.2.4** Elevator lobby exit access door locking in accordance with 7.2.1.6.3 shall be permitted. | New provision |
| **30.2.6 Travel Distance to Exits.** Travel distance shall be measured in accordance with Section 7.6. | New provision — no technical change |
| [former] ~~**30.3.4.1.3** A fire alarm system shall not be required in buildings that are protected throughout by an approved automatic sprinkler system in accordance with 30.3.5.1, that do not exceed 4 stories in height, and that contain not more than 16 dwelling units.~~ | Provision deleted |
| **30.3.4.5* Smoke Alarms.** Smoke alarms shall be installed in accordance with 9.6.2.10 in every sleeping area, outside every sleeping area in the immediate vicinity of the bedrooms, and on all levels of the dwelling unit, including basements. | Provision revised to require smoke alarms in all sleeping areas |
| **30.3.4.6* Protection of Fire Alarm System.** The provision of 9.6.1.8.1.3 shall not apply to the smoke detection required at each fire alarm control unit by 9.6.1.8.1(1). | New provision |
| **30.3.5.1** All buildings shall be protected throughout by an approved, supervised automatic sprinkler system installed in accordance with 30.3.5.2.<br>[former] ~~**30.3.5.2** Sprinkler systems shall not be required in buildings where every dwelling unit provides one of the following:~~<br>~~(1) Exit door opening directly to the street or yard at ground level~~<br>~~(2) Direct access to an outside stair that complies with 7.2.2 and serves a maximum of two units, both located on the same floor~~<br>~~(3) Direct access to an interior stair serving only that unit and separated from all other portions of the building by fire barriers having a 1-hour fire resistance rating with no openings therein~~ | Provision revised to require new apartment buildings to be sprinklered, without exception |
| **30.4.1.2*** Emergency plans in accordance with Section 4.8 shall be provided and shall include the following: | New provision |

| Subject / 2009 Edition Text | Notes |
|---|---|
| (1) Egress procedures<br>(2) Methods<br>(3) Preferred evacuation routes for each event, including appropriate use of elevators | |
| **Chapter 31 Existing Apartment Buildings**<br>**31.2.2.2.2.4** Elevator lobby exit access door locking in accordance with 7.2.1.6.3 shall be permitted. | New provision |
| **31.2.6 Travel Distance to Exits.** Travel distance shall be measured in accordance with Section 7.6. | New provision — no technical change |
| **31.2.7 Discharge from Exits.** Exit discharge shall comply with Section 7.7.<br>[former] ~~**31.2.7.2** Any required exit stairway that is located so that it is necessary to pass through the lobby or other open space to reach the outside of the building shall be continuously enclosed to a level of exit discharge or to a mezzanine within a lobby at a level of exit discharge.~~<br>[former] ~~**31.2.7.3** The distance of travel from the termination of the exit enclosure to an exterior door leading to a public way shall not exceed 150 ft (46 m) in buildings protected throughout by an approved automatic sprinkler system and shall not exceed 100 ft (30 m) in all other buildings.~~ | Provisions deleted |
| **31.3.4.1.1** Apartment buildings four or more stories in height or with more than 11 dwelling units, other than those meeting the requirements of 31.3.4.1.2, shall be provided with a fire alarm system in accordance with Section 9.6, except as modified by 31.3.4.2 through 31.3.4.6. | Provision revised from "more than three stories" to "four or more stories in height" for correlation with new 4.6.3 |
| [former] ~~**31.3.4.1.3** A fire alarm system shall not be required in buildings that are protected throughout by an approved, automatic sprinkler system in accordance with 31.3.5.3 with listed quick-response or listed residential sprinklers installed throughout all dwelling units, that do not exceed four stories in height, and that contain not more than 16 dwelling units.~~ | Provision deleted |
| **31.3.4.5.3** In buildings other than those equipped throughout with an existing, complete automatic smoke detection system or a complete, supervised automatic sprinkler system in accordance with 31.3.5, smoke alarms shall be installed in every sleeping area in accordance with 9.6.2.10, as modified by 31.3.4.5.4.<br>**31.3.4.5.4** Smoke alarms required by 31.3.4.5.3 shall be permitted to be battery powered. | New provisions |
| **31.3.4.6* Protection of Fire Alarm System.** The provision of 9.6.1.8.1.3 shall not apply to the smoke detection required at each fire alarm control unit by 9.6.1.8.1(1). | New provision |
| **31.3.7 Subdivision of Building Spaces — Smoke Partitions.** In buildings other than those meeting the requirements of 31.3.7.1, 31.3.7.2, 31.3.7.3, 31.3.7.4, or 31.3.7.5, the following criteria shall be met:<br>(1) Smoke partitions in accordance with Section 8.4 shall be provided in exit access corridors to establish not less than two compartments of approximately equal size.<br>(2) The length of each smoke compartment, measured along the corridor, shall not exceed 200 ft (61 m).<br>**31.3.7.1** Smoke partitions shall not be required in buildings using Option 4.<br>**31.3.7.2** Smoke partitions shall not be required in buildings having exterior exit access in accordance with 7.5.3 that provides access to two exits.<br>**31.3.7.3** Smoke partitions shall not be required in buildings complying with 31.2.4.2, 31.2.4.3, 31.2.4.4, or 31.2.4.5.<br>**31.3.7.4** Smoke partitions shall not be required in buildings with exits not more than 50 ft (15 m) apart.<br>**31.3.7.5** Smoke partitions shall not be required where each dwelling unit has direct access to the exterior at the finished ground level. | Provisions revised to require smoke partitions rather than smoke barriers |

| Subject / 2009 Edition Text | Notes |
|---|---|
| **31.4.1.2*** Emergency plans in accordance with Section 4.8 shall be provided and shall include the following:<br>(1) Egress procedures<br>(2) Methods<br>(3) Preferred evacuation routes for each event, including appropriate use of elevators | New provision |
| **Chapter 32 New Residential Board and Care Occupancies** | |
| **32.1.2.2** The requirement of 32.1.2.1 shall not apply to apartment buildings housing residential board and care occupancies in conformance with Section 32.4. In such facilities, any safeguards required by Section 32.4 that are more restrictive than those for other housed occupancies shall apply only to the extent prescribed by Section 32.4. | New provision |
| **32.2.3.4.4* Protection of Fire Alarm System.** The provision of 9.6.1.8.1.3 shall not apply to the smoke detection required at each fire alarm control unit by 9.6.1.8.1(1). | New provision |
| **32.3.1.3 Minimum Construction Requirements.** Large board and care facilities shall be limited to the building construction types specified in Table 32.3.1.3 *(see 8.2.1)*, based on the number of stories in height as defined in 4.6.3.<br>**Table 32.3.1.3 Construction Type Limitations** | New provisions replace the referencing of requirements of NFPA 5000 |
| **32.3.2.1.1** Means of egress from resident rooms and resident dwelling units to the outside of the building shall be in accordance with Chapter 7 and this chapter.<br>**32.3.2.1.2** Means of escape within the resident room or resident dwelling unit shall comply with Section 24.2 for one- and two-family dwellings. | New provisions |
| **32.3.3.4.9* Protection of Fire Alarm System.** The provision of 9.6.1.8.1.3 shall not apply to the smoke detection required at each fire alarm control unit by 9.6.1.8.1(1). | New provision |
| **32.7.5.3*** Newly introduced mattresses within board and care facilities shall comply with 32.7.5.3.1 or 32.7.5.3.2.<br>**32.7.5.3.1** Newly introduced mattresses shall be tested in accordance with the provisions of 10.3.2.2 and 10.3.4. | Provisions revised from "new mattresses" to "newly introduced mattresses" |
| **32.7.7 Inspection of Door Openings.** Door assemblies for which the door leaf is required to swing in the direction of egress travel shall be inspected and tested not less than annually in accordance with 7.2.1.15. | New provision |
| **Chapter 33 Existing Residential Board and Care Occupancies** | |
| **33.2.3.4.4* Protection of Fire Alarm System.** The provision of 9.6.1.8.1.3 shall not apply to the smoke detection required at each fire alarm control unit by 9.6.1.8.1(1). | New provision |
| **33.3.1.3 Minimum Construction Requirements.** Large facilities shall be limited to the building construction types specified in Table 33.3.1.3. *(See 8.2.1.)*<br>**Table 33.3.1.3 Construction Type Limitations** | Provisions revised to include tabular format |
| **33.3.2.1.1** Means of egress from resident rooms and resident dwelling units to the outside of the building shall be in accordance with Chapter 7 and this chapter.<br>**33.3.2.1.2** Means of escape within the resident room or resident dwelling unit shall comply with Section 24.2 for one- and two-family dwellings. | New provisions |
| **33.3.3.4.9* Protection of Fire Alarm System.** The provision of 9.6.1.8.1.3 shall not apply to the smoke detection required at each fire alarm control unit by 9.6.1.8.1(1). | New provision |
| **33.7.5.3*** Newly introduced mattresses within board and care facilities shall comply with 33.7.5.3.1 or 33.7.5.3.2.<br>**33.7.5.3.1** Newly introduced mattresses shall be tested in accordance with the provisions of 10.3.2.2 and 10.3.4. | Provisions revised from "new mattresses" to "newly introduced mattresses" |

| Subject / 2009 Edition Text | Notes |
|---|---|
| **33.7.7 Inspection of Door Openings.** Door assemblies for which the door leaf is required to swing in the direction of egress travel shall be inspected and tested not less than annually in accordance with 7.2.1.15. | New provision |
| **Chapter 36 New Mercantile Occupancies**<br>**36.1.3 Special Definitions.** A list of special terms used in this chapter follows:<br>. . .<br>(4) **Major Tenant.** See 3.3.157.<br>(5) **Mall.** See 3.3.158.<br>(6) **Mall Building.** See 3.3.32.9.<br>. . . | New references to Chapter 3 definitions |
| **36.1.4.2.1** Mercantile occupancies shall be subclassified as follows:<br>. . .<br>(2) Class B, as follows:<br>(a) All mercantile occupancies of more than 3000 $ft^2$ (280 $m^2$), but not more than 30,000 $ft^2$ (2800 $m^2$), aggregate gross area and occupying not more than three stories for sales purposes<br>(b) All mercantile occupancies of not more than 3000 $ft^2$ (280 $m^2$) gross area and occupying two or three stories for sales purposes<br>. . . | Item (2)(b) is new |
| **36.2.2.2.3** Elevator lobby exit access door-locking arrangements in accordance with 7.2.1.6.3 shall be permitted. | New provision |
| **36.2.4.3** A single means of egress shall be permitted in a Class C mercantile occupancy, provided that the travel distance to the exit or to a mall pedestrian way (*see 36.4.4.2*) does not exceed 75 ft (23 m). | Provision revised from "or to a mall" to "or to a mall pedestrian way" |
| **36.2.5.11** Exit access in Class A and Class B mercantile occupancies that are protected throughout by an approved, supervised automatic sprinkler system in accordance with 9.7.1.1(1), and exit access in all Class C mercantile occupancies, shall be permitted to pass through storerooms, provided that the following conditions are met:<br>. . .<br>(4) The path of travel through the storeroom shall be defined, direct, and continuously maintained in an unobstructed condition. | Item (4) revised to delete requirement for fixed barriers |
| **36.2.7.2*** Fifty percent of the exits shall be permitted to discharge through the level of exit discharge in accordance with 7.7.2 only where the building is protected throughout by an approved, supervised automatic sprinkler system in accordance with 9.7.1.1(1).<br>[former] ~~and the distance of travel from the termination of the exit enclosure to an outside street door shall not exceed 50 ft (15 m).~~ | Provision deleted |
| **36.3.4.3.1 Occupant Notification.** During all times that the mercantile occupancy is occupied, the required fire alarm system, once initiated, shall activate an alarm in accordance with 9.6.3 throughout the mercantile occupancy, and positive alarm sequence in accordance with 9.6.3.4 shall be permitted.<br>[former 36.3.4.3.1(2)] ~~(2) It shall activate an alarm signal in a continuously attended location for the purpose of initiating emergency action, by personnel trained to respond to emergencies, as follows:~~<br>~~(a) Emergency action shall be initiated by means of live voice public address system announcements originating from the attended location where the alarm signal is received, unless otherwise permitted by 36.3.4.3.1(2)(c).~~<br>~~(b) The live voice public address system shall be permitted to be used for other announcements, provided that the emergency action use takes precedence over any other use.~~<br>~~(c) In lieu of live voice public address system announcements, any other occupant notification means in accordance with 9.6.3 shall be permitted.~~ | Option deleted to provide occupant notification via building public address system |

| Subject / 2009 Edition Text | Notes |
|---|---|
| **36.4.4.2.1** The travel distance within a tenant space to an exit or to the mall shall not exceed the maximum travel distance permitted by the occupancy chapter. | Provision revised to delete reference to 200 ft (61 m) |
| **36.4.4.2.2** An additional 200 ft (61 m) shall be permitted for travel through the mall space, provided that all the following requirements are met:<br>. . .<br>(4) The mall, and all buildings connected thereto, except open parking structures, shall be protected throughout by an approved, supervised automatic sprinkler system in accordance with 9.7.1.1(1), which shall be installed in such a manner that any portion of the system serving tenant spaces can be taken out of service without affecting the operation of the portion of the system serving the mall.<br>(5)*Walls dividing tenant spaces from each other shall have a fire resistance rating of not less than 1 hour, and the following also shall apply:<br>(a) The partition shall extend to the underside of the ceiling or to the roof or floor above.<br>(b) No separation shall be required between a tenant space and the mall.<br>(6)* Malls with a floor opening connecting more than two levels shall be provided with a smoke control system. | Item (4) revised to exempt open parking structures<br>Item (5) revised to require 1-hour rated barrier between tenants but the barrier is permitted to stop at underside of ceiling<br>Item (6) revised to require smoke control only where mall floor opening connects more than two levels |
| **36.4.4.3.2.2** A single means of egress shall be permitted in a Class C mercantile occupancy or a business occupancy, provided that the travel distance to the exit or to a mall pedestrian way (*see 36.4.4.2*) does not exceed 100 ft (30 m). | Provision revised from "or to a mall" to "or to a mall pedestrian way" |
| **36.4.4.3.6** Each individual major tenant of a mall building shall be permitted to have a maximum of one-half of its means of egress independent of the mall. | New provision |
| **36.4.4.4.3.1 Occupant Notification.** During all times that the mall is occupied, the required fire alarm system, once initiated, shall perform one of the following functions:<br>. . .<br>(3) Occupant notification shall be permitted to be made via a voice communication or public address system in accordance with 9.6.3.9.2.<br>[former 36.4.4.4.3.1(3)] ~~(3) It shall activate an alarm signal in a continuously attended location for the purpose of initiating emergency action, by personnel trained to respond to emergencies, as follows:~~<br>~~(a) Emergency action shall be initiated by means of live voice public address system announcements originating from the attended location where the alarm signal is received, unless otherwise permitted by 36.4.4.4.3.1(3)(c).~~<br>~~(b) The live voice public address system shall be permitted to be used for other announcements, provided that the emergency action use takes precedence over any other use.~~<br>~~(c) In lieu of live voice public address system announcements, any other occupant notification means in accordance with 9.6.3 shall be permitted.~~ | Item (3) revised to reference new provisions of 9.6.3.9.2 rather than detailing the public address system features for occupant notification; former details deleted |
| **36.4.4.4.3.2*** Visible signals shall not be required in malls. *(See 9.6.3.5.7 and 9.6.3.5.8.)* | New provision |
| **36.4.4.9* Smoke Control.** Smoke control in accordance with Section 9.3 and complying with 8.6.7(5) shall be provided in a mall with floor openings connecting more than two levels. | Provision revised to require compliance with Section 9.3 (i.e., NFPA 92B) |
| **36.4.5.4.3 Occupant Notification.** During all times that the mercantile occupancy is occupied, the required fire alarm system, once initiated, shall activate an alarm in accordance with 9.6.3 throughout the mercantile occupancy, and positive alarm sequence in accordance with 9.6.3.4 shall be permitted.<br>[former 36.4.5.4.3(2)] ~~(2) It shall activate an alarm signal in a continuously attended location for the purpose of initiating emergency action, by personnel trained to respond to emergencies, as follows:~~ | Option deleted to provide occupant notification via building public address system in bulk merchandising retail buildings |

| Subject / 2009 Edition Text | Notes |
|---|---|
| ~~(a) Emergency action shall be initiated by means of live voice public address system announcements originating from the attended location where the alarm signal is received, unless otherwise permitted by 36.4.5.4.3(2)(c).~~<br>~~(b) The live voice public address system shall be permitted to be used for other announcements, provided that the emergency action use takes precedence over any other use.~~<br>~~(c) In lieu of live voice public address system announcements, any other occupant notification means in accordance with 9.6.3 shall be permitted.~~ | |
| **36.7.1 Emergency Plans.** Emergency plans complying with Section 4.8 shall be provided in high-rise buildings. | New provision |
| **Chapter 37 Existing Mercantile Occupancies**<br>**37.1.3 Special Definitions.** A list of special terms used in this chapter follows:<br>. . .<br>(4) **Major Tenant.** See 3.3.157.<br>(5) **Mall.** See 3.3.158.<br>(6) **Mall Building.** See 3.3.32.9.<br>. . . | New references to Chapter 3 definitions |
| **37.1.4.2.1** Mercantile occupancies shall be subclassified as follows:<br>. . .<br>(2) Class B, as follows:<br>(a) All mercantile occupancies of more than 3000 $ft^2$ (280 $m^2$), but not more than 30,000 $ft^2$ (2800 $m^2$), aggregate gross area and occupying not more than three stories for sales purposes<br>(b) All mercantile occupancies of not more than 3000 $ft^2$ (280 $m^2$) gross area and occupying two or three stories for sales purposes<br>. . . | Item (2)(b) is new |
| **37.2.2.2.3** Elevator lobby exit access door-locking arrangements in accordance with 7.2.1.6.3 shall be permitted. | New provision |
| **37.2.4.3** A single means of egress shall be permitted in a Class C mercantile occupancy, provided that the travel distance to the exit or to a mall pedestrian way (*see 37.4.4.2*) does not exceed 75 ft (23 m). | Provision revised from "or to a mall" to "or to a mall pedestrian way" |
| **37.2.5.11** Exit access in Class A mercantile occupancies that are protected throughout by an approved, supervised automatic sprinkler system in accordance with 9.7.1.1(1), and exit access in all Class B and Class C mercantile occupancies, shall be permitted to pass through storerooms, provided that the following conditions are met:<br>. . .<br>(4) The path of travel through the storeroom shall be defined, direct, and continuously maintained in an unobstructed condition. | Item (4) revised to delete requirement for fixed barriers |
| **37.2.7.2*** Fifty percent of the exits shall be permitted to discharge through the level of exit discharge in accordance with 7.7.2 only where the building is protected throughout by an approved automatic sprinkler system in accordance with 9.7.1.1(1).<br>[former] ~~and the distance of travel from the termination of the exit enclosure to an outside street door shall not exceed 50 ft (15 m).~~ | Provision deleted |
| **37.3.4.3.1 Occupant Notification.** During all times that the mercantile occupancy is occupied, the required fire alarm system, once initiated, shall perform one of the following functions:<br>. . .<br>(2) Occupant notification shall be permitted to be made via a voice communication or public address system in accordance with 9.6.3.9.2.<br>[former 37.3.4.3.1(2)] ~~(2) It shall activate an alarm signal in a continuously attended location for the purpose of initiating emergency action by personnel trained to respond to emergencies, as follows:~~ | Item (2) revised to reference new provisions of 9.6.3.9.2 rather than detailing the public address system features for occupant notification; former details deleted |

| Subject / 2009 Edition Text | Notes |
|---|---|
| ~~(a) Emergency action shall be initiated by means of live voice public address system announcements originating from the attended location where the alarm signal is received, unless otherwise permitted by 37.3.4.3.1(2)(c).~~<br>~~(b) The live voice public address system shall be permitted to be used for other announcements, provided that the emergency action use takes precedence over any other use.~~<br>~~(c) In lieu of live voice public address system announcements, any other occupant notification means in accordance with 9.6.3 shall be permitted.~~ | |
| **37.4.4.2.2** An additional 200 ft (61 m) shall be permitted for travel through the mall space, provided that all the following requirements are met:<br>. . .<br>(4) The mall, and all buildings connected thereto, except open parking structures, shall be protected throughout by an approved, supervised automatic sprinkler system in accordance with 9.7.1.1(1).<br>. . .<br>(6)* Malls with a floor opening connecting more than two levels shall be provided with a smoke control system. | Item (4) revised to exempt open parking structures<br><br>Item (6) revised to require smoke control only where mall floor opening connects more than two levels |
| **37.4.4.3.2.2** A single means of egress shall be permitted in a Class C mercantile occupancy or a business occupancy, provided that the travel distance to the exit or to a mall pedestrian way *(see 37.4.4.2)* does not exceed 100 ft (30 m). | Provision revised from "or to a mall" to "or to a mall pedestrian way" |
| **37.4.4.3.6** Each individual major tenant of a mall building shall be permitted to have a maximum of one-half of its means of egress independent of the mall. | New provision |
| **37.4.4.4.3.1 Occupant Notification.** During all times that the mall is occupied, the required fire alarm system, once initiated, shall perform one of the following functions:<br>. . .<br>(3) Occupant notification shall be permitted to be made via a voice communication or public address system in accordance with 9.6.3.9.2.<br>[former 37.4.4.4.3.1(3)] ~~(3) It shall activate an alarm signal in a continuously attended location for the purpose of initiating emergency action, by personnel trained to respond to emergencies, as follows:~~<br>~~(a) Emergency action shall be initiated by means of live voice public address system announcements originating from the attended location where the alarm signal is received, unless otherwise permitted by 37.4.4.4.3.1(3)(c).~~<br>~~(b) The live voice public address system shall be permitted to be used for other announcements, provided that the emergency action use takes precedence over any other use.~~<br>~~(c) In lieu of live voice public address system announcements, any other occupant notification means in accordance with 9.6.3 shall be permitted.~~ | Item (3) revised to reference new provisions of 9.6.3.9.2 rather than detailing the public address system features for occupant notification; former details deleted |
| **37.4.5.4.3 Occupant Notification.** During all times that the mercantile occupancy is occupied, the required fire alarm system, once initiated, shall perform one of the following functions:<br>. . .<br>(2) Occupant notification shall be permitted to be made via a voice communication or public address system in accordance with 9.6.3.9.2.<br>[former 37.4.5.4.3(2)] ~~(2) It shall activate an alarm signal in a continuously attended location for the purpose of initiating emergency action, by personnel trained to respond to emergencies, as follows:~~<br>~~(a) Emergency action shall be initiated by means of live voice public address system announcements originating from the attended location where the alarm signal is received, unless otherwise permitted by 37.4.5.4.3(2)(c).~~<br>~~(b) The live voice public address system shall be permitted to be used for other announcements, provided that the emergency action use takes precedence over any other use.~~ | Item (2) revised to reference new provisions of 9.6.3.9.2 rather than detailing the public address system features for occupant notification; former details deleted |

| Subject / 2009 Edition Text | Notes |
|---|---|
| ~~(c) In lieu of live voice public address system announcements, any other occupant notification means in accordance with 9.6.3 shall be permitted.~~ | |
| **37.4.6 Retail Sales of Consumer Fireworks, 1.4G.** Mercantile occupancies in which the retail sale of consumer fireworks, 1.4G, is conducted, other than approved existing facilities, shall comply with NFPA 1124, *Code for the Manufacture, Transportation, Storage, and Retail Sales of Fireworks and Pyrotechnic Articles.* | New provision for consistency with 36.4.6 |
| **37.7.1 Emergency Plans.** Emergency plans complying with Section 4.8 shall be provided in high-rise buildings. | New provision |
| **Chapter 38 New Business Occupancies**<br>**38.2.2.2.3** Elevator lobby exit access door-locking arrangements in accordance with 7.2.1.6.3 shall be permitted. | New provision |
| **38.2.3.3** Street floor exits shall be sufficient for the occupant load of the street floor plus the required capacity of open stairs and ramps discharging through the street floor. | Provision revised to have applicability only where the stairs or ramps are open |
| **38.2.6.1** Travel distance shall be measured in accordance with Section 7.6. | New provision — no technical change |
| **38.3.4.3 Occupant Notification.** During all times that the building is occupied, the required fire alarm system, once initiated, shall activate a general alarm in accordance with 9.6.3 throughout the building, and positive alarm sequence in accordance with 9.6.3.4 shall be permitted.<br>[former 38.3.4.3(2)] ~~(2) It shall activate an alarm signal in a continuously attended location for the purpose of initiating emergency action, by personnel trained to respond to emergencies, as follows:~~<br>~~(a) Emergency action shall be initiated by means of live voice public address system announcements originating from the attended location where the alarm signal is received, unless otherwise permitted by 38.3.4.3(2)(c).~~<br>~~(b) The live voice public address system shall be permitted to be used for other announcements, provided that the emergency action use takes precedence over any other use.~~<br>~~(c) In lieu of live voice public address system announcements, any other occupant notification means in accordance with 9.6.3 shall be permitted.~~ | Option deleted to provide occupant notification via building public address system |
| **38.3.4.4 Emergency Forces Notification.** Emergency forces notification shall be provided and shall include notifying the following:<br>(1) Fire department in accordance with 9.6.4<br>(2) Local emergency organization, if provided | New provision |
| **38.4.3 Air Traffic Control Towers.**<br>**38.4.3.1** Air traffic control towers shall comply with the requirements of this chapter and Section 11.3.<br>**38.4.3.2** The requirements of Section 11.8 shall not apply to air traffic control towers. | New provisions |
| **38.7.1 Emergency Plans.** Emergency plans complying with Section 4.8 shall be provided in high-rise buildings. | New provision |
| **Chapter 39 Existing Business Occupancies**<br>**39.2.2.2.3** Elevator lobby exit access door-locking arrangements in accordance with 7.2.1.6.3 shall be permitted. | New provision |
| **39.2.2.2.4** The re-entry provisions of 7.2.1.5.7 shall not apply to the following:<br>(1) Existing business occupancies that are not high-rise buildings<br>(2) Existing high-rise business occupancy buildings that are protected throughout by an approved automatic sprinkler system in accordance with 9.7.1.1(1) | Provision revised as it formerly exempted all existing business occupancies from the requirement for re-entry |

| Subject / 2009 Edition Text | Notes |
|---|---|
| (3) Existing high-rise business occupancy buildings having approved existing means for providing stair re-entry | |
| **39.2.6.1** Travel distance shall be measured in accordance with Section 7.6. | New provision — no technical change |
| **39.3.4.3 Occupant Notification.** During all times that the building is occupied *(see 7.2.1.1.3)*, the required fire alarm system, once initiated, shall perform one of the following functions:<br>. . .<br>(2) Occupant notification shall be permitted to be made via a voice communication or public address system in accordance with 9.6.3.9.2.<br>[former 39.3.4.3(2)] ~~(2) It shall activate an alarm signal in a continuously attended location for the purpose of initiating emergency action, by personnel trained to respond to emergencies, as follows:~~<br>~~(a) Emergency action shall be initiated by means of live voice public address system announcements originating from the attended location where the alarm signal is received, unless otherwise permitted by 39.3.4.3(2)(c).~~<br>~~(b) The live voice public address system shall be permitted to be used for other announcements, provided that the emergency action use takes precedence over any other use.~~<br>~~(c) In lieu of live voice public address system announcements, any other occupant notification means in accordance with 9.6.3 shall be permitted.~~ | Item (2) revised to reference new provisions of 9.6.3.9.2 rather than detailing the public address system features for occupant notification; former details deleted |
| **39.4.3 Air Traffic Control Towers.**<br>**39.4.3.1** Air traffic control towers shall comply with the requirements of this chapter and Section 11.3.<br>**39.4.3.2** The requirements of Section 11.8 shall not apply to air traffic control towers. | New provisions |
| **39.7.1 Emergency Plans.** Emergency plans complying with Section 4.8 shall be provided in high-rise buildings. | New provision |
| **Chapter 40 Industrial Occupancies**<br>**40.3.4.1 General.** A fire alarm system shall be required in accordance with Section 9.6 for industrial occupancies, unless the total occupant load of the building is under 100 persons and unless, of these, fewer than 25 persons are above or below the level of exit discharge. | Provision revised from "total capacity" to "total occupant load" |
| **Chapter 42 Storage Occupancies**<br>**42.8.2.2.3.2** In open-air parking structures, stairs complying with 7.2.2.5.1 shall not be required. | New provision |
| **42.8.2.2.9.2** In open-air parking structures, the area of refuge requirements of 7.2.12.1.2(2) shall not apply. | New provision |
| **42.8.2.6.2** In open parking structures, travel distance shall comply with one of the following:<br>(1) The travel distance to an exit shall not exceed the travel distance specified in Table 42.8.2.6.1.<br>(2) The travel distance to a stair that does not meet the provisions for an exit enclosure shall not exceed the travel distance specified in Table 42.8.2.6.1, and travel along the stair shall not be limited. | New provision |
| **Chapter 43 Building Rehabilitation**<br>**43.2.2.1.4* Reconstruction.** The reconfiguration of a space that affects an exit or a corridor shared by more than one occupant space; or the reconfiguration of a space such that the rehabilitation work area is not permitted to be occupied because existing means of egress and fire protection systems, or their equivalent, are not in place or continuously maintained. | Provision revised from "shared by more than a single tenant" to "shared by more than one occupant space" |

| Subject / 2009 Edition Text | Notes |
|---|---|
| **43.4.2 Capacity of Means of Egress.** The capacity of means of egress, determined in accordance with Section 7.3, shall be sufficient for the occupant load thereof, unless one of the following conditions exists:<br>(1) The authority having jurisdiction shall be permitted to establish the occupant load as the number of persons for which existing means of egress is adequate, provided that measures are established to prevent occupancy by a greater number of persons.<br>(2)* The egress capacity shall have been previously approved as being adequate.<br>[former] ~~**43.6.2.2 Capacity of Means of Egress.** The capacity of means of egress, determined in accordance with the Section 7.3, shall be sufficient for the occupant load thereof, unless one of the following conditions exists:~~<br>~~(1) The authority having jurisdiction shall be permitted to establish the occupant load as the number of persons for which existing means of egress is adequate, provided that measures are established to prevent occupancy by a greater number of persons.~~<br>~~(2)* The egress capacity shall have been previously approved as being adequate.~~ | Provision moved from 43.6 Reconstruction so as to apply to Renovation, Modification and Reconstruction |
| [former] ~~**43.6.2.3 Dead-End Corridors.** Newly constructed dead-end corridors shall comply with the requirements of other sections of this *Code* applicable to new construction for the occupancy.~~ | Provision deleted |
| **43.6.2.2 Illumination and Emergency Lighting of Means of Egress.**<br>**43.6.2.2.1** Means of egress in rehabilitation work areas shall be provided with illumination and emergency lighting in accordance with the requirements of other sections of this *Code* applicable to new construction for the occupancy.<br>**43.6.2.2.2** Where the reconstruction rehabilitation work area on any floor exceeds 50 percent of that floor area, means of egress throughout the floor shall be provided with illumination and emergency lighting in accordance with the requirements of other sections of this *Code* applicable to new construction for the occupancy, unless otherwise specified in 43.6.2.2.4.<br>**43.6.2.2.3** In a building with rehabilitation work areas involving more than 50 percent of the aggregate floor area within the building, the means of egress within the rehabilitation work area and the means of egress, including the exit and exit discharge paths, serving the rehabilitation work area shall be provided with illumination and emergency lighting in accordance with the requirements of other sections of this *Code* applicable to new construction for the occupancy, unless otherwise specified in 43.6.2.2.4.<br>**43.6.2.2.4** Means of egress within a tenant space that is entirely outside the rehabilitation work area shall be permitted to comply with the requirements for illumination and emergency lighting applicable to the existing occupancy in lieu of the requirements for illumination and emergency lighting applicable to new construction required by 43.6.2.2.2 and 43.6.2.2.3. | Provisions expanded to address emergency lighting, as well as illumination of means of egress |
| [former] ~~**43.6.2.5 Exit Signs.**~~<br>~~. . .~~<br>[former] ~~**43.6.2.6 Handrails.**~~<br>~~. . .~~ | Provisions deleted |
| **43.7.1 Change of Use or Occupancy Classification.**<br>**43.7.1.1** A change of use that does not involve a change of occupancy classification shall comply with the requirements applicable to the new use in accordance with the applicable existing occupancy chapter, unless the change of use creates a hazardous contents area as addressed in 43.7.1.2.<br>**43.7.1.2** A change of use that does not involve a change of occupancy classification but that creates a hazardous area shall comply with the requirements applicable to the new use in accordance with the applicable occupancy chapter for new construction. | New provision<br><br>New provision |
| **43.7.2.1** Where a change of occupancy classification occurs within the same hazard classification category or to an occupancy classification of a lesser hazard classification category (that is, a higher hazard category number), as addressed by Table 43.7.3, the building shall meet both of the following:<br>. . . | |

| Subject / 2009 Edition Text | Notes |
|---|---|
| (2)* Automatic sprinkler and detection, alarm, and communications system requirements and the requirements for hazardous areas applicable to new construction for the occupancy created by the change *(see Chapters 12, 14, 16, 18, 20, 22, 24, 26, 28, 30, 32, 36, 38, 40, and 42)* | Item (2) revised to include hazardous area protection as an additional feature that must be provided in accordance with the requirements applicable to new construction |
| [former] ~~**43.7.2.5** Portions of the building in which the occupancy classification is not changed shall be permitted to comply with the requirements of the applicable existing occupancy chapters, provided that one of the following criteria is met:~~<br>~~(1) The occupancies are separated as required by 6.1.14.4.~~<br>~~(2) The occupancies are separated via approved compliance alternatives.~~ | Provision deleted |
| **Table 43.7.3 Hazard Categories and Classifications** | Hazard category 1 description changed from "high hazard contents" to "industrial or storage occupancies with high hazard contents" |
| **43.8.3 Fire Protection Systems.** In other than one- and two-family dwellings, existing compartment areas without an approved separation from the addition shall be protected by an approved automatic sprinkler system where the combined areas would be required to be sprinklered by the provisions applicable to new construction for the occupancy. | Provision revised to exempt one- and two-family dwellings; and by addition of "where the combined areas would be required to be sprinklered by the provisions applicable to new construction for the occupancy" |
| **43.8.4 Smoke Alarms.** Where an addition is made to a one- or two-family dwelling or a small residential board and care occupancy, interconnected smoke alarms, powered by the electrical system, meeting the requirements of the other sections of this *Code* shall be installed and maintained in the addition.<br>[former 43.8.4(2)] ~~(2) Smoke alarms shall be provided in the existing building in accordance with 9.6.2.9.~~ | <br><br><br><br>Provision deleted |

# Code Index

## -A-

## -B-

## -C-

## -D-

## -E-

## -F-

## -G-

## -H-

## -I-

## -J-



## -K-



## -L-

## -M-

## -N-

## -O-

## -P-

## -S-

## -T-

# Commentary Index

## -B-

## -C-

## -D-

## -E-

## -F-

## -G-



## -H-

## -Q-



## -R-

## -X-



## -Z-

# IMPORTANT NOTICES AND DISCLAIMERS CONCERNING NFPA® DOCUMENTS

## NOTICE AND DISCLAIMERS OF LIABILITY CONCERNING THE USE OF NFPA DOCUMENTS

NFPA codes, standards, recommended practices, and guides, including the documents contained herein, are developed through a consensus standards development process approved by the American National Standards Institute. This process brings together volunteers representing varied viewpoints and interests to achieve consensus on fire and other safety issues. While the NFPA administers the process and establishes rules to promote fairness in the development of consensus, it does not independently test, evaluate, or verify the accuracy of any information or the soundness of any judgments contained in its codes and standards.

The NFPA disclaims liability for any personal injury, property or other damages of any nature whatsoever, whether special, indirect, consequential or compensatory, directly or indirectly resulting from the publication, use of, or reliance on these documents. The NFPA also makes no guaranty or warranty as to the accuracy or completeness of any information published herein.

In issuing and making these documents available, the NFPA is not undertaking to render professional or other services for or on behalf of any person or entity. Nor is the NFPA undertaking to perform any duty owed by any person or entity to someone else. Anyone using these documents should rely on his or her own independent judgment or, as appropriate, seek the advice of a competent professional in determining the exercise of reasonable care in any given circumstances.

The NFPA has no power, nor does it undertake, to police or enforce compliance with the contents of these documents. Nor does the NFPA list, certify, test or inspect products, designs, or installations for compliance with these documents. Any certification or other statement of compliance with the requirements of these documents shall not be attributable to the NFPA and is solely the responsibility of the certifier or maker of the statement.

## ADDITIONAL NOTICES AND DISCLAIMERS

### Updating of NFPA Documents

Users of NFPA codes, standards, recommended practices, and guides should be aware that these documents may be superseded at any time by the issuance of new editions or may be amended from time to time through the issuance of Tentative Interim Amendments. An official NFPA document at any point in time consists of the current edition of the document together with any Tentative Interim Amendments and any Errata then in effect. In order to determine whether a given document is the current edition and whether it has been amended through the issuance of Tentative Interim Amendments or corrected through the issuance of Errata, consult appropriate NFPA publications such as the National Fire Codes® Subscription Service, visit the NFPA website at www.nfpa.org, or contact the NFPA at the address listed below.

### Interpretations of NFPA Documents

A statement, written or oral, that is not processed in accordance with Section 6 of the Regulations Governing Committee Projects shall not be considered the official position of NFPA or any of its Committees and shall not be considered to be, nor be relied upon as, a Formal Interpretation.

### Patents

The NFPA does not take any position with respect to the validity of any patent rights asserted in connection with any items which are mentioned in or are the subject of NFPA codes, standards, recommended practices, and guides, and the NFPA disclaims liability for the infringement of any patent resulting from the use of or reliance on these documents. Users of these documents are expressly advised that determination of the validity of any such patent rights, and the risk of infringement of such rights, is entirely their own responsibility.

NFPA adheres to applicable policies of the American National Standards Institute with respect to patents. For further information, contact the NFPA at the address listed below.

### Law and Regulations

Users of these documents should consult applicable federal, state, and local laws and regulations. NFPA does not, by the publication of its codes, standards, recommended practices, and guides, intend to urge action that is not in compliance with applicable laws, and these documents may not be construed as doing so.

### Copyrights

The documents contained in this volume are copyrighted by the NFPA. They are made available for a wide variety of both public and private uses. These include both use, by reference, in laws and regulations, and use in private self-regulation, standardization, and the promotion of safe practices and methods. By making these documents available for use and adoption by public authorities and private users, NFPA does not waive any rights in copyright to these documents.

Use of NFPA documents for regulatory purposes should be accomplished through adoption by reference. The term "adoption by reference" means the citing of title, edition, and publishing information only. Any deletions, additions, and changes desired by the adopting authority should be noted separately in the adopting instrument. In order to assist NFPA in following the uses made of its documents, adopting authorities are requested to notify the NFPA (Attention: Secretary, Standards Council) in writing of such use. For technical assistance and questions concerning adoption of NFPA documents, contact NFPA at the address below.

### For Further Information

All questions or other communications relating to NFPA codes, standards, recommended practices, and guides and all requests for information on NFPA procedures governing its codes and standards development process, including information on the procedures for requesting Formal Interpretations, for proposing Tentative Interim Amendments, and for proposing revisions to NFPA documents during regular revision cycles, should be sent to NFPA headquarters, addressed to the attention of the Secretary, Standards Council, NFPA, 1 Batterymarch Park, Quincy, MA 02169-9101.

For more information about NFPA, visit the NFPA website at www.nfpa.org.